ON MORAL MEDICINE

On Moral Medicine

Theological Perspectives in Medical Ethics

THIRD EDITION

Edited by

M. Therese Lysaught & Joseph J. Kotva Jr.

with

Stephen E. Lammers & Allen Verhey

William B. Eerdmans Publishing Company

Grand Rapids, Michigan / Cambridge, U.K.

First edition 1987
Second edition 1998
Third edition 2012

Published by
Wm. B. Eerdmans Publishing Co.
2140 Oak Industrial Drive N.E., Grand Rapids, Michigan 49505 /
P.O. Box 163, Cambridge CB3 9PU U.K.

Printed in the United States of America

18 17 16 15 14 13 12 7 6 5 4 3 2 1

Library of Congress Cataloging-in-Publication Data

On moral medicine: theological perspectives in medical ethics. — 3rd ed. /
edited by M. Therese Lysaught . . . [et al.].
p. cm.
ISBN 978-0-8028-6601-1 (pbk.: alk. paper)
1. Medical ethics. 2. Medicine — Religious aspects.
I. Lysaught, M. Therese.

R724.O58 2012
174.2 — dc23

2012003539

www.eerdmans.com

Contents

II: Christianity and the Social Practice of Health Care

III: Patients and Professionals

CHAPTER NINE

Care of Patients and Their Suffering 445

IV: Vulnerable Persons

CHAPTER TEN

Persons with Mental Illness 487

CHAPTER ELEVEN

Aging and the Elderly 533

CHAPTER TWELVE

Persons with Disabilities 583

VI: The End of Life

Preface to the Third Edition

How does one "update" a classic as outsized in reputation and length as *On Moral Medicine?* When Allen Verhey and Steve Lammers approached us seven years ago with the idea, how could we say no? Along the way, we occasionally asked ourselves, "What did we get ourselves into?" But finally, the third edition of *On Moral Medicine* has come to fruition, and we are grateful for the journey that has made it possible.

Longtime users of *On Moral Medicine* will note similarities and differences between the second and third editions. With the original vision of *On Moral Medicine,* we continue to highlight essays that bring theological reflection to bear on issues in medicine, technology, and health care. We likewise continue to bring together a mix of "classic" essays and contemporary voices. Even more than in earlier editions, authors in the third edition speak with specifically Christian voices, using more overtly theological language. And the third edition joins its predecessor in being designed specifically to be a resource for those in the church, the clinic, and the academy who must wrestle with the relevance of the Christian tradition to questions of medical ethics. But, if the first edition was big and the second edition bigger, the third edition is . . . well, even bigger, though the fine editorial staff at Eerdmans Publishing Co. has masterfully contrived to fit the greater number of essays and volume of text into less than 1,200 pages.

One challenging aspect of revising a large and widely used anthology is deciding what to keep and what to add. Of the 156 essays now included in *On Moral Medicine,* 93 are new, as are all but one of the chapter introductions. Changes in medicine have proceeded apace, and new theoretical and theological questions and foci have emerged. With the second edition, stem cell research and "therapeutic" cloning had yet to explosively reshape public debate, and attention to aging and the demographic shift had only just gained a footing on the field's radar. Likewise, theologians are now attending more carefully and explicitly to questions surrounding mental illness and disability. Chapters on these, and other topics, had to be added.

We also include even more robust suggestions for further readings. These suggestions are more than a list of essays that "didn't make the cut." Given the ever-growing scope of the literature in theology and medical ethics, hard calls were made at every juncture. Many essays that we initially hoped to include had to be put aside because they were too long, were too expensive (permission fees occasionally proved insurmountable), overlapped with other essays, or were not sufficiently theological. For topics covered in this edition, the reading lists should provide a good start for further research and reflection. We also encourage all readers to continue to reference earlier editions of *On Moral Medicine* and the important essays contained therein. The earlier editions remain wonderful resources that we routinely consult in our own research and teaching.

While *On Moral Medicine,* third edition, is similar to its predecessors in key ways, differences are notable throughout. Readers will find many more essays that directly work from a virtue ethics perspective. We also integrated a greater diversity of voices, including more women and people of color and a few more authors from outside North America. The notion of the health care professional is intentionally expanded to include more essays regarding nurses, chaplains, and clergy. We sought to frame issues more biblically, as seen in the selection of articles that work with biblical texts as well as the greater number of scripture readings that open many of the chapters. So too, expanding on a theme detectable in earlier editions, several essays provide an even greater caution that technology is not morally neutral — that technology assumes and reinforces certain moral perspectives. And readers will find a few more stories, since some aspects of both ethics and medicine are conveyed only through narrative display.

The structure of the text itself evidences a significant change. As with the first two editions, Chapters One and Two (now under the new heading "Method") attend to the questions of religion and medicine and theology and medical ethics, respectively. Beyond that opening, however, we have restructured the former division between the second edition's Part II, "Concepts in Religion and Medicine," and Part III, "Issues in Medical Ethics," into five integrated sections, each of which provides a broader theological and methodological context for the sections that follow. (Think of the last five "Parts" of the book as five concentric circles, with Part II being the broadest and most all-encompassing.) Thus, discerning readers will note that we have framed the rest of the volume with the new section on the social responsibility of Christian health care (Part II). We intend to suggest by this structure that the social and economic dimensions of health care — and the attendant theological convictions — are visible in the way that we look at everything from questions of health care access in the U.S. to how authors treat issues of newer and emergent technologies (like genetics) or end-of-life care. That is, the social responsibility framework influences nearly every chapter in some way. The social dimension of health care is no longer primarily framed as "scarcity." It is instead more thickly construed along the lines of stewardship, fidelity, and generosity. It also questions the often invisible economic assumptions and infrastructure that shape many dilemmas and "issues" within bioethics as well as health care delivery overall. And it is no longer limited to responsibility within the U.S.; rather, it gives more attention to the intersections of North American health care and bioethics and its implications for the Two-Thirds World.

Designating Part III "Patients and Professionals" indicates additional important shifts in this edition. As with Chapter Six, "The Patient-Physician Relationship," we have altered the traditional order of this pairing away from prioritizing the professional, calling attention instead to the central character in all medical encounters: the patient. Commensurate with calling attention to the patient, we include in Part III chapters on personhood, embodiment, and care of patients and their suffering. Each of these chapters provides an angle from which to understand better the patient side of the relationship. By referring in the plural to "professionals," the designation of Part III also foreshadows the inclusion of essays dealing with actors beyond physicians who "profess" the goods and ends of medicine, such as nurses and chaplains. And by pairing patients and professionals in Part III, the designation alludes to the conviction running throughout the included authors that morally worthy medicine is intrinsically relational.

Another significant change is the inclusion of another entirely new section, "Vulnerable Persons" (Part IV). Here we bring together previous chapters on research subjects and psychiatry with new chapters on persons with disability, aging and the elderly, and human embryonic stem cell research. Again structure is important: by grouping these essays together we underline the obvious but too often overlooked realization that medicine and health care engage vulnerable individuals and populations. Christian theological ethics offers rich reflections about such engagements.

The book closes with seemingly more traditional sections on the beginning of life and end of life. But even here we have endeavored to reflect the best of explicitly Christian theological reflection on medicine. Thus, for example, Part V's chapter on children attempts to understand theologically and narratively the moral place of children in our lives together. Along with considerations of life and its sanctity, this chapter on children necessarily precedes theological reconsiderations of contraception, assisted reproductive technologies, and abortion. Issues of genetics are only then considered, having been framed by the more fundamental considerations of children and pregnancy.

Likewise, Part VI, "The End of Life," continues to be overtly Christian and theological. It is here that the reader finds reflections on what Christians mean by seeking to "die well" and its connection to "living well." Similarly, it is here that the reader finds essays dealing with how faithful Christians and discerning communities approach the mystery of death, including how they approach distinctions between choosing death (Chapter Twenty-Two) and accepting death (Chapter Twenty-Three).

How might readers work with this text? We know that teachers and scholars developed many creative and insightful ways to use previous editions of *On Moral Medicine;* we hope that the third edition proves as amenable to a variety of pedagogical and scholarly innovations. We certainly recommend reading the book front to back, as it starts by considering questions of method, reminds us of our social context and social responsibilities, and ends by highlighting the deep connections between how we live and how we die. Alternatively, one might read an entire "Part" at a time, which enables one to see the interconnections of themes and concerns across the material. Of course, the most common approach is to read a chapter at a time. With all approaches, but especially with this latter approach, we strongly encourage reading the respective chapter introductions. The introductions provide essential background and context for grappling with the associated essays. Whichever route is chosen, we (as editors) contend that Parts I ("Method"), II ("Christianity and the Social Practice of Health Care"), and VI ("The End of Life") are especially critical for understanding the nature of *Christian theological* reflection on medical ethics, and we strongly encourage all readers to engage these sections as part of their exploration of theology and medical ethics.

Technology not only changes medicine and raises new questions in medical ethics; it also provides new avenues for utilizing *On Moral Medicine.* With this third edition, we are delighted that electronic versions of the text are now available through a variety of commercial and library-based e-book options. When we set out to revise the second edition, e-book technologies were barely in their infancy, and we spent significant time exploring ways to include an electronic — and searchable — component with the third edition. Such a component, we reasoned, would helpfully stand in lieu of an index (an item often requested by users of the book) and would enable students and scholars to find relevant materials in other chapters or parts of the book. New e-book formats obviated the need for such a component, not to mention making this behemoth much more transportable! We recognize that for many students an e-book copy will be sufficient, but fellow scholars or those who wish to use *On Moral Medicine* for research purposes might consider purchasing both a paper and an electronic copy of the work. Many of us find that physical books better enable us to "sit with" and "digest" a text, but the merits of a searchable, electronic version of this text are also undeniable.

Allen and Steve have yet to agree about which of them had the initial idea for this anthology; both insist on crediting the other and neither archival research nor personal quizzing of them while consuming good beer seems destined to unearth the answer. Whatever the truth of its origin, we thank them together for creating such a unique and influential book, for providing an invaluable service to the medical and theological communities, and for giving us the great privilege of continuing that tradition.

We could not, of course, have completed this revision without the communion of saints that assisted us in this project. We are grateful to Jon Pott and many others at Wm. B. Eerdmans Publishing Co. for their patience with us and for their help with this project; Jon has been involved in all three editions of this great work. We are grateful to the authors and publishers who have permitted us to utilize their material, especially those who requested reasonable permission fees. We are grateful to our many colleagues who gave advice and counsel — particularly Keith Meador, M.D., now at Vanderbilt University Medical Center, who at the outset of this project organized a small gathering of physicians and theologians to advise us on the revision. We are grateful to our many graduate students at the University of Dayton and Marquette University — Juliana Vazquez, Thomas Bridges, Timothy Cavanaugh, Aaron James, Maria Morrow, and others — who provided important assistance at many points along the way. And we are grateful for the many colleagues who have long used *On Moral Medicine* and have asked again and again for the new edition, encouraging our work on this project. In this latter regard, Kotva wants to thank Willard Swartley, who encouragingly asked about the book's progress too many times to count, turning a potentially isolating task into a communal adventure. We also want to thank Rebecca Slough, the academic dean at AMBS (Associated Mennonite Biblical Seminary), who freed up office space and academic support for Kotva after his stint with ACHE (the now-extinct Anabaptist Center for Healthcare Ethics).

Scholars are also indebted in incalculable ways to their families. We are keenly aware of this truth now. Our families encouraged us and allowed us unreasonable quantities of time, space, and expense. They also provided wonderful family "distractions," which indirectly, but continually, challenged us to put this work within the broader context of the Christian life. All these signs of love were visible one summer as we worked on the book during a Lysaught family vacation in upper Michigan. But they were also visible as our families freed us to meet at retreat centers, at coffee shops, and during numerous Skype calls. To Carol, Joseph, Matthew, Bill, Meg, and Sam: we love you and are ever in your debt.

As each edition of *On Moral Medicine* has shown, theological reflection on health care is vibrant, rich, and growing. Along with an ever-changing social context and with technological developments, it appears that there will continue to be a need for new editions of *On Moral Medicine*. We do not know what book publishing will look like by then, but we look forward to the wonderful authors and enlivening ideas we will encounter as we start the journey toward the next edition.

M. Therese Lysaught
Joseph M. Kotva Jr.

Preface to the Second Edition

The opportunity to prepare a new edition of this anthology has been both gratifying and daunting. It has been gratifying because it comes as confirmation of the success of the first edition. A decade ago it had been our hope to assemble a collection of readings that would display something of the richness of theological reflection on the issues within medical ethics when the field had been quite thoroughly secularized, that would help initiate students into this literature when most anthologies were neglecting it, and that would be a resource for those in the church, the clinic, and the academy who were curious about the relevance of the Christian tradition to questions of medical ethics. It is only fitting that in the preface to this edition we thank those who welcomed the first edition, those who used it creatively and successfully as a text or as a resource volume.

With the opportunity to do a new edition, however, came the task of revision, and it has been a daunting one. It has been daunting both because the medicine that prompts moral commentary has continued to change and because the literature that provides moral commentary has continued to grow.

The changes in medicine have required changes in many of the chapters. A decade ago there was no Human Genome Project, assisted reproductive technologies were in their infancy, physician-assisted suicide was not openly practiced or advocated, and managed care had just begun to shape medicine.

The literature in medical ethics had grown huge, and it has been enriched in the last decade by a revival of interest in religious perspectives and traditions. Among the signs of that revival have been a series of publications by The Park Ridge Center for the Study of Health, Faith, and Ethics, a new series of volumes called Theology and Medicine, and a new journal called *Christian Bioethics.* There has been much to choose from in revising this anthology, and the choices have been sometimes very difficult. We want to thank those who recommended changes and selections for this edition, even though we did not always follow their advice. We have retained the format of the first edition, moving from "Perspectives on Religion and Medicine" to "Concepts in Religion and Medicine" to "Issues in Medical Ethics." Some colleagues have reported that they have used the text from the back to the front, allowing the "issues" to prompt student interest in the "concepts" and "perspectives." Some colleagues have paired certain chapters in Parts I and II with consideration of the "issues" in Part III. We decided to retain both the format and our appreciation of the creativity of our colleagues who use the book in ways that fit their courses and teaching styles.

The most frequent judgment about the first edition was also the most obvious: it was big. This edition is a little bigger. Some colleagues complained about the size, and many admitted that they did not assign everything in the text, but most were glad for the size and for the opportunity to make their own selections from the readings.

We have also tried to preserve a mix of "classic" and contemporary pieces, and of course, we continue to focus on theological reflection on the issues raised by medical research and technology.

The changes include a number of new selections (67), revisions to the introductions to the chapters, and additional selections for further reading. Some of the new selections respond to new developments in health care. Some of them attend to the care of patients with AIDS. Some of them recognize the importance of nurses to health care (and the use of the first edition by nursing students and professionals).

We continue to disagree about which of us had the initial idea for this anthology, each thinking it was the other, but we agree that we would not have been able to have completed it or to have revised it without the help of many others. We are grateful to Jon Pott — and many others — at Wm. B. Eerdmans Publishing Co. for their patience with us and for their help with this project; we are grateful to authors and publishers who have permitted us to utilize their material; we are grateful to colleagues who gave advice, encouragement, and counsel; we are grateful to our secretaries, Yvonne Osmun and Karen Michmerhuizen, who supported our efforts with their own; and we are grateful to our students who continue to test our ideas of a text.

Stephen E. Lammers
Allen Verhey

Preface to the First Edition

A little over two decades ago Kenneth Boulding first suggested that the twentieth century would witness a "biological revolution" with consequences as dramatic and profound as those of the industrial revolution of the eighteenth century.[1] The years since Boulding made his prophetic remark have seen advances in medical science and technology which have made his words seem almost reserved. Not all of the advances have been as dramatic as "cracking" the genetic code or the birth of a "test-tube baby"; not every advance has been as striking as the implantation of an artificial heart into a human patient or the electrical stimulation of the brain; but each of the advances has contributed to a rapidly expanding human control over the human and natural processes of giving birth and dying, over human genetic potential, and over behavioral performance. With the help of biological and behavioral sciences, human beings are seizing control over human nature and human destiny. That is what makes the biological revolution "revolutionary"; the nature now under human dominion is *human* nature. We are the stakes as well as the players.[2]

The new powers have raised new moral questions, and the public discussion of the complex issues raised by developments in medicine has been vigorous (and sometimes rancorous). Although the questions are raised by the developments in science and technology, they are not fundamentally scientific and technological questions. They are inevitably moral and political. Science can tell us a lot of things, but it cannot tell us what ends we ought to seek with the tools it gives us or how to use those tools without morally violating the human material on which they work. Answers to the novel questions posed by new developments in medicine always assume or contain some judgments both about the good to be sought and done and about the justice of certain ways of seeking it.

1. Kenneth Boulding, *The Meaning of the Twentieth Century* (New York: Harper and Row, 1964), p. 7.

2. Pierre Teilhard de Chardin, *The Phenomenon of Man* (New York: Harper and Row, 1959), p. 229: "We must have become aware that, in the great game that is being played, we are the players as well as being the cards and the stakes."

Thus among reflective people the novel questions posed by developments in medicine lead quickly to some of the oldest questions of all. The new powers have raised new moral problems, but any attempt to deal with them soon confronts fundamental questions about the meaning of life, death, health, freedom, and the person, and about the goals worth striving for and the limits to be imposed on the means to reach them. And these questions inevitably raise the most ancient question of all: What are human beings meant to be and to become? It could hardly be any different, for the nature now under human dominion is human nature.

Public discussion of the novel questions raised by these new powers has seldom candidly raised the ancient and fundamental questions about human nature and human flourishing, however. The public debate has tended to focus instead on two issues: freedom or autonomy and the weighing of risks versus benefits. This is not accidental. Many contemporary moral philosophers have identified the moral point of view with the so-called impartial perspective and have defended either a right to equal freedom or the principle of the greatest number as required by that perspective. Since the Enlightenment the project of philosophical morality has been to identify and justify some impartial and rational principle — some principle which we can and must hold on the basis of reason alone, quite apart from our loyalties and identities, quite apart from our particular histories and communities with their putatively partial visions of human flourishing.[3] The development of bioethics as a discipline, as a branch of applied philosophy, in the last two decades has led many to the task of applying that impartial perspective with its purely rational principles to the concrete and complex quandaries posed by the new developments in medical science and technology. The literature has become increasingly governed by (and limited to) utilitarian and formalist accounts of morality. There remains considerable practical discussion about which impartial principle is the *right* impartial principle, whether respect for auton-

3. Alasdair MacIntyre, *After Virtue* (Notre Dame: University of Notre Dame Press, 1981).

omy or the greatest good for the greatest number, but the assumption still seems to be that public discourse must be limited and governed by an impartial rational principle. That assumption has affected the anthologies in medical ethics, too.

This anthology starts from different assumptions. It is our conviction that theological reflection on the issues raised by advances in medical research and technology is critically important. It is important, first, of course, for communities of faith with visions of what it means for human beings to flourish, for they want to live in faith, and to live with integrity to the identity they have been given and to which they are called. But it is also important for the broader community, for a genuinely pluralistic society requires the candid expression of different perspectives. Candid attention to the religious dimensions of morality, including medical morality, could prevent the reduction of morality to a set of minimal expectations necessary for pluralism and could remind all participants in the public discourse of broader and more profound questions about what human beings are meant to be and to become.

Classes and programs in medical ethics have sprung up all over the country in response to the new developments in medicine and the public controversy concerning them. Many of the courses are in religious studies departments; many more are in institutions which preserve and nurture a lively sense of the Christian tradition. It is primarily for such courses that we produced this anthology, but we hope it will be useful as well to a broader audience as a demonstration of the possibility and promise of candidly theological reflection about these issues.

The criteria for selection of articles for inclusion in this anthology have been these: First, the article should articulate a theological perspective; short of that, it must at least be of significant theological interest. Second, the article should be readable and interesting. Third, the articles should be representative of the diversity of theological opinion and approaches. And fourth, the articles should be either recent pieces or "classic" pieces. It was still difficult to decide what to include and what to leave out, and many of the articles listed in the suggestions for further reading in each chapter are worthy of inclusion. Nevertheless, we think we have assembled a collection which can be used in reading and in teaching to become acquainted with and appreciative of the contributions of theological reflection to medical ethics.

To produce an anthology is to be reminded of one's indebtedness to others, not only to the authors of the essays included in the anthology but also to those who have assisted us in preparing it.

We are especially grateful to Robert Burt and Richard Mouw for permission to print previously unpublished essays.

Jon Pott of William B. Eerdmans Publishing Company has been consistently patient with us and ready with his encouragement and help. Many other friends and colleagues have encouraged us in the project and advised us concerning it: Jim Childress, Rich Mouw, Stan Hauerwas, Lisa Cahill, and David Cook. A special debt of gratitude is due David H. Smith, the director of the National Endowment for the Humanities seminar in medical ethics at which we met and began to collaborate on this project and a good friend and valued colleague ever since.

Our institutions have been helpful to us not only by providing leaves and sabbaticals and faculty grants, but also by supplying colleagues and support personnel and students. To mention any names means that many more whose help and support deserve acknowledgment are slighted, but we must risk at least mentioning our secretaries, Karen Michmerhuizen at Hope College and Jacqueline Wogotz at Lafayette College. And all teachers know they are indebted to their students for the simple possibility of owning the identity of teacher — and for a good deal more besides. So, thanks are due the students in IDS 454, Medicine and Morals, at Hope College, and in Religion 302, Medical Ethics, at Lafayette, on whom we have tried some of our ideas and some of these articles.

Stephen E. Lammers
Allen Verhey

I. Method

CHAPTER ONE

Religion and Medicine

Medicine is modern, clinical, scientific, objective, and rooted in empirical facts, measurable outcomes, data, and observation. Religion, on the other hand, is private, subjective, personal, individual, based on believing things that we cannot see. This, at least, is the conventional wisdom. These assumptions about medicine and religion deeply shape those of us who inhabit contemporary Western culture.

How we have come to think about religion and medicine in these ways is a long story, one best told by historians of medicine.[1] Suffice it to say that the differences between religion and medicine may not be as clear-cut as we believe. In fact, the connections between them are far deeper than we tend to imagine.

Take, for example, the very words we use. "Salvation" — clearly a "religious" term — derives from the Latin root *salus,* which means health, safety, and well-being, a meaning captured in the Spanish-speaking world in their word for health, *salud.* Or consider the French term for health, *santé,* which comes from the Latin root *sanctus,* meaning holy, whole, consecrated. The English word *health* also derives from Anglo-Saxon roots meaning wholeness *(hail),* which in archaic usage also conveyed salvation and spiritual, moral, or mental soundness or well-being *(Oxford English Dictionary).*

Are these connections embedded in our language simply archaic holdovers from a pre-modern age, quaint reminders of a benighted past, before human rationality had learned to disenchant nature and separate religion, science, politics, economics, society, and law into their proper spheres? Or does our language point toward essential and important dimensions of medicine, Christianity, and the relationship between them? The essays in Chapter One argue for the latter claim. They demonstrate the complex and subtle ways that medicine in the first decade of the twenty-first century continues to exhibit deeply religious dynamics. They likewise push readers to rethink common assumptions about religion or more particularly Christianity, especially in its interface with medicine.

Roy Branson maps these connections in his essay "The Secularization of American Medicine" (selection 1). Writing in 1973, before the explosive growth of the industry of contemporary health care in the final quarter of the twentieth century, Branson approaches medicine with the eye of a sociologist and demonstrates the variety of ways in which medicine functions as "a kind of religious system with its own symbols, values, institutions and rituals." Moreover, he rightly notes how science and scientific medicine have in many ways replaced religion as the unifying focus of modern culture. Branson prophesied, in 1973, that with the advent of patient-rights and informed consent, the days of medicine-as-a-religion are coming to an end. Yet thirty-five years later the religious dimension of medicine described by Branson seems, if anything, more powerful. Should anyone doubt his claims, one need look no further than contemporary news stories, especially in venues like the Sunday *New York Times Magazine, Harper's Magazine,* or the ubiquitous pharmaceutical ads for precisely the kinds of theological language, concepts, assumptions, and practices Branson identifies as operative in the early 1970s. A useful exercise to accompany Branson's essay is to ask students to review contemporary media with an eye to these religious dynamics.

At the turn of the new millennium, "alternative medicine" has become big business and has entered the mainstream of U.S. culture. Eminent psychologist and commentator Sidney Callahan shows, in her essay "A New Synthesis: Alternative Medicine's Challenge to Mainstream Medicine and Traditional Christianity" (selection 2), how this new movement in medicine challenges both traditional medicine and traditional religion. She believes rapprochement among these three players will eventually take place. But central to many variants of alternative medicine are rituals, spirituality, and the transcendent, suggesting not simply that alternative medicine is better

1. A thorough understanding of medical ethics requires attention to the history of medicine. The past two decades have seen an increasing number of excellent studies of the history of medicine, both in the U.S. and in relation to Christianity. We include a few titles under "Suggestions for Further Reading." One of the best histories of the relationship between medicine and Christianity is Guenter B. Risse's *Mending Bodies, Saving Souls: A History of Hospitals* (New York: Oxford University Press, 1999).

able to incorporate religion but that it may itself be coming to function as an alternative religion.

George Khushf pushes these connections one step further and gives them a twist. He argues, in "Illness, the Problem of Evil, and the Analogical Structure of Healing" (selection 3), not only that there are religious dimensions of medicine (even to the point of the idolatry of health) but also that medicine itself provides an analogy for Christian claims about sin, suffering, sickness, death, renewal, and redemption. Indeed, "analogy" might be too weak a word for the claim he is making. For Khushf does not simply suggest that we can learn about Christian convictions by looking at medicine and saying "this is like that." Nor is he looking for ways in which Christian convictions can find a place within the world of medicine. Rather, Khushf inverts the picture, locating medicine within the overarching framework of God's redemption. He argues that only when medicine is practiced within a Christian matrix can it find its proper place and direction; it is then that medicine provides a window from which to understand sin and redemption.

The first three essays, then, challenge us to see the thick interconnections between religion and contemporary medicine. William F. May, in his essay "Money and the Medical Profession" (selection 4), turns the lens in a different angle. May, a theologian, knows well that a main candidate for idolatry in the Gospels is none other than Mammon. Here he highlights the myriad of ways that money (the ecumenical, almighty dollar, complete with graven images, and more) continues to have religious dimensions, even in the twentieth century. This theological sensibility lies behind the critical questions May raises on the relationship between money and the medical profession.

This issue remains one of the most vexing yet unaddressed questions in medical ethics. Total health care spending in the U.S. in 2007 reached $2.4 *trillion* annually or 17 percent of the gross domestic product. Concerns have surfaced about physician relationships with the pharmaceutical and biotech industries, be it through perks supplied by sales personnel or physicians acting as consultants or speakers. A growing number of voices have begun to question the astounding amounts of money community-based physicians can make for enrolling patients in clinical trials.[2] Yet, as a culture, we lack a nuanced, careful, critical means to talk about money. Religion and politics remain taboo subjects at cocktail parties and family gatherings, but equally taboo are questions of money. How many people know, would ask, or would discuss their salaries with colleagues, neighbors, or members of their church?

This taboo reaches beyond personal conversations to bioethics. Like the broader culture, contemporary bioethics — generally centered around philosophical principles — lacks the tools to analyze or address the economic, industrial infrastructure that drives many "quandaries" in bioethics. Genetic testing, *in vitro* fertilization, stem cell research — these are not only practices that raise moral questions; they are big business. How ought the fact that these endeavors are highly profitable industries enter into one's ethical analysis and evaluation? This edition of *On Moral Medicine* endeavors to make more visible the economic dimensions of what have long been treated as merely "ethical," philosophical, or theological questions. We do so not only because they are largely invisible yet powerfully operative; we do so also because, with May, we hold that economic questions are essentially ethical/theological concerns.

While public interest in alternative medicine has been on the rise over the past two decades, interest in the connections between "religion" and "health" have equally captured public attention, and research into these connections has become a discipline in its own right. In "Conceptualizing 'Religion'" (selection 5), three physicians — Daniel E. Hall, Harold G. Koenig, and Keith G. Meador — argue that much of this research is bound to fail. It is not that they believe such connections are not to be found — Koenig remains one of the leading figures in the field of religion and health. They argue, however, that most research in religion and health misunderstands religion. Most research in this area operates with what they call a "functional" or "instrumental" view of religion. Such a view is utilitarian, since it sees religion as positive only when it is a useful tool for achieving some other end (like health). Such a view also presumes that "religion" is a universal category — that all faith traditions are essentially the same and can be evaluated from an objective, external perspective. This concept of religion, they argue, has little to do with the way that religions are actually practiced. Thus they call for a different model: "religion as a second first language." Religious traditions, they contend, must be understood from the "inside"; researchers must gain "fluency" in particular religions if they are to adequately understand them. Until they do, their research will necessarily be plagued by fundamental design flaws and will not produce meaningful results.

Stanley Hauerwas, in the final essay in this chapter — "Salvation and Health: Why Medicine Needs the Church" (selection 6) — concurs with Hall et al., and takes their argument one step further. Not only do contemporary attempts to "relate" medicine and religion misconstrue religion; they also misunderstand and distort the nature and character of medicine. Hauerwas does not want to follow Khushf in arguing that medicine needs to be dependent on theology; instead, he reframes the question. Medicine, he claims, is that social practice whereby society sets aside certain people (physicians, nurses, chaplains, and others) for the vocation of being present to the ill and suffering. Medicine is, at its core, a human presence in the face of suffering. To be such a presence can be a profound privilege, but it still presents real burdens. How, he asks,

2. Jill A. Fisher, *Medical Research for Hire: The Political Economy of Pharmaceutical Clinical Trials* (New Brunswick, N.J.: Rutgers University Press, 2009); Marcia Angell, *The Truth about Drug Companies: How They Deceive Us and What to Do about It* (New York: Random House, 2005).

can practitioners be sustained in their commitment to such a practice, especially in the face of the burdens it inevitably presents? The church, Hauerwas believes, provides such a resource, "a resource of the habits and practices necessary to sustain the care of those in pain [as well as those who care for them] over the long haul."

It has been said that the first question of ethics is not "what should I do?" but "what is going on here?"[3] This is another way of saying that the most important step in ethical analysis is getting the description of the situation right. We hope these essays in Chapter One begin to dislodge oversimplified understandings of medicine and religion and provide a more accurate, nuanced, and multifaceted description of their complex interrelationships.

SUGGESTIONS FOR FURTHER READING

Ferngren, Gary B. *Medicine and Health Care in Early Christianity* (Baltimore: Johns Hopkins University Press, 2009).

Foucault, Michel. *The Birth of the Clinic* (New York: Vintage, 1994).

Marty, Martin E., and Kenneth Vaux, eds. *Health/Medicine and the Faith Traditions: An Inquiry into Religion and Medicine* (Philadelphia: Fortress Press, 1982). See also individual volumes in the Health/Medicine in the Faith Traditions series published by the Park Ridge Center.

Pellegrino, Edmund D. *Helping and Healing: Religious Commitment in Health Care* (Washington, D.C.: Georgetown University Press, 1997).

Risse, Guenter B. *Mending Bodies, Saving Souls: A History of Hospitals* (New York: Oxford University Press, 1999).

Rosenberg, Charles E. *The Care of Strangers: The Rise of America's Hospital System* (Baltimore: Johns Hopkins University Press, 1995).

Shuman, Joel, and Keith Meador. *Heal Thyself: Spirituality, Medicine, and the Distortion of Christianity* (New York: Oxford University Press, 2002).

Shriver, Donald W., Jr., ed. *Medicine and Religion: Strategies of Care* (Pittsburgh: University of Pittsburgh Press, 1980).

Starr, Paul. *The Social Transformation of American Medicine* (New York: Basic Books, 1984).

Tournier, Paul. *A Doctor's Casebook in the Light of the Bible,* trans. Edwin Hudson (London: SCM Press, 1954; New York: Harper & Row, 1960).

3. H. Richard Niebuhr, *The Responsible Self: An Essay in Christian Moral Philosophy* (Louisville: Westminster John Knox, 1999; originally published in 1962).

1 The Secularization of American Medicine

Roy Branson

Physicians have reason to be frightened. The American Medical Association opposes national health insurance because it knows voting on such a proposal by Congress will mark the end of medicine's privileged status among professions in America. It will memorialize the transferring of power from the professional in medicine to the layman. Under the pressure of increasingly powerful outside forces, America's most cloistered profession has already begun conforming to the values, norms and practices of the society around it. Physicians know that with comprehensive health insurance Congress will be celebrating nothing less than the secularization of American medicine.

Enough has been written by sociologists and historians to demonstrate that health and disease are not purely physiological, but conditions defined by the whole matrix of human expectations, beliefs and habits. Medicine has always been practiced within the context of what a society conceived as normative in thought and action. The enormous prestige of medicine in the recent history of America derives, to a large extent, from its adherence to values and norms that have been central to American society. The problem for medicine today is that these values sometimes stand in opposition to other values, equally fundamental to American society.

Medicine continues to have faith in the inherent value of reason to discover order in empirical facts, continues to believe scientific and technological knowledge testify to a rational order.[1] It is an unquestioned good that man

1. Paul Tillich, *Systematic Theology,* I (Chicago: University of Chicago Press, 1951), pp. 53-54, 72-74. Reason here refers to what Tillich called *technical reason.* "By the technical concept of reason, reason is reduced to the capacity for reasoning. Only the cognitive side of reason remains and within the cognitive realm only those cognitive acts which deal with the discovery of means for ends" (pp. 72, 73). Tillich contrasts technical reason with ontological reason. "According to the classical philosophical tradition reason is the structure of the mind which enables the mind to grasp and to transform reality. It is effective in the cognitive, aesthetic, practical and technical functions of the mind" (p. 72). Elsewhere, he identified ontological reason with ecstatic and existential reason. "Ecstatic reason is reason grasped by an ultimate concern" (p. 53). What Tillich calls ontological reason could not be opposed to a sense of equality and freedom; but rationality, narrowly defined as

From the *Hastings Center Studies* 1, no. 2 (1973): 17-28. © The Hastings Center. Used by permission of the publisher and the author.

should know this order. Medicine believes man should not only discern order intellectually, but he should also act according to rationally ordered patterns. Because it adheres to the value of order in both thought and action, medicine acts according to the criterion of effectiveness. Medicine could not help but flourish in an America loyal to scientific rationality and bureaucratic efficiency.

But now values as basic to America as rationality and order are being powerfully articulated. There are increasing demands that the self-evident truths of freedom and equality of all men be extended throughout American society. It is being argued that no group has the right, because of its knowledge and effectiveness — no matter how impressive — to dictate the terms of life and death to the rest of society. Every group of experts, including medical doctors, must recognize the basic equality of all men to set the conditions of their existence. Doctors are faced with the norm they so treasure — effectiveness — losing precedence to free participation of equals as the criterion society follows in deciding problems of medical care.

This fundamental shift in emphasis from order and technical knowledge to equality and freedom, from efficiency of the expert to participation of the citizen, will affect the roles of doctor and patient. As much as loss of revenue, this is what frightens the physician. Patients will not as easily allow themselves to be treated as deviants from the doctor's marvelously rational world. They will not revere the physician as the mediator of special knowledge. Patients will quite likely regard themselves as fellow-citizens demanding technical information. Certainly any sense that medical care is a privilege that the physician mediates to those he chooses will give way to the community asserting, indeed enforcing, its right to medical care.

The Religion of Medicine

Alterations in medical care have been analyzed from the perspectives of economics and political theory. But if the controversy and deep emotion accompanying basic alterations in medical practice are to be understood, it must be realized that medicine in America has not been merely one more occupation in our economic system or an effective power bloc in American polity. Medicine's roots go deeper. If we are to understand why the conflicts over federal health care legislation have been so passionate, we must realize that medicine has acted in America as a kind of religious system, with its own symbols, values, institutions and rituals.

---

technical reason, can be. Cf. Langdon Gilkey, *Religion and the Scientific Future* (New York: Harper & Row, 1970), p. 96. "Knowing for Greek philosophy, was not *techne,* knowing how to do something; it was rather *wisdom,* knowledge of the self. . . . Modern knowing is science, on the other hand; it represents objective knowledge of external structure unrelated to the self, or to the mystery of its freedom."

Robert Bellah defines religion "as a set of symbolic forms and acts which relate man to the ultimate conditions of his existence."[2] Thomas O'Dea concurs: "Religion is a response to the ultimate which becomes institutionalized in thought, practice and organization."[3] Agreement with his fellow sociologists on a functional definition of religion allows J. Milton Yinger to describe science as an attempt to deal with ultimate questions, to characterize science as a religious enterprise.

> Few men can avoid the problem of struggling with questions of salvation (how can man be saved from his most difficult problems?), of the nature of reality, of evil (why do men suffer?), and the like. Science as a way of life is an effort to deal with these questions.[4]

Science affirms that there is an ideal natural order, a set of laws or patterns, and that, as Stephen Toulmin puts it, "these ideals of natural order have something absolute about them."[5] Science has believed that ultimate questions could be answered by knowing the order it affirms. The scientist has seemed to say to his fellow men that "if we know or are aware of everything, if we understand all relevant causes and factors, we can control everything." The scientist, quintessential modern man, has genuinely believed and committed his life to what Langdon Gilkey calls "faith in the healing power of knowledge."[6]

Medicine, of course, is the healing knowledge par excellence. Medicine assumes that disorders can be treated by relying on the order science proclaims. "The science of medicine depends on the faith that it is not chance which operates, but cause."[7]

Talcott Parsons argues that while the cosmos proclaimed by traditional religion no longer dominates modern culture, society depends for its very existence on some sense of order. He suggests that the pattern of beliefs and values integrating contemporary culture is maintained by the "intellectual disciplines," among which science is pre-eminent.[8] If Parsons is right that science has replaced religion (narrowly defined) as the uni-

2. Robert Bellah, "Religious Evolution," *American Sociological Review* 29 (June 1964): 359.

3. Thomas O'Dea, *The Sociology of Religion* (Englewood Cliffs, N.J.: Prentice-Hall, Inc., 1966), p. 27; cf. Milton J. Yinger, *The Scientific Study of Religion* (New York, N.Y.: Macmillan Co., 1970), p. 7. "Religion, then, can be defined as a system of beliefs and practices by means of which a group of people struggle with these ultimate problems of human life."

4. Yinger, *The Scientific Study of Religion,* p. 12.

5. Stephen Toulmin, *Foresight and Understanding* (New York: Harper & Row, 1961), p. 57.

6. Gilkey, *Religion and the Future,* p. 52. "Use of knowledge for control over physical nature has until the present raised few moral problems, and so the model taken from engineering and medicine has seemed to validate over and over this hope for a better scientific technology" (p. 85). Cf. pp. 79, 85-89, 95, 96.

7. Lester S. King, *The Growth of Medical Thought* (Chicago: University of Chicago Press, 1963), p. 36.

8. Talcott Parsons, *The System of Modern Societies* (Englewood Cliffs, N.J.: Prentice-Hall, Inc., 1971), p. 99.

fying focus of modern culture, then medicine is part of the central faith of our times.

Because medicine has identified itself so closely with science it has gained great authority as a profession. One of America's foremost sociologists of medicine, Eliot Freidson, is convinced that

> medicine is not merely one of the major professions of our time. Among the traditional professions established in the European universities of the Middle Ages, it alone has developed a systematic connection with science and technology. . . . Medicine has displaced the law and the ministry from their once dominant positions.[9]

Much of the credit physicians receive for knowing the true order of things, for being experts, comes from medicine's widely proclaimed commitment to the scientific ideals of knowledge and order.

Medicine, of course, is not a purely scholarly profession. It would not be supported by the public for simply possessing knowledge. Medicine is expected to transmute science into therapy, knowledge into action. As they move from theory to practice, physicians adhere strictly to their scientific faith, trying not only to think but act in orderly fashion. Physicians who believe in a reality that is coherent regulate their actions by strict patterns of behavior. Medical doctors are committed to following procedures that have the least waste motion, that cure in the shortest amount of time. Physicians believe they should move as directly as possible from symptom to cause, from cause to treatment. The profession of medicine combines the values of scientific faith — knowledge and order — with concrete norms for regulating medical practice — effectiveness and efficiency. Medicine, then, not only conforms to what has been the fundamental perspective of modern, scientific culture, but energetically follows some of the guiding principles of pragmatic, American society. It is no wonder medicine has enjoyed enormous prestige in America.

So great has been the respect accorded medicine by American society that some commentators have come to describe it as more than an ordinary profession. Freidson believes "medicine's position today is akin to that of the state religions yesterday — it has an officially approved monopoly of the right to define health and illness and to treat illness."[10]

It is understandable that medicine would achieve such an exalted status in American society; that it would be trusted not only to control but define deviancy. What would be more appropriate than a group so obviously dedicated to order and effectiveness deciding what constitutes deviance from these values and standards?

Talcott Parsons, who has done as much as anyone to show disease to be not simply a physical condition but a social role, goes so far as to call disease the primary type of deviance in American society.[11] He does so because a person in a diseased condition cannot be effective, cannot achieve.[12] Of course, the diseased person not only violates norms regulating behavior in society. He is at fundamental odds with the natural order. Parsons follows the logic of his reasoning. He explicitly correlates illness with original sin.[13]

Freidson agrees that the stigma of having been a deviant stays with the diseased person, even after he has recovered; that someone who has received grace remains in some sense a sinner, or at least an ex-sinner. But Freidson insists that there are still important variations in society's abhorrence of disease. He suggests that two independent criteria, personal responsibility and seriousness of condition, are used to distinguish, for example, among a careless youngster sniffling from a cold, a drunk bleeding from a brawl, a bachelor suffering from venereal disease, and a gunman critically wounded in an attempted homicide.[14] Freidson's clarifications do not contradict Parsons' basic point. Indeed, both men assume the same premise. "Quite unlike neutral scientific concepts like that of 'virus' or 'molecule,' the concept of illness is inherently evaluational. Medicine is a moral enterprise."[15]

Indeed, in a scientific age, where illness becomes the most ubiquitous label for deviance, medicine emerges as a crucial agent in the application of the scientific creed to a variety of problems. Consider the importance of medical testimony in courts and the influence of medical opinion in defining alcoholism and drug addiction as not strictly ecclesiastical or legal issues but as health problems. Imperceptibly, physicians, as loyal defenders of rationality, order and effectiveness, become the group that defines normality, that arbitrates orthodoxy in modern culture.[16]

Of course, physicians are not content to identify sin. They have the ability to combat it. Their knowledge of science and their extended training in applying that knowledge in a rational, disciplined manner give them

9. Eliot Freidson, *Profession of Medicine* (New York: Dodd, Mead & Co., 1970), p. xviii; cf. Talcott Parsons, "A Sociologist Looks at the Legal Profession," in *Essays in Sociological Theory* (New York: Free Press, 1949), p. 376. "Established scientific knowledge *does* constitute a highly stable point of reference. Hence the 'authority' of the relevant professional groups for interpretations can always be referred to such established knowledge."

10. Freidson, *Profession of Medicine,* p. 5.

11. Talcott Parsons, "Definitions of Health and Illness in the Light of American Values and Social Structure," in *Patients, Physicians and Illness,* ed. by E. Gartley Jaco (New York: Free Press, 1958), p. 186.

12. Ibid., p. 185; cf. Talcott Parsons, *The Social System* (New York: Free Press, 1951), pp. 437-39.

13. Parsons, "Definitions of Health and Illness," p. 175; cf. Freidson, *Profession of Medicine,* p. 231.

14. The specific examples are mine, not Freidson's.

15. Freidson, *Profession of Medicine,* pp. 208, 233, 236, 252; cf. pp. 339-40. "Furthermore, an essential component of what is said to be knowledge is the designation of illness, which, I have insisted, is in and of itself evaluative and moral rather than technical in character."

16. Ibid., pp. 244, 248-49; cf. Parsons, *The Social System,* p. 445.

confidence that evil can be purified. Men who are not in harmony with the basic order of existence can be restored. Those who have capitulated, who believe they cannot perform according to acceptable standards, can be rehabilitated. Medicine has the means.[17]

For those means to be effective the agents of order and rationality must be trusted. The sick and those responsible for them must realize that they cannot find restoration by their own efforts. They must rely on those who are competent in these matters; those who possess the proper knowledge. Furthermore, it is impossible for each practitioner to be asked to prove and re-prove his merit every time he heals. Patients must come to trust physicians as such; not the admittedly fluctuating worth of individual doctors, but the office of physician.[18] It will not do for patients to take their own medical records from one waiting room to another demanding evidence of a doctor's competence. The sick must put themselves in the hands of the professional. Patients must believe in physicians. "Their therapy depends upon faith. And we may be wise to recognize that there is a faithful quality to medical practice."[19]

The most obvious way for the diseased to show their trust in the representatives of science and their desire to return to a life of rationality and order is for patients to follow the procedures outlined for them by their physicians. It is "the patient's obligation faithfully to accept the implications of the fact that he is 'Dr. X's patient' and so long as he remains in that status he must 'do his part' in the common enterprise."[20] The patient is out of harmony with the basic order of existence. He suffers from the power of disruptive forces distorting his life. Through the course of action outlined by the physician, the patient can experience the power of rationality in his own life. By means of carefully planned actions the physician mediates the mysteries of scientific research for the benefit of ordinary, diseased patients. In the process, medicine creates a ritual system, and the doctor becomes a priest.

As is the case in all religious systems, medicine's symbols are effective because they arise from generally accepted truths. The impact of these symbols is familiar. With the separation of the priest from the layman, the mystery enshrouding the priest expands and his authority increases.

A desire to avoid contamination may be the basis for the physician's dress, but their spotless white apparel instantly conveys an aura that divides the diseased from the holy. Even when their attire cannot contribute to asepsis, physicians cling to their peculiar vestments.[21] Traditional clerics and theologians have begun to refer to their new colleagues and rivals as "the men in the white coats."[22] Technical language may be precise and convenient, but it also allows conversations among physicians which the laymen are not ready to hear. If the laymen did understand, their questions would impede the efficiency of efforts to rescue them from their grave condition.[23]

Asking a deviant for the location of records of his past actions, requiring him to give a recital of his previous deeds and present attitudes, demanding that he disrobe for a careful examination of the visible signs of his polluted state, all have good, scientific justification. They also comprise an interrogation as old as Egyptian medical rites and as intimidating as any confession taken in the Inquisition.[24] After this ritual there is no question as to where authority in the doctor-patient relationship lies.

If any doubt lingers, it is soon expelled. The fully robed, impressively self-contained examiner pronounces a verdict on the condition of the diseased. He may grant complete absolution, saying that the problem is imaginary, or he may absolve the diseased of any guilt for his present condition; none of his past actions have led to his present deplorable state. Quite likely the inquisitor points out where there have been some past transgressions contributing to the present turmoil, and prescribes a series of penitential acts by which purity may be regained.[25] The discipline may include the purchase of objects with special powers to assist in achieving full release.[26] If the condition is serious a sentence of separation from the healthy may be pronounced. Those untouched by the corruption deserve protection, and the diseased must be encouraged to seek a new life.[27]

The authority of the physician reaches its heights when men face the ultimate threat of death. The terror is greatest because the secrecy is absolute. Nothing is more mysterious or tremendous than death, nothing more daunting. Before this final specter men become desperate for reliable knowledge of science. They gladly deliver themselves into the hands of its representative, pleading for him to effectively impose rational order on lives being drawn into chaos. As Parsons observes,

> It is striking that the medical is one of the few occupational groups which in our society have regular, expected contact with death in the course of their occupational roles. . . . It is presumed that this association with death is a very important factor in the emotional toning of the role of the physician.[28]

17. Parsons, "Definitions of Health and Illness," p. 178.
18. Parsons, *The Social System,* p. 439.
19. Yinger, *Study of Religion,* p. 77; cf. Eliot Freidson, *Professional Dominance: The Social Structure of Medical Care* (New York: Atherton Press, 1972), pp. 119, 143.
20. Parsons, *The Social System,* p. 465.
21. Julius A. Roth, "Ritual and Magic in the Control of Contagion," *American Sociological Review* 20 (June 1957): 310-14; cf. Freidson, *Profession of Medicine,* p. 9.
22. Gilkey, *Religion and the Future,* p. 79.
23. Raymond S. Duff and August B. Hollingshead, *Sickness and Society* (New York: Harper & Row, 1968), pp. 132, 327.
24. Erwin H. Ackerknecht, *A Short History of Medicine* (New York: Ronald Press, 1968), p. 16; cf. Henry E. Sigerist, *A History of Medicine* (New York: Oxford University Press, 1951), pp. 188, 196.
25. Freidson, *Profession of Medicine,* p. 228.
26. Yinger, *Study of Religion,* p. 77.
27. Freidson, *Profession of Medicine,* pp. 228, 313-14; cf. Talcott Parsons and Renée Fox, "Illness, Therapy and the Modern Urban American Family," *Patients, Physicians and Illness,* pp. 241, 244.
28. Parsons, *The Social System,* pp. 444-45.

He goes on to say that while he believes the physician is not identical to a clergyman, he "has very important associations with the sacred."[29] Certainly the patient, desperate to achieve salvation from death, regards a physician offering him medicine with the same awe as he does a priest extending the wafer. The physician is providing a visible means by which man may receive salvation.

Parsons' own illustrations of the sacred within clinical training and practice point less in the direction of internal medicine and more towards surgery.

> Dissection is not only an instrumental means to the learning of anatomy, but is a symbolic act, highly charged with affective significance. It is in a sense the initiatory rite of the physician-to-be into his intimate association with death and the dead.[30]

If dissection of an already dead cadaver is an initiatory rite, how is cutting into a living body to be regarded? Clearly, at the present time, the medical profession itself looks on this act with the greatest awe. Medical students list surgery as a desirable specialty because it is "one which offers a wide variety of experience and in which responsibility is symbolized by the possibility of killing or disabling patients in the course of making a mistake."[31] Training to become a surgeon is the longest in medicine, and the profession has agreed that performing an operation should bring the highest financial reward of any single act in medical practice.

As for the sick, nothing in medicine frightens them more than surgery.[32] They know that the potential benefits are great. Patients feel that an operation, if survived, promises the fastest and most efficient recovery from a major illness.[33] But the sick also know that for a major operation, they must knowingly relinquish to the doctor complete control over their destiny. On previous occasions the patient has been dependent on the physician, but at no other time is the act of submission into the hands of a doctor so carefully considered, so self-conscious.

Once the decision is made, a prescribed, carefully planned sequence of actions is set in motion. The force of these lengthy preparations comes from the knowledge that they are required by the rational, orderly faith of science. Deviations will bring evil consequences, severe complications.

Days before the operation the patient enters a rigid discipline. His actions are restricted. His diet becomes even more controlled than before. The day of the operation he receives special, cleansing ministrations.

Few know exactly what transpires within the secluded area where surgery is performed. Ordinary functionaries are not allowed entrance; only those with special training. Even these enter only after purifying themselves. The surgeon himself must unvaryingly observe necessary ablutions before approaching the body. Reports indicate that drugs administered to the patient bring a deep sleep. Special ointments applied to the body complete the rituals anticipating the climactic act. Then, according to the requirements of science, the knife falls.

Of course, some are lost though their death often advances the cause of science. But sacrifice is not the culminating rite of this religion. Many recover from surgery. When they do, the religion of medicine has been able to do nothing less than ritualize the miracle of miracles. Through the surgeon's knowledge of the fundamental order of reality and his performance in the most efficient manner possible, a body has been laid to rest, and risen again.[34]

Not surprisingly, no believer testifies more zealously to his faith than the newly-recovered surgical patient. In his previous, broken condition he felt himself the least knowledgeable, least effective member of the medical community. Within the medical hierarchy it seemed appropriate that he occupy the lowest position. Grateful for his astonishing recovery, the patient regards the surgeon as high priest.

Profanation of the Religion

Except for the years from the Renaissance to the nineteenth century in the West, the physician has always been regarded as a priest. Only during the relatively brief period when faith in miraculous healing through incantation and prayer was being lost and trust in a substitute authority had not yet emerged, did the physician lose his aura of possessing sacred powers. In primitive tribes, in the high cultures of Mesopotamia, Egypt, China, India, Greece and Rome, right into the Christian Middle Ages, the physician was a religious functionary.[35]

Universally, disease was considered an evidence of sin. Not only in primitive tribes, but in Mesopotamia, Egypt, India, Mexico and Christian countries, confession necessarily preceded cure.[36] Potions with mysterious powers and rituals with guaranteed purgative effect have been prescribed by all civilizations. In Egypt, India and Greece, incubation was a central part of medical treat-

29. Ibid., p. 445.

30. Ibid.

31. Eliot Freidson, "Medical Personnel," *International Encyclopedia of the Social Sciences,* 2nd edition, 10, p. 107; based on data from Howard S. Becker et al., *Boys in White: Student Culture in Medical School* (Chicago: University of Chicago Press, 1961).

32. Duff and Hollingshead, *Sickness and Society,* p. 273.

33. Ibid., p. 294.

34. For a concurring analysis of surgery (though the two analyses were developed independently of each other) see Robert N. Wilson, "Teamwork in the Operating Room," *Human Organization* 12 (Winter, 1954): 9-14.

35. In addition to the works of Ackerknecht and Sigerist already cited, I am especially indebted for the historical background given by the following authors: Lester S. King, *The Growth of Medical Thought* and George Rosen, "The Hospital: Historical Sociology of a Community Institution," in *The Hospital in Modern Society,* ed. by Eliot Freidson (Glencoe, Ill.: Free Press, 1963).

36. Ackerknecht, *History of Medicine,* pp. 27-28, 31, 38; Sigerist, *History of Medicine,* pp. 188, 196.

ment.[37] The buildings to which the patient traveled for his healing sleep (when he was visited by the gods) were temples, presided over by physicians who were priests.[38] Especially charismatic physicians evolved from mediators of the sacred into its incarnation; for example, Akhnaton in Egypt and Aesculapius in Greece.[39]

As late as the seventeenth century the clergy were the principal healers in America.[40] Even today in America, there are hospitals with religious sponsorship, operated by ecclesiastical orders.

However, it is undeniable that from the Renaissance into the nineteenth century, medicine in the West suffered a crisis of confidence. No potion, no priesthood, no prayers, could stay the ravages of the Plague. As many people died under medical care as survived. Increasingly, the masses were unwilling to dismiss this record as the all-wise will of God. Hospitals, far from being temples, were shunned as repositories of those already enduring the final agonies of death.[41]

The recovery of medicine's influence and authority followed the rise of a new confidence in science. Though it came late, long after basic scientific discoveries, medicine finally discovered vaccines for immunizing mass populations and developed aseptic and anesthetic procedures, allowing the performance of extensive surgery.[42] Medicine had found the effective means to mediate the new, scientific world view.

The buildings where the new scientific wonders were discovered or performed ceased to be shunned as charnel houses. The population, as they had not since perhaps the days of Egypt and Greece, were awed by the new mysterious power active in these edifices. They flocked to them, seeking release from their grievous condition. Once again, in the twentieth century, the physician found amidst the marvels of scientific technology, the appropriate setting for his traditional role of wonder-worker. Never has he been more revered.

But medicine faces a crisis as challenging to its authority as the Renaissance and Enlightenment's diminished faith in the efficacy of prayer and miracle. Just as men's reliance on their own ability to think and act during that time undercut the influence of priestly physicians, so today's demand for self-determination in every sector of society threatens medicine's independence of action. The process by which the laity in some parts of the West seized control of the church in the sixteenth century, the state in the eighteenth and nineteenth centuries and the economy in the twentieth, is now threatening the autonomy of science and technology. Medicine, so proudly identified as a bastion of scientific orthodoxy, must brace itself for this latest wave of reformation.[43]

Talcott Parsons identifies the present stage of reformation as an "education revolution" that insists that all institutions, groups and professions must operate in accordance with wider cultural values. Groups can find their own special areas of concern, but they must conform to the culture's general values. If they do not, if a group insists on remaining isolated, acting according to its own idiosyncratic principles, it is falling into a fundamentalism. Examples could include the American Amish, the Roman Catholic Curia, as well as such twentieth-century political movements as Fascism and Stalinism.[44] If the scientific community rejects the basic values of a culture, it too is fundamentalist.

Reformers of contemporary culture, concerned about segments of society resisting universal values, understandably concentrate their attention on the professions. From Emile Durkheim on, social philosophers have regarded the professions as pivotal elements in modern society. With the disappearance of the tribe and the weakening of the family and church, the professions have become crucial as moral orders, drawing men not only into common tasks, but common interpretations of life.[45] Parsons goes so far as to say that

> the professional complex, though obviously still incomplete in its development, has already become the most important single component in the structure of modern societies . . . the massive emergence of the professional complex, not the special status of capitalistic or socialistic modes of organization is the crucial development in twentieth-century society.[46]

As we have already noted, with the waning of faith, the clergy has differentiated into distinct professions. These

37. Ackerknecht, *History of Medicine,* pp. 21, 41, 50.

38. Rosen, *Hospital in Society,* pp. 26, 29.

39. Ackerknecht, *History of Medicine,* pp. 21, 50.

40. Ibid., pp. 219, 220.

41. Rosen, *Hospital in Society,* pp. 26-29.

42. Ackerknecht, *History of Medicine,* p. 171; King, *Growth of Medical Thought,* p. 221; Freidson, *Profession of Medicine,* p. 16.

43. Parsons, *System of Modern Societies,* p. 99. Although Parsons does not interpret changes within medicine as a process of secularization, he does note that significant developments within the field are taking place. He analyzes the changes in medicine in terms that he elsewhere uses to describe developments in religious structures; developments which he calls secularization. See in particular, Parsons, "Some Theoretical Considerations Bearing on the Field of Medical Sociology," *Social Structure and Personality* (New York: Free Press, 1964), p. 257. "A further highly significant feature of the general process of change which has been going on is the generalization of the value complex involving health problems. This is a relatively intangible matter to which little explicit research attention has been devoted." Ibid., p. 355. Freidson does put changes within medicine in a historical continuity with secularization of institutional religion. See *Profession of Medicine,* pp. xviii, 250.

44. Parsons, *Systems of Modern Societies,* p. 100.

45. Emile Durkheim, *On the Division of Labor in Society,* trans. by George Simpson (New York: 1893); Cornelia Brookfield, *Professional Ethics and Civic Morals* (London: 1898-1900); Theodore M. Steeman, "Durkheim's Professional Ethics," *Journal for the Scientific Study of Religion* 2 (April 1963): 163-81; C. P. Wold, "The Durkheim Thesis: Occupational Groups and Moral Integration," *Journal for the Scientific Study of Religion* 2 (Spring 1970): 17-32.

46. "Professions," *International Encyclopedia of the Social Sciences,* 2nd edition, 12, p. 545.

newer orders of service within society have gained recognition because of their technical knowledge, their mastery of a particular set of facts and skills, but the professions have also become influential because they have been relied upon to continue the traditional function of the clergy: inculcating within individuals the overarching values of a culture.

Max Weber quite consciously called the scientific professions a "calling," with the clear religious overtones that word carries, to underline the central role of these particular professions in mediating the values of the modern, scientific age.[47] If our previous analysis is correct, medicine is the profession within the scientific callings that has most clearly assumed the function of the clergy.[48]

Protestants against this new priesthood do not dispute the technical expertise of physicians, but they do object to medical doctors thinking that mastery of scientific data qualifies them to act as moral arbiters. Influence and leadership within a society, they say, should result from adherence to universally acknowledged moral principles.

Of course physicians, and others in the scientific callings, have thought that they already lived according to the basic beliefs of the age. Certainly science has kept faith with rationality and order. It is startling to hear contemporary reformers inveighing against science as a new orthodoxy blind to more inclusive concerns. Today's reformers declare that knowledge is not sacrosanct. They demand that science recognize the priority of equality and freedom.

Appeals to equality and freedom may initially seem harmless enough. But when the reformers begin to draw out the implications of these values physicians become aware that a full-dress challenge is under way to their profession and its hallowed status. Equality means extension of power beyond the privileged few. Today's laity, like their predecessors in previous centuries, claim that equality gives them the right to participate in making decisions affecting their own lives and destiny.

Participation in medicine means invading the heart of its authority: defining the nature of disease.[49] Physicians can list a set of symptoms, but it is up to the general population to decide whether or not the condition described by the physician is normal or abnormal, acceptable or unacceptable. Definition of sin cannot be the exclusive preserve of those ordained by the community to wage war against evil.[50]

If equality means the laity involves itself to the point of defining illness, it certainly means laymen can set priorities as to which diseases are especially abhorrent, and which will receive less attention. Allocation of medical resources is the prerogative of the donors, not the functionaries receiving funds to perform designated services. Equality, for many reformers, even means that laymen retain the right to decide whether or not the method by which a physician treats a deviant conforms to generally accepted standards of behavior and practice.[51] Regional medical programs, comprehensive health planning, public review boards, and even the courts, are all ways in which laymen are already beginning to exercise authority over professionals in medicine.[52]

As this process of secularization continues, the roles of the patient and doctor will be affected. The patient will approach the physician, not as a suppliant, but as a fellow-citizen. He will not request expiation of his condition, but affirm his right, as a member of the community, to medical care. The physician can continue to have authority, but in a much more limited sphere. The function of the physician will be much more specific. He will provide information concerning the etiology and rehabilitation of various physical disorders.

Secularization seems always to affect ritual last. As long as death, or the possibility of death, continues to strike fear in human beings, actions that are able to ward it off, or at least postpone its advent, will elicit confidence. No doubt the rite of surgery will continue to create a response of dread and awe. Certainly individual acts of healing will result in grateful patients according respect to their own physician.

But as medicine enters a new era, the rituals of cure are less impressive than the cooperative efforts of a community trying to improve its general health. The citizenry is becoming less inclined to measure the adequacy of medicine by miraculous deeds in the temple, and more interested in finding a way of life that makes spectacular cures unnecessary. Participation is moving beyond citizens asserting their control over the processes of cure to their assuming responsibility for bettering the conditions for health. The goal is not simply reforming the ministrations of physicians, but improving the health of the community to the point where their mediation is almost unnecessary.[53]

47. *From Max Weber,* ed. and trans. by H. H. Gerth and C. Wright Mills (New York: Oxford University Press, 1963), pp. 129-56; Robert M. Veatch, "Medical Ethics: Professional or Universal?" Working Paper for the Institute of Society, Ethics and the Life Sciences, Hastings-on-Hudson, New York, p. 2. A comparison of professional to universal ethics in medicine.

48. Freidson, *Profession of Medicine,* pp. 335, 348.

49. Ibid., p. 206.

50. Ibid., pp. 252, 342-43, 345.

51. Ibid., pp. 345, 374; Veatch, "Medical Ethics," pp. 16-18.

52. See Barbara Ehrenreich, *American Health Empire* (New York: Random House, 1970), for criticisms of these programs and arguments for more radical proposals for community control of health care.

53. See Bellah's article "Religious Evolution" for helpful periodization of religious change. Within Bellah's stages of primitive, archaic, historic, early modern and modern, medicine might be described as in transition from historic to early modern. There is a shift from an emphasis on sacrifice to morality, from dependence on the rituals of the temple to a kind of "inner-worldly" maintenance of health. As medicine moves on from its present point of maturation there will likely be increased emphasis on each person maintaining his own health through measures that heretofore have

Of course, the majority of American physicians stress the dangers of this secularization of medicine. As the goal of medicine moves from cure to health, they warn that medicine's task will become much more diffuse and ill-defined. It will be less easy to integrate into a coherent pattern the knowledge needed for this expanded enterprise. It will be impossible to rely on a stable body of information to achieve specific ends. Furthermore, as the task broadens, individuals from increasingly diverse disciplines will be needed. The process of coordinating these increasingly differentiated roles will make medicine less precise. As the widened goal of health is pursued, previous standards of effectiveness in cure will be impossible to maintain. When these developments coincide with common citizens insisting on exercising their influence in medical matters, barbarism will have engulfed the orderly, scientific practice of medicine in America.[54]

The American medical community may be correct that the efficacy of their expertise is threatened by present trends. If our analysis is correct, the changes coming in American medicine are so thoroughgoing, affecting, as they do, its values, norms, roles and practices, that no one can guarantee that the future will improve on the past. However, for better or worse, one thing is certain about American medicine: it must either narrow its understanding of itself or broaden its vision.

Medicine can become one occupation among many dealing with the improvement of a community's health; that occupation responsible for the technical question of finding the physical causes and cures of disease. It can remain committed exclusively to rationality, order and effectiveness. Physicians can become ever more efficient in performing their unending round of therapeutic rituals. There is no doubt that a culture needs these tasks performed.

Or, medicine can accept the vast challenge of improving America's health. It can embrace the values of equality and freedom, and recognize the right of the whole population to involve itself in determining the nature of disease and the priorities of medical care. Medicine can redefine its task as not exclusively ceremonial, but increasingly educational. To a population with rising expectations of participation it can respond with full disclosure concerning the facts of health and cure. If physicians want to continue to enjoy the enormous respect and influence they have heretofore received in American society, they must consider assuming the crucial job of dramatizing, for the public, conditions preventing a general improvement in health.

The days when the mysteries of science could be relied upon to awe the credulous are fading quickly. Faith in the power of technical reason to save man is dead. Physicians cannot survive as mediators of the holy. With the secularization of medicine, doctors will most likely endure as civil-service technicians.

The only alternative is for physicians to launch themselves into a life where scientific knowledge gives no automatic advantage, where worth depends on sensitivity to principles known to all. Among the most highly respected individuals in American society today are those who point out to the community those places where its disregard for basic values maims and kills; those who arouse the citizenry to correct injustices and thereby improve and save the lives of thousands.[55]

Recognition that science can no longer be a religion will lead physicians to realize that they can no longer be priests performing mysterious healing rites. Instead, physicians adopting the role of pointing out the relevance of universal values and norms to particular evils will have found a new way of life. They will be demonstrating a loyalty to the freedom, dignity and worth of man. They will have put their trust in the enduring validity of morality. They will have become prophets. The secularization of medicine may prove to be its salvation.

---

not been considered "medical." Living a well-rounded life, with its appropriate measure of recreation, reflection and aesthetic endeavors will all be seen as part of the good, healthy life, with each person free to combine the various elements according to what is best for him. At that point, medicine will have reached Bellah's modern stage of religion, where each man echoes Jefferson's statement that "I am a sect myself." Cf. Parsons, *Social Structure and Personality*, p. 355.

54. Freidson, *Profession of Medicine*, pp. 352-53.

55. Robert F. Buckhorn, *Nader: The People's Lawyer* (Englewood Cliffs, N.J.: Prentice-Hall, Inc., 1972), p. 276. "Pollster Louis Harris ran a survey of 1,620 families in March, 1971, asking a nationwide cross-section this question: 'Do you feel that in his attacks on American industry, consumer-advocate Ralph Nader has done more good than harm, or more harm than good?' The result: a lopsided 53 percent to 9 percent agreed that Nader was doing more good than harm. . . . Louis Harris said the survey showed that, basically, the efforts of Nader 'have been extremely well received by the American public.' A poll by George Gallup taken in the same month showed that out of 1,571 persons sampled, Nader was known to 50 percent of American men and 37 percent of the women. That would be a recognition factor at the time higher than most of the announced presidential candidates."

2 A New Synthesis: Alternative Medicine's Challenge to Mainstream Medicine and Traditional Christianity

Sidney Callahan

Alternative medicine's increasing popularity challenges conventional scientific medicine as well as mainstream religion. Both challenges to the status quo arise from the focus on spirituality that alternative medicine manifests in its beliefs and practice. Emphasizing the spiritual dimension of healing and health provides the "alternative" perspective of alternative medicine, also known as "holistic," "mind-body," "integrated," "complementary medicine," or "spiritual healing." The spirituality of alternative medicine accounts for much of its popular appeal.[1]

The statistics of the U.S. boom in alternative medicine are by now familiar. In 1997 more than 42 percent of Americans used some form of alternative medicine. During the same year the country's consumers made 629 million visits to alternative practitioners. More people visited alternative providers than primary care physicians, and they paid more than $27 billion out of pocket to do so.[2] Such a widespread social movement can be analyzed through many different lenses: economic, legal, sociological, political, anthropological, or as a media phenomenon. Here I examine some of the fundamental intellectual claims in conflict, first between alternative medicine and mainstream medicine and then between holistic medicine's spirituality and mainstream Christianity. Paying more attention to these basic differences should help resolve many of the political, legal, and practical problems that await if and when mainstream medicine and culture accept alternative medicine.

Most of alternative medicine gradually will be integrated into conventional medicine, and the spirituality underlying much of alternative medicine can be welcomed by mainstream Christianity, albeit with some reservations.

Challenges to Conventional Medicine

Given the diversity of beliefs and practices that are called "alternative medicine" a skeptical observer could safely define it as what is not currently being taught in medical schools. This negative approach is inadequate. There really are common characteristics and a common core of beliefs and assumptions that underlie the movement's diverse manifestations.[3]

Insisting on a holistic approach to health, alternative medicine consistently rejects the tenets of secular modernistic dogmas adopted during the Enlightenment. No whole person can be reduced to his or her organic subsystems or be categorized as a set of symptoms of a disease. A human being consists of a mind/body/spirit unity energized by a vital healing life force that strives for health and wholeness.

Moreover, other transcendent healing forces exist in the universe, and prayer, imagery or other rituals can invoke them for healing. The healer's role becomes one of encouraging people to take responsibility for the processes of their own healing. While many of the healing techniques employed in holistic medicine originated within a specific religious perspective, today the practices' religious origins have faded. Some observers see the evolving spirituality of alternative medicine as a synthesized, stripped down, or "secular" spirituality that is pragmatic and eschews doctrinal and institutional boundaries.[4] Practitioners employ various syntheses of Eastern and Western spiritual traditions, but all the beliefs underlying alternative medicine oppose the secular modernism of conventional scientific medicine, with its fundamental assumptions of reductive materialism, empiricism, atomism, and universally applicable laws.[5]

1. Ted J. Kapichuk, OMD, and David M. Eisenberg, "The Persuasive Appeal of Alternative Medicine," *Annals of Internal Medicine* 129, no. 12 (1998); Michael S. Goldstein, "Medicine and the Spirit," *Alternative Health Care: Medicine, Miracle, or Mirage* (Philadelphia: Temple University Press, 1999) 74-109.

2. David M. Eisenberg et al., "Trends in Alternative Medicine Use in the United States, 1990-1997: Results of a Follow-up National Survey," *JAMA* 280:1569-1575; Goldstein, *Alternative Health Care.*

3. National Institutes of Health, "Classification of Alternative Medicine Practices — What Is CAM? National Center for Complementary and Alternative Medicine Practices" (http://altmed.od.nih.gov/nccam/what-is-cam/index.shtml); "Defining and Describing Complementary and Alternative Medicine" (panel on definition and description, CAM Research Methodology Conference, April 1995); *Alternative Therapies* 3, no. 2 (1997) 49-57; see also Goldstein, "The Core of Alternative Medicine," *Alternative Health Care,* 40-73.

4. Goldstein, "Medicine and the Spirit," *Alternative Health Care;* John Shea, "Health Care's Transformation: Spirituality Expands the Horizons of Medicine," *Park Ridge Center Bulletin,* January/February 1999, 5-8; Larry Dossey, *Healing Words: The Power of Prayer and the Practice of Medicine* (HarperSanFrancisco, 1993).

5. Meredith B. McGuire, "Mapping Contemporary American Spirituality: A Sociological Perspective," *Christian Spirituality Bulletin: Journal for the Study of Christian Spirituality* 5, no. 1 (1998) 1-8; Beatrice Bruteau, "Global Spirituality and the Integration of East and West," *Cross Currents,* Summer/Fall (1985) 190-205.

From Sidney Callahan, "A New Synthesis: Alternative Medicine's Challenge to Mainstream Medicine and Traditional Christianity," *Second Opinion* 1 (Sept. 1999): 57-78. Permission to use and reprint given by The Park Ridge Center, the copyright holder.

In alternative medicine health and illness exist on a continuum and health amounts to more than the absence of illness. The balance of health over illness depends to a large extent on the individual's own life choices and environmental factors. Thus, holistic medicine focuses on the underlying causes and not just on removing symptoms. The sick person can view her illness as an opportunity to reassess her life and change it for the better. Only progress on her spiritual path toward balance and wholeness brings true healing. Individuals transcend their parts and experience healing spiritual actions which, like prayer, can work at a distance.

Alternative health practitioners generally consider the "spirit" to be, at a minimum, that aspect of the whole person which consists of core beliefs, deep aspirations, and cognitive and emotional powers of will and desire. The holistic and dynamic self-conscious choices of a person's spirit are as important to health as the physiological systems. Most alternative practitioners don't deny the effect of the body on the mind and spirit, but they view the mind and spirit's effect upon the body as more important in restoring and maintaining health. Even if a physiological cure of an illness is not possible, spiritual healing and holistic growth can take place.

Naturally many opponents of alternative medicine object most forcefully to the focus on immaterial spiritual causation. Such skeptics charge that alternative medicine is an antiscientific and dangerous retreat from reason. The debunkers feel duty bound to defend science and reason by attacking the claims and practices of alternative medicine as "a variety of snake oil," or a "holistic hoax."[6] The skeptics warn the public that there is no scientific evidence for the effectiveness of most of alternative medicine and plenty of reason to worry about the gullibility of people who can be defrauded, if not harmed physically.

Here it is important to point out that methodologies of research and inquiry are never neutral or theory free.[7] Research methods are not simply transparent ways to explore reality but are themselves theory driven and infused by theoretical assumptions. Research methods always embody their own assumptions about the reality of the world; these foundational assumptions determine which procedures will be used and what kind of results will count as valid. The materialistic presumption that measurements must be made and functions explained makes it difficult to study subjective consciousness or interpersonal relationships. Obviously you cannot see or touch a person's faith, hope, love, beliefs, trust, or feelings of being cared for. How can you objectively measure a sense of inner healing and wholeness? Complex realities that transcend physiology and operate only in unique circumstances may not be detected by medicine's gold standard of research, the randomized double-blind experiment.

Considering the way the core beliefs of alternative medicine diverge from conventional medicine's worldview and methods, accommodation might seem impossible.

Paths and Strategies for Pluralistic Accommodation

Despite these disagreements, alternative medicine's assimilation into conventional medicine has already begun.[8] This assimilation is likely to increase as three different intellectual processes of validation take place.

First, by establishing the Office of Alternative and Complementary Medicine, the National Institutes of Health has made more funding available to conduct conventional scientific testing of holistic medicine's diverse claims. Open-minded physicians and scientists will accept those practices and treatments that are tested and found effective because conventional medicine's own standards of research will have validated them.

While materialistic research methods may be unable to detect or explain subtle human processes of activated self-consciousness, certain physiological health outcomes and behavioral effects will be robust enough to be measured empirically. Already conventional physicians are gradually and grudgingly accepting the positive health benefits from practices of meditation, stress-reduction techniques, regular religious worship, social support, optimism, hardiness, disclosure of secrets, massage, perceived control, and positive expectations (the powerful placebo effect).[9] Negative health outcomes are

6. An example of such an attack by the former editor in chief of *The New England Journal of Medicine,* and professor emeritus of medicine and social medicine at Harvard Medical School, can be read in Arnold S. Relman, "Andrew Weil, the Boom in Alternative Medicine, and the Retreat from Science: A Trip to Stonesville," *The New Republic,* December 14 (1998) 28-37; see also Stephen Barren, M.D., "'Alternative' Medicine: More Hype Than Hope," *Alternative Medicine and Ethics,* James M. Humber and Robert F. Almeder, eds. (Totowa, NJ: Humana Press, 1998) 3-42.

7. Brent D. Slife, Carolen Hope, and R. Scott Nebeker, "Examining the Relationship Between Religious Spirituality and Psychological Science," *Journal of Humanistic Psychology* 39, no. 2 (1999) 51-85; see also National Institutes of Health, "How Should We Research Unconventional Therapies? A Panel Report from the Conference on Complementary and Alternative Medicine Research Methodology," *International Journal of Technology Assessment in Health Care* 13, no. 1 (1997) 111-121.

8. Goldstein, "Recognition by Conventional Medicine," *Alternative Health Care,* 124-130; Nancy C. Elder, M.D., M.S.P.H.; Amy Gillerist, M.D.; Rene Minz, M.D., "Use of Alternative Health Care by Family Practice Patients," *Archives of Family Medicine,* March/April (1997) 6, 181-184; John A. Astin, Ph.D., et al., "A Review of the Incorporation of Complementary and Alternative Medicine by Mainstream Physicians," *Archives of Internal Medicine* 158 (1998) 2303-2310.

9. Vimal Patel, Ph.D., "Understanding the Integration of Alternative Modalities into an Emerging Healthcare Model in the United States," in *Alternative Medicine and Ethics,* op. cit., 45-95; David J. Hufford, Ph.D., "Integrating Complementary and Alternative Medicine into Conventional Medical Practice," *Alternative Therapies* 3, no. 3, 81-83; Conference at Park Ridge Center Report from two health care systems.

correlated with stress, cynicism, hostility, mania, depression, loneliness, and grief.

While no one in any discipline can explain how human consciousness emerges, how it relates to the brain's physical material, human attitudes, beliefs, emotions, and interpersonal relationships clearly affect the body. The new field of psychoneuroimmunology, for example, studies how mental and emotional states affect the immune system, and vice versa.[10]

Second, much of conventional medicine and conventional research techniques have not kept up with advances in other scientific fields. Conventional scientific medicine is still based on a Newtonian model of science, while physics itself has become much more complex.[11] When new findings of physics and the human sciences become integrated into medicine, many of the holistic claims of alternative medicine will not appear so far-fetched. The universe appears to be much weirder and more holistically constituted, at least at the micro level, than the assumptions of the Newtonian worldview. (Even nonlocal activity and causation at a distance seems to occur in physics.)

Certainly psychology's "consciousness revolution" has transformed the discipline in the last three decades. Behaviorism's materialistic contention that the mind, self, and consciousness are irrelevant epiphenomena has been overturned. New understandings of the power of subjective consciousness, human emotion and cognition have created new subdisciplines and the interdisciplinary field of cognitive science.[12] Brain imaging techniques offer evidence of the mind's active power to process information and direct behavior. Scientists have also advanced the study of altered states of consciousness such as hypnosis, trance, sleep, and dreams.[13] Many of these phenomena have long been considered important and useful in non-Western spiritualities and alternative therapies.

An expanded science of psychology and neuropsychology focusing on consciousness will continue to develop, supporting many of alternative medicine's claims about the mind's effects on the body. New and more subtle research techniques, some involving brain imagery and new qualitative methods, hover on the horizon. These techniques will make it easier either to validate or finally to refute certain claims resulting in mind-body medicine's incorporation into science. At the same time, the "human spirit" may be demystified because it will be identified with psychological capacities of human consciousness. If this occurs, it will have the ironic effect of subsuming much of what has been called alternative medicine's spirituality into the psychology of consciousness. The stripped-down and secular spirituality characterizing holistic medicine will be assimilated into a beefed-up psychobiosocial science of the mind. A harbinger of this development can be seen in alternative practitioner Jon Kabat-Zinn's resistance to using the word "spirituality"; he prefers to talk of his work teaching stress-reduction meditation and mindfulness, as practicing a "consciousness discipline."[14]

Even the transcendent healing forces assumed in much of alternative medicine's spirituality may be understood as naturally occurring group effects and species interconnections. Already, ecology and other studies of field forces point to the ways all life is interdependent and affected by socioenvironmental conditions. A Navajo healing ceremony which includes the whole community in complex rituals will not seem alien or superstitious when science recognizes the power of subjective and interconnected group consciousness.

At the same time, conventional scientific medicine will continue to progress and remain a powerful and accepted part of any new integrated approach to healing. Scientific medicine has been successful because its perspectives on physiology and the material world's biological and chemical operations have largely been accurate. In fact, modern technological medicine is one of the great achievements of human reason, validating the scientific method and exemplifying the human will to relieve suffering. It is misguided to assign the power and popularity of scientific medicine solely to the continuing social dominance of Western elites who impose their perspective on reality. No, modern scientific medicine persists because it works and has brought benefits to millions. Laws of matter and nature exist, but to say that this is all that exists is too narrow a perspective. Once scientific medicine gives up an outmoded mind-body dualism inherited from Descartes, it can expand its perspectives and effectiveness.

In the history of ideas and theories, in and out of science, we have seen concepts move from the fringe to the center and back out. Socioeconomic factors and changing cultural interpretations play a part in the acceptance of new ideas, but human reasoning and the experience of reality hold greater weight. Theories win because their arguments accord with reason, factual evidence, and experience. In the future, integration of alternative medicine into traditional medicine will take place when rea-

10. S. F. Maier, L. R. Watkins, M. Fleshner, "Psychoneuroimmunology: The Interface Between Behavior, Brain, and Immunity," *American Psychologist,* 49, no. 12, 1004-1017.

11. Joseph F. Rychlak, *In Defense of Human Consciousness* (Washington, DC: American Psychological Association, 1996); John R. Searle, *The Rediscovery of the Mind* (Cambridge, MA: MIT Press, 1992); Giulio Tononi and Gerald M. Edelman, "Consciousness and Complexity," *Science* 4, vol. 282, 1846-1851.

12. Howard Gardner, *The Mind's New Science: A History of the Cognitive Revolution* (New York: Basic Books, 1987); Owen Flanagan, *Consciousness Reconsidered* (Cambridge, MA: MIT Press, 1992).

13. J. Allan Hobson, M.D., *The Chemistry of Conscious States: How the Brain Changes Its Mind* (New York: Little Brown, 1994); Harry T. Hunt, *The Multiplicity of Dreams: Memory, Imagination, and Consciousness* (New Haven: Yale University Press, 1989); Peretz Lavie, *The Enchanted World of Sleep* (New Haven: Yale University Press, 1996).

14. Jon Kabat-Zinn, *Wherever You Go There You Are: Mindfulness Meditation in Everyday Life* (New York: Hyperion, 1994) 264.

soned judgments conclude that integrating the two approaches best reflects the universe's material and spiritual complexities.

But if alternative medicine is gradually winning acceptance in science and society, will its underlying spiritual beliefs also be accepted by mainstream Christianity?

Challenges to Mainstream Christianity

Alternative medicine and the underlying spirituality of its worldview challenge mainstream Christianity. This spirituality de-emphasizes particular doctrines and institutional ties while incorporating elements from Eastern, Western and Native American practices.[15]

Here I will use Roman Catholicism as my example of a traditional mainstream Christian faith that possesses a highly developed doctrinal and institutional character as well as its own traditions of spirituality. I write as a Catholic committed to the reforms of Vatican II and to its ideal of an ever-evolving church that is loyal to its life-giving Gospel tradition. I am also engaged in American Catholic intellectual life and am particularly interested in the dialogue between religion and science.[16] As a psychologist, I am most intrigued by the relationship of psychology to religion. The following opinions are my own, but I doubt they are at variance with other mainstream Catholic thinkers.

Mainstream Christianity should welcome, with certain reservations, the new spirituality of alternative medicine. On the whole, the rise of alternative medicine in American culture brings good news for the faith. The spiritual worldview underlying alternative medicine challenges a secular establishment that has for too long dismissed religion. Reductionistic materialism and doctrinaire antireligious assumptions have reigned among certain elites. In the present climate of intellectual ferment and cultural change it is no longer quite so easy to arrogantly dismiss spiritual realities and the transcendent capacities of human consciousness.

Happily, alternative medicine's emphasis on positive, transcendent healing forces in the universe is in accord with many traditional Christian doctrines, including the idea of a benevolent God of love Who creates, sustains, and redeems the world. Healing hearts and minds is the Holy Spirit's work, in all places and at all times, so although a non-Christian spirituality may not explicitly identify the powers of healing as orthodox Christianity does, the Spirit still works.[17]

Other beliefs and practices of alternative medicine also echo Christian tradition. The power of prayer to effect good, and the potency of group prayer for healing others, are long-held Christian beliefs. Holistic medicine's avowal of the interconnections of all elements of reality resonates with Christianity's teaching that humankind exists as one interdependent family, one body, embedded in a communion of saints both living and dead that transcends time. The healing power of vicarious and face-to-face prayer and the laying on of hands have always been central to Christian beliefs and sacramental practices.

In the Christian scriptures a God of love is revealed as the divine healer of all wounds. Christ's example and teaching inspire the historic Christian ministries of healing and works of mercy, including hospitals and religious orders dedicated to caring for the sick and indigent. The rise of spiritual healing in alternative medicine can only revive and encourage the Church's own healing ministries.

Alternative medicine's assertion that spiritual healing can take place even if a physiological cure cannot be effected affirms the power of the spirit in the same manner that Christianity sees the Holy Spirit at work. Christians believe that the gifts and fruits of the Holy Spirit can coexist with suffering and illness, as well as with persecution and other tragic life events. The Spirit's gift of joy can be received in the midst of the world's ills. (Psychology helps explain this with new research that demonstrates how the sources and pathways of positive and negative emotions may be independent and therefore can be simultaneously activated.)[18] Joy and suffering are not always a zero-sum game but can be felt simultaneously in complex configurations of multidimensioned human persons. Thus, as much of alternative medicine affirms, to struggle toward health and wholeness is not simply a matter of removing symptoms and impairments; the spiritual path may have triumphs, even if disease and death cannot be cured.

Christians believe that God's Spirit works to bring the best outcomes possible whenever illness and other evils

15. Mary Farrell Bednarowski, "Theological Creativity: Personalizing Religious Traditions Can Help the Healing Process," *Park Ridge Center Bulletin,* January/February (1999) 3, 10; Peter Van Ness, "A Paradox on the American Landscape: 'Secular Spirituality' Affects Contemporary Health Care," *Park Ridge Center Bulletin,* 11; John A. Coleman, S.J., "Exploding Spiritualities: Their Social Causes, Social Location and Social Divide," *Christian Spirituality Bulletin* (Spring 1997) 9-15.

16. Sidney Callahan, *In Good Conscience: Reason and Emotion in Moral Decision Making* (HarperSanFrancisco, 1991); Sidney Callahan, *With All Our Heart and Mind: The Spiritual Works of Mercy in a Psychological Age* (New York: Crossroad, 1988).

17. Catherine Mowry LaCugna, *God For Us: The Trinity & Christian Life* (HarperSanFrancisco, 1992); David S. Cunningham, *These Three Are One: The Practice of Trinitarian Theology* (Oxford: Blackwell, 1999).

18. Joseph LeDoux, "The Power of Emotions," *States of Mind: New Discoveries about How Our Brains Make Us Who We Are,* ed. Roberta Conlan (New York: John Wiley & Sons, 1999); Richard J. Davidson, "The Neuropsychology of Emotion and Affective Style," in *Handbook of Emotions,* Michael Lewis and Jeannette M. Haviland, eds. (New York: The Guilford Press, 1993) 143-154; J. T. Cacioppo and G. G. Berntson, "Relationship Between Attitudes and Evaluative Space: A Critical Review, with Emphasis on the Separability of Positive and Negative Substrates," *Psychological Bulletin* 115, 401-423; E. Diener and R. A. Emmons, "The Independence of Positive and Negative Affect," *Journal of Personality and Social Psychology* 47 (1984) 1105-1117.

befall human beings. Unfortunately, in the past the experience of God's Spirit striving to heal, mend and comfort sufferers after tragedy often led to a mistaken belief that since believers can spiritually grow from suffering and pain, then God must send suffering to perfect human beings.[19] The healing that takes place with God's help after the fact of illness and tragedy was interpreted as a sign of God's intentions before the fact. God's providential plan and will were thought to include every detail that happened in the universe; thus persons should either be resigned to the illness that God sends or welcome the suffering as a sign of God's favor. Such a pessimistic glorification of suffering needs correcting, and the positive emphasis of alternative medicine upon healing and wellness can help the process.

New optimistic theological reflections that are appearing affirm that God created the universe as free, open and engaged in dynamic processes of evolution.[20] A free and open universe is governed by natural laws but also includes chance and indeterminacy. God sustains and infuses the universe but has embraced a self-limitation of power for the sake of human freedom.[21] God's actions and influences in the world are totally beneficent, but they can operate only if the freedom of created human beings is not violated. God can also work through chance and within the consciousness (or spirits) of human co-creators redeeming and healing the world. Human beings in their freedom can be viewed as co-creators and healers of self, others and the rest of creation.

Illness and suffering need never be viewed as directly sent by God for our own good. Illness can be seen as the result of chance and evolving processes in an independent, incomplete universe. But since the universe is open to change and growth, there always exist possibilities for positive transformations. Hope for healing is appropriate, and human co-creative work in the world can be effective, views that have undergirded the development of conventional technological medicine. Self-healing alternative practices simply extend the human response to the divine call for human co-creation. God's healing powers can be invoked through prayer, action, and consciousness disciplines as well as through science-based medicine.

When prayer does not work cure at the physical level, Christians can attribute this to the fact that evil exists, and that illness and death have accrued real power in our free but incomplete universe. Christians affirm that in some way human nature resists Divine influence; this results from living in a fallen or wounded world. Powerful physical and social evils springing from chance, incomplete development and evil human choices actually exist and plague humankind. They will continue to exist until the Kingdom comes and every tear is wiped away. Thus in this interim time, God's self-limitation is real and God's loving goodness does not omnipotently direct every outcome of every event in the creation. In the same way the human mind and spirit cannot completely control the embodied dimensions of the self or possess the power to overcome illness and death. We remain in all too many ways "at the will of the body."[22] Only the sting of death can be conquered, promised by those who love God and exist as embodied beings.

As conventional medicine must give up its dualistic view of human existence, so must Christians give up the vestiges of soul-body dualisms. But what will take the place of a worldview in which spirit and mind constitute separate realities? Philosophically we can safely assume the fall of Descartes, but the existence of embodied human consciousness remains an unexplained mystery. Alternative medicine provides one refutation of a reductionistic belief in the world as "nothing but matter." On the other hand those believers who affirm that only mind and spirit exist seem equally misguided. Perhaps the future lies with what has been called "nonreductive physicalism," or "dual-aspect monism."[23] Nonreductive physicalism grants that persons *are* their bodies, not souls and minds that inhabit bodies, because the mind/self depends upon an embodied brain. At the same time something more, some emergent property of self-consciousness gives human beings their spiritual identity. Dual-aspect monism claims that while reality is unified, it employs either a spiritual-mental or material-physical perspective — one reality, two different lenses. At any rate, the contemporary resurgence of holistic mind-body medicine ensures that believers, philosophers and scientists will continue to struggle with the perennial problem of our embodied human consciousness.

Christian theologians, for their part, will continue the growing dialogue between religion, science, and medicine, a dialogue that will be engaged by believers who worship God as Truth and affirm that the creation is one central way God reveals GodSelf to humankind.[24] Christians find God revealed in scripture, tradition, reason and our experience in and of the world. Using these sources of authority, Roman Catholic Christians develop and grow in their secular and religious commitments as reason is informed by faith. Vatican II ushered in a newly

19. C. S. Lewis expresses this traditional view in *The Problem of Pain* (New York: Macmillan, 1962).

20. Elizabeth A. Johnson, C.S.J., "Does God Play Dice? Divine Providence and Chance," *Theological Studies* 57, no. 1 (1996) 3-18; William R. Stoeger, S.J., and John Polkinghorne, "Natural Science, Temporality, and Divine Action," *Theology Today* 55, no. 3 (1998) 329-343; Michael Welker, "God's Eternity, God's Temporality, and Trinitarian Theology," *Theology Today* 55, no. 3 (1998) 317-328.

21. Lucien Richard, *Christ the Self-Emptying of God* (New York: Paulist Press, 1996).

22. Arthur Frank, *At the Will of the Body: Reflections on Illness* (Boston: Houghton Mifflin, 1991).

23. Nancey Murphy, "Nonreductive Physicalism: Philosophical Issues," *Whatever Happened to the Soul? Scientific and Theological Portraits of Human Nature,* Warren S. Brown, Nancey Murphy and H. Newton Malony, eds. (Minneapolis, MN: Augsburg Fortress Press, 1999) 127-148.

24. Bruce G. Epperly, *Crystal & Cross: Christians and New Age in Creative Dialogue* (Mystic, CT: Twenty-Third Publications, 1996).

vigorous dialogue with science, the humanities and other religions.

Incompatibilities and Reservations

Are there then any conflicts between the stripped-down, synthetic, secular spirituality of alternative medicine and a mainstream Christian religion such as Roman Catholicism? Yes, certainly. Some of the core beliefs underlying some forms of alternative medicine make claims and assertions that are not compatible with Christian beliefs. (It should be noted, however, that many of the spiritual healing movement's unacceptable elements are found in its published popularizers and may not be representative of the everyday pragmatic activity of most alternative practitioners.) As one would expect, often the spiritual beliefs that clash with Christianity are imported from non-Christian Eastern religions and mixed together with ancient gnostic spiritual traditions, transmitted by way of Jungian transpersonal psychology and/or nineteenth-century theosophy and spiritualism. A claim, for example, that an individual's eternal spirit soul pre-exists this life and progresses through many reincarnations conflicts with the orthodox Christian doctrine of creation and redemption. Thus Christians would reject the belief that in an illness a person could be in need of past life therapy. In fact, Christians would find unacceptable any implications in alternative spiritualities that individuals choose their illnesses or are living out their karma.

Two or three examples of the claims appearing in bestsellers give the general picture. Louise Hay is a popular California healer who asserts that "We create every so-called illness in our body."[25] But many of these negative processes are due to the soul's past choices in its endless journey through eternity. A certain omnipotence of the mind and spirit is affirmed when she says,

> We come to this planet to learn particular lessons that are necessary for our spiritual evolution. We choose our sex, our color, our country; and we look around for the perfect set of parents who will mirror our patterns.[26]

In such a spiritual system every illness and misfortune is caused by past actions; even the presence of AIDS reflects some cosmic reason.

Another more intellectual and even more popular exponent of alternative medicine's spirituality is Deepak Chopra, a physician trained in both Western and ancient Hindu Ayurveda medicine. He also believes in a timeless, eternal spiritual reality, which means that many so-called objective material realities are merely the result of illusory beliefs. Diseases are mostly the results of individual errors of consciousness. Thus,

> the physical manifestation of a disease is a phantom . . . while the real culprit, the persistent memory that creates the cancer cell goes undetected. . . . Ayurveda tells us to place the responsibility for disease at a deeper level of consciousness, where a potential cure could also be found.[27]

In later works Chopra explains that the body is not a frozen sculpture but a river of eternally recycling energies; the body is ageless and the mind is timeless. By an intentional training of consciousness one can use the power of awareness to reverse entropy, undo aging and above all overcome the debilitating fear of death.[28]

In this kind of spirituality, individuals and their choices reign supreme; the good news is that individuals have the spiritual power to change and heal their bodies by changing their awareness, their beliefs, and the way they live and deploy attention. Unfortunately, the positive hope that this spiritual approach to healing engenders is often bought at the price of attributing people's illnesses to their unenlightened state of consciousness. To see illness as caused by individual choices seems as wrong as the idea that God chooses to send human beings pain and suffering for their own good.

Christians must remember that when Christ healed a man born blind he made the point that the man's blindness was not caused by sin, neither on his part nor on the part of his parents. The man's blindness was no one's fault but was able to serve as an opportunity for God to demonstrate His healing power. In all of Christ's healing, we never find Christ blaming the ill for their diseases but only offering acceptance and remedy.

Yet even some Christian exponents of spiritual healing remain ambivalent on whether sin can cause an illness. John Sanford, a noted writer on Christian spiritual healing, interprets (or in my opinion misinterprets) the Gospel story of Christ healing the thirty-eight-year illness of the man lying by the Bethsaida pool. Sanford claims the man's illness was a self-inflicted, egocentric clinging to infirmity.[29] While he generally denies that every illness arises from sin, Sanford also asserts that "some people prefer illness to health because they don't want to pay the price of health."[30]

This judgment is similar to accusations that those who seek spiritual healing do not receive it because their faith is not strong enough. These arguments falsely exaggerate the power of individual spiritual autonomy. Christian healers, along with other alternative medicine practitioners, do well to encourage people to take re-

25. Louise Hay, *You Can Heal Your Life* (Santa Monica, CA: Hay House, 1984) 128.

26. Ibid., 36.

27. Deepak Chopra, M.D., *Quantum Healing: Exploring the Frontiers of Mind/Body Medicine* (New York: Bantam Books, 1989) 265.

28. Deepak Chopra, M.D., *Ageless Body, Timeless Mind* (New York: Crown Publishers, 1993), see especially Part Five, "Breaking the Spell of Mortality," 279-334.

29. John A. Sanford, *Healing Body and Soul: The Meaning of Illness in the New Testament and Psychotherapy* (Westminster: John Knox Press, 1992) 26-29.

30. Ibid., 29.

sponsibility for much of their health, but it seems incorrect, if not immoral, to hold people responsible for having become ill or for not being able to heal themselves. To see illness as the result merely of error, sin or wrong thinking denies the independent power of the material world that is not only ordered but also filled with chance, chaos and intractable, destructive forces.

The key incompatibility of Christianity and many of the new spiritualities centers on their different views of material reality and the status of creation. For Christians the healing powers of the Holy Spirit are always at work, but because creation is free and separate from God, evil can exist. Sin, illness, death, and suffering are real and not illusory. Embodied selves are also created by God as real, eternal, unique beings; human individuals will not be absorbed into the eternal recycling of universal spiritual forces. Human beings are destined for an eternal, transformed life in God, but they are not divine. Beliefs that deny the existence of matter, evil, or the body easily lead to denying the validity of conventional medical interventions. When such denial leads to rejecting conventional treatment for ill children, it can be criminal.

Believers in the Christian God will be forced to reject all spiritual systems with claims that reality is Divine Consciousness. Nor can individuals create their own reality through their subjective consciousness. When this train of thought becomes widely accepted and simplified you end up with true believers like Shirley MacLaine, who can say:

> I realized I created my own reality in everything. I must therefore admit that, in essence, I was the only person in my universe. I went on to express my feeling of total responsibility and power for all events that happen in the world, for the world is happening only in my reality.[31]

Exalting the self and subjective consciousness results in a pantheism that sees God as a name for a transcendent spiritual force rather than as a Divinely transcendent personal Creator. In a typical expression of this idea, the psychiatrist Thomas Hora says:

> We like to speak of God not only as Life Principle but also as Love-Intelligence. . . . All these adjectives help us to gain a more precise understanding of God which is not a person but a power, a Reality, an "Is."[32]

When God is only a spiritual force, the important thing is to be "in harmony with what is." It then follows that, "Since God is infinite consciousness, enlightenment means conscious union with Cosmic Consciousness, or at-one-ment with Love-Intelligence."[33] Behavior and actions are secondary, if not beside the point.

In this extreme belief in an individual's spiritual creation of reality, one ends up with moral relativism and a denial of objective truths that can be known by science and human reason. Traditional Christians, along with most scientists, cannot accept the collapse of all reality into subjective consciousness. One can grant the power of human consciousness but affirm the existence of a real world out there beyond one's own perceptions and projections. I advocate "critical realism," which affirms that human beings can by reasoned inquiry gradually approximate more adequate knowledge of the universe.[34] As a traditional believer I also affirm that God is not an impersonal force or cause but an ineffable, perfect, personal being that transcends all other realities.

Finally, Christians will believe that the worship of God can transcend the need for health, happiness, and joy, as good as these gifts of God are. Worship of the God revealed in Christianity demands justice, charity, and moral actions that may require sacrifice of other goods. Taking up a cross out of love for others in order to relieve their suffering may not lead to good health or long life. In other words, Christian spirituality must include an allegiance to altruistic communal values that are not limited to an individual's private spirituality and well-being. Privately following your bliss and enjoying good health will not suffice to fulfill a Christian's commitment to charity and justice.

Accommodation in Practice

What pragmatic responses should Christians make to the challenge of the stripped-down, secular spirituality and practice of alternative medicine? Since Christians believe that a God who endows His creation with freedom certainly desires freedom of conscience and religion for all persons, they will on principle uphold a stance of openness and tolerance toward alternative medicine and its beliefs. And this openness will be supported by the reliable Scriptural criteria for practical judgments that "by their fruits you shall know them." Already, we can see benefits arising from the way holistic medicine has encouraged a return to spirituality in secular culture and the revival of spiritual healing ministries. This turn to spirituality has been a corrective for a secularized world.

In addition, alternative medicine often works and relieves the suffering of many. Americans patronize both alternative and conventional medicine because they receive benefits from both. Even if Christians do not accept the core beliefs or worldview of some practitioners, they should feel free to use alternative healthcare practices as long as they are not harmful or illegal. Certainly the underlying secular materialistic beliefs of much modern medicine and its clinicians do not deter Christian believers from making use of science-based medicine.

31. Shirley MacLaine, *It's All in the Playing* (New York: Bantam Books, 1987) 174.

32. Thomas Hora, M.D., *Beyond the Dream: Awakening to Reality* (New York: Crossroad, 1996) 293.

33. Ibid.

34. Susan Haack, *Evidence and Inquiry: Towards Reconstruction in Epistemology* (Oxford: Blackwell, 1995); Thomas Nagel, *The Last Word* (New York: Oxford University Press, 1997).

However, as with conventional medicine, there may be some limits to openness. Any practices in any kind of medicine which seem only to be serving the practitioners' purse, or power, or ego-driven desires to gain fame or followers should be suspect.

Another danger can also come from adhering to an alternative approach that dogmatically refuses to countenance conventional medical treatment. Most alternate medical practitioners recognize that for certain kinds of medical problems conventional medicine is necessary. Yes, people are victims of modern medicine and die from drugs and surgery, but people can also die from refusing conventional interventions.

Another limitation to openness could arise if some alternative practices actively and explicitly conflict with Christianity's faith commitments. Many Christians find certain conventional medical practices immoral, such as abortion, euthanasia and certain fertility treatments. In alternative medicine some healing practices might also have to be avoided. Some healing practices might also be so integral to another religion's worship service that a Christian could not participate in good faith. Would a Christian approve of an unbeliever who took communion at Mass because of a notion that it might heal? Modern Westerners have not scrupled to co-opt and take up Eastern and indigenous religious practices, but respect for the integrity of another religious community's worship should be shown.

In order to make adequate moral and religious judgments about alternative medicine, more guidance should be made available to Christian believers. Traditional Christian theologians, scholars, teaching authorities, and healers should learn more about alternative health care and its spiritualities. The churches could then provide leadership by welcoming what is compatible with Christianity and pointing out which beliefs or practices they judge suspect or incompatible with the faith.

Reservations about the practical use of alternative medicine by Christians would be rare, for the most part. Pragmatic openness is appropriate upon principle but also because the stripped-down spiritualities underlying alternative medicine are themselves open, flexible, eclectic, and pragmatic. Holistic medicine's focus on individual choice works against imposing any authoritative approach as the one and only path. Alternative medicine judges by the fruits of practice, so its practitioners and clients tend to endorse whatever works in a particular case.

In an open, pluralistic society that values freedom of conscience and free inquiry, primary values will exist that include tolerance and progress, self-correction and progressive revision. Western science prides itself on its rational, self-correcting capacities. The scientific goal is to creatively generate ideas, test them rigorously by methods of critical doubt, and never fool oneself. By these methods, science moves from less adequate to more adequate understanding of the universe. Conventional science-based medicine must therefore in principle endorse change and progress. In a different way Christianity too seeks to evolve better and better understandings of God's truth, engaging in "the endlessness of making sense" of the good news, as theologian Nicholas Lash phrases it.[35] Over the centuries Christians have developed, elaborated, refined and furthered their understanding of God and nature. Surely too Western society's pragmatic practitioners of alternative medicine will find themselves joining in the process of testing, self-correction, and change. Both conventional medicine and alternative medicine will continue to develop as they converge into an expanded and truly integrated medicine.

Traditional religious believers need not worry that the growing popularity of new spiritualities and spiritual healing will mean the end of mainstream Christianity. As popular as they are, new spiritualities will not replace traditional religions. For one thing, life presents more problems and concerns than individual health and illness. Death is unlikely to disappear, nor vulnerability to old age and disease to be conquered. As evolutionary medicine pessimistically assures us, new diseases continually emerge because microbes and viruses constantly evolve new ways of evading medical treatments.[36] Their selective processes race against the growth of human ingenuity.

The continuing presence of disease, vulnerability and death ensure that the great eternal religious questions about the existence of God and evil will remain. And from those who worship the God revealed in the Bible, the call will still go out to come and join the struggle for other goods besides health. Social structural injustices, or social sin, require corporate and institutional measures to combat them. Persons will still respond to the Christian challenge to love one's neighbor as oneself. Followers of Christ then must work for all kinds of human flourishing, such as peacemaking, education, art, politics, science, ethics, economics, and humanistic inquiry. Certainly, human beings need to be spiritually and physically healed, but they also need to live in just communities in an economically and ecologically balanced world.

To fulfill all these strivings for personal and social transformation, individuals will continue to turn to religious communities that provide developed theologies of social justice, public corporate spiritualities, and communal support for change. As the Benedictine monk Sebastian Moore once commented, the Roman Catholic Church is the only worldwide and world-old institution dedicated to changing the world. Traditional Christianity holds its own because it continues to meet the criteria William James sets out for a valid religion. It provides cognitive meaning to the world, is morally helpful to its adherents, and provides immediately luminous experi-

35. Nicholas Lash, *Believing Three Ways in One God* (Notre Dame: Notre Dame Press, 1992) 10.

36. R. M. Nesse and G. W. Williams, *Why We Get Sick: The New Science of Darwinian Medicine* (New York: Vintage Books, 1995).

ences.[37] Stripped-down spiritualities that individuals choose to construct to achieve private healing, harmony and well-being too easily avoid the larger religious imperatives and struggles. While traditional Christians may welcome the growth of spiritual healing, they should still affirm that rational beings need developed theological grounding, moral reflection, and institutionally organized, stable communities of worship. Institutions and structures provide the doctrinal backbone and social continuity that encourage mature individual spiritualities that persist from one generation to another.

37. William James, *The Varieties of Religious Experience: A Study in Human Nature* (New York: The Modern Library, 1902).

3 Illness, the Problem of Evil, and the Analogical Structure of Healing: On the Difference Christianity Makes in Bioethics

George Khushf

We must take great care to employ this medical art, if it should be necessary, not as making it wholly accountable for our state of health or illness, but as redounding to the glory of God.

Basil the Great[1]

From the start, Christians subordinated physical healing (even the miraculous sort) to the deeper spiritual healing that was given in Jesus Christ's redemptive act. The most significant human problem was not the lack of health, but rather the alienation from God, humanity, and self; i.e. not illness but sin. However, this did not mean that Christians were callous to the needs of those who were physically ill. To the contrary, as Henri Sigerist notes, the sick person "assumed a preferential position," just as did the hungry, homeless, and ostracized (Sigerist, 1943, p. 70). The task of the Christian bioethicist must be to place this concern with the sick in the broader context of the Church's understanding of the human condition and God's redemptive work. In this way the legitimate role as well as limits of medicine can be properly appreciated, and concrete direction can be found for the explication of content-full bioethical norms.

For the Christian, physical problems such as sickness and poverty relate to the deeper spiritual predicament of sin in the same way that symptoms relate to a disease. This does not mean that a poor or sick person is a worse sinner than others. Rather, the physical afflictions are an expression of a brokenness in the human race (Amundsen and Ferngren, 1986, p. 45; Augustine, 1983b, book xiv, ch. 3; book xxii, ch. 22). Sin, generically understood, introduced a disorder into material creation. However, creation is not evil, and the material aspects of life cannot be ignored. Unlike gnostics, who divide the material from the spiritual and view the former as evil, Christians ad-

1. This is from Basil the Great's Long Rule 55, quoted in Amundsen (1982, p. 338).

From George Khushf, *Christian Bioethics,* Volume 1, No. 1, pp. 102-20. Slightly abridged and edited from the original. Used by permission.

vance a doctrine of creation that sees body and material existence as an essential part of human identity (Amundsen and Ferngren, 1986, p. 46). Although a person's own body does indeed seem alien in the experience of illness, this does not indicate that it is evil and separable from spirit. The alienation manifests a rupture in the created identity; it reveals an assault on the unity of body and soul, not their essential difference. This assault has even been understood in terms of demonic forces; malevolent forces directly undermine the harmony of God's creation (Amundsen and Ferngren, 1986, p. 54). Care for the sick amounts to assistance of the wounded, fallen in a grand cosmic battle. The problem of sickness is thus seen as an instance of a more radical problem of evil.

Although the physical problems cannot be ignored, they also cannot take center stage, just as symptomatic care cannot be given priority over treatment of disease. While it is good to relieve a patient's pain, it is better to treat an underlying infection that is causing the pain. In some cases it may even be necessary to make symptoms worse; for example, a leg may need to be broken in order to be properly reset. In the same way, healing of sickness is good, but it is subordinated to the spiritual healing that is at the heart of the Christian witness (Amundsen and Ferngren, 1986, pp. 58-59).

For the early Church, the most important role played by ministering to the sick lay not in the immediate end of physical healing, but rather in the way such healing could serve as a means through which the "good news" about God's act in Jesus Christ could be conveyed. The analogy between physical and spiritual health provided Christians with an opportunity to convey symbolically through concrete deeds of service their message of life.[2] As a physician relates to illness, so Jesus Christ relates to sin. When people see how Christians reach out to the poor and needy physically, they will be able to understand how God reaches out to sinful humanity, and they will be able to see the importance of submitting to spiritual healing as the sick submits to a physician. Through this analogical structure, people can understand that Jesus is the "Great Physician" (Augustine, 1983a, p. 90; 1980, p. 373).

Historically, the Church has thus had a twofold interest in medicine. (1) It has been concerned with assisting those who struggle in the battle of earthly life, helping them to recover so that they can continue to persevere. Medicine is here an expression of care and solidarity with the sick, and its direct concern is to confront that rupture and assault on human identity that is seen in the illness experience. Analogously, medicine is symptomatic care of the human condition, where sin is the underlying disease. (2) Medicine also can be a particular, concrete form of conveying the gospel. In this case, analogously, it is a way of treating the disease of the human condition. Through the deeds of service, medicine makes God's healing manifest in visible terms. In this case, when it is viewed as evangelism, medicine calls for reflection on the praxis of physical healing, using words to convey the manner in which the deeds are symbolically understood. The two types of medicine — symptomatic and disease oriented; i.e. the care and cure models — are thus extended analogously into two ways in which medicine can be appropriated by the Church.

Unfortunately, Christians today have lost sight of the second function of medicine, and many do not even appreciate the relativity of physical health. As noted by Numbers and Amundsen (1986, p. 3), evangelization has been displaced by a "humanitarianism" that eschews the use of medical practice as a means of conveying the gospel, arguing that such a use is "subtly coercive" and thus improper.[3] Here we clearly see a bioethic at work; one that is implicated in the broad secularization process that led to an increasing emphasis on material ends at the expense of spiritual ones. Is it coercive for a physician to move beyond symptomatic care in order to treat an underlying pathology? If not, then why is it coercive for a Christian physician in a Catholic or religiously affiliated hospital to move beyond medical care in order to address sin, which is the deeper pathology of the human condition? Although a Christian bioethic would need to carefully consider how a physician's evangelistic zeal may lead to abuses of authority, one can only dismiss the evangelistic concerns outright in a context where Christian priorities have been subverted, and where sight has been lost of the broader theological, analogical framework in which medicine and human bodily existence are rightly understood — that is, where they are understood in the framework of a Christian worldview.

The task of a Christian bioethic is to reestablish the appropriate priorities, provide the analogical framework, and work out the implications of these priorities in terms of concrete norms and virtues. This will involve placing concerns with human sickness, suffering, and death associated with medicine in the broader context of the Christian concern with redemption and renewal of humanity in the image of God. In this essay, I will sketch an outline for such a bioethic. I will begin by challenging the idolatry of health that is found in modern secular approaches to medicine. Then, I will consider how the illness experience manifests the insufficiency of fallen individuals and brings them beyond themselves to community. In the medical community one finds a knowledge base for healing that follows certain "natural"

2. For an early use of this analogy, see John 9. The healing of the blind man is used analogously to show how God gives sight to those who are in the darkness of sin. For Augustine this blind man symbolizes the human race, and the blindness is rooted in sin (1983, tractate xliv). This passage in John is especially instructive since it explicitly raises the question about an individual's personal responsibility for sickness, and it points to sickness as an opportunity to manifest the works of God (9:2-3).

3. This shift from evangelization to humanitarianism can be found among most Christian denominations, especially the more liberal, mainline ones. For a discussion of the shift among Baptists, see Weber (1986, esp. p. 305).

patterns that, in turn, can provide helpful analogies for the way in which spiritual sickness is healed. At the boundaries of human life, in the face of death, the insufficiency of medicine becomes apparent, and the deeper spiritual brokenness of humanity is existentially experienced. This is the root of the "problem of evil," and its "solution" is not found in theoretical theodicies, but rather in the concrete witness of the Christian community; in deeds of service coupled with proclamation about the import of such deeds. Through Christian service the true nature of healing can be understood, and the limits of medicine can be rightly appreciated. The norms that direct this particular form of service will be constitutive of a Christian bioethic, and they will guide medicine to its higher end. In this way, as Basil the Great so eloquently exhorts, the medical art will redound to the glory of God.

The Idolatry of Health

Today there is a cult of health (Skrabanek, 1994). Advertisements by national health-spa chains speak of a "baptism by sweat." Youth and strength are idealized, aging is transformed into a disease, and any form of dependence is eschewed as contrary to the dignity of the human person (Goodwin, 1991). In this context, sickness becomes the primary evil. In response to this evil, humanity mobilizes all of its resources, and "progress" is understood in terms of the development of medical knowledge and skills. "Science" becomes the savior (Herberg, 1983, ch. 4). However, in those cases where science cannot save, and where individuals fall into dependency and diminished competence, one should "die with dignity," perhaps by euthanasia or suicide (Humphrey and Wickett, 1990). In this way the myth of the self-sufficient individual is maintained until the end.

Although the technological armamentarium of modern medicine is a recent phenomenon and it raises unique bioethical issues, the idolatry of health is not new. In a masterful discussion of the relation of ancient philosophy to medicine, Ludwig Edelstein (1967) shows how philosophers like Plato and Aristotle confronted a similar cult. Physicians of the time set forth health as the *summum bonum,* and they laid out a full regimen of diet and exercise, along with rules — can we say "norms" — about what could and could not be done (pp. 357-59). In response, philosophers argued that medicine is unable to address which ends are the appropriate ones. Medicine begins with a relative end, health, and then determines what furthers or hinders the realization of this end. But it can say nothing about how its end is to be ranked relative to other important ends (p. 360). The valuation of medicine and its ends thus depends on the supreme good of humanity, and this is determined independently of medicine (pp. 349-56).

The Christian answer to the idolatry of health and the rampant medicalization of reality will follow the same line of argumentation as that of Plato and Aristotle (McCormick, 1985, pp. 97, 106-7). However, the specificity of the Christian response will be governed by the particular end it advances; namely, by fellowship with God, and this involves renewal in the image of God, which is manifest in the person of Jesus Christ (Amundsen and Ferngren, 1986, pp. 48-49). This particular end will determine the unique content of a Christian bioethic.[4]

Edelstein also addresses another area where an interesting parallel can be drawn between the ancient and modern world. He notes that "the greatest debt of philosophy to medicine" lay in the analogy that medicine provided of the philosophical endeavor (1967, p. 360). By using medicine as a means to convey philosophical ideas, it is further relativized, the idolatry of health is undermined, and people are brought to contemplate the more important ends, which transcend the medical domain. Thus for example,

> In the beginning of the *Nichomachean Ethics,* Aristotle parallels his teaching concerning moral qualities with the teaching concerning health, because, he says, it is necessary to explain what is invisible by means of visible illustration. The soul is invisible; knowledge about it is elusive. By comparing the soul and body, that which is seemingly unreal is translated into comprehensible language. . . . In referring to medical insight the philosopher speaks of something that people can be expected to possess and that will help them to grasp the new kind of insight that they are expected to acquire through philosophy. (Edelstein, 1967, p. 361)

Christianity relates to medicine in a similar way, using it to convey a knowledge of redemption. However, in the Christian case, the capacity of medicine to provide such an analogy will be rooted in (1) a doctrine of creation, which accounts for the manner in which created things — especially human act, e.g. medical intervention — can convey a knowledge of the Creator's Act (this is the doctrine of the *analogia entis* set in the context of the *analogia fidei*), and (2) the contention that illness is at its root a manifestation of the brokenness introduced by sin and thus manifests the structure of sin. These two theological assumptions provide the conditions of the Christian use of medicine as an analogy, and they specify the unique way in which that analogy will be used to convey the "good news."

Illness as General Revelation

For the Christian, sickness is ultimately rooted in sin, individually, communally, and cosmically conceived. This

4. In this essay I will not consider why a person would want to accept this end. Here it is simply assumed that one is working within the framework of Christian commitment, and one is considering what implications such commitment has for the norms of a Christian bioethic.

does not mean sickness is the result of the personal sin of the individual who is suffering. Rather, sickness is tied to the fallenness of the human race as a whole (Amundsen and Ferngren, 1986, pp. 45-46; Augustine, 1983b, Book xxii, ch. 22).

Will Herberg summarizes the Judeo-Christian understanding of evil, when he speaks of it as "a certain spiritual perversity which tempts man to try to throw off his allegiance to the Absolute and to make himself the center of his universe" (1983, p. 54). Sin is then the "self-absolutization in rebellion against God" (p. 51). It introduces a rupture between the self and God, and this rupture then is extended into an alienation from others and self, as well. The individual becomes blind to the deeper meaning of life, trapped within an illusory, empty world of self (Niebuhr, 1953, pp. 12-18, chs. vii-viii; Niebuhr, 1984). The disordered relationships with self, others, and God are then extended into disordered communities and skewed relationships with nature. Poverty, hunger, war, and sickness, as well as destroyed environments follow. The egocentricity of sin is well exhibited in the idolatry of health, as well as the radical individualism where each person assumes self-sufficiency.

In addition to being ultimately caused by sin, illness manifests the structure of sin. The phenomenology of the illness experience reveals an experienced alienation from self, others, and God. S. Kay Toombs nicely sketches the way in which "[b]odily dysfunction necessarily causes a disturbance in the various and varying interactions between embodied consciousness and world" (1992, p. 62). Time and space shrink upon the here and now, as the lived world collapses upon the isolated self (Toombs, 1992, pp. 15, 66-70). The description Toombs gives of the way in which bodily intention is frustrated could be taken as an account of the bondage of the will, associated since Augustine with human sinfulness (Toombs, 1992, pp. 62-63, 70-76; Augustine, 1980b; see also Paul's Epistle to the Romans 7:14-24). As possibility constricts, individuals lose the power to deliver themselves. Drew Leder elaborates on this in his account of the phenomenology of pain, which is associated with illness, showing how "when beset by pain, the body surfaces as Other, something disharmonious with mind" (Leder, 1992, p. 98). Further, "[p]ain forces itself between self and other, introducing an existential rift" (p. 99). As pain increases, one's ability to interact in community decreases, even as pain makes painfully clear one's dependency on others and community. "Pain recalls us to our finitude and dependency, dragging us back into the mundane world" (p. 98). The illusion of self-sufficiency is shattered, and one is brought to self-transcendence; motivated to move beyond self to the others who can help.

Illness thus is revelatory of the human condition in general, although the specific content of that revelation is ambiguous, and thus is in need of interpretation by those who understand its deeper import. Because illness is related in its ultimate cause to sin and manifests, albeit ambiguously, its structure and thus the human predicament, illness comes within the purview of the activity of the Church and provides unique opportunities for Christian witness.

Medicine as Analogy

Through illness individuals become aware of their insufficiency and turn to others for help. However, most people do not appreciate the full revelatory function of illness — that it discloses a deep brokenness that is there already, and not brought about for the first time by the sickness. Instead, people think of the dis-integration of self and the alienation from community and God as a consequence of sickness, rather than as something unveiled in and by sickness. For them, the loss of self-sufficiency is an aberrant state; a fall from the "normal" independence of the individual. The need to turn to community for assistance is thus viewed as a temporary lapse, necessitated by the individual's inability to maintain somatic integrity.

Many people look to medicine as the primary way of combating the dis-integration that attends illness. Through the physician one finds the mediation of the communal knowledge by which wholeness can be restored. However, paradoxically, the physician heals by way of a process that initially exacerbates the alienation of the patient from self and others (Khushf, 1992). In modern medicine, "health" is understood in terms of "normal" anatomy and physiology (Foucault, 1973), as well as the negation of those natural forces that negate normal function (Mainetti, 1992). By identifying the pathoanatomical or pathophysiological truth value of a given clinical manifestation of illness, the physician can map the patient's condition on to the body of knowledge possessed in the medical domain, and thereby determine the appropriate intervention needed to restore somatic function, minimize the debilitating effects if such function cannot be restored, or at least provide prognosis (Englehardt, 1986, ch. 5). Through the diagnostic process the patient's illness experience is translated into a disease description, which accounts for all factors in terms of a closed world of material, interrelated causes (Englehardt, 1992; Khushf, 1992). The living subject is thereby transformed into an object — what Toombs refers to as body-as-scientific-object — and placed in the totalizing world of science (Toombs, 1992, pp. 76-81). The biological substratum of personal life is then manipulated in a way that brings it into accord with statistical norms of acceptable function (Boorse, 1975).

This process of objectivization and manipulation is distancing and dehumanizing, further intensifying the experience of alienation that attends illness (Leder, 1992, p. 96). In a sense, the patient is killed, divested of soul (Khushf, 1992, p. 294). This point regarding the metaphorical death of the patient has been well made by Michel Foucault and Richard Zaner, when they note how the "anatomical body" into which physicians transform their patients has the status of a corpse; namely, that corpse in gross anatomy laboratory on which all physicians receive their initial training (Toombs, 1992, p. 78). "[A]s a scientific object, a particular body is simply an exemplar of *the* human body (or of a particular class of human bodies) and, as such, it may be viewed independently from the person whose body it is" (Toombs, 1992, p. 79). Once the dysfunction of "body" is appropriately addressed, then it is often assumed that the physician's responsibility qua physician is finished, and the integration of personal life is expected to follow naturally thereafter. Following the metaphorical death comes a renewed integration, a resurrection (Khushf, 1992, p. 294).

In this account of medicine we find a rich analogy for understanding the Christian message. Instead of the anatomical and physiological archetype, one has the image of God that is manifest in Jesus Christ. The knowledge of this standard is found in the Christian community, and it is mediated by those who have been themselves transformed from the old ways of sin into the new way that is according to the Image of God. Likewise, the way of this transformation involves death; a giving up of self, and a submission to others, ultimately to an Other, God, who works for individuals a work that they are not able to accomplish by themselves.

In a more extensive discussion it would be fruitful to develop the analogy in some detail, showing what I think are very significant parallels between the process of modern medicine and the way of salvation that is at the heart of the Christian message. The analogy between medicine and spiritual healing make the medical discipline an important profession for the Christian, especially when services are offered freely to those who cannot otherwise afford them (as God's grace is offered freely). When the charitable act of physical healing is coupled with confession that makes clear how the deeds symbolically convey God's salvific work, medicine can obtain a sacramental character.[5] For the purpose of this essay, however, it will be enough to identify the analogy, and to note again that, for the Christian, priority of importance will be given to the deeper spiritual concerns. Suffering, sickness, and medicine will be understood within the broader theological framework. Instead, our question will be: what implications does this parallel have for the practice of medicine and the norms of a Christian bioethic? Before we can answer this question we will first need to consider an approach to medicine that is different from the disease-oriented one outlined above.

Today many people in the field of medicine are criticizing the disease-oriented approach to medicine, and they are advocating a "care ethic" that puts greater emphasis on addressing the disruption of the lived body associated with the illness experience. There is a call for "holistic medicine" that goes beyond the "disease" and ministers to the "illness," including the altered relation of the patient to self and community. Medicine will then focus on "the process of reconstructing the shattered domain" (Leder, 1992, p. 102; see also Toombs, 1992, p. 82).

The emphasis on "care" resonates well with an attempt to alleviate symptoms, which has always been a part of medical practice. However, "the care ethic" also arises as a response to perceived deficiencies in the dehumanizing objectivization of the patient that is, as discussed above, at the heart of modern scientific medicine.[6] The disease-oriented approach seems especially inappropriate in cases of chronic illness or where it is unlikely that such treatment will be successful and the patient is near death. In these cases, the metaphorical killing of the patient becomes the final word; it is not followed by the re-integration that arises naturally from restored physiological function. Rather, it is followed by literal death. For this reason, the indignity of the disease-oriented approach — the dehumanization that is a part of its method — does not seem warranted, and one looks for another response to the illness experience; one that addresses the needs of the whole person and does not simply focus on the biological substratum.

While the disease-oriented approach is closely tied to the scientific worldview and it will be relatively constant across cultures (at least in principle, because the anatomy and physiology is relatively constant across cultures), the care-oriented approach will be much more dependent on the particular cultural understandings of self, community, and God (Khushf, 1992, pp. 283-88; Hauerwas, 1978, p. 148). For this reason, Christians can accept much of what is found in the disease-oriented approach to medicine. They can openly acknowledge a degree to which all are implicated within a closed world of interrelated causes. As long as the scientific account of the world recognizes its limits, it is fully in accord with Christianity (Jockey, 1978; Herberg, 1983, p. 21). However, when one focuses on the lived body disruption and not just the body-as-scientific-object, then uniquely Christian values, especially the understanding of sickness, suffering, and death, will play a constitutive role in defining an ethic of care.

There will be a conflict between Christianity and the more naturalistically oriented approaches to the alienating experiences that attend illness. Many of the care-oriented approaches to medicine do not appreciate the revelatory function of illness — that it discloses a disruption at the heart of the human condition. Instead, they view the alienation from self, other, and God as caused by the biological dysfunction. Although there will be an attempt to minister to the person as a whole, the personal problems are still given a material, physiological etiology. In this way they are medicalized. The response will often involve coping strategies that seek to eliminate the

5. Hauerwas points to this sacramental function when he outlines the way in which the healer makes God present (1985). However, he does not sufficiently address the nature or "what" of presence, focusing purely on the fact or "that" of presence.

6. On the ambiguities of care and the different needs to which an ethic of care responds, see Hauerwas (1978).

awareness of the alienation or dull its perception; e.g. pain relief becomes a central focus (Skelly, 1994). The intent is to restore as much as possible of the illusion of self-sufficiency; an illusion that often goes under the name of "autonomy." In contrast, Christianity reverses the relation between the spiritual and material. Instead of taking the dis-integration of self and community as an epiphenomenon of physiological dysfunction, the latter is understood as a symptom of sin, which is the deeper personal dis-integration. Christianity will thus resist the medicalizing of human reality associated with the attempts to develop a "holistic" medicine.[7] Instead, it will seek to appropriately place the limits of medicine, and it will develop the revelatory function of the illness experience so that it discloses the deeper import of sickness and suffering. A Christian "ethic of care" will not be primarily a form of medicine, but rather a broader ministry, which accounts for and appropriates medicine within its concern with spiritual well-being.

Just as individuals must recognize their insufficiency in certain illness experiences and go beyond self to others (the medical community), so too the insufficiency of medicine must be recognized. This is something many are unwilling to do. However, when one moves from the center of everyday medicine to its boundaries, where the reality of death cannot be escaped and the inability of medicine to alleviate suffering becomes apparent, then the plight of the human condition can be glimpsed. At these boundaries, illness and death are again revelatory, and they point to an answer that lies beyond self and the medical community.

The "Problem of Evil" as the Human Predicament

The brokenness manifest in the illness experience and made especially apparent at the boundary conditions of human life is not just that of the one who is ill. It is a brokenness that is also experienced by those who are intimately related to the ill person, and even by those who observe the plight and seek to understand it. Parents and close friends, for example, also experience an alienation from self and from others as they are implicated in the sufferings of their child or friend. This alienation manifests a need to go beyond self and secular community, although the character of the answer does not become apparent in a natural way. A Christian ethic of care must appreciate the way in which the disruptions associated with the illness experience open outward to the broader disruptions associated with the problem of evil. Without the proclamation that properly diagnoses the human predicament and conveys the "good news" about what God has done to heal, there is an ambiguity and absurdity in certain experiences of "natural evil" (such as a child's suffering) that cannot be overcome medically or philosophically. This is because there is an alienation from God that can only be bridged from beyond self, in the community of faith, which extends God's mediation of true life.

To appreciate the full character of the human predicament, consider the following situation: there is a young girl, burnt from head to foot, racked with pain and looking with unwillingly dry eyes to her father, who is sitting as near as he can, but afraid to touch her bandaged body; afraid that his embrace will cause more pain than comfort. This is a God-fearing family, simple in belief but faithful. Now, however, as the father looks helplessly upon his child, perceiving the "why?" in her stare, he is confused, unable to place his present experience in the broader context of understanding that attends his faith, and he is groping for the spiritual source and help that can minister to the hurt of his suffering daughter. In this father's particular, very concrete experience, where the surdity of unwarranted pain confronts the simple understanding of belief, the "problem of evil" finds its existential source (Hauerwas, 1990).

In this account of father and daughter we have a dis-integration of self and community that extends beyond the immediate consequences of the physiological etiology. There is a sense of meaning and human purpose that is shattered by the very existence of a child's suffering, and it cannot be healed simply by treating the burn. This sense of absurdity is intensified in the case of terminal illness — for example, when a child is dying of leukemia, as recounted so powerfully in Peter DeVries' *The Blood of the Lamb* (1969). A true ethic of care will minister to this deep crisis in meaning, and not simply attempt to dull or view the physical, emotional, and spiritual pain associated with the experience.

Philosophers have attempted to conceptually articulate the existential crisis through the classical formulation of the problem of evil. "How can an omnipotent, omnibenevolent God permit such evil?" "Is this experience not the refutation of theism?" In the "classical theodicies" one begins with the three propositions regarding God's omnipotence, omnibenevolence, and the presence of evil, and then one qualifies their meaning and seeks to establish a conceptual framework in which contradiction is overcome (Hick, 1978). Or, in the same general vein, one can soften the paradox by denying one of the conceptually articulated propositions in the collision — for example, one can deny God's omnipotence, as does Harold Kushner in his popular *When Bad Things Happen to Good People* (1981), or, with the Christian Science practitioner, one can deny the reality of evil. In each case, one assumes that we are in a position where we can in principle understand; where we can conceptually resolve the paradox and determine the context that rightly

7. Holistic medicine is often a substitute for a content-full tradition in a contemporary, pluralistic culture where one does not want the commitment associated with a tradition like Christianity. It then involves a rival account of human flourishing — an account that is often rooted in the myths of self-sufficiency outlined earlier in this essay. It should also be noted that there are many different types of holistic medicine, each with a different understanding of the human good.

"places" pain and suffering. Why make this assumption? Further, it is assumed that the "existential crisis" is sufficiently captured in the philosophical articulation, so that one can answer the crisis by answering the philosophically formulated "problem of evil." This implies that the deep healing humanity needs is conceptual. The healer is then the person who provides the right ideas and conceptual framework for overcoming the absurdity.

This approach fails to do justice to our full humanity. Just as certain medicalizing, naturalist approaches err by focusing on the body at the expense of the broader spiritual and intellectual dimensions, this approach ignores the concrete needs of human material existence; it ignores body, emotions, and much more. How many really would be satisfied with a nice conceptual framework when confronted with the suffering of their little child? In such moments all ideological solutions are empty and shallow. Offering such solutions involves a fundamental misapprehension about the character of the problem. The pain and suffering that confronts belief is not just that physiological pain that is, for example, in the child. That pain particularizes a deep brokenness that is not just here or there, but lies behind and confronts every and all human endeavors, including the endeavor to conceptually grasp and address the problem of evil. The deep suffering is not just the pain and suffering that one seeks to reconcile with omnipotence and omniscience, conceptually understood. It is the very absurdity, experienced in the contradiction that is the problem of evil. It is this contradiction that challenges the broader framework of meaning and existentially confronts individuals with the absence of an omnipotent, omnibenevolent God. The conceptual aporia called "the problem of evil" and the disrupted life-world associated with the illness experience each particularize in their own way that "problem of evil" called "sin" that is at the heart of the human predicament. An ethic of care that ministers to this primordial disruption should not focus only on the conceptual dimension, just as it should not focus only on the somatic dimension. By appreciating the congruence of the somatic and conceptual forms of disruption, one can move beyond those attempts that address the human predicament in a fragmented way and one can turn to the root problem.

From the Christian perspective it must be affirmed that one will only be able to fully understand when God's Kingdom has come. Only then will we be in a position where we no longer see through a glass dimly, and where the deep contradictions of the present life are overcome. To use a Hegelian idiom, it is important to remember that the Owl of Minerva takes flight at dusk, after a given form of life has fully blossomed (Hegel, 1967, p. 13). Only then can philosophy paint its conceptual grey on grey, and only then will the question and answer to the problem of evil obtain its philosophical form. Until then we live in the absurdity of a human condition that is both redeemed and yet to be redeemed. In this context, the role of the healer is not to convey a purely conceptual reconciliation, nor is it to simply restore somatic function. It is rather to convey an existential reconciliation, which anticipates and proleptically makes present the coming perfection of the Kingdom of God. Theodicy, as an appropriate response to the need seen in and as the problem of evil, must thus be Christian healing.[8]

Christian Healing

Healing involves the mediation of life. In Christianity the paradigm of such healing is found in Jesus Christ, "the one mediator between God and men" (1 Timothy 2:5). He provides the Image of God, the archetype of spiritual health. Through the cross, Christ took on the brokenness that humanity could not bear, redeeming those who could not redeem themselves. He entered into the condition and suffering, even the sinfulness, of those who had become alienated from spiritual life, and thereby mediated that life. Through the resurrection it became manifest that such self-giving was not futile, but bore within it the hope of a new, deeper existence, one that goes beyond that which is presently experienced (Khushf, 1993b, pp. 29-33).

In faith — the simple confidence in the prospect of that new life — the followers of Jesus emulate "the way" of death and resurrection (John 14:6). They too enter into the sufferings of others and thereby convey the life of Christ, just as Christ conveyed the life of God (Khushf, 1993a, ch. 4). When one enters into another's suffering, one takes that suffering upon oneself. For example, one comes and cries with the father whose child is dying of leukemia. Rather than stay at a distance and provide conceptual answers, one comes down into the confusion and uncertainty of the situation, never knowing exactly how to respond or what one can do (this is part of the uncertainty, and makes many people unwilling to visit those in grief or suffering). But one comes with a paradigm of life; namely, the gospel of Jesus Christ. Through this message, hope is brought into a situation where there is no hope. One comes with a confidence that the seemingly unredeemed and unredeemable suffering (in human terms) is overcome in a form of life that cannot yet be grasped, or, to the degree it is now seen, it is only seen "through a glass dimly" (1 Corinthians 13:12). By following this way of humility, the witness becomes conformed to the Image of God, and as a reflection of that Image makes the way of healing known to the one who is suffering. This is the form of Christian care. By entering

8. Hauerwas (1990) is moving toward such an approach to the problem of evil when he recognizes that modern medicine has been viewed as a theodicy (ch. iii), and when he suggests that we need to move beyond medical solutions and come to a practice that is rooted in Christian community. Unfortunately, he does not say much about what such practice would involve other than being present to the sick person. How does this "Christian" presence distinguish itself from all the ways in which non-Christians are present to the sick?

into the suffering of the sufferer, by suffering-with *(mitleiden)* the alienated other, the healer establishes a community that transcends the form of community from which the sufferer became alienated in the illness experience (Hauerwas, 1985, p. 223).

Since the problem of evil that characterizes the human condition has material, intellectual, and spiritual dimensions, the Christian response will not just involve the spiritual dimension by itself. Christianity is concerned with the whole person, and there is a "preferential love" for those who experience misery. Thus the proclamation in words and deeds of the message about healing (salvation) will also involve the use of natural means to respond to physical needs (*Catechism of the Catholic Church*, 1994, p. 588). Food will be gathered for the hungry, money for the poor, and medicine will be used to heal the sick. By "caring" for the needy physically, the Church will witness to the way God cares for humanity. The invisible will be made visible in the works of mercy. This essay has elaborated on the way this can take place in medicine.

It is important, however, for the Christian to appropriately direct the concern with physical misery such as sickness so that it does not veil its central concern with the healing of sin. Unfortunately, in many of the "Christian" hospitals and for many physicians a sense of their deeper calling has been lost. They have forgotten that the rupture in human identity does not first take place when one is ill or when a loved one is suffering. Rather, the fallen condition becomes manifest in these experiences. By disclosing the fallen character of humanity and thus the need for grace, "natural evils" provide a special opportunity for the Church to bear witness (John 9:3; 11:4). They make people more receptive to accepting the message of life. The task of a Christian bioethic should be to order the practice of medicine so that it responds to this opportunity; so that it unveils rather than veils the deeper healing offered by the Church.

In this essay I have considered the basic framework for the development of this bioethic. The task is now to work out its implications in the many particulars that constitute the content of a bioethic. Thus one will need to consider the dynamics between physician and patient, noting as well the way in which this relation is extended into one between Christian witness and hearer of the Word, and the way the physician can coordinate with other healers such as the minister or priest. One will need to consider the withholding and withdrawing of treatment, framing the debate with a recognition of the higher end of humanity and thus the limits of medicine. At an institutional level, one will need to ask what it means to develop a Christian hospital, or perhaps a Christian managed care plan. In each case one will not just look at supererogatory acts or motivation that is separate from norms (McCormick, 1995). Neither will one just consider the type of community needed to sustain medical practice (Hauerwas, 1985). One will be concerned with a fundamental, radical transformation of all acts so they are reordered toward their higher ends. The result will be an ethic of care that takes seriously the call of Christ on all those in the health care arena who would live their lives in his service.

References

Amundsen, D. W. (1982). "Medicine and faith in early Christianity," *Bulletin of the History of Medicine* 56, 326-50.

Amundsen, D. W., and Ferngren, G. (1986). "The Early Christian Tradition," in R. L. Numbers and D. W. Amundsen (eds.), *Caring and Curing: Health and Medicine in the Western Religious Traditions,* Macmillan Publishing Company, New York, pp. 40-64.

Augustine (1980a). "On the Creed: A Sermon to Catechumens," in P. Schaff (ed.), *Nicene and Post-Nicene Fathers of the Christian Church,* First Series, Vol. III, Wm. B. Eerdmans Publishing Company, Grand Rapids, Michigan, pp. 369-75.

Augustine (1980b). "On the Spirit and the Letter," in P. Schaff (ed.), *Nicene and Post-Nicene Fathers of the Christian Church,* First Series, Vol. V, Wm. B. Eerdmans Publishing Company, Grand Rapids, Michigan, pp. 80-114.

Augustine (1983a). "Expositions on the book of Psalms," in P. Schaff (ed.), *Nicene and Post-Nicene Fathers of the Christian Church,* First Series, Vol. VIII, Wm. B. Eerdmans Publishing Company, Grand Rapids, Michigan.

Augustine (1983b). "The City of God," in P. Schaff (ed.), *Nicene and Post-Nicene Fathers of the Christian Church,* First Series, Vol. II, Wm. B. Eerdmans Publishing Company, Grand Rapids, Michigan, pp. 1-511.

Boorse, C. (1975). "On the distinction between disease and illness," *Philosophy and Public Affairs,* 5, 49-68.

Catechism of the Catholic Church (1994). Liguori Publications, Liguori, Montana.

Curzer, H. J. (1993). "Is Care a Virtue for Health Care Professionals?," *Journal of Medicine and Philosophy,* 18, 51-69.

De Vries, P. (1969). *The Blood of the Lamb,* Little, Brown and Co., Boston.

Edelstein, L. (1967). "The Relation of Ancient Philosophy to Medicine," in O. Temkin and C. L. Temkin (eds.), *Ancient Medicine: Selected Papers of Ludwig Edelstein,* The Johns Hopkins University Press, Baltimore, pp. 349-66.

Engelhardt, H. T. (1986). *The Foundations of Bioethics,* Oxford University Press, Oxford.

Engelhardt, H. T. (1992). "Observer Bias: The Emergence of the Ethics of Diagnosis," in J. L. Peset and D. Gracia, *The Ethics of Diagnosis,* Kluwer Academic Publishers, Dordrecht, pp. 63-71.

Foucault, M. (1975). *The Birth of the Clinic,* A. M. S. Smith (trans.), Vintage Books, New York.

Goodwin, J. S. (1991). "Geriatric Ideology: The Myth of the Myth of Senility," *Journal of the American Geriatrics Society* 39 6, 627-31.

Hauerwas, S. (1978). "Care," in W. T. Reich, *The Encyclopedia of Bioethics,* Vol. I, Free Press, New York, pp. 145-50.

Hauerwas, S. (1985). "Salvation and Health: Why Medicine Needs the Church," in E. Shelp (ed.), *Theology and Bioethics,* D. Reidel Publishing Company, Dordrecht, pp. 205-24.

Hauerwas, S. (1990). *Naming the Silences: God, Medicine, and the Problem of Suffering,* Wm. B. Eerdmans Publishing Company, Grand Rapids, Michigan.
Hegel, G. W. F. (1967). *Hegel's Philosophy of Right,* T. M. Knox (trans.), Oxford University Press, London.
Herberg, W. (1983). *Judaism and Modern Man,* Atheneum, New York.
Hick, J. (1978). *Evil and the God of Love,* Harper & Row, New York.
Humphrey, D., and Wickett, A. (1990). *The Right to Die,* The Hemlock Society, Eugene, Oregon.
Jockey, S. (1978). *The Road of Science and the Ways of God,* University of Chicago Press, Chicago.
Khushf, G. (1992). "Post-modern Reflections on the Ethics of Naming," in J. L. Peset and D. Gracia (eds.), *The Ethics of Diagnosis,* Kluwer Academic Publishers, Dordrecht.
Khushf, G. (1993a). *Deconstructing General Hermeneutics/(Re)Constructing a Biblical Hermeneutic,* University Microfilms International, Ann Arbor, Michigan.
Khushf, G. (1993b). 'Die Rolle des "Buchstabens" in der Geschichte des Abendlands und im Christentum," in H. U. Gumbrecht and K. L. Pfeiffer, *Schrift,* Wilhelm Fink Verlag, München.
Kushner, H. S. (1981). *When Bad Things Happen to Good People,* Schocken Books, New York.
Leder, D. (1992). "The Experience of Pain and Its Clinical Implications," in J. L. Peset and D. Gracia (eds.), *The Ethics of Diagnosis,* Kluwer Academic Publishers, Dordrecht, pp. 95-105.
Mainetti, J. A. (1992). "Embodiment, Pathology, and Diagnosis," in J. L. Peset and D. Gracia (eds.), *The Ethics of Diagnosis,* Kluwer Academic Publishers, Dordrecht, pp. 79-93.
McCormick, R. (1985). "Theology and Bioethics: Christian Foundations," in E. Shelp (ed.), *Theology and Bioethics,* D. Reidel Publishing Company, Dordrecht, pp. 95-113.
Niebuhr, R. (1953). *The Nature and Destiny of Man,* Vols. I and II, Charles Scribner's Sons, New York.
Niebuhr, R. (1984) "Sin," in A. Cohen and M. Halverson (eds.), *A Handbook of Christian Theology,* Abingdon Press, Nashville.
Sigerist, H. (1943). *Civilization and Disease,* Ithaca, New York.
Skelly, F. J. (1994). "Price of Pain Control," *American Medical News* (May 16), 13-15.
Skrabanek, P. (1994). *The Death of Humane Medicine,* St. Edmundsbury Press Ltd., Bury St. Edmunds, Suffolk.
Toombs, S. K. (1992). *The Meaning of Illness: A Phenomenological Account of the Different Perspectives of the Physician and Patient,* Kluwer Academic Publishers, Dordrecht.
Weber, T. P. (1986). "The Baptist Tradition," in R. Numbers and D. Amundsen (eds.), *Caring and Curing,* Macmillan Publishing Company, New York, pp. 288-316.

4 Money and the Medical Profession

William F. May

The theme of money and the professions triggers the imagination. Money is many-faced, and I do not mean the grave and graven images (of the dead presidents — Washington, Lincoln, and Jackson) who gaze somberly out as we handle our bills. Rather, many-faced in that money performs variously and importantly and positively in our lives, and we had better, at the outset, acknowledge that varied performance. How do I need thee? How do even professionals need thee? Let me count the ways.

1. Money feeds. Except in the world of barter, one needs money to live. We need it to buy our daily bread. Amateurs may do it for love. But a professional, alongside all other workers, does it for money, and it would be a species of angelism to deny that fact. Since money feeds, it also supplies some stability to the relationship between the professional and the customer or the client. If professional services depended entirely on love, then they might falter. Love (at least emotionally) would tend to rise and fall, wax and wane. Money supplies a bit of constancy to the relationship. Philanthropy is flighty. Adam Smith knew this when he noted that the fellow who can be counted on to get up at 3:00 A.M. to tend to a sick cow either owns it or gets paid to take care of it. Norman Mailer put it another way when he said, the professional writer is the person who can keep at it, even on a bad day. Money keeps us from being dilettantes; it steadies the attention.

2. Money thus motivates. Above and beyond the bread it supplies, money often marks personal worth, especially when the good being sold is not simply a commodity but one's own skill. It certainly is no perfect marker of worth, but even those professionals whom the marketplace usually underpays, such as teachers and members of the clergy, recognize money, in their own inner markets, as indicators of worth.

3. Money connects us to the stranger. Families, friends, and neighbors meet in enclosed spaces, in the house, the church, and the synagogue; but the marketplace puts us out into the open; it throws us into contact with the stranger. From the seventeenth century forward, professionals — the doctor and the lawyer — hung out their

---

From William F. May, "Money and the Medical Profession," *Kennedy Institute of Ethics Journal* 7.1 (1997): 1-13.

shingles on the street. The professional shingle, jutting out for every passerby to see, signals that a professional is making a skill available not simply to the enclosed world of friends and relatives and neighbors, but to the stranger. Money, in a sense, is ecumenical; it breaks out beyond the boundaries of the parochial. The pressures for free trade reflect the inherently expansive nature of the market. It transcends even national boundaries as it opens out toward the faraway, the strange.

4. Money talks. Whether it barks out commands or courts with sweet-talk, money mobilizes and organizes resources and talent. It is not inert. Since it feeds, since it powerfully motivates and persuades, and since it overcomes barriers — as we say, it opens doors — it is remarkably fluid. We can move it easily and it moves other things easily; it lubricates and keeps societies moving. It is dynamic, seizing on the inventive, the novel. It also lets one adapt rapidly to change, readjusting and reconfiguring the markets.

Baron de Montesquieu pointed out that the spring of action in an aristocratic society is the aspiration to honor and excellence and the spring of action in a despotic society is fear (De Montesquieu 1949, pp. 19-28). Clearly, the spring of action in a commercial society is money, which supplies us with the objects of our desiring and gratifies our self-interest. Thus, while the pictures on the face of money may be grave and engraven, money itself is dynamic and protean, so much so that when we celebrate it, we can border on the blasphemous and idolatrous. We refer to the almighty dollar, a reference that moves us toward the dark side of money, a side so dark and deep, that Scripture once referred to the love of money as the root of all evil (1 Tim. 6:10).

If not the root of all evil, money certainly fertilizes the roots. While money feeds, motivates, breaks down barriers, commands, and organizes, it also can vulgarize, distract, corrupt, distort, and banish as it excludes people from basic goods. It can vulgarize, distract, and corrupt professionals as they offer their services; it can distort the services they have to offer; and it can exclude the needy from access to professional services. The dangers of money thrive on the complicated double relationship of the marketplace and the professions: they grew together and yet they differ (or they ought to differ) in their essence.

The increased power of the professions in the modern world coincides and intertwines with the emergence of the modern marketplace and with the still later emergence of the winner in the marketplace, the modern, large-scale corporation. I see the connections as follows. Aristotle once referred to the good community, the *polis,* as a community of friends, people who share needs and goals. Aristotle's ideal city was quite small, small enough to be a community of well-known, familiar names and to engage every one (well, not exactly everyone, not women, not slaves) in civic responsibilities. The city remained relatively small until the eighteenth century. This cameo scale let people in the city associate chiefly within the framework of family, neighbors, and friends. From the eighteenth century forward, the West and particularly the United States increasingly shifted from a community of neighbors to a society of strangers.

(In Dallas, where I live now, the house-attached garage completes the process of separating the self from the neighbor. I drive home along an alley, flick the garage door open to avoid getting out of the car, park inside, and then flick the garage door shut and enter the kitchen. If kids are out in their front yards playing, if neighbors are out mowing the grass, I wouldn't know it. We live in a society of strangers, sometimes friendly strangers, but still strangers.)

How do persons in the modern setting connect? Mostly not through shared interests, but through *cash,* which temporarily connects people who otherwise may share few common interests. Professionals are part of that platoon of paid strangers who partly substitute for the families, neighbors, and friends who provided services in earlier societies.

Aging patients (their children in distant cities) now look to the physician and nurse as the fixed stars in their lives. Young women look to Ob-Gyn specialists rather than to the experienced aunt or the competent neighbor for assistance in birth. At one time, disputes were resolved through the mediations of friends and neighbors acquainted over a lifetime with the parties to a conflict. They now end up in the courts. Since the parties to the dispute and those who will conduct and judge the proceedings do not know the principals, one needs lawyers to follow the strict rules of evidence and the paper trails that lead to a judgment, if not justice, in a particular case. Litigation flourishes in a society of strangers, and trained experts handle the proceedings and preside, like the furies, over outcomes. Moreover, the several sets of experts intersect. Precisely because the doctor/patient relationship today chiefly connects strangers linked by money and because it points toward a desperately hoped-for favorable outcome, the relationship is increasingly unstable and, thus today, sometimes erupts into enmity. The disappointed patient resorts angrily to the court, which in its own right and turn is controlled by strangers to both parties; strangers attempt to bring closure to the disputes between strangers, with money at issue at every point.

Nevertheless, although the professions and the marketplace (and money) grew together in the modern world, the identity of the first does not tidily fuse with the second. For, in fact, the professional has a double identity. The professional has one foot in the marketplace. She is paid for her work. That distinguishes her from the amateur. But, at the same time, a commitment transcending the marketplace defines the professional.

We express this transcendence least satisfactorily by pointing to the aristocratic origins of the professional in the West. "Having a profession" provided a social location in life for the second, third, and fourth sons of aristocrats, who, in a society committed to primogeniture, could not inherit the land (the family property went exclusively to the eldest son), and yet, who, as children of the aristocracy, could not submit to the vulgarities of the marketplace by working for a living. Thus the professions — the law, civil service, the military, and medicine — provided the great families with an honorable social location, a parking lot, for their surplus gentlemen.

The aristocratic ideal of *noblesse oblige* deserves criticism. It smacks of the condescension of the superior to the inferior. It bends low with benevolence. And it operated within the circle of the old boy's network. But it also deserves some praise. It avoided the illusions of the self-made man or woman. It recognized that the privileged largely inherit and receive what they are; a receiving that generates obligations to others. The moral ideal that those who have received much, owe much carried over into the nineteenth-century ideal of *pro bono publico* service. This ideal applied not only to the law and medicine but also to those professions explicitly and directly aimed at some aspect of the public good: civil service, military service, and service to the church.

In any event, the vestigial remains of the aristocratic ideal persist in professional complaints that:

1. Money vulgarizes, and therefore professionals should not advertise, least of all their fees, lest they tarnish the moral elegance of the *honorarium*. The courts, beginning with the Virginia decision in the 1970s, banned professional guilds from prohibiting advertising on the grounds that such prohibitions led to monopolistic price fixing. The cost of professional services had been rising much faster than the rate of inflation. Thus the professions, while invoking an ethic superior to the marketplace, in effect, behaved in a fashion morally inferior to the marketplace. Understandably, the courts wanted to put a stop to this hypocrisy. But rampant advertising does make one wince. Money vulgarizes. "Two root canals for the price of one until the end of the month." "Radial keratotomy at $1250 an eye, with $500 off for the two procedures if you make your decision before you leave our seminar room." "If you need a lawyer's help on your traffic ticket, just dial 9-GOTCHA, credit cards accepted."

Recoiling from all money matters, professionals daintily hand over to their office staffs the task of collecting money from their patients and clients so as not to brush up too close to cash. But the polite conventions of professional billing do not fool. Professional schools increasingly require courses in business management; they do not enroll as many students in purely elective courses in professional ethics. Moreover, the social profile of the recruits for the professions has changed massively and for good social reasons. The professions no longer serve as the parking place for the younger sons of the aristocrats, but as the social escalator that carries sons and daughters — those previously without clear public identities and often without resource — upward to earn their entire living from their profession. Thus the modern professional seems to have both feet planted in the marketplace.

The question grows more acute. Does the professional have any further identity that transcends the cash nexus? Is the professional simply a combination of technician plus entrepreneur, someone who sells a skill in the law, medicine, accounting, engineering, teaching, or pastoring? Or is the professional something more?

Roscoe Pound, the great jurist, sought to illuminate this further reach of professional identity by invoking the old religious term, a "calling." In an oft quoted line, he said:

> The term [profession] refers to a group . . . pursuing a learned art as a common calling in the spirit of public service — no less a public service because it may incidentally be a means of livelihood. Pursuit of the learned art in the spirit of public service is the primary purpose. (Pound 1953, p. 5)

Pound thus defines a profession as a calling, and he links a calling with the pursuit of the common good. Much earlier, the religious tradition of the West made this connection in its Scriptures, as did William Perkins, a seventeenth-century Puritan who was influential on the American scene. He defined a calling as that "kind of life, ordained and imposed on man by God, for the common good" (Perkins 1965, p. 36). So conceived, all lines of work, but especially those callings that serve goods basic to our common life, such as law, medicine, and religion, ought to contribute to the common good.

However, in our time the notion of a calling has tended to deteriorate into a career. A career refers to that wherein I invest myself, on the basis of PSAT, SAT, GRE, LSAT, and MCAT scores, to pursue my own private goals. Etymologically, a career derives from the same root as a car. A career is an automobile, literally, a self-driven vehicle through life, in and through which we enter into the public thoroughfares for the purposes of reaching our own private destinations.

But if a profession is a calling to serve a public good and not simply a vehicle for serving our own private, careerist aims for money and fame, then we have arrived at a second danger and temptation of money, more serious than the first.

2. Money not only vulgarizes, it also distracts. The moralist Alasdair MacIntyre distinguishes between the goods internal to a practice — such as the arts of lawyering, healing, and preaching — and the goods external to a practice — such as the fame or fortune that those practices may generate (MacIntyre 1981, p. 178). If someone chooses medicine, law, or the ministry only for the prestige or the cash, she has lost that single-mindedness, that purity of heart, that allows all else to burn away, as the practice shines through. The love of money and fame distracts; it focuses attention elsewhere. The professional loses that purity of heart that the Epistle of James and, later, Kierkegaard reminded the world, is "to will one thing."

In Kingsley Amis's 1954 novel, *Lucky Jim*, a college history professor answers his phone saying, "History here." What a wonderful line! Better than "Historian here" or "Dr. Toynbee here." "History here" points to the activity, pure and simple, not to the office or to the attainment of the person. Isn't that what a distressed patient wants when he calls the doctor about a baffling symptom? "Healing here." Isn't that what the distressed client or parishioner needs, when calling the lawyer or the priest? "Sanctuary here." But money distracts the professional from what should be his or her single-minded professional purpose (the client's welfare) by focusing a wall-eye on some external good.

3. Money corrupts. Eventually, a distracted focus on the goods external to a practice corrupts the practice itself. The actress interested only in her Nielsen ratings and the advertising revenue they generate repeats the tricks of the trade that worked for her last week, and at length her show deteriorates into a series of running gags, tired repeated cliches that corrupt the good of the original performance.

The specific corruption of money in the case of the professional transaction can be stated as follows. A marketplace transaction, as distinct from a professional exchange, presupposes two self-interested and relatively knowledgeable parties engaged in the act of buying and selling. Each party attempts primarily to protect his or her own self-interest. The seller does not feel particularly constrained to watch out for the buyer's interests and well-being. That is up to the buyer who, by comparative shopping and other means, has ways of becoming knowledgeable.

But a basic asymmetry exists in the relation of the professional to her client. The professional possesses knowledge (and the power that knowledge generates), while the troubled client is often too ignorant, powerless, anxious, and dependent to protect his or her interests. A medical crisis, moreover, usually leaves little time for comparative shopping, even if the patient knew how to assess the professional's skills. Patients, students, clients, and parishioners cannot readily obey the marketplace warning, *caveat emptor* — buyer beware. Their lack of knowledge and their neediness require that the professional exchange take place in a fiduciary setting of trust that transcends the marketplace assumptions about two wary bargainers. The importance of this trust should determine our view of what the professional has to sell.

I am very fond of a Volvo automobile and thus have often walked into a Volvo showroom, but I have never yet had a salesman say to me, "Professor May, do you really need this car? In the total economy of your life, as a professor, wouldn't it make more sense for you to trot across the highway and buy a Toyota Tercel at half the price?" Instead, the salesman does his best to serve his own self-interest and sell me the car. When I enter the showroom, I am a pork chop for the eating. That's part of the game.

But if I visit a physician, I must be able to trust that he or she sells two items, not one. First the physician, to be sure, sells a procedure. But, second, she must also offer her professional judgment that I need the treatment she offers. The surgeon is not simply in the business of selling hernia jobs. She also sells the cold, detached, disinterested, unclouded judgment that I need that wretched little procedure. If she sells me more operation than I need, she abuses her disproportionate power and poisons the professional relationship with distrust. Instead of sheltering, she takes advantage of the distressed. She reduces me merely to a profit-opportunity. And, if I discover her pushing her own interests at my expense, I will resent her for exploiting my ignorance and powerlessness.

Herein lies the ground for all professional strictures against conflicts of interest. The professional must be sufficiently distanced from his own interests and that of other clients to serve the client's well-being. Money does not alone tempt the physician to compromise the interest or welfare of his or her patient. The lure of fame can also undercut loyalty to the patient, as, for example, when a clinical researcher recruits patients for research protocols that are not particularly in their interest. But money creates by far the most cases of conflict of interest and corrodes most aggressively professional responsibility.

Under the until recently prevailing fee-for-service system in medicine, money has worked, on the whole, to create temptations to overtreat patients. Coupled with third-party insurance coverage, the system has led to the overuse of medical services and sometimes to the abuse of patients, pummeled as they were by often irrelevant or unnecessary tests.

> A primary care internist can increase his or her net income by a factor of almost three by prescribing a wide but not unreasonable set of tests. The term not unreasonable is a reflection that the use of such tests is so common as to be almost standard practice; yet some clinicians would argue that few of the tests are actually necessary. (Harold Tuft, cited in Rodwin 1953, p. 55).

Closely related to, but distinct from, fee-for-service practice lie a range of other financial incentives to physicians. Marc A. Rodwin (1953, pp. 56-94) has detailed six of the most important of these lures in his book on *Medicine, Money, and Morals.* The practices themselves pose a conflict of interest even though, in a particular case, the practice may not have broken a law or injured a patient:

(1) Kickbacks for referrals; that is, payments either received by physicians from other parties or institutions or given by physicians to other parties or institutions;
(2) Self-referrals, in which physicians refer patients to facilities from which they profit (either in-house or external facilities in which they have invested);
(3) Income that physicians derive from dispensing drugs, selling medical products, and performing ancillary services that they themselves have prescribed;
(4) The sale to a hospital of a physician's medical practice;
(5) Payments from hospitals to recruit or bond physicians;
(6) Gifts from medical suppliers.

Money can corrupt the medical exchange by creating incentives not only for excessive treatment under a fee-for-service system, but also for inadequate treatment under prepayment systems. Physicians profit under many prepayment systems from the surplus of income over medical costs (Rodwin 1953, pp. 56-94). This time, money tempts physicians to do too little rather than too much. One moves from the sins of the overbearing to the sins of the underbearing. Undertreatment takes various forms, including insufficient medical care, tardy treatment, and inappropriate treatment settings. E. Haavi Morreim (1995, chs. 3–5) has detailed at length the ways in which the new economics of medicine has sharply curtailed professional loyalty to the best interests and well-being of patients. Meanwhile, the so-called "gag rules," imposed upon doctors (and nurses) by some health maintenance organizations (HMOs), further compound the offense against patients. Some HMOs prohibit their doctors or nurses from informing patients that the services available under a given contract do not offer the patient the best or most needful services in a particular case. They may also prohibit professional members of the HMO from disclosing to their patients both the fact and the degree to which they profit from economizing both on treatments and on referrals to specialists in the HMO. In effect, this institutional gagging of doctors further disempowers patients; it frustrates patients' efforts to make good on the old marketplace warning, buyer beware.

4. Money distorts, as well as corrupts, distracts, and vulgarizes the professional relationship. That claim requires us to identify a further way, in addition to its disinterestedness, in which the professional exchange should differ from a marketplace transaction.

The commercial transaction between buyer and seller seeks to gratify the buyer's wants. The professional exchange should be, when circumstances require, transformational, and not merely transactional. The practitioner in the helping professions must respond not simply to the client's self-perceived wants but to his deeper needs. The patient suffering from insomnia often wants simply the quick fix of a pill. But if the physician goes after the root of the problem, she may have to help the patient transform the habits that led, in the first instance, to the symptom of sleeplessness. The physician is slothful if she dutifully jumps to acute care but neglects preventive medicine.

Most of the incentives in conventional fee-for-service medicine favor acute care, at the expense of preventive, rehabilitative, long-term, and terminal care; they favor physical, at the expense of mental, health care. The physician who hands the patient what he wants — the sleeping pill — gets him out of the office faster. His basic office costs of receptionist, secretary, and nurse come out roughly the same, whether he handles more or fewer patients. Thus the temptations are great to become an artful people mover.

To question the patient about his deeper problem takes time. What gives with your Atlas syndrome that you can't let go of the world for seven hours? Have you thought about your perfectionist tendencies that make you lie in bed at night, reliving painfully the gaffes of the previous day or worrying about the overload of duties that fill the morrow? Such counseling takes time. It demands effective teaching of the patient, and teaching is slow boring through hard wood.

The reward system in medicine has undercompensated those engaged in primary care and overcompensated those engaged in piece-work medicine. Money has distorted and skewed the goods delivered. We are acute care gluttons and preventive care and rehabilitative care anemics. As one expert put it, "We give millions for acute care and not one cent for preventive medicine." Those words were written in 1886 (Hutchinson 1886, p. 478). Robert Morisson, the thoroughly secular Cornell scientist, said before his death that what the last years of the twentieth century needed for the improvement of its health was another John Wesley, whom he described as the greatest public health officer of the eighteenth century. Wesley and the Methodist movement were crucial in transforming the health habits of the working class in eighteenth-century England.

Sensitive to the importance of addressing our deeper needs, thoughtful reformers have argued that a national health care package ought to include less emphasis on acute care and offer more help in preventive, rehabilitative, long-term, and terminal care.

5. Finally, money excludes. It sets up barriers. Money opens doors, but usually only to those who can pay for a key. Those who cannot pay their way into the marketplace cannot acquire the good. That arrangement works out acceptably enough in the purchase of optional commodities — like a "walkman," a tie, or a scarf, but professionals presumably generate and offer not optional commodities, but basic goods — goods needed for human security and flourishing. When physicians heal, lawyers defend, the military and the police protect, the clergy guide and console, and academics teach, they help others to secure the basic goods of health, justice, defense, and intellectual and spiritual flourishing. Something has gone deeply awry when these fundamental goods do not reach all. We do not expect people to be able to afford to hire a lieutenant colonel and his battalion to secure the good of defense, but it sometimes can take at least that to purchase the goods of medicine.

Without the good of medicine people suffer a triple deprivation: the misery of their trouble, the desperation of no treatment, and the cruel proof on the part of the society that they do not really belong. The untreated ill, the undefended client, become aliens in their own land. So even while money leaps over and seeps under boundaries and enclaves, it also excludes and expels. The principle of universal access derives from the conviction that health care is a fundamental good, not an optional commodity. Universal access goes to the soul of health care reform. Currently, we are the only industrial nation, other than

South Africa, that fails to offer universal access to health care.

So much for the subject of money as it vulgarizes, distracts, corrupts, distorts, excludes, and thus endangers the integrity of the professions.

I have not sent up these warning signals about money in order to dismiss it, but in order to let money do its proper but limited work: as it feeds and motivates professionals, as it connects them to the stranger, and as it mobilizes their resources and talents in the huge institutions where they most often work. Money is a useful but unruly servant. We need to take care that it sustains rather than obscures what we profess on behalf of patients, clients, students, and parishioners when we dare to cut, burn, or laser their bodies or advise them. What we profess ought to come down to what our patients surely hope for: "Healing here." What our clients and parishioners surely hope for: "Sanctuary here."

But why care about all this? Why not treat our professions merely as a means to a livelihood? Why take seriously Roscoe Pound's insistence that the primary purpose of a profession is "the pursuit of [a] learned art in the spirit of public service"?

Let me close with just two reasons: First, going to a professional school in a society like ours gives young people a shot at becoming members of the ruling class. Traditional societies transmitted power largely on the basis of blood, their rulers inherited their power. But we transmit power chiefly on the basis of knowledge, largely acquired at a university. That is why parents — rich or poor, successful or drifting — worry about whether their children will get into good universities. Through education, the young will acquire their power base in life; as power wielders, in effect, they will rule, and the task of rulers, if they stick to their proper goal, is the pursuit of the common good. (Aristotle once noted severely that the specific corruption of tyranny is the wielding of public power for one's own private purposes. The modern careerist, in pursuing exclusively his own private goals, may not engage in the tyrant's melodramatic sins of commission, but he cumulatively and relentlessly defects from his duties to the common good through his sins of omission.)

Second, the power that professionals acquire at a university is not a power that they have picked up on their own. No one can go through a university and think of him- or herself simply as a solo entrepreneur gathering up a private stockpile of knowledge to be sold on the market to the highest bidder. No one can think of him- or herself as a self-made man or woman. A huge company of people have contributed to the shaping of professionals as they zigzag their way through college and professional schools: the janitors who clean the johns, the help in the kitchen, the secretaries who make the operation hum, the administrators who wrestle with the institution's problems, the faculty who share with students what they know, the vast research traditions of each of the disciplines that set the table for that sharing, and the patients and clients who lay their bodies and souls on the line, letting young professionals practice on them in the course of perfecting their art. And behind all that, the public moneys and the gifts that support the enterprise, so much so that tuition money usually pays for only a fraction of the education. When physicians and other health care professionals treat education as a merely private asset, they systematically distort and obscure the social origins of knowledge and therefore the power that that knowledge places within their grasp and the end that that power ought to serve — the nation's health and flourishing.

Acknowledgment

This article is based on the 1996 Edmund D. Pellegrino lecture at the Kennedy Institute of Ethics.

References

De Montesquieu, Baron. 1949. *The Spirit of the Laws*, tr. Thomas Nugent, Book III. New York: Hafner Press, a division of Macmillan Publishing Co., Inc.

Hutchinson, W. 1886. Health Insurance, On Our Financial Relation to the Public. *Journal of the American Medical Association* 7 (30 October): 477-81.

MacIntyre, Alasdair. 1981. *After Virtue.* Notre Dame, IN: University of Notre Dame Press.

Morreim, E. Haavi. 1995. *Balancing Act: The New Medical Ethics of Medicine's New Economics.* Washington, DC: Georgetown University Press.

Perkins, William. 1965. A Treatise of the Vocations or Callings of Men, with Sorts and Kinds of Them, and the Right Use Thereof. In *Puritan Political Ideas,* ed. Edmund S. Morgan, pp. 35-59. Indianapolis: Bobbs-Merrill Co., Inc.

Pound, Roscoe. 1953. *The Lawyer from Antiquity to Modern Times.* St. Paul, MN: West Publishing.

Rodwin, Marc. 1953. *Medicine, Money and Morals.* New York: Oxford University Press.

Much of the controversy about religion and health is rooted in the fact that most medical debates presume a homeostatic understanding of human well-being. This concept of human well-being is a product of a secular worldview, but even for the confirmed secularist, it is rarely treated as the ultimate end of human life. Differing worldviews foster different conceptions of the human good, and as such, worldview may have measurable health repercussions. However, worldviews are not amenable to surgical or pharmacological intervention. Consequently, it may be that worldviews (religious or otherwise) and the practices of living formed by such worldviews should simply inform the practice of medicine like other important demographic variables. Because each worldview fosters particular ways of valuing homeostatic health, there may be patterns of disease (or health) that correlate with specific worldviews in much the same way that Japanese men are predisposed to gastric cancer. Precise knowledge of such correlations would only improve the capacity to make informed medical decisions. Furthermore, to the extent that clinicians can recognize (if not fluently speak) languages of various worldviews, they may become better equipped to engage both the science of curing and the art of caring for the sick and suffering.

Conclusion

In an attempt to stimulate debate over the conceptual basis for the scientific study of religion, we have presented a critique of the dominant paradigm of studying religion as a frosting added to the generic cake of secular human experience. This approach presumes the universality of the secular worldview, distorting the coherence of independent religious worldviews. We suggest that religion is better conceived as a cultural-linguistic system that must be studied from the inside rather than by forcing religion to speak in secular terms. In tracing the implication of this critique, we have argued that (1) there is no objective frame of reference from which to study religion; (2) studying a religion is most like learning a foreign language; (3) measurement of religiousness is most like assessing fluency in a language and implies the assessment of the skill by someone skilled in that language; (4) the scientific study of religion may be important even if religion doesn't "work"; and (5) this critique leads to the dangerous possibility that there may in fact be health consequences associated with specific worldviews. We contend that meaningful research regarding the associations between religion and health will depend on applying these ideas in the design, conduct, and analysis of future research.

Acknowledgment

The authors wish to thank Jeffrey Bishop, Adam Cohen, Farr Curlin, Cynthia Linkas, and several anonymous reviewers for their helpful comments on this manuscript.

References

Aspinwall, L. G., and S. M. Brunhart. 2000. What I do know won't hurt me: Optimism, attention to negative information, coping and health. In *The science of optimism and hope: Research essays in honor of Martin E. P. Seligman,* ed. J. E. Gillham, 162-200. Philadelphia: Templeton Foundation Press.

Bahm, A. J. 1946. Humanism: A religion for scientists. *Scientific Monthly* 62 (4): 310-15.

Bellah, R., et al. 1985. *Habits of the heart: Individualism and commitment in American life.* New York: Harper and Row.

Denett, D. C. 1996. *The intentional stance.* Cambridge: MIT Press.

Derrida, J. 1973. *Speech and phenomena,* trans. D. B. Allison. Evanston: Northwestern Univ. Press.

Feinstein, A. R. 1999a. Multi-item "instruments" vs. Virginia Apgar's principles of clinimetrics. *Arch Int Med* 159 (2): 125-28.

Feinstein, A. R. 1999b. Statistical reductionism and clinicians' delinquencies in humanistic research. *Clin Pharmacol Ther* 66 (3): 211-17.

Feinstein, A. R. 2002. Appraising the success of caring. In *The lost art of caring,* ed. L. Cluff and R. Binstock, 201-18. Baltimore: Johns Hopkins Univ. Press.

Fetzer Institute/NIA Working Group (Fetzer/NIA). 1999. *Multidimensional measurement of religiousness/spirituality in health research.* Kalamazoo: John E. Fetzer Institute.

Fogelin, R. J. 1980. *Wittgenstein.* London: Routledge & Kegan Paul.

Foucault, M. 1971. *The archeology of knowledge,* trans. A. M. Sheridan Smith. New York: Pantheon Books.

Foucault, M. 1994. *The order of things: An archeology of the human sciences.* New York: Random House.

Frei, H. W. 1974. *The eclipse of biblical narrative: A study in eighteenth and nineteenth century hermeneutics.* New Haven: Yale Univ. Press.

Gadamer, H. 1975. *Truth and method,* trans. G. Barden and J. Cumming. New York: Seabury Press.

Hare, R. M. 1999. *Objective prescriptions, and other essays.* New York: Oxford Univ. Press.

Hatch, R. L., et al. 1998. The spiritual involvement and beliefs scale: Development and testing of a new instrument. *J Fam Pract* 46 (6): 476-86.

Hill, P. C., and R. W. Hood, Jr., eds. 1999. *Measures of Religiosity.* Birmingham, AL: Religious Education Press.

Hummer, R. A., et al. 1999. Religious involvement and U.S. adult mortality. *Demography* 36: 273-85.

Idler, E. L., and S. V. Kasl. 1997a. Religion among disabled and nondisabled persons I: Cross-sectional patterns in health practices, social activities, and well-being. *J Gerontol B Psychol Sci Soc Sci* 52 (6): S294-305.

Idler, E. L., and S. V. Kasl. 1997b. Religion among disabled and nondisabled persons II: Attendance at religious services as a predictor of the course of disability. *J Gerontol B Psychol Sci Soc Sci* 52 (6): S306-16.

Idler, E. L., et al. 2003. Measuring multiple dimensions of religion and spirituality for health research: Conceptual background and findings from the 1998 General Social Survey. *Research on Aging,* 25 (4): 327-65.

Jones, J., and D. Hunter. 1995. Consensus methods for medical and health services research. *BMJ* 311 (7001): 376-80.

Kalb, C. 2003. Faith and healing. *Newsweek,* Nov. 10, 44-56.

King, M. 1995. The royal free interview for religious and spiritual beliefs: Development and standardization. *Psychol Med* 25: 1125-34.

Koenig, H. G. 2002. An 83-year-old woman with chronic illness and strong religious beliefs. *JAMA* 288 (4): 487-93.

Koenig, H. G., M. E. McCullough, and D. B. Larson. 2001. *Handbook of religion and health.* New York: Oxford Univ. Press.

Ku Klux Klan. 2003, The Knights home page, http://www.kukluxklan.org. Accessed March 5, 2003.

Kuhn, T. 1962, *The structure of scientific revolutions.* Chicago: Univ. of Chicago Press.

Larson, D. B., J. P. Swyers, and M. E. McCullough. 1998. *Scientific research on spirituality and health: A consensus report.* Monograph sponsored by the John M. Templeton Foundation. R[ockville, MD: National Institute for Healthcare Research.]

Lash, N. 1996. *The beginning and the end of "religion."* New York: Cambridge Univ. Press.

Levin, J. S. 1996a. How prayer heals: A theoretical model. *Altern Ther Health Med* 2 (1): 66-73.

Levin, J. S. 1996b. Religious attendance and psychological well-being in Mexican Americans. *Gerontologist* 36: 454-63.

Levin, J. S., L. M. Chatters, and R. J. Taylor. 1995. Religious effects on health status and life satisfaction among Black Americans. *J Gerontol Sec Sci* 50B: S154-S163.

Levin, J. S., and H. Y. Vanderpool, 1987. Is frequent religious attendance really conducive to better health? Toward an epidemiology of religion. *Soc Sci Med* 24 (7): 589-600.

Lindbeck, G. 1984. *The nature of doctrine: Religion and Theology in a postliberal age.* Philadelphia: Westminster.

MacIntyre, A. 1984. *After virtue: A study in moral theory,* 2nd ed. Notre Dame: Univ. of Notre Dame Press.

MacIntyre, A. 1988. *Whose justice? Which rationality?* Notre Dame: Univ. of Notre Dame Press.

McCullough, M. E., et al. 2000. Religious involvement and mortality: A meta-analytic review. *Health Psychol* 19: 211-22.

Meador, K. G., and S. C. Henson. 2000. Growing old in a therapeutic culture. *Theology Today* 57 (2): 185-202.

Neeleman, J. 1997. Tolerance of suicide. *Psychol Med* 27: 1165-71.

Pargament, K. I. 1997. *The psychology of religion and coping: Theology, research, practice.* New York: Guilford.

Plantinga, A. 1999. *Warranted Christian belief.* Oxford: Oxford Univ. Press.

Polanyi, M. 1964. *Personal knowledge: Towards a post-critical philosophy.* New York: Harper & Row.

Shuman, J. J., and K. G. Meador. 2003. *Heal thyself: Spirituality, medicine, and the distortion of Christianity.* New York: Oxford Univ. Press.

Slater, W., T. W. Hall, and K. J. Edwards. 2001. Measuring religion and spirituality: Where are we and where are we going? *J Psychol Theol* 29 (1): 4-21.

Sloan, R. P., and E. Bagiella. 2002. Claims about religious involvement and health outcomes. *Ann Behav Med* 24 (1): 14-21.

Sloan, R. P., E. Bagiella, and T. Powell. 1999. Religion, spirituality, and medicine. *Lancet* 353 (9153): 664-67.

Sloan, R. P., et al. 2000. Should physicians prescribe religious activities? *N Eng J Med* 342 (25): 1913-16.

Snibbe, A., and H. Markus. 2002. The psychology of religion and the religion of psychology. *Psychol Inquiry* 13 (3): 229-34.

Stark, R., L. R. Iannaccone, and R. Finke. 1996. Religion, science, and rationality. *Am Econ Rev* 86 (2): 433-37.

Strawbridge, W. J., et al. 1997. Frequent attendance at religious services and mortality over 28 years. *Am J Public Health* 87 (6): 957-61.

Strawbridge, W. J., et al. 2001. Religious attendance increases survival by improving and maintaining good health behaviors, mental health, and social relationships. *Ann Behav Med* 23 (1): 68-74.

Swinburne, R. 2001. *Epistemic justification.* Oxford: Clarendon Press.

Taylor, S. E., and L. G. Aspinwall. 1996. Mediating and moderating processes in psycho-social stress: Appraisal, coping, resistance, and vulnerability. In *Psychosocial stress: Perspectives on structure, theory, life-course and methods,* ed. H. G. Kaplan. San Diego: Academic Press.

Underwood, L. G., and J. A. Teresi. 2002. The daily spiritual experience scale: Development, theoretical description, reliability, exploratory factor analysis, and preliminary construct validity using health-related data. *Ann Behav Med* 24 (1): 22-33.

Wittgenstein, L. 1969. *On certainty.* Oxford: Basil Blackwell.

Wolterstorff, N. 1984. *Reason within the bounds of religion,* 2nd ed. Grand Rapids: Wm. B. Eerdmans.

Wolterstorff, N. 2001a. Rethinking the place of the religious voice in the so-called secular university. From Religion in the University: The 2001 Taylor Lectures, presented at the 2001 Yale Divinity School Convocation, New Haven, CT.

Wolterstorff, N. 2001b. Why the traditional view must be rethought. From Religion in the University: The 2001 Taylor Lectures, presented at the 2001 Yale Divinity School Convocation, New Haven, CT.

6 Salvation and Health: Why Medicine Needs the Church

Stanley Hauerwas

A Text and a Story

While it is not unheard of for a theologian to begin an essay with a text from the Scripture, it is relatively rare for those who are addressing issues of medicine to do so. However I begin with a text, as almost everything I have to say is but a commentary on this passage from Job 2:11-13:

> Now when Job's friends heard of all this evil that had come upon him, then came each from his own place, Eliphaz the Temanite, Bildad the Shuhite, and Zophar the Na'amathite. They made an appointment together to come console with him and comfort him. And when they saw him from afar, they did not recognize him; and they raised their voices and wept; and they rent their robes and sprinkled dust upon their heads toward heaven. And they sat with him on the ground seven days and seven nights, and no one spoke a word to him, for they saw that his suffering was very great.

I do not want to comment immediately on the text. Instead, I think it best to begin by telling you a story. The story is about one of my earliest friendships. When I was in my early teens I had a friend, let's call him Bob, who meant everything to me. We made our first hesitant steps toward growing up through sharing the things young boys do — i.e., double dating, athletic activities, and endless discussions on every topic. For two years we were inseparable. I was extremely appreciative of Bob's friendship, as he was not only brighter and more talented than I, but also came from a family that was economically considerably better off than my own. Through Bob I was introduced to a world that otherwise I would hardly know existed. For example, we spent hours in his home playing pool in a room that was built for no other purpose; and we swam in the lake that his house was specifically built to overlook.

Then very early one Sunday morning I received a phone call from Bob requesting that I come to see him immediately. He was sobbing intensely, but through his crying he was able to tell me that they had just found his mother dead. She had committed suicide by placing a shotgun in her mouth. I knew immediately I did not want to go to see him and/or confront a reality like that. I had not yet learned the desperation hidden under our everyday routines and I did not want to learn of it. Moreover I did not want to go because I knew there was nothing I could do or say to make things even appear better than they were. Finally I did not want to go because I did not want to be close to anyone who had been touched by such a tragedy.

But I went. I felt awkward, but I went. And as I came into Bob's room we embraced, a gesture that was almost unheard of between young men raised in the Southwest, and we cried together. After that first period of shared sorrow we somehow calmed down and took a walk. For the rest of the day and that night we stayed together. I do not remember what we said, but I do remember that it was inconsequential. We never talked about his mother or what had happened. We never speculated about why she might do such a thing, even though I could not believe someone who seemed to have such a good life would want to die. We did what we always did. We talked girls, football, cars, movies, and anything else that was inconsequential enough to distract our attention from this horrible event.

As I look on that time I now realize that it was obviously one of the most important events in my life. That it was so is at least partly indicated by how often I have thought about it and tried to understand its significance in the years from then to now. As often as I have reflected on what happened in that short space of time I have also remembered how inept I was in helping Bob. I did not know what should or could be said. I did not know how to help him start sorting out such a horrible event so that he could go on. All I could do was be present.

But time has helped me realize that this is all he wanted — namely, my presence. For as inept as I was, my willingness to be present was a sign that this was not an event so horrible that it drew us away from all other human contact. Life could go on, and in the days to follow we would again swim together, double date, and generally waste time. I now think that at the time God granted me the marvelous privilege of being a presence in the face of profound pain and suffering even when I did not appreciate the significance of being present.

Yet the story cannot end here. For while it is true that Bob and I did go on being friends, nothing was the same. For a few months we continued to see one another often, but somehow the innocent joy of loving one another was gone. We slowly found that our lives were going in different directions and we developed new friends. No doubt the difference between our social and cultural opportunities helps explain to some extent our drifting apart. Bob finally went to Princeton and I went to Southwestern University in Georgetown, Texas.

But that kind of explanation for our growing apart is not sufficient. What was standing between us was that day and night we spent together under the burden of a

---

From *Suffering Presence: Theological Reflections on Medicine, the Mentally Handicapped, and the Church,* by Stanley Hauerwas, pp. 63-83.

profound sadness that neither of us had known could exist until that time. We had shared a pain so intense that for a short period we had become closer than we knew, but now the very pain that created that sharing stood in the way of the development of our friendship. Neither of us wished to recapture that time, nor did we know how to make that night and day part of our ongoing story together. So we went our separate ways. I have no idea what became of Bob, though every once in a while I remember to ask my mother if she has heard about him.

Does medicine need the church? How could this text and this story possibly help us understand that question, much less suggest how it might be answered? Yet I am going to claim in this essay that it does. Put briefly, what I will try to show is that if medicine can be rightly understood as an activity that trains some to know how to be present to those in pain, then something very much like a church is needed to sustain that presence day in and day out. Before I try to develop that thesis, however, I need to do some conceptual groundbreaking to make clear exactly what kind of claim I am trying to make about the relationship of salvation and health, medicine and the church.

Religion and Medicine: Is There or Should There Be a Relation?

It is a well-known fact that for most of human history there has been a close affinity between religion and medicine. Indeed that very way of putting it is misleading, since to claim a relation suggests that they were distinguished, and often that has not been the case. From earliest times, disease and illness were not seen as matters having no religious import but rather as resulting from the disfavor of God. As Darrel Amundsen and Gary Ferngren have recently reminded us, the Hebrew scriptures often depict God promising

> health and prosperity for the covenant people if they are faithful to him, and disease and other suffering if they spurn his love. This promise runs through the Old Testament. "If you will diligently hearken to the voice of the Lord your God, and do that which is right in his eyes, and give heed to his commandments and keep all his statutes, I will put none of the diseases upon you which I put upon the Egyptians; for I am the Lord, your healer" (Exod. 15:26). ([2], p. 92)

This view of illness was not associated only with the community as a whole, but with individuals. Thus in Psalm 38 the lament is

> There is no soundness in my flesh because of thy indignation; there is no health in my bones because of my sin. . . . My wounds grow foul and fester because of foolishness. . . . I am utterly spent and crushed; I groan because of the tumult of my heart. . . . Do not forsake me, O Lord! O my God, be not far from me! Make haste to help me, O Lord, my salvation! (vv. 3, 5, 8, 21-22)

Amundsen and Ferngren point out this view of illness as accompanied by the assumption that acknowledgment of and repentance for our sin was essential for our healing. Thus in Psalm 32:

> When I declared not my sin, my body wasted away through my groaning all day long. For day and night thy hand was heavy upon me; my strength was dried up. . . . I acknowledged my sin to thee, and I did not hide my iniquity; I said, "I will confess my transgressions to the Lord"; then thou didst forgive the guilt of my sin (vv. 3-5). ([2], p. 93)

Since illness and sin were closely connected it is not surprising that healing was also closely associated with religious practices — or, put more accurately, healing was a religious discipline. Indeed Amundsen and Ferngren make the interesting point that since the most important issue was a person's relationship with God the chief means of healing was naturally prayer. That clearly precluded magic and thus the Mosaic code excluded soothsayers, augurs, sorcerers, charmers, wizards, and other such figures who offered a means to control or avoid the primary issue of their relation to Yahweh ([2], p. 94). They also suggest that this may have been why no sacerdotal medical practice developed in Israel particularly associated with the priesthood. Rather, the pattern of the Exodus tended to prevail, with illness and healing more closely associated with prophetic activity.

The early Christian community seems to have done little to change these basic presuppositions. If anything it simply intensified them by adding what Amundsen and Ferngren call the "central paradox" in the New Testament:

> Strength comes only through weakness. This strength is Christ's strength that comes only through dependence upon him. In the Gospel of John, Christ says: "I have said to you, that in me you may have peace. In the world you have tribulation; but be of good cheer, I have overcome the world" (16:33). "In the world you have tribulation." It is simply to be expected and accepted. But for the New Testament Christian no suffering is meaningless. The ultimate purpose and meaning behind Christian suffering in the New Testament is spiritual maturity. And the ultimate goal in spiritual maturity is a close dependence upon Christ based upon a childlike trust. ([2], p. 96)

Thus illness is seen as an opportunity for growth in faith and trust in God.

Because of this way of viewing both the positive and negative effect of illness, Amundsen and Ferngren note that there has always been a degree of tension in the way Christians understand the relation between theology and secular medicine, between the medicine of the soul and the medicine of the body.

> According to one view, if God sends disease either to punish or to test a person, it is to God that one must turn for care and healing. If God is both the source and

> healer of a person's ills, the use of human medicine would circumvent the spiritual framework by resorting to worldly wisdom. On another view, if God is the source of disease, or if God permits disease and is the ultimate healer, God's will can be fulfilled through human agents, who with divine help have acquired the ability to aid in the curative process. Most Christians have asserted that the human agent of care, the physician, is an instrument of God, used by God in bringing succor to humankind. But in every age some have maintained that any use of human medicine is a manifestation of a lack of faith. This ambivalence in the Christian attitude, among both theologians and laity, has always been present to some degree. ([2], p. 96)

Nor is it possible to separate or distinguish religion and medicine on the basis of a distinction between soul and body. For as Paul Ramsey has reminded us, Christians affirm that God has created and holds us sacred as embodied souls ([14], p. xiii). Religion does not deal with the soul and medicine with the body. Practitioners of both are too well aware of the inseparability of soul and body — or perhaps better, they know the abstractness of both categories. Moreover when religion too easily legitimates the independence of medical care by limiting medicine to mechanical understanding and care of the body, it has the result of making religious convictions ethereal in character. It may be that just to the extent Christianity is always tempted in Gnostic and Manichean directions it accepts too willingly a technological understanding of medicine. Christians, if they are to be faithful to their convictions, may not ever be able to avoid at least potential conflict between their own assumptions about illness and health and how the ill should be cared for and the assumptions of medicine. One hopes for cooperation, of course, but structurally the possibility of conflict between church and medicine cannot be excluded, since both entail convictions and practices concerned with that same subject.

Put differently, given Judaism and Christianity's understanding of humankind's relation with God — that is: how we understand salvation — health can never be thought of as an autonomous sphere. Moreover, insofar as medicine is a specialized activity distinguished from religious convictions, you cannot exclude the possibility that there may well be conflict between religion and medicine. For in many ways the latter is constantly tempted to offer a form of salvation that religiously may come close to idolatry. The ability of modern medicine to cure is at once a benefit and potential pitfall. Too often it is tempted to increase its power by offering more than care, by offering in fact alleviation from the human condition — e.g., the development of artificial hearts. That is not the fault of medical practitioners, though often they encourage such idolatry; rather the fault lies with those of us who pretentiously place undue expectations on medicine in the hope of finding an earthly remedy to our death. But we can never forget that the relation between medicine and health, and especially the health of a population, is as ambiguous as the relation between the church and salvation.

In the hope of securing peace between medicine and religion, two quite different and equally unsatisfactory proposals have been suggested. The first advocates a strong division of labor between medicine and religion by limiting the scope of medicine to the mechanism of our body. While it is certainly true that medicine in a unique way entails the passing on of the wisdom of the body from one generation to another, there is no way that medical care can be limited to the body and be good medicine [10]. As Ramsey has reminded us again and again, the moral commitment of the physician is not to treat diseases, or populations, or the human race, but the immediate patient before him or her ([14], pp. 36, 59). Religiously, therefore, the care offered by physicians cannot be abstracted from the moral commitment to care based on our view that every aspect of our existence is dependent upon God.

By the same token the clergy, no less than physicians, are concerned about the patient's physical well-being. No assumptions about technical skills and knowledge can legitimate the clergy retreating into the realm of the spiritual in order to claim some continued usefulness and status. Such a retreat is as unfaithful as abandoning the natural world to the physicist on the grounds that God is a God of history and not of nature. For the church and its officeholders to abandon claims over the body in the name of a lack of expertise is equivalent to reducing God to the gaps in scientific theory. Such a strategy is not only bad faith but it results in making religious convictions appear at best irrelevant and at worse foolish.

The second alternative to accepting the autonomy of medicine from our religious convictions seeks to maintain a close relationship by resacralizing medical care. Medicine requires a "holistic vision of man" ([7], p. 9), because the care it brings is but one aspect of salvation. Thus the church and its theology serve medical care by promoting a holistic view of man, one that can provide a

> comprehensive understanding of human health [that] includes the greatest possible harmony of all man's forces and energies, the greatest possible spiritualization of man's bodily aspects and the finest embodiment of the spiritual. True health is revealed in the self-actualization of the person who has attained that freedom which marshals all available energies for the fulfillment of his total human vocation. ([7], p. 154)

Such a view of health, however, cannot help but pervert the kind of care that physicians can provide. Physicians rightly maintain that their skill primarily has to do with the body, as medicine promises us health, not happiness. When such a general understanding of health is made the goal of medicine, it only results in making medical care promise more than it can deliver. As a result, we are tyrannized by the agents of medicine because we have voluntarily vested them with too much power. It is already a difficult task in our society to control the expectations people have about modern medicine; we only compound that problem by providing religious legitimacy to this overblown understanding of health. Certainly we believe that any account of salvation includes questions of our health, but that does not mean that medicine can or ever should become the agency of salvation. It may be a fundamental judgment on the church's failure to help us locate wherein our salvation lies that so many today seek a salvation through medicine.

Can Medical Ethics Be Christian?

The already complex question of the relation between religion and medicine only becomes more confusing when we turn our attention to more recent developments in medical ethics. For even though religious thinkers have been at the forefront of much of the work done in the expanding field of "medical ethics," it is not clear that they have been there as religious thinkers. Joseph Fletcher [5], Paul Ramsey [13], James Gustafson [6], Charles Curran [4], and Jim Childress [3], to name just a few, have done extensive work in medical ethics, but often it is hard to tell how their religious convictions have made a difference for the methodology they employ or for their response to specific quandaries. Indeed it is interesting to note how seldom they raise issues of the meaning or relation of salvation and health, as they seem to prefer dealing with questions of death and dying, truth-telling, etc.

By calling attention to this fact by no means do I wish to disparage the kind of reflection that has been done concerning these issues. We have all benefited from their careful analysis and distinctions concerning such problems. Yet one must wonder if, by letting the agenda be set in such a manner, we have already lost the theological ball game. For the very concentration on "issues" and "quandaries" as central for medical ethics tends to underwrite the practice of medicine as we know it, rather than challenging some of the basic presuppositions of medical practice and care. Because of this failure to raise more fundamental questions, concerns that might provide more access for our theological claims are simply never considered.

There are at least two reasons for this that I think are worth mentioning. The first has to do with the character of theological ethics itself. We tend to forget that the development of "Christian ethics" is a relatively new development [8]. It has only been in the last hundred years that some have styled themselves as "ethicists" rather than simply theologians. It is by no means clear that we know how to indicate what difference it makes conceptually and methodologically to claim our ethics as Christian in distinction from other kinds of ethical reflection. In the hopes of securing great clarity about their own work many who have identified their work as Christian have nonetheless assumed that the meaning and method of "ethics" was determined fundamentally by non-Christian sources. In a sense the very concentration on "medical ethics" was a godsend for many "religious ethicists," as it seemed to provide a coherent activity without having to deal with the fundamental issue of what makes Christian ethics Christian.

This can be illustrated by attending to the debate among Christian ethicists concerning whether Christian moral reasoning is primarily deontological or consequential. This debate has been particularly important for medical ethics, as obviously how you think about nontherapeutic experimentation, truth-telling, transplants, and a host of other issues seems to turn on this issue. For instance, Joseph Fletcher, who wrote one of the first books by a Protestant in medical ethics, has always argued in favor of a consequential stance, thus qualifying the physician's commitment to an individual patient in the name of a greater good [5]. In contrast, Paul Ramsey has emphasized that the "covenant" of the physician with the patient is such that no amount of good to be done should override that commitment [14].

It is interesting to note how each makes theological appeals to support his own position. Fletcher appeals to love as his basic norm, interpreting it in terms of the greatest good for the greatest number, but it remains unclear how his sense of love is theologically warranted or controlled. Ramsey provides a stronger theological case for his emphasis on "covenant" as a central theological motif, but it is not clear how the many "covenants of life with life into which we are born" require the covenant of God with a particular people we find in Scripture. Ramsey's use of covenant language thus underwrites a natural law ethic whose status is unclear both from a theological and/or philosophical perspective.[1]

What is interesting about the debate between Fletcher and Ramsey is that it could have been carried on completely separate from the theological premises that each side claimed were involved. For the terms of the debate — *consequential* and *deontological* — are basically borrowed from philosophical contexts and are dependent on the presuppositions of certain philosophical traditions. Of course that in itself does not mean that such issues and concepts are irrelevant to our work as theologians, but what is missing is any sense of how the issue as presented grows, is dependent on, or informed by our distinctive commitments as theologians.

The question of the nature of theological ethics and its relation to the development of ethical reflection in and about medicine is further complicated by our current cultural situation. As Ramsey has pointed out, we are currently trying to do the impossible — namely, "build a

1. Ramsey's position is complex and I certainly cannot do it justice here. His emphasis on "love transforming natural law" would tend to qualify the point made above. Yet it is also true that Ramsey's increasing use of covenant language has gone hand in hand with his readiness to identify certain "covenants" that need no "transformation." Of course he could object that the covenant between doctor and patient is the result of Christian love operating in history.

civilization without an agreed civil tradition and [in] the absence of a moral consensus" ([13], p. 15). This makes the practice of medicine even more morally challenging, since it is by no means clear how one can sustain a non-arbitrary medicine in a genuinely morally pluralistic society. For example, much of the debate about when someone is "really" dead is not simply the result of our increased technological power to keep blood flowing through our bodies, but witnesses to our culture's lack of consensus as to what constitutes a well-lived life and the correlative sense of a good death. In the absence of such a consensus our only recourse is to resort to claims and counterclaims about "right to life" and "right to die," with the result of the further impoverishment of our moral language and vision. Moreover, the only way to create a "safe" medicine under such conditions is to expect physicians to treat us as if death is the ultimate enemy to be put off by every means. Then we blame physicians for keeping us alive beyond all reason, but fail to note that if they did not we would not know how to distinguish them from murderers.

Alasdair MacIntyre has raised this sort of issue directly in his "Can Medicine Dispense with a Theological Perspective on Human Nature?" Rather than calling attention to what has become problematic for physicians and surgeons — issues such as when it is appropriate to let someone die — he says he wants to direct our attention to what is still taken for granted, "namely, the unconditional and absolute character of certain of the doctor's obligations to his patients" ([12], p. 120). The difficulty is that modern philosophy, according to MacIntyre, has been unable to offer a persuasive account of such an obligation.

> *Either* they distort and misrepresent it *or* they render it unintelligible. Teleological moralists characteristically end up by distorting and misrepresenting. For they begin with a notion of moral rules as specifying how we are to behave if we are to achieve certain ends, perhaps *the* end for man, the *summum bonum.* If I break such rules I shall fail to achieve some human good and will thereby be frustrated and impoverished. ([12], p. 122)

But MacIntyre notes that this treats moral failure as if it is an educational failure and lacks the profound guilt that should accompany moral failure. More importantly, such an account fails entirely to account for the positive evil we know certain people clearly pursue.

Moral philosophers who tend to preserve the unconditional and absolute character of the central requirements of morality, however, inevitably make those "oughts" appear as if they are arbitrary. What they cannot do is show how those oughts are rationally entailed by an account of man's true end. Kant was only able to do so because he continued the presupposition (which he failed to justify within his own philosophical position) that "the life of the individual and also of that of the human race is a journey toward a goal" ([12], p. 127). Once that presupposition is lost, however, and MacIntyre believes that it has been lost in our culture, then we lack the resources to maintain exactly those moral presuppositions that seem essential to securing the moral integrity of medicine.

Such a situation seems ripe for a theological response, since it might at least be suggested that it thus becomes our task as theologians to serve our culture in general and medicine in particular by supplying the needed rationale. Yet, MacIntyre argues, such a strategy is doomed, since the very intelligibility of theological claims has been rendered problematic by the ethos of modernity. Therefore, just to the extent theologians try to make their claims in terms offered by modernity, they only underwrite the assumption that theological language cannot be meaningful.

This kind of dilemma is particularly acute when it comes to medicine. For if the theologian attempts to underwrite the medical ethos drawing on the particular convictions of Christians, just to the extent those convictions are particular they will serve only to emphasize society's lack of a common morality. Thus theologians, in the interest of cultural consensus, often try to downplay the distinctiveness of their theological convictions in the interest of societal harmony. But in the process we only reinforce the assumption on the part of many that theological claims make little difference for how medicine itself is understood or how various issues are approached. At best theology or religion is left with justifying a concern with the "whole patient," but it is not even clear how that concern depends on or derives from any substantive theological conviction that is distinguishable from humanism.

Almost as if we have sense that there is no way to resolve this dilemma, theologians and religious professionals involved in medicine have tended to associate with the patients' rights movement. At least one of the ways of resolving our cultural dilemma is to protect the patient from medicine by restoring the patient's autonomy over against the physician. While I certainly do not want to underestimate the importance of patients recovering a sense of medicine as an activity in which we play as important a role as the physician, the emphasis on the patient's rights over against the physician cannot resolve our difficulty. It is but an attempt to substitute procedural safeguards for what only substantive convictions can supply. As a result our attention is distracted from the genuine challenge we confront for the forming of an ethos sufficient to sustain a practice of medicine that is morally worthy.

Pain, Loneliness, and Being Present: The Church and the Care of the Ill

I can offer no "solution" to the issues raised in the previous section, as I think they admit of no solution, given our social and political situation. Moreover, I think we will make little headway on such matters as long as we try to address the questions in terms of the dichotomies of religion and medicine or the relation between medical ethics and theology. Rather, what is needed is a restatement of the issue. In this section I will try to do that by returning to my original text and story to suggest how they may help remind us that more fundamental than questions of religion and morality is the question of the kind of community necessary to sustain the long-term care of the ill.

Indeed, part of the problem with discussing the question of "relation" in such general terms as "medicine" and "religion" is that each of those terms in its own way distorts the character of what it is meant to describe. For example, when we talk in general about "religion" rather than a specific set of beliefs, behaviors, and habits embodied by a distinct group of people, our account always tends to be reductionistic. It makes it appear that underlying what people actually believe and do is a deeper reality called "religion." It is as if we can talk about God abstracted from how a people have learned to pray to that God. In like manner we often tend to oversimplify the nature of medicine by trying to capture the many activities covered by that term in a definition or ideological system. What doctors do is often quite different from what they say they do.

Moreover, the question of the relation of theology to medical ethics is far too abstract. For when the issue is posed in that manner it makes it appear that religion is primarily a set of beliefs, a world view, that may or may not have implications for how we understand and respond to certain kinds of ethical dilemmas. While it is certainly true that Christianity involves beliefs, the character of those beliefs cannot be understood apart from its place in the formation of a community with cultic practices. By focusing on this fact I hope to throw a different perspective on how those who are called to care for the sick can draw upon and count on the particular kind of community we call the church.

I do not intend, for example, to argue that medicine must be reclaimed as in some decisive way dependent on theology. Nor do I want to argue that the development of "medical ethics" will ultimately require the acknowledgment of, or recourse to, theological presuppositions. Rather all I want to try to show is why, given the particular demands put on those who care for the ill, something very much like a church is necessary to sustain that care.

To develop this point I want to call attention to an obvious but often overlooked aspect of illness — namely, that when we are sick we hurt and are in pain. I realize that often we are sick and yet not in pain — e.g., hardening of the arteries — but that does not ultimately defeat my general point, since we know that such an illness will lead to physical and mental pain. Nor am I particularly bothered by the observation that many pains are "psychological," having no real physiological basis. Physicians are right to insist that people who say they have pain, even if no organic basis can be found for such pain, are, in fact, in pain, though they may be mistaken about what kind of pain it is.

Moreover I am well aware that there are many different kinds of pain, as well as intensity of pains. What is only a minor hurt for me may be a major trauma for someone else. Pain comes in many shapes and sizes, and it is never possible to separate the psychological aspects of pain from the organic. For example, suffering, which is not the same as pain since we can suffer without being in pain, is nonetheless akin to pain inasmuch as it is a felt deficiency that can make us as miserable as pain itself.[2]

Yet given these qualifications it remains true that there is a strong connection between pain and illness, an area of our lives in which it is appropriate to call upon the skills of a physician. When we are in pain we want to be helped. But it is exactly at this point that one of the strangest aspects of our being in pain occurs — namely, it is impossible for us to experience one another's pain. That does not mean we cannot communicate to one another our pain. That we can do, but what cannot be done is for you to understand and/or experience my pain as mine.

This puts us under a double burden because we have enough of a problem learning to know one another in the normal aspects of our lives, but when we are in pain our alienation from one another only increases. For no matter how sympathetic we may be to the other in pain, that very pain creates a history and experience that makes the other just that much more foreign to me. Our pains isolate us from one another as they create worlds that cut us off from one another. Consider, for example, the immense gulf between the world of the sick and the healthy. No matter how much we may experience the former, when we are healthy or not in pain we have trouble imagining and understanding the world of the ill.

Indeed the terms we are using are still far too crude. For we do not suffer illness in and of itself, but we suffer this particular kind of illness and have this particular kind of pain. Thus even within the world of illness there are subworlds that are not easily crossed. Think, for example, of how important it is for those suffering from the same illness to share their stories with one another. They do not believe others can understand their particular kind of pain. People with heart disease may find little basis of communion with those suffering from cancer. Pain itself does not create a shared experience; only pain from a particular kind and sort. Moreover the very commonality thus created separates the ill from the healthy in a decisive way.

Pain not only isolates us from one another, but even from ourselves. Think how quickly people with a terribly diseased limb or organ are anxious for surgery in the hope that if it is just cut off or cut out they will not be burdened by the pain that makes them not know themselves. This gangrenous leg is not mine. I would prefer to lose the leg rather than face the reality of its connection to me.

2. For a fuller account of the complex relation between pain and suffering see [11].

The difficulties pain creates in terms of our relation with ourselves is compounded by the peculiar difficulties it creates for those close to us who do not share our pain. For no matter how sympathetic they may be, no matter how much they may try to be with and comfort us, we know they do not want to experience our pain. I not only cannot, but I do not want to, know the pain you are feeling. No matter how good willed we may be, we cannot take anther's pain as our pain. Our pains divide us and there is little we can do to restore our unity.

I suspect this is one of the reasons that chronic illness is such a burden. For often we are willing to be present and sympathetic with someone with an intense but temporary pain — that is, we are willing to be present as long as they work at being "good" sick people who try to get well quickly and do not make too much of their discomfort. We may initially be quite sympathetic with someone with a chronic disease, but it seems to be asking too much of us to be compassionate year in and year out. Thus the universal testimony of people with chronic illness is that their illness often results in the alienation of their former friends. This is a problem not only for the person who is ill but also for those closely connected with that person. The family of a person who is chronically ill often discover that the very skills and habits they must learn to be present to the one in pain creates a gulf between themselves and their friends. Perhaps no case illustrates this more poignantly than a family that has a retarded child. Often they discover it is not long before they have a whole new set of friends who also happen to have retarded children [9].

Exactly because pain is so alienating, we are hesitant to admit that we are in pain. To be in pain means we need help, that we are vulnerable to the interests of others, that we are not in control of our destiny. Thus we seek to deny our pain in the hope that we will be able to handle it within ourselves. But the attempt to deal with our pain by ourselves or to deny its existence has the odd effect of only increasing our loneliness. For exactly to the extent I am successful, I create a story about myself that I cannot easily share.

No doubt more can be and needs to be said that would nuance this account of pain and the way it tends to isolate us from one another. Yet I think I have said enough that our attention has been called to this quite common but all the more extraordinary aspect of our existence. Moreover, in the light of this analysis I hope we can now appreciate the remarkable behavior of Job's friends. For in spite of the bad press Job's comforters usually receive (and in many ways it is deserved!), they at least sat on the ground with him for seven days. Moreover they did not speak to him, "for they saw that his suffering was very great." That they did so is truly an act of magnanimity, for most of us are willing to be with sufferers, especially those in such pain that we can hardly recognize them, only if we can "do something" to relieve their suffering or at least distract their attention. Not so with Job's comforters. They sat on the ground with Job doing nothing more than being willing to be present in the face of his suffering.

Now if any of this is close to being right, it puts the task of physicians and others who are pledged to be with the ill in an interesting perspective. For I take it that their activity as physicians is characterized by the fundamental commitment to be, like Job's comforters, in the presence of those in pain.[3] At this moment I am not concerned to explore the moral reason for that commitment, but only to note that in fact physicians, nurses, chaplains, and many others are present to the ill as none of the rest of us are. They are the bridge between the world of the ill and the healthy.

Certainly physicians are there because they have been trained with skills that enable them to alleviate the pain of the ill. They have learned from sick people how to help other sick people. Yet every physician soon learns of the terrible limit of his/her craft, for the sheer particularity of the patient's illness often defies the best knowledge and skill. Even more dramatically, physicians learn that using the best knowledge and skill they have on some patients sometimes has terrible results.

Yet the fact that medicine through the agency of physicians does not and cannot always "cure" in no way qualifies the commitment of the physician. At least it does not do so if we remember that the physician's basic pledge is not to cure, but to care through being present to the one in pain. Yet it is not easy to carry out that commitment on a day-to-day, year-to-year basis. For none of us have the resources to see too much pain without the pain hardening us. Without such a hardening, something we sometimes call by the name of professional distance, we fear we will lose the ability to feel at all.

Yet the physician cannot help but be touched and, thus, tainted by the world of the sick. Through their willingness to be present to us in our most vulnerable moments they are forever scarred with our pain — a pain that we the healthy want to deny or at least keep at arm's length. They have seen a world we do not want to see until it is forced on us, and we will accept them into polite community only to the extent they keep that world hidden from us. But when we are driven into that world we want to be able to count on their skill and their presence, even though we have been unwilling to face that reality while we were healthy.

But what do these somewhat random and controversial observations have to do with helping us better understand the relation between medicine and the church and/or the story of my boyhood friendship with Bob? To begin with the latter, I think in some ways the mechanism that was working during that trying time with Bob is quite similar to the mechanism that works on a day-to-day basis in medicine. For the physician, and others concerned with our illness, are called to be present during times of great pain and tragedy. Indeed physicians, be-

3. I am indebted to a conversation with Dr. Earl Shelp for helping me understand better the significance of this point.

cause of their moral commitments, have the privilege and the burden to be with us when we are most vulnerable. The physician learns our deepest fears and our profoundest hopes. As patients, that is also why so often we fear the physician, because she/he may know us better than we know ourselves. Surely that is one of the reasons that confidentiality is so crucial to the patient-physician relation, since it is a situation of such intimacy.

But just to the extent that the physician has been granted the privilege of being with us while we are in pain, that very experience creates the seeds of distrust and fear. We are afraid of one another's use of the knowledge gained, but even more deeply we fear remembering the pain as part of our history. Thus every crisis that joins us in a common fight for health also has the potential for separating us more profoundly after the crisis. Yet the physician is pledged to come to our aid again and again, no matter how we may try to protect ourselves from his/her presence.

The physician, on the other hand, has yet another problem, for how can anyone be present to the ill day in and day out without learning to dislike, if not positively detest, our smallness in the face of pain. People in pain are omnivorous in their appetite for help, and they will use us up if we let them. Fortunately the physician has other patients who can give him distance from any patient who requires too much. But the problem still remains how morally those who are pledged to be with the ill never lose their ability to see the humanity that our very suffering often comes close to obliterating. For the physician cannot, as Bob and I did, drift apart and away from those whom he or she is pledged to serve. At least they cannot if I am right that medicine is first of all pledged to be nothing more than a human presence in the face of suffering.

But how can we account for such a commitment — the commitment to be present to those in pain? No doubt basic human sympathy is not to be discounted, but it does not seem to be sufficient to account for a group of people dedicated to being present to the ill as their vocation in life. Nor does it seem sufficient to account for the acquiring of the skills necessary to sustain that presence in a manner that is not alienating and the source of distrust in a community.

To learn how to be present in that way we need examples — that is, a people who have so learned to embody such a presence in their lives that it has become the marrow of their habits. The church at least claims to be such a community, as it is a group of people called out by a God who, we believe, is always present to us, both in our sin and our faithfulness. Because of God's faithfulness we are supposed to be a people who have learned how to be faithful to one another by our willingness to be present, with all our vulnerabilities, to one another. For what does our God require of us other than our unfailing presence in the midst of the world's sin and pain? Thus our willingness to be ill and to ask for help, as well as our willingness to be present with the ill, is no special or extraordinary activity, but a form of the Christian obligation to be present to one another in and out of pain.

Moreover, it is such a people who should have learned how to be present with those in pain without that pain driving them further apart. For the very bond that pain forms between us becomes the basis for alienation, as we have no means to know how to make it part of our common history. Just as it is painful to remember our sins, so we seek not to remember our pain, since we desire to live as if our world and existence were a pain-free one. Only a people trained in remembering, and remembering as a communal act, their sins and pains can offer a paradigm for sustaining across time a painful memory so that it acts to heal rather than to divide.

Thus medicine needs the church not to supply a foundation for its moral commitments, but rather as a resource of the habits and practices necessary to sustain the care of those in pain over the long haul. For it is no easy matter to be with the ill, especially when we cannot do much for them other than simply be present. Our very helplessness too often turns to hate, both toward the one in pain and ourselves, as we despise them for reminding us of our helplessness. Only when we remember that our presence is our doing, when sitting on the ground seven days saying nothing is what we can do, can we be saved from our fevered and hopeless attempt to control others' and our own existence. Of course to believe that such presence is what we can and should do entails a belief in a presence in and beyond this world. And it is certainly true many today no longer believe in or experience such a presence. If that is the case, then I do wonder if medicine as an activity of presence is possible in a world without God.

Another way of raising this issue is to ask the relation between prayer and medical care. Nothing I have said about the basic pledge of physicians to be present to the ill entails that they should not try to develop the skills necessary to help those in pain and illness. Certainly they should, as theirs is an art that is one of our most valuable resources for the care of one another. But no matter how powerful that craft becomes, it cannot in principle rule out the necessity of prayer. For prayer is not a supplement to the insufficiency of our medical knowledge and practice; nor is it some divine insurance policy that our medical skill will work; rather, our prayer is the means that we have to make God present whether our medical skill is successful or not. So understood, the issue is not whether medical care and prayer are antithetical, but how medical care can ever be sustained without the necessity of continued prayer.

Finally, those involved in medicine need the church as otherwise they cannot help but be alienated from the rest of us. For unless there is a body of people who have learned the skills of presence, the world of the ill cannot help but become a separate world both for the ill and/or those who care for them. Only a community that is pledged not to fear the stranger — and illness always makes us a stranger to ourselves and others — can welcome the continued presence of the ill in our midst. The hospital is, after all, first and foremost a house of hospitality along the way of our journey with finitude. It is our sign that we will not abandon those who have become ill simply because they currently are suffering the sign of that finitude. If the hospital, as too often is the case today, becomes but a means of isolating the ill from the rest of us, then we have betrayed its central purpose and distorted our community and ourselves.

If the church can be the kind of people who show clearly that they have learned to be with the sick and the dying, it may just be that through that process we will better understand the relation of salvation to health, religion to medicine. Or perhaps even more, we will better understand what kind of medicine we ought to practice, since too often we try to substitute doing for presence. It is surely the case, as Paul Ramsey reminds us, "that not since Socrates posed the question have we learned how to teach virtue. The quandaries of medical ethics are not unlike that question. Still, we can no longer rely upon the ethical assumptions in our culture to be powerful enough or clear enough to instruct the profession in virtue; therefore the medical profession should no longer believe that the personal integrity of physicians alone is enough; neither can anyone count on values being transmitted without thought" ([14], p. xviii). All I have tried to do is remind us that neither can we count on such values being transmitted without a group of people who believe in and live trusting in God's unfailing presence.

References

[1] Amundsen, D., and Ferngren, G. 1982. "Medicine and Religion: Pre-Christian Antiquity." In M. Marty and K. Vaux, eds., *Health/Medicine and the Faith Traditions,* pp. 53-92. Philadelphia: Fortress Press.

[2] Amundsen, D., and Ferngren, G. 1982. "Medicine and Religion: Early Christianity Through the Middle Ages." In M. Marty and K. Vaux, eds., *Health/Medicine and the Faith Traditions,* pp. 93-132.

[3] Childress, J. 1981. *Priorities in Biomedical Ethics.* Philadelphia: Westminster Press.

[4] Curran, C. 1978. *Issues in Sexual and Medical Ethics.* Notre Dame, Ind.: University of Notre Dame Press.

[5] Fletcher, J. 1954. *Morals and Medicine.* Boston: Beacon Press.

[6] Gustafson, J. 1975. *The Contributions of Theology to Medical Ethics.* Milwaukee: Marquette University Press.

[7] Haring, B. 1973. *Medical Ethics.* South Bend, Ind.: Fides Publishers.

[8] Hauerwas, S. 1983. "On Keeping Theological Ethics Theological." In A. MacIntyre and S. Hauerwas, eds., *Revisions: Changing Perspectives in Moral Philosophy,* pp. 16-42. Notre Dame, Ind.: University of Notre Dame Press.

[9] Hauerwas, S. 1982. "The Retarded, Society and the Family: The Dilemma of Care." In S. Hauerwas, ed., *Responsibility for Devalued Persons.* Springfield, Ill.: Charles C. Thomas.

[10] Hauerwas, S. 1982. "Authority and the Profession of Medicine," In G. Agich, *Responsibility in Health Care,* pp. 83-104. Dordrecht, Holland: Reidel.

[11] Hauerwas, S. 1979. "Reflections on Suffering, Death, and Medicine," *Ethics in Science and Medicine* 6:229-37.

[12] MacIntyre, A. 1981. "Can Medicine Dispense with a Theological Perspective on Human Nature?" In D. Callahan and H. Englehardt, eds., *The Roots of Ethics,* pp. 119-38. New York: Plenum Press.

[13] Ramsey, P. 1973. "The Nature of Medical Ethics." In R. Neatch, M. Gaylin, and C. Morgan, eds., *The Teaching of Medical Ethics,* pp. 14-28. Hastings-on-Hudson, N.Y.: Hastings Center.

[14] Ramsey, P. 1970. *The Patient as Person.* New Haven: Yale University Press.

CHAPTER TWO

Theology and Medical Ethics

Chapter One makes clear that medicine and religion have a long and intertwined, if complicated and recently contested, relationship. It should come as no surprise, therefore, that the relationship between the second-order discourses — theology and medical ethics — is equally long, intertwined, complicated, and contested. Chapter Two explores this relationship, providing some historical background and focusing on the question of method: How ought (or ought not) one engage in theological reflection on medicine? What fundamental dynamics shape the interaction between theology and contemporary medical ethics? What role might race, gender, class, and social location play in how one participates in this interaction?

First, a bit of background: the discipline that we now know as "medical ethics" or bioethics began to emerge in the late 1960s. Yet this hardly marks the beginning of moral reflection on medicine. For almost two millennia, a lively and substantive discussion on the obligations of physicians and patients, on caring for the sick, and on the meaning of life and death was carried on within the Roman Catholic and Jewish traditions, as well as within the profession of medicine itself.[1] Catholicism also boasted a two-millennia-long practice of care for the sick, sustained by a broad infrastructure of institutions; it was joined in this work in the nineteenth and twentieth centuries by various Protestant traditions, including the Methodists, Lutherans, Anabaptists, and Adventists.

Thus, when a variety of cultural factors began to converge in the 1960s, it is not surprising that theologians — Roman Catholic, Jewish, and Protestant — were among the first to join physicians and scientists in examining the moral dimensions of human subjects research, organ donation, genetics, the personhood of the patient, and more. So significant a role did theologians play that LeRoy Walters speaks of "Religion and the Renaissance of Medical Ethics."[2] Lisa Sowle Cahill (selection 8) names the major theological figures in this renaissance and gives a succinct summary of this history.

After the "renaissance," however, came the "enlightenment" of medical ethics, and the role of theology in the nascent field of medical ethics quickly became contested. As the new questions and cases of medical ethics moved from the scholarly community to the courtroom and the realm of public policy in the early 1970s, philosophers argued that the language of bioethics must be the language of the public sphere, accessible to anyone in a pluralistic culture. Case law and public policy could not be based on reasons rooted in particular religious traditions, it was argued; a secular language was needed.

The culminating point in this process of secularization can be marked with the publication of the *Belmont Report*. Issued in 1979 by the National Commission for the Protection of Human Subjects, the *Belmont Report* sought to articulate an ethic of universal principles designed to guide the conduct of research with human subjects. These principles — respect for persons, beneficence, and justice — were taken to transcend particular communities and specific religious identities. They were principles with which all rational people of goodwill the world over could agree. They were principles that could secure agreement among diverse perspectives in a pluralistic democratic culture.

Although the principles of respect for persons, beneficence, and justice were developed in the context of the oversight of human subjects' research, they immediately became the privileged ethic for the growing field of bioethics. For 1979 also saw the publication of what quickly became the defining textbook in the field of bioethics, Tom Beauchamp and James Childress's *The Principles of Biomedical Ethics*.[3] Here the principles of *Belmont* (slightly modified to comprise four principles, respect for autonomy, beneficence, nonmaleficence, and justice)

1. For good, succinct accounts of this history see Edmund D. Pellegrino, "The Metamorphosis of Medical Ethics: A Thirty-Year Retrospective," *Journal of the American Medical Association* 269, no. 9 (March 3, 1993): 1158-62; and LeRoy Walters, "Religion and the Renaissance of Medical Ethics in the United States: 1965-1975," in *Theology and Bioethics*, ed. Earl E. Shelp (Dordrecht: D. Reidel, 1985), pp. 3-16.

2. Walters, cited in note 1 above.

3. Tom Beauchamp and James Childress, *The Principles of Biomedical Ethics* (New York: Oxford University Press, 1979).

were transferred from the context of experimentation to the clinical setting.[4]

A number of histories of bioethics have been written since the mid-1990s. One of the most important accounts of this history, especially for those interested in the relationship between theology and medical ethics, is John Evans's *Playing God? Human Genetic Engineering and the Rationalization of Public Bioethical Debate.*[5] Bringing the eye of a sociologist to the topic, he documents the declining fortune of religious voices in bioethics through the 1970s and 1980s. But more importantly, he offers a compelling sociological account of the Weberian dynamics at play in the rise of bioethics. Rejecting the thesis on pluralistic democracy, he demonstrates how the principles of bioethics are particularly suited to a bureaucratic form of society, one in which substantive rationality gives way to formal instrumental rationality embedded in a legal framework as the dominant method for the distribution of power. For Weber, such a system is efficient, yet traps individuals within the iron cage of rational control. The controlling function of bioethics is difficult to notice, given the rhetoric of freedom captured in the hallmark principle of autonomy. Evans's book is recommended background reading for anyone interested in these questions.[6]

Evans plots these developments with the aid of hindsight. Yet some recognized the shift as it unfolded. In his classic piece from 1978, "Theology Confronts Technology and the Life Sciences" (selection 7), James Gustafson lays the blame for the marginalization of theology squarely at the feet of theologians. In this essay, he takes theologians or "religious ethicists" to task for not being more explicitly and rigorously theological. He grants that in our contemporary context it can be difficult to speak in a rigorously theological manner for a variety of reasons: that the audience is not interested in theology, and non-theologians define the problems and do so in such a way that there are no obvious theological answers. Nevertheless, he demonstrates the variety of ways in which theological convictions have a fundamental bearing on how we understand technology and the life sciences — in terms of anthropology, eschatology, our understanding of nature and grace, and more. Gustafson argues that "ethicists" need to again become theologians and that, if nothing else, one of the most important gifts theology provides to medical ethics is the ability to identify hidden aspects of the discussion and to reframe the questions.

4. For an analysis of this shift from *Belmont* to Beauchamp and Childress, see M. Therese Lysaught, "Respect: Or, How Respect for Persons Became Respect for Autonomy," *Journal of Medicine and Philosophy* 29, no. 6 (2004): 665-80.

5. John Evans, *Playing God? Human Genetic Engineering and the Rationalization of Public Bioethical Debate* (Chicago: University of Chicago Press, 2002).

6. For an allied sociological reading of the development of bioethics, see M. Therese Lysaught, "And Power Corrupts . . . : Theology and the Disciplinary Matrix of Bioethics," in *Handbook of Bioethics and Religion,* ed. David Guinn (New York: Oxford University Press, 2006), pp. 93-123.

Lisa Sowle Cahill in "Theologians and Bioethics: Some History and a Proposal" (selection 8) takes up Gustafson's argument twenty-five years later. She provides a succinct history of the field of bioethics, fleshing out the story to which Gustafson and Evans refer, and adds the next chapter. Cahill maintains that while theology might have been marginalized *vis-à-vis* mainstream, public, secular bioethics, theological engagement with questions of medicine and ethics have continued to flourish elsewhere. Importantly, however, she takes Gustafson's analysis one step further. Cahill argues convincingly that the marginalization of theology *vis-à-vis* bioethics has occurred not only because of the failure of theological nerve and language on the part of theologians. She shows how, contrary to their claims to neutrality, "secular" bioethics, along with their allied disciplines of science, economics, and liberalism, are in fact "thick" worldviews deeply and extensively rooted in traditions. Moreover, she makes clear the ways in which science and the market function, often with religious overtones — grounded in communal practices, replete with mythologies and saints and warnings regarding demons and sinfulness, surrounded with language of salvation and eschatology. Theology has been marginalized from secular bioethics not because one is religious and the other secular, but because what we have is a clash of two thick theological perspectives.

While the "thick" worldview of secular bioethics will continue to make it difficult for religious perspectives to gain a real hearing, Cahill is optimistic about the future of what she names "theological bioethics." The source of her optimism does not lie, however, in the academy. Instead, she sees the real work of theological bioethics being done by those Christians engaged in caring for the sick and marginalized in their local settings, tying their care for the sick to local, grassroots politics. As she goes on to argue in her essay, it is by allying itself to these practices of "participatory democracy" that (academic) theological bioethics will be able to influence both the public square and public policy.

Cahill is not alone in recognizing that the primary space where theological engagement with medicine flourishes is, in many ways, off our usual radar. As one might discern from the histories provided by Gustafson, Evans, and Cahill, the discipline of bioethics has, for most of its history, been done from a very narrow social location — that of academics and policy makers, physicians, administrators, theologians, and philosophers. The official discipline has long been very white, very upper-class, very U.S. Equally marginal to the official discipline of bioethics have been the perspectives of race, of different socioeconomic locations, and of perspectives from outside of the U.S. The next two essays — "European-American Ethos and Principlism: An African-American Challenge" by Cheryl J. Sanders (selection 9) and "Bioethics in a Liberationist Key" by Márcio Fabri dos Anjos (selection 10) — make this clear. These essays broaden the discourse; they also illustrate the centrality of theology to the perspectives they articulate. Sanders, for example, highlights the central role of Black

Theology in the framework of African-American thought and analysis. Dos Anjos's categories of a liberationist perspective are, likewise, deeply theologically rooted.[7]

Cognizant of the arguments in the foregoing essays, Stephen E. Lammers in his "Bioethics and Religion: Some Unscientific Footnotes" (selection 11) comes at the question of theology and medical ethics from yet a different angle. Suddenly our setting is the clinic, where he argues that, at least on the surface, religious belief and practice have fared quite well. Echoing the concerns of Hall et al., from Chapter One, Lammers argues that religious beliefs continue to be honored in the clinical setting only because they have been misconstrued under the rubric of "choice." "The choice model," he notes, "that is normative and supportive of religion turns out to lead to misunderstanding of the situation of many believers. Further, this understanding is often a function of class and power. Finally, choice as the central metaphor is not true to the experience of disease for those who are ill."

We close with a final methodological question. For those who take Gustafson's challenge seriously, who wish to confront technology and the life sciences from a thickly theological perspective, who understand Christianity to be a thick tradition that one inhabits rather than simply a "choice," where does one begin? Allen Verhey, in "The Bible and Bioethics: Some Problems and a Proposal" (selection 12), makes clear that Christians must engage Scripture. But how? How one goes about using Scripture with regard to contemporary medicine is a significant issue — one will not find "stem cell research" in one's concordance. Verhey's essay carefully outlines the difficulties Scripture presents *vis-à-vis* questions in medicine, identifies problematic approaches to using Scripture in medical ethics, and then offers a constructive proposal.

As bioethics moves into its fifth decade as a discipline, its relationship to theology remains contested yet as vibrant as ever, strengthened by renewed attention to the theological character of science, bioethics, and the market itself; by new voices from the margins for whom theological traditions are central; and by seasoned reflections on the nature of religion, Scripture, and theological method. Contemporary theologians reflecting on the moral dimensions of medicine have heeded Gustafson's challenge — theological perspectives on bioethics are, increasingly, theological. In doing so, theology continues to challenge and advance the field, providing substantive and authentic perspectives far richer than the concepts and authentic perspectives far richer than the framework provided by four formal principles. Stephen Toulmin once argued that medical ethics saved the life of philosophy; it may well be that as the twenty-first century proceeds, theology might well save the life of bioethics.[8]

7. Paul Farmer and Nicole Gastineau Campos take dos Anjos's argument one step further and ask what difference it might make to approach questions in medical ethics from the perspective of the poor, in their essay "Rethinking Medical Ethics: A View from Below," *Developing World Bioethics* 4, no. 1 (2004): 17-41.

8. Stephen Toulmin, "How Medicine Saved the Life of Ethics," *Perspectives in Biology and Medicine* 25, no. 4 (1982): 736-50.

SUGGESTIONS FOR FURTHER READING

Callahan, Daniel, and Courtney S. Campbell. *Hastings Center Report* Special Supplement on "Theology, Religious Traditions, and Bioethics" 20, no. 4 (July/August 1990).

Campbell, Courtney S. "Religion and Moral Meaning in Bioethics." *Hastings Center Report,* Special Supplement 20, no. 4 (July/August 1990): 4-10.

Elliott, Carl. "Where Ethics Comes from and What to Do about It." *Hastings Center Report* 22, no. 4 (1992): 28-36.

Evans, John. *Playing God? Human Genetic Engineering and the Rationalization of Public Bioethical Debate* (Chicago: University of Chicago Press, 2002).

Flack, Harley, and Edmund Pellegrino. *African-American Perspectives on Biomedical Ethics* (Washington, D.C.: Georgetown University Press, 1992).

Fox, Renee C., and Judith W. Swazey. "Medical Morality Is Not Bioethics — Bioethics in China and the United States." *Perspectives in Biology and Medicine* 27 (Spring 1984): 336-60.

Guinn, David E. *Handbook of Bioethics and Religion* (New York: Oxford University Press, 2006).

Jonsen, Albert R. *The Birth of Bioethics* (New York: Oxford University Press, 1998).

Kelly, David F. *The Emergence of Roman Catholic Medical Ethics in North America: An Historical-Methodological-Bibliographical Study* (New York: Edwin Mellen, 1979).

Verhey, Allen D. *Reading the Bible in the Strange World of Medicine* (Grand Rapids: Eerdmans, 2003).

Verhey, Allen D. *Religion and Medical Ethics: Looking Back, Looking Forward* (Grand Rapids: Eerdmans, 1996).

7 Theology Confronts Technology and the Life Sciences

James M. Gustafson

That persons with theological training are writing a great deal about technology and the life sciences is clear to those who read *The Hastings Center Report, Theological Studies* and many other journals. Whether *theology* is thereby in interaction with these areas, however, is less clear. For some writers the theological authorization for the ethical principles and procedures they use is explicit; this is clearly the case for the most prolific and polemical of the Protestants, Paul Ramsey. For others, writing as "ethicists," the relation of their moral discourse to any specific theological principles, or even to a definable religious outlook is opaque. Indeed, in response to a query from a friend (who is a distinguished philosopher) about how the term "ethicist" has come about, I responded in a pejorative way, "An ethicist is a former theologian who does not have the professional credentials of a moral philosopher."

Much of the writing in the field is by persons who desire to be known as "religious ethicists" if only to distinguish themselves for practical reasons from those holding cards in the philosophers' union. Exactly what the adjective "religious" refers to, however, is far from obvious. If it refers to something as specific as "Christian" or "Jewish," or even "Protestant" or "Catholic," presumably writers would be willing to use the proper term. Again Ramsey is to be commended; one can ask for nothing more forthright than his 1974 declaration, "I always write as the ethicist I am, namely a Christian ethicist, and not as some hypothetical common denominator." If "religious ethicists" would even say what the "religious dimensions" of the problems were, we could place the adjective in some frame of reference: Tillichian, Deweyan, Luckmannian, Geertzian or what have you.

The difficulties in formulating a theological (and not merely moral) confrontation with technology and the life sciences are real, and not just apparent, as any of us who have written in this area knows. Unless the intended readership is one internal to the theological community, communication problems are exacerbated beyond the ordinary. Much of the writing is done for persons who are making policy or choices in the areas of technology, biological experimentation and clinical medicine. While there is a self-consciously Catholic constituency among these professional persons (for example, the member of the National Federation of Catholic Physicians' Guilds who sponsor *The Linacre Quarterly*), and while there may well be constituencies from the evangelical wing of Protestantism, most of the professional persons the writers seek to influence are judged not to be interested in the theological grounds from which the moral analysis and prescription grows. (I recall attending a party after a day of meetings with biologists and physicians at which a biologist, made friendlier by the ample libations provided, said to me, "Say something theological, Gustafson." I had the presence of mind to utter a guttural and elongated "Gawd.")

Not only is the audience frequently uninterested in the theological principles that might inform moral critique, but also the problems that are addressed are defined by the non-theologians, and usually are problems that emerge within a very confined set of circumstances. Should one cut the power source to a respirator for patient *y* whose circumstances are *a, b,* and *c?* Although the stakes are much higher, this is not utterly dissimilar to asking whether $8.20 an hour or $8.55 an hour ought to be paid to carpenters' helpers in Kansas City. Even a clear and well-developed principle of distributive justice would not easily answer the latter question. To ask what "theology" might say to that question is patently more difficult. Obviously it is not easy to give a clearly theological answer to a question that is formulated so that there are no theological aspects to it. To make the practical moral question susceptible to any recognizably theological answer requires nursing, massaging, altering, and maybe even transforming processes. When these processes are completed one might discover that a different set of issues are under discussion from those that originated the interaction.

To respond to specific questions requires more acumen in moral reasoning than it requires theological learning and acumen. I am sure that the writers of the manuals in medical moral theology were well schooled in the tractates on the Trinity; the bearing of those texts on their medical moral discussions, however, is at best remote. It is quite understandable, then, that theology (either as doctrine from an historic tradition, or ideas about the "religious dimensions" of life) tends to be displaced in the attention of the writer by ethical theory and by procedures of practical moral reasoning.

In the Catholic tradition with its continued development of natural law as a basis for ethics an intellectual legitimation for the autonomy of moral theology developed; the natural moral order was itself created by God, so the natural order was God's order. Ethical analysis and prescription were theological in principle; moralists were theologians by being moralists. Enough said about theology. Unfortunately, in this tradition the resources and dimensions of theological reflection became confined to a basic theological authorization for ethics, and almost nothing more. And the ethical questions were stirred by particular acts about which judgments of moral rightness

From *Commonweal* 105 (June 16, 1978): 386-92. Used by permission.

or wrongness could be made. It did not occur to these moralists, for example, to wonder if the prophets' critiques of the worship of Baal might not provide, by an act of imagination if not by well-developed analogy, some basis for a theological criticism of the excessive scrupulosity that the moral enterprise itself might promote.

A brute fact, and a source of some embarrassment in discourse with the professionals in technology and the life sciences, is the lack of consensus among theologians on some rather simple matters. What is it that theologians think about and write about? What is the subject matter of theology? The high degree of *anomie* among practicing theologians, and the uncertainty among some as to what defines their work as theological, is hardly an asset to any interaction between "theology" and technology and the life sciences. A tired old story from the years of the banquet circuit of the National Conference of Christian and Jews comes to mind. A priest, a Protestant minister and a rabbi were asked to respond to the same question. The priest began, "The Church teaches that. . ." The rabbi began, "The tradition teaches that. . ." The minister began, "Now I think that. . ." There are very good historical and intellectual explanations for the extension of a kind of Protestant *anomie* to the theological enterprise as a whole, but explanations of why it is hard to answer the simple question "what is the subject matter of theology?" do little to identify a melody in a collective cacophonous response. I can readily cite coherent passages from Tillich on technology, Barth on clinical medical moral problems, Rahner on the uses of genetic knowledge, and Ramsey on why Richard McCormick's Jesuit probabilism requires a rigorist response, but I see no way in which I can find among them a basis for a generalization about how theology confronts technology and the life sciences.

We know what many of the *moral* issues are in technology and the life sciences; we are not sure what the "religious" or *theological* issues are. While debate continues about what moral principles ought to be decisive in determining courses of action in the life sciences and technology, at least the principles under debate can be formulated with some conceptual precision. Much of the literature deals with such matters as the rights of individuals, the preservation of individual self-determination, the conditions under which others might exercise their own self-determination, and the consideration of what benefits and whose good might justify overriding the rights of individuals. Certain principles are invoked constantly: informed consent, risk-benefit ratios, distributive justice, and so forth. There are procedures for justifying particular judgments; there are complex prescriptions like double-effect.

Nothing of comparable detail and precision exists in the more strictly theological realm of discourse; and for various theological reasons the sorts of questions a previous generation asked — such as "What is God doing in these circumstances?" or "What is God saying to us through these crises?" — appear to be very odd and unanswerable. Ethics provides a basis for a new casuistry that is indispensable as long as the issues are framed by the professional persons who have to make particular choices, and as long as the terms of discussion are those on which there can be some consensus, namely ethical terms. No doubt there can be a theological justification for the casuistry, but then there can also be a lot of other, non-theological justification for it. The ethical questions have become fairly clear, and to an ethical question one gives an ethical answer, whether one is a physician, engineer, philosopher or theologian. The theological questions are not clear, and as a result frequently even those writers trained in theology neither attempt to make them clear, nor attempt to answer those that can be asked.

Matters of Belief

I have long believed, and often said, that many of the debates that are passionately conducted within the framework of ethics are misplaced, and that the issues that divide persons are matters of beliefs (whether theological in function or in fact, or whether moral or something else we need not decide here) and loyalties which determine our value choices. Paul Ramsey's Beecher Lectures at Yale, from which came the widely read *The Patient as Person,* provoked a discussion between an internist and surgeon both of whom worked in the renal program. The internist was much taken by Ramsey's argument and vehemently supported the Uniform Anatomical Gifts Act, an act stipulating in precise detail the consent procedures for using an organ from a corpse. The surgeon strongly expressed the opinion that hospitals and their staff ought legally to be authorized to "salvage" from corpses any usable organs that might benefit the health and prolong the life of patients. There certainly are ways to deal with the controversy between these two that might lead to some agreement — that might determine whether to pay the carpenters' helpers $8.20 or $8.55 an hour. The precision of the debates at the level of casuistry is not to be demeaned. But the difference between these two physicians really stemmed from more general beliefs and valuations, and these divergences will not be settled, or even addressed, by the latest refinement of the principle of double-effect and its application to cases in the operating room.

Who ought to address these differences? What is the agenda for exploring them? What are the grounds for convictions about the "limit questions," to use Stephen Toulmin's phrase? In a most technical sense, perhaps, these are not yet "theological" questions; but surely they demand a response that is more "theological" than casuistic. And surely there are resources in the religious traditions, in speculative natural theologies, and in the discussions of "religious dimensions" that can be used at least to frame the questions and explore answers to them.

A different example reveals the need for another kind of discourse which at least approaches "theology" if it is not theology. How one understands the relation of self and society, how this relationship is interpreted and conceptualized has profound effects upon the outcome of very specific answers to specific questions. I shall illustrate this too simply by suggesting that the competing metaphors used to depict this relationship are the mechanistic and the organic. The first understands society basically in contractual terms; society is a structure that individuals voluntarily agree to institute and develop. The second understands society, obviously, in organic terms; society is a network of interrelatedness and interdependence in which the relations of the parts are "internal" (I do not intend to invoke a whole Hegelian view by using this term), and in which the development of the well-being of the whole must be considered, if not supreme, at least on par with the well-being of its individual members. The population geneticist tends to take the latter view; when he or she speaks of "benefits," the reference is to the human species. When the ecologist speaks of benefits, the reference is to the well-being of life on the planet. Physicians and most persons writing about ethical issues in medicine and the life sciences have consciously or implicitly adopted the more mechanistic metaphor, and not without some good reasons. Those who use the organic metaphor are more ready to justify overriding an individual "right." If there is any plausibility to my observations, it is fair to ask who is responsible to think about such matters of basic perception, in this case of the relations of individuals to society. What data and warrants support alternative views, and which view in the end appears more adequate?

Another example refers more specifically to Christians and their doctrinal differences. I have argued elsewhere that Karl Rahner's apparent openness to certain kinds of experimentation on humans is a reasonable conclusion from his philosophical and theological anthropology, and from his understanding of the relations of grace and nature. This openness so alarmed Paul Ramsey that he described it as "remarkably like a priestly blessing over everything, doing duty for ethics," and yet Rahner's attitude rests firmly on theological and philosophical grounds.

If one does not like Rahner's openness (which is really very guarded and has several severely restraining principles) one has to argue with his theological and philosophical anthropology and with his views of the relations of grace and nature. If one is persuaded that Rahner's theology is the best available for the Catholic Church today (and the number of dissertations sympathetically exploring his thought suggest that quite a few people are so persuaded), then one ought to come out in moral theology somewhere within the range of his conclusions. If one is concerned that Rahner's openness is morally dangerous in its potential consequences, perhaps one ought to examine one's own theological anthropology, and one's own views of grace and nature. The proper argument is not to be confined to the consequences of relatively closed or open positions but must pursue the question further, to the adequacy of doctrines of God and different anthropologies. A *real* theological discussion then becomes unavoidable.

In the course of such an argument an apparently astounding matter might be seen, namely that one's theological convictions and their articulation in principles about the character of ultimate reality and about human life have a fundamental bearing on one's attitude toward the life sciences and technology. This bearing, in fact, might be more significant in determining one's particular moral preferences than the specific principles chosen to justify a particular decision. It might turn out that passionate ethical debates about technology and the life sciences are missing the crucial point where the real differences lie, and (my goodness!) "ethicists" might have to become theologians! They might find an agenda that would give them something distinctive to do!

To be trained in theology should alert one to aspects of discussion that are otherwise hidden. Several years ago a number of us participated in an intensive conference with research and clinical geneticists. One of the papers was rather more utopian in outlook than the others; its author limned out a vision of the vast benefits to the human race that would accrue from vigorous pursuit of genetic research. I call such scientists "hawks." The paper generated a very passionate discussion, mostly by other scientists and clinicians. Among them were the "doves." Indeed, the rhetoric in the discussion was what those of us alert to religious language could only call apocalyptic. One could interpret the whole discussion as a contest between competing eschatologies: prospects for a universal salvation pitted against prospects for eternal annihilation. The arguments were finally not about matters of hard science; there were some discussions about whose extrapolations from the known to the unknown were most reliable, and about the time frame in which certain possibilities (such as cloning of humans) might occur. But what really divided the disputants were questions that traditionally have been judged to be religious in character.

Most apparent was the question "For what can we hope?" And that could not be answered without asking, in effect, "In whom can we trust?" and "In what can we trust?" Also in dispute were answers to the question "What is desirable?" — which to my mind, incorrigibly saturated with biblical and theological language, becomes "What are proper objects of our love?" I feel I do not unduly alter what went on there if I say we were in the midst of a discussion of hope, faith and love. We were also in a discussion of the proper objects of hope, faith and love. No one proposed the Pauline answer, "Your hope is in God." Or the more general Christian answer, "Trust in God." Or the Augustinian answer, "God is the proper object of desire." But the discussion was about whether one should trust chance, or the evolutionary process with minimal intervention, or scientists and statesmen who have power to intervene. The house could readily have been divided between the Augustinians and Pelagians on other questions: the extent of "free will" and the depths of human corruption. It cannot be said that my intervention, in which I pointed out these themes, turned the conversation to one about theology, and certainly about Christian theology, as a subject in itself. I do believe, however, that something dawned in the consciousness of some participants: theology might not provide answers you like to accept, but it can force questions you ought to be aware of. To paraphrase the title of an article by H. Richard Niebuhr, in these circumstances theology is not queen, but servant.

This article ought to have made clear my criticisms of the interchange between theology and technology and the life sciences as long as that interchange is confined merely to the "ethical." With equal severity I would criticize those who confine the theological discussion to *Zeitgeist,* ethos and other comparably general terms. To be honored in such theologians is their radically prophetic stance. They know golden calves when they see them, and they see them sooner than persons preoccupied with how to get from one oasis to the next in the Sinai of contemporary culture and society. I have been accused, in my preoccupation with some matters of a casuistic sort, of "rearranging the deck chairs on the *Titanic.*" Valid charge. My equally nasty retort to those critics is that they think the only proper response is to jump in the North Atlantic and push the icebergs away.

Whether or not one uses the religious language of idolatry, the attack on ethos and *Zeitgeist* implies a call to radical repentance, to a turning away from the Baals of technology whose reliability is bound to fail, and to whom cultural devotion can only lead to desolation for the coming generations. What the culture is to turn from is clear; that it is to return to Yahweh is not necessarily proclaimed. That persons and society are in bondage to the powers of technology, that they are looking for a "salvation" in medical therapy that therapy cannot give them, these are poignantly indicated by the contemporary prophets. That the need is for liberation from bondage, and that some fundamental conversion of individuals and of ethos is required, these points are well made. The sickness is "global" and the antidote must be sufficient for the poison. The creative and exasperating French Protestant Jacques Ellul is one such prophet; he works out of a highly biblical and confessional theology. Not only technology and science, but programs of social revolution and churches feel the sting of his prophetic rhetoric. For him and others like him, technology tends to become reified as a demonic power which only the power of the crucifixion can overcome.

Myopic casuists need strong enough lenses to see the point of the radical theological critics. On the other hand, the perspectives of the radical prophets make conversation with persons who specialize in technology and the life sciences very difficult. If they cannot address the specific and concrete manifestation of the ethos (if it can be said to exist independently) in the particularities of cases and policy choices, if they cannot show how their theologies address the issues as they arise out of specific activities, conversation never gets down to the ground. Many theologians who are critics of culture write for other theologians and for a half-converted religious readership even when they are writing as theologians of culture — technological culture, "modern" culture, or what have you. Indeed, often when they write about the *need* for theology to be engaged in criticism of technological and scientific culture, they are addressing a like-minded group. Why not *test* the need and the practice on an endocrinologist who researches testosterone levels?

Sometimes it turns out that those who are famous as prophetic critics of culture have nothing very specific to say about any particular event in technology and the use of the life sciences. We are told, for example, that a theology of hope addresses social and cultural issues. It turns out that the principal point of the address is that present institutions and cultural values are ephemeral and relative, and we ought not to absolutize them. Thanks a lot! Any student of the history of science and technology knows that. That does not assist the committees on experimentation on human subjects on which I sit to decide whether protocol #6172 is acceptable from a moral perspective. That particular *Titanic* has not yet sunk, and there is merit in arranging things so that it can stay afloat for some time in the future, or at least in organizing things so the lifeboats can be used effectively. Theology cannot push the icebergs away. It might at least help to develop the radar technology that aids in avoiding them.

The moralists find a vocabulary enabling them to interact with the professionals from technology and the life sciences; this tends to limit the theological questions. The prophetic theologians find a vocabulary that is somewhat "theological" in some sense which enables them to interact with other theologians and with other prophetic critics of the ethos; this tends to limit their capacities to relate to the specific occasions in which critical choices have to be made.

Since this is my occasion for broadsides, yet another group of writers can be noted. They are those concerned about the relations between "religion" and "science." Frequently both terms are abstractions: these writers are not concerned about the relations of Judaism to human genetics. They frequently publish in that very interesting journal called *Zygon.* Their intention is to humanize technology and science with some sense of the sacred, and to scientize theology with arguments that presumably support "religion." While it is the case that all modern theology continues to reel from the impact of the Enlightenment, and that theologians continue to find philosophical bases on which to justify the existence of religion (or "the religious" as some like to call it), on the whole this synthetic enterprise is not in the best of repute philosophically, scientifically, or theologically and for some substantial reasons.

"Sciences are a fundamental resource for theology," writes Ralph Wendell Burhoe, a person seldom cited by professional theologians but more widely known than

Van Harvey or Gordon Kaufman or David Tracy by groups of scientists interested in the relations of science and religion. Burhoe is confident. He writes, "I suggest that before this century is out we shall see all over the world an increasing integration of information from the sciences into the heart of the belief systems of traditional religions. I prophesy human salvation through a reformation and rehabilitation of religion at a level superior to any reformation in earlier histories, a level high above that of Jasper's axial age as that was above the primitive religions of 10,000 B.C. . . . The new religious and theological language will be as high above that of five centuries ago as contemporary cosmology is above the Ptolemaic, as contemporary medicine, agriculture, communications and transportation concepts are above those of the fifteenth century." Burhoe's program is in sharpest contrast with those theologians that Kai Nielsen has called "Wittgensteinian fideists" who separate religious consciousness and language from scientific consciousness and language in such a way that the former is virtually rendered immune from any criticism by the latter.

In effect the writers of whom Burhoe is fairly typical aspire to develop both theology and ethics on the basis of science, and the life sciences seem to have a privileged place in these proposals. The enterprise is not novel, and different proposals come forward from it about the biological bases for ethics, for knowledge of ultimate reality, and for other matters. Now, no less than in previous decades, it is fraught with difficulties that have frequently been indicated by philosophers of science, philosophers of religion, and moral philosophers. Inferences from scientific data and theories to theological and ethical conclusions are often weakly warranted. The enterprise has the merit of a challenge, however. Can we think theologically and ethically on the basis of what we know about biology? If we find an affirmative answer to the question unacceptable, at least we have to give our reasons for that, and we are left with the chore of figuring out just how knowledge of biology relates to ethics and theology. That is a philosophical and theological problem as important for one aspect of culture as the relation of Marxist theory to ethics and theology for another.

What can be anticipated about theology's "confrontation" with technology and the life sciences? I have amply distributed my criticisms so that few, if any, theologically trained writers in this field are exempt, including myself. I have not described the social, historical and institutional contexts in which the discussions increasingly occur. As far as the ethical responses are concerned, what was a lively, interdisciplinary enterprise even a decade ago has increasingly become a separate profession, if only because the volume of literature has exponentially increased so that it takes a full-time effort to be in control of it. Theologically trained writers had a prominence a decade ago that is receding and will continue to do so. Their prominence was in part the effect of the concern that religious communities had for practical moral questions, a concern that moral philosophers, until very recently, looked upon with haughty disdain. Now philosophers, physicians and many other professions are contributing a larger portion of the literature than was the case. Separate institutes, national commissions, advisory committees and other organizations have come into being. Theologically trained persons have not been excluded from participation in these, and indeed continue to be significant contributors, but insofar as the contribution of the "theologians" has been and continues to be "practical moral philosophy," the basis of their being attended to is shared by practitioners who are at least as skillful as they are. Competence in argumentation is the criterion by which their contributions will be judged, and a number of them will continue to be highly respected.

Usage and Interpretation

But what if "theologians" choose to be clearer about what the theological issues, or the "religious dimensions," are in the life sciences and technology? I grant that some anxieties will arise. There is not a wide world waiting to hear about these ideas, since they do not immediately assist in determining what constitutes a just distribution of health care resources. There may, however, be more people out there who are interested than we presently recognize. Traditional theological language, and perhaps also the efforts to decontaminate its historical particularities with the language of natural theology or of religious dimensions, will require some skillful usage and significant interpretation. Timidity might be as much a restraining factor as are the objectively real problems in undertaking such discourse. Theologians and other religious thinkers seem highly self-conscious of their own cultural relativity; they often forget that other areas of thought share the same plight. It will have to be accepted that not everyone in that highly esteemed secular technological culture will be interested in the contributions of theologians, but that some persons (even some with social power) might.

In the meantime there are still a large number of people who attend churches, and who seem not fully alienated from traditional religious language and practice. They fall sick, have unexpected pregnancies, vote for legislators who in turn vote on health insurance plans and funding of research. Catholic moral theologians are more conscious of that constituency than are Protestants. Perhaps there is quite a bit to be done to help these persons understand technology in the light of their religious faith and convictions!

In the matters I have been discussing as in so many others, my impression is that much theological or "religious" writing is directed to the justification of an enterprise in the eyes of persons who are not really interested enough to care whether the justification is adequate or not. (I worked for years on a book *Can Ethics Be Christian?* with the nagging sense that most persons who answer in an unambiguous affirmative would not be interested in my supporting argument, that a few fellow professional persons might be interested enough to look at it, and that for those who believe the answer is negative the question itself is not sufficiently important to bother about.) While theologians ought to continue to participate competently in the public debates about matters of technology and the life sciences, they would also do well to attend to the home folks who *might* care more about what they have to say. I am not suggesting that theologians are the best retail communicators, but that the historically identifiable religious communities are fairly obvious loci to be taken into account in writing theology and theological ethics in relation to technology and the life sciences.

It is the "religious ethicists" who have most to be anxious about, in my judgment. They will have either to become moral philosophers with a special interest in "religious" texts and arguments, or become theologians: Christian theologians, or natural theologians, or "religious dimensions" theologians. Only indifference to what they are writing, or exceeding patience with inexcusable ambiguity, can account for the tolerance they have enjoyed.

8 Theologians and Bioethics: Some History and a Proposal

Lisa Sowle Cahill

The contemporary discipline of bioethics arose as part of efforts in the 1960s and 1970s specifically to change social practices in medicine and research. One key agenda item was experimentation that exploited vulnerable populations, especially by subjecting them, without their consent, to research projects that were harmful. The names Tuskegee and Willowbrook symbolize the failure of U.S. researchers to meet the moral requirements of the Nuremberg Code.[1] Another was the need to find a way to deal with the use and allocation decisions necessitated by new technologies. The Seattle dialysis lottery, heart transplants, and the removal of Karen Ann Quinlan from a respirator made worldwide news and raised public consciousness of the ethical quandaries modern medicine rapidly introduced.[2]

Theological luminaries such as Paul Ramsey, Richard McCormick, and James Gustafson were visible figures in the shaping of the new bioethics. As a result of their efforts, in cooperation with philosophers, medical doctors, and researchers, the practice of biomedicine in the United States shifted directions. It moved decisively toward respect for patient autonomy and informed consent and toward the formation of public policies, laws, and judicial precedents to govern aspects of practice such as research on human subjects and decisions about life-sustaining treatment.

Two of the most prominent early voices, Ramsey (a Methodist) and McCormick (a Roman Catholic), were often in good-natured conflict with one another. Other important players were Joseph Fletcher (an Episcopalian

1. These are infamous research projects, in which African American men were left untreated for syphilis even after treatments had been shown effective (Tuskegee syphilis study), and in which mentally retarded children were exposed to hepatitis (Willowbrook State School). See Jeffrey P. Kahn, Anna C. Mastroianni, and Jeffrey Sugarman, *Beyond Consent: Seeking Justice in Research* (New York: Oxford University Press, 1998) 3-4; and Warren T. Reich, "Bioethics in the United States," in *Bioethics: A History*, ed. Corrado Viafora (Bethesda, MD: International Scholars Publications, 1996) 83-87. The Nuremberg Code may be found in Tom L. Beauchamp and LeRoy Walters, *Contemporary Issues in Bioethics* (Belmont, CA: Wadsworth, 1978), 404-5.

2. Reich, "Bioethics," 88.

Excerpted from Lisa Sowle Cahill, *Theological Bioethics: Participation, Justice, and Change* (Washington, D.C.: Georgetown University Press, 2005). Used by permission of the publisher.

and a situation ethicist) and James Gustafson (a Reformed theologian who increasingly attended to the importance of the natural and human sciences for Christian bioethics). Karen Lebacqz (a Congregationalist) has been a key thinker both in feminist bioethics and in policy discussions. Jewish voices include Fred Rosner, Immanuel Jakobovitz, Elliott Dorff, and David Bleich. Though more names could be mentioned,[3] these clearly illustrate the engagement of theologians in bioethics debates throughout the 1980s.

Topics of central concern included abortion, reproductive technologies, genetic engineering, human experimentation, termination of treatment, direct mercy killing, and the allocation of scarce medical resources. Theologians joined in debates about how medicine and research are institutionalized in U.S. society and about law and public policy. Theologians such as Ramsey, Gustafson, McCormick, and Lebacqz not only served on important policy bodies like the National Commission on the Protection of Human Subjects (1974) and the President's Commission (1979), but were major players in formation of the field of bioethics — helping to establish centers such as The Institute of Religion at the Texas Medical Center in Houston (1954); the Institute of Society, Ethics, and the Life Sciences, later to become the Hastings Center, in New York State (1961); the Kennedy Institute of Bioethics at Georgetown University (1971); and the Park Ridge Center in Chicago (1985). The first edition of the *Encyclopedia of Bioethics,* whose very existence and title lent substance to the new field, was filled with entries by theologians and articles written from religious perspectives.[4] Theologians have continued to hold membership on national commissions, such as the National Bioethics Advisory Commission (NBAC; under President William Clinton) and the President's Council on Bioethics (PCB), formed by George W. Bush in 2001, initially to advise him on stem cell policy.[5]

Richard McCormick provides an especially good example of multifaceted involvement, as he was a commentator on Catholic Church teaching as it affected not only individuals but the policies of numerous Catholic health facilities. In fact, one of his books on theological bioethics is styled as a revised set of guidelines for Catholic health care.[6] He also commented frequently on court cases, especially regarding end-of-life decisions.[7] McCormick's work illustrates the opportunity that theologians have to affect social practices by means of the infrastructure and networks of civil society, such as religious bodies, health care institutions, and professional organizations and norms, as well as by influencing the processes of legislative change and judicial precedent.

"Theology" is essentially a process of reflection on religious experience, in which the systematic coherence of religious narratives and symbols is clarified and their practical ramifications developed. Theological ethics is the explication and defense of the personal moral and the social behavior required or idealized by a religious tradition. Theologians were particularly well-equipped to advance bioethics at its inception because religious communities had cultivated long-standing traditions of reflection on life, death, and suffering and had given more guidance on the specifics of moral conduct than had moral philosophy at that time.[8] Thomas Shannon notes that theologians entered the early bioethics debates so effectively because they — in contrast to most philosophers of the day — were prepared to take on issues of practical decision making.[9] They sometimes, but not always, used religious language and stories in the process.

The early theological bioethicists used religious language, imagery, and teaching to advance discourse within their faith traditions. In public settings they sometimes sought expressions that were more philosophical, but occasionally used religious imagery to destabilize cultural assumptions and suggest a different

3. Students of Gustafson who entered the field early on included James Childress (a Quaker, who usually writes from a philosophical perspective), Allen Verhey (developing biblical ethics within the Reformed tradition), Stanley Hauerwas (a Methodist, whose proposal of a communitarian, narrative ethics has been immensely influential), and Margaret Farley (a Roman Catholic and major contributor to feminist bioethics). David Smith (an Episcopalian) has worked at the intersection of theology, philosophy, and policy; Warren Reich (a Catholic) edited the *Encyclopedia of Bioethics.* Charles E. Curran argued that Catholic moral theology in general should be more historical and applied this to norms in bioethics. William E. May (also a Catholic) defended Catholic Church teaching on bioethics, while William F. May (a Methodist) turned his attention more to the social and professional roles and obligations of physicians than to practical problem solving. Robert Veatch has expanded the interreligious dialogue among many traditions. For further discussion, see LeRoy Walters, "Religion and the Renaissance of Medical Ethics in the United States," in *Theology and Bioethics: Exploring the Foundations and Frontiers,* ed. Earl E. Shelp (Dordrecht, Neth.: Kluwer, 1986), 3-16; Warren Thomas Reich, "Bioethics in the United States," in *History of Bioethics: International Perspectives,* ed. Roberto Dell'Oro and Corrado Viafora (San Francisco, CA: International Scholars Publications, 1996), 83-118; and James F. Childress, "Religion, Theology and Bioethics," in *The Nature and Prospects of Bioethics: Interdisciplinary Perspectives,* ed. Franklin G. Miller (Totowa, NJ: Humana Press, 2003), 43-67.

4. Warren T. Reich, *Encyclopedia of Bioethics* (New York: Macmillan, 1978).

5. The theologian on NBAC was James Childress; the theologian on the PCB is Gilbert Meilaender.

6. Richard A. McCormick, *Health and Medicine in the Catholic Tradition* (New York: Crossroad, 1984).

7. One of his more famous and influential pieces in this regard was "To Save or Let Die: The Dilemma of Modern Medicine," *Journal of the American Medical Association* 229 (1974): 172-76. The essay was published simultaneously in *America* 131 (July 1974).

8. See Walters, "Religion and the Renaissance," 3-16; and Warren T. Reich, with the assistance of Roberto Dell'Oro, "A New Era for Bioethics: The Search for Meaning in Moral Experience," in *Religion and Medical Ethics: Looking Back, Looking Forward,* ed. Allen Verhey (Grand Rapids, MI: Eerdmans, 1996), 96-115.

9. Thomas A. Shannon, "Bioethics and Religion: A Value-Added Discussion," in *Notes from a Narrow Ridge: Religion and Bioethics,* ed. Dena S. Davis and Laurie Zoloth (Hagerstown, MD: University Publishing Groups, 1999), 31.

context for considering biomedical choices. Even explicitly theological language and religious symbols or stories (such as creation in the image of God, the story of the Fall, the healings performed by Jesus, the parable of the Good Samaritan, the ideal of covenant community) can evoke patterns of individual existence and social life that are similarly shared, abhorred, or admired in nonreligious associations. Examples are the universal human vulnerability to illness and need for health; the inevitability of death and the preciousness of life; the reality of social exploitation and the ideal of social cooperation and respect; and the reality of violent ideologies, contrasted with religious and moral traditions of other-concern and altruism.

Theologians participated then and do now in many circles of expression and influence, including teaching, academic and popular publishing, media commentary, conferences (theological and interdisciplinary, national and international), and membership on the bodies and committees that produce the "official" positions and teachings of religious traditions and denominations. Theology is mediated to the public in a variety of ways, including the representative positions of institutional religious bodies; pastors, teachers, and congregations; religiously sponsored educational systems; activist organizations and movements; and representation on public commissions. The bioethicist and audience or constituency are interdependent.

While some thinkers are influenced by their settings to be more concerned about the integrity of their shaping traditions and values, and to resist what they perceive as threatening cultural trends, others are more concerned about adequacy to contemporary experience and challenges and welcome innovative practices. A biblical image or theological concept such as creation may be invoked to rule out certain biomedical acts or practices as "playing God"; that same image can also underwrite human freedom as part of what it means to be cocreator with God.[10] The uses of images depend in part on the practices and communities in which they are embedded and the practices and policies they are meant to encourage or discourage.

Religious imagery and theological language can be harnessed either to "conservative" or "progressive" social and political agendas, and this is true of theological bioethics. The proposal to be developed in this book [*Theological Bioethics*], especially in chapter 2, affirms the importance and the effectiveness of the political participation of religious communities and theologies in shaping bioethical practices and policies. However, I do not see all types of religious advocacy as morally equal or equally representative of the ideals of the Christian biblical and theological traditions. Biblically and theologically grounded norms of justice, as the inclusion of all in the common good with a preferential option for the poor, should energize and renew a theological ethics of inclusion, participation, equality, and empowerment, especially for the least well-off.[11]

Theological Bioethics in the Public Forum

From the end of the 1970s until the last decade of the century, bioethics enjoyed great cultural credibility. But theological participation in public debates had to contend with the objection that such debate ought to occur on "neutral" ground and to ward off the idea that theological interventions are attempts to impose religious dogma on those of differing convictions. Such complaints can be rebutted fairly easily if theologians are willing to agree that positions inspired by religious commitment have to be "translated" into moral terms that can be accepted by all in order to have public viability. In other words, they have to sink or swim on the basis of their appeal to secular thinkers and philosophers. According to Daniel Callahan, founder, with Willard Gaylin, of the Hastings Center, most theological bioethicists enjoyed success because they adopted an "interesting and helpful" approach to biomedical dilemmas, rather than railing against the establishment.[12] They "were quite willing to talk in a fully secular way." In fact, bioethics may even have become popular because it was able "to push religion aside."[13]

Making themselves heard in pluralistic debates, often touching on public policy, some theological bioethicists began to operate like moral philosophers, ceding power to a "thin" and "secular" discourse that limits its moral claims to minimal requirements of procedural justice — or so goes a common critique.[14] This became more and more true in the 1980s, as more aspiring bioethicists,

10. See Philip Hefner, "The Evolution of the Created Co-Creator," in *Cosmos as Creation: Theology and Science in Consonance*, ed. Ted Peters (Nashville, TN: Abingdon, 1989), 211-33. For an example of this sort of argument about genetic technology, and a discussion of some alternatives, see Ted Peters, *For the Love of Children: Genetic Technology and the Future of the Family* (Louisville, KY: Westminster/John Knox Press, 1996).

11. For some grounds for this approach to theological ethics, see [the introduction to *Theological Bioethics*,] notes 1, 4, and 5.

12. Daniel Callahan, "Why America Accepted Bioethics," *The Hastings Center Report* 23, no. 6 (1993): S8.

13. Ibid.

14. Daniel Callahan, "Religion and the Secularization of Bioethics," *Hastings Center Report* 20 (July/August 1990): 2-10; Courtney Campbell, "Religion and Moral Meaning in Bioethics," *Hastings Center Report* 20 (July/August 1990): 4-10; Hauerwas, *Suffering Presence: Theological Reflections on Medicine, the Mentally Handicapped, and the Church* (Notre Dame, IN: University of Notre Dame, 1986); Hauerwas, "How Christian Ethics Became Medical Ethics: The Case of Paul Ramsey," in *Religion and Medical Ethics: Looking Back, Looking Forward*, ed. Allen Verhey (Grand Rapids, MI: Eerdmans, 1996), 61-80; Brent Waters, "What Is the Appropriate Contribution of Religious Communities in the Public Debate on Embryonic Stern Cell Research?" in *God and the Embryo: Religious Perspectives on Stem Cells and Cloning*, ed. Brent Waters and Ron Cole-Turner (Washington, DC: Georgetown University Press, 2003), 19-28.

even those pursuing theological degrees, were educated specifically for this new field of endeavor and assumed roles in clinical settings. Moreover, many seemed to pay more attention to crises and dilemmas than they did to their theological or even philosophical foundations. Consequently, specifically as theologians, they became marginalized in a field that came increasingly to rely on the kind of moral principles that could plausibly be claimed to be universal, rational, and "secular" and that sought the kind of decision-making and policy resolutions that could be squared with U.S. legal traditions and command public support.[15]

The sociologist John H. Evans offers an interpretation of theological bioethics that resembles the previous description. Focusing especially on genetic science, he laments the ascendancy of an approach to bioethics centered on the four "secular" principles of autonomy, beneficence, nonmaleficence, and justice.[16] Evans employs a distinction between "thick" and "thin" theories of the good that ultimately goes back to John Rawls.[17] Rawls distinguished between "thin" and "fuller" theories of the good in order to get people to come to the table of public decision making and agree that certain primary goods should be secured for all in a just society. He maintained that social inequalities are just only insofar as they work to secure these primary goods for society's least-favored members.[18] Evans's complaint is that the consequent "thinning" of public debate has "eviscerated" the discourse needed to make important decisions about whether human genetic engineering is compatible with worthy societal ends, because discussion of those ends is ruled out of bounds in the first place.

In his view, the policy discourse on genetic engineering in the United States is both exemplified and shaped by *Splicing Life,* a report of a presidential advisory commission on genetic engineering (President's Commission for the Study of Ethical Problems in Medicine and Biomedical and Behavioral Research, 1983). The commission entertained the concerns of theologians and religious leaders about the aims of genetic engineering and its ultimate effects on human life and on societies. Yet the final report termed the theological concerns "vague" and focused on more concrete problems (e.g., creating animal-human hybrids) that the theological objections could not definitively resolve. Thus the concerns that the creation of new life forms oversteps the boundaries of prudence and humility, or that the poor are being left behind in the development of genetic technologies, are left out of the final reckoning of the ethics and legality of genetic engineering.[19] Evans maintains that more recent debates over cloning have served to consolidate the formal rationality of "bioethics" and to further eliminate "thick" traditions and perspectives on the larger ends of biomedicine from public debate. Instead, autonomy has become an unexamined end in itself, and few if any limits have been imposed by law or regulation on the adventures of science.[20]

As a result of theologians' infatuation with public influence, it would seem, they capitulated to a procedural bioethics that reduced all substantive moral values to autonomy and informed consent. Some even see theological bioethics as having "sold out" to the gatekeepers of thin, abstract bioethics debate. As a result, theology lost its power to identify, expose, and challenge social problems stemming from the misuse of medicine and technology. For example, while theological bioethicists have joined the cause of individual autonomy, health care dollars are increasingly directed away from underserved populations; scientists and investors proceed with threats to "human dignity," such as stem cell research and human cloning, anticipating profit-making benefits for the wealthy.

While it is true that many liberal and progressive theologians have backed away from public religious arguments, it is not true that the discourse they have joined is neutral. In fact, it is governed by the values of individualism, science, technology, the market, and profits. By not engaging these other value traditions from the standpoint of their own distinctive commitment to justice and the common good, theologians fail to make any great impact on cultural norms.

The challenge to theology is to recover its religiously distinctive prophetic voice and enter into policy debates as an energetic adversary of the liberal consensus. Theologians ought to stick to their own convictions, remain unapologetically theological in orientation, while still seeking common cause and building a common language with all who are similarly committed to health care justice.

Theological bioethicists, including those backing progressive social causes, must reassert their religious identity while not giving up moral credibility and social impact. Theologians searching for a new model of thinking

15. See Tom L. Beauchamp and James P. Childress, *Principles of Biomedical Ethics,* 5th ed. (Oxford, UK: Oxford University Press, 2001). The first edition of this work appeared in 1979. (See n. 16.)

16. John H. Evans, *Playing God? Human Genetic Engineering and the Rationalization of Public Bioethics Debate* (Chicago: University of Chicago Press, 2002), 88. These four principles were first given a philosophical explanation and defense in Beauchamp's and Childress's *Principles of Biomedical Ethics* (1979), which has subsequently seen five editions. However, they had been earlier articulated as principles for public policy at a conference convened in 1974 by the National Commission for the Protection of Human Subjects of Behavioral and Biomedical Research (created by Congress in 1973). This conference or "retreat" issued recommendations in the form of the 1978 *Belmont Report,* named after the conference center, Belmont House. The report was submitted to the Department of Health, Education, and Welfare, which adopted it as public law governing federally funded research. (See Evans, *Playing God?,* 83-89; and Callahan, "Religion and the Secularization of Bioethics," S3.)

17. John Rawls, *A Theory of Justice* (Cambridge, MA: Harvard University Press, 395-99; see also Rawls, *Political Liberalism* (New York: Columbia University Press, 1993), 178-95.

18. Rawls, *Theory of Justice,* 396.

19. Evans, *Playing God,* 127-31.

20. Ibid., 158-65.

bioethically should recall postmodernism's insight that even abstract and supposedly universal principles always come to be articulated out of particular and historical communities of practice and discernment. Every political value system or agenda has a past, a context, and a set of investments, whether it be liberal democracy, the scientific research imperative, free market economics, communitarianism, or socialism.

On the one hand, contextuality may limit the applicability range of values and principles. But on the other hand, the practical context is what gives the principles "legs." Context-generated moral insights and proposals can gain a public hearing if they can prove themselves relevant and useful in the various contexts that together make up the common good of interest to the public in question. "Particularistic" references to the originating context need not be abandoned, though they should be introduced with respect for interlocutors and their differences. Conversation partners from other contexts may find these illuminating in light of shared values and commitments and especially in light of the immediate practical contexts of problem solving and decision making that bring the different traditions together around a common need or goal.

Jeffrey Stout has recommended to theologians a style of "immanent criticism" that "claims no privileged vantage point above the fray."[21] This type of social criticism can still manage to unite "people with diverging conceptions of the good to identify the same moral problems and collaborate in common concern," working within "specific social practices and institutions."[22] Sometimes shared problems and the need for mutually agreeable resolutions can lead people toward consensus about the good life and just social relationships, even when their theoretical or conceptual frameworks do not seem to converge. Theological claims, arguments, and conclusions in bioethics are not primarily intellectual products to be deployed scientifically. They are tradition-based and contextual strategies for uniting and concretizing a number of concerns and goals having to do with biomedical trends and behavior patterns. Theories of bioethics have to be understood in relation to the social worlds of their origin; likewise, their public influence depends on the social responses they can generate. The field of such responses is not limited to legislation and public commissions; it extends to nearly every corner of civil society.

Theological Bioethics: Public and Socially Engaged

A premise of [my] book is that "theological bioethics" is not so nerveless and enervated an enterprise as some of its critics make out, nor is it as marginal to current biomedical practice and policy as some imply. The real conflict is not between "thin" and "thick" moral languages and views of the good, but between competing "thick" worldviews and visions of intimacy, complete with concepts of sin and salvation, good and evil, saints and sinners, liturgies and moral practices. Several theologians on a spectrum seek a middle path between a seemingly "secular" voice for bioethics that essentially capitulates to the liberal market ethos of modern Western democracies and a richer, more nuanced discourse that coheres with communal religious identities but seems to become less compelling in the public sphere.[23] The impact and potential of theological bioethics can only be seen and appreciated if one's vision is broadened beyond the realms of academia and high-level government regulation. Although these are the spheres in which early bioethics made its name, today they do little to deter the profit-driven race for biotech innovation. The reality of theological bioethics certainly includes scholarship and policy, but its roots and much of its potential influence lie in broader and deeper networks that can exert pressure on research science, health care policy, and biotech investment.

Evans's ideal, for which he believes the prospects to be bleak, is for citizens to listen to professional debates about genetic engineering, take their concerns back to their "thick" communities of belief and value, and then bring the "demands" of their group regarding ends "to the public's elected officials."[24] Evans cites the burgeoning "participatory democracy" literature to bolster his case.[25] In my view, Evans is on the right track in suggesting that greater public participation in bioethical debates would more fully engage the members of religious traditions and other groups whose perspectives do not find a comfortable home in the discourse of "professional" bioethics. I also affirm his interest in maintaining a vital connection between faith communities and public policy. For national commissions, for example, to be truly democratic and representative, they would need to enact much more aggressive and broad-reaching mechanisms to engage the publics they supposedly address or represent. Rather than providing "expert" answers, they should be setting agendas for further public debate and acquiring legitimacy by connecting with "broad, ground-level forms of moral discourse" and "the practical con-

21. Jeffrey Stout, *Ethics after Babel: The Languages of Morals and Their Discontents* (Boston: Beacon Press, 1988), 282 and 283, respectively.

22. Ibid., 284 and 285, respectively.

23. David H. Smith, "Religion and the Roots of the Bioethics Revival," in Verhey, *Religion and Medical Ethics,* 2-18; Gustafson, *Intersections: Science, Theology, and Ethics;* Gustafson, "Styles of Religious Reflection in Medical Ethics," in *Religion and Medical Ethics,* ed. Verhey, 81-95; Reich, "New Era for Bioethics," 96-115; Richard A. McCormick, "Theology and Bioethics: Christian Foundations," in *Theology and Bioethics: Exploring the Foundations and Frontiers,* ed. Earl Shelp (Dordrecht, Neth.: Kluwer, 1986), 95-113; and Cahill, *Bioethics and the Common Good.*

24. Evans, *Playing God,* 197.

25. He cites the groundbreaking work of Amy Gutmann and Dennis Thompson, *Democracy and Disagreement* (Cambridge, MA: Harvard University Press, 1996).

texts of moral decision-making faced by most Americans."[26] These contexts will often or even usually involve religious experiences, values, practices, and theological explanations. But broad consultation and public legitimacy are very unevenly represented in national commissions to date.

Hence it is striking that Evans and other critics of the secularization of bioethics keep their gaze so firmly fixed on governmental bodies such as public commissions, regulatory agencies, and legislatures. Not only are the decisions and policies of such bodies the ultimate target of influence, but they are also expected to play a major role in the reinvigoration of the discourses that they are claimed to have suppressed. No wonder Evans's expectation of change is modest. And Evans is not alone; in fact, he represents the general assumptions of most of the literature on theology, bioethics, and policy.[27]

In an interesting discussion of John Evans's book, several theologians express varying levels of displeasure and dismay at his analysis of their "public" marginalization. Nevertheless, they fall into line behind the "thin" and "thick" distinctions with which Evans frames his characterization of the public and "religious" spheres and proceeds to argue that theologians are not taken seriously in the former.[28] On closer inspection, though, the description given by some of the theologians of what their work actually does militates against an easy distinction between "thin" public and "thick" religious discourse. It also tacitly links public and religious-theological discourse to practical settings and interests that are complex and interactive.

This is especially true of the interventions of Gilbert Meilaender and James Childress, both of whom have served on presidential and governmental policy bodies (in Childress's case, quite a number).[29] Meilaender seems to accept the "story line" Evans has plotted, in which advisory commissions have moved from substantive to formal rationality. Yet Evans and Meilaender both agree that advisory commissions were created in the first place "as a device to keep science free of regulation" by funneling ethical concerns through professional bioethicists who would keep their sights narrowly set on a few basic principles and not raise any radical questions about "scientific" objectives.[30] This description of the practical activities of bioethics commissions — their membership, their language, and their ritual hearings — should be enough to at least raise the suspicion that their public discourse is not as "thin" as one might suppose.

Indeed, Jeffrey Stout characterizes most such commissions as "the modern, bureaucratic equivalent of feudal councils, with professionals in place of noblemen."[31] A few further questions from Stout bring home the fact that theologians can become involved in languages, symbolic occasions, and social practices that are quite "thick," if not "theological," when they take on the role of bioethicist for "governments, courts, hospitals, universities, and the press. 'What sort of expertise or authority is one claiming to have when one accepts these roles? Who is supposed to defer to the ethicist's findings and for what reasons? What sort of society are we becoming complicit in when we encourage our fellow citizens to defer to our alleged expertise?'"[32] Stout seems fairly convinced of the pernicious effect of bioethical expertise on the theologian, as it works toward the submergence of the exercise of theological ethics in the practices and languages of foreign institutions.

This does not have to be the case. A theological bioethicist may enter the practice and the "thick" multilayered discourse of the hospital, the court, or the government commission. Still, as a theologian, he or she can and should remember to exercise the critical functions of the worldview, symbols, and distinctive practices that he or she brings to each setting and not become overwhelmed by the dominant (and "thick") discourse that typically controls there. Theological bioethics will represent and lift up for attention and endorsement a variety of alternative discourses and practices concerning health and biomedicine that have an impact on the same areas of life that policymakers envision in a more top-down manner.

James Childress warns Evans and others not to underplay the role and effect that theology has had in shaping

26. Albert W. Dzur and Daniel Levin, "The 'Nation's Conscience': Assessing Bioethics Commissions as Public Forums," *Kennedy Institute of Ethics Journal* 14, no. 4 (2004): 351.

27. Mark Hanson concludes his Introduction to a set of Hastings Center papers on the engagement of religious groups and theologians with the critics of gene patenting and cloning with the observation that "policy discourse was impoverished by an inability to accommodate religious insights in productive ways." Mark J. Hanson, ed., *Claiming Power over Life: Religion and Biotechnology Policy* (Washington, DC: Georgetown University Press, 2001), x. In the same volume Courtney Campbell rightly urges religious thinkers and communities to put up "meaningful resistance" to the dominant focus on autonomy, but envisions the audience of such appeals primarily as "public policy" and "the policy process." Campbell, "Meaningful Resistance: Religion and Biotechnology," in *Claiming Power over Life, Religion and Biotechnology Policy,* ed. Hanson, 26. The identification and development of other avenues of religious and theological influence on social practices is important. In the same volume, Andrew Lustig and Audrey Chapman push further in this direction. Lustig, "Human Cloning and Liberal Neutrality: Why We Need to Broaden the Public Dialogue," in *Claiming Power over Life: Religion and Biotechnology Policy,* ed. Hanson, 30-52; Chapman, "Religious Perspectives on Biotechnology," in *Claiming Power over Life: Religion and Biotechnology Policy,* ed. Hanson, 112-43.

28. John H. Evans, "John H. Evans Responds," *Journal of the Society of Christian Ethics* 24, no. 1 (2004): 216.

29. Meilaender serves on the PCB. Childress has served on NBAC (1996-2001), as well as on the Human Fetal Transplantation Research panel, the National Organ Transplantation Task Force, and the Recombinant DNA Advisory Committee.

30. Gilbert Meilaender, "Comments of Gilbert Meilaender," *Journal of the Society of Christian Ethics* 24, no. 1 (2004): 192.

31. Jeffrey Stout, "Comments of Jeffrey Stout," *Journal of the Society of Christian Ethics* 24, no. 1 (2004): 190.

32. Ibid.

"the public culture," presumably beyond or below the "thin" air of policy advisory bodies.[33] Moreover, he believes that theologians have been influential even in the latter, pointing as evidence to the theologian members of these bodies and to testimony given by theologians. However, the issue for theological bioethics is the dominant language of the "practice" of advisory commissions — rights, autonomy, and cost-benefit ratios stated in terms of demonstrable harm or risk. This practice-embedded language can govern debates about reproduction, health care, and research in a way that drowns out talk about who has access, who will benefit, and who will profit from any given option or innovation, as well as about practical ways to change the status quo without waiting for formal policy adjustments. The language and practices of modern science, market economics, and liberal individualism are generally unreceptive to consideration of distributive justice and a "preferential option for the poor."

Evans's view that (liberal) theologians are not taken seriously on public commissions is really a way of saying that the practices represented by the commissions and their members have by and large been able to edge out practical and verbal challenges from the theologians invited to participate, especially if they threaten scientific privilege, profits, or the freedom of those who already have control of the resources. One reason some politically conservative varieties of bioethics (e.g., against abortion and stem cell research) have enjoyed more political success in recent years is that they have been abetted by effective grassroots organizing and networking among organizations. But another reason is that they pose little serious challenge to neoliberal economic policies, to the idea that health care should go to those who can pay for it, or even to the idea that any research that can make a profit should be allowed. For instance, even "conservative" policies about *federal* funding of stem cell research in no way limit the freedom of *private* corporations to create, buy, use, or destroy embryos. . . .

Participatory Theological Bioethics: A Proposal

We have seen that, while theologians such as James Gustafson, Paul Ramsey, and Richard McCormick were active and influential in the emergence of bioethics as a field, their counterparts in the next generation of scholars have sometimes struggled to gain a voice in the public sphere. Theological bioethicists have been criticized for having yielded the floor of public debate to a thin, secular, philosophical discourse that excludes and demeans theology and that is incapable of a truly prophetic or transforming contribution to health care, health policy, or research ethics.

On the other hand, the election of George W. Bush as U.S. president in 2000 (and for a second term in 2004) brought into power a leader who is an avowed evangelical Christian and who specifically invoked divine guidance and religious imagery in pursuing his domestic and international policies. His administration is generally viewed as being under the influence of the bioethical concerns and values of the so-called religious right.[34] Bush's reelection showed that many in the American mainstream were at least open to religious influences on the public life of the country. Bush supporters sought to appoint Supreme Court justices who favored modification or reversal of the permissive abortion policy established by *Roe v. Wade,* sought to severely limit federal funding of embryonic stem cell research, and sought to define marriage legally and constitutionally as a union between a man and a woman, with a concomitant curtailment of protections and benefits for same-sex unions. The Bush administration did not seek to extend universal health care coverage to all members of U.S. society or to raise its level of support for the fight against worldwide "diseases of the poor" to the levels achieved by other wealthy societies.[35] The Bush campaigns and reelection show that religious denominations and theologians can have a public voice. But not all varieties of theological bioethics are equal either in effectiveness or in moral values and outcomes.

Effectiveness requires both the deployment of a vocabulary and imagery with broad cultural appeal and the cultivation of grassroots practices and communities that display and reinforce that imagery. For instance, early in the 2004 election season, evangelical political organizers were already appearing in local congregations in Oregon, Michigan, Montana, Arkansas, and Ohio to collect signatures for state ballot measures against their signature issue, gay marriage.[36] Progressive activists, who were much more interested than the religious right in health care reform, typically tried to advance this and other goals through the national media, national figures, and publications aimed at a college-educated public. In so doing, they failed to engage religious values and theological interpretations to the degree necessary to advance this goal culturally and win votes. According to Jim Wallis, the 2004 campaign showed that the politically conservative "moral values" agenda virtually excluded

33. James Childress, "Comments of James Childress," *Journal of the Society of Christian Ethics* 24, no. 1 (2004): 200.

34. This is confirmed by the fact that Bush's reelection was perceived by Christian conservatives as vindication of their social goals and as an encouragement to push forward with state and local initiatives on same-sex marriage, public education, and abortion. See Neela Banarjee, "Christian Conservatives Press Issues in Statehouses," *New York Times,* December 13, 2004, A18.

35. In 2005, the United States gave 15 hundredths of 1 percent to foreign aid, the smallest percentage among major donor countries. See Celia W. Dogger, "U.N. Proposes Doubling of Aid to Cut Poverty," *New York Times,* January 18, 2005, A6. See also a U.N. Millennium Project report on global poverty, *Investing in Development,* released in January 2005, at www.unmillenniumproject.org

36. Sarah Linn, "Gay-'marriage' foe takes petition to churches," *Washington Times,* June 19, 2004, C10.

the issue of poverty, to which the Bible devotes thousands of verses. On the other hand, "Democrats seem uncomfortable with the language of faith and values, preferring in recent decades the secular approach of restricting such matters to the private sphere." He asks, "Where would we be if Martin Luther King Jr. had kept his faith to himself?"[37]

As [my] next chapter discusses, progressive causes have been advanced successfully under religious and theological auspices in the past, and positive examples can be found today, especially in the realm of Catholic health care institutions, advocacy, and moral theology. However, such measures are underrecognized and underutilized in the preponderance of theological scholarship in bioethics. Theological bioethics should strengthen already existing practices "on the ground" and broaden and deepen the vocabulary of solidarity and care of neighbor, both religiously and by appeal to shared political traditions.

I propose an alternative understanding of public theological bioethics, as *participatory*. Participatory theological bioethics operates simultaneously in many spheres of discourse and activity, from which it is possible to affect the social relationships and institutions that govern health care. Participatory theological bioethics can be either conservative or progressive, right or left, pro-life or pro-choice, market oriented or social-welfare oriented, or some combination of any of these. In my view, the promotion of progressive causes in bioethics through grassroots organizing, participation in the networks of civil society, and the partnering of explicitly religious and faith-based organizations with counterparts from other religious or nonreligious counterparts has been underappreciated.

What Is "the Public Sphere"?

It is a mistake to think that the "public sphere" is a sphere of argument and debate rather than action and that, when public debate does occur, it has legitimacy only when participants engage one another in respectful yet emotionally detached rational argument, offering warrants that are "secular," pragmatic, and nonparticularistic, and, where possible, empirically sustained. The public sphere so defined is inhabited largely by experts and elites. By lamenting their exclusion from this sphere, theologians tacitly validate its authority and importance in defining health care ethics and in constituting the "public" arena above all others in which it is crucial to be heard.

The notion of the public sphere must be reenvisaged to include action as well as argument and to include integral reference to the contexts and interests of those communicating within it. A definition of the public sphere by Charles Taylor serves as a useful point of departure, because it both embodies standard assumptions about the legitimacy of public debates and implies the need for a different approach.

> What do I mean by a *public sphere?* I want to describe it as a common space in which the members of society are deemed to meet through a variety of media: print, electronic, and also face-to-face encounters; to discuss matters of common interest; and thus to be able to form a common mind about these.[38]

Taylor goes on to specify that the common space of discussion that makes up the public sphere is "nonlocal" or "metatopical"; that it is "extrapolitical" or "not an exercise of power"; and that it is "secular" or having to do with "profane," historical time rather than a transcendent realm.[39]

Like many others, Taylor tends to envision the arena of public exchanges as a metaphorical "space," above and beyond the realities of ordinary life and beyond the particular interests and relationships that have created the identities of the conversation partners. But, in fact, parties to public debate continue to participate in the practices and purposes of their lives, including "local" and "transcendent" ones, even as they interact with others about the meaning and goals of practices and interests they share in common. This is indeed implied by Taylor's references to necessary "media" of communication to bridge locations, as well as by the fact that "matters of common interest" engage those who join in the conversation. Matters of common interest exist and come into focus if and when the debaters share practical concerns — when they come together in certain communities, identities, practices, interests, goals, or fears, even as they retain differences in others.

The factor left out in Taylor's definition, then, is that the common meeting space of society's members is filled not only by "discoursing" individuals in the abstract but also by the intersecting groups to which they belong — families, neighborhoods, churches, ethnic groups, age cohorts, political parties, citizens groups, sports teams, schools, professions, types or sites of employment, and more. No individual enters in disconnection from the communities of belonging and worldview formation that are constitutive for his or her particularity and agency. Moreover, it is precisely converging communities and identities that bring people together around "public" concerns. Mediating between individuals and the public sphere and lending coherence to social agency are insti-

37. Jim Wallis, "'After the Election . . .': Neither Republicans nor Democrats Have a Clue," *Boston Theological Institute Newsletter* 34, no. 19 (2005): 1-2. See also Jim Wallis, *God's Politics: Why the Right Gets It Wrong and the Left Doesn't Get It* (San Francisco, CA: HarperSanFrancisco, 2005).

38. Charles Taylor, "Politics and the Public Sphere," in *New Communitarian Thinking: Persons, Virtues, Institutions, and Communities*, ed. Amitai Etzioni (Charlottesville: University Press of Virginia, 1995), 85-86,

39. Ibid., 190-96.

tutions. Institutions are patterns of social relationship that give normative definition to practices, structure experience, and shape individual character and commitments. Practices and institutions make up the infrastructure of society and are a necessary component of the public sphere.[40]

While the common space evoked by Taylor may be "metatopical" in that it is not limited to participants in any one place, the identities of participants and their concrete conditions of participation bring a variety of physical and social locations into the mix. The public sphere is never outside of or immune to the dialectics of power. Although the common space may not be identified with any one manifestation of institutionalized political power or government, the participants in discourse will have differentials of influence along a number of different axes — income, education, race, gender, age, profession — and so will the practices and institutions in which they participate. The public sphere is a space in which power is exercised and mediated, resulting both in conflict and in shifting equilibria. Although the public sphere may not be the one in which transcendent meaning is most directly addressed, the individuals and groups coming into it will often if not always integrate their actions and expressions with a grounding view of the human condition that refers to ultimate origins or purposes.[41]

The narrow, liberal understanding of what makes up public discourse deters theologians and others from appreciating the integral relation of public ethical debates to practices and institutions. Ethical arguments and their ability to persuade are rooted in and rely on such practices, not just on intellectual cogency and verbal rhetoric. In fact, the debate over whether religious discourse should be "allowed" into the public sphere is virtually beside the point, given that religious persons, groups, and institutions have always interacted on myriad levels with other actors, dialectically constituting the playing field on which cultural interactions about uses and abuses of modern biomedical science take place. All these agents contribute to a common discourse, and potentially to the development of consensuses, by acting individually and collectively, as well as by speaking in public. More socially conservative bioethics grasps the political potential of activism and works hard to reinforce, heighten, and extend the kind of specifically religious identity that provides thick opposition to abortion and the destruction of embryos. Socially progressive theological bioethicists, on the other hand, who see the "secular political sphere" as the important sphere of influence, tend to overlook the potentially expansive appeal of religious symbols and especially to neglect the opportunities for cooperative action and collective power that civil society provides.

The real issue is which tradition has priority, precedence, and presumed authority within the patterns of social exchange about ethics and ethical behavior. The three main contenders in twenty-first-century postindustrial societies are science, economics, and liberalism. Theological bioethics should and can confront these thick traditions with persuasive counterstrategies, symbolic systems, and narratives, as well as with ethical "reasons." The challenge before theologians is not to cast aside a thin discourse for a richer one, but to dislodge the thick discourses that are so widely entrenched that their constituting narratives and practices are no longer directly observed.

Although socially conservative bioethics rightly fights the instrumentalization and commercialization of innocent or vulnerable life (even in its earliest and last stages), merely defending the rights of embryos, fetuses, the handicapped, or the comatose does not do enough to counteract the individualism of health care in this country or, increasingly, worldwide. It also does not offer a strong enough and broad enough challenge to a general "medicalization" and "technologization" of human life and human problems, advanced by the worship of modern science or of the profits it brings.

"Thick" Traditions: Science, Economics, Liberalism

The quasi-religious overtones of scientific ideals and the quest for scientific knowledge have been identified before. Carolyn Merchant was one of the first to search out the religious motivations behind Francis Bacon's drive to restore "man's" dominion over nature for the sake of the human race, and so to redeem humanity from the consequences of the Fall.[42] Geneticists have described the genome as "the 'Bible,' the 'Book of Man,' and the 'Holy Grail,'" viewing it as a "sacred text" with great explanatory power and even as "the secular equivalent of the human Soul."[43] Opponents of genetic engineering are thus cast as the enemies of human self-transcendence. Andrew Lustig notes that in debates about cloning, ostensibly nonreligious and explicitly religious arguments for and against cloning can function in analogous ways, placing aesthetic and moral concerns against a backdrop of ultimate meaning.[44] Lustig's main point is to show that

40. William M. Sullivan, "Institutions as the Infrastructure of Democracy," in *New Communitarian Thinking,* ed. Etzioni, 175.

41. According to Nicholas Wolterstorff, a good number of citizens exercise their religious convictions and identities by basing their contributions to political issues on them, whether they are directly expressed or not. Hence the "liberal" idea of a religion-free zone is unworkable and unfair. Wolterstorff, "The Role of Religion in Political Issues," in *Religion in the Public Square: The Place of Religious Convictions in Political Debate,* Robert Audi and Nicholas Wolterstorff (Lanham, MD: Rowman & Littlefield, 1997), 77.

42. Carolyn Merchant, *The Death of Nature: Women, Ecology and the Scientific Revolution* (San Francisco, CA: Harper and Row, 1980), 164-71.

43. Dorothy Nelkin and M. Susan Lindee, *The DNA Mystique: The Gene as a Cultural Icon* (New York: W. H. Freeman and Co., 1995), 39, 198.

44. Lustig, "Human Cloning and Liberal Neutrality: Why We Need to Broaden the Public Dialogue," in *Claiming Power over Life: Religion and Biotechnology Policy,* ed. M. J. Hanson, 33-36.

religious objections to cloning can converge with secular concerns, helping to build consensus. I want also to stress that "secular" justifications of cloning and other genetic techniques often rely on the same kind of framework of transcendence that backs religious arguments but that is labeled unacceptable if put forward in explicitly religious or theological terms.

Science is not the only symbol system of ultimacy, morality, and meaning competing to define the cultural role of the new genetics. Ronald Cole-Turner astutely noted a decade ago that genetic engineering "involves nations, corporations, individual researchers, investors, and consumers" and thus "cannot be said to serve the interests of humanity" as such, as is so often claimed.[45] Cole-Turner's concern is that it would be naïve for theologians to accept the eschatology of genetics, in which the new knowledge serves the future of humanity as a species. But his observation also exhibits why neither beneficence nor the quest for scientific knowledge fully accounts for the direction, claims, and power of the new genomics. New discoveries and patented techniques for cloning, genetic testing, and pharmacogenomics promise prestige for researchers and profits for biotech corporations, pharmaceutical companies, and even research universities. The mystique of science is reinforced and perhaps even co-opted by the ideology of market capitalism as the driving force of liberal democracy's global expansion.

Biotechnology is big business, and industry advocates present it as having a moral role in shaping humanity's future. According to the Biotechnology Industry Organization's (BIO) website, BIO is the "largest trade organization to serve and represent the emerging biotechnology industry in the United States and around the globe." As envisioned by this self-defined "leading voice for the biotechnology industry," "biotechnology's future is bright." BIO's website assures visitors that its "leadership and service-oriented guidance have helped advance the industry and bring the benefits of biotechnology to the people of the world."[46] BIO's projects in 2003 (the fiftieth anniversary of the discovery of DNA) included an ad campaign to guarantee that pharmaceutical companies would be paid for drugs for the elderly, under Medicare, to support President George W. Bush's assertion that genetically modified foods can help end hunger in the third world (not displace subsistence farming and create dependency on corporate seed manufacturers, as critics claim), and to celebrate the "modern era of molecular biology" in which the initiative and creativity of scientists have led to the industry's profitable yet humanitarian endeavors. In a publicity statement, BIO president Carl B. Feldbaum celebrates the sacred traditions, search for ultimate meaning, salvific potential, humanistic ethic, and saints of genetic science:

> No doubt in another 50 years we will look back in wonder at just how much suffering will have been alleviated through a chain of events that began in the early 1950s with a couple of scientists looking for "the secret of life" in X-ray diffraction photos and ball-and-stick chemical models.[47]

Unfortunately, according to Dan Eramian, BIO's vice president for communications, "some in the religious community," including "fundamentalists" and "radical anti-abortionists," are trying to "obstruct attempts to further embryo cloning and stem cell research in the United States." Interference would undermine the lead such research has already achieved, thanks to a government that "pumps millions of dollars into basic research." That would mean disaster for the country's biotechnology industry, because the "largest pharmaceutical companies . . . have continued to partner with biotechnology companies to develop new drugs based on this [stem cell] science." Eramian calls for "dialogue" with religious representatives as part of a program to "manage controversy" and permit research, development, marketing, and sales to go forward.[48] The implication is that, while religious objections to BIO's investment agenda are obstructionist and irrational, BIO's advocacy for research dollars is unbiased and backed by sound data.

In a functionalist view at least, this is not a competition between religion and a "secular," "scientific," or "business" worldview, but a contest between missionary agendas. It has been argued that the most powerful explanation of the world is science; the most attractive value system, consumerism; the largest religious denomination, "our" economic system; the theology in service of that religion, the discipline of economics; and the god whom all serve, the market.[49] Traditional religions have been deplorably unable to offer "a meaningful challenge to the aggressive proselytizing of market capitalism, which has already become the most successful religion of all time, winning more converts more quickly than any previous belief system or value-system in human history."[50] The appeal of this new religion lies in its promise of salvation from human unhappiness through commodities, a promise that can never be fulfilled even for the few who enjoy the ability to purchase almost unlimited quantities.

Theological critics likewise have unveiled the "religion of the market" in ways that are instructive for bioethics. The vitality of this religion depends on several myths, nicely laid out in a critique of globalization by

45. Ronald Cole-Turner, *The New Genesis: Theology and the Genetic Revolution* (Louisville, KY: Westminster/John Knox Press, 1993), 54.

46. See the BIO website, www.bio.org.

47. Statement by BIO president Carl B. Feldbaum, Washington, DC, April 14, 2003, PRNewswire, retrieved from www.bio.org.

48. Dan Eramian, "Stem Cell Research: The Dialogue between Biotechnology and Religion," speech delivered during "Managing Controversy in Science and Health" at the Global Public Affairs Institute, Dublin, Ireland, May 7, 2002, retrieved front www.bio.org.

49. David R. Loy, "The Religion of the Market," *Journal of the American Academy of Religion* 65, no. 2 (1997): 275.

50. Ibid., 276.

Cynthia Moe-Lobeda.[51] First, growth benefits all. The way to growth is through free trade and investment, which in turn lead to greater economic well-being for everyone. The fallacies within the myth are that economic activity translates into social and cultural health; that economic growth brings general welfare, regardless of income distribution; and that the environment and future generations can sustain the costs of current growth. Second, freedom means the right to own and dispose of private property. This notion of freedom disregards the impact of market freedom on the limits posed to human freedom by deprivation of basic necessities for those who cannot find a reliable livelihood, compete in the market, or accumulate property. It also disregards the fact that, especially in a globalized economy, most market exchanges are not "voluntary." Most important, freedom as market freedom dismisses or represses other notions of freedom, including the freedom to participate in a community that includes the common good of all.

Third, the religion of the market depends on the myth that human beings are essentially autonomous agents, who find ultimate fulfillment in acting individually or by contract to maximize self-interest, with "self-interest" defined in terms of acquisition and consumption. Like the previous myth, this one eliminates aspects of life in community and in solidarity with others that most religious and cultural traditions have defined as fundamental. It "dehumanizes" the human and subjects the less competitive to the more competitive and dominating persons, groups, and economies. Fourth, and most dangerously for the fate of theological bioethics, is the myth that market expansion and the growth of transnational corporations (including the major pharmaceutical companies) is inevitable and "evolutionary, a contemporary form of manifest destiny, a step in modernity's march of progress."[52] On the contrary, the market economy can be resisted and changed, both locally and internationally, as can a rapidly globalizing biotech industry.

Along with the "religions" of science and market capitalism, the traditions, symbols, and practices of liberal individualism provide a framework of meaning and transcendence that deserve a challenge from theology. Liberal philosophy and politics are even more deeply entrenched in the U.S. cultural ethos than science and the market and much more explicitly linked to claims of "ultimacy." Liberalism provides a rationale for the ways in which the science and economics of health care and research are institutionalized and discussed. Liberalism, "the political theory of modernity," begins from the proposition that persons have different conceptions of the good life that cannot be reconciled without violence. They therefore must be accommodated within a rational legal system that favors none and allows all to flourish. Hence, a key liberal value is "tolerance." Classical liberalism upholds a political order that aims to ameliorate the human condition "by the peaceful competition of different traditions." According to defenders of liberalism, "the classical liberal advocacy of the free market is, in effect, only an application in the sphere of economic life of the conviction that human society is likely to do best when men are left free to enact their plans of life unconstrained except by the rule of law."[53] Liberalism, in other words, is not in reality "neutral," "pluralistic," or even "tolerant." Its core value — individual freedom — is a foundational dogma that is highly intolerant of any limits imposed for the sake of marginal persons or the common good.

Liberalism is strangely oblivious, for a theory of political economy, of the effects that differences in economic and social class will have on basic material and social goods and hence on the ability of citizens to "enact their life plans." Thus liberalism as a philosophy and political theory has been attacked from almost too many directions to enumerate: Marxist, feminist, liberationist, and more. Its continuing hold on the North American imagination and culture is partly explained by our founding myths of independence and partly by the strength of the economic interests with which liberalism is symbiotic. Yet the irreversible reign of liberal autonomy within the market, within science, and within health care is another myth that can be uncovered. The narratives, moralities, liturgies, and institutions created by the religion of liberal democratic capitalism can be challenged and perhaps reformed.

Each of these cultural traditions owes its strength partly to an important value it advances: the power of science to illumine the world we live in and avoid some of its dangers, the usefulness of efficient production to maximize quantity and circulation of goods, and the recognition of the intrinsic value of every individual person as well as the importance of respecting differences. However, all of these values can be and are distorted by social, political, and economic systems that give only some people access to their promised benefits or rights, then permit the privileged few to have unbalanced power over the well-being of those who are excluded.

Because of their positive value, all of these traditions have been adapted to some extent and in a variety of ways by bioethicists. Among them, liberalism has seemed the most favorable to bioethicists seeking to modify health care and biotechnology in order to reflect the needs of those who are excluded from present systems. Liberalism seems to offer a theory that coincides with basic cultural values (in the United States at least), that allows for the interaction of different parties in a spirit of mutual respect, and that is premised on equality. Some philosophical theories of bioethics adapt the liberal principles of John Rawls in a way that affirms the basic good of health care as a good in which all members of so-

51. Cynthia Moe-Lobeda, *Healing a Broken World: Globalization and God* (Minneapolis, MN: Fortress Press, 2002), 48-65.

52. Ibid., 62.

53. John Gray, *Liberalism* (Minneapolis: University of Minnesota Press, 1986), 90-91.

ciety have a right to participate.[54] From a common good point of view, such theories are welcome challenges to a culturally widespread attitude that individuals and families need be morally concerned only about their own access. However, even modified liberalism in health care ethics tends to accept the status quo of modern medical technology and to limit its critical analysis of market-based health care to "our own" society.

For example, an important book on new innovations in genetics uses a Rawlsian framework to urge that health care is a basic primary good that should be provided to all, insofar as it is a prerequisite of normal human functioning.[55] However, when the analysis reaches the point of recognizing that newly developed techniques for modifying genes will almost certainly be used by wealthy consumers to their own advantage, the book's authors incredibly propose that some day gene modifications will be available to all as part of a "basic package" of health care.[56] The weakness of this suggestion lies in the fact that it is advanced more or less within the same cultural parameters that have created exclusive health care institutions and is directed theoretically to philosophers involved in or analyzing national policy discourse in "a liberal society." There is little or no practical incentive for those now benefiting from the system to change the access patterns; those lacking access have little power to make sure their needs are represented. Under these circumstances, health care resources will certainly continue to be allocated according to market advantage, while the "liberal" values of free choice and tolerance sidetrack any serious critique of the ways the choices of some constrain the biomedical realities of others.

Another work, by theologian Richard Miller, proposes that liberalism can serve as a useful "political theory," if not as a "comprehensive" one. Liberalism as a political tool permits theologians to join with others in provisionally setting aside "metaphysical claims" and "particular religious and philosophical doctrines."[57] They can then participate in a consensus about basic principles of fairness, including access to some primary goods. But the question is whether political liberalism actually leads to significant social changes that match these theoretical principles of justice. Although I affirm Miller's desire for consensus on basic goods, I question whether "thin" and "neutral" theorizing[58] can accomplish much change in institutions whose injustice feeds off the liberal groundbed of individual autonomy.

Miller's specific focus is the care of grievously ill and suffering children receiving treatment in an intensive care unit (ICU) in the United States. He sensitively and poignantly renders case studies and offers compassionate and persuasive moral analyses, given the parameters of critical care in major medical facilities. He modifies liberal autonomy to the extent that family privacy must be subject to the limiting criterion of the welfare of the child.[59] Miller also examines pressures on families to participate in drug trials for which pharmaceutical companies have a financial incentive, which suggests the larger problem of the interaction of medicine and business.[60] However, liberalism invoked as a "political theory" does not ultimately lead to more radical questions about why the many agonized children and families described are subjected to "aggressive" treatment rather than provided with hospice, about what happens to children and families without health insurance, or about why medical centers in North America institutionalize pediatric "intensive care" to excess, while millions of children perish worldwide from preventable diseases.

A much more direct, specific, and critical confrontation with liberal political philosophies, and the practices with which they are symbiotic, is necessary to achieve any real progress toward health care justice. Science, the market, and liberalism all underwrite their cultural status with ideologies of reasonableness and beneficence that conceal the harm and injustice perpetrated by their exaggerated and imperialistic forms, especially in terms of global health inequities. What is needed is a critique that creates or connects with alternative, subversive, or transformative practices, practices that go beyond academia and "official" policymakers.

Public Theological Bioethics

Theological bioethics is, then, not embedded in a free-standing religious "silo" from which it must struggle to be heard in a post-Christian, postreligious, "modern," and "secular" policy world, where the natural sciences and economics have claim to a more "objective," "inclusive," "persuasive," and publicly "appropriate" language. Science, economics, theology, and "liberal democratic" political norms all depend on analogous worldviews that define human nature, human meaning, human goods and goals, and the good society.[61] All invoke symbols of

54. See, e.g., Norman Daniels, *Just Health Care* (Cambridge: Cambridge University Press, 1985); and Richard B. Miller, *Children, Ethics and Modern Medicine* (Bloomington and Indianapolis: Indiana University Press, 2003).

55. Allen Buchanan, Dan W. Brock, Norman Daniels, and Daniel Winkler, *From Chance to Choice: Genetics and Justice* (Cambridge: Cambridge University Press, 2000), 80, 147, 314.

56. Ibid., 97-98.

57. Miller, *Children, Ethics, and Modern Medicine,* 123-25.

58. Ibid., 125

59. Ibid., 269, 274.

60. Ibid., 254.

61. Brian Stiltner argues that liberalism, feminism, communitarianism, and other "philosophical schools," such as religion and theology, make "substantive" and not merely procedural arguments and that these imply "comprehensive accounts of human beings and what is of value to them." Hence, all can and should contribute to policy formation, as part of the common good. Brian Stiltner, "Morality, Religion, and Public Bioethics: Shifting the Paradigm for the Public Discussion of Embryo Research and Human Cloning," in *Cloning and the Future of Human Embryo Research,* ed. Paul Lauritzen (Oxford: Oxford University Press,

ultimacy that capture the imagination, convert desires, direct practical reason, and motivate action. Perhaps even more important, these worldviews and symbols do more than inspire action consequently; they are themselves nourished and shaped by action continuously. Practices, institutions, moral orientations, and symbolic expressions are co-originate and interdependent.

Several years ago, Roger Shinn wrote that the formation of public policies on genetics necessarily represents an interaction of human values and faiths, scientific information and concepts, and political activity. Religious communities are part of the body politic, advocating their political convictions within the political process. They are especially committed to exposing ideological biases and to speak for "the oppressed and those too often despised by elites." The convictions of theologians seek and often find "wide resonance" in a pluralistic society, especially regarding the value of community and of freedom and the concern for justice.[62] Biomedicine, ethics, policy, religion, and theology engage one another in the public sphere in many more and deeper ways than the display of rational, verbal argumentation by individual spokespersons. Practices, institutions, and issue-oriented activism also make up the dialectical common space where bioethics is negotiated as theory, policy, and implementation.

For example, within bioethics, rights language comes from Western political and constitutional traditions, cost-benefit language comes from market economics, the research imperative comes from enlightenment science, and the call for scientific knowledge to be used for human benefit and the relief of suffering owes much to modern evolutionary views of society as well as modern democracy. The "preferential option for the poor" comes from religious traditions, is reflected in philosophical traditions about equal respect and solidarity, can be backed up by democratic politics, and has some roots in Karl Marx's critique of industrial capitalism and others in scripture.

Even religiously indebted images such as "care for the poor" or "we are all children of God" can stimulate the imaginations of those from diverse traditions so that common ground can be amplified. To the degree that any one image, story, moral principle, or concrete moral analysis can appeal to a variety of associational values and commitments, it can have a chance to influence public life by raising the profile of one pattern of associational behavior over another. For instance, when reformers call for universal access to health care over the present U.S. market-based system, they are appealing to fellow citizens to prioritize solidaristic experiences of social life over capitalism and class, and they can use many rhetorical and symbolic incentives to do this. Theological voices should not be ruled out of court simply because they emerge from traditions that are not completely shared by all other participants in civil society.

Five Modes of Discourse

Since the 1960s, virtually all bioethics has been dialectical in its stance toward society and public debate, rather than strictly autonomous or separationist or totally assimilated to and continuous with nonreligious worldviews and language. But theology moves into public bioethics in a variety of modes and languages. Theology's influence arises in large part from its ability to interface effectively with social problems (here, in biomedicine) that have been identified as important across a broad swath of society. James M. Gustafson has identified four varieties of moral discourse in which theology engages: ethical, policy, prophetic, and narrative.[63] I propose a fifth be added: participatory discourse. Although these are intertwined and have all been represented by theologians since the 1960s, the accent falls on different forms of discourse at different times and for different purposes.

First, the definitions. The aim of *ethical discourse* "is to decide how one ought to act in particular circumstances"[64] by finding moral justification linked to a basic theory of morality focused around such concepts as rights, duties, obligations, and justice. In a theological theory, these concepts will be interpreted in relation to a concept of God and God's purposes or claims regarding humanity. Ethical discourse also requires and relies on an interpretation of the circumstances of action, for instance, as provided by the natural and social sciences.

Policy discourse is closely related to ethical discourse. It involves decisions about what kinds of general practices, institutions, permissions, and constraints should guide social behavior or the behavior of individual agents within social institutions. Compared to ethical discourse, however, policy discourse is more driven by the need to acknowledge and accommodate to the conflicts and limitations inherent in any particular situation of decision. "The 'ought' questions are answered within possibilities and limitations of what resources exist or can be accumulated or organized."[65] Theology can bring to policy discourse a sense that all human enterprises are relative and marked by finitude and sinfulness. Theology can also further a commitment to prioritize and defend some basic values, such as the value of human life, the dignity of every person, and the obligation to advocate for those who are most vulnerable and those who suffer most. However,

2001), 184. Stiltner is right, but the resemblances among these approaches go beyond the kinds of contributions they make to philosophical argument, and the sphere of their influence goes beyond public policy in the narrow sense.

62. Roger Lincoln Shinn, *The New Genetics: Challenges for Science, Faith, and Politics* (Wakefield, RI: Moyer Bell, 1996), 92.

63. James M. Gustafson, *Varieties of Moral Discourse: Prophetic, Ethical, and Policy* (Grand Rapids, MI: Calvin College, 1988); and *Intersections.*

64. Gustafson, *Intersections,* 39.

65. Ibid., 54.

in a public policy setting, theologians will usually seek expressions of conviction that can communicate effectively with their interlocutors. Sometimes this includes explicitly religious stories or references; usually it does not.

A third type of discourse follows from the fact that theology, along with other value systems and outlooks, prioritizes certain values over others and attempts to see that these values are embodied in social practices and institutions. This is *prophetic discourse.* "Prophetic discourse is usually more general than ethical discourse and sometimes uses narratives to make prophetic points."[66] Prophetic discourse can also be used in a policy setting, although its aim is less to settle specific questions and more to widen horizons of vision. It takes the form either of indictment or of utopia (a visionary inspiration of human hopes and aspirations). Like the prophets of the Hebrew Bible, theological prophets today often forward a critique of economic systems that exclude the poor from basic goods such as health care. They combat an overly pragmatic and individualist approach to biomedical decision making and insist that not all human problems can be resolved by more technology. Though their utopia is ultimately eschatological, they hold up a vision of a more equitable society characterized by the virtues of solidarity and compassion and of justice inspired by love of God and neighbor. Narratives that might bring home these points include biblical accounts and stories, such as the ancient Israelite mandate to care for the widow and orphan (Isaiah 10:1-2), the Gospel of Matthew's parable of judgment (Matthew 25:31-46), or Luke's story of the Good Samaritan (Luke 10:25-37).

The fourth type of discourse uses such stories not just to make theological and ethical points but to form communities and persons in the virtues necessary to enact the points as ways of life. It is called *narrative discourse.* "Narratives function to sustain the particular moral identity of a religious (or secular) community by rehearsing its history and traditional meanings, as these are portrayed in Scripture and other sources."[67] Narratives shape the ethos of a community and the moral character of participants so that they construe the world and envision appropriate action in ways that are suitable to the narrative. Narrative discourse is dialectical in that it forms agents who interact in multiple communities at once. Narratives do not aim to provide clear answers to moral quandaries. They engage the emotions and the imagination to illuminate what is at stake in a certain kind of moral choice or way of life.

By means of both prophetic and narrative discourse, theology moves beyond the theoretical identification of ideals, principles, rules, and resolutions to problems and conflicts. Through prophesy and narrative, theology helps reorient the worldviews of persons and communities and forms them with the virtues that will dispose them to act on their ethical understandings and conclusions. By recalling and living within the story of Yahweh's liberation of the people from bondage, or the sacrifice of Christ on the cross, a religiously and theologically informed people will become better prepared to take action on behalf of those without health care or dying of AIDS. When confronted with public policy choices about new biotechnology, they will be more inclined to ask who will have access, who will profit, and who is likely to bear any associated risks or harms. Recalling that religious communities coexist with other kinds of associations in patterns of interdependence and that people in society participate in many communities and associations at once, it is key to stress that theology's prophetic and narrative roles are not limited to the internal life of religious communities, strictly defined. Illuminating insights can be generated even for those who do not share the entire worldview and symbol system of the speaker.[68] Prophetic critique and narrative formation can extend to other groups or activities in which theologians associate with people on the basis of more limited unifying factors.

The use of distinctively religious and theological language and symbols in the public bioethical realm is not always appropriate or appropriate in the same way. But neutral language in public and strong theological language in community (or in a communal "witness" against cultural assumptions) are not the only options. Theological language and religious stories and images are sometimes effective in public settings — not to dominate, alienate, or condemn, but to stimulate the emotions and imaginations of discussion partners. If a "public" theological participant suggests a symbol, value, or principle from his or her specific tradition, the suggestion may resonate with aspects of the experiences and traditions of other participants, either distinctive or common, leading to agreement on certain values, bonds, practices, and decisions, even in the public realm. Theology can tip sensibilities in a certain direction, disposing participants to consider a line of argument more favorably. In such cases, the role of theology is both narrative and prophetic, creating both an ethos and a set of practical dispositions to act that can combat the technology-driven refusal of death or the control of health care by market economics. Religious and theological language can foster better understanding of the human condition and more humane, just, and beneficent practices and policies of biomedicine.

The types of ethical, policy, narrative, and prophetic discourse identified by Gustafson are not easily separable, nor are they ever abstracted from ways of life and patterns of action in which their speakers are involved. Attempts to advance moral ideals and standards and to transform behavior and social relationships depend on active, participatory engagement, as well as on speech. Therefore, as I indicated earlier, to Gustafson's four types can be added a fifth: theology as *participatory discourse.* Participatory discourse refers to a mode of theological and ethical speech in which its practical roots and out-

66. Ibid., 41.

67. Ibid., 19.

68. See Childress, "Religion, Theology, and Bioethics," 56-57.

comes are intentionally acknowledged. Theological ethics in the participatory mode recognizes that its persuasive value derives only in part from its intellectual coherence. It derives in equal or greater measure from its power to allude to or induce a shared sphere of behavior, oriented by shared concerns and goals, and its power to constitute relations of empathy and interdependence among the "arguers." To name theological-ethical discourse as participatory discourse is to hold up as an explicit goal the creation of connective practices among interlocutors in order that shared social practices may be transformed in light of religiously inspired (though not necessarily tribalistic) visions and values.

Gustafson's four types — ethical, policy, prophetic, and narrative discourse — all refer primarily to language and verbal or textual expressions — concepts, principles, stories, statements, and so on. To name the participatory mode is to direct our attention explicitly to the kinds of joint activities that give rise to these types of language, bringing interlocutors together in a common practical space or enterprise where the language is mutually understood. Participatory practices are, of course, already implied by Gustafson's scheme. For example, those engaged in an "ethical" exchange will share or potentially share a terrain of values and priorities — such as respect for persons, the common good, or the obligation to do no harm — on which debates about specific applications can proceed. They will also share a cultural or scholarly setting in which the field of "ethics" is acknowledged, even if that setting is created cross-culturally, for example, by publications, conferences, and visiting lectureships.

Those engaged in policy discourse share or potentially share common social and legal institutions, precedents, and expectations that enable mutually intelligible argument about "best" policies — such as self-determination, informed consent, proportion of cost to benefit, or the right to profit by one's labor. These will have already been made explicit by a framing tradition of policy, regulation, judicial precedents, and law. Contemporary theological bioethics rightly engages in policy discussions and the requisite social practices (presidential bioethics commissions, lobbying in Washington, D.C., court testimony). But this is only one sphere of social action and influence open to religion and theology. Theological bioethicists too readily concede the playing field to those who define it in "policy discourse" terms, essentially the terms of liberal democratic capitalism. This means that theologians become captives to the practice of policy making as the exclusive way to engage others on bioethical matters and forget about equally or more important avenues of reform.

Theological bioethics as participatory must explicitly link religion and theology to practices and movements in civil society that can have a subversive or revolutionary impact on liberalism, science, and the market. The public and social effects of prophetic and narrative discourse should be integrated with participatory, inclusive practices. Prophetic naming of injustice and the enhancement of narratives of resistance and empowerment can unite persons of a variety of religious and moral faiths. It is especially critical to recognize that real-world coalitions around shared purposes and goals are a means of rooting and furthering theological bioethics as participatory discourse. The theoretical apparatus of theological bioethics must include specific attention to the public impact of participatory practices.

Social distortions and social reform need to be understood in light of a more comprehensive and multifaceted interpretation of knowledge, moral commitment, and action. The next chapter [in *Theological Bioethics*] will build on the dialectical character of early theological bioethics and propose that theological bioethics participate more self-consciously in reformist practices today. Participatory theological bioethics connects public discourse and influence to a variety of political movements and institutions of civil society in which religious groups can be effective.

Moving Ahead: Feminist Bioethics

Most theological bioethicists today are dialectical in that they engage with cultural problems and increasingly do so in a global sphere of concern. They are also committed to maintain intact those tenets of the Christian tradition that they perceive to be essential. Many believe that the dialectical relation of theology and culture cuts both ways in the sense that religious traditions must sometimes be corrected on basic issues in light of contemporary experience. But still needed is a theological bioethics that explicitly connects theories and worldviews to cooperative social action, combating systemic social distortions with reformist or revolutionary practices that create or join coalitions in civil society.

In theological bioethics, feminist authors have been ahead of the curve on this issue, as on that of making a preferential option for the poor definitive of the contribution of theology to bioethics. Feminist bioethics, religious and nonreligious, arose in close connection with struggles for women's social equality in the 1960s and 1970s. Because the stereotyping of women's roles as defined by sex and reproduction was the target of the feminist movement, these also were the focus of the earliest ventures in feminist bioethics. From the beginning, debates about the ethics of reproductive medicine, such as birth control, sterilization, abortion, and reproductive technologies, were carried out by feminists with a close eye to their practical significance and in coordination with practical activism to change women's opportunities.

Many of the first feminist bioethicists, representatively theologian Beverly Harrison, adopted a "liberal" defense of women's autonomy, advocating for a right to abortion.[69] Yet Marxist and radical feminists soon posed

69. Beverly Wildung Harrison, *Our Right to Choose: Toward a New Ethic of Abortion* (Boston: Beacon Press, 1989).

a challenge to the idea that a liberal model of women's choice would necessarily free women from patriarchal scientific institutions and the pervasive influence of the profit motive. Remarked one bioethicist with theological training, "Perhaps the most confusing message about the new reproductive technologies is that they are a gift to women, because they appear to give so-called infertile women the ability to reproduce. However . . . more and more areas of female living have been colonized by medical intervention, and staked out as medical territory."[70]

Particularly as feminist bioethics grew to include the testimony of Latina and African American women and of women from the "two-thirds world," the significance of biomedical practices for women's concrete reality was focused on issues of socioeconomic and racial-ethnic as well as gender oppression. This focus has become much more central as feminist ethicists confront the challenges of globalization. In the words of Karen Lebacqz, the "first thing" theology brings to public discourse is "justice as a crucial category," assessed in terms of "the plight of the poor" and requiring "a willingness to let go of the landscape as we know it in order to permit justice to be done."[71]

Some general directions for feminist theology and bioethics are captured by Margaret Farley and Barbara Andolsen. In 1985, Farley grounded feminist theology in the experience and well-being of women and lifted up three central themes: human relational patterns, human embodiment, and human interpretation of "nature."[72] Farley insists that patterns of relationship not be hierarchical and oppressive, especially to women; that women can reclaim their bodies as personal subjects active in the world; and that the domination of nature that goes along with domination of women can be overcome in the name of a sacramental view of creation. Important interdependent principles for Farley are autonomy and relationality, equality and mutuality.[73]

Andolsen gives special attention to issues of race and class, observing that, ultimately, feminist theology is concerned about "the well-being of all persons, including men, and about the good of the entire natural world."[74] In accordance with her interest in the intersection of race and class with gender, Andolsen corrects a theory of justice as detached impartiality with an ethic of care sensitive to the particular circumstances and forms of oppression suffered by women and others. Seeking to jar religious sensibilities into a new way of seeing the relation between the divine and the world, she suggests a reinvigorating use of the image of God as mother, both to empower women as patients and health care practitioners and to foster a belief in "the God/dess who will tolerate no excluded ones."[75]

Conclusion

Two important trends must be emphasized. First, the practice of medicine and the provision of health care are in our culture increasingly scientific rather than humanistic enterprises, and they are even more quickly being directed by marketplace values. Participants in biomedicine — whether providers or patients — are finding this situation ever less satisfactory at a personal level, and many are raising questions about the kind of society that is sponsoring these shifts, in turn to be re-created by them. Because they deal in the elemental human experiences of birth, life, death, and suffering, the biomedical arts provide an opening for larger questions of meaning and even of transcendence. Religious themes and imagery can be helpful in articulating these concerns and addressing them in an imaginative, provocative, and perhaps ultimately transformative way. Religious symbolism may be grounded in particular communities and their experiences of God and community, but perhaps it can also mediate a sensibility of transcendence and ultimacy that is achingly latent in the ethical conflicts, tragedies, and triumphs that are unavoidable in biomedicine. The immense current interest in the spiritual dimensions of health care exemplifies this trend.[76]

A second, not unrelated, trend is toward investment in the social and even global picture of health care ethics by theologians. In religious perspective, justice in medicine and access to preventive and therapeutic care are increasingly seen not only in terms of autonomy but in communal terms. While philosophical and public policy bioethics in this country is still dominated by considerations of autonomy and informed consent, theological bioethics, even when "translated" into more general, nonreligious categories, tends to prioritize distributive justice and social solidarity over individual rights and liberty. This makes theological bioethics more resistant to the market forces that so often control what research is funded, where it is conducted and on whom, who has ac-

70. Janice Raymond, "Preface," in *Man-Made Women: How New Reproductive Technologies Affect Women,* Gena Corea et al. (Bloomington and Indianapolis: Indiana University Press, 1987), 12.

71. Karen Lebacqz, "Theology, Justice and Health Care: An International Conundrum" (paper presented at the University of Uppsala, Uppsala, Sweden, April 2002), 6.

72. Margaret A. Farley, "Feminist Theology and Bioethics," in *Theology and Bioethics,* ed. Earl E. Shelp (Dordrecht, Neth.: D. Reidel Publishing Company, 1985), 163.

73. Ibid., 174.

74. Barbara Hilkert Andolsen, "Elements of a Feminist Approach to Bioethics," in *Feminist Ethics and the Catholic Moral Tradition, Readings in Moral Theology, No. 9,* ed. Charles E. Curran, Margaret A. Farley, and Richard A. McCormick (New York: Paulist Press, 1996), 142-43. This essay first appeared in *Religious Resources and Methods in Bioethics* in 1994.

75. Ibid., 378.

76. See Daniel P. Sulmasy, *The Healer's Calling: A Spirituality for Physicians and Other Health Care Professionals* (New York: Paulist, 1997); Benedict Ashley and Kevin O'Rourke, *Health Care Ethics: A Theological Analysis,* 3rd ed. (St. Louis, MO: Catholic Health Association, 1978), 389-412; and Vigen Guroian, *Life's Living toward Dying* (Grand Rapids, MI: Eerdmans, 1996).

cess to the benefits, who profits from new knowledge and its implementation, and how health care is organized within a society as a whole. Biblical foundations can be found for such a perspective, especially in the Hebrew prophets and in the teaching and example of Jesus about love of neighbor and serving the poor and vulnerable. Warrants can also be found in religious traditions of practice, where care of the sick has often been institutionalized as a work of devotion and self-offering to the divine and where morality has been communal in nature and definition. In today's world, the community in which the neighbor is served and goods shared is increasingly international and global, and theological bioethics is responding directly to these new global realities.

9 European-American Ethos and Principlism: An African-American Challenge

Cheryl J. Sanders

Introduction

One of the most significant contributions thinkers of European-American descent have made to the field of bioethics is the development of a deductive approach that applies ethical theory and principles to a broad range of problems and cases. The work of Tom Beauchamp and James Childress perhaps represents the best of this line of thought, lifting up such principles as autonomy, nonmaleficence, beneficence, and justice, and rules regarding veracity, confidentiality, fidelity, and the like. Still, notably absent from their *Principles of Biomedical Ethics* (1983) is any discussion of the perspectives, writings, thought, or experience of African-Americans as theorists or participants in the American health care system. Moreover, the authors' apparent marginalization of race or religion as noteworthy factors in the thirty-five cases they cite in their book indicates a devaluation of the community and belief systems characteristic of African-American ethical discourse and social life. As a specific cultural phenomenon, principlism in bioethics seems to fall short in the effort to posit a body of knowledge that is intellectually rigorous and universally applicable cross-culturally.

In the April 1989 issue of the Kennedy Institute of Ethics *Newsletter,* Harley Flack and Edmund Pellegrino presented an exploratory discussion of the importance of African-American perspectives in biomedical ethics. This brief article (1989) offers insightful reflections on data gathered during a February 1987 conference of African-American scholars, educators, health professionals, and philosophers. It suggests that African-Americans and Anglo-Americans differ significantly in their ideas about morality and ethics. It further offers a credible account of the dominant ideas of the African-American perspective on morals in terms of the greater importance ascribed to community, religion, the ethics of virtue, and personal life experiences in comparison to

---

From Cheryl J. Sanders, "European-American Ethos and Principlism: An African-American Challenge," in *A Matter of Principles? Ferment in U.S. Bioethics,* ed. Edwin R. DuBose and Ronald P. Hamel (Valley Forge, PA: Trinity Press International, 1994), 148-63. Reproduced by kind permission of Continuum International Publishing Group

Western value systems. The authors called for further dialogue on the question of how these two moral systems differ in relation to biomedical ethics.

However, that article made a couple of problematic assertions that have influenced my own critical analysis of the problems and limitations of an African-American perspective on biomedical ethics. First is their explanation of the unique nature of the African-American experience, as manifested in norms such as the dominant value of community, the importance of religion and ethics of virtue, and the weight given to personal life experiences:

> Slavery, segregation, discrimination, poverty and a disadvantaged position with respect to education, health and medical care sensitize African-Americans in specific ways. These experiences evoke a more empathetic response to the social-ethical questions — justice in the distribution of resources, sensitivity to the vulnerability and dependence of the sick person, and a sense of responsibility for the poor and rejected members of society. (Flack and Pellegrino 1999: 2)

While their description of the norms of the African-American perspective seems accurate enough, they seek to account for this distinctiveness in terms that seriously understate the issue. In their view, what makes the African-American experience unique is a greater empathy for social-ethical concerns. What they leave unsaid is that the social injustice, insensitivity, and irresponsibility that have created this empathy are direct manifestations of a racist Anglo-American ethos that is itself uniquely indifferent to community, religion, virtue, and personal experience. In other words, it seems absurd to speak of the unique moral context of the African-American experience of suffering without at the same time addressing the cause of this suffering in the broader moral context of European-American racism.[1]

A second problem is the call for dialogue and the parenthetical observation that "so few African-Americans are involved in scholarly work in biomedical ethics and how their number might be increased" (Flack and Pellegrino 1989: 2). Again, I take issue not with what they say but rather with what they don't say. Clearly, African-Americans are engaging in biomedical ethical discourse on a daily basis, but not necessarily in ways that European-Americans would regard as scholarly or even noteworthy. Further, it may be that African-Americans have thoughtfully concluded that Western biomedical ethics is not useful or applicable to their dilemmas precisely because their data and input have not been taken into account. In other words, the dialogue being called for may have already taken place in other quarters, and the lack of scholarly work by African-Americans in the field may indicate an informed judgment that biomedical ethical discourse is an esoteric and exclusive enterprise where African-American participation is not really welcome on any level.

I don't dispute that there is a distinctive African-American ethos that has a direct bearing upon how biomedical ethics is done. But the real question is not *whether* such a perspective exists but *why* it exists and whether its continued existence is predicated upon the persistence of racist oppression of African-American people. Given the reality of racism, we must not fall into a trap and let the discussion of uniqueness divert attention from the universals, where the African-American perspective is strictly valued on the ground of uniqueness and not fully appreciated for its universal significance as a critique of the destructive inhumanity of the dominant ethos. In my opinion, the authentic dialogue begins when we realize that both perspectives are operating within one moral universe and not two, and that each brings a valid critique to bear upon the other. Both must be subjected to scrutiny by similar standards — it is as erroneous to romanticize (uncritically) African-American culture as it is to overlook the racism that is endemic to European-American culture. The point is not that the African-American ethos is unique, but that it is *characteristically human* in ways that the European-American ethos is not. I will discuss the problems and limitations of principlism in bioethics from an African-American perspective — that is, taking into account the distinctive ethos, theology, and ethics of the African-American people, with a view toward understanding how honest dialogue among African-Americans and European-Americans can move us all toward a bioethics that is truly ethical.

The African-American Ethos

Based upon my own teaching and research in the area of African-American ethical discourse, I would like to offer a list of seven features that describe the African-American ethos or lifestyle and contrast them with opposite features that characterize the European-American ethos. I am indebted to one of my former doctoral students, Fr. George Ehusani, for helping me to understand and describe distinctive features of both African and African-American cultures. Although the following characterization of the African-American ethos is my own, these and other humanistic aspects of traditional African culture are discussed in detail in Ehusani's book, *An Afro-Christian Vision: "Ozovehe!" Toward a More Humanized World* (1991), with specific reference to his own ethnic group, the Ebira of Nigeria.

First, the African-American ethos is holistic, not dualistic, emphasizing that most matters are better understood in terms of "both-and" rather than "either-or." Second, it is inclusive, not exclusive, accepting of difference rather than seeing difference as grounds for dis-

1. I prefer to use the term *European-American* in place of *Anglo-American* because it compares more consistently with *African-American* with reference to continent of origin, and it avoids the typically American bias that regards *Anglo* as superior to and/or representative of the rest of Europe.

crimination or exploitation. Third, it is communalistic, not individualistic, especially valuing family and community over the individual in moral importance. Fourth, it is spiritual, not secular, rejecting any ultimate dichotomization of the sacred and the secular and acknowledging the pervasive presence and power of the unseen realm over what is seen. Fifth, it is theistic, not agnostic or atheistic, affirming not only the existence of God but also the relevance of belief to every aspect of life. Sixth, its basic approach or method is improvisational, not forced into fixed forms, with an openness to spontaneity, flexibility, and innovation, particularly in the realm of music and art. Seventh, it is humanistic, not materialistic, valuing human life and dignity over material wealth or possessions.

These features of the African-American ethos are largely derived from traditional African cultures, yet in America as well as in Africa, this life-affirming perspective is not always strictly adhered to or applied. However, the African-American ethos, notwithstanding the many exceptions and abuses that can readily be cited, is essentially holistic, inclusive, communalistic, spiritual, theistic, improvisational, and humanistic in ways that the European-American ethos is not, though exceptions would apply there as well. Moreover, even if it is an exaggeration to say that the European-American ethos is dualistic, exclusive, individualistic, secular, atheistic, inflexible, and materialistic, these characteristics are necessary and sufficient conditions for the propagation of racism, which can be regarded as the logical consequence of a worldview that readily expends both soul and spirit in the pursuit of wealth. The roots of the African-American ethos predate by centuries the exploitative schemes Europe brought to Africa, Asia, and the New World in the form of slavery, imperialism, and colonialism. Still its best fruits are yet to emerge if and when African-Americans can resist cultural and ethical assimilation of European-American values that have spelled death to our ancestors and our children and can persuade ourselves and others to embrace African-American values that are more humane and life affirming.

The Problem of a Black Theology

Black theology is a term first popularized some twenty years ago by James Cone, an African-American theologian who authored *Black Theology and Black Power* in 1969, followed by numerous other books and articles on the subject. It is one of several specific cultural expressions of a broader genre known as liberation theology. Liberation theologies all begin with the analysis of oppression, affirm the personhood of oppressed people, and advocate social and political change to liberate the oppressed. Black theology, in particular, analyzes the oppression of black people, affirms the personhood of black people, and advocates their social and political liberation.

In his 1984 volume *For My People: Black Theology and the Black Church,* Cone critically assesses the development of black theology during the 1960s and 1970s, with a view to influencing its direction for the 1980s and beyond. His critique includes a series of generalizations concerning the dialogue between black theology and the liberation theologies of the world, each of which has direct relevance to the problem of principlism in relation to African-American thought. First, Cone asserts that "every theology is a product of its social environment and thus in part a reflection of it" (1984: 172). Thus, European-American theology, as well as philosophy, brings a unique set of collective experiences and biases to scholarly discourse, despite any disclaimers to the contrary offered (or implied) in the interest of objectivity and universalism. The same is true for black theology and philosophy, except that African-Americans can more self-consciously accept the limitations of discourse that reflects social environment. Specifically, African-Americans are more aware of the limitations of their own voices and have a heightened sensitivity to the social context of others who seek to do theology and philosophy for the whole.

The second general statement Cone makes speaks even more specifically to the problem of principlism:

> Every theology ought to move beyond its particularity to the concrete experiences of others. No theology should remain enclosed in its own narrow culture and history. That has been the awful mistake of the dominant theologies of Europe and North America. They talk about God as if Europeans are the only ones who can think, and that is why they still have difficulty taking seriously liberation theologies in Asia, Africa, and Latin America, or that of minorities in the U.S.A. (1984: 173)

Third, Cone concludes that:

> Every theology needs instruments of social analysis that will help theologians define the causes of injustice. How can we participate in the liberation of the poor from poverty if its causes are not clearly understood through social analysis? Social analysis is nothing but a way of uncovering the causes of evil and exploitation. It helps us to see more clearly and thus to know the nature of the evil we are fighting against. As long as theology remains ignorant of the causes of exploitation, it will not be able to effectively fight it. (1984: 174)

Here he reveals participation in the liberation of the poor as the essential agenda of black and other liberation theologies. Of course, just as no theological or philosophical consensus exists as to what constitutes justice in the society, so also it may be difficult or impossible to agree upon how evil can be discerned. In any case, for Cone, evil is measured most precisely by the suffering of the oppressed. From the vantage point of bioethics, the social manifestations of that suffering include lack of access to health care resources and the inattentiveness of the dominant society to the special health needs of minority communities.

In view of our concern here for the cultural parochialism of principlism, it must be admitted that a strictly black or African-American theological perspective could have similar limitations. If there is only One God, in whose image all human beings are made, then reflection upon the nature of God is severely restricted in any theological discourse that only takes account of the experience of one race, culture, or gender. The African-American experience may provide an appropriate starting point for theology, because all theological reflection is grounded in the particularities of race, class, gender, and culture. Indeed, all theologies have a contextual point of departure and are rooted in the particularities of human experience, even if their conclusions point toward universal revelation and eschatological considerations. But the basic message and implications of black theology ought not be exclusive to the African-American community simply because historically the experience of suffering, rejection, and exploitation in relation to the dominant culture has been a major hermeneutical concern of African-American religion. In other words, African-American religion never intended to isolate itself morally from the dominant culture, but rather sought to stand as a witness against racism in the name of God. And to the extent that blacks and whites identify themselves as Christians, the relevant scriptural mandate to love one's neighbor as oneself has been habitually violated — whites have despised their black neighbors, and blacks, insofar as they have internalized this racial hatred and animosity, have not loved themselves. Cone addresses some of these issues in detail in his most recent book, *Martin & Malcolm & America: A Dream or a Nightmare* (1991), in the course of his theological analysis of the life and thought of Martin Luther King, Jr., and Malcolm X. Cone's closing exhortation draws on his evaluation of the joint contributions of these two great African-Americans to American religion and politics: "As Americans we (blacks, whites, Latinos, Asians, and Indians) should create a society which contributes to the well-being of all citizens, not just to the well-being of some" (1991: 317-18). Indeed, this call to accountability ought to be extended to the whole community of bioethicists, African-American and European-American alike.

I accept as established historical fact that the black churches emerged in response to racism — not because African-Americans chose to exclude European-Americans from their worshiping communities, but because they were denied full participation in virtually every aspect of American life, including religion. Ironically, the black churches were forced into existence by white churches that excluded blacks from participation in worship on the basis of racism and related ideas concerning the inferiority of African-American religion and culture on the one hand, and the superiority of European-American religion and culture on the other. It is tragic that racism overruled love in the justification of racial separation in the religious realm. And since it remains true today — as Martin Luther King, Jr., claimed many years ago — that 11 o'clock on Sunday morning is the most segregated hour in America, then both black and white Christians must be held accountable for allowing racism, or the response to racism, to dictate their behavior and systems of values in relation to each other.

While it may be valid to uphold the particular cultural traditions associated with religious worship, any theology that exclusively addresses the perspectives of one group without giving attention to the interests and concerns of others is suspect. For example, it became characteristic of European-American religion to dichotomize and relativize any theological considerations that would question white hegemony. Rather than face the fact that slavery, terrorism, discrimination, and other manifestations of racism contradict the central teaching of the Christian faith — which is to love God and neighbor as oneself — in the interest of logical consistency, it became more convenient to invalidate any association between what one believes about God and what one does to others. While it is rare to find overt pronouncements of racist ideology in white religion, many seem to understand that songs, sermons, and liturgies about love of neighbor are not to be taken seriously with reference to blacks. Praxis and principle are necessarily divorced from each other. On the other hand, historically it has been in the best interest of African-Americans to lay full claim to the relevance of praxis to principle in a theological context where God exercises sovereignty over all peoples in all situations, and not only during worship or on Sundays. Also, it makes more sense to identify the separation of the sacred from the secular as an expression of the peculiarity or deviance of white religion than to single out the merger of the same as indicative of the distinctiveness of black religion.

If black theology and black churches have brought a distinctive perspective to American life, it grows out of their courage to address questions of theodicy brought to the fore by the experience of racism and their willingness to respond theologically to the reality of unmerited suffering by affirming the goodness of God, the evil capacities of humanity, and the promise of salvation offered through Jesus Christ to bring redemption, reconciliation, and wholeness to a broken world. Yet, the fact remains that any theology or any church whose existence is justified primarily on the basis of racism or its effects will bring serious deficiencies and liabilities to the ethical dialogue needed to formulate a bioethics that promotes justice, healing, and human dignity for all.

There are other black theologians whose work bears critically upon the prospects for increased dialogue between European-American and African-American bioethics. One is James Evans, president and professor of systematic theology at Colgate Rochester Divinity School and author of *We Have Been Believers: An African-American Systematic Theology*. In the book's introduction, Evans proposes a procedure for establishing an understanding of justice based on criteria developed by black theologians:

> One must have a set of criteria by which one can determine whether the present social order is just. These criteria must themselves be drawn from the content of African-American Christian faith, rather than from any extraneous philosophical norms of good and evil, right and wrong. Therefore, one cannot introduce a notion of justice, for example, as central to ethical behavior if the notion itself is not central to the theological affirmations of African-American faith. (1992: 8)

This method of resolving the question of whether or not there is justice in the social order speaks directly to the problem of principlism. Perhaps justice takes priority over every other ethical norm in this regard, where the European-American philosophical notion of justice is subject to correction or affirmation by the collective experience of African-American people, who know firsthand the consequences of justice ill-conceived, misapplied, and flatly denied.

A second significant work grounded in the norms of black theology is *Empower the People: Social Ethics for the African-American Church,* by Theodore Walker of the Perkins School of Theology at Southern Methodist University. This book presents an outline of a contemporary black social ethics, offering the symbol of "breaking bread" as a guide to interpreting and applying biblical and religious principles to the ethical dilemmas faced by the African-American community. Citing the title of a well-known Negro spiritual as a backdrop for the ritual mediation of meanings communicated by the symbol, Walker explains:

> Our understanding of the witness of Scripture is that we ought to break bread together (bread being understood as a symbol for the various resources that nourish wholesome social existence), and moreover we understand from the biblical witness that this is the absolutely essential aspect of right relation to God — indeed, it is the ethic of breaking bread that in God's final judgment separates righteousness from unrighteousness. (1991: 102)

His prescriptive analysis for the whole of African-American life draws on the African holistic emphasis in black theology and extends beyond the purview of blacks in the U.S. to embrace an ecological concern for the health and well-being of the entire world:

> We know that the bread we ought to break internationally, nationally, and locally includes leadership, money, food, jobs, land, housing, righteous education, and socialization (including the use of such resources as religious ritual, music, and dance), vastly increased attention to male-female-family-church relations, health care, child care, home care, family care, elder care, power, and other opportunities and resources essential to the nurture, survival, fruitful increase, and empowerment of all the people . . . the ecological sensitivity that we can harvest from the cultural gardens of traditional African and native American peoples, and from the gardens of other traditional peoples, calls us to see that the well-being of people is fully related to the well-being of other life. In order to contribute to the well-being of all the people, including those who are not yet born, we must contribute to the nurture and fruition of the whole living planet. (1991: 120)

Although Walker does not give a great deal of specific attention to bioethics, he clearly conceptualizes the global context in which bioethical dilemmas need to be analyzed and resolved, further affirming the need for African-American ethicists to work out both principle and praxis in creative dialogue with European-Americans and others who may not hold the same point of view with regard to what constitutes human well-being and who must take responsibility for it.

The Problem of a Black Ethic

The idea of a uniquely black ethic entails some of the same problems and limitations of black theology if it does not transcend its particularity at some points in order to bring critical commentary to bear upon the society at large. Although a number of ethicists and philosophers have sought to characterize the African-American ethic as it compares to and contrasts with its European-American counterpart, one of the most insightful analyses was published in 1971 by African-American ethicist Preston Williams. In "Ethics and Ethos in the Black Experience," Williams offers a three-part typology to describe the life experiences of blacks in a racist America: (1) victimization, based upon "the fact that every Black person in America is injured or cheated by the conscious and unconscious notions of white superiority in the American mind and social system"; (2) integration, achieved as an exception to the rule of racial exclusion by "the unusual Black who by the power of his intellect, drive or personality has forced his way into mainstream America in spite of the color of his skin"; and (3) black awareness, which goes "beyond integration to ask that all men recognize the existence of a spirit, a set of social structures and norms in Black life that are worthy of acquisition by Blacks and whites" (1971: 104-5).

All three aspects of this typology — victimization, integration, and black awareness — should be taken into account when evaluating the relevance of African-American ethical discourse to biomedical concerns. Still, the fundamental assumption of the black awareness ideal, namely that black values and norms ought to be shared with and acquired by others, especially commends itself as a worthwhile point of departure for African-American participation in bioethics. Ultimately, the ethical question is not one of African-American perspective as much as it is a matter of African-American participation and inclusion. Perspective suggests a particular point of view, a unique angle or approach, while participation assumes an unqualified stake and role within the whole discourse. It must not be forgotten that the hyphen in the term *African-American* connects two irreducible dimensions of experience: first, the retention of vestiges of African identity, and second, the struggle for acceptance as Americans. Moreover, what is arguably the most distinctive ethical claim that African-Americans have made against a racist America — that is, the fundamental affirmation of human dignity regardless of social condition — is clearly worthy of adoption by bioethicists who are conscientiously concerned with transcending the particularities of race and culture in the pursuit of justice and human wholeness. Walker's ethic of "breaking bread" suggests ways black theological ethicists can produce a prescription for human wholeness in dialogue with more secular European-American thinkers.

> This black God-conscious social ethical prescription — that we break bread together — is understood to apply to every social circumstance. It is at this point that black theological social ethics can offer a prescriptive word to the whole world . . . the ethic of breaking bread calls black theological social ethics to affirm the bread-breaking aspects of liberal and radical and other secular social ethical thought. (1991: 102)

Can Bioethics Be Ethical?

An African-American perspective is ultimately a human perspective — a concrete, particular witness to universal truth. The African-American ethos should not merely be regarded as an interesting minority perspective or contribution, but rather as a perspective that informs the shape and content of the whole discourse. In order to be truly ethical, bioethics must be holistic, inclusive, communalistic, and humanistic, if not also spiritual, theistic, and improvisational, which is to say that it ought to reflect both the particularity and universality of the African-American experience and not be grounded solely in the thought of European-American philosophers.

To take a holistic approach in bioethics, emphasizing that most matters are better understood in terms of "both-and" rather than "either-or," would enable the pursuit of a harmonizing relationship between Afrocentric and Eurocentric thought rather than rejecting one and replacing it with the other. Such an approach would seek to augment and humanize the deductive, rationalistic, individualistic ethics of European-American thinkers to take into account some of the religious, historical, and cultural factors that characterize African-American collective experience. Many African-Americans have no problem combining modern medicine with such remedies as prayer and folk cures in their own personal health care decision making; on the level of bioethical discourse, the same notion can be applied to include what appeals simultaneously to the rational faculties and to the religious sensibilities in pursuit of human wholeness. While the principlism of European-American bioethics seems not to allow for the peculiarities of African-American exceptions and examples in the decision-making process, a holistic bioethics that embraces both principle and praxis, African-American bioethicists can more easily envision harmonizing Eurocentric and Afrocentric thought since most African-Americans have by necessity acquired the habit of holding European-American perspectives in tension with our own experiences. An inclusive bioethics is ethical insofar as it sees difference as an opportunity to enhance the whole rather than as grounds for discrimination or exploitation. There is a critical distinction to be made here between the terms *inclusive* and *holistic.* A *holistic* bioethics seriously questions the characteristic dualisms of Western culture, whereas an *inclusive* bioethics promotes the self-conscious and intentional rejection of racist, sexist, or classist biases and practices. Therefore, to be inclusive is not the same thing as seeking diversity as an end in itself; rather, the desired outcome of inclusivity in bioethics is fruitful dialogue, genuine mutuality, and the sharing of power and resources.

It is no simple matter to move from exclusion to inclusion. In fact, inclusivity can emerge as a more sophisticated form of oppression when the morally problematic assumptions that produced the exclusive practices in the first place remain unexamined as "others" are invited to become assimilated into the dominant group.

One of the most important distinctions to be made between the European-American bioethics of principlism and the proposed African-American bioethics is that the former is highly individualistic, while the latter would be more communalistic. The failure to give attention to the moral importance of both the individual and the community in which that individual is situated is a serious shortcoming of much of modern bioethical discourse in the U.S. While some attention is normally given in such thought to the roles of family members in making treatment decisions and resolving ethical dilemmas, not much weight tends to be given to the influence of extended family, faith communities, neighbors, and peer groups, in such matters. For example, the subject in just two of thirty-five cases in the Beauchamp and Childress text is identified by race — a white male lawyer dying from emphysema who carried on his legal practice from his hospital bed (1983: 301-4), and an unmarried white woman forced by court order to undergo a cesarean section (1983: 312-13). It is unclear why race was a factor in either case. Although it could be that the editors made no decision to report or not report race consistently, given that the cases were drawn from a variety of sources, one wonders how race is to be understood as relevant to these cases. Is race mentioned in these cases to make a point about their social location or moral values? Or does the reference merely serve to reinforce racist assumptions that only white males work hard or only white infants are worth saving? Ethnicity is a key factor in defining and valuing community among African-Americans, so a communalistic bioethics would give attention to race in order to enhance understanding of the individual in relation to the group, and at the same time, would take care not to use racial referents to evoke unsubstantiated judgments against individuals.

A bioethics that acknowledges the pervasive presence and power of the unseen realm over what is seen and rejects any ultimate dichotomization of the sacred and the secular seems to me to have greater authenticity than the strictly secular European-American bioethics. Although African-Americans are not demonstrably more "religious" than other Americans as measured by church attendance, denominational affiliation, and the like, the health and justice issues of the African-American community cannot intelligently be discussed without specifically referring to the pervasive influence of religious institutions, leadership, and belief systems on people inside and outside the church. Typically, European-American bioethicists lift up religious affiliation as important only on the abstract level of individual belief rather than in the context of a community of persons giving support to each other in collective ethical practice. Furthermore, religion tends to be raised as a factor only when a serious conflict emerges between religious belief and medical advice. For example, in the thirty-five cases listed in the Beauchamp and Childress text, religion is only mentioned in relation to noncompliant, deviant, or criminal behavior, including two Jehovah's Witnesses who refused blood transfusions, an involuntary mental patient who mutilated himself upon direct orders from God, and the finding that among men committing impersonal sexual acts with one another in public restrooms, most of the married men were Catholic (1983: 298-300; 295-96; 285-87).

Thus, one is drawn to the conclusion that religion is only noteworthy as a negative factor in bioethical discourse. It would be preferable for bioethicists to devote more careful and respectful attention to religion as context and as resource for persons engaged in health care decision making. Perhaps this can occur only if we return to a more theistic frame of reference for doing bioethics. Even if the agnostic or atheistic biases of individual European-American bioethicists must remain unchallenged, it seems necessary to cultivate an intellectual awareness of the ways African-Americans affirm the existence of God and the relevance of belief to every aspect of life. To reconsider the significance of the sacred in bioethics seems to be an essential step toward increased insight into a whole range of human attitudes and behavior with respect to health issues.

While it may seem far-fetched to expect European-American bioethicists to adopt improvisational approaches or methods in keeping with the African-American ethos, the question remains as to what extent justice can be served by rigid adherence to fixed forms and structures. Given the very difficult fiscal dilemmas now being encountered by public-policy makers on the federal, state, and local levels with regard to the allocation of health care resources, particularly for the uninsured poor, an openness to spontaneity, flexibility, and innovation is something to be desired and not to be feared or guarded against if bioethicists are to make any effective contribution to the creation of viable and just cost-cutting measures. Much of the improvisational ethic in African-American life derives precisely from the challenge of "making do" with limited resources to meet the needs of the individual or the community. It may be that the insights and proposals of those who have understood the conditions of poverty and oppression will provide a distinctive reality base for European-American bioethicists who are accustomed to doing scholarly analysis without taking assumptions other than those of the white middle class into account.

If the African-American ethos is truly humanistic, valuing human life and dignity over material wealth or possessions, then incorporation of this perspective into the bioethics of the dominant culture should result in the development of more humane and less materialistic approaches to health care dilemmas. This humanistic point of view seems to be missing from many systems now in place to administer health care in the U.S. How many medical schools prepare their graduates to understand ethics, culture, and religion in relation to the administration of medical care? To what extent are research and development priorities geared exclusively toward technological advances that will benefit a small segment of the society? If bioethics embraces the "bottom-line" logic of measuring human outcomes primarily in terms of social costs and benefits, how can a high regard for human dignity on its own terms be cultivated so as to humanize public policy? Commitment to the concept of human dignity on the part of bioethicists can help to counteract the American penchant toward applying inhumane measures to human problems, so that some members of the society are deemed more worthy than others to receive its benefits and blessings.

Conclusion

The African-American ethos can serve as a rich resource for ongoing research and dialogue with regard to pressing issues such as health care resource allocation, treatment-nontreatment decisions, patient-physician relationships, and management of reproductive technologies and interventions. Without a doubt, African-American ethicists have much to gain through continued conversations with European-Americans who remain firmly committed to principlism. It is hoped that this discussion will foster meaningful partnerships between bioethicists of European-American and African-American backgrounds as they undertake the common task of addressing the ethical dimensions of medical practice, resource allocation, and public policy. It remains my conviction that any bioethics that does not give priority to justice, equality, and human dignity in administering health care is unethical, regardless of how much care is taken by whom to be racially, culturally, or intellectually inclusive.

References

Beauchamp, Tom L., and James F. Childress. 1983. *Principles of Biomedical Ethics.* 2d ed. New York: Oxford University Press.

Cone, James H. 1991. *Martin & Malcolm & America: A Dream or a Nightmare,* 317-18. Maryknoll, N.Y.: Orbis Books.

———. 1984. *For My People: Black Theology and the Black Church.* Maryknoll, N.Y.: Orbis Books.

———. 1969. *Black Theology and Black Power.* New York: Harper and Row.

Ehusam, George Omaku. 1991. *An Afro-Christian Vision: "Ozovehe!" Toward a More Humanized World.* Lanham, Md.: University Press of America.

Evans, James H., Jr. 1992. *We Have Been Believers: An African-American Systematic Theology.* Minneapolis: Fortress Press.

Flack, Harley, and Edmund D. Pellegrino. 1989. "New Data Suggests African-Americans Have Own Perspective on Biomedical Ethics." Kennedy Institute of Ethics *Newsletter* 3 (April): 2.

Walker, Theodore, Jr. 1991. *Empower the People: Social Ethics for the African-American Church.* Maryknoll, N.Y.: Orbis Books.

Williams, Preston N. 1971. "Ethics and Ethos in the Black Experience." *Christianity and Crisis* (31 May): 104-5.

10 Bioethics in a Liberationist Key

Márcio Fabri dos Anjos

By and large, bioethics in the United States is concerned with the problems raised by high-cost and high-tech medicine and experimentation. Other issues, however, await the attention of bioethics, issues that affect a vast proportion of the world's population who live and die far from the resources of sophisticated medical techniques. Against this backdrop, I want to introduce the question of the poor: what chance do poor people have of seeing their problems dealt with by bioethics? Once raised, this question immediately takes on a methodological coloring: how does one go about doing bioethics immersed in the world as it is lived in and perceived by the poor? How does one at least include on the agenda a treatment of their problems? Are these problems of interest to bioethics?

My intention is to offer a Latin American perspective on these questions. The enormous contrasts between rich and poor undoubtedly provoke the development of such a perspective. It is necessary to recognize, however, that a treatment of bioethics in a liberationist key, in Latin America, is as yet but sketchy. Broad methodological principles can be found that apply to bioethics, but it is much more difficult to locate studies that take this broad approach systematically. Thus the embryonic state of bioethical reflection in Latin America leads me to be cautious in treating the theme at hand.

Still, we can describe the general shape of a bioethics elaborated in a liberation key. One characteristic of the liberationist methodology is its propensity to bring into close relationship theory and practice. In that spirit, I have taken lived experience in Latin America as the backdrop for my reflection, a move that should not be construed as a desire to project our problems uncritically into the North American bioethical scene. Rather, it should be seen as a demonstration of an applied methodology that may help, at least indirectly, in the rethinking of U.S. bioethics.

Furthermore, I am working within the context of an effort in Latin America to develop a particular Christian, theological vision. The relevance of theology's contribution to bioethics, I believe, goes beyond any sectarian in-

From Márcio Fabri dos Anjos, "Bioethics in a Liberationist Key," in *Matter of Principles? Ferment in Bioethics,* ed. Edwin R. DuBose, Ronald P. Hamel, and Laurence J. O'Connell (Valley Forge, PA: Trinity Press International, 1994), 130-47. Reproduced by kind permission of Continuum International Publishing Group.

terest. At the same time, I recognize the legitimacy of other convictions and the richness that dialogue with them brings.

Basic Inspiration

A suitable starting point for outlining a vision of bioethics in a liberationist key is its basic inspiration. Inspiration? For a long time, the sciences have assumed principles without considering themselves obliged to prove them. Currently, many authors alert us to the nonneutrality of the sciences and point to the world of convictions that constitute the *credo* presiding over every one of them.[1] It is what lies behind these convictions that we refer to as *inspiration.*

Bioethics finds its fundamental inspiration in seeking answers to some of the basic questions about human life and its end, the deeper meaning of suffering and death, and the rationality of human relationships in these circumstances. The answers that one gives to these questions determine the various models of bioethical practice. Therefore, not just religious interests are at stake. Facing the question of the fundamental inspiration of bioethics carries a requirement for safeguarding its academic seriousness. These remarks not only indicate areas in which theology can legitimately contribute to bioethics, but also make clear the wealth of cultural and scientific dialogue to be explored in the attempt to answer these basic questions.

Let us first consider several ideas that have inspired a liberationist bioethics and then look at some practical consequences that can be drawn from them.

Life as a Gift

The affirmation that human life is a gift rings ironic when one considers the bitter experience of death and the various forms in which life is denied in Latin America. It is not even necessary to have recourse to history, recalling the genocide of indigenous peoples and the violence of slavery, to illustrate this. Even today, in many places in Latin America life expectancy barely reaches the fifty-year mark, and the mortality rate for children between the ages of one and five is above 10 percent per year.[2] The drama of this experience of death is heightened when we see it legitimized by some as being *the will of God.*

Christian theology nonetheless affirms that God is the God of life and not of death. Life is a *gift* that we receive and is intended to be shared and developed responsibly. We receive life from God, and by God's power we transmit it. Implicit in this clearly religious affirmation is the recognition that we do not wish to suffer and die.

Another statement, which complements the previous one, is that God is Father and that makes all of us brothers and sisters. This affirmation commits us, on the one hand, to affirm the basic equality of all human life as a foundational ethical principle, and, on the other, to recognize a responsibility that unites us in a mutual promotion and defense of life, without appeal to privileges or discrimination against individuals or groups. In practical terms, statements about God are, in this context, ethical proposals for the governance of our vital relationships: be committed to one another in the search for life and in the overcoming of death; because we have God as a common "father," we should treat each other as brother and sister; and because we experience "God as the God of Life," this should impel us to overcome the processes that generate death (Gutiérrez 1989).

The Reality of Death

It would be naive to attempt a reflection on life without any reference to death. The harsh reality of violent death immediately shatters any such romanticism. Within the Christian perspective, life and death are not to be understood as two single-sense, mutually exclusive concepts. The notion of the transcendence of justice, for example, permeates the concept of life. If this were not so, death in any form, but particularly the death of the poor person who has suffered injustice, would be unredeemably absurd. By means of the concept of transcendence, death is transposed into an ethical key. It is total death only for the one who produces it unjustly.[3]

For the Christian, death and suffering negate life to the extent that they proceed from injustice, which is understood as any violation of the fundamental rule that the other is brother or sister. Grounded in such a rule, liberationist bioethics presupposes a critical reading of sickness, of suffering, and of death; it examines not only their *biological* but also their *ethical* roots. Expressions of this injustice are the *lack of commitment* that ignores or excludes people; *violence* that inflicts suffering and death; *dominion* that simply uses human beings, exploiting the life-force within them. The principal enemy faced by bioethics is thus not simply death but *premature death* and *suffering* as the *fruits of injustice.*

In a certain sense death has its own place on the horizon of life, as have also sickness and suffering. First, inasmuch as we all suffer and die, we can feel the solidarity

1. The theology of liberation exploits extensively this notion of a fundamental *credo* in its assessment of the political and economic sciences, noting in their structure a close analogy with religion. See, for example, Assman and Hinkelammert 1989.

2. UNICEF 1992.

3. There exists an extensive biblical tradition which affirms: "God did not make death, and he does not delight in the death of the living. For he created all things that they might exist, and the generative forces of the world are wholesome, and there is not destructive poison in them; and the dominion of Hades is not on earth. For righteousness is immortal" (Wisdom 1:13-15, RSV).

with others by which human life is woven. Second, in death and suffering we are pointed to the places where human life reaches its limits. In the first case, the end of one person's life generates life for another. In the second case, the end of a life forces us to confront that critical moment in which we must re-elaborate the sense of our own lives. These moments allow us to comprehend pain and death as profound experiences of life and not simply as evils to be avoided at all costs. Such a broadened horizon of meaning raises pointed questions for a bioethics that confines itself to the challenges of killing pain and keeping death at bay.

A Consciousness of the "Other"

A consciousness of the "other" is a third notion that inspires bioethics in a liberationist key. The "other," leaving aside for the moment the question of the transcendence of God, is our fellow human being, and the faith dimension allows us to perceive the other as brother or sister. Solidarity with those who suffer, who are sick or close to death follows. By means of this first step, one breaks with the individualism that allows one to act as if one's own interests were the only interests. We make ourselves capable of seeing the other with the eyes of the heart.

This faith dimension of consciousness is complemented by a *critical* dimension of consciousness of the other. In this critical dimension, consciousness awakens, in the most scientific way possible, to the situation in which the other is found; one is aware of how that other is being treated and of what needs must be met if he or she is to be treated truly as brother or sister. This double consciousness constantly returns to concrete experience as a starting point for the elaboration of ethics. It also frees ethical reflection from the temptation of making faith a hiding place for lack of commitment or a pretext for exploiting one's fellow.

Gratitude

From a Christian perspective, an ethical consciousness would be incomplete and even incorrect if gratitude were lacking. In our very existence we carry the marks of gratuity: no one is born or grows up without the intervention of others. Thus life is affirmed not merely as a gift from God to the individual to do with as he or she would wish. Life is also a gift that one weaves in solidarity with others in a circulating gratitude that builds life, even if, in the process, one passes through suffering and death. This perception lies behind the great synthesis made by the Christian faith in its passage through the violent death and resurrection of Jesus.

Derived from this perception is a concept of justice that is important for a liberationist bioethics. We are used to understanding justice as *distributive equity,* and that is undoubtedly one of its fundamental meanings. But experience of the God of life, the Father of all, shows that "justice alone does not have the last word" (Gutiérrez 1987: 142). The fundamental discovery is the gratuity that we learn from the very affirmation of life as a gift of God. To exclude gratuity would be to undermine the ground on which we walk.[4]

This perspective opens up an alternative path for bioethics, precisely when society in general seems to be accepting competitiveness as the rule of the game of life, leaving behind the "vanquished." It questions not only the legitimacy of lack of commitment to the life of the other but also the mentality of those who are content with strictly legal relationships.

A Vision of Liberation

Because the vision that coheres around the concepts of justice, solidarity, and gratuity seems unrealizable, many of the poor and marginalized abandon their hopes, pragmatically bending before the demands of individualism. One aspiration, therefore, is important in any discussion of bioethics in a liberationist key. It is the aspiration to *liberate bioethics* itself,[5] so that it may avoid being merely a legitimizer of practices that fail to promote commitment between people and avoid being a bioethics that serves the currently dominant social system, without any capacity for criticizing it.

Bioethics inspired by the desire for liberation takes as its task not only the eminently practical challenge of discerning ethical norms for action in the medical field, but also a more theoretical reflection on the general values that are the basis for human solidarity. Such reflection involves a serious critique of human relationships as they exist and the development of new forms of human relationship capable of transforming the exploitation, discrimination, and individualism. Without this reflection and transformation, the poor and excluded are not likely to find their place in bioethical reflection, and what is produced is not likely to be a liberationist bioethics.

The Challenges That Practice Poses for Theoretical Reflection

A close relationship between theory and practice characterizes the method used by those who share in the liberationist vision, and reflection on experience is a critical and obligatory moment in the reflective process. The concepts described above point bioethics in a direction that is unsettling on both the theoretical and the practical level.

It is important to study the implications of these con-

4. See Moser and Leers 1987: 121-26.

5. This notion is borrowed from Segundo 1975.

cepts for the methodology of bioethics. First, though, I wish to focus on the practices that challenge bioethics as theory elaborated from a liberationist perspective: from what, and starting from where, does one liberate?

The Challenge of Concrete Practices

The way we treat human life in practice is the basic point of departure and the raw material for our reflection. When we do bioethics, the vantage point from which we initiate reflection affects the quality of our reflection. It is one thing to do bioethics in the tranquility and relative isolation of a university study; it is quite another to elaborate one's thoughts within earshot of the cries of the suffering sick in a Rio de Janeiro *favela.*

For a liberationist bioethics, our *locus, our vantage point,* is not simply a matter of geography. It has to do with our network of social relationships, the people to whom we attribute importance, the necessities or problems to which we give priority. It signifies at once the point from which we gaze and the perspective with which we "read" and interpret our experience and project possible lines of action.

The perspective adopted normally points toward a community that nourishes our options and our practices. For example, a Latin American liberationist is rooted in a community of persons who develop a preferential solidarity with those who are impoverished and marginalized by society. Hearing cries of suffering in the midst of sickness and death, the listener is led to consider, in terms pertinent to bioethics, the root causes of the suffering and death of the poor and marginalized.

What topics emerge when we consider bioethics from a point of view that corresponds to that of the poor within our society?

1. The Degradation of Life

Despite the sophistication of medical technology, the devaluation and degradation of life is a tangible fact among those in Latin America. It is evident — to give only a few examples — in the high levels of infant mortality, in the low levels of life expectancy for adults, in the number of diseases that are endemic, in the number of accidents in the workplace. And these facts are but the tip of the iceberg. They show that the path leading to the doctor and the hospital, in our context, passes first through an acute social degeneracy. Sickness and death have their social roots in hunger, in unhealthy living conditions, in the lack of sewage systems and running water, in precarious working conditions, in the lack of education about basic health precautions, and in the lack of economic resources to put them into practice.

A few statistics help to summarize this situation. For example, the percentage of the population (urban and rural) that subsists below the level of absolute poverty is 46 and 83 percent in Peru; 40 and 65 percent in Ecuador; 32 and 70 percent in Colombia.[6] These figures send one back to the economic realities behind health policy options. Sickness and premature death bear all the marks of hunger and unhealthy conditions, which themselves can be linked with subemployment and low wages.[7] The social and economic policies of a nation, in their turn, depend on international political and economic systems. The sickness and premature death of the poor person in Latin America are therefore closely linked with both the foreign and domestic debt of his or her country.

The logic of the degradation of life that appears in this macrosocial scheme of things shows itself equally in the ecological problems that we face today. There is a growing conviction that these problems cannot be dealt with without concerted action from society as a whole. This complexity of social relationships within which sickness and death occur challenges bioethics to face up to one fact: the majority of viruses that the doctor scrutinizes under the microscope not only feed and develop on the biological body of the patient, but also nurture themselves in the body politic.

2. The Discrediting of Folk Medicine

It is illuminating to consider the relationship between technological advances in medicine and health care and the culture of the poor. Poor people in Latin America have developed their own ways of interpreting, resisting, and facing sickness and death. Certainly exaggerated claims for their results should not be made. On the other hand, advanced technology, while demonstrating to the poor a high level of efficiency in the medical and pharmaceutical fields, ends up discrediting the health care interpretations and resources of their culture. That in itself would not be a serious problem. The difficulty arises when, having deprived the poor of the resources provided by their folk medicine, the health care system also denies them access to the more technologically advanced forms of medicine. The poor are made culturally dependent in the area of health care, and then they are distanced and even excluded from access to its technologies by means of economic filters.

3. The Preference for Curative Medicine over Preventive Medicine

Social health policies, on a large scale, give preferential treatment to curative medicine at the expense of preventive medicine. This is not an innocent preference. Behind it lies a string of interrelated interests. For example, hospital systems and pharmaceutical and health insurance

6. UNICEF 1992: 72-73.

7. The average wage of 50 percent of Latin American workers is less than 100 U.S. dollars a month. In Brazil nearly 41 percent of the workers earn between 45 and 135 U.S. dollars for a whole month's work. See Anuário Estatístico do Brasil 1990: 104; also UNICEF 1992: 72-73.

companies, while undoubtedly providing social services, are also highly lucrative ventures. Clearly, sickness must exist so that profit can be made from it. The search for health is organized according to the demands of the market economy; paradoxically, health needs disease so it can offer itself as a "product" (Macedo 1981).

These economic realities help to explain the general lack of interest in seeking out the socially rooted causes of disease. Measures of public health more frequently indicate the lack of disease rather than the presence of health (Dallari 1987: 18). More serious, however, is the fact that a lack of concern for the close relationship between health and quality of life leads to a falsification of the statistics, which fail to portray the true state of the health of the population: a pile of percentages obscures the huge inequalities in quality of life and health (Laurentie 1985). Even worse is the Malthusian cynicism that says, "Only disease and hunger are capable of controlling the South's mad demographical situation."[8]

4. The Objectification of the Patient

The most common experience for someone who falls sick is to be treated as an object, as someone to whom things are done. Further, within the hospital complex, the "patient" is isolated from the cultural and affective ties of his or her everyday world. Death in the hospital thus becomes a drama. To the extent that medicine becomes a technique for curing disease and not a science that helps treat people who are sick, those who are incurably ill or who are old become highly problematic.

5. The Dispensability of Persons

The social and interpersonal practices that characterize medicine and health care among the poor add up to a frightening pragmatism. People become dispensable. The macro-political and economic level reflects this sense as well, where certain Third World countries are considered "dispensable" in the international economic scheme. Technological advances have reached a point where the rest of the world can do without the labor and even the raw materials from the Third World.[9]

This logic, which is beginning to be called the "logic of dispensability," has in its own way already penetrated the hospital, with the result that the claims of certain people to health care are simply discarded. A text on liver transplants in children crudely illustrates this pragmatism. The words are of a doctor and researcher: "The queue of children waiting for a liver transplant is long, and the criteria used for discarding a candidate are variable. Automatically one eliminates, for example, a child that wouldn't have the minimum sociocultural conditions, who lives in a miserable hovel, in subhuman living conditions. . . . On his first day home, back in contact with poor quality sanitation, he would quite likely end up with diarrhea, for example, and the operation would have been a waste of time."[10]

The influence of social factors in these cases needs no commentary. What is certain is that ethical reflection cannot afford to ignore these data.

The Challenge of Producing an Adequate Theory of Practice

Bioethical theory is itself a form of practice, expressed concretely in the principles, systematizations, and arguments that bioethics uses and in the proposals that it produces. The question is whether the theory sheds adequate light on concrete procedures and whether it can help in the transformation of the current situation. Before treating the question of method, we should note some of the challenges involved in the liberation of bioethics itself.

Bioethics, as a discipline, has received a great deal of attention lately, especially because of the interdisciplinary way in which its fundamental concepts are treated. Certain questions, however, persist, not the least of which concern the very concept of bioethics. In the Latin American historical context, there is a strong tendency to reduce bioethics to a mere deontology for the doctor, taught as an appendix to forensic medicine and mainly concerned with defending the interests of the medical profession.

In this situation, the scope of bioethical reflection frequently is restricted to the individualist concerns of the doctor or of the patient and rarely escapes beyond the boundaries of the hospital or the laboratory; the problems attended to have their origins in intensive care units or in the use of advanced laboratory techniques. These issues are not without merit, but bioethics should not isolate itself from the real context of life and health, death and disease that goes on in the world outside the hospital walls.

For example, in an article about the tendencies of bioethics in the last twenty years, the author included an item on those who confuse bioethics with social questions (Elizari 1991: 103-16). But the current patterns of thinking testify predominantly to a *disassociation* between bioethics and serious social problems. One reason for this, quite possibly, is that bioethical reflections are being elaborated by people who have no experience of these social problems. Another possible reason is the tendency to isolate the context in which one does bioethics from political and economic questions. I have critiqued these tendencies elsewhere: "In the first case we have a bioethics that is inadequate for the Third World.

8. See Rufin 1991,

9. Hinkelammert 1991: 1-6. The quotation is from an interview given by J. C. Rufin to *Paris Match* (15 October 1992): 40.

10. "Transplante de figado infantil: 85 percento de êxito. O trabalho do Prof. Maksoud e sua equipe," in *Prática Hospitalar* 6 (1991): 9.

In the second case arises the question of how one could possibly think through a bioethics without reference to politics and economics. On the level of anthropology it would signify neglecting the political, social, and economic dimensions of the body, while on the level of the reality of the social systems in which we live, it would signify ignoring the interplay of political and economic interests which underlie the themes treated by bioethics" (Anjos 1988: 219).

Thus we see that one must view bioethics more holistically if one is to avoid the danger of reducing it to an individualist vision of things. Further, it is necessary to attend to two dimensions of this holistic approach. One dimension permits us to understand the human person in the totality that constitutes his or her subjectivity. Consequently, one cannot arrive at an adequate bioethics without taking into account the horizons of meaning of human life, of suffering, of death — the horizons of the motivations and convictions that drive the subject or that may be proposed to him or her.

Second, one cannot possibly avoid the social dimension. A consideration of this dimension would start from a reflection on human solidarity as a necessary condition for the flourishing of the subjective life. In this way, bioethics rediscovers the social commitment that presides over our lives and our potentialities, concurrently being energized so that it does not become a simple legitimizer of selfish and subjective individualism.

A third and final challenge for the practice of bioethical theory arises from reflecting on these questions: For whom does one do bioethics? Who benefits? The theology of liberation alerts us to a vice that frequently occurs in ethical discourse: the tendency to legitimize ethically the status quo, with its dominant social, economic, and political system, forgetting to question whether the presuppositions of the system are antiethical.[11] The underlying question is whether and to what extent bioethics is capable of self-criticism so that it does not become a cluster of principles and systematizations at the exclusive service of people powerfully installed in society.

All these considerations converge to reinforce the necessity of an interdisciplinary approach to the doing of bioethics. Obviously, the social sciences which analyze society, its cultural traditions, and its structures, and the sciences of religion play an important role.

Some Methodological Principles

Here I propose some methodological principles for a bioethics conceived within a Latin American theological perspective. Of interest is not so much the religious convictions in themselves but rather their impact on the method used.

See, Judge, Act

The methodological procedure I propose includes three steps, popularly known as "see, judge, and act." This method aims at concretizing a strict relationship between theory and practice, drawing conclusions from the theoretical phase concerning the appropriate action. It seeks, at the same time, to maintain a certain dynamism by means of a circularity: new practices provoke a new way of seeing the world, which in turn provokes a revision of theory, from which derives a revision of one's practical proposals. This methodological circularity works its effect on the level of concrete practices, on the level of the practice of theory and, in our case, on the practice of theory that we call bioethics. Specifically in the case of bioethics, we can note the following.

During the *first moment* in the process, one looks at and analyzes the realities that would be a challenge in the field of bioethics. Specifically, the sciences examine the various dimensions of that reality. On the empirical level, it falls to bioethics to seek the help of the sciences that study the structures and mechanisms of the medical and health care world; on the philosophical level, to seek the aid of sciences that analyze the horizons of meaning of human life. This first moment is, therefore, one of interdisciplinary activity, during which bioethics opens itself to a broad field of concern both in terms of individuality and in terms of society. Obviously, it is not possible to investigate exhaustively all facets of this moment before taking subsequent steps. Precisely because of this limitation, however, we see the importance of the inspiration that presides over bioethics and that generates the options that we necessarily choose as we proceed with our analysis of reality. A Latin American, liberationist vision tends to lead preferentially to a search for the root causes of disease and of the suffering and death of the poor and excluded.

The *second moment,* methodologically speaking, is devoted to ethical and theological discernment. Here one confronts the options chosen during the process of analysis, and the initial conclusions to which one may have come with the criteria of faith. The spiritual faith tradition, enriched especially by biblical hermeneutics, nourishes fundamental convictions about human life in all its dimensions: historical, transcendent, individual, and communitarian. It offers criteria for choosing liberating practices as a response to the reality analyzed during the first phase.

In the *third moment,* one begins to develop practices of liberation that flow from the reflection elaborated during the first two moments. In the case of bioethics, it is a question of developing a new theory of practice that would be at the service of concrete liberating practices in the area of biomedicine.

The Question of Subjects

This liberating characteristic is made clearer if we look at some of its more constant preoccupations. The first of

11. E. Dussel calls this way of elaborating ethics "infra-systemic morals." Cf. *Etica Comunitaria* 1986: 43-44.

these preoccupations concerns the subjects of bioethics. Here, we cease giving privileged status to the social classes whose interests have tended to predominate until now, while at the same time discovering *new subjects* in the faces of the impoverished and the excluded. These new partners in dialogue even confront the more academic discourse of bioethics, at least to the extent that it (a) considers their problems and health needs, and (b) takes seriously their cultural world and their sentiments. This question concerning the subjects of bioethical discourse is indispensable if we are to liberate bioethics from a possible cynicism and hypocrisy in its choice of whom to exclude from the benefits of its service.

Microsocial, Midisocial, and Macrosocial Levels

The liberationist method is also constantly preoccupied with the extent of its social scope — with the extent and quality of the relationships between the subjects involved in the issues treated by bioethics. At times, these relationships are merely interpersonal, scarcely going beyond the interests of the individual patient or doctor. Three levels of activity are crucial in the doing of bioethics: the microsocial, the midisocial, and the macrosocial levels.

The *microsocial level* extends principally to interpersonal relationships that involve the doctor, the sick person, and his or her family. Case studies and a variety of questions raised by medical ethics frequently treat problems exclusively on this level.

The *midisocial level* refers to relationships that extend to the interests and necessities of groups, as, for example, doctors as a social class, or high-risk groups, such as AIDS victims.

The *macrosocial level* focuses attention on the great social systems and political, economic, or cultural structures, with their implications for a huge variety of relationships within the field of bioethics.

I indicated above the importance of these levels when I spoke of the need to consider the impact of macropolitics and macroeconomics in bioethical practice. In general, most bioethicists agree on the importance of reflecting on the subjective and interpersonal dimensions of issues treated. But reflection on the right of a sick person to die with dignity is not the only moving concern of bioethics. Just as significant is reflection on the quality of life and on the right to health for segments of the population who are often denied this right because of their social and economic exclusion. Various types of discrimination, especially in health care, are relevant topics for bioethicists. All these dimensions, however, escape scrutiny if bioethics does not reflect upon them at an appropriate level.

The necessity to bear in mind the social dimensions of our existence leads us finally to a preoccupation with discerning, with regards to human life, the values that are *most important* and *most urgent.* This means a commitment to recognizing a strongly relational character both in health in general and in the life of the individual. The health interests of the individual need to be confronted with the interests of the general public, and vice versa.

Challenges for Bioethics Today

Several important challenges must be recognized before one attempts to elaborate bioethics in a liberationist key. In addition, it may be helpful to locate points of contact between the Latin American way of seeing things and the critical re-reading of bioethics that is under way in the United States.

Our sharp criticism of the technicalization in biomedicine should not be confused with a rejection of scientific and technological advances. Human life and its complexity constantly require some scientific decoding and some technology to give it direction. Liberation does not and cannot signify naiveté in the face of vital processes; the conquests made in the area of medical care should not be despised.

Ethical criticism of technicalization in biomedicine has other sources, however, and it is there that we find the current major challenges for bioethics: to reconsider the subjects of bioethics; to be open to new *horizons of meaning* in the field of bioethics; to recognize the importance of social context for bioethics, and to appreciate the necessity for bioethics to have its own *mystique.*

Reconsideration of New Subjects in Bioethics

The question of the subjects of bioethical discourse arises as a prerequisite for doing bioethics effectively. This question challenges us to make people and not technological casuistry the focus for reflection. It also challenges us to reflect on our situation, which is one of being in relationship with others. This means that we must be prepared to open ourselves to questions about life that come from the poor and the needy; we must overcome, as a response to this questioning, a discriminatory and selective bioethics that merely concerns itself with the problems of a particular class of people who have access to the sophisticated world of well-equipped hospitals and laboratories. Here we identify a further challenge: the need to overcome a narrow view that reduces bioethics to the professional problems of the doctor and that tends to justify the treatment of the sick person as a "patient-object." A final challenge in this context relates to a consciousness of the cultural boundaries within which one develops one's reflections, a factor that leads to respect for forms of bioethics that are found in other cultural contexts.

Facing up to this group of challenges is a complex task. No matter how close our fellow human beings may be physically, it is at times a long haul truly to perceive the other as our fellow and our equal. It is undoubtedly true that in the United States, whole groups of people are excluded from access to health care. Thus one of the challenges for U.S. bioethics is precisely to make evident and unmask the mechanisms of such inequality. As a next step, it could then examine seriously the question, for whose benefit is bioethics being done?

Recognition of the Sociopolitical Dimension

Closely linked with the question of the *subjects* is another: the question of developing a sociopolitical dimension within bioethics. Bioethics would lose its critical sense if it did not consider the wide social context in which its problems and solutions interweave with political and economic problems and options. Even admitting that epistemological objections may make the evolution of bioethics on the level of politics and economics difficult, the necessity of, at the very least, conducting bioethical reflection in dialogue with social ethics persists.

Social ethics today makes strong criticisms of the political and economic systems that currently predominate in the West. In view of this, bioethics, if its field of activity is reduced to the hospital or the laboratory, ends up being a domesticated prisoner, and the risk constantly grows that it will be co-opted by an anti-ethical system. Bioethicists must examine what is going on outside the hospital and be aware of the factors that lead people to need a doctor. The challenge, then, is to introduce into bioethics the questions that have been identified by macrosocial ethics. It is true that some studies have led bioethics to concern itself with the problem of the distribution of health care resources,[12] but the question is much broader than that, and one should look directly at the national and international relations themselves that have an impact on bioethics. Precisely on that point, even in countries like the United States, bioethics must begin to reflect on its national options, bearing in mind the quality of life of all its citizens but also the implications of its international options for the life and health of other peoples and nations.

Openness to New Horizons of Meaning

It is vitally important for bioethics to reconsider the horizon of meaning within which we understand life, suffering, and death itself. For example, in the present horizon of meaning characterizing modern medicine, we see first that technological efficiency increasingly transforms death into a dehumanizing, a lingering, and often, for the people involved, a senseless horror. Second, an emphasis on strong individualism discards the bond of solidarity between people and insists on *individual well-being* as an indispensable prerequisite for meaningful life. Within such a narrow horizon of meaning, bioethics tends to be reduced to an ethics of efficiency applied predominantly on the individual level. This is surely an important limitation to overcome.

The opening up to new horizons of meaning challenges us to recover elements of our humanistic heritage, for example, a sense of the transcendence of life. Such a sense can confer on suffering and on death itself a meaning that embraces a life shared and transformed. Intercultural dialogue can reveal these new horizons with a certain facility, and undoubtedly the same can occur in dialogue with theology. As a science, theology has among its principal tasks precisely that of reflecting on and systematizing the questions and answers concerning the meaning of our lives.

The Challenge of Evolving a Mystique for Bioethics

It may seem strange to a way of thinking marked by pragmatism and the cult of efficiency to suggest that bioethics needs a *mystique.* In a liberationist vision of things, however, there is no way of escaping from this proposal. Bioethics needs a horizon of meaning, no matter how narrow it may be, in order to develop its reflections and its proposals. At the same time, one cannot do bioethics without selecting a series of options within the world of human relationships. That in itself is an indication of the need for some form of *mystique* or set of fundamental meanings that we accept and by means of which we cultivate our idealisms, weave our options, and organize our concrete practices.

It is not possible to define in a few words a liberationist *mystique* for bioethics. It would, however, include a conviction of the transcendence of life that rejects the notion that sickness, suffering, and death are unbearable absolutes. It would also include a perception of the others as partners capable of living in solidarity and of accepting life as a gift. It would witness the central emphasis on individual interests giving way to a willingness to hear the voice of *others,* to hear the cry of the needy and the excluded. It would witness a new willingness to redefine the values, principles, and norms that constitute bioethics. It may even herald the coming of a biomedicine that explicitly accepts being ruled by the demands of human solidarity.

As I present this vision of bioethics, I am of course aware of a much greater complexity to be explored in the terms here used. Moreover, a great deal of idealism is necessary if one is to forge ahead with developing a bioethics that allies itself with so many "losers" and with so many people who are excluded from the onward march of society. At the same time, it is encouraging to know that many people and groups, in different social and cultural contexts, are making enormous efforts to guarantee a life in which all are called to share and participate.

12. An early interesting article on the subject is Outka 1976: 373-95.

References

Anjos, Márcio Fabri dos. 1988. "Bioética a partir do Terceira Mundo." In *Temas Latino-americanos de ética,* 219. Aparecida: Ed. Santuario.

Aquinas, Thomas. *Summa Theologica* 1, q. I, a. 8.
Assman, Hugo, and Franz Joseph Hinkelammert. 1989. *A Idolatria do Mercado. Ensaio sobre Economia e Teologia,* 114-17. São Paulo: Ed. Vozes.
Dallari, Sueli Gandolfi. 1987. *A Saúde do Brasileiro,* 18. São Paulo: Ed. Moderna.
Dussel, Eduardo. 1986. *Etica Communitaria.* Petropolis: Ed. Vozes.
Elizari, Javier. 1991. "Veinte Añios de Bioética." In *Moralia* 13, no. 49: 103-16.
Gutiérrez, Gustavo. 1987. *Falar de Deus a partir do sofrimento do Inocente,* 142. Petropolis: Ed. Vozes.
———. 1989. *El Dios de la Vida.* Lima: CEP.
IBGE. 1990. *Anuario Esiatistico do Brasil.*
Hinkelammert, Franz Joseph. 1991. "La crisis del socialismo y el tercer mundo." In *Pasos,* no. 30: 1-6.
Laurentie, R. 1985. *Estatísticas de saúde.* São Paulo: EDUSP.
Macedo, Carmen Cinira. 1981. "A produção social de saúde." In *Vida Pastoral* 22: 9-12.
Moser, A., and Bernadine Leers. 1987. *Teologia Moral: Impasses e alternativas,* 121-26. Petropolis: Ed. Vozes.
Prática Hospitalar. 1991. 6, no. 5: 9.
Outka, Gene. 1976. "Social Justice and Equal Access to Health Care." In *Bioethics,* ed. T. A. Shannon, 373-95. New York: Paulist Press.
Rufin, J. C. 1991. *L'Empire et les nouveaux Barbares.* Paris: J. C. Lattes.
Segundo, Juan Luis. 1975. *Liberación de la teología.* Buenos Aires: Ed. Carlos Lohlé.
UNICEF. 1992. *Situação Mundial de Infáncia — 1992.*

11 Bioethics and Religion: Some Unscientific Footnotes

Stephen E. Lammers

Introduction

Bioethicists might well raise questions about the existence of collections like this one [*Notes from a Narrow Ridge: Religion and Bioethics*]. "Why another collection of articles speaking about religion or religious studies and bioethics?" After all, on one reading, religious belief and practice have fared rather well at the hands of the bioethics community. Religious choices, as they become clear as genuine choices, are honored. For example, bioethicists defended Jehovah's Witnesses when they refused blood or blood products, and today no one argues that physicians should not respect the wishes of adult Jehovah's Witnesses when no one depends upon them. In addition, bioethics centers and programs sponsor seminars on cultural differences, and among the differences religious ones are always noted. Bioethicists may be children of the Enlightenment, at least in their academic origins, but they insist that physicians and other medical care personnel respect the choices that people make. Among those choices are choices that flow from the religious commitments of persons who seek medical treatment.

The clinical side of the bioethics community might even speak up more strongly. Not only were they not formally involved in the Enlightenment project of trying to get past religious divisiveness to develop an ethic that would be universal, but clinicians generally have noted the religious differences of their patients and the effects of those differences. Further, many hospitals in this country have a religious community in their background, and a respect for religious beliefs and practices has long been a part of the clinic. Even many secular hospitals have pastoral care departments that are involved intimately in the care of patients. As a "lurker" on the Medical College of Wisconsin Bioethics Bulletin Board, I must say that I am often impressed with the sensitivity with which the religious beliefs of patients are often treated (there are exceptions) and the realization that the

From Stephen E. Lammers, "Bioethics and Religion: Some Unscientific Footnotes," in *Notes from a Narrow Ridge: Religion and Bioethics,* ed. Dena S. Davis and Laurie Zoloth (Hagerstown: University Publishing Group, 1999), pp. 151-63. Used by permission of University Publishing Group.

sensitive treatment of those beliefs sometimes increases the difficulty for the medical caregivers.

In addition, the influence of bioethicists upon medical and nursing personnel has been considerable — much of it positive. As a person who started "hanging around" hospitals 15 years ago, I can attest that physicians have become more sensitive to informing their patients and more careful to listen to their patients. Realistically, one might attribute some of these changes to the influence of patterns of litigation and state and federal legislation, but this does not explain all of these changes. In short, bioethics has had an influence upon the practice of medicine that, some would say, is praiseworthy. At the same time, some of the problems with contemporary bioethics flow from these very successes.

There are thinkers who are members of religious communities who are satisfied with bioethics as it is currently being practiced in this country. So the question of what this chapter and this collection might be about would be reasonable.

I cannot speak for other writers in this present collection of essays [*Notes from a Narrow Ridge*]. Nor can I, in what follows, pretend to speak from anywhere. I cannot claim to be other than a teacher of religious studies who does Christian ethics informed by a particular understanding of the Roman Catholic tradition. From within that perspective, let me give voice to my worries about bioethics, in particular a philosophical bioethics that relies primarily upon principles. Many of the points that follow have been made by persons with religious commitments different from mine or persons with no religious commitments whatsoever. The following concerns are seen as growing out of one interpretation of a particular community's vision of what a good life might be and what role medicine might play in that good life. One might make the same judgments from another starting point. At the same time, one might have very different reasons for these judgments.

How Bioethics Came into the Clinic

Bioethics came upon the scene when American medicine was losing its way. In particular, medicine had lost its service orientation. No longer intimately connected to the communities of service that had sustained it earlier in the United States, medicine had become technologically sophisticated and socially powerful. It also had become the place of arrogant behavior toward patients.

The field of bioethics began to develop in that context, and it appeared to be "prophetic." Many writers in bioethics reminded physicians of who they were and what they should become. In that setting, many welcomed bioethics as a corrective to what was happening in medicine. One example of a thinker influenced by his own religious tradition who was important in early bioethics was Paul Ramsey. Ramsey was clear that he expected better of physicians, that they should treat the "patient as [a] person," to paraphrase the title of his influential work.[1]

At the same time, other thinkers were not interested in restoring medicine to the service orientation it once had; they wished to rethink the relationship between physician and patient in the new circumstances of late 20th-century medicine. This reformulation usually took place under the rubric of patient rights and a contractual relationship between physician and patient.[2] Both philosophical and legal analysis would be applied to the rights of patients.

It was in this context that the case became important as a focus of discussion in bioethics. Cases here should be understood in two ways, medical and legal. Briefly, the legal matter first.

In the Anglo-Saxon philosophical tradition, there is an interest in law and legal regulation. In addition, in American culture, contentious events often turn into legal issues. Bioethics simply reflects these two phenomena. The consequence is that it is assumed that one should know the relevant law as part of one's expertise in bioethics and, in particular, one should know case law. Significant cases such as *Dax, Quinlan, Cruzan,* and *Wanglie* all are part of the knowledge base of bioethics. This attention to legal cases is simply reinforced by the use of medical cases in the clinical setting.

What then happens in the clinical setting with respect to cases? The typical case that is constructed for teaching purposes usually has a number of individuals who are involved around a patient. The patient may or may not be able to make decisions for her- or himself; what is relevant is that something must be decided for and/or with this patient. How to proceed is the question of the day. The conflicts in the case come in at a number of different levels. The patient or the patient's spokesperson may desire care the medical team thinks is inappropriate. Then again, the patient or spokesperson may wish to discontinue care that the medical team thinks is vital. An industry has grown up around the process whereby cases are resolved, and it is a requirement of the Joint Commission on Accreditation of Healthcare Organizations that hospitals have in place a process for the resolution of such conflicts.

Now it is not surprising that much of modern bioethics is preoccupied with cases so constructed. Many persons in bioethics work in or around teaching hospitals, and they were sometimes brought to those hospitals to help clinicians think about the difficulties of their work. The case is a typical device for teaching in medicine and nursing; it is useful for a discussion of the ethical issues that arise in the practice of modern nursing and medicine. What it is important to realize here is that, for clinicians, cases are one of the ways in which they learn.

1. P. Ramsey, *The Patient as Person: Explorations in Medical Ethics* (New Haven, Conn.: Yale University Press, 1970).

2. R. Veatch, *A Theory of Medical Ethics* (New York: Basic Books, 1991).

It was in the context of cases that claims about physicians' arrogance were articulated. It was by using cases to show how physicians proceeded with their patients that bioethics made its mark in the modern period. The enemy was the paternalistic physician; the object of the paternalistic behavior was the presumably competent patient whose wishes, especially wishes about the discontinuation of treatment, were being ignored. Bioethics became important by providing tools for analyzing cases where the paternalistic physician played an important role. Not so incidentally, in terms of hospital culture, bioethics became allied with various forces within hospitals that wished to limit physicians' power and authority. The choice of the patient was put over against the claims of the physician.

In many important ways, the introduction of bioethics into the clinical setting has been to the good. Physicians' behavior is probably less arrogant than it was in the past. More often than before, physicians and patients have conversations about what is important to the patient and what physicians think their obligations are. Still, it is not often enough.[3]

Note, however, what is not discussed in such a situation. What is not discussed is how the individual came into the healthcare system in the first place. What is not discussed are the ethical issues surrounding the care, or lack of it, for the patient before he or she came into the hospital. The social context within which decisions about the patient have been made are, generally speaking, not part of the conversation. Of course, one does not need to be working out of a religious tradition to make this observation.[4]

The tool that bioethics has used in order to make a difference in the clinic was its understanding of choice. Choice became a key concept of modern bioethics. Physicians claimed that they wanted to seek the good of patients, as the physicians understood that good. Without denying that physicians sought the good as they saw it, many bioethicists focused on the centrality of the patient's choice as determining what should be done. Much of what has happened in modern bioethics can be understood as the attempt to think out the implications of making choice the central datum in medical care. Religions were seen as one more choice that a patient might make.

The Metaphor of Choice

Religion as Choice

Thus the place to begin this inquiry is with the assumption that one can understand religious belief or religious commitment primarily as a lifestyle choice. Treating religion as a choice might be a positive development for clinicians in that they are supposed to respect patients' choices and, if one is consistent, one recognizes that consequences flow from those choices. Sometimes these consequences are of the type that clinicians are trained to resist and reverse. This is what happened in the discussion of the refusal to accept blood and blood products by Jehovah's Witnesses. Although many perceive this choice as irrational, and the risks of mortality or morbidity are sometimes high, it is argued that this choice should be respected. Note that it is not *religious* choice that is to be respected, but religion as *choice* that is to be respected.

Now it is not surprising that the bioethics community respects religiously based choice insofar as this community is part of American culture. Bellah and colleagues document how many people in the United States think that they can not only choose but constitute their own religious system.[5] But that is only part of the story of religion in American culture.

For many religious believers, their primary experience is not one of choices but of being called or being chosen. The important choice is not theirs but the deity's. Thus, the experience of some believers is that they cannot do other than they now do. To treat religion primarily as a choice is to misconstrue believers' understanding of who they are and what they are called to become. What is perceived by many on the outside as a choice is seen by the believer as being chosen. Jon Levenson does an excellent job of presenting this issue, and the political implications of it, in a discussion of "covenant" in the *Harvard Divinity Bulletin*. He points out that to understand the covenant between God and the Jewish people solely as the consequence of the choice of the Jewish people is to distort the textual evidence. This is not to say that choice was not involved; it is to say that it was a choice with no realistic alternative.[6]

The point here for Levenson is that the experience of choice is presumed to be one in which there are options. I might have bought car *A* instead of car *B*. This type of experience is simply not the experience of many believers. They are called or chosen to be who they are. They may refuse that call, but the choice is not neutral. To refuse the call is to be unfaithful. It should be obvious that this discussion is based on "Western" religious systems, ones dependent upon Judaism. Stanley Hauerwas has made this point in the context of speaking about bioethics from a Christian perspective in reviewing the work of H. Tristram Engelhardt, Jr.[7] But this is not only a Western religious view. The point could be made about

3. J. Teno et al., "Do Formal Advance Directives Affect Resuscitation Decisions and the Use of Resources for Seriously Ill Patients?" *The Journal of Clinical Ethics* 5, no. 1 (Spring 1994): 23-30.

4. S. Benetar, "Just Healthcare Beyond Individualism: Challenges for North American Bioethics," *Cambridge Quarterly of Healthcare Ethics* 6, no. 4 (1997): 397-415.

5. R. Bellah et al., *Habits of the Heart: Individualism and Commitment in American Life* (Berkeley, Calif.: University of California Press, 1985).

6. J. Levenson, "Covenant and Consent: Biblical Reflections on the United States Constitution," *Harvard Divinity Bulletin* 3, no. 3 (1995): 1-4.

7. S. Hauerwas, *Wilderness Wanderings* (Boulder, Colo.: Westview Press, 1997).

adherents to other religious traditions. Buddhists know that one "could" choose otherwise than to affirm the Four Noble Truths. To do so for Buddhists, however, is to continue in illusion.

Choice and the Poor

The difficulties of the model of choice in modern bioethics do not end with its failure to comprehend the experience of many believers. This model of choice is not the experience of people of limited education and income. For many persons in the United States, their lives are shaped not by their choices but by forces around them that they do not understand and of which they are (often rightfully) suspicious. To thrust them into an environment in which choice is presumed to be dominant is to put them in a situation where they will be hostile. Why should they trust anyone offering them choices? Physicians and bioethicists are perceived to be from the community of the educated and the powerful, which has been taking choices out of their hands for years.

For example, persons in poverty know that they do not have choices about the kind of medical care they will receive. There is a "system" of healthcare available to them that is not as good as that available to individuals who have employer-paid healthcare. Anyone who has spent time in the clinics that serve many of the poor people in this country knows that, if the poor had a choice, they would not be there in those clinics.

Given that many people in poverty do not have any choices about the kind of healthcare they receive, they wonder why they should believe they are being given a choice at some critical juncture in the care of themselves or a loved one. Choice, as they understand the world, is simply not the most important reality, and to pretend that it is to misunderstand their lives. This is one of the reasons that sometimes there is so much miscommunication between physicians and ethics committees and poor people. In the circumstances in which these parties often meet, the care of a loved one at the end of life, the only real choice of the poor is to resist. Often that means to refuse to do what the physicians are recommending, especially if the physicians are recommending discontinuing treatment. That recommendation may appear to all in the medical community as not only reasonable but required in order to minimize the patient's pain and suffering. However, for the child or the spouse of the patient, that recommendation appears to be one more way in which their lives are declared less meaningful.

Choice and Disease

Disease is another area in medicine where the metaphor of choice is not helpful. The discussion that follows does not deny that persons can make choices that are deleterious to their health. What is being argued here is that often these are not the most important factors.

Some of us are born genetically predisposed to certain diseases. A woman with a family history of breast cancer has certain choices, to be sure; however, her experience is not that of someone who is empowered to make choices but that of a person who has to deal with factors she did not choose. To focus on her possible choices is to miss an important part of her experience. But our genetic inheritance is not the only place where metaphors of choice are not helpful. Disease often comes to us because of causal factors over which we have no control. This lack of control may be due to causes that are unique to the individual, such as an airborne virus, or because of social arrangements that the person did not choose and from which he or she cannot escape, such as living next to a former toxic landfill site. In both cases, individuals have choices. Yet when choice becomes the central organizing feature of the discussion, much of what is important is missed. How one deals with tragedy, how one lives with events over which one has no control, the stance one takes toward these events — all of this is pushed into the background if choice about what to do about a particular matter becomes central. Further, how one might organize and join with others to effect change is often ignored. Yet, in the case of a toxic landfill, for example, changing those circumstances will probably have more to do with good health than any medical intervention.

In summary, the choice model that is assumed to be normative and supportive of religion turns out to lead to misunderstandings of the situation of many believers. Further, this understanding of choice often is a function of class and power. Finally, choice as the central metaphor is not true to the experience of disease for those who are ill.

Religion as a "Private" Choice

The model of choice is part of a larger project, that of the Enlightenment, within which certain phenomena are identified as "public" and "rational" and others as "private" and "a-rational." John Milbank has made this point in *Theology and Social Theory.*[8] Not surprisingly, medicine belongs to the public world and religion to the private one. This construction of reality privileges medical discourse.

Milbank points out how new religious claims are introduced *sub rosa.*[9] The consequences of this for bioethics are quite important. First, bioethicists are unable to appreciate and critique the functioning religious commitments of the Enlightenment project itself. Insofar as bioethicists participate in that project, they are unaware of their own religious commitments. Second, religion is pushed into the sphere of the private. Because bioethicists imagine themselves involved in public discourse, religious language must be excluded because it is

8. J. Milbank, *Theology and Social Theory* (Oxford, England: Basil Blackwell, 1990).

9. Ibid.

not a language of public discourse. An important corollary is that any statement coming out of a religious perspective is perceived to be public and relevant only if the thinker chooses to make it so, and on other grounds. By thus compartmentalizing religious language, religion is protected and at the same time neutralized.

In another place I have commented upon the marginalization of religious voice in academic bioethics.[10] The general issue here remains the construction of the public and the private spheres of discourse. Religious voices — whether they are the voices of an individual or of a religious organization or institution — have been marginalized when they are assumed to be private voices that are allowed to have their say as long as they do not influence public discussion. The Enlightenment forefathers of bioethics imagined a world in which there were "positive" religions (by which they meant Christianity and Judaism) that were "particular," and a "universal" religion that could be the basis of a civil religion. That entire construction of religion has been subject to critique in the work of thinkers like Nicholas Lash. One point stands out. The Enlightenment thinkers did not realize that they themselves were particular, that their constructions were just as historically limited as were the religions that they wished to overcome. But if that is the case, there is no reason to marginalize religious discourse to the realm of the private on the grounds that there is some language that is not particular but universal. Without that assumption, much of modern bioethics has to change its view, not only of religion, but of itself. Persons working in bioethics would have to attend to the historical circumstances in which they find themselves now and the implications of those circumstances for their task at hand. In short, they would have to enter into history instead of pretending to be above it.[11]

This is not to assert that arguments that rely upon assumptions not widely shared should win the day in public discourse simply because they are religious arguments. However, everyone's assumptions need to be understood, and everyone's voice should be part of the conversation. When voices are excluded simply because they are religious, there has been a confusion between the process of public discussion and the justifications for arguments in public discussion.

Religiously Based Critiques of Healthcare

It is at the level of the public world that members of religious communities have generated critiques of the healthcare system in this country. One example from the Roman Catholic community would be Andrew Lustig's essay on healthcare reform and healthcare rationing. Lustig reports that what is often taken as conventional wisdom on healthcare in this country has come in for critical comment from the Roman Catholic bishops.[12] He points out that the Roman Catholic bishops have articulated a position on what we owe one another in terms of healthcare that is markedly different from that of the U.S. healthcare community. Insofar as the bioethics community participates in that larger healthcare community and does not critique that community on this point, the bioethics community becomes marginal to the discussion of how healthcare should be organized in this country. One does not have to be Roman Catholic to make this point, of course. Indeed, at least one thinker proposes that religious communities have not done enough here. Yet the silence of the bioethics community has been noted.[13]

There is, of course, an alternative interpretation. Bioethicists have benefited greatly from the current medical care system. In their unwillingness to engage in systematic critique of that system and to use religious language here, the bioethics community begins to look like priests who are celebrating the beliefs of the powerful, and the religious communities begin to look like the outsiders. But that religious critique is generally not heard or attended to within the bioethics community.

Why might this be so? When discussion comes from the religious community directed to the larger community, it is difficult for members of the bioethics community to understand it. This is because bioethicists generally share the assumptions of the Enlightenment about religious discourse. First, such discourse can lead to great conflict. This assumption is, of course, true. Second, religious discourse can be a mask for self-interest. That, of course, is also true. Yet these two truths become translated into an attitude that manages to marginalize all sorts of religious critiques of the larger society and of modern medicine as part of that society.

Let us start with the second assumption first, that religious critique can be a mask for self-interest. Modern bioethics owes part of its heritage to the Nuremberg trials; one cannot talk about modern bioethics without talking about the Holocaust. It appears that much of what passes for reflection on the Holocaust is reflection from the perspective of those who did not suffer from it. This does not make it invalid. What it does, however, is to limit the influence of the victims, the majority of whom were Jews. If Jewish communities speak about experimentation upon human beings, for example, they speak out of the memory of this experience. The speech

10. S. E. Lammers, "The Marginalization of Religious Voice in Bioethics," in *Religion and Bioethics: Looking Backward, Looking Forward,* ed. A. Verhey (Grand Rapids, Mich.: William B. Eerdmans, 1996), 19-43.

11. N. Lash, *The Beginning and End of Religion* (Cambridge, Mass.: Cambridge University Press, 1996), 183-98.

12. A. Lustig, "Reform and Rationing: Reflections on Health Care in Light of Catholic Social Teaching," in *Secular Bioethics in Theological Perspective,* ed. E. Shelp (Dordrecht, The Netherlands: Kluwer, 1996), 31-50.

13. D. Fox, "America's Ecumenical Health Policy: A Century of Consensus," *Mt. Sinai Medical Journal* 64, no. 2 (1997): 72-74.

may have elements of self-interest, in that they do not want to see future persecutions of Jewish communities. But the speakers may see themselves as doing a service to the larger community, a service that the larger community may or may not desire. A perspective that can only hear that speech as self-interested or irrelevant for public discourse is going to miss important elements of that speech.

All of this flows with the difficulty of taking religious systems seriously as potential resources for discussion. It is obvious that they can be barriers, but the possibility of using religious systems as a resource is rarely explored. In following a recent discussion of caring and the altruistic caregiver and the ensuing debate on the Medical College of Wisconsin Bioethics Bulletin Board, I was reminded of debates that have occurred within many religious traditions concerning how one sustains persons who care for others so that they do not become self-righteous. One commentator said something like, "Being a child of or a spouse of a super-altruistic person would be very difficult." The proposal being made was that one had to switch to a model of caring in which there is explicit attention to the needs of the caregiver. This, of course, is not news to most religious traditions, which have long worried about how one sustains care in the face of adversity without either being overcome by the adversity or becoming absorbed in the care of some to the detriment of one's obligations. The solutions of the past are not recommended here. However, a familiarity with the literature might give us food for thought, as we struggle today to think about how to care for the sick and for those who care for them.

It is the responsibility of scholars of religion to remind persons in bioethics that these resources exist and might be used as part of the conversation. It is a hopeful sign that some scholars in bioethics appear to be willing to consider what thinkers who proceed out of religious commitments are saying.

One final example. Bioethics has had difficulty doing anything about the lack of universal healthcare in the United States. Although a small number of persons have worked on this issue, it does not seem to exercise the bioethics community as a whole.[14] There seems to be a kind of passivity among bioethicists that has received some notice. Given the fascination with choice as the central organizing metaphor for ethics, the importance of the case for medicine in general and with its choice dilemma for bioethics in particular, and the individualism of our culture, it should not be surprising that there is relatively little interest in the issue of universal healthcare. In this sense, bioethics simply reflects the culture instead of commenting critically upon it.

I am suggesting that there are grounds for a critique of the bioethics community from within the religious community where I stand. As I observe those who call themselves bioethicists, it is not clear to me that this critique is even known; the more worrisome alternative is that it might be known but it is being ignored. I have waited, for example, for a lively discussion of the debate going on within American Catholicism over the selling of formerly not-for-profit, religiously affiliated hospitals to for-profit hospital chains. That conversation, which could be a lively one, has largely not occurred. Where it has occurred, it has been around the issues of rights and not of social justice. Rights are important, but fascination with them leads to a minimalist account of healthcare. Such a minimalist account is incapable of raising the more important issues of social justice.

14. S. Miles, "Is Bioethics One of Kitty Genovese's Neighbors?" *Bioethics Examiner* 1, no. 2 (1997): 1-2.

Some Final Remarks

This essay is only an introduction to the issues within religion and bioethics. Other thinkers working out of the Christian tradition have made more radical claims about the nature of modern bioethics. Stanley Hauerwas of Duke University thinks of medicine as part of the Baconian project whereby humans pretend that they are gods and are in control of the universe. Medicine's power is hidden from us under the guise of its supposed neutrality and its scientific authority. Hauerwas's view is that medicine assists the "liberal project," which involves helping people put off death as long as possible. It is that liberal project that should be critiqued. Unfortunately, in Hauerwas's view, bioethics as it is currently constituted simply affirms that project.[15]

Gilbert Meilaender takes a different but every bit as radical a stance. Bioethics as it is practiced in the United States, according to Meilaender, has forgotten that human persons are beings with bodies. Modern bioethics is the latest form of dualism in Western thought, drawing, as it does, such a clear distinction between being a person and having a body. Meilaender claims that bioethics has in fact become "angelic ethics" and needs to return to the concept of person that is rich enough to include the histories of persons as we know them, from fetus to old age.[16]

There are other critiques of bioethics that arise out of religious perspectives, as well as celebrations of bioethics that arise out of religious perspectives. What is needed now is some attention to these critiques and celebrations. Without that attention, the bioethics community will continue to be entirely too self-referential and will fail to take seriously perspectives that offer fundamental challenges to it. Ironically, that is what some in that community might have said about historic religious communities. Often, in fact, that observation is on target when speaking about religious communities. It is becoming more and more true of the bioethics community as well.

15. S. Hauerwas, *Suffering Presence* (Notre Dame, Ind.: University of Notre Dame Press, 1986).

16. G. Meilaender, *Body, Soul, and Bioethics* (Notre Dame, Ind.: University of Notre Dame Press, 1996).

12 The Bible and Bioethics: Some Problems and a Proposal

Allen Verhey

Once upon a time I had a wise and wonderful teacher who said that in the simplest acts of piety — in prayer and reading Scripture, for example — we find new strength, new virtue, for daily life.[1] That teacher's remark is something like the North Star for the chapters in this book [*Reading the Bible in the Strange World of Medicine*]. I simply want to take that reminder of the significance of simple acts of piety to the hospital, to the doctor's office, to all the places we endure and care in the face of sickness and suffering and death. I want to find new strength, new virtue, for bioethics in the practice of reading Scripture.

To search the Scriptures and to attend to God in the context of bioethics, and to think about bioethics in the context of the churches' practice of reading Scripture — that is what this book attempts. Such an undertaking may well seem daunting and unpromising to the secular practitioner of medicine. Modern medicine, after all, seems thoroughly "religionless." The technologically well-equipped hospital seems emblematic of a "world come of age," to use Bonhoeffer's term for our secular world and its accomplishments. And such an undertaking will surely seem strange (at best) to the secular philosopher who prefers a bioethics that quite deliberately and self-consciously brackets talk of God. So let it be said again that the context for this undertaking is the church. It is first and finally and fundamentally the church with whom theologians talk of God. This project is a project for the church and of the church, for and of the church as a community of moral discourse, for and of the church gathered around Scripture, confident that reading it together may be a source of renewal and reform.[2]

Even there, however, even in the church, an effort to join bioethics and the Bible may sometimes seem daunting and unpromising. Even there, or especially there, cautionary tales are sometimes told. Precisely because the churches acknowledge the authority of Scripture, stories will be told that warn of the abuse of Scripture and invoke care in reading. Perhaps it would be wise to begin with one such cautionary tale.

A Cautionary Tale: Psalm 51:10, the Jarvik Seven, and Psalm 50:9

There was, so the tale is told, a heart patient who was both quite sick and quite pious. He had the habit of opening his Bible at random and, without looking, putting his finger upon the page. He would take any passage thus identified to be a word from God for him in whatever circumstances he found himself. After he had been admitted to the hospital, and after the initial round of tests and procedures, when he was finally left alone in his room, he took his Bible and let it fall open upon his lap. It fell open to the Psalms, and he put his finger down upon Psalm 51:10. He opened his eyes to read it; "Create in me a clean heart, O God," it said. And then he looked up with rapture that God should speak so directly to his condition. It was a word from God, surely — a message, a sign. And he knew what it meant. It could only mean that he should receive a Jarvik Seven, the artificial heart that he had recently read of in the newspaper. He summoned the nurse to report this remarkable event, and he sent a message to his doctor that he needed a Jarvik Seven.

The physician stopped by in the morning, and when she had heard the patient's story, she refused to take Psalm 51:10 as an indication of a need for a Jarvik Seven.

1. The teacher was Henry Stob. He said something similar in print: "Through prayer and scriptural meditation we hold communion with our God and find new strength for daily tasks" ("Justification and Sanctification: Liturgy and Ethics," in *Marburg Revisited,* ed. Paul C. Empie and James I. McCord [Minneapolis: Augsburg, 1966], pp. 105-17, at p. 116). That line was the "text" for the lectures I was honored to be invited to give in the remarkable series of lectures honoring Henry Stob, now published together as *Seeking Understanding: The Stob Lectures, 1986-1998* (Grand Rapids: Eerdmans, 2001).

2. Because the context for this work is the Christian church, obviously the Scripture to be searched is the Christian Scripture. There are other communities, of course, and other scriptures, other collections of writings acknowledged in other communities of faith as somehow having authority for reflection concerning the moral questions prompted by the practice and use of medicine. Islam, for example, has the Qur'an, and Islamic reflection about medical ethics frequently appeals to texts of the Qur'an as normative. (See Frazur Rahman, *Health and Medicine in the Islamic Tradition* [New York: Crossroad, 1987].) Hinduism also has its scripture. The oldest and most sacred of Hindu writings are the Vedas, but Hinduism also has the Upanishads and the Ayurvedic literature, the latter of which even contains two medical oaths. (See H. G. Coward, J. J. Lipner, and K. K. Young, *Hindu Ethics: Purity, Abortion, and Euthanasia* [Albany: State University of New York, 1989].) And Judaism, of course, has the Torah and a tradition of interpretation and application of the Torah to questions of medical ethics. (See David M. Feldman, *Health and Medicine in the Jewish Tradition* [New York: Crossroad, 1986].) This, however, is not a book about the relationship of the Qur'an or the Upanishads or even the Torah to bioethics. I am a Christian, and I write as a member of the community that acknowledges the Christian Scriptures as "canon," as a rule for its faith and practice. Moreover, I write for the Christian community, for those who make a practice of reading these writings as their Scripture and who struggle somehow to perform them.

From Allen Verhey, "The Bible and Bioethics: Some Problems and a Proposal," in *Reading the Bible in the Strange World of Medicine* (Grand Rapids: Eerdmans, 2003), pp. 32-54.

"A Jarvik Seven is probably not what the psalmist had in mind," she said. The patient was not easily convinced; he kept pointing to the still-open Bible and to Psalm 51:10. As the doctor got up to leave the room and to quit the argument, she put her finger down upon that same Bible, upon the psalm before Psalm 51, upon its ninth verse, and she read its words: "I will accept no bull from your house."[3] That sort of "bull" is probably not what the psalmist had in mind either, of course, but the patient was suddenly a little less confident about his method of "searching the Scriptures." And so should we be.

He should have known better, of course. This way of "searching the Scriptures" — as if they are a magical text that provides oracular advice upon request — is not the church's way to read Scripture or to exercise moral discernment. And to caution against such a way of reading Scripture is the reason, of course, for the telling of such a cautionary tale within the Christian community. But the tale also invites us to ask whether there are better habits of "searching the Scriptures." How can we read Scripture faithfully? And how does a faithful reading of Scripture illumine faithfulness in sickness and in caring for the sick? The cautionary tale reminds us that "searching the Scriptures" can be done badly, but it also invites us to consider more carefully how the Christian community can join the Bible to bioethics. There are some obvious problems with any effort to join them, and the cautionary tale suggests the wisdom of acknowledging them.

Some Problems

The Silence of Scripture

There is, for one thing, the *silence* of Scripture about bioethics. Scripture simply does not speak of the new powers of medicine or the new moral problems that they pose. No law code of Israel attempted to write legislation on human cloning. No biblical sage ever commented on the wisdom of in vitro fertilization or on the prudence of another round of chemotherapy and radiation. The prophets who beat against injustice with their words never mentioned the issue of national health-care insurance. No scribe ever asked Jesus about the use of human subjects in medical research, nor did any early Christian community ask Paul about physician-assisted suicide. The creatures of Revelation may seem to a contemporary reader to be the result of a failed adventure in genetic engineering, but the author does not speak to the issue of the Human Genome Project. The Bible simply does not answer many of the questions that new medical powers have forced us to ask. The authors of Scripture, even the most visionary of them, never dreamt of these new powers, and it is folly to "search the Scriptures" looking for veiled references to them.[4]

The Strangeness of Scripture

But the silence of Scripture about the novel powers and problems of medicine is not the only reason — or even the main reason — to be cautious about joining the Bible and bioethics. Besides the silence of Scripture, there is the *strangeness* of Scripture. When Scripture does speak of sickness and of healing, its words are, well, quaint. We should admit, I think, that the world of sickness and healing in Scripture is strange and alien to us.

Consider King Asa. "In the thirty-ninth year of his reign Asa was diseased in his feet, and his disease became severe; yet even in his disease he did not seek the LORD, but sought help from physicians" (2 Chron. 16:12). None of us, I presume, would chide a friend — as the Chronicler chided Asa — for consulting physicians about what was probably gangrene; on the contrary, we would insist that the friend get to a doctor.

Or imagine that we stand before a priest with one the Bible calls a leper. He is probably not a victim of Hansen's bacillus, or of what we would call leprosy today. He has some chronic skin disease, characterized by red patches covered with white scales, perhaps what we would call "the heartbreak of psoriasis."[5] The priest makes a diagnosis in accordance with Leviticus 13–14, but it leads to no medical therapy. Instead, as prescribed in Leviticus, the priest declares the man ritually impure; he tells the man of his exclusion from the community and instructs him to cry "Unclean, unclean" to any who pass by (Lev. 13:45). If our hearts do not break at that, they should at least shudder a little.

Or, consider David in Jerusalem worrying about the child born to Bathsheba and assuming the posture of penitence after "the LORD struck the child" (2 Sam. 12:15). It may seem odd to us, but in any sickroom of Scripture you are likely to hear the sounds of penitence. The "sick role"[6] in ancient Israel evidently involved as-

3. The patient's Bible must have been a Revised Standard Version (RSV).

4. This silence of Scripture is taken by some secularists to discredit the Bible. Carl Sagan, for example, has said, "The fact that so little of the findings of modern science is prefigured in Scripture to my mind casts further doubt on its divine inspiration" (*The Demon-Haunted World* [New York: Random House, 1995], p. 35). One might, however, equally well suppose that to expect Scripture to provide a text, or even a pre-text, for "modern science" is to entertain unreasonable expectations of Scripture. Whatever inspiration means, it does not mean that the Bible may be read (or judged) as if it were a science text or a medical handbook. Some questions are inappropriate to Scripture. If we ask the wrong question of Scripture, of course we will get a wrong answer, but the fault is not in Scripture but in our question.

5. Hansen's bacillus, or modern leprosy, was probably first brought to the Near East by the troops of Alexander the Great; see Klaus Seybold and Ulrich B. Mueller, *Sickness and Healing* (Nashville: Abingdon, 1978), pp. 67-74, and Stanley G. Browne, "Leprosy in the Bible," in *Medicine and the Bible*, ed. Bernard Palmer (Exeter: Paternoster, 1986), pp. 101-27.

6. There was a "sick role" in Israel as surely as there is a "sick role" today, but it was quite a different role. Today when we identify someone as "sick," we exempt them from blame for their condition, exempt them largely from normal social responsibilities, expect them to seek competent medical help and to cooperate in the

suming the posture of a penitent before God, pleading with God for forgiveness and healing. "There is no soundness in my flesh because of your indignation; there is no health in my bones because of my sin," the psalmist said (Ps. 38:3), joining confession to his lament. From our world of sickness there are many unanswered questions: What's the diagnosis? What's the prognosis? Is there a doctor in the house? But in the strange world of sickness in Scripture there is evidently no concern with a medical diagnosis, no effort to secure the aid of a physician or even to send for some aspirin (which had been discovered by the Sumerians a thousand years earlier).

It is a strange world of sickness in Scripture. It would not be difficult to multiply examples. We may as well admit it: Much of what Scripture says about sickness and healing is alien to us, and honest Christians are driven to admit that the words of Scripture are human words, words that they may not simply identify with timeless truths dropped from heaven or repeat without qualification as Christian counsel in bioethics today.

The Diversity of Scripture

Scripture is sometimes silent, sometimes strange, and frequently *diverse.* That's the third problem in joining the Bible to bioethics: Scripture does not speak with one voice about sickness or about healing. If, as we have seen, the sick were sometimes blamed for their condition and expected to assume the posture of a penitent, the book of Job rejects that familiar paradigm that sickness is a punishment for sins. Job suffers not only from his sickness but also from the confidence of his friends in that paradigm. He holds fast to his conviction that God is healer, but he struggles against the conventional assumption that the role of penitent and supplicant is appropriate to him because he is sick. Instead he insists upon his innocence and brings suit against the Lord (for divine malpractice, I suppose). Jesus himself rejects the putative connection between a man's blindness and either his own sin or the sin of his parents (John 9:2-3).

And as we have seen, while the Chronicler evidently rejected physicians and their medicines, in the deuterocanonical book of Sirach (also known as Ecclesiasticus) the sage Jesus ben Sirach effortlessly integrated physicians and their medicines into Jewish faith in God the healer (Sir. 38:1-15). "Honor physicians for their services," he said, "for the Lord created them. . . . The Lord created medicines out of the earth, and the sensible will not despise them" (Sir. 38:1, 4). King Asa would have loved it. And so, of course, would Luke, "the beloved physician" (Col. 4:14).

And if the Israelites in the wilderness and the Philistines at Ashdod and David in Jerusalem thought sickness was the hand of God striking, others could attribute disease to a variety of other causes. The Wisdom Literature, for example, could begin to trace sickness to natural causes (e.g., Sir. 31:20-22; 37:27-31). Apocalyptic literature attributed sickness to the power of demons or to the rule of death. The power of demons — at the periphery of explanations of sickness in the Hebrew Scriptures (e.g., Ps. 91:5-6) — took center stage in the New Testament's stories of exorcism (e.g., Mark 1:21-28, 5:1-20, 9:14-29).[7]

It will hardly do, of course, to respond to this diversity (or the diversity of interpretations of Scripture) by treating Scripture (and its interpretation) as though we were at some literary garage sale, looking for something we like, something that strikes our fancy, something that will not cost us much, while we regard most of the literary material as white elephants.[8]

The Abuse of Scripture

Scripture is sometimes silent, sometimes strange, and frequently diverse — but the biggest problem in joining the Bible to bioethics is not so much a problem with Scripture as a fault in the readers of Scripture. Readers are sometimes arrogant, and in that arrogance they have used Scripture in self-serving ways, twisting it into the service of the conclusions they had previously reached on other grounds. Scripture has sometimes been *abused* — and then people have also been sometimes abused with Scripture as the instrument. Appeals to Scripture, it must simply be admitted, have sometimes done a great deal of harm.

When Genesis 3:16, "in pain you shall bring forth children," was quoted to oppose pain relief for women in labor, a great deal of harm was done.[9] When some Dutch Calvinists, the "Old Reformed," refused to have their

process of getting well. So, at least, runs Talcott Parsons' famous account of the "sick role" (Talcott Parsons, "The Sick Role and the Role of the Physician Reconsidered," *Milbank Memorial Fund Quarterly* 53 [Summer 1975]: 257-78). The sick role in Israel was quite different: Far from being exempted from blame for one's condition, the sick person was very largely blamed for it. Far from being expected to seek competent medical advice, the sick evidently were, as a result of Israel's faith in God, cut off from the developing medical arts. Not only were the use of magic and charms forbidden, but the fairly sophisticated and rational medicines of the Egyptians and Sumerians were not to be welcomed, not even into the courts of the king. To be sure, there is evidence of folk remedies and salves and techniques for treating wounds, but medicine seems a heathen art in most of the Hebrew Scriptures.

7. The demonological view of sickness grew in importance in the post-biblical writings of Judaism. See further Seybold and Mueller, *Sickness and Healing,* pp. 112-13.

8. The "white elephant" image is from Victor Paul Furnish, *The Moral Teachings of Paul,* revised ed. (Nashville: Abingdon, 1985), p. 18. He contrasts regarding Scripture as white elephant with regarding it as "sacred cow."

9. See Ronald L. Numbers and Ronald C. Sawyer, "Medicine and Christianity in the Modern World," in *Health/Medicine in the Faith Traditions: An Inquiry into Religion and Medicine,* ed. Martin Marty and Kenneth Vaux (Philadelphia: Fortress, 1982), pp. 133-60, at p. 134. Numbers and Sawyer also observe, however, that Scripture was also cited to justify the use of anesthetics, notably Genesis 2:21, where God mercifully caused "a deep sleep to fall upon Adam" before removing his rib.

children immunized against polio because Jesus said, "those who are well have no need of a physician" (Matt. 9:12),[10] then a great deal of harm was done. When some prohibit transfusions because of a curious reading of a curious set of texts about blood, a great deal of harm is done.[11] When the Bible was pointed to by those who said AIDS was God's punishment for homosexual behavior, a great deal of harm was done. And when faith-healers cite Matthew 7:7, "Ask, and it will be given you; search, and you will find; knock, and the door will be opened for you," as if faith worked like a charm against sickness, as if it were only the littleness of one's faith that left one susceptible to mortality and vulnerable to disease, as if the sick should condemn themselves for their failure to get well, then a great deal of harm is done.[12]

It may be said, and rightly said, that these uses of Scripture are all abuses of Scripture, but people have nevertheless been harmed — notably women and children and other patients on the margins, seldom "righteous" adult males. The abuse of Scripture, and the abuse of people with Scripture as weapon, should give us pause before we attempt to join the Bible to bioethics. The silence of Scripture about the novel moral problems posed by the new powers of medicine, the strangeness of Scripture when it deals with problems of sickness and healing, the diversity of Scripture on these issues, and the abuse of Scripture, which has done real harm to real people — all of these conspire to suggest that there might be wisdom in simply refusing to connect the Bible to bioethics. Given all the problems, perhaps it would be best simply to ignore Scripture. It is little wonder, perhaps, that even those who know Scripture hesitate to read it as relevant to bioethics.

The Problem

On the other hand, there is that famous commendation of Scripture by the author of Second Timothy: "All scripture is inspired by God and is useful for teaching, for reproof, for correction, for training in righteousness, so that everyone who belongs to God may be proficient, equipped for every good work" (3:16). There is that commonplace affirmation of the creeds and confessions of the churches that Scripture is somehow normative for the churches' faith and life.[13] And there is, moreover, the practice of Christian communities; they continue to read the biblical materials not simply as an interesting ancient Near Eastern library but as Christian Scripture, not only as curious literary artifacts but as canon, not only as scripted, as written, but also as script to be somehow performed.

That practice is not an optional one in Christian community; it is essential to Christian community. "Scripture" and "church" are correlative concepts. Part of what we mean when we call a community "church" is that this community uses Scripture *somehow* as normative for its identity and its common life. To say "church" is to name a community that gathers around Scripture and uses it *somehow* to form and reform its walk and its talk. And part of what we mean when we call certain writings "Scripture" is that these writings ought to be used *somehow* in the common life of the church to nurture and reform it. To say "Scripture" is not simply to name a little collection of ancient religious texts; it is to name the writings that Christian churches take as "canon," as the rule *somehow* for their thought and life.[14] Ignoring Scripture is not an option for the church, at least not if it is to continue to be the church.

Granted, then, the problems of the silence and strangeness and diversity and abuse of Scripture, the real problem for the Christian community is not *whether* Scripture is somehow normative but *how* it is, *how* Scripture is to be performed in bioethics, *how* it guides us through the new powers of medicine and through the ancient human events of giving birth, suffering, dying, and caring.

If we allow the problems we have identified to overwhelm us, if we push Scripture to the margins of congregational life because of them, we put ourselves at risk of

10. See Richard Mouw, "Biblical Revelation and Medical Decisions," in *Revisions: Changing Perspectives in Moral Philosophy,* ed. Stanley Hauerwas and Alasdair MacIntyre (Notre Dame, Ind.: University of Notre Dame Press, 1983), pp. 182-202, at pp. 197-98. Mouw puts the best possible face on this foolishness, construing it as resistance against the tendency to reduce the human struggle with suffering to the medical model for that struggle.

11. I refer, of course, to the prohibition of blood transfusions by the Jehovah's Witnesses on the basis of Genesis 9:4, Leviticus 17:13-14, and Acts 15:29. See W. H. Cumberland, "The Jehovah's Witness Tradition," in *Caring and Curing: Health and Medicine in the Western Religious Traditions,* ed. Ronald L. Numbers and Darrel W. Amundsen (New York: Macmillan, 1986), pp. 473-78.

12. It is not just faith-healers who are guilty of abusing this particular passage. The Methodist Hospital in the Texas Medical Center painted this verse on an outside wall as part of a mural that celebrated the triumphs of medical technology. A visitor who noticed it (and not many did) might be forgiven for concluding that Matthew was advising them to seek the help of medical technology. I may be forgiven, I hope, if I suspect they were using the passage to baptize the triumphalist expectations of technology in modern medicine.

13. To give just one example, the Belgic Confession, Article 7: "We believe that this Holy Scripture contains the will of God completely and that everything one must believe to be saved is sufficiently taught in it. . . . Therefore we reject with all our hearts everything that does not agree with this infallible rule" (quoted from the *Psalter Hymnal* [Grand Rapids: CRC Publications, 1987], p. 821).

14. David Kelsey, *The Uses of Scripture in Recent Theology* (Philadelphia: Fortress, 1975), pp. 89-119. "Part of what it means to call a community of persons 'church' . . . is that use of 'scriptures' is essential to the preservation and shaping of their self-identity [and] part of what it means to call certain writings 'scripture' is that . . . they ought to be used in the common life of the church to nourish and reform it" (p. 98). Of course, as Kelsey also made plain, to say that Scripture ought to be used "somehow" does not say precisely how Scripture should be used to shape the church's faith and life. The agreement *that* Scripture has authority does not entail agreement about *how* Scripture should function as authoritative.

forgetfulness. Without the practice of reading Scripture, the church suffers amnesia; she forgets who she is and what she is called to be and to do. There is no Christian life that is not shaped somehow by Scripture. There is no Christian moral discernment that is not tied somehow to Scripture. There is no Christian ethics — and no Christian bioethics — that is not formed and informed somehow by Scripture.

Granted, Scripture is sometimes silent about the particular moral questions in bioethics that Christians face today. Granted, the worlds of sickness and healing in Scripture are sometimes strange and alien. Granted, Scripture is sometimes diverse and sometimes difficult. But in spite of the problems Christian communities turn again and again to Scripture, and they find in Scripture a resource to renew their life, to retrieve their identity and vocation, and to reform their practices. The fundamental problem is finally not *whether* to continue to read Scripture as "useful for teaching, for reproof, for correction, and for training in [bioethics]" but *how.* A contemporary Christian ethic will not simply be identical with Scripture, but it must somehow be informed by it.[15] *Somehow* — but *how?* That is the problem of joining the Bible and bioethics.

Somehow — but *How?* A Proposal

It is not the sort of problem, however, that, given a little time and giving a little effort, we can figure out and set aside as solved. It is more a mystery than a puzzle. The formation of a community and its moral life by the reading of its Scripture is a mystery that transcends our puzzling over it, eludes our efforts at mastery of it, and evokes not just curiosity but wonder. That mystery is admitted and celebrated when Christians point toward the Spirit of God as the One who both inspires Scripture and illuminates it.

The mystery should keep methodological reflection humble, but it does not eliminate the need for it. The Spirit did not simply overrule the human authors of Scripture. They spoke and wrote with their own voices. And the Spirit does not simply overrule the human readers of Scripture. We hear and interpret with our own ears. And as there were many prophets who claimed to speak a word from the Lord, so there are many interpreters who claim to hear a word from God in Scripture. The community that gathers around Scripture needs to think hard and humbly about *how* Scripture is "useful" for the moral life.

"Humbly" would indeed seem to be the first rule for the use of Scripture. *We must read and use Scripture humbly.* That first rule, of course, applies also to proposals for the use of Scripture. If we must read Scripture humbly, then surely we must make proposals for the use of Scripture humbly. This proposal is not offered as the last word about the use of Scripture in Christian ethics, as if this problem were merely a puzzle waiting for solution. It is offered in recognition of the mystery at work in creating and reading Scripture. It is intended not to be the last word but to be a helpful word, a humble contribution to the Christian community that gathers around Scripture in the conviction that it must somehow be "useful" to the community's conversations about bioethics.

Humility requires that any proposal for joining the Bible and bioethics acknowledge that decisions about how to use Scripture are reached not so much at the end of an argument as in the context of a religious community and as a result of an experience of the authority of Scripture within such a community. The authority of Scripture is recognized in and with what David Kelsey calls an "imaginative construal" of the way God is present among the faithful, of the way God is related to Scripture and to the community through Scripture.[16] And that "imaginative construal" of Scripture and of God's relationship to us through Scripture is enabled (and finally tested) by the common life of the community of faith; it is enabled (and finally tested) by practices like prayer and proclamation, liturgy and service, and — not least — by the practice of moral discourse.

To say that proposals for the use of Scripture depend on some "imaginative construal" of Scripture is not to say that there are no controls, no limits, on the moral imagination of those who would join Scripture to bioethics. It is not to say that proposals for the use of Scripture are finally arbitrary. It is not to say that there is nothing to prevent individuals with an imaginative brainstorm from twisting Scripture to their own and their community's destruction. These are old and legitimate concerns, of course. The author of 2 Peter expressed them early on: "There are some things in them [i.e., in the letters of Paul] hard to understand, which the ignorant and unstable twist to their own destruction, as they do the other scriptures" (3:16). We point toward the controls and limits when we return to the point made just a moment ago: Imaginative construals of Scripture — and proposals for the use of Scripture which have their beginning in such construals — are not only enabled by participation in the common life of the churches *but also finally tested* by the common life of the community of faith. They are not only enabled *but also finally tested* by practices like prayer and proclamation, liturgy and service, and — not least — by the churches' practice of moral discourse. A humble proposal submits itself to the community and to its practices. It makes itself publicly accountable. That requires, of course, that an account be given. Proposals for the use of Scripture must

15. See also the "important two part consensus" identified by Bruce Birch and Larry Rasmussen that "Christian ethics is not synonymous with biblical ethics" and that "for Christian ethics the Bible is somehow normative" (*Bible and Ethics in the Christian Life* [Minneapolis: Augsburg, 1976], pp. 45-46).

16. Kelsey, *Uses of Scripture,* p. 98.

be able to bear examination in the discourse of the community, must be "patient of reasoned elaboration" and "consistent formulation."[17]

Reading Scripture Humbly

The first rule for the use of Scripture, we said, was that *we must read and use Scripture humbly.* To read Scripture humbly is to read it with a readiness to be formed — and reformed — by it and by God speaking through it. To read Scripture humbly is to reject the pride or the "interpretative arrogance" that reads Scripture to defend our own righteousness and to condemn others as "sinners." When we use Scripture as a weapon against others and in defense of our own interests, we do not read Scripture humbly. When we called attention to the problem of the abuse of Scripture, we called attention to the fact that the abuse of Scripture frequently leads to the abuse of people, and we observed that it was usually women, children, and those on the margins who ended up hurt. Let the rule that we read Scripture humbly, therefore, make us suspicious of those readings of Scripture, including those that claim to be "objective" readings, that hurt or abuse the weak and powerless among us. Let the rule that we read Scripture humbly prompt us rather to identify with them in our readings. At the very least, let this rule prompt us to listen carefully to them and to *their* readings of Scripture.

Scripture is "inspired by God," the author of Second Timothy reminds us, but all our efforts to "use" it in moral instruction remain human efforts. We may not substitute our reading of Scripture for Scripture itself. We may not presume to speak the divine Word, or the last word, simply because our argument makes some use of Scripture. And we may not be so arrogant as to insist upon our own way in reading it, claiming for ourselves some "right to private interpretation." Love "does not insist on its own way" (1 Cor. 13:5), even when it is a way of reading Scripture. We read Scripture humbly when we read it in community with those who are different from us. We read it humbly when we are part of a community that silences neither Scripture nor each other, when we are part of the whole people of God attentive to the whole of Scripture. *We must read and use Scripture in Christian community.* That is the second rule for our use of Scripture, and all the rest are simply implications of it.

Reading Scripture in Christian Community

This second rule comes as no surprise, I suppose, for we have observed that "Scripture" and "church" are correlative concepts. Part of what we mean when we call a community "church" is that this community uses Scripture *somehow* as essential to its identity and to its common life. And part of what we mean when we call certain writings "Scripture" is that these writings ought to be used *somehow* in the common life of the church to nourish and reform it. Without the church the writings we call "Scripture" are simply a little library of ancient Near Eastern religious texts. And without the Scriptures the church loses its identity and its way.

Reading the Scripture as "Canon" Without the church, as we have noted, the writings of Scripture are simply a little library of ancient Near Eastern texts. Within the church, however, they are "canon." To read Scripture within Christian community means, therefore, that *we must read it as canon.*

"Canon" is correlative to "church," not to the university. Within the university, at least within the university formed by the Enlightenment of the eighteenth century, these writings *are* regarded as simply a miscellaneous collection of ancient religious texts. Within such universities, moreover, the interpretation of Scripture was and is required to be "scientific." A "scientific" reading of Scripture requires objectivity and neutrality; it requires that Scripture be treated like any other text. The historian's inquiry is limited to the historical situation about which (or in which) the texts were written. When the historians assume hegemony over the reading of Scripture, they conscientiously bracket consideration of the contemporary significance of the text.[18]

Moreover, because the Enlightenment regarded public order as founded on rational and universal principles rather than on the particular traditions of specific communities, the university formed by the Enlightenment undercut the "public" significance of Scripture. Part of that rational public order, after all, was the guarantee of freedom of choice in things "publicly indifferent." And the Enlightenment regarded the interpretation of Scripture as one such "publicly indifferent" thing. Individuals were authorized to interpret it in a publicly indifferent way — as addressed, as Hobbes insisted, to the "inward man" about the inward man,[19] or, following Kant, as a naive and mythical account of a morality that the "en-

17. Kelsey, *Uses of Scripture,* p. 171.

18. The historical study of these texts has, to be sure, provided important information about them, information that those who would read Scripture in Christian community may not simply dismiss. The historian's methods have provided quite valuable information and quite interesting theories about the history of Israel and of Jesus and of the early church, about the historical circumstances of the texts. The "objective" historian, however, is, ironically, always at risk of forgetfulness. There is plenty of recollection of data, but — without surrendering "objectivity" and joining the confession of the church that these writings are canon — there is no owning this story as our story, no remembering in which we can find identity and community. The "objective" historians are always at risk of reducing Scripture (and so, the memory of the church) to a (biased) recollection of historical data. The methods and results of post-Enlightenment historians fragmented the canon and drove a wedge between the historical meaning of Scripture and its continuing significance, and the wedge quickly opened up an "ugly ditch" between the past and the present.

19. Thomas Hobbes, *Leviathan* (Harmondsworth: Penguin, 1968), IV, chap. 47, pp. 710-11.

lightened" could now recognize and approve as rational.[20] Thus the Enlightenment sanctioned and sustained "the right of private judgment."[21]

In Christian community, however, the Bible is "canon," not just a miscellaneous collection of texts. The Christian community reads Scripture not to serve the task of historical recollection but to serve the task of memory — and the task of memory is to form identity and community. Christian community, moreover, authorizes no "right of private judgment." That would be to violate the rule against reading Scripture in Christian community. The Bible as canon is not the book of the Enlightenment university nor the book of the autonomous individual; it is the book of the church. And while the church puts the book in the hands of individuals, it does not surrender the task of interpretation to "private" individuals. We read Scripture — and perform it — as "members one of another."

The church is the community of interpretation. It does not license "private interpretation" nor substitute the interpretation of some ecclesiastical or academic hierarchy for Scripture itself. In the communal conversation and interpretation, of course, ecclesial leaders and academic scholars have an important role to play and a contribution to make, but the church does not gather around them. It gathers around Scripture, and it listens to the diversity of voices in the congregation.

And Scripture is the book of the church. It was, after all, the church that canonized certain writings and not others. Of course, the churches that made the decision to canonize these writings had already received these writings, had made a habit of reading them, and had discovered in them the authority they acknowledged in the decision to canonize them. It is fair to say that the church did not so much create Scripture as acknowledge it; these were the texts within which the Spirit moved to give life and to guide. Even so, that decision was obviously of critical importance to the construction of Scripture. And it was of no less importance to the identity of the church! If we are to read Scripture as "canon," then we may be instructed by the story of the church's decision.

The Story of Scripture: Reading without Dualism The history of the canon is, of course, a complicated history, but any account of it that fails to acknowledge the significance of Marcion is a flawed account. Marcion came to Rome around A.D. 140. There he proclaimed the gospel as he understood it, and there the church said that he misunderstood it, misunderstood it so thoroughly as to destroy it. Marcion (mis)understood Paul's contrast between Law and gospel to entail an antithesis between the Hebrew Scriptures and the good news of Jesus. Indeed, Marcion proclaimed that Jesus, far from being an agent of the God who had created the world and covenanted with Israel at Sinai, had delivered humanity from that Creator God, from Israel's lawgiver, from that vindictive judge. Jesus, Marcion insisted, had delivered us from the world that God made and from the hold that God has on us through our bodies. Marcion rejected the Hebrew Scriptures and proposed instead a new Scripture, a collection of the ten Pauline epistles and an abridged Gospel of Luke. Correlative with such a canon and with such a view of God was Marcion's anthropology. He (mis)understood Paul's contrast between "flesh" and "spirit" to imply a dualism between body and spirit and to entail indifference, indeed, animosity, toward the body. Accordingly, his version of Luke's Gospel left out the nativity narratives and began when Jesus "came down to Capernaum" (from heaven presumably). It comes as no surprise that Marcion demanded of his followers a rigorous asceticism.

The church said "no" to Marcion — "no" to his theology, "no" to his anthropology, and "no" to his canon. And when Marcion insisted on his own Scripture and on his own way of reading it, the church excommunicated him in 144. The response hastened the development of both canon and creed. The canon would (continue to) include the Hebrew Scriptures as Christian Scripture, and it would include a larger collection of "New Testament" writings. The creed summarized the story of that Scripture and guided the reading of it.

To read Scripture as canon, therefore, is to read it without Marcion's dualism — and to read it *against* any similar dualism. We must read Scripture without animosity to the world God made or to the bodies God created. We must read Scripture not as good news about deliverance *from* the world God made but as deliverance *for* the world God made. We must not reduce its significance to an address to some "inner man" about some otherworldly realities. We must acknowledge its worldly and "public" significance. And we must remember the rootedness of Christian proclamation in Hebrew Scripture.

The (Short) Story of Scripture: Reading according to the Creed Also entailed in the story of the canon is this: to read Scripture as canon is to read it according to the "Rule of Faith," according to the creed. The Apostles' Creed can be thought of as the "short story" of the canon.[22] It begins,

20. Immanuel Kant, *Religion within the Limits of Reason Alone,* bk. 3.

21. See John Milbank, *Theology and Social Theory: Beyond Secular Reason* (Oxford: Basil Blackwell, 1990), pp. 17-20.

22. "What the Scriptures say at length, the creed says briefly" (Nicholas Lash, *Believing Three Ways in One God: A Reading of the Apostles' Creed* [London: SCM, 1992], p. 8). The Apostles' Creed — or any creed — may not be *substituted* for Scripture. Lash goes on to insist that one can "only discover the meaning of the creed in the measure that the Bible stays an open book" (*Believing Three Ways,* p. 9). The creed provides the "rule" for reading Scripture, but it is to Scripture that the church continually returns and must continually return. The Apostles' Creed can hardly be traced, as the legend goes, to the work of the apostles on the tenth day after the Ascension, but it can be traced to a creed that developed in Rome about the end of the second century (John Leith, ed., *Creeds of the Churches,* third ed. [Louisville: John Knox, 1982], p. 22). The "Rule

as the canon begins, with the Creator. Against Marcion and other dualists the creed insisted that the Creator is the Redeemer, that the God who made this world, these bodies, and covenant promises is the very God who sent Jesus, "his only begotten Son," into the world. The center of the creed, and the center of the Christian canon, is the story of that Jesus, who "suffered under Pontius Pilate, was crucified, died, and was buried. . . . On the third day he arose again from the dead. . . ." And the end of the creed is the end of the story, the work of the Spirit; the creed, like the canon, concludes with the confident hope that the Spirit who gives life will bring "life everlasting, and the resurrection of the dead." The creed is a Cliff's Notes for our reading of Scripture. It may not be substituted for Scripture, but it may guide our reading of it. Indeed, unlike Cliff's Notes, the creed *must* guide our reading of Scripture.

Scripture As Script and As Scripted: Reading with Exegetical Care As "canon" Scripture is recognized both as scripted and as script.[23] It is scripted — that is to say, it was written. The texts of Scripture were written once upon a particular time by authors who did certain things with words. And it is script — that is to say, it is to be performed. Scripture is performed again and again by those who set these writings aside as "canon." It is performed again and again in the life of the churches, in their worship, in their organization, in their moral choices. Indeed, as Nicholas Lash has observed, "the fundamental form of the *Christian* interpretation of Scripture" is the life of the believing community.[24]

Every performance of any script is, of course, an interpretation. A performance can be improved if someone in the troupe attends carefully to what the author did once with the words at his or her disposal. To be sure, such study is hardly a guarantee of a good performance. Lacking other gifts, a troupe will give a wooden and spiritless performance of a carefully studied text. Moreover, careful study of the script is not even strictly necessary for an excellent performance. A troupe may have seen (or heard) enough fine performances in the past to perform not just adequately but splendidly. Even so, even though careful study of the original script is neither sufficient nor strictly necessary, it remains important — and important both for those who would check the "integrity" of a performance and for the troupe, for those who have the responsibility to perform. Moreover, because there are different performances, and because no performance definitively captures the meaning of the script, study of the script as scripted, as written, remains critically important as a test for and guide to performance. If this is true of, for example, Shakespeare's *Hamlet,* how much more is it true of Scripture as script and as scripted. The implication is obvious, I hope. It is a case for careful exegesis, for consideration of what the authors of Scripture did with the words at their disposal. To read Scripture as script to be performed we must read it carefully as scripted, as written once upon a particular time by authors who did certain things with words. The rule that we must read Scripture in Christian community is not a license to neglect exegesis, as though we could simply substitute some particular tradition of interpretative performance for the script. On the contrary, to read Scripture in Christian community requires that we nurture and sustain biblical scholarship as an important contribution to the communal effort to understand and perform Scripture. We must read Scripture with exegetical care and skill.

The canon itself recognizes that the writings gathered there have a history. Scripture is quite candid about the fact that it did not simply fall from heaven as some timeless document. Luke, for example, reported that he made use of the oral tradition and of other narratives in putting together his Gospel. Paul's letters are quite clearly letters, concrete addresses to particular congregations dealing with specific problems in a timely way. To read Scripture with exegetical care and skill will mean to attend not only to the grammatical construction of the words authors had at their disposal but also to literary issues like genre, to issues of audience and occasion, to the use of sources and traditions, and to the social and historical location of the text as written.

Reading Scripture among Diverse Gifts and Voices To read Scripture with exegetical care and skill is a daunting task, and as we have said, careful attention to the script as scripted does not ensure a lively and spirited performance. So, we come back to the rule about reading Scripture in Christian community, now to celebrate the diversity of gifts within the community. Some are gifted with exegetical learning and skills. They bring their knowledge of Hebrew and Greek, or their training in the tools of historical, literary, or social investigation, not just to the texts but to the community. And the community may be glad for their contribution to the communal task of interpretative performance. Others are gifted with an awareness of the traditions of interpretation and performance within that particular community — or within a different particular community. Some are gifted with moral imagination. Some are gifted with a passion for righteousness, a hunger for justice. Some are gifted with sweet reasonableness, peacemakers among us. Some are gifted with intellectual clarity, and some with simple piety. Such gifted people — including those gifted with exegetical learning — may not boast of their gifts, or

of Faith" of Irenaeus (in the late second century) was not exactly a creed, but it did quite deliberately provide a guide for the interpretation of Scripture (and a basis for catechetical instruction), so that the church would not be misled by Gnosticism and its dualism.

23. Or, to use a distinction made by Nicholas Wolterstorff, Scripture is both "object" and "instrument"; it is the effect of the action of writing texts and the instrument that we use to perform certain other actions. See Nicholas Wolterstorff, *Art in Action: Toward a Christian Aesthetic* (Grand Rapids: Eerdmans, 1980), p. 80.

24. Nicholas Lash, "Performing the Scriptures," in *Theology on the Way to Emmaus* (London: SCM, 1986), p. 40.

claim to have no need of the other members of the community. The task of interpretative performance is a communal one. We must read Scripture in Christian community, glad for the diversity of gifts we find there.

There is a diversity of gifts — and there will likely remain also a diversity of interpretations, diverse ways of using Scripture as morally instructive. Reading Scripture in Christian community does not mean that we will always agree. There have been diverse ways of using Scripture in moral discourse for as long as there have been Christian communities. Jewish Christians did not all read Scripture one way, but they read it differently than many Gentile Christians did. Within the New Testament canon there are diverse ways of interpreting the Hebrew Scripture and the traditions concerning Jesus, of using them for moral instruction. Matthew, for example, has Jesus say of the Torah that "whoever breaks one of the least of these commandments, and teaches others to do the same, will be called least in the kingdom of heaven" (Matt. 5:19). Mark, on the other hand, reports not only that Jesus broke the Sabbath commandment (Mark 2:23–3:6; cf. Matt. 12:1-14) but also that he taught others to disregard the commandments concerning kosher (Mark 7:18-19). To read Scripture in Christian community, to read Scripture as canon, is not to insist upon unanimity in reading it. It is to insist that, together with those with whom we differ, we hand down existing traditions — *and continue to assess existing traditions* — of interpretative performance of Scripture, of those works written by authors and recognized as canon.

Reading Scripture Prayerfully To read Scripture in Christian community is to read it in ways informed by the practices of Christian community, and finally tested by those practices. Consider, for example, the practice of prayer. There is an obvious — but often overlooked — connection between reading Scripture and prayer. The churches recognize the connection in the intimate association between Scripture and prayer in most Christian liturgies. When Scripture is read, a prayer for illumination is close at hand. We read Scripture in the context of prayer. Wisely so, for we must read Scripture prayerfully.

Moreover, to pray is itself a performance of Scripture. When we say the Lord's Prayer, following the advice of Scripture, "Pray then in this way . . ." (Matt. 6:9), or when we cry "Abba!" (Rom. 8:15) or "*Maranatha*" (1 Cor. 16:22), or when we simply groan in pain toward God's good future (Rom. 8:22-27), we perform Scripture. We pray in the context of reading Scripture, and we must read Scripture in the context of the practice of prayer.

Prayer is a part of the Christian life. Indeed, it is, as John Calvin said, the most important part, "the chief exercise of faith,"[25] the part of the whole Christian life that cannot be left out without the whole ceasing to *be* the Christian life. And as Karl Barth said, the Christian life is a life of prayer, a life of "humble and resolute, frightened and joyful invocation of the gracious God in gratitude, praise, and above all, petition."[26] Prayer is a practice of the Christian life; it is, to use Alasdair MacIntyre's important (but complex) definition of a practice, a

> socially established cooperative human activity through which goods internal to that form of activity are realized in the course of trying to achieve those standards of excellence which are appropriate to, and partially definitive of, that form of activity with the result that human powers to achieve excellence and human conceptions of the ends and goods involved are systematically extended.[27]

To be sure, not many Christians at prayer are likely to quote Calvin or Barth or MacIntyre, but some Christians at prayer would be likely to make Calvin and Barth and MacIntyre nod their heads and say, "Yes, that's what I meant."

Prayer is learned in Christian community, and it is learned not only as an idea but as a human activity that engages one's body as well as one's mind, one's affections and passions and loyalties as well as one's rationality. Prayer is an activity that focuses one's whole self on God. In learning to pray, one learns the good that is "internal to that form of activity"; one learns, that is, to attend to God, to look to God.[28] To attend to God is not easy to learn — or painless. Given our inveterate attention to ourselves and to our own needs and wants, we frequently corrupt the practice. We corrupt prayer whenever we turn it into a means to accomplish some other good than the good of prayer, whenever we make of it an instrument to achieve wealth, happiness, health, or even moral improvement. In learning to pray, we learn to look to God; and after the blinding vision, we begin to look at all else in a new light.

In learning to pray, we learn as well certain standards of excellence[29] that belong to prayer and its attention to God, standards of excellence that are appropriate to prayer and partially definitive of prayer. In learning to pray, we learn *reverence,* the readiness to attend to God as God and to all else in relation to God. In learning to

25. John Calvin, *Institutes,* III.xx.1.

26. Karl Barth, *Church Dogmatics,* IV/4: *The Christian Life,* trans. Geoffrey Bromiley (Grand Rapids: Eerdmans, 1981), p. 43.

27. Alasdair MacIntyre, *After Virtue: A Study in Moral Theory* (Notre Dame, Ind.: University of Notre Dame Press, 1981), p. 175. On prayer as a practice, see further Allen Verhey, "The Practices of Piety and the Practice of Medicine: Prayer, Scripture, and Medical Ethics," in *Seeking Understanding: The Stob Lectures, 1986-1998* (Grand Rapids: Eerdmans, 2001), pp. 191-250.

28. On prayer as attention see especially Iris Murdoch, "On 'God' and 'Good,'" in *Revisions: Changing Perspectives in Moral Philosophy,* ed. Hauerwas and MacIntyre, pp. 68-91; Craig Dykstra, *Vision and Character* (New York: Paulist, 1981), pp. 45-98; and Simone Weil, *Waiting on God,* trans. E. Craufurd (London: Routledge and Kegan Paul, 1951), p. 51.

29. Consider, for example, John Calvin's attention to the "rules" of prayer in *Institutes,* III.xx.4-16. Calvin's "rules" are reverence, a sincere sense of want (that is, to pray earnestly), humility, and confident hope.

pray, we learn *humility,* the readiness to acknowledge that we are not gods but the creatures of God, cherished by God but finite and mortal and, yes, sinful creatures in need finally of God's grace and God's future. In learning to pray, we learn *gratitude,* the disposition of thankfulness for the opportunities within the limits of our finiteness and mortality to delight in God and in the gifts of God. We learn *hope,* a disposition of confidence and courage that comes not from trusting oneself and the little truth one knows well or the little good one does well, but from trusting the grace and power of God. And we learn *care;* attentive to God, we grow attentive to the neighbor as related to God. These standards of excellence form virtues not only for prayer but also for daily life — and for the reading of Scripture. Prayer-formed persons and prayer-formed communities — in the whole of their being and in the whole of their living — will be reverent, humble, grateful, hopeful, and caring. One does not pray in order to achieve these virtues. They are not formed when we use prayer as a technique. They are formed in simple attentiveness to God, and they spill over into new virtues for daily life and discernment.

What would a prayer-formed reading of Scripture look like? There are some hints, I think, in these standards of excellence, but consider also the forms that such attention to God takes. Prayer attends to God in the forms of invocation and adoration, confession, thanksgiving, and petition. *Invocation* is remembrance.[30] We invoke (and revere) not just any old god, not some nameless god of philosophical theism, not some idolatrous object of somebody's "ultimate concern." We invoke the God "rendered" in Scripture, and a prayer-formed reading of Scripture will serve remembrance and invocation. So the practice of prayer both performs Scripture and forms the practice of reading Scripture in Christian community. We remember God; and, as we do, we are reoriented to God and to all things in relation to *that* God.

This reorientation to all things is called *metanoia,* repentance. Invocation evokes repentance. Attention to God in prayer, therefore, also takes the form of (humble) *confession.* Prayerful readings of Scripture will serve confession. Prayer will form a readiness to read Scripture over-against ourselves and not just for ourselves; over-against our lives and our common life and not simply in self-serving defense of them; over-against even our conventional readings of Scripture, subverting our efforts to use the texts to boast about our own righteousness or to protect our own status and power. Confession is good for the soul, but it is also good for hermeneutics; it can form a hermeneutic humility. Such humility will attend carefully but without anxiety to the readings of saints and strangers (especially to the readings of the poor and the powerless and those whom it has been too much our impulse to shun and neglect), and it will attend to the whole church attending to the whole Scripture.

Attention to God also takes the form of (grateful) *thanksgiving.* Gratitude to God can form in readers the readiness not to count what is given as "ours to dispose of as if we created it nor ours to serve only our own interests."[31] Prayers of thanksgiving can train us to stewardship of our gifts, including Scripture and the skills to read it. They train readers to share their gifts, to use them in service to the community, without the conceit of philanthropy. The conceit of philanthropy divides the community of readers into two groups, the relatively self-sufficient benefactors (or scholars) and the needy beneficiaries of their interpretative skill. Prayer-formed readers of Scripture will share their gifts (including the scholarly gifts of some readers) and serve the community, acknowledging that we are each and all recipients of God's gifts. Such service is no less a response to gift than the prayers of thanksgiving themselves. Gratitude, moreover, trains readers to gladness, to delight in the gifts of God, including Scripture. It forms an attitude toward Scripture that is itself a "performance" of the psalmists' delight in Torah. Moreover, as prayers of thanksgiving are a form of attention to God, the gifts are celebrated not so much because they serve our interests as because they manifest God's grace and glory and serve God's cause. Prayers of thanksgiving, then, this form of attention to God, form in the community of readers a readiness to reform their reading habits and their "performances" that God may be manifest and God's cause served.

Finally, simple attentiveness to God takes the form of (hopeful and caring) *petition.* It is easy, of course, in petition to attend to ourselves rather than to God, to our wishes rather than to God's cause. The practice of prayer is corrupted when we use it as a kind of magic to get what we want, whether a fortune, or four more healthy years, or a resolution to an interpretative or moral dispute. When petition is a form of attention to God, however, then we pray — and pray boldly — that God's cause will be displayed, that God's good future will be present. We pray — and pray boldly — as Jesus taught us, for a taste of that future, for a taste of it not in an ecstatic spiritual experience but in such ordinary things as everyday bread and everyday forgiveness, in such mundane realities as tonight's rest and tomorrow's work, in such earthy stuff as the health of mortal flesh and the peace and justice of our communities. We govern our petitions — and our deeds, including the acts of reading and interpreting Scripture — by a vision of God's good future and by the aching acknowledgment that it is not yet. That vision is evoked by remembrance and formed by reading Scrip-

30. On prayer as an act of remembrance see Nicholas Wolterstorff, *Until Justice and Peace Embrace* (Grand Rapids.: Eerdmans, 1983), pp. 152-56. Donald Saliers, "Liturgy and Ethics: Some New Beginnings," *Journal of Religious Ethics* 7 (Fall 1979): 173-89, also emphasizes that "the shape and substance of prayer is anamnetic" (p. 178).

31. James M. Gustafson, "Spiritual Life and Moral Life," in *Theology and Christian Ethics* (Philadelphia: Pilgrim, 1974), p. 170.

ture, but it also must govern our readings. A prayer-formed reading of Scripture attends to God and to the cause of God, and it forms in turn both our words in petition and our works in everyday attention to God. So, the practice of prayer may form both the practice of reading Scripture and the Christian life.

Prayer is not a technique to get what we want, and it does not rescue us from ambiguity. It does not free us from the necessity of thinking hard about moral cases, sorting out various principles, identifying the various goods at stake, and listening carefully to different accounts of the situation. It does not liberate us from the tasks of reading texts carefully, attending to genre and to grammar, to historical and social contexts. Prayer does not rescue us from all of that, but it does permit us to do all of that while attentive to God and to be attentive to all of that as related to God. Moreover, the standards of excellence for prayer — reverence, humility, gratitude, hope, and care — may spill over into both our reading and our living when our reading is remembrance and our lives are attentive to God.

The Practice of Reading Scripture To read Scripture in Christian community is, as we have said, to read it in ways informed — and tested — by the practices of Christian community. Prayer is such a practice, but so is reading Scripture itself.[32] Christians learn to read Scripture (and to read Scripture as important to the moral life) by being initiated into the practice of reading Scripture in Christian community, not by being taught that a creed calls Scripture an "infallible rule," nor by being taught by a biblical scholar that the Bible is a little library of ancient Near Eastern literature. The creed and the scholar may both be right, and Christian communities should affirm their creeds and be hospitable to scholars, but Christians learn this practice of reading Scripture in Christian community.

In learning to read Scripture as a practice of Christian community, Christians learn as well the good that belongs to reading Scripture, the "good internal to that form of activity." They learn, that is, *to remember.*[33] They learn to remember not only as an intellectual exercise, not just as a mental process of recollection, not just as disinterested recall of historical facts. They learn to own a past as their own past in the continuing church, and to own it as constitutive of identity and determinative for discernment.

That remembered past is not simply a series of events that can be described objectively but rather events to be celebrated in repentance and jubilee, to be rehearsed in ritual and festival. That past, moreover, is not simply gone; we do not live in the past, but it lives in us. Neither we nor our communities live in simple transcendence over time. Against Kant and Kierkegaard, it must be said that we do not discover ourselves as "noumenal" selves in moments of radical freedom cut off from past and future. On the contrary, we find ourselves by remembering. By remembering we interpret the present, make sense of it. And by remembering we sustain certain possibilities and nurture certain expectations; by remembering we learn to hope. Without memory there is no hope. We are not "fated" by our past (not as long as repentance remains a possibility sustained by our memory, at any rate). On the contrary, the freedom we have we have by marshalling memories, by learning to tell a different story of our lives, to interpret our present situation differently, and by sustaining other possibilities.

Without remembering, there is no identity. In amnesia, one loses oneself. In memory, one finds an identity. And without common remembering, there is no community. It is little wonder that the church sustains this practice of reading Scripture and is itself sustained by it. The practice of reading Scripture is not the only way the church has to remember, but Scripture is surely the critical document for the church's remembering.

There are temptations to forgetfulness in public life, when Enlightenment assumptions demand generic principles and "scientific" knowledge, pushing "god" to the margins. There are temptations to forgetfulness in personal life, when the private realm is construed as a space for the self-centered quest to satisfy desire. And there are temptations to forgetfulness, ironically, in the sort of historical reading of Scripture that treats these writings simply as the (more or less reliable) record of a figure of the past whose life ended with his death. Then the memory of Jesus is "merely a memory,"[34] an intellectual process of recollection, a disinterested reconstruction of some historical facts, not the memory that is constitutive of identity and community and determinative for discernment. In Christian community Scripture is read on the Lord's Day, in celebration of resurrection, and in the confidence that the remembered Jesus lives. Forgetfulness threatens a loss of identity, but the remedy for forgetfulness is remembrance, and remembrance is served by reading Scripture.

Moreover, in learning to read Scripture and to remember (just as in learning to pray), Christians learn as well certain standards of excellence appropriate to and partially definitive of this practice — three pairs of virtues for reading Scripture: holiness and sanctification, fidelity and creativity, discipline and discernment.

Holiness is the standard of excellence for reading Scripture in Christian community that sets these writings apart from others, and also sets apart a time and a place to

32. On reading Scripture as a practice, see further Verhey, "The Practices of Piety," pp. 41-51, and "The Holy Bible and Sanctified Sexuality," *Interpretation* 49, no. 1 (1995): 41-45.

33. For the notion of remembrance as the "good" of reading Scripture, I am indebted to Hauerwas, "The Moral Authority of Scripture: The Politics and Ethics of Remembering," in *A Community of Character* (Notre Dame, Ind.: University of Notre Dame Press, 1981), pp. 53-71. See also James M. Gustafson, *Treasure in Earthen Vessels* (New York: Harper and Brothers, 1961), pp. 71-78.

34. See Luke Timothy Johnson, *Living Jesus: Learning the Heart of the Gospel* (San Francisco: HarperSanFrancisco, 1999), pp. 3-11.

read them and to remember.[35] *Sanctification* is the standard of excellence in reading Scripture that is ready to set this canon alongside our lives and our common life as their rule and guide. If holiness sets the Bible apart, and sets apart a time to read and to remember, sanctification is the readiness to set the remembered story not just apart but *alongside* all the stories of our lives — stories of sexual desire, stories of sickness and healing, stories of wealth and poverty, stories of our politics — until our conduct and character and communities are judged and made new by the power of God, are formed in remembrance and hope, and themselves render the story rendered by Scripture.[36] Sanctification invites and welcomes attention to the saints as the best interpreters.

Remembrance provides identity, and *fidelity* is simply the standard of excellence in reading and performing Scripture that is ready to live with integrity, ready to live faithfully in the memory that the church has owned as its own and in the hope that memory endues. Fidelity, however, requires a process of continual change, of *creativity;* for the past is past and we do not live in it, even if we remember it. We do not live in David's Jerusalem or in Pontius Pilate's, and an effort to "preserve" the past is doomed to the failure of anachronistic eccentricity. Nicholas Lash makes the point quite nicely with respect to the traditions and ecclesiastical dress of the Franciscans:

> If, in thirteenth-century Italy, you wandered around in a coarse brown gown, . . . your dress said you were one of the poor. If, in twentieth-century Cambridge, you wander around in a coarse brown gown, . . . your dress now says, not that you are one of the poor, but that you are some kind of oddity in the business of "religion."[37]

Fidelity to a tradition of solidarity with the poor requires creativity and change. Fidelity to the identity provided by remembrance must never be confused with anachronistic, if amiable, eccentricity. Moreover, God's good future is not yet, still sadly not yet. We do not live in John's "new" Jerusalem either, and an effort to read Scripture that neglects the continuing power of sin is condemned to the failure of utopian idealism. Creativity is the standard of excellence (nurtured in and limited by particular communities and traditions) that is ready to find words and deeds fitting both to Scripture and to our own time and place, in order to live in the present with memory and hope and fidelity. The practice of reading Scripture and the good of remembrance that belongs to it require both

35. See Stephen E. Fowl and L. Gregory Jones, *Reading in Communion: Scripture and Ethics in Christian Life* (Grand Rapids: Eerdmans, 1991), pp. 31-33. The church sets these writings apart as "holy" Bible, sets them apart as a whole as canon. To read any text as canonical is to read it in Christian community and in the light of that "whole." The canon itself, however, as we have seen, reminds its readers that texts have genre, authors, and audience, that they involve a process of tradition, that they have social and historical location. To read any text as canonical, therefore, does not license reading it as if it stood in timeless transcendence over its own time and place. On the contrary, holiness invites and welcomes attention to the textual, grammatical, literary, historical, and social investigations. "Holy" Bible is set apart as the Word of God, but it remains, of course, human words. The conjunction of the divine and the human has always been difficult to be precise about — whether the conjunction is relevant to the church's confession concerning Jesus of Nazareth, the sacraments, or Scripture. At the Council of Chalcedon (451) the church struggled with the conjunction of the divine and human in Jesus of Nazareth. It did not so much make a positive statement as a series of negative ones about this conjunction. We apprehend Jesus, it said, in two natures, "without confusing the two natures, without transmuting one nature into the other, without dividing them into two separate categories, without contrasting them according to area or function" (Leith, *Creeds of the Churches,* p. 36). There is, I think, an instructive analogy to the conjunction of the divine and human with respect to Scripture. The human words should not be simply identified with (or "confused" with) the Word of God. But neither should we divide the Bible into two categories, divine and human (perhaps putting the divine words in red letters), or contrast the human words with the Word of God. On the one side there are some heirs of fundamentalism who understand the conjunction to signal an identification of the human words with the words of God, whose confusion of the Word of God and the human words of Scripture leads them to use the Bible as a revealed medical text and timeless moral code. John M. Frame, *Medical Ethics: Principles, Persons, and Problems* (Phillipsburg, N.J.: Presbyterian and Reformed, 1988), and Franklin E. Payne, *Biblical/Medical Ethics* (Milford, Mich.: Mott Media, 1985), for example, start with such claims about Scripture in their efforts to join the Bible and bioethics; they stand ready to appeal directly to biblical statements and rules as "inerrant" medical and moral propositions. As Frame puts it, "Scripture says it, we believe it, and that settles it" (p. 2). On the other side are some heirs of liberalism who understand the conjunction to signal a contrast, who so emphasize "human words" that they are obliged to decide what it is in them that has any abiding value. Charles Hartshorne, "Scientific and Religious Aspects of Bioethics," in *Theology and Bioethics: Exploring the Foundations and the Frontiers,* ed. E. E. Shelp (Dordrecht, Netherlands: D. Reidel, 1985), pp. 27-44, for example, rejects not only "scriptural literalism" but most appeals to these writings of "human hands" (p. 27). He does accept "the two great commandments," but the selection of these is controlled less by Scripture itself than by a "philosophical rationality." Between these extremes there are various emphases, of course, but there is also a consensus, I think, that the conjunction of the Word of God and human words must be understood without either confusing and identifying the one with the other or dividing and contrasting them.

36. Our practice here is frequently better than our theology. Our theology tends to construe God's relation to Scripture and to us through Scripture simply as "revealer." Then the content of Scripture can simply be identified with revelation, and the theological task becomes simply to systematize and republish timeless biblical ideas or doctrines or principles or rules. In the practice of reading Scripture in Christian community, however, we learn, I think, to construe God's relation to Scripture and surely to us through Scripture as "sanctifier." Then what one understands when one understands Scripture in remembrance is the creative and re-creative power of God to renew life, to transform identities, to create a people and a world for God's own glory and for their flourishing. See further Allen Verhey, *The Great Reversal: Ethics and the New Testament* (Grand Rapids: Eerdmans, 1984), pp. 180-81, and David Kelsey, "The Bible and Christian Theology," *The Journal of the American Academy of Religion* 68, no. 3 (1980): 385-402.

37. Lash, *Theology on the Way to Emmaus,* p. 54.

fidelity and creativity.[38] To treat Scripture, then, as a revealed medical text or as a timeless moral code for bioethics is a corruption of the practice of reading Scripture. It allows the tradition to petrify, to fossilize. It confuses fidelity with an anachronistic — and sometimes less than amiable — eccentricity. And to treat Scripture as simply dated and as irrelevant to contemporary medical practice and bioethics is also a corruption of the practice. It turns remembrance into an archivist's recollection, and runs the risk of alienating Christian community from its own moral tradition and from its own moral identity. It invites amnesia. The narrow path between anachronism and amnesia requires both discipline and discernment.

Discipline is the standard of excellence for reading Scripture that marks one as ready to be a disciple, ready to follow the one of whom the story is told, ready to order one's life and the common life to fit the story. Discipline, of course, requires a community of disciples, people who are together ready to submit to and to contribute to the mutual admonition and encouragement of Christian community, to its interpretative and moral discourse. Discipline is the humility not to insist that Scripture be read "for ourselves," either by insisting on a "right to private judgment" in interpretation or by demanding that any interpretation serve our interests. It is the humility to read Scripture "over-against"[39] ourselves and our communities, in judgment upon them and not in self-serving defense of them — to read it, as we have noted, over-against even our conventional reading of biblical texts, subverting our own efforts to use Scripture to boast about our own righteousness or to protect our own status and power. It is the humility of submission. The remedy for forgetfulness is still to tell the old, old story, and remembrance still takes the shape of obedience. A costly discipleship tests character and conduct by the truth of the story we love to tell. Discipline holds both individuals and ecclesial communities to their responsibilities to read and to perform Scripture, to form their lives and their common life by the truth of the story they love to tell.

Yet, the shape of that story and of lives formed to it requires *discernment*. Discernment is the standard of excellence that is able to recognize "fittingness."[40] In reading Scripture, discernment is the ability to recognize the plot of the story, to see the wholeness of Scripture, and to order the interpretation of any part toward that whole. It is to recognize how a statute, a proverb, or a story "fits" the whole story. And in reading Scripture as "useful . . . for training in righteousness" (2 Tim. 3:16), discernment is the ability to recognize whether an action or a practice "fits" the story of Scripture. It is the ability to plot our own lives in ways that "fit" the whole of Scripture, the skill to order our lives toward that whole. The question discernment asks is not whether the strange world of Scripture can be fit into our modern and enlightened world of medicine; the question is, rather, whether our own strange stories of sickness and healing can be made "fitting" to Scripture, can be made "worthy of the gospel."[41]

We began by acknowledging that the world of sickness and healing in Scripture is strange and alien to us; we end by claiming that reading Scripture may help us to discern the strange world of sickness and healing in modern medicine, may help us to name the strangeness, may help us to form and to reform the ways we use and practice medicine. To make good on such claims is the agenda of this book, but permit me to foreshadow what is to come.

It is a strange world of sickness when we look to medicine to deliver us from our finitude, from our mortality and our human vulnerability to suffering. Reading the Bible may help us to see the strangeness of that and to name it not only "the Baconian project" but "idolatry." Reading the Bible may help us to keep medicine in its (modest) place and then to celebrate it as good, without extravagant and idolatrous expectations of it. It is a strange world of medicine when modern medicine reduces the person to body and the body to manipulable nature. Reading the Bible may help us to see the folly of reducing our knowledge of persons and their bodies to the objective and objectifying gaze of science. It may help us to form and inform a medicine capable again of seeing and treating persons as embodied and communal selves, capable indeed of recognizing a patient's suffering (as well as the patient's disease) and responding to it with compassion. It is a strange world of medicine when it pretends to be value-

38. Again, the practice of reading Scripture is sometimes better than our theology for it. There are some theologians who insist on continuity, who are suspicious of creativity, and who think of themselves as embattled defenders of a tradition threatened by change. These stand ready to accuse others of "accommodation" (i.e., Franklin E. Payne, introduction to *Biblical/Medical Ethics*). There are other theologians (or philosophical theists) who insist on change, who minimize the significance of continuity, and who stand ready to accuse others of "irrational conservativism" (i.e, Charles Hartshorne, "Scientific and Religious Aspects of Bioethics," p. 28). The practice of reading Scripture, however, rejects both extremes; it insists on both fidelity and creativity, on both continuity and change. Again, although emphases vary, there is, I think, a consensus among theologians that would insist on both continuity and change, both fidelity and creativity.

39. Dietrich Bonhoeffer, *No Rusty Swords*, trans. E. H. Robertson and John Bowden (New York: Harper and Row, 1965), p. 185; see also pp. 308-25, and Fowl and Jones, *Reading in Communion*, p. 42.

40. On discernment see especially James M. Gustafson, "Moral Discernment in the Christian Life," in *Norm and Context in the Christian Life*, ed. Gene H. Outka and Paul Ramsey (New York: Charles Scribner's Sons, 1968), pp. 17-36.

41. One is reminded, I hope, of Karl Barth's "The Strange New World of the Bible" in *The Word of God and the Word of Man*. Consider also the observation of Nicholas Lash: "In the self-assured world of modernity, people seek to make sense of the Scriptures, instead of hoping, with the aid of the Scriptures, to make some sense of themselves" ("When Did the Theologians Lose Interest in Theology?" in *Theology and Dialogue: Essays in Conversation with George Lindbeck*, ed. Bruce D. Marshall [Notre Dame, Ind.: University of Notre Dame Press, 1990], pp. 131-47, at p. 143).

free, a set of skills available on the marketplace, and stranger yet when it becomes what it pretends, prepared to do the bidding of the one who pays, a hired hand, a hired gun. It is a strange world of medicine when the dying are not permitted to die, and stranger yet when compassion kills. It is a strange world of medicine when children are not begotten but made, and when those begotten are casually destroyed. It is a strange world of medicine when it fails the tests of both justice and charity. Reading the Bible may help us to see and to name the strangeness of modern medicine and to discern what might "fit" the story of Scripture a little better, what might be a little more "worthy of the gospel."

Discernment is a complex but practical wisdom. It does not rely on the simple application of general principles (whether of hermeneutics or of ethics) to particular cases by neutral and rational individuals. As there is no theory of memory in Scripture, neither is there any theory of discernment. There is no checklist, no flowchart for decisions, no tidy instructions about how to read and perform Scripture in "fitting" ways. Still, as there is memory in Scripture and in the community that reads it, so there is discernment in Scripture and in the community that struggles to live it.

Discernment regards decision as the recognition of what is fitting, coherent, to the kind of person one is and hopes to become. It asks not just "What should a rational person do in a case like this one?" but "What should *I* do in this case?" It recognizes that serious moral questions are always asked in the first person, and it insists on the moral significance of the question, "Who am I?" The practice of reading Scripture and the good of remembrance that belongs to it give us identity and form character and conduct into something fitting to it.

Discernment regards decisions as the recognition of what is fitting, or coherent, to the circumstances, to what is going on. It recognizes that the meaning of circumstances is not exhausted by objective observation and public inspection. Life is not like a can of peas, with a label telling us what the ingredients are. But reading Scripture trains us to see the religious significance of events, to read the signs of the times in the things that are happening about us, and to locate events and circumstances — as well as our selves — in a story of God's power and grace.[42] Reading Scripture trains us to answer the question "What is going on?" with reference to the remembered story, fitting the parts of our lives into the whole of Scripture.

Decisively, however, in Christian community discernment regards decisions as the recognition of what is fitting, or coherent, with the cause of God. It is that cause that God has made known in a narrative in which Christ is the center. It is that cause that is known in memory and in hope and expressed in both petition and mundane decision.

Discernment is learned and exercised in the community gathered around the Scriptures, and it involves the diversity of gifts present in the congregation. Some, as we said, are gifted with the scholarly tools of historical, literary, and social investigation; others, with moral imagination or with a passion for justice or with sweet reasonableness. But all are gifted with their own experience, and each is gifted with the Spirit that brings remembrance (John 14:26). Discernment requires a dialogue with the whole church gathered around the whole of Scripture; it requires reading Scripture with those whose experience is different from our own and whose experience of the authority of Scripture is different from our own. It requires a dialogue in which people listen both to Scripture and to one another, muting neither Scripture nor one another. In that dialogue and discernment, the authority of Scripture is "nonviolent."[43] The moment of recognition of Scripture's wholeness and truthfulness comes before the moment of submission to any part of it and prepares the way for it. Discernment enables us to see in the dialogue with Scripture and with saints and strangers that our readings of Scripture do not yet "fit" Scripture itself, and that our lives and our communities do not yet "fit" the story we love to tell and long to live. Then discernment is joined to discipline again, and the recognition of a more fitting way to tell the story and to live it prepares the way for humble submission and discipleship.[44]

To be sure, in the community some are blinded by fear, and some are blinded by duty, and the perception of each is abridged by investments in their culture or in their class. To be sure, whole communities are some-

42. H. Richard Niebuhr, *The Meaning of Revelation* (New York: Macmillan, 1974), p. 109: "What concerns us at this point is not the fact that the revelatory moment shines by its own light but rather that it illumines other events and enables us to understand them. Whatever else revelation means it does mean an event in our history which brings rationality and wholeness into the confused joys and sorrows of personal existence and allows us to discern order in the brawl of communal histories."

43. Margaret Farley, "Feminist Consciousness and the Interpretation of Scripture," in *Feminist Interpretation of the Bible,* ed. Letty M. Russell (Oxford: B. Blackwell, 1985), pp. 41-51; see esp. pp. 42-44. She cites Paul Ricoeur, *Essays in Biblical Interpretation,* ed. L. S. Mudge (Philadelphia: Fortress, 1980), p. 95.

44. Once again, the practice is sometimes better than our theology for it (and sometimes sadly not). The slogan *"sola scriptura"* is sometimes used to deny or ignore the relevance of other voices and other sources, to discount natural science or "natural" morality. And talk of the "authority" of Scripture is sometimes used to end discussion, as though we could beat into silence or submission those who speak from some other experience or for some other source. The practice can become corrupt, we said, but it can also sometimes be better than our theology. Discernment, or the perception of what is fitting, cannot demand that people violate what they know they know in other ways. It cannot demand that they violate either the experience of oppression or the assured results of science or the rational standards of justice. Of course, there can be disagreements — and discussion — about how to read and interpret one's experience or the "assured results" of science or some minimal notion of justice as there can be disagreement — and discussion — about how to read and interpret Scripture. On the relevance of other sources see further Verhey, *The Great Reversal,* pp. 187-96.

times blinded by idolatrous loyalties to their race, their social standing, or their power. Witness, for example, the "German Christians" during Hitler's rule or the Dutch Reformed Church in South Africa during apartheid. And to be sure, the practice of reading Scripture is corrupted then. Frequently the habits of reading Scripture do not measure up to the standards of excellence given with the practice, and communities can stand at risk of forgetfulness even when they call Scripture an "infallible rule" and treat it as an icon.

The remedy for forgetfulness is still to hear and to tell the old, old story, and to hear it now and then from saints[45] and now and then from strangers.[46] In the struggle against forgetfulness we read Scripture in Christian community and struggle to meet these standards of excellence for reading it, both holiness and sanctification, both fidelity and creativity, both discipline and discernment.

Scripture and Moral Discourse in the Church

The practice of reading Scripture is not a substitute for the practice of moral discourse, but by now it should be clear that the two are intimately related. As in prayer we learn to be attentive to God and to all things as related to God, so in reading Scripture we learn to remember the story of God's work and way and to exercise discernment. In reading Scripture we remember a story that stretches from the creation of all things to "all things made new" (cf. Rev. 21:5) through the story of Jesus of Nazareth, and we learn to do ethics "by way of reminder" (Rom. 15:15).

The practice of moral discourse is evidently as old as the church itself. Paul described the Christian churches at Rome as "full of goodness, filled with all knowledge, and able to instruct one another" (Rom. 15:14). Nevertheless, he wrote "rather boldly" to the congregations he praised "by way of reminder" (Rom. 15:15), reminding them of the gospel of God in order to encourage "the obedience of faith" (Rom. 1:5; 16:26). The reading of Scripture in the context of moral discourse will also proceed "by way of reminder." Its good is remembrance. Its form is evangelical, remembering and telling "the gospel of God." And the standards of excellence are holiness and sanctification, fidelity and creativity, discipline and discernment.

Continuing churches are still — by tradition and vocation — communities of moral discourse. They talk together about what they ought to do. And not only about *what* they ought to do, but also about *why* they ought to do it. They give and hear reasons. And they weigh the reasons, they test them against the story they love to tell and long to live. That is to say, continuing churches are also still — by tradition and vocation — communities of moral deliberation, discernment, and memory.

The church's moral discourse, of course, frequently integrates deliberation, discernment, and memory into one conversation. They are not a set of sequential steps, as though any conversation had to proceed through these stages in sequence in order to count as a good conversation. Even so, permit me to divide them into stages or levels of discourse for the sake of analysis, for at the different stages of the church's discourse Scripture is "useful" in different ways. At the different levels of its conversation Scripture's authority is different.

When we are simply talking about our concrete choices, about what we should do or leave undone, Scripture is hardly "useful." We do not live in the first century. Our choices are different. Even a choice that would have some external similarity to a choice in the first century will be a different choice because the social context for it is different. The choice, for example, to take interest on a loan is a different choice in our world than it was in the economic world of the first century.

At the stage of deliberation, however, when reasons are given and heard, Scripture can be cited (and frequently is cited) as part of the process of deliberation in Christian communities. It is "used" to say why something was done or left undone. And, of course, among the passages of Scripture which can be cited (and frequently are cited) there are rules and "prescriptions." When we are talking about why something should be done, we sometimes appeal to one or another of these biblical rules. Or we may appeal to a particular piece of advice that Paul gave to the Corinthian Christians — in ways not unlike the ways some members of that early church appealed to the Hebrew Scripture. We may appeal to some biblical rule as a reason that something should be done or left undone in the contemporary church — say, to Matthew's prohibition of divorce "except for unchastity" (Matt. 19:9) as a reason to license (or prohibit) a certain divorce.

Notice, however, that at the deliberative stage there are also appeals to a wide variety of other sources of moral insight and wisdom. As in the early church, Christians today may give reasons that appeal to the witness of a charismatic prophet or to the authority of an official leader of the community. They may appeal to the moral commonplaces of the surrounding culture or to the traditions of the community, to conventional wisdom or to sociological information. They may appeal to their own experience, or to what they know that they know in some other way than that it is found in Scripture.

It is altogether appropriate that deliberation involve a variety of sources. In the deliberative dialogue, we may not demand that people violate what they know that they know in other ways. We may not use the slogan *sola scriptura* to silence other voices and other sources, to discount the experience of oppression or natural science or "natural" morality. We may not use the "authority of

45. Fowl and Jones, *Reading in Communion*, pp. 62-63. They quote Athanasius, *The Incarnation of the Word of God* (New York: Macmillan, 1946), p. 96: "Anyone who wishes to understand the mind of the sacred writers must first cleanse his own life, and approach the saints by copying their deeds."

46. Fowl and Jones, *Reading in Communion*, pp. 110-34.

Scripture" to put a stop to conversation, to beat into silence and submission those who speak from some other experience or for some other source. Of course, in the community gathered around Scripture it will always be appropriate to invite each and all to the reconsideration of what we know that we know, but that is an invitation to the next level, to discernment. In the Christian community it will always be appropriate to exhort each other to interpret our experience, or the "assured results" of science, or some minimal notion of morality in the light of Scripture, but that is a call to engage in the next stage, in discernment.

At the deliberative stage it is appropriate that there be appeals to a wide variety of sources — and at the deliberative stage it is also altogether appropriate that Scripture be counted simply as one of many sources! The rules and laws of Scripture have a limited "usefulness" and authority at the level of deliberation. The prescriptions and prohibitions that are found within Scripture ought to be considered in deliberation, but the ability to cite a biblical rule does not put a stop to the community's deliberative conversation. Fidelity to Scripture requires creativity. We may repeat Paul's word to the Corinthians, "Does not nature itself teach you that if a man wears long hair, it is degrading to him" (1 Cor. 11:14), but we may not repeat it as the last word in a conversation about proper coiffure for men. We may repeat Matthew's account of Jesus' word concerning divorce, "whoever divorces his wife, except for unchastity, and marries another commits adultery" (Matt. 19:9), but we may not repeat it as a timeless rule that puts a stop to a community's conversation about, for example, divorce following abuse. To be sure, there are many biblical rules that we do well to regard as normative rules for ourselves. But we do well to regard them as such not because they have the status of biblical rules but because they have been tested and validated by the community's experience and discernment. *The point is this: appeals to Scripture at the deliberative level remain subject to the communal process of discernment, just as subject as appeals to the wide variety of other sources.* A prescription or prohibition lifted from Scripture may be and must be tested and accepted or qualified or rejected by the discernment of the community gathered around Scripture and exercising discernment. Reasons are given and heard in the community, but any and all reasons must finally be tested in the community and defended, discarded, or qualified by their coherence with the gospel. Every judgment and every reason given in deliberation — *even when it involves the citation of Scripture* — is to be tested and qualified by a communal discernment of the shape and style of life "worthy of the gospel of Christ" (Phil. 1:27).

At the stage of discernment, when we are testing the reasons, Scripture is "useful" and authoritative because by reading Scripture we remember the story against which we test all the little good we do well and all the little wisdom we think we know well. Discernment, or the perception of what is "fitting" or "worthy," is — as already noted — a complex human enterprise, and there is no recipe for it in Scripture or in the community. Discernment is clearly neither simply reliance on intuition nor simply the deductive application of generic principles. Communal discernment is not just a matter of sharing the little moral wisdom each member knows well or of compensating for the abridgments (major or minor) of each one's moral vision. Discernment is always in the church to be the discernment of what is fitting or worthy of the story Christians love to tell and long to live. It is that story which makes them a community, and it is that story which calls them to a discernment not conformed to this age, but transformed by the renewal of their mind (Rom. 12:1-2).[47] It is that story that forms community and character, identity and perspective, fundamental values and commitments, into something coherent with the remembered story and capable of testing the reasons given in deliberation, even "scriptural" ones.

I do not deny the presence of prescriptions in Scripture, nor do I propose that they be torn from the canon, from that collection of writings (in all their "great variety") which (as a whole) can and should rule the churches' life and speech. I do not deny that citations of scriptural prescriptions can be appropriate in the deliberative process of giving reasons for specific moral judgments and rules. What I deny is this: that the fact that one can cite a scriptural prescription or prohibition is *sufficient* for the justification of a contemporary judgment or rule. One cannot simply and definitively answer the question "What ought I (or we) do?" by citing a scriptural prescription or prohibition. The Christian community is a community of discernment by testing rules — even rules that are formally identical to scriptural prescriptions — by their creative fidelity to the whole story, by their ability to nurture and sustain a contemporary "performance" not of a little piece of the canon but of Scripture as a whole. Indeed, the rules within Scripture are finally normative for the church less as rules than as part of the whole story.

The churches are communities of moral discourse and moral deliberation, "able to instruct one another," because they are communities of moral discernment, and they are communities of moral discernment by being communities of memory. Discernment in Christian community depends finally on remembering the story of Jesus. And Scripture is "useful" for that remembering. It is by reading Scripture that the church remembers! Remembering is the good that the Christian community aims at in its practice of reading Scripture. The greatest danger for the Christian life is still forgetfulness, and reading Scripture together is still the remedy for it.

47. Wayne A. Meeks, *The Origins of Christian Morality: The First Two Centuries* (New Haven: Yale University Press, 1993), p. 17: "The moral life has a plot, and it is a plot that implicates not merely each individual, but humankind and the cosmos. It may be that what most clearly sets Christian ethics apart from all the other ethical discourse of late antiquity, with which it otherwise shares so much, is just the creation of this peculiar story in which each of us is called on to be a character, and from which character itself and virtue take their meaning." See further pp. 189-210.

Somehow — but how? That is the question. It is less a puzzle to solve than a mystery to live with. Even so, we can hardly avoid making some effort to answer it. Christians must read and use Scripture humbly. We must read and use Scripture in Christian community. We must read it as canon. We must read it without Marcion's dualism. We must read it according to creed, the "Rule of Faith." We must read it with exegetical care and skill. We must continually assess existing traditions of interpretation and performance. We must read Scripture prayerfully. A prayer-formed reading of Scripture will serve invocation and remembrance. It will serve repentance by reading Scripture over-against ourselves. It will serve thanksgiving to God by the sharing of gifts. And it will serve petition by governing both our petitions and our readings by the vision of God's good future born of remembrance — and by the aching acknowledgment that that future is not yet. We must read Scripture in order to remember. We must set these writings aside as "holy" and set aside a time and a place to read them. We must set all the stories of our lives alongside the story of Scripture, that they may be made new. We must read Scripture and perform it both faithfully and creatively. We must read it with a readiness to be disciplined by it, to be disciples of the remembered Jesus. We must read it with (and for) discernment. We must read it not as a timeless moral code but as the story of our lives.

The subsequent parts of this book [*Reading the Bible in the Strange World of Medicine*] are an effort to read Scripture within the context of the Christian community and for it, and especially within the context of the churches as communities of moral discourse about bioethics and for their discernment. I do not presume to have the last word about any issue in bioethics because I am reading Scripture. It is still the church, not the Bible, and surely not this little book, which Paul described as "full of goodness, filled with all knowledge." Nevertheless, I will proceed "boldly," for I will proceed "by way of reminder" (Rom. 15:15). The subsequent parts of this book will attempt to read Scripture for the sake of remembrance. Together we will remember Jesus, and we will remember the early church remembering Jesus, in the strange world of sickness and healing. The good we seek in reading Scripture is remembrance. The standards of excellence we aim at are holiness and sanctification, fidelity and creativity, discipline and discernment.

Acknowledgment

This essay draws on material previously published in Allen Verhey, "Scripture and Medical Ethics: Psalm 51:10, the Jarvik 7, and Psalm 50:9," in *Religious Methods and Resources in Bioethics*, ed. Paul Camenisch (Dordrecht, Netherlands: Kluwer Academic, 1994), pp. 261-88; and Allen Verhey, *Remembering Jesus: Christian Community, Scripture, and the Moral Life* (Grand Rapids: Eerdmans, 2002).

II. Christianity and the Social Practice of Health Care

CHAPTER THREE

Christianity and the Social Responsibility of Health Care

Part I explored questions of "method." The essays examined how we, as a society, think about medicine, how we think about its relationship to religion, and how we think about the relationship between theology and medical ethics. We now turn to two chapters located under the more general heading of "Christianity and the Social Practice of Health Care." In doing so, we are making a significant claim: that the study of the ethics of medicine — whether undertaken from a secular or a theological perspective — must start with the question of the social context of health care.

This is a novel methodological claim for a book on medical ethics. Most textbooks or monographs start with the question of personhood, physician-patient relationship, moral theory, or processes for decision making. Most of the analyses in the field, beginning with Paul Ramsey's *The Patient as Person* (the preface of which you can read in Chapter Seven below), assume that most of the pertinent ethical questions in medicine are questions of individual decision making almost completely circumscribed within the confines of the dyad of patient and physician. Consequently, the main principles of analysis in bioethics remain autonomy, beneficence, and non-maleficence. Attempts to introduce the principle of "justice" into the analyses are often ambiguous.

By the structure of this third edition of *On Moral Medicine,* we wish to push the field of medical ethics to overcome the artificial distinction between bioethics and social ethics. We take a cue from an important document within the Catholic tradition, the U.S. Catholic Bishops' *Ethical and Religious Directives for Catholic Health Care Services* (4th ed., 2001) (selection 13; this document is also referred to as the ERDs).[1] This document marks an innovative moment within medical ethics and within Catholic reflection on medicine: the bishops structure the ERDs so as to begin in part one with "The Social Responsibility of Catholic Health Care Services." In doing so, they effectively claim that all subsequent questions in medicine — the physician-patient relationship, beginning of life, end of life, and so on — must be contextualized within the larger questions of the social role of health care.

Such a claim is grounded both theologically and epistemologically. Theologically, it is supported by almost two thousand years of Christian history and fundamental theological convictions. Since its inception, the church has reached out to care for the sick, who were most often, simultaneously, the poor. It has fostered a long and rich history of being the *place* of health care delivery — through monasteries, religious orders, the building of hospitals, and more.[2] The Catholic Church in particular has been deeply invested in the delivery of health care in the U.S. since the earliest days of this country, mostly through the mission work of small orders of tireless women religious who lived among the poor and cared for the sick.[3] As a result, Catholic health care currently comprises approximately six hundred hospitals, or 12 percent of the health care infrastructure in the U.S., an infrastructure augmented by the presence of facilities allied with the Methodist, Lutheran, Jewish, and Seventh-Day Adventist traditions, as well as other Christian traditions.

This practical commitment to care for the sick and poor grew in part from the church's ongoing commitment to continue Jesus' healing ministry. It is also rooted in fundamental Christian christological, ecclesiological, and an-

1. We excerpt here the introduction and part one of the *Ethical and Religious Directives for Catholic Health Care Services.* The document in its entirety can be found at: http://www.usccb.org/bishops/directives.shtml (accessed January 31, 2009). Those interested in the sections "The Professional/Patient Relationship," "Issues in Care for the Beginning of Life," "Issues in Care for the Dying," as well as information on how Catholic health care institutions can partner with other-than-Catholic institutions are encouraged to read through the entire document.

2. Guenter B. Risse, *Mending Bodies, Saving Souls: A History of Hospitals* (New York: Oxford University Press, 1999).

3. See Suzy Farren, *A Call to Care: The Women Who Built Catholic Healthcare in America* (Catholic Health Association, 1996). A DVD documentary is also available from the Catholic Health Association at: https://servicecenter.chausa.org/ProductCatalog/Product.aspx?ID=489.

thropological convictions. Per Matthew 25:31-46, Christians are called not only to "visit the sick" (one of the basic corporal works of mercy) but also to understand the sick and poor *as Christ.* As members of the body of Christ, Christians proclaim that they are "members of one another" such that they share in each other's sufferings (1 Corinthians 12; Romans 12; Galatians 6:2). And beyond the church, Christians hold to a thickly social anthropology, understanding all persons to be interconnected through their creation in the image of the Triune God, a God who is in essence and action relational. These fundamental theological convictions have long driven Christianity to recognize medicine as a basic human and social good, like food, clothing, and shelter. This commitment to health care as a fundamental human good led Pope John XXIII to name health care as a fundamental human right (1961),[4] a claim first made in the United Nations' Universal Declaration on Human Rights (1948), which was heavily influenced by the tradition of Catholic social thought.[5]

Yet the claim that all questions in medical ethics must be situated within the larger social context of health care is also an epistemological claim. An adequate analysis of any question in medical ethics must take into account all relevant data; in the contemporary context this requires attention to the social and economic infrastructure of sickness and health care in the U.S. and globally — attention that until recently has been sorely lacking. Over the past two decades, health care has been transformed into a corporate, now global, industry. As mentioned in the introduction to Chapter One, total health care spending in the U.S. in 2007 reached $2.4 *trillion* or 16 percent of the gross domestic product (GDP).[6] Hospitals have merged to form systems to garner greater market share. Health insurance and pharmaceutical companies are publicly traded, posting record profits, even in down markets. The administrative costs of U.S. health care due to our insurance system are estimated at $50 billion per year; executive compensation has become excessive, and the size and funding of the health care lobby are sobering. Analyses that fail to attend to these infrastructural questions serve only to mask operative ethical dynamics, those that lie in the power exerted by the ever-growing bio-pharmaceutical-technological-medical-industrial complex. The pharmaceutical industry provides an excellent window into this complex, as detailed by former editor-in-chief of the *New England Journal of Medicine,* Marcia Angell, M.D., in her book *The Truth about Drug Companies: How They Deceive Us and What to Do about It.*[7]

This economic transformation of health care was well under way in 1986 when David Schiedermayer, M.D., penned his parody of the Hippocratic Oath, "The Corporate Physician's Oath" (selection 14), published in the *New England Journal of Medicine.* Schiedermayer succinctly captures the fact that health care in the U.S. has become a business, whose purpose is to maximize profit. (The original Hippocratic Oath can be found in Chapter Five below, for those interested in comparing the two.)

Schiedermayer's voice of the physician-as-corporate-profit-center is contrasted with the voice of one sick, poor woman, Teresa Maldonado, in "Sick of Being Poor" (selection 15). Maldonado's first-person account, a view from below, poignantly details the obstacles faced by the poor — especially poor women — as they attempt to access the few health care resources available to them and their children. Her story echoes those told by David Hilfiker in his important book, *Not All of Us Are Saints: A Doctor's Journey with the Poor.*[8] Early on in his work in inner-city Washington, D.C., Hilfiker came to see how the systems that are, putatively, in place to provide health care to the poor and underserved in fact put up barriers to that care. Maldonado captures this dynamic from the patient's perspective, detailing the many ways in which the system dehumanizes, impersonalizes, belittles, and even blames the poor as they try to care for their own health or that of their families. Her story of what happens when she finally secures health insurance illuminates why health care costs in the U.S. continue to spiral without a correlative impact on health outcomes.

These two pieces illustrate how deeply the patient-physician relationship is embedded in its wider social context and how critical that context is for analysis. They also illustrate a fundamental question: Is health care a consumer product, governed by the rules of profit and the market, or is it a fundamental human good, to which all persons have a right? The remaining selections in this chapter marshal theological responses to this question and show that the response is equally analytical and practical.

Willard Swartley and John Roth succinctly summarize the history and heritage of the Christian tradition with regard to health care and healing in their essays "The Bible and Christian Convictions" and "The Christian and Anabaptist Legacy in Healthcare" (selections 16 and 17). Beginning with the Jewish tradition's call to *shalom,* they show how the Christian practice of caring for the sick indeed constituted one of the central activities of the church, complementing the usual story with additional examples of how this practice of discipleship has played out within the Anabaptist traditions. The involvement of the church

4. John XXIII, *Mater et Magistra* (1961). Available at: http://www.vatican.va/holy_father/john_xxiii/encyclicals/documents/hf_j-xxiii_enc_15051961_mater_en.html (accessed February 23, 2010).

5. The Universal Declaration on Human Rights (1948). Available at: http://www.un.org/en/documents/udhr/index.shtml (accessed February 23, 2010). Health care is identified as a human right in Article 25. Mary Ann Glendon details the Catholic contribution to the 1948 Universal Declaration on Human Rights in her essay in *Believing Scholars: Ten Catholic Intellectuals,* ed. James L. Heft (New York: Fordham University Press, 2005).

6. See, e.g., http://www.kff.org/insurance/snapshot/oecd042111.cfm (accessed March 4, 2012).

7. Marcia Angell, *The Truth about Drug Companies: How They Deceive Us and What to Do about It* (New York: Random House, 2005).

8. David Hilfiker, *Not All of Us Are Saints: A Doctor's Journey with the Poor* (New York: Hill and Wang, 2004).

in the delivery of health care, and, indeed, its integral role in this work until the seventeenth century, is a long, rich, and fascinating story, one important to reclaim in our contemporary situation.

The Christian tradition, therefore, boasts a long and deep history of involvement in caring for the sick. It equally brings a powerful tradition of analysis by which contemporary health care could be transformed. One piece of this tradition is Catholic social thought. The Catholic Bishops' Joint Bioethics Committee provide a helpful introduction to this tradition in their essay "Catholic Social Teaching and the Allocation of Healthcare" (selection 18). Here they examine each principle of Catholic social thought, show how each principle is grounded scripturally and theologically, and then use it to analyze the question of allocation.

The tradition of Catholic social thought has continually evolved, largely in response to changing social conditions. One of the most recent developments in this tradition is the field known as liberation theology (helpfully outlined by dos Anjos in Chapter Two above). In "Health, Healing, and Social Justice" (selection 19) physician Paul Farmer describes what medicine might look like if approached from the point of view of liberation theology. Farmer carefully shows what the potentially abstract principles of the preferential option for the poor, solidarity, the common good, human dignity, and subsidiarity mean for thinking about the practice of medicine and the crafting of health care policy. Farmer pulls no punches: to take Christianity seriously means to move beyond our comfortable relativism to action. He also demonstrates that, confounding conventional wisdom, such an approach is often more realistic and more clinically effective than current approaches to health care both in the U.S. and in situations of poverty around the world.

We close this section with a chapter from Joel Shuman and Brian Volck's book *Reclaiming the Body: Christians and the Faithful Use of Modern Medicine.*[9] In this book, Shuman (a theologian) and Volck (a physician) challenge Christians to take seriously what the tradition has to say about "the body" — both our own non-dualistic embodiment as persons and the claim that Christians belong to a corporate body, the body of Christ, a membership mediated through the practices of baptism and eucharist. What might this mean for how Christians think about and live with contemporary medicine? The chapter we have selected — "A Body without Borders" (selection 20) — argues that to take these theological claims seriously means that, if nothing else, a Christian practice of medicine must first refuse to submit to the usual "borders" that isolate our bodies from one another and fragment the body of the church — especially the borders of race, class, and nationality. They offer three examples of what the practice of medicine looks like when it understands those borders to be false constructs.

We will continue to explore this question of Christianity and the social context of health care in Chapter Four. But we hope that readers of this third edition of *On Moral Medicine* will keep these essays in Chapters Three and Four in mind as they work through subsequent chapters. For the questions, for example, of stem cell research or euthanasia cannot be studied in isolation from the socioeconomic infrastructure of contemporary health care, from the principles of Catholic social teaching or liberation theology, or from the fundamental Christian commitment to understand medicine and health care always as a social practice.

SUGGESTIONS FOR FURTHER READING

Cahill, Lisa Sowle. "National and International Health Access Reform." In *Theological Bioethics* (Washington, D.C.: Georgetown University Press, 2005), pp. 131-68.

Hall, Amy Laura. "Whose Progress? The Language of Global Health." *Journal of Medicine and Philosophy* 31 (2006): 285-304.

Hughes, Edward. "The Current Medical Crises of Resources: Some Orthodox Christian Reflections." In *Allocating Scarce Medical Resources: Roman Catholic Perspectives,* ed. H. Tristram Engelhardt Jr. and Mark J. Cherry (Washington, D.C.: Georgetown University Press, 2002), pp. 237-62.

Outka, Gene. "Social Justice and Equal Access to Health Care." In *On Moral Medicine,* 2nd ed., ed. Stephen E. Lammers and Allen Verhey (Grand Rapids: Eerdmans, 1998), pp. 947-59.

Plantak, Zdravko. "Universal Access to Health Care and Religious Basis of Human Rights." *Update* (Loma Linda Center for Bioethics) 20, no. 2 (June 2005): 1-11.

Stoneking, Carole Bailey. "A Communion of Saints . . . Maybe." *Christian Bioethics* 2, no. 3 (1996): 346-54.

Sulmasy, Daniel. "Do the Bishops Have It Right on Health Care Reform?" *Christian Bioethics* 2, no. 3 (1996): 309-25.

Verhey, Allen. "A Protestant Perspective on Access to Healthcare." *Cambridge Quarterly of Healthcare Ethics* 7 (1998): 247-53.

9. Joel Shuman and Brian Volck, *Reclaiming the Body: Christians and the Faithful Use of Modern Medicine* (Grand Rapids: Brazos, 2006).

13 General Introduction and Part One of *Ethical and Religious Directives for Catholic Health Care Services,* Fourth Edition

U.S. Conference of Catholic Bishops

General Introduction

The Church has always sought to embody our Savior's concern for the sick. The gospel accounts of Jesus' ministry draw special attention to his acts of healing; he cleansed a man with leprosy (Mt 8:1-4; Mk 1:40-42); he gave sight to two people who were blind (Mt 20:29-34; Mk 10:46-52); he enabled one who was mute to speak (Lk 11:14); he cured a woman who was hemorrhaging (Mt 9:20-22; Mk 5:25-34); and he brought a young girl back to life (Mt 9:18, 23-25; Mk 5:35-42). Indeed, the Gospels are replete with examples of how the Lord cured every kind of ailment and disease (Mt 9:35). In the account of Matthew, Jesus' mission fulfilled the prophecy of Isaiah: "He took away our infirmities and bore our diseases" (Mt 8:17; cf. Is 53:4).

Jesus' healing mission went further than caring only for physical affliction. He touched people at the deepest level of their existence; he sought their physical, mental, and spiritual healing (Jn 6:35, 11:25-27). He "came so that they might have life and have it more abundantly" (Jn 10:10).

The mystery of Christ casts light on every facet of Catholic health care: to see Christian love as the animating principle of health care; to see healing and compassion as a continuation of Christ's mission; to see suffering as a participation in the redemptive power of Christ's passion, death, and resurrection; and to see death, transformed by the resurrection, as an opportunity for a final act of communion with Christ.

For the Christian, our encounter with suffering and death can take on a positive and distinctive meaning through the redemptive power of Jesus' suffering and death. As St. Paul says, we are "always carrying about in the body the dying of Jesus, so that the life of Jesus may also be manifested in our body" (2 Cor 4:10). This truth does not lessen the pain and fear, but gives confidence and grace for bearing suffering rather than being overwhelmed by it. Catholic health care ministry bears witness to the truth that, for those who are in Christ, suffering and death are the birth pangs of the new creation. "God himself will always be with them [as their God]. He will wipe every tear from their eyes, and there shall be no more death or mourning, wailing or pain, [for] the old order has passed away" (Rev 21:3-4).

In faithful imitation of Jesus Christ, the Church has served the sick, suffering, and dying in various ways throughout history. The zealous service of individuals and communities has provided shelter for the traveler; infirmaries for the sick; and homes for children, adults, and the elderly.[1] In the United States, the many religious communities as well as dioceses that sponsor and staff this country's Catholic health care institutions and services have established an effective Catholic presence in health care. Modeling their efforts on the gospel parable of the Good Samaritan, these communities of women and men have exemplified authentic neighborliness to those in need (Lk 10:25-97). The Church seeks to ensure that the service offered in the past will be continued into the future.

While many religious communities continue their commitment to the health care ministry, lay Catholics increasingly have stepped forward to collaborate in this ministry. Inspired by the example of Christ and mandated by the Second Vatican Council, lay faithful are invited to a broader and more intense field of ministries than in the past.[2] By virtue of their Baptism, lay faithful are called to participate actively in the Church's life and mission.[3] Their participation and leadership in the health care ministry, through new forms of sponsorship and governance of institutional Catholic health care, are essential for the Church to continue her ministry of healing and compassion. They are joined in the Church's health care mission by many men and women who are not Catholic.

Catholic health care expresses the healing ministry of Christ in a specific way within the local church. Here the diocesan bishop exercises responsibilities that are rooted in his office as pastor, teacher, and priest. As the center of unity in the diocese and coordinator of ministries in the local church, the diocesan bishop fosters the mission of Catholic health care in a way that promotes collaboration among health care leaders, providers, medical professionals, theologians, and other specialists. As pastor, the diocesan bishop is in a unique position to encourage

---

National Conference of Catholic Bishops. From "General Introduction" and "Part One: The Social Responsibility of Catholic Health Care Services," in *Ethical and Religious Directives for Catholic Health Care Services* by the National Conference of Catholic Bishops, fourth ed., 2001, pp. 4-11.

1. United States Conference of Catholic Bishops, *Health and Health Care: A Pastoral Letter of the American Catholic Bishops* (Washington, DC: United States Conference of Catholic Bishops, 1981), p. 5.

2. Second Vatican Ecumenical Council, *Decree on the Apostolate of the Laity (Apostolicam Actuositatem)* (1965), no. 1.

3. Pope John Paul II, Post-Synodal Apostolic Exhortation *On the Vocation and the Mission of the Lay Faithful in the Church and in the World (Christifideles Laici)* (Washington, DC: United States Conference of Catholic Bishops, 1988), no. 29.

the faithful to greater responsibility in the healing ministry of the Church. As teacher, the diocesan bishop ensures the moral and religious identity of the health care ministry in whatever setting it is carried out in the diocese. As priest, the diocesan bishop oversees the sacramental care of the sick. These responsibilities will require that Catholic health care providers and the diocesan bishop engage in ongoing communication on ethical and pastoral matters that require his attention.

In a time of new medical discoveries, rapid technological developments, and social change, what is new can either be an opportunity for genuine advancement in human culture, or it can lead to policies and actions that are contrary to the true dignity and vocation of the human person. In consultation with medical professionals, church leaders review these developments, judge them according to the principles of right reason and the ultimate standard of revealed truth, and offer authoritative teaching and guidance about the moral and pastoral responsibilities entailed by the Christian faith.[4] While the Church cannot furnish a ready answer to every moral dilemma, there are many questions about which she provides normative guidance and direction. In the absence of a determination by the magisterium, but never contrary to church teaching, the guidance of approved authors can offer appropriate guidance for ethical decision making.

Created in God's image and likeness, the human family shares in the dominion that Christ manifested in his healing ministry. This sharing involves a stewardship over all material creation (Gn 1:26) that should neither abuse nor squander nature's resources. Through science the human race comes to understand God's wonderful work, and through technology it must conserve, protect, and perfect nature in harmony with God's purposes. Health care professionals pursue a special vocation to share in carrying forth God's life-giving and healing work.

The dialogue between medical science and Christian faith has for its primary purpose the common good of all human persons. It presupposes that science and faith do not contradict each other. Both are grounded in respect for truth and freedom. As new knowledge and new technologies expand, each person must form a correct conscience based on the moral norms for proper health care.

Part One: The Social Responsibility of Catholic Health Care Services

Introduction

Their embrace of Christ's healing mission has led institutionally based Catholic health care services in the United States to become an integral part of the nation's health care system. Today, this complex health care system confronts a range of economic, technological, social, and moral challenges. The response of Catholic health care institutions and services to these challenges is guided by normative principles that inform the Church's healing ministry.

First, Catholic health care ministry is rooted in a commitment to promote and defend human dignity; this is the foundation of its concern to respect the sacredness of every human life from the moment of conception until death. The first right of the human person, the right to life, entails a right to the means for the proper development of life, such as adequate health care.[5]

Second, the biblical mandate to care for the poor requires us to express this in concrete action at all levels of Catholic health care. This mandate prompts us to work to ensure that our country's health care delivery system provides adequate health care for the poor. In Catholic institutions, particular attention should be given to the health care needs of the poor, the uninsured, and the underinsured.[6]

Third, Catholic health care ministry seeks to contribute to the common good. The common good is realized when economic, political, and social conditions ensure protection for the fundamental rights of all individuals and enable all to fulfill their common purpose and reach their common goals.[7]

Fourth, Catholic health care ministry exercises responsible stewardship of available health care resources. A just health care system will be concerned both with promoting equity of care — to assure that the right of each person to basic health care is respected — and with promoting the good health of all in the community. The responsible stewardship of health care resources can be accomplished best in dialogue with people from all levels of society, in accordance with the principle of subsidiarity and with respect for the moral principles that guide institutions and persons.

Fifth, within a pluralistic society, Catholic health care services will encounter requests for medical procedures contrary to the moral teachings of the Church. Catholic health care does not offend the rights of individual conscience by refusing to provide or permit medical proce-

4. As examples, see Congregation for the Doctrine of the Faith, *Declaration on Procured Abortion* (1974); Congregation for the Doctrine of the Faith, *Declaration on Euthanasia* (1980); Congregation for the Doctrine of the Faith, *Instruction on Respect for Human Life in Its Origin and on the Dignity of Procreation: Replies to Certain Questions of the Day (Donum Vitae)* (Washington, DC: United States Conference of Catholic Bishops, 1987).

5. Pope John XXIII, Encyclical Letter *Peace on Earth (Pacem in Terris)* (Washington, DC: United States Conference of Catholic Bishops, 1963), no. 11; *Health and Health Care*, pp. 5, 17-18; *Catechism of the Catholic Church*, 2nd ed. (Washington, DC: Libreria Editrice Vaticana — United States Conference of Catholic Bishops, 2000), no. 2211.

6. Pope John Paul II, *On Social Concern, Encyclical Letter on the Occasion of the Twentieth Anniversary of "Populorum Progressio" (Sollicitudo Rei Socialis)* (Washington, DC: United States Conference of Catholic Bishops, 1988), no. 43.

7. United States Conference of Catholic Bishops, *Economic Justice for All: Pastoral Letter on Catholic Social Teaching and the U.S. Economy* (Washington, DC: United States Conference of Catholic Bishops, 1986), no. 80.

dures that are judged morally wrong by the teaching authority of the Church.

Directives

1. A Catholic institutional health care service is a community that provides health care to those in need of it. This service must be animated by the Gospel of Jesus Christ and guided by the moral tradition of the Church.
2. Catholic health care should be marked by a spirit of mutual respect among care-givers that disposes them to deal with those it serves and their families with the compassion of Christ, sensitive to their vulnerability at a time of special need.
3. In accord with its mission, Catholic health care should distinguish itself by service to and advocacy for those people whose social condition puts them at the margins of our society and makes them particularly vulnerable to discrimination: the poor; the uninsured and the underinsured; children and the unborn; single parents; the elderly; those with incurable diseases and chemical dependencies; racial minorities; immigrants and refugees. In particular, the person with mental or physical disabilities, regardless of the cause or severity, must be treated as a unique person of incomparable worth, with the same right to life and to adequate health care as all other persons.
4. A Catholic health care institution, especially a teaching hospital, will promote medical research consistent with its mission of providing health care and with concern for the responsible stewardship of health care resources. Such medical research must adhere to Catholic moral principles.
5. Catholic health care services must adopt these Directives as policy, require adherence to them within the institution as a condition for medical privileges and employment, and provide appropriate instruction regarding the Directives for administration, medical and nursing staff, and other personnel.
6. A Catholic health care organization should be a responsible steward of the health care resources available to it. Collaboration with other health care providers, in ways that do not compromise Catholic social and moral teaching, can be an effective means of such stewardship.[8]
7. A Catholic health care institution must treat its employees respectfully and justly. This responsibility includes: equal employment opportunities for anyone qualified for the task, irrespective of a person's race, sex, age, national origin, or disability; a workplace that promotes employee participation; a work environment that ensures employee safety and well-being; just compensation and benefits; and recognition of the rights of employees to organize and bargain collectively without prejudice to the common good.
8. Catholic health care institutions have a unique relationship to both the Church and the wider community they serve. Because of the ecclesial nature of this relationship, the relevant requirements of canon law will be observed with regard to the foundation of a new Catholic health care institution; the substantial revision of the mission of an institution; and the sale, sponsorship transfer, or closure of an existing institution.
9. Employees of a Catholic health care institution must respect and uphold the religious mission of the institution and adhere to these Directives. They should maintain professional standards and promote the institution's commitment to human dignity and the common good.

8. The duty of responsible stewardship demands responsible collaboration. But in collaborative efforts, Catholic institutionally based health care services must be attentive to occasions when the policies and practices of other institutions are not compatible with the Church's authoritative moral teaching. At such times, Catholic health care institutions should determine whether or to what degree collaboration would be morally permissible. To make that judgment, the governing boards of Catholic institutions should adhere to the moral principles on cooperation. See Part Six [in *Ethical and Religious Directives for Catholic Health Care Services*].

14 The Corporate Physician's Oath

David Schiedermayer

I swear by Humana and Columbia HCA and Cigna and Prudential and FHP and Wellpoint and HMO and PPO and IPA, making them my witnesses, that I will fulfill according to my ability this oath and this covenant:

To hold the one who has taught me this business as equal to my corporation president, and to live my life in partnership with him or her, and if he or she is in need of capital to give him or her some of mine, and to regard his or her offspring as equal to my colleagues and to teach them this business — if they desire to learn it — for a fee and under contract; to give a share of my practice management techniques and computer systems and all other business acumen to my children and the children of those who have taught me, and to students who have signed the contract and have taken an oath according to Medicare law, but to no one else.

I will apply dietetic measures for the benefit of the obese, the alcoholic, the smoker, and the drug addict, but in this culture and in this political climate I will seldom be able to keep them from self-harm and injustice.

I will neither give a deadly drug to anybody if asked for it, nor will I make a suggestion to that effect (depending on the outcome of Oregon's Ballot Measure 16). As an internist I will not do an abortion, leaving that to the obstetricians. In fear of malpractice I will guard my life and my business.

I will not use the knife, but I will try to learn some form of endoscopy.

Into whatever clinics I may enter, I will come for the benefit of the members, required to remain clear of all except capitated care for the indigent.

Things which I may see or hear in the course of treatment, or even outside of treatment regarding the life of human beings, things which one should never divulge outside, I will report to government commissions, immigration officials, hospital administrators, or use in my book.

If I fulfill this oath and do not violate it, may it be granted to me to enjoy life and business, being able to retire at age 50 in the sunbelt. If I transgress it and swear falsely, may Milwaukee be my lot.

Used with permission of the author. An earlier version was published as "The Hippocratic Oath — Corporate Version," in the *New England Journal of Medicine,* Jan. 2, 1986, p. 62.

15 Sick of Being Poor

Teresa Maldonado

I woke up early one morning with strong pains in my stomach. As I lay in bed, the pain would come and go. When it came, I doubled over and broke out in a sweat. My husband was out of town, and I was at home with my five children. After about an hour, I realized I had to do something.

I thought about what I could do. I thought of walking to one of the medical clinics just around the corner from my house, but we were broke. I thought of going to a hospital emergency room, but we didn't have health insurance. If I couldn't pay a doctor, I certainly couldn't pay a hospital emergency room bill either. My only remaining choice was to go to the Board of Health clinic.

I panicked. Although I was a registered patient there and had taken my children there many times, I had gone there only once or twice for myself. I was afraid because I knew I needed help, yet I knew that getting into the clinic might not be easy.

If I called and made my condition sound too serious, they would say, "Honey, don't come in. You're too sick. Go straight to the hospital." If I didn't communicate how sick I was, they would say, "Sure you can come in. How about a week from Friday?"

The pain was too intense to ignore, so I took a deep gulp and called. A gentleman in the Adult Medicine department answered. I explained my situation and asked for permission to come in. His response was, "You've called the wrong place. You belong in Family Planning."

Family Planning! The effort I was making to hide my pain kept me from blowing up. "I know the difference between my stomach and my uterus," I said. He got flustered and put me on hold.

Within a few minutes a nurse was on the line. I had to start all over. When I was through, she said the same thing: "You belong in Family Planning."

"I am a registered patient with Adult Medicine. I do not belong in Family Planning," I repeated. "I'm not going to have any more babies. Please let me come in."

The nurse put me on hold again. When she came back, she was clearly annoyed with me. I could not come in until 1:00 p.m., she said. And if I did come in, she

From David Caes, *Caring for the Least of These: Serving Christ Among the Poor* (Scottdale, Penn.: Herald Press, 1992), pp. 17-24. Reprinted by permission of the Christian Community Health Fellowship, 803 N. 64th Street, P.O. Box 12548, Philadelphia, Penn. 19151-0548.

wouldn't guarantee I would see the doctor, even if I waited until closing time that evening.

After hanging up, I decided my pain wasn't bad enough to be worth enduring such treatment all day. I was powerless. I never did go in. The pain eventually subsided.

To be poor is to be powerless, to be boxed in, to have no choices. The professionals who live and work in my community are there by choice. They have the option of walking away into the regular job market and earning more somewhere else. The very fact that professionals are providing services implies a position of power. Such people are not poor, no matter how frugally they choose to live.

Those of us who receive those services are powerless, perhaps because we lack education, good communication skills, or marketable job skills. We cannot walk away from our neighborhood into the land of success and prosperity.

The health care system illustrates the lack of options for the poor. I am forced to seek health care for myself and my children in a system that is dehumanizing, impersonal, belittling, and blaming.

Health Care Which Dehumanizes

A typical visit to the Board of Health Clinic includes at least six, and sometimes as many as ten, lines to wait in. When one of my children gets sick and I call to ask permission to bring my child in, I brace myself for a three-to-five-hour ordeal.

When I arrive, I go to the nurse's desk and wait my turn. When I see the nurse, I assure her that I called and let her know that I have arrived. She puts a check next to my name and sends me to the records counter.

I then wait my turn to get my records. When I receive my child's medical records, I shuffle back to the nurse's station and wait my turn again. She pulls out a computer sheet that will be filled out by every person who sees my child and attaches it to the records.

I go back to the first desk to see the person who will prepare my bill. I go to the other side of the clinic and wait my turn to pay the fee. Next I go to a waiting room to get my child's weight and temperature checked.

After that I gather everything together and wait in the waiting room for the doctor. If the doctor feels a lab test is necessary, I go to the lab. I have to wait longer there than in all the other lines combined. When I am through at the lab, I go back to the doctor and wait for her to see me again.

If the doctor feels a prescription and follow-up visit are needed, I must go to the other side of the center to wait for my prescription, then back to the records counter for the clerk to give me another appointment.

Through all this I am juggling my infant and two toddlers as I shuffle from line to line. If it is winter, I'm also toting four sets of hats, coats, scarves, and gloves. As if there weren't enough waiting in line already, during my first visits I got in wrong lines several times.

By the time I leave the clinic, I feel exhausted, disgusted, and worthless. At every station I have had to endure intolerance, indifference, and impatience from those "helping" me. Through body language, tone of voice, or lack of eye contact, I get the message loud and clear that I am a nobody. It seems every time I go in at least one person is angry with me for daring to ask for service. When a child is sick, my only choices are to endure this treatment or decide that I can't handle it that day and stay home with my sick child.

When you have to go through this dehumanizing process time after time, it eventually becomes a part of you. You begin to believe you really *are* nobody.

When I shared my experiences with a friend, she pointed out that Dr. Martin Luther King, Jr., had said, "They no longer have to tell us to go to the rear of the bus; we will fight to get there." In other words, when you are treated like that again and again, it becomes a part of your being, and you begin to do only what is expected of you.

Health Care Which Is Impersonal

When I go to the corner store, the grocer knows me, my children, and my husband. She knows my neighbors and their families. If I haven't been to each of the businesses in my neighborhood at least a dozen times, I have passed them on my way to the others. If I don't know the owners by name, I at least know them by sight. I know them and they know me.

During the warm weather we live outside our houses as much as we do inside. I have a neighbor who always sits outside his house. He is our neighborhood patriarch — a solid, consistent fixture. I see him whenever I get my mail. I see him when I go outside to call my children. I see him when I open my door to see what the weather is like. He knows everybody — who they are, where they live, who lives with them, and what is going on in their lives.

Impersonal service is foreign to my community, where I know I belong. But this security withers when I have to go to the Women, Infants, and Children program (WIC), the Public Aid office, or the Board of Health Clinic. Once inside these offices, I am anonymous. I become a number, and that anonymity hurts.

When I am in touch with that pain, all I want to do is run out and go home. Whatever I am there to get doesn't seem worth it. I avoid those places if at all possible. After two years on WIC, I got to the point where I couldn't stand the dehumanizing treatment any more; I gave up my benefits.

Health Care Which Belittles

When I go to the clinic, any of ten doctors could be on duty. The doctor doesn't know me and may not see me again for a year. To the doctor, I am just another face.

Because I don't have money, I am treated as though I cannot think for myself, or make appropriate choices for my family. It would seem that relating to a child's mother would be a key part of diagnosing the child's illness. After all, I know my child better than she does. But when I say, "I think my child has this," the doctor doesn't listen and treats me as if I don't count.

I don't go to the clinic unless my child is very sick, so that at least they will believe me when I say my child is ill. I have a daughter who just turned five years old. Before her third birthday, she had pneumonia twelve times. She never had a cold or flu; whenever she got sick she got pneumonia, and that would eventually be verified at the clinic.

After her second or third bout with pneumonia, I began to recognize the symptoms. I would call for permission to go into the clinic and plan on being there for three to five hours. I thought going in before the pneumonia got bad was the responsible thing to do.

Each time all I would hear was, "Yes, your daughter has a fever. Yes, she is coughing. But no, she does not have pneumonia."

In my mind I'd say, *Yes, but give her a day or two.* I'd get Sudafed and Tylenol and be sent home. Two days later, my daughter would be sicker. I would have to hold my limp, little girl in my arms while I tried to work the system. That is powerlessness.

One year we actually had health insurance. When our daughter started to have trouble breathing one evening, my husband and I were pleased to realize we didn't have to wait until the next day to go to the clinic — we could take her to the hospital emergency room for a shot of adrenaline. After the doctor finally examined her two hours later, he said she had asthma and gave her a shot. He also said she had a touch of pneumonia; he wanted to hospitalize her.

That confused me. Hospitalize her for a touch of pneumonia? I said that I knew how to take care of her at home. My husband said there was no way we would leave her in the hospital because all they would do was give her an antibiotic and some Tylenol. We said no.

The doctor left. When he came back five minutes later, he dropped a bomb. "We think your daughter has cystic fibrosis." What could we do? We gave in and let them hospitalize her.

My husband and I took turns staying with her days and evenings. By the fifth day, we still had not seen the doctor. He somehow managed to examine my daughter in the ten minutes it took one of us to get a sandwich. She was never tested for cystic fibrosis.

When we called the doctor, he said, "I don't have confidence in this hospital's ability to test for cystic fibrosis. When I release her, I'll give you an order, and you can take her to Children's Memorial Hospital."

My daughter was in the hospital for ten days. During that time she got Tylenol regularly and an antibiotic every eight hours. A respiratory therapist came and pounded on her back once a day. I could have done that! When we got the bill, the insurance company refused to pay $3,000 because it was a preexisting condition. This kind of experience is belittling.

Health Care Which Blames the Victim

When our children get sick, we parents naturally feel responsible. But when we take our children in for care, it is devastating to be told it is all our fault.

When my son was six months old, he got a high fever. When I took him in, I found out he had an ear and throat infection. That infection and fever seemed to last until after his first birthday. As I think back on that time, my only memories are of being in the bathroom with my son in the tub (trying to bring his fever down), or at the doctor's office getting him a prescription for an antibiotic. Toward the end of those six months, the doctor looked me squarely in the face. He said if I could not get my child well and keep him well, he was going to have my son taken away from me.

Now I know children get sick in the suburbs. Why else would there be so many pediatricians and hospitals out there? Do the pediatricians in the suburbs blame the child's mother every time a child is sick? Do pediatricians in the suburbs threaten to take a child away from its mother because the child is sick? Why am I always to blame when my child is sick? I am told that decisions I make, the food I prepare, the way I dress my children, and where we live is all my fault. That is why my child is sick.

When I was asked to share my experiences, I was afraid. What if people agreed with the doctor at the clinic? But as I was working on this, I showed it to some of my neighbors and relatives. As they read about my experiences, their mouths fell open. They were amazed that I had been able to name something deep inside of them — something that was tearing them up. "That's me," they said. "Go ahead and say it."

So I decided to risk it. And what I have to say is that most of the time the health care system's treatment of the poor in this county is dehumanizing, impersonal, belittling, and blaming. But it doesn't have to be. Empowered by God's Spirit, people can learn to serve the poor with compassion and without paternalism.

16 The Bible and Christian Convictions

Willard M. Swartley

What are our basic biblical and Christian convictions about healthcare? Do all people have the right to healthcare access? When we address this issue as Anabaptist Christians, should we advocate "rights" language or basic biblical and Christian moral teachings? I contend that the Christian passion for issues of healthcare access are less rooted in seeking our "rights" than in a missional concern for others.

Jesus taught his disciples to love all people, including their enemies, not because they belong to our group, believe as we do, or choose the good instead of evil. Rather, because the heavenly Father gives rain and sun to the good and evil alike, so we should love all people, even our enemies (Matthew 5:43-48; Luke 6:27-36). Such care for others certainly includes seeking to make healthcare accessible for all.

Five biblical themes and early Christian practices underline the urgency of improving healthcare access for all:

1. Scripture identifies shalom as God's will and gift for people.

Shalom, the Hebrew word for *peace* (210 occurrences; over 350 uses, including derivatives) has many dimensions of meaning: wholeness, well-being, peace, salvation, and justice. Shalom occurs often in inquiring about one's *welfare* (Genesis 29:6; 37:14; 43:27; Exodus 18:7; 1 Samuel 10:4; 17:18, 22; 25:5; 30:21; Jeremiah 15:5 for shalom of Jerusalem; 38:4). This inquiry about one's "welfare includes everything necessary to healthful living: good health, a sense of well-being, good fortune, the cohesiveness of the community, relationship to relatives and their state of being, and anything else deemed necessary for everything to be in order" (Claus Westermann, "Peace [*Shalom*] in the Old Testament," in *The Meaning of Peace,* ed. Perry B. Yoder and Willard M. Swartley [Elkhart, Ind.: IMS, 2001], 49). English versions may translate shalom as prosperity (Psalm 30:6; Isaiah 54:13). Shalom also has moral connotations: it is opposed to deceit (Psalm 34:13-14; Jeremiah 8:22–9:6). The notion of *well-being* shades over into shalom's cognate, *sholem* (used 33 times), which denotes holistic health.

Shalom assumes relationship with God and meaningful relationships with fellow-humans. Cheating others, hurting others in any way, violating covenants, and living selfishly deprive the community of shalom. When certain people are disqualified from healthcare benefits, they are excluded from experiencing shalom. When a healthcare system excludes the weakest and most vulnerable citizens from basic, non-emergency healthcare coverage it deprives the people excluded of fullness of shalom. Such exclusion obstructs God's moral shalom purpose for humans.

2. Old Testament Scripture emphasizes justice.

Justice describes God's moral nature (Psalm 89:14), and justice often occurs in parallel to righteousness (Psalm 72:1-2; Proverbs 2:9; 8:20; Isaiah 5:7b; 32:16; 33:5-6; 54:13-14; 60:17b) and shalom/peace (Isaiah 32:16-17; 59:8; cf. Psalm 85:10b; Isaiah 60:17). But the meaning of justice *(mishpat)* in Hebrew thought is not the same as the Greek view, popular in western society, that each person receives *equal* due. But in the biblical understanding of justice, the needs of the poor, widows, and orphans must be met (Psalm 72:4, 12-14; 146:6b-9).

Assisting the needy is linked often to "the fear of the Lord" (Deuteronomy 10:10-20; cf. Leviticus 25:35-43; 19:14, 32; Isaiah 33:5-6). Pursuit of this radical justice in communal life was a condition for living in the land God promised to the covenant people: "Justice, and only justice, you shall pursue, so that you may live and occupy the land that the Lord your God is giving you" (Deuteronomy 16:20).

Hear Amos, "Let justice roll down like waters, and righteousness like an ever-flowing stream" (5:24).

The prophets ranted and raved because Israel failed to practice God's justice. Read the following texts and ponder their significance for healthcare access: Isaiah 5:5-10; Amos 8:4-10; Micah 6:1-8; and Nehemiah 5:1-13. These texts indicate that nothing stirs God's wrath against his people more than failure to practice justice by caring for the needy. The same moral priority continues in the New Testament. James says, "Religion that is pure and undefiled before God, the Father, is this: to care for the orphans and widows in their distress, and to keep oneself unstained by the world" (1:27).

3. Jesus modeled healthcare inclusion of the poor and marginalized.

Jesus's healing ministry had an unusual access policy. Most people Jesus healed from illness or delivered from demons were not persons with standing in the religious community or people of means. Jairus' daughter was an exception, since Jairus was a ruler of the synagogue. Approximately a third of those Jesus healed were women.

From *Healing Healthcare: A Study and Action Guide on Healthcare Access in the United States,* pp. 10-12, edited by Joseph J. Kotva Jr.

Some were ritually defiled, unclean. Another third were socially ostracized, lepers, Gentiles, and "sinners." There were no exclusions in Jesus's healing ministry. Nor were there exclusions in what Jesus taught about caring for the sick. For example, Jesus says he will separate the sheep from the goats in the judgment of the nations. The sheep (nations?) are those who cared for the hungry, thirsty, naked, and the *sick* (Matthew 25:31-40).

When we consider Jesus's teaching and the social, economic, and political profile of the people he healed, we must conclude that exclusionary policies in healthcare are wrong. As Christians, we cannot morally accept the present U.S. distribution pattern of healthcare services. Indeed, Christian witness to national government on healthcare policy can testify to Jesus's Lordship and can be part of the manifold witness to the powers that Paul speaks about in Ephesians 3:9-10.

4. Sharing material resources was a basic teaching and practice of the New Testament church.

After Pentecost the early church had all things in common (Acts 2:42-45; 4:32-37). Another model of sharing, more applicable to us now, involved collecting money from wealthier Jewish-Gentile Christian churches throughout Asia Minor and Macedonia for the poorer Jewish Christians in Jerusalem. Paul speaks of this relief gift extensively (2 Corinthians 8–9), grounding it in "the grace given me by God" (Romans 15:15). Paul likewise prays that this "offering of the Gentiles may be acceptable, sanctified by the Holy Spirit" (15:16).

Paul describes his relief work at length: "At present, however, I am going to Jerusalem in a ministry *(diakonia)* to the saints; for Macedonia and Achaia have been pleased to share their resources with the poor among the saints at Jerusalem. They were pleased to do this, and indeed they owe it to them; for if the Gentiles have come to share in their spiritual blessings, they ought also to be of service to them in material things" (Romans 15:25-27). Because the assistance was *mutual,* it would be returned if the situation was reversed (2 Corinthians 8:13-15). Such mutual care manifested God's gift of grace in the community. It bonded formerly alienated people into one in Jesus Christ, their peace (Ephesians 2:13-17).

Paul gave his life to practice mutual aid, despite prophesy that he would encounter arrest and imprisonment in Jerusalem (Acts 21:7-14). Paul says, ". . . I am ready not only to be bound but even to die in Jerusalem for the name of the Lord Jesus Christ" (v. 13b). Paul regarded his relief gift to Jerusalem as the crowning achievement of his apostolic calling since it proved the unity of the Gentiles and the Jews in Christ (read 2 Corinthians 8–9 and Acts 21:7-14 in light of Romans 15:25-31 and Galatians 2:10)! Such material caring for one another created *shalom.* It expressed true love for one another (2 Corinthians 7–8; cf. John 13:34-35). Love of God showed itself in love for the needy brother and sister (cf. 1 John 3:17-18).

5. The Christian church in the next centuries continued to assist in healthcare needs of its own members and those outside the church.

Virtually everyone in the Roman Empire was poor (99 percent); only a few were wealthy. Likewise, the church was composed largely of poor people (1 Corinthians 1:26-28). By A.D. 251, the church in Rome had a massive program of care for widows and the poor. With numerous house churches throughout the city, 1500 people were on the church's support role. Bishop Cornelius was aided by seven deacons, seven more sub-deacons, and ninety-four more working in minor roles to aid the needy (Eusebius, *Ecclesiastical History* 6.43.11). Poor people outside the church community were also helped by the Christians. In light of this model, we ask: how many deacons (or similar caregivers) does your congregation have?

The Roman world treated the poor cruelly, allowing female infants to die with their bodies decaying in open sewers running down the middle of the city streets. Rodney Stark, in his sociological study of early Christianity, says, "We've unearthed sewers clogged with the bones of newborn girls." The early Christians "had to live with a trench running down the middle of the road, in which you could find dead bodies decomposing" (Stark, "A Double Take on Early Christianity," *Touchstone* 13/1 [2000]: 44, 47). Christians did not put sewer systems in the cities, but they spoke against infanticide; they cared for each other and those abandoned in a social order blinded to human need.

Though agnostic toward Christianity, Stark is convinced that early Christians made a striking difference in their world: standing for life against death, caring for each other, and valuing women and children, granting them dignity. They lived a counterculture, manifesting God's kingdom values amid a morally bankrupt society. Early Christianity fostered shalom amid horrid healthcare conditions.

Attending to the above five biblical themes and early Christian practices intensifies our concern for the failed U.S. healthcare system. We live in a society where high-tech healthcare innovations are in abundance, often in overlapping availability and competing for the same demographic groups. Yet, skewed distribution of resources, almost endless beginning and end of life expectations, and a for-profit, market-driven system deprive the needy of healthcare. Is that shalom?

At "Dialogue 1992: The Church Confronts Its Mission in Health and Healing," Dr. Willard Krabill used the image of a "devil's triangle" that exacerbates the healthcare crisis:

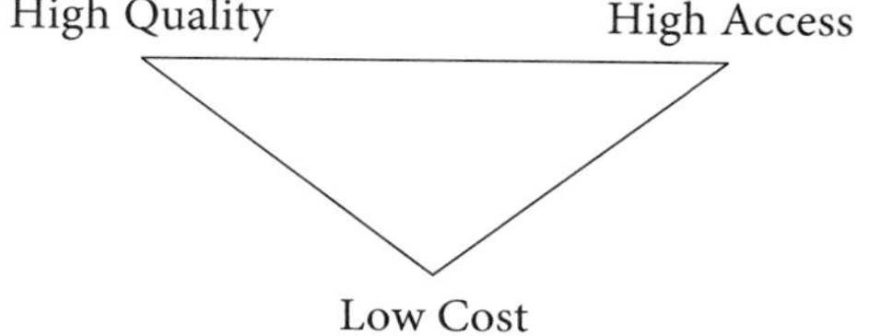

Krabill noted that many argue that only by dropping *quality* can *costs* be contained and *access* improved. If we want access for all and/or lower costs, then we must sacrifice quality. Krabill countered the argument, maintaining that all three are possible. To achieve this he called for restraint in high-tech procedures and medical fees, lowering lawyer's fees in malpractice suits (and fewer of them), converting insurance priorities from economic gain to wider coverage policies, breaking the stranglehold of costly pharmaceutical and medical equipment, and conversion from selfish consumerism.

For such a shift to occur, I propose that we view healthcare through new lenses, what I call "God's triangle":

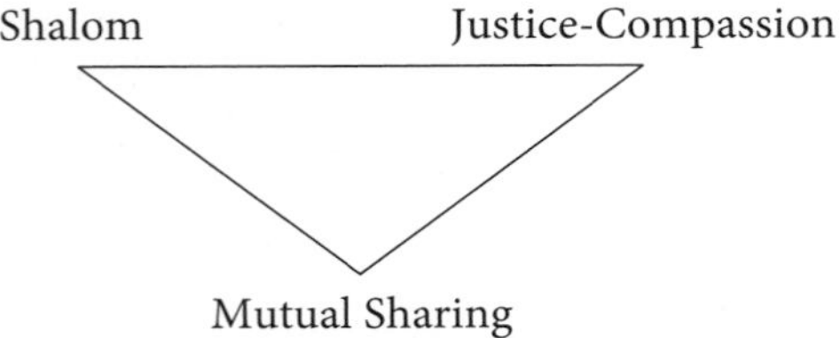

As we assess the healthcare crisis through these lenses, it becomes an engaging *challenge*. What steps might your church take to wear these glasses?

17 The Christian and Anabaptist Legacy in Healthcare

John D. Roth

"In the name of Jesus Christ of Nazareth, walk!" . . . Instantly the man's feet and ankles became strong. He jumped to his feet and began to walk. Then he went with them into the temple courts, walking and jumping, and praising God.

Acts 3:6-8

The Early Church: Continuing Christ's Healing Ministry

From the Christian church's beginning, miraculous stories, such as Peter's curing the man outside the temple gates (Acts 3:1-10), make it clear that Jesus's healing ministry would continue through his followers. Accounts of Jesus curing the sick, casting out demons, and restoring life to the dead fill the Gospels. By continuing this ministry of healing, the early church testified to Christ's living presence in their midst. Throughout Acts, "miraculous signs and wonders" of healing frequently accompanied the apostles' call to repentance (Acts 5:12-16; Acts 8:47; Acts 9:40-42). Clearly, the ministry of healing — of minds, bodies, spirits, and relationships — was a defining characteristic of early Christianity. Concern for the sick was not unique to early Christians. After all, the Hippocratic Oath originated in Greek culture five centuries before Christ, and the Romans were famous for their curative purges and healing baths. But unlike healthcare in Greco-Roman society, the Christian community's concern for the sick extended beyond the wealthy to include the poor, the orphan, and the stranger. Moreover, the Christian tradition brought an institutional expression to its pastoral concern for the sick that led to a flourishing of hospices, orphanages, and respite centers. Already in 325, the Council of Nicaea commanded that a building dedicated to the care of the sick be constructed in every cathedral town. The hospice of St. Basil at Caesarea in Cappadocia, for example, completed by 370, was renowned for its treatment of the sick and as a place of refuge for travelers and poor people.

From *Healing Healthcare: A Study and Action Guide on Healthcare Access in the United States,* pp. 13-15, edited by Joseph J. Kotva Jr.

Early Christians built similar hospices at Constantinople and Alexandria in Egypt and in cities throughout Syria and Asia Minor.

In Europe, monasteries played a vital role in the care of the sick. Committed to the practice of "hospitality" (from the Latin *hospes,* or host), most monasteries set aside part of their facility as an infirmary for the sick. These early "hospitals" did not so much promise to cure illnesses as to provide a place of relative comfort where the sick could "die a good death" amidst the prayers and ministrations of the pious. Some monastic infirmaries became widely known for the quality of their care. The Hôtel Dieu, for example, founded by the bishop of Paris in the seventh century and still in operation today, was among the most famous of these early hospitals. These more specialized facilities spread rapidly from the eleventh through the fourteenth centuries, often founded as philanthropies of the crusading orders such as the Knights Templars and the Teutonic Knights. During periods of devastating epidemics in Europe — such as the spread of leprosy during the twelfth century or the bubonic plague in the fourteenth century — these church-based hospices provided the afflicted with a small measure of Christian charity and comfort.

Following the Reformation, Catholic monasteries were frequently dissolved in Protestant countries, the secular ruler confiscating their properties. As a consequence, healthcare in Europe increasingly moved from the church's control into the secular hands of the state or private foundations.

The Anabaptist Tradition of Mutual Aid: Communities of Compassion

Born in the tumult of the Reformation, the Anabaptists shared the general Protestant rejection of monasticism. But the monastic ideal of a radical commitment to Christ lived on in Anabaptist communities, as did the monastic tradition of extending hospitality to the poor and the sick. Although Anabaptists in the sixteenth and seventeenth centuries did not establish formal institutions for healthcare, they were deeply committed to the New Testament principle of "bearing one another's burdens." That commitment inevitably found expression in dealing with physical health and well-being.

In many communities, Anabaptists gained local renown for their skills as midwives, physicians, or healers. In Moravia, for example, the Hutterites were noted for their healing potions, and Hutterite physicians often found employment in the courts of local lords. Mennonites in Switzerland and South Germany frequently found favor with the local population, even during times of severe persecution, as trustworthy midwives, herbalists and veterinarians. The Dutch Mennonites, who enjoyed toleration already in the 1570s, frequently sent their university students to medical school rather than the theological faculties of the state churches; thus, many of their educated pastors in the seventeenth and eighteenth centuries were trained as physicians. One famous Mennonite physician, Govert Bidloo (1649-1713), published an anatomical textbook and served as a professor of medicine in the Dutch town of Leiden.

Why did so many Anabaptists-Mennonites, as a persecuted religious minority, gravitate to the healing arts? Historians have offered several suggestions: unlike farming, medicine was an occupation that did not require heavy investments in land and could easily be "transported" from one region to another; it was a highly valued skill that brought them into favor with the local population even during times of persecution; and it was a pursuit that arose naturally out of their commitment to a life of practical morality and love of neighbor.

The commitment to show Christ's love in daily human relations found more general expression in the Anabaptist-Mennonite tradition of mutual aid — a concern for the needy that went beyond poor relief to include care for the weak, injured, sick, and dying members in their midst. Following the model of the early church, Mennonite congregations appointed deacons whom they charged with the task of addressing the needs of the sick. Mennonite deacons in the urban congregations of the Netherlands were especially attentive to the medical concerns of poor people in their congregations. One congregation in Amsterdam paid a local surgeon a flat fee to treat anyone in the congregation who was ill. The physician was to provide his own "salve, plasters, gargling fluid, waters and cooling-draughts" while the deacons pledged to provide any necessary medicines from the apothecary. Already in the early seventeenth century, Dutch Mennonites took the lead in establishing hostels *(hofjes)* to provide living quarters and assistance to the chronically ill, the aged, or to members with physical or mental disabilities.

The Dutch Mennonite impulse toward more formal or institutionalized forms of healthcare found even more vigorous expression among related groups of Mennonites who migrated across northeast Germany to Poland and then, in the early nineteenth century, to Russia. In their highly independent colonies in South Russia, healthcare among the Mennonites flourished during the late nineteenth century. Indeed, by the early twentieth century, Russian Mennonites had established several well-equipped hospitals, a mental hospital, several schools for the deaf and blind, a training institute for nurses, and various mutual aid programs that became the forerunners of modern forms of health insurance.

Twentieth-Century Anabaptist-Mennonite Attitudes and Practices

Twentieth-century North American Mennonites have also shown the love of Christ through healing ministries. In the fall of 1908, for example, Mennonites established their first hospital in North America — a sanitarium for the treatment of tubercular patients at La Junta, Colorado, which later expanded into a nurses training college. As North American Mennonites entered vigorously into mission work, a focus on health — including numerous clinics in India, a hospital in Tanzania, and a leprosarium in Paraguay — always accompanied the evangelistic message.

These concerns took on even more public and dramatic expression in the aftermath of World War II. Among the many Mennonite conscientious objectors who chose to enter Civilian Public Service (CPS) camps during the early 1940s, some 1,500 served as attendants in various state institutions for the mentally ill. Deeply troubled by the conditions they witnessed in many facilities, a group of CPSers in Philadelphia began to collect information and concerns, along with constructive ideas for changes, from their fellow workers. Inspired by these reports, *Life* magazine published an expose of conditions in U.S. mental hospitals (May 1946). Other exposes followed, galvanizing a public outcry that eventually led to the creation of National Mental Health Foundation and a fundamental transformation in American legal and cultural attitudes toward mental illness. The CPS experience in mental health reform also profoundly influenced the Mennonite church. Sponsored by the newly-formed Mennonite Mental Health Services (MMHS), Mennonite-related groups had five mental health centers by the mid-1960s, with another three facilities working in close affiliation with MMHS (now MHS Alliance). "What seems clear," wrote William Klassen, "is that the Mennonites would never have established mental hospitals had they not been spurred on by a corps of dedicated and visionary men who had worked in mental hospitals and become convinced that something could be done for the mentally ill and that the church do something for them."

Since then, the Mennonite commitment to healthcare has continued to flourish. Organizations such as Mennonite Mutual Aid, Mennonite Medical Association, Mennonite Nurses Association, the Mennonite Health Association (1980) and many others have given various visible expressions to the ministry of healing. Increasingly, these organizations have broadened their focus from care for the sick to a more proactive emphasis on wellness — physical, emotional, and spiritual — throughout all stages of life.

As more people are without access to healthcare, as healthcare costs continue to spiral upward, as new technology leads to progressively complex ethical questions, as Mennonite young people increasingly enter health-related professions, and as Mennonites in general become more acculturated into modern society, the call to participate in Christ's ministry of healing remains clear. How Mennonites will continue to answer that call requires careful and thoughtful discernment. But the complexities of the issues ahead should not distract us from the imperative to be ministers of healing.

18 Catholic Social Teaching and the Allocation of Healthcare

The Catholic Bishops' Joint Bioethics Committee

The foregoing chapters, in the interests of promoting common understanding, all appeal to reasoned considerations the force of which may be recognised without benefit of Christian faith. But Christian faith itself gives powerful support to those considerations. This is because answers to questions about healthcare resource allocation must make underlying assumptions about the nature and dignity of the human person, and about the nature of human community and how people should relate to each other. Catholic Christianity has a developed body of teaching about these fundamental matters as well as about the ethics of healthcare. A fully adequate understanding of the human situation and of the truths we need to grasp if we are to live well is available to us only in virtue of revelation and, in particular, of our revealed knowledge of human destiny. So this chapter sets the main elements of the moral framework developed in previous chapters within the broader context of understanding provided by divine revelation.

15.1 Introduction

Much of this Report has been built upon 'common morality': those principles and approaches common to people of all religions and none, articulated in documents ranging from great religious texts to international human rights documents, and described by many thinkers both secular and religious. We have adopted points of departure, methods of argumentation, and language common to many outside our faith tradition in order better to provide an exposition which may appeal to, and engage in dialogue, people of all religions and none. We are confident that all human beings share a 'moral sense which enables them to discern by reason the good and the evil, the truth and the lie.'[1]

1. *Catechism of the Catholic Church* (hereafter *Catechism*) para. 1954; cf. *Catechism* paras. 1954-1960; Finnis, *Natural Law and Natural Rights.*

From Anthony Fisher and Luke Gormally, eds., "Catholic Social Teaching and the Allocation of Healthcare," in *Healthcare Allocation: An Ethical Framework for Public Policy* (London: The Linacre Centre, 2001), 145-61.

Nonetheless we believe that specifically Catholic thinking in this area has a unique contribution to make because of the strong association of the Church with healthcare, its centuries of accumulated experience and wisdom in dealing with healthcare dilemmas, and the particular gifts of inspiration, sensitivity and reason which it brings to bear on moral questions more generally. Healthcare allocation is a theological matter every bit as much as it is an issue for philosophy, medicine or public policy — for it goes to the heart of attitudes toward the dignity of the human person, the nature of community, and right relations between people under God.[2] Decisions about healthcare allocation have implications beyond the obvious ones for effective and efficient healthcare management: they contribute to or hinder a greater reality which, by virtue of God's promise and grace, can begin in this life and extend into the completed kingdom and family of God in heaven.[3]

Furthermore, while a sound ethic can in principle be recognised and lived by anyone of good will and right reason, reason's full implications, and morality's practical applications, are well understood only when full account is taken of the human situation. Catholics believe that the human situation is only adequately and reliably illuminated by the life and teachings of Jesus Christ, mediated to us in the Church's Scriptures and tradition. A theologically-informed ethic thus assists the agent to live a 'fully human life' by educating conscience, shaping character, and facilitating wise choices in particular cases; it also helps people respond to their divine calling and prepares them for eternal life.[4]

Lastly, Catholic tradition offers an especially rich collection of resources in the areas of social ethics[5] and bioethics[6] — the very two areas which intersect in our present investigation. The following are among the points made repeatedly in the teaching on social ethics: the dignity of the human person; the consequent rights (reasonable expectations) of persons to those things necessary for their flourishing (including rights to life, food and shelter, healthcare and education, work and a worthy standard of living . . .); the nature of persons as social and political animals who must co-operate to achieve their good; the consequent duties to respect civil rights, collaborate mutually, and act responsibly with respect to others; the intimate link between love and justice; the consequent special care for the poor and marginalized and opposition to attitudes such as racism; the notions of community, common good, needs, rights and duties as the context for the establishment of social, political and economic relations; and 'subsidiarity' or supportive decentralisation of decision-making and opportunities. In the official documents on Catholic bioethics, respect for the dignity of the human person is again emphasised, especially in the face of contemporary threats to human life and health even in healthcare situations. Nothing can lessen the intrinsic goodness and inviolability of human life; no personal or social benefit can justify its destruction or abandonment. These documents show an acute awareness of the very real pressures presently faced by health planners, health workers and patients, such as limited resources; but the Church remains committed to preaching 'the Gospel of Life' and to championing the cause of the victims of 'the culture of death', opposing all disrespectful, uncaring and especially homicidal healthcare decisions, including those made in the interests of 'more efficient' resource allocation.

15.2 The Dignity of the Human Person and the Right to Live and Flourish

Catholic reflection upon the appropriate level and allocation of healthcare begins with the claim that every human being has intrinsic, equal and inalienable dignity or

2. Cf. Catholic Health Association of the United States, *No Room in the Marketplace: The Healthcare of the Poor.* St. Louis, MO: The Catholic Health Association 1986, and *idem, With Justice for All? The Ethics of Healthcare Rationing.* St. Louis, MO: The Catholic Health Association 1991; J. M. Finnis and A. Fisher, 'Theology and the four principles: a Roman Catholic view'. In R. Gillon (ed.), *Principles of Health Care Ethics.* Chichester: Wiley, 1993: 31-44.

3. Grisez, *Christian Moral Principles:* 115-140, 459-476; cf. Vatican II, *Gaudium et Spes,* paras. 38-39; Pope John Paul II, Encyclical Letter *Sollicitudo Rei Socialis* 1987: sec. 47.

4. Finnis and Fisher, 'Theology and the four principles: a Roman Catholic view'.

5. E.g. Pope Leo XIII, Encyclical Letter *Rerum Novarum* 1891; Pope Pius XI, Encyclical Letter *Quadragesimo Anno* 1931; Pope John XXIII, Encyclical Letter *Mater et Magistra* 1961, and Encyclical Letter *Pacem in Terris* 1963; Vatican Council II, *Gaudium et Spes* 1965; Pope Paul VI, Encyclical Letter *Populorum Progressio* 1967, and Apostolic Letter *Octogesima Adveniens* 1971; Synod of Bishops 1971, *Justice in the World;* Pope John Paul II, Encyclical Letter *Laborem Exercens* 1981, Encyclical Letter *Sollicitudo Rei Socialis* 1987, and Encyclical Letter *Centesimus Annus* 1991; National Conference of Catholic Bishops of the USA, *Economic Justice for All: Pastoral Letter on Catholic Social Teaching and the US Economy* 1986. These documents were commonly occasioned by the concerns of their day: the condition of workers; the rise of totalitarian governments; the arms race and threats to world peace; the aspiration to a new international order in which peace is protected and peoples given opportunities to develop; problems with both Marxist and capitalist worldviews. Nonetheless they established some enduring principles. Repudiating approaches which reduce justice to non-interference with others, or fulfilling agreements, or treating everyone the same, Catholic social teaching has proposed a rich conception of the nature, purposes and obligations of community life, and the need for moral rectitude, fairness and commitment to the common good ('solidarity') among the members of a community.

6. E.g. Congregation for the Doctrine of the Faith, *Declaration on Procured Abortion* 1974, *Declaration on Euthanasia* 1980, and *Instruction on Respect for Human Life in Its Origin and on the Dignity of Procreation* 1987; Pontifical Council for the Pastoral Care of Health Care Workers, *Charter for Health Care Workers* (hereafter *Charter*) 1994; United States Catholic Conference of Bishops, *Ethical and Religious Directives for Catholic Health Services* 1994 (henceforth: USCC, *Ethical and Religious Directives*); Pope John Paul II, Encyclical Letter *Evangelium Vitae* 1995.

worth, deserving uncompromising reverence and respect. Persons are created 'in the image of God' (Gen 1:26) as free and rational beings with a divine calling, and restored to that image by Christ's redemptive work (Eph 1:10; 1 Tim 2:46), making them children of God.[7] The Author and Lord of life commands reverence and love for every person. Their life and health are precious gifts — 'talents' — entrusted to human beings by God to be cherished and well used.[8] We have an inalienable responsibility to take reasonable care of our own health and that of our dependents, without selfishly ignoring the needs of others and the demands of the common good.[9] And because much healthcare is beyond our personal capacities to provide, we must co-operate with others if we are to fulfil this responsibility.[10] Above all, then, any healthcare system must be consistent with respect for and indeed positively serve 'the primary and absolute value of life: of all human life and the life of each and every human being'.[11]

Furthermore, as the Second Vatican Council noted,

> Human persons by their very nature stand completely in need of life in society. . . . Life in society is not something accessory to human persons: through their dealings with others, through mutual service, and through fraternal dialogue, people develop their talents and are enabled to rise to their destiny.[12]

Social by nature and grace, persons are bound together as a community by birth as 'children of the first Adam and the first Eve' and by redemption as 'children of the new Adam and the new Eve'. As members of one human family and the community of disciples, they are called to love one another and to collaborate in providing for the means for each other's proper development, especially where individuals cannot provide for their needs by themselves.[13] Opposing 'the luxury of a merely individualistic morality' Christians insist upon the obligations of justice and mercy which are only satisfied by contributing to the common good according to one's means and the needs of others.[14] Their love is to exceed the ordinary limitations of affection, overcome the hopelessness evoked by the enormity of some social problems, and the partiality, indifference and individualism common in the face of competing interests. As Vatican Council II declared:

> Everyone should look upon their neighbour (without exception) as another self, bearing in mind above all the neighbour's life and the means necessary for living it in a dignified way (Jas 2:15-16) lest he follow the example of the rich man who ignored Lazarus, the poor man (Lk 16:19-31).[15]

Thus the impetus behind Christian healthcare down through the ages has been a high regard for the human person and a concern to love one's neighbour as oneself (Mt 19:19), spending oneself for them (Mt 5 and 6; Jn 13:34; 15:13), thereby seeking first God's Kingdom and trying to be like him (Mt 5:48; 6:33). The model of this self-sacrificing love is, of course, Jesus, who 'went about doing good and healing everyone' (Acts 10:38).[16] Care

7. *Gaudium et Spes,* sec. 29: 'All people are endowed with a rational soul and are created in the image of God; they have the same nature and origin and, being redeemed by Christ, they enjoy the same divine calling and destiny; there is here a basic equality between all persons and it must be given even greater recognition.' On the dignity of the human person: see e.g. *Gaudium et Spes,* Part 1; Vatican Council II, *Dignitatis Humanae.*

8. Congregation for the Doctrine of the Faith, *Instruction on respect for human life in its origin and on the dignity of procreation (Donum Vitae)* I, 1987; *Catechism,* paras. 2259E ; Pope John Paul II, *Evangelium Vitae* 1995.

9. *Catechism,* paras. 2288-91.

10. On the duty of the community to assist the family in caring for the young, the old, the sick, the handicapped, and the poor: *Catechism,* paras. 2208-9.

11. *Charter,* Preface. Cf. *Charter,* para. 1, citing *Catechism,* para. 2288 and various addresses by John Paul II: 'The work of health care professionals is a very valuable 'service to life'. It expresses a profoundly human and Christian commitment, undertaken and carried out not only as a technical activity but also as one of dedication to and love of neighbour. It is 'a form of Christian witness'. 'Their profession calls for them to be guardians and servants of human life.' Life is a primary and fundamental good of the human person. Caring for life, then, expresses, first and foremost, a truly human activity in defence of physical life. It is to this that professional or voluntary health care workers devote their activity.'

12. *Gaudium et Spes,* sec. 25. Cf. St. Thomas Aquinas, *Commentary on Aristotle's Nicomachean Ethics* 1, 1; *Catechism,* para. 1879.

13. E.g. *Gaudium et Spes,* secs. 24-26, 32: "Scripture teaches us that love of God cannot be separated from love of one's neighbour: 'Any other commandment is summed up in this sentence: You shall love your neighbour as yourself; therefore love is the fulfilling of the law' (Rom 13:9-10; cf. 1 Jn 4:20). It goes without saying that this is a matter of the utmost importance to people who are coming to rely more and more on each other. . . . The human person is and ought always to be the beginning, the subject and the object of every social organization. . . . The human person stands above all things and their rights and duties are universal and inviolable. . . . The social order and its development must constantly yield to the good of the person, since the order of things must be subordinate to the order of persons and not *vice versa.* . . . God did not create humankind to live as individuals but to come together in the formation of social unity. . . . In his preaching Christ clearly outlined an obligation on the part of the children of God to treat each other as brothers and sisters. In his prayer he asked that all his followers should be 'one'. . . . This solidarity must be constantly increased until that day when it will be brought to fulfilment. . . ." *Catechism,* para. 1880: "A society is a group of persons bound together organically by a principle of unity that goes beyond each one of them. . . . By means of society, each man is established as an 'heir' and receives certain 'talents' that enrich his identity and whose fruits he must develop. He rightly owes loyalty to the communities of which he is part, and respect to those in authority who have charge of the common good." On friendship, community or solidarity as a direct demand of human and Christian brotherhood see Pope John Paul II *Sollicitudo Rei Socialis* (1987) and *Centesimus Annus* (1991); *Catechism,* paras. 1939ff. On the necessity of the state for human flourishing: *Catechism,* para. 1882.

14. *Gaudium et Spes,* sec. 30.

15. *Gaudium et Spes,* sec. 27; cf. *Catechism,* para. 1931.

16. *Charter,* para. 4.

for the sick and the weak, the suffering and the sinful, was a major focus of his life and served alongside his words and mighty deeds to proclaim the coming of God's kingdom.

He restored sight to the blind (Mk 8:22-26; 10:46-52; Mt 20:29-34), hearing to the deaf (Mk 7:32-37; Mt 11:5) and speech to the mute (Mt 9:32-33; 12:22; Lk 11:14). He cured the woman with a haemorrhage (Mk 5:25-34), lepers (Mk 1:40-45; Lk 17:12-19) and the paralysed and lame (Mk 2:3-12; Mt 8:6-13; 21:14; Jn 5:3-8). He even restored dead people to life (Mk 5:35-43; Lk 7:12-17; Jn 11; cf. Mk 9:17-29). For Mark Jesus is very much the exorcist-healer. Luke records that in initiating his ministry, Jesus declared programmatically that he had been anointed not only to bring good news to the poor but also sight to the blind (Lk 4:17) and that he later compared himself with a physician (of bodies and souls: Lk 5:31), with a miraculous preacher-healer (Lk 7:22-23), and with a Good Samaritan nursing a Jew mugged and left for dead (Lk 10:29-37). His many cures are summed up by Luke (14:40): 'Now when the sun was setting, all those who had any sick with various diseases brought them to him; and he laid his hands on them and healed them.' Likewise Matthew (15:30-31; cf. Mk 7:37) tells us: 'Great crowds came to him, bringing with them the lame, the maimed, the blind, the mute, and many others. They put them at his feet, and he cured them, so that the crowd were amazed when they saw the mute speaking, the maimed whole, the lame walking, and the blind seeing. And they praised the God of Israel.' Indeed, so replete was his life with the cure of every kind of ailment and disease (Mt 9:35) that Matthew interpreted Jesus' mission as the fulfilment of the prophecy of Isaiah: 'He took away our infirmities and bore our diseases' (Mt 8:17; cf. Is 53:4).[17]

At Christ's own invitation, Christians are to see in every suffering person a brother or sister in need, indeed Christ himself, and know that what they do for this person they do also for Christ and for Christ's sake (Mt 25:31-40).[18]

In faithful imitation and continuation of that ministry, Christians have served the sick, suffering and dying in various ways throughout history: monastic pharmacies and infirmaries; hospitals, nursing homes, hospices for the dying, and medical and nurse training schools run by religious orders; lay faithful committed to healthcare as their vocation; sacramental and other pastoral care for the sick; systematic reflection on healthcare ethics. Modeling their efforts on Jesus' own work, these men and women have demonstrated the power of healthcare as an authentic expression of neighbourliness toward those in need.[19]

> The mystery of Christ casts light on every facet of Catholic health care: to see Christian love as the animating principle of health care; to see healing and compassion as a continuation of Christ's mission; to see suffering as a participation in the redemptive power of Christ's passion, death and resurrection; and to see death, transformed by the resurrection, as an opportunity for a final act of communion with Christ.[20]

Here, as elsewhere, Christians have opposed unjust discrimination,[21] and have sought to make healthcare an integral part of the Church's mission to preach and live the Gospel.[22]

Health is not, however, an exclusive, dominant value[23] or healthcare the only good goal of persons; nor are life, health and resources infinite.[24] Pain and death will not be eliminated in this life. Suffering must be faced head-on, against the pervasive temptation of contemporary secular societies to demand an immediate technological 'fix' for every discomfort and to devote endless resources to the futile quest to extend life indefinitely or to achieve perfect health and comfort throughout life. Part of the specifically Christian contribution to consideration of what is appropriate in healthcare will therefore be reflection upon the meaning of sickness and death and the human encounter with both in healthcare situations.[25] Christians believe that suffering can be united to the Redeemer's cross (Col 1:24) and so share in its salvific efficacy.

> On the Cross, the miracle of the serpent lifted up by Moses in the desert (Jn 3:14-15; cf. Num 21:8-9) is renewed and brought to full and definitive perfection. Today, too, by looking upon the one who was pierced, every person whose life is threatened encounters the sure hope of finding freedom and redemption.[26]

17. This paragraph is drawn from Anthony Fisher, OP, 'Is there a distinctive role for the Catholic hospital in a pluralist society?' In L. Gormally (ed.), *Issues for a Catholic Bioethic.* London: The Linacre Centre 1999: 200-229, at pp. 212-213.

18. *Charter,* para. 4, quoting from a 1980 address by Pope John Paul II: "What a stimulus for the desired 'personalization' of medicine could come from Christian charity, which makes it possible to see in the features of every sick person the adorable face of the great, mysterious Patient, who continues to suffer in those over whom your profession bends, wisely and providently!"

19. Cf. USCC, *Ethical and Religious Directives,* 1994.

20. USCC, *Ethical and Religious Directives.*

21. *Gaudium et Spes,* sec. 29.2: 'Every form of social or cultural discrimination in fundamental personal rights on the grounds of sex, race, colour, social conditions, language or religion, must be curbed and eradicated as incompatible with God's design.' On the scandalous and sinful nature of some inequalities of access see: *ibid.,* sec. 29.3; *Catechism,* para. 1938.

22. *Charter,* para. 5.

23. Against the cult or idolisation of the body and of physical health see: *Gaudium et Spes,* sec. 41; *Catechism,* para. 2289.

24. The virtue of temperance ought to moderate the consumption of medicine as of other goods: cf. *Catechism,* paras. 1809, 2290, 2407.

25. See *Charter,* paras. 53-55; Pope John Paul II, Apostolic Letter *On Suffering (Salvifici Doloris),* 1984. See also D. A. Jones, OP, 'The encounter with suffering in the practice of medicine in the light of Christian revelation'. In L. Gormally (ed.), *Issues for a Catholic Bioethic.* London: The Linacre Centre, 1999: 159-172.

26. Pope John Paul II, *Evangelium Vitae,* sec. 50.

Thus without in any way minimizing or exaggerating the reality of human suffering, they acknowledge it not with blind resignation but with the serene knowledge that the human spirit under grace can triumph even over sickness, pain and death and that God can bring good out of any evil.[27] The limitations of healthcare and of health resources are, therefore, no ultimate tragedy, but merely the field in which people of good will are called to do all that is practically and morally possible under grace, entrusting the rest to the God of love.

15.3 The Right to Healthcare

In addition to being a manifestation of Christian love and concern for suffering others, healthcare has been viewed by the Christian tradition as an entitlement in justice — but under a view of justice which is about right relations between persons and an imaginative, generous, merciful application of the Golden Rule (Mt 7:12), rather than the narrow contractual conception all too common today.[28] The right of individuals to live and to flourish, and the duty of communities to assist their members in achieving these goals, are the foundations of the Catholic claim that there is a right to healthcare.

Thus Pope John XXIII taught in *Pacem in Terris:*

> Man has a right to live. He has the right to bodily integrity and to the means necessary for the proper development of life, particularly food, clothing, shelter, medical care, rest, and finally, the necessary social services. In consequence, he has the right to be looked after in the event of ill-health, disability [and] old age.[29]

Similarly, John Paul II has said that 'as regards necessities — food, clothes, housing, medical and social assistance . . . — there must be no privileged social strata',[30] for every individual has a 'primary right . . . to what is necessary for the care of his health and therefore to adequate health services'. The *Catechism of the Catholic Church* echoes these sentiments, insisting that communities must provide the conditions for the well-being and development of their members, including access to adequate healthcare.[31] The US Bishops have argued that

> Every person has a basic right to adequate healthcare. This right flows from the sanctity of human life and the dignity that belongs to all human persons, who are made in the image of God. It implies that access to that healthcare which is necessary and suitable for proper development and maintenance of life must be provided for all people, regardless of economic, social, or legal status. Special care should be given to meeting the basic health needs of the poor.[32]

15.4 The Option for the Poor and Sick

Catholic reflection upon the duty of communities to provide adequate healthcare to their members is further enriched by the social doctrine of the 'option' or 'preferential love' of God and his Church for the poor, sick and otherwise disadvantaged.[33] This doctrine has a long history, stretching back well into the Old Testament period. The prophets, for instance, commonly focussed their critical gaze upon idolatry of various kinds — not just of foreign gods, but of wealth, power and privilege — and upon the quality of relationships between individuals, between communities, and with God. They preached *hesed* (love or mercy) and *sedaqah* (justice, or righteousness), which included harmonious community life, distributive justice, honesty and fair dealing. The litmus test of this mercy and justice was how the *anawim* (widows, orphans, the poor, refugees . . .) were treated; the prophets spoke for God in condemning the predatory rich and powerful for their oppression or hard-heartedness towards the deprived.

Jesus took up this notion himself, teaching his disciples to be compassionate to all (as is their heavenly Father: Lk 6:36) but especially to the 'marginalised'. His parable of the feast of the kingdom of God began with the instruction: 'When you hold a banquet, invite the poor, the crippled, the lame, the blind' (Lk 14:13),[34] and these were the very sorts of people whom Jesus most often healed and associated with. It was by how each of us treats the least advantaged that he proposed to judge us (Mt 25:40).[35]

The Fathers of the Church and its great scholastic Doctors echoed Christ's words in their 'radical' claims that 'not to share with the poor is to steal from them, indeed to kill them', whereas 'to attend to their needs is to give them what is rightly theirs, not ours'.[36] This ancient theme has been restated and amplified in various ways in modern Catholic social teaching dating from Pope Leo XIII (*Rerum Novarum* 1892).

The so-called 'preferential option for the poor' is a counsel of justice perfected by Christian mercy, and applies as much to healthcare allocation as elsewhere in life. Thus Christians themselves, individually or co-operating as charitable organizations, have established healthcare

27. Cf. *Charter,* para. 54.

28. *Catechism,* paras. 2213, 2407, 2443ff.

29. Pope John XXIII, *Pacem in Terris,* sec. 11.

30. John Paul II, Homily at Mass in Recife, Brazil, 4 August 1980, in 72 (1980) *Acta Apostolicae Sedis:* 929.

31. *Catechism,* paras. 1908, 2211, 2288.2.

32. United States Catholic Conference, *Health and Healthcare: A Pastoral Letter of the American Bishops.* Washington, DC: United States Catholic Conference, 1981. 11 (1981) *Origins:* 396-402.

33. Pope John Paul II, *Centesimus Annus,* sec. 57; Congregation for the Doctrine of the Faith, *Instruction on Christian Freedom and Liberation* 1986, sec. 68; *Catechism,* secs. 2443ff.

34. Cf. Mt 5:42; 6:2-4; 8:20; 10:8; 25:31-46; Mk 12:41-44; Lk 3:11; 6:20-22; 11:41; Eph 4:28; Heb 13:3; Jas 2:15-16; 5:1-6; 1 Jn 3:17.

35. Cf. *Catechism,* para. 1932.

36. See, e.g., the texts from St. John Chrysostom and St. Gregory the Great cited in *Catechism,* para. 2446.

institutions and programmes targeted at the poor and otherwise disadvantaged; and they have also sought to ensure the social conditions, including government programmes, necessary to complement these efforts if those who cannot provide for themselves are to be guaranteed access to adequate healthcare. The US Bishops observed a few years ago that:

> In accord with its mission, Catholic healthcare should distinguish itself by service to and advocacy for those people whose social condition puts them at the margins of our society and makes them particularly vulnerable to discrimination: the poor, the uninsured and the underinsured; children, the unborn, single parents and the elderly; those with incurable diseases and chemical dependencies; and racial minorities, immigrants and refugees. In particular, the person with mental or physical disabilities, regardless of the cause or severity, must be treated as a unique person of incomparable worth, with the same right to life and to adequate healthcare as all other persons.[37]

If traditional distributions of healthcare or contemporary trends in allocation further disadvantage such people — and put their health and very lives at risk — the Catholic community can be expected to oppose such distributions and seek reform. And their own healthcare institutions must give a lead in this respect.

A growing and increasingly disadvantaged group which the Catholic Church has been especially keen in recent times to commend to the attention of those who distribute health resources has been the elderly[38] — a group for whom 'filial piety' would commend special consideration in any case.[39] In *Evangelium Vitae* Pope John Paul renewed this call, pointing to the danger in cultures such as ours that the elderly will be regarded as 'a useless burden' and consequently abandoned or even killed. In place of such 'intolerable' neglect of the elderly, he exhorts us to reestablish a sort of 'covenant' between generations in which there is mutual respect and support of various kinds — including, of course, healthcare.[40]

15.5 The Responsibility of the Community to Respond to Healthcare Needs

The sources of communal responsibility for healthcare are thus several: reverence for the goodness of life and health not only as experienced by ourselves but by all others; our nature as social beings, interdependent by nature and called by grace to the service of others; the obligation to express such care and respect in concrete acts such as the provision of healthcare; the need for the community's contribution towards, and participation in, healthcare to be large-scale if it is to be achieved at the level which can reasonably be expected in the contemporary world; the natural expectation on the part of members of a community that such assistance will be available to them in order that they might live, flourish and participate in the life of their society; and the particular concern of Christians that the most disadvantaged as 'God's little ones' be given special care. As the *Catechism of the Catholic Church* observes:

> On coming into the world, man is not equipped with everything he needs for developing his bodily and spiritual life. He needs others. Differences appear tied to age, physical abilities, intellectual or moral aptitudes, the benefits derived from social commerce, and the distribution of wealth. These 'talents' are not distributed equally. These differences belong to God's plan, who wills that each receive what he needs from others, and that those endowed with particular 'talents' share the benefits with those who need them. These differences encourage and often oblige persons to practise generosity, kindness and sharing of goods; they foster mutual enrichment. . . .[41]

Two fundamental ideas here are 'the common good' and 'distributive justice'. The common good is described variously in Catholic social teaching as the range of economic, political and social conditions necessary for the flourishing of individual members of a community, for respect for fundamental rights, and/or for achieving appropriate common goals.[42] Co-responsibility for the common good — 'love of neighbour' or 'solidarity' — is the basis of the duties to pay taxes,[43] to show loyalty to

37. USCC, *Ethical and Religious Directives,* 1994. Cf. Catholic Health Association, *With Justice for All? The Ethics of Health Care Rationing,* p. 24: 'Those who are marginalized by society — those who cannot speak for themselves, the powerless, the disenfranchised, the vulnerable — have the most urgent claim on healthcare because they are among the least fortunate in our society. Rationing schemes should not be devised to the detriment of these people. Given the life-threatening conditions in which they are often forced to live, their claims on the healthcare system are ethically more compelling, not less. Development of healthcare policy should always proceed from the perspective of disadvantaged persons, with a bias toward improving their health status first.'

38. E.g. *Gaudium et Spes,* sec. 27; John Paul II, *Salvifici Doloris,* 1981; John Paul II, *Christifideles Laici,* 1988: sec. 48; John Paul II, 'Letter to the elderly', *L'Osservatore Romano,* 1 October 1999.

39. Ex 20:12; Dt 5:16; cf. Lk 2:51; Mk 7:8-13; Eph 6:1-3; *Catechism,* paras. 2197ff.

40. Pope John Paul II, *Evangelium Vitae,* sec. 94; cf. Pontifical Council for the Laity, *The Dignity of Older People and Their Mission in the Church and in the World* in *L'Osservatore Romano* [weekly edition] 10 February 1999.

41. *Catechism,* para. 1936.

42. E.g. Pope John XXIII, *Mater et Magistra; Gaudium et Spes,* secs. 26.1 and 74.1; Pope Paul VI *Populorum Progressio;* United States Catholic Conference of Bishops, *Economic Justice for All. Catholic Social Teaching and the US Economy,* 1986, sec. 8; and *Catechism,* paras. 1905-6: the common good is 'the sum total of social conditions which allow people, either as groups or as individuals, to reach their fulfilment more fully and more easily'. Vatican Council II, *Dignitatis Humanae,* sec. 6: 'The common good of society consists in the sum total of those conditions of social life which enable people to achieve a fuller measure of perfection with greater ease.' Cf. USCC, *Ethical and Religious Directives,* 1994.

43. *Catechism,* paras. 2240 and 2465 (cf. Mt 22:21; Rom 13:7).

the group and respect for its authority,[44] to show respect for human rights,[45] to co-operate to provide the necessities for the flourishing of all,[46] to seek (only reasonable) assistance from the community with respect to achieving one's own fulfilment. It requires fellow-feeling, genuine self-giving, joint effort with others to promote the flourishing of all, encouragement and support for the efforts of others, and various interventions by the state in accordance with a just hierarchy of values.

The provision of healthcare, whether by individual health professionals[47] or by the community as a whole,[48] is an expression of this virtue of solidarity. And people have an ethical claim on the community in general, and the health professions in particular, for help in the maintenance of their health. This is, in the Christian view of things, part of what society is for and a large part of what (private) property and (medical) education are for. But it has its limits: we have no right to expect that everyone else go without so that we can have the best of everything.

We have examined secular conceptions of distributive justice in previous chapters. In chapter 11 (11.4) we proposed that distributive justice in healthcare might be judged by a test something like this: *would I think the healthcare budget and its distribution was fair if I (or someone I loved) were in healthcare need, especially if I were among the weakest in the community (i.e. sick with a chronic, disabling and expensive ailment, elderly, poor and illiterate)? Would I think it were fair if I were one who would go without under the proposed arrangements?* This approach is strongly supported by Jesus' own enunciation of the Golden Rule (Mt 7:12),[49] his explication of its radical demands in the Sermon on the Mount (e.g. Mt 5:40-42; 6:2-4; cf. 10:8), and his repeated insistence on the duties of those with power and wealth to redistribute to the poor and to see things from their perspective (e.g. Mt 19:23-26; Lk 6:24; 12:16-21; 16:19-31).[50] Jesus' is certainly a much richer conception of justice than those 'liberal' accounts we analysed in chapters 7 and 8.

44. *Catechism,* para. 1880.

45. *Dignitatis Humanae,* sec. 3: 'Since the common welfare of society consists in the entirety of those conditions of social life under which people enjoy the possibility of achieving their own perfection in a certain fullness of measure and also with some relative ease, it chiefly consists in the protection of the rights, and in the performance of the duties, of the human person.'

46. *Gaudium et Spes,* sec. 26: 'The common good is the sum total of social conditions which allow people, either as groups or as individuals, to reach their fulfilment more fully and more easily. . . . The human person ought to have ready access to all that is necessary for living a genuinely human life: for example, food, clothing, housing. . . . The social order requires constant improvement: it must be founded in truth, built on justice, and enlivened by love: it should grow in freedom towards a more humane equilibrium.'

47. Cf. *Catechism,* paras. 1942 and 2447.

48. Catholic Health Association, *With Justice for All? The Ethics of Health Care Rationing,* pp. 15-16: "The common good cannot be reduced simply to the will of the majority, and it is not synonymous with 'the greatest good for the greatest number'. Rather, the common good is achieved when communities of mutual concern and responsibility work on behalf of all. In healthcare, the common good is an ideal that presupposes initiatives from all sectors of society, including healthcare providers, the insurance industry, and government. In practice, the common good calls for solidarity, that is, an ethical commitment to do whatever is necessary to create constructive forms of social, political and economic interdependence."

49. Cf. *Catechism,* paras. 1939 and 2407.

15.6 The Limits to Autonomy in Property Ownership and Healthcare

Implicit in the claim that the community has duties to provide a certain level of healthcare, especially to those unable to provide for themselves, is a limit to the rights of private property: otherwise no-one would be morally required to give up what is 'theirs' by paying just taxes or by appropriate 'charitable' donations. Catholic teaching upholds the usefulness of private ownership but insists upon the universal destination of the goods of the earth (i.e. that the world's resources were created for the flourishing of all) and the consequent duty of those who 'have' to share with those who 'have-not'. This puts it very much at odds with liberal ideologies which absolutize private property, talents and energies, and the right to dispose of these benefits as one wishes. As Vatican II declared:

> In their use of things people should regard the external goods they legitimately own not merely as exclusive to themselves but common to others also, in the sense that they can benefit others as well as themselves. Therefore everyone has the right to possess a sufficient amount of the earth's goods for themselves and their family. This has been the opinion of the Fathers and Doctors of the Church, who taught that people are bound to come to the aid of the poor and to do so not merely out of their superfluous goods.[51]

Against the background of this traditional teaching, the Church has criticized 'excessive economic and social disparities' between individuals and societies as 'a source of scandal' which also 'militates against social justice, equity, human dignity, as well as peace'[52] and called for 'every effort to be made to put an end as soon as possible to these immense inequalities'.[53] Instead of a view of property as a thing to be accumulated, profited from, used and disposed of as the owner wishes, the Christian tradition promotes the notion of 'responsible stewardship' for the goods of creation, circumscribed by proper commit-

50. *Catechism,* para. 2446.

51. *Gaudium et Spes,* sec. 69; here the Council cites St. Basil, Lactantius, St. Augustine, St. Gregory the Great, St. Bonaventure and St. Albert the Great. See also: St. Thomas Aquinas, *Summa Theologiae* IIa IIae 32, 5; 66, 2; Pope Leo XIII, *Rerum Novarum;* Pope John XXIII, *Mater et Magistra;* Pope John Paul II, *Sollicitudo Rei Socialis* and *Centesimus Annus; Catechism,* paras. 2402ff.

52. *Gaudium et Spes,* sec. 29; cf. sec. 63.

53. *Gaudium et Spes,* sec. 66.

ments (e.g. to one's own family or patients), the needs of particular others, and the requirements of the common good.[54] Recent Catholic social teaching has been especially critical of the risks of avarice, acquisitiveness and waste in consumerist societies, the indifference of many affluent people toward the poor, and the swing of governments away from redistributive taxation, welfare 'safety nets', and foreign aid to poor nations, towards a kind of 'economic rationalism' which encourages and enacts hard-heartedness and selfishness.

Healthcare resources are like all other goods in this respect: those with access to or control of them have duties of responsible stewardship over them, ensuring that such resources are not squandered uselessly nor hoarded meanly, and that they are distributed justly and efficiently with respect for each person's needs and the good health of all the community.[55] The Church has consistently called for a redistribution of medical resources from the richer to the poorer, both within and between societies,[56] and for an 'integrated and comprehensive' view of public health and healthcare which encourages not only cure but prevention also.[57]

15.7 The Principle of Subsidiarity

'Subsidiarity' is a word which had some currency in the political rhetoric of the 1980s. As a principle of Catholic social teaching it means that each should be encouraged, enabled and willing to take responsibility for their own sphere (for themselves, their dependents . . .) and be given assistance *(subsidium)* to do so, rather than having that responsibility taken over by individuals and groups with greater power and resources. This doctrine favours a 'decentralisation' of decision making and resource allocation, with governments and other larger or more powerful groups avoiding usurping such functions where they can be adequately achieved by individuals and smaller and less powerful associations.[58] Pope John Paul II articulates the principle thus:

> A community of a higher order should not interfere in the internal life of a community of a lower order, depriving the latter of its functions, but rather should support it in case of need and help co-ordinate its activity with the activities of the rest of society, always with a view to the common good.[59]

Applied to healthcare allocation this doctrine suggests that larger units (such as central government) ought not to assume functions that smaller units (such as health authorities, primary care groups, charities, individual healthworkers or, most importantly, patients themselves) could effectively perform. In chapter 16 we shall see that recent NHS reforms have sometimes been attributed, at least in part, to this principle. Whether a commitment to subsidiarity is really behind these moves is debateable, but it might represent a useful corrective to any previous tendencies to undue paternalism, authoritarianism, or unnecessary centralisation. Two points should be noted about the application of the principle of subsidiarity: first that recent changes have been accompanied by the growth of an increasingly large and complex health bureaucracy; and secondly, that the principle should not be invoked by larger, more powerful and better resourced bodies, such as central government, as a reason for withdrawing from responsibility (e.g. devolving responsibility for care of the elderly to local councils or to families) where the smaller, less powerful and poorer unit cannot adequately fulfill this responsibility or is not being resourced to do so.

15.8 The Model of the Good Samaritan

After criticizing a number of long-established and contemporary approaches to healthcare allocation (chapters 5 to 8) we proposed a more substantive, 'natural law' alternative which attends more adequately to the goods of the human person and community, and to the norms and virtues which follow therefrom (chapters 9 to 11). On this basis we argued that a just health service will (as far

54. On the inadequacy of profitability and efficiency tests of the appropriate use of property see: Pope John Paul II, *Centesimus Annus:* sec. 24; *Catechism,* paras. 2423-25.

55. The United States Bishops *(Ethical and Religious Directives)* make the point that this applies to Catholic health care institutions, especially hospitals. 'Catholic health care ministry exercises responsible stewardship of available health care resources. A just health care system will be concerned both with promoting equity of care — to assure that the right of each person to basic health care is respected — and with promoting the good health of all in the community. The responsible stewardship of health care resources can be accomplished best in dialogue with people from all levels of society, in accordance with the principle of subsidiarity and with respect for the moral principles which guide institutions and persons.'

56. E.g. Pope John Paul II, *Evangelium Vitae,* sec. 26: 'a just international distribution of medical resources is still far from being a reality'.

57. 'The benefits provided in national healthcare policy should be sufficient to maintain and promote good health as well as treat disease and disability. Emphasis should be placed on the promotion of health, the prevention of disease, and adequate protection against environmental and other hazards to physical and mental health. If health is viewed in an integrated and comprehensive manner, the social and economic context of illness and healthcare must be an important focus of concern and action. . . . Public policy should provide incentives for preventive care, early intervention and alternative delivery systems.' (United States Catholic Conference of Bishops, *Pastoral Letter on Health and Healthcare.* Washington, DC: United States Catholic Conference 1981.)

58. *Catechism,* paras. 1883, 2208-9; Pope Pius XI, *Quadragesimo Anno;* Pope John XXIII, *Mater et Magistra,* sec. 53. Cf. Boyle, 'The concept of health and the right to health care'; Finnis, *Natural Law and Natural Rights:* 146-147, 168-169; Grisez, *Living a Christian Life:* 847-848. In this respect Catholic teaching sympathizes with liberal suspicion of creeping bureaucracy and hostility toward attempts to regulate all of human society by government.

59. Pope John Paul II, *Centesimus Annus,* sec. 48.4.

as possible) ensure access for all members of the community to care sufficient to meet their healthcare needs; and we specified what this level and these needs may be. We suggested some ways in which needs may be identified, moderated, sorted and reasonably satisfied. We argued further (in chapters 12 to 13) that healthcare should be allocated according to need, irrespective of factors such as race, religion, social contribution, age, consciousness, intelligence, quality of life, provider-whim and ability to pay. We noted a possible exception to a strictly needs-egalitarian approach: preference in favour of the disadvantaged, a choice which would be supported by the Catholic social doctrine elaborated in 15.4, the 'option for the poor'.

At several points in the present Report we have suggested that the Gospel parable of the Good Samaritan (Lk 10:25-37) is a useful model for good practice in healthcare allocation. The Good Samaritan is the story of one person's ready response to the suffering of another human being before him; it tells of the recognition of claims which rest on our common humanity, of the character of the virtuous person, of the 'common humanitarian duty of care' and, particularly, of the norm that one ought (where possible and reasonable) to assist 'neighbours' who are gravely and immediately in need of care. It is a model of human relating which, while manifestly concerned with practicalities — the Samaritan intervenes to provide very practical assistance, seeks help from others (the inn-keeper) to do so, and ensures that the latter is justly paid — does not reduce such relationships to utilitarian transactions, to be assessed in the light of cost-benefit considerations. It is a story, above all, of rescue and inclusiveness: God's rescue of damaged, abandoned, desperate humankind; Christ the Physician, healer of bodies and souls, responding to crying need wherever it is heard; and the Christian imitating this, participating in God's continuing work of rescue and inclusion, and responding to Christ's command to 'Go and do likewise' (Lk 10:37). As awareness of needs and ability to assist increase, so do the scope and opportunities for good neighbourliness: as the Second Vatican Council suggested, 'today there is an inescapable duty to make ourselves the neighbour of every person, no matter who they are, and if we meet them, to come to their aid in a positive way'.[60]

The Good Samaritan parable has long inspired the vocation of Christian healthcare: the response to a transcendent call to care lovingly for the sick person, to treat all those in need of such care, and to do one's best to save, heal and care.[61] Only the consciousness of such a divine 'calling' or 'mission' 'can motivate and sustain the most disinterested, available and faithful commitment' of health-workers, and it is this that gives their work a saving, 'priestly' value.[62]

The Good Samaritan model of rescue and inclusiveness stands in stark contrast to certain alternative bases for healthcare allocation which we have examined in this Report: discrimination against certain patients on the basis of undesired characteristics (the Samaritan's unlikely patient was a Jew for whom Samaritans were aliens); preference on the basis of social contribution or ability to pay (the Samaritan does not inquire into these); punishment for self-destructive behaviour (he likewise does not ask whether the victim 'brought it upon himself'); or QALY maximisation (we cannot imagine the Good Samaritan assessing whether the man beaten and left for dead will derive enough quality-adjusted life-years to justify the investment of two healthcare denarii).

In chapter 11 we proposed that health systems, like the Good Samaritan's acts of rescue and care, can be symbolic demonstrations of crucial values, such as generosity, respect for the dignity and equality of persons, for the inviolability of human life and the good of health, special concern for the vulnerable and powerless, solidarity with and compassion for those who suffer. 'Every society's judgments and conduct' — including its healthcare allocations — 'reflect a vision of the human person and their destiny.'[63] Thus health systems can tell the story of the kind of people we are and wish to be.

The Good Samaritan model does *not* counsel that we should give all our attention or spend all our resources on any one case of need. Indeed, while the compassionate Samaritan delays his travels so as to care for the beaten and abandoned stranger, he then hands him over to an inn-keeper and continues his own work, promising to make good the hospitaler's expenses on his return. The rescuer, then, has other responsibilities too, and these properly make their demands on his or her time and resources. Nor is the Good Samaritan the only model offered us by Christ: the wise steward is also praised (Mt 24:45; cf. Mt 10:16; 25:1-13; 25:14-30) and preventative healthcare strategies — no part of the Good Samaritan's work — are increasingly commended by the Church.[64] Thus Christians are recommended to combine the roles of both merciful healer and wily steward.

15.9 Conclusion

As citizens Christians are obliged to take an active part in public affairs, promoting social goods such as: civil and economic justice — often a powerful determinant of health; respect, protection and promotion of basic human goods — including life and health; and access to appropriate social assistance — including healthcare. To achieve this they have various responsibilities: to vote

60. *Gaudium et Spes,* sec. 27.

61. Examples of recent texts include: Pope John Paul II 1995, *Evangelium Vitae,* sec. 27; *Charter,* paras. 3, 5.

62. *Charter,* para. 3, citing Pope John Paul II, Address to the Association of Catholic Doctors, 28 December 1978 (*Insegnamenti* 1: 436) and Discourse for the 120th Anniversary of the Bambini Gesu Hospital, 18 March 1989 (*Insegnamenti* XII/1: 605-8, sec. 2).

63. *Catechism,* para. 2257.

64. *Charter,* paras. 50-52.

conscientiously — taking into account the attitude of candidates to the fundamental requirements of justice (and most particularly the absolute prohibition on killing the innocent) as well as their attitude to specific health policies; to obey just laws and pay just taxes — thereby contributing to a good health service, among other things; to make no unreasonable demands of government and society — including immoderate claims upon the health service; to contribute personally and to associate with others in complementing any government programmes to promote human flourishing — by, for instance, contributing to Church and other charity hospitals; and (sometimes) to participate more actively in politics — e.g. lobbying for the basic requirements of justice and for good health policies, or even standing for election with a view to securing justice in the practice of healthcare.

Many of the principles proposed to us in Catholic social and bioethical teaching, and which we have outlined in this chapter, provide only general orientations and bases for criticism, rather than specific directions on the best allocative mechanisms and healthcare programmes. Within these confines there may be legitimate differences between communities and between individuals over such things as: the extent to which access to provision for needs is a right; the proportion of a nation's national income which should be given over to healthcare as compared to other worthwhile purposes; the best balance between government, the market and the individual in healthcare provision; the appropriate response to particular kinds and cases of sickness; and the very urgency of healthcare rationing. Catholic teaching allows room both for the objective, universal requirements of the moral law and a range of culturally particular responses to the demands of that law. Above all it calls individuals and communities to conversion and to a genuinely Christian life, without which the virtues necessary for meeting healthcare needs are hardly likely to flourish.

19 Health, Healing, and Social Justice: Insights from Liberation Theology

Paul Farmer

If I define my neighbor as the one I must go out to look for, on the highways and byways, in the factories and slums, on the farms and in the mines — then my world changes. This is what is happening with the "option for the poor," for in the gospel it is the poor person who is the neighbor par excellence. . . .

But the poor person does not exist as an inescapable fact of destiny. His or her existence is not politically neutral, and it is not ethically innocent. The poor are a by-product of the system in which we live and for which we are responsible. They are marginalized by our social and cultural world. They are the oppressed, exploited proletariat, robbed of the fruit of their labor and despoiled of their humanity. Hence the poverty of the poor is not a call to generous relief action, but a demand that we go and build a different social order.

Gustavo Gutiérrez,
The Power of the Poor in History

Not everything that the poor are and do is gospel. But a great deal of it is.

Jon Sabrino, *Spirituality of Liberation*

Making a Preferential Option for the Poor

For decades now, proponents of liberation theology have argued that people of faith must make a "preferential option for the poor." As discussed by Brazil's Leonardo Boff, a leading contributor to the movement, "the Church's option is a preferential option *for the poor, against their poverty*." The poor, Boff adds, "are those who suffer injustice. Their poverty is produced by mechanisms of impoverishment and exploitation. Their poverty is therefore an evil and an injustice."[1] To those concerned with health, a preferential option for the poor offers both a challenge and an insight. It challenges doc-

1. Boff 1989, p. 23.

From Paul Farmer, "Health, Healing, and Social Justice: Insights from Liberation Theology," in *Pathologies of Power: Health, Human Rights, and the New War on the Poor* (Berkeley: University of California Press, 2004), 139-59. Used by permission of University of California Press.

tors and other health providers to make an option — a choice — for the poor, to work on their behalf.

The insight is, in a sense, an epidemiological one: most often, diseases themselves make a preferential option for the poor. Every careful survey, across boundaries of time and space, shows us that the poor are sicker than the nonpoor. They're at increased risk of dying prematurely, whether from increased exposure to pathogens (including pathogenic situations) or from decreased access to services — or, as is most often the case, from both of these "risk factors" working together.[2] Given this indisputable association, medicine has a clear — if not always observed — mandate to devote itself to populations struggling against poverty.

It's also clear that many health professionals feel paralyzed by the magnitude of the challenge. Where on earth does one start? We have received endless, detailed prescriptions from experts, many of them manifestly dismissive of initiatives coming from afflicted communities themselves. But those who formulate health policy in Geneva, Washington, New York, or Paris do not really labor to transform the social conditions of the wretched of the earth. Instead, the actions of technocrats — and what physician is not a technocrat? — are most often tantamount to managing social inequality, to keeping the problem under control. The limitations of such tinkering are sharp, as Peruvian theologian Gustavo Gutiérrez warns:

> Latin American misery and injustice go too deep to be responsive to palliatives. Hence we speak of social revolution, not reform; of liberation, not development; of socialism, not modernization of the prevailing system. "Realists" call these statements romantic and utopian. And they should, for the reality of these statements is of a kind quite unfamiliar to them.[3]

Liberation theology, in contrast to officialdom, argues that genuine change will be most often rooted in small communities of poor people; and it advances a simple methodology — *observe, judge, act.*[4] Throughout Latin America, such base-community movements have worked to take stock of their situations and devise strategies for change.[5] The approach is straightforward. Although it has been termed "simplistic" by technocrats and experts, this methodology has proven useful for promoting health in settings as diverse as Brazil, Guatemala, El Salvador, rural Mexico, and urban Peru. Insights from liberation theology have proven useful in rural Haiti too, perhaps the sickest region of the hemisphere and the one I know best. With all due respect for health policy expertise, then, this chapter explores the implications — so far, almost completely overlooked — of liberation theology for medicine and health policy.[6]

Observe, judge, act. The "observe" part of the formula implies analysis. There has been no shortage of analysis from the self-appointed apostles of international health policy, who insist that their latest recipes become the cornerstones of health policy in all of Latin America's nations.[7] Within ministries of health, one quickly learns

2. The literature on the correlation between poverty, inequality, and increased morbidity and mortality is massive. For reviews, see, for example, Farmer 1999b; Kim, Millen, Irwin, and Gershman 2000; and Wilkinson 1996. Other major reviews include Leclerc, Fassin, Grandjean, et al. 2000; World Health Organization 1999, 2000; World Bank 2000; Bartley, Blane, and Smith 1998; Sen 1998; Coburn 2000; and Fiscella, Franks, Gold, et al. 2000. Other articles review case studies of inequality in access to treatment of specific diseases; see, for example, Rathore, Berger, Weinfurt, et al. 2000; and of course the sizable body of literature on inequality of access to HIV therapy.

3. Gutiérrez 1983, p. 44.

4. For a concise history of liberation theology, its historical relevance, and an explanation of key themes and motivations, see Leonardo and Clodovis Boff's slim and helpful volume, *Introducing Liberation Theology* (1987).

5. Base-community movements, also known as "basic ecclesial communities," are disparate and sociologically complex, and I do not aspire to review their idealized or actual impact. But, as this movement has been felt throughout Latin America, I would encourage further reading. For an insider account, see the volume by Father Alvaro Barreiro (1982). A study by John Burdick (1993) contains a complementary, scholarly examination of such communities in urban Brazil.

6. There are other clues that liberation theology might have something to offer the healing professions: for one, the more destructive forces hate it. In 1982, for example, advisers to U.S. President Ronald Reagan argued that "American foreign policy must begin to counterattack (and not just react against) liberation theology" (quoted from the Santa Fe Document, a Reagan administration working paper; cited in Boff and Boff 1987, p. 86).

7. Recent health care "reforms" in Latin America and other developing regions have followed a neoliberal framework that favors commercialization, corporatization, and privatization of health and social welfare services. Most notable is the enthusiastic exportation of the U.S. model of "managed care." As Neill notes in his critique of these developments, "managed health care is touted by many experts — usually found in USAID, the World Bank, and various havens of academia — as a tangible model which can be of immense value to developing countries if applied wisely and efficiently" (2001, p. 61). This position, of course, ignores the growing body of evidence challenging the unabashed claims that managed-care organizations (MCOs) provide quality care with efficiency and cost-effectiveness — evidence that also points to managed care's role in exacerbating the already large inequities that characterize health care in the United States (Anders 1996; Andrulis and Carrier 1999; Farmer and Rylko-Bauer 2001; Ginzberg 1999; Himmelstein, Woolhandler, and Hellander 2001; Lewin and Altman 2000; Maskovsky 2000; Pellegrino 1999; Peterson 1999; Schneider, Zaslavsky, and Epstein 2002).

In fact, Waitzkin and Iriart note that, as the U.S. market has become saturated and MCOs face growing criticism, these corporations

> have turned their eyes toward developing countries, especially those in Latin America. In the tradition of tobacco and pesticides, U.S. corporations are exporting to developing countries — in the form of managed care — products and practices that have come under heavy criticism domestically. The exportation of managed care is also receiving enthusiastic support from the World Bank, other multilateral lending agencies, and multinational corporations. . . . developing countries are experiencing strong pressure to accept managed care as the organizational framework for privat-

not to question these fads, since failure to acknowledge the primacy of the regnant health ideology can stop many projects from ever getting off the ground. But other, less conventional sources of analysis are relevant to our understanding of health and illness. It's surprising that many Catholic bishops of Latin America, for centuries allied with the elites of their countries, have in more recent decades chosen to favor tough-minded social analysis of their societies. Many would argue that liberation theology's key documents were hammered out at the bishops' conventions in Medellín in 1968 and in Puebla in 1978. In both instances, progressive bishops, working with like-minded theologians, denounced the political and economic forces that immiserate so many Latin Americans. Regarding causality, the bishops did not mince words:

> Let us recall once again that the present moment in the history of our peoples is characterized in the social order, and from an objective point of view, by a situation of underdevelopment. Certain phenomena point an accusing finger at it: marginalized existence, alienation and poverty. In the last analysis it is conditioned by structures of economic, political, and cultural dependence on the great industrialized metropolises, the latter enjoying a monopoly on technology and science (neocolonialism).[8]

What began timidly in the preparation for the Medellín meeting in 1968 was by 1978 a strong current. "The Puebla document," remarks Boff, "moves immediately to the structural analysis of these forces and denounces the systems, structures, and mechanisms that 'create a situation where the rich get richer at the expense of the poor, who get even poorer.'"[9] In both of these meetings, the bishops were at pains to argue that "this reality calls for personal conversion and profound structural changes that will meet the legitimate aspirations of the people for authentic social justice."[10]

As Chapter 1 [in *Pathologies of Power*] noted, liberation theology has always been about the struggle for social and economic rights. The injunction to "observe" leads to descriptions of the conditions of the Latin American poor, and also to claims regarding the origins of these conditions. These causal claims have obvious implications for a rethinking of human rights, as Gutiérrez explains:

> A structural analysis better suited to Latin American reality has led certain Christians to speak of the "rights of the poor" and to interpret the defense of human rights under this new formality. The adjustment is not merely a matter of words. This alternative language represents a critical approach to the laissez-faire, liberal doctrine to the effect that our society enjoys an equality that in fact does not exist. This new formulation likewise seeks constantly to remind us of what is really at stake in the defense of human rights: the misery and spoliation of the poorest of the poor, the conflictive character of Latin American life and society, the biblical roots of the defense of the poor.[11]

Liberation theologians are among the few who have dared to underline, from the left, the deficiencies of the liberal human rights movement. The most glaring of these deficiencies emerges from intimate acquaintance with the suffering of the poor in countries that are signatory to all modern human rights agreements. When children living in poverty die of measles, gastroenteritis, and malnutrition, and yet no party is judged guilty of a human rights violation, liberation theology finds fault with the entire notion of human rights as defined within liberal democracies. Thus, even before judgment is rendered, the "observe" part of the formula reveals atrocious conditions as atrocious.

The "judge" part of the equation is nonetheless important even if it is, in a sense, pre-judged. We look at the lives of the poor and are sure, just as they are, that *something is terribly wrong*. They are targets of structural violence. (Some of the bishops termed this "structural sin.").[12] This is, granted, an a priori judgment — but it is seldom incorrect, for analysis of social suffering invariably reveals its social origins. It is not primarily cataclysms of nature that wreak havoc in the lives of the Latin American poor:

> ization of their health and social security systems. . . . this experience is serving as a model for the exportation of managed care to Africa and Asia (2001, p. 497).

There is, of course, much money to be made by tapping into the health care and social security funds of the public sector even in poorer developing nations, under the guise of rescuing these countries from inefficient bureaucracies and rising costs by importing neoliberal managed-care solutions. Large segments of the population in Latin America live in poverty and often have minimal or no access to formal health care. The consequences of such health care transformations for the poor and the oppressed in developing countries, as well as for the public health systems they might rely on, are dire, to say the least. "As public health systems are dismantled and privatized under the auspices of managed care, multinational corporations predictably will enter the field, reap vast profits, and exit within several years. Then developing countries will face the awesome prospect of reconstructing their public systems" (Waitzkin and Iriart 2001, p. 498). For more on health care reforms in Latin America, see Armada, Muntaner, and Navarro 2001; Barraza-Lloréns, Bertozzi, González-Pier, et al. 2002; Iriart, Merhy, and Waitzkin 2001; Laurell 2001; Pérez-Stable 1999; and Stocker, Waitzkin, and Iriart 1999.

8. Segundo 1980, p. 16; quoted from Segunda Conferencia General del Episcopado Latinoamericano, Medellín 1968.

9. Boff 1989, p. 20.

10. Eagleson and Sharper 1979, p. 118.

11. Gutiérrez 1983, p. 87.

12. Sobrino explains the link between structural violence and structural sin:

> God's creation is being assaulted and vitiated. . . . because this reality is not simply natural, but historical — being the result of action taken by some human beings against others — this reality is sinful. As absolute negation of God's will, this sinfulness is very serious and fundamental (1988, p. 15).

> All these aspects which make up the overall picture of the state of humanity in the late twentieth century have one common name: oppression. They all, including the hunger suffered by millions of human beings, result from the oppression of some human beings by others. The impotence of international bodies in the face of generally recognized problems, their inability to effect solutions, stems from the self-interest of those who stand to benefit from their oppression of other human beings. In each major problem there is broad recognition of both the moral intolerableness and the political non-viability of the existing situation, coupled with a lack of capacity to respond. If the problem is (or the problems are) a conflict of interests, then the energy to find the solution can come only from the oppressed themselves.[13]

Rendering judgment based on careful observation can be a powerful experience. The Brazilian sociologist Paulo Freire coined the term *conscientization,* or "consciousness raising," to explain the process of coming to understand how social structures cause injustice.[14] This "involves discovering that evil not only is present in the hearts of powerful individuals who muck things up for the rest of us but is embedded in the very structures of society, so that those structures, and not just individuals who work within them, most be changed if the world is to change."[15] Liberation theology uses the primary tools of social analysis to reveal the mechanisms by which social structures cause social misery. Such analysis, unlike many fraudulently dispassionate academic treatises, is meant to challenge the observer to judge. It requires a very different approach than that most often used by, say, global health bureaucrats. It requires an approach that implicates the observer, as Jon Sobrino notes:

> The reality posed by the poor, then, is no rhetorical question. Precisely as sin, this reality tends to conceal itself, to be relativized, to pass itself off as something secondary and provisional in the larger picture of human achievements. It is a reality that calls men and women not only to recognize and acknowledge it, but to take a primary, basic position regarding it. Outwardly, this reality demands that it be stated for what it is, and denounced. . . . But inwardly, this same reality is a question for human beings as themselves participants in the sin of humankind. . . . the poor of the world are not the causal products of human history. No, poverty results from the actions of other human beings.[16]

How is all of this relevant to medicine? It is more realistic, surely, to ask how this could be considered irrelevant to medicine. In the wealthy countries of the Northern hemisphere, the relatively poor often travel far and wait long for health care inferior to that available to the wealthy. In the Third World, where conservative estimates suggest that one billion souls live in dire poverty, the plight of the poor is even worse. How do they cope? They don't, often enough. The poor there have short life expectancies, often dying of preventable or treatable diseases or from accidents. Few have access to modern medical care. In fact, most of the Third World poor receive no effective biomedical care at all. For some people, there is no such thing as a measles vaccine. For many, tuberculosis is as lethal as AIDS. Childbirth involves mortal risk. In an age of explosive development in the realm of medical technology, it is unnerving to find that the discoveries of Salk, Sabin, and even Pasteur remain irrelevant to much of humanity.

Many physicians are uncomfortable acknowledging these harsh facts of life and death. To do so, one must admit that the majority of premature deaths are, as the Haitians would say, "stupid deaths." They are completely preventable with the tools already available to the fortunate few. By the criteria of liberation theology, these deaths are a great injustice and a stain on the conscience of modern medicine and science. Why, then, are these premature deaths not the primary object of discussion and debate within our professional circles? Again, liberation theology helps to answer this question. First, acknowledging the scandalous conditions of those living in poverty often requires a rejection of comforting relativism. Sobrino is addressing fellow theologians, but what he writes is of relevance to physicians, too:

> In order to recognize the truth of creation today, one must take another tack in this first, basic moment, a moment of honesty. The data, the statistics, may seem cold. They may seem to have precious little to do with theology. But we must take account of them. This is where we have to start. "Humanity" today is the victim of poverty and institutionalized violence. Often enough this means death, slow or sudden.[17]

A second reason that premature deaths are not the primary topic of our professional discussion is that the viewpoints of poor people will inevitably be suppressed or neglected as long as elites control most means of communication. Thus the steps of observation and judgment are usually difficult, because vested interests, including those controlling "development" and even international health policy, have an obvious stake in shaping observations about causality and in attenuating harsh judgments of harsh conditions. (This is, of course, another reason that people living in poverty are cited in this book as experts on structural violence and human rights.)

Finally, the liberation theologians and the communities from which they draw their inspiration agree that it is necessary to *act* on these reflections. The "act" part of

13. Pixley and Boff 1989, p. 242.

14. In the English translation of *Pedagogy of the Oppressed,* the original Portuguese term is retained. In Freire's own words, "*Conscientizaçãdo* is the deepening of the attitude of awareness characteristic of all emergence" — in other words, critical consciousness (1986, p. 101).

15. Brown 1993, p. 45.

16. Sobrino 1988, p. 31.

17. Ibid., pp. 13, 15.

the formula implies much more than reporting one's findings. The goal of this judging is not producing more publications or securing tenure in a university: "in order to *understand* the world, Latin American Christians are taking seriously the insights of social scientists, sociologists, and economists, in order to learn how to *change* the world."[18] Sobrino puts it this way: "There is no doubt that the only correct way to love the poor will be to struggle for their liberation. This liberation will consist, first and foremost, in their liberation at the most elementary level — that of their simple, physical life, which is what is at stake in the present situation."[19] I could confirm his assessment with my own experiences in Haiti and elsewhere, including the streets of some of the cities of the hemisphere's most affluent country. What's at stake, for many of the poor, is physical survival.

The results of following this "simple" methodology can be quiet and yet effective, as in the small-scale project described in the next section. But careful reflection on the inhuman conditions endured by so many in this time of great affluence can of course also lead to more explosive actions. Retrospective analysis of these explosions . . . often reveals them to be last-ditch efforts to escape untenable situations. That is, the explosions follow innumerable peaceful attempts to attenuate structural violence and the lies that help sustain it. The Zapatistas, who refer often to early death from treatable illnesses, explain it this way in an early communiqué:

> Some ask why we decided to begin now, if we were prepared before. The answer is that before this we tried other peaceful and legal roads to change, but without success. During these last ten years more than 150,000 of our indigenous brothers and sisters have died from curable diseases. The federal, state, and municipal governments' economic and social plans do not even consider any real solution to our problems, and consist of giving us handouts at election times. But these crumbs of charity solve our problems for no more than a moment, and then, death returns to our houses. That is why we think no, no more, enough of this dying useless deaths, it would be better to fight for change. If we die now, we will not die with shame, but with the dignity of our ancestors. Another 150,000 of us are ready to die if that is what is needed to waken our people from their deceit-induced stupor.[20]

Applying Principles of Liberation Theology to Medicine

To act as a physician in the service of poor or otherwise oppressed people is to prevent, whenever possible, the diseases that afflict them — but also to treat and, if possible, to cure. So where's the innovation in that? How would a health intervention inspired by liberation theology be different from one with more conventional underpinnings? Over the past two decades, Partners In Health has joined local community health activists to provide basic primary care and preventive services to poor communities in Mexico, Peru, the United States, and, especially, Haiti — offering what we have termed "pragmatic solidarity." Pragmatic solidarity is different from but nourished by solidarity per se, the desire to make common cause with those in need. Solidarity is a precious thing: people enduring great hardship often remark that they are grateful for the prayers and good wishes of fellow human beings. But when sentiment is accompanied by the goods and services that might diminish unjust hardship, surely it is enriched. To those in great need, solidarity without the pragmatic component can seem like so much abstract piety.

Lest all this talk of structural violence and explosive responses to it seem vague and far-removed from the everyday obligations of medicine, allow me to give examples from my own clinical experience. How does liberation theology inform medical practice in, say, rural Haiti? Take tuberculosis, along with HIV the leading infectious cause of preventable adult deaths in the world. How might one observe, judge, and act in pragmatic solidarity with those most likely to acquire tuberculosis or already suffering from it?

The "observation" part of the formula is key, for it involves careful review of a large body of literature that seeks to explain the distribution of the disease within populations, to explore its clinical characteristics, and to evaluate tuberculosis treatment regimens. This sort of review is standard in all responsible health planning, but liberation theology would push analysis in two directions: first, to seek the root causes of the problem; second, *to elicit the experiences and views of poor people* and to incorporate these views into all observations, judgments, and actions.

Ironically enough, some who understand, quite correctly, that the underlying causes of tuberculosis are poverty and social inequality make a terrible error by failing to honor the experience and views of the poor in designing strategies to respond to the disease. What happens if, after analysis reveals poverty as the root cause of tuberculosis, tuberculosis control strategies ignore the sick and focus solely on eradicating poverty? Elsewhere, I have called this the "Luddite trap," since this ostensibly progressive view would have us ignore both current distress and the tools of modern medicine that might relieve it, thereby committing a new and grave injustice.[21] The destitute sick ardently desire the eradication of poverty, but their tuberculosis can be readily cured by drugs such as isoniazid and rifampin. The prescription for poverty is not so clear.

18. Brown 1993, p. 45.

19. Sobrino 1988, p. 32.

20. "Communiqué from the CCRI-CG of the EZLN, January 6, 1994," in Marcos and the Zapatista Army of National Liberation 1995, p. 58.

21. See Farmer 1999b, chap. 1; and Farmer and Nardell 1998.

Careful review of the biomedical and epidemiological literature on tuberculosis does permit certain conclusions. One of the clearest is that the incidence of the disease is not at all random. Certainly, tuberculosis has claimed victims among the great (Frederic Chopin, Fyodor Dostoyevsky, George Orwell, Eleanor Roosevelt), but historically it is a disease that has ravaged the economically disadvantaged.[22] This is especially true in recent decades: with the development of effective therapy in the mid-twentieth century came high cure rates — over 95 percent — for those with access to the right drugs for the right amount of time. Thus tuberculosis *deaths* now — which each year number in the millions — occur almost exclusively among the poor, whether they reside in the inner cities of the United States or in the poor countries of the Southern hemisphere.[23]

The latest twists to the story — the resurgence of tuberculosis in the United States, the advent of HIV-related tuberculosis, and the development of strains of tuberculosis resistant to the first-line therapies developed in recent decades — serve to reinforce the thesis that *Mycobacterium tuberculosis,* the causative organism, makes its own preferential option for the poor.[24]

What "judgment" might be offered on these epidemiological and clinical facts? Many would find it scandalous that one of the world's leading causes of preventable adult deaths is a disease that, with the possible exception of emerging resistant strains, is more than 95 percent curable, with inexpensive therapies developed decades ago. Those inspired by liberation theology would certainly express distaste for a disease so partial to poor and debilitated hosts and would judge unacceptable the lack of therapy for those most likely to become ill with tuberculosis: poverty puts people at risk of tuberculosis and then bars them from access to effective treatment. An option-for-the-poor approach to tuberculosis would make the disease a top priority for research and development of new drugs and vaccines and at the same time would make programs to detect and cure all cases a global priority.

Contrast this reading to the received wisdom — and the current agenda — concerning tuberculosis. Authorities rarely blame the recrudescence of tuberculosis on the inequalities that structure our society. Instead, we hear mostly about biological factors (the advent of HIV, the mutations that lead to drug resistance) or about cultural and psychological barriers that result in "noncompliance." Through these two sets of explanatory mechanisms, one can expediently attribute high rates of treatment failure either to the organism or to uncooperative patients.

There are costs to seeing the problem in this way. If we see the resurgence or persistence of tuberculosis as an exclusively biological phenomenon, then we will shunt available resources to basic biological research, which, though needed, is not the primary solution, since almost all tuberculosis deaths result from lack of access to existing effective therapy. If we see the problem primarily as one of patient noncompliance, then we must necessarily ground our strategies in plans to change the patients rather than to change the weak tuberculosis control programs that fail to detect and cure the majority of cases. In either event, weak analysis produces the sort of dithering that characterizes current global tuberculosis policy, which must accept as its primary rebuke the shameful death toll that continues unabated.

How about the "act" part of the formula advocated by liberation theology? In a sense, it's simple: heal the sick. Prompt diagnosis and cure of tuberculosis are also the means to prevent new infections, so prevention and treatment are intimately linked. Most studies of tuberculosis in Haiti reveal that the vast majority of patients do not complete treatment — which explains why, until very recently, tuberculosis remained the leading cause of adult death in rural regions of Haiti. (It has now been surpassed by HIV.) But it does not need to be so. In the country's Central Plateau, Partners In Health worked with our sister organization, Zanmi Lasante, to devise a tuberculosis treatment effort that borrows a number of ideas — and also some passion — from liberation theology.

Although the Zanmi Lasante staff had, from the outset, identified and referred patients with pulmonary tuberculosis to its clinic, it gradually became clear that detection of new cases did not always lead to cure, even though all tuberculosis care, including medication, was free of charge. In December 1988, following the deaths from tuberculosis of three HIV-negative patients, all adults in their forties, the staff met to reconsider the care

22. Even at the dawn of the era of antibiotics, when streptomycin was already available, class divisions were sharp inside Europe's sanatoriums. George Orwell's journal entries from the year before his death of tuberculosis are telling:

> Curious effect, here in the sanatorium, on Easter Sunday, when the people in this (the most expensive) block of "chalets" mostly have visitors, of hearing large numbers of upper-class English voices. I have been almost out to the sound of them for two years, hearing them at most one or two at a time, my ears growing more & more used to working-class or lower-middle-class Scottish voices. In the hospital at Hairmyres, for instance, I literally never heard a "cultivated" accent except when I had a visitor. It is as though I were hearing these voices for the first time. And what voices! A sort of over-fedness, a fatuous self-confidence, a constant bah-bahing of laughter abt [*sic*] nothing, above all a sea of heaviness &c richness combined with a fundamental ill-will — people who, one instinctively feels, without even being able to see them, are the enemies of anything intelligent or beautiful. No wonder everyone hates us so (journal entry from April 17, 1949; Orwell 1968, p. 578).

For more on the history of tuberculosis in North America, see Georgina Feldberg's (1995) helpful review; see also the classic study by Dubos and Dubos (1952). Unfortunately, little has been written of the history of tuberculosis in the regions of the world where it has taken its greatest toll.

23. For an overview of the burden of disease and death caused by *M. tuberculosis,* see Farmer, Walton, and Becerra, 2000.

24. These "twists" are reviewed in Farmer 1999b, chap. 9.

these individuals had received. How had the staff failed to prevent these deaths? How could we better observe, judge, and act as a community making common cause with the destitute sick?

Initially, we responded to these questions in differing ways. In fact, the early discussions were heated, with a fairly sharp divide between community health workers, who shared the social conditions of the patients, and the doctors and nurses, who did not. Some community health workers believed that tuberculosis patients with poor outcomes were the most economically impoverished and thus the sickest; others hypothesized that patients lost interest in chemotherapy after ridding themselves of the symptoms that had caused them to seek medical advice. Feeling better, they returned as quickly as possible to the herculean task of providing for their families. Still others, including the physicians and nurses, attributed poor compliance to widespread beliefs that tuberculosis was a disorder inflicted through sorcery, beliefs that led patients to abandon biomedical therapy. A desire to focus blame on the patients' ignorance or misunderstanding was palpable, even though the physicians and nurses sought to cure the disease as ardently as anyone else involved in the program.

The caregivers' ideas about the causes of poor outcomes tended to coalesce in two directions: a *cognitivist-personalistic* pole that emphasized individual patient agency (curiously, "cultural" explanations fit best under this rubric, since beliefs about sorcery allegedly led patients to abandon therapy), and a *structural* pole that emphasized the patients' poverty. And this poverty, though generic to outsiders like the physicians from Port-au-Prince, had a vivid history to those from the region. Most of our tuberculosis patients were landless peasants living in the most dire poverty. They had lost their land a generation before when the Péligre dam, part of an internationally funded development project, flooded their fertile valley.[25]

More meetings followed. Over the next several months, we devised a plan to improve services to patients with tuberculosis — and to test these discrepant hypotheses. Briefly, the new program set goals of detecting cases, supplying adequate chemotherapy, and providing close follow-up. Although they also continued contact screening and vaccination for infants, the staff of Zanmi Lasante was then most concerned with caring for smear-positive and coughing patients — believed to be the most important source of community exposure. The new program was aggressive and community-based, relying heavily on community health workers for close follow-up. It also responded to patients' appeals for nutritional assistance. The patients argued, often with some vehemence and always with eloquence, that to give medicines without food was tantamount to *lave men, siye até* (washing one's hands and then wiping them dry in the dirt).

25. This story is told more fully in Farmer 1992, chap. 2, pp. 19-27.

Those diagnosed with tuberculosis who participated in the new treatment program were to receive daily visits from their village health worker during the first month following diagnosis. They would also receive financial aid of thirty dollars per month for the first three months; would be eligible for nutritional supplements; would receive regular reminders from their village health worker to attend the clinic; and would receive a five-dollar honorarium to defray "travel expenses" (for example, renting a donkey) for attending the clinic. If a patient did not attend, someone from the clinic — often a physician or an auxiliary nurse — would make a visit to the no-show's house. A series of forms, including a detailed initial interview schedule and home visit reports, regularized these arrangements and replaced the relatively limited forms used for other clinic patients.

Between February 1989 and September 1990, fifty patients were enrolled in the program. During the same period, the clinical staff diagnosed pulmonary tuberculosis in 213 patients from outside our catchment area. The first fifty of these patients to be diagnosed formed the comparison group that would be used to judge the efficacy of the new intervention. They were a "control group" only in the sense that they did not benefit from the community-based services and financial aid; all tuberculosis patients continued to receive free care.

The difference in the outcomes of the two groups was little short of startling. By June 1991, forty-six of the patients receiving the "enhanced package" were free of all symptoms, and none of those with symptoms met radiologic or clinical diagnostic criteria for persistent tuberculosis. Therefore, the medical staff concluded that none had active pulmonary tuberculosis, giving the participants a cure rate of 100 percent. We could not locate all fifty of the patients from outside the catchment area, but for the forty patients examined more than one year after diagnosis, the cure rate was barely half that of the first group, based on clinical, laboratory, and radiographic evaluation. It should be noted that this dismal cure rate was nonetheless higher than that reported in most studies of tuberculosis outcomes in Haiti.[26]

Could this striking difference in outcome be attributed to patients' ideas and beliefs about tuberculosis? Previous ethnographic research had revealed extremely complex and changing ways of understanding and speaking about tuberculosis among rural Haitians.[27] Because most physicians and nurses (and a few community health workers) had hypothesized that patients who "believed in sorcery" as a cause of tuberculosis would have higher rates of noncompliance with their medical regimens, we took some pains to address this issue with each patient. As the resident medical anthropologist, I conducted long — often very long — and open-ended interviews with all patients in both groups, trying to delineate

26. For a more detailed discussion of this study, see Farmer 1999, pp. 217-25.

27. Farmer 1990.

the dominant explanatory models that shaped their views of the disease. I learned that few from either group would deny the possibility of sorcery as an etiologic factor in their own illness, but I could discern no relationship between avowal of such beliefs and compliance with a biomedical regimen. That is, the outcomes were related to the quality of the program rather than the quality of the patients' ideas about the disease. Suffice it to say, this was not the outcome envisioned by many of my colleagues in anthropology.

Although anthropologists are expected to underline the importance of *culture* in determining the efficacy of efforts to combat disease, in Haiti we learned that many of the most important variables — initial exposure to infection, reactivation of quiescent tuberculosis, transmission to household members, access to diagnosis and therapy, length of convalescence, development of drug resistance, degree of lung destruction, and, most of all, mortality — are all strongly influenced by *economic* factors. We concluded that removing structural barriers to "compliance," when coupled with financial aid, dramatically improved outcomes in poor Haitians with tuberculosis. This conclusion proved that the community health workers, and not the doctors, had been correct.

This insight forever altered approaches to tuberculosis within our program. It cut straight to the heart of the compliance question. Certainly, patients may be noncompliant, but how relevant is the notion of compliance in rural Haiti? Doctors may instruct their patients to eat well. But the patients will "refuse" if they have no food. They may be told to sleep in an open room and away from others, and here again they will be "noncompliant" if they do not expand and remodel their miserable huts. They may be instructed to go to a hospital. But if hospital care must be paid for in cash, as is the case throughout Haiti, and the patients have no cash, they will be deemed "grossly negligent." In a study published in collaboration with the Zanmi Lasante team, we concluded that "the hoary truth that poverty and tuberculosis are greater than the sum of their parts is once again supported by data, this time coming from rural Haiti and reminding us that such deadly synergism, formerly linked chiefly to crowded cities, is in fact most closely associated with deep poverty."[28]

Similar scenarios could be offered for diseases ranging from typhoid to AIDS. In each case, poor people are at higher risk of contracting the disease and are also less likely to have access to care. And in each case, analysis of the problem can lead researchers to focus on the patients' shortcomings (for example, failure to drink pure water, failure to use condoms, ignorance about public health and hygiene) or, instead, to focus on the conditions that structure people's risk (for example, lack of access to potable water, lack of economic opportunities for women, unfair distribution of the world's resources). In many current discussions of these plagues of the poor, one can discern a cognitivist-personalistic pole and a structural pole. Although focus on the former is the current fashion, one of the chief benefits of the latter mode of analysis is that it encourages physicians (and others concerned to protect or promote health) to make common cause with people who are both poor and sick.

28. Farmer, Robin, Ramilus, et al. 1991, p. 260. For more on this project, see Farmer 1999b, chap. 8.

A Social Justice Approach to Addressing Disease and Suffering

Tuberculosis aside, what follows next from a perspective on medicine that is based in liberation theology? Does recourse to these ideas demand loyalty to any specific ideology? For me, applying an option for the poor has never implied advancing a particular strategy for a national economy. It does not imply preferring one form of development, or social system, over another — although some economic systems are patently more pathogenic than others and should be denounced as such by physicians. Recourse to the central ideas of liberation theology does not necessarily imply subscription to a specific body of religious beliefs; Partners In Health and its sister organizations in Haiti and Peru are completely ecumenical.[29] At the same time, the flabby moral relativism of our times would have us believe that we may now choose from a broad menu of approaches to delivering effective health care services to the poor. This is simply not true. Whether you are sitting in a clinic in rural Haiti, and thus a witness to stupid deaths from infection, or sitting in an emergency room in a U.S. city, and thus the provider of first resort for forty million uninsured, you must acknowledge that the commodification of medicine invariably punishes the vulnerable.

A truly committed quest for high-quality care for the destitute sick starts from the perspective that health is a

29. Indeed, one does not need to ascribe directly to the religious tenets of liberation theology in order to make a "preferential option for the poor." Pixley and Boff summarize the widespread starvation, malnutrition, and poverty that are a daily reality for millions (remarking that one does not need "socio-scientific instruments" to prove this) and conclude that "this state of affairs is *morally intolerable,* for those who do not believe in the God of the Bible as much as for those who do" (1989, pp. 238, 239). They note the simple facts of the situation and what our response — whether one imbued with faith, or one relying solely on reason — must logically be:

> The energy to find the solution can come only from the oppressed themselves. Wherever there is oppression, there will be struggles to win life-sustaining conditions — struggles between classes, between races, between nations, between sexes. This is simply an observable fact, not a moral imperative or a scientific conclusion. We can see the just struggles of the oppressed going on around us, and we cannot see any other way out of the vast problems that afflict humanity at the close of the twentieth century (p. 242).

For a more in-depth discussion of these matters, refer to the full argument made by Pixley and Boff (1989, pp. 237-43).

fundamental human right. In contrast, commodified medicine invariably begins with the notion that health is a desirable outcome to be attained through the purchase of the right goods and services. Socialized medicine in industrialized countries is no doubt a step up from a situation in which market forces determine who has access to care. But a perspective based in liberation theology highlights the fundamental weakness of this and other strategies of the affluent: if the governments of Scandinavian countries and that of France, for example, then spend a great deal of effort barring noncitizens from access to health care services, they will find few critics within their borders. (Indeed, the social democracies share a mania for border control.) But we will critique them, and bitterly, because access to the fruits of science and medicine should not be determined by passports, but rather by need. The "health care for all" movement in the United States will never be morally robust until it truly means "all."

Liberation theology's first lesson for medicine is similar to that usually confronting healers: There is something terribly wrong. Things are not the way they should be. But the problem, in this view, is with the world, even though it may be manifest in the patient. Truth — and liberation theology, in contrast to much postmodern attitudinizing, believes in historical accuracy — is to be found in the perspective of those who suffer unjust privation.[30] Cornel West argues that "the condition of truth is to allow the suffering to speak. It doesn't mean that those who suffer have a monopoly on truth, but it means that the condition of truth to emerge must be in tune with those who are undergoing social misery — socially induced forms of suffering."[31]

The second lesson is that medicine has much to learn by reflecting on the lives and struggles of poor or otherwise oppressed people. How is suffering, including that caused by sickness, best explained? How is it to be addressed? These questions are, of course, as old as humankind. We've had millennia in which to address — societally, in an organized fashion — the suffering that surrounds us. In looking at approaches to such problems, one can easily discern three main trends: *charity, development,* and *social justice.*

Each of these might have much to recommend it, but it is my belief that the first two approaches are deeply flawed. Those who believe that charity is the answer to the world's problems often have a tendency — sometimes striking, sometimes subtle, and surely lurking in all of us — to regard those needing charity as intrinsically inferior. This is different from regarding the poor as powerless or impoverished because of historical processes and events (slavery, say, or unjust economic policies propped up by powerful parties). There is an enormous difference between seeing people as the victims of innate shortcomings and seeing them as the victims of structural violence. Indeed, it is likely that the struggle for rights is undermined whenever the history of unequal chances, and of oppression, is erased or distorted.

The approach of charity further presupposes that there will always be those who have and those who have not. This may or may not be true, but, again, there are costs to viewing the problem in this light. In *Pedagogy of the Oppressed,* Paulo Freire writes: "In order to have the continued opportunity to express their 'generosity,' the oppressors must perpetuate injustice as well. An unjust social order is the permanent fount of this 'generosity,' which is nourished by death, despair, and poverty." Freire's conclusion follows naturally enough: "True generosity consists precisely in fighting to destroy the causes which nourish false charity."[32] Given the twentieth century's marked tendency toward increasing economic inequity in the face of economic growth, the future holds plenty of false charity. All the recent chatter about "personal responsibility" from "compassionate conservatives" erases history in a manner embarrassingly expedient for themselves. In a study of food aid in the United States, Janet Poppendieck links a rise in "kindness" to a decline in justice:

> The resurgence of charity is at once a *symptom* and a *cause* of our society's failure to face up to and deal with the erosion of equality. It is a symptom in that it stems, in part at least, from an abandonment of our hopes for the elimination of poverty; it signifies a retreat from the goals as well as the means that characterized the Great Society. It is symptomatic of a pervasive despair about actually solving problems that has turned us toward ways of managing them: damage control, rather than prevention. More significantly, and more controversially, the proliferation of charity *contributes* to our society's failure to grapple in meaningful ways with poverty.[33]

30. Perhaps it goes without saying that no physician who bases his or her practice on clinical trials can in good faith buy into the postmodern argument that all claims to truth are merely "competing discourses." But, as Christopher Norris writes, in both the social sciences and the humanities, the conviction that we ought to find out what really happened is proof

> that we hadn't caught up with the "postmodern" rules of the game, the fact that nowadays things have moved on to the point where there is no last ground of appeal to those old, self-deluding "enlightenment" values that once possessed authority (or the semblance thereof), at least in some quarters. Anyone who continues to invoke such standards is plainly in the grip of a nostalgic desire for some ultimate truth-telling discourse — whether Platonist, Kantian, Marxist or whatever — that would offer a delusory refuge from the knowledge that we are nowadays utterly without resources in the matter of distinguishing truth from falsehood (1992, p. 13).

Norris's devastating account of intellectuals and the Gulf War (1992) is one of the best critiques of the postmodern foolishness that has gained quite a foothold in universities on both sides of the Atlantic. See also Norris 1990.

31. West 1993, p. 4.

32. Freire 1986, p. 29.

33. Poppendieck 1998, p. 5.

It is possible, however, to overstate the case against charity — it is, after all, one of the four cardinal virtues, in many traditions. Sometimes holier-than-thou progressives dismiss charity when it is precisely the virtue demanded. In medicine, charity underpins the often laudable goal of addressing the needs of "underserved populations." To the extent that medicine responds to, rather than creates, underserved populations, charity will always have its place in medicine.

Unfortunately, a preferential option for the poor is all too often absent from charity medicine. First, charity medicine should avoid, at all costs, the temptation to ignore or hide the causes of excess suffering among the poor. Meredeth Turshen gives a jarring example from apartheid South Africa:

> South African paediatricians may have developed an expertise in the understanding and treatment of malnutrition and its complications, but medical expertise does not change the system that gives rise to malnutrition nor the environment to which treated children return, an environment in which half of the children die before their fifth birthday. Malnutrition, in this context, is a direct result of the government's policies, which perpetuate the apartheid system and promote the poor health conditions and human rights violations.[34]

Second, charity medicine too frequently consists of second-hand, castoff services — leftover medicine — doled out in piecemeal fashion. How can we tell the difference between the proper place of charity in medicine and the doling out of leftovers? Many of us have been involved in these sorts of good works and have often heard a motto such as this: "the homeless poor are every bit as deserving of good medical care as the rest of us." The notion of a preferential option for the poor challenges us by reframing the motto: the homeless poor are *more* deserving of good medical care than the rest of us.[35] Whenever medicine seeks to reserve its finest services for the destitute sick, you can be sure that it is option-for-the-poor medicine.

What about development approaches?[36] Often, this perspective seems to regard progress and development as almost natural processes. The technocrats who design development projects — including a certain Péligre dam, which three decades ago displaced the population we seek to serve in central Haiti — plead for patience. In due time, the technocrats tell the poor, if they speak to them at all, you too will share our standard of living. (After a generation, the reassurance may be changed to "if not you, your children.") And certainly, looking around us, we see everywhere the tangible benefits of scientific development. So who but a Luddite would object to development as touted by the technocrats?

According to liberation theology, progress for the poor is not likely to ensue from development approaches, which are based on a "liberal" view of poverty. Liberal views place the problem with the poor themselves: these people are backward and reject the technological fruits of modernity. With assistance from others, they too will, after a while, reach a higher level of development. Thus does the victim-blaming noted in the earlier discussion of tuberculosis recur in discussions of underdevelopment.

For many liberation theologians, developmentalism or reformism cannot be rehabilitated. George Pixley and Clodovis Boff use these terms to describe what they consider an "erroneous" view of poverty, in contrast to the "dialectical" explanation, in which the growth of poverty is dependent on the growth of wealth. Poverty today, they note, "is mainly the result of a contradictory development, in which the rich become steadily richer, and the poor become steadily poorer." Such a poverty is "internal to the system and a natural product of it."[37] Developmentalism not only erases the historical creation of poverty but also implies that development is necessarily a linear process: progress will inevitably occur if the right steps are followed. Yet any critical assessment of the impact of such approaches must acknowledge their failure to help the poor, as Leonardo and Clodovis Boff argue:

> "Reformism" seeks to improve the situation of the poor, but always within existing social relationships and the basic structuring of society, which rules out greater participation by all and diminution in the privileges enjoyed by the ruling classes. Reformism can lead to great feats of development in the poorer nations, but this development is nearly always at the expense of the oppressed poor and very rarely in their favor. For example, in 1964 the Brazilian economy ranked 46th in the world; in 1984 it ranked 8th. The last twenty years have seen undeniable technological and industrial progress, but at the same time there has been a considerable worsening of social conditions for the poor, with exploitation, destitution, and hunger on a scale previously unknown in Brazilian history. This has been the price paid by the poor for this type of elitist, exploitative, and exclusivist development.[38]

In his introduction to *A Theology of Liberation*, Gustavo Gutiérrez concurs: we assert our humanity, he argues, in "the struggle to construct a just and fraternal

34. Turshen 1986, p. 891.

35. Samuel Johnson once observed that "a decent provision for the poor is the true test of civilization." Surely this is true, and it serves as an indictment of affluent society. But liberation theology delivers an even more damning indictment, since its proponents argue that we should reserve our highest standards for the poor.

36. My critique of development is by no means original; it draws heavily on a very large literature reaching back almost thirty years. From André Gunder Frank to Immanuel Wallerstein, the more refined versions of dependency theory cannot be lightly dismissed. For more recent reviews of the limitations of development approaches to health care, see Meredeth Turshen's wonderful book *Privatizing Health Services in Africa* (1999).

37. Pixley and Boff 1989, pp. 6-7.

38. Boff and Boff 1987, p. 5.

society, where persons can live with dignity and be the agents of their own destiny. It is my opinion that the term *development* does not well express these profound aspirations."[39] Gutiérrez continues by noting that the term "liberation" expresses the hopes of the poor much more succinctly. Philip Berryman puts it even more sharply: "'Liberation' entails a break with the present order in which Latin American countries could establish sufficient autonomy to reshape their economies to serve the needs of that poor majority. The term 'liberation' is understood in contradistinction to 'development.'"[40]

In examining medicine, one sees the impact of "developmental" thinking not only in the planned obsolescence of medical technology, essential to the process of commodification, but also in influential analytic constructs such as the "health transition model."[41] In this view, societies as they develop are making their way toward that great transition, when deaths will no longer be caused by infections such as tuberculosis but will occur much later and be caused by heart disease and cancer. But this model masks interclass differences *within* a particular country. For the poor, wherever they live, there is, often enough, no health transition. In other words, wealthy citizens of "underdeveloped" nations (those countries that have not yet experienced their health transition) do not die young from infectious diseases; they die later and from the same diseases that claim similar populations in wealthy countries. In parts of Harlem, in contrast, death rates in certain age groups are as high as those in Bangladesh; in both places, the leading causes of death in young adults are infections and violence.[42]

The powerful, including heads of state and influential policymakers, are of course impatient with such observations and respond, if they deign to respond, with sharp reminders that the overall trends are the results that count. But if we focus exclusively on aggregate data, why not declare public health in Latin America a resounding success? After all, life expectancies have climbed; infant and maternal mortality have dropped. But if you work in the service of the poor, what's happening to that particular class, whether in Harlem or in Haiti, always counts a great deal. In fact, it counts most. And from this vantage point — the one demanded by liberation theology — neither medicine nor development looks nearly so successful. In fact, the outcome gap between rich and poor has continued to grow.

In summary, then, the charity and development models, though perhaps useful at times, are found wanting in rigorous and soul-searching examination. That leaves the social justice model. In my experience, people who work for social justice, regardless of their own station in life, tend to see the world as deeply flawed. They see the conditions of the poor not only as unacceptable but as the result of structural violence that is human-made. As Robert McAfee Brown, paraphrasing the Uruguayan Jesuit Juan Segundo, observes, "unless we agree that the world should not be the way it is . . . there is no point of contact, because the world that is satisfying to us is the same world that is utterly devastating to them."[43] Often, if these individuals are privileged people like me, they understand that they have been implicated, whether directly or indirectly, in the creation or maintenance of this structural violence. They then feel indignation, but also humility and penitence. Where I work, this is easy: I see the Péligre dam almost every week.

This posture — of penitence and indignation — is critical to effective social justice work. Alas, it is all too often absent or, worse, transformed from posture into posturing. And unless the posture is linked to much more pragmatic interventions, it usually fizzles out.

Fortunately, embracing these concepts and this posture do have very concrete implications. Making an option for the poor inevitably implies working for social justice, working with poor people as they struggle to change their situations. In a world riven by inequity, medicine could be viewed as social justice work. In fact, doctors are far more fortunate than most modern professionals: we still have a sliver of hope for meaningful, dignified service to the oppressed. Few other disciplines can make this claim with any honesty. We have a lot to offer right now. In Haiti and Peru and Chiapas, we have found that it is often less a question of "development" and more one of redistribution of goods and services, of simply sharing the fruits of science and technology. The majority of our efforts in the transfer of technology — medications, laboratory supplies, computers, and training — are conceived in just this way. They end up being innovative for other reasons: it is almost unheard of to insist that the destitute sick receive high-quality care as a right.

Treating poor Peruvians who suffer from multidrug-resistant tuberculosis according to the highest standard of care, rather than according to whatever happens to be deemed "cost-effective," is not only social justice work but also, ironically enough, innovative. Introducing antiretroviral medications, and the health systems necessary to use them wisely, to AIDS-afflicted rural Haiti is, again, viewed as pie-in-the-sky by international health specialists but as only fitting by liberation theology. For example, operating rooms (and cesarean sections) must be part of any "minimum package" of health services wherever the majority of maternal deaths are caused by cephalopelvic disproportion. This is obvious from the perspective of social justice but controversial in international health circles. And the list goes on.

A preferential option for the poor also implies a mode

39. Gutiérrez 1973, p. xiv.

40. Berryman 1987, p. 91.

41. For an introduction to the notion of health transition, see Caldwell, Findley, Caldwell, et al. 1990; Gutiérrez, Zielinski, and Kendall (2000) have more recently qualified this concept by placing it in broader social context. See also the discussion by Mosley, Bobadilla, and Jamison (1993) on the implications of this model for developing countries.

42. McCord and Freeman 1990.

43. Brown 1993, p. 44.

of analyzing health systems. In examining tuberculosis in Haiti, for example, our analysis must be *historically deep* — not merely deep enough to recall an event such as that which deprived most of my patients of their land, but deep enough to remember that modern-day Haitians are the descendants of a people enslaved in order to provide our ancestors with cheap sugar, coffee, and cotton.

Our analysis must be *geographically broad*. In this increasingly interconnected world ("the world that is satisfying to us is the same world that is utterly devastating to them"), we must understand that what happens to poor people is never divorced from the actions of the powerful. Certainly, people who define themselves as poor may control their own destinies to some extent. But control of lives is related to control of land, systems of production, and the formal political and legal structures in which lives are enmeshed. With time, both wealth and control have become increasingly concentrated in the hands of a few. The opposite trend is desired by those working for social justice.

For those who work in Latin America, the role of the United States looms large. Father James Guadalupe Carney, a Jesuit priest, put his life on the line in order to serve the poor of Honduras. As far as we can tell, he was killed by U.S.-trained Honduran security forces in 1983.[44] In an introduction to his posthumously published autobiography, his sister and brother-in-law asked starkly: "Do we North Americans eat well because the poor in the third world do not eat at all? Are we North Americans powerful, because we help keep the poor in the third world weak? Are we North Americans free, because we help keep the poor in the third world oppressed?"[45]

Granted, it is difficult enough to "think globally and act locally." But perhaps what we are really called to do, in efforts to make common cause with the poor, is to think locally *and* globally and to act in response to both levels of analysis. If we fail in this task, we may never be able to contend with the structures that create and maintain poverty, structures that make people sick. Although physicians and nurses, even those who serve the poor, have not followed liberation theology, its insights have never been more relevant to our vocation. As international health experts come under the sway of the bankers and their curiously bounded utilitarianism, we can expect more and more of our services to be declared "cost-ineffective" and more of our patients to be erased. In declaring health and health care to be a human right, we join forces with those who have long labored to protect the rights and dignity of the poor.

44. Carney is said to have been killed after being captured when he participated in an ill-fated guerrilla incursion from Nicaragua into Olancho Province, Honduras.

45. Carney 1987, p. xi. Carney goes on to criticize the United States directly, citing the U.S.-backed 1973 military coup d'état in Chile, in which tens of thousands were killed, as his own moment of realization about the extent of the often brutal U.S. involvement in the political and economic affairs of the region:

> After the bloody military coup of 1973 in Chile, *it was obvious that the United States would never allow a country that is economically dependent on it to make a revolution by means of elections* — through the democratic process directed by the majority — at least as long as the country has an army that obeys the capitalist bourgeoisie of the country (p. 311).

For an examination of U.S. policy toward progressive movements in Guatemala, El Salvador, and Haiti in a similar light, see Farmer 1994.

Works Cited

Anders, G. 1996. *Health Against Wealth: HMOs and the Breakdown of Medical Trust.* Boston: Houghton Mifflin.

Andrulis, D. P., and B. Carrier. 1999. *Managed Care in the Inner City: The Uncertain Promise for Providers, Plans, and Communities.* San Francisco: Jossey-Bass.

Armada, F., C. Monomer, and V. Navarro. 2001. "Health and Social Security Reforms in Latin America: The Convergence of the World Health Organization, the World Bank, and Transnational Corporations." *International Journal of Health Services* 31 (4): 729-68.

Barraza-Lloréns, M., S. Bertozzi, E. González-Pier, et al. 2002. "Addressing Inequality in Health and Health Care in Mexico." *Health Affairs* 21 (3): 47-56.

Barreiro, A. 1982. *Basic Ecclesial Communities: The Evangelization of the Poor.* Maryknoll, N.Y.: Orbis Books.

Bartley, M., D. Blane, and G. D. Smith. 1998. "Introduction: Beyond the Black Report." *Sociology of Health and Illness* 20 (5): 563-77.

Berryman, P. 1987. *Liberation Theology: Essential Facts about the Revolutionary Movement in Latin America and Beyond.* New York: Pantheon Books.

Boff, L. 1989. *Faith on the Edge: Religion and Marginalized Existence.* 1st ed. San Francisco: Harper and Row.

Boff, L., and C. Boff. 1987. *Introducing Liberation Theology.* Maryknoll, N.Y.: Orbis Books.

Brown, R. M. 1993. *Liberation Theology: An Introductory Guide.* Louisville: Westminster/John Knox Press.

Burdick, J. 1993. *Looking for God in Brazil: The Progressive Catholic Church in Urban Brazil's Religious Arena.* Berkeley: University of California Press.

Caldwell, J. C., S. Findley, P. Caldwell, et al. 1990. *What We Know about Health Transition: The Cultural, Social, and Behavioural Determinants of Health. The Proceedings of an International Workshop, Canberra, May 1989.* Canberra: Health Transition Centre, Australian National University.

Carney, J. G. 1987. *To Be a Revolutionary.* San Francisco: Harper and Row.

Coburn, D. 2000. "Income Inequality, Social Cohesion, and the Health Status of Populations: The Role of Neo-Liberalism." *Social Science and Medicine* 51 (1): 135-46.

Dubos, R., and J. Dubos. 1952. *The White Plague: Tuberculosis, Man, and Society.* Boston: Little, Brown.

Eagleson, J., and P. Sharper. 1979. *Puebla and Beyond: Documentation and Commentary.* Maryknoll, N.Y.: Orbis Books.

Farmer, P. E. 1990. "Sending Sickness: Sorcery, Politics, and Changing Concepts of AIDS in Rural Haiti." *Medical Anthropology Quarterly* 4 (1): 6-27.

———. 1992. *AIDS and Accusation: Haiti and the Geography of Blame.* Berkeley: University of California Press.

———. 1994. *The Uses of Haiti.* Monroe, Maine: Common Courage Press.

———. 1999. *Infections and Inequalities: The Modern Plagues.* Berkeley: University of California Press.

Farmer, P. E., and E. Nardell. 1998. "Nihilism and Pragmatism in Tuberculosis Control." *American Journal of Public Health* 88 (7): 4-5.

Farmer, P. E., S. Robin, S. L. Ramilus, et al. 1991. "Tuberculosis, Poverty, and 'Compliance': Lessons from Rural Haiti." *Seminars in Respiratory Infection* 6 (4): 254-60.

Farmer, P. E., and B. Rylko-Bauer. 2001. "L''exceptionnel' système de santé américain: Critique d'une médecine à vocation commerciale" (The "exceptional" American health care system: Critique of the for-profit approach). *Actes de la Recherche en Sciences Sociales* 139: 13-30.

Farmer, P. E., D. A. Walton, and M. C. Becerra. 2000. "International Tuberculosis Control in the 21st Century." In *Tuberculosis: Current Concepts and Treatment,* 2d ed., edited by L. N. Friedman, pp. 475-96. Boca Raton: CRC Press.

Feldberg, G. 1995. *Disease and Class: Tuberculosis and the Shaping of Modern North American Society.* New Brunswick, N.J.: Rutgers University Press.

Fiscella, K., P. Franks, M. R. Gold, et al. 2000. "Inequality in Quality: Addressing Socioeconomic, Racial, and Ethnic Disparities in Health Care." *Journal of the American Medical Association* 283 (19): 2579-84.

Freire, P. 1986. *Pedagogy of the Oppressed.* New York: Continuum.

Ginzberg, E. 1999. "The Uncertain Future of Managed Care." *New England Journal of Medicine* 340 (2): 144-46.

Gutiérrez, E. D., C. Zielinski, and C. Kendall. 2000. "The Globalization of Health and Disease: The Health Transition and Global Change." In *The Handbook of Social Studies in Health and Medicine,* edited by G. Albrecht, R. Fitzpatrick, and S. Scrimshaw, pp. 84-99. London: Sage.

Gutiérrez, G. 1973. *A Theology of Liberation: History, Politics, and Salvation.* Maryknoll, N.Y.: Orbis Books.

———. 1983. *The Power of the Poor in History.* Maryknoll, N.Y.: Orbis Books.

Himmelstem, D., S. Woolhandler, and I. Hellander. 2001. *Bleeding the Patient: The Consequences of Corporate Health Care.* Monroe, Maine: Common Courage Press.

Iriart, C., E. E. Merhy, and H. Waitzkin. 2001. "Managed Care in Latin America: The New Common Sense in Health Policy Reform." *Social Science and Medicine* 52 (8): 1243-53.

Kim, J. Y., J. V. Millen, A. Irwin, and J. Gershman, eds. 2000. *Dying for Growth: Global Inequality and the Health of the Poor.* Monroe, Maine: Common Courage Press.

Laurell, A. C. 2001. "Health Reform in Mexico: The Promotion of Inequality." *International Journal of Health Services* 31 (2): 291-321.

Leclerc, A., D. Fassin, H. Grandjean, et al. 2000. *Les inégalités sociales de santé.* Paris: Éditions la Découverte et Syros.

Lewin, M. E., and S. Altman, eds. 2000. *America's Health Care Safety Net: Intact but Endangered.* Washington, D.C.: National Academy Press.

Marcos, S., and the Zapatista Army of National Liberation. 1995. *Shadows of Tender Fury: The Letters and Communiqués of Subcomandante Marcos and the Zapatista Army of National Liberation.* New York: Monthly Review Press.

Maskovsky, J. 2000. "'Managing' the Poor: Neoliberalism, Medicaid HMOs, and the Triumph of Consumerism Among the Poor." *Medical Anthropology* 19: 121-46.

McCord, C., and H. Freeman. 1990. "Excess Mortality in Harlem." *New England Journal of Medicine* 322 (3): 173-77.

Mosley, W. H., J. L. Bobadilla, and D. T. Jamison. 1993. "The Health Transition: Implications for Health Policy in Developing Countries." In *Disease Control Priorities in Developing Countries,* edited by D. T. Jamison, W. H. Mosley, A. R. Measham, and J. L. Bobadilla, pp. 673-99. New York: Oxford Medical Publications.

Neill, K. G. 2001. "Dancing with the Devil: Health, Human Rights, and the Export of U.S. Models of Managed Care to Developing Countries." *Cultural Survival Quarterly* 24 (4): 61-63.

Norris, C. 1990. *What's Wrong with Postmodernism: Critical Theory and the Ends of Philosophy.* Baltimore: Johns Hopkins University Press.

———. 1992. *Uncritical Theory: Postmodernism, Intellectuals, and the Gulf War.* Amherst: University of Massachusetts Press.

Orwell, G. 1968. *The Collected Essays, Journalism, and Letters of George Orwell.* Vol. 4, *In Front of Your Nose, 1945-1950.* New York: Penguin Books.

Pellegrino, E. 1999. "The Commodification of Medical and Health Care: The Moral Consequences of a Paradigm Shift from a Professional to a Market Ethic." *Journal of Medicine and Philosophy* 24 (3): 243-66.

Pérez-Stable, E. J. 1999. "Managed Care Arrives in Latin America."*New England Journal of Medicine* 340 (14): 1110-12.

Peterson, M. A., ed. 1999. "Managed Care Backlash." *Journal of Health Politics, Policy, and Law* 24 (5): 873-1218 (theme issue).

Pixley, G. V., and C. Boff. 1989. *The Bible, the Church, and the Poor.* Maryknoll, N.Y.: Orbis Books.

Poppendieck, J. 1998. *Sweet Charity? Emergency Food and the End of Entitlement.* New York: Viking Press.

Rathore, S. S., A. K. Berger, K. P. Weinfurt, et al. 2000. "Race, Sex, Poverty, and the Medical Treatment of Acute Myocardial Infarction in the Elderly." *Circulation: Journal of the American Heart Association* 102 (6): 642-48.

Schneider, E. C., A. M. Zaslavsky, and A. M. Epstein. 2002. "Racial Disparities in the Quality of Care for Enrollees in Medicare Managed Care." *Journal of the American Medical Association* 287 (10): 1288-94.

Segundo, J. L. 1980. *Our Idea of God.* Dublin: Gill and Macmillan.

Sen, A. 1998. "Mortality as an Indicator of Economic Success and Failure." (Text of the Innocenti Lecture of UNICEF, delivered in Florence, March 1995.) *Economic Journal* 108 (446): 1-25.

Sobrino, J. 1988. *Spirituality of Liberation: Toward Political Holiness.* Maryknoll, N.Y.: Orbis Books.

Stocker, K., H. Waitzkin, and C. Iriart. 1999. "The Exportation of Managed Care to Latin America." *New England Journal of Medicine* 340 (14): 1131-36.

Turshen, M. 1986. "Health and Human Rights in a South African Bantustan." *Social Science and Medicine* 22 (9): 887-92.

———. 1999. *Privatizing Health Services in Africa.* New Brunswick, N.J.: Rutgers University Press.

Waitzkin, H., and C. Iriart. 2001. "How the United States Exports Managed Care to Developing Countries." *International Journal of Health Services* 31 (3): 495-505.

West, C. 1993. *Prophetic Thought in Postmodern Times.* Monroe, Maine: Common Courage Press.

Wilkinson, R. G. 1996. *Unhealthy Societies: The Afflictions of Inequality.* London: Routledge.

World Bank. 2000. *The Burden of Disease among the Global Poor: Current Situation, Future Trends, and Implications for Strategy.* Washington, D.C.: World Bank.

World Health Organization. 1999. *World Health Report 1999 — Making a Difference.* Geneva: World Health Organization.

World Health Organization. 2000. *World Health Report 2000. Health Systems: Improving Performance.* Geneva: World Health Organization.

20 A Body without Borders

Joel Shuman and Brian Volck

In a culture bedazzled by electronic entertainment, "good old stories, plainly told" get little hearing. Jesus told plain stories in his lifetime, some of which the evangelists found important enough to record.[1] But Jesus was no stand-up comic headlining nightly shows with two performances on Saturday.[2] He told stories to instruct, and for a first-century Palestinian audience as stuck in their ways as we are in ours, he told them both to intrigue and discomfort. Unfortunately, like the theatergoer who complained Shakespeare was only a patchwork of clichés, Christians have heard Jesus's stories too often truly to listen. Through overuse, Jesus's stories have lost much of their power to disturb and convict.

Consider the familiar tale that Jesus, in good rabbinical tradition, tells in the middle of an edgy debate over the essence and fulfillment of the law (Luke 10:25-37). A man lies half dead at the side of the road.[3] A priest happens by but quickly crosses to the other side of the road and heads on. We have no window into his head — Jesus is more interested in the social than the psychological — though we can infer that the priest is connected to the cultic life of the temple. Touching a body which may be Gentile, dead, or both, would render this honored man defiled under the law.

A Levite, a student of the law, passes along as well and, perhaps for similar reasons, does the same. A third traveler — a Samaritan — sees the injured man and provides medical assistance, takes him to shelter on his own beast, and pays for the injured man's care. Anyone who knows how to tell a joke knows the "rule of threes": three situations, three tries, three people, with the punch line held out until the end. For his first hearers, Jesus pushes this joke to the border of poor taste, and our pious modern

1. Matthew says, "Indeed . . . (Jesus) . . . said nothing to them without a parable" (Matt. 13:34).

2. Jesus was an observant Jew. Except for healing the sick, Saturday was his day off. (See Matt. 12:9-13.)

3. Since he's half dead, there's still a story to be told. If he were completely dead, there would be nothing left to do but "look through his pockets for loose change," as Miracle Max in *The Princess Bride* advises. Completely dead bodies figure prominently in mystery stories. As we will soon see, this too is a mystery story, but of a different sort, offering more possibility of redemption than the typical detective tale.

habit of calling it "the Good Samaritan" ruins the punch line.[4] Samaritans were despised by first-century Palestinian Jews as enemies, outside the law and alien to God's people, but this Samaritan goes beyond what might be expected even for a friend. Jesus's verbal sparring partner, a lawyer who came to test Jesus and justify himself (vv. 25-29), can't even bring himself to say the word *Samaritan* when prompted. To his first hearers, a "Good Samaritan" was an oxymoron, which of course was Jesus's point: the God of Israel is Lord of all creation, Samaria included, and the demands of the Torah are universal. That a Samaritan can observe the law better than those who constantly study it reinforces the universal validity of the law — the love of neighbor (Lev. 19:18) in particular — while extending its obligations past boundaries Jesus's hearers thought uncrossable.

Luke's Gospel is also full of stories *about* Jesus, often taking the following form: a person is separated from the life of the community by some socially defined mark: foreignness, gender, disease, or sinful activity.[5] Jesus encounters this person, frequently touching him or her or permitting himself to be touched, and welcomes him or her back into full relationship. The marginalized and excluded are, through an embodied encounter, reunited with the people of God. These reclamation stories are far more social than individual and generally occur in one of two settings: healings and meals.[6] Both serve the life and health of the community, addressing physical needs and spiritual distress in the same embodied action. We know no better summation of reclaiming of the body than this sequence of aphorisms by Wendell Berry:

> The grace that is the health of creatures can only be held in common. In healing the scattered members come together. In health the flesh is graced, the holy enters the world.[7]

These gospel themes should prod us into greater discernment, finding the body — both gift and gathering — in unexpected places, especially among the marginalized, those cut off from the whole. This requires recognizing the bodily needs of the marginalized: healing, of course, but also the physical and spiritual nourishment shared in community. In traditional Mediterranean cultures, meals were about much more than just food. They were also social markers, declaring openly with whom one associated, and with whom one did not. In his First Letter to the Corinthians, which we examined in chapter 3, Paul makes explicit the intimate connection between meals, the gathered body, and bodily health: "For any one who eats and drinks without discerning the body eats and drinks judgment upon himself. That is why many of you are weak and ill, and some have died" (I Cor. 11:29-30). As Luke Timothy Johnson explains, Christians of the New Testament and succeeding generations understood the eucharistic meal as dining together in the presence of Christ and sharing in the power of the risen Lord.[8] Jesus's invitation to the table always includes a demand for painful and complete transformation, but his invitation is nonetheless radically inclusive.[9] If we share in the power of that risen Lord, how can we not wish to properly discern the body and reach out to those separated from us by social barriers?

Rival Visions

What keeps us from seeing and touching our own world's "lepers," the marginalized whom our economy and culture prefer to keep invisible, flailing about among the tombs? One obstacle, curiously enough, is the power of medicine, which, echoing the thrust of Western liberal

4. Once again, our complacent piety emasculates Jesus's stories, shielding the modern hearer from the bitter tasks of conversion by rendering divine demand impotent. Jesus's parables are masterpieces of edgy social commentary, and in that sense at least, Jesus can be understood as the Lenny Bruce of first-century Palestine. That Jesus's social criticism arises from the heart of Torah places him in the perilous tradition of the prophets, whom Abraham Joshua Heschel calls "the most disturbing people who ever lived" (Abraham Joshua Heschel, *The Prophets: An Introduction,* vol. 1 [New York: Harper and Row, 1962], ix).

5. We realize Luke's Gospel is the reigning favorite among socially conscious exegetes, though it was not ever thus. John Howard Yoder's masterpiece, *The Politics of Jesus* (Grand Rapids: Eerdmans, 1972), provides a close reading of Luke precisely because the dominant reading of Luke in the 1950s and 1960s saw Luke's editorial purpose as "apologetic," reassuring his reader that Christians were not a threat to the empire (2nd ed., 53). Since our purpose in this chapter is to prophetically widen the body's vision beyond borders, Luke is a logical fit. Were we to emphasize the perilous tasks of discipleship or the authority of Christ and his church, we may well have turned to Mark or Matthew, respectively.

6. Space limitations preclude a thorough survey here. Exemplary healings can be found in Luke 5:12-24, 7:1-10, 7:11-16, 8:26-39, 9:37-43, and 17:11-19. Note the absence of distinction between healings and the exorcisms in Luke 4:40-41, 6:18, 8:26-39, and 9:37-43; Luke builds no Cartesian wall between body, mind, and spirit. Meal stories in Luke include 6:27-32, 7:36-50, 14:1-24, 19:1-10, 22:14-23, 24:13-35, and 24:36-53. The other synoptic Gospels include parallel themes. Charles Amjad-Ali observes that healing miracles in Mark bring the marginalized back into full political, economic, social, and religious participation within the community. See Charles Amjad-Ali, *Passion for Change: Reflections on the Healing Miracles in Saint Mark* (Rawalpindi: Christian Study Centre, 1989). Meals and healings are signs of the eschatological "kingdom of heaven" in Matthew, as in Matthew 22:1-14 and 12:22-28. Special thanks to Father Greg Schaffer for helping us set Lukan accounts in broader synoptic context.

7. Wendell Berry, "Healing," in *What Are People For?* (New York: North Point Press, 1990), 9.

8. See his chapter, "Meals Are Where the Magic Is," in Luke Timothy Johnson, *Religious Experience in Earliest Christianity* (Minneapolis: Fortress Press, 1998).

9. As Matthew's Gospel tells it, the kingdom's banquet extends an invitation to many. Sadly, few respond, and even among these few, at least one is turned out for not changing into a wedding garment. As we once heard J. Glenn Murray, S.J., say, "Jesus was promiscuous about whom he ate with, but he invited tax collectors, prostitutes, and sinners to the table precisely so they would not leave as tax collectors, prostitutes, and sinners."

political and economic thought, speaks an almost uninterrupted language of individualism. To be sure, there are university departments of social medicine and entire schools of public health, but these are hardly central to the medical-industrial complex in North America, even though much of what we consider the "blessings of modern medicine" — significantly decreased infectious disease mortality, longer lives, etc. — come more directly from public health efforts (clean water, improved sanitation and nutrition, and immunizations, among others) than from technologically enhanced individual care. Nonetheless, the "developed nations," the United States in particular, show increasing disregard for the health of populations as opposed to individual selves.[10]

In medical ethics, there is a flourishing strain of utilitarian thought, with its maxim concerning "the greatest good for the greatest number," though that "number" is understood as a summation of individual selves, particularly those with the resources necessary for "agency," that is, the power to make choices. Arguments are typically framed, often under the cloak of "cost-effectiveness," to value some people (able-bodied "contributors to society") over others (the severely impaired).[11] Within the "deontological" strain of medical ethics (i.e., the study of moral obligations or rules), the two most commonly used principles are beneficence (doing or at least intending good) and autonomy.[12] Doctors are supposed to direct their efforts toward a patient's "good" — a conspicuously vague term — while the patient exercises her autonomy largely by choosing among various options in a process called "informed consent." Through such mysteries and rituals, we — or at least the fortunate — are left to pursue our individual lives in freedom.[13]

Thus, when most of us hear the phrase "medical ethics," we think of difficult *individual* cases, often at life's margins: the terminal cancer patient, sick both from her tumor and chemotherapy, asking her physician to help her die; the pregnant woman pondering late-term abortion versus fetal surgery for her deformed child; or the dizzying technological manipulations aimed at the human zygote. Those who have worked in so-called developing countries or the inner-city slums and rural backwaters of the United States know these issues rarely arise there. Such highly individualized questions are almost exclusively the concern of the well-off, since ethical dilemmas at life's margins usually involve uncommon material and financial resources. An enormous chasm gapes between the topics explored in most medical ethics curricula and the realities and health and disease endured by most of the world's population. Physician Paul Farmer notes:

> Conventional medical ethics, mired as they are in the "quandary ethics of the individual," do not often speak to these issues, because the bulk of their attention is focused on individual cases where massive resources are invested in delivering services unlikely to ever benefit most patients.[14]

Consider only a few of the immensities about which "quandary ethics of the individual" has nothing to say. We noted in the previous chapter that 10 million children die globally each year, mostly from preventable or easily treatable causes no longer considered problems in the "developed world."[15] In 2004, there were 3.1 million AIDS deaths, half a million of which were children.[16] The vast majority of these deaths were once again in "developing countries," since in the "developed world" Highly Active Antiretroviral Therapy (HAART) turns HIV from a death sentence into a manageable, if life-threatening, chronic disease. Nor are health disparities limited to "developing nations." In 1990, mortality rates for persons between the ages of five and sixty-five years were higher in Harlem than in Bangladesh, one of the poorest countries in the world.[17] In 2003, 15.6 percent of the United States population — 45 million people! — had no health insurance coverage, making even the most basic medical

10. See Laurie Garrett, *Betrayal of Trust: The Collapse of Global Public Health* (New York: Hyperion, 2001), and Paul Farmer, *Infections and Inequalities: The Modern Plagues* (Berkeley: University of California Press, 2001).

11. As in the estimated "cost to society" for raising a child with Down syndrome we mentioned in the previous chapter [of *Reclaiming the Body*].

12. We readily acknowledge that contemporary medical ethics is far more complicated than this brief taxonomy suggests. One happy arrival on the scene is so-called intrinsic ethics, owing much to the work of Alasdair MacIntyre. As we read the literature, though, highly individualistic accounts of utilitarianism and deontology dominate the field, with the ghosts of John Stuart Mill and Immanuel Kant still haunting the machine of medical ethics.

13. Having been on both the giving and receiving end of the highly ritualized legal transaction of informed consent, we find the claims made about the process largely illusory. One of us once heard a seasoned clinician warn, "if you're not a little frightened about what you can persuade a patient or her representative to do, you're not very observant." Real consent is a much longer, far more complicated relational process than a rehearsal of "risks and benefits" followed by a signature at the bottom of a printed form — rather like marriage, actually! Graduate medical education rarely acknowledges this. The bare ritual is followed by the respective parties, leaving "each in the cell of himself . . . almost convinced of his freedom" (from "In Memory of W. B. Yeats," W. H. Auden, *Collected Poems* [New York: Random House, 1976], 197).

14. Paul Farmer, *Pathologies of Power, Health, Human Rights, and the New War on the Poor* (Berkeley: University of California Press, 2003), 21. Farmer and Nicole Gastineau Campos provide a sustained, withering critique of medical ethics' neglect of the world's poor in "Rethinking Medical Ethics: A View from Below," *Developing World Bioethics* 4, no. 1 (2004): 17-41.

15. Black, Morris, and Bryce, "Where and Why," *Lancet* 361 (2003): 2226-34.

16. *AIDS Epidemic Annual Report 2004,* U.N. Programme on HIV/AIDS, www.unaids.org/wad2004/report.html.

17. Colin McCord and Harold P. Freeman, "Excess Mortality in Harlem," *New England Journal of Medicine* 322 (1990): 173-77. Similar statistics for infant or neonatal mortality should be viewed with caution. Very different approaches to premature infants in the United States and in "developing countries" skew the numbers significantly.

services financially burdensome.[18] Most considerations of the health effects of such disparities treat them as social or political problems in search of "cost-effective" solutions, entering the territory of modern medicine only through the neglected hinterlands of public health. As to any moral obligations of the medical-industrial complex to rectify these inequities, standard medical ethics is largely silent.[19]

The Christian understanding of the body should — though often fails to — shatter this silence. For starters, every body on the planet is a gift. Peter tells Cornelius and his household, "Truly I perceive that God shows no partiality" (Acts 10:34). Christians worldwide eat at the same table, are served by the same Lord, and live as neighbor to non-Christians, whom we are called to love as self. As with the Samaritan in Luke's Gospel, faithfulness leaves no choice but to reach across boundaries of human design. Discerning the body Christ gathers, while recalling how Jesus explicitly identifies with "the least of these" (Matt. 25:40), makes denying our responsibility to the world's poor a rejection of Christ himself. Certainly Christians have cultivated such denial over the centuries, often blaming God for the misfortunes of others and engineering calamities in God's name, but to pin the suffering of millions of God's children on "God's will" — rather than on human deafness to God's call — makes God a capricious sadist.

Compared to the quandary structure of standard medical ethics — the beneficent or maleficent aims of medical technology brought against the individual patient's sacred autonomy — Christian "body ethics" is vastly more complicated. For the Christian, all things are seen first in the light of God, the maker of all gifts. Furthermore, the patient cannot be understood as an isolated individual, but as a person within a larger whole, defined by family, friendships, and various interpenetrating communities.[20] "Health" is similarly redefined within such communities to include far more than pharmaceutical needs: food — remember the social importance of meals in Luke's Gospel — as well as water, housing, jobs, and a reasonable amount of safety. Understood in this way, no medical interaction concerns a single autonomous patient, nor does it place moral obligations only on medical personnel. An entire web of relationships must be considered and constantly reevaluated.

What might standard medical ethics say about the health inequities we mentioned above, if they were to speak of them at all? Using the bourgeois liberal categories of contemporary ethical thought, that which can't be reduced to the private world of contractual interaction or voluntary association typically falls to the nation-state and its governmental apparatus. Alternatively, one might employ alternate bureaucracies, such as the International Red Cross and the World Health Organization. Such nongovernmental organizations (NGOs) — a category name that makes explicit the normative place of nation-state governments in the secular world — often act more effectively than states, though they sometimes are less publicly accountable. Unfortunately, such NGOs grow into bureaucratic mirror images of the governments they are supposed to be so unlike. Thus, the chasms separating the health care of rich and poor are turned over to bureaucratically administered policies and programs, acting as much or more in their own interests than in the interests of those they claim to serve. By adopting the state model, medicine also adopts the logic of envy, rivalry, and competition characterizing the state when the tactics of co-option fail and those of coercion become "necessary." Not only did "progressive medical science," allied with the state, forcibly sterilize over 60,000 in the United States and purposely export eugenicist theory and practice to the rest of the world — including pre-Nazi Germany[21] — it also conducted the Tuskegee Syphilis Study, following but not treating syphilis-infected African American males in Alabama from 1932 to 1972, even though effective treatment for syphilis became available in 1947.[22] While various governmental entities have apologized for such mistakes, similarly troubling research continues in resource-poor, often disease-rich countries, invariably among the people least able to say no.[23]

18. Carmen DeNavas-Walt, Bernadette Proctor, and Robert J. Mills, *Income, Poverty, and Health Insurance Coverage in the United States: 2003* (Washington, DC: U.S. Government Printing Office, 2004), 14.

19. Though not entirely so. Márcio Fabri dos Anjos, who tellingly writes from the perspective of liberation theology (of which we will say more in our discussion of Paul Farmer), asks, "To what level of quality can medical ethics aspire, if it ignores callous discrimination in medical practice against large populations of innocent poor? . . . How effective can such theories be in addressing the critical issues of medical and clinical ethics if they are unable to contribute to the closing of the gap of socio-medical disparity?" (Márcio Fabri dos Anjos, "Medical Ethics in the Developing World: A Liberation Theology Perspective," *Journal of Medicine and Philosophy* 21 [1996]: 629-37).

20. See Wendell Berry's short story "Fidelity" in *Fidelity: Five Stories* (New York: Pantheon, 1992) and his less mordant, downright funny "Watch with Me," in *Watch with Me and Six Other Stories of the Yet-Remembered Ptolemy Proudfoot and His Wife, Miss Minnie, Née Quinch* (New York: Pantheon, 1994).

21. See again Edwin Black, *War against the Weak* (New York: Four Walls Eight Windows, 2003).

22. See Susan M. Reverby, ed., *Tuskegees Truths: Rethinking the Tuskegee Syphilis Study* (Chapel Hill: University of North Carolina Press, 2000), and Allan M. Brandt, *No Magic Bullet: A Social History of Venereal Disease in the United States since 1886* (New York: Oxford University Press, 1987).

23. See Thomas C. Quinn, Maria J. Wawer, Nelson Sewankambo, et al., "Viral Load and Heterosexual Transmission of Human Immunodeficiency Virus Type 1," *New England Journal of Medicine* 342 (2000): 921-29, a study that identified and observed couples in Uganda in which only one partner was HIV-positive, in an effort to see which factors contributed to heterosexual transmission of the virus. Marcia Angell's editorial in the same issue noted, with dismay, "it is important to be clear about what this study meant for the participants. It meant that for up to 30 months, several hundred people with HIV infection were observed but not

In emulating the state, medicine further adopts the utilitarian, zero-sum calculus of scarcity that decides some people are worth saving while others are too costly to bother about, and there is little comfort in the knowledge that such exclusionary decisions are now being made individually — at least in "developed" countries. What little we seem to have learned from American and Nazi eugenics amounts to this: quality control of human "stock" ought to rest in the hands of the individual consumer, not in the bureaucratic state. Marketing itself as a supplier of technological options, medicine claims the messianic role of savior, softening the harsher edges of the state in a false promised land of individual choice, never mentioning the extent to which individual choice has been formed by available options and prevailing fashions.

Bridging the divides of care between rich and poor will surely require the power that is the nation-state as much as the power that is medicine, but Christians must not be content with merely voting persons or parties with the best policy into power. Our responsibility to the body can never be delegated. We are personally and corporately responsible to the marginalized, and the shape of that obligation is embodied in the life of Jesus: we are required to reach out to the marginalized and reincorporate them into the community, the body that Christ gathers.

Solidarity with the Poor

What shape might medicine take if lived according to gospel demands? To begin with, such medical practice would look odd enough to annoy medicine's entrenched Pharisees. One group doing precisely this is Partners in Health (PIH), led by its cofounder Paul Farmer, the physician whose observations on "quandary ethics" we noted above. Farmer is best known to the general public as the subject of Tracy Kidder's compelling biographical study, *Mountains beyond Mountains.*[24] Dr. Paul Farmer, internist, infectious disease specialist, and professor of medicine and medical anthropology at Harvard Medical School, spends the majority of each year living and working in Cange, Haiti, located in the heartbreakingly poor central plateau region of the poorest country in the western hemisphere. In a world of health disparities, Haiti is an extreme:

> Haiti has the highest infant and maternal mortality, the worst malnutrition and the worst AIDS situation in the Americas. The general mortality rate . . . (is) also the highest in the Americas. A quarter of children suffer from chronic malnutrition, 3 to 6 percent from acute malnutrition. . . . Acute respiratory infections and diarrhea cause half of the deaths in children under five years of age. There are complications in a quarter of deliveries. . . . 40% of the population has no real access to basic health care, 76% of deliveries are made by non-qualified personnel, and only half the children are vaccinated.[25]

In such an unpromising place, Farmer's organization, Zanmi Lasante (Haitian Creole for "Partners in Health"), has built a general hospital with ambulatory and women's clinics, a tuberculosis treatment center, a school, and a kitchen serving 2,000 meals a day, all in the immediate vicinity of an Anglican church. While the clinics and hospital charge nominal fees, no one is refused service for inability to pay, which means many patients receive much-needed care for free. What makes Zanmi Lasante work, however, is less the incredible drive of Paul Farmer than the solidarity and community ownership embodied in its many activities and institutions. Money, medicines, and supplies come from donors in the United States and elsewhere, but it is the people of Cange who make them count. As just one example, locally trained community health workers carry out regular home visits to the many tuberculosis and HIV patients, identifying along the way those who need food, transportation, housing, or access to clean water. The health shared in common here transcends individual therapeutic intervention: there is as much meal as medicine at Zanmi Lasante.

The results are clear: mother-child transmission of HIV has been reduced to 4 percent, significantly lower than the current U.S. rate. More than 700 area patients receive HAART, the antiretroviral drug regimens most HIV patients in the United States now receive but that is largely unavailable in impoverished Haiti. Infant mortality and malnutrition have been drastically, reduced. Tuberculosis is treated in systematic, communally based fashion at a fraction of U.S. costs, with no TB deaths in the Cange region since 1988.

Farmer and his colleagues work in other impoverished areas of the world, taking on similarly "impossible" projects. One of Farmer's early supporters was Father Jack Roussin, pastor at St. Mary of the Angels in an impoverished neighborhood of Boston. After Father Jack succumbed to multidrug-resistant tuberculosis (MDR-TB), contracted during his work in the slums of Lima, Peru, Farmer and fellow PIH-er Dr. Jim Yong Kim demonstrated to the World Health Organization that WHO's deliberate neglect of MDR-TB was based on faulty assumptions and false economies. Using expen-

treated" ("Investigators' Responsibilities for Human Subjects in Developing Countries," *NEJM* 342 [2000]: 967-69). See also a troubling chapter in contraceptive research in Ana Regina Comes Dos Reis, "Norplant in Brazil: Implantation Strategy in the Guise of Scientific Research," *Issues in Reproductive and Genetic Engineering: Journal of International Feminist Analysis* 3 (1990): 111-18.

24. While we shall soon see how explicitly Farmer grounds his work in theological language and convictions, we owe a great debt to M. Therese Lysaught for providing a larger theo-political framework in which to understand those convictions. Lysaught's unpublished lectures delivered at the Church and Culture Conference at Valley Covenant Church, Eugene, Oregon, in 2004, entitled "Anointing the Sick: A Christian Politics of Medicine," are particularly helpful in this regard.

25. Paul Farmer, "Political Violence and Public Health in Haiti," *New England Journal of Medicine* 350, no. 15 (2004): 1483-86.

sive "second-line" medications — those typically reserved for patients in wealthier "developed" countries and used only when first choices fail — in a carefully monitored approach, Farmer and Kim were able to achieve an astounding 85 percent cure rate among people most TB experts had written off as "beyond hope." WHO has since changed its MDR-TB guidelines to incorporate this newer approach and — for those focused on the bottom line — reduced treatment costs by 90 percent in five years.[26]

What we find so interesting about Farmer is that this baptized Roman Catholic who never considered the religion of his birth very compelling, lacked suitable language to describe his vision for health care until, following the assassination of Salvadoran Archbishop Oscar Romero, he discovered liberation theology. Through his reading and growing familiarity with the struggles of the poor, he increasingly made common cause with impoverished Haitians as well as the nuns and "church ladies" who championed their cause. Kidder describes Farmer's process:

> He was already attracted to liberation theology. "A powerful rebuke to the hiding away of poverty," he called it. "A rebuke that transcends scholarly analysis." In Haiti, the essence of the doctrine came alive for him. Almost all the peasants he was meeting shared a belief that seemed like a distillation of liberation theology: "Everybody else hates us," they'd tell him, "but God loves the poor more. And our cause is just." . . . (Farmer) felt drawn back to his Catholicism now, not by his own belief but in sympathy with theirs, as an act of what he'd call "solidarity."[27]

It would be easy to construe Farmer's work as that of a secular physician-anthropologist who merely exploits "church connections" or employs religious language to do "mercenary work" for his causes. On the contrary, Farmer uses explicitly theological language to describe the reality he sees, opposing that vision to the one embraced by the powerful, who, if they responded to the poor at all, did so with cast-off materials and substandard "cost-effective" therapies:

> The fact that any sort of religious faith was so disdained at Harvard and so important to the poor — not just in Haiti but elsewhere, too — made me even more convinced that faith must be something good. . . . I know it sounds shallow, the opiate thing, needing to believe, palliating pain, but it didn't feel shallow. It was more profound than other sentiments I'd known, and I was taken with the idea that in an ostensibly godless world that worshipped money and power and, more seductively, a sense of personal efficacy and advancement, like at Duke and Harvard, there was still a place to look for God, and that was in the suffering of the poor.[28]

26. Kidder, *Mountains beyond Mountains,* 241-60.
27. Ibid., 78.
28. Ibid., 85.

Farmer, who speaks French, Haitian Creole, and Spanish, is also multilingual when it comes to social thought. He seems comfortable using the language of liberation theology or that of human rights, depending on his audience.[29] Even so, in his book *Pathologies of Power: Health, Human Rights, and the New War on the Poor,* he characterizes his descriptive narratives as "bearing witness," and he begins his more theoretical second half with chapters entitled "Health, Healing, and Social Justice: Insights from Liberation Theology" and "Listening for Prophetic Voices: A Critique of Market-Based Medicine."

The unofficial but incessantly used motto of Partners in Health is "O for the P," "Option for the Poor," a phrase brought into the theological lexicon at the 1979 Latin American Bishops conference in Puebla, Mexico, after much social, biblical, and ecclesial reflection.[30] Partners in Health claims this option not because the poor are better or more loved by God, but rather because the powers preferentially serve the powerful, rendering the poor and powerless invisible. The poor are where we find Christ (per Matthew 25), who demands far more than donations from our cash surplus or obsolete equipment and cast-off medicines sent abroad to salve guilty consciences. As Farmer puts it:

> Many of us . . . have heard a motto such as . . . : "the homeless poor are every bit as deserving of good medical care as the rest of us." The notion of a preferential option of the poor challenges us by reframing the motto: the homeless poor are *more* deserving of good medical care than the rest of us. Whenever medicine seeks to reserve its finest services for the destitute sick, you can be sure that it is option-for-the-poor medicine.[31]

Farmer directly takes on the alliance of medicine and state by reminding the reader how much medical "scarcity" is an invention of the nation-state. Global health resources are in fact not scarce at all, but inequitably distributed with national borders often acting as barriers to access. In *Pathologies of Power,* Farmer makes explicit the connection between the structural violence that the pow-

29. Rights talk and God talk aren't mutually exclusive, but they are, in Wittgensteinian terms, very different language games.

30. The history of this phrase is briefly recounted by one of its leading proponents, Gustavo Gutiérrez, in an interview in Daniel Hartnett, "Remembering the Poor: An Interview with Gustavo Gutiérrez," *America,* Feb. 3, 2003, available online at: www.americamagazine.org/gettext.cfm?articleTypeID=1&textID=2755&IssueID=420.

31. Farmer, *Pathologies of Power,* 155. While we retain a healthy skepticism toward governmental solutions in health matters, we acknowledge the remnants of goodness within the powers and seek to further that goodness without becoming enthralled. Consider how the debate over universal health care might play out in the United States (which, except for South Africa, is the only "developed" nation that does not guarantee some level of health care to its citizens) if Farmer's vision were more common. Rather than complaining about long waits for certain procedures (as in Canada), we might rather focus on finally making such procedures available to the millions of Americans now denied them.

ers encourage us to accept as necessary and the immensity of human suffering across the globe. The zero-sum logic of scarcity leads to highly predictable patterns of violence, deprivation, and illness. In contrast, Farmer calls his readers to engage in "pragmatic solidarity," reaching beyond borders to recognize a larger community to which we are responsible.

Getting Out of the Way

Partners in Health, while using Christian language and theory, is nonetheless not a Christian organization. What it does provide Christians, however, is a model for healing outside the powers that rule the world. Those seeking a more ecclesial approach might consider the remarkable history of the San Lucas Toliman Mission along the shore of Lake Atitlan in Guatemala.

For forty years, the people of San Lucas Toliman, with the assistance of Father Greg Schaffer and the support of the Diocese of New Ulm, Minnesota, have answered the needs of many by simply being the church. When most Americans hear the word *mission,* the image conjured is of well-intentioned white Middle-Americans invading the jungle to convert naked heathens. Having been schooled by his Guatemalan colleagues, Father Schaffer describes this proselytizing model as "the struggle to fill the tent," contrasting that with evangelism, which he understands as "bringing what the Creator wants to God's creation."[32] "What we've learned to do," he admits, "is give the people a chance and then get out of the way."[33] After forty years in one place, "getting out of the way" clearly means something other than offering a handout and walking away. Perhaps it is better understood as being present without hindering. If anything, it serves as a reminder to all involved that each person is a channel of grace, serving the others as called upon, but never unnecessarily encumbering the other with an ego-driven need to be "helpful."

Since 1964, "La Parroquia" in San Lucas Toliman has moved from distributing relief aid in the form of food to building a communal farm to cultivating beehives, growing and selling "fairly traded" coffee, securing farmland for families, and engaging in reforestation and conservation projects.[34] Health care was first provided in a small room in the parish office, while the new two-story clinic provides modern inpatient and outpatient care, including pediatric, adult, obstetric, and eye and dental clinics, as well as a nutrition center, emergency room, and operating room. Primary and secondary schools have been built and staffed, land has been more equitably distributed, and houses and farms have been constructed with access to reliable drinking water. Every step in this process has come about because of the expressed needs of the people, with the church acting both as catalyst and the embodiment of the people. Perhaps most amazing is that all these things were accomplished despite a thirty-six-year civil war, which, while sparing San Lucas Toliman from the most horrific atrocities, nonetheless did not leave it untouched.[35]

Like Partners in Health, the San Lucas Toliman Mission cannot survive without patrons from the "developed nations," busy people who have many worthy causes from which to choose. Father Greg is in Guatemala because his religious superior asked him to go, but as he now admits, the Christian understanding of the body of Christ emphasizes that we have no actual choice with whom we associate. Rather like family, we are all brothers and sisters, dependent upon the same God. What his work teaches him, he says, is the prophets' continual reminder to the people of Israel: we are all abjectly dependent upon God, and this primary relationship to God defines our relation to everyone else. When we lose sight of this, we stray from the kingdom of God.

Father Greg shared with us the story of Celestino, a once witty and jesting neighbor in San Lucas Toliman who grew discouraged with his overbearing employer, his poor housing, and the many things he could not afford for his family.[36] In medical terms, Celestino looked clinically depressed. When Father Greg asked why he looked so downtrodden, Celestino replied: "(I) found out something today, Padre. I am an animal." Whatever had made

32. From remarks made at an International Health Medical Education Consortium Conference, La Antigua, Guatemala, February 2004. In the larger context of the health of the body, we hear echoes of Wendell Berry here: "To be creative is only to have health: to keep oneself fully alive in the Creation, to keep the Creation fully alive in oneself, to see the Creation anew, to welcome one's part in it anew. . . . The most creative works are all strategies for this health" (Wendell Berry, "Healing," in *What Are People For?* 9).

33. Dr. Greg Schaffer, from a personal telephone conversation with one of the authors.

34. Much of this information comes from Encarnacion Ajcot's delightful *Maltiox Tat: A History of Father Gregory Schaffer and the San Lucas Toliman Mission,* privately published and available through the Diocese of New Ulm, Minnesota.

35. The sad and disturbing history of United States involvement in the coup that precipitated the civil war can be found in Stephen Schlesinger and Stephen Kinzer's *Bitter Fruit: The Story of the American Coup in Guatemala,* expanded ed. (Cambridge, MA: Harvard University Press, 1999), and Nicholas Cullather's *Secret History: The CIA's Classified Account of Its Operations in Guatemala, 1952-1954* (Stanford, CA: Stanford University Press, 1999). Daniel Wilkinson explores the unspeakable violence of the ensuing war in his *Silence on the Mountain: Stories of Terror, Betrayal, and Forgetting in Guatemala* (Boston: Houghton Mifflin, 2002). In the 1950s, the Roman Catholic hierarchy in Guatemala supported the U.S. forces. By the 1990s, that — and quite a few other things — had completely changed. In April 1998, seventy-five-year-old auxiliary bishop Juan Jose Gerardi Conedera released the 1,440-page church report on the war, "Guatemala: Nunca Mas" (Never Again). It estimated that, of the 200,000 casualties in the civil war, more than 80 percent had been killed or "disappeared" by the U.S.-supported (and often U.S.-trained) Guatemalan military. Two days after the report reached the public, Bishop Gerardi was murdered in his garage, beaten to death with a concrete block used to crush his skull.

36. Related to us by personal communication from Father Greg Schaffer.

him so resilient through years of bitter poverty was at last buckling under the weight of the powers. Soon after, at a meeting of potential parish catechists, Father Greg asked who could help turn out hand-sawn lumber for the local building projects. To Father Greg's surprise, Celestino tentatively raised his hand, saying, "Don't know if I can, Padre, but I sure will try." Celestino sought out an old craftsman who knew how to use the seven-foot pit saw, with which he soon grew skilled enough to begin training others. About the same time, he and his wife learned how to read and write through evening classes offered at the mission. Their oldest daughter was one of the first Maya-Cakchiquel girls to attend the church-sponsored school, which she later returned to as an auxiliary teacher to encourage other girls in their education. One of her brothers is also a teacher, and another went on to study medicine and now serves his people as a physician. A sister helps with the fair-trade coffee program.

Celestino helped friends and neighbors build houses before finally building one for his family — one he could at last be proud of. He also received three acres from the parish "Land for the Landless" program, from which he feeds his family and raises a small crop of coffee. Now he jokingly shows how much better his hand-sawn boards are than the milled lumber available elsewhere. In relating Celestino's story, Father Greg concludes: "A proud man, and rightly so! He had his chance, made the most of it, and we just had to get out of his way!"

This is no standard American rags-to-riches story, an individual rising above circumstances to achieve material success. Celestino's story is communal — growing out of the people's shared needs — in this case, not only lumber for building, but land to farm, schools to attend, and work to be proud of. And it started because someone (in this case, Father Greg, but it could have been anyone) saw, wondered, and asked what was wrong.[37] Celestino's material and spiritual poverty ceased to be invisible, and he was reclaimed by the community. As in Luke, there is no bright line between physical disease, material want, and spiritual distress: all must be addressed within community for any true healing to occur.

Not everyone can devote a lifetime's work to the people of Haiti or Guatemala, but every year, hundreds work short-term in these and similar endeavors, while thousands offer monetary and material support. Christians never satisfy their obligation to the body merely by writing checks, but recognizing the shared body across national borders may at least begin here.

Not Just for Saints

Not everyone can travel to developing countries. Not everyone is Mother Teresa. Many well-intentioned Christians write off such service as "saintly," by which we mean, "for other people who don't have to live in the real world." But the honor Christians have shown the saints becomes theologically incoherent if they are placed in a superhuman category. The saints are honored because, through each of them, God reveals yet another way to share the life of Christ. Through them, we get a glimpse of what God can do through our own lives if we only open ourselves to God's power. By putting saints "over there," we effortlessly escape their disturbing demand upon the way we live. Dorothy Day, no pushover herself, shot down claims that she was a living saint by insisting, "I don't want to be dismissed so easily."

The chasms in medical care we tacitly encourage through our excessive concern with the individual and his or her sacred autonomy are easily found within the borders of a country such as the United States. What makes matters worse, the invisible proximity of the indigent to the exorbitantly wealthy, as is the case in most American cities, is only exacerbated by media portrayals of what constitutes "normal": large vehicles, jewelry, the leisure time necessary to engage in self-help regimens. David Hilfiker, a family physician who left rural Minnesota to work in inner-city Washington, D.C., observes that poverty can be cruelly internalized in such circumstances.[38] Among many of the "dirt poor" here and abroad, simply lifting the yoke of economic and political oppression is sufficient — do that, and the poor will do well. For others, even the tools for sustenance have been lost, and creative economic and educational assistance is necessary. For a third group, however, even the hope of escape from poverty has been lost — they no longer believe things can be any different.[39] Drugs, alcohol, abusive relationships, and indiscriminate violence only cement this despair. Simply "getting out of the way" no longer works when people are possessed by something very much like demons.

In the capital city of the United States, Hilfiker practiced something very different from the medicine that generally worked well in Minnesota. In D.C., Hilfiker was practicing a new specialty: "poverty medicine," in which "the 'strictly medical' is not the most crucial factor in most healing."[40] By his own admission, Hilfiker's prac-

37. "What is wrong with you?" is, of course, the question Parzival, the Grail Knight, finally asks the wounded King Anfortas, but only after long suffering following his (much regretted) missed opportunity. That hospitality and compassion lie at the heart of this medieval epic speaks volumes about the poverty of virtue in the tales we tell today. The adventurous might well seek out Chretien de Troyes's *Perceval,* or Wolfram von Eschenbach's *Parzival,* though shorter attention spans will be rewarded by reading Katherine Paterson's delightful retelling, *Parzival: The Quest of the Grail Knight* (New York: Lodestar Books, 1998).

38. Hilfiker's Minnesota experiences and his decision to move to Washington are documented in his book *Healing the Wounds: A Physician Looks at His Work* (New York: Pantheon, 1985). Two of the chapters originally appeared in the *New England Journal of Medicine.*

39. David Hilfiker, "The New American Hopelessness: A Kingdom Response," in *Upholding the Vision: Serving the Poor in Training and Beyond,* 2nd ed., David Caes, ed. (Philadelphia: Christian Community Health Fellowship, 1996).

40. David Hilfiker, *Not All of Us Are Saints: A Doctor's Journey with the Poor* (New York: Ballantine, 1994), 11 (hereafter *NAUAS*).

tice and writing are less about medicine than they are about race, culture, and "medical helplessness before drugs lodged . . . deeply in our society" (*NAUAS,* 13). They are less about

> bold prescriptions for political or societal change than about what it's like to find oneself suddenly enmeshed in the crumbling relationship between government and the poor. It's about the grim consequences of two decades of governmental withdrawal and the deliberate underfunding of social agencies, about the helplessness of helpers running into closed doors and cul-de-sacs of social policy. It is about the wholesale abandonment of the poor. (*NAUAS,* 13)[41]

But, like Paul Farmer and the missionaries of San Lucas Toliman, Hilfiker sees the violence done to the poor in theological terms:

> If one dismisses spiritual (or even explicitly religious) motivation for medical work with the inner-city poor — in Washington, at least — there's not much left to talk about in the 1990s except the leaching of all care from the ever-growing worlds of poverty and homelessness. . . . Often all that was left were church groups and other parareligious organizations trying against overwhelming odds to address even the barest, most basic needs of the poor. . . . The "liberal" inclination to see in economic and political oppression the causes of poverty must not blind us to the fact that an unjust society produces a kind of brokenness that cannot always be addressed by removing the injustice. (*NAUAS,* 21-22)

What Hilfiker, strengthened by his church community, finds himself called to do is live with the poor to whom he provides medical care, in their own neighborhood, in a residence just above the inpatient facilities for "Christ House." He reclaims the poor into community less by healing wounds than by being present, by entering, in the limited ways available to him, into the community of the poor. Hilfiker may not be as accomplished a writer as Paul Farmer's biographer, but his story is compelling nonetheless, in part because of his unsettling honesty: Hilfiker picks apart the bourgeois defenses most of us employ whenever responsibility to the poor is mentioned. He unflinchingly examines the divides of race, class, and life experience that inevitably distance him from those he serves. He devotes as much attention to his failures as to his successes:

> Perhaps the deepest pain involved in living among the poor is the juxtaposition of my own limitations and woundedness with theirs. . . . The demands of justice, at least in this city, are endless. And it is precisely in trying to respond in some small way that I find my own damaged heart, my own limits. (*NAUAS,* 168)

But the limits he embraces in practicing "poverty medicine" are not only personal. The power of medicine imposes many of its own: urban hospitals creaking under the weight of patients unable to pay a fraction of what their care actually costs, a system of medical education that uses the urban poor for training purposes, and doctors who applaud Hilfiker's work even as they question his decision to "waste your professional education" on something better suited for "a social worker or nurse practitioner" (213). We are all broken people working under the influence of the powers. Only by God's grace and strengthened by the community into which we are gathered can any of us hope to persevere.

Practices of Presence

Hilfiker ultimately left Christ House to establish a similar residential facility for HIV-infected patients. What remains unchanged in his new setting is the uncomfortable bodily closeness to the poor, the direct encounter resisting the power of medicine to dissolve the poor into abstraction — a patient who goes home (if he has a home) to a place most of us, in more comfortable surroundings, choose not to think about. Others, both in and outside the medical professions, are called to be present in their own way. If we can't move to the inner city and practice "poverty medicine," we can be present through other practices of hospitality: soup kitchens, food banks, housing assistance, drug treatment programs, and halfway houses. We can also witness, as Christians, to secular powers, encouraging them to consider the needs of the poor to be at least as important as the needs of the fortunate.

Within the systems of medical education, a greater awareness of the needs of the poor is essential. Christian Community Health Fellowship encourages such awareness and calls students, nurses, therapists, and physicians to pay attention.[42] Many sustained endeavors, such as Crossroad Health Center, located in one of the most poverty-stricken neighborhoods of Cincinnati, have been inspired by the work of John Perkins. Perkins's reflections on his work with impoverished and oppressed communities stresses the responsibility for Christians to relocate, reconcile, and redistribute: living and working among the people we serve, loving God and neighbor properly, and putting our lives, education, and talent in the service of the community. The goal is, with God's

41. Any critique of medical care for the poor in the United States must take this abandonment into account. Anyone who has worked within the bureaucracies meant to serve the poor knows how quickly the best of hearts grow heavy with cynicism arising when, despite one's best effort, things do not change. The people working within such systems are, for the most part, truly compassionate and willing to sacrifice something of their own material comfort for the good of others. As a people, though, the United States has permitted the poor to be abandoned. We trust God will judge us accordingly.

42. See David Caes, ed., *Caring for the Least of These: Serving Christ among the Poor* (Scottdale, PA: Herald Press, 1992), and David Caes, ed., *Upholding the Vision: Serving the Poor in Training and Beyond,* 2nd ed. (Philadelphia: CCHF, 1996).

grace, to address the universal needs so often unmet in poor and oppressed communities: the need to belong, the need to be significant and important, and the need for a reasonable amount of security.[43]

The goal for Christians is not a world where everyone can afford cosmetic surgery or use medical technology in purely individual terms, but rather a community where our webs of connection are recognized and nurtured in faithfulness to God. Such communities require bodily presence, not "telescopic philanthropy" or acts of drive-by charity. Bodily presence opens mind and spirit to the senses, enabling us to truly see the poor, hear the suffering, touch the sick — and for them to see, hear, and touch us. What Paul Farmer, Father Greg, David Hilfiker, and countless others have undergone is no less than a conversion, guided by the very people the powers encourage us not to see, hear, or touch. By being present to the poor, we learn how to inhabit our own bodies, recognizing ourselves in places we did not expect, across borders we once imagined uncrossable.

43. See John Perkins's *Restoring At-Risk Communities: Doing It Together and Doing It Right* (Grand Rapids: Baker, 1995) and *Beyond Charity: The Call to Christian Community Development* (Grand Rapids: Baker, 1993). Perkins plays an important role in Charles Marsh's *The Beloved Community: How Faith Shapes Social Justice from the Civil Rights Movement to Today* (New York: Basic Books, 2005).

CHAPTER FOUR

The Christian Social Practice of Health Care

The essays in Chapter Three outlined a series of fundamental principles and theological convictions that must shape any theological perspective on medical ethics. The essays in Chapter Four take these principles and convictions, flesh them out, and show what they look like in practice. Given the connections between these two chapters, we strongly urge those interested in working through the essays in Chapter Four also to read the materials in Chapter Three.

The question of access to health care animated the essays in Chapter Three. Access has been seen as one of the primary moral questions of health care delivery since calls for health care reform began in the late 1960s with the instituting of the Medicare and Medicaid programs. Yet today, proposals for reform of the U.S. health care system cannot be considered in isolation from questions of the infrastructure of health care delivery globally. On the one hand, the U.S. remains the only democratic country and one of only a few industrialized countries that does not offer some form of universal health care to all its citizens.[1] Approximately 47 million Americans lack health insurance (a figure that has increased during the recession of 2008-2012 as unemployment has reached 10 percent), and an additional 9 million lack insurance at some point every year. Despite the enormous sums of money the U.S. spends on health care each year, a study released by the World Health Organization in 2000 ranked the U.S. 37th out of 191 countries in terms of performance, taking last place among industrialized countries.[2] The Institute of Medicine estimates that 18,000 Americans die every year because of lack of health insurance.[3] On the other hand, approximately 10 million children die every year from preventable or easily treatable causes in "resource poor" or "developing" countries, and the morbidity and mortality borne by adults in these contexts are likewise significant.

Increasing access to health care services for U.S. citizens, while important, will address only one aspect of the larger social infrastructure in which Schiedermayer and Maldonado (whom we encountered in Chapter Three) might meet. For disparities exist even among those with access to health care. The Institute of Medicine, in its 2002 report *Unequal Treatment: Confronting Racial and Ethnic Disparities in Health Care,* details the ongoing effects of the racial and ethnic infrastructure of the U.S. on the delivery of health care.[4] Both the Institute of Medicine documents and continuing studies confirm that ongoing health disparities among various racial and ethnic groups, as well as between men and women, are the result not only of unequal access but of differences in treatment quality in the clinical setting. Providers all too often bring with them unconscious racial and gender biases they have absorbed from their cultural context. These biases can translate into differential treatment and disparate health outcomes.

Thus, any consideration of the social context of medicine must address not only questions of economics and class, but also the interrelated questions of race and gender. Aana Vigen argues that such questions must be attended to not only from the level of statistical analysis, but, again, from below. In her two-part essay, "Listening to Women of Color with Breast Cancer: Theological and Ethical Insights for U.S. Healthcare" and "'Keeping It Real' While Staying Out of the 'Loony Bin': Social Ethics for Healthcare Systems" (selection 21), Vigen employs ethnographic methods, listening to the voices of African-American and Latina women with breast cancer. She does so with two ends in mind. First, she allows the theological insights of these women to enflesh the principles of Cath-

1. See T. R. Reid, *The Healing of America: A Global Quest for Better, Cheaper, and Fairer Health Care* (New York: Penguin Press, 2009).

2. World Health Organization, *World Health Report 2000 — Health Systems: Improving Performance* (Washington, D.C.: World Health Organization, 2000).

3. Committee on the Consequences of Uninsurance, Institute of Medicine, *Care without Coverage: Too Little, Too Late* (Washington, D.C.: National Academy Press, 2002).

4. Brian D. Smedley, Adrienne Y. Stith, and Alan R. Nelson, eds., *Unequal Treatment: Confronting Racial and Ethnic Disparities in Health Care* (Washington, D.C.: National Academies Press, 2002).

olic social teaching outlined in Chapter Three by Fisher and Gormally. For example, a first principle of Catholic social teaching is the dignity of the human person. Vigen asks each woman "how her faith in God informs what dignity and respect means." Rather than speaking of anthropology, the women thicken the principle theologically, speaking, for example, of "gratitude." Vigen then uses the theological and practical insights provided by these women to suggest structural changes in U.S. health care and to illuminate the operative dynamics of race, gender, and class in our current system.[5]

As Vigen makes clear, the relationship between theology and medicine does not involve principles alone; it is equally about persons and practices. How does a theological perspective on medicine get concretized in action? What do these principles and convictions look like in practice? How, churches ask themselves, can we care for the sick and poor in our own congregation or in our communities? We include in this section three essays that highlight Shuman and Volck's challenge in Chapter Three to be "a body without borders" — exemplars of the historic Christian practice of caring for the sick today. We do not think these three stories are unique. Hundreds of similar stories could have been told: stories of Christians, congregations, community development organizations, and others working to care for the sick and poor in their midst. We highlight these as three possibilities and encourage the reader to search for more.

First, William Grimes, M.D., D.Min., talks about his experience in "Starting a Free Clinic in a Rural Area" (selection 22). Discussions of underserved populations in the U.S. often focus on the plight of persons living in inner-city, urban settings. Such a focus, while important, fails to note that an equally underserved population is those persons who live in rural communities in the U.S. Grimes's essay brings this to light. His story starts with the principle of solidarity: "Go to the people. Live among them. Learn from them. Love them. Start with what they know. Build on what they have. . . ." The story of building the clinic in Kentucky brings the principles of Catholic social teaching to life, showing what it means to treat persons as persons, to honor their dignity, to work with a vision of the common good, to call for participation from all members of the community, to value subsidiarity — all in the context of health care.

While starting a clinic is one incarnation of the Christian tradition of caring for the sick, parish nursing is a second. Parish nursing has been called one of the best-kept secrets of contemporary health care. We include Abigail Rian Evans's essay "Parish Nursing: A New Specialty" (selection 23) to bring this movement to the attention of readers of *On Moral Medicine*. Through parish nursing programs, congregations attend to the health of their members in a distinctive way.

One does not need to be a physician or a nurse to practice the Christian call to care for the sick and poor. One does not even need to have a physician or nurse in one's parish. Kyle Childress, in "Austin Heights and AIDS" (selection 24), tells the story of what happened when one small Baptist church in East Texas (with a membership of forty) accepted the challenging prospect of addressing the food needs of local men with AIDS. While standard utilitarian reasoning would have argued against taking on this project, Childress makes clear how following biblical convictions and the challenge to overcome fearsome borders resulted — in good Gospel fashion — in outcomes that never could have been imagined. Grace abounds and abounds and abounds.

The Childress piece — as well as those by Grimes and Evans — demonstrates what is possible. Such stories may be difficult to universalize, though that might be one piece of the wisdom they impart: that just as important as systemic health care reforms are practices of local congregations in addressing the health needs of those among them through face-to-face, person-to-person encounters. This is not to say, however, that congregational attention to healing and the hurly-burly realm of health care policy occupy two different worlds of discourse, such as "action and legislation" or "action and theory."

The question of the just allocation of scarce health care resources was, one could argue, the first issue that contributed to the development of the contemporary field of medical ethics. Shana Alexander's exposé in *Life* magazine of the Seattle Kidney Transplantation Committee in the early 1960s was the first medical ethics "case" brought to public attention by the media. Thus, the question of allocation has been with medical ethics from the beginning. Which criteria ought society to use to allocate scarce resources fairly: merit, social contribution, supply and demand, need, or the rule to treat similar cases similarly?[6]

B. Andrew Lustig, in his essay "Reform and Rationing: Reflections on Health Care in Light of Catholic Social Teaching," analyzes a more contemporary attempt to address the question of just allocation (selection 25). Lustig succinctly summarizes the principles of Catholic social teaching, highlighting their theological underpinning, and demonstrates how differently an issue like health care rationing looks when viewed through a lens supplied by these principles. He looks specifically at the 1989 Oregon Basic Health Services Act, an attempt to simultaneously increase access to basic health services while reining in costs by providing "limited coverage to every poor person" in Oregon rather than simply "providing extensive medical coverage for only some of the poor." Lustig carefully demonstrates how Oregon's program,

5. Vigen expands her findings in these essays in her book *Women, Ethics, and Inequality in U.S. Healthcare: "To Count among the Living"* (New York: Palgrave Macmillan, 2006).

6. Gene Outka's classic 1974 essay, "Social Justice and Equal Access to Healthcare," provides one of the best summaries of these criteria. He reviews the assumptions behind each of these criteria as well as their implications in a way that remains relevant thirty years later. Outka's essay can be found in both the first and second editions of *On Moral Medicine*.

though much maligned in the press, met many of the principles of Catholic social teaching (though not by design) and would be improved by embodying them more fully. If nothing else, Oregon's proposal aimed to promote the common good and involved an honest and open public discussion of limits, unlike the covert process of rationing that operates in our current system of profit-driven, insurance-governed health care delivery.

The principles of Catholic social teaching — or any theological principle, for that matter — not only concern questions of justice at the macro-level of health care infrastructure but are also applicable within particular institutions. We include here a selection from Philip S. Keane's book *Catholicism and Health-Care Justice* (2002), on the just treatment of health care employees (selection 26).

A useful exercise to attend the readings in this chapter would be to study the various forms of universal health care currently in operation globally. PBS's *Frontline* feature, *Sick Around the World,* provides an excellent starting point for classroom exploration, documenting the different approaches to universal health care in five capitalist democracies in five ten-minute video segments available online.[7] Journalist T. R. Reid, who narrates the documentary, has now also published a book-length version of his study in his 2009 text, *The Healing of America: A Global Quest for Better, Cheaper, and Fairer Health Care.*[8] As Reid makes clear, and as the various essays in this chapter confirm, there is no one-size-fits-all answer to the moral imperative of universal health coverage. The challenge for those with Christian commitments is to discover those models that will work in the U.S. context as well as *via* our local congregations to promote and protect the health — and therefore dignity — of the human person and thereby promote the common good. In so doing, we shall continue to fulfill the biblical mandate and constant witness of the Christian tradition to care for the poor and the sick.

SUGGESTIONS FOR FURTHER READING

Birrer, R. B., and Ann Stango. "Strengthening Charity Care: One Catholic Hospital Has a Method for Providing More — Not Less — Care for the Uninsured." *Health Progress* (May-June 2005): 39-43.

Farley, Margaret A. "Partnership in Hope: Gender, Faith, and Responses to HIV/AIDS in Africa." *Journal of Feminist Studies in Religion* 20, no. 1 (Spring 2004): 133-48.

Farmer, Paul. *Pathologies of Power: Health, Human Rights, and the New War on the Poor* (Berkeley: University of California Press, 2004).

Farmer, Paul, and David Walton. "Condoms, Coups, and the Ideology of Prevention: Facing Failure in Rural Haiti." In *Catholic Ethicists on HIV/AIDS Prevention,* ed. James F. Keenan (New York: Continuum Press, 2000), pp. 108-19.

Kaveny, M. Cathleen. "Distributive Justice in the Era of the Benefit Package: The Dispute Over the Oregon Basic Health Services Act." In *Critical Choices and Critical Care,* ed. K. Wm. Wildes (Dordrecht: Kluwer Academic Publishers, 1995), pp. 163-85.

McConnaha, Scott. "Catholic Teaching and Disparities in Care: Our Ministry Is Perfectly Positioned to Lead the Struggle Against Inequities in Care." *Health Progress* (January-February 2006): 46-50.

Pellegrino, Edmund. "Ethical Issues in Managed Care: A Catholic Christian Perspective." *Christian Bioethics* 3, no. 1 (1997): 55-63.

Repenshek, Mark. "Stewardship and Organizational Ethics: How Can Hospitals and Physicians Balance Scarce Resources with Their Duty to Serve the Poor?" *Health Progress* (May-June 2004): 31-35, 56.

Rutledge, Everard O. "Removing Bias from Health Care." *Health Progress* (January-February 2003): 33-37, 57.

7. Videos are available online at: http://www.pbs.org/wgbh/pages/frontline/sickaroundtheworld (accessed January 31, 2009).

8. Reid, *The Healing of America.*

21 Listening to Women of Color with Breast Cancer: Theological and Ethical Insights for U.S. Healthcare; and "Keeping It Real" While Staying Out of the "Loony Bin": Social Ethics for Healthcare Systems

Aana Vigen

Part 1: Listening to Women of Color with Breast Cancer: Theological and Ethical Insights for U.S. Healthcare

I am a Christian social ethicist who contends that adequate moral inquiry necessarily involves interdisciplinary reflection and conversation. In my view, the proper place of a professional ethicist is not only in the library or at the computer, but is also found in dialogue with others who have key insights to share. And many times, these persons are not formal academics. Early on in graduate work, I realized that I wanted to explore healthcare disparities. Confronting the troubling statistics about the numbers of uninsured (now up to 45 million, according to the U.S. Census) along with evidence of persistent racial-ethnic inequalities in health and healthcare preoccupied much of my scholarly attention.

Yet, what I also came to realize was that consulting the current literatures related to these questions would not suffice as a method of moral analysis. In addition to that research, I sought to learn from people who have had substantive experience seeking healthcare themselves. Consequently, from June through December of 2003, I interviewed eight Black and/or Latina women who have had, or currently have, breast cancer.[1] I met the women with cancer primarily through women's cancer support group networks in New York City.[2] During this time, I also interviewed six healthcare providers, five of whom work primarily with cancer patients.[3]

This article will share theological insights of these women with breast cancer who make visceral connections between what they know of God and what they know about what human beings owe one another. I will also describe the qualities of a patient-provider relationship that these women most prize. [Then] I will take these theological and practical insights seriously as I consider what has to be in place — structurally — for such wisdom to be heeded within U.S. healthcare.

"God Has to Live in Each One of Us": Theo-ethical Insights of Women with Breast Cancer

As part of the ethnographic research, I asked each of the women if and how her faith in God informs what dignity and respect mean; how human beings ought to treat one another; and how they try to treat others. Seven of the women identified explicitly as Christians.[4]

Before articulating how faith in God informs their sense of what dignity and respect mean, I need to touch upon another term: gratitude. This gratitude to God was voiced so often that it seems fundamental to understanding anything else the women said regarding the relationship between God and humanity. Even as several of them were/are contending with cancer and uncertain futures, these women effusively thanked God and emphasized that they felt accompanied by God throughout their

1. These participants range in age from thirty-three to sixty-seven years old. Seven of them explicitly express a Christian faith. One has Christian roots in the Black Church and notes that although she does not attend anymore, she has a belief in a higher power than humankind. The women vary in how they describe their racial-ethnic backgrounds. Two identify as Black and two as African American; two identify as Latina; one prefers the term Hispanic (of these three, one specifically identifies as Puerto Rican and two as Dominican). One woman identifies as Black Puerto Rican, underscoring the fact that one can be both Black and Latina.

One woman first had cancer of the cervix and uterus in the 1980s before having subsequent diagnoses of breast cancer in the 1990s and in 2003. For the others, breast cancer was their first diagnosis. They have received cancer care at several different sites — private specialty hospitals, public hospitals and clinics, and teaching hospitals. Seven are presently insured: one has Medicaid; another has Medicaid and Medicare; five have employer or school-based insurance. One woman had lost her employer-based insurance and was uninsured at the time of the interview.

2. All names have been changed. Hospital names will not be used. Seven of the eight women with cancer chose their own pseudonym.

3. I interviewed an oncologist, two social workers, one nurse, one nurse case manager, and one third-year medical student.

4. Sandra Gavin explained that she was raised in the Black church, but is no longer an active member. She did not specifically identify herself as Christian. Sandra said that she believes in a higher power, but that she has a lot of issues with the church, particularly the Black church. She explained that she has problems with how many ministers are male while most of the active members are women and how ministers use women — she emphasized that she "uses the term 'use' loosely" — to serve a variety of functions in the church. She shared with me that her form of prayer is to ask her mother, as if she were still alive, to pray for her.

Part 1 from Aana Vigen, "Listening to Women of Color with Breast Cancer: Theological and Ethical Insights for U.S. Healthcare," *Journal of Lutheran Ethics,* Oct. 2005. Used by permission of the publisher and the author.
Part 2 from Aana Vigen, "'Keeping It Real' WHile Staying Out of the 'Loony Bin': Social Ethics and Healthcare Systems." *Journal of Lutheran Ethics,* Mar. 2006. Used by permission of the publisher and the author.

lives. They expressed ardent confidence in God and acknowledged that God is ultimately in control — that they live in dependence upon God and God's goodness. Slimfat Girl expressed her faith this way: "It's like this — He's always been there. He has never left my side. I have been in some situations, and I always thank God, and I thank the Lord that they pulled me through. So I do believe. I do believe there's a higher power than myself."[5] And Marcela: "And I thank God that I feel, that I am feeling really, really well — thanks to God. I appreciate this God that is up above because I ask Him for this every day."[6] She then added this description of the divine: "I think that He is support, where we find refuge, that if one looks, if we look for God day after day, He will unconditionally support us always."[7]

This theme of gratitude and thankfulness came up in the three breast cancer support groups that I attended as well. In each of these cases, I heard many and varied women in challenging life circumstances unreservedly thank God and "give God all the praise and glory": Immigrant women; undocumented women; Black and Latina women born and raised in New York City; women with limited economic means; women who have lost all their hair; women who were feeling poorly (some who had just had chemotherapy); women with poor prognoses. Through their tears, whether shed out of happiness or out of fear and worry, still they thanked God.

This gratitude was not a form of denial of their illness, nor did it seem at all superficial or cliché. I saw fear and strength — doubt and hope — in many pairs of eyes. I understand their words of gratitude to God to serve as *both* expressions of their active hope and faith *as well as* reassurance that there are reasons to have faith — as a way to combat the fear that gnaws away at hope. As a white, educated, physically-well woman who has been discouraged by surveying all that is wrong in this world, I am humbled by their ability to stay rooted in hope in the midst of concrete suffering and reasons for despair.

Their praise did not mean that they never got angry with God or struggled with faith. Sophia openly acknowledged that having faith can be really difficult, that sometimes she felt like she was "faking it." I am sure that these and other women with cancer struggle so much and can be so angry or sad that they go to the point of losing any scrap of hope or faith. Yet what struck me about the dozens of women I met or observed was that both their faith in God and their hope for their own lives had grit. These inter-connected hopes gave them staying-power to endure the suffering and the uncertainty — at least in the moments that I have known them.

It can be hard to find words to describe the divine-human relationship. When I asked Slimfat Girl how God wants people to treat each other, she exclaimed, "He wants everything — oh, boy! That's why Adam and Eve *did not* stay in the garden, okay? Because they didn't listen to what He said. And if they hadda' listened, if they had of listened, you know, maybe the — our world would be a better place" (emphasis hers). The question of how faith in and knowledge of God informs how people are to treat one another can be daunting. The complexities and brokenness of this world can make it hard to imagine what human beings can and ought to do.

Despite the mammoth problems of this world, however, Marcela eloquently expressed her understanding of who God is and of what this means for human relationships:

> God says that He is love, right? And so, God has to live in each one of us. If one says that they love, one can assume it is because he/she knows God. Therefore, God says we are going to love one another. . . . Love is so important that it is, how to tell you, something that one cannot even define. So, we are going to love one another, respect one another, support one another so that this way God is reflected in each one of us.[8]

Her logic is compelling: God is love — something so important that it defies the boundaries of any definition. Human beings love. To the extent that we love, God lives in each one of us. In fact, we are only able to love *because* we know God who is love itself. This radical incarnational understanding of the divine means for Marcela that in our concrete activities and lives, human beings are able and supposed to image God — to reflect this love and to be a refuge and support to others. Wanda made a similar connection. "I want to always treat people the way that they're supposed to be treated, with respect and dignity and the love of Christ and having them see that Christ-like example within me."[9] Wanda wants others to see divine love alive within her.

5. Given that the women are speaking of their personal faith and out of respect for it, I will not alter their language for God.

6. In Spanish, Marcela said: "Y gracias a Él me siento, me estoy sintiendo bien de bien, gracias a Dios. Yo agradezco este Dios que está arriba porque a eso todos los días le pido." The Spanish used when speaking about God and faith is more beautiful than my translation renders. So I have decided to include original phrasings in places so that Spanish speakers may compare it with my translation.

7. "Pienso que Él es el apoyo, donde nosotros nos refugiamos, que si uno lo busco, si nosotros lo buscamos dia tras día, Él nos va a apoyar siempre — incondicionalmente."

8. "Siempre o sea Dios dice que Él es amor, ¿verdad? Y por lo tanto tiene que vivir en cada uno de nosotros. Si uno dice que uno ama supone es porque cononce a Dios. Entonces, Dios dice vamos a amarnos uno a otro, querernos. El amor es tanto significado que es, como te digo, algo no se puede ni siquiera definir. Entonces, vamos a amarnos, respetarnos, apoyarnos uno a otro para que así Dios se refleje en cada uno de nosotros."

9. Wanda credited being raised in the church for grounding her in an ability to love and respect others. She articulates this connection this way:

> I've always had a strong background in the church and been raised in the church since I was a little girl, and have always been raised to try to do, you know, the right thing, and treat other people with dignity and with the love of God. And so I think that that plays an important part for me because I want to always treat people the way that they're supposed to

Reflecting on Marcela's and Wanda's words, I realized that their emphasis is the reverse of what I usually articulate as my aim; namely, to see Christ (or the divine) in the other. While both ways of putting it are important, their vision is an important corrective for me because it inspires creative moral agency, in addition to respectful listening to and recognition of others. In an emphasis on seeing the divine in others, it is possible to forget or deemphasize the crucial insight that *by my own* actions and decisions, I can reflect and embody (if only very partially) God's love for the others I encounter in any given day. What matters is not only *seeing* the divine in others, but *expressing* divine love and justice in relation to others.

When I asked a couple of the women to define dignity, I again heard an emphasis on self agency. Marcela told me, "Dignity is something that lifts your self esteem. . . . What you think of yourself is what helps you have dignity." I clarified, "So dignity is not something that others give a person, it is what one has inside oneself?" Marcela readily agreed. Indeed, while she agreed that others in society do not have the right to make a person feel bad, she was quick to add, "But it is not them who will resolve this problem for me, it is me." I commented that if one has dignity in oneself it will be a kind of protection — to protect one against these influences — that others cannot rob this dignity because it is one's own internal property. Marcela concurred: "[Dignity] doesn't depend on them; *it depends on you.* But above all, you have to maintain it always no matter what happens, you have to go on (her emphasis)."[10]

I was surprised by her words. They place a great deal of weight on an individual to guard and maintain one's own dignity.[11] I felt she was letting social and structural inequalities off the hook too easily. As I continued to ponder her thoughts, I recalled Luz's perspective. Even as Luz recalled her mother's words, that she was born with "three strikes against her" — namely, being born Black, Dominican, and a woman — she, too, placed great emphasis on individual agency — speaking of how important it is to "be feisty" — to learn English, to get an education, to be assertive and to prove them wrong. Marcela and Luz's point was that people who experience discrimination and prejudice must not internalize either. For persons and communities who regularly face racism, one way to contend with it is to deny and resist its power to determine their future or sense of self. "Dignity is yours to protect. It is not dependent upon others." In these words, I heard a strong refusal to see themselves or be seen by others as victims — as persons utterly dependent upon systems and forces outside of their control. While I maintain it is essential to hold systems and individuals accountable for the ways in which they eat away at the dignity of certain identities and communities, their insight chastened any inclination on my part to deny their agency out of misplaced pity or sympathy.

I learned something else about dignity. Its flip side is respect for others. What makes dignity genuine and what keeps it from devolving into narcissism or egocentrism is holding self-respect in dynamic tension with love and concern for others — being attentive to others as persons who also have dignity. From these women with breast cancer, I heard in a powerful way that part of respecting others *and* one's self involves humility. Maria commented that an inner balance is needed among humility, respect and consideration for others. "None weighs more than another, the three all weigh (count) the same." Her words caused me to reflect that if one has authentic self-respect, she will be more humble with regard to others. Humility does not mean an absence of self-respect, but rather, having a grounded sense of one's importance — not having to inflate one's ego because one knows she is truly loved and worthy of love. Therefore, she can be less egocentric and instead turned more outward to face and address the needs and personhoods of others. Here I sensed a resonance with that pre-modern man Luther.

Maria gave an example of how gratitude to God and humility within herself help her to notice and respond to

---

be treated, with respect and dignity and the love of Christ and having them see that Christ-like example within me. And that helps me to just be able to really work with people and to deal with people and to relate to people, just having a spiritual upbringing.

10. In Spanish, the dialogue went like this:

MR: Bueno, por lo menos la dignidad de uno es yo digo como algo . . . que levanta a tu auto estima. . . . Pero por lo menos tú tienes este auto estima alto, eso te levanta todo — lo que tú piensas de ti misma es lo que ayuda tener buena dignidad.

AV: Entonces dignidad no es de otra persona, que ellos le dan. Es lo que tiene dentro de si misma.

MR: Claro, porque yo pienso que por lo menos tú . . . tienes que seguir en como ellos te van a tratar. Por eso, yo no sé, no me quiero definir como una persona diferente a todo los demás. Pero, si yo, por lo menos, trato de cuando tengo mi derecho — saber como voy a seguir para que esa persona no tenga el derecho de ofenderme de hacerme sentir mal . . .

AV: Pero ellos no tienen el derecho de hacerlo tampoco.

MR: No, no tienen el derecho de hacerlo, hacer sentir mal. Pero no son ellos que me van a solucionar ese problema, soy yo.

AV: Y usted tiene que tener la dignidad dentro de si misma que no — que es una forma de proteccíon — para protegerse contra estas influencias y es — no pueden robar esta dignidad porque es properidad de usted.

MR: Sí exactamente.

AV: Y pueden enseñar respeto o no, pero la dignidad es su cosa — parte de su identidad — no depende de ellos.

MR: Sí, exactamente. No depende de ellos. Depende de tí. La dignidad depende de tí. Pero sobre todo, tienes que manterla siempre aunque pase lo que pase, ir para allá.

11. When I subsequently asked Marcela to elaborate more upon her perspective, she said, "If you think you're garbage, how will that animate you? If you think you are intelligent, this will animate you. . . . Even if they look at you negatively, you have to be strong, you can say no — and not let it offend you."

the needs of others. She said that when she sees hungry people on the street and she has two or three dollars, she often goes and buys the person something to eat. She does this, she says, not so that God will appreciate her, but because she is grateful to God. "I am very grateful to God, first of all, and then to my family and to [the second hospital]." She added that she is also grateful to the cancer support organizations and to their volunteers and staff.[12] And because she is so grateful for all the information and support she has received and for her life, she wants to give back. "God's given me a second chance and if someone is in the shoes I was in, I will try to help." In terms of giving back to the organizations that have helped her, she tries to be present for the events, walk-a-thons and the marches on Washington — "as long as God permits." Both her cancer support volunteering and her feeding of hungry people are expressions of her self-respect and her humility.

In a similar vein, Sophia explained that cancer has made her acutely aware of human fragility — that life can be gone in the blink of an eye. She vividly sees what really matters in life. She said that cancer has changed things in a positive way in this sense because it helped her get her priorities in order and to see what is truly important. She reflected, "Cancer made me stronger in a lot of ways. It made me more vulnerable in a lot of ways. I'm more open than I was before. . . . Now I kind of want to do more, help more. Not just with cancer, but with anything, anything I can do. . . . I listen more to people, too. It's less about me, you know?"

Self-respect and respect for others go hand in hand. Wanda brought this fact into full light for me. I asked her to define dignity. After a long pause, she said:

> I think just treating others the way that you would want to be treated, just with respect, not looking down on people, not — because a person, for example, may have, like, HIV, and, you know, not treating them with disrespect, but treating them like a human being, like they're somebody. And I use that example because that was a population that I worked with. And I used to see how people would treat them and just wouldn't want to be bothered or touch them or anything like that. And, you know, once I became educated about the illness, you know, it didn't frighten me. You know, I was, like, they're a human being too, you know. . . . (T)hey have a disease; but they're a human being, you know, they need to be treated with respect and not looked down upon or thrown away.

What struck me about this comment is that when I asked Wanda to define dignity, she did so not only in abstract terms, but reflected on a change she had experienced in herself as she worked with a stigmatized population. Said differently, she did not speak about how others ought to respect *her* dignity, but rather focused on how in one instance she herself had become more attuned to the *dignity of others.* This insight conveyed a great deal of self-reflexivity.

Moreover, Wanda explained how confronting her own biases and assumptions has not only helped her to respect others more, but to also have a grounded sense of dignity and self respect in herself. Specifically, she said that working with people with HIV has helped her to speak up for herself. "And I just think having the job of working with the HIV population has really helped me, you know? Not only did it help me empower my clients, but it helped empower myself, and to speak up for myself." Working with a community of people who are vulnerable in their own way gave her a window into her own life. In getting to know people with HIV and seeing what they go through, Wanda learned how to look out for herself *and* how to be more genuinely compassionate to others.

In all, in articulating what dignity in oneself and respect for others mean, these women also saw how far human beings are from what God wants for us. Yet this knowledge did not stop them from offering a vision of what ought to be. Several emphasized that it is important to strive for what is possible in one's life. To recall again Marcela's insight, God has to live in each of us. When we love, it is because God is in us. And because God's love and grace make it possible for God to dwell within humanity, we had better get busy. Because we are loved so intimately and profoundly — because God has searched and dwells within all human hearts, knew each of us in our mother's wombs and cherishes every one beyond description — we too can and must do all that we can to cherish one another.

"I Didn't See [a] 'Doctor.' I Just Saw a Woman": Patient Expectations of Healthcare Providers

That's how Hannah sees her breast surgeon — as a woman first. And that is how Hannah feels seen by her as well. This quality of relationship seems so fundamental. Yet it is not so easy to achieve in actual patient-physician relations. In what follows, I want to explore what I have learned from these women with breast cancer about what ingredients form the basis for high quality patient-provider relationships. I will touch upon four.

Above all other remarks, when asked what they most want from their doctors and/or other primary care providers, all of the women repeatedly emphasized authentic listening, empathy and understanding. I cite Sandra to illustrate the point. She explained that the most important thing care providers and systems need to do in terms of showing respect and honoring the person is hearing — *genuinely* hearing — without being compromised by an impatience to move on. "Listening is the biggest thing. I don't know if it's an acquired skill, but it certainly diminishes and affects the dignity and respect of the person when they don't listen." The basic yet crucial act of listening may be the most direct way of respecting another person. Sandra went on to comment,

12. Specifically, Maria named Share and Cancer Care as two organizations that have been very important to her.

"Those who did not hear forced me to seek more information so that I could feel comfortable." Indeed, when doctors or nurses rush the listening, they may end up having to spend more time with the patient and being less efficient in the long run. Being in a hurry, or overly relying on impersonal protocols for processing people, especially in the initial stages of a professional relationship, can inhibit trust and delay relationship-building.

Antonia Morales, a 3rd year medical student, also understood that listening well makes the work easier for the provider:

> And I see amazing doctors. And I see some that are not. . . . (T)hose that are amazing are the ones that drive me. Because they are so much better physicians in what they do. And it is obvious. If you want to do a better job . . . communicate better with your patients. They're going to tell you what's going on if they feel they can trust you. If not, you know, I think it's going to be harder for you. Your patients are going to come back . . . or they're going to have problems, and you're always going to see them sick. . . . I'm following an amazing doctor now. And even though she runs around, and she has a lot of work, when she comes into a room, the patient, I mean, shines. Because all she needs to do is come next to their bed, you know, come down to their level, and hold their hand, and talk to them face to face, smile at them, let them know everything's going to be okay, let them know what's going on. It doesn't take that much time. . . . Come down, sit down next to them by the bed, you know, apologize for anything that's going on, you know, because things happen, nurses you know, or whatever. Apologize. Doesn't hurt, you know, and it makes them feel like you care about what's going on with them while they're [in the hospital]. Apologize for it. "I'm sorry." And "We'll try our best to do better."

Antonia points out that adequate listening is not only a function of the ears and brain, but of one's quality of presence. Sitting down next to a patient can indicate that a doctor is truly present to the condition of the person in the bed. Even more, Antonia signals the importance of empathy — even to the point of apologizing. The act of offering an apology — communicating that one is sorry that another is uncomfortable or that things have not gone smoothly — seems something so obvious and yet may be the last thing a care provider thinks to say to a patient.

Finally, genuine listening involves not being put off by questions. Sandra noted the importance of this quality by pointing out its absence in her relationships with her first two physicians. Interestingly, she noted that in her case, being educated did not make a difference in terms of being listened to or treated with respect. In fact, she felt her education had worked against her. She felt treated as a "dumb nurse" by the first physician because she did not already know all the medical information, asked a lot of questions and had let her insurance lapse. The second doctor, while less abrasive, also seemed threatened by her educated questions.

A second quality of healthcare providers that I heard the women desire is honesty. Slimfat Girl implored: "And just be honest with me. *Be honest, just be honest.* You know?" (emphasis hers). Honesty was also of paramount importance to Luz, who poignantly articulated this need by explaining that part of the problem with her first doctor was that he was not honest with respect to what he did not know. He assured her that she was fine (or would be fine) before having test results to support this claim. Luz adamantly stated:

> A doctor tells you the truth of your illness. A doctor is professional enough to tell you, "This is what I understand from my studies, from the books — not from my feelings. . . ." And not a doctor that would tell you, "Oh, you're ok, that's nothing." A doctor should never tell a patient "That's nothing," or "This looks like" — no. A doctor should say, "Let's take whatever it is, send it to a lab, let's see what it is."

Rather than saying, "I don't know what you have," or "We have to wait and do all the tests before we will know," this doctor tried to reassure Luz. Attempts at reassurance that are not based in facts quickly diminish in their value to a patient. Even if the words sound good at first, their hopefulness is eventually unmasked for what they are: empty attempts to keep the patient from being upset (at least in the provider's presence). In this way, Luz explained that such attempts to be caring actually do the opposite:

> [E]ven though he spoke the same language, he was not like caring because he didn't understand my feelings. For example, you know that what you are telling me is from you, it's not from medicine. It's not like you have tested this and know that this is a fact. You just see a worried person and you are going to tell me something to make me feel better, not something that is medically correct. When I sat down with the doctor [at the second care setting], he told me, "Your cancer is aggressive. It's a bad cancer." He told me. He told me the truth about my cancer. He did not tell me something I wanted to hear. . . . Coat it with honey, coat it with sugar, do something, but tell me the truth, not something that I want to hear. So I have to do what I have to do to take care of my body . . . so I can make my decisions. (emphasis hers).

According to Luz, the most caring thing to do is to give the patient the most accurate information possible. To reassure someone without knowing all the facts undermines respect for the person as well as one's agency. Luz needed to know the truth so that she could make the best decisions of what to do next to take care of herself. "Coat it with honey . . . but tell me the truth."

While Maria agrees that honesty is important, she would emphasize the need for honey. Genuine compassion is the third ingredient. Just as compassion without information has serious deficiencies, so does being candid without having tact. Maria felt her doctors were incredibly brusque with her — "frío." Providers need to be honest and they need to convey information in a caring and compassionate manner. It is a delicate, but crucial balance.

Compassion and honesty need to be joined in a provider's relating to patients. Most nursing and medical school textbooks would emphasize this point. The harder question is how to achieve such a balance. I asked Wanda how she knows when compassion is genuine — and providers are not simply going through the textbook motions. She responded:

> I look at body language, the way they're talking, how they're expressing themselves. Body language is really important to me. If someone is — if I'm asking a question, and they're like, you know, shrugging their shoulders, and as if they don't care or it's not important, or, you know, trying to brush me off, then I look at that. I also look at just the way they speak, their voice, how they talk to me, and not talking down to me.

Patients are able to read their providers as thoroughly as their providers read their charts and test results. Feigning interest or concern rarely works. Wanda also commented that her primary cancer physician (a white woman) "really loved her job. She loved working with people." Her love both for her work *and* people showed through in her words and actions. In dramatic contrast to two of Sandra's doctors, Wanda's physician enthusiastically (and without defensiveness) encouraged her to get a second opinion and gave her all her records to take with her. They have had an ongoing relationship since Wanda's diagnosis; they have come to know and trust one another. This relationship has been built on consistently good (honest) communication and positive rapport (genuine compassion and sensitivity).

Wanda underscored the weight of such qualities on patient-provider relationships. They are not mere courtesies; they can affect the patient on a profound level:

> I think that that can help soothe a person or help the healing process, if you have a very compassionate doctor working with you, or staff working with you. . . . Because if a patient has to come back, and they'd be worried about how you're treating them, their immune system is already weakened, so that's stress on them. I mean, that's just going to bring them down even more.

While a brusque exchange with a person in authority can irritate a healthy person or cause her stress, it may not as easily threaten her well-being. Wanda introduces an important possibility that might be overlooked. An absence of honesty, compassion or listening may very well beat down an already compromised immune system. The critically ill are in a weakened position — physically, emotionally — with respect to their caregivers. They have more to lose than their care providers.

Finally, I heard the women emphasize their need for their providers to be skilled clinicians. They want thorough work-ups and tests. This point, while obvious, ought not be taken for granted. Maria's story represents one example of what can happen when the work-up is not done, but deferred over the course of several months and visits. In delaying the biopsy, her tumor grew significantly and was joined by a second.

Luz and Marcela also emphasized the importance of having comprehensive and prompt testing. Marcela grew impatient with how long her providers were taking at the first hospital and so took her files to a second in order to speed up the determination of a diagnosis and to get a second opinion in the process. For her part, Luz was pleased with how fast and thorough her providers were when she got into the second care setting. There, in just three days, they did additional tests and performed the mastectomy because they found her cancer to be so aggressive. They took her and her medical situation seriously.

While everyone wants a skilled doctor, some experience more ease in finding one. Although she expressed overall satisfaction with her cancer care, Marcela (a woman insured by Medicaid) had no choice in providers. In less than a year, she had three different primary cancer physicians and was given little explanation for the changes. Luz was only able to access the second care site because of a friend who is a nurse who happened to work for one of their prominent cancer physicians. Luz called ten times over two days before asking this nurse's help. During this time, she was told again and again that there were no available appointments and that they would not accept her insurance. Indeed, all of the women were well aware of the role money and insurance play. They either open up doors or close them. Similarly, all expressed an awareness of how financial dynamics/assumptions can get in the way of good patient-provider relationships.

In all, the most poignant thing I heard from these women regarding what they want from healthcare providers is this: to be seen as a person. They used different expressions to get at this request, from positive statements such as Slimfat Girl wanting to be treated "as you would somebody else" to negative statements regarding how they do *not* want to be treated, such as not being a "bill." While some of these statements explicitly used financial metaphors, all made reference to not wanting to be objectified.

For example, Hannah is grateful that her doctor does not see her as a check or as income. Slimfat Girl expressed a similar sentiment when she said that she does not want to be treated as a "a paycheck," "money in the bank" or as a "guinea pig." And Marcela commented that it is important that providers do not treat patients "like a piece of furniture." She described that the best scenario is when providers "forget it's a job":

> [I] think that at least, even though it is a place of employment, one must think, if one is going to relate to another person as a human being and that this human being is going through a difficult situation, in this moment, one ought to forget it's a job. Do you understand me? This person is going through a difficult moment and needs help, above all, support. One cannot think that this [work] is as it were — as if I were making,

hum, furniture. "I am going to make furniture and I will throw the furniture there." That — no. It is as if you take a piece of furniture and put it there — to take a person and check them and go — no.

"Forget it's a job." That may seem like an odd or unrealistic request. Yet, perhaps her words offer an important reminder to healthcare professionals. While Marcela does not use the terminology, these comments speak to the difference many theological scholars have noted between a "job" and a "vocation." A job is something one does to survive financially — to bring in the paycheck. In contrast, a vocation is one's "calling" into which one puts one's heart, mind, talents, and energy because one senses in a profound way that this is what "I was put on the planet to do." Of course, while living out one's vocation, making a living is still a basic necessity. The key difference is that the work is done out of a sense of purpose and service, not only for one's own financial sustenance or enrichment. To build upon Marcela's illustration, if one is working in healthcare primarily out of a sense of vocation, and not employment, he or she will not think of it as a paycheck so much as a way of serving and being present to others. In the process, Marcela thinks, patients will be less likely to feel objectified, "treated like furniture."

Marcela added that doctors need at least a bit of psychology background to realize what all is going on in their patients. She explained:

> I think that the doctors have to co-penetrate [the situation] with the patient. In one way or another, many times the patient does not say exactly what [the problem] is, just what they feel. Sometimes [the patient] does not want to talk, is sometimes timid. For one or another reason, [the patient] does not want to say exactly what she/he is feeling.[13]

Marcela later explained that what she means by "conpenetrar" is that the doctor enters the experience of the person in order to understand both it and the person more fully. Womanist ethicist and theologian Emilie Townes defines empathy in a way that resonates with Marcela's understanding of "copenetrar": "As a moral virtue, empathy means that we put ourselves in the place of another. This means sharing and understanding the emotional and social experiences of others and coming to see the world as they see it. We move away from 'those people' and 'they' language and behavior to 'we' and 'us' and 'our' ways of living and believing."[14] Again, to relate in this way to patients, providers may very well need to be deeply invested in their work as a calling. To be authentically present to suffering on a daily basis is an exhausting task for which the tangible rewards can seem paltry. Moreover, it takes courage to possess and express empathy.

In sum, genuine listening, honesty, compassion and technical skill all facilitate trust. And trust is perhaps the most essential foundation upon which quality patient-provider relationships are built. Yet there is another way of describing this quality. To conclude, I want to draw attention back to the notion at which it began. What patients most integrally need may be personhood. Hannah glowed when she told me that she sees her breast specialist "as one of the girls." Her experience is a wonderful illustration of what is possible for patient-doctor relationships when the baggage of racial and socio-economic assumptions, bureaucracies and financial bottom lines do not interfere. It is not insignificant that Hannah had excellent health insurance and that she and this doctor shared a similar racial-ethnic background. Her words convey so much of what each of the women I spoke with would like from their primary caregivers:

> HJ: [My breast surgeon]'s so down to earth, too, you know. When I saw her, I didn't know she was a surgeon [laughs] . . . you know . . . just the way she, you know, just my experience with others, you know, doctors.
>
> AV: She didn't come in, total, all, "I'm the doctor."
>
> HJ: No. She was just one of the girls. She just had that air about her that, you know. . . . I didn't see her, I didn't see, you know, "I'm a medical doc," you know. No, I didn't see "Doctor." I just saw a woman, you know. She's a woman first, you know. Yes, she's a doctor, but she's also a woman.
>
> AV: And maybe that's how she saw you first, not as patient.
>
> HJ: Not as a patient, but just as a woman, you know, like you and I, just sitting here talking. . . . You know, she didn't see . . . "here's another bill." [laughs]
>
> AV: Right. "Here's another check."
>
> HJ: Right . . .
>
> AV: That shows a lot right there, you know.
>
> HJ: Yes, it does.
>
> AV: That you saw her as a woman, and she saw you as a woman, first. And that's where you connected.
>
> HJ: And that's where we connect.

13. This and the previous quotation in Spanish: Sí, pero pienso que por lo menos áun sea un sitio de empleo hay que pensar si va a relacionar con la otra persona, como ser humano y que este ser humano está pasando por una situación dificil, en este momento deber olividarse que es un empleo. ¿Me entiendes? Esta persona está pasando por un momento dificil y necesita ayuda, sobre de todo apoyo. No se puede pensar que eso es como si fuera — que estoy haciendo eh — mueble. "Voy a hacer mueble, voy a tirar mueble allí." Eso no, es como cuando usted coge un mueble y ponerlo allí — coger a una persona checquerla y vete — no. Yo creo que los doctores tienen que conpenetrarse con el paciente. Por de una u otra manera, muchas veces el paciente no dice exactamente lo que es, simplamente lo que se siente. A veces no quiere hablar, a veces es timido. Por una u otra razón, no quiere decir exactamente lo que esta sintiendo. . . . Y tiene [el doctor] por lo menos un poco de psycologia — se puede dar cuenta de algo pero si no, si se ve simplamente como un mueble que está fabricando — pues, tira el mueble para allí y coger otro mueble. . . .

14. Emilie M. Townes, *Breaking the Fine Rain of Death* (New York: Continuum, 1998), 175.

In this relationship, Hannah and her doctor were first and foremost women — persons — in one another's eyes. In a society where human interactions are often structured by and filtered through external roles and internal expectations, it is no small matter to be seen simply as a woman by one's doctor and to have the courage and self-confidence to see one's doctor in the same way.

Part 2: "Keeping It Real" While Staying Out of the "Loony Bin"

These women who have survived or are living with breast cancer shared a great deal of embodied wisdom with me. They know a lot because they have been through a lot. They see and appreciate what is good in some healthcare contexts and what is problematic in others, and they offered up descriptions of what most matters to them as particular persons. What I have learned from them has significant implications for healthcare quality discussions. My questions now are: "What has to be in place in healthcare institutions for these themes to be more adequately addressed within the cultures and practices of healthcare than they are now? How might healthcare organizations and providers heed the wisdom of these women?"

As a way to explore these questions, I will use the four themes as guideposts (the interplay of racial and socio-economic assumptions, the imbalance of power dynamics in the patient-provider relationship, the role and necessity of advocates and self-advocacy, the impact of bureaucratic processes and financial bottom lines) in order to reflect upon what they mean for the doing of healthcare. In making connections between these themes and ethical implications, I will touch upon four constructive possibilities for healthcare and medical ethics.

Racial and Socio-Economic Assumptions and Power Imbalances

The combination of these assumptions with the imbalance of power dynamics inherent in patient-provider relationships is potent and potentially deeply alienating. Undeniably, all breast cancer patients are in a position of relative vulnerability to their oncologists given that the patients are physically compromised by cancer and depend on their doctor for care and help. However, it is clear that communities of color, along with those who are poor and/or who lack health insurance (or who have inadequate medical coverage), experience additional forms of vulnerability. Indeed, they are doubly or triply at risk because they may not be able to access care as easily and they may carry the burden of providers' assumptions related to race and/or socio-economics.[15]

Race and class are distinct but interwoven realities within U.S. mind-sets and social structures. While they cannot be conflated, their intersections need to be understood. The combination of racial-ethnic and class assumptions can make a huge difference in terms of the degree of both access and visibility that darker skinned women have when negotiating healthcare as compared with lighter skinned women. Having excellent insurance coverage does not magically dispel these assumptions from the minds of care providers.

Sophia's sense that providers expect her to change their minds reveals a lot. There is something seriously — systemically — wrong when patients such as Sophia feel the burden to change provider assumptions — to demonstrate that they are "different," "one of the good Black Puerto Ricans" so that providers will be deeply invested in doing the absolute best they can for them. It is an unjust burden for her and others to bear. Given the relative power differences, the burden ought to fall on the providers — to work harder to know, understand and care for the patients who are most different from them. For it is in these scenarios where misunderstandings, mistrust and poor communication are most likely to fester and cripple patient-provider relationships, treatment plans and cure rates. In considering the weight and prevalence of these assumptions within a context of unequal power dynamics, two specific suggestions for change surface.

Conclusion #1: Educating Providers to See Their Own Assumptions

Providers need to be attuned to the peril of compartmentalizing people. Seeing patients primarily though the lens of their physiological condition, insurance status or through assumptions based on racial-ethnic and/or class background diminishes and limits the quality of their care. Such narrow vision can render the actual persons invisible.

Healthcare systems and practitioners need to understand that it is unjust to hoist the burden of changing provider assumptions onto patients. Instead, healthcare institutions and practices can and ought to support the seeing and understanding of the social contexts in which these lives are situated. Simply put, we — as providers, ethicists, healthcare practitioners and professionals, and theologians — need to do our homework. For holistic care to be comprehensive, appreciation of the person as embedded within a network of socio-economic, cultural, familial and political relationships and structures is needed in addition to attending to her physical, spiritual and intellectual dimensions.

15. Since I began this research, it has been pointed out to me a few times (interestingly always by white academics or professionals) that the white working class, the white poor, and whites living in rural areas also suffer a lack of healthcare due to socio-economic assumptions and barriers. Undeniably, these lighter skinned populations are at risk and merit attention. However, the fact that they too are vulnerable ought not be used to deny or obscure the particular vulnerabilities of darker skinned communities.

Antonia spoke to these qualities when she described the kind of doctor she hopes to become:

> The kind of doctor that I want to be is a doctor who . . . truly, truly wants what's best for the patient, and is not just looking at the patient as an illness, but is learning about who that patient is, learning about their background, about the family home life, what's going on with them. . . . You're constantly learning about diseases and illness [in medical school]. And a lot of times, you're not exposed to patients. And, but when you are, and you get that little piece of information about them which fascinates you — something you find out about them, and you're like, "Wow, this is a person who has a life, this is a person who has dreams." And you just learn so much more about them.

Rather than using such contextual information to stereotype a person, the provider can use it to be attentive to the complexity and richness of every human life. When doctors possess these skills, they stand out. Antonia observes: "But I personally have seen many, no, I've seen a few white doctors who are amazing to all their patients. . . . [T]hese physicians who are amazing were culturally competent. They were respectful. They were understanding. And it's interesting how that can cross over all cultures." I take heart in knowing that at least a few of Antonia's white mentors get it.

Antonia mentions an important and increasingly discussed concept: cultural competence.[16] There are many possible strategies for enculturating such understanding. I would like to highlight the need for *intensive* cultural competency training. By cultural competence education, I mean integrated attention to racial-ethnic, socio-economic, linguistic, cultural and religious particularities that shape patient needs, perceptions, experiences of health and illness, needs and fears with which they contend. Such education must teach both appreciation of the complexity of others' lives as well as critical self-reflection. Said differently, ethicists and providers need to analyze in-depth the socio-economic contexts of healthcare provision, and we need to articulate and attend to our own internal assumptions and biases.

The word "integrated" is important. One course or class segment devoted to "cultural diversity" will not suffice. Instead, a cultivation of these skills ought to be integrated throughout courses as well as be reflected in how clinical training is taught and modeled. Moreover, some curricula are better than others in this regard. Some amount to little more than cataloging a list of generalized (and sometimes stereotypical) descriptions of certain cultural or linguistic habits, preferences, practices, etc. Others require prolonged critical self-reflection, analysis of power dynamics and privilege, and the unmasking of stereotypes and assumptions. Thus, the quality and ethos of the training and curriculum matters a great deal.[17]

Antonia worked for a not-for-profit organization before going to medical school and still volunteers with women of color cancer support programs. In light of these experiences, she suggested that immersion in a racial, socio-economic and cultural context that is different from the student's be a part of one's professional development:

> I think that everybody, before they go to medical school, should really spend a year someplace where they wouldn't see themselves. Just someplace where they really have no clue about those people, or that group of people. . . . Yeah, just to sort of, you know, go away, go somewhere, go to the Caribbean maybe, or go to Puerto Rico, or the Dominican Republic, go to Cuba, come up to Harlem. They'll go to East Harlem, spend time in a small HIV clinic. That's what I did. I was a — I went to an HIV clinic for about six months, and I volunteered there. It's putting yourself in the position to learn from others. . . . And just seeing something from a different view, and being around people [who have a different view].

Antonia is right that such experiences are a wonderful way to prepare for medical school. However, given that all students may not seek out these experiences on their own before gaining entrance into a formal medical program, the schools need to provide them as well. Immersion experiences, mentoring programs and clinical experience in socio-economic and racial-ethnic contexts that differ significantly from the student's are all ways in which assumptions and beliefs might be questioned in ways which enrich understanding and care. Sophisticated methods for critical self-reflection must be a part of such curricular programs. Additionally, greater emphasis on speaking and understanding second languages is needed both at undergraduate and graduate curricular levels than is currently oftentimes present.

However, such suggestions may be hard to realize. The cultures of many medical programs are predominately focused on the important matters of learning the physiological and technical dimensions of healthcare. Antonia herself does not expect her formal education to teach her the skills of relating to patients:

> I wouldn't say there's an actual push for us to really bond with patients — you know, to really learn about the patient. But there are bits and pieces, sort of to remind us, you know, that you — you're going into this medical profession. . . . You need to know how to communicate with your patients, and that's very important. But I think it's something within you. It's . . . very diffi-

16. There is a fast-growing body of texts and curricula on this topic. Here are just two examples: Larry D. Purnell and Betty J. Paulanka, *Transcultural Health Care: A Culturally Competent Approach,* 2nd ed. (Philadelphia: F. A. Davis Co., 2003); Bette Bonder, Laura Martin, and Andy Miracle, *Culture in Clinical Care* (New Jersey: Slack Inc., 2002).

17. In a future project, I would like to analyze various cultural competency models utilized by medical and nursing schools in order to discern what may be the most rigorous and transformative models.

> cult to learn. It's not going to be part of your medical education. You've got to either develop it through experience or have it.

Antonia is right that such things are challenging to teach and instill in another. Yet it gives me pause that she does not expect such values to be part of her formal education. I wonder how many medical students have similar experiences and expectations of their curricula. I believe that some medical and nursing programs do foreground an ethos of service to and understanding of our diverse society; however, I am not at all certain of how widespread this pattern is.

There are opportunities to gain such skills after graduation. Many hospitals periodically offer diversity trainings to their staff. However, brief diversity trainings held for current healthcare professionals can fall short of what is needed. Staff sometimes view them as nothing more than a bureaucratic hoop for accreditation. Indeed, a couple of the care providers were clear that short diversity trainings do little to alter provider assumptions. Beef Stew, a nurse case manager, was pointedly candid in her criticism of them:

> That's a bunch of bullshit. Okay. Because how it is conveyed is not from a person of color. It's from a person who says, "Okay, these people are complaining about there's a problem. Okay, how do we be nice to them? Okay, this is how we're going to be nice to them." . . . That's putting a Band Aid on it. That's not, like, "Okay, well, let's try to understand the problem, okay? This is a problem. Why is this problem happening? . . . All right, now, how are we going to change this to improve the dialogue between us, to improve the communication so this doesn't happen again?" That's not the spirit that it's coming from. It's coming from, "Look, okay, the Department of Labor says we have to do this."

The impetus behind the training matters. It also matters if the hospital and practitioners are open to rigorous self-critique, or if they want to apply "Band Aids" that give an appearance of serious attention to the issues. Indeed, interpersonal communication techniques cannot be employed as "tricks" to build trust with a patient. Attempts at understanding and compassion need to be sincere. If not, none of the strategies will help much because they are motivated by self-interest rather than concern for others.

Moreover, the narrow scope of these trainings and cultural sensitivity courses can limit the scope of the analysis as well. Some researchers contend that the culture of medicine and the medical gaze may make it difficult for communities of color and/or lower socioeconomic classes to be seen as persons. For example, Good and Good add that such classes often focus on the culture of patients without incorporating social analysis:

> Until recently, when cultural analyses were proposed, the focus was largely on patient culture. Burdens of difference were on patient communities, and medicine and health professionals were expected to learn to be culturally competent in attending to the diverse populations that make up American society. When we are challenged to examine the culture of medicine and of our healthcare institutions, we are also challenged to bring a critical perspective that has largely been ignored by most research to date or that has circumscribed cultural inquiry to the differences between patients' and physicians' "beliefs." Disparities in medical treatment are not simply matters of differences in "beliefs." Clearly, political and economic factors that shape our medical commons and our larger society are implicated in the production of these disparities.[18]

Culturally competent care involves more than learning about different foods, beliefs and religious practices of patients. It must also rigorously and self-critically analyze the socio-economic and political forces that structure healthcare institutions and practices themselves.

I asked Wanda who has been both a patient in and an employee of hospitals how hospitals can engender respect for persons:

> I think you have those culture sensitivity courses. And you stay on that. You — not just have the courses, and then, okay, they've got the training, but see how the staff is treating the patients. Walk around, you know, be involved in something. Because what I think tends to happen is that people will go — some hospitals offer the culture sensitivity course. And then the staff will go. But then what happens after that? How do you follow up and how do you make sure that they're doing what they're supposed to do? Because, like I said, I worked in a hospital, and I've see what happens. And even if you take culture sensitivity classes, people don't follow, follow those things. So I think having the higher-up staff oversee it, making sure that it's being done, instilling that in their staff. . . .

Wanda understands that periodic trainings will not change the culture of institution. Real change must be consistently promoted and instilled at all levels within the organization. In particular, Wanda notes the importance of those in leadership positions. Akin to mentoring medical and nursing students, administrative managers, senior physicians and nurse managers need to see the value and need for such efforts and change.[19]

18. Mary-Jo DelVecchio Good, Byron J. Good, et al., "The Culture of Medicine and Racial, Ethnic, and Class Disparities in Healthcare," in Brian D. Smedley, Adrienne Y. Stith, and Alan R. Nelson, eds., *Unequal Treatment: Confronting Racial and Ethnic Disparities in Healthcare,* Institute of Medicine (Washington: National Academy Press, 2002), 620.

19. Wanda emphasized that hospital leadership needs to take a lead in making the changes part of the institutional culture:

> (W)hen I worked in a hospital, we used to speak with the interns. And the first thing the social workers would do was, you know, give them a speech. And then, you know, they would leave and go to their — through their own same old stuff. But then they had doctors who were over them, teach-

While a simplistic "top down" approach can alienate staff, so too will efforts flounder at the staff levels if change is not supported by the leadership of a hospital. Both levels need to be engaged for cultural competence to take hold within the practices and sensibilities of care settings. Instilling such awareness and sensitivity is a complex process of moral and professional formation to which both honest self-criticism and social analysis are integral.

Conclusion #2: Emphasizing Healthcare Leadership of Color

Affirmative Action

Apart from the ability to cross cultures to build trust and understanding, there is also the matter of increasing the number of providers of color. More leadership of darker skinned people within healthcare will transform the cultures of institutions in ways that no number of diversity trainings can. Some quantitative studies have found that race concordance between patients and doctors aids patient satisfaction. Undeniably, many patients and doctors succeed in creating strong bonds regardless of race concordance or its absence. However, having more staff of various racial-ethnic backgrounds will affect medical cultures and assumptions in ways that are both broader and deeper than a singular focus on cross-cultural patient-provider relations. For example, care providers of color might propose changes for how various religious traditions are accommodated, for how language translation services are provided and for how a hospital connects with its surrounding neighborhoods and communities through education and prevention programs.

Such diversity among healthcare providers is especially needed at leadership levels — senior physicians and medical school faculty. Beef Stew observes that there are numerous staff of color at her hospital, even doctors, but not in leadership roles: "(T)here's plenty of doctors of color. I'm talking managers. I'm talking head honchos. I'm talking calling the shots. I'm talking, you know, nurse managers, vice presidents, CEOs, board of trustees. That is what'll make an impact." For substantive changes to take hold, it is not sufficient to have a diverse staff at the level of technicians, nurses, nurse assistants and clerical support.[20]

Presently, the racial-ethnic diversity represented within the general population is not reflected in the population of healthcare providers. Latinos represent fourteen percent of the total population and Blacks represent thirteen percent of the total population. Yet Latinos "make up 2% of registered nurses, 3.4% of psychologists, and 3.5% of physicians . . . and while one in 8 Americans is black, fewer than 1 in 20 physicians or dentists is black."[21] The Association of American Medical Colleges reports that as of 2000, nine percent of all medical school graduates are members of one of these four communities: African American, Asian American, Latino, and Native American. One current estimate is that within this total percentage, Latino graduates comprise 2.25 percent of the total population of medical graduates.[22] Latinos now constitute the largest and fastest-growing ethnic community (comprised of many differing racial-ethnic and cultural communities) in the United States. Yet their numerical growth within the ranks of healthcare professionals continues to sputter.

Unfortunately, change in this reality does not look promising. *The New York Times* recently reported that the current administration's budget does not see leadership of color as a priority: "President Bush's budget would cut spending for the training of health professionals and eliminate a $34 million program that recruits blacks and Hispanics for careers as doctors, nurses and pharmacists."[23] It is disturbing that such cuts are being proposed even as the administration has been criticized for trying to downplay the realities of racial-ethnic disparities in healthcare.[24]

Having drawn this conclusion, it is also important to not see the problem only as one of numbers. Good and Good make the case that the medical gaze is potent in training students to focus in upon certain information relevant when listening to and giving care to patients. In short, students of whatever color are taught to "speak the language of medicine." They argue that this culture is strong and pervasive even though there has been "a sea change in the gender, and to a lesser extent, the racial and ethnic profile of medical students. In addition, extraordinary developments in medical technology, biomedical science, and the political economy and financing of medicine and the delivery of healthcare appear to be subsumed into this culture and way of learning medicine."[25] Having more

---

ing them, who didn't have bedside manners. So, I mean, you would need to get to the root of it, you know, the top doctors who are doing the teaching.

20. Beef Stew later commented:

> When you put money, and when you put power behind that change? . . . When you make the price high enough that when you don't do it, you're going to feel it, guess what, change is going to come. And that change will happen when you get a black head nurse, when you get a Hispanic CEO, when you get an Asian board of trustees. . . . Okay, when you start reflecting diversity that way, on a high level, then guess what, that's when the change is going to come. Until then, you can put all the black staff nurses and all the Asian doctors and Hispanic whatever, anywhere you want.

21. *Associated Press,* "Report Urges Diversity in Health Jobs," 5 February 2004. They cite from the newly published Institute of Medicine Report, *In the Nation's Compelling Interest: Ensuring Diversity in the Health Care Workforce,* available online.

22. Brian D. Smedley, Adrienne Y. Stith, and Alan R. Nelson, eds., *Unequal Treatment: Confronting Racial and Ethnic Disparities in Healthcare,* 114.

23. Robert Pear, "Taking the Spin Out of Report that Made Bad into Good Health," *New York Times,* 22 February 2004, online: www.nytimes.com.

24. Recall the article: H. Jack Geiger, "Why is HHS Obscuring a Health Care Gap?" *Washington Post,* 27 January 2004, A17.

25. Good and Good, et al., "The Culture of Medicine and Racial, Ethnic, and Class Disparities in Healthcare," 599.

providers of color is essential, but it is not a simple solution to the complex nest of problematic disparities. The very way in which medicine and healthcare are taught needs substantial revision as well. Furthermore, ongoing race and socioeconomic class analysis is needed on the part of healthcare providers, students and educators.

The Imperative of Advocacy and the Impact of Bureaucracies and Bottom Lines

After surveying the extensive and growing medical sociological literature on healthcare quality disparities and interviewing a few patients and care providers, I have come to the conclusion that radical changes are needed in the structures of U.S. healthcare provision. Piecemeal approaches cannot sufficiently address systemic problems. A system where doctors are reimbursed different amounts for different patients — or even worse where they are compensated to attend to some but not others — already sets up structural care disparities in which some lives are more valued than others. Indeed, the political economy embedded within the financing, organization, and delivery of healthcare dehumanizes some by making available to others (those with the financial, political, and social resources) healthcare that is more comprehensive and better matched to their health needs and cultural backgrounds. Simply put, initiatives aimed at making individual providers more sensitive will falter miserably if they do not address the economic systems and institutional cultures in which the providers are supposed to learn and practice this sensitivity.

To make this case does not mean that no poor person or person of color receives good care. In fact, many, many do — the women with whom I spoke testify to this fact. Rather, the point is that regardless of the fact of whether or not some individuals encounter exceptional care, skill and compassion, an intrinsically unjust system is in place which contradicts the egalitarian principles and ideals to which it aspires. As Leonard Orlando, a white oncologist, put it to me in our conversation, "I'm very idealistic, and it's very important for me to be a human, humanistic. But I don't think the environment supports that. . . . (T)he system promotes — encourages us to be otherwise." Cavernous disparities in care due to combinations of access and quality issues mock and transgress the moral obligations of a democratic society. Therefore, the fact that some lives are more fully seen, valued and respected than others represents a serious moral problem with which ethicists, healthcare policymakers and theologians all must wrestle. In response to the failings of present structures, I offer two specific recommendations.

Conclusion #3: Funding and Support of Community Networks

Several of the women told me stories of how they were only able to access acceptable care because of a friend or a contact in a healthcare network that helped them make a change: Maria's daughter sought out care at another hospital; Luz would not have been able to get into a site of care she preferred without the help of a friend and the friend's sister-in-law (a nurse). As a nurse case manager, Beef Stew acknowledged that while she does her job for every patient, she takes additional time to educate patients who do not have many resources at their disposal.[26]

In short, without advocating for themselves along with the advocacy of others, many would have remained in care settings with which they were neither satisfied nor comfortable. Quite literally, advocacy and connections help you be seen. Consequently, I find that community not-for-profit support and information networks provide vital services to women. They help them process everything they are going through and make informed decisions.

I shudder when I contemplate the traps in which those who are ill and who do not have these networks or connections — those who are timid or isolated — may find themselves.[27] One of the breast cancer support group facilitators coordinates a Latina group to which predominately new immigrants come. Many of the participants speak only Spanish and some are undocumented. Many have no benefits or health insurance and find it difficult to attend the support groups after they are well enough to work. They cannot afford to stay at

26. Beef Stew confided:

> I will say — and maybe this is a bias — but I will say that, when I see a person of color, and it doesn't have to be a African American, can be Hispanic, Asian, you know, Middle Eastern person, anyone, a person of color who is especially disadvantaged, like may have Medicaid, no insurance, worker's comp, no fault, I tell you, I do go out of my way and work a little harder in regards to making sure that they understand the process. Because usually people that may be disadvantaged or indigent, poverty-stricken, maybe not educated and affluent, they don't know the process. And sometimes they're lost in it. Versus people who have really good insurance, you know, and who are rich and everything, and are affluent, well, they know the system.

27. A recent investigative reporting article by Katherine Boo recounts the story of Juana, an uninsured woman in Texas who died at the age of 36 of cervical cancer, two years following her diagnosis. Because she had no insurance, she was shut out of all of the for-profit hospitals near her in Cameron County, Texas. From the article, I believe Juana was not an undocumented inhabitant. Boo reports:

> While federal law requires those hospitals to treat the uninsured in emergencies — gun shot wounds, heart attacks — the institutions usually decline to accept uninsured supplicants who need chemotherapy, radiation, or other longer-term treatments. Juana, like most uninsured patients with advanced cancer in Cameron County, had to travel back and forth to the state public hospital in Galveston. It is an eleven-hour bus trip each way. (Katherine Boo, "Letter from South Texas: The Churn," *The New Yorker* 29 March 2004, 72.)

Texas has the highest rate of uninsured of any state in the union.

home during their recovery because of their need of the income, however meager.

This facilitator explained to me that many of these immigrants are scared — because of the cancer, because of their immigration status, and because of their very limited income levels. She observed that many of them come from cultures in which it is expected that patients trust their doctors and do not ask questions. These insights gave me a sense of why I may not have heard more immigrants complain about the quality of their care when I spoke to them at the support meetings. Indeed, the facilitator said that many of the Latina immigrants she has worked with are so afraid of dying or being deported that they are simply grateful for whatever care they do receive — even if there are no translators or doctors are rude, inattentive or hurried. Without groups such as The Witness Project of Harlem, Share, Cancer Care and Gilda's Club, many women would not have a safe place to ask questions, learn about their disease and treatment options and receive emotional support.

Moreover, these organizations intensively work to create deep connections in the communities they serve. Rather than using a white staff person coming to facilitate a group in Harlem or Queens, for example, all of the above organizations make it a priority to have group facilitators who share the cultural and racial backgrounds of the communities in which the groups take place. More ample funding and support of such community networks is essential.[28]

Unfortunately, these non-profit organizations, which rely heavily upon volunteers and donations, are not prioritized in healthcare funding budgets. Community health programs — community-oriented prevention and educational services — tend not to be emphasized by either government or private healthcare institutions. Many of the organizational representatives spoke to me how strained their budgets are and how precarious their futures can be from one year to the next.

Conclusion #4: The Value of Continuity and Choice

All patients benefit from the opportunity to work with the same provider over time so that trust and rapport can develop. On the other hand, they also benefit from being able to switch providers if they are uncomfortable with their care in a given setting. Given the social, economic and structural power imbalances, patients of color and/or lower socio-economic status need to be able to keep or change a given provider without fear of losing healthcare coverage. Hannah's story describes the experience of one woman who, because of the comprehensive and generous nature of her health plan, has felt free to interview prospective doctors as needed before settling on one. And once she has made her choice, she has not had to worry about a change in doctors being made without her involvement.[29] What amazes me is that Sandra, temporarily without insurance, forged ahead and switched doctors until finding one to whom she could relate to as a person. And it is important to note that she was able to do this both because she is a strong woman who is also a well-educated nurse and because she had nurse friends *and* contacts helping her to navigate her way through this harrowing time.

While having excellent health insurance is not a guarantee of receiving excellent care, what it *can* do (both literally and metaphorically) is buy more time. Not having to worry about what services and tests will be reimbursed or how many visits will be covered can create a context in which there are sufficient opportunities for women of color to break down provider assumptions and to build up relationships. Sophia's story represents one example of this transformation. She was clear that when her breast cancer was first diagnosed, she was able to get through to her doctors because she and they knew that they would be working together over time. There was continuity of care. She developed a strong relationship not only with her breast surgeon, but with her oncologist and the nurses and nurse practitioners as well. As a team of providers and as individuals, they crossed their cultural, racial, and socio-economic differences to come to know Sophia as a unique and valuable person.

The point is that such transformations take time. When I asked Sophia how it is possible for providers of differing backgrounds from a patient to create genuine relationships and to see the patient as a person instead of as a stereotype, she remarked that: "Unfortunately, it's not something that you can go in and change off the bat, like with people of the same race. Like if a white person goes in to see the doctor, there are no defenses. You know. Unfortunately, with me personally, it's something that comes in time." I then added, "So it's kind of like you have to work harder." Sophia responded: "Yeah. It's something that you — that, in time, kind of works itself hopefully and just disappears. And there's always the little underlining of, 'When are they going to show their true colors?' . . . Yeah, like, you know, I don't think now they think that there are any true colors. You know? I

28. Emilie Townes explores models of care that developed within and are particularly attuned to African American communities. Her analysis offers important alternatives to western cultural productions of health and also includes several constructive examples of African American community programs and education strategies. See Townes, *Breaking the Fine Rain of Death*, 147-167.

29. It is important to note that as of this writing, Hannah Jacobs lost her job after over twenty years of service due to corporate down-sizing. While I do not know the specifics of her prior company's situation or firing, it is reasonable to entertain the possibility that the high costs of health insurance for full-time employees figured in, at least in part, to the company's decision to cut back on staff numbers. If this were the case, it highlights the fact that in present healthcare and business climates, even those who are presently insured are not exempt from the threat of losing such coverage at any time.

think they see this is her true color. But I, you know, that took — that takes a little longer."

Ultimately, this need for continuity and choice means that universal healthcare needs to get back on the table as a serious topic for healthcare policy reform. Since the 2000 election, the bulk of congressional healthcare debate has taken the form of prescription drug coverage for seniors and what to do with respect to the internet availability (and substantially lower prices) of Canadian prescription drugs. Prescription drug coverage is a topic worthy of public debate. By itself, however, it makes for anemic healthcare reform. Current political platforms are a far cry from the healthcare reform agenda on which Clinton and Gore ran in 1992. Twelve years later, a comprehensive approach to healthcare reform is sorely absent from the public scene.

A form of universal healthcare may help to make healthcare less of a private commodity purchased by some and more of a public service provided to all. Without universal coverage, providers are compensated differently for different patients. Leonard, the white oncologist, laments that he cannot take Medicaid patients because the rates do not adequately compensate his services. Even as he defended the free market economy, he cautiously noted: "[C]ancer care is so complicated and comprehensive that it's hard to do a lot of pro bono work. But it wouldn't matter, a patient's economic status, if [doctors] had full-time positions. You know? With just a set salary."[30]

Leonard also noted that there ought to be fewer administrative hassles in order to give more time and better care. He complained that his days are too occupied by the piles of paperwork — not done only as medical charting — but as formulaic, duplicative documentation for insurance companies. Rebecca Williams, a white oncology social worker, also commented that her main frustration is that she has to spend an inordinate amount of time on paperwork, instead of offering psycho-social support to patients. Discharge planning has a tangible benefit to the hospital's finances; sitting with and listening to patients do not. Again, Leonard expressed a similar sentiment: "(M)y salary is very much tied to my productivity. . . . And the reality is . . . that insurance companies [don't] pay for an emotional investment, really. . . . You know, not that one wants to, you know, bill, you know, for compassion. . . . But the point is that there are constraints that are very much in place that force one to kind of keep moving forward and moving ahead."

Of all these collaborators who shared enlightening insights and experiences, Sophia spoke with the most candor and critical reflection. She had no trouble naming the fact that human beings arbitrarily create systems of meaning (such as those focused on wealth) and that in doing so, we have fashioned a world light-years away from what God wants for us. In not shying away from stark honesty, her words took on a prophetic quality for me. Akin to all genuine prophets, she knows that being real and speaking truth can put one in danger — they can "end up in the loony bin." I heard this prophetic voice most clearly at the end of our interview when Sophia described the ideological framework in which U.S. healthcare is conceived and given. Her incisive analysis needs no further introduction or commentary from me. Its wisdom speaks for itself. Indeed, without realizing its Greek meaning, Sophia chose her pseudonym well.

SA: It's this world that we've created. And money is something that's created. And, you know, gold is in the ground, I mean, that's, like, free, really, when you think of it. You know, we've made this — we've given it so much importance. And when you think about the rest of the world, like the backwoods, and we think that they're really primitive, but places in Africa and places in Nicaragua and places all the way back in the hills, they have medicine men who cure people. And they would never think of taking a dime for doing what is the most natural thing to do in this world, which is make you well if you are sick. People will give them food and give them donations. And . . . but they would never think of taking money for something that, in their eyes, is a God-given gift. And, you know, I think, you know, there are a lot of healthcare providers and healthcare facilities that try, you know, to do things. But in the math, in the math of it, you know, medicine is a corporate business. It's not a business of sacrifice like that anymore. I'm not saying that everybody's like that. And there's healthcare professionals out there who do. But I think self-sacrifice is, like, such a big thing. And I think that God would like that.

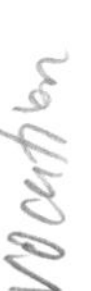

AV: But the context of the institution or the system isn't set up to facilitate that.

SA: No, no. And it all comes down to the almighty dollar that we ourselves have given all this importance to. Well, we still have to pay our bills and all that. I mean, there's got to be — I guess for people who don't have the same kind of faith, they have to have something to hold onto, and something that is important. So you can make up anything and make it important. I can make that picture important. I can make it the most important thing in this house, you know. But it really — that's what it is. It's not real.

30. Leonard's internal conflict on the matter of universal health coverage was apparent:

> (I)f everyone is flatly salaried, then regardless of what you do, either in quantity or quality, then the forces are in place to do as little as possible. . . . However, having said that, I think that we really all should be salaried, that there should be some kind of universal infrastructure, so that as physicians we are adequately compensated, and then have a little bit less or fewer administrative hassles. So, I do think that we need some type of national, you know if not, you know, national health insurance, some type of national healthcare system where we are adequately and appropriately compensated. . . .

AV: No.

SA: And I think that's what God wants. I think that's what God wants from all of us. You know?

AV: Yeah.

SA: It's really, really out there, though.

AV: No. But it's also just right here.

SA: Yeah. It's right here, which is why nobody's going to do anything about it.

AV: It's too close.

SA: It's too close. It's too real. And people that tend to be too real are the ones that end up in the loony bin.

Why These Stories Matter: Methodological Implications for the Doing of Ethics

Before drawing this work to a tentative close, I would like to discuss one last relevant area of analysis: implications this research has for the doing of social ethics itself. The conclusion I draw is simply this: It matters who is at the table. My research does not portend to solve the various problems related to healthcare disparities. Neither my desk nor brain is big enough to bear such weight. In other words, no single person or group is able to arrive at such a resolution. Indeed, well apart from offering the above constructive points for changes in healthcare delivery, I seek to contribute to changing the way in which we as academics search out these answers. Not only does the content of decisions fundamentally matter, *but the process used to come to them* matters as well. It is my conviction that adequate and dynamic understandings of dignity, respect or personhood only happen through the course of sustained and broad relationships and conversations in particular communities — and out of profound dialogue across difference. Moral deliberation and formation are neither one-time nor individual events. Even more, they are not the sole property of scientists, policymakers or academics.

This insight is as true for theology, the social sciences and healthcare policy as it is for social ethics. Across disciplines, a shift is needed in how we think about and tackle the pressing problems and questions facing us. With respect to healthcare quality disparities, those who have most directly confronted healthcare quality disparities ought to be at the tables and involved in setting the terms of the conversations convened to eradicate them. We need to find the answers together. Ethicists, physicians, social scientists, healthcare policy analysts and theologians all need the knowledge of those who may be laypersons with respect to our fields, but who know viscerally what it means to feel disrespected and disregarded in society.

James Spradley begins *The Ethnographic Interview* with a basic but crucial distinction: "Rather than *studying people,* ethnography means *learning from people.*"[31] In order to learn from people, you need to assume you do not already know what they are going to teach you. Spradley goes on to acknowledge: "Ethnography starts with a conscious attitude of almost complete ignorance."[32] The value of this insight is multifold and it is not limited to those in academia. First and foremost, I — whether I am a white scholar, activist, teacher, social worker, doctor, friend, or church member — will learn more if "what I think I know" does not get in the way of actual learning and listening. An even bigger payoff, especially in terms of the formation of a white scholar, is that when one is not overly focused on being an expert, but rather on being a person, there is great potential to cultivate humility both within one's vocational endeavors and inner spirit.

Moreover, there are ramifications here not only for individual scholars, but for entire disciplines. To put it bluntly: White scholars may profit greatly if/when we spend significant, sustained time and energy *outside* of libraries/offices and *inside* a variety of relationships and activities. I came upon inequalities in healthcare not primarily by deducing the problems from books of social theory, ethics and theology, but by listening — to patients, loved ones, and staff — and by working in relationship with them.

In a related vein, it would be helpful if more academics would push ourselves to speak and hear fluently second and third languages — not only to read or translate them. Even if English is a common language between a researcher and the people with whom she is working, meanings cannot be taken for granted. Semantic differences, even when the same language is being spoken, ought not be overlooked.

For example, especially when I, a white person, attempt qualitative research within communities of color, I do not want participants to translate meanings for me, to cease speaking their own language and begin to speak in ways that are more familiar to the white and/or professional ear. If I want to hear people in their own voices, then they need to not alter what they are saying to overly-accommodate me. The burden is upon me, the white scholar, to understand (or to learn to understand) what others are saying — their experiences, culture, worldview — in the fullest sense possible.[33] Of course, the persons with whom I am working will always be accommodating me to a degree, and every description is a translation. But the important point is that I must make every attempt possible to ensure that my descriptions flow as directly as possible from the concepts and meaning of the people with whom I am working or interviewing.[34]

For white academics to engage racism and white privilege adequately in our scholarship, we need to find avenues of contact and relationship with the people who most directly confront racial inequalities. Learning from

31. James P. Spradley, *The Ethnographic Interview* (New York: Holt, Rinehart and Winston, 1979), 3.

32. *Ibid.*, 4.

33. *Ibid.*, 18-22.

34. *Ibid.*, 24.

scholars of color is vital, and we need to ever expand our treatment of their texts. Yet we ought not stop here. The incorporation of works by scholars of color will be stronger and more credible if it bears out in relation to concrete movements, projects and experiences. It not only matters whom I have read, but with whom I worship, eat lunch, volunteer on weekends or evenings, lobby politicians and canvass the neighborhood. It takes time and effort to cultivate the sensibilities and skills within white academics that will curb the presumptuous and self-righteous qualities often present in white identity.

While not all white scholars will do formal qualitative fieldwork in their research, more ought to consider it. Moreover, there are other avenues for similar involvement (volunteering with grassroots organizations that address housing, poverty, education, environmental racism, prison reform, healthcare or migrant labor issues). I am well aware of the pressure to increase one's scholarly credentials, namely to publish books and articles. But perhaps an additional measure of an accomplished scholar ought to be given more weight: The hours one spends working with community programs dedicated to social, economic and racial transformation. Perhaps seminaries, colleges and universities might more intentionally promote and support the notion of a public scholar, whose task in whatever field is not only to advance knowledge, but to contribute concretely to the shaping of people and communities in which the scholar lives and works.

In sum, there is a claim upon all scholars in whatever field (and of whatever racial-ethnic background) to envision and create even a small corner of the good society. Intrinsic to any such creation is a specific claim upon me, as a white person and scholar, to cultivate sustained, concrete relationships with communities of color in entirely different life situations and vocations from myself. These kinds of practical engagements and relationships are of paramount importance especially for white scholars and other scholars of privilege. For if we do not get it right in our day-to-day interactions and relationships, we won't get it right in our scholarship either.

Catching a Glimpse of the Reign of God: What Solidarity Means

The theological case made by this [article] is this: For any theological description of what it means to be a child of God, or made in the image of God *(imago dei),* to be adequate, it needs to be concrete — incarnate — and reflective of the needs and experiences of the most vulnerable — in a city, in a region, in the world. From this theological starting point, I have argued in the language of ethics that for any positive change in healthcare quality to take place and last in institutional and interpersonal ways of being, we need attuned and sustained listening to those who occupy vulnerable positions in both society and healthcare settings. I am trying to envision and articulate what justice and solidarity mean and how they might be realized more fully, even if imperfectly.

Sustained and self-critical attention to those marginalized by systems of injustice is the only basis upon which efforts at solidarity are possible. Those in relative privilege (white, middle- and upper-socio-economic classes, the well-insured, the presently healthy, the educated, members of the First World) need to not only "care" or "feel badly" about the plight of those less privileged, but must also understand that we are both implicated and accountable for their life situations. In responding to economic globalization, Cynthia Moe-Lobeda defines solidarity this way:

> Solidarity entails seeing, hearing, and heeding what is obscured by privilege: people and other parts of creation destroyed, degraded, or impoverished by five centuries of globalization, culminating in the contemporary form. Said differently, people of economic privilege will seek out and hear the stories of those who experience globalization as a threat to life and will respond to those voices.[35]

Whether the topic is globalization or healthcare disparities, Moe-Lobeda's emphasis upon *seeing, hearing and responding to* the stories and peoples most threatened by present structures is crucial. Calls to solidarity ring hollow if they are not accompanied by profound efforts to listen, perceive, understand and respond. Listening on the part of the relatively privileged ought to involve a cost to the hearers — and a fundamental change in their dispositions and practices.

Moreover, solidarity necessarily involves recognition of others in their particularity and uniqueness. Differences are honored, not erased. No one is left unaccounted for or rendered voiceless. No one is superfluous. Everyone's unique heart, perspective, and abilities are needed. This is how I envision the reign of the divine. Rather than holding an autonomous and individualist notion of the self, Roman Catholic and Womanist theologian M. Shawn Copeland understands personhood only within the context of complex and diverse peoples living and working together. Indeed, such efforts at solidarity offer a glimpse of the dominion of God in which everyone in bright and varied array is present and participating. Copeland casts solidarity in an explicitly theological light by contending that attempts at solidarity are a way to worship God.[36]

Copeland's conceptualization of the relationship between personhood and solidarity calls those of us in positions of privilege to radical accountability: "If personhood is now understood to flow from formative living in

35. Cynthia Moe-Lobeda, *Healing a Broken World: Globalization and God* (Minneapolis: Fortress), 121.

36. She writes: "In this solidarity, the Creator is worshipped, the *humanum* honored, particularity engaged, difference appreciated. Solidarity affirms the interconnectedness of human be-ing in common creatureliness. . . . Humanity is one intelligible reality — multiple, diverse, varied and concrete, yet one." M. Shawn Copeland, "The New Anthropological Subject at the Heart of the Mystical Body of Christ," *CTSA Proceedings* 53 (1998): 42.

community rather than individualism, from the embrace of difference and interdependence rather than their exclusion, then we can realize our personhood only in solidarity with the exploited, despised, poor 'other.'"[37] The significance of solidarity is found not only in the possibility of social transformation or in an embodied respect for exterior differences, but also in its potential for inner transformation. Not only is the care of vulnerable communities at stake, but so is the moral formation of those less vulnerable — the affluent, the lighter skinned, the healthy, the well-insured. If we do not push ourselves and our communities to live and act in ways that are in solidarity with those socio-economically, politically and physically at risk, we stand to lose our own humanity.[38] When we put ourselves above such struggles or denying that we are inherently implicated, the formation of white and privileged beings continues to be woefully misshapen. The consequences are both devastating to others and shame-producing for us.

Indeed, we can be downright ugly and mean-spirited. Two of the care providers I interviewed, Beef Stew and Lucy Bristol, spoke of a personality characteristic that they would like to see disappear, which seems prevalent among both their white patients and colleagues. Lucy explained how she has noticed that white and/or affluent patients can be less appreciative of and feel more entitled to healthcare. She observed that they are less likely to say "please" and "thank you," whereas less fortunate patients "are so grateful for any little thing you do for them." She found that in the city hospital where she once worked, the patients (the vast majority of whom were impoverished and persons of color) were more respectful of the nurses than some of her white and affluent patients at the well-respected private hospital where is currently employed.

More than Lucy, Beef Stew was sharp in her description of this trait:

> It's amazing how people believe that they have this white card, and they can do anything that they want. . . . And I would really love . . . to find out how that has happened, so that we can knock that down. Because once someone gets taken down a peg, not to humiliate, but to understand that, look, you are not privileged because your skin is white, you're a blonde. . . . You're a human — take that off . . . you bleed the same way I do.[39]

I have started to refer to this pernicious disposition noted by Lucy and Beef Stew as a "white entitlement syndrome." Beef Stew makes a very important distinction: Calling white and other privileged people into accountability for our presumption is not done to humiliate us, but rather to stop allowing white persons and communities to be the center — the standard and the norm. "Taking us down a peg" is done so that we might be who we most truly are: human beings intrinsically interrelated and accountable to other varied, but equally beloved human beings.

Ultimately, combating white entitlement, privilege, discrimination and bias involves not only education, but conversion. People of privilege, perhaps especially the ones who espouse and cling to "good intentions," need vehicles for honest self-reflection. For example, I commented to Wanda that most likely healthcare providers do not want to/intend to look down on anyone. Yet when there are differences between providers and patients — race, socioeconomic class, HIV status, culture, religion, language — it is complicated to meet the other as a person. I then asked her how care providers might learn to more fully understand and respect people within such particularity. She responded:

> I think it takes a lot of soul searching within the individual self, you know, because I know people, they know that they're doing something wrong because I'm pretty sure they're getting complaints, you know, the way they may have treated a patient or something like that. They get complaints on that so they know. . . . But I think you have to be willing to accept that you did that, and be willing to make that change. But a lot of people are not willing to do that because they think, "Oh, it's not me, I'm not like that."[40]

Both hearts and minds of the privileged must turn in new directions in order to see and appreciate the humanity of others. This [article] has tried to articulate methodological steps that may facilitate the soul-searching and intellectual analysis needed. A combination of different and sharp tools are needed to cut through the tough, encrusted layers of denial that keep people's eyes, intellects and souls from seeing how our assumptions and sites of privilege wound the well-being of others.

The Possibility and Necessity of Making Normative Claims

All human beings will always have to re-evaluate the world we are creating or want to create. We must always be on the lookout for who is not among us, who has not spoken and who has been left out or put aside. Revision

37. *Ibid.*, 31-32.

38. See Jennifer Harvey, Karin Case, and Robin Hawley Gorsline, eds., *Disrupting White Supremacy from Within: White People on What WE Need to Do* (Cleveland, OH: Pilgrim, 2004).

39. On this point, Beef Stew encouraged me to see the film *A Day in Black and White,* which treats the differences in perception between Black and white people.

40. Wanda continued:

> And I think that's what helps me, that I can look at myself and say I don't want to be like that; or if I did something, I can just, you know, pray about it, and ask God to forgive me for that, and change, you know, work towards the changing, you know, because I am not perfect. And I pray every day that when I walk out of my house, that I could, you know, I would treat people with respect, that I will not look down upon people, you know, wherever — wherever I'm working and wherever I'm going. . . . Or, if I did something to someone, you know, that may have offended them, I can go to them and just, you know, apologize or something like that.

does not equal relativism in ethics. However, it does mean that all our expressions of justice, faith, right relationship, grace and love are approximations — finite and imperfect and ever in need of critical re-evaluation.

When we think we arrive at the last word or the final and complete sense of a value, virtue, principle or theological concept, we have fallen into idolatry. This statement does not mean there can be no norms. For me, to love one another as our self and to love God with everything we've got transcends time, space and context. Yet its meaning must always be worked out in the particular and in concrete relationships. What loving the neighbor means in one context may not look or translate exactly the same in another. Appreciation of this reality helps to keep the norms vibrant within embodied relationships and structures, rather than eroding into "pretty" but abstracted concepts that fail to be manifest in lived reality.

We cannot deny the impartiality of all knowledge or the particularity of social locations. Ironically, recognizing particularity may actually open the door to a kind of universality. In Carter Heyward's words, "Knowing our particular social locations and our limits . . . is intellectually empowering as a lens through which we may catch a glimpse of what is, paradoxically, universally true — that all people are limited by the particularities of their life experience."[41] The reality that all people are particular and limited in their knowledge and perspectives is something shared by all humanity. This fact shows again how deeply we need one another's stories, experiences and wisdom in order to arrive at adequate social norms. The descriptions, philosophies, theologies and perspectives of an individual or a relative few will not suffice. Human beings are forever and inescapably interdependent creatures.

Having said this, it is also imperative to recognize that some forms of relationality and interdependence are more desirable than others. Some structures and practices actively promote justice, health and right-relation. Others capriciously prey upon the needs of some while simultaneously profiting from the resources they possess. Undeniably, suffering, abuse and exploitation occur across cultures, societies, and nations. In the case of this research, U.S. healthcare quality disparities are a problem for which lighter skinned and affluent communities (found at all levels of government, healthcare institutions, insurance companies and lobbyists) are most pointedly accountable.

While the process of arriving at normative conclusions is arduous and fraught with thorny complexity, theological and social ethicists nonetheless have a responsibility to offer persuasive and compelling visions that carry normative weight and that hold privileged communities accountable. What is needed now, both in academic circles and also in the larger society, are thorough descriptions of present social realities along with constructive proposals for what ought to be and for how people ought to be regarded. Roman Catholic white feminist ethicist Margaret Farley understands that:

> An obligation to respect persons requires . . . that we attend to the concrete realities of our own and others' lives. . . . We can risk considering seriously the meaning the other gives to the world; building communities of support that have openness to the other at the center of their strength; surrendering our tendencies to omniscience without surrendering to despair; learning the particular content of just and fitting care.[42]

Respect for persons and difference does not negate the possibility of making normative claims. Human beings — as moral agents facing daunting and myriad injustices — dare not give up on creating pragmatic strategies and conceptual frameworks which foster right relationship among human communities living in a fragile and precious creation. Ventures into theological and social ethics are not sufficient if they stop at the place of description and deconstruction of present realities. We must also take the risk of offering constructive, bold and hope-filled vision.

As Copeland asks questions about differences, commonalities and solidarity, she articulates concrete measures by which to assess if the full humanity of persons is being respected or not. For insight into these questions, she turns to an understanding of the demands and obligations, which human beings (specifically Christians) must bear as fitting responses to the incarnation of the divine. In doing so, she offers the following description of human identity that is inextricably woven together with human responsibility:

> Our search for the humanum is oriented by the radical demands of the incarnation of God. . . . [T]o be a human person is to be (1) a creature made by God; (2) a person-in-community, living in flexible, resilient, just relationships with others; (3) an incarnate spirit, i.e., embodied in race, sex, and sexuality; (4) capable of working out essential freedom through personal responsibility in time and space; (5) a social being; (6) unafraid of difference and interdependence; and (7) willing daily to struggle against "bad faith" and resentment for the survival, creation, and future of all life. . . . Taken together, the various theologies for human liberation push us, in self-giving love, to forward this realization in "the forgotten subject" — exploited, despised poor women of color. Only in and through solidarity with them, the least of this world, shall humanity come to fruition.[43]

41. Carter Heyward, *Touching Our Strength: The Erotic as Power and the Love of God* (San Francisco: Harper & Row, 1989), 9-10.

42. Margaret Farley, "A Feminist Version of Respect for Persons," in *Feminist Ethics and the Catholic Moral Tradition, Readings in Moral Theology,* edited by Charles Curran and Margaret Farley (New York: Paulist Press, 1996), 179.

43. Copeland, "The New Anthropological Subject at the Heart of the Mystical Body of Christ," 34-35.

In this description, Copeland makes the connections between theology, anthropology, social analysis and ethics explicit. The full meaning and implications of these points may only be spelled out in particular communities of dialogue and action. What is clear is who is the normative anthropological subject. The test, then, will be if social, theological and medical ethics can remember this "forgotten subject" and if, in doing so, transformative practices, institutions and communities are creatively fashioned by imperfect yet beloved human beings working together for the sake of those most in need of love and care.

Sophia's words show the kind of contribution theological language can make in shifting the terms and frameworks for healthcare discussions. She spoke eloquently about what God wants from and for human beings. I asked her how she thinks God wants human beings to treat each other. She answered:

> What does God want human beings to do for each other? That's an easy one, although it's hard to practice sometimes. Everybody is supposed to be more Christlike. . . . That means that we're supposed to . . . treat each other kind. We are each other's keeper. And everything that I feel I deserve, you deserve. I mean, that's what God wants us to do. We're supposed to treat each other with humility. We're supposed to treat each other with kindness, with sympathy, with affection. This is what we're supposed to do. . . . And we're here to take care of each other. And if somebody — if we don't take care of each other, we're not taking care of ourselves. There's no way around it. We're all one people. There's no way around it. Anything that you do to me that isn't right, you're saying that it's okay — you're saying it's okay for it to be done to you. Right? I mean, okay, we have all this medical profession, and it's all well and done. The world in itself was made perfect, and there's a natural remedy for everything anyway. So we made up all of these other things around it, and we're wrapped up around it. But let's just keep it real. And that's what God wants us to do. And all of our creation, and all of our man-made things, we still, at the end, as human beings, have to keep it real.

I asked, "And how do we keep it real?" Sophia answered:

> By not getting caught up in all of that, and remembering at the end what it is that matters, and that is life. That is human life. And how it is that we're treated, and how fragile it is, and how much we can just lose it. At a blink of an eye we can be gone. And it all revolves around love. And love is, you know, a big thing when you think of everything that's thrown in there. It's hard to have unconditional love for strangers. You know? In a perfect world, that's exactly what it should be, though. Because we are — we're all blue blood until it comes out of our body. I mean, it's just — but that's in a perfect world. I mean, that's like, in this world right now, that's a fantasy. But that would be ideal, right? And I think that's what God would want. And He gave us the power of choice . . .

While she clearly sees the harshness of this world, Sophia also stays grounded in what is most real and in what most matters. She has not allowed the language and structures of meaning within corporate healthcare define ultimate meaning for her. Even if it means swimming upstream against strong financial, cultural and ideological currents, human beings have a choice. Sophia reminds us that God has given us all a crucial choice regarding how we will live, what we will value and how we will treat others. No singular entity — whether philosophical, scientific, bureaucratic, or biomedical — has the right to dominate the terms and frameworks for discussion of such critical matters.

The breadth and depth of healthcare quality disparities for darker skinned peoples and members of lower socio-economic classes communicate something important about how we as a society value human life. These disparities affect people when they are not only generally vulnerable within the structures of society, but when they are acutely vulnerable — when they are seriously ill. Those of us who are Christians profess faith in a God who knows and loves each strand of hair on each human head. We are called to love God and to love one another as ourselves. Thus, such disparities in care represent both a moral and theological crisis. Simply put, we are not seeing or loving our neighbors as fully as we ought.

A distinctive and important kind of learning can happen when human beings faithfully and descriptively hear and re-tell stories — whether they are scriptural, their own, or from another's life experience. Such listening can facilitate a kind of transformation within both the intellect and the heart of the hearer. In short, what I have attempted to do is to help close what can be a cavernous gap between abstracted numerical realities and the concrete lives of people with respect to healthcare quality disparities.

To do so, I have listened to just a few stories from a very few people, from Latina and Black women with breast cancer and from healthcare providers. My prayer is that my re-telling of their stories and perspective has been faithful and that it has neither idealized nor demonized any of them. The critical thing is that they are neither heroic exemplars nor utter failures, but human. The beauty is that they are unique and ordinary members of the human species. I hope that substantive reflection on these few individuals might help those who read this text to not lose particular peoples in the generalities and statistics of our times.

Indeed, I have seen professionals pass over statistics without being moved by them. One of my questions has been, "How do you get through to people?" It is relatively easy to post a set of principles on the wall which lists every patient's bill of rights to respect and to being treated with dignity. It is not as easy to embody them consistently — on both interpersonal and structural levels. While policies and laws can regulate much (never all) external behavior, they cannot legislate the kinds of interactions, relationships, attitudes and efforts that will make such respect and concern for dignity most deeply embodied and concrete. A genuine commitment to seeing people in a new light is a fundamental part of creating justice and social transformation.

While I have learned much from these collaborators, I cannot offer any perfect solutions for safeguarding human dignity across time and location. It is wise to recognize, as Ivone Gebara does, "We have no consistent record of humanity's progressing in virtues and moral values. Instead we have the impression that at each moment of our history, we have to learn all over again the meaning of giving and receiving respect."[44] My goal is not to create a universal ethical framework, but rather to add one additional way for individual and communal moral formation and discernment to happen that helps us to keep re-evaluating our tentative embodiments of larger ethical norms. Again, in Gebara's poetic words:

> To love the other as oneself has to be understood in concrete situations in which each individual, whether among community, friends, family, or work associates, is ethically obliged to place himself or herself within the skin of the other. A mutuality takes hold and transcends any principle or judgment deriving from already established dogmatic laws. We have to construct among different groups provisional agreements, always capable of revision, in order to allow the common good to be effective, not just a beautiful expression stated in a document, like the Universal Declaration of Human Rights, that lacks any force.[45]

Time and time again, human beings — moral agents — have to translate and implement what it means to love truly and deeply our neighbor as ourselves. This is our common gift and task. While humbling, it seems most honest to stay grounded in the dust, joy and particular dynamics of the times and places in which we find ourselves.

To discover anew what respect and love mean in the concrete is not simply an intellectual assent; rather, a conversion to love is required. Through meaningful encounters with those who most directly confront healthcare disparities and inequalities, perhaps we — social, theological and bio-medical ethicists along with those who work in healthcare — might not only learn about the disparities, but might also turn anew to our neighbor and glimpse the sacred. Equally important, perhaps this kind of learning will contribute not only to the amelioration of human suffering, but also to our own moral and vocational re-formation. Perhaps we will discover more concretely what it means for us to be responsible, accountable and present to another.

Latina and Black women with breast cancer have much to teach the larger society about healthcare quality. This knowledge embedded within their particular experiences may contribute a vital measurement for assessing the adequacy of healthcare policies and practices. Knowing one counts among the living can mean the difference between life and death, between healing and alienation, between redemption and despair. My deep hope is that attentive listening to those most vulnerable might make U.S. healthcare more humane for all persons.

44. Ivone Gebara, *Out of the Depths: Women's Experience of Evil and Salvation* (Minneapolis: Fortress Press, 2002), 96.

45. *Ibid.*, 142.

22 Starting a Free Clinic in a Rural Area: People in a Small Kentucky Town Pool Their Talents to Solve the Access Problem

William R. Grimes

Today millions of Americans lack regular access to health care. Although we usually think of such people as city dwellers, the fact is that many can be found in our nation's rural areas.

What can be done to help the uninsured and disadvantaged? If people are truly made in the image of God, and, as his children, have a right to his gifts, including health care; and if we as Christians and ministers of the compassion of God really have the desire to care for those most in need — what should we do?

One set of answers is offered by the Christian Community Development Association (CCDA), a Chicago-based organization that specializes in training Christian community leaders for impoverished areas. Born in rural Mississippi in the 1960s, the organization now has members around the world. (For more information about the CCDA, go to www.ccda.org.) The CCDA describes the plight of the uninsured as a "desperate condition" that calls "for a revolution in our attempts at a solution. . . . These desperate problems cannot be solved without strong commitment and risky actions on the part of ordinary Christians with heroic faith."

To its members the CCDA says: "Go to the people. Live among them. Learn from them. Love them. Start with what they know. Build on what they have. But of the best leaders, when their task is done, the people will remark, 'We have done it ourselves.'"

My own introduction to the plight of the uninsured came from one of my good friends, a nurse practitioner named Julia Maness. Julia was concerned about the fact that the hard-working poor of our area — rural eastern Kentucky — were not getting the health care they needed. Because of her concern, she had taken a job on a mobile clinic operated by St. Joseph Hospital in Lexington. The clinic, which travels around the area, specializes in treating the urban poor and uninsured in Lexington.

"We can do the same thing right here, in the hills of eastern Kentucky," she said to me one day. "Just imagine: We could have a mobile clinic and go from community to community with health care and spread the 'good news' at the same time."

From then on, each time we met (usually following services at St. Julie Catholic Church in Owingsville, KY), she brought up the idea. "When are we going to do this? It needs to be done now. Let's get it on the road."

Then, one day in December 1999, I was standing on the sidewalk in Owingsville, waiting to watch the town's annual Christmas parade, when my friend Dave Daniels happened to come by. Owingsville, a village of about 1,000 people, is in the mountains some 45 miles east of Lexington. Dave is a planner for the district's health department. I told him that I was concerned about the area's growing number of uninsured people. He was concerned, too, and he had the demographics to back up his concern.

Not long after this, Julia, Dave, and I began meeting regularly in the church basement to discuss the problem. We knew from our reading that it is necessary, before tackling such problems, to analyze the community involved and see what assets are available. According to one source, community development must start from within the community. "Development of policies and activities [should be] based on the capacities, skills and assets of lower income people and their neighborhoods."[1] Every community needs its "movers and shakers." But in order for a community to mobilize, everyone involved must participate to one degree or another. "Community builders soon recognize that these groups [composed of people with low incomes] are indispensable tools for development, and that many of them can in fact be stretched beyond their original purposes and intentions to become full contributors to the development process."[2]

Creating a Free Clinic

Here's how we went about "stretching" the Owingsville community to fulfill the promise of a free health care clinic.

Jeff, a carpenter who is himself uninsured, came first to our assistance and offered help with the planning. A local bank had given us the use of an empty store, but the building was in bad shape. The building had to be gutted and rebuilt. Jeff helped put up the new walls that would divide the structure into a waiting room, offices, a laboratory, and examination rooms. Charlie, a semiretired hardware store manager and electrician, put in new wiring. Danny, a contractor, directed the drywalling. Since

From William R. Grimes, "Starting a Free Clinic in a Rural Area: People in a Small Kentucky Town Pool Their Talents to Solve the Access Problem." *Health Progress* (St. Louis) 85.2 (Mar.-Apr. 2004): 23-25, 51. Copyright © 2004 by the Catholic Health Association. Reproduced from *Health Progress* with permission.

1. John P. Kretzman and John L. McKnight, *Building Communities from the Inside Out: A Path toward Finding and Mobilizing a Community's Assets,* Northwestern University Press, Evanston, IL, 1993, p. 5.

2. Kretzman and McKnight, p. 6.

Danny was uninsured as well, he became one of our first patients when the clinic finally opened.

Ron, who works at a local lumber company, got us discounts on building material. Scott, a journeyman plumber, put in all new plumbing, including five sinks and new water lines. Scott, who also has no insurance, has significant heart disease. We have been taking care of him for a year now.

Roy, who owns a heating and air-conditioning company, thinks I saved his life. Some years ago he came into the clinic where I worked complaining of chest pain. I started him on life support and sent him to the hospital in an ambulance. Now he is always eager to help and will get involved with me on any project. He installed a whole new heating and air-conditioning system in our building.

John, who does carpeting and other flooring, came to show us how to use the nail gun to put down the subfloor. He wound up doing most of the job and also donated the flooring. Mike, a retired judge who has spent his retirement putting in computer systems, asked if he could help. "Sure," we told him. "We need a server and five work stations so that our medical records will all be computerized." It was done. And all the labor and equipment were donated.

Many other people volunteered hours of painting, plastering, cleaning, sweeping, nailing, drilling — and in general made themselves available for other duties as well.

With two very important partners, St. Claire Medical Center, Morehead, KY, and the Gateway District Health Department (a consortium of four county health departments), we formed a coalition that we called NewHope Ministries, Inc. Our partners not only donated equipment to the clinic; as established not-for-profit health care entities, they also provided us with access to other equipment and materials.

Today, St. Claire Medical Center renders us technical support and does our lab work at a reduced rate. The district health department assists us by providing specialty care such as mammograms and pap smears. Another local health care facility, Mary Chiles Hospital in nearby Mount Sterling, KY, does our x-rays at cost and one of its radiologists interprets them for us. St. Joseph Hospital, which is sponsored by the Sisters of Charity of Nazareth, Nazareth, KY, has given us equipment and supplies as well as financial and spiritual support.

Money was sent to us by local people — some from "haves," but more from "have-nots." In a few months, we collected $25,000 from such sources. Other funding was provided in the form of grants, mostly from local organizations: the Kiwanis Club, local churches, banks, and other businesses. Some congregations of women and men religious also provided grants to help us get under way. The renovations cost $4,500 (about a tenth of their estimated market worth); the equipment for the clinic was free except for transportation costs.

We began renovating the building in July 2000. On October 19 of that year, we opened the doors of the NewHope Clinic to the public. We were warmly greeted by, among others, the local ministerial association, whose members circled the building holding hands and praying for our success. A reporter from the *Lexington Herald Leader* attended the opening, later telling his readers: "The whole thing has been thrown together over the last few months with a modest amount of donated money, a ton of volunteer labor, and more than a few prayers."[3]

But the best thing about the project was that we were able to get the community involved in — and excited about — the effort. The clinic is the child not of NewHope Ministries, Inc., but rather of the community of Owingsville, Bath County, KY.

Grace and Healing

As the Kentucky poet Wendell Berry so eloquently put it:

> The grace that is the health of creatures can only
> be held in common.
> In healing the scattered members come together.
> In health the flesh is graced, the holy enters
> the world.[4]

What have we created? We have created a tapestry (or perhaps, considering the region, a quilt) of individuals who have come together as a community to work toward a goal of helping others by creating a free clinic. We have taken a diverse group of people and formed them into a unified whole, one that represents all that is good and noble in this community. We have organized a group who, as disparate individuals, had a deep longing for unity and only needed a project under which to blossom.

Each time a needy person comes to the clinic for help and we are able to provide him or her with healing and caring, we do it in the name of the community. Each time someone longs to be of assistance to another, we give them a venue in which to do so. Each time a church group wants to answer the call to help those in need, we open a spot for them to share and care and give of themselves. NewHope Clinic is not the property of NewHope Ministries, Inc. It is the property of all the people of this area who have assisted us, or who need our help, or who have sent us donations, or who have helped us to create it.

In trying to organize my thoughts on "health care as ministry," I have found especially helpful the writings of Thomas Droege, associate director of the Interfaith Health Program at the Carter Center, Emory University, Atlanta. In an article about faith-based initiatives in health care, entitled "Congregations as Communities of Health and Healing," he urges "praxis, not theory."[5] Droege maintains that "we have a window of opportu-

3. Jim Warren, "Free Clinic Opens in Owingsville," *Lexington Herald Leader,* October 29, 2000, p. B1.

4. Wendell Berry, *What Are People For?* North Point Press, New York City, 1990, p. 9.

5. Thomas A. Droege, "Congregations as Communities of Health and Healing," *Interpretation,* April 1995, p. 119.

nity at this juncture of history to make a major contribution to health reform by recommitting ourselves to health ministry in congregations and communities and by giving priority to the needs of those who bear the greatest burden of suffering from preventable disease. We can meet the challenge with both vision and hope, confident of the presence and power of the One who said, 'I came that they may have life, and have it abundantly' (Jn 10:10)."[6]

Sojourners

After three years of service to this community, we have accumulated more than 1,350 patients and responded to more than 7,000 patient visits. In the beginning, we saw patients from 9 am to 5 pm on Thursdays; recently we have held clinic hours on Monday as well. We generally see from 30 to 40 patients a day.

Two key staff members receive minimal pay for their work. Fortunately, the clinic also has many volunteers, both professional and nonprofessional, who provide everything from medical care and nursing to administration and cleaning.

Because there is so much poverty in the Owingsville area, we offer care at no charge to anyone in the range of 200 percent of poverty. Seldom have we had an uninsured patient who was not eligible for our clinic's care. We consider persons with Medicare or Medicaid coverage to be insured and do not accept them as patients; however, we do help many Medicare recipients get their prescription medications through indigent drug programs.

After the clinic's opening, an editorial about it appeared in the *Lexington Herald Leader.* "Various studies suggest that the uninsured receive less medical care and are in poorer health than those who have health insurance," the writer said. "The health care safety net is broad, though fraying, in this country. The volunteers who are trying to shore up the safety net in Bath County by operating the NewHope Clinic are heroes. So are countless health professionals who provide free care."[7]

But we who had launched the clinic knew we weren't really "heroes." We were only doing what, as Christians, health care providers, and concerned people, we should be doing. We had decided that, as a group, we would serve others with the talents God has given us. Service to others is thus an exercise in justice. And justice is the first step toward peace. I have seen a bumper sticker that summarizes it quite nicely: "If you want peace, work for justice" (Pope John Paul II).

Jim Wallis, a social activist and editor of *Sojourner* magazine has written: "We don't have any blueprints for a new system. . . . At best, what we have are some spiritual guideposts and road maps. The process of change will feel more like a journey than a policy conference or board meeting. And the sojourn itself is a part of the solution."[8]

So those of us who seek health care reform are on a "sojourn" of faith and hope, love, and promise. Where will the sojourn lead us? How will we respond to the ever-growing need for health care? How can we overcome the obstacles that make modern-day health care such a bureaucratic quagmire? Seen this way, genuine reform looks almost Sisyphean.

The answer to this conundrum is to be found in faith. As one writer has said, "True faith — the only actually salvific faith — is faith informed by love, faith that becomes the practice of solidarity and liberation: orthopraxy."[9] Faith, in regard to service, is characterized by love in action. We who work in the NewHope Clinic are determined to help provide loving caring service to the marginalized of our society. We are on a mission to bring God's tender care and loving mercy to the working poor of Owingsville and the surrounding area. We are determined to be people for whom faith is more than a word, people who believe that faith is primarily a praxis.

How do we as health care providers look at our role in an ethical manner? I have come to believe that, ethically, we as providers of care are obligated to become the persons we were meant to be. But how do we become what we already are? How do we determine not only what God wants of us, but also what we are in actual fact in God's eyes? Thomas Merton wrote: "God utters me like a word containing a partial thought of Himself. A word will never be able to comprehend the voice that utters it. But if I am true to the concept that God utters in me . . . I shall be full of His actuality and find Him everywhere in myself."[10] Merton, it seems to me, is saying that in order to be myself I must abandon any idea of who I am and seek my identity in God alone. Only in absence of self and presence of the Self, can I truly act, and only then will my actions be completely honest and true. When I serve others, I do so at the very center of my self, and God does the work, not in me or in spite of me, but through me.

So I've come to believe that in order to be the best possible health care provider, person, activist, missionary, Christian, and parent, I must become fully what God wants me to be; I must allow myself to be discovered by God. "Our discovery of God is, in a way, God's discovery of us," Merton wrote. "We cannot go to heaven to find Him because we have no way of knowing where heaven is or what it is. He looks at us . . . and His seeing us gives us a new being and a new mind, in which we also discover Him. We only know Him insofar as we are known by Him."[11]

6. Droege, p. 128.

7. "Reality Check," *Lexington Herald Leader,* October 21, 2000, section A.

8. Jim Wallis, *The Soul of Politics,* New Press, New York City, 1994, p. 147.

9. Leonardo Boff, *Cry of the Earth, Cry of the Poor,* Orbis Books, Maryknoll, NY, 1997, p. 5.

10. Thomas Merton, *New Seeds of Contemplation,* New Press, New York City, 1995, p. 37.

11. Merton, p. 39.

23 Parish Nursing: A New Specialty

Abigail Rian Evans

Although the church has been involved for centuries in a health and healing ministry, as indicated in chapter I [of *Healing the Church*], now is the fullness of time for the church to develop new directions for its health ministries. The parish nurse movement has had a tremendous impact in the late 1980s and 1990s in helping congregations to begin a health ministry and provide the necessary leadership. Hence, it is important to understand something about it and how a parish nurse may revitalize a church's mission in health.

The experience and vision of these new health ministers are truly amazing. They collectively represent a large cross-section of the church in terms of age, geography, theology and, to some extent, racial-ethnic background. The energy, commitment, and vibrant faith are contagious. The annual Westberg Symposium sponsored by the International Parish Nurse Resource Center focuses on creative worship and an inspiring exchange of ideas.

The significance of the parish nurse has been documented in numerous sources. It is perhaps the fastest growing specialty within nursing today. The movement was conceptualized by Rev. Granger Westberg, a Lutheran clergyman. Parish nursing is a professional model of health ministry with the health minister being a registered professional nurse. A health minister does not have to be a parish nurse because it is a broader term inclusive of other disciplines. Here the focus is more narrowly on the parish nurse.

What follows is not a definitive description of parish nursing but some impressions based on personal experience over the past fifteen years.[1] In the mid-1980s, as director of National Capital Presbytery Health Ministries, I wrote parish nurse job descriptions; cohosted a television special in Washington, D.C., in 1990 on the subject; discussed parish nursing in my courses and lectures on health ministry; and was involved in setting up some of the early training programs. These experiences are supplemented by a review of the body of literature on the subject, conversations with health care professionals and pastors in the United States and the United Kingdom, and travel with my research assistant, Jane Ferguson, to selected parish nursing sites on the East and West Coasts of the United States.

1. This more definitive task is being accomplished by the International Parish Nurse Resource Center in Chicago, and potentially by the members and elected officials of the Health Ministries Association whose information is based on firsthand experience as practitioners in the field.

From Abigail Rian Evans, "Parish Nursing: A New Specialty," in *Healing the Church: Practical Programs for Health Ministries,* by Abigail Rian Evans (Cleveland, OH: United Church Press, 1999), pp. 153-175. Used by permission of the publisher.

Specialization in Nursing

The development of this new nursing specialty follows that of the clinical nurse specialist, which is recognized as a profession and legal designation for advanced nursing practice. The growth of nursing as a profession accelerated after World War I, necessitating differentiation and specialization. Specialization first occurred informally as nurses selected specific areas for practice and, through independent study and practice, became knowledgeable and skillful in caring for persons with specific needs.

Role definition is achieved through the development of norms, attitudes, standards, and new expectations that must be integrated through observation and participation. In the early years of parish nursing, since there were only a handful of nurses practicing this yet-to-be-designated specialty, a source to assist in role definition was the Parish Nurse Resource Center. The center was founded for the purpose of taking that learning of the original six parish nurses, the congregations they served, and Lutheran General Hospital, the partnering hospital, and making this learning available to all interested parties. One group of interest was the clinical nurse specialist (CNS). Some have cited it as an illustration of how nursing specialties began, which helps us to understand parish nursing.[2]

After World War II, Hildegard Peplau recognized the need for formal advanced preparation for clinical specialists and started the first clinical nurse specialist graduate program at Rutgers University in 1954.[3] She cited three reasons for initiating the clinical nurse specialist role: (1) increased knowledge germane to the field of specialization; (2) development of new technology; and (3) response to a hitherto unrecognized public need or interest. Sociological literature cites that changes in the complementary characteristics of a system or roles (such as in the health care system) are stimulated by technology, increased organizational complexity, and new output demands. Role differentiation implies the reallocation of existing role expectations to meet new organizational expectations.[4] The parish nurse movement is responding to these professional and sociological criteria for instituting a new nursing role, as well as being grounded in the theological framework described earlier.

2. Norma Small and Abigail Rian Evans, "Parish Nurses as Integrators of Health" (paper presented at the annual Parish Nurse Conference, Chicago, Illinois, September 1989), 19.

3. Ibid., 20.

4. Ibid.

The evolution of a new specialty has predictable and observable phases: role identification and differentiation, role definition, setting standards, educational preparation, justification, and certification. Most current nursing specialties have passed through these phases, but not all have followed this sequence.

Development of the Parish Nurse Specialty

Identification of a new role develops from the "soil of social organization."[5] The "soil" that has fostered the germination of the parish nurse role has been the need for an integrated approach to health and healing in response to soaring health care costs, a decrease in the overall health of the nation, and the absence of the religious community, especially the church, in health care. The increased health costs result from, among other factors, medical advances and increased technology, which prevent death from acute illness but do little to promote healthy lifestyles that prevent acute and chronic disease and injury. (See chapter 2 [of *Healing the Church*] for further discussion of this point.) The key to improving health lies with the individual and his or her lifestyle choices and in society's need to provide a safe and healthy environment. These issues are best addressed from the whole person definition of health and the responsibility of each individual to be a "good steward" of one's body. This also includes being one's brother's or sister's keeper in the areas that affect the abilities of others to fulfill health potential.

History of Parish Nursing

The historical roots of parish nursing stem from several sources. First, the early work of the Nurses Christian Fellowship by members such as Shelly Fish, Ruth Stoll, Norma Small, and others who affirmed the appropriate role of the nurse in the spiritual dimensions of health. The spiritual wellness inventory developed for use by nurses was one of the earliest instruments of its kind based on an integrated understanding of what constitutes health.

Second, as mentioned previously, the work of Granger Westberg in the 1960s in founding Wholistic Health Centers for primary health care, which included pastors, family practitioners, social workers, and nurses as a health team, created the aegis for parish nursing. Since the nurse was recognized as the health professional who most often held the team together, by the 1980s when economics and practicality inhibited the expansion of these Wholistic Centers, the idea of parish nurses was born. It began ecumenically in hospitals and parishes, and embraces an interfaith style.

Third, the black Baptist and Pentecostal churches' "church nurse" contributed to the historical precedent for the two terms coming together. The church nurse, who was not a trained nurse, was quite limited in her functions, for example, reviving those "slain in the spirit" with smelling salts — ministering to members becoming ill during a service. The fact that these churches recognized the church nurse in a generic sense as a part of the ministerial staff was an important contribution, though it was a nonprofessional nurse model.

In addition, deaconess nursing in Kaiserwerth, Germany, and Scandinavia through the Lutheran Church provided a model of parish nursing in the early 1800s that is still flourishing.

> Some schools, including the Lahti College of Parish Social Services in Lahti, Finland, incorporate diaconal education into the basic baccalaureate nursing curriculum. The curriculum at Lahti includes courses in parish social services, theology, ethics, caring science and caring theology. Diaconal studies are also available at the graduate level in both Norway and Finland. For twenty years the deaconesses were the only nurses in Norway. As the century turned, about 400 of them worked in various capacities.[6]

The most recent phase of parish nurse development is the establishment of the International Parish Nurse Resource Center and the publication of the *Parish Nurse Newsletter* and numerous books and articles. With experienced and strong leadership this center has provided the resources needed for such a fast-growing movement. It is now under the umbrella of Advocate Health Care, and its crucial place is (hopefully) secured. In addition, the founding of a national Health Ministries Association, a professional organization for parish nurses and other health ministers, testifies to the importance of parish nurses.

The parish nurse movement is timely as health care changes its main venue from the hospital to the community. The technological focus of the medical model has meant that medicine has mainly been practiced in the hospital setting for much of this century. But as managed care makes hospitals less profitable, the focus is moving to preventive health in the community, including the church.

With increased awareness that lifestyle is a personal responsibility, people are encouraged to take an active role in promoting their own health by learning more about health and illness and by practicing self-care behaviors, such as diet modification, exercise, and stress reduction. These activities are largely outside the formal health care institutions and health care reimbursement systems. They appropriately should be assumed within the mission of faith communities with their theological mandate to promote wholeness in the image of God and their breadth and depth in reaching all age, socioeconomic, racial, and ethnic segments of society.

5. Ibid.

6. Joan Zetterlund, "Kaiserwerth Revisited: Putting the Care Back into Health Care," *Journal of Christian Nursing* 14, no. 2 (spring 1997): 12.

The need for parish nurses is evident from their rapid growth in numbers from a handful in 1984 to more than 2,000 today.[7] The national Health Ministries Association has more than 650 parish nurses on its mailing list. In 1984 there were only six nurses working in six congregations — two Roman Catholic churches, and four Lutheran and Methodist churches.[8] How carving out this role from within and without the current health care system will impact on other legally and ethically defined healing roles, health institutions, including the church, and the health care system is one of the future questions.

Parish Nursing — a New Specialty

A reenvisioned understanding of health propels the church to an enhanced role in a health and healing ministry. The parish nurse is the best professional to help the church assume its central role. Nursing, which prepares and socializes its members into a whole-person, health-promotion, continuing-care-practice model, is the profession best prepared to integrate health and wholeness into the faith community's worship, education, and ministry. This is a practical way of including the church as a part of the health care system. Specifying a parish nurse signifies that she is not just a generic nurse located in a church but one who has additional nursing knowledge and skills and theological understanding of health and wholeness. Defining the role of the parish nurse and implementing this new concept have been the challenges facing the parish nurse movement today.

The American Nurses Association (ANA) in 1997 recognized parish nursing as a specialized practice of professional nursing, and the ANA adopted the *Scope* and acknowledged the *Standards of Parish Nursing Practice.* On the one hand, the definition of the parish nurse role is broad enough in scope to encompass the diversity in size, location, composition, and values of faith communities in which the parish nurse role may be implemented. The parish nurse is more than a community health nurse. On the other hand, in order to achieve clear identity and acceptance within the professional and health care communities, the definition is specific enough to allay territorial concerns of other specialties as well as give a clear picture to the consumers and employers of their expectations concerning investment of time and the church's resources. Parish nurses can only do the independent practice of nursing for which they are licensed. The uniqueness of parish nursing is its focus on the faith community, its members (families and individuals), and its ministry to the larger community. Several excellent curriculum models have been developed by the International Parish Nurse Resource Center and other institutions to address this scope of practice.[9]

Now that the specialty is defined and standards of practice developed, it must be justified through research based on practice and health outcomes. While we would like to think that the concept and goals of parish nursing are sufficient to secure economic support, even faith communities must translate their faith into economic reality. By means of analyzing cost-benefit ratios and measuring outcomes, churches can be good stewards of the resources entrusted to them by their members. Sources for funding of parish nurses are emerging as an important topic as their contribution is becoming more and more valued.

The last phase in a new specialty is attaining national recognition of the expertise demonstrated by practitioners of the role. In nursing this process, called professional certification, requires the demonstration of advanced knowledge and skill beyond the competent standards of the practice. The criteria for professional certification may be established by the American Nurses Association or other nursing specialty organizations and require a certification examination in addition to education and practice criteria. The next step will be developing a certification examination, but the cost, estimated to be $100,000, is currently inhibiting this step. Professional certification is frequently confused with "institutional certification." Institutional certification is established by an institution such as a denomination or health care agency to insure the qualification of those practices within the institution (such as clergy). These criteria may be standards of care and/or professional performance that are higher than the "competent" standards of practice recognized by the profession, but may not be recognized nationally as professional certification, the mark of excellence.

Now that the parish nurse has been accepted as legitimate within the profession of nursing, it must be embraced by the health care system, which includes the church, community agencies, and acute long-term care institutions. The task of defining and interpreting the parish nurse's role in relation to other healers and to the clients it will serve is crucial to role implementation.

The International Parish Nurse Resource Center has facilitated the definition process through its networking functions, annual meetings, curriculum, and resource materials and helped in launching the organization of the Health Ministries Association (HMA). As the preparation of nurses for the parish nurse specialty has become more formalized, their role is even more crucial. The HMA, which expanded from several dozen members at its organizational meeting in 1989 to more than a thousand members in 1999, both provides a society to establish educational standards and serves as a professional

7. Ann Solari Twadell, interview by author, December 1997, International Parish Nurse Resource Center, Chicago, Illinois. There are five thousand on their mailing list, but because of the loose use of the term "parish nurse," it is difficult to determine exact numbers.

8. "History of Parish Nursing," bookmark, International Parish Nurse Resource Center, Chicago, Illinois.

9. Practice and Education Committee of the Health Ministries Association, Inc., *Scope and Standards of Parish Nursing Practice* (Washington, D.C.: American Nurses Publishing, 1998).

membership organization. This may foster more cohesion within the specialty in the future.

From the norms and attitudes that have evolved thus far, identification of competencies has been determined so that education programs, whether continuing education or academic, can be developed. There has been extensive discussion about the need for a formal degree program versus continuing education to be a parish nurse. I was involved in piloting a master of arts in parish nursing at the Georgetown University School of Nursing in the mid-1980s, but the costs and time required to complete the degree made it prohibitive for nurses. These questions are being more and more debated but are not yet resolved. However, those calling themselves parish nurses are required by the "Standards of Professional Performance" to acquire the knowledge and skills to meet the competency level of the "Standard of Care."

Profile of a Parish Nurse

Parish nurses typically feel "called" to their profession, articulating the need to use the gifts God gave them by incorporating their faith with their healing profession. In the age of managed care, parish nursing offers a welcome relief to the mechanization and bureaucratization of health care. "One of the reasons we enjoyed parish nursing so much was that we didn't have to spend so much time with paperwork," remembers one seasoned parish nurse. "We had the freedom to 'be' with people in their joy and pain, and not be locked into time-consuming documentation."[10]

Parish nurses are registered professional nurses. They come to churches with different stories. Some are retired. Some are burned out by the medical profession after years of working in intensive care units. Others, in states where social services have been cut, are hard-pressed to find work in hospitals upon graduation from nursing school, and look to churches as an alternative source of employment. Still others have started to raise a family and are interested in part-time work. Common to all is a religious faith they bring to bear on the healing art they practice.

The parish nurse may be a member of the church she or he serves. When the church has not had a nurse to draw from its ranks, it has found that having a nurse who is not a member of the church, or even the same denomination, can be beneficial. Sometimes church members talk more comfortably about their concerns to a parish nurse who is not a church member because they are less worried about confidentiality.

Overwhelmingly, parish nurses are women. They range in age from their twenties, if they have just graduated from nursing school, to their sixties, if they are retired. Most parish nurses are of a mature age, more spiritually seasoned than younger nurses, who naturally tend to be more ambitious, eager to acquire new skills and advance in their profession.

In an age of malpractice suits and criticism of managed care, the parish nurse blows as a fresh wind or one might even say the breath of the Holy Spirit, offering compassionate care and nursing competence. The caring style of the parish nurse engenders confidence and trust on the part of parishioners, which may not exist between professional and patient in other avenues of the health care system. This spontaneous, wholistic approach to health, enhanced by the movement of the Holy Spirit, is the province of the parish nurse and signals what is missing in the current health care system. She or he can provide the catalyst for the church to rediscover its unique healing ministry. Granger Westberg, the pioneer of parish nursing, observed,

> A congregation willing to test out the idea of a parish nurse on their staff soon learns that this is an entirely new kind of nurse. She has entered this kind of nursing because she is convinced that traditional nursing makes it difficult for a spiritually motivated nurse to treat her patients holistically. Hospital protocol keeps her very busy doing mechanical kinds of good deeds, leaving no time for a listening ministry — to say nothing of a teaching ministry in which the Christian way of life can be understood as health enhancing.[11]

The distinguishing characteristic of nursing is its emphasis on care, not just cure, and on prevention through health education. Parish nursing forms the bridge between the medical establishment and the church/synagogue. Indeed, parish nurses find they must listen with a "third ear" to detect the deeper spiritual wound that may be behind a congregant's stated physical complaint. The calling card may be that the "scratch is getting red," but the parish nurse soon finds herself listening to problems about the person's marriage, stress at work, or sadness and depression. Her wholistic approach, which embraces a concern for body, mind, and spirit, offers the opportunity to uncover the deeper issues some people might be too intimidated to announce to the pastor or even admit to themselves.

Whereas most nurses usually see patients only when they are ill, the parish nurse sees congregants over a continuum of good times and bad, so she has a keener sense of when intervention is needed. In time of crisis, when a mother is grieving the loss of a child, the parish nurse is there to remind the mother to drink lots of water, the simple health habits a traumatized individual forgets and a pastor may overlook. By encouraging congregants to take care of their physical needs, the parish nurse helps

10. Anne Marie Djupe, R.N.C., M.A., "Documentation: Tracing Our History — Underlining Our Future," *Perspective in Parish Nursing Practice* 3, no. 4 (Park Ridge, Ill.: Parish Nurse Resource Center, winter 1993): 4. Of course, it is true that as the parish nurse movement has matured, they too are required to provide documentation for their work.

11. Granger E. Westberg, "The Church as Health Place," *Dialog: A Journal of Theology* 27 (winter 1988): 191.

them rally their own spiritual forces to deal with a crisis. She reminds people they have a body when they are in spiritual crisis and links them to the spiritual realm during times of physical illness.

Qualifications for Parish Nurses

The qualifications to be a parish nurse are partly related to the job description or self-defined role that she assumes. Her roles obviously affect the necessary qualifications. Generally, to date there has not been much rigor in required qualifications. In many cases being a registered nurse with a desire to work in a church either in a paid or in a volunteer capacity is considered sufficient. However, now that the scope and standards of parish nursing have been developed, that situation will change.[12]

The eight standards of professional performance, as set forth by the Health Ministries Association, accompany what one would generally expect from nurses, including proposed measurement criteria.[13] They cover quality of care, performance appraisal, education, teaching and sharing with colleagues, respecting of values and beliefs of others following professional ethics, collaboration with agencies and other health providers, continued research on parish nursing practice, and utilization of effective resources to achieve desired outcomes.

Early on, Iowa Lutheran Hospital spelled out several qualifications necessary for a parish nurse as it initiated positions and training in this new specialty:

The first qualification relates to *education.* The person should be a registered professional nurse with a current nursing license, BSN or RN, and active in a continuing education program relating to parish nurse responsibilities. David Carlson, Director of Parish Nursing, Meriter Hospital, Madison, Wisconsin, recognized this opportunity in the way his training programs were established when he was at Iowa Lutheran Hospital. He stressed the "pastoral model" rather than a "medical model." This experience-based education program is one year in length.

It begins with three weeks of intensive clinical pastoral education at the hospital, followed by an internship in a congregation(s). During the internship the candidate returns at regular intervals to Iowa Lutheran Hospital for seminars and collegial interchange. The curriculum seeks to develop competencies in pastoral care, community health nursing, wholistic health and wellness, psychological concepts, assertiveness training, and marketing and salesmanship.[14]

Second, in terms of *experience,* three to five years of nursing experience were suggested as a minimal standard, preferably in one or more of the following areas: public health, education, public schools, medical/surgical nursing, and/or emergency room outpatient nursing.

Third, the category of *personal* qualifications received the greatest emphasis. These included a broad range of qualifications: knowledge of healing/health ministry of the church; the practice of wholistic health philosophy; skill in communication and teaching techniques; knowledge in health promotion and of health services and resources in the community, including public health and hospice; motivation to grow personally and professionally with a knowledge of current nursing and health care issues; participation in church and community activities that contribute to professional growth and to the promotion of wholistic philosophy; knowledge of and compliance with the Code of Ethics of Nursing and the Nurse Practice Act of Iowa, including the practice of confidentiality and professional standards; membership in professional organizations; and individualized study programs. In addition, they suggested that a person should be willing to donate time as a parish nurse for a year with the possibility that the church would consider making the parish nurse a salaried person after a one-year pilot project.[15]

Salary of a Parish Nurse

The salary, unlike that of other professions, is correlated not with years of experience or training but with the available funds for these newly created positions. Funding for parish nursing is available through some church denominations, resulting in a church-based health ministry. But many hospitals also are eager to fund hospital-based parish nursing programs in churches. The hours and pay for parish nurses vary. Some work from five hours to twenty hours a week at the rate of roughly twenty dollars an hour. Others who are not sponsored by hospitals volunteer for the first few years; later their church may start paying them. However, if a volunteer parish nurse is doing an effective job, a congregation may realize her importance only after she leaves and not recognize the need for financial support. The majority of parish nurses still work as unpaid staff.

Style of Parish Nursing

Not only because it is a new specialty but also because of the grassroots development of the ministry, parish nurses must be flexible. Some have church offices with regular hours. Others prefer to go where the parishioners are, in their homes, at their church committee meetings, or after services on Sunday. One parish nurse began with office hours and found that no one came, so she went to the Sunday coffee hours, attended women's meetings,

12. The Parish Nurse Resource Center, Park Ridge, Illinois, and the national Health Ministries Association, with offices throughout the United States, work with the ANA to interpret the standards.

13. *Scope and Standards of Parish Nursing Practice,* 15-22.

14. Granger E. Westberg and Jill Westberg McNamara, *The Parish Nurse: How to Start a Parish Nurse Program in Your Church* (Park Ridge, Ill.: Parish Nurse Resource Center, 1987), 11.

15. Ibid., 61.

and started a Bible study group. Usually, the parish nurse combines office hours with a roving visitation schedule in the community.

Parish nurses network by going to parish nurse support groups organized either by the hospitals that sponsor them or by the Health Ministries Association chapter in their area. There they swap ideas and help one another solve problems they have encountered in their ministry. Parish nurses assert that the uniqueness of each program leads to collegiality. It is important that parish nursing continues to reflect individuality and creativity in its different styles that meet the local needs.

There is no such thing as a typical day in the life of a parish nurse. Unhampered by the exigencies of bureaucracy, parish nurses operate with a flexibility that allows them to respond to the moment. Consider, for example, the parish nurse who was called upon to distribute communion to a depressed and homebound elderly mother of five grown children who were their mother's caretakers. Taking the time to talk to the weeping mother, the parish nurse discovered that the source of the elderly woman's depression was a power struggle between her and her children. Much to her children's distress, she was refusing to take the medication that was keeping her alive because, as she saw it, her children were trying to force the medicine on her without respecting her desire not to take it. The parish nurse observed the psychological dynamics of an elderly woman unwilling to give up control to her children because of her pride and the deeper spiritual wounds caused by her feeling that her children no longer respected her. Acting on her medical knowledge, the parish nurse was able to determine that three of the four pills the mother was taking were essential for her life; the fourth pill was a painkiller that the mother could decide whether she wanted or not: giving the mother the choice to take this last pill gave back her self-respect. The parish nurse then did a role-play to teach the mother and the daughter how to communicate in a respectful way through listening and paraphrasing to each other what they had said in order to let the other know she had been heard.

Parish Nurse as Initiator of Health Ministry

Sometimes the parish nurse is a catalyst for a health ministry within her or his church, and at other times the needs of the church dictate the type of health ministry that unfolds. In some cases, a hospital will launch a parish nurse program in a church and provide financial support under community outreach before the church builds a budget for the program. Hospitals have found parish nurses to be much more effective in teaching preventive health than any mass marketing campaign. The parish nurse builds trust with patients and visits them one-on-one in their homes and in the church, where people feel safe and comfortable. It is not unusual to find a nucleus of interdenominational and even interfaith groups supported by a local hospital to implement a parish nursing program.

At one parish nurse support group sponsored by a local hospital, a salesperson for a health care company was there to promote the sale of a remote calling device for use by elderly persons in their homes to alert their families and the medical establishment for help in case they fell or were disabled. The danger of some hospitals' enthusiasm to launch parish nurse programs in churches as a way to market to their clients in the community is that they might be too overeager. Churches may take on parish nursing before they have had time to lay the groundwork for a health ministry program into which the parish nurse fits. However, this may be a moot point, considering that health ministries are often sparked by the start-up of a parish nurse program or at least simultaneous with it.

The churches may also launch parish nurse programs and then lodge them in the community after they have gained acceptance. When parish nurses start a health ministry program at their church, they ideally approach the pastor and church council armed with facts and an argument. They define health ministry and explain how it fills the gaps of the U.S. health care system, which has fewer financial resources and time to care for the poor, the elderly, and the unemployed. They point out that the majority of health care problems can be adjusted by lifestyle changes — a natural niche for the church. They quote Scripture that calls the disciples of Christ to address health. They speak of the need for advocacy, especially for the elderly who find the present health care system exceedingly complicated and difficult to negotiate. They present the idea of bringing the concept of the unity of body, mind, and spirit to the congregation. They can help to reenvision good health as a community responsibility, not an individual achievement, and propose a health ministry/parish nurse program supported by a commission of selected members from the congregation (including the pastor) who would serve as advisors to the parish nurse and evaluate her activities.

In many cases, parish nurse proposals have been enthusiastically accepted by the church governing body, but on occasion they are rejected. Confident in her call, one parish nurse whose request had been spurned asked the church to let her volunteer for six months, and then the church could decide whether to support a health ministry or not. The church was completely won over after six months and has been operating a thriving health ministries program for several years. In other cases, the nurse's ideas are readily accepted because the pastor is already aware of the benefits of the whole person health approach because she has practiced alternative healing techniques before becoming a pastor.

Pastor and Parish Nurse Collaboration

It is crucial for a parish nurse to be part of the church staff in order to give her credibility with the congregation: committees may come and go, but a staff member is viewed more seriously. A parish nurse knows she has arrived when her name is listed under the names of the pastor and the deacons in the church bulletin and on the church letterhead. Some parish nurses meet with the pastor on a weekly basis, especially to discuss whom they have visited, and attend staff meetings and retreats. Together they decide the course of action, working as a team to try to bring a person to a healthier place both spiritually and physically. As a team, the pastor and the parish nurse can ride on each other's coattails: if the parish nurse sees a patient she thinks is in need of deeper spiritual direction than she is equipped to provide, she alerts the pastor; if after a home visit the pastor is concerned that a person is not receiving proper care, or has a physical ailment, the pastor can call the situation to the attention of the parish nurse.

This need for a collaborative style was precisely the motivating factor to start a parish nursing program at one church in Pennsylvania where the pastor was making regular visits to a homebound church member only to discover that she was missing the cues of the church member's failing eyesight, which signaled advanced diabetes. The church member needed her legs amputated because of her untreated diabetes, a situation that might have been prevented had a parish nurse been on staff to recognize the red flags. However, it is not always the parish nurse who saves the day.

The pastor can offer the parish nurse perspective on what it means to heal, curbing the nurse's desire to cure and helping her negotiate the thorny theodicy questions. When the physician can do no more to heal the ill person, the task of caring for the patient is not over. As the patient struggles to adapt to limitations and pain, the parish nurse and the pastor are there to assist in that adaptation. In the face of suffering, all healers need one another's support. The doctor who pronounces the illness to be incurable, the patient who must adjust to the news, the parish nurse who cares, and the pastor who prays for healing are equally in need of God's grace. The key element that separates the parish nurse from other public health or community health educators may be her freedom within the religious community to emphasize and enhance the spiritual dimensions of health. At that point the cooperation between the parish nurse and the pastor is most fruitful.

The Parish Nurse as Part of the Health Care Team

The parish nurse does not do all of this work by herself. Though a nurse might be approached by the pastor to handle all the suffering and grief-stricken people in the church by herself, the wise pastor and parish nurse know that it takes a team to make a health ministry work; one person would be crushed by the challenge. Ideally, a parish nurse is part of an overall health ministries program. The standards of practice define her clients as the faith community, a family and the individual. There might be several health ministry programs in addition to parish nursing, such as grief support groups, parenting support groups, healing liturgies, and home visitation. Each group has a volunteer leader from the congregation who enlists the volunteers for that group.

The parish nurse is the glue that holds the health ministry program together by offering support and training to volunteer leaders and their volunteer recruits. For example, as part of the goal to integrate health into the spiritual teaching of the church, the parish nurse may need to work closely with the Christian educator. Her goal is to integrate health and wholeness concepts into the existing curriculum for all ages as well as to arrange special education programs dealing with specific problems such as teenage pregnancy. If the Christian education director perceives the parish nurse as competition for time and resources, the collaboration may be inhibited unless the director is knowledgeable about the overall health ministry team.

Since promoting self-care requires health education about diet and medication, professional nutritionists and pharmacists may feel that clients should come to them instead of the parish nurse for this information. Incorporating members of the congregation with health-related expertise into the health and healing program will not only enrich the program but also provide another source of integration rather than conflict. The role of the parish nurse must be well defined as integrating spiritual aspects of health and healing with the noninvasive, medical functions of nursing as prescribed by state regulation, lest physicians and nurses in the community become wary that the parish nurse will "take away their patients." Enlisting physicians and nurses in the congregation to help interpret the parish nurse role to community physicians may allay their fears.

Promotion of self-care and a whole person approach to health is viewed by some professionals in the medical community as anti-physician. But it is less threatening when viewed as the ethical right and spiritual responsibility of an individual to be informed and to make choices about health and health care according to a person's level of development and ability. The intervention by others when there is a deficit in self-care may reassure physicians that people needing medical diagnosis and treatment will be referred as appropriate. The parish nurse must know her limits and refer to specialists and qualified practitioners when the resources are not available within the congregation. In case management and referral of individuals and families the parish nurse may be perceived as infringing on the domain of the social worker. Once more, collaboration is the ideal in order to help the members of the congregation to reach their highest level of self-care in their journey toward wholeness.

Though a church can have a health ministries program without a parish nurse, or vice versa, churches may find each is weakened by the loss of the other. Without a health ministries program and a cabinet, the parish nurse finds it difficult to get the support she needs; without a parish nurse, the church misses out on the professional expertise the nurse affords the programs. Usually, the parish nurse reports to a health ministry committee, which may be organized according to the polity of the church into a commission, a committee, or a cabinet. At a United Church of Christ program, for example, the parish nurse first reported to a Mission and Service Commission but became so successful that a Health Ministry Commission was formed all on its own with a seat on the church governing body.

The Functions of Parish Nurses

There are an expanding number of models and functions of parish nursing. They range from an empowerment for health model to direct health care services, such as the measurement of blood pressure, to preventive, educational approaches. Parish nurses generally follow a preventive rather than a crisis model. A referral system is especially important for the maximum use of a parish nurse. She can fulfill various functions, enriching the church's health ministry and serving the health needs of the community.

Parish nurses typically offer services that fall into the seven categories of advocacy, empowerment, prevention, training, personal health counseling, liturgical and direct health care services, described below.[16] Besides these activities, the parish nurse organizes church health fairs where congregants can go from booth to booth and get anything from flu shots, to a cholesterol screening, to a foot massage. To help with large events such as health fairs and home visitation programs, the parish nurse draws on the doctors, nurses, and wholistic practitioners who are members of the church and are willing to volunteer their time. At one of these health fairs, the pastor of one church attended a booth offering stroke awareness in order to encourage parishioners to do the same. During the course of the screening, he discovered he had an atrial fibrillation, which prompted him to seek further testing that revealed he was heading for a stroke. Medication was prescribed along with a change in lifestyle that resulted in a loss of thirty pounds. He informed the parish nurse that he had renewed energy and felt better than he had in ages, an example that the parish nurse can serve an essential purpose by saving the life of the church pastor!

The functions described here reflect the variety of activities in which a parish nurse may be involved, although not every parish nurse offers all of these services since the congregation determines the needs. Sometimes these categories overlap. In advocating for parishioners, for example, a parish nurse models what people have the right to demand of a doctor, thus empowering them to stand up for themselves in the future.

Advocate

Often, parish nurses will advocate for the elderly or newly arrived immigrants in their congregation who have difficulty with English as they try to wend their way through the cumbersome and often complicated corridors of the medical establishment. Parish nurses will accompany parishioners into the doctor's office and explain what the doctor is prescribing. In many instances, parish nurses are able to secure patients extended stays in the hospital, occupational therapists, or a health care worker to take care of them at home. Because of their medical vocabulary and knowledge of how the system works, they are effective in accessing the health care system. In many ways, they bridge the gap between the health care system and the patient.

Parish nurses may be advocates for the family of a patient. For example, a wife who could not get her husband to go to the doctor asked him to see the parish nurse, and she was able to persuade the man to visit a physician. On a broader level, parish nurses may help the church advocate the rights of mentally ill or disabled persons or others in the community marginalized by their health condition.

Functional and ethical aspects of the advocacy role may bring the parish nurse into conflict with some physicians. Physicians may not welcome the parish nurse's flagging undetected health problems or changes in health status that they missed. Unresponsiveness by a physician may require the parish nurse to offer the patient other alternatives for care. As a health educator, the parish nurse will provide information about diseases and treatments and encourage the patient to ask questions about treatment and medications. These nursing functions that encourage patient independence may be viewed as interfering with the practice of medicine and create areas of conflict.

Empowerer

A key function of the parish nurse is to empower people to take charge of their own health. She can do this in a myriad of ways. Perhaps the most important is to serve as a resource about the health care services available in the community, from twelve-step programs to complementary health care practitioners, nutritionists, and medical specialists. By networking with other health care providers in the community (to locate free mammogram services and other preventive treatments), the parish nurse can open doors for people who then will be able to take healing into their own hands.

The parish nurse serves as a liaison between the church and a variety of community resources and services and often advocates on behalf of parishioners with these agen-

16. Some of these functions are mentioned in *Beginning a Health Ministry: A "How to" Manual,* ed. Maureen Ahrens and Joni Goodnight, produced by the Health Ministries Association, 3d ed., November 1995, funded by a grant from Lutheran Brotherhood Foundation, Minneapolis, Minnesota, containing photocopied materials from many sources around the country, and in the International Parish Nurse Resource Center material on the functions of the parish nurse.

cies. The complexity of the current health care system may overwhelm the average person, and parish nurses can help keep their parishioners from getting lost in the system. Parishioners have reported that they are tremendously grateful to the parish nurses for introducing them to many types of care they did not know existed. This may be especially true for those who are suffering from addictions and need self-help and support groups as well as information about treatment facilities; victims of domestic violence who are afraid to talk to anyone else can unburden themselves to the parish nurse.

Empowerment to heal by serving as a resource can take many forms. One parish nurse was asked to conduct a vigil service for a baby in her church who had died from SIDS (sudden infant death syndrome). The parish nurse prepared her sermon by calling the national hot line to find out all the medical facts about SIDS. By sharing information about SIDS during the vigil service, she communicated to family and friends that no one had neglected the baby. She conveyed to the parents that it was not their fault that their baby had died and they should not blame themselves. The parish nurse empowered the parents to be healed by supplying them with the medical facts to release them from their own sense of culpability. Hearing the facts from a nurse provided the parents with confidence in the information they could not have obtained from a preacher. This combination of the scientific with the spiritual and psychological was a healing moment for the family.

Health Educator

The parish nurse can fulfill the function of prevention by being a health educator. The nurse teaches or uses others to lead courses, seminars, and workshops for the congregation on a wide variety of health-related topics such as health maintenance, disease prevention, early detection through screening, the role of emotions in illness and, most important, an introduction to the interrelation of body and soul.

Through a variety of formats — seminars, conferences, classes, workshops, small discussion groups, individual sessions, newsletters, printed educational materials, and bulletin boards — the parish nurse seeks to raise the health awareness of the parish community and to foster an understanding of the relationship between lifestyle, personal habits, attitudes, faith, and well-being. She can offer workshops on a wide range of bioethical dilemmas and other health-related topics.

The nurse supplements her teaching with programs that feature qualified speakers from medicine, public health, physical therapy, social work, nutrition, and psychology, as well as ethics and theology. Physicians from the congregation also speak on their own specialties or general health concerns.

The nurse organizes and finds facilitators (possibly herself) for groups centered on particular issues such as weight loss, diabetes, divorce, stress management, arthritis, youth problems, problems of loss and grief, children of aging parents, and so forth.

Through health education, a parish nurse may highlight a monthly theme that conforms to the theme being promoted by the local health department or the American Medical Association. For example, a theme on the healthy heart prompted a man in a congregation who knew CPR (cardiopulmonary resuscitation) to come forward and volunteer to give free CPR classes to church members. Another monthly theme on nutrition inspired a long-time parishioner who had recently lost seventy-eight pounds to share his joy and regimen with other church members struggling with their weight. The individual formed a Weight Watchers group and called it "Soul Weights" (as a takeoff on Soul Mates), which now meets every two weeks at the church. Some people weigh in; others do not. Some have formed a walking group. About fourteen church members attend.

Of course, not every educational attempt is a success. Even though the parish nurse got an oncology nurse to launch a breast cancer awareness month one Sunday at her church, no one came. At another church, some church members walked out of a video presentation on how to do self-breast examinations because they were troubled by what they perceived as immodesty.

Often a parish nurse can spot a misdiagnosis. An active church member who complained of insomnia had been prescribed Benadryl by a doctor. Encountering the individual at church, the parish nurse first prayed with the man and then talked to him as they sat on a pew at the back of the church. The man soon disclosed his problems: he was sending money to his son who was in a drug rehabilitation center; he did not know what to do, and the problem was keeping him up at night. It was disturbing him so much that he was drinking heavily. Then the man revealed he was an alcoholic. His wife had been asking him to stop drinking for some time, but he could not see his wife's point of view. He needed another view. By listening to the man, the parish nurse helped him see his problem from another perspective, after which he started attending Alcoholics Anonymous.

Grief support groups are another avenue parish nurses use to help prevent disease and addictive and destructive behavior. Grief support groups are essential for children and adults going though divorce, death in the family, or a change of job to take them through the stages of grief and relieve the stress that results in disease. Grief support groups are invaluable to help immigrants name their unclaimed sorrow that stems from the pain of immigration, the confusion of a new language and who they are in a new land. The lack of support in this area explains why so many immigrant adolescents are in gangs and involved in drugs.

Trainer

One of the parish nurse's functions is to find volunteers who are naturally warm, understanding, and willing to listen to hurting people. These volunteers can be instructed to do even better what they are already doing naturally. They can become additional hands, ears, and eyes for the nurse as they make house calls on the sick, serve as small group study leaders, and participate in many other tasks. In large congregations the nurse by herself cannot begin to respond to all the needs, so trained volunteers can add tremendously to her effectiveness.

The parish nurse may guide volunteers to reach out, for example, to individuals who have recently sustained a loss or to families attempting to care for a family member recently discharged from the hospital. The services needed and provided are as varied as the human needs encountered.[17]

This training function is distinguished from the empowering one because the nurse is training church volunteers to be health workers with members of the congregation. The parish nurse's training function is central to home visitation programs that many churches have successfully launched with a cadre of volunteers under the direction of a volunteer leader, who in turn is trained by the parish nurse. The parish nurse at one church, for example, holds potlucks twice a year for the leader and twenty-two volunteers of her home visitation program. There, the volunteers are trained on how to listen effectively, start conversations, and pray with the people they visit. More technical training is required for the volunteers who agree to help the parish nurse with blood pressure screenings and inoculations. Often, the parish nurse trains pastoral staff in health education so they can minister more effectively to congregants. A priest asked the parish nurse, for example, to explain to him why babies are stillborn so that he could better counsel a family who was grieving in this situation. (One might wonder if he should have simply sent the parish nurse to meet with them.)

Personal Health Counselor

Creating an atmosphere in which parishioners are comfortable in sharing concerns, the parish nurse is available to all parishioners to discuss personal health problems, to recommend medical intervention when necessary, and to make home, hospital, and nursing home visits. This may be especially important in a medical emergency when family members are out of town.

The parish nurse usually works with members of the congregation, but also works with some nonmembers. She fills a missing ingredient in the health care system by providing a professional listening ear, assessing health problems, recommending and/or providing minor health care measures, and making referrals to physicians and/or community support services. She educates individuals in specific ways that they might better care for themselves and communicates good health concepts as a role model. She may also help people with instructions about their medications.

Minor health problems, when detected early, can be prevented from developing later into major illnesses. Likewise, individuals may be unaware of the relationship between their lifestyle and personal habits and their health problems. The visibility and availability of a parish nurse help parishioners recognize, acknowledge, and seek treatment for symptoms they might otherwise have ignored or denied. Also, the presence of the parish nurse may encourage parishioners to take more responsibility for their own health.

Often church members will approach the parish nurse with a physical ailment only to confess spiritual or psychological problems. At one parish in San Jose, California, an elderly woman came for a blood pressure screening. Her reading was alarmingly high, and the parish nurse suggested she see a doctor nearby. The woman said she had no problems, and the parish nurse invited her for lunch. It was over lunch that the woman opened up and told a story of benign neglect. She had recently arrived in the United States from Peru to be with her youngest son and his family, but they considered her meddlesome and said they did not want her to be so involved in their lives. The elderly woman was distraught. The parish nurse listened to the woman tell her story for five hours and then took her blood pressure; it was back to normal. The parish nurse counseled the woman to return to her homeland to be with her eldest son; there she would be happier, well cared for in a culture that honors the elderly.

Spiritual Counselor

This function is not to be a counselor in the technical sense of the word but to assist people to explore matters of health and faith. Unaddressed grief is believed to be one of the primary causes of people's mental and physical diseases, and it often manifests itself in anger. Parish nurses can help address this by encouraging people to cry and not to hold back their tears at funerals. One parish nurse considers her work with grieving families at funerals to be central to her health ministry. At the vigil service the night before a funeral, she helps the family plan the funeral and makes sure that each member of the family has a role to play in the service.

The parish nurse may assist overwrought people to decide what they should do and how to work with the pastor/priest/rabbi to plan the service. At a Catholic church in California, there had been a suicide/murder in which the husband had poured gasoline on himself and his wife and lit the flames that killed them as their two children, ages six and eight, watched. The parish nurse saw the children being excluded from the funeral planning process. She saw the critical need for them to be involved so they could find an outlet for their trauma. She adapted the existing liturgy to more fully incorporate

17. Anne Marie Djupe, R.N.C., M.A., Harriet Olson, R.N., M.S.N., Judith A. Ryan, R.N., Ph.D., F.A.A.N., with Jane C. Lantz, *An Institutionally Based Model of Parish Nursing Services* (Park Ridge, Ill.: International Parish Nurse Resource Center, n.d.).

and respond to the family needs. The children sprinkled the holy water on the coffins of their parents and took the flowers off their parents' coffins in order for the pall to be placed on the father's coffin by his brother and on the mother's coffin by her two sisters. These small acts made a great difference to the grieving children.

Some parish nurses are directly linked to the worship service by being trained to be chalice bearers at communion. Quite a few churches have healing stations where the parish nurse and trained volunteers stand on communion Sundays, either to the side of the pulpit or at the back of the church in the narthex, to hear the concerns of the people and pray for them while anointing them with consecrated oil in the name of Christ.

One parish nurse, Jean Wright-Elson, tells of the woman who said to her, "I wish to be healed of my breast lump." Alarmed that the woman might think prayer alone would address her problem, the nurse whispered that the woman should see her after the service. The woman did, and the parish nurse counseled her to see a doctor, which the woman had been avoiding because of her fear of the medical establishment. Through more prayer and the assurance that the parish nurse would accompany her to the doctor, the woman went to the hospital and discovered the lump was malignant and needed to be treated with chemotherapy. A radical mastectomy was not necessary because the lump was detected at the early stages.

Provider of Health Services

Within the limits of nursing education and licenses, parish nurses can provide some health services. Blood pressure screenings are very popular because they are noninvasive. They are also highly effective tools in preventive medicine; the three top killers — strokes, heart attacks, and diabetes — can be detected with a blood pressure reading. Churches are ideal locations for flu and other inoculations.

Some parish nurses have medical equipment for loan such as walkers, wheelchairs, crutches, commodes, and beds. The borrowers sign a liability form stating that they are borrowing the equipment from the church as a service to parishioners, and they will not sue the church if it does not work. In one church, the request for equipment was so great that the parish nurse said the place looked like Lourdes.

A related ministry may spring from direct services. In visiting a church member who had diabetes, for example, a parish nurse discovered the man had to stand on the corner and jump in a truck to get work as a migrant worker — work for which he often was not paid or which resulted in abuse. The parish nurse wrote a grant and received $200,000 to start a job center for migrant workers where they could find one of the few public showers in the city and decent work at a fair wage. General concern with welfare reform has led other churches to band together to combine resources in order to feed the poor.

Some churches have care teams that parish nurses organize and coordinate to respond to people who have been hospitalized and then are homebound upon release. One group of volunteers on the care team prepares food for a week to take to the patient; another group focuses on providing volunteers to pray with the individual on a daily basis; still another group helps around the house and gardens; if she can, the parish nurse tries to find someone who has suffered the same ailment in order to encourage the patient.

The Future of Parish Nursing

Parish nursing is developing so rapidly that future projections are hard to chart. As more parish nurses become incorporated into the health care system, they may become bureaucratized with reports and forms. If this serendipitous response to health needs becomes overly institutionalized, the unique contribution of parish nursing may be lost.

Joni Goodnight, a former president of Health Ministries Association, wrote, "Most of us in parish nursing love it because we're able to speak about Christ. We're encouraged to pray with our clients, and we're rewarded by seeing the peace that envelops them when they feel God's spiritual healing in their lives."[18] Parish nursing has become the ideal way of bringing together professional skills and one's faith. If parish nurses become public health nurses, they will have lost a valuable opportunity to change the face of health care in this country — not simply health education with a spiritual overlay.

Another challenge facing parish nursing is whether it can become truly interfaith. Although the movement has been ecumenical from the outset, it has been strongest in Lutheran, Presbyterian, Methodist, and Roman Catholic parishes. By the late 1990s, some Jewish congregations hired parish nurses, and those from Eastern religions are exploring this model. The question is whether the raison d'être of this specialty will lose its uniqueness and theological dimension in seeking the lowest common religious denominator or be enriched by those of different faiths.

18. Joni Goodnight, facsimile to author, 21 January 1999.

24 Austin Heights and AIDS

Kyle Childress

Fifteen years ago our congregation found out how true the old saying is: "Be careful what you pray for, because you may get it." We also discovered that God answers prayer in surprising ways. Austin Heights Baptist Church is a small congregation, but back in 1991 we were a lot smaller, running around forty people in worship on Sunday mornings. Even then we were half again larger than just two years before when, between pastors, the congregation had reached its low ebb and considered closing its doors. In other words, the word "survival" was a frequent part of congregational conversations, and we looked longingly at every young-family-filled minivan that passed our church on its way to somewhere else.

On a Sunday morning a church member handed me the front page of the local newspaper telling the story of a local organizing effort to provide food for some men who had been diagnosed with AIDS. These men had lost their jobs, many had lost their homes and apartments, and some even had been turned away by their families, all because they had AIDS. As a result, their most immediate need was simply finding enough to eat. They did not have enough money to buy food and in a few cases did not have the health and strength to go to the grocery store. The paper quoted a couple of these men as saying, "We've gone to almost every church in town and had the door slammed in our face every time."

When I read the story I knew what we were to do and I knew that God was calling us to meet this need. I just knew. And some of our church members knew as well since we gathered after the service to talk about it. Here were some people who were sick and in need of food, with no one else helping them. We knew what we had to do.

I knew all of this but I did not want to do it because it was going to be hard; it was going to take enormous effort and deep commitment and be full of grief and pain. These men with AIDS were going to die and we were going to be among those helping them die and I didn't know if we could do that or not. And I also knew that this was going to be full of controversy. Not only was AIDS a disease surrounded by fear and ignorance, but it was associated with men who were homosexual or were intravenous drug users, not exactly the constituency by which one grows a Baptist church in East Texas and certainly not the way to attract young families driving minivans.

From Kyle Childress, "Austin Heights and AIDS," in Health, *Christian Reflection: A Series in Faith and Ethics,* 22 (Waco: The Center for Christian Ethics at Baylor University, 2007): 70-73. Reprinted by permission. Available online at www.ChristianEthics.ws.

Beginning with a Food Drive

I met with the two young men trying to organize the food drive. They came to my office ready to fight. After having so many rejections from churches, they were not all that eager to have another conversation with a Baptist preacher. But after we listened to one another they said, "If you're willing to work alongside gay men then we're willing to work alongside a Baptist church."

So it began with leading a food drive, but of course it did not end there. Before long delivering food to men with AIDS turned into visiting the men, which turned into the most basic forms of care: taking them to the doctor (when we could find one who would see HIV/AIDS patients), running errands, going to the pharmacy, and so on. All of this led to the discovery that not all persons with AIDS were men: we met and began helping support families in which the mother had received an IV during pregnancy and the baby was born with HIV. We also discovered families, especially older East Texas couples whose sons were diagnosed with AIDS, upon whom the toll of caring in an atmosphere of ostracism was overwhelming.

We were involved in helping put together a fledgling organization called the East Texas AIDS Project (ETAP). At a party hosted by the ETAP board, I met Barbara Cordell, who had a PhD in nursing and public health. She had recently moved to Nacogdoches with her husband and she was writing the first Texas Department of Health grant proposal for money to fund ETAP. I walked through the kitchen where Barbara was making coffee; she turned to me and said, "Aren't you the pastor of Austin Heights Baptist Church?" After I nodded a "yes," she said, "My husband and I are going to join your church." I was taken aback; after having several prospects politely decline to join our church because of our AIDS ministry, this was a new experience having someone join our church because of it.

With Barbara in our congregation we were able to accelerate and improve the level of training of the congregation in caring for persons with AIDS. We learned how to prepare meals for persons with AIDS, our church nursery workers were trained in the care of HIV infants, and we organized the first of several special worship services "for persons whose lives have been touched by AIDS."

Gathering for Worship

We prepared and trained and planned for this first worship service, and we also prayed. We prayed a lot. We prayed because we were scared, partly because we did not know who would come or if anyone would come and partly because we were still trying to learn what to do when someone with AIDS did come to our church. We prayed because we wanted to practice the hope and hospitality of Jesus Christ for persons and families caught in a downward spiral of despair and ostracism. In other words, even though we knew that Jesus did not slam the door in people's faces, we were nervous about what would happen when the door was opened.

What happened is that we had people from the highways and the byways streaming in. This side of the New Testament I had never seen anything like it. Almost everyone in our own congregation showed up because we knew it was going to take all of us to do this. And though we expected a few people with either HIV or full-blown AIDS, we did not expect fifty. We certainly did not expect the large numbers of parents and grandparents and siblings and babies, families who had members with AIDS but could not talk about it.

Through the door people came, packing our little church. Bobby literally had to be carried by friends because he was so weak from being in the last stages of AIDS. Carl and Tim began crying when they came in the door because it had been so long since they were welcomed into a church. Bill confessed to me that his stomach had been in knots over the fear of walking back into a Baptist church. Brandy, sitting with a six-month-old in her arms, cried because her baby son had HIV from a blood transfusion she had received during pregnancy.

For the next two hours we sat together and sang hymns: "Amazing grace, how sweet the sound. . . . I once was lost, but now am found"; and, "What have I to dread, what have I to fear, leaning on the everlasting arms."

We read Scripture: "The LORD is my shepherd; I shall not want. . . . Yea, though I walk through the valley of the shadow of death, I will fear no evil; for thou art with me; thy rod and thy staff they comfort me"; and, "What man of you, having a hundred sheep, if he lose one of them, doth not leave the ninety and nine in the wilderness, and go after that which is lost, until he find it?"

And we prayed. We prayed out loud and silently. We prayed for one another, passing out index cards so people could write their requests down and share them. And we prayed lined up at four stations in corners of the sanctuary, where we put our hands on shoulders, and hugged necks, and cried together.

After almost two hours we were ready to eat. So we gathered around tables and ate together a potluck supper of epic proportions. Everyone had brought food, and at the conclusion sacks full of leftovers were carried out the door for folks to eat for days to come.

Understanding Our Prayers

Our congregation looks back at that worship service as the time when God answered our prayers. Since that night, we really do not worry over whether the congregation will survive or not. Many of the men who came to that first AIDS service ended up becoming active members of our church and we came to know them as our brothers in Christ and friends rather than someone with AIDS or someone who is gay.

I won't lie to you; it wasn't easy. We had frank discussions about AIDS and about sexuality and sexual behavior, heterosexual as well as homosexual. The hardest thing was that over the next few years we buried almost all of our friends who had AIDS and who had come to that first worship service.

Yet God answered our prayers. All the time when we were praying for God to help us survive as a church, we assumed that the operative word was "survive." Now we know that the operative word was "church." God helped us be the church of Jesus Christ. We were not called to survive, but to be the Church. All the rest was and is in God's hands. Thanks be to God.

One more thing: we came to be known locally as "the AIDS church." But one day the chair of the physics department at nearby Stephen F. Austin State University and a charter member and deacon of our congregation met the young family of the new astronomy professor. The wife, with her two-year-old in tow, asked, "Don't you go to the church with the AIDS ministry?" He said, "Yes, I do." "We want to join your church," she said. Well, they did join, and yes, they drove a minivan. Within a few years she was instrumental in starting the local affiliate of Habitat for Humanity. But that is another story.

25 Reform and Rationing: Reflections on Health Care in Light of Catholic Social Teaching

B. Andrew Lustig

Introduction

In this essay, I analyze two issues at the forefront of recent policy discussion — health care reform and health care rationing — in light of Roman Catholic social teaching.[1] It is important, as I begin, to identify and critique a position often deemed to be the conventional wisdom on the place of religion in policy debates. Many would assert that the claims of particular religious communities are irrelevant or unnecessary to the formulation and justification of public policy in a secular and pluralistic society. However, their easy dismissal of religious voices can be questioned on two grounds. First, they assume, with little or no argument, that the claims of religious communities cannot be justified in more general terms. If such common ground were indeed absent, it would seemingly follow that religious communities could not fully participate in policy formation because of constitutional concerns regarding the separation of church and state. However, this first assumption is demonstrably false. The facts of overlapping consensus, despite the varied theological, philosophical, and political viewpoints of those who achieve practical agreement, play a pivotal role in legislative pronouncements and judicial reasoning. Shared moral and legal conclusions on particular issues and common policy conclusions on appropriate societal remedies are possible despite the lack of agreement about the first principles at work in particular perspectives, whether religiously informed or not. Second, the tendency to disqualify the claims of religious communities from debates on public policy confuses the *process* of public discussion and debate, where the views of particular communities may exercise legitimate influence, with the *warrants* for and *justification* of policy choices, where parochial appeals are inappropriate.

The present essay is offered as an exercise meant to illustrate, through the lens of debates on health care reform and rationing, how Roman Catholicism has engaged the problematic of particularism in public debate and discussion. The essay falls naturally into three parts. After this brief introduction, I consider, in Part I, the theological warrants in modern Catholic social teaching on the nature and scope of health care as a positive right. In Part II, I consider the legitimacy of health care rationing in light of Catholic social principles that constrain health care as an individual entitlement according to the requirements of the common good. In Part III, I assess the relevance of Catholic arguments on health care reform and rationing to the broader secular debate on those issues. I conclude by suggesting that the Roman Catholic approach, while sharing affinities with consensus principles that can be developed on other grounds, also brings a distinctive perspective to issues of health care policy.

I. Health Care in Catholic Social Teaching

In Catholic social teaching since Vatican II, access to health care is seen as a positive right, i.e., a justified entitlement claimable by individuals against society. The warrants for that position are expressly theological, involving a number of themes and principles that, while interconnected, can be analyzed separately. The first is an appeal to the dignity of the individual made in the image of God. The second is an understanding of the common good, which, in contrast to secular liberal understandings, presents an organic vision of society with duties incumbent on institutions according to the purposes of society as established by God. The third theme, which is developed in the modern encyclical literature as an extension of the traditional emphasis upon the common good, is the regulative ideal of social justice. Social justice is a specific notion that enjoins institutions and, increasingly, governments to guarantee the basic material concomitants of individual dignity. The fourth theme involves an appeal to the principle of subsidiarity, first enunciated by Pius XI, which speaks to the intrinsic and instrumental value of meeting the basic needs of persons at the lowest or least centralized level of association and authority possible. Finally, certain Catholic writers have emphasized distributive justice as a decisive appeal that functions, in important respects, independently of the general institutional focus expressed in the language of social justice. Each of these themes or principles merits careful attention.

In Catholic social teaching, every individual has dignity because he or she is made in the image and likeness of God (Genesis 1:26) and has been redeemed by Christ (Ephesians 1:10). By the time of John XXIII, the material conditions required by individual dignity have been enumerated into a list of specific individual rights, including the right to health care, which must be safeguarded by responsible institutions. John says in *Pacem in Terris*:

1. Significant sections of this essay closely parallel my analysis of recent Catholic documents on health care in "The Common Good in a Secular Society," *The Journal of Medicine and Philosophy* 18 (1993): 569-87.

From Earl E. Shelp, *Secular Bioethics in Theological Perspective* (Dordrecht: Kluwer Academic Publishers, 1996), pp. 31-50. Used with kind permission from Kluwer Academic Publishers.

> . . . we see that every man has the right to life, to bodily integrity, and to the means which are necessary and suitable for the proper development of life. These means are primarily food, clothing, shelter, rest, *medical care,* and finally the necessary social services [emphasis mine]. Therefore, a human being also has the right to security in cases of sickness, inability to work, widowhood, old age, unemployment, or in any other case in which he is deprived of the means of subsistence through no fault of his own ([5], p. 167).

In John's successor, Paul VI, one finds a renewed emphasis on a theme central to the writings of Pius XI, namely, that "material well-being is not simply instrumental in value. It is not a means of a dignified life. It is, rather, *integral* to the standard of all moral value, human dignity" ([8], p. 79).

Throughout this discussion, one is struck by the general nature of papal pronouncements about what individual dignity requires. That level of generality is not surprising. The encyclicals are statements of theological and moral vision rather than policy recommendations. They provide more than a mere statement of ideals but less than a blueprint for specific choice and action. Nonetheless, the expressly theological basis of human dignity provides, albeit in quite general terms, a different and richer context for understanding the usual arguments about liberty and equality in secular debates about the right to medical care. In Catholic social teaching, although individuals are endowed with freedom, theirs is a freedom to be exercised in community. The latter emphasis is surely to be expected, given the trinitarian nature of the God whom Christians worship and in whose image they are made. That trinitarian understanding has specific moral implications. In the words of one commentator:

> . . . our trinitarian theology becomes a radical challenge to community. How can Christians say they believe in God if they are unwilling to put together structures that build human community and meet fundamental human needs? How can someone really claim to believe in the triune God and not feel a sense of outrage about the quarter of the U.S. population which lacks or is inadequately supplied with such a basic good as health care coverage? If we believe in the triune God as the very ground of community, the problem of our health care system is not just an ethical or economic or political problem. The problem is ultimately a religious or theological problem ([10], p. 105).

In light of the belief in God as Trinity, and in contrast to the polarities one often finds in secular debates about positive rights, Catholic social teaching elevates neither liberty nor equality to a position of unchallenged priority. Rather than seeing either value as trumping the other, Catholic teaching, especially since the time of John XXIII, presents liberty and equality as mutually accommodating principles.

The notion of the common good is a second characteristic emphasis in recent Catholic social teaching. Again, this appeal, much like the theological grounding for arguments about individual dignity, offers an alternative to those secular versions of political theory that emphasize liberty as either a side-constraint or as a primary positive value. Unlike approaches that begin (and often end) with an emphasis upon individualism, the common good is fundamentally social and institutional in its focus. It stresses human dependence and interdependence. However, the common good should not be interpreted as a Roman Catholic analogue to a utilitarian calculus. Rather, the common good is the "set of social conditions which facilitate the realization of personal goods by individuals" ([8], p. 64). The common good

> insists on the conditions and institutions . . . necessary for human cooperation and the achievement of shared objectives as decisive normative elements in the social situation, elements which individualism is both unable to account for in theory and likely to neglect in practice ([11], p. 102).

The common good need not be viewed as being in necessary tension with the rights of individuals, at least in encyclicals since the time of John XXIII. Rather, the common good functions in two important senses: first, it is invoked to temper and correct the inequities often associated with secular individualism; and second, it incorporates guarantees for personal rights and duties ([12], pp. 429-36). Still, in contrast to individualistic theories, a fundamentally social understanding infuses Catholic social thought. This social perspective is especially evident in Catholic teaching on the nature and scope of property, with implications for a number of positive rights, including the entitlement to health care. Theologically, men and women are imagers of a trinitarian God. Practically, this suggests that the claims of individuals to resources are limited by the claims of others for the satisfaction of basic needs. In hard cases, where choice is inevitable, John Paul II characterizes the conclusions of the tradition as follows:

> Christian tradition has never upheld [private property] as absolute or untouchable. On the contrary, it has always understood this right within the broader context of the right common to all to use the goods of the whole of creation: the right to private property is subordinated to the right to common use, to the fact that goods are meant for everyone ([9], # 43).

In this emphasis on property in common as a regulative notion, the common good emerges as fundamental. Individual rights and duties are seen as constitutive of the common good, but there are no absolute or unmediated claims to private ownership of property. Unlike perspectives that begin with the distinction between private and public resources as the unassailable datum from which moral analysis proceeds, the Catholic tradition does not deem individual ownership to be sacrosanct. Rather, common access according to use remains the relevant criterion according to which social arrangements and practices must be assessed, especially in the circumstances of a developed economy.

As a third theme, the Catholic tradition has emphasized, since its enunciation by Pius XI in *Quadragesimo Anno,* the so-called principle of subsidiarity. In one respect, this principle can be seen as following logically from the idea of the common good ([I], p. 132). Drew Christiansen describes subsidiarity as "another dimension" of the common good; subsidiarity, then, involves "the notion that responsibility is rightly exercised at the smallest appropriate level" ([3], pp. 46-47). Thus, problems that can be addressed by the small-scale initiatives of individuals or voluntary associations should be handled at those levels. Matters that can be solved by lower levels of governmental involvement (city rather than state, state rather than federal) should also be addressed at the lowest level possible to achieve effective results. As a functional corollary of the common good, such a prudential concern with efficiency is quite appropriate. Subsidiarity implies that "the first responsibility in meeting human needs rests with the free and competent individual, then with the local group" ([I], p. 132). Moreover, there is essential, not only instrumental, value in the moral involvement of individuals in the interpersonal forms of association that subsidiarity commends as a functional aspect of the common good. The common good, as I noted, involves the good of persons. Subsidiarity, as an expression of the common good, involves the intrinsic value of direct and immediate forms of the individual's responsibility to others.

However, since the papacy of John XXIII, there has been an increasing emphasis in the Church's social teaching on the necessity of governmental involvement in meeting the basic needs of persons. The principle of subsidiarity, then, bears two implications for health care reform proposals. As Keane observes:

> . . . Catholic social teaching on subsidiarity . . . can tell us two important things. First, we really do need to find a health care system which offers us some balance between private management and public management. . . . Second, in view of the increasingly complex character of health care delivery, it is only to be expected (and clearly "catholic") that more and more government management of health care will in fact be necessary. Thus we ought not to be afraid on religious/moral grounds of the fact that many of the major health care reform proposals which are being discussed in the United States today are calling for a significantly increased level of government involvement, at least in the financing of health care. In the end, Catholic social teaching may well help us to decide which of the current reform proposals seem best, by challenging us to consider carefully which proposal best mixes subsidiarity and socialization in our current health care context ([10], pp. 149-50).

To be sure, given the complex features of modern social and economic life, the links between property in common and the common good cannot be understood literally. Thus, since the time of Pius XI, the common good is usually linked with another idea characteristic of recent social teaching, viz. social justice. Pius XI invokes the notion of social justice as a "conceptual tool by which moral reasoning takes into account the fact that relationships between persons have an institutional or structural dimension" ([8], p. 54). In contrast to atomistic understandings of individual rights, Pius emphasizes social justice as a regulative institutional principle. As societies develop, as medicine progresses, institutions, especially at the governmental level, are morally required to mediate the claims of human dignity and to shape the content of human rights, including the right to medical care.

Another emphasis in recent Catholic social teaching has been the so-called "preferential option for the poor." Although this option is sometimes invoked as a separate appeal, it can be viewed as a practical implication of the three broader themes discussed above: the positive rights of individuals, the common good, and social justice. In service to these values, institutions are required to respond to those inequities between and among individuals that particularly threaten the dignity of the most disadvantaged in society. Whether one views the preferential option for the poor as an implication of more fundamental values, or as having independent standing, the practical results at the level of social policy, about health care and other social goods, are likely to be the same.

Finally, some recent perspectives have emphasized the need to invoke distributive justice as an appeal that functions somewhat independently of the more general focus of social justice. Philip Keane is representative of this trend, especially in relation to arguments about health care reform. Although Keane is sympathetic to the broad critique of health care institutions afforded by the language of social justice, he is skeptical about the precision it affords regarding the practical questions associated with health care reform and rationing. Thus he says:

> . . . reform of the structures of society so that society can more effectively deliver health care still depends on society's having a clearer focus on just what health care goods it ought to be delivering to people. Thus, while the social structures question, like the equality question, is a pivotal aspect of all justice including health care justice, my judgment is that the distribution question (i.e., What health care benefits must we provide?) is the most central of all the justice questions which relate to health care ([10], p. 138).

Keane continues in a cautious vein:

> If we focus too much on social justice, the risk is that we will emphasize the structures necessary to furnish health care instead of first focusing on the human need of real persons to have real health care crises adequately addressed. Such emphasis on structures without a prior commitment to genuine human needs can raise all the

> fears of complex bureaucracies without really substantial goals ([10], p. 139).

For these reasons, Keane believes that the principle of distributive justice should assume moral priority in debates about reform and rationing. In developing this claim, he appeals to the work of Protestant theologian Gene Outka on the requirements of distributive justice in health care [13]. Outka views health care needs as discontinuous from other basic needs. According to Outka, medical needs are randomly distributed, to a significant degree "unmerited," often catastrophic, and to a great extent unpredictable. Outka therefore sees critical health care emergencies as having an immediacy and urgency that distinguishes them from other sorts of deprivation. Given that distinctiveness, Outka concludes that "similar treatment for similar cases," based on a criterion of medical need, is the fairest canon of distributive justice among various alternatives that have been proposed for health care delivery. Keane characterizes Outka's conclusions in this way:

> . . . with careful reflection and dialogue, we should determine those health care needs which we as a society must meet as a minimum standard, and then provide those needs for everyone, regardless of merit, usefulness, economic ability, etc. Such an approach means that there will be some possible health services which will not be provided because they are not truly needs or because they are beyond our capacity as a society of mortals who must face the fact of death ([10], p. 142).

II. Two Recent Catholic Documents on Health Care

I now turn my attention to two recent Catholic documents that focus specifically on health care, one the U.S. Bishops' "Resolution on Health Care Reform," the other a moral analysis of health care rationing by the Catholic Hospital Association entitled *With Justice for All?* I have several reasons for analyzing these documents in some detail: first, to discuss the warrants at work in their arguments; second, to scrutinize and critique several conceptual and practical tensions in their respective recommendations for public policy; and finally, to use the documents as points of reference for Part III's brief overview of the relevance of theologically based arguments to secular policy debates.

A. The U.S. Bishops' Resolution on Health Care Reform

The recent "Resolution on Health Care Reform" by the U.S. Roman Catholic bishops provides the occasion for a closer look at the way that basic principles of Catholic social teaching on the right to health care have been brought to bear on general issues of health care reform. In its introduction, the resolution identifies the fundamental problems that beset present health-care delivery: excessive costs, lack of access for many Americans, and questions about the quality of the care provided. The bishops address the document to the "Catholic community" *and* to "the leaders of our nation" ([15], p. 98). The document, although at times expressly theological, also attempts to speak to the broader public, primarily through its appeals to human dignity, which can be justified for both theological and non-theological reasons, and by its expressions of concern about the plight of those presently underserved by the U.S. health care system.

The resolution appeals to the recent tradition by rooting its approach to health care in the three fundamental themes I discussed in Part I. First, "[e]very person has a right to adequate health care. This right flows from the sanctity of human life and the dignity that belongs to all human persons, who are made in the image of God." Health care is a "basic human right, an essential safeguard of human life and dignity." Moreover, the bishops' call for reform is rooted in "the priorities of social justice and the principle of the common good." In light of these fundamental values, the bishops judge that "existing patterns of health care in the United States do not meet the minimal standard of social justice and the common good." Indeed, "the current health care system is so inequitable, and the disparities between rich and poor and those with access and those without are so great, that it is clearly unjust" ([15], p. 99).

The bishops also appeal to a preferential option for the poor as a particular implication of the common good. Pointing out that the "burdens of the system are not shared equally," the bishops conclude that we must "measure our health system in terms of how it affects the weak and disadvantaged." Fundamental reform must be especially concerned with "the impact of national health policies on the poor and the vulnerable." In this context, the bishops quote with approval a recent ecumenical statement on the common good; to wit:

> More than anything else, the call to the common good is a reminder that we are one human family, whatever our differences of race, gender, ethnicity, or economic status. In our vision of the common good, a crucial moral test is how the weakest are faring. We give special priority to the poor and vulnerable since those with the greatest needs and burdens have first claim on our common efforts. In protecting the lives and promoting the dignity of the poor and vulnerable, we strengthen all of society ([15], p. 98).

As a final appeal in Section I of the Resolution, the bishops invoke the prudential notion of "stewardship." The cost of present health care in the United States "strains the private economy and leaves too few resources for housing, education, and other economic and social needs." In response, "[s]tewardship demands that we address the duplication, waste and other factors that make our system so expensive" ([15], p. 99).

The practical focus of Section II of the bishops' resolution raises the same cluster of thematic concerns in more focused fashion. In this section, the bishops set forth eight practical criteria by which to judge the moral adequacy of proposals for reform. The criteria are as follows: (1) respect for life, (2) priority concern for the poor, (3) universal access, (4) comprehensive benefits, (5) pluralism, (6) quality, (7) cost containment and controls, and (8) equitable financing. Given the brevity of the resolution, these criteria are not adequately developed, but as a whole, they emerge as practical expressions of the fundamental theological values that inform the Catholic tradition on health care. At the same time, because the bishops clearly intend these criteria as useful guides for assessing public policy, it is important to note certain conceptual and practical tensions between and among the various criteria. For purposes of the present discussion, I will focus on the first four.

Overall, the criteria are based on considerations of human dignity that are theologically based: thus, "reform of the health care system which is truly fundamental and enduring must be rooted in values which reflect the essential dignity of each person, ensure that basic human rights are protected, and recognize the unique needs and claims of the poor" ([15], p. 100).

The first principle, respect for life, speaks to the need for any reform proposal to "preserve and enhance the sanctity and dignity of human life from conception to natural death" ([15], p. 100). Nonetheless, "sanctity of life" does not, of itself, shed light upon *how* to proceed in cases when "hard choices" involving allocation of resources must be made between and among individuals, all of whom might at least marginally benefit from continued provision of care. Moreover, the relevance of this first principle to certain "hard cases" (including abortion and the status of persistently vegetative patients) is unclear, since the grounding of "personhood" claims in these instances may depend on theological understandings of "ensoulment" or capacities to "image" God that are not available as warrants for secular policy.

The second principle — priority concern for the poor — implies, according to the resolution, that any reform proposal should be judged as to "whether it gives special priority to meeting the most pressing health care needs of the poor and underserved, ensuring that they receive quality health services" ([15], p. 100). Here the difference between according the "preferential option for the poor" independent weight or interpreting it as a particular implication of the common good may significantly affect how one assesses a particular reform proposal. While it is doubtless true that working correlations between overall indices of poverty and poorer health can be drawn, it is not the case that for any particular indigent individual, health outcomes will necessarily be correlated with access to health care. Indeed, there are strong arguments, doubtless of a more prophetic sort, that reform of health care as a discrete sector may be one of the least effective ways of improving the *general* health outcomes of the poor as a class. Overall poverty, not simply limited access to medical care, may be a far more relevant determinant of health than the bishops' second criterion suggests.

With regard to medical care, then, the preferential option for the poor will require greater attention to a definition of the "poor" for whom preference is to be shown — those who are "generally poor," according to most indices, or those who are "medically indigent." To the extent that the unclarity persists, the relevance of the criterion for any particular patient, as compared with its relevance as a working generalization about classes of persons, will not be obvious. Indeed, for any particular patient, the first criterion, "respect for life," might suggest that general indices of poverty, in contrast to criteria relating specifically to medical need or medical indigence, may discriminate unfairly against a needy patient who would not (at least initially) qualify according to the former indices.

By contrast, if the "preferential option for the poor" does not have independent weight but instead is seen as a particular application or implication of the common good, then determinations of medical indigence or medical need might proceed apace with difficult judgments about basic social goods other than medical care. On this account of the preferential option, the common good might be invoked as a systematic consideration to limit the availability of resources for particular individuals as the result of prior social choices, independent of individual circumstances of need. In this scenario, one might then be able to distinguish circumstances that are admittedly unfortunate from those that are unfair ([4], pp. 342ff.).

According to the bishops' third criterion, any morally acceptable proposal must provide "universal access to comprehensive health care for every person living in the United States." A number of practical questions arise here. How shall the system be reformed in order to provide genuinely universal access to comprehensive benefits? What implications might this principle have for conscripted medical service to presently underserved areas, especially in rural America? Alternatively, if one relies on market mechanisms and incentives to expand access and availability, how will such competitive economics work to ensure entitlement on a universal basis? In addition, should citizenship be morally decisive in determining access to available services? The wording of this criterion would suggest that health care coverage be limited to those within the United States but also that all persons within U.S. borders (not only citizens) be provided care. Practically, this may pose significant difficulties, since the costs of such care, indiscriminately provided, may undercut the willingness and/or ability of taxpayers to fund a basic level of health care for all.

The fourth criterion offers a benchmark of "comprehensive benefits" for any morally acceptable reform proposal. Comprehensive benefits include those "sufficient to maintain and promote good health, to provide preventive care, to treat disease, injury, and disability appropriately and to care for persons who are chronically ill or dying" ([15], p. 100). Again, the choices and tradeoffs required among these various goods might well conflict with the focus on particular individuals seemingly implied in such principles as "respect for life" or "universal access." Health care "sufficient to maintain and promote good health" for a given individual may be, in effect, a black hole, since that person's needs, according to the fourth criterion, might swallow an inordinate amount of resources to which others with lesser needs might otherwise have access. Moreover, as noted above, medical services may be fairly low among overall indices for health. Thus criteria for "health care" reform, if invoked without sufficient attention to the multifactorial nature of good health as an outcome, may be coopted by tendencies already present in technology-driven medicine to misallocate funds that could be better spent on primary or preventive care. Finally, only "caring for" those who are chronically ill or dying might involve a number of rationing choices that, while supported on grounds of the common good or social justice, fail to comport with the individual focus of other criteria.

As noted above, Section II of the resolution sets forth a number of other practical criteria for assessing reform proposals, which, while interesting, emerge as fairly "commonsensical" in tone. By contrast, Section III lists four "essential priorities" that the bishops urge upon their readers in applying their eight criteria of assessment: (1) priority concern for the poor and universal access; (2) respect for human life and human dignity; (3) pursuing the common good and preserving pluralism; and (4) restraining costs ([15], pp. 100-101). Although each of these priorities merits scrutiny in its own right, I will focus on key tensions generated by the bishops' discussion of the first and third priorities.

In their discussion of the first priority — concern for the poor and universal access — the bishops voice strong support for "measures to ensure true universal access and rapid steps to improve the health care of the poor and underserved" ([15], p. 100). In light of that commitment, they "do not support a two-tiered health system since separate health care coverage for the poor usually results in poor health care. Linking the health care of poor and working class families to the health care of those with greater resources is probably the best assurance of comprehensive benefits and quality care" ([15], pp. 100-101). Nonetheless, in discussing their third priority — preserving pluralism — the bishops emphasize the following:

> We believe the debate can be advanced by a continuing focus on the common good and a healthy respect for genuine pluralism. A reformed system must encourage the creative and renewed involvement of both the public and private sectors. . . . It must also respect the religious and ethical values of both individuals and institutions involved in the health care system ([15], p. 101).

While it is true that both priorities, as normative generalizations, may help frame policy discussions on health care reform, the potential for tensions between a commitment to a single-tiered system and a respect for pluralism of individuals and institutions is, as a matter of practical policy choice, enormous. Moreover, in light of the theological convictions central to the broader Catholic discussion of health care, considerations of individual liberty and dignity, as well as of the common good, might reasonably lead to a different practical conclusion; viz., that two tiers of health care delivery are both morally appropriate and practically preferable, so long as universal access to comprehensive basic care is assured. Consider, for example, basic education as a useful analogy to health care: a tax-based commitment to education for all citizens does not prevent individual parents from paying for alternative "basic" schooling for their children. It is not obvious, at least without a great deal more argument than the bishops provide, that health care should be viewed differently. Nor is it obvious, in light of the general theological warrants analyzed in Part I of this essay, that the common good would necessarily dictate the priority of equality over liberty in the delivery of health care.

The bishops' tendency to ignore or underemphasize conceptual and practical tensions among criteria and normative priorities is instructive for several reasons. First, it indicates that the bishops often conflate hortatory and pragmatic concerns in their discussion. Second, it suggests that a great deal more by way of careful, practically oriented, argument will be necessary before their assessment criteria and normative priorities can be viewed as significant contributions to the policy debate. Third, as I will conclude in Part III, the conceptual and practical tensions in the bishops' discussion will require the discriminating reader to identify the various modes of moral discourse at work in their recommendations in order to appreciate the different ways that Catholic themes and principles may be relevant to secular discussions.

B. The Ethics of Health Care Rationing

In Part I we discussed a number of relevant theologically grounded principles in Catholic social teaching on health care. We have seen how the bishops' resolution addresses general issues of health care reform. I turn now to a consideration of how Catholic themes and principles may function in judgments about the legitimacy of health care rationing. Here, because I am considering rationing along the lines developed by the Health Services Commission in Oregon, a brief review of the Oregon plan is in order.

1. The Oregon Model of Health Care Rationing In 1989, the Oregon State legislature passed the Oregon Basic Health Services Act. The Act established a Health Services Commission, which was charged to develop a "priority list of health services, ranging from the most important to the least important for the entire Medicaid population." The purpose of the Act was to permit expansion of Medicaid coverage to all Oregonians up to 100 percent of the federal poverty level, and to do so by covering only those services judged to be of sufficient importance or priority. In effect, rather than providing extensive medical coverage for only some of the poor, Oregon chose to provide limited coverage to *every* poor person, as measured by the federal poverty standard.

The most recent version of the Oregon list ranks about 700 medical procedures according to their effectiveness. Depending on how many procedures can be financed from the Medicaid budget, the state will draw a line — paying for every procedure above the line but none below. Initially, Oregon has agreed to underwrite the first 568 procedures — thereby excluding, for example, treatment of common colds and infectious mononucleosis.

There are a number of important features to the Oregon proposal that require attention. First, the Oregon Basic Health Services Act of 1989, if its proponents are to be believed, was meant not as an effort to institutionalize rationing of health care for the poor, but to begin a *process* that will, if successful, establish a unified system of setting health care priorities that will eventually cover the vast majority of Oregon's citizens. There are three separate bills that comprise the approach. The Basic Health Benefits Act expands coverage and access by extending Medicaid eligibility to Oregonians below the federal poverty line. Priorities will be set for preferentially funding services that are judged to be the most effective in contributing to length and quality of life. If funding restrictions occur, procedures with the least potential for benefit will not be offered. The Act will establish statewide managed care through prepaid plans and other mechanisms designed to contain costs while ensuring access and coordination of care. A second Senate bill, the State Health Risk Pool Act, would establish a Medicaid Insurance Pool program for "medical uninsurables," that is, persons who do not qualify for Medicaid and who cannot now qualify for coverage because of preexisting conditions. The Act sets out the ways that state and private insurers will subsidize the pool. Finally, the so-called Health Insurance Partnership Act, if passed, will mandate that four years after the implementation of the Basic Act, employers must provide health benefits that can be purchased through the state insurance pool. The benefits package offered by employers must offer coverage equal to or greater than that provided in the Medicaid benefits package. Any employer who does not provide insurance to all permanent employees and their dependents by a specified date will be taxed at a rate that approximates what would otherwise be the employer's contribution toward insurance.

2. With Justice for All? The Ethics of Health Care Rationing Beyond the general development of health care as a right constrained by common good requirements in the encyclicals, there has also been a recent focused discussion of health care rationing offered by the Catholic Health Association (CHA). The CHA document, *With Justice for All? The Ethics of Health Care Rationing*, provides the most focused analysis to date of health care rationing, in light of Catholic principles.

Chapter Three of *With Justice for All?* on "The Public Policy Context" develops eight criteria for assessing the "ethics of rationing." These criteria can be summarized as follows. First, the need for health care rationing must be demonstrable. Second, health rationing must be oriented toward the common good. Third, a basic level of health care must be available to all. Fourth, rationing of health care should apply to all. Fifth, rationing should result from an open and participatory process. Sixth, the health care of disadvantaged persons has an ethical priority. Seventh, rationing must be free of wrongful discrimination. Finally, the social and economic effects of health care rationing must be monitored ([2], pp. x-xi).

Several of these criteria might, at first glance, appear to justify Oregon-like efforts to devise acceptable strategies for Medicaid rationing, while others would seem to disallow such selectively targeted efforts. Although the need for rationing may be "demonstrable," given the rise in health care inflation and the lack of coverage for so many uninsured and underinsured persons, Catholic principles would appear to dictate rationing as a last rather than a first or even intermediate resort. Thus easy or early recourse to rationing as the only practical solution to issues of cost, quality of care, and access may undercut prior efforts to eliminate inefficiencies and waste. Nonetheless, if Oregon's priority-setting is the first step in a more comprehensive process that will lead to systematic scrutiny of the efficacy and cost-effectiveness of medical services, Medicaid "rationing" may work in tandem with practical efforts toward more comprehensive reform.

Moreover, Oregon's plan, again if seen as a first step toward more systematic reform, seems, relative to the status quo, to be oriented toward the common good. As the CHA document notes:

> Clinical medicine must always be oriented to the best interests of every individual patient. However, public policy choices governing the distribution of health care services beyond the level determined to be each person's right must consider the common good. An ethically acceptable rationing scheme must limit expensive medical services, when necessary, in a way that is fair to all ([2], p. 21).

Again, assuming the best case scenario for the eventual passage of all three bills, Oregon's priority-setting will define for the vast majority of all state residents, beginning with the Medicaid population, what the right to basic care means. Rather than rhetoric, the scope of the entitlement to basic care will be specified. Every poor person, and ultimately all those who, while not poor, are uninsured or uninsurable, will be able to claim a meaningful entitlement. That willingness to set priorities — denying access to low-rated services and procedures while expanding access to cost-effective and efficacious care — appears at least in principle to be oriented to the common good. So too, assuming that the Oregon Medicaid experiment is in fact a first step toward comprehensive reform, the Basic Health Services Act will do much to help establish a basic level of health care for all who are presently marginalized — the poor, the uninsured, the underinsured.

However, Oregon-like proposals are problematic in light of two other criteria set forth in the CHA document. According to the fourth criterion, rationing should apply to all: "Those who construct and implement a health care rationing system are likely better to understand its effects on others if they, too, are required to live within the limitations they construct" ([2], p. 22). And again:

> Only when rationing applies to all can it be the occasion for sharing a common hardship rather than an occasion for deepening the gaps between wealthy and poor, old and young, healthy and sick, and among racial groups. Equity in rationing would suffer if a significant minority of the public obtained their care outside the health care system while acquiescing to limitations on services for those who were economically less secure ([2], p. 23).

This suggestion — that rationing should apply to all — is a criterion obviously at odds with our usual assumptions about two tiers of health care delivery being an inevitable part of health care in the United States. Given the general Catholic discussion of private property and its limits, this criterion is perhaps unsurprising, and indeed, there are two points that might be mustered in its defense. First, the criterion challenges us to reconsider our working assumptions about two tiers of health care. A casual acceptance of two tiers of health care delivery, in respect of the freedom of those better off to obtain more expensive care, may undercut the sense of solidarity that the common good emphasizes. Second, even if the criterion is not implemented, it may encourage us to consider our mutual responsibilities for one another; by so doing, it might serve to broaden the package of basic services that are seen as sufficiently comprehensive, by most citizens, to make "buying out" of basic coverage less appealing. Indeed, in contrast to the U.S. bishops' call for a single tier of health care, the CHA document discusses a first approximation of satisfying this criterion in a realistic footnote:

> Practically speaking, this criterion could be satisfied if those "buying out" of a rationed health care system constituted a very small percentage of Americans. If too many choose to "buy out," the rationed system would be disproportionately composed of the economically disadvantaged and would be more likely to decline in scope and quality. A large proportion of Americans "buying out" would also send a strong political signal that the rationed system is insufficiently comprehensive or seriously deficient in other respects ([2], p. 22).

Still, the criterion that rationing should apply to all, even granting the realism expressed in the above footnote, suggests that the Catholic Health Association would deem the present exclusion of certain large groups — especially the Medicare population — as unacceptable, even on prudential grounds. So long as some groups are deemed to be "untouchable" relative to general standards of rationing that apply to other large populations, there emerges a perception, at the very least, of serious inequity that fails to comport to recent Catholic social teaching on property. After all, a large percentage of Medicare coverage draws upon common resources, as with Medicaid. To be sure, there are differences in the initial moral appeals that were made in creating Medicare and Medicaid as legal entitlements: Medicare was, to a large extent, seen as a merit-based entitlement due the elderly poor for their years of service, while Medicaid was perceived as an entitlement based on grounds of charity. Nonetheless, though I cannot develop a full argument here, I have concluded elsewhere that Catholic social teaching places moral priority on property in common, based upon use criteria according to need [12]. Consequently, arbitrary exclusion of the Medicare population from the scope of rationing would seem to require something more than prudential judgments to be morally compelling in light of Catholic social principles.

A final criterion might also call Oregon's process into question, the criterion that "the health care of disadvantaged persons has an ethical priority." As with the bishops' resolution, it is difficult to specify the target of this principle; i.e., are we speaking of those generally indigent, or the medically indigent? Although these groups overlap, the principle might well be applied differently, depending upon how that determination is made. One way to consider the issue would be to pose it in Rawlsian terms: does the impact of the Oregon Basic Health Services Act make the worst off better or worse off as a group? On the one hand, the basic Act does not seem to require much from better-off Oregonians. Providers will be reimbursed more for their services. Unless and until taxes rise to expand coverage for Medicaid (which appears quite unlikely), businesses and taxpayers will not pay much more. Moreover, those who are privately covered will continue to enjoy benefits, with tax-subsidized insurance, not available to their poorer Oregonian neighbors. Neither of these results seems in accord with the Catholic emphasis upon the common good and the need for a broader understanding of social justice.

On the other hand, if the Basic Health Benefits Act ultimately functions in tandem with the other two bills, extension of the priority setting beyond the Medicaid population will do much, as a comprehensive strategy, to improve the lot of all who would gain access, finally, to a meaningful entitlement to basic care. If one reads the future more optimistically, benefits to those presently disadvantaged by gaps in coverage would emerge, and this CHA criterion would be more clearly satisfied.

III. The Relevance of Catholic Principles to the Secular Debate

In Part I, I discussed the principles of Catholic social thought on medical care as an individual right, but one constrained by considerations of the common good, as well as of social and distributive justice. In Part II, I assessed two recent Catholic documents — one on health care reform, the other on rationing. In this section, I will conclude by posing a series of related questions about how, or whether, a particular theological understanding — here the Catholic tradition on health care — can have resonance with and relevance to the formation and justification of secular policy? What good might a specifically Catholic perspective do in our public discussion of the nature and scope of health care as a right? How might a Catholic perspective further the public debate on such a large and controversial issue as health care rationing?

To revisit an earlier point: we should not assume, at least without argument, that a particular religious voice is irrelevant to policy choices simply because we insist on finding secular and pluralistic warrants for policy formulation. A more full-blooded reading of secular pluralism would celebrate, rather than discourage, the vibrancy of various voices in the public dialogue about difficult issues. James Gustafson reminds us that moral discourse, whether theologically inspired or not, may function in a number of ways. He discusses four "modes" of moral discourse — what he calls ethical discourse, prophetic discourse, narrative discourse, and policy discourse. Each of these, he suggests, is at some level necessary to the moral deliberations of particular communities and society at large but none is, of itself, sufficient [6].

These days, of course, "ethical discourse" may be the mode most familiar to us — the so-called "Georgetown mantra" of principles, the appeals to various rights, the vocabularies of consequentialism and deontology. Ethics is an important language, for it serves to frame our reflections as we justify choices in a pluralistic society where a common narrative cannot be assumed. But ethics, according to Gustafson, tends to be micro-focused, small in scale, working within the status quo, not concerned, much of the time, with the larger cultural or social picture. Ethical discourse may also be rather dry, often trading on technical or legal niceties. Ethics may talk more about the patient's right to refuse treatment than it does about the cultural worship of medical technology that may pose such a quandary in the first place. Ethics may speak exhaustively (and exhaustingly) about the autonomy of individuals in making their own decisions even as it gives short shrift to the discussion of the individual's responsibilities to the larger society.

Prophetic discourse, by contrast, is often passionate in its sweeping indictment of larger cultural trends and social sins. Such discourse makes up in vision what it lacks in precision. It forces us to notice the forest through the trees, to see those large-scale background features that the ethical mode in the foreground often tends to underplay.

The discourse of narrative is the language of story, the story that shapes a community — in the Christian tradition, the centrality of the good news, the complexity of the parables, the attitudes and ethos shaped by the story the community tells, the faithfulness of the community to its own shaping narrative. Narrative is not the language of argument, of precise moral reasoning, of premises and conclusions. Narrative is more full-blooded, less skeletal. The bare bones of argument so dear to secular philosophers are covered with the flesh and blood of tradition. Narrative, before all else, is about inspiration, about the formation of character. We are shaped by the stories that we tell.

Finally, there is policy discourse. Policy discourse, rather than focusing on ideal theories or grand conceptions, usually functions within the constraints of history and culture. It works with the values already embedded in the choices that we have made. It seldom, if ever, is prophetic; its horizon is limited. It generally asks not, "What is the good or the right choice?" but, within a range of alternatives, "What is the reasonably good and feasible choice?"

It is useful, in light of Gustafson's distinctions, to consider in which mode or modes Catholic social teaching belongs in debates about health care reform and rationing. With all the appropriate caveats in place concerning the differences between the formation and the justification of public policy in a secular pluralistic society, Roman Catholic discussions of health care might contribute to policy formation in a number of different, perhaps complementary, ways. As ethical discourse, Catholic thought might call us to achieve a better balance between the language of "rights" and "obligations." Individuals have rights, but the language of the common good provides a useful counter to the usual stridency of rights language. As prophetic discourse, the Catholic understanding of the limits on private property might call into question the unexamined assumptions of a secular society about the seemingly sacrosanct status of individual acquisition and private property. Moreover, the CHA criterion that rationing should apply to all — however impracticable it may be — might force us to reconsider our status quo assumptions about separate and unequal forms of care.

So too, the Catholic voice, by emphasizing certain themes in the Christian story — especially the universalizing tendency of Christian love — might invite broader reflections about what we owe one another and how we are responsible to one another for the meeting of our basic needs. In addition, the richer narrative voice would surely reinforce distinctive emphases in Catholic institutions, perhaps about the sorts of services that they will or will not ration. Finally, the Catholic policy voice, proclaimed by the bishops in their resolution and by the CHA in its statement on rationing, will challenge Catholics, and perhaps others, to consider their own best moral instincts and values, especially those already embedded in earlier policy choices about expanding access and improving care, as exemplified by the passage of Medicare and Medicaid.

None of these modes of moral discourse, as I have suggested, is likely to provide, in itself, a specifically "Roman Catholic" warrant for secular social policy or public choices on health care reform. Indeed, in the two documents that I analyzed in Part II, the mixture of modes is quite striking, even as it leaves one uncertain about how to interpret the authority of particular conclusions. However, because Roman Catholic social ethics continues to invoke natural law categories of reflection, one would not expect Catholic policy discourse to be unique (although on some issues it will retain a distinctive cast). After all, the strength of natural law, in principle, is its availability as a source of natural moral insight to persons of goodwill. Yet it is worth remarking, as I close, that the persuasiveness of natural law in Catholic arguments has been quite variable, even to those still somewhat sympathetic to that methodology. As Bryan Hehir observes, recent Catholic policy statements argued in natural law terms have been received more favorably on general matters of social ethics than on specific issues in bioethics and sexual ethics. For example, in their pastoral letters in the 1980s on the economy and war and peace, the U.S. Catholic bishops invoked a recognizable version of natural law. In Hehir's judgment:

> Even though such a position is not well known or widely used in American academic or social policy debate, the positions of the bishops catalyzed a broad public discussion and found support beyond the boundaries of the Catholic community. [Moreover] [t]he bishops' philosophical perspective often found more support than the specific policy conclusions they drew from it ([7], p. 357).

By contrast, on particular biomedical and sexual issues, "it has been very difficult to get a hearing for either the philosophical foundation or the conclusions espoused by the bishops" ([7], p. 357).

The reasons for that difference in reception are complex, but they involve, most crucially, the way that general principles and particular policy conclusions are distinguished or conflated in social ethics and bioethics respectively. The counsels of prudence usually feature more prominently in social teaching than in the strict moral conclusions traditionally reached on sexual and bioethical issues, primarily, as Hehir notes, because the latter involve judgments about "intrinsically evil acts" ([7], p. 358). To be sure, the recent stance taken by the U.S. bishops against support for any package of basic health care benefits that includes abortion exemplifies a point of intersection between two ordinarily distinct approaches. Indeed, the policy arguments required to sustain that position will offer an instructive challenge for Catholics who wish to speak appropriately in the policy mode. While one would clearly expect religious values to be invoked as focal elements of prophetic or narrative discourse, policy arguments, on abortion and other issues, require nonparochial, i.e., public, reasons. This, indeed, remains the central drama of being a public church: to witness by persuasion as well as by example, to speak to similarities as well as differences, to discover and celebrate those commonalities of experience and reflection that allow religious values, albeit indirectly, to work their leaven upon the world.

Institute of Religion/
Center for Ethics
Texas Medical Center

Bibliography

1. Ashley, B. M. and O'Rourke, K. D., 1978, *Health Care Ethics*, Catholic Hospital Association, St. Louis.
2. Catholic Hospital Association (CHA), 1991, *With Justice for All? The Ethics of Health Care Rationing*, St. Louis, Mo.
3. Christiansen, D., 1991, "The Great Divide," *Linacre Quarterly* 58 (May), 40-50.
4. Engelhardt, H. T., 1986, *The Foundations of Bioethics*, Oxford University Press, New York.
5. Gremillion, J. (ed.), 1976, *The Gospel of Peace and Justice: Catholic Social Teaching Since Pope John*, Orbis Books, Maryknoll, New York.
6. Gustafson, J., 1990, "Moral Discourse About Medicine: A Variety of Forms," *The Journal of Medicine and Philosophy* 15 (April): 125-42.
7. Hehir, J. B., 1992, "Policy Arguments in a Public Church: Catholic Social Ethics and Bioethics," *The Journal of Medicine and Philosophy* 17 (June): 347-64.
8. Hollenbach, D., 1979, *Claims in Conflict: Retrieving and Renewing the Catholic Human Rights Tradition*, Paulist Press, New York.
9. John Paul II, 1981, *On Human Work*, United States Catholic Conference Office of Publishing Services, Washington, D.C.
10. Keane, P., 1993, *Health Care Reform: A Catholic View*, Paulist Press, New York.
11. Langan, J., 1986, "Common Good," in James Childress and John Macquarrie (eds.), *The Westminster Dictionary of Christian Ethics*, Westminster Press, Philadelphia, p. 102.
12. Lustig, B. A., 1990, "Property and Justice in the Modern Encyclical Literature," *Harvard Theological Review* 83, 415-46.
13. Outka, G., 1974, "Social Justice and Equal Access to Health Care," *The Journal of Religious Ethics* 2 (Spring), 11-32.
14. Treacy, G. C. (ed.), 1939, *Five Great Encyclicals*, Paulist Press, New York.
15. United States Bishops, 1993, "Resolution on Health Care Reform," *Origins* 23, 98-102.

26 A Summary of Catholic Principles for Health-Care Justice

Philip S. Keane

Catholic Teaching and the Just Treatment of Health-Care Employees

No presentation of the Catholic principles of health-care justice would be complete if it did not reflect on the Catholic commitment to the just treatment of employees. In the United States there are millions of persons employed in health care. In these days of the Balanced Budget Act, when billions of dollars of public funding are being withdrawn from health care each year, health-care providers can be sorely tempted to make ends meet through strategies such as the reduction or elimination of cost-of-living increases for employees. But how can a health-care system be just if it does not treat its employees justly? And how could Catholic thought, with its historic commitment to working people, not see justice to employees as an essential component of just health care?

To summarize Catholic thinking on justice for health-care employees, five issues will be reviewed: (1) the right of working people to just earnings and benefits, (2) the right of working people to a genuine experience of participation in their work and to ongoing development of their abilities, (3) the responsibility of working people to share in the mission of their work, particularly in the special mission of health care, (4) the right to non-discrimination, and (5) the right to unionize.

Just Earnings and Benefits

The main beginning point of modern Catholic social teaching in the 1890s was the idea that working people had a right to be paid a living wage, that is, an earning level that enabled them to live in a reasonable and frugal comfort.[1] Certainly, those who work in health care deserve to earn enough to live in the reasonable comfort and security envisioned by Catholic teaching. Any pressure to respond to the financial burdens of health care today by underpaying health-care employees must be strictly resisted. Especially when we consider that healthcare executives earn very large incomes, the injustice of underpaying employees becomes very clear. The minimum wage provided for in U.S. legislation does not deserve to be considered a living wage. At current price levels, how can anyone be expected to live in reasonable and frugal comfort (with adequate food, clothing, shelter, and health care) for only about $10,000 per year?

Three issues can be raised in order to fill out the context of the right of health-care employees to a just wage. *First,* the exact specifics of what constitutes a living wage may vary in different economic times and settings. To show how much the level of a just wage can shift in changing economic times, we need only recall that some of the first serious scholarship on the living wage proposed that in the early 1900s a family in the United States needed to earn $600 annually in order to be said to have a living income.[2] While no one would dream of this figure today, economic factors influencing the cost of living can change rapidly, meaning that health-care leaders need to maintain an ongoing vigilance to be sure that they are paying just wages.

Second, just benefits are an intrinsic part of the concept of a living wage. The major elements in a just benefits package are retirement security and health-care coverage. On the topic of health-care benefits, there is a special obligation on health-care providers to construct truly just packages of health-care benefits for health-care employees. I am not implying that every conceivable service need be offered (for example, merely cosmetic plastic surgeries). But the package of benefits must be just, based on criteria that both employers and employees can accept. If a health-care provider offers a great many extra health benefits to its higher level employees, or if the higher level employees who can afford it very frequently seek treatments beyond the basic package, there may be significant questions about the justice of the basic package of health-care benefits. Also, there is a need for special care in the administering of health-care benefits for health-care employees. Health-care employees are likely to seek care from the health-care provider for whom they work. Hence there are important obligations to make sure that the confidentiality of employee-patients is properly protected and to make sure that employees with complicated health issues suffer no prejudice in the workplace because of their illness. There are also special considerations needed on the theme of employee health and the safe treatment of patients.

Third, in the earlier history of just wage theory, there was often a tendency to focus on the need to pay a just wage to heads of families, who were usually men.[3] Per-

1. *Rerum Novarum* no. 34 (*Catholic Social Thought: The Documentary Heritage,* David J. O'Brien and Thomas A. Shannon, eds. [Maryknoll, New York: Orbis Books, 1992], 31 [hereafter *CST*]).

Philip S. Keane, "A Summary of Catholic Principles for Health-Care Justice." Excerpts from *Catholicism and Health-Care Justice: Problems, Potential, and Solutions* by Philip S. Keane, S.S., pp. 27-40.

2. This was the figure (actually $601.03) given by John A. Ryan in 1906 in his *The Living Wage: Its Ethical and Economic Aspects* (New York: The Macmillan Company, 1912), 123-30.

3. This was a clear theme in Ryan's work, but we would view the matter very differently today.

haps this approach was understandable in a former time, when relatively few women, especially married women, worked outside the home, and when it seemed a reasonable social objective to ensure that each family had enough income to live comfortably. But this earlier approach had the undeniable side effect that persons — very often women — who were not heads of households frequently earned significantly less than heads of households. Partly due to the two world wars of the twentieth century, the world is very different today, and in many cases it is an economic necessity for married women to work. There has been some progress in recent decades in moving to pay all employees — including women — equally and justly when they perform tasks of equal worth to those performed by men. But the issue has not gone away completely, and women remain statistically likely to be paid less than men for work of equal value. These considerations are especially important in a field like health care, which employs many women. Wages cannot be just unless they are gender just.

Genuine Participation and Ongoing Development of Employees

For many people, Catholic thought on employees is almost synonymous with the idea of just compensation. But Catholic thought on employees goes far beyond the topic of financial compensation. The employee is far more than a mere commodity whose function is to get some specific task accomplished. The employee is a human person with all the rights and dignity inherent in human personhood. For this reason, Catholic thought understands human work as a noble action. When a human person works, she or he adds an element of transcendence to the task, an element that cannot be described in quantifiable terms. As a specifically human activity, work is endowed with a human dignity and worth that goes far beyond economic or utilitarian values. The human working person must therefore be honored and respected in the workplace. What she or he thinks about the work should be attended to carefully by employers, and if employee suggestions about the work or the workplace are feasible, they should be implemented.

A term that helps express all this is "participation." Employees ought to have a genuine sense of participation in their work.[4] With a genuine sense of participation, the employee will feel heard, honored, and respected in the workplace, even if the work itself is difficult and demanding, as is often the case with work in health care. In September 1999, the Domestic Policy Committee of the United States Catholic Conference issued an important statement on justice for workers in Catholic health care. Participation emerged as a very important theme in that statement.[5]

It would be wrong to understate the classic Catholic commitment to just wages and benefits. Still, there are ways in which genuine participation in one's work may be even more important than wages and benefits. People need to be paid enough money. But we should ask why employees become especially loyal to their work, or why it is that sometimes employees stay with the same work situation for many years, even in the face of other, perhaps financially more attractive options. This kind of loyalty is generated more through participation than through financial incentives. And this kind of loyalty can be pricelessly important in a field such as health care.

A climate of true participation ought to include opportunities for both human and professional development. If there is true participation, there will be natural opportunities for the building of meaningful human relationships and for the ongoing human development of both employers and employees. Some critics argue that many people today have almost too much of their human development based in the workplace. This happens because the pace of modern life can restrict time for the building up of family relationships. Family life should retain its traditional importance. But this does not take away the importance of human development in the workplace. Development in the workplace needs to include the creation of opportunities for employees to move ahead in their work. Opportunities to learn new skills and take on new responsibilities are highly important, both humanly and professionally. People in the workplace will not all possess the same potential for professional growth and career advancement. But a climate of opportunity needs to be present, especially for employees at lower levels.

The Mission Responsibility of Health-Care Workers

One of the main cautions in Catholic thinking about human rights is that rights can never be an occasion for an attitude of "I demand my rights," with its implication that no one else's rights matter. Instead the Catholic vision is that rights always involve correlative responsibilities. In the context of employment, the correlative responsibility is that employees are to do the work for which they are employed to the best of their ability. Without this commitment and effort on the part of the employees, work loses its nobility and human meaning. The responsibility of employers to furnish compensation, participation, and development becomes empty and meaningless.

These comments about the responsibility of employees have their force in any employment situation. But the notion of employee responsibility takes on a unique

4. NCCB, *Economic Justice for All*, nos. 68-76 (*CST*, 595-96).

5. United States Catholic Conference Domestic Policy Committee, "A Fair and Just Workplace: Principles and Practices for Catholic Health Care," *Origins* 29 (1999), 181, 183-88 [hereafter *FJW*]. Cf. also John Paul II, *Laborem Exercens*, nos. 24-27 (*The Encyclicals of John Paul II*, edited with introductions by J. Michael Miller [Huntington, Indiana: Our Sunday Visitor Press, 1996], 206-14).

dimension in the health-care context. Shortly we will discuss the point that dying stands as perhaps the most basic existential challenge of human living and that therefore one of the most basic of all human responsibilities is the responsibility we humans have to stand by one another as we confront serious illness and the journey toward death. While every human person shares in this responsibility, those who work in health care share in it in a very special way. This is true not only for nurses and doctors but also for those whose work in health care requires lesser training or is removed from the locus of the patient, for example, persons who clean rooms, wash linens, fix meals, or work as accountants or computer programmers. Even these health-care workers have a special connection with the human mystery involved in serious illness and dying.

In this context, everyone who works in health care is called upon to have a special sense of *mission,* of commitment to stand by the sick and the dying, so as to make the experience of serious illness and dying as human an experience as possible. The environment of the health-care workplace should be palpably different because of this sense of mission. While many themes can be stipulated as part of this sense of mission, it might help to highlight the quality of presence that health-care workers are called to have to patients and families and to one another. In the end, health care is about caring, and gestures such as a welcoming presence and a genuine compassion and respect for all, especially the sick, serve to put flesh and blood on the mission of caring. Yes, employers are to treat health-care workers well, but the workers in their turn have a clear mission responsibility.

The issue of mission is a two-way street. Because a sense of mission is pivotally important for the successful provision of health-care services, I have argued that employees in health care are obligated to develop a sense of mission. But also because of the importance of mission, employers have an added responsibility to meet all the demands of employee justice (compensation, participation, and so on). If the employers fail to meet these needs, how will employees be able to develop a sense of mission, and how in the end will health care be able to be truly successful in reaching out to patients and families?

Health-Care Workers and Non-Discrimination

For the student of Catholic social teaching, Vatican II's *Pastoral Constitution on the Church in the Modern World (Gaudium et Spes)* contains many important highlights. One of these highlights is No. 29's forceful assertion that discrimination in any form — whether on the basis of sex, race, color, social condition, language, or religion — is to be rejected as contrary to the will of God.[6] To help buttress *Gaudium et Spes's* position, many authors quote Galatians 3:28: "There is neither Jew nor Greek, there is neither slave nor free person, there is not male and female; for you are all one in Christ Jesus."[7] Vatican II's words against discrimination were written in the mid-1960s, against the backdrop of worldwide concern about racial justice. But the words remain remarkable today. What seems especially refreshing and inspired about the words is that they are not limited to any one form of discrimination. Instead the words reject *all* discrimination.

In the context of health care, the obligation to avoid discrimination touches all the usual issues. There should be no discrimination based on race, gender, or other circumstances in hiring, pay scales, health and retirement benefits, promotion, recognition, opportunities for additional learning, termination, and support for those who are being terminated. Health-care providers are expected to put into place personnel systems that protect the rights of all employees (and also all patients) on any matters related to discrimination. It should also be added that, because of health care's special focus on human frailty and human illness, health-care providers have a unique obligation not to discriminate against employees because of developmental disabilities or problems of physical or mental health. I am not implying that health-care employers are obligated to retain employees who simply cannot do their work. But frequently the employees I have just mentioned can do their work, perhaps with some adjustments. Or they can be shifted to some other tasks that they are able to manage.

In raising these issues about discrimination, I want to note that I have personally seen many strong anti-discriminatory stances taken by hospitals and other health providers. In these complicated times for health care, it is not unusual for a health provider to need to reduce its work force. I have seen such workforce reductions accomplished with a great deal of care for those involved, and with a real effort to help those who lose their jobs prepare for and find meaningful work elsewhere. I have also seen health-care providers implement highly effective policies for the hiring of special people. But discrimination can have a pernicious way of creeping in if we fail to be vigilant. The challenge for health care is to maintain a constant watchfulness, so that the richness of the mission of health care is not tainted by any discrimination.

The Right of Health-Care Employees to Join Labor Unions

Both the *Ethical and Religious Directives for Catholic Health Care Services (ERD)* and the United States Catholic Conference's September 1999 statement are clear in their insistence on the right of health-care workers to form and join unions. The *ERD* in No. 7 affirms "the rights of employees to organize and bargain collectively

6. *CST,* 183.

7. Vatican II quotes Gal 3:28 most notably in its assertion of the equality of all the members of the church in *Lumen Gentium,* no. 32 (*The Documents of Vatican II,* Walter Abbott, ed. [New York: America Press, 1966], 58 [hereafter *DV2*]).

without prejudice to the common good."[8] The September 1999 statement, entitled *A Fair and Just Workplace: Principles and Practices for Catholic Health Care,* says that "workers have the right to organize themselves for collective bargaining and to be recognized by management for such purposes."[9] The directness of these two statements leaves no doubt about the Catholic openness toward unions as a matter of basic principle. But these two statements do not answer all of the practical follow-up questions about whether a union is appropriate in a given situation or whether, and under what conditions, strikes might be justifiable in the health-care context.

Some historical background may help explain the nature and depth of the Catholic commitment to unions, especially in the United States. In the late nineteenth century, the combination of *laissez-faire* economics and the Industrial Revolution left many workers, both in Europe and in the United States, in a very difficult position. In response, workers in a number of places sought to form labor unions as a means of improving their lot. The original attitude of the Vatican was to oppose labor unions, which were understood, in the context of the growth of Marxism, as secret societies with an anti-religious, even atheistic outlook. Some of the early union leaders in the United States were Catholics who were concerned about the situation of coal miners in states such as Pennsylvania. Cardinal James Gibbons of Baltimore had the opportunity to meet with these early Catholic union leaders, especially with leaders of the union known as the Knights of Labor. Cardinal Gibbons became convinced of the justice of the Knights' cause, and the rest is history.

In the 1880s, Gibbons made his famous trip to the Vatican during which he succeeded in getting the Vatican to drop its opposition to unions.[10] The results of Gibbons's trip were very significant both for working Catholics in the United States and for the Catholic Church in the United States. Many of the millions of Catholics then migrating to the United States became part of union families, and their earnings helped send their sons and daughters to college. Catholics became an upwardly mobile group in the United States. This upward movement was due in part to the success of the labor movement. By the mid- and late twentieth century, Catholics were able to assume many prominent positions in the social, economic, and political structures of U.S. society.

If the results of the Catholic commitment to unions were notable for Catholics in the workplace, the results were also very significant for the church itself. In Europe, after the Industrial Revolution, vast numbers of Catholics stopped practicing their faith, and they have never really returned to the practice of the faith. But working Catholics in the United States did not leave the church in great numbers. They stayed and became the basis for the church's twentieth-century expansion that saw the establishment and/or development of many parishes, schools, hospitals, and colleges and universities. Commitment to unions became part and parcel of the Catholic tradition of social liberalism that I described earlier. Indeed, virtually every stage of the Catholic tradition of social liberalism included support for trade unions. For someone who understands this tradition, there can be no surprise that the *Ethical and Religious Directives* say what they say about unions.

But what does Catholicism's strong historical support for unions have to say about health-care providers and the unions of today? While the church's support for unions at the level of principle is unquestionable, what about unions in practice? Surely it is wrong for any health-care provider to reject unions as a matter of principle. A health-care employer cannot simply forbid employees to form or join unions. Nor should an employer create a climate of undue duress around the union question. Similarly, a health-care employer could not be said to be acting with justice if the employer refuses to bargain in good faith with legitimately recognized unions.

But are unions always the best answer from the viewpoint of the employee? Not necessarily, especially in our times, which have seen changes in labor legislation as well as other factors that are quite different from the original context in which Cardinal Gibbons elicited Catholic support for unions. The real bottom line for employees is that the employer meet all the issues of justice that have been outlined in the past few sections: compensation, participation, development, and nondiscrimination. If a given health-care employer is truly just in addressing all of these issues, so that the employees do not experience a need to unionize, all well and good. If the issues of employee justice are not met, the case for unionization becomes all the more compelling.

Geography is a large factor in assessing how necessary unions are as agents of justice for health-care employees. In some locales, unions have played a strong historical role in health care, and they will surely continue to do so. In other geographical areas, there may be a stronger custom of healthcare employers and employees working out true employee justice with lesser or even no union involvement. Because of these geographical factors, it is wrong for large national health-care systems to agree to national union contracts for all their employees in a given field. Instead, these systems should work out suitable approaches to the union question that are tailored to the diverse local areas in which these national systems are present. What seems crucial is that in all geographical areas health-care providers maintain an attitude of genuinely open dialogue on the union question. I understand this commitment to true dialogue to be a key element in

8. *Ethical and Religious Directives for Catholic Health Care Services,* 4th ed. (Washington, D.C.: United States Conference of Catholic Bishops, 2001), no. 7.

9. *FJW,* 185.

10. Charles Morris's *American Catholic: The Saints and Sinners Who Built America's Most Powerful Church* (New York: Random House, 1997) is a very helpful new history of the Catholic Church in the United States. Morris treats the Knights of Labor issue (including Gibbons's impact on *Rerum Novarum*) on pages 88-93.

the *Fair and Just Workplace* statement. If the dialogue is present, and if the result is true employee justice, the objectives of the church's principled stance on unions will be met in the health-care context, regardless of the specific decisions made about unions in the many various and diverse health-care settings.

Doctors, Nurses, and Health Care as a Profession

In addition to the comments on health-care employees in general, there is a need to focus on the specific question of health-care professionals. This focus must address the responsibilities of these professionals to their patients and to the health-care systems in which they serve. This focus must also address the legitimate expectations of professionals, expectations of the systems in which they serve, and expectations of the patients and families for whom they care. Many critics feel that the role of the professional is under severe threat in today's health-care context, so it is important to review the traditional thinking about professionals in both Catholic and related sources.

When we use the term "professionals" in the health-care context, we most often think about doctors. While doctors surely are professionals, modern health care embraces many other professionals as well. Nurses, physical therapists, social workers, pastoral counselors, health-care administrators, and several other groups can be legitimately described as health-care professionals. Here there will be a special emphasis on the doctor as a professional, because of the unique character of the doctor-patient relationship. But this emphasis should not obscure the clear professional role of others who are involved in the provision of health-care services.

There is an intersection but not a complete overlap between health-care employees and health-care professionals. Some health-care professionals are employees, and some are self-employed. Historically, a great many doctors owned their own medical practices and were given privileges to practice medicine at one or several hospitals. While this still happens in some cases, large numbers of physicians today work for medical practices that are owned by hospitals or by managed-care organizations. So today's physicians are often employees instead of being self-employed. But whether they are employees or independent, the standards of professionalism apply to all physicians, as well as to other health-care professionals.

Several themes in classic Catholic social and moral teaching help shape the concept of the professional person, whether in medicine or in other fields such as law, public service, science, or engineering. The very word *professional* has important roots in medieval Catholic thought. The theme of professional confidentiality has roots in the ancient world, for instance in the oath of Hippocrates. A basic theme in traditional Catholic thought is the idea that the secular realm is autonomous in its own sphere.[11] The implication of this notion of autonomy is clear: even though the church expects that Catholics who are professionals will be committed to Catholic teaching and values, the church recognizes that the professional has a legitimate autonomy. He or she has a specific and proper knowledge that is best challenged on the basis of a competent professional assessment of the issues which are at stake. Religious authorities should maintain a stance of respect for the place of professional competence.

Closely related to this theme of autonomy is the Catholic position that qualified[12] lay persons, clearly including professionals, possess a lawful freedom to inquire into the specific areas in which they are competent.[13] Such a freedom to inquire surely implies a place for legitimate professional judgment. The new *Code of Canon Law* reasserts these traditional themes about the secular order and about those who exercise secular professions. The new code also makes the notable statement that lay persons who are qualified are expected to make their views known, not only to church leaders, but also to others who need to hear what the qualified person has to say.[14]

These Catholic themes rather clearly set forth a foundation for a theology of the professions. Other traditional sources can be conjoined to these themes so as to articulate a more developed concept of the professions. In the context of medicine, probably the most important ancient source is the oath of Hippocrates, with its insistence that the doctor never harm the patient, that the doctor always act for the patient's benefit, and that the doctor always maintain confidentiality about anything he or she learns while caring for the patient.[15] It is no surprise that from very early days, Christianity, with its incipient concept of professionalism, felt a strong compatibility with the Hippocratic oath. Almost at the beginning of the Christian era, there were Christianized versions of the Hippocratic oath in which the oath was taken in the name of the Father, Son, and Holy Spirit instead of in the names of the Greek gods.[16]

11. For an explanation of this concept of autonomy, cf. Jacques Maritain, *Man and the State* (Chicago: University of Chicago Press, 1951), esp. 153, 159. Maritain roots his treatment of autonomy in Leo XIII's encyclical *Immortali Dei.*

12. I hesitate to give a full definition of the term "qualified." More normally it involves high-level study and practice in a field such as law or medicine. But sometimes persons go through a unique set of life experiences and/or nontraditional learning modes that can render them qualified to speak on a given subject.

13. *Gaudium et Spes,* no. 62 (*DV2,* 270).

14. *Code of Canon Law,* Latin-English edition, new English translation (Washington, D.C.: The Canon Law Society of America, 1998), no. 212, §63.

15. Quoted in *Ethics in Medicine: Historical Perspectives and Contemporary Concerns,* Stanley Reiser, Arthur Dyck, and William Curran, eds. (Cambridge, Massachusetts: MIT Press, 1977), 5 [hereafter *EM*].

16. W. H. S. Jones, "From the Oath According to Hippocrates in So Far as a Christian May Swear It," *EM,* 10.

In today's health-care context, three key questions concerning the role of the doctor as a health-care professional come to the surface. *First,* what about the legitimate autonomy of the doctor as a professional to arrive at her or his own best medical judgment about the proper course of treatment for a given patient? Obviously no doctor (or other professional) is so totally autonomous as to be completely free of external accountability. But physician autonomy does seem to be under particular stress in our times, and we will need to inquire as to whether the solid tradition of professional medical autonomy is sufficiently protected in the current climate. *Second,* what about the long-standing tradition of the doctor, as a professional, having a strong obligation to speak her mind to those who have a right to hear her judgment? Do doctors have sufficient freedom to do this today? *Third,* what about the doctor's basic obligation to avoid all harm to her or his patient and only to act in the patient's best interest? Is there sufficient protection of this physician responsibility in today's health-care world? Or are there too many financial incentives that may undermine the physician's professional judgment?

The point about the obligation to act in the best interest of the patient opens up the more explicitly Christian theme of covenantal loyalty. There are several possible images out of which a doctor might understand herself: as the advancer of scientific knowledge, the fighter against disease, the conqueror of death, and so on. In light of the tradition of professionalism, the doctor is best understood as the person who is radically committed to caring for the patient and doing only what is good for the patient. This radical commitment suggests that the doctor owes the patient a special loyalty, a loyalty sometimes described as a "covenantal loyalty." William F. May very helpfully develops this theme of covenantal loyalty in his book *The Physician's Covenant,* but the term also has echoes in the work of the late Paul Ramsey, who did so much to help shape the entry of Protestant thought into a disciplined approach to medical ethics.[17]

The richness of the term "covenantal loyalty" opens up a very profound question. Granted the long historical rooting of the concept of the doctor as a professional, does the theme of professionalism ultimately go far enough in identifying who the doctor is? Once we grant the special covenant of trust that ought to exist between doctors and patients, and as we begin to explore the powerful existential meaning of serious illness and dying, I believe it can be said that the doctor's committed presence to the seriously ill and the dying has about it an even deeper meaning, so that the practice of medicine should be described as a vocation. This theme of medicine as vocation does not take away professionalism and professional standards, but it does suggest that the doctor — and some of the other health-care professionals as well — has an even more profound vocational identity. If this is true, the questions about today's threats to the identity of the physician become all the more serious.

17. William F. May, *The Physician's Covenant* (Philadelphia: Westminster Press, 1983). Paul Ramsey, *The Patient as Person* (New Haven: Yale University Press, 1970).

III. Patients and Professionals

CHAPTER FIVE

The Professions

We refer to the "health professions" and we think of those who work in the field of health care as "professionals," but what does this term really mean? Where did this way of thinking about practitioners of health care come from? Does the notion of "professional" matter to medicine?

These are not simply theoretical questions. In 2002, the American Board of Internal Medicine (ABIM), the American College of Physicians–American Society of Internal Medicine (ACP-ASIM), and the European Federation of Internal Medicine (EFIM) promulgated a new charter on medical professionalism.[1] These three internal medicine organizations contend that an explosion of technology, changing market forces, problems in health care delivery, and globalization are threatening the practice of medicine. They believe that a reaffirmation of professional commitments to their patients and to the public is essential in the face of these challenges. Specifically, they challenge physicians to affirm a professional commitment to the principles of patient welfare, patient autonomy, and social justice. From these principles, the charter goes on to derive various responsibilities, including competence, honesty, patient confidentiality, a commitment to scientific knowledge, improving both quality and access to care, and setting standards of professional behavior. For these organizations, the very practice of medicine hinges on our understanding of and commitment to what it is to be a professional.

In contemporary jargon, seemingly everyone is a "professional." Mechanics and plumbers, hairstylists and personal trainers, physicians and lawyers all tout their professional credentials. Likewise, we see ads for "professional-grade" products ranging from trucks and tools to hair care products, computer laptops, and digital cameras. Thus, "professional" seems a remarkably broad term meant to indicate the excellence or high standard of one's skill set, product, or services.

1. ABIM Foundation, ACP-ASIM Foundation, and European Federation of Internal Medicine, "Medical Professionalism in the New Millennium: A Physician Charter," *Annals of Internal Medicine* 136, no. 3 (February 5, 2002): 243-46. The charter is also available online at the web site for the *Annals of Internal Medicine:* http://www.annals.org/content/136/3/243.full (accessed June 8, 2010).

Sociologists sometimes use a more restricted understanding of "professional." Here professionals are those with specialized skills and knowledge, including a vocabulary that is at least partially incomprehensible to those outside the guild. Moreover, entrance into a profession is controlled and regulated by those within the profession itself. Under this understanding, the term "professional" is in part a designation of social power: professionals are those who control skills and knowledge that others need.

Largely owing to this control of needed skills and knowledge, professionals and professional organizations also exercise substantial autonomy and receive extensive status from the wider society. The larger society implicitly and explicitly grants autonomy, status, and centralization of power to the professions because they are seen as providing something society needs, such as legal protection or health, something that is not readily achieved in some other way. But in exchange for this centralization of freedom and power, and directly connected to the perception that society is thereby served by them, the professions accept various obligations, including obligations of profession-specific competency, service, and levels of sacrifice. Thus, "professional" designates social power, but that power is usually seen as linked to profession-specific duties or obligations.

In *Ethics in Pastoral Ministry,* Richard Gula reminds us of a third meaning of "profession": "the oldest use of the term 'profession' carried fundamentally a religious meaning. The professions derive from the religious setting of monks and nuns making a religious 'profession' of their faith in God by taking the vows of poverty, celibate chastity, and obedience. . . . Organized groups of professed religious reached out to respond to the immediate needs of people for education, legal rights, health care, and salvation."[2] By the late Middle Ages, many of these tasks had been taken over by non-religious institutions, but the basic notion of "professional" remained.

Leon R. Kass also appeals to an older, classic notion of professional in his pivotal essay, "Professing Medically:

2. Richard M. Gula, *Ethics in Pastoral Ministry* (New York: Paulist Press, 1996), p. 12.

The Place of Ethics in Defining Medicine." Many years before the new charter on medical professionalism, Kass argued that the field's moral direction depends significantly on the understanding of medicine as "a unique and intrinsically moral profession."[3] Medicine, says Kass, is distinguished from the skilled handicraft of the trade by its public profession to a way of life that is devoted to others and that serves the higher goods of human health and wholeness. As with other learned skills or arts, medicine requires virtues such as honesty, industry, and reliability. But as a healing art, medicine also addresses the threat posed to embodied humanity by illness. As such, medicine requires the physician to honor and remain present amidst the patient's inevitable vulnerability and exposure: "When one professes medicine, one offers the healing, comforting, and encouraging hand, which, when it is grasped, may not be pulled away."[4]

The older, classic notion of the professional to which those like Gula and Kass appeal involves at least six interrelated qualities that are particularly pertinent to understanding what it might mean to call health care a "profession." First, a profession is focused on serving human need. Thus, artisans and blacksmiths would not be among the professions, in part because their work, while valuable, less directly attends to human need. Second, the profession serves a specific end or good — for instance, the physician serves health, clergy serve salvation, the lawyer attends to justice, and the educator promotes knowledge. Third, the professional has acquired the expert knowledge and skills needed to serve that end or good. Clergy need to know theology and Scripture; lawyers must know the law; physicians study the body. Fourth, integrity and various qualities of character are as essential as expert knowledge to serving the profession's ends. For example, one cannot serve justice without honesty, and one cannot serve health without the courage and compassion to be among the sick. Fifth, there exist structures of accountability among those within a given profession. Classic notions of professions include internal mechanisms to assure that human need is served, the requisite knowledge and skill acquired, and character exhibited. The sixth feature is an open avowal or promise — that is, an act of professing — of the ends or goods that professionals serve and the character they strive to maintain. To be a professional is to make a profession.

Reviewing these three notions of what it means to be a professional — (1) excellence of one's product or services; (2) a designation of social power and corresponding duties; (3) a profession to serve specific goods — raises complex questions in the context of medicine and health care. For example, to what extent do those involved in medicine still have something distinctive to profess or avow, and to what extent is the designation "professional" simply a marker for the high standards of techniques and skills available for purchase or a designation of the social power associated with modern medicine? This question matters in part because the moral obligations associated with these disparate notions of professional differ greatly. For instance, if "professional" is a broad term meaning "excellent," then physicians have a duty to develop and maintain relevant skills, but they are no more obligated than the excellent auto mechanic or beautician to make those skills available to those who cannot afford to purchase them. By contrast, the "professing" notion of medicine entails a commitment to serving human need, which may mean that the more vulnerable members of society are to be given a kind of priority apart from their ability to pay. Medicine as social power likely falls somewhere between no-obligation and a prioritizing-obligation to those who cannot afford medical care.

Another set of questions asks about the relationship between medicine and the profession or avowal of Christian faith. Is there a neat harmony or significant tension between these professions? Does the Christian profession add to, challenge, or complement the profession of medicine? Or perhaps the skills, knowledge, and techniques of medicine are morally neutral commodities to which the profession of Christian faith adds little. Consider, for example, the issue of physician specialization. Due in some measure to school debt, medical students are increasingly moving into specialties where they can be assured a higher income. This trend likely means an inadequate number of primary and family care physicians in the near future.[5] How does the Christian profession, with its story of the Good Samaritan (Luke 10:30-37) and the charge to care for "the least of these" (Matthew 25:31-46), inform the trend toward specialization? How might the medical profession as excellence or social power or service to the good of health inform the trend? Do these notions of profession fit together nicely? Or does the issue of specialization illustrate the tension between professing Christian faith and certain notions of medicine as profession?

Especially over the past few decades, as contemporary health care has shifted from a more physician-centered model to a more team-based approach, medicine and medical ethics have come to understand the notion of "the profession" to include more than just physicians. Nurses, chaplains, and clergy — long involved in health care but relegated to second-class status — are now regularly understood to be key members of the health care team and professionals in their own right. Of course, who should be counted among health care professionals depends in part on the understanding of "professional." Depending on which of the three accounts of profession is primarily in view, physical, occupational, and respiratory

3. Leon R. Kass, "Professing Medically," in *Toward a More Natural Science* (New York: The Free Press, 1985), p. 213.

4. Kass, "Professing Medically," p. 223.

5. PBS Newshour, "States Face Shortages of Primary Care Doctors" (January 6, 2009), http://www.pbs.org/newshour/bb/health/jan-june09/doctors_01-06.html (accessed February 28, 2010); Mary Whitley, "Obama Administration Concerned about Growing Shortage of Primary-Care Doctors," *The Plain Dealer* (April 26, 2009), http://www.cleveland.com/nation/index.ssf/2009/04/obama_administration_concerned.html (accessed February 28, 2010).

therapists, as well as radiologic and diagnostic lab technicians, pharmacists, social workers, and health information technicians, are arguably all medical professionals. In this third edition of *On Moral Medicine*, we expand this chapter beyond the usual essays on physicians to include important articles on nursing, chaplaincy, and clergy. This selection of essays is meant to be representative, not necessarily exhaustive, of those who should be counted among medical professionals.

Each essay in this chapter offers support for the more historically rooted understanding of profession. The Hippocratic Oath (selection 28) and the explicitly Christian reconstruction of that oath ("The Hippocratic Oath Insofar as a Christian May Swear It," selection 29) assert that medicine has goods and ends that the physician is called to embody and profess. This classic sense is equally pronounced when Allen Verhey ("The Doctor's Oath — and a Christian Swearing It," selection 30) and Mary Doornbos, Ruth Groenhout, Kendra Hotz, and Cheryl Brandsen ("A Christian Vision of Nursing and Persons," selection 33) describe medicine and nursing as social practices, with ends and virtues internal to those practices. William May's use of the biblical image of covenant as opposed to a contract ("The Physician's Covenant," selection 31) likewise indicates the conviction that physicians still possess much to profess. May's reservations about a contractual view of medicine also highlight some of the limitations of a strictly sociological view of the professional.

Joseph Kotva's "Hospital Chaplaincy as Agapeic Intervention" (selection 34) and Kristina Robb-Dover's "Spiritual Morphine" (selection 35) also presume a more traditional account of the professions in their discussions of chaplaincy. They worry that chaplains are too often pressured into the first notion of professional, with their skills simply another product available for consumption. In part because chaplains are expected to bring comfort, they often are also expected to offer a kind of generic spiritual blessing on whatever transpires in medicine and on whatever a patient believes or desires. Kotva and Robb-Dover instead argue that such behavior amounts to a failure to profess the goods internal to Christian ministry, and as such amounts to a betrayal of those they serve, both human and divine. Similarly, from a congregational point of view, Joseph Kotva's "The Christian Pastor's Role in Medical Ethics" (selection 36) pushes in the same direction: Christian clergy must help Christians be Christians, whose convictions and practices are sometimes coherent with and sometimes at odds with modern medicine.

Most of the essays included here also help address the question of the relationship between the professions of medicine and the profession of Christian faith. The readings from Sirach 38:1-15 (selection 27) and Florence Nightingale ("The Nurse's Profession," selection 32) assume the greatest coherence between professing faith and medicine. For Jesus ben Sirach, since God is the creator of the world and all that is in it, God can act in and through the actions of physicians and pharmacists. For Nightingale, nursing is a service of love to God and neighbor. By contrast, Kotva's "The Christian Pastor's Role" envisions significant potential (but ultimately fruitful) tension between these professions. Verhey, May, and Doornbos/Groenhout/Hotz/Brandsen offer aspects of the biblical narrative that can helpfully inform the goods and practices of medicine, suggesting that the Christian profession and the profession of medicine are not far removed from each other. Altogether, the essays here assume neither a facile harmony nor an irreparable divide between modern medicine and the Christian profession.

SUGGESTIONS FOR FURTHER READING

Baker, Robert, and Linda Emanuel. "The Efficacy of Professional Ethics: The AMA Code of Ethics in Historical and Current Perspective." *Hastings Center Report* 30, no. 4 Suppl. (July-August 2000): S13-17.

Baker, Robert B., et al. *The American Medical Ethics Revolution: How the AMA's Code of Ethics Has Transformed Physicians' Relationships to Patients, Professionals, and Society* (Baltimore: Johns Hopkins University Press, 1999).

Barnard, David. "The Physician as Priest." *Journal of Religion and Health* 24 (Winter 1985): 272-86.

Beauchamp, Tom L., and Laurence B. McCullough. *Medical Ethics: The Moral Responsibilities of Physicians* (Englewood Cliffs, N.J.: Prentice-Hall, 1984).

Brody, Howard. *The Healer's Power* (New Haven: Yale University Press, 1992).

Cameron, Nigel de S. *Life and Death After Hippocrates: The New Medicine* (Wheaton, Ill.: Crossway Books, 1991).

Campbell, Alastair V. *Professional Care: Its Meaning and Practice* (Philadelphia: Fortress, 1984).

Cassell, Eric. *The Healer's Art* (New York: Lippincott, 1976).

DuBose, Edwin R. *The Illusion of Trust: Toward a Medical Theological Ethics in the Postmodern Age* (Dordrecht: Kluwer Academic Publishers, 1995).

Etziony, M. B. *The Physician's Creed: An Anthology of Medical Prayers, Oaths and Codes of Ethics Written and Recited by Medical Practitioners Through the Ages* (Springfield, Ill.: Charles C. Thomas, 1973).

Gustafson, James M. "Professions as Callings." *Social Science Review* 5 (December 1982): 501-15.

Hauerwas, Stanley. "Authority and the Profession of Medicine." In *Suffering Presence: Theological Reflections on Medicine, the Mentally Handicapped, and the Church* (Notre Dame: University of Notre Dame Press, 1986), pp. 39-62.

Hilfiker, David. *Not All of Us Are Saints: A Doctor's Journey with the Poor* (New York: Hill and Wang, 1994).

Kass, Leon R. "Professing Medically." In *Toward a More Natural Science* (New York: Free Press, 1985), pp. 211-23.

Lebacqz, Karen. *Professional Ethics: Power and Paradox* (Nashville: Abingdon, 1985).

Lifton, Robert Jay. *The Nazi Doctors: Medical Killing and the Psychology of Genocide* (New York: Basic Books, 1989).

May, William F. *The Physician's Covenant* (Philadelphia: Westminster, 1983).

McKenny, Gerald M., and J. R. Sande, eds. *Theological Analysis of the Clinical Encounter* (Dordrecht: Kluwer Academic Publishers, 1994).

Pellegrino, Edmund D. *The Christian Virtues in Medical Practice* (Washington, D.C.: Georgetown University Press, 1996).

Pellegrino, Edmund D. *The Philosophy of Medicine Reborn: A Pellegrino Reader*, ed. H. Tristram Engelhardt Jr. and Fabrice Jotterand (Notre Dame: University of Notre Dame Press, 2008).

Siegler, Mark A. "Professional Values in Modern Clinical Practice." *Hastings Center Report* 30, no. 4 Suppl. (July-August 2000): S19-22.

Smith, Harmon M., and Larry R. Churchill. *Professional Ethics and Primary Care Medicine* (Durham, N.C.: Duke University Press, 1986).

Spencer, Edward M., et al. *Organization Ethics in Health Care* (New York: Oxford University Press, 2000), pp. 69-91.

Welie, Jos V. M. "The Relationship Between Medicine's Internal Morality and Religion." *Christian Bioethics* 8, no. 2 (August 2002): 175-98.

27 Honor the Physician

Sirach 38:1-15

Honor the physician with the honor due him,
according to your need of him,
for the Lord created him;

for healing comes from the Most High,
and he will receive a gift from the king.

The skill of the physician lifts up his head, and
in the presence of great men he is admired.

The Lord created medicines from the earth,
and a sensible man will not despise them.

Was not water made sweet with a tree
in order that his power might be known?

And he gave skill to men that he
might be glorified in his marvelous works.

By them he heals and takes away pain;
the pharmacist makes of them a compound.

His works will never be finished; and from him
health is upon the face of the earth.

My son, when you are sick do not be negligent,
but pray to the Lord, and he will heal you.

Give up your faults and direct your hands
aright, and cleanse your heart from all sin.

Offer a sweet-smelling sacrifice, and a memorial
portion of fine flour,
and pour oil on your offering, as much as you
can afford.

And give the physician his place, for the Lord
created him;
let him not leave you, for there is need of him.

There is a time when success lies in the hands of
physicians,
for they too will pray to the Lord

that he should grant them success in diagnosis
and in healing, for the sake of preserving life.

He who sins before his Maker,
may he fall into the care of a physician.

28 The Hippocratic Oath

The Hippocratic Oath

I swear by Apollo Physician and Asclepius and Hygieia and Panaceia and all the gods and goddesses, making them my witnesses, that I will fulfil according to my ability and judgment this oath and this covenant:

To hold him who has taught me this art as equal to my parents and to live my life in partnership with him, and if he is in need of money to give him a share of mine, and to regard his offspring as equal to my brothers in male lineage and to teach them this art — if they desire to learn it — without fee and covenant; to give a share of precepts and oral instruction and all the other learning to my sons and to the sons of him who has instructed me and to pupils who have signed the covenant and have taken an oath according to the medical law, but to no one else.

I will apply dietetic measures for the benefit of the sick according to my ability and judgment; I will keep them from harm and injustice.

I will neither give a deadly drug to anybody if asked for it, nor will I make a suggestion to this effect. Similarly I will not give to a woman an abortive remedy. In purity and holiness I will guard my life and my art.

I will not use the knife, not even on sufferers from stone, but will withdraw in favor of such men as are engaged in this work.

Whatever houses I may visit, I will come for the benefit of the sick, remaining free of all intentional injustice, of all mischief and in particular of sexual relations with both female and male persons, be they free or slaves.

What I may see or hear in the course of the treatment or even outside of the treatment in regard to the life of men, which on no account one must spread abroad, I will keep to myself holding such things shameful to be spoken about.

If I fulfil this oath and do not violate it, may it be granted to me to enjoy life and art, being honored with fame among all men for all time to come; if I transgress it and swear falsely, may the opposite of all this be my lot.

From Ludwig Edelstein, "The Hippocratic Oath: Text, Translation and Interpretation," in Oswei Temkin and C. Lillian Temkin, eds., *Ancient Medicine* (Baltimore: Johns Hopkins University Press, 1967), pp. 3-63. Used by permission.

29 The Hippocratic Oath Insofar as a Christian May Swear It

Blessed be God the Father of our Lord Jesus Christ. Who is blessed for ever and ever; I lie not.

I will bring no stain upon the learning of the medical art. Neither will I give poison to anybody though asked to do so, nor will I suggest such a plan. Similarly I will not give treatment to women to cause abortion, treatment neither from above nor from below. But I will teach this art, to those who require to learn it, without grudging and without an indenture. I will use treatment to help the sick according to my ability and judgment. And in purity and holiness I will guard my art. Into whatsoever houses I enter, I will do so to help the sick, keeping free from all wrongdoing, intentional or unintentional, tending to death or to injury, and from fornication with bond or free, man or woman. Whatsoever in the course of practice I see or hear (or outside my practice in social intercourse) that ought not to be published abroad, I will not divulge, but consider such things to be holy secrets. Now if I keep this oath and break it not, may God be my helper in my life and art, and may I be honoured among all men for all time. If I keep the faith, well; but if I forswear myself may the opposite befall me.

From W. H. S. Jones, *The Doctor's Oath: An Essay in the History of Medicine* (New York: Cambridge University Press, 1924), pp. 23-25. Used by permission.

30 The Doctor's Oath — and a Christian Swearing It

Allen Verhey

The Hippocratic Oath is the most familiar of that long line of oaths, prayers, and codes by which doctors have transmitted an ethos to members of their profession. Indeed, it is sometimes simply called "the doctor's oath." In our age, however, enamored of novelty and confident of its technological powers, familiarity seems to have bred, if not contempt,[1] at least the sort of quaint regard which relegates ancient documents to the historian's museum of curiosities. It is my intention, nevertheless, to suggest that there are lessons to be learned — or relearned — from this oath and its history, lessons which can be instructive concerning a professional ethic for physicians and the possible contributions of theology to that ethic.

The intention ought not be misunderstood. I will not suggest that the Hippocratic Oath is an adequate and comprehensive foundation for a professional ethic today. I will not call upon doctors and moralists concerned with medical ethics to swear it again. I will not deny that the invocation of Apollo, Asclepius, Hygeia, Panacea, and all of the gods and goddesses sounds quaint to modern ears or claim that such an invocation can be made with Christian integrity. I will not deny that the ancient institutions presupposed in the oath for the learning and practice of medicine differ from their contemporary counterparts. And I will not recommend the stipulations of the oath as a code to simplify the address to the dilemmas and quandaries posed by medical practice.

1. The attitude of Robert Veatch toward the oath can only be characterized as contempt. He argues that the oath is morally "dangerous." See Robert Veatch, *A Theory of Medical Ethics* (New York: Basic Books, 1981), pp. 18-26, 79-107, and especially 141-69. See also his "The Hippocratic Ethic: Consequentialism, Individualism, and Paternalism," *No Rush to Judgment*, ed. by David Smith and Linda M. Bernstein (Bloomington, Ind.: Poynter Center, 1978), pp. 238-64; "Medical Ethics: Professional or Universal?" *Harvard Theological Review*, 65:4 (Oct., 1972): 531-39; and *Death, Dying, and the Biological Revolution* (New Haven: Yale University Press, 1976), pp. 171, 172. Veatch criticizes both the basis and the content of the oath. The basis is criticized because the oath is based on a special professional ethic rather than on universal rational moral norms. The content is criticized because the oath is construed as consequentialist, individualist, and paternalistic.

Reprinted with permission from *Linacre Quarterly*, vol. 51, no. 2, pp. 139-58. 850 Elm Grove Road, Elm Grove, WI 53122. Subscription rate: $20 per year; $5 per single issue. Slightly abridged and edited from the original. Used by permission.

That list of disclaimers, it may easily be observed, involves every part of the oath. It may prompt the question of what is to be salvaged. But the lessons to be gleaned from this ancient document are not to be found in its content so much as in certain features of its history and its method. I want to suggest that there are lessons to be learned (1) from its reformist intention; (2) from its treatment of medicine as a practice with intrinsic goods and standards; and (3) from setting these standards in a context which expressed and evoked an identity and recognized one's dependence upon and indebtedness to a community and to the transcendent. Finally, I want to suggest (4) that there is a lesson for Christians who would contribute to the discussions of bioethics in the early Church's adoption and revision of the doctor's oath. In an age when medicine's powers flourish, but its ethos flounders, the ancient oath may help us to attend to ways of doing medical ethics which are not currently popular. I undertake, therefore, both to describe certain features of the ancient oath and to defend them as having some promise for the contemporary consideration of medical ethics in comparison to certain features of the current literature.

The Reformist Intention

According to Ludwig Edelstein, interpreter of the oath, the Hippocratic Oath was not formulated by the great Hippocrates himself, but by a small group of Pythagorean physicians late in the fourth century B.C. Edelstein observes that the oath was a minority opinion, "a Pythagorean manifesto," written against the stream and intending the reform of medicine.[2]

For centuries before the oath, ancient physicians had provided poison for those whom they could not heal, had counted abortifacients among the tools of their trade, and had been disposed to the use of the knife instead of the less invasive use of dietetics and pharmacology. Moreover, they had sometimes been guilty of injustice and mischief toward their patients, and sometimes quite shamelessly broken confidences.

When the little sect of Pythagoreans set out to reform the condition of medicine, they found no help in the law, which forbade neither suicide nor abortion. They could plainly find no help in the conventional behavior of physicians in antiquity. Nor did they find help in any "philosophical consensus," for, insofar as there was any agreement about these issues, it worked against the Pythagorean position. Platonists, Cynics, and Stoics could honor suicide as a courageous triumph over fate. Aristotelians and Epicureans were much more circumspect, but they did not forbid suicide. And abortion was typically considered essential for a well-ordered state. The arguments between Pythagoreans and other Greek philosophers must have seemed as interminable and as conceptually incommensurable as any contemporary moral argument. The minority status of their opinions, however, did not dissuade the Pythagoreans.

The point is not to defend the oath's absolute prohibitions of abortion and euthanasia and surely not to defend Pythagorean philosophy or the premises it might supply to defend such prohibitions.[3] The point is rather to call attention to this feature of the oath's method and history, that in spite of their minority position, the convictions of this community led them and moved them to reform. They refused to be satisfied with the medicine they saw around them. They refused to reduce medical morality to what the law allowed or what some philosophical consensus determined. They intended the reform of medicine.

The lesson, I suggest, for the contemporary discussion of medical ethics is that some, at least, should take courage to investigate and articulate a medical ethic which may stand at some remove from conventional behavior and attitudes within the profession and which may be based on convictions and standards more particular and profound than legal and contractual obligations or some minimal philosophical consensus. Communities with convictions about what human persons are meant to be and to become, with visions of what it means for embodied persons to flourish and thrive, have an opportunity and vocation to think through the art of medicine from their own perspectives.

The recent literature on medical ethics has not owned such an agenda. Indeed, the moral convictions and visions of particular communities typically have been tolerated and trivialized in the literature. On the one hand, there is an insistence that everyone's moral point of view should be respected. On the other hand, there has been an insistence that the only arguments which may count publicly are those which can be made independent of a distinctive moral point of view. This simultaneous tolerance and trivialization is accomplished by making the autonomy of the agent the highest human good, by making contracts between such autonomous agents the

2. Edelstein, Ludwig, "The Hippocratic Oath: Text, Translation and Interpretation," *Ancient Medicine* ed. by Oswei Temkin and C. Lillian Temkin (Baltimore: Johns Hopkins University Press, 1967), pp. 3-63. I am convinced by Edelstein concerning the Pythagorean origins of the oath. Even if it originated in some other community, however, it would still have had the intention to reform ancient medicine, and that is the feature of the oath to which I would call attention.

3. For example, the Pythagorean premise concerning the status of the fetus was supplied by a physiology which took the seed to be clot of brain containing the warm vapors whence came soul and sensation. The Pythagorean asceticism, which justified intercourse only as the necessary condition for procreation, surely affected their perspective on abortion. See Edelstein, op. cit. It is important to observe, however, that the oath, while coherent with Pythagorean doctrines and beliefs (as Edelstein shows), does not simply apply Pythagorean doctrine *to* medicine (as Edelstein presumes to have shown). The oath draws *from* medicine the morality to guide and limit the behavior of physicians. See section 2, "Medicine as a Practice," and reference 6 below.

model of human relationships, and by focusing almost exclusively on the procedural question of who should decide.[4] The ancient enterprise of attempting to understand and communicate the intrinsic good of human persons and of some human relationships and activities has been largely abandoned. Attempts to articulate communities' or traditions' address to those ancient questions may be tolerated if the "good" is kept to themselves, relegated resolutely to a "private" arena and, thus, trivialized. It may not even be tolerated if the "good" is announced as "public" good, for then it threatens to restrict and subvert autonomy. Such recent literature on medical ethics has provided — and can provide — only a "thin theory of the good,"[5] only a shriveled and dangerously minimal construal of the moral life in its medical dimensions. We find, in much contemporary medical ethics, for example, a readiness to insist on procedures to protect autonomy but a reticence to provide any advice about the morally proper uses of that autonomy and a dismissal of the idea that physicians should be the ones to give such advice.

The Hippocratic Oath, however, can remind us that the current focus on autonomy and contracts and procedural questions provides only a minimal account of medical morality. It can encourage us to own a fuller vision of medical morality and to seek the reform of medicine in the light of that vision.

The Pythagoreans' reform movement finally triumphed. The oath gradually moved from the status of a countercultural manifesto to a historic document which formed and informed the ethos of physicians for centuries. The explanation for this triumph was not any philosophical triumph by the Pythagoreans; their influence, never great, waned. Their reform, however, articulated not just Pythagorean moral premises and conclusions, but standards inherent in medicine when it is seen as a practice with certain intrinsic goods. They situated these standards in a context which provided and formed identity and which recognized dependence and indebtedness to a community and to the transcendent. These standards finally won the support of another minority community, a community which did move to dominance in Western culture — the Christian Church. These features of the oath explain its triumph. They are still instructive and, after more than two millennia, again innovative. They can help form the "fuller vision" of medical morality which may once again call for and sustain the reform of medicine.

4. So, for example, Robert Veatch, *A Theory of Medical Ethics.* See the review by Allen Verhey, "Contract — or Covenant?" *Reformed Journal* 33:9 (Sept. 1983): 23, 24.

5. The phrase, of course, is John Rawls's. See, e.g., *A Theory of Justice* (Cambridge, Mass.: Harvard University Press, 1971), pp. 396ff. The complaint about "the thin theory of the good" in the contemporary literature echoes Daniel Callahan, "Minimalist Ethics," *Hastings Center Report* 11:6 (Oct. 1981): 19-25.

Medicine as a Practice

The Pythagoreans began with their own convictions about human flourishing. But one of these convictions concerned the moral significance of the crafts, the arts, the *technē*.[6] The Pythagoreans honored the arts, especially music and medicine, as having moral and, indeed, ontological significance. Therefore, they did not simply apply Pythagorean premises to morally neutral medical skills; instead, they tried to educe and elucidate the moral significance of the craft, the art, the *technē* of medicine itself. Because this Pythagorean attitude to the crafts came to be dominant in late philosophical schools, notably the Stoics,[7] the Pythagorean reform of medicine flourished while Pythagorean philosophy waned.

In striking an intriguing contrast to most contemporary literature on medical ethics, which so often picks an ethical theory (whether Mill's or Rawls's or Nozick's or . . .) and applies it to dilemmas faced by medical practitioners, the Pythagorean conviction about the crafts allowed and required one to identify the good implicit in the craft and to articulate the standards coherent with the good of the craft. According to the oath, then, the doctor is obligated not because he is a Pythagorean, but because he is a doctor, and his obligations consist not only of standards based on Pythagorean doctrine but also of standards implicit in medicine.

The oath treats medicine as a craft, an art, a *technē*, or, to use Alasdair MacIntyre's terms,[8] as a practice, not simply a set of technical skills. That is to say, it treats medicine as a form of human activity with goods internal to it and standards of excellence implicit in it, not simply as an assortment of skills which can be made to serve extrinsic goods with merely technological excellence.

The goal of medicine, the good which is intrinsic to the practice, is identified by the oath as "the benefit of the sick." To benefit the sick is not simply the motive for taking up certain ethically neutral skills nor merely an extrinsic end to be accomplished by ethically neutral technical means.[9] It is, rather, the goal of medicine as a

6. Edelstein recognizes the importance of the Pythagorean attitude toward the crafts (e.g., "the Professional Ethics of the Greek Physician" in his *Ancient Medicine*, pp. 319-48, p. 327), but he fails to recognize that it warrants construing medicine as a practice of intrinsic goods and implicit standards (e.g., ibid., n. 21). The same failure marks Veatch's use of Edelstein (e.g., *A Theory of Medical Ethics*, p. 21).

7. *Precepts* and *On Decorum*, later writings in the Hippocratic corpus, are probably Stoic in origin; see Edelstein, op. cit.

8. On the notion of a practice, see Alasdair MacIntyre, *After Virtue* (Notre Dame: University of Notre Dame Press, 1981), pp. 175-78.

9. Veatch's criticism of the oath's "consequentialism" relies heavily on the oath's commitment to "the benefit of the sick." Veatch's understanding of the oath at this point makes "benefit" an extrinsic good and, moreover, renders benefit definable in terms of the physician's (or the patient's) private preferences. I am convinced that this is a misunderstanding. The *technē* of medicine is not construed in the oath as morally neutral skills accessible to

practice, and so it governed the physician's use of his skills in diet, drugs, and surgery, and the use of his privileged access to the patient's home and privacy. This intrinsic good entailed standards of professional excellence which could not be reduced to technological excellence.

The pattern is repeated again and again in the oath. Its prohibitions of active euthanasia, of assisting in suicide, and of abortion, for example, were not argued on the basis of Pythagorean premises; they were given as standards of a practice whose goal is to benefit the sick. Because the ends intrinsic to medicine are to heal the sick, to protect and nurture health, to maintain and restore physical well-being, limits could be imposed on the use of skills within the practice. The skills were not to be used to serve alien ends, and the destruction of human life — either the last of it or the first of it — was seen as an alien and conflicting end. The point was not that one would fail to be a good Pythagorean if one violated these standards, although that is true enough, but rather that one would fail to be a good medical practitioner. The good physician is not a mere technician; he is committed by the practice of medicine to certain goods and to certain standards.

The notoriously difficult foreswearing of surgery, even on those who stand to benefit from it, is also founded on the notion of medicine as a practice. Edelstein is probably right in tracing this stipulation to the Pythagorean preference for dietetics and pharmacology as modes of treatment,[10] but the foreswearing in the oath did not appeal to any uncompromising Pythagorean position about either the appetitive and dietetic causes of illness or the defilement of shedding blood. It rather articulated a standard for medical practice whose goal is to benefit the sick: namely, don't attempt what lies beyond your competence. To benefit the sick was not merely a motive, but the good intrinsic to medicine, and to put the patient at risk needlessly — even with the best of intentions — can be seen to violate medicine understood as such a practice. There was, therefore, no universal prohibition of surgery, only the particular prohibition of surgery by those ill-equipped to attempt it. That standard may well have been of particular relevance to Pythagorean physicians, but one need not have been a Pythagorean to accept its wisdom as a standard of practice.

The stipulations concerning decorum are yet another example. They can be readily understood against the background of Pythagorean asceticism and the proverbial "Pythagorean silence,"[11] but again, the oath presented them not as Pythagorean stipulations, but as standards of medicine understood as a practice. The goal of the practice, "the benefit of the sick," was repeated in this context even as the (necessary) intrusion into the privacy, the homes, of the sick was acknowledged. The physician's access to the intimacies of the patient's body and household and his exposure to the vulnerability of the patient and his household were granted and accepted for the sake of the goal intrinsic to medicine. To use such access for any other end or to make public the vulnerability to which the physician was made privy was seen to subvert the relation of such access and such exposure to the end of medicine. It debased the patient who should be benefited. It vitiated medicine as a practice and, therefore, the standards prohibiting sexual relations with patients and prohibiting breaches of confidentiality were implicit in medicine as a practice.

These standards could be further explicated,[12] and, if the point of this essay were to treat the oath as a code, then the further explication would be necessary. But that is not the point. It is not my claim that the oath provides an unexceptionable code of conduct. The standards of a practice at any particular time are not immune from criticism. The point is to call attention to this feature of the oath's method, that it construes medicine as a practice. It does not provide a timeless code for medicine, but there are standards of excellence appropriate to and partly definitive of the practice, whose authority must be acknowledged, and there is a good intrinsic to the practice which must be appreciated and allowed to govern the skills and to form and reform the standards. The lesson, I suggest, for the contemporary discussions of medical ethics is that those who seek the constant reform of medicine should also construe medicine as a practice with implicit goods and standards.

That is a hard but important lesson in a culture as bullish on technology and as pluralistic in values as our own. There is a constant tendency to reduce medicine to a mere — but awesome — collection of techniques that may be made to serve extrinsic goods, themselves often reduced to matters of taste.

The technology of abortion is a telling example. In *Roe v. Wade,* the Court declared that a woman's decision with respect to abortion was a private matter between herself and her physician. It recognized that the moral status of the fetus was controverted, but it held that the fetus is not a *legal* person and so is not entitled to the protection the law extends to persons. It wanted to leave the moral controversy about the status of the fetus within

consumers; it is not just a "means" even to health; it is a human activity of inheriting and learning and teaching and applying a wisdom about living with a finite body. See further E. Pellegrino and D. Thomasma, *A Philosophical Basis of Medical Practice* (New York: Oxford University Press, 1981); and Stanley M. Hauerwas, "Authority and the Profession of Medicine" (Manuscript). That Veatch misunderstands the oath at this point is obvious when he suggests — quite against the oath's own straightforward prohibition — that the oath's concern for benefit of the patient could permit participation in bringing about the death of an infant (*A Theory of Medical Ethics,* pp. 15-26).

10. Edelstein, "The Hippocratic Oath," op. cit., pp. 21-33.

11. Ibid., pp. 33-39.

12. See especially Leon Kass, "The Hippocratic Oath: Thoughts on Medicine and Ethics," a lecture given on Nov. 12, 1980, in the seminar series sponsored by the program in the Arts and Sciences Basic to Human Biology and Medicine and the American Medical Students' Association, at the University of Chicago.

that private arena of the decision a woman and her doctor would make. The court presumed (and suggested by calling the decision to abort a "medical decision") that the professional ethos of physicians would limit abortions, even if abortion were legalized and it might have been, if there had been a vivid sense of medicine as a practice.[13] The legal license was interpreted by many (both women and physicians) as a moral license, and the outcome has been a callous and frightening disregard for fetal life and welfare. The protests — usually applying some extrinsic good or extrinsic standard — have been long and loud and have sometimes exhibited callous disregard for the rights of women with respect to their own bodies and ignored the legitimate controversy about the status of the fetus. The opportunity for medicine to reassert itself as a practice, different from the practice of politics or the marketplace, has almost been lost. But the lesson of the oath is that the attempt is both possible and worthwhile.

The notion of medicine as a practice stands in marked contrast to a good deal of the current literature concerning the professions in general and medicine in particular. Michael Bayles, for example, would reject the normative characteristics of the professions, including medicine.[14] He reduces the professions to skills learned by training and made accessible to consumers. The professions, on this view, are not justified or guided by any intrinsic good but by "the values of a liberal society."[15] Thus, there are no standards implicit in the practice but only "ordinary norms" to be applied in professional contexts.

The problems with such a view are manifold. One is linguistic. "Professional" and "unprofessional" continue to be used evaluatively and, moreover, with respect to excellences not merely technical.

The notion of applying ordinary norms to medical dilemmas is also problematic. It is naive and presumptuous to suppose that a moral philosopher or theologian can boldly put to flight a moral dilemma by expertly wielding a sharp principle or some heavy theory.[16] And how shall we select the "ordinary norms" to apply? Justice is surely relevant, but there is more than one theory of justice. Good ends surely ought to be sought in medicine, too, but shall we use St. Thomas Aquinas or John Stuart Mill to define a good end? The values of society may be important, but none of us, I trust, has forgotten the atrocities committed when Hitler's vision of a "third reich" was applied to medicine.

I am much more comfortable with Bayles's "values of a liberal society" than with Hitler's "third reich," but I am not so much more confident about the practice of politics than the practice of medicine that I would make the professional ethic dependent upon our political ethic. Indeed, I wonder whether a society is truly "liberal" if it tailors the professions to a liberal society's (minimal) vision of the good. A liberal society can be guilty of trivializing ancient wisdom about human flourishing when it renders the professions, including medicine, merely instrumental skills to satisfy consumer wants.

Bayles's application of his "ordinary norms" to medicine leads to minimal moral claims and, because the minimal character of the claims is not acknowledged, to a truncated and distorted medical ethic. There is, for example, no limit to "professional services" when a profession is basically skills accessible to consumers: laetrile, genetic testing for sex determination, plastic surgery to win the Dolly Parton look-alike contest, all become the sphere of the professional entrepreneur. Immoral clients cannot be refused on the basis of "professional integrity," for there is no such thing. Bayles is aware of the problem posed by clients who would use professional skills for ends which are morally questionable but which do not clearly violate the "ordinary norms," and he presents two options for dealing with such clients. The "no difference" option quite candidly leaves no room for integrity of any kind and renders the professional the "animated tool" of the consumer.[17] The second option permits the physician to refuse services to such clients on the basis of "moral integrity," but this "moral integrity" is represented as strictly personal and private rather than professional.[18]

Bayles's attempt to reduce professional norms to "ordinary norms" applied in a medical context, to give one more example, leads to a minimal and truncated version of the prohibition of sexual intercourse with patients.[19] The ordinary norm he provides, that sexual intercourse requires the free consent of both parties, is itself a dangerously minimal account of sexual ethics. It does provide a justification for the prohibition, but it does not discount either the possibility or the importance of a "professional" justification, that the (necessary) access to the patient's privacy and vulnerability must be guided by and limited to the "good" of medicine and not be used for extrinsic ends (even when they are freely chosen or consented to).

The debate about the crafts, about the professions, is

13. The court's use of Edelstein's study of the Pythagorean origins of the Hippocratic Oath, unfortunately, tended to reinforce the position that extrinsic goods and standards may be applied to medicine but that goods and standards intrinsic to medicine do not exist. At the very time the court laid a heavy burden on physicians by calling abortion a "medical decision," it weakened physicians' resolve and ability to resist this culture's tendency to construe medicine as a set of skills to satisfy consumer wants.

14. Michael Bayles, *Professional Ethics* (Belmont, Calif.: Wadsworth Publishing Co., 1981). See also Alan Goldman, *The Moral Foundations of Professional Ethics* (Tutowa, N.J.: Rowman and Littlefield, 1980).

15. In Goldman's view, op. cit., the justification and guidance are provided by a modified utilitarianism.

16. See further Arthur L. Caplan, "Ethical Engineers Need Not Apply: The State of Applied Ethics Today," *Science, Technology and Human Values*, 6:33 (Fall, 1980): 24-32.

17. This is, of course, Aristotle's definition of a slave. See Paul Ramsey, *Ethics at the Edges of Life* (New Haven: Yale University Press, 1978), pp. 45-158.

18. Bayles, op. cit., pp. 52ff.

19. Ibid., p. 21.

an ancient and an enduring one. The lesson of the oath is that we should not too readily accept the notion of medicine as a collection of skills accessible to consumers. We should not identify our task as simply applying universal and rational norms of conduct to medicine and to the quandaries faced within it.[20]

If the *technē* of medicine is construed simply in terms of its techniques or skills, learned by training and accessible to consumers, then, of course, it is morally neutral. Skill in pharmacology enables one to be a good healer or a crafty murderer. But if a *technē* is more than technique, if it has its own goal and its own virtues, then it is hardly morally neutral. Then some moral wisdom about living as a finite body may exist within the practice of medicine and within those communities and traditions which learn and teach medicine as a practice. Then medicine's fragile capacity to resist being co-opted by an alien ideology, even a liberal ideology (not to mention the "third reich"), can be strengthened and nurtured. The lesson of the oath, I suggest, is that for some, at least, the task should be to defend the vision of medicine as a practice while educing and elucidating the goods and standards implicit in that practice.

The Hippocratic Oath had its origins among the Pythagoreans who had the courage to attempt the reform of medicine and the wisdom not merely to apply Pythagorean premises to medicine but to construe it as a practice. It was handed down not as legislation but as voluntary rule imposing voluntary obedience. Its power to reform was not coercive or simply rationally persuasive; its power to reform was its power to form character and a community which nurtured it. It did not set its standards in a context of legal sanctions or in a context of impartial rationality. It set these standards in a context which expressed and evoked an identity and recognized one's dependence upon and indebtedness to both a community and the transcendent. To those features of the oath we turn next.

Identity, Community, and the Transcendent

The oath, like all oaths and promises, was a performative declaration rather than a descriptive one. It did not just describe reality; it altered it. The one who swore this oath was never the same "one" again. The one swearing this oath adopted more than a set of rules and skills; he or she adopted an identity. The goods and standards of medicine as a practice were owned as one's own and gave shape to integrity with one's identity. Therefore, "physician" was a description not only of what one knew or of what one did or of what one knew how to do, but of who one was. Henceforth, one examined questions of conduct in this role not as an impartial and rational agent, calculating utility sums, say, but as a physician. Integrity with this identity called for the physician to exert himself on behalf of the patient at hand, even the patient-scoundrel at hand, without calculating the greatest good for the greatest number. Indeed, to allow that question, to bear toward the patient the kind of impartial relation which makes it plausible, was to lose one's identity, to forfeit one's integrity.

This feature of the oath calls our attention to the moral significance of "identity." Once again the lesson of the doctor's oath sets a different agenda than the one contemporary medical ethics has generally undertaken. Contemporary medical ethics usually adopts the perspective of impartial rationality, either in the form of utilitarianism or in the form of contract theory.[21] To adopt any such impartial perspective, however, requires the doctor's alienation from his own moral interests and loyalties *qua* physician, from himself and from his special relationship to his patient. Doctors are asked, indeed, obliged, by this perspective to view the project and passion of their practice as though they were outside objective observers.

They are asked by this approach to disown — and for the sake of morality — the goods and standards they possess as their own and which give them their moral character as physicians.[22]

The perspective of impartial rationality is not to be disowned. It can enable conversation between people with different loyalties and the adjudication of conflicting interests, and it can challenge the arbitrary dominance of one perspective over another. To be made to pause occasionally and, for the sake of analysis and judgment, to view things as impartially as we can is not only legitimate, but also salutary. But such an ethic remains minimal at best, and if its minimalism is not acknowledged, it can distort the moral life. Physicians — and patients — cannot consistently live their moral lives like that with any integrity. The Hippocratic Oath calls our attention to the importance of a physician's identity, character, and integrity. Such an approach might recover the importance of performative rituals like swearing an initiatory oath, and it would surely attend not only to the ways in which acts effectively realize ends, but also to the ways in which acts express values and form character.[23]

The oath expressed and evoked an identity, but it was an identity which recognized its dependence upon and indebtedness to a community and the transcendent.

The oath bound one to a community where not only the requisite skills were taught, but where the requisite

20. Veatch, *A Theory of Medical Ethics,* op. cit., is a case in point.

21. Again, Veatch, ibid., is a case in point.

22. See further Stanley Hauerwas, *Truthfulness and Tragedy: Further Investigations in Christian Ethics* (Notre Dame: University of Notre Dame Press, 1977), pp. 23-25; and Bernard Williams, "A Critique of Utilitarianism," in J. J. C. Smart and Bernard Williams, *Utilitarianism: For and Against* (New York: Cambridge University Press, 1973), pp. 100-118.

23. Childress, James, *Priorities in Biomedical Ethics* (Philadelphia: Westminster Press, 1981), p. 82, citing Max Weber, *Max Weber in Economy and Society,* nicely distinguishes "goal-rational" and "value-rational" conduct.

character and identity were nurtured. The doctor swore to live in fellowship (Gk.: *koinosasthai*) with his teacher, to share a common life with him. He pledged, moreover, to teach the art to his teacher's sons, to his own sons, and to all who wanted to learn not simply the skills, but also the practice. Here was not an autonomous individual practitioner, utilizing his skills for his private good and according to his private vision of the good or as contracted by another to accomplish the other's "good." The doctor who swore the oath stood self-consciously in a community and in a tradition. He acknowledged gratefully his dependence upon this community and tradition, his indebtedness to his teacher, and his responsibility to protect and nurture the practice of medicine.[24]

This section of the oath is often criticized.[25] It is accused of fostering a medical guild where obligations to colleagues take priority over obligations to patients, so that medical incompetence and malpractice are usually covered up and the incompetent and unscrupulous (protected by the guild) do further harm to patients. The charge is a serious one, and the profession's reluctance to discipline its members makes it cogent. The fault is not with the oath, however, but with the corruption of the oath in the absence of a commitment to medicine as a practice. When there is such a commitment, it governs relations with colleagues as well as patients, and protecting and nurturing the practice — both the requisite skills and the requisite character — enable and require communal discipline. The failure of the profession to discipline itself adequately may be traced not to the perspective of the oath but to the dismissal of the perspective of the oath.

Today the training for medicine has shifted to university-based medical schools, which pride themselves on their scientific detachment from questions of value in their dispassionate pursuit of the truth. Such a context can virtually sponsor the construal of medicine as a collection of skills and techniques to be used for extrinsic goods which are not matters of truth but matters of taste.[26] Then there is no community of people committed to a practice and under its standards; there is only the camaraderie of those who have undergone the same arduous routine. Then the profession lacks both a commitment to a practice which makes discipline possible and a genuine enough community to make discipline a nurturing as well as a punishing activity.

The stress on community in the oath can help call our attention to the moral necessity of attending to the institutions, communities, and traditions within which the physician's identity is nurtured. Adding courses in medical ethics taught by philosophers or theologians to the curricula of medical schools may be important, but it is neither essential nor sufficient. Indeed, if such courses are co-opted as token evidence of the moral concern of the institution, or if clinical instructors abdicate the responsibility for difficult decisions to "the moral expert," the results could be counter-productive. It is more important to have teachers chosen and rewarded not only for their excellent skills but also for their excellence in medical practice — chosen and rewarded not only for their ability to teach the skills, but also for the ability to model the practice. The philosopher or theologian may then have an important role as participant in — and mid-wife for — a continuing dialogue between such teachers and their students about the goods and standards implicit in medicine as a practice. In such a continuing dialogue there will surely be continuing conflicts, but so any living tradition is passed down.

No less important than institutions where doctors are trained are institutions within which they practice and the communities within which they live, including the religious communities. That religious communities might nurture and sustain the identity of physicians is, of course, suggested by the doctor's oath itself. The physician acknowledged his dependence upon and indebtedness to not only the community of doctors, but also the transcendent.

The opening line called all the gods and goddesses as witnesses to this oath, and the last line puts the doctor at the mercy of divine justice. The invocation of the gods and their divine retribution served, of course, to signify the solemnity of the oath and the stringency of the obligations. More than that, however, was accomplished by the oath's piety, by its recognition of our dependence upon and indebtedness to transcendent power which bears down on us and sustains us. A narrative is provided, a narrative which helps inform identity and helps sustain community, a narrative which supports and tests the practice of medicine. The deities named are a lineage. Apollo, the god of truth and light, here invoked as

24. Veatch's charge that the oath is "individualistic" (*A Theory of Medical Ethics*, pp. 154-59, and "The Hippocratic Ethic," pp. 255-59) fails to recognize this communal character of the practice of medicine in the oath. The oath, indeed, seems much more cognizant of the social and historical character of medicine than Veatch himself for whom independent and autonomous individuals contract for medical services. Veatch's accusation cannot stand; it can, in fact, be turned against Veatch's own position, for it is Veatch's contract model which protects and perpetuates the individualism of modern liberalism and sets medicine in the ethos of the marketplace. Veatch's contract theory may provide a minimal amount of medical morality, but unless its minimalism is acknowledged, it can distort medical morality into the most arid form of individualism, quite incapable of nurturing or supporting other than contractual relationships. See further James Childress, "A Masterful Tour: A Response to Robert Veatch," *Journal of Current Social Issues* 4:12 (Fall 1975): 20-25.

25. See, e.g., William F. May, "Code and Covenant or Philanthropy and Contract?" in *Ethics in Medicine: Historical Perspectives and Contemporary Concerns*, ed. by Stanley J. Reiser, Arthur J. Dyck, and William J. Curran (Cambridge, Mass.: MIT Press, 1977), pp. 65-76 (an expanded and revised form of an essay first published in *Hastings Center Report* [Dec. 1975]: 29-38).

26. See further William F. May, *Notes on the Ethics of Doctors and Lawyers*, a Poynter Pamphlet (Bloomington, Ind.: Poynter Center, 1977), pp. 16-21; and his "Normative Inquiry and Medical Ethics in Our Colleges and Universities," in *No Rush to Judgment*, pp. 332-61.

"Apollo Physician," is the father of Asclepius. Asclepius, the father of medicine and the patron of physicians and patients, had two daughters, Hygeia and Panacea, or "Health" and "All-heal," the goddesses of health maintenance and therapy.[27] It is a story of the divine origins and transmission of the work physicians are given and gifted to do. To undertake the work of a physician was to make this story one's own story, to continue it and embody it among human beings. They were not tempted to "play God" or to deny their subordinate role, but they were supported and encouraged in their ministrations by this story. In serving patients in their practice, they continued a narrative that had its beginnings among the gods. They were not tempted to magic by this story,[28] but they were enabled to acknowledge the mystery of healing, the subtle and profound connections of the spirit and the body.[29]

This feature of the oath can remind us of the religious dimensions of medicine and medical morality. It is a hard but important lesson for an age as noisily secular as ours. The oath, I think, is an example of the moral significance of a natural piety, the importance of what Calvin would call a *sensus divinitatis,* the sense of the divine. This natural piety includes the sense of gratitude for the gifts of life and of the world, a sense of dependence upon some reliable, but dimly known order, a sense of some tragic fault in the midst of our world, and a sense of responsibility to the inscrutable power Who stands behind the gifts and the order and Who judges the fault.[30] One can do worse, I think, than name this other wrongly; one could understand (misunderstand) this other as the "enemy" of his own work, as a deluding power, or one could deny or (like so much of the contemporary literature) ignore this other and these senses. The oath adopted neither of those forms of distrust;[31] rather, it set the practice of medicine in the context of a natural piety, in the context of a sense of gratitude, of dependence, of tragedy, and of responsibility to the transcendent. Such a natural piety can still nourish and sustain the physician's calling. Its responsiveness to the transcendent can protect the physician both from the presumption of "playing God" and from the reductionism of plying the trade for hire. It remains part of the fuller vision of medicine.

The Christian's Swearing It

The triumph of the doctor's oath may finally be attributed to the triumph of a new religion in the ancient world. Christianity adopted it as its own, finally presenting it in a Christian form, "The Oath According to Hippocrates Insofar as a Christian May Swear It." There were certain revisions, to be sure, but the continuity of the Christian version with the ancient oath is undeniable. Both the continuity and the revisions are instructive for Christian theologians and communities who take part in the current discussions of bioethics.

First, note the adoption and reiteration of the standards of the Hippocratic Oath. There are some minor variations in the stipulations governing the practice — the operation clause is omitted, even "unintentional" harm (negligence) is forbidden, the prohibition of abortion is amplified — but the similarity is the striking thing. The claim is not that here finally we have a Christian code to be used and applied to current dilemmas. The claim is rather that there is a lesson here for those Christians who would contribute to the conversations about medical ethics. The lesson is that Christian ethics does not disown "natural" morality. It does not construct an ethic *ex nihilo,* out of nothing. It selects and assimilates the "natural" moral wisdom around it in terms of its own truthfulness and in terms of its integrity with the Christian vision. The theologians who would contribute to the conversation about bioethics must first listen attentively and respectfully to "natural" moral wisdom concerning medicine. Then they can speak responsively and responsibly about the adoption and selection of certain standards as coherent with reason, with medicine construed as a practice, and with the Christian vision.

"The Oath Insofar as a Christian May Swear It" offers a second lesson for theologians interested in medical ethics. Note the two obvious changes. The first is that the practice and its standards were set in the context of a Christian identity and of the Christian story. God, the Father of our Lord Jesus Christ, was invoked rather than Apollo et al.; the physician cast himself on the mercy of His justice. Once again, the invocation of God and His retribution served not only to signal the solemnity of the oath and the stringency of the obligations, but also to set the physician's identity and practice in the context of a story which has its beginnings with God. This feature was expressed visibly as well. "The Oath Insofar as a Christian May Swear It" — or at least some copies of it — was written in the shape of a cross.[32] The one who swore such an oath adopted the physician's identity as a follower of Christ, "Who took our infirmities and bore our diseases" (Matt. 8:17; cf. Is. 53:4). A Christian identity nurtured, sustained, and shaped the physician's identity for those who took such an oath seriously.

The second obvious change is the reduction of duties to one's teacher. Historically, this change is understandable. Medical instruction had shifted from artisan fami-

27. Kass, op. cit.

28. See Edelstein, "Greek Medicine in Its Relation to Religion and Magic," op. cit., pp. 205-46.

29. Kass, op. cit.

30. See further James M. Gustafson, "Theocentric Interpretation of Life," *The Christian Century,* July 30-Aug. 6, 1980, p. 758; and *Ethics from a Theocentric Perspective* (Chicago: Chicago University Press, 1981), pp. 129-36.

31. See H. R. Niebuhr, *The Responsible Self* (New York: Harper & Row, 1963), pp. 115-18.

32. W. H. S. Jones, *The Doctor's Oath: An Essay in the History of Medicine* (New York: Cambridge University Press, 1924), pp. 23-25. See facsimiles in W. H. S. Jones, *The Doctor's Oath,* frontispiece and p. 26.

lies and guilds to universities and eventually to faculties of medicine. The Church itself was, for centuries, the nurturing and sustaining institution and community for medicine. It chartered and administered the universities; it dominated the curriculum; its pervasive ethos ruled the professions.[33] Morally, the change was required by setting the oath in the context of the Christian story, for that story makes service the mark of greatness as well as of gratitude. So, it was inevitable that service to the patient was emphasized rather than obligations to teachers. The Christian story of breaking down the barriers that separate people, moreover, made it inevitable that the emphasis shifted from professional elitism to open access to the community of service.

What Is the Lesson Here?

The lesson here is not that we should attempt to reintroduce "Christendom" or even the patterns of medical instruction of that time. Notwithstanding the impossibility of such an attempt, the dominion of the Church was marked by parochialism as well as majesty, by pettiness as well as grandeur, by obscurantism as well as learning. The reformist intention does not lead back to Christendom for either medicine or the Church. There is little hope for a Christian medical ethic that proceeds by way of a theological triumphalism, that claims to have truth, if not captive, at least cornered. The lesson is rather that Christian medical ethics cannot proceed with integrity if it always restricts itself to articulating and defending standards of the practice or certain applications of impartial principles of philosophy or law to medical dilemmas. It is lamentable that so little of the work in medical ethics by Christian theologians candidly and explicitly attends to the Christian story and its bearing on medicine.[34] It is lamentable for the communities of faith out of which these ethicists work, for they want to live in faith, to live in integrity with the identity they have been given and to which they are called. But it is also lamentable for the broader community, for a pluralistic society profits from the candid expression of different perspectives. Candid attention to the theological dimensions of morality could prevent the reduction and distortion of morality to a set of minimal expectations necessary for pluralism and remind all participants in such a culture of broader and more profound questions about what human persons are meant to be and to become. The integrity to think about and talk about the relevance of the Christian story is the second lesson of "The Oath Insofar as a Christian May Swear It."

The first lesson of "The Oath Insofar as a Christian May Swear It" was that Christian ethics does not disown "natural" morality. The Christian story does not force those who own it to disown either medicine as a practice or human rationality. The second lesson of "The Oath Insofar as a Christian May Swear It" is that Christians concerned with medical ethics should have the integrity to set medicine in the context of the Christian story, to form, inform, and reform medicine. The first lesson stands against any premature sectarian stance, against opting prematurely for either a sectarian community or a sectarian medicine.[35] The second lesson stands against any simple identification of a Christian ethic either with universal and rational principles or with a professional ethic, against, for example, sanctifying contract theory by identifying it with "covenant."[36] The task is to transform or, to put it less presumptuously, to qualify[37] a rational ethic and a professional ethic by candid attention to the Christian story.

There will be tensions, of course. With respect to decisions about the refusal of treatment, for example, a universal and rational ethic may emphasize the patient's autonomy, but a professional ethic may emphasize the physician's commitment to the life and health of his or her patient, and a theological ethic may emphasize dispositions formed and informed by a story where the victory over death is a divine victory, not a technological victory, where people need not stand in dread of death, but may not practice hospitality toward it.[38] These tensions and their resolution will require the careful attention of those who make it their task to think about medicine and who care about the Christian story as the story of our life, our whole life.

Finally, it may be observed that theological reflection, even when it is presumptuous enough to talk about "transformation," does not represent an alien imposition upon the practice of medicine. As we have seen, the tradition of medicine as a practice is at home in piety. Loyalty to God, the Father of our Lord Jesus Christ, fulfills and redeems natural piety. The native senses of gratitude and dependence, of a tragic fault in the midst of our world, and of responsibility, are not disowned by a theological approach, but informed and reformed by the

33. May, *Notes on the Ethics,* op. cit., pp. 16, 17; and "Normative Inquiry," op. cit.

34. See James M. Gustafson, "Theology Confronts Technology and the Life Sciences," *Commonweal* 2:5 (June 1978): 386-92. See also Stanley Hauerwas, "Can Ethics Be Theological?" *Hastings Center Report* 5:8 (Oct. 1978): 47, 48. To his credit, Robert Veatch introduces the notion of "covenant" into his *A Theory of Medical Ethics.* Unfortunately, it is unclear how, if at all, the religious significance of covenant affects his understanding of the contract between physician and patient. Indeed, the meaning of "covenant" seems to be reduced to the notion of "contract." For some of the differences between contract and covenant (and for an outstanding example of theological reflection on medical ethics focusing on the notion of covenant), see William May, "Code and Covenant," op. cit.

35. Stanley Hauerwas calls for the formation of "a sectarian community" ("Authority and the Profession of Medicine," p. 22).

36. As Robert Veatch, *A Theory of Medical Ethics,* op. cit.

37. See James M. Gustafson, *Can Ethics Be Christian?* p. 173 *et passim.*

38. See further Allen Verhey, "Christian Community and Identity: What Difference Should They Make to Patients and Physicians Finally?" *Linacre Quarterly* 52:2 (May 1985).

Christian story. The current literature on bioethics stands at risk of ignoring that story, of neglecting those resources. Christians have a vocation to identify and articulate the significance of the Christian story for medicine not only because that agenda stands comfortable in an ancient tradition, but also because it will serve both integrity within the Christian community and humanity with medical practice. To renege on this opportunity and vocation will diminish not only the communities of faith, but the art of medicine as well.

31 The Physician's Covenant

William F. May

Ernest Hemingway's works illuminate a professional ethic that prizes technique as a shield against ties. William Faulkner's novels and stories create a bonded world. Faulkner's characters take their bearing from a promissory event. He usually wrote about the ties of marriage and the family, the bond between the races and the generations, or the primordial tie to the land. Hemingway and Faulkner both wrote about men who kill animals; Hemingway used such deaths as climaxes to end a poem ("and then it was over"); Faulkner used them as a sacrifice to establish a covenant, as in "Delta Autumn":

> I slew you; my bearing must not shame your quitting life. My conduct forever onward must become your death.[1]

Isaac McCaslin made this unspoken promise as he killed his first deer under the tutelage of old Sam Fathers, the Indian who taught him to hunt. Some seventy years later, old Isaac McCaslin still returns annually to that sacred place where, as a boy, he learned to hunt. During the annual trek back into the delta, he recovers that moment, seven decades ago, when he first slew his deer, what Faulkner calls elsewhere the "binding instant":

> . . . and the gun leveled rapidly without haste and crashed and he walked to the buck lying still in the shape of that magnificent speed and bled it with Sam's knife and Sam dipped his hands into hot blood and marked his forehead forever.[2]

The event alters his being: It binds and judges the rest of his life, whatever its content. From then on, just as the marked Jew, the errant, harassed, and estranged Jew, recovers through ritual renewal the covenant of the exodus and Mount Sinai, Isaac returns to the delta every autumn to renew the hunt and to suffer there his own renewal despite the alienation he has subsequently known across a lifetime.

This promissory event shapes his future morally as well as ritually. The covenant details duties that give specific content to the future, while enjoining a comprehensive fidelity that extends beyond particulars to unforeseen

1. William Faulkner, "Delta Autumn," in *Go Down Moses* (Vintage Books, 1973), p. 351.
2. Ibid., pp. 350-51.

and unforeseeable contingencies. The hunter's specific duties in this case include learning how to use a rifle to bring down game and a knife to kill. More broadly, he must also protect the species on which the hunt depends; this obligation demands that he protect the doe and the wilderness so crucial to its flourishing. Metaphorically, the covenant broadens still further to enjoin fitting ways to use land and respect for the human community that uses it. (In the story, Faulkner nicely juxtaposes obligations to the nonhuman and the human worlds through the metaphor of the doe. A faithless hunter violates covenantal fidelity not only by killing a doe but by abandoning a black woman who has borne his child.) The duty to protect the weak and the vulnerable eventually expands into a comprehensive fidelity that exceeds specification. It includes the contingent needs of others that the original covenant could not specifically anticipate.

Finally, a future-shaping covenant centers on a promise, but it does not begin with that promise. It begins, still earlier, with what the initiate received and assumed as a gift:

> He seemed to see the two of them — himself and the wilderness as coevals, his own span as a hunter, a woodsman not contemporary with his first breath but transmitted to him, assumed by him gladly, humbly, with joy and pride, from that old Major de Spain and that old Sam Fathers who had taught him how to hunt.[3]

The gifts are several: the wilderness and its game, but also the gift of instruction by mentors, who have taught him how to respect the wilderness and to hunt. These gifts precede the promise — just as the gifts of courtship precede a marriage vow, and, in the Scriptures of Israel, the exodus precedes Mount Sinai. The Jews bind themselves to God at Mount Sinai as those who have already received an astonishing gift, the deliverance from Egypt. A covenantal ethic positions human givers in the context of a primordial act of receiving a gift not wholly deserved, which they can only assume gratefully. God tells the Israelites: When you harvest your crops, leave some for the sojourner. For you were once sojourners in Egypt. Givers themselves receive. Benefactors ultimately benefit.

The biblical understanding of covenant defines the world about which Faulkner writes. The Scriptures of ancient Israel are littered with such covenants and covenantal duties: between men and women (the covenant of marriage), between men and men (the covenants of friendship), between nations (treaties and covenants of conquest), between a people and the stranger in the midst (duties to the sojourner), and between the generations (the transmission of a blessing, with its filial duties). But these secondary covenants derive from and reflect imperfectly that singular covenant that embraces all others, the covenant of the people with God.

The primary religious covenant includes the aforementioned elements: first, an original gift between the soon-to-be covenanted partners (the deliverance of the people from Egypt); second, a promise based on the original or anticipated gift (the vows at Mount Sinai). These two aspects of covenant, taken together, alter the being of the covenanted people (God "marks the forehead" of the Jews forever) so that fidelity to the covenant defines their subsequent life. Third, the covenanted people accept an inclusive set of ritual and moral obligations by which they will live. These commands are both specific enough to make the future duties of Israel concrete (e.g., the dietary laws and laws governing protection of the weak), yet summary enough (e.g., "Love the Lord thy God with all thy heart . . .") to require a fidelity to the intent as well as to the letter.

This brief summary of the structural features of a covenantal ethic does not yet suggest how it would work out in a professional setting — except to contrast starkly with an ethic that eschews ties and commitments. Just how it grounds obligations to patients, colleagues, the profession, and the wider society unfolds in due course as we compare the ethic with an ideal and a mechanism that in some particulars it resembles: the philanthropic ideal enshrined in the written codes of the profession and the marketplace mechanism of contractual agreements.

The Hippocratic Oath

Although the notion of covenant originates and develops primarily in the biblical tradition, a covenantal ingredient also figures in the classical physician's oath. The Hippocratic Oath includes three parts: first, codal duties to patients; second, covenantal obligations to one's teacher and his family; and, third, the setting of both in the context of an oath to the gods.

The physician's duties to his patients, as noted earlier, include a series of absolute prohibitions and positive injunctions largely philanthropic in their origin (and partly technical in their content). The second set of obligations, directed to the physician's teacher, his teacher's children, and his own, require him to accept full filial responsibilities for his adoptive father's personal and financial welfare and to transmit without fee his art and knowledge to the teacher's progeny and his own and to other pupils, but only those others who take the oath according to medical law. The setting and the spirit of the second set of obligations differ from those of the first.

In his study of the Hippocratic Oath, the historian Ludwig Edelstein characterizes those duties that a physician undertakes toward patients as an ethical code and those assumed toward the professional guild (one's teachers) as a covenant. Edelstein traces this difference to the Pythagorean convention of adopting the student by oath into the "family" of the teacher.[4]

In my judgment, the fact of indebtedness constitutes

3. Ibid., p. 354.

4. Ludwig Edelstein, *Ancient Medicine*, ed. by Owsei Temkin and C. Lillian Temkin (Johns Hopkins Press, 1967), pp. 40-48.

the chief reason for using the term "covenant." The word conveniently describes the distinctive obligations to one's teacher. Physicians undertake duties to their patients, but they *owe something* to their teachers. They have received goods and services for which they owe their filial services. Toward their patients, they function as benefactors, but toward their teachers, they relate as beneficiaries. This responsiveness to gift characterizes a covenant. Both the Hammurabic Code and the Mosaic Law state those laws and statutes that will shape their respective civilizations; but the biblical covenant differs from the Hammurabic and other codes. It places the moral duties of the people in the all-important context of a divine gift of deliverance. When the people of Israel promise to obey God, they respond to goods already received. Analogously, in the Hippocratic Oath, the physician undertakes obligations to the teacher and the teacher's progeny out of gratitude for services already rendered. The modern practice of medicine has tended to reinforce this ancient distinction between code and covenant and has opted for code as the ruling ideal in relationships to patients, but not with altogether favorable consequences for the moral health of the profession.

The countless exchanges between colleagues — referrals, favors, personal confidences, tips, training, consultations, and collaborative work on cases — strengthen, amplify, and intensify this ancient bond with the teacher (colleague). Loyalty to colleagues grows as a response to gifts already received and to those anticipated. Rules governing behavior toward patients have a different ring to them from that fealty which physicians owe their colleagues. The medical codes do not interpret duties to patients as a partly responsive act for gifts and services received. This element of covenantal indebtedness does not figure in the interpretation of professional duties to patients from obligations of the Hippocratic Oath to the modern codes of the AMA.

The Hippocratic Oath, of course, includes a third element: a vow, or religious oath proper, directed to the gods. "I swear by Apollo Physician, and Asclepius and Hygieia, and Panaceia and all the gods and goddesses, making them my witnesses, that I will fulfill according to my ability and judgment this oath and this covenant."[5] A religious reference appears again in the statement of duties to the patient: "In purity and holiness I will guard my life and my art." And the promise maker finally petitions: "If I fulfill this oath and do not violate it, may it be granted to me to enjoy life and art . . . ; if I transgress it and swear falsely, may the opposite of all this be my lot."[6]

This religious oath, in the literal sense of the term, made a "professional" out of the man who subscribed to it. He professed or testified thereby to the power of healing, which his duties to his patients and his obligations to his teacher made specific. Swearing by Apollo and Asclepius affirmed the ontological root of his life. He professed, in effect, those powers that altered his own state of being. Henceforth he was a professional, a professor of healing.

This third element in the Hippocratic Oath, so interpreted, expands the covenant to refer not simply to a limited indebtedness to one's teachers but also, more broadly, to those transcendent powers on which healing depends. The religious oath partly resembled a covenant in that the physician made a promise that referred to the gods from whose power the profession of healing ultimately derives. To this degree, it put the physician in the position of a recipient. This religious promise supported that secondary promise that the physician made to care for his teacher and to fulfill his duties to his patients.

Yet in two important respects, the vow itself differs from a biblical covenant: It offers no prefatory statement about the actions of the divine to which the human promise responds; and its form deemphasizes the responsive nature of the physician's action, for he swears *by* the gods instead of promises to the gods to fulfill his professional duties. His promise by the gods simply gives gravity and shape to the details of the oath.

Detached altogether from this religious vow, both the Hippocratic Oath and the profession that it helped to shape move further toward a purely codal definition of duties to patients. These duties, as transmitted in a clinical setting, largely prize the ideal of technical efficiency. But, as engraved in the written tablets of the profession, they elevate into the compensatory and ultimately pretentious ideal of philanthropy.

Philanthropy versus Covenantal Indebtedness

The philanthropic ideal of service to humankind, inscribed in the written codes, cannot be faulted for its material content. It succumbs, however, to what might be called the conceit of philanthropy when it assumes that the professional's commitment to patients is a wholly gratuitous rather than a responsive act. The codes acknowledge, in modern times, neither an indebtedness to a transcendent source nor the physician's substantial indebtedness to the community. As a result, the odor of condescension taints the documents. The American code of 1847, for example, asserts that the patients' duties derive from what they have received from their doctors:

> The members of the medical profession, upon whom is enjoined the performance of so many important and arduous duties toward the community, and who are required to make so many sacrifices of comfort, ease, and health for the welfare of those who avail themselves of their services, certainly have a right to expect and require that their patients should entertain a just sense of the duties which they owe to their medical attendants.[7]

5. Ibid., p. 6.
6. Ibid.

7. "American Medical Association — First Code of Medical Ethics" (1847), in Stanley J. Reiser et al. (eds.), *Ethics in Medicine: Historical Perspectives and Contemporary Concerns* (MIT Press, 1977), p. 30, Sect. 2, Art. 11.

In like manner, the section "Obligations of the Public to Physicians" emphasizes those many gifts and services that the public has received from, and that create its indebtedness to, the medical profession.

> The benefits accruing to the public, directly and indirectly, from the active and unwearied beneficiaries of the profession, are so numerous and important that physicians are justly entitled to the utmost consideration and respect from the community.[8]

But turning to the preamble on the physician's duties to the patient and the public, we find no corresponding section of the code of 1847 (or 1957) that acknowledges, or even partly derives, physicians' duties from those gifts and services that they have received from the community. Thus the code offers the picture of a relatively self-sufficient monad, who out of the nobility and generosity of his disposition and the gratuitously accepted conscience of his profession has taken on himself the noble life of service. The false posturing in all this is blurted out in one of the opening sections of the 1847 code. Physicians "should study, also, in their deportment so as to unite tenderness with firmness, and condescension with authority, so as to inspire the minds of their patients with gratitude, respect, and confidence."[9]

Significantly, the code shifts its terms, depending on the direction in which it moves. It refers not to the "Obligations of Patients to Their Physicians" but the "Duties of Physicians to Their Patients." The shift from "Obligations" to "Duties" may seem slight, but, in fact, it reveals a differing source and intensity to moral claim. "Obligation" has the same root as the words "ligament" and "religion"; it emphasizes a bind, a bond, a tie. The AMA viewed the patient and public as bound and indebted to the profession for its services but viewed the profession as accepting *duties* to the patient and public out of a noble conscience rather than a reciprocal sense of indebtedness.

The profession parodies God not so much because it exercises power of life and death over others, but because it does not really think of itself as beholden, even partially, to anyone for those duties to patients that it lays on itself. The profession claims the godlike power to draw its life from itself alone and to act wholly gratuitously.

In fact, however, the physician owes a very considerable debt to the community. The original Hippocratic Oath adumbrates the first of these. The physician owes someone or some group for his or her education. In ancient times, this led to a special sense of covenantal obligation to one's teacher. Under the conditions of modern medical education, the profession owes obligations both substantial (far exceeding the social investment in the training of any other professional) and widely distributed (including not only teachers but those public monies that provide for medical education, the teaching hospital, and massive research into disease).

Because many more qualified candidates apply to medical school than can be admitted and because, until recently, the society needed many more doctors than the schools could train, physicians incur a second order of indebtedness for the privilege of practice that has almost arbitrarily come their way. Although the 1847 code refers to the "privileges" of being a doctor, it does not specify the social origins of those privileges. Third, and not surprisingly, the codes do not refer to that extraordinary social largesse that befalls the physician, in payment for services, especially in a society suffering from a limitless fear of death and, until recently, a limited supply of personnel. Furthermore, the codes do not concede the indebtedness of the physician to those patients who have offered themselves as subjects for experimentation or as teaching material (either in teaching hospitals or in the early years of practice). Early practice includes, after all, the element of increased risk for patients who lay their bodies on the line as the apprentice doctor practices on them. The pun in the word "practice" but reflects the inevitable social price of training.

Judah Folkman, M.D., in a class day address to young graduates at Harvard Medical School, eloquently acknowledged this indebtedness to the patient, which, he suggests, physicians must repay, much "like tithing." Such *pro bono publico* work might take various forms: a willingness to see Medicaid patients; attending continuing education courses and taking recertification examinations; carrying out investigation or research; or perhaps even doing volunteer work for national or philanthropic services.[10]

Physicians not only owe their patients for a start in their careers but remain unceasingly in their debt. The power and authority that mature professionals exude somewhat obscure this reciprocity of need. They seem self-sufficient virtuosos whose life derives from their competence, whereas others appear before them in their indigence, their illness, their crimes, or their ignorance, for which the professional, as doctor, lawyer, or teacher, offers remedy.

In fact, however, a reciprocity of giving and receiving nourishes the professional relationship. The professional does not function as benefactor alone but also as beneficiary. In teaching, for example, students need a teacher, but the teacher also needs students. They provide the teacher with a regular occasion and forum in which to work out what he or she has to say and to rediscover the subject afresh through the discipline of sharing it with others. Likewise, the doctor needs patients. No one can watch a physician nervously approach retirement without realizing how much the doctor has needed the patients to be himself or herself.

A covenantal ethic helps acknowledge this context of need and indebtedness in which professionals undertake and discharge their duties. It also relieves professionals of the temptation and pressure to pretend that they are

8. Ibid., p. 34, Sect. 3, Art. 11.

9. Ibid., p. 29, Sect. 1, Art 1.

10. Published in *The New York Times,* June 6, 1975, Op-Ed page.

demigods exempt from human exigency. In addition to the specific ways in which they owe their patients, professionals stand unceasingly exigent and needy before God. The derivation of the notion of professional covenant from a divine-human covenant should not seduce us into slotting healers (and other professionals) into the position of God. God is not to humankind as the healer is to his or her patients. Despite all flattering impressions to the contrary, professionals undertake their responsibilities not as godly benefactors but as those who, first and foremost, benefit. The human activities of healing, teaching, parenting, and the like do not create — that is God's work — but, from beginning to end, respond. Only within a fundamental responsiveness do professionals undertake their secondary little initiatives on behalf of others.

Contractor Covenant

While criticizing the ideal of philanthropy, I have emphasized the elements of exchange and reciprocity that mark the professional relationship. Should we therefore eliminate the element of the gratuitous in professional ethics? Do physicians merely respond to the social investment in their training, the fees paid for their services, and the terms of an agreement drawn up between themselves and their patients, the element of the gratuitous altogether disappearing?

Does covenant simply act as a commercial contract in which two parties calculate their respective best interests and agree on some joint project from which both derive roughly equivalent benefits for good contributed by each? If so, covenantal ethics would support those theorists who would interpret the doctor-patient relationship as a legal agreement and assimilate medical ethics to medical law.

The notion of the physician as contractor has obvious appeal. First, it breaks with more authoritarian models (such as parent or priest). It emphasizes informed consent rather than blind trust; it encourages respect for the dignity of the patient, who does not, because of illness, forfeit autonomy as a human being; it also encourages specifying rights, duties, conditions, and qualifications that limit the contract. In effect, it establishes some symmetry and mutuality in the relationship between doctor and patient as they exchange information and reach an agreement, tacit or explicit, to exchange goods (money for services).

Second, a contract provides for the legal enforcement of terms on both parties and thus offers each some protection and recourse under the law to make the other accountable under the contract.

Finally, a contract does not rely on the pose of philanthropy or condescend as "charity." It frankly presupposes that self-interest primarily governs people. When two parties enter into a contract, they do so because each cuts a deal that serves his or her own advantage. Self-interest motivates not only private contracts but also that primordial contract in and through which the state came into being. So argued the contractarians of the seventeenth and eighteenth centuries. The state does not derive from some heroic act of sacrifice by gods or men. Rather men and women "left" the state of nature and entered into the political contract because each served thereby his or her own advantage. They surrendered some liberty and property to the state to escape the evils that would beset them individually apart from the state's protection. The state arises as a defensive reaction, on behalf of self-interest, against the threat of murder, anarchy, theft, and other forms of the threat of violent death.

Subsequent enthusiasts about the social instrument of contracts[11] have measured human progress by the degree to which a society bases its life on contracts rather than on status. By this measure, the ancient Romans made the most striking progress when they used commercial contracts where custom previously ruled. The modern bourgeoisie extended the use of contracts still further into economics and politics and even into religion with the free-church emphasis on voluntary choice rather than received religious traditions. Some educators today have used the device of contracts in the classroom (as they encourage students and teachers to reach explicit agreements about units of work for levels of grade). More recently, some liberationists would extend it into marriage; and still others would prefer to see it define the professional relationship. The movement, on the whole, intends to laicize authority, legalize relationships, activate self-interest, and encourage collaboration.

Some of these aims of the contractualists appeal strongly, but it would be unfortunate if professional ethics folded into a commercial contract alone. First, the notion of contract suppresses the element of gift in human relationships. Earlier I verged on denying the importance of this ingredient in professional relationships when I criticized the medical profession for its conceit of philanthropy, its self-interpretation as the great giver. In fact, I do not object to the notion of gift but to the moral pretension of professionals who see themselves as givers alone.

The contractualist approach tends to reduce professional obligation to self-interested minimalism, quid pro quo. Do no more for your patients than what the contract calls for: specified services for established fees. A commercial contract may be a fitting instrument in the purchase of an appliance, a house, or services that can be specified fully in advance of delivery. A legally enforceable agreement in professional transactions may also protect the patient or client against the physician or lawyer whose services fall below a minimal standard. But reducing duties to the specifics of a contract alone fails to honor the full scope of professional obligation.

Professionals in the so-called helping professions serve unpredictable needs. The professional deals with

11. See, for example, Henry Sumner Maine, *Ancient Law*, rev. ed. (Oxford University Press, 1931).

the sickness, ills, crimes, needs, and tragedies of humankind. No contract can exhaustively specify in advance for each patient or client. The professions must be ready to cope with the contingent and the unexpected. Calls on services may exceed those needs anticipated in a contract or the compensation available in a given case. Services, moreover, are more likely to achieve the desired therapeutic result if they come in the context of a relationship that the patient or client can really trust.

Contract and covenant, materially considered, appear to be first cousins; they both include an agreement and an exchange between parties. But in spirit, contract and covenant differ markedly. Contracts are external; covenants are internal to the parties involved. We sign contracts to discharge them expediently. Covenants cut deeper into personal identity. A contract has a limited duration, but the religious covenant imposes change on all moments. A mechanic can act under a contract, and then, when not fixing a piston, act without regard to the contract; but a covenantal people acts under covenant while eating, sleeping, working, praying, cheating, healing, or blundering.

Paul remarks, in effect: When you eat, eat to the glory of God, and when you fast, fast to the glory of God, and when you marry, marry to the glory of God, and when you abstain, abstain to the glory of God (1 Corinthians 10). Initiation into a profession means, in effect, that the physician is a healer when healing and when sleeping, when practicing and when malpracticing. In the modern world, this dedication has deteriorated into the macho ethic of residency training, particularly in surgery: twelve hours a day, six days a week, and night service every other night, on and off for five years. But such training (despite its morally and professionally dubious aspects) does bespeak a deep claim on the person's identity.

Covenants also have a gratuitous, growing edge to them that springs from this ontological change and builds relationships. No one has put this contrasting feature of a contract and a covenant better than Faulkner in his comic novel *Intruder in the Dust*.

At the outset of the novel, a white boy, hunting with young blacks, falls into a creek on a cold winter day. While thrashing about in the icy water, he feels a long pole jab at his body and hears a commanding black voice say, "Boy, grab hold." After the boy clambers out of the river, Lucas Beauchamp, a proud, older black man, brings him shivering to his house, where Mrs. Beauchamp takes care of him. She takes off his wet clothes and wraps him in "Negro blankets," feeds him "Negro food," and warms him by the fire.

When his clothes dry, the boy dresses to go, but, uneasy about his debt to Lucas, he reaches into his pocket for some coins and offers 70 cents compensation for Beauchamp's help. Lucas rejects the money firmly and commands the two black boys to pick up the coins from the floor where they have fallen and to return them to the white boy, who thus fails in his effort to get rid of his feeling of indebtedness.

Shortly thereafter, still uneasy about the episode at the river and his frustrated effort to pay off Lucas for his help, the boy buys some imitation silk for Lucas's wife and gets his black friend to deliver it. Now he feels better. But a few days later, the white boy goes to his own backdoor stoop only to find a jug of molasses that Lucas has left for him. The gift puts him back where he started, again beholden to the black man.

Several months later, the boy passes Lucas on the street and scans his face closely, wondering whether the black man remembers the incident between them — a little like the high school boy who spies the girl in the hall the morning after and reads her face to see what registers from the evening before. He can't be sure. Four years pass, and town authorities falsely accuse Lucas of murdering a white man. They take him to the jailhouse, where a crowd gathers to watch. The boy goes early, watches the proceedings, and ponders whether the old man remembers their past encounter; just as Lucas is about to enter the jailhouse, he wheels and points his long arm in the direction of the boy and says, "Boy, I want to see you." The boy obeys and visits Lucas in the jailhouse, and eventually he and his aunt succeed in proving Lucas's innocence.

Faulkner's story serves as a parable for the relationship of whites to blacks in the South. Black people have labored in white people's fields, built and cared for their houses, fed, clothed, and nurtured their children. In accepting these labors, the whites have received their life and substance from the blacks over and over again. But they resist this involvement and try to pay off the blacks with a few marketplace coins. They try to define their relationship as transient and external, to be managed at arm's length.

For better or for worse, blacks and whites in this country share a common life and destiny. They cannot resolve the problem between them until they accept the covenant that the original receipt of labor entails.

The story emphasizes the donative element in the upbuilding and nourishing of covenant — whether the covenant of marriage, friendship, or professional relationship. Quid pro quo characterizes a commercial transaction, but covenantally, each partner must serve and draw on the deeper reserves of the other. Contractual exchanges of buying and selling can expand into further episodes of giving and receiving, but then they deepen toward a covenantal bond.

This donative element should infuse not only the healer's care of the patient but also other aspects of health care. In his fascinating study *The Gift Relationship*, the late economist Richard M. Titmuss compared the voluntary British system of obtaining blood with the American system, which relies heavily on buying blood.[12] The British system obtains more and better blood without exploiting the indigent, which the Ameri-

12. Richard M. Titmuss, *The Gift Relationship: From Human Blood to Social Policy* (Pantheon Books, 1971).

can system has condoned and which our courts encouraged when they refused to exempt nonprofit blood banks from the antitrust laws. By court definition, blood exchange becomes a commercial transaction in the United States. Titmuss extended his critique beyond the limited subject of human blood to general social policy by offering a sober comment on the increased commercialism of American medicine (and American society at large). Recent court decisions have tended to shift more and more professional services into the category of commodity transactions, with negative consequences — Titmuss believed — for health care delivery systems. Quite apart from court decisions, physicians have contributed to this commercialization of medicine by their strong support for a fee-for-service system of compensation, as opposed to systems that rely on salaried professionals. A piecework payment system tends to reduce the professional transaction even further in the direction of closely calibrated, self-interested exchange.

The minimalism that a purely contractualist understanding of the professional relationship encourages produces a professional too grudging, too calculating, too lacking in spontaneity, too quickly exhausted to go the second mile with patients along the road of their distress.

Contract medicine not only encourages minimalism; it also provokes a peculiar maximalism, "defensive medicine." Under the pressure of the fear of disease and death, patients often push for the maximum in tests and procedures, and physicians often yield to (or exploit) these fears, because they fear malpractice suits. Paradoxically, contractualism tempts the doctor simultaneously to do too little and too much for the patient — too little in that one extends oneself only to the limits the contract specifies, and too much in that one orders procedures that are useful in pampering the patient and protecting oneself, even though the patient's condition does not demand them. The emphasis on self-interest in contractual decisions provides the link between these apparently contradictory strategies of too little and too much. The element of gratuitous service vanishes.

Given its emphasis on self-interest, a contractualist ethic must rely too heavily on several external restraints to keep the supplier of services within moral limits. In commerce, consumers presumably protect themselves by acquiring knowledge about the products they purchase. Insofar as contract medicine encourages increased knowledge on the part of the patient, well and good. But relying exclusively on the injunction "Let the buyer beware" to keep the seller within bounds does not work. A latent antinomianism underlies this conventional marketplace control. It suggests that the seller has few obligations above and beyond those that the knowledge or skepticism of the buyer enforces. This marketplace mechanism alone will not suffice in medical practice. The physician's knowledge so exceeds that of the patient that the patient's knowledgeability alone will not satisfactorily constrain the physician's behavior. One must, at least in part, cultivate some internal fiduciary checks that physicians (and their guilds) will honor.

The consumer's freedom to shop and choose among various vendors provides another self-regulating mechanism in the traditional contractual relationship. Certainly this freedom of choice needs expansion by the better distribution of physicians, the provision of alternative delivery systems, and the proper development of paramedical personnel. However, the crises under which many patients press for medical services do not always provide them with the leisure or calm required for discretionary judgment. Thus normal marketplace controls will never wholly protect the consumer in dealings with the physician.

Finally, the reduction of ethics to contractualism alone fails to judge the more powerful of the two parties (the professional) by transcendent standards. Normally conceived, ethics establishes rights and duties that transcend the particulars of a given agreement. The standards then measure the justice of any specific contract. If, however, such rights and duties inhere only in the contract, then a patient or client might legitimately waive his or her rights. The contract determines only what is required, not necessarily what is just. That arrangement simply augments the power of the more preponderant of the two bargainers. A contract cannot demand an illegal act and should not allow an unethical act. Professional ethics should not permit a professional to persuade his or her patient to waive rights that transcend the particulars of their agreement.

As opposed to a marketplace contractualist ethic, the biblical notion of covenant obliges the more powerful to accept some responsibility for the more vulnerable and powerless of the two partners. It does not permit a free rein to self-interest, subject only to the capacity of the weaker partner to protect himself or herself through knowledge, shrewdness, and purchasing power. Faulkner's novels have highlighted this feature of covenantal ethics. The background for Faulkner's sense of covenant lies in Scripture: The Mount Sinai covenant requires the Israelites to accept responsibility for the widow, the orphan, the stranger, and the poor in their midst. Still earlier, the covenant with Noah set forth a responsibility for the nonhuman creation. And Jesus later insisted that God will measure his people by their treatment of the sick, the imprisoned, the hungry, and the thirsty; God joins himself to the needy and makes their cause his own. Contractualism, on the contrary, builds few constraints on action other than those that prudent self-interest and explicit legislation impose.

Robert Veatch, in *A Theory of Medical Ethics*,[13] has responded to the criticisms I have directed against the notion of contract as a basis for medical ethics by distinguishing between a commercial contract and a primor-

13. Robert M. Veatch, *A Theory of Medical Ethics* (Basic Books, 1981).

dial social contract that provides a transcendent standard of moral judgment.[14] Veatch largely draws his view of the latter, not from the earlier contractarian theorists Hobbes and Locke, but from a conflation of John Rawls's theory of justice[15] and Roderick Firth's theory of the ideal observer.[16] Thereby Veatch tries to rescue the idea of contract from the cruder features of self-interest and recommend it as a kind of secular equivalent to the religious notion of covenant.[17] Purged of crude self-interest, the notion of contract provides some protection for the powerless. Rawls, for example, invites us to play a game whereby we withdraw from the world as we know it, including knowledge of our peculiar slot in life — as doctor, lawyer, car washer, or unemployed person — and assume an imaginary "original position" of ignorance in which we do not yet know our actual power, talents, or fate. Given this veil of ignorance, all prudently self-interested persons, Rawls argues, will agree to a fundamental social contract that will insist on equality of treatment for all participants (excepting those inequalities that work to the advantage of the least advantaged). Thus a social contract emerges — based on rational self-interest — that protects the interest of all, including the poor. Such principles of fairness ought to govern the fundamental institutions of the land, including, Veatch believes, the professional relationship. Social contract theory thus offers a secular surrogate for covenant, free of the crass forms of self-interest that sully marketplace contracts. Reason, rather than religious tradition, seems to arrive at a transcendent standard of judgment that protects the powerless.

Such contractarianism fails at two points. First, its conception of humankind is insufficiently communal. Its original appeal to an isolated self-interest generates, to be sure, principles of fairness, but self-interest alone does not suffice to carry over those principles from a fictitious original position into the actual world. It may well be that an isolated self — under the conditions of ignorance about its own position in the lottery of life — would self-protectively choose social principles of fair distribution. But if it carries that self-interest and nothing more over into the actual world, what would give the self the motivation not to compromise the rules of the game whenever those rules no longer served its wants and interests? Does not the original self require a more communal sense of humankind, a more spacious sense of the common good, in order to sustain its commitment to a principle of fair distribution under the pressured conditions of existence?

Second, recent contractarianism does not reckon with the full destructive force of the actual world, which tempts us to abandon the ideal of rational self-interest.[18] We drive hard bargains and give the needy short shrift because we find ourselves not in an original position of ignorance but in the thick of the race — beleaguered by competitors, creditors, deadlines, demanding patients, and threats of disaster, disease, and death. Imagining an ideal state does not curb the beast of self-interest within us or the dread on which it feeds: the fear that our competitors will do us in or that we will slide into the vortex of decay and death with the powerless if we get too close to them. Aggressive self-interest rules us because it seems to answer the threat of death. It appeals by virtue of its apparent metaphysical realism.

Ultimately the steadfast commitment to protect, nourish, and heal the needy will falter unless we have some resource for reckoning with the harsh world of which needy people so palpably remind us, with the threat of poverty, failure, and death. A steadfast commitment to the needy and their cause requires more than an appeal to an ideal of rational self-interest abstracted from the world that we know. It requires placing that harsh world in the context of yet another world, more powerful, plausible, and gripping, that both deals with the sting of suffering and death and makes it possible, tolerable, imperative, and inviting for us to deal with the needy (and our own needs) in a better way. To describe contract as a secular version of covenant reduces religion to a matter of dispensable trimming. It fails to reckon with religion in its metaphysical substance, that is, its attempt in faith to delineate, in ritual to re-present, and in ethics to honor the real.

This discussion of contract and covenant, then, forces a return to the world that the biblical covenant presents as it attempts to deal with the sting of disease, suffering, and death. Without discussion of that threat, a covenantal imperative to serve the needy will seem just as marginal to the real world as the moral ideal of rational self-interest.[19]

14. William F. May, "Code, Covenant, Contractor Philanthropy," *Hastings Center Reports* (Dec. 1975): 29-38.

15. John Rawls, *A Theory of Justice* (Harvard University Press, 1971).

16. Roderick Firth, "Ethical Absolutism and the Ideal Observer Theory," *Philosophy and Phenomenological Research* 12 (1952): 317-45.

17. Veatch is willing to use the words "contract" and "covenant" interchangeably, but he ignores the differences that a religious setting makes. His theory tilts in the direction of the view of contract generally available through John Rawls.

18. The earlier contractarians, Hobbes and Locke, differ from the Rawls/Veatch version of contractarian thought. They never asked us to engage in a thought project that prescinds from the fact of evil. In fact, they see the state as arising purely as a defensive reaction to the fact of evil, the threat of theft, murder, and violent battle. Criticism of this line of contractarian thought takes a different tack, which I tried to explore in an essay, "Adversarialism in America and the Professions," *Center Magazine* 14, no. 1 (Jan.-Feb. 1981): 47-58.

19. Paul Ramsey of Princeton University, following the theologian Karl Barth, first applied the term "covenant fidelity" to the problems of medical ethics in this country in his impressive and influential *The Patient as Person* (Yale University Press, 1970). As brilliantly, however, as Ramsey marks out the ramifications of the moral ideal for decision making, he spends only two pages in the preface (pp. xii and xiii) acknowledging the theological origins of the notion. Without a firm sense of the religious setting for cov-

Covenant in the Christian Setting

The healer nurtured in the Christian understanding of covenant affirms the Holy of Holies as creative, nurturant, and donative rather than destructive. This affirmation does not deny the reality of disease, pain, suffering, and deat but puts them in the setting of a power that persists and endures in the very midst of them. God ultimately encompasses suffering and death; they are *real* but not *ultimate;* they do not speak the last word about the human condition. The Christian sees in Jesus an event that does not eliminate suffering and death (How could it? The Savior himself experienced the full range of human need; he suffered under Pontius Pilate, was crucified, dead, and buried) but instead exposes destructive power in its final impotence to separate men and women from God.

The term "new covenant" describes the peculiar gift of this self-expending love, its human reception, and promissory ties to it. In laying down his own life, Jesus takes up death itself into the power of donative love. He himself gives and receives in the midst of his own dying and allows others to participate in the selfsame power. This love does not extricate men and women from the arena of human need, suffering, and death, but relieves this arena of its terror. The covenant in Christ, in effect, locates the self, the beleaguered, fearful self, within the dynamics of giving and receiving — gift love and need love — and thus allows the Christian to sit loose to the world: to enter the world without panicking before it or getting mired in it. The covenant deepens ties to the world precisely because it has lightened them. The bond to the world and the patient becomes bearable because, strictly speaking, the covenanted cannot take the ideals and terrors of the ordinary world with ultimate seriousness. The covenantal setting frees us from the need to avoid ties to the perishing. The dying — and we ourselves in the midst of them — are no longer marked by the absence of God. That nonchalance of which the apostle Paul speaks in Romans provides the setting for a truly serious-lighthearted medical practice.

> Neither death, nor life, nor angels, nor principalities, nor things present, nor things to come, nor powers, nor height, nor depth, nor anything else in all creation, will be able to separate us from the love of God. (Rom. 8:38-39)

That primordial tie makes other ties bearable.

Detached from this setting, however, the ideals of technical proficiency, philanthropy, and contract tend to deteriorate into devices whereby healers, beset by pain, pettiness, and suffering, shield themselves from patients and their perishing life. Professionals who prize technique alone find in their technique a protection against the terrible disorder of war, disease, and death and their emotional reaction to it. The philanthropist solves the problem of neediness by adopting the pose of the self-sufficient giver who extends a hand while figuring out how to wriggle free. Philanthropy offers a doctrine of love without ties. It deteriorates into condescension, not because philanthropists harbor a conviction of their ultimate superiority to petitioners, but because they fear that they will drown in a sea of need if they step down from their promontory. Contractors, similarly, seek to solve the problem of perishing by keeping their commitments limited — so much piecework for so much pay, whether directly or indirectly compensated under a third-party payment system. Contractors thus dart in and out of the patient's world of need, shoring up their own life through the transaction of selling. Contractors guard their own interest, carefully specifying the precise amount of time and service for sale. Thus code, philanthropy, and contract, within the context of death, are all devices for evading ties. All have in common a fear of perishing, of drowning in the plight of the other. Ties suck one down into the vortex of death. To call contract, or any other of these devices, merely a secular version of covenant overlooks the important question of metaphysical setting.

Covenantal ethics, despite its advantages over the ideal of philanthropy and the legal instrument of contract, generates difficulties that only a setting in the transcendent resolves. As opposed to the ideal of philanthropy that pretends to wholly gratuitous altruism, covenantal ethics is responsive. As opposed to the instrument of contract that presupposes agreement reached on the basis of self-interest, covenantal ethics requires an element of the gratuitous. A potential conflict, however, emerges between the two characteristics of responsiveness and gratuitous service. Response to debt and gratuitous service seem to be opposed principles of action.

This conflict results when one abstracts the concept of covenant from its original context in the transcendent. One cannot fully appreciate the indebtedness of a human being by toting up the varying sacrifices and investments made by others in his or her favor. The sense that one inexhaustibly receives presupposes a more transcendent source of donative activity than the sum of gifts received from others. In the biblical tradition this transcendent source secretly gives root to every gift between human beings, a source that the human order of giving and receiving can only (and imperfectly) signify. Jewish farmers obedient to the injunction to leave something for the sojourner did not simply respond mathematically to earlier gifts received from Egyptians or from strangers drifting through their own land. At the same time, they did not act gratuitously. Their ethic of service to the needy flowed from Israel's original and continuing state of neediness and indebtedness before God. Thus action that at a human level appears gratuitous, in that a specific gratuity from another human being does not provoke it, still, at its deepest level, as gift, answers to gift. The New

enant (that reckons with suffering and death in the context of the divine fidelity), the moral ideal of fidelity fades before the exigencies of the real world or threatens merely to torture the unduly conscientious.

Testament expresses this responsivity theologically as follows: "In this is love, not that we loved God but that he loved us. . . . If God so loved us, we also ought to love one another" (1 John 4:10-11). In some such way, covenantal ethics, grounded in the transcendent, shies away from the idealist assumption of wholly gratuitous professional action and also from the contractualist assumption that quotidian self-interest should govern every exchange.

A transcendent reference may also help lay out not only the larger horizon in which human service takes place but also the specific standards by which we should measure it. Earlier we noted some dangers in reducing rights and duties to the terms of a particular contract. We observed the need for a transcendent norm that measures and limits contracts. By the same token, rights and duties should not wholly derive from the particulars of a given covenant. What limits ought to be placed on the demands of an excessively dependent patient? At what point does the keeping of one covenant do an injustice to obligations entailed in others? These questions warn against a conventional ethic that sentimentalizes any and all involvements, without reference to a transcendent that both justifies and measures them.

Covenantal Ethics Applied

If a covenantal ethic is responsive, what goal or goals define the content of that response? What human good does (or should) the medical profession pursue? Our discussions on the shaman, the parent, and the fighter cumulatively suggest that neither resistance, avoidance, nor the quietistic acceptance of suffering and death should define the healer's task, but rather pursuit of health and, let it be noted, the extension of a healing care in the midst of disintegrating health. An ancient and positive etymological link exists between "holy," "healing," and "making whole"; between "salve" and "salvation." Leon Kass emphasizes health as the determinative goal of medicine, which he defines in its classical sense as the well-working of an organism as a whole.[20] To promote this "well-working" is the healer's fundamental goal. It emphasizes preventive and rehabilitative care as well as crisis intervention. Edmund Pellegrino rightly contends that health cannot be the exclusive goal of practice without undercutting the physician's responsibility for care in the midst of the patient's failing health. The organism may never work well again as a whole, but the physician still must "heal" in the sense of helping to keep the distracted patient whole in the face of ineliminable adversity. Either way, the tasks of the healer define themselves positively.

Needless to say, this more positive vision of the healer's role does not altogether eliminate a military component in the healing process. The fight against suffering and death has an important and contributory, but subordinate, relation to the positive goal of health. The biblical position does not imply that the three responses to death of flight, fight, and acceptance have no validity whatsoever. Although the avoidance of death becomes unwholesome when it assumes the proportions of frantic denial, the prudent avoidance of harm and injury is an obligation for those who take seriously a creative and nurturant God. Although a resistance to death takes a grim toll on patients and families alike when it escalates into unconditional warfare, the fight against death has a subordinate, but positive, place in a faith that would respect and conserve life. Although Christians and Jews should not worship death ("You shall have no other gods before me"), they should prepare for it fittingly. The anticipation of death need not mean worship of it; and such anticipation and preparation, with God's grace, may help to make the avoidance of death a little less desperate and the fight against it a little less grim. Released from a metaphysically desperate sense of the human condition, the professional may pursue a little more freely the primary goal of health care.

Questions still remain about the quality control and tenor of that care. This chapter closes, therefore, with a discussion of the implications of a covenantal ethic for relationships to colleagues (the issue of professional self-regulation) and to patients (the virtue of fidelity).

1. Professional Self-Regulation and Discipline

The problem of lax professional self-regulation and discipline dates to the Hippocratic tradition, with which this chapter began. The ancient oath distinguished between codal duties to patients and covenantal obligations to the physician's teacher and his progeny. The latter acquire a gravity that gives them precedence over obligations to patients, because they flow from the student's indebtedness to the teacher. When concern for the teacher (or, by extension in the modern world, professional colleagues) dominates, professional ethics reduces itself to courtesy within a guild. Responsibilities to patients (such as informing them about incompetent treatment) do not simply disappear; professionals deny them; professionals view such reports as a breach of the discretionary bonds that pertain in the guild. Thus an inversion occurs. A report on incompetent or unethical behavior to patients becomes a breach in "professional ethics," that is, a breach in courtesy.

For many reasons, social, religious, and cultural, doctors in the modern world duck responsibility for professional self-criticism and regulation. First, like any professional group, doctors find themselves in a complex, interlocking network of relationships with fellow professionals: They extend favors; incur debts; exchange referrals; intertwine personal histories. The bond with fellow professionals grows, while ties with patients seem transient. Furthermore, an organization directed to specific ends tends to generate a sense of community among pro-

20. Leon R. Kass, "Regarding the End of Medicine and the Pursuit of Health," *Pubic Interest* 40 (Summer 1975): 27-29.

fessional staff members serving those ends. The experience of collegiality can become an end in its own right and subtly take precedence over the needs of the population served. Hence, professional life inevitably mutes criticism.

Second, doctors, more than other professionals, may find self-regulation more difficult to achieve because public criticism seems somewhat more natural to lawyers and academicians, whose work goes on in an adversarial or at least a disputatious setting. The doctor, however, plays a special role in relation to his or her patients, the quasi-priestly-parental; public criticism would seem to subvert this role. Even if one breaks free of the parental-priestly model, trust remains an important ingredient in the relationship; free-ranging criticism erodes trust.

Third, the physician's authority, while great, is precarious. The analogy often drawn between the authority of the modern doctor and the traditional power of parent and priest obscures an important difference between them in the security of their status. The modern doctor walks a high wire. Many patients apotheosize the doctor, but they bitterly resent him if his hand slips publicly but once.

The reason for this precariousness of status lies in differing sources of authority. Parents and priests in traditional society derive their authority from sacred powers perceived as largely creative, nurturant, and beneficent. Given this derivation from positive power, laypeople could tolerate some human defect in the religious authority figure. The power of good would prevail despite human lapse. The modern doctor's authority, however, derives reflexively from a grim negativity, that is, from the fear of death. The same power of death that exalts physicians and makes them the most highly paid and authoritative professionals in the modern world threatens to bring them low if through their own negligence, unscrupulousness, or incompetence they endanger the life of a patient. Thus although modern physicians enjoy much more prestige and authority than contemporary teachers or lawyers, they risk a nasty fall. Resentment against them can flare out. Professional self-criticism in academic life or in the law seems like child's play compared with medicine. The mediocre teacher deprives me merely of the truth; the negligent lawyer forfeits my money or, at worst, my freedom; but the incompetent doctor endangers my life. The stakes seem much higher in the case of medicine. The profession draws its wagons into a circle to protect its members when challenged.

Fourth, Americans in all walks of life have a morally healthy suspicion of officiousness. They press charges against their neighbors or colleagues only reluctantly. They do not like the hypocrisy of those zealous about the sliver in their neighbor's eye while unmindful of the beam in their own. One ought to tend to one's own professional conduct, but beyond that, live and let live. After all, who can tell the difference between an honest mistake and culpable negligence? Who can know enough about a particular medical case to second-guess the physician in charge? Better to keep one's mouth shut. Must a physician be his or her colleague's keeper?

This revulsion against officiousness deserves sympathy, but it fails to respect fully the special covenantal obligations of the professional. Professionals always claim the right to pass judgment (in professional matters) on colleagues or would-be colleagues. The society supports this right when it establishes licensing procedures under the control of professionals and backs up these procedures by prosecuting imposters and pretenders. In effect, the state sanctions a monopoly (a limitation on the supply of professionals). To be sure, patients profit from this through higher standards, but the profession also profits — handsomely — financially. If the professional were, in fact, engaged in a freelance competition (as the myth would have it) without the protection of the monopoly, he or she would not fare nearly so well.

Professional accountability, therefore, must extend beyond the question of one's own personal competence to the competence of other guild members. Duty requires professionals to pass judgment on colleagues; otherwise they profit from a monopoly established by the state without enforcing those standards the need for which alone justifies the monopoly. The individual's license to practice derives ultimately from a prior license to license. If the license to practice carries with it the duty to practice well, the license to license carries with it the duty to judge and monitor well. In professional ethics today, the test of moral seriousness may depend not simply on personal compliance with moral principles but on the courage to hold others accountable. Otherwise the doctor's responsibility to patients yields to the somewhat tarnished privilege of the guild.

The effort to deepen a sense of responsibility for professional self-regulation by appeal to covenantal responsibilities to the profession, to patients, and to the society at large should not lead to the exclusion of some of those values best symbolized by code and contract. Those who live by a code of technical proficiency have a standard on the basis of which to discipline their peers. As noted earlier, Hemingway's novels emphasize discipline. Those who live by a code know how to ostracize deficient peers. Medicine, no exception, relies chiefly on the power of the referral system to isolate the incompetent colleague and contain that person's power to harm.

Defenders of an ethic based on code might argue further that deficiencies in enforcement today result largely from a too strongly developed sense of covenantal obligations to colleagues than from a too weakly developed sense of code. From this perspective, a covenantal ethic creates a problem for professional discipline rather than providing the basis for its amendment. Covenantal obligations to colleagues inhibit the enforcement of duties to patients.

A code alone, however, does not in and of itself solve the problem of professional discipline. It provides only a basis for excluding from one's own inner circle an incompetent physician. But, as Eliot Freidson has pointed out in *Professional Dominance*, the incompetent professional today, when excluded from a given hospital, group practice, or circle of referring colleagues, simply moves his or her practice and finds another circle of equally incompetent colleagues with whom it is possible to function.[21] Given a mobile society with a scarcity of doctors — at least in some areas — the device of local ostracism simply passes on problem physicians to other patients elsewhere. It does not address them. It would take a much more active comprehensive sense of covenantal obligation to all patients on the part of the profession to enforce standards in the guild beyond the locally limited and informal patterns of ostracism.

Codal patterns of discipline, moreover, not only fall short of adequate protection for the patient, they also fail in collegial responsibility to the troubled physician. Those who ostracize handle a colleague lazily when they fail altogether to make a first attempt at remedy and to address the physician personally in his or her difficulty.

At the same time, the indispensable interest and pride of the medical profession in technical proficiency should not lapse because of an expressed preference for a professional ethics based on covenant. Covenantal fidelity to the patient remains unrealized if it does not include proficiency. A rather sentimental existentialism unfortunately assumes that it morally suffices for human beings to be "present" to one another. But in crisis, the ill person needs not simply presence but skill, not just personal concern but highly disciplined services targeted to specific needs. Covenantal ethics, then, must include rather than exclude the interests of the unwritten codes of the profession in the refinement of technical skills.

Neither should a preference for a covenantal ethic lead to the exclusion of the interests of an enforceable contract. Although the reduction of medical ethics to a contract alone incurs the danger of minimalism, patients should have recourse against those physicians who fail to meet minimal standards. They should not depend entirely on disciplinary measures undertaken in the profession. They should retain the right to appeal to the law in cases of malpractice or breaches of contract, explicit or implied.

On the other hand, a legal appeal cannot correct an injustice without assistance and testimony from physicians who take their obligations to patients and their profession seriously. If, in such cases, fellow physicians simply mill around and protect their colleague like a wounded elephant, the patient with just cause probably will not secure redress in the courts. Thus the instrument of contract and other avenues of legal redress rely on physicians who have a deep sense of obligation to the patient and the profession. Needless to say, professional discipline and continuing education vigorously pursued within the profession could cut down drastically on the number of cases that need to reach the courts. But this takes a depth of commitment to the profession and the patients that exceeds minimalist demands under the law. In brief, covenantal fidelity includes the codal duty to become technically proficient; it includes the obligation to meet the minimal terms of contract, but it also requires much more. This more intense obligation, moreover, may finally help not only patients but also troubled colleagues.

21. Eliot Freidson, *Professional Dominance: The Social Structure of Medical Care* (Atherton Press, 1970), p. 94.

2. *Fidelity to the Patient*

The foregoing contrast between a contract and a covenant points toward fidelity as the defining professional virtue. The physician and other health care practitioners owe a double fidelity, both to a body of knowledge that aids and abets healing and to the patient who benefits from the healer's art. Physicians receive pay for their work. The professional exchange partly conforms to a marketplace exchange of buying and selling. But the professional exchange also transcends, or ought to transcend, the cash nexus; it must be disinterested rather than self-interested, and, where necessary, transformational rather than merely transactional.

Buyers and sellers in the marketplace meet as two frankly self-interested and relatively knowledgeable parties. Both sides are justifiably wary. However, patients cannot obey the marketplace warning, "Buyer beware." Their very limited medical knowledge and often confused perception of self-interest hardly protect them. An asymmetry exists between the professional's knowledge and therefore power and the patient's relative ignorance and powerlessness. This imbalance requires that the professional exchange take place in a fiduciary setting of trust that transcends the marketplace assumptions about two wary bargainers. Only the physician's fidelity to the patient in the disposition of his or her knowledge and power justifies that trust. Fidelity requires disinterested discernment, judgment, and action on behalf of the patient's best interest and well-being.

The temptation to depart from disinterested fidelity to the patient takes two forms: overtreatment and undertreatment. The fee-for-service system generally tempts the practitioner to overtreat the patient, especially with acute-care interventions. Fee-for-service, a contracted piecework payment system, says, in effect, the more discrete pieces of work, the more compensation. Hospitals and doctors alike tend to dice up work into distinct, identifiable procedures, each qualifying for compensation, the cumulative effect of which is to overtreat patients with acute-care services, precisely those services that the system can identify as separate, objective procedures. In a sense, the fee-for-service system also tempts the practitioner to undertreat or mistreat by failing to compensate adequately for those sometimes more thoughtful, sometimes less dramatic, modes of care that the ill and the dying may need. Recent adjustments in the federal fee schedules, which now pay less to the doers and more to the thinkers in medicine (less to surgeons, radiologists, and anesthesiologists, more to internists and deliverers of primary care), increase the rewards for the reflective work patients need. The fee-for-service system also fails to compensate sufficiently those many unglamorous caregivers who provide services for patients in their homes or in nursing homes where care for the chronically ill and the dying might more humanely take place. Disinterested professional service should not mean undercompensated professional service.

The current trends in the third-party payment system have moved the United States increasingly in the direction of undertreatment. The burgeoning growth of for-profit health maintenance organizations (HMOs) and preferred provider organizations (PPOs), which often contract to compensate physicians with bonuses based on the difference between a standard capitation payment per patient and the cost of health services delivered, tends to encourage timely preventative medicine. Early treatment generally tends to reduce the costs of care. But the profit incentives that some HMOs and PPOs tie to reduced costs can tempt practitioners, hospitals, and delivery organizations to undertreat patients and thus compromise fidelity to the patient. This temptation affects not simply the delivery of acute care but also some of those services that might reduce the suffering of the elderly, the dying, and their families. For example, some HMOs and PPOs deny payment for adequate mental health services. (This omission led the American Psychiatric Association to state at its annual meeting in 1994 that the psychiatrist has an ethical obligation to tell the patient [or family in the case of the marginally competent] that a treatment is indicated, whether or not the HMO or PPO will approve of the care. But the HMO or PPO can often drop without cause the psychiatrist who has presented the organization with this awkwardness! Systemic pressures of this sort can make it difficult to practice the virtue of disinterested fidelity to the patient: A system that imposes martyrdom on ordinary virtue is, to say the least, somewhat faulty.)

The covenantal professional exchange differs in a second way from a contractual, marketplace transaction. In addition to its disinterestedness, it is, for want of a better word, transformational, not merely transactional. The healer must respond not simply to the patient's self-perceived wants but to his or her deeper needs. The patient suffering from insomnia often wants simply the quick fix of a pill. But if the physician goes after the root of the problem, then he or she may have to help the patient transform the habits that led to the symptom of sleeplessness. The physician is slothful if he or she dutifully offers acute care but neglects to look for the beginning of an illness and offer preventive medicine. Rehabilitative medicine and long-term and terminal care also engage the healer in the task of transforming patients. The victim of a heart attack, cancer, or a stroke suffers major changes in body and circumstance, which reflexively call for changes in habits and skills in the course of rehabilitative and long-term care.

As covenantal fidelity requires and inspires healers to engage in responding to patients' deeper needs, the conventional quandary of truth-telling in medicine takes on a different look. Moralists usually reduce the quandary of telling the truth to the question of whether to tell the truth. Consequentialists seek to answer the question by calculating the goods and harms produced by the truth, evasion, or lying. They prize the virtue of benevolence. Duty-oriented moralists tend to argue for the truth irrespective of consequences. A lie wrongs the patient even when it does no harm. Managing the patient, even for benevolent reasons, subverts the patient's dignity. Only the truth respects the patient as a rational creature. Such moralists thus prize foremost the virtue of honesty.

The virtue of covenantal fidelity expands the question of truth-telling in the moral life. Truth becomes a question not only of telling the truth but of being-true. This assertion rests on more than a play on words. The foundational truth of God in Scripture is that God is faithful to his promises. His covenant faithfulness grounds and sustains the world, makes possible our knowledgeable access to it and our performance in it. The very possibility of making truthful assertions rests ultimately on a being-true, a steadfastness that creates and sustains the world. Fidelity on the human scene in all its imperfection reflects in a small way this more spacious ontological setting.

J. L. Austin once drew the distinction, now famous, between two kinds of utterances: descriptive and performative. In ordinary descriptive sentences, one points to or characterizes a given item in the world. (It is raining. The tumor is malignant.) In performative utterances, however, one alters the world by introducing an ingredient that would not be there apart from the utterance. Promises make such performative declarations. (I, John, take thee, Mary. We will defend your country in case of attack. I will not abandon you.) To make a promise alters the world of the person to whom one extends the promise. Conversely, defecting from a promise can be world shattering.

Medical ethics treats the question of truth-telling entirely at the level of descriptive speech. Should the doctor tell the patient that he or she has a malignancy? If not, may one lie, or must one merely withhold the truth?

The notion of performative speech expands the question of truth-telling in professional life. Physicians and nurses face the moral question not simply of telling the truth, but of being true to their word. Conversely, the total situation for a patient includes not only the disease one has but also whether others desert or stand by a person in this extremity. The fidelity of others does not eliminate the disease, but it mightily affects the human context in which the disease runs its course. The doctor offers a patient not simply proficiency and diagnostic accuracy but also fidelity.

Thus the virtue of fidelity begins to affect the resolution of the dilemma itself. Perhaps more patients and clients could accept the descriptive truth if they experienced the performative truth. The anxieties of patients in terminal illness compound because they fear that professionals will abandon them. Perhaps patients would be more inclined to trust the doctor's performative utterances if they trusted diagnoses and prognoses. That is why a cautiously wise medieval physician once advised his colleagues: "Promise only fidelity!"

Furthermore, truth-telling raises not merely the substantive question as to *whether* one tells the truth, but *how* one tells it directly or indirectly, personally or with a sparing impersonality. As the saying goes, "It is not only what you say, but when and how you say it." The theologian Karl Barth once observed that Job's friends were metaphysically correct in what they had to say, but existentially false in their timing, and therefore ultimately false theologically. They chose a miserable moment to sing their theological arias on the subject of suffering.

Prudence in these matters demands much more than shrewdness in knowing how to package what one has to say. Discretion depends on metaphysical perception, a sense for what the Stoics called the fitting, a discretion that discerns more deeply than mere tact, a feel for behavior congruent with reality. Death may not be ultimate, but its sting nevertheless hurts. One must respect that fact. Without *discretion* professionals do not reckon with the whole truth. They may tell the truth, but they do not serve the truth when they tell it. They may use the truth to serve their own vanity; or to satisfy their own craving for power over their patients; or to indulge themselves in the role of nag, policeman, pedant, or judge.

The physician finds telling the truth easier in those cases where the patient and physician can do something together to prevent a disease or cure it, but it also matters as a part of healing in terminal illness. Healing "makes whole." The physician and the patient may not be able to knock out the cancer that kills. But they may still go a long way toward keeping the patient whole or intact even in extremity. This is part of the hard opportunity in truth-telling. But it depends on much more than the readiness of the physician to dispense sentence pellets of the truth about the patient's condition. Such pellets, unsupported by faithful care and by care that takes the form of sensitive teaching, can be lethal and anything but respectful of patients. Thus the question of the truth expands beyond decision bits and raises the question of the healer's readiness to accept his or her role as teacher in the therapeutic enterprise.

32 The Nurse's Profession

Florence Nightingale

. . . Does not the Apostle say: "I count not myself to have apprehended: but this one thing I do, forgetting those things which are behind, *and reaching forth unto those things which are before, I press toward* the mark for the prize of the *high calling* of God in Christ Jesus"; and what higher "calling" can we have than Nursing? But then we must "press forward." . . .

When the head and the hands are very full, as in Nursing, it is so easy, so very easy, if the heart has not an earnest purpose for God and our neighbour, to end in doing one's work only for oneself, and not at all — even when we seem to be serving our neighbours — not at all for them or for God. . . .

But "can we not see ourselves as God sees us?" is a still more important question. For while we value the judgments of our superiors, and of our fellows, which may correct our own judgments, we must also have a higher standard which may correct theirs. We cannot altogether trust them, and still less can we trust ourselves. And we know, of course, that the worth of a life is not altogether measured by failure or success. We want to see our purposes, and the ways we take to fulfil such charge as may be given us, as they are in the sight of God. "Thou God seest me."

And thus do we return to the question we asked before — how near can we come to Him whose name we bear, when we call ourselves Christians? How near to His gentleness and goodness — to His "authority" over others?

And the highest "authority" which a woman especially can attain among her fellow women must come from her doing God's work here in the same spirit, and with the same thoroughness, that Christ did, though we follow him but "afar off."

Lastly, it is charity to nurse sick bodies well; it is greater charity to nurse well and patiently sick minds, tiresome sufferers. But there is a greater charity even than these: to do good to those who are not good to us, to behave well to those who behave ill to us, to serve with love those who do not even receive our service with good temper, to forgive on the instant any slight which we may have received, or may have fancied we have received, or any worse injury.

From Rosalind Nash, ed., *Florence Nightingale to Her Nurses: A Selection from Miss Nightingale's Addresses to Probationers and Nurses of the Nightingale School at St. Thomas's Hospital* (London: MacMillan and Co., Limited, 1914).

If we cannot "do good" to those who "persecute" us — for we are not "persecuted": if we cannot pray "Father, forgive them, for they know not what they do" — for none are nailing us to a cross: how much more must we try to serve with patience and love any who use us spitefully, to nurse with all our hearts any thankless peevish patients! . . .

Let us be on our guard against the danger, not exactly of thinking too well of ourselves (for no one consciously does this), but of isolating ourselves, of falling into party spirit — always remembering that, if we can do any good to others, we must draw others to us by the influence of our characters, and not by any profession of what we are — least of all, by a profession of Religion. . . .

We have been, almost all of us, taught to pray in the days of our childhood. Is there not something sad and strange in our throwing this aside when most required by us, on the threshold of our active lives? Life is a shallow thing, and more especially *Hospital* life, without any depth of religion. For it is a matter of simple experience that the best things, the things which seem as if they most would make us feel, become the most hardening if not rightly used.

And may I say a thing from my own experience? No training is of any use, unless one can learn (1) to feel, and (2) to think out things for oneself. And if we have not true religious feeling and purpose, Hospital life — the highest of all things *with* these — *without* them becomes a mere routine and bustle, and a very hardening routine and bustle.

. . . Without deep religious purpose how shallow a thing is Hospital life, which is, or ought to be, the most inspiring! For, as years go on, we shall have others to train; and find that the springs of religion are dried up within ourselves. The patients we shall always have with us while we are Nurses. And we shall find that we have no religious gift or influence with them, no word in season, whether for those who are to live, or for those who are to die, no, not even when they are in their last hours, and perhaps no one by but *us* to speak a word to point them to the Eternal Father and Saviour; not even for a poor little dying child who cries: "Nursey, tell me, oh, why is it so dark?" Then we may feel painfully about them what we do not at present feel about ourselves. We may wish, both for our patients and Probationers, that they had the restraints of the "fear" of the most Holy God, to enable them to resist the temptation. We may regret that our own Probationers seem so worldly and external. And we may perceive too late that the deficiency in their characters began in our own.

For, to all good women, *life* is a prayer; and though we pray in our own rooms, in the Wards and at Church, the end must not be confounded with the means. We are the more bound to watch strictly over ourselves; we have not less but more need of a high standard of duty and of life in our Nursing; we must teach ourselves humility and modesty by becoming more aware of our own weakness and narrowness, and liability to mistake as Nurses and as Christians. Mere worldly success to any nobler, higher mind is not worth having. Do you think Agnes Jones, or some who are now living amongst us, cared much about worldly success? They cared about efficiency, thoroughness. But that is a different thing.

We must condemn many of our own tempers when we calmly review them. We must lament over training opportunities which we have lost, must desire to become better women, better Nurses. That we all of us must feel. And then, and not till then, will *life* and *work* among the sick become a prayer.

For prayer is communion or cooperation with God: the expression of a *life* among his poor and sick and erring ones. But when we speak with God, our power of addressing Him, of holding communion with Him, and listening to His still small voice, depends upon our will being one and the same with His. *Is* He our God, as He was Christ's? To Christ He was all, to us He seems sometimes nothing. Can we retire to rest after our busy, anxious day in the Wards, with feeling: "Lord, into Thy hands I commend my spirit," and those of such and such anxious cases; remembering, too, that in the darkness, "Thou God seest me," and seest them too? Can we rise in the morning, almost with a feeling of joy that we are spared another day to do Him service with His sick? —

> Awake, my soul, and with the sun,
> Thy daily stage of duty run.

Does the thought ever occur to us in the course of the day, that we will correct that particular fault of mind, or heart, or temper, whether slowness, or bustle, or want of accuracy or method, or harsh judgments, or want of loyalty to those under whom or among whom we are placed, or sharp talking, or tale-bearing or gossiping — oh, how common, and how old a fault, as old as Solomon! "He that repeateth a matter, separateth friends"; and how can people trust us unless they know that we are not talebearers, who will misrepresent or improperly repeat what is said to us? Shall we correct this, or any other fault, not with a view to our success in life, or to our own credit, but in order that we may be able to serve our Master better in the service of the sick? . . .

This is the spirit of prayer, the spirit of conversation or communion with God, which leads us in all our Nursing silently to think of Him, and refer it to Him. When we hear in the voice of conscience *His* voice speaking to us; when we are aware that He is the witness of everything we do, and say, and think, and also the source of every good thing in us; and when we feel in our hearts the struggle against some evil temper, then God is fighting *with* us against envy and jealousy, against selfishness and self-indulgence, against lightness, and frivolity, and vanity, for "our better self against our worse self." . . .

And let me say a word about self-denial: because, as we all know, there can be no real Nursing without self-denial. We know the story of the Roman soldier, above fourteen hundred years ago, who, entering a town in France with his regiment, saw a sick man perishing with cold by the wayside — there were no Hospitals then — and, having nothing else to give, drew his sword, cut his own cloak in half, and wrapped the sick man in half his cloak.

It is said that a dream visited him, in which he found himself admitted into heaven, and Christ saying, "Martin hath clothed me with his garment": the dream, of course, being a remembrance of the verse, "When saw we thee sick or in prison, and came unto thee?" and of the answer, "Inasmuch as ye have done it unto one of the least of these my brethren, ye have done it unto me." But whether the story of the dream be true or not, this Roman soldier, converted to Christianity, became afterwards one of the greatest bishops of the early ages, Martin of Tours. . . .

Suppose we dedicated this "School" to Him, the Divine Charity and Love which said, "Inasmuch as ye do it unto one of the least of these my brethren" (and He calls all our patients — all of us, His brothers and sisters) "ye do it unto me" — oh, what a "Kingdom of Heaven" this might be! Then, indeed, the dream of Martin of Tours, the soldier and Missionary-Bishop, would have come true! . . .

When a Patient, especially a child, sees you acting in all things as if in the presence of God — and none are so quick to observe it — then the names he or she heard at the Chaplain's or the Sister's or the Night Nurse's lips become names of real things and real Persons. There *is* a God, a Father; there *is* a Christ, a Comforter; there *is* a Spirit of Goodness, of Holiness; there *is* another world, to such an one.

When a Patient, especially a Child, sees us acting as if there were *no* God, then there but too often becomes no God to him. Then words become to such a child mere words. . . .

Above all, let us pray that God will send real workers into this immense "field" of Nursing, made more immense this year by the opening out of London *District* Nursing at the bedside of the sick poor at home. A woman who takes a sentimental view of Nursing (which she calls "ministering," as if she were an angel) is of course worse than useless. A woman possessed with the idea that she is making a sacrifice will never do; and a woman who thinks any kind of Nursing work "beneath a Nurse" will simply be in the way. But if the right woman is moved by God to come to us, what a welcome we will give her, and how happy she will soon be in a work, the many blessings of which none can know as we know them, though we know the worries too! . . .

Nurses' work means downright work, in a cheery, happy, hopeful, friendly spirit. An earnest, bright, cheerful woman, without that notion of "making sacrifices," etc., perpetually occurring to her mind, is the real Nurse. Soldiers are sent anywhere, and leave home and country for years; *they* think nothing of it, because they go "on duty." Shall *we* have less self-denial than they, and think less of "duty" than these men? A woman with a healthy, active tone of mind, plenty of work in her, and some enthusiasm, who makes the best of everything, and, above all, does not think herself better than other people because she is a "Nightingale Nurse," that is the woman we want. . . .

I must have moral influence over my Patients. And I *can* only have this by *being* what I appear, especially now that everybody is educated, so that Patients become my keen critics and judges. My Patients are watching me. They know what my profession, my calling is: to devote myself to the good of the sick. They are asking themselves: does that Nurse act up to her profession? This is no supposition. It is a fact. It is a call to us, to each individual Nurse, to act up to her profession.

We hear a good deal nowadays about Nursing being made a "profession." Rather, it is not the question for *me: am I* living up to my "profession"?

33 A Christian Vision of Nursing and Persons

Mary Molewyk Doornbos, Ruth E. Groenhout, Kendra G. Hotz, and Cheryl Brandsen

Being a Christian nurse is not only about what one does but also about who one is. So who are nurses? How do they become the sorts of persons who are suited to nursing practice? What kinds of contexts shape their work? What kinds of assumptions do they make about what it means to pursue and promote the health and well-being of their clients? In many ways, Christian nurses will find that their assumptions about the nature of nursing practice, or health, or the like are shared with non-Christian nurses. We share a common created nature and should expect to find such agreement. But there are also ways in which the perspective of the Christian nurse enriches or deepens his or her understanding of these foundational concepts, and it is important to note this as well. Christianity qualifies and shapes the people who become nurses, the ways in which they interpret their circumstances, and the values that guide their actions. In this chapter we examine more specifically how it does so.

It is common in introductory nursing textbooks to refer to four concepts that are foundational for understanding professional nursing practice. These are sometimes called the four defining or "metaparadigm" concepts, namely: *nursing, person, health,* and *environment.* This chapter offers a fresh and distinctively Christian interpretation of the foundational concepts of *nursing* and *person.* These two basic concepts are then situated in the next chapter in terms of a Christian understanding of *health* and *environment,* the second pair of metaparadigm concepts of nursing theory.

Nursing: Practitioners and Their Institutions

If we went out and asked most nurses what it is that they do, they would be likely to answer in terms of specific kinds of nursing. "I'm an acute care nurse," one might say, "with a primary specialization in ICU nursing." Or "I'm a visiting nurse with a Hospice program. I do a combination of community nursing and end-of-life care in the context of a Hospice setting." Or "I'm a nurse in an Ob-gyn practice where I do client education." If we pressed a bit harder, these same nurses might go into more detail in terms of the specific techniques and practices involved in their work, whether monitoring client status in the ICU or working on pain management techniques with clients facing terminal illness. And of course these are all accurate descriptions of what a specific nurse might find himself or herself doing in a particular nursing role.

But we might be asking a slightly different question here when we ask what nurses do. We might be asking less about the actual specifics of a particular aspect of nursing and more about what it means to be a nurse. That is, we might be asking questions about what it is that makes nursing a specific profession, rather than a subset of some other profession (such as medicine or social work). And we could also be asking questions about what the ideals of nursing are, both in terms of the profession as a whole and in terms of the practitioners. Every profession has some sense of what it should be and what its practitioners should be like, and though the ideal is generally not realized in every particular, it nonetheless shapes the way professionals understand themselves and their identity.

Nursing as a Social Practice

When we ask questions of this sort, we are treating nursing as a social practice. That is, we are thinking of nursing not just as a job someone might have but as an identity in some sense. For the purposes of this book [*Transforming Care*], we will be defining nursing as a social practice, oriented toward a holistic understanding of health, practiced by professionally educated and licensed practitioners. As is the case with almost any profession, undergoing education and becoming licensed as a nurse involves more than just passing certain courses and being able to answer certain questions on exams. Becoming a nurse is a process of professionalization that partly defines one's identity as a person and that shapes one's character in important ways. When I am introduced to someone and ask what he does, if he tells me that he is a nurse I am likely to make certain assumptions about what sort of person he probably is, and many of those assumptions will turn out to be correct.

This notion of a social practice is one that has been developed and analyzed by the philosopher Alasdair MacIntyre, and it has been enormously influential in thinking about how we organize social life, how we understand identity, both of self and other, and what it means to be a particular kind of person. MacIntyre's account of a social practice is helpful for thinking about what nursing is and about how nursing as a profession shapes the identities of nurses, so we will borrow certain aspects of it for our discussion here. MacIntyre's definition of a social practice reads as follows:

Mary Molewyk Doornbos, Ruth E. Groenhout, Kendra G. Hotz, and Cheryl Brandsen, "A Christian Vision of Nursing and Persons," in *Transforming Care: A Christian Vision of Nursing Practice* (Grand Rapids: Wm. B. Eerdmans Publishing Company, 2005), 40-66.

> By a "practice" I am going to mean any coherent and complex form of socially established cooperative human activity through which goods internal to that form of activity are realized in the course of trying to achieve those standards of excellence which are appropriate to, and partially definitive of, that form of activity, with the result that human powers to achieve excellence, and human conceptions of the ends and goods involved, are systematically extended. (MacIntyre 1984, 187)

This definition begins with the notion that a social practice is a coherent and complex form of socially established cooperative human activity, and nursing certainly exemplifies this aspect of a practice. The contemporary practice of nursing is a coherent whole (otherwise it couldn't be taught as a specialized area of study), but it is also enormously complex (as anyone involved in developing a nursing curriculum will tell you!). These two aspects of a practice do tend to generate a certain internal tension in most practices, since any definition of the practice that emphasizes the coherence will tend to deemphasize the complexity and vice versa.

But it is not enough to note that nursing is both internally coherent and complex. It is also, as MacIntyre's definition suggests, a socially established cooperative human activity. Nursing exists as a particular sort of activity, engaged in by practitioners whose right to call themselves nurses is not a matter of (merely) individual choice, but a matter of meeting the standards of the profession and engaging in the right sorts of education and activities to meet standards for licensing and the like. No one could have been a nurse (for example) in the mid-1600s in Mexico, though there were certainly people in that setting who performed some of the tasks that are associated with contemporary nursing. In the absence of a social system of health care, a body of knowledge about human health, and a system of determining who can legitimately call herself or himself a nurse, there aren't nurses in the sense in which we use the term today. This means that nursing as a practice has a history. What counted as "nursing" a century ago is no longer what counts as nursing today; but at the same time, contemporary nursing would not be what it is without those practitioners who set the standards in former times.

These characteristics establish that nursing fits the general schema MacIntyre offers of a practice, but clearly more specific characteristics are required to make it nursing. What is it that identifies nursing as the specific sort of practice that it is? MacIntyre notes that a practice is defined in part by the goods that are "internal to that practice." There are certain central values or goods or aims that are the main focus of nursing and that define it as a practice. Health is the most central of these, since nursing is a health care practice that aims at the alleviation of pain; at restoring physical, psychological, and emotional functioning; at attending to the well-being of the whole person; and so on. While these latter aims may coincide with physical health, they also may diverge in certain cases. A terminally ill client, for example, is unable to achieve full physical health, but she can certainly look to her caregivers for the alleviation of pain and for concern for her emotional well-being.

These central goods can be redefined over time. In the past, nursing tended to think of itself as a matter of service work. Training as a nurse involved learning to change dressings and bedpans in the hospital setting, and nursing education involved learning to carry out physician's orders (McKenna 1997, 87). But nursing no longer defines itself in this way. It now defines itself as a science-based practice and as an independent profession, and it requires practitioners to master knowledge of the scientific basis of nursing practice and to internalize professional standards of behavior that include responsibility and client advocacy (Group and Roberts 2001, 344). This is an important change in the professional self-definition of nurses, and it involves a shift in the central goods of nursing from a more service-based model to a science-based model of nursing, though historical studies demonstrate that nursing has never been entirely service based (Nelson 2001, 31; Lewenson 1993, 5).

These goods, or central values, are what MacIntyre calls "internal" goods of a practice. He calls them internal for two reasons. The first is that they define the central identity of nursing as a practice, so that without them it would not be nursing. The second is that they are distinctive from other goods that might be incidentally connected to the practice but do not define it. So nursing is a job, and it involves a salary, various benefits, and often certain schedules for working. These are good things, and important things, but by themselves they don't identify what nursing is all about. A nurse's salary may change as she moves from one health care system to the next, but her goals as a nurse remain focused on health. Further, we can envision changing, say, the normal schedule nurses work without changing their identity as nurses. But if we ask nurses to focus on the profitability of the health care system rather than on the promotion of health, we are making a change in the nature of nursing itself and in the nature of what it is to identify oneself as a nurse.

This notion of the internal goods of a practice becomes more complex when we combine it with the notion, discussed earlier, that practices have a history. The definition of nursing that we find in Florence Nightingale is significantly different from the definition of nursing that we find in contemporary textbooks in some ways, though her definition clearly sets the tone for the later development of nursing (McKenna 1997, 86). This is not so much because Nightingale somehow got nursing wrong, but rather because nursing as a practice has developed and refined its notion of what nursing is all about to the point where it now defines itself differently than it did, as a practice, many years ago. Presumably, as health care continues to develop and change, nursing will continue to develop and refine the notion of what it means to be a nurse. Part of what makes it a practice (rather than just a job) is that these revised understandings come from inside the practice itself as those who engage in it gain a better understanding of what its goals are. This is what MacIntyre means by his claim that in engaging in a practice the goods of that practice are systematically extended.

But let's shift our focus now, from nursing as a profession to the professionals who engage in nursing. Earlier the claim was made that when someone identifies himself or herself as a nurse, we are likely to make certain assumptions about that person's character and identity. For example, if I meet a new member of my church, and he introduces himself to me as a nurse, I am likely to assume that he will be a reliable and level-headed individual and one who will not panic in an emergency. Is this legitimate? MacIntyre would argue that it is. We noted that a practice such as nursing involves collective activity. One can't just decide to be a nurse. One has to have had the right education, one's grasp of that education needs to be validated by licensing, and certain social structures must be in place before one can be a nurse in the contemporary sense of the word. How does this affect the individual's character and identity?

At the most basic level, the internal goods of nursing shape the character of the nurse because they shape the goals and structure of nursing education. Imagine, for a moment, that we see a faculty member teaching students how to draw blood. Instead of teaching them the proper techniques for assuring sterile conditions and for causing the minimum of pain, however, our professor teaches them how to draw blood from several clients with the same needle because that saves money, and she endorses a certain amount of pain because that ensures that clients will be taught to fear the students and be properly submissive to them. What such a horrible professor is teaching is not nursing, but another practice that shares some techniques with nursing. This is quite different from saying that this professor is a bad nurse. Instead, the point here is that she is not teaching nursing at all, but some quite different practice, organized around internal goods of control and power. It isn't nursing because its internal goods are not those of nursing. The standards of this alternative practice are quite different because the internal goods of the practice are different, so that what makes someone a bad nurse would actually make them good at whatever this professor is teaching.

But now think as well of how this professor is shaping the character of the students she teaches. What she inculcates in them is quite different from the traits that a nursing professor should try to inculcate in students. The internal goods of the practice of nursing are not just external goals that people educated as nurses happen to go along with. Instead, education as a nurse develops the whole person and shapes one's character in some obvious ways and in others that aren't so obvious. Nurses learn to deal with crises in a calm and rational manner; they learn to be tremendously efficient in their use of time and energy; and they learn to provide emotional support and care while maintaining healthy boundaries (Chambliss 1996, 30-41). Further, nurses internalize the values of the health care system of which they are a part, placing a high value on health, on economic efficiency, and on protecting human life.

Both of these aspects of nursing practice, then, coincide with the role that Christian faith plays in an individual's life. Nursing qualifies and shapes a person's character and values. And there is a natural overlap between some of the ways Christian commitments and nursing training shape character and values, since both are focused on the well-being of others. This overlap is due in part to the fact that nursing as a practice was originally developed by women who were deeply motivated by their Christian faith. In fact, though the profession now distances itself from this history, Christian faith has qualified and shaped nursing practice from its inception. Nursing, then, is not a practice that is somehow intrinsically alien to Christian faith, and that makes the task of identifying the ways in which Christian faith shapes and qualifies it much simpler. For example, the Christian nurse's character is shaped in part by her or his commitment to the good of the other because the other is seen as bearing the image of God, and this adds a depth to her or his response to the other that is an important part of the Christian nurse's character. Further, the Christian nurse acts out of a hope that is grounded in faith in the Creator and Sustainer of all that exists. This means that, both in terms of character and in terms of what he or she values, the Christian nurse knows that the suffering, pain, and dying that call for care are not the end of the story. They are an occasion for grief and lament, surely, when they cannot be cured or mitigated, but our grief is not absolute because we live in a world where death is not final.

Character and values are not the only things shaped by a nursing education, however. Becoming a nurse is clearly a matter of knowledge. Nursing is a science-based practice, and to be educated as a nurse requires learning the content and practices of that science. But nursing is more than this knowledge, and that "more" involves becoming the sort of person who can respond to clients in the right way, the sort of person who recognizes pain as needing alleviation, or who respects and encourages a client's attempts at self-care. Developing the character of a nurse involves developing habits of action (efficiency, prioritization), skilled knowledge or "knowing how" (knowing how to start an IV, recognizing an unusual level of confusion in a client with Alzheimer's), and theoretical knowledge (understanding the physiology of blood gases). In addition to these, the nurse develops personal characteristics that permit him or her to respond empathetically to a client, without trying to take over the client's life (Halpern 2001, 113). Because nursing, like other professions, requires character formation in addition to knowledge and skills, it is more than a science; it is an art as well.

All of these patterns of character formation shape the identity of the practitioners in a profession. Some practitioners will lack certain aspects of this character, of course; but taken as a group, practitioners will show a definite pattern of character. Those who are educated and licensed as nurses will have been inducted into a profession that encourages and even requires certain characteristics in its practitioners. These characteristics are certainly not those that sometimes have been associated with nursing in the past (being a "nice girl," for example); rather, they are characteristics such as having an aptitude for science, having a quick intellectual grasp of theories and being able to see how they apply in real world conditions, and being capable of self-control when faced with an obstreperous client.

It is also worth noting that tensions can arise between professional standards of behavior and socialized patterns developed in the context of particular health care systems. Because a significant part of the education of nurses takes place in particular hospital or clinic settings, the social context of those settings can either support or subvert the education a nurse receives in school. If a school had high professional standards, but the unit has a history of practices that are less professional, it is difficult for students to maintain the standards of the education. A gap of this sort, between the ideal standards of the profession and the actual behavior of practitioners, is not unusual in the professions, but in the best-case scenario the gap is a minor one.

As is often the case, the very characteristics that are the strength and pride of nursing can sometimes also contribute to problems in nursing. As sociologist Daniel Chambliss notes, the knowledge and professional education of nurses makes it hard for them to be understanding toward clients who choose to remain ignorant about their own condition and who make choices that seem trivial and silly from the perspective of a health professional (Chambliss 1996, 124). The very virtues of professional education can make it hard to avoid treating such a client patronizingly. It remains a challenge for the contemporary nurse to discern when the characteristics that are inculcated by contemporary nursing sometimes create blind spots.

But the identity of a nurse is formed by more than just the education she or he has received. It is also the case that the practice of nursing shapes who someone is in important ways. We (the authors of this book) had an interesting example of this as we met to begin writing. One of the philosophers in the group mentioned that health care practitioners tended to assume automatically that physical health is an individual's highest priority in making life decisions, while philosophers might sometimes be more concerned about logical consistency than health. The remark occasioned a certain amount of amusement among the nurses, and several of the nurses thought that this showed just how irrational philosophers really are! If this sort of assumption is true, then becoming a nurse is likely to shape one's character in deep and important ways. When one becomes a health care professional, one devotes one's life to the pursuit of human health in general, and health then becomes one of the central values of one's life. This good of health, however, is not the only one that a person can value, and many people do not consider it to be so central. Like the philosopher mentioned earlier, they may have a different set of goods that structure their lives.

So in addition to encouraging the development of particular character traits such as responsiveness, nursing also will tend to structure the basic set of values a practitioner holds. In this way, it is a practice that shapes the professional's life and values in central and important ways. It is important to see this so that nurses (and other professionals) recognize that what they value most highly may not be the central concern for others. But it is also important to see this because it allows the nurse to examine her or his values critically and to reflect on whether those should be values that shape her or his life. The Christian nurse may occasionally find that she or he needs to place the value of health in its proper perspective as a very important good, but not the ultimate meaning of life (Mohrmann 1995, 15).

Up to this point we have been discussing the nature of nursing education and the relationships nurses have with clients. Nurses work in a context that shapes and structures that relationship because providing nursing care always occurs in an institutional or organizational context. A Christian perspective does not end when one moves from personal to institutional contexts, so it is worthwhile to think about how faith shapes our understanding of the systemic and organizational aspects of nursing practice as well. In the next section we'll focus on two features of institutional organization. The first involves the connections between central values of the nursing profession and institutional values. The second examines connections between the nurse's professional responsibility and the professional responsibility of the other actors in the institutional setting.

Nursing and Institutional Context

Nursing is a profession that involves the organization of certain caring tasks in society. The social organization of these tasks is vital, since the education of nurses, their licensing, and the structure and responsibilities of their jobs are decided collectively. Imagine the chaos society would experience if individuals had to find their own care-givers before they entered the hospital, negotiate wages and working conditions, evaluate competency, and ensure compliance. Hospitalization would be an even more harrowing experience than many find it to be now. Organizing nursing care needs to be done at a professional level so that competent care is provided in a regular, continuing, and efficient manner. And because this is accomplished through professional organization, nurses can monitor themselves to a large degree. This is one of the hallmarks of professionalization, and it is also the reason why many professional organizations require members to take an oath or pledge, making a public promise that they will use their knowledge and skills for the well-being of those who call on them (Koehn 1994, 56-59). The professional organization of nursing practice is built into the contemporary health care system.

This both shapes and constrains nursing practice in important ways. One obvious way it shapes nursing practice is by providing both the financial structure necessary to offer nursing care and the financial limitations of providing that care. Without institutional structures, even the structures nurses complain about most (insurance companies! government agencies!), there would be no consistent way to provide the care that makes up the heart of nursing practice.

As Christians, we may be tempted to become cynical at this point, mutter "render unto Caesar," and pretend that financial issues have no relevance to Christian life and thought. But ignoring the financial structures of contemporary nursing is a mistake. Nursing practice is fundamentally affected by economic structures, whether at basic levels of staffing and salaries or at more general levels of what treatments are funded for which clients. And because nurses are the health care professionals most constantly involved in the day-to-day care of clients, nurses often find that they have to explain to clients what insurance will or will not cover; they may even negotiate with insurance companies as to what, exactly, is meant by a term such as "life-threatening."

Given this central role for the nursing profession as a whole, then, it is vital for nursing to be vocal in advocating for financial structures that support rather than prevent good care. But what does this mean for the Christian nurse? We will discuss issues of social justice at greater length in subsequent chapters, but it is worth noting here that an important part of being a professional involves active participation in shaping the organizations of one's profession. Christian nurses have a responsibility to participate in productive ways in professional organizations, to speak out on issues on which they have expertise, and to contribute to the internal development and growth of the profession.

Participating in professional organizations, while important, is not the most obvious aspect of institutional structures that the nurse confronts on a day-to-day basis, however. The organization that structures the nurse's life in ways that can be both rewarding and frustrating is the health care campus within which much care is given. For the acute care nurse, and some types of mental health nursing, this may be the site of professional practice. For the parish nurse this may be the location where clients are sent for care, from which they come needing arrangements for home health care, and the like, but few nurses work in contexts where their practice is not structured by the demands of the health care system.

Working in the health care system also involves working with other health care professionals: physicians, technicians, aides, and administrators. The complexities of the nurse/physician relationship have been noted by many researchers and cannot all be examined in detail here, but a few aspects are worth noting in the context of considering how Christian faith influences nursing practice. Nurses often find themselves in a frustrating or difficult situation due to the organizational role they play as mediator between client and physician (Engelhardt 1985, 62-79). The frustrations that can accompany this role are described and analyzed in some of the later chapters of this book, but a few general comments are worth making here.

First, the Christian nurse has a sense of confidence in her or his role. Nursing involves advocacy for the client, often the most vulnerable and weakest individual involved in any controversy. The use of professional status and knowledge for the benefit of the vulnerable is one important part of the Christian life, and the nurse occupies an institutional role that allows her or him to do this. Further, a Christian perspective can give nurses a sense of freedom from some of the status fights that often go on in the health care setting over who has the authority to do what. From a Christian perspective it is clear that what is central is that good care be provided in ways that are consistent and fair. Work that involves dealing with the less pleasant aspects of embodiment and sickness are not, from a Christian perspective, inherently demeaning or lower in status. In fact, Jesus specifically names caring for basic bodily needs as the service that is proper to those who would be his followers. Recognizing this, the Christian nurse operates from a position of confidence in negotiating with other professionals. What he or she does is important and worthy of respect. If others consider it less valuable because it sometimes requires getting messy, then that reflects badly on others' values.

It is important to be clear about what this does not imply. Being a Christian nurse does not require the nurse to give up on basic claims of justice or to cheerfully accept mistreatment or abusive relationships. The knowledge that one is a beloved child of God should always provide a sense of confident expectation that professional relationships will be structured fairly and in ways that protect the basic dignity of everyone involved. We consider some of the aspects of justice with regard to institutional structures in Chapter Four [of *Transforming Care*] and will say more on this topic later. But the point to be made here is that when nurses are involved in work that others may be tempted to dismiss as "mere service work" or as unimportant because it involves hands-on care, nurses can confidently reply that this work is central to human life and well-being. It is not menial; it does not deserve disrespect; and those who do it deserve societal gratitude and a fair salary.

Noting that organizational structures sometimes treat hands-on, caring work as trivial or unimportant provides an important transition to our next topic. What is it that allows the Christian nurse to see such labor as valuable and worthy of respect? In part, the Christian nurse can draw on a Christian understanding of what it is to be a person. The Western tradition has tended to define persons in terms of independent existence and rational intellect, while downplaying or ignoring their embodied, emotional, interrelational nature (Benner and Wrubel 1989, 29-54). It can be easy to see caring for bodily needs as a mark of subordination in part because we do not always value or respect our embodied nature. As Christians we have resources for seeing persons in another way, however, and seeing them in that way gives us better insight into what nursing itself is.

Persons: Embodied and Made in the Image of God

In the previous chapter [of *Transforming Care*] we met a nurse, Janet, whose client, Ann, suffered from congestive heart failure and edema. Being a competent nurse, Janet took diagnostic information with practiced hands and showed genuine concern for Ann by greeting her warmly and honoring her request to have her hair combed despite the complications this made for Janet.

The story of Janet and Ann suggests that an adequate picture of human persons starts with the notion of embodiment: persons are bodily beings. Nursing practices, from the taking of diagnostic information to combing hair, demonstrate the bodily character of the persons involved and the interactions between them. Embodiment involves both independence and dependence related in interesting ways. A full understanding of what it is to be a person requires us to go beyond embodiment and recognize that persons are created in God's image. In turn, this leads to understanding persons as characters in a narrative, co-authors of the stories in which they are embedded. We'll deal with each of these three concepts — embodiment, the image of God, and the narrative structure of human life — in the sections that follow.

Embodiment and Independence

We'll begin with the idea of embodiment. To say that a person is embodied implies two things about being a person. The first is subjectivity, the sense of being a concrete, particular "I," someone who is able to consciously experience her or his life. The second is wholeness. We sometimes elaborate this by saying that a person is an integral unity of a variety of interrelated dimensions: physical, emotional, mental, social, moral, and spiritual. Wholeness and subjectivity are connected to each other. The unity or integrality of being a person is what makes it possible for someone to speak of himself or herself in the first person, as an "I." We sometimes call this concrete unity of being subjectivity, or being a "subject."

These two notions of unity and subjectivity are central components of being a human person, but when we start with them we run the risk of implying that all persons have this sort of wholeness and sense of self. This clearly isn't true. Some people lack any sense of self, perhaps because they suffer from Alzheimer's or some other cognitive dysfunction. Others lack physiological wholeness because their bodies have been ravaged by disease or they've been badly burned. So how do we maintain our sense that being a person involves wholeness and subjectivity, while recognizing that some persons lack both of these to some degree? What we need to recognize is that wholeness and subjectivity are part of the way humans are supposed to be. When we recognize another as a person, we recognize that both of these features should be attributes of his or her life. One of the aspects of health that nurses often work toward is the restoration of wholeness and subjectivity when these have been diminished by disease or accidents. In some cases we deal with persons who will never gain or regain these capacities, as when we work with people with severe developmental disabilities. In such cases we recognize the capacity only in its absence, and this can be cause for lament.

There is another danger in starting our discussion of personhood with the notion of embodiment. When we think of embodiment we often first think of the body as it is portrayed in anatomy and physiology textbooks: as a system of cells organized into tissues, organs, and organ systems that function together as a body. The body is portrayed as a physical something that can be operated on, studied by science, and so forth. This picture of the body is extremely useful and important for nursing practice, and it produces what we might call an objective account of the body, an account that is the result of focusing on the body as an object of study. The result of such study is a picture of the body as a sophisticated but purely physical mechanism.

We need to recognize, however, that this picture of the body as an object is an abstraction. Our first experience of the body is our own lived experience of being embodied, of seeing the world from this particular location, reaching out for a cup of coffee, waking up and stretching in the morning. To begin to see bodies as objects rather than people requires us to abstract the body from its immediate context of the concrete, living person and to focus solely on its physical (physiological, biological) aspects, as an object. This process of abstraction is part of the process of education as a nurse, and although it feels natural once one has been socialized into nursing, it is worth remembering that it is not natural for those outside the health care context (Chambliss 1996, 26-28). Although this abstraction is both important and necessary for scientific study of health and disease processes, we should keep in mind that abstractions are always partial and that the concrete person is more than physiological processes.

Keeping this cautionary note in mind, we will use the term *embodied* to refer to the concrete person: the embodied subject. Embodiment does not refer to only one aspect of the person, namely his or her physical dimension, abstracted from the other dimensions (emotional, social, moral, spiritual, and so forth) or abstracted from the fact that such a person is an "I," a subject. Instead, embodiment refers to a unified, integral someone who can say "I," an embodied subject, the concrete person before any abstraction occurs. Embodiment is, first of all, the person as a unified, particular "I."

Part of the character of embodiment involves the occupation of a location, here and now. This means that as a creature I am not just any old where, nowhere in particular; certainly I am not, more fancifully, everywhere in general. Thinking back to our example, Janet was in a particular location, Ann's room, standing beside her, with the early morning sun shining on the floor and wall. Being finite, being creatures, means that we are always located in a particular place and time. Spatial and temporal location is what makes being a human "I" possible at all. And it is also a central aspect of the recognition of another person as an "I" in her own right. Janet recognizes this particularity when she addresses Ann by name. To call another by name is tacitly to recognize that person as an "I," a concrete person, rather than as an abstraction or a role. When we refer to someone as "the congestive heart failure in room 3574" or "the complainer down the hall" we diminish that person's subjectivity. Names are important precisely because they recognize our embodied specificity, the particular person that we are rather than the interchangeable occupants of a hospital bed.

In addition to location in space and time, embodiment also implies that I have some independence from my surroundings and can interact with them in ways that are satisfying and meaningful for me. Enjoying the taste of freshly baked bread or the warmth of a cozy house on a cold winter's evening offers evidence of my relative independence and ability to interact with my environment in ways that are satisfying and pleasurable (Levinas 1961, 110). The senses of rightness and well-being that we discussed in the last chapter are related to enjoyment. Enjoyment is one way in which we feel those senses in our everyday lived experience. In other words, we become aware of our sense of rightness in moments when we experience enjoyment.

When we are not able to interact in satisfying ways, we experience this as a lack of independence and find it frustrating and sometimes painful. Enjoyment, then, is an integral, interior aspect of the subjectivity of embodiment. We see this even in situations where one might not expect to see much joy. Ann's desire to have her hair combed is a small request, but it touches the core of her subjectivity and offers evidence of her ability to experience some of the basic physical pleasures of life. The caring nurse, in fact, notices when such requests diminish or disappear. This is a bad sign, an indicator that a client is losing a sense of self. In these cases the client has a diminished sense of subjectivity, manifest in the lack of enjoyment of minor bodily processes. Enjoyment is a delight that comes with well-being, and its absence is always a danger signal.

Even when well-being is no longer robust enough to sustain much independence as we normally think of independence, in terms of directing the course of one's life and activities, it is still possible for an individual to experience the small physical activities of the day as a source of satisfaction. The enjoyment of embodiment constitutes the standing possibility for thanksgiving: a heartfelt thanks for goodness, delight, and life. And so we return to themes developed in our first chapter, as we see that for the Christian nurse even the most mundane activities can be experienced as participating in worship and gratitude and delight.

But there is more to our relative independence than enjoyment. Separation from our environment as bodily creatures makes us beings that can have certain amounts of control over what we do, where we go, what we will eat, who we will talk to, what we will say, and what we will decide. Janet's activities in the hospital room were actions, the activity of a being with agency, as was Ann's request. Being an embodied person, an "I," means to be a point of origin of deliberate, voluntary, particular actions; in other words, it means having agency (Merleau-Ponty 1962, 137). To be an "I" is to have agency with respect to my surroundings. Again, of course, we need to recognize that this is a description that begins with how things ought to be. Too often in life we experience a frustrating lack of agency in our own case or that of others. Sometimes this is merely temporary, other times it is lifelong, and always it is cause for a certain level of frustration and lament. This brings us to a second aspect of being an embodied person, namely dependency.

Embodiment and Dependence

Ann's situation indicates ways in which she is capable of acting as an embodied agent, but it also points to the other side of embodiment — dependence. Dependence is universal. We are dependent on the ground on which we walk and on the air we breathe. These universal dependencies remind us of our constant dependence on God's continuing creative and sustaining work. We also depend on the other people and the social institutions that provide the context within which we act and live. Human life makes sense only within an interdependent web of relationships. As embodied, dependent, and interdependent creatures, then, we are vulnerable. Embodiment is a fragile state; enjoyment is always precarious. And because we are embodied and vulnerable, we cannot ignore the environment within which we function. When we discuss health and environment in the next chapter we will see how dependent we are on environmental factors, but for now it is important to note that embodiment always involves a tension between agency and dependency. We are always vulnerable because we are always dependent. In fact, part of embodiment involves our knowledge that there will come a time when each of us ceases to be an "I," when the elements out of which we are composed no longer make up a person. The vulnerability of embodiment constitutes the standing possibility for lament: an anguished cry against suffering, degradation, and untimely death.

There is yet another side to being an embodied person, related to both vulnerability and agency — namely, openness (Levinas 1987, 146). Embodiment means permanent exposure to incoming disruptions. Because we are located in space and time and in relations of interdependence with other people, we are always in a position to be interrupted by other things and, more importantly, other people. This is not something we have any choice about. Right from the start of life we find ourselves constantly in relationships where others make decisions that affect us. As we grow and gain some relative independence we have more control over some of these mutual interactions, but especially in occupations such as nursing that involve constant attentiveness to others' needs we are never free from the demands of others. And though a bit more time away from others' demands generally sounds attractive, none of us really wants to be isolated and completely alone; there are few things more damaging to selfhood than extended solitary confinement. A basic part of embodied personhood is this openness to other selves.

Openness means that persons are always formed by reciprocal interdependence. Janet competently took information from an objective body — blood pressure, oxygen levels, pulse, urine output — but while she was doing that she also attended to Ann as a whole person. Janet greeted her warmly, asked an open-ended question, listened for the answer, complied with the request, and didn't draw attention to its complications. This suggests a fundamental openness, an attunement to others. It also requires that we set aside expectations and prejudgments so that we can be open to others as the vulnerable, enjoying, embodied beings that they are (Olthuis 2002, 128). Openness thus also points to the responsibility we have to and for the other person. While we generally begin with an assumption of our own freedom and agency, part of being an interdependent person is to feel the need to relativize one's own freedom because of responsibility to another person. To be a person is to be called to put one's agency to work for the good of the other person, to care for that other person. We experience our own openness when we recognize that we have a responsibility, here and now, in this relationship, to care.

Being a person involves having a responsibility to care for others, and this responsibility is a part of the interdependence that marks the human condition. Most nurses, of course, have no trouble remembering that they have a responsibility to care for others, particularly clients, since that is built into their professional identity. But this relationship of responsibility is a reciprocal one, not a one-way street. At the same time that the nurse cares for his or her client, we frequently find that the client responds by trying to take care of the nurse. The client denies her pain because she doesn't want her care-giver to feel distress. Or the client makes sure he asks about the nurse's life and family. These gestures can be awkward, but they indicate that the client feels a need to be in a reciprocal relationship. Sometimes it is tempting for the nurse to brush these gestures aside as impertinent, and they can be inappropriate and intrusive. But at the same time, recognition that the client is not an entirely passive object of the nurse's care is an important part of the relationship between these two embodied persons. It is a relationship of interdependence, though not of equal dependency. Failure to recognize this interdependence and reciprocity of the nurse-client relationship can result in what William May has described as the "conceit of philanthropy," which assumes that the world can be neatly divided into care-givers and care-receivers, which lends an air of superiority to the care-giver (May 1975, 37).

Persons as Image-Bearers

This recognition that being a person always involves interdependence and responsibility naturally brings the discussion for Christians to the notion of persons as bearers of the image of God. One way we bear the image of God is in being God's stewards — representatives, co-workers, co-authors, signs of God's reign — here on earth. To be an image-bearer is also to be oriented toward our neighbor (Berkouwer 1959, 151). In discipleship, life becomes a truly human life, lived in service of God through attending to one's neighbor.

This means, of course, that there are at least two image-bearers in any relationship: the one who is being neighborly and the person to whom one is neighborly. Recalling our discussion earlier about location, we can say that the term *neighbor* involves a closeness that includes openness and care for the other. So the call to be a neighbor is the call to image God in caring action. Using our freedom to respond to others' vulnerability in responsible action shows us to be image-bearers. In our example, Janet shows God's image by her attunement to Ann, by showing her respect and care. And Ann, reciprocally, images God to Janet, so that Janet finds herself in the presence of the sacred as she ministers to Ann's physical, emotional, and social needs. The call from God that I experience when I see another's vulnerability and need is a fundamental part of what it is for me to be a subject (Bloechl 2000, 46).

Thus the other person also bears God's image. In fact, the very suffering and pain of another reflect the image of God in that person. The reason we call it *suffering* is related to the dignity and sacredness of life and the recognition that concrete, individual lives ought to exhibit well-being. We can recognize the absence of something as tragic only when we know that its presence is part of the proper ordering of a good creation. This recognition of sacredness is not a respect for "dignity of life" generally, as an abstract principle, but recognition of the concrete dignity of this particular person, here and now. The dignity of Ann's particular, individual life bears the image of God, the Provider and Sustainer of life, and her suffering is painful precisely because it is a breakdown of the rightful well-being of the other as a living person. The task of neighborliness is not blindly or abstractly directed at humanity in general. It is directed to the other person precisely because the other bears God's image in his or her vulnerability and need.

Because being a person is always a matter of reciprocal interrelatedness, the giving and receiving of care flows in both directions. In our example, despite Janet's role as care-giver, she not only gives but also receives from Ann. Conversely, despite Ann's need for care, she not only receives but also gives to Janet. The reciprocity is not an economic exchange of equal and comparable goods. What is given and received may well be quite different for each person in the relationship and will depend in part on what each needs. Nurses receive gifts of all sorts from the clients they care for, from the gift of service as a "guinea pig" that a client gives to a nursing student as he learns to start an IV to the gift of respect that a client gives to a practiced, professional nurse for her expertise and experience. It would be a mistake to think that in giving care nothing is traveling in the reverse direction. In fact, without the reciprocal gifts of respect, gratitude, warmth, and humanity that clients can offer, nursing would be an unattractive profession. And as scheduling pressures and lack of funds have made this reciprocity harder and harder to maintain in acute care settings, nursing has become more stressful and less rewarding. The problem of mid-career burnout has clear connections to the structures that prevent reciprocity in the nurse/client relationship.

Persons as Co-authors

We have described embodiment as enjoyment and vulnerability, freedom and responsibility, all drawn together in the image of God; but this still leaves something unsaid because it treats persons as if they were complete at any given instant. Such a description omits the ways in which identity involves being a character in a narrative with a past, present, and future plot (MacIntyre 1984, 206). Ann and Janet are not abstract embodied agents. Each of them also has a history that has determined the shape of her character and makes sense of her choices and actions. Part of this story is composed of the social roles into which we are born. None of us enters society as a generic human being. We begin our lives as someone's son or daughter, as a citizen of a nation and a member of a particular society and civilization. Each of these roles involves expectations and responsibilities. We enter the world as members of ethnic groups with particular languages, concepts, assumptions, rules for the proper use of humor, and so forth, all of which constrain the shape that the story of our lives can take, while providing the necessary context within which those stories can be told. Without membership in those larger social groupings I would have no particular identity — which is to say, no identity at all, for identity is always particular.

To be a person is to be historically and socially situated. Each person has a character informed by social expectations about gender, social class, nation, race, and ethnicity as well as by assumptions about duties, rights, goods, dangers, temptations, evils, and obligations. Both Janet and Ann enter their interactions with each other from the midst of such social presuppositions about identity and roles. Their identities as characters, including their social roles as nurse and client, only make sense against the backdrop of the narratives of the communities — family, society, nation, civilization — in which they are embedded. Most of the time we simply assume that these identities exist, without paying them much attention, but when we find ourselves working in a context where groups with critical cultural differences must interact, we suddenly become aware of how deeply our assumptions of identity structure our lives.

However, the social situation in which one is a character is not the only feature that marks personal identity. One is always a character in a narrative in two ways: first, passively, to the extent that one's life is scripted by historical and social conditions; and second, actively, to the extent that one affirms or rejects those conditions. Just as independence is always relative to vulnerability and dependence, so active determination of the direction and meaning of one's life always takes place against the background of social and historical possibilities. Both Janet and Ann exhibit this mixture of activity and passivity, albeit in different ways. Janet, we might think at first glance, is largely the agent in this narrative fragment, the one who has the freedom to come into the room, actively checking diagnostic information, initiating conversation, deciding to get the comb, and so forth. Yet she is also constrained in at least two ways. First of all, she is constrained by the setting — namely, the institutional procedures and her workload, as well as currently accepted nursing practices, including expectations of efficiency and thoroughness. Second, she is constrained by the person of Ann, to whom she attends, listens, and complies. Janet's sense of herself as a nurse will be partly determined by the response she receives from Ann. Being a nurse is an important part of Janet's identity, so Ann's response can be quite powerful.

Ann, we might also think at first glance, is (literally) the patient, the passive one who suffers, who receives the care that Janet gives her, who is constrained by the rules and expectations of the particular institution she is in, and who acquiesces to the health care system of which she is part. Yet her request to have her hair combed shows agency, a continuing expression of freedom. And her expression of freedom gains its meaning from the part it plays in the continuing story of her life. We can imagine that she has always been careful of her personal appearance, and the request then fits into a story of continued care for propriety in the context of a world that feels in disarray. On the other hand, Ann may be the sort of person who goes through life with a cheerful disregard for the finer points of personal hygiene. In that case her request has a different sort of meaning, and it may prompt Janet to inquire whether she is expecting visitors or some special event.

This indicates why we speak of persons as characters in a narrative. The meaning of their actions and of the events that occur in their lives always relates back to the particular narrative structures that make sense of what they do. For Christians, individual life stories are always embedded in the greater narrative of God's creative and redemptive activity, a story we learn in Scripture. And just as we come to knowledge and relationship with God through the stories of Scripture, we also come to a knowledge and relationship with other persons through the stories those persons tell us of their lives.

Because people are agents, they have some control over how the story of their life goes. Sometimes we might speak of this as being the author of one's life, or determining how the plot will play out. But simply to speak of authorship is too one-sided. An author of a book has total control over the story's path or trajectory. But the person writing her or his life has only partial control. Because she or he is constrained by circumstances and by other people who are not under her or his control, we need to speak of the individual as the co-author rather than the author of her or his life. A person is a character who co-authors the narrative.

Furthermore, it is as a character in a particular story that an agent finds herself with the obligation to act in particular ways and not others. Janet's recognition that she needs to respond to Ann with respect and care, and her understanding that part of that respect requires her to go through the cumbersome process of leaving and then reentering Ann's room without burdening Ann with a sense of having asked too much, are shaped by the context in which she provides nursing care. The context of a narrative gives the actions chosen by an agent their meaning and their moral status. Actions are judged right or wrong, wise or foolish, in or out of character against a background composed of social practices and roles, professional and personal life plans, and the narrative unity of a whole life (Ricoeur 1992, 157; MacIntyre 1984, 205). We can evaluate how and when actions are to be approved or disapproved, or how and when characters are to be praised or blamed for their actions, only in the context of the stories, including the story of God's self-revelation through Scripture, of which those actions are a part.

Persons in Community

Very few stories are written with only one character. We've already noted that being a person involves interdependence and openness to others, and this is true of the stories of our lives as well. Every story has multiple characters made up of the other people in the communities of which one is a member. We have already noted how a person's identity is shaped by the societal and communal stories of which she or he is a part. But the fact of communal existence brings us to another aspect of personhood as well. Whenever there are multiple members of a community, we face the issue of determining how the benefits, resources, and burdens of that community will be distributed among them. This points our attention forward to Chapter Four [of *Transforming Care*], in which we will discuss ethical principles in more detail, but it warrants some mention here as well.

To return to our example, Janet's competent interaction with Ann is shaped not only by the structure of nursing practice but also, more concretely, by clients in other rooms who also are under her care. While Ann as an image-bearer of God deserves to be treated with dignity and respect, Janet has other clients who also are image-bearers and who also deserve to be treated with dignity and respect. These other clients are tacitly present in the room as Janet competently cares for Ann in her decisions about how long to stay, whether she has time to fetch the comb, and so forth. Furthermore, Janet's fellow nurses on the unit also are tacitly present, as a team of care-givers of which she is a member, in which she has to carry out a fair share of the workload. Part of her competence in responsibly nursing Ann is her tacit responsibility to her fellow workers to "pull her weight" on the entire unit. The reverse is true as well. Janet must be tacitly present in the work of the other nurses on the unit, and they must do their part so that Janet is treated fairly and given the space to do her work well. Each of the members of this small and fluid community deserves to be treated as a neighbor, to be offered respect, to receive care that permits her or his life to go well, and to experience her or his membership as a matter of equality and fairness. What we are dealing with here, then, is a question of justice. Justice involves structuring responsibilities and practices in ways that make it possible to treat all members of the community fairly, with equity, giving each her or his due.

Justice, absolute fairness, is never fully realized, of course, and decisions about equitable sharing of resources are always contestable. Even when a care facility has rules and regulations that are intended to be equitable, to treat both clients and care-givers fairly, we might find that they lack effectiveness or have imperfections or limitations. As we will note when we discuss environmental factors such as the Medicare system, even when a system is designed to contribute to justice and fairness for all the members of that society, we might still find that it falls short in important ways. Concrete social practices, plans, and policies are always limited, fallible, and reflective of their makers' self-deception and sinfulness.

That is not to say that all rules or regulations or practices are equally unjust. On the contrary, the recognition that no regulations embody perfect justice does not rule out the simultaneous recognition that some regulations fall much farther short of justice than others. For example, nursing practice is better structured when it makes care its central concern than when it instead makes efficiency or profit its central goal. This is not to suggest that a nurse should be inefficient or that an institution ought to finance itself into bankruptcy. However, a health care system that aims to remain solvent to facilitate care is a very different system from one that aims for profit as a primary motive, just as being efficient in caring for others and aiming at efficiency as one's primary goal are two different things. And, we might say, the call to justice in the area of health care is precisely the call to aim not at profit or efficiency, but at an equitable distribution of competent care — money, time, staffing, equipment — so that all within the reach of the community can flourish. We will return to this question of justice in Chapter Four [of *Transforming Care*], but for now we can note that being a person always places one into the context of moral relationships that require judgments about justice and fairness and about how we respond to the weak and vulnerable among us. For the Christian nurse, this moral dimension of personhood is what we would expect to find, given our understanding of persons as created by, loved by, and imaging a God of justice.

From a Christian perspective we might say that justice forms the communal horizon for particular characters whose social roles include being health-care providers. Here we can return briefly to the discussion of embodiment, one that we have never quite left. Embodiment, as it turns out, means many things. It means being in a location, here and now, being a character in a narrative. Embodiment means having relative freedom with respect to one's surroundings, being both an agent in the story and a co-author of the narrative. It means enjoyment of life, being oriented toward well-being and flourishing. Embodiment means being vulnerable, not only to suffering but also to being informed by the expectations of the community into which one is born. And it means openness, the ethical call to responsibility in the context of community. Justice is the shape that the ethical call takes in a communal context, as we together engage in the social practices that allow embodied persons to care for other embodied persons.

Conclusion

Because nursing is a profession in the fullest sense of the word, it is a practice oriented toward important human goods, and it is a practice that shapes the lives of its practitioners in important ways. It is a moral practice, carrying within it certain values and encouraging the development of certain character traits in its practitioners. The identity of nurses is shaped by the education they receive and by the institutions within which they practice. The identity of nursing is also shaped by assumptions about the nature of the persons who become nurses and the clients for whom they care. As we have seen, both the nature of nursing and the identity of persons are shaped and qualified in important ways by the Christian nurse's faith commitments. This does not mean that the Christian nurse and the non-Christian nurse disagree about what nursing involves; it means instead that although there is broad agreement about what nursing is, the Christian nurse comes to that practice shaped by her or his faith and seeing the privileges and responsibilities of that role in terms of the grand story of God's creating, sustaining, and redeeming activity.

In the same way that Christian faith shapes one's understanding of the practice of nursing and the meaning of personhood, it also shapes the fundamental orientation nursing has toward the good of health. It is fairly commonplace to define nursing as a practice oriented toward health. This orientation is a part of the very earliest history of nursing. The health in question is not an abstract idea of health, however, but the health and well-being of concrete people with whom the nurse works. And these people live, work, and sometimes suffer in the midst of particular environments. Because all of these concepts are so inescapably interconnected with nursing practice, they are often called the metaparadigm concepts of nursing. The next chapter [of *Transforming Care*] examines the two concepts we have not yet discussed — health and environment — from the perspective of an understanding of nursing and personhood shaped by Christian faith.

Works Cited

Benner, Patricia, and Judith Wrubel. 1989. *The Primacy of Caring: Stress and Coping in Health and Illness.* Menlo Park, CA: Addison Wesley Publishing Company.

Berkouwer, G. C. 1959. The reformed faith and the modern concept of man. *International Reformed Bulletin* 2, no. 3.

Bloechl, J. 2000. *Liturgy of the Neighbor.* Pittsburgh: Duquesne University Press.

Chambliss, D. 1996. *Beyond Caring: Hospitals, Nurses, and the Social Organization of Ethics.* Chicago: University of Chicago Press.

Engelhardt, H. Tristram, Jr. 1985. Physicians, patients, health care institutions — and the people in between — nurses. In *Caring, Curing, Coping: Nurse, Physician, Patient Relationships,* edited by Anne Bishop and John D. Scudder, 62-79. Birmingham: University of Alabama Press.

Group, Thetis M., and Joan I. Roberts. 2001. *Nursing, Physician Control, and the Medical Monopoly: Historical Perspectives on Gendered Inequality in Roles, Rights, and Range of Practice.* Indianapolis: Indiana University Press.

Halpern, Jodi. 2001. *From Detached Concern to Empathy: Humanizing Medical Practice.* Oxford: Oxford University Press.

Koehn, D. 1994. *The Ground of Professional Ethics.* London: Routledge.

Levinas, Emmanuel. 1961. *Totality and Infinity.* Pittsburgh: Duquesne University Press.

Levinas, Emmanuel. 1987. *Collected Philosophical Papers.* Pittsburgh: Duquesne University Press.

Lewenson, Sandra Beth. 1993. *Taking Charge: Nursing, Suffrage, and Feminism in America, 1873-1920.* New York: Garland Publishing, Inc.

MacIntyre, Alasdair. 1984. *After Virtue.* 2nd edition. Notre Dame: University of Notre Dame Press.

May, William F. 1975. Covenant, contract, or philanthropy. *Hastings Center Report* 5:29-38.

McKenna, Hugh. 1997. *Nursing Theories and Models.* New York: Routledge.

Merleau-Ponty, M. 1962. *Phenomenology of Perception.* London: Routledge and Kegan Paul.

Mohrmann, Margaret E. 1995. *Medicine as Ministry: Reflections on Suffering, Ethics, and Hope.* Cleveland: Pilgrim Press.
Nelson, Sioban. 2001. *Say Little, Do Much: Nurses, Nuns, and Hospitals in the Nineteenth Century.* Philadelphia: University of Pennsylvania Press.
Olthuis, J. 2002. *The Beautiful Risk.* Grand Rapids: Zondervan.
Ricoeur, P. 1992. *Oneself as Another.* Chicago: University of Chicago Press.

34 Hospital Chaplaincy as Agapeic Intervention

Joseph J. Kotva Jr.

I am ambivalent about hospital chaplaincy. I know several fine chaplains whose ministries are vehicles for God's grace and mercy. Yet, I worry that chaplaincy is often more about cheap grace than gospel, more about compromise than conviction.

My ambivalence is captured in the very designation 'hospital chaplain.' 'Hospital' remains a positive word, although reservedly so. Hospital sounds like hospitality, a virtue to which Christians aspire. Indeed, the term 'hospital' derives from the Latin word *"hospitalis,* meaning 'guest,' and the early hospitals were an outgrowth of the guest houses attached to monasteries in the Middle Ages" (Javitt, 1998). Thus, the modern hospital is rooted in a centuries-long tradition of extending hospitality to travelers, the sick, the elderly, and the poor — a tradition that Christian clergy should seek to extend by their presence. The hospital is also where most Americans take their first and last breath — occasions for Christian clergy to affirm both God's gift of new life and God's continuing care through death. The word 'hospital' is therefore basically positive, reflecting a tradition of care for the sick and indicating a place where we greet newborns and comfort the dying.

The word "chaplain" is less positive. Most definitions of chaplaincy refer to the appointment of a non-parochial cleric to the private chapel of someone of wealth and power, such as a monarch, nobleman, or bishop (Smith, 1990; see also *Oxford Dictionary of the Christian Church*). The *Encyclopedia of Religion* similarly uses the designation "chaplain" to describe "the many cases in which the priest is a functionary attached to the ruling circles" (Eliade, 1995, p. 532). From my Mennonite tradition's perspective, this definition is suspicious since it removes clergy from the call and life of the believing community and places them in the direct service of individuals from the wealthy or privileged social classes that often distort the gospel and oppress the poor.

Even worse, the term 'chaplain' is inextricably tied to military chaplaincy. Attachment or service to a military unit is always included in definitions of chaplaincy, while service in a hospital is not always similarly listed. This priority makes sense since military chaplaincy signifi-

From Joseph J. Kotva Jr., "Hospital Chaplaincy as Agapeic Intervention," *Christian Bioethics* 4 (1998): 257-75. Used by permission.

cantly antedates hospital chaplaincy and since the English term 'chaplain' has a military background. The term derives from the Middle Ages, by which time St. Martin of Tours (a former soldier) was regarded as the patron saint of French kings. The church allowed those kings to carry St. Martin's cloak into battle, but as a church relic, the cloak itself was cared for by the priest who served as the king's pastor. The priest was called *"capellanus"* — keeper of the cloak. It is from this title that we get the English word 'chaplain' (Starling, 1990). The word 'chaplain' is thus inherently tied to warfare.

Several features of military chaplaincy are troubling to me as a Mennonite pastor. First, military chaplains have divided loyalties. They are accountable to both ecclesiastical and military authorities. A chaplain must be ordained or otherwise endorsed by his or her religious body, but that clergyperson is also commissioned as a military officer. Denominational endorsement and military commissioning "symbolize the chaplain's ongoing accountability to two institutions" (Starling, 1990). Such divided loyalties make it easy for the chaplain to confuse the military's agenda for the church's agenda. Divided loyalties also make it less likely that the chaplain will challenge inhuman aspects of the military culture.

Second, the mere presence of clergy lends the military the impression of divine validation. Clergy serve the symbolic role of representing both the church and, in many minds, God's presence. Thus, by maintaining a constant presence in the Armed Forces — institutions whose reason for being is killing or the threat of killing — chaplains imply divine approval of the military and its objectives.

Third, chaplaincy helps the Armed Forces cultivate better soldiers. When chaplains ease consciences by hearing confessions and call for personal virtues such as temperance, courage, and obedience, they help cultivate better soldiers. That is, they help produce soldiers who do what they are told, function even in fearful situations, keep disruptive habits in check, and perform/kill with clear consciences.

Of course, hospital chaplaincy is not military chaplaincy. The parallel between the two forms of chaplaincy is limited by the fact that hospitals aim at curing, not killing. Still, it seems to me that military chaplaincy provides a historical paradigm which hospital chaplaincy may be following too closely. As with the military chaplain, the hospital chaplain's loyalties are divided. Although he or she is ordained or commissioned by a denominational body, "the chaplain's daily interactions are in the hospital, as well as are the chaplain's accountability to and salary from the hospital" (Holst, 1985, pp. 8, 229). These divided loyalties make it less likely that the chaplain will perceive, let alone confront, issues that conflict with the hospital's social interests or reputation. Unethical behavior, systematic problems, and structural injustice are simply more difficult to recognize when such recognition threatens the institution to which you are accountable and from which comes your pay.

As with the military chaplain, the hospital chaplain's presence lends the perception of divine validation. This perception is acceptable, even warranted, as long as hospitals are caring and just, but the perception of divine validation becomes deeply problematic as our dual infatuation with technology and profit makes hospitals less humane and medical spending turns increasingly unjust.

Parallel to shaping good soldiers, hospital chaplains help us to be good patients by reinforcing traits such as trust, humility, and patience. Such reinforcement is appropriate only so long as hospitals deserve our trust, humility, and patience.

In short, I am ambivalent about the notion of hospital chaplaincy. The hospital is a place for Christian clergy to maintain a presence. Yet I worry that hospital-sponsored presence is unable to challenge wrongs. I further worry that such presence actually validates and helps to sustain an institution that may no longer deserve that support.

Reflecting my ambivalence about hospital chaplaincy, the remainder of this paper proceeds in two sections. The first section focuses on an especially troubling aspect of contemporary hospital chaplaincy: the tendency toward a generic chaplaincy that downplays the chaplain's own particular perspective and denominational allegiance. The second section then argues that, despite reservations, Mennonites should serve as hospital chaplains. Instead of generic service, however, Mennonite chaplains should view their task as analogous to relief and development work and thus as a form of what C. Norman Krause calls "agapeic intervention" (1994).

I. Generic Chaplaincy

Although I suspect that military chaplaincy also tends to be generic, I now leave that comparison to focus on the instances and dangers of that tendency in hospital chaplaincy. Several features incline hospital chaplains to downplay theological convictions and denominational allegiance. Take, for instance, the history of Clinical Pastoral Education (C.P.E.). According to Lawrence Holst, "four major intellectual streams provided the context and impetus for C.P.E in the 1920s and 1930s" — theological liberalism, philosophic pragmatism, psychology, and religious existentialism (1985, p. 16). Holst says that C.P.E. borrowed certain emphases from these streams. From theological liberalism and religious existentialism, C.P.E. garnered antiauthoritarian and individualistic tendencies. From pragmatism, C.P.E. learned to attend more to function than to the content of convictions. And psychology taught C.P.E. to emphasize "the inner dynamic world" of the unconscious (p. 18). C.P.E. is thus historically rooted in several strains of thought that depreciate theological convictions and denominational allegiance.

Another factor feeding the tendency toward a generic chaplaincy derives from the multiple roles hospital chaplains often fill. Many of these roles — such as those of group therapy leaders, alcoholism counselors, marriage therapists, program coordinators, hospital ethicists — do not require pastoral office and draw primarily on non-theological disciplines (Holst, 1985, p. 47). At a minimum, these multiple roles "often may sidetrack their [hospital chaplains'] primary role as spiritual leader" (Phillips, 1993, p. 100; see also Eyer, 1985, pp. 208-209). In addition, chaplains are employees of (often secular) hospitals that serve patients from a variety of denominational and religious backgrounds, many of whom share the broad-based cultural view that treats religion as a supermarket where people have "a vast array of choices of how to meet their many spiritual needs" (Sawatsky, 1995, p. 33).

The combination of these features implicitly, if not explicitly, discourages chaplains from focusing on the content of their own beliefs and encourages a way of interacting with patients that reflects a (supposedly) more neutral, objective, and open-minded stance. This de-emphasizing of one's own particularity is what I call a generic chaplaincy.

To my mind, the biggest problem with a generic, supposedly neutral, hospital chaplaincy is that it isn't neutral at all; rather, a particular perspective is smuggled in and authorized under the guise of something more universal and open-minded. Consider, for example, Don S. Browning's discussion of the case of "Margaret and the Will of God." Browning notes that Margaret and her family held "to a rigid version of reformed Christianity . . . in which all life's fortunes, good or bad, were regarded as the direct will of God." Browning says that these beliefs were not "just idle chatter. Margaret did not comply well with even the simple routines of her everyday care" (1986, p. 69). After all, why should she? If God decides that she will be sick, she will be sick. And if God decides that she should get better, then she will get better.

For our purposes, the response of the chaplain in this case (Chaplain Carr) is noteworthy. Chaplain Carr acknowledged God's potential governance, but challenged Margaret's understanding of that rule by using scriptural arguments to show that God's providence does not mean that God wills particular sicknesses. Instead, argued Carr, God's providence is such that we can strive with it toward health. The chaplain's caring conversation and skillful use of scripture profoundly affected Margaret. Her attitude changed and she started to cooperate with treatment.

While I support Chaplain Carr's interaction with Margaret as a form of loving intervention, Browning's interpretation of that interaction is disturbing. According to Browning,

> Chaplain Carr does not attempt to convert Margaret or make her a better Christian . . . the purpose was not to change Margaret's beliefs to fit more closely his own. The purpose was to detect elements in Margaret's beliefs that were working against the possibility of her becoming well. The value of improved health was the aim of the conversation; conversion, salvation, justification, or sanctification as such were not Chaplain Carr's immediate concerns (1986, p. 70).

Browning thus interprets Chaplain Carr's interaction as a form of generic chaplaincy. Chaplain Carr is not, according to Browning, advancing his own particular beliefs but is advocating for the more objective or neutral value of health.

Browning is wrong to suggest that the chaplain is not trying to change Margaret's beliefs to fit his own. No doubt, Chaplain Carr is advocating for Margaret's health, but that advocacy is intimately tied to his understanding of human agency and divine providence. Chaplain Carr viewed Margaret and her family as having an inadequate understanding of God's providence and therefore helped them, through theological/scriptural discussion, toward a new understanding of providence — an understanding more like the chaplain's own view.

Browning later admits that "Chaplain Carr's own religious views doubtless led him to believe that there were more adequate ways to speak of God's providence . . . than Margaret and her family had received." Yet, according to Browning, this does not mean that the chaplain was trying to move Margaret toward his particular perspective, since "rather than giving Margaret and her family a lecture about his views of the Christian faith, the chaplain helped them grasp a more classic expression of their own Calvinist faith" (p. 71).

Browning fails to appreciate that framing the discussion in terms of Margaret's own Calvinist heritage does not alter the fact that the chaplain is trying to move her toward his viewpoint. If I as a Mennonite pastor argue with my Catholic friends for a pacifist position by appealing to dynamics within Catholic theology and social teachings, I am still trying to make their beliefs more closely fit my own. Such an argument might be merely tactical or it might reflect a healthy respect for the Catholic tradition, but in either case I am trying to move them closer to my particular perspective. So too, Chaplain Carr's appeal to the Calvinist tradition might be merely tactical or more respectful, but either way the chaplain's own beliefs are being advanced.

Given that I approve of Chaplain Carr's intervention, my argument with Browning's description of that intervention might seem unimportant. But I believe that Browning's description is deceptive and dangerous. Browning's description hides the chaplain's own beliefs and agenda under the lofty goal of "health." Concealing the chaplain's goal from both chaplain and patient alike, Browning's account makes it more likely that the chaplain will advance his or her convictions with the authority and impunity accorded such a noble idea as health. Thus, chaplains who accept that description are more likely to violate (unintentionally) the patient's trust than are chaplains who forthrightly admit their convictions and denominational allegiance.

If this danger seems overstated, consider what happens when the issue is abortion and we accept Browning's description of the chaplain's neutral adherence to the priority of health. Kent Richmond's account of his encounter with a young Roman Catholic woman contemplating abortion is instructive here. Richmond depicts a woman who

> faced the dilemma of giving birth to a seriously deformed infant. Amid great soul searching, she elected to terminate the pregnancy. A strong Roman Catholic, her upbringing had taught her that, apart from its being done to save her own life, abortion was morally wrong in all cases. Now, on the eve of the termination, she tearfully talked with me about her decision and the despair and guilt that filled that decision with pain (1992, p. 57).

Richmond uses this case to open a discussion of abortion and does not tell us what the woman finally decides. Richmond's own participation in the case is potentially disturbing, however. Noting that the woman is a strong Roman Catholic, Richmond never acknowledges that his being a United Methodist minister was equally significant to this encounter. Indeed, Richmond never directly acknowledges that he is United Methodist. We must infer Richmond's denominational commitment from a much later comment where he observes, citing *The Book of Discipline of the United Methodist Church,* that his "own faith tradition" permits abortion "only after thoughtful and careful consideration by the parties involved, with medical, pastoral, and other appropriate counsel" (1992, p. 60).

Richmond's failure to acknowledge his tradition may suggest that he accepts a generic description of his role as chaplain. He may, like Browning, assume that his task concerns health, not his personal convictions. Yet, Richmond is probably more accepting of abortion than is the woman's Roman Catholic tradition. We see this probability both in the quotation from *The Book of Discipline* and in his own description of what is a "moderate" approach to abortion (1992, p. 60). The problem then becomes this: Richmond's failure to acknowledge explicitly his denominational commitments makes it more likely that his tradition's greater openness to abortion will enter the conversation under the guise of a neutral concern for the woman's health — a concern that is, after all, fundamental to many pro-choice arguments.

In Richmond's case, perhaps he could find a Catholic priest to talk with the young woman. If that solution is impractical or inappropriate, he could gently, but firmly and repeatedly, remind himself and the young woman that he does not share her tradition's convictions on this matter and suggest that she evaluate his comments accordingly. Such an approach is far more honest and far less dangerous than implying that a chaplain has no agenda other than health. Perhaps Richmond offered these kinds of qualifying remarks to the young woman, but his account of the encounter leaves one wondering.

Additional illustrations of a tendency toward a generic chaplaincy are found in two sets of guidelines distributed by the Bioethics Committee of the College of Chaplains: *Guidelines for the Chaplain's Role in Bioethics* (1992) and *The Chaplain's Role in Bioethics Consultation* (1993). We see an inclination toward a generic chaplaincy when, for instance, the latter document implies that chaplains should be exponents of everyone's position except their own. The 1993 guidelines say that "the chaplain respects and advocates for the expression of views and values of bioethics committee members as it pertains to the ethical discussion of matters brought before the committee." The chaplain also "serves *as an advocate* for the spiritual values and religious beliefs held by the patient even when those values and beliefs *are not those of the chaplain*" (1993, p. 3, emphasis added). The guidelines combine these assertions about advancing the views of others with solely negative comments about the chaplain's own convictions. Chaplains are told to refrain from "making comments that reflect rigid personal or value biases that may be disruptive to the committee's deliberations." We are similarly told that chaplains risk disrupting committee deliberations when their own "rigid biases, based on personal theological perspectives, *are raised*" (p. 3, emphasis added) or the clergy-person attempts "to force . . . [his or her] own doctrinal belief system *into the dynamics of the process*" (p. 1, emphasis added). The cumulative effect of these comments is overwhelming. Chaplains are said to advance viewpoints with which they disagree, and their own convictions are only referred to as "rigid biases" which they are not even to raise or insert into the deliberative process.[1] The desire to be open-minded, fair, and non-particular thus results in a document that makes chaplains advocates of all positions except their own.

We see a similar tendency toward a generic chaplaincy in the emphasis on general bioethical principles, an emphasis especially visible in the 1992 guidelines. The guidelines expect chaplains both to "have basic training in bioethical principles" and to "teach bioethical principles." Similarly, the committee on which the chaplain serves is to "clarify various ethical options through reflective discussion in the context of bioethical principles" (1992, p. 2).[2] Chaplains surely need to know the language of bioethics. But in context, this emphasis on bioethical principles reflects the push toward a generic chaplaincy. The guidelines do not envision chaplains as representing the theological wealth and moral wisdom of specific religious traditions. They instead see chaplains as promoters of general principles assumed accessible and compelling to all. I challenge this assumption below, but it is sufficient now to note that instead of valuing chaplains as

1. Although not as developed, the 1992 *Guidelines for the Chaplain's Role in Bioethics* shows similar tendencies. For example, "chaplains have the responsibility to be advocates for the particular spiritual values of the patient, family and also staff" (p. 3).

2. A similar emphasis on bioethical principles is apparent in the 1993 guidelines where theoretical constructs of beneficence, autonomy, etc. are advanced as more reliable for ethical decision-making than the values which one inherits from culture and upbringing. See *The Chaplain's Role in Bioethics Consultation,* p. 2. A corresponding emphasis on principles is seen in Hinrichs and Nelson (1985).

gateways to particular viewpoints, the guidelines instruct them to use and teach the principles that (presumably) render appeal to those distinct viewpoints secondary, if not altogether unnecessary.

These two bioethical guidelines thus exhibit the tendency toward a generic chaplaincy — a chaplaincy that advances all positions as equal, withholds personal convictions, and teaches general principles. As argued above, such a generic stance includes the potential to smuggle in personal convictions under the guise of something more neutral. Vulnerability to this danger is seen in the 1992 guideline's claim that "Chaplains serve as resource persons concerning the spiritual dimensions of illness and health, both to community clergy and to the bioethics committee — even when patients or their families have no apparent religious affiliation" (p. 1).

The problem, of course, is that there are no general or neutral understandings of "the spiritual dimensions of illness and health" — a fact that the guidelines fail to acknowledge. A particular view of illness and health must be represented. Some understand or experience illness as divine punishment or as proof of God's absence or nonexistence. Others dutifully accept sickness as predetermined. Still others regard illness as an evil that stands against God's will and thus as something to be battled. Many see in illness an occasion for personal growth in virtues such as patience and hope or as an occasion to deepen their walk with God. And still others will regard illness in other ways. So, when the chaplain serves as a resource person "concerning the spiritual dimensions of illness," whose view of illness is represented? More specifically, whose view is expressed when the patient has "no apparent religious affiliation?" One possibility is that the chaplain's own theology of illness will surface here. This possibility is unproblematic if the chaplain acknowledges those convictions as his or her own. The guidelines' push toward a generic chaplaincy and the consequent devaluing of particularity makes such honesty less likely, however.

Another, potentially more insidious, danger of generic chaplaincy is that the chaplain merely becomes a mouthpiece for the broadly accepted, but no less historically particular, views of our culture. This is a version of the problem I have been discussing: a particular perspective is smuggled in and authorized under the guise of something more universal and open-minded. The difference is that instead of the chaplain's own theological tradition exercising covert influence, the influence derives from our culture's largely relativistic emphasis on the individual. This danger is evident in two, already discussed, facets of the bioethics guidelines: chaplains as advocates for the views of others and as proponents of bioethical principles.

The guidelines' emphasis on serving as advocate for the diverse views of individual patients is a reflection of our culture's value system. Most eras and most cultures would not see such advocacy as vital or even justified. When, for example, authority rests with the community or is vested in the priest, medicine man, or doctor, there is little need to consult (let alone advocate for) the individual's particular divergent views. Indeed, such advocacy is recent even in our culture's practice of medicine, which used to place virtually unquestioned confidence in the physician's benevolent authority. Thus, when chaplains accept advocacy as central to their role, they advance a distinct value system — specifically, our culture's focus on the individual.

I, too, support taking individuals seriously. Various Mennonite convictions — such as freedom of conscience and nonviolence — require fully listening to the individual and his or her commitments. Still, we should be aware that the bioethics guidelines' view of chaplaincy advances a particular set of moral convictions. Moreover, the guidelines reflect a set of convictions that go further than merely respecting individual conscience: they reflect our culture's obsessive, ostensibly relativistic, focus on the individual.

Consider, for example, the 1993 guidelines' claim that chaplains are to "serve as an advocate" for the patient's beliefs, no matter the chaplain's own convictions. The guidelines never acknowledge, let alone wrestle with, the possibility that the patient might be wrong. I would firmly support asking chaplains to be agents of communication, helping all parties genuinely understand each other. But instead of agents of communication, the 1993 guidelines make chaplains advocates of the patient's convictions, no matter their merit. The 1993 guidelines thus reflect our culture's essentially relativistic focus on the individual where few norms exist other than the inviolability of the individual's convictions.

The potential outcome of a generic chaplaincy is more troubling to me than the consequences of Browning's view. I worry that Browning's description permits the chaplain's own theological tradition to exercise a kind of covert influence. But at least Browning's view allows the chaplain in certain circumstances to question, even challenge, patient convictions that the chaplain believes to be errant. It is unlikely, however, that the 1993 guidelines' individualistic focus allows for the kind of engagement seen with Chaplain Carr. Browning's description may enable chaplains to smuggle in their convictions. But such smuggling is preferable, it seems to me, to the 1993 guidelines' hidden importation of our culture's relativistic individualism.

I also worry about what happens to chaplains who follow the 1993 bioethics guidelines. What kind of people do they become? What happens to the character and convictions of someone who continually serves as an advocate of various positions regardless of whether he or she holds them? Such a practice will likely undermine virtues such as integrity and courage. Such advocacy subverts the strong sense of self necessary to the honesty and consistency of convictions exhibited by a person of integrity. Similarly, the practice of continually advancing one position and then another hardly trains the chaplain to hold courageously to his or her faith when facing opposition or ridicule or apathy. It also seems to me that chaplains following these guidelines will likely acquire characters more befitting lawyers (i.e., advocates) than clergy.

Turning our attention to the 1992 guidelines' emphasis on bioethical principles does not improve matters. The standard medical ethics principles — autonomy, nonmaleficence, beneficence, justice — are not universally available, general principles, equally compelling to all. Rather, they are the norms of a particular group (primarily later 20th-century, liberal, white North American males) that gained hegemony in medical circles. Consider, for instance, that the principle of autonomy, which fits American culture, is not well-suited to the moral vision of the Amish or Mennonites or various monastic communities or Orthodox Moslems. In these contexts, social connections and duties often carry greater moral weight than individual autonomy.

We can see the ultimately provincial nature of the principles from many directions. For instance, many Christian traditions would view beneficence — the positive duty to help others further their interests if this can be done without extensive risk or inconvenience to oneself — as an inadequate substitute for Christian notions about self-sacrifice. Similarly, as Sondra Wheeler notes, while "Christian convictions provide a foundation for a strong obligation not to harm . . . Christian moral thought does not always share common medical ethical assessments of what count as harms, or how they are to be compared to one another" (1996, p. 52). Medicine treats death as the ultimate harm and concentrates on avoiding physical, and perhaps psychological, harms. Christian convictions are at least equally concerned with moral and spiritual harms, viewing "not death but final separation from God [as] . . . the evil to be avoided at all costs" (p. 53). Also absent from the principles are matters such as the place of prayer in moral discernment, an account of divine providence, the role of the virtues, the way that deep emotions enlighten (not merely hinder) decision-making, casuistry as a tool of prudential reasoning, and so on (see, for example, DuBose *et al.*, 1994).

The point is that bioethical principles provide a particular framework for working on medical ethical issues. Yet, without acknowledging the principles' particularity or encouraging chaplains to evaluate those principles from their respective theological traditions, the guidelines insist that chaplains use and promote bioethical principles. The result is that under the pretext of something more universal and open-minded, chaplains become the mouthpiece for a distinct value system often at odds with specific Christian convictions.

In short, the problem with a generic chaplaincy is that a particular perspective is smuggled in and authorized under the guise of something more universal and open-minded: either the chaplain's own convictions and tradition sneak in or, even worse, the chaplain becomes the uncritical representative for other contemporary moral influences.

II. Agapeic Intervention

Despite the above reservations, I want to argue that Mennonites should serve as hospital chaplains. There is, I will contend, abundant biblical warrant and historical precedent for being present in the hospital. However, due to concerns about generic chaplaincy, I will propose "agapeic intervention" as a model to guide that presence.

Eighteen years ago, Erland Waltner — now Professor and President Emeritus at Associated Mennonite Biblical Seminary — reviewed the biblical and historical foundations for Mennonites serving as hospital chaplains (1980). As far as I can tell, that presentation is the first and only sustained theological justification for Mennonite participation in hospital chaplaincy. In that presentation, Dr. Waltner argues that "the widest and deepest ground for hospital chaplaincy ministries" rests in God's concern for our salvation — a concern that includes wholeness and health. Indeed, the concern for human health and wholeness is suggested by the Hebrew term *shalem* (healthy, whole), a cognate of the central biblical term *shalom* (peace) (p. 3).

Waltner also observes Jesus' involvement in ministry to the sick. The Gospels report more than two dozen individual healings and almost a dozen more references to many being healed. Those stories make no sharp distinction between physical and spiritual healing. Thus, for example, the story of the paralytic whose friends lower him through the roof brings together physical and spiritual healing. Recognizing their faith-filled concern for their friend, Jesus offers a word of forgiveness and then physical healing (Mark 2:1-12). As Waltner notes, the Gospels so interconnect physical and spiritual restoration "that Jesus' word, 'Your faith has saved you' can also be rendered 'Your faith has made you well' (Luke 7:50; 8:48)" (p. 4).

Both the interconnection between physical and spiritual restoration and the understanding of salvation as including physical well-being are apparent when Jesus identifies his healing ministry as a sign of the kingdom of God (Luke 11:20). They are similarly evident when John the Baptist asks through his disciples whether Jesus is the Messiah. Jesus answers by pointing primarily to his ministry of physical healing (Luke 7:22-23). The text immediately goes on, however, to describe John, and his baptism of repentance, as a forerunner to Jesus (vs. 24-30). The text then designates Jesus "a friend of tax collectors and sinners" (v. 34) (p. 31). Thus, the text includes elements of physical healing, repentance, forgiveness, and fellowship.

The New Testament makes clear that Jesus' disciples are to continue his ministry to the sick. Jesus commissions his disciples to heal the sick (Luke 9:2, 6; 10:9), and ministry to those who are ill is visible throughout the New Testament — such as when Peter and John heal the "lame man" (Acts 3:1-10) or Paul lists gifts of healing as *charismata* of the Spirit (1 Cor. 12:10, 28). Such healing involves more than mere physical improvement, as is evident, for instance, when James 5:16 "calls for the use of confession, prayer, and oil (medicine?)." The kind of ministry that disciples are to undertake is even prefigured in the power of Jesus' name, which Acts associates with proclamation (4:18; 5:40; 9:27), baptism and forgiveness (2:38; 10:48), and physical healing (3:6; 16:18).[3]

As Waltner's comments intimate, even a cursory examination of Scripture underscores the importance of standing with those who are sick. However, in my judgement, Waltner's scriptural overview omits a key text: the judgment scene where the Son of Man separates people "as a shepherd separates the sheep from the goats" (Matt. 25:32, NRSV). This scene virtually lists hospital chaplains as among those welcomed into the kingdom of God. Invited into the kingdom are those who take care of and visit the sick (vs. 36, 39). Similarly commended are those engaged in activities related or analogous to hospital chaplaincy, such as welcoming the stranger and visiting the prisoner (vs. 35-36, 38-39).

This text combined with Waltner's comments indicates ample scriptural warrant for hospital chaplaincy. Hospital ministry can be an extension of Jesus' own ministry to the sick. According to Scripture, such a ministry values physical healing; it also visits with and tends to those who are sick. Such ministry will attend to matters of faith, listen to confession, offer prayer and anointing, welcome those who feel turned into strangers or prisoners by their illnesses, and so on.

Beyond the scriptural witness, Waltner sees "striking precursors" of some chaplaincy ministry in Mennonite history. For example, he discusses two letters written by Menno Simons that foreshadow a kind of chaplaincy: the letter of Consolation to a Sick Saint (1557) and the Pastoral Letter to the Amsterdam Church (Nov. 14, 1558).

In the former letter, Menno writes a married woman believed to be his sister-in-law. Much of the letter "seeks to reassure her that while she seems to have added the burden of a guilty conscience to the burden of her illness, it is not appropriate for her to do so. If there has been sin in her life, she is to remember that all are sinners, and that in any case the forgiveness of God is assured 'by the perfect righteousness, atonement and intercession of Christ'" (1980, pp. 5-6). Menno also frankly acknowledges the seriousness of her illness and calls for her to accept suffering as a reality and as a potential asset to those of faith. The letter then moves toward having her accept in faith whatever lies ahead, whether life or death. Menno wrote the second letter during a major pestilence in the city of Amsterdam. He writes to urge members "not to stop visiting each other during this time of danger, but to look at the presence and prospect of death calmly . . . 'For your whole life and death is lodged in the hands of the Lord'" (p. 7). Although hardly qualifying as hospital chaplaincy, these letters from Menno exhibit rich pastoral care of those who are sick and those seriously affected by the illness of others.

3. I owe this insight to a comment by Dr. Mary Jo Iozzio on an earlier draft of this paper.

Waltner also sees precursors to hospital chaplaincy in various Mennonite confessions of faith. Particularly striking is the Dordrecht confession of 1632. Article IX of the confession concerns church offices. Among those offices are ordained deacons and deaconesses whose role includes visiting the feeble, sick, and grieving (p. 7).[4]

Waltner mentions in passing another precursor to a Mennonite chaplaincy that I believe deserves greater attention than he affords it: the Civilian Public Service (CPS) ministries in mental hospitals (1942-1946) (p. 11). During World War II, the United States provided an unpaid alternative to military service for conscientious objectors. Most of these CPS men came from the historic peace churches — Mennonite, Brethren, and Quaker — and many (more than 3000) were assigned to work in mental hospitals (usually as attendants). The physical and hygienic state of these hospitals was deplorable. The patients were often kept in conditions little better than concentration camps. In time, however, the CPS men began to influence the character of these hospitals. This influence came from several directions: (1) They worked hard and displayed genuine care for the patients. (2) CPS men provided evidence for the media to expose the dreadful conditions. (3) They formed the Mental Hygiene Program, which became the National Mental Health Foundation, to help better prepare them for their hospital work and to take steps toward long-range reform.[5]

The CPS case is relevant to our discussion in several ways. To start, the event of placing conscientious objectors to serve in hospitals reminds us that standing with those who suffer in such institutions is itself valuable as an expression of God's mercy. The CPS workers embodied a level of personal, concrete concern for the patients that was not part of those patients' ordinary experience. Such embodiment is surely one way in which God's own concern is expressed to and experienced by those who suffer.

The CPS case also shows that such presence can, over time, influence the shape of care in hospitals. Although the changes were often gradual, CPS helped to transform mental hospitals into more humane and caring institutions.

The CPS experience further suggests that one can be lovingly, respectfully present in a secular hospital without downplaying one's particular faith commitments and denominational allegiance. Even if they had wanted to, CPS workers could not hide their distinctive convictions. They were, after all, serving in those hospitals because they held minority views about Christian participation in warfare. The CPS case demonstrates, however, that being explicit about one's faith commitment need not jeopar-

4. Similar to the Dordrecht language, the deaconess movement was introduced into General Conference Mennonite Church in 1890. This movement's attention to physical and spiritual care was especially directed toward the sick.

5. For a brief description of CPS's impact on mental hospitals, see Elmer M. Ediger, 'Roots' (1983, pp. 21-25).

dize one's relationship with patients or necessitate heavy-handed proselytizing.

CPS, the Dordrecht confession, and the letters of Menno Simons illustrate the types of precedent to be found within Mennonite history for hospital chaplaincy. When we combine this precedent with the biblical call to minister to the sick, the appropriateness, even necessity, of Mennonites serving as hospital chaplains is evident.

Such chaplaincy should not be generic, however. My concerns about a generic chaplaincy might be overruled were there no other way to be present. But Scripture's mingling of faith and healing, Menno's explicitly theological language in his pastoral care, and (especially) the CPS experience point to a non-generic way of being present to the infirm.

I suggest that this non-generic hospital presence is appropriately described as "agapeic intervention." C. Norman Krause, a theologian and missionary, uses this phrase to depict the work of the Mennonite Central Committee (MCC) — the relief and development arm of the Mennonite Church. I believe that this apt depiction of MCC's activity also provides a fitting description of a respectful but non-generic hospital chaplaincy.

MCC is present with the poor and suffering of the world. But that presence is not neutral. Instead, argues Krause, MCC

> is an institution for agapeic intervention in situations of need. It does not send service workers into the various parts of the world merely to be respectfully and sympathetically present, but to be *catalytic* and *dialogical* change agents. This is fundamentally implicit in its explicit Christian identity as a part of the God-Movement (Kingdom) inaugurated by Jesus Christ (Krause, 1994, p. 3).

The idea of catalytic and dialogical change requires unpacking. Krause loosely draws on chemical catalysis to provide a metaphor for thinking about agents of social change. Krause describes "a social catalyst as a change agent that induces desired modifications in the host culture which are integral and intrinsic to its well-being." The language of catalyst implies, however, that while the changes are desirable, certain inhibiting elements prevent change from taking place. Thus, the social catalyst "attempts to work respectfully and unobtrusively to induce changes that will enhance the host culture" (1994, p. 3).

The second term, "dialogical," refers to the method of social change, to the way of being a catalyst. Dialogue seeks mutual understanding, and, at its heart, says Krause, involves an open and respectful relationship. It is a relationship in which the partners engage in courteous "but frank and sincere . . . communication in order to establish voluntary human community on its highest possible moral and spiritual level" (1994, p. 4). This genuine, community-seeking dialogue requires several factors.

> First, the dialogical partners must have clear self-identities. It is extremely difficult to dialogue with a "nobody." Second, they must be willing to sincerely identify with the partner and listen to her/him. Such identification does not mean uncritical agreement. Rather, it means an empathetic willingness to put oneself in the other's place and see from their perspective.
>
> And third, dialogical partners must be willing to share frankly and intelligently from their own experience. Remember, the goal of catalytic dialogue is not to find the lowest common denominator, but to generate change toward the highest common denominator (1994, p. 4).

In short, "catalytic" change directed at well-being through "dialogical" presence is what Krause means by agapeic intervention. Still missing from my summary of Krause's notion, however, is the phrase's thoroughly Christian overtone. Krause is, after all, trying to depict a Christian agency that explicitly seeks to be present with people "in the name of Christ." Hence, Krause observes that

> When I used the word agape I am referring to a specifically Christian concept which was embodied in the life and ministry of Jesus Christ. When I say that we are interventionist, I am simply identifying MCC as an institution representing the continuing mission of God begun in Christ's incarnational ministry. Jesus Christ is God's intervention into the human scene, and the church through the presence and empowerment of the Spirit of Christ continues that intervention ministry (1994, p. 8).

Agapeic intervention is an unapologetically Christian notion. Consciously dependent on the Spirit, it seeks to continue God's loving intervention through Christ.

Although Krause does not discuss the virtues, agapeic intervention clearly requires virtuous practitioners. The dialogical presence aimed at change that Krause describes requires a host of virtues. For example, genuine listening requires the humility to believe that the other person has something valuable to say, the patience to hear them out fully, and the empathy to sense how things look and feel from the other's perspective. But, since dialogue is more than listening, the virtues of honesty and courage are also needed. Real dialogue requires an honest evaluation of the other's position and an equally honest expression of one's own position. Real dialogue similarly requires the courage to remain steadfast to one's convictions or tradition even when they are unpopular or represent a minority perspective, but it also requires the courage to change long-held positions when such change is warranted. In addition, because agapeic intervention aims at more than dialogue for dialogue's sake, the virtue of hope is essential. Agapeic intervention clings to the hope that dialogical presence can move the conversation partners closer to the truth and can transform the situation toward the Kingdom of God.

Agapeic intervention also has a complex relationship to self-identity. Genuine dialogue requires clear self-identities. I cannot engage in real dialogue unless I know who I am. Yet, it is equally true that self-identity emerges or is strengthened in such conversation. Conversation with non-Christians and Christians of other traditions helps to crystallize my Mennonite identity, for instance. I become clearer about my tradition as I learn to explain it to others. I also discover in conversation with non-Mennonites what is distinctive, or not so distinctive, about Mennonites, and I learn which features of my tradition I appreciate and which features I wish were otherwise. Dialogue thus both presupposes and enhances self-identity.

To summarize, agapeic intervention is an explicitly Christian, Spirit-dependent, notion of "catalytic" change directed toward God's Kingdom through "dialogical" presence. Such presence requires people of virtue. It also depends on and strengthens self-identity.

I suggest that this description of MCC as an institution of agapeic intervention provides a fitting model for a loving, non-coercive, but non-generic hospital chaplaincy. Like Browning's description of Chaplain Carr, this model recognizes the need for intervention and change to promote genuine well-being. Yet unlike Browning's description, agapeic intervention requires clear self-identities and a willingness to share frankly and intelligently from one's own perspective. Like the College of Chaplains bioethics guidelines, this model requires fully listening to and respecting the other. Yet unlike those guidelines, agapeic intervention does not automatically capitulate to the other's point of view or serve as a mouthpiece for our culture's obsessive individualism.

This notion of agapeic intervention is not too idealistic and impractical. Events such as CPS (mid-1940s) and institutions like MCC (since 1920) model a way of being present that is loving and non-coercive without being generic. However imperfectly, they model agapeic intervention. Other Christian traditions have similar or related experiences and institutions that offer corresponding models. Following such models will, I believe, prove more faithful and less prone to violating trust than a generic chaplaincy.

It is, however, an open question whether most secular hospitals will want to employ non-generic chaplains. I hope so. If not, perhaps we need to rethink how chaplains are paid and placed. Such rethinking would encourage a non-generic chaplaincy; it might also address the problem of divided loyalties with which we began this paper.

Works Cited

Bioethics Committee of the College of Chaplains, Inc. (1992). *Guidelines for the Chaplain's Role in Bioethics,* American Protestant Hospital Association, Schaumburg, IL.

Bioethics Committee of the College of Chaplains, Inc. (1993). *The Chaplain's Role in Bioethics Consultation,* American Protestant Hospital Association, Schaumburg, IL.

Browning, D. S. (1986). 'Hospital chaplaincy as public ministry,' *Second Opinion* 1 (1) (March), 69.

Cross, F. L. (ed.) (1997). 'Chaplain,' *The Oxford Dictionary of the Christian Church,* Oxford University Press, New York.

DuBose, E. R., Hamel, R., and O'Connell, L. J. (eds.) (1994). *A Matter of Principles: Ferment in U.S. Bioethics,* Trinity Press International, Valley Forge.

Ediger, E. M. (1983). 'Roots,' in *If We Can Love: The Mennonite Mental Health Story,* V. H. Neufeld (ed.), Faith and Life Press, Newton.

Eliade, M. (ed.) (1995). *Encyclopedia of Religion,* Macmillan Publishing Co., New York.

Eyer, R. (1985). 'Clergy's role on medical ethics committees,' *The Journal of Pastoral Care* 39/3 (September), 208-209.

Hinrichs, S. W. and Nelson, W. (1985). 'Biomedical ethics and clinical pastoral education,' *The Journal of Pastoral Care* 39/3 (September), 201-203.

Holst, L. (ed.) (1985). *Hospital Ministry: The Role of the Chaplain Today,* Crossroad, New York.

Javitt, S. M. (1998). 'Hospital,' in *Collier's Encyclopedia* (Electronic Edition), Collier, New York.

Krause, C. N. (1994). 'A theological basis for intervention ministries,' MCC Occasional Paper, No. 20 (May) (available from Mennonite Central Committee, 21 South 12th Street, P.O. Box 500, Akron, PA 17501).

Phillips, D. F. (1993). 'Pastoral care: Finding a niche in ethical decision making,' *Cambridge Quarterly of Healthcare Ethics* 2, 100.

Richmond, K. D. and Middleton, D. L. (1992). *The Pastor and the Patient: A Practical Guide for Hospital Visitation,* Abingdon Press, Nashville.

Sawatsky, E. (1995). 'Helping dreams come true: Toward wholeness — Articulating the vision,' in *Understanding Ministerial Leadership,* J. Esau (ed.)., Institute of Mennonite Studies, Elkhart.

Smith, K. W. (1990). 'Chaplain/Chaplaincy,' in *Dictionary of Pastoral Care and Counseling,* R. Hunter (ed.), Abingdon Press, Nashville.

Starling, I. C., Jr. (1990). 'Military service and military chaplaincy,' *Dictionary of Pastoral Care and Counseling,* R. Hunter (ed.), Abingdon Press, Nashville.

Waltner, E. (1980). 'Toward an anabaptist theology of chaplaincy in health care institutions,' paper presented at the Mennonite Health Assembly, St. Louis, MO., March 11 (Available from the Associated Mennonite Biblical Seminary Library, 3003 Benham Avenue Elkhart, IN 46517).

Wheeler, S. E. (1996). *Stewards of Life: Bioethics and Pastoral Care,* Abingdon Press, Nashville.

35 Spiritual Morphine: The Delusory Hope of Dying on Your Own Terms

Kristina Robb Dover

The doctors had said she had little more than six months to live. Since then, the cancer had aggressively metastasized, but not enough to destroy her insatiable will to live. Esther, 72, talked confidently about God's power to heal both the pain and the cancer.

When I asked her where she drew her inspiration from, she cited the teachings of Joel Osteen and his mother, Dodie Osteen, who, in a little book titled *Healed from Cancer,* attributed her own miraculous recovery to a strict, daily regimen of reciting particular "healing" verses from Scripture. Invoking God's Word "against the devil" in the guise of aches and pains took its place next to a special diet of pureed fruits and vegetables and occasional rounds of chemotherapy.

I decided that I would check out the Osteens' teachings for myself. What I found was an innocuous, pain-free form of faith with a quid pro quo for its adherents. "Claim God's Word in your thoughts and speech, and you will be healed, because God's will for you is to be healthy and happy" is a good summary.

With the exception of a few scarce references to Jesus Christ, Joel Osteen's *Your Best Life Now* reads more like a secular self-help manual than a Christian work. It offers "seven simple, yet profound, steps to improve your life": "enlarge your vision; develop a healthy self-image; discover the power of your thoughts and words; let go of the past; find strength through adversity; live to give; and choose to be happy." Nothing about pain, or dying, or death, about lives that can't be "improved" but have to be endured.

Pain-Killing Care

Osteen's teachings reflect one incarnation of a gospel touted for its painkilling properties. But Esther's enthusiastic conversion to the Osteens' teaching points to a larger phenomenon of religion as pain relief that both intrigues and disturbs me: its role in care for the dying.

As a hospice chaplain, in weekly meetings convened to discuss patients' care, I took my seat next to doctors, nurses, and social workers, all of whom had made it their single, greatest aim to relieve the pain of terminally ill clients. This place at the table for religious faith deserves celebration: first, because it signifies a growing appreciation for the spiritual dimensions of health and, in turn, significant advances in understanding how to care for whole persons; and second, because it may be an example of how science and religion are learning to converse with one another in a shared language.

Yet the highest, governing value presumed in these meetings was the necessity of freeing the patient from pain, physical, emotional, or spiritual. It is this presumption that gives cause for concern. In my experience as a hospice chaplain — and I know that others may have a very different and more extensive experience — this value has become an implicit, guiding principle that directs chaplains in their ministry of "pain relief."

Some will dispute this interpretation. They argue that hospice is less about pain relief and more about patient autonomy, but I am not so sure these are two different things. If the customer is "always right" (as he usually is in the privatized hospice setting with which I am most familiar), the overriding goal of palliative care is to keep the customer as comfortable as possible. Eliminating sources of pain and discomfort is the most obvious way to do so.

If I am right about this principle, I think it relies on two unspoken, common assumptions.

Redemptive Death

The first is that the terminally ill patient is always right. Because he is on the threshold of death, he is presumed to enjoy greater access to virtue and judgment than is attainable by those who dwell in the land of the living. He attains a kind of sanctified status.

This attitude of reverence towards the dying is one that the journalist Ron Rosenbaum describes as "an increasingly cultlike exaltation, sentimentalization and even worship." He attributes its prominence at least in part to the work of Elisabeth Kübler-Ross. Her books have become the standard texts for the dying and those who care for them — as I discovered, having received many "recommended reading" lists during chaplain residencies at two separate sites.

It may be true that while pain relief is a large part of hospice care, it is not an end in itself, but a means of helping patients resolve various emotional and spiritual end-of-life conflicts. Even so, the use of palliative medicine as a way to encourage the pursuit of emotional and spiritual wholeness is still about helping the patient achieve his best death on his own terms.

The measure by which the success of this endeavor is evaluated is the degree to which the patient expresses pain, physical, emotional, or spiritual. The standard for

"Spiritual Morphine: The Delusory Hope of Dying on Your Own Terms" originally appeared in the January/February 2008 issue of *Touchstone: A Journal of Mere Christianity* magazine, www.touchstonemag.com.

success, in other words, is whether the patient "feels good" physically, emotionally, and spiritually.

The second assumption is that death, embodying a "natural" transition to a carefree afterlife, is a good in itself. After reportedly studying some 20,000 cases of "near-death experiences," Kübler-Ross concludes that life after death is universally a "glorious experience" and a "pleasant reunion" of sorts: "There will be a total absence of panic, fear, or anxiety"; "you will be very beautiful, much more beautiful than you see yourself now"; and you "will always experience a physical wholeness."

Everyone experiences this happy transition to a blissful new way of being. "Even the angriest and most difficult patients, very shortly before death, begin to deeply relax, have a sense of serenity around them, and begin to be pain free in spite of, perhaps, a cancer-ridden body full of metastases."

Given this reassuring paradigm, it is no exaggeration to suggest that death attains an almost divine status for its ability to redeem human beings from the sufferings of life.

To commemorate the life of a patient known by his children as a delinquent father and by the medical staff as an ornery old man, the chaplain presiding at his memorial service played, in celebratory fashion, the Frank Sinatra hit, "I Did It My Way." Tears were wept in reverence for a man who lived and died "his" way, even though it may have been a wrong and destructive way.

The suggestion? That through death, an otherwise less-than-exemplary and miserable person had become a kind of sage whose way of life called for emulation from his students, and that dying would be as triumphant and carefree for this man as living *his* way had been.

Disturbing Implications

For the chaplain who is a "mere Christian," this underlying principle of pain relief contains some disturbing theological implications.

The first is that God is a God of grace only, not of judgment, with the implication that an orthodox Christian understanding of human sin and our need for divine pardon is outmoded and inadmissible. Guilt, regret, or a conviction of divine wrath only fosters unnecessary discomfort, and must therefore be eliminated.

Where this belief plays out practically at the bedside of the dying patient is in the prescribed omission of prayers of confession and petitions for God's forgiveness: Unless the patient makes a specific request, the chaplain is forbidden to suggest it, even if the patient is a Christian. Unless a patient clearly professes a particular faith — the chaplain's job is to summon a Catholic priest to perform last rites for Catholics, for example — such religious practices are in fact discouraged.

In this context, the "meaning" that a patient derived from hosting cocktail parties or playing golf is as significant for patient and chaplain as are expressions of his relationship with God. (After all, as the commonly occurring assumptions go, the patient is always right, and death for all is nothing but a sublime passage to a better place.) "Spirituality" in turn is reduced to little more than a list of personal preferences and hobbies.

When I met him in the months before he died, Mr. Z. was a self-described "backslidden" Christian. He had made a lot of mistakes in his life, and was notorious in his last days as the angry old man who had it in for the hospital staff. Even his daughter spoke with ambivalence and regret about the way her father had lived his life.

In the moments before he died, moments preceded by desperate cries for a quick end to his life, I was at his bedside, and in a final prayer that included thanksgiving for his life, I asked God to "forgive the things" he had "done and left undone." Afterwards, I noted (among the "spiritual" interventions that chaplains are required to chart for each patient) that I had "prayed for the patient's forgiveness."

After reading my notes, a fellow chaplain and supervisor zealously interrogated me about why I had felt it necessary to pray for forgiveness for Mr. Z. Unless Mr. Z. had vocalized in his dying moments that he *wanted* forgiveness — which would have been nearly impossible in those last minutes of fleeting consciousness — I was not to pray such a prayer. "You need to set your theology aside in interactions with patients," I was told.

Such a reprimand leads us to the second disturbing implication of this principle of palliative care: The chaplain must leave his "theology" at the door before entering a patient's room. The chaplain's primary purpose is to embrace the *patient's* definitions of truth and salvation, whatever they might be, with the goal of helping him feel affirmed and, in turn, pain-free and comfortable.

One colleague confidently declared that "no Evangelical Christian would ever be hired for a chaplaincy position, because an Evangelical is not capable of leaving his views out of patient interactions." The presumption here that a chaplain can indeed set aside the system of beliefs that has shaped his life fails to recognize the inextricable link between theology and practice — namely, that the practice of "leaving one's beliefs at the door" is in fact a manifestation of a particular theology.

Jesus' Pain

In a great stroke of irony, then, the principle of freeing the patient from pain offers a version of Christianity that, while vastly different in content, shares the same fundamental motivation to relieve pain and promote happiness that drives Osteenism. While Osteen would have us eliminate pain with the mantra, "Your best life now," proponents of the hospice culture seek to conquer it with the advertisement, "Your best death now."

But is "feel-good faith" really in keeping with the church's charter story? There I read of a life of pain and discomfort for the man named Jesus and his band of followers. From his birth in a filthy stable, to the scorn of his hometown and the rejection of his own people, to his grisly death on a cross, Jesus chose a life full of pain and discomfort.

His disciples did the same, rejecting easier ways to embrace the Way. Their path was not one of pain purely for pain's sake, or martyrdom for the sake of martyrdom. Pain was not their highest and governing value, but neither was pain relief. They had come face to face with something more worthy of joyful worship: rescue from the meaninglessness of existence and a claim on their life in the person of Jesus Christ. For that, they would gladly suffer.

So I ask if we haven't gotten Christianity just a little wrong when we turn it into just another means of escape from what we all must face some day. Pain, after all, is itself not only inevitable but a necessity for us: It is a reality check, a reminder of mortality, something anesthetic belief categorically denies.

Simone Weil goes so far as to say that in the same way that the natural phenomenon of a sunset reminds us of the order and beauty of creation, so too does affliction — it is written into the delicate structure of the universe to which human beings belong and ultimately must give heed. In her essay, "The Love of God and Affliction," she writes:

> Each time that we have some pain to go through, we can say to ourselves quite truly that it is the universe, the order and beauty of the world, and the obedience of creation to God that are entering our body. After that, how can we fail to bless with tenderest gratitude the Love that sends us this gift?

By agreeing with Weil that even pain can minister God's grace to us, I do not intend to glorify suffering purely for suffering's sake. There is nothing redemptive in suffering *alone.* Nor do I wish to suggest that death is a good. The Bible is clear from start to finish that just as death did not belong to God's original plan for creation, death will not have a place in the heavenly resurrected life that God promises to those who love him.

My unease is with a Christianity that in a highly therapeutic, health-obsessed Western culture genuflects before the idols of comfort and happiness. A religion that assigns greater value to pain relief in the here and now than to the lordship of Jesus Christ has only succeeded in erecting another golden calf, with the damaging result that health and comfort and a pain-free death are falsely proclaimed as the answer to the riddle of human existence.

Such misplaced worship is a far cry from "true religion," understood as that "which binds us to God as the one and only God," in the words of John Calvin (a man, incidentally, racked with illness his whole life). It falls prey to the kind of utilitarianism that Friedrich Schleiermacher once bewailed: religion that exists not for its own sake, but as a means to an end — in this case, the relief of pain.

The Only Comfort

This brings me back to the quandary of my role as a chaplain to Esther, Mr. Z., and the many like them who, through either the empty promises of Osteenism or the misleading claims of hospice culture, cling to the empty promises of a spiritual anesthesia with the hope that I, as their chaplain, would alleviate their suffering once and for all.

Should I, like the good and able medical professionals with whom I work, attend to the bedsides of the sick with the sole purpose of easing their pain? Is my role to administer a spiritual morphine drip? Or am I called to deliver another proclamation, one that serves a greater, more life-giving end?

Perhaps the beginning of an answer to this question lies in the prayer that Jesus uttered in Gethsemane on the eve before his crucifixion. "Father, if you are willing," he pleads, "remove this cup from me; yet not my will but yours be done." In those words is the acknowledgment that no one is the ultimate master of his destiny but that we live, rather, in submission to the will of the Creator.

And perhaps this reality is consolation enough, for in the words of the sixteenth-century landmark document of the Protestant Reformation, *The Heidelberg Catechism,* there is but one clear answer to the question, "What is your only comfort, in life and in death?" and it is "that I belong — body and soul, in life and in death — not to myself but to my faithful Savior, Jesus Christ."

36 The Christian Pastor's Role in Medical Ethics: In the Pew and at the Bedside

Joseph J. Kotva Jr.

Since discussions of medical ethics often focus on a case, consider Eve. Eve was a fixture at Christ Church. She married and buried her husband there. She raised her children there. For fifty years she sat in the same pew and joined with fellow members in offering prayers of invocation, thanksgiving, confession, and petition. For fifty years she looked at the stained glass windows of the Good Shepherd, Jesus blessing the children, and the resurrected Christ welcoming all. For fifty years she sang hymns about God's providential care and listened to countless sermons about God's grace and how we are to respond with faith, hope, trust, and love. For most of those years she read the scriptures with her Sunday School class while facing pictures of Christian martyrs.

At eighty-four years old, Eve elected to have major surgery despite her age and a significant chance that she would not survive the operation. She chose surgery because her heart had become so bad that she could no longer participate in the church and family activities that she loved.

Paul, Eve's pastor, visited the night before surgery. They talked about her faithful life and the hope and risks of surgery. Eve responded that God had been good to her and that matters were now in God's hands, as they had always been. They read Psalm 16 together: "Protect me, O God, for in you I take refuge."

Although surgery went well, Eve's recovery did not. She looked and felt good initially. But her heart would not stay in sinus rhythm, her kidneys began to fail, and her lungs filled with fluid. Two weeks after surgery Eve was on a respirator and maximum doses of heart and kidney medications. The doctor told the family that there was some chance that Eve would recover and recommended starting dialysis. The family agreed.

At that point, Pastor Paul, who stayed with Eve and her family throughout the two weeks, intervened. Paul pressed the doctor to explain to the family what "some chance" of recovery meant. The doctor responded that Eve probably had a two or three percent chance of getting significantly better. Although chilled by this news, the family was still inclined to start dialysis. Paul then gently suggested that continuing treatment seemed inconsistent with Eve's life and with the family's own trust in God.

After prayerful consideration, Eve and her family decided against dialysis and asked for the respirator's removal. Christ Church was filled for Eve's funeral service. The service itself was filled with tears and laughter — the latter celebrating the well-lived life of one who trusted that we are in God's hands.

Unlike typical case studies in medical ethics, Eve's case starts long before and separate from hospitalization and culminates after her death. I begin with this case because it illustrates my contention that for Christians the pastor's relationship to medical ethics extends from the pew to the bedside.

Reflecting the dual focus on pew and bedside, my argument has two distinct sections. The first section does not deal with what first occurs to most of us when we hear someone say "ethics" or "medical ethics" — that is, a forced choice between undesirable alternatives or a violation of moral norms or the principles and procedures we adhere to in making decisions. Instead, the first section directs our attention to concerns that are antecedent to this type of ethics by contending that, for Christians, medical ethics is an outgrowth of congregational life. More specifically, I argue that both moral medical decision making and medicine as a morally worthwhile social practice are dependent on preceding theological convictions and qualities of character. I then argue that the pastoral responsibilities of communicating Christian convictions and helping shape Christian character constitute a significant pew-based, that is, congregation-based, relationship to medical ethics.

Many will recognize this first section as an argument for concerns arising from character or virtue ethics. Central to virtue ethics is a shift in the focus of ethical reflection. Since the eighteenth century, moral theory has tended to focus on moral quandaries, rules, principles, and methods for determining the moral status of specific acts. By contrast, virtue ethics shifts the focus by concentrating on "background" issues, such as character traits, personal commitments, community traditions, and the conditions for humans to excel and flourish.[1] The first section of this paper argues for this shift in focus. However, instead of an extended technical discussion of virtue theory, I use Eve's case to argue for the importance to medical ethics of background issues, such as convictions and character. And, consequently, I locate much of the pastor's role in medical ethics in the background.

Without losing sight of these background concerns, the second section deals more directly with what most understand when they think of medical ethics. This section discusses the pastor's role at the bedside by sketch-

From Joseph J. Kotva Jr., "The Christian Pastor's Role in Medical Ethics: In the Pew and at the Bedside." *Second Opinion* 5 (Mar. 2001): 22-48. Permission to use and reprint given by The Park Ridge Center, the copyright holder.

1. See also Joseph J. Kotva Jr., *The Christian Case for Virtue Ethics* (Washington, D.C.: Georgetown University Press, 1996), 5.

ing interconnected images of ministry: the pastor as priest, theological interpreter, medical translator, prophet, and friend. I use these images to highlight aspects of the pastoral bedside task and to suggest how that task intersects with medical ethics. Thus, for instance, I argue that the pastor's priestly role of representing the faith community's and God's presence to the patient helps limit medicine to its proper authority.

A caveat about the scope of this project is in order. Due largely to my own social location, this paper addresses how the pastor in the Christian congregation or parish intersects with and informs aspects of medical ethics. How these issues work out for leaders in other faith traditions is not my explicit concern. Further, while some aspects of the second section are applicable to Christian clergy in noncongregation-based ministries — hospital chaplains, for example — I do not directly address these ministries.[2]

Congregational Life

Christian Convictions

In her wonderful book *Stewards of Life,* Sondra Wheeler observes that virtually "every serious decision about the treatment of the sick has theological implications."[3] Wheeler is right. In Eve's case, for example, the decisions to not start dialysis and to remove the respirator presumed certain theological convictions, including the need to "honor your parents." Remembering the serenity with which Eve approached this risky surgery, the family realized, with help from the pastor, that continuing to deny death's approach was to dishonor their mother and her convictions.[4]

The family also shared Eve's belief that her life was in God's hands and that death is not the last word. Eve raised her family in the church. They always attended Good Friday and Easter services. They grew up with that window of the resurrected Jesus and those same pictures of the martyrs. They knew that suffering and death are not the worst evils. With Pastor Paul's help, they gradually realized that to deny death not only dishonored their mother, it belied their own faith in God.[5]

This contrasts sharply with the physician who recommended dialysis while suggesting that Eve might still recover. It is possible, indeed likely, that the physician made the recommendation in part because he viewed death as the end and final defeat. Although seldom explicit, this view is common in our culture. When death is viewed as the ultimate defeat, fighting death to the bitter end becomes the medical imperative. Thus, when we compare the doctor's actions to those of Eve and her family, we see that convictions about death that are at heart theological lead to different medical decisions.

Like the decision to forgo dialysis, Eve's decision to pursue surgery rested on theological convictions, specifically about the purpose of life. As a Christian, Eve viewed life as a good directed to God and others. Life is for relationship to God, worship of God, and serving God through the church; life is for relating to and caring for others. Yet Eve's health left her unable to participate in church or to join in family activities. Eve cherished life and would never have aimed at her own death.[6] Her decision for surgery aimed instead at getting well enough to participate more fully in the purposes of life: worship, relationships, service.

End-of-life decisions are not the only ones to rest on theological beliefs. Other examples include abortion and issues of justice. Two years ago, a young woman, still in high school, told me and some of her peers that she was pregnant. Someone soon raised the question of abortion. The young woman responded immediately, "Oh, I couldn't do that." When pressed for a reason, she offered religious convictions, talking about the limits of human freedom and about the unborn being precious to God. Her religious convictions ruled out abortion. So too, when medicine wrestles with questions of justice — such as who gets the transplant or how health care should be distributed — it wrestles with "an area that the prophets and epistle writers persist in viewing as a theological matter."[7]

Medical decisions presume beliefs that are at bottom theological, although these convictions are often implicit and unconscious. They assume that we are essentially autonomous or interdependent, that life is merely a personal project or necessarily involves vocation and service, that we are embodied selves or merely bodies or trapped in our bodies, that our worth derives from our social contribution or our being-in-relation to God.

To realize this dependence on theological premises is to recognize that, for Christians, medical ethics is all outgrowth of congregational life and pastoral leadership, for it is in our churches that we discuss and learn, or fail to discuss and learn, Christian theology. It was in the church that Eve learned the convictions that led to her surgery and then to forgoing further treatment. Lacking a congregational context like Eve's, or failing to talk explicitly in church about beliefs and their real world im-

2. For my reflections on hospital chaplaincy, see: "Hospital Chaplaincy as Agapeic Intervention," *Christian Bioethics* (December 1999): 257-75 [selection 34 in this volume].

3. Sondra Ely Wheeler, *Stewards of Life: Bioethics and Pastoral Care* (Nashville: Abingdon Press, 1996).

4. Honoring a parent is very different from acknowledging another's autonomy. Honoring parents is an intrinsically relational notion that presumes interdependence and responsibility. By contrast, autonomy is an individualistic notion that leaves us responsible only to accept another's autonomous wishes.

5. See also Allen D. Verhey, *The Practices of Piety and the Practice of Medicine: Prayer, Scripture, and Medical Ethics* (Grand Rapids: Calvin College and Seminary, 1992), 59-60.

6. For the importance of this distinction, see Joseph Kotva, "A View from Two Sides: The Principle and Its Cases," *Christian Bioethics* 3/2 (1997): 158-72, especially 167-71.

7. Wheeler, *Stewards of Life.*

plications, Christians slowly adopt assumptions that are often at odds with Christian beliefs.

Christian Character

Although our beliefs are important, moral decision making requires more than mere intellectual assent to certain claims. Determining and doing the right requires our having developed the appropriate tendencies, dispositions, and capacities; it requires our having developed the requisite virtues. Some examples will clarify what I mean.

Over a lifetime, Eve acquired virtues she drew on in her decision for surgery. We see hope both in her desire for healing and in the serenity with which she approached death. Truthfulness is visible both in Eve's description of her current life, its value and its limits, and in her recognition that surgery might fail.

Contrast Eve with Harold, another member at Christ Church. Harold successfully hid his fifty years of heavy smoking from fellow church members. To those few who knew his secret, Harold insisted that it was a harmless habit. Harold developed serious lung and circulatory problems, but he continued to smoke, claiming that smoking had nothing to do with his "minor" problems. As things progressed, Harold's physician frequently hinted that there was little point in additional treatments or therapies, but Harold could not hear this limit. Indeed, for the last six months of his life, Harold was repeatedly rushed to the hospital, admitted to various treatment and rehabilitation programs, and then sent home again. Harold continued to insist that he was getting better and would often note, "I just don't know what is wrong with me."

The difference between Eve and Harold does not rest on their beliefs. They believed the same things. The difference is that those shared beliefs were not rooted in Harold's character in the form of the virtue of truthfulness. Harold never intentionally lied; he simply did not have the ability to look at himself and the world honestly. He lacked the quality of truthfulness. Deficient in this characteristic, Harold never faced his impending death. The result was that instead of getting ready to die, instead of having those important conversations with family, instead of getting his house in order, Harold spent much time and money (private and public) in treatment programs that provided marginal improvement at best.

In the stories of Eve and Harold we see that moral decision making requires well-formed character. It is important to recognize, however, that moral decisions depend on character at multiple levels: our character informs not only how we handle the decisions that we confront but also what decisions we confront.

I treat the latter point first. Character significantly influences what we see as choices before us. In Harold's case, character not only informed his decisions, it determined what he encountered as a choice. Harold's inability to be truthful about his impending death meant that he never encountered or viewed treatment as an option that might be declined.

Our virtues and vices enable us to perceive certain choices and incline us to overlook others. A physician or nurse who has internalized a concern for justice will notice when someone is being treated unfairly or when the real underlying question is one of distribution. Those who lack the virtue of justice are unlikely to recognize when it is at stake.

Similarly, I notice that some nurses quickly sense when a patient does not understand the doctor's explanation of treatment options, while other equally caring nurses never recognize the patient's confusion. The difference, I suspect, is that the former have acquired characteristics and skills — that is, virtues such as patience, sympathy, and the ability of imaginative listening — that enable them to recognize when communication and patient understanding are amiss.

Beyond influencing what decisions we confront, well-formed character is vital to deciding well. Lacking the requisite virtues, we are far less likely to find the right course or to see it through. Consider how vital the virtue of courage is to moral medical decisions. In our litigious age, doctors often need courage to reject unnecessary tests. Lacking courage, the tests will be ordered, perhaps under the guise of thoroughness or patient autonomy. Nurses need courage when deciding whether to approach a doctor who discounts a patient's wishes or when contemplating whether to submit an incident for ethics review. Patients need courage when they consider asking for another opinion or contemplate rejecting their doctor's recommendation.

Moral medical decisions rest on character: character informs both what moral choices we confront and how we decide them. Yet to realize the importance of character is to realize that congregational life and pastoral leadership are related to medical ethics. Church life and pastoral leadership are, or ought to be, eminently concerned with shaping Christian character, for the church is the principal place in which Christians seek to become the kind of people God is calling them to be.

Medicine Needs the Church

The argument that medical ethics is, for Christians, an extension of congregational life can be extended to suggest that the practice of medicine needs the church or church-like communities. Stanley Hauerwas claims that what we value about medicine depends on health workers and patients alike belonging to communities like the church.[8] It is in the church and church-like communities where people acquire the convictions and character

8. Stanley Hauerwas, *Suffering Presence: Theological Reflections on Medicine, the Mentally Handicapped, and the Church* (Notre Dame, Ind.: University of Notre Dame Press, 1986), 75-82; see also Allen Verhey and Stephen E. Lammers, *Theological Voices in Medical Ethics* (Grand Rapids: Wm. B. Eerdmans, 1993), 67.

necessary to sustain medicine as a morally worthwhile activity.[9]

Consider, for example, the commitment to stay with the sick in the midst of pain, fear, and helplessness, even when we cannot cure or they cannot pay. I take it that most Christians, perhaps most people in our society, would accept this commitment as one of medicine's central purposes.

Note, however, that this commitment assumes certain convictions and qualities of character: we are essentially social creatures who need each other, and we owe each other care even when it is uncomfortable, financially unprofitable, or risky. This commitment also assumes a host of virtues, including courage, fidelity, and hope. It takes courage not to flee when we are confronted with disease, sickness, and death. And we cannot trust our doctors and nurses to remain with us in crucial moments if they lack fidelity and hope.

The problem is that these convictions and virtues are not supported by the broader culture. Our culture prizes autonomy and freedom above interdependence and obligations. Our culture idolizes effectiveness and the technological control of nature. Ours is an ethos of the marketplace, where skills are commodities to be purchased by autonomous consumers. We Americans share few socially accepted examples of courage — except perhaps the soldier, who may not be the best role model for health workers. Our culture's notion of fidelity is seen in the divorce rate and the preponderance of absentee fathers.

The commitment to remain with the sick assumes convictions and character that are increasingly at odds with this dominant ethos. To the extent that medicine still exhibits this commitment, it exhibits a morality that is out of step with our culture. To the extent that medicine is becoming something less morally worthy, we need look no further than the society shaping the convictions and character of those who practice medicine.

There are, in fact, good reasons to be distressed about medicine's direction. The doctor/patient relationship is starting to look more like a contract than a covenant. Patients increasingly sue physicians for failing to meet their expectations. Hospitals compete over patients, cut staff to improve profit margins, and send people home before they are ready. And, in a great irony, medicine's technologically driven imperative to cure is now being resisted with appeals to autonomy that would force another — the very one we have asked to cure us — to help us die.

Yet, as Stanley Hauerwas and Charles Pinches point out, we should not ascribe

> blame to the institution of medicine for our present state of ill health. . . . The simple fact is that we are getting precisely the kind of medicine we deserve. Modern medicine exemplifies a secular social order shaped by mechanistic economic and political arrangements, arrangements that are in turn shaped by the metaphysical presumption that our existence has no purpose other than what we arbitrarily create.[10]

The problem with modern medicine is not the institution of medicine itself but the wider society that shapes medicine and its practitioners.

Our society cannot be trusted to form the kind of people necessary to sustain medicine as a morally worthwhile activity. This is why Hauerwas suggests that medicine needs communities, like the church, whose convictions and practices might shape a people capable of morally worthy medicine.[11]

Pastoral Implications

This dependence on well-formed people has profound implications for pastoral moral leadership. Pastors help shape the convictions and character of their parishioners and help their congregations become the kind of communities that facilitate the formation of Christian beliefs and virtues.[12] The following discussion illustrates how the pastor facilitates the formation of Christian convictions and character by attending to everyday matters, such as funerals, prayer, and visual images. This discussion also highlights the connection between such formation and medical ethics.

Communicating Convictions To consider the importance of clearly communicating Christian theological convictions and their possible moral implications in medical settings, let us return to Eve's case. Besides the biblical prescription to honor your parents, Eve's case includes the beliefs that: (1) God cares about us and can be trusted; (2) death is not the end; and (3) we are created

9. To be fair to Hauerwas, his claim focuses more on character than convictions. Indeed, Hauerwas says that he does not believe that "medicine necessarily requires theological presuppositions in order to subsist" (*Suffering Presence,* 75). What Hauerwas means by this, however, is unclear. His central claim is that "medicine needs the church not to supply a foundation for its moral commitments, but rather as a resource of the habits and practices necessary to sustain care of those in pain over the long haul." Nevertheless, in the same paragraph, Hauerwas admits that believing that we can and should be present with the sick "entails a belief in a presence in and beyond this world" (*Suffering Presence,* 81). Similarly, Hauerwas's final comment is that we cannot count on the values necessary to medicine "being transmitted without a group of people who believe in and live trusting in God's unfailing presence" (*Suffering Presence,* 82). Medicine therefore appears to need the church as a character-forming community whose convictions have taken root in the community's common life and practices.

10. Stanley Hauerwas and Charles Pinches, *Christians Among the Virtues: Theological Conversations with Ancient and Modern Ethics* (Notre Dame: University of Notre Dame Press, 1997), 170.

11. That institutionalized medicine is shaped by the larger ethos is also why authors such as Hauerwas and Allen Verhey question whether the vision of medicine as a caring presence is still sustainable in our culture, e.g., Verhey, *Practices of Piety,* 62; Hauerwas and Pinches, *Christians Among the Virtues,* 217, no. 31.

12. Joseph Kotva, "The Formation of Pastors, Parishioners, and Problems: A Virtue Reframing of Clergy Ethics," *The Annual of the Society of Christian Ethics* 17 (1997): 271-90, especially, 283-386.

for the purposes of worship, fellowship, and service. These beliefs are not rules or prescriptions for action, nor are they commonly discussed in standard works on medical ethics. Yet Eve's case turned on such obviously theological notions.

Pastors need to be aware that such basic theological convictions do real work in parishioners' lives outside of worship. Knowing this, it behooves pastors to be explicit about what Christians believe and to illustrate how those beliefs function in shaping lives and informing decisions, including medical decisions.

For example, funerals and Ash Wednesday offer opportunities to remind parishioners that they are made of dust and should be unashamed of their finitude. Christians know that it is fine to be finite, that it is okay to be dust, because God views these earthen vessels as good, and because they commune with a God who breathes life into their clay bodies.

To illustrate how these convictions function in the life of a Christian, the pastor can allude to their implications in end-of-life decisions. Much of modern technological medicine is a denial of our finitude. We pour as much as 80 percent of medical dollars into the last two years of life, because we do not know that the end of life is at hand and because we deny our finitude and the propriety of death. People who know themselves to be divine breath-filled dust do not need to so deny death.

Another example of Christian convictions and their potential medical implications is the apostle Paul's vision of the church as a body.[13] Pastors can rightly highlight the implications of this image for Christian medical decision making. If Christians are as interdependent as the parts of a body, then they should seek the counsel of other parts of the body when making major medical decisions. So too, in making those decisions, they need to ask whether the contemplated course is commensurate with building up the body.[14]

Shaping Character Pastors must also attend to character formation. Here the issue is broader and subtler than merely explicating Christian beliefs from the pulpit or in Sunday School. Pastors must consider matters as diverse and mundane as prayer, visual images, music, and church potlucks because every choice, experience, and relationship has "some effect — no matter how small — on the person we are in process of becoming."[15]

To illustrate let us again return to Eve's case. She offered prayers with the same congregation for fifty years. If Eve learned to pray well during those fifty years, if she learned to attend to and wait on God, then in the process she acquired virtues such as humility, patience, and solidarity.

When we pray well we cease to be preoccupied with ourselves and cease to be the center of our own attention. We thereby begin to acquire humility. So too, as we rightly learn prayers of confession, we learn to own our limitations, failures, and rebellion. And as we learn to pray prayers of petition, we are reminded of our needs and our dependence on God and others. Humility is therefore a virtue of prayer. In learning to pray rightly — learning to attend to God, learning to confess and petition properly — we also grow in humility.

Humility is also essential to moral medicine. Humility is part of what enables physicians to recognize their limits and part of what prevents them from taking advantage of vulnerable patients. Humility enables patients to recognize honest, human mistakes by doctors and nurses for what they are: the normal consequences of well-intentioned but limited people endeavoring to offer care. Lacking humility, patients will sue for any perceived mistake or failure, irrespective of genuine incompetence or negligence. Finally, patients require humility to open their bodies to strangers and to grant these caregivers invasive authority. When patients lack humility, medicine loses its authority and starts to look like one commodity among others from which we may pick and choose.

Other prayer-formed, medically relevant virtues include patience and solidarity. As Michael Duffey notes, prayer teaches the prayerful to wait:

> Prayer is the suspension of time and the adoption of a patient and quiet heart in order that we might be led into deeper communion with God. Praying requires stepping out of the current of activities in which we are caught up. . . . Prayer is first of all the intention to create an opening, a space where we might wait for the stirrings of God.[16]

Learning to pray thus means learning to wait, learning patience.

Prayer also teaches solidarity. This is seen in the Lord's Prayer, where Christians are taught: pray to *our* Father, ask for *our* daily bread, and seek forgiveness for *our* debts. Solidarity is also learned in intercessory prayers, where one presents another's need to God.

Morally worthy medicine also needs these virtues. It is difficult to imagine how one could be a good doctor, patient, or nurse without patience. How can we remain with each other in our sickness if we have not learned to wait? Similarly, how can medicine expect to stand with those who cannot pay or cannot be cured unless health workers have acquired a deep sense of solidarity with those whom they serve?

Prayer is thus relevant to medical ethics. It is also an issue of pastoral leadership, for Christians learn how to pray from and with others in the church. They learn how to pray as they stand in the liturgy and pray prayers of in-

13. 1 Cor. 10:17; 12:12-31; Rom. 12:4-5, New Revised Standard Version.

14. E.g., 1 Cor. 8:1ff; 10:23ff; 12:7; 14:12, 26, NRSV.

15. David L. Norton, "Moral Minimalism," in *Midwest Studies in Philosophy XIII Ethical Theory: Character and Virtue,* ed. Peter A. French, Theodore E. Uehling, and Howard K. Wettstein (Notre Dame, Ind.: University of Notre Dame Press, 1988), 186.

16. Michael K. Duffey, *Be Blessed in What You Do: The Unity of Christian Ethics and Spirituality* (New York: Paulist Press, 1988), 38.

vocation, confession, petition, and so on; as the Psalms are read aloud and as the congregation recites the Our Father; as prayer is modeled by teachers, friends, and those viewed as saints. They learn to pray as others teach them how.[17]

Congregational life involves many other character-shaping practices besides prayer, for example, viewing the windows of Jesus and pictures of Christian martyrs. Such images have power to shape. They provide pictures of the ends and purposes of life, present role models to be emulated, and "create assumptions about how the world really is."[18] Routinely viewing pictures of martyrs would lead one to expect suffering as part of faithful Christian existence. The image of Jesus the Good Shepherd could affirm one's self-worth, while the image of the resurrected Christ might make one less anxious about death.

This ability to shape is relevant to medical ethics. One who expects suffering is likely to respond differently to end-of-life decisions than is one who views suffering as an evil to be avoided at all costs.[19] The person who has learned his or her self-worth is less likely to be bullied into or out of medical procedures. And Eve is a perfect example of what happens when death is less feared.[20]

Prayer and images are only two aspects of congregational life that bear character-shaping implications. Nevertheless, it should already be clear that pastoral moral leadership requires attention to mundane, everyday matters. There is nothing earthshaking about prayer and pictures of martyrs. Such matters present no obvious dilemmas or conflicts. Indeed, they are so mundane that they usually escape our attention. Yet, it is in and through them that Christians become, or fail to become, the kind of people they should be. Thus, pastoral moral leadership includes such seemingly insignificant matters as helping parishioners learn to pray well, evaluating the images to which they are exposed, testing whether music cultivates emotions and desires befitting Christians, asking whether potlucks encourage Christian friendships, exploring how the Lord's Supper might train the believer in community and forgiveness, and so on.

These everyday pastoral concerns are indirectly relevant to medical ethics. Patients, nurses, and doctors will confront the right questions, choose the right answers, and engage in the right actions only if they are rightly formed. Moreover, medicine's moral value as an expression of solidarity with the sick depends on character-shaping communities whose ethos is at odds with our culture's.

Pastor's Role In short, the pastor's role in medical ethics is neither cursory nor centered at the bedside, and it has surprisingly little to do with medical moral dilemmas or the four standard principles of medical ethics. The focal point of the pastor's relationship to medical ethics is the pew: pastors help or fail to help parishioners acquire the requisite convictions and character.

This conclusion does not mean that pastors should spend an enormous amount of time thinking about medicine's requirements. The foremost reason for teaching Christian convictions is not that medicine needs them but that we believe them to be true and relevant to our whole lives. Likewise, serving medicine is not the primary reason for cultivating Christian character; the primary reason is that God calls and enables us to become a certain kind of people.

Nevertheless, pastors must remain cognizant of medicine. As any active pastor or priest can attest, medicine suffuses the lives of parishioners. Indeed, institutionalized medicine seems to have become more culturally powerful and "pervasive in our lives than the church ever was and surely far more powerful than it is today."[21] Since Christians cannot and should not avoid medicine, they need to help each other acquire the convictions and character required to meet medicine as Christians.

Medicine pervades the lives of parishioners — whether as patients, families of patients, or health workers. Pastors do not teach and seek to cultivate character because of medicine, but since virtually all North American Christians confront Western medicine and medical decisions, pastors must ask whether church teaching and practices equip parishioners to morally navigate contemporary medicine well.

Pastors can, for instance, ask whether they sufficiently teach Christian convictions about the purposes and nature of life, and they can use medical examples to illustrate the repercussions of such convictions. Pastors can similarly ask whether the congregation provides sufficient opportunities to grow in patience, humility, solidarity, and so on. So too, when privileged to stand with a patient like Eve, the pastor can ask what convictions and practices enabled her to make the choices she did. When standing with a patient

17. I am not suggesting that we learn to pray in order to become better people. Prayer is about attending to God, and if we engage in prayer for some other purpose than waiting on God, it quickly ceases to be prayer. Nevertheless, learning to pray well shapes character. And if character is left unchanged by prayer, we should ask about the quality of our prayers.

18. Michael Warren, "The Material Conditions of Our Seeing and Perceiving: Religious Implications of the Power of Images," *New Theology Review* 7, no. 2 (May 1994): 45; see also Gregor Goethals, "TV's Iconic Imagery in a Secular Society," *New Theology Review* 6, no. 1 (February 1993): 40-53.

19. See also Wheeler, *Stewards of Life,* 32-35.

20. The power of images to shape us is not lost on corporate America. Their willingness to spend millions of dollars on beer, toothpaste, and truck commercials only makes sense if images shape behavior. Corporations spend this money because they know that images inform our desires and that people copy what they see. They spend this money because they know that we will buy their products if we envision the purpose of life in the back of a pickup, with our teeth white and a beer in one hand. Wall Street does not underestimate the power of images; neither should we.

21. Hauerwas and Pinches, *Christians Among the Virtues,* 168; see also Bonnie J. Miller-McLemore, "Thinking Theologically About Modern Medicine," *Journal of Religion and Health* 30, no. 4 (Winter 1991): 289.

like Harold, the pastor can ask how the congregation may have failed to help Harold become more truthful.

At the Bedside

Although the pastor's greatest contribution to medical ethics is in the pew, Eve's case reminds us that pastors also play an important role at the bedside. Pastor Paul read scripture with Eve the night before surgery, visited her and her family throughout the ordeal, and intervened in the family's discernment process. This extensive involvement is common when parishioners know and trust their pastors. I unpack this involvement at the bedside by using a series of partial, interconnected images of ministry: priest, theological interpreter, medical translator, prophet, and friend.[22]

Priest

Perhaps the central dimension of the pastor's role at the bedside is that of priest.[23] This dimension is not limited to churches with formal liturgies or an officially sanctioned priesthood. Even in less formal traditions, such as Baptist or Mennonite, the pastor's presence has a symbolic and ritual function. Specifically, the pastor represents the church community and often represents God's own loving and faithful presence.[24] As many pastors can attest, parishioners often view the church as virtually absent — irrespective of how many congregational members visit — until the pastor appears. Yet when the pastor makes himself or herself readily available, those same parishioners see the church as overwhelmingly present. Moreover, the extraordinary comfort that many find in unhurried pastoral visits is understandable once we grant that those visits symbolize God's own presence.

This priestly function includes the rituals of prayer, scripture reading, confession, and Communion. Pastors offer prayers of invocation, gratitude, and intercession; they sometimes also offer prayers that voice the feelings, thoughts, and fears that patients themselves dare not express. Such prayers console and often strengthen the patient's resolve to cling to God. Sometimes they even bridge the chasm that patients sense between themselves and a seemingly distant God. Similarly, the pastor's reading of Scripture allows patients to affirm the faith that they share with the biblical writers and to listen to God's Word for comfort and encouragement.[25] Although many would not call it "confession," patients often acknowledge their sins in the pastor's presence. In these moments, the "priest" is especially evident: the pastor both verbally expresses God's promise of forgiveness and physically demonstrates the patient's reconciliation to God and the church by remaining present.[26] In many traditions, the patient's participation in Communion is a comparably powerful reminder of God's love and presence in the midst of suffering.

Pastors fulfill this priestly function to serve God, not to serve medicine. But this dimension of the pastor's role does affect medical ethics. Minimally, Christian patients will make more consistently Christian decisions when they experience their faith community's support and know themselves reconciled to God. It is easier to calmly and honestly face uncertain or even life-threatening decisions when we know that we are not alone.

This priestly function serves another task vital to medical ethics; it helps to counteract medicine's excessive authority. In our day, medicine and psychology provide the major metaphors for healing, and laity often heed medical advice "with the kind of deference given religious disciplines in earlier centuries."[27] My personal experience is that many parishioners, especially older ones, obediently accept "doctor's orders" without questioning or understanding those orders. This excessive authority is visible in Eve's case: Eve's family initially accepted without question the physician's recommendation to start dialysis and still inclined to dialysis even after hearing that Eve's chance of recovery was slim. This reaction reflects their unquestioning acceptance of the physician's authority. If they were looking for a medical miracle, then it also reflects medicine's hegemonic control of healing metaphors. The pastor's priestly function helps curb this immense authority. By symbolically representing God's presence, calling in prayer on the one true redeeming God, and reading passages wherein God through Christ is healer, the pastor helps the patient take medicine and his or her doctor a little less seriously.

H. Phil Gross, a retired orthopedic surgeon and professed Christian, writes that he only prayed silently for himself and his patients. The major reason for not praying aloud, he says, is that such prayer can be construed as a lack of authority and confidence.[28] I believe that Dr. Gross was wrong never to pray aloud, but he was right about prayer's ability to rein in a physician's authority. As Allen Verhey points out,

22. I chose these particular images to organize the following discussion and call our attention to specific aspects of the pastor's bedside task. The images are helpful on both counts, but I make no theological or biblical claim for these particular images beyond these simple objectives. Moreover, I doubt that the images chosen here provide a comprehensive picture of ministry at the bedside, let alone a full picture of pastoral ministry in its entirety. Others may choose different images with equal effectiveness.

23. See also Richard Bondi, *Leading God's People: Ethics for the Practice of Ministry* (Nashville: Abingdon Press, 1989), 38-40.

24. Richard M. Gula, *Ethics in Pastoral Ministry* (New York: Paulist Press, 1996), 12, 57, 60, 71-73; Kent D. Richmond and David L. Middleton, *The Pastor and the Patient: A Practical Guidebook for Hospital Visitation* (Nashville: Abingdon Press, 1992), 16, 21, 26; Wheeler, *Stewards of Life,* 111-12.

25. See also Richmond and Middleton, *The Pastor and the Patient,* 101.

26. Richmond and Middleton, *The Pastor and the Patient,* 98.

27. Miller-McLemore, "Thinking Theologically About Modern Medicine," 289.

28. H. Phil Gross, "Is It Appropriate to Pray in the Operating Room?" *The Journal of Clinical Ethics* 6, no. 3 (Fall 1995): 273-74.

> One cannot invoke the one true God and take a presumptuous medicine too seriously. . . . When we invoke God as redeemer, we are freed from the vanity and illusion of wielding human power to defeat mortality or to eliminate the human vulnerability to suffering. An honest prayer could . . . restore a modest medicine to its rightful place alongside other measures that protect and promote life and health.[29]

I concur with Verhey. Prayer's ability to restrain medicine's authority is enhanced when combined with the pastor's priestly representative function.

Theological Interpreter

The pastor's task as theological interpreter includes two related elements: helping patients search for theological meaning and helping patients properly understand their traditions. Regarding the former point, hospitalization often occasions a search for meaning. Whether faced with a life-threatening procedure or merely with the strangeness and inconvenience of hospitalization, many ask questions of meaning. Am I being punished? Do I somehow deserve this suffering? Where is God in this? What am I to learn from this experience?

The pastor can gently guide the parishioner in this search for meaning.[30] This guidance takes various forms. Pastors can point out appropriate scriptures or discuss the role of suffering in the life of a disciple or ask what it means to believe in a God who suffers. Pastors can also suggest worthy lessons that can be learned from the experience. For example, I suggested to a parishioner that her frequent but not serious hospital stays were an occasion for her to grow in patience — a virtue she recognized was not well developed in her life. So too, pastors can sometimes legitimately suggest that a parishioner view his or her illness as an opportunity for growth in humility, trust, or hope.

In guiding the search for meaning, pastors must sometimes challenge a patient's theological assumptions. If a parishioner assumes too simple a connection between sin and suffering, for instance, then the pastor may need to challenge this linkage — perhaps by pointing to Job or to Jesus' explicit rejection of a simple correlation between sin and suffering or to Jesus' own innocent death. Of course, the pastoral goal in pointing to Job and Jesus is not merely to challenge assumptions but to offer a more profound engagement with suffering — that is, an invitation to wrestle with the meaning of suffering and to cling to God's presence, even when such meaning eludes us.

In addition to guiding the search for meaning, the pastor also helps the patient or family properly understand their tradition. Faithful adherents of a tradition often misconstrue its beliefs or implications. Consider as examples the cases offered by Don Browning and William O'Brien.

Browning's case is that of "Margaret and the Will of God." Browning notes that Margaret and her family held "to a rigid version of Reformed Christianity . . . in which all life's fortunes, good or bad, were regarded as the direct will of God." Browning says that these beliefs were not "just idle chatter. Margaret did not comply well with even the simple routines of her everyday care."[31] After all, why should she? If God decides that she will be sick, then she will be sick. And if God decides that she should get better, then she will get better.

For our purposes, it is the chaplain's response that makes this case noteworthy. The chaplain acknowledged God's providential governance, but challenged Margaret's understanding of that rule by using scriptural arguments to show that God's providence does not mean that God wills particular sicknesses. Instead, argued the chaplain, God's providence is such that we can strive with it toward health. The chaplain must have been caring in his conversation and skillful in his use of scripture, for the effect on Margaret was profound. Her attitude and behavior changed; she started to cooperate with her treatment.

O'Brien's case concerns sixty-five-year-old Thelma.[32] Thelma was ventilator dependent. Thelma had a large, growing, inoperable tumor in her face and sinus cavity. She had a history of pulmonary embolism, heart disease, asthma, lupus, and diabetes. Thelma was lucid, but she grew understandably frustrated and asked for the ventilator's removal.

Thelma's request sounds unremarkable, given the circumstances. But Thelma and her loving family were devoted Catholics who worried that withdrawal, and the resulting death, amounted to suicide or euthanasia. They feared that Thelma's death would leave her rejected by God and by her church. Thelma's family had cared for her the past eight years and was willing to continue that care. They strongly resisted Thelma's request.

As a Catholic priest, Father O'Brien helped Thelma and her family move toward a more accurate understanding of their shared tradition. By clarifying the distinction between "killing" and "letting die," O'Brien helped them to see that, from a Catholic perspective, Thelma was neither committing suicide nor asking for euthanasia. Thelma was instead asking to be allowed to die. Once relieved of their fears about suicide, the family, guided by Father O'Brien, directed their energy toward caring for and assuring each other.

We see the theological interpreter at work in both Browning's and O'Brien's cases. The chaplain helped Margaret and her family come to a more classic expression of their Calvinist faith. O'Brien helped Thelma and

29. Verhey, *The Practices of Piety*, 22.

30. Richmond and Middleton, *The Pastor and the Patient*, 27, 41, 48.

31. Don S. Browning, "Hospital Chaplaincy as Public Ministry," *Second Opinion* 1 (March 1986): 69.

32. William J. O'Brien III, "Dialogue Between Faith and Science: The Role of the Hospital Chaplain," *The Journal of Clinical Ethics* 6, no. 3 (Fall 1995): 280-84.

her family move toward a fuller and more accurate understanding of Church teaching. In both cases, the person responsible for pastoral care did more than help an individual in her private search for meaning. Accepting the authority of their respective traditions, the pastors directed patients and their families toward more complete understandings of those traditions.

As with the priestly image, pastors do not fulfill their function as theological interpreters to serve medical ethics. If they fulfill this function well, they serve God and their parishioners, and they do so in the belief that the theological claims are true. Nevertheless, this aspect of the pastor's role is relevant for medical ethics. The pastor as theological interpreter is primarily concerned with beliefs and convictions, although the search for meaning sometimes also includes character growth. But as we saw earlier, convictions and character matter to medical ethics.

The moral implications of the interpretive function are obvious in the cases discussed by Browning and O'Brien. Margaret's care and Thelma's death hinged on their gaining better understanding of their respective theological heritages. Without this understanding, Margaret had no reason to comply with her treatments and Thelma's family had every reason to resist her decision.

Note too that the standard principles of medical ethics — such as the principles of autonomy and beneficence — could not substitute for this interpretive function. Granting Margaret's autonomy or talking about beneficence does nothing to address her lack of self-care.[33] Indeed, the lack of self-care could be claimed as an autonomous right. Even worse, to emphasize Thelma's autonomy would disregard the moral claims that her family rightly makes on her. As a good Catholic, Thelma may not make her decision in isolation. Her faith and her family have a voice that she is morally obligated to hear. Unlike those who make a generic appeal to autonomy, Father O'Brien recognized these moral connections. He also recognized that Thelma and her family were misunderstanding their faith. Attending to either the principle of autonomy or the pastor's interpretive function might have arrived in Thelma's case at the same physical action — removing the respirator. The latter, however, honored Thelma's existing moral commitments in a way that the former could not.

Translator

The pastor's role at the bedside also includes translation, where he or she works toward mutual understanding between all parties, including the patient, family, and hospital staff.[34] As translator, the pastor helps patients and their families "hear" each other, asks questions of medical personnel that patients and families find difficult to voice, and ensures that patients and their families understand what they are being told about tests or treatment options.[35]

Pastor Paul acted as a translator, as an agent of communication, when he pressed the doctor to explain Eve's chance of recovery. Suspecting that relevant information was being left out, Paul asked the doctor a question that the family could not bring themselves to ask.

The chaplain in Browning's case also acted as translator. Margaret was hospitalized with severe kidney problems when dialysis was still scarce and kidney transplantation was new. Seeing Margaret's lack of self-care, the hospital committee charged with determining her course of treatment concluded that she lacked the intelligence and background to follow the routines and procedures that would make such treatments effective. The chaplain objected to this conclusion. He realized that Margaret's behavior, which was perfectly consistent with her world view, was being interpreted by the committee as a lack of intelligence. The chaplain argued that what the committee saw as signs of mental deficiency were actually signs that Margaret looked at the world differently. Thus, besides helping Margaret reinterpret her tradition, the chaplain acted as translator by helping the committee to understand Margaret's view of God's providence.[36]

Facilitating open communication is a task shared with others in the health care setting, including nurses, social workers, and ethics consultants.[37] People in these roles are often positioned to recognize breaks in communication and understanding. Nevertheless, there are several reasons that pastors are especially well situated to this task.

First, there is a good chance that the pastor and the patient already know and trust each other. In contrast, the patient experiences the hospital as a virtual "universe of strangers."[38] Amid those strangers, the pastor offers an established relationship of trust in which the patient may explicitly or implicitly confess questions and concerns that he or she would not otherwise admit. Moreover, because the pastor knows the patient as a real person outside the hospital, the pastor may notice when the patient's care, mannerisms, or decisions seem unbefitting his or her identity.

Second, it is socially acceptable to acknowledge need and express vulnerability to a minister. There is a social stigma attached to admitting need; yet, many who would never admit need or questions to a doctor, nurse,

33. Aspects of the theological interpreter role undoubtedly fall within the broad principle of beneficence as a role-specific obligation for clergy. However, discussion of the principle does not automatically alert us to the need for a theological interpreter nor does the principle by itself provide the skills of communication, imagination, theological knowledge, and situation-specific perception necessary to the interpretive role.

34. For this section, see Wheeler, *Stewards of Life*, 97-101.

35. Richmond and Middleton, *The Pastor and the Patient*, 67.

36. Browning, "Hospital Chaplaincy as Public Ministry," 69, 71-72.

37. E.g., Joseph J. Fins, "A Secular Chaplaincy," *Journal of Religion and Health* 33, no. 4 (Winter 1994): 373-75; Wheeler, *Stewards of Life*, 100.

38. Wheeler, *Stewards of Life*, 100.

social worker, or ethics consultant are free to talk to their pastor.

Third, the pastor and parishioner operate out of the same world view. They share beliefs and convictions that health workers may not share. As Browning's case suggests, understanding each other's convictions is no small matter. Behavior or wishes that seem odd to hospital staff may be perfectly comprehensible to one who shares the patient's world view.[39]

To fulfill this function of translator well, the pastor must cultivate a climate of trust, security, and openness to human vulnerability. The pastor also must exhibit a basic familiarity with the clinical and moral language used in the hospital setting. For example, it helps to know the difference between a nasogastric and a PEG tube. It helps to know what a respirator does or how violent — and often futile — resuscitation is. It helps to know what is meant by DNR (do not resuscitate) or PVS (persistent vegetative state) or EEG (electroencephalogram). Pastors do not need a technical understanding about such matters, but a modest level of understanding is essential if they are to help bridge communication gaps.[40]

Similarly, pastors need a basic working knowledge of matters such as living wills, health care proxies, informed consent, and the four principles of bioethics: autonomy, nonmaleficence, beneficence, and justice. As translators, pastors take these notions and relate them to language and convictions that are more natural for their Christian parishioners. Conversely, pastors sometimes need (as best as possible) to translate patient and family concerns into the moral language of modern medicine.

Prophet

In invoking the image of prophet, I suggest two aspects of the pastor's role at the bedside: (1) challenging parishioners to live and die in a way consistent with what they profess, and (2) explicitly advocating for patients whose voices are ignored or drowned out.

Pastor Paul acted as prophet when he gently suggested to Eve's family that continuing treatment was not in keeping with their trust in God. Paul's gentle suggestion reminds us that being a prophet at the bedside does not require harsh, caustic, or demanding speech. The words may be gentle, the tone quiet. What is required is hard honesty about making decisions that are faithful to what one believes. Pastor Paul exhibited this honesty in Eve's case.

Such hard honesty is conspicuously absent, however, from Harold's case. Harold lived and died his last few months in a way that belied his faith in God. Harold never admitted the harmful effects of his addiction or that he was dying. Perhaps the pastor should have been more prophetic in Harold's case. Perhaps he should have reminded Harold that Christians need not deny their sinfulness or their mortality. Perhaps what Harold needed was a soft but clear word from his pastor: "Harold, you are dying. Spend your time with your family. Spend your time getting things in order."

Being a bedside prophet also means advocating for the patient whose voice is unheard. The chaplain in Browning's case not only translated Margaret's world view, he championed her cause. The chaplain challenged the committee's conclusion that Margaret lacked the mental resources for treatment. He also challenged their assumption that perceived intellectual capacity should determine treatment: "He argued that Margaret was a human being and for that reason alone was deserving of treatment."[41]

Pastors should not underestimate the need for prophetic patient advocates. Institutional medicine is still basically benevolent, but the cultural and economic forces shaping a different, less caring kind of medicine are strong. Pastors need to watch out for patients who are poor and for patients who lack family as advocates.

I pastor a small urban church, and my parishioners go to any of four local hospitals. I see much good care at these hospitals. But in the last few years I have also seen the grossly inadequate pain management of an elderly person afraid to complain; the discharge to an unsupervised apartment of a scared, elderly, confused woman who was both incontinent and unable to walk; the failure to determine proper medication levels before discharge, resulting in multiple readmissions; nursing assistants who repeatedly failed to close the door, pull the curtain, or cover an unconscious, naked patient; technicians and support personnel who allow patients to believe that they are trained nurses; physicians who do not present patients with all their treatment options; and doctors and families who ignore a patient's advance directives.

The patients in these instances were unable to advocate for themselves and lacked family to advocate for them. With the current cultural and economic pressures on medicine, pastors will need to fulfill their prophetic function in part by becoming patient advocates.

This prophetic function at the bedside may, of course, inform the pastor's prophetic role beyond the hospital walls. Many difficulties confronted within the hospital are systemic. The second-rate or shortened care a patient receives often has more to do with limited or absent health insurance or a health maintenance organization's focus on the bottom line than it does with the particular doctors and nurses involved. Nurse or physician error is often ultimately rooted in hospital organization, not health worker incompetence. So too, patient care is directly influenced by the exorbitant cost of medications and indirectly influenced by the way drugs are marketed

39. See also Deborah Whisnand, "An Enhanced Methodology for Conflicts in Ethics Consultation," *Clinical Ethics Report* 9, no. 4 (Winter 1995): 7.

40. Nurses in the congregation are an excellent resource for such pastoral self-education.

41. Browning, "Hospital Chaplaincy as Public Ministry," 73.

to physicians and public alike. I believe that when such systemic issues emerge in the pastor's advocacy at the bedside, they should inform aspects of the pastor's prophetic task outside the patient's room, outside the hospital walls. These experiences within the hospital could prompt us, for instance, to ask how the church should voice its concerns within public debates about universal health coverage, error reporting, Medicare, drug costs, and so on.

The reach of the pastor's prophetic task beyond the bedside is a reminder that his or her influence is not unidirectional. What happens at the bedside also informs our activity within the congregation and in "the world."

Friend

Sometimes pastors are fortunate enough to have their parishioners also become their friends. I do not mean that they pal around together or that it is a peer relationship. Rather, I refer to that deep connection between people who share common values and goals, who have come to know, respect, and trust each other, and who desire each other's well-being.

This image of friendship hints at moral aspects of care at the bedside that do not easily fit within the other images. Consider, for instance, what it means for a friend to visit, or hold your hand, or cry with you. Friends do not visit out of duty or obligation or because they fill a specific social role. Friends visit because they care about you — with all your particular needs, wants, commitments, experiences, and idiosyncrasies. Friends visit because they prize what you bring to the relationship.

There is something deeply affirming and solidifying about a visit from a friend that is not encompassed by the images of priest, interpreter, translator, and prophet. When the pastor is lucky enough to be a friend, the visit involves mutual care, even though it is more focused on the patient. When the pastor is a friend, the patient is affirmed as an utterly unique individual who knows that he or she has received and given more than a priestly visit.

Relatedly, friends listen. Careful, empathetic, and imaginative listening skills are also vital to the pastoral dimensions of interpreter and translator, but good friends listen in a way that is not entirely captured by those images. Good friends often understand what we mean even though our words are not carefully chosen. Friends are frequently the best at understanding what we mean, not what we say. Conversely, friends are sometimes called upon to listen even when they do not understand what we mean or what we are talking about. At such times, what is important is not the understanding but the personal affirmation implied by the act of listening. Indeed, sometimes we need our friends to listen even when we are not speaking at all.

Friends are also those whom we are most likely to invite into our moral discernment. Pastors are often involved in a patient's moral deliberation, but that involvement is most profound when the pastor is a friend. In deliberating with true friends, we do not need to ask about what some abstract rational person would do. When deliberating with friends, we are not even limited to asking what a believing Christian should do. When friends discern together they ask a different question: "What should you — my friend, an individual whom I value, a person with a unique story — do?"

Conclusion

The Christian pastor's relationship to medical ethics extends from the pew to the bedside. It starts in the pew, for it is in the church that we acquire the convictions and character vital both to deciding well and to sustaining medicine as a praiseworthy practice. It extends to the bedside since pastors are, or sometimes become, priests, interpreters, translators, prophets, and friends.

CHAPTER SIX

The Patient-Physician Relationship

There is an inherent power imbalance in the relationship between patients and physicians. The patient is often ill, a position of vulnerability. The patient shares detailed, personal information with the physician; the physician does not reciprocate. The patient is often naked and sometimes even unconscious, heightening defenselessness and dependency. The physician has knowledge and access to pharmaceuticals and medical technology that the patient lacks. The relationship is thus uneven: the patient's illness, nakedness, and self-disclosure in the face of the physician's access to knowledge and technology combine to create a significant power discrepancy. This imbalance is often accentuated by the complex social and cultural dynamics surrounding race, gender, economic status, and religion.[1]

For many who write about medical ethics, this power imbalance is a point of concern. In a society preoccupied with autonomy, this inherent inequity risks dependency and undue physician control. At a minimum, this imbalance can allow for the kind of paternalistic physician-patient relationship that was until recently the norm in medicine. At its worst, it could allow the physician to control, even exploit, the patient. The dominant responses to such concerns are partially tied to the Nuremberg trials, but they appear even more connected to aspects of the civil rights movement of the late 1960s and early 1970s. As such, these responses to patient/physician inequalities emphasize patient autonomy, choice, and rights. Such responses often encourage a confrontational image of physician control versus patient autonomy. Other responses make the relationship sound like a contract, where the physician is in a contractual relationship with the patient to provide certain services. Still other responses underline the patient's freedom to leave the relationship at any time; occasionally, they underline the freedom of both patient and physician to leave the relationship. In general, concerns about physician-patient power imbalance engender responses that depersonalize, and often conflictualize, the relationship, describing both patients and physicians in terms of autonomy, contracts, freedom, and independence.

While the movement toward depersonalization is driven in part by concerns over a power imbalance, many health care access proposals in the U.S. also assume a depersonalized relationship. For example, "consumer driven health care" assumes that physicians and patients are strangers, as well as entrepreneurs and consumers, respectively. In part, the idea is that if we arm consumers (patients) with the right tools (for instance, information about physician charges and performance) and make them feel the true financial costs of health care, the power of the market will direct patient choice of providers (physicians) and drive down costs while rewarding quality. If the physician is given sufficient freedom, the same market forces will encourage the entrepreneur/provider (physician) to keep down costs and keep up quality. The model forgoes any notion of long-standing relationships of trust directed toward a common good. Instead, it assumes that physicians and patients are well-intended strangers and that a key to controlling health care costs and improving quality is to give both parties more freedom and give patients more power (principally in the form of information).

The way health care is reimbursed in the U.S. likewise pushes toward depersonalization. The combination of fee-for-service and managed care severely limits the amount of time physicians can spend with patients in order to maximize "efficiency" and profit — sometimes as little as seven minutes per patient — and encourages physicians to view their practice primarily in business terms.[2] Similarly, by interjecting extensive paperwork and

1. The accentuated power imbalance between providers and patients due to race, gender, economic status, and religion is a persistent subtheme in this volume; see especially the essays in Chapter Three, "Christianity and the Social Practice of Health Care."

2. The literature on length of physician-patient consultations is extensive, varied, and in no way limited to the U.S. As examples, see the following: Hernan C. Doval et al., "Perception of Consultation Length in Cardiology and Its Ethical Implications," *Revista Panamericana De Salud Pública = Pan American Journal of Public Health* 24, no. 1 (July 2008): 31-35; David A. Gross et al., "Patient Satisfaction with Time Spent with Their Physician," *Journal of Family Practice* (August 1998), http://findarticles.com/p/articles/mi_m0689/is_n2_v47/ai_

middle-persons between patients and physicians, managed care efforts to control costs often reinforce the notion that patients and physicians are simply strangers purchasing and providing services. And the now-common business practice of employers trying to control premium costs by routinely changing insurance providers forces both employees and patients to frequently change physicians — again encouraging depersonalization.

Additional historical and social factors have changed the patient-physician encounter, in terms of both power dynamics and the nature of the relationship. For example, until comparatively recent history, most physicians were itinerant or community-based, and practices such as home visits were a routine part of medicine. This social setting enabled physicians and patients to know each other in ways that are difficult to replicate in today's primarily institutional encounters.[3] Similarly, the secularization of medicine in the nineteenth and twentieth centuries has changed this relationship. For example, throughout the history of Western medicine, physicians were commonly encouraged to enquire into the patient's spiritual state and religious convictions. The practice of such enquiry remained an important component of medicine until after World War II, at which point religion began to be construed as private and unscientific.[4] But bracketing off from the patient-physician encounter such important matters, which are so deeply tied to identity, necessarily makes the participants a bit more like strangers.

The authors in this chapter reject the move toward depersonalization and help us rethink the power relationship between patients and physicians. For example, as can be seen in our first essay, "Strangers or Friends?" (selection 37), there is renewed interest in patient-physician conversations about religious matters. In this essay, physicians Farr Curlin and Daniel Hall suggest that the conversation between patients and physicians need not be that of strangers who are limited to discussing patient ills and purely physiological issues. They instead contend that patients and physicians can talk together about religious concerns as "moral friends." The language of "moral friends" implies a far deeper relationship than do more standard patient-physician images that either rule out religious talk or frame such conversations as a matter of therapeutic technique. Such conversations, say Curlin and Hall, must move to include notions of human flourishing and must be marked by seeking "the patient's good through wisdom, candor, and respect."

The story "Daniel" (selection 38) by Margaret E. Mohrmann, also a physician, implicitly challenges depersonalization by helping us see that the quality of the patient-physician relationship depends in part on the moral formation of the physician. It likewise helps us to see that the relationship is not confined to the patient and physician but extends outward to family members and other physicians. By highlighting the limits of physician-prognosticating skills and a mother's advocacy for and defense of her newborn, Mohrmann's short story also indirectly challenges our assumptions about the power relationship between physicians and patients.

Like Mohrmann, Stephen Lammers, in "AIDS and the Professions of Healing" (selection 39), invites us to consider the context of physician moral formation. Lammers reminds us that the kind of physician commitment to patients we desire cannot be sustained by our society's dominant utilitarian, individualistic, and contractarian modes of speech. Lammers instead challenges us to consider what type of broader community commitments are needed to sustain the moral art of medicine and its corresponding relationships.

"Exousia" (selection 40), Daniel Sulmasy's essay, specifically rejects notions that view the patient-physician relationship primarily as a struggle for power. Instead, Sulmasy, a physician and Franciscan friar, offers the biblical notion of *exousia* as requiring a covenant relationship between patient and physician that is itself subsumed under a greater good and directed to a common end. Sulmasy thus rejects the depersonalization that is increasingly prevalent as medicine is conceived in entrepreneurial (from the physician side) or consumerist (from the patient side) terms. Sulmasy equally rejects both a paternalistic medicine which believes that "authority has to do with knowledge and control that properly belong to the medical profession," and an "autonomism" which believes that control belongs to the patient but the patient grants it "to the physician only because the patient lacks knowledge." The biblical notion of *exousia* instead suggests a model of a trusting relationship between doctor and patient that is oriented to a shared *telos*. In biblical and Christian terms, that *telos* is the glory of God. But, following Edmund Pellegrino, M.D., and David Thomasma, Sulmasy contends that "the good of the patient" can provide a secularly credible orienting *telos* for medicine.

Karen Lebacqz, "Empowerment in the Clinical Setting" (selection 41), challenges us to rethink power in the patient-physician relationship by broadening the context to see how the clinical setting itself is often disempowering and invalidating to the patient. For example, patients lose their "normal status" in the world and are instead set aside by location (hospital room) and dress (hospital gown), where they are seldom allowed to see their own charts, and where their own voice or story is often discounted. As ways of ameliorating this situation of disempowerment, Lebacqz focuses on "the communication that comes from empathy, the centering power of music

---

21086292/?tag=content;col1 (accessed December 19, 2009); Peter Salgo, "The Doctor Will See You for Exactly Seven Minutes," *The New York Times* (March 22, 2006), http://www.nytimes.com/2006/03/22/opinion/22salgo.html?_r=1 (accessed December 19, 2009).

3. The story "House Calls on Cardinal Jackson" by David Schiedermayer, reprinted below in Chapter Twenty-three, is instructive for reminding us about how much is learned and shared in a home visit.

4. Cynthia B. Cohen, Sondra E. Wheeler, and David A. Scott, "Walking a Fine Line," *Hastings Center Report* 31, no. 5 (September 2001): 29-39.

and art, the adequacy of religious language and the solidarity of religious ritual and community."

But Lebacqz challenges us to rethink the patient-physician relationship even further by framing that relationship within the power dynamics of a broader social context, including access to health care and research priorities. While commending changes in the patient-physician relationship such as more thoughtful listening, Lebacqz contends that structural change is needed. In a social setting where women's issues are often ignored and the poor lack access to health care, changes in the patient-physician relationship are insufficient by themselves. Instead, empowering patients (at least those who are comparatively powerless) requires fundamental changes to the system.

This chapter is rounded out by two further essays. The first is Karl Barth's "The Will to Be Healthy" (selection 42). Barth reinforces and expands themes seen in the other authors here. Health, says Barth, is the desire and vitality to exercise our full potential as human beings, including a relationship to God. As such, health is a good that enables other goods, but it must never become an idol. And while Barth says many positive things about physicians, they must know the limits of their powers. Both Barth's optimism and his cautions regarding health and the patient-physician relationship are instructive. Like Karen Lebacqz, Barth also helps us situate discussions of the patient-physician relationship within a broader concern for public health and social justice, including living conditions and living wages.

Finally, "Thorn-in-the-Flesh Decision Making" (selection 43), by Richard Mouw, challenges our preoccupation with autonomy in these discussions, arguing that the desire for autonomy is too often the sinful desire to be a self-legislator. Mouw reminds us that dependency on expertise is common to the human experience. This acceptance of a kind of dependency is married to Mouw's insistence that the medical profession respect the patient as an image-bearer. This acceptance of dependency and the corresponding insistence on respect is a long way from the depersonalized struggle over power that characterizes many discussions of the patient-physician relationship.

All the essays in this chapter frame the patient-physician relationship in terms other than a business exchange between strangers or a conflict between paternalistic physician control (however benevolent) and patient autonomy. Thus, for example, the language of "moral friends" offered by Curlin and Hall, Sulmasy's image of a trusting relationship directed to a shared *telos,* and Mouw's combination of dependency and respect resist depersonalization and seek richer, non-conflictual (but also non-subservient) accounts of the power dynamics at work in the relationship. While sharing these concerns, the other essays also reframe the patient-physician relationship by reminding us that it occurs within larger contexts, including other relationships (Mohrmann), sustaining and forming communities (Lammers), and social, economic, and health care structures (Lebacqz and Barth).

Long-time readers of *On Moral Medicine* will notice that we have changed the name of this chapter. Earlier editions of *On Moral Medicine* followed traditional nomenclature in referring to the *physician*-patient relationship. We have flipped the terms, referring instead to the *patient*-physician relationship. By this change, we do not imply a struggle for power or depersonalization in a different form. We instead mean to call attention to the central player in all medical encounters — the patient. Unlike most television medical dramas — which depict the medical staff in heroic terms but seldom portray patients as real people with real stories — we recall Sulmasy's claim that the organizing reason for this relationship is "the good of the patient," as well as Margaret Mohrmann's claim in Chapter Nine of this volume that the real "heroes" of the clinical encounter are the patients. Such is not a relationship between equals in power, but it can be a good deal more than a commercial exchange between strangers or a competition for control.

SUGGESTIONS FOR FURTHER READING

Albury, W. R., and G. M. Weisz. "The Medical Ethics of Erasmus and the Physician-Patient Relationship." *Medical Humanities* 27, no. 1 (June 2001): 35-41.

Aquinas, Thomas. *Summa Theologica* 2.2 q. 110.

Barnard, David. "The Physician as Priest, Revisited." *Journal of Religion and Health* 24 (Winter 1985): 272-86.

Benner, P. "A Dialogue Between Virtue Ethics and Care Ethics." *Theoretical Medicine* 18, nos. 1-2 (March-June 1997): 47-61.

Bloom, Samuel W. "Professional-Patient Relationship: Sociological Perspectives." In *Encyclopedia of Bioethics,* vol. 4, 3rd ed., ed. Stephen G. Post (New York: Macmillan Reference USA, 2004), pp. 2141-50.

Burt, Robert A. "The Suppressed Legacy of Nuremberg." *Hastings Center Report* 26, no. 5 (September 1996): 30-33.

Cassell, Eric J. *The Healer's Art* (Cambridge, Mass.: MIT Press, 1985).

Cohen, Cynthia B., Sondra E. Wheeler, and David A. Scott. "Walking a Fine Line." *Hastings Center Report* 31, no. 5 (September 2001): 29-39.

Dyck, Arthur J. "Being a Physician and Being a Christian." *Second Opinion* 17 (October 1991): 135-38.

Entralgo, Pedro Laín. "Professional-Patient Relationship: Historical Perspectives." In *Encyclopedia of Bioethics,* vol. 4, 3rd ed., ed. Stephen G. Post (New York: Macmillan Reference USA, 2004), pp. 2132-41.

Gert, H. J. "Avoiding Surprises: A Model for Informing Patients." *Hastings Center Report* 32, no. 5 (September-October 2002): 23-32.

Gunderman, R. "Illness as Failure: Blaming Patients." *Hastings Center Report* 30, no. 4 (July-August 2000): 7-11.

Hall, Daniel E., and Farr Curlin. "Can Physicians' Care Be Neutral Regarding Religion?" *Academic Medicine: Journal of the Association of American Medical Colleges* 79, no. 7 (July 2004): 677-79.

Haring, Bernard. "The Physician-Patient Relationship." In *On Moral Medicine: Theological Perspectives in Medical Ethics,* 2nd ed., ed. Stephen E. Lammers and Allen Verhey (Grand Rapids: Eerdmans, 1998), pp. 793-95.

Justin, R. G. "Can a Physician Always Be Compassionate?" *Hastings Center Report* 30, no. 4 (July-August 2000): 26-27.

Kilner, John F., Robert David Orr, and Judy Allen Shelly, eds. *The Changing Face of Health Care* (Grand Rapids: Eerdmans, 1998).

May, William F. *The Physician's Covenant: Images of the Healer in Medical Ethics* (Philadelphia: Westminster, 1983).

McCormick, Richard A. "Beyond Principlism Is Not Enough: A Theologian Reflects on the Real Challenge for U.S. Biomedical Ethics." In *A Matter of Principles? Ferment in U.S. Bioethics*, ed. Edwin R. DuBose et al. (Valley Forge, Pa.: Trinity International Press, 1994), pp. 344-61.

McKenny, Gerald P., and Jonathan R. Sande, eds. *Theological Analyses of the Clinical Encounter* (Dordrecht: Kluwer Academic Publishers, 1994).

Owens, Dorothy M. *Hospitality to Strangers: Empathy and the Physician-Patient Relationship* (American Academy of Religion, 1999).

Pellegrino, Edmund D. "Self-Interest, the Physician's Duties, and Medical Ethics." In *Duties to Others*, ed. Courtney S. Campbell and B. Andrew Lustig (Boston: Kluwer Academic Press, 1994).

Peppin, J. F. "The Christian Physician in the Non-Christian Institution: Objections of Conscience and Physician Value Neutrality." *Christian Bioethics* 3, no. 1 (March 1997): 39-54.

Purtilo, Ruth. "Professional-Patient Relationship: Ethical Issues." In *Encyclopedia of Bioethics*, vol. 4, 3rd ed., ed. Stephen G. Post (New York: Macmillan Reference USA, 2004), pp. 2150-58.

Schiedermayer, David. "Honor Thy Patient." In *On Moral Medicine: Theological Perspectives in Medical Ethics*, 2nd ed., ed. Stephen E. Lammers and Allen Verhey (Grand Rapids: Eerdmans, 1998), pp. 771-77.

Shelp, Earl E. *The Clinical Encounter: The Moral Fabric of the Patient-Physician Relationship* (Boston: Kluwer Academic, 1983).

Siegler, M. A. "Professional Values in Modern Clinical Practice." *Hastings Center Report* 30, no. 4 Suppl. (July-August 2000): S19-22.

Spiro, Howard M., ed. *Empathy and the Practice of Medicine* (New Haven: Yale University Press, 1993).

Thielicke, Helmut. "The Truthfulness of a Physician." In *On Moral Medicine: Theological Perspectives in Medical Ethics*, 2nd ed., ed. Stephen E. Lammers and Allen Verhey (Grand Rapids: Eerdmans, 1998), pp. 785-93.

Veatch, Robert M. *The Patient-Physician Relation: The Patient as Partner* (Bloomington: Indiana University Press, 1991).

Zaner, Richard M. *Ethics and the Clinical Encounter* (Englewood Cliffs, N.J.: Prentice Hall, 1988).

37 Strangers or Friends? A Proposal for a New Spirituality-in-Medicine Ethic

Farr A. Curlin and Daniel E. Hall

Both professional[1-6] and popular[7] literature document revitalized interest in the intersection between faith and health. A growing body of evidence in medicine,[8] psychology,[9] and sociology[10] describes empirical associations between faith and health, and although this "faith-health connection" remains controversial,[8, 11-13] there is emerging consensus that religion is important to many patients, particularly in the context of suffering and illness.[13-15] In response, the medical literature has supported a lively debate about how physicians should and should not address the religious commitments of their patients.[13, 16-18] Although not always acknowledged as such, this debate is ultimately a moral debate because it concerns what physicians should and should not do. We suggest that thus far the debate has focused only on a limited range of the possible moral questions, and in this article we will attempt to expand the debate to better encompass the experience of both patients and physicians.

Reviewing the Current Debate

Despite the widespread consensus that physicians should be attentive to and respectful of the religious commitments of their patients, there is little agreement on how physicians should ascertain or address religious concerns. Should a physician try to discern them passively or should she actively inquire? Should she simply acknowledge and respect religious commitments or should she go further and attempt to clarify their implications? And if clarified, should they be validated, taken into account, supported, or challenged? Should a physician ever suggest or even recommend alternative ways of understanding religious commitments? Should she proselytize? At some point along this spectrum, most physicians grow uncomfortable saying "yes," but there is no agreement on where the line should be drawn.

Proponents of what is called "spiritual inquiry"[1-3] ar-

From Farr A. Curlin and Daniel E. Hall, "Strangers or Friends? A Proposal for a New Spirituality-in-Medicine Ethics," *Journal of General Internal Medicine: Official Journal of the Society for Research and Education in Primary Care Internal Medicine* 20.4 (2005): 370-74. Used by kind permission from Springer Science and Business Media.

Table 1. Current and Proposed Approaches to Dialogue Regarding Religion

Current Approach		Proposed Approach	
Ideal	**Question**	**Ideal**	**Question**
Competence	Are physicians competent to engage patients in dialogue regarding religious concerns?	Wisdom	How might a physician learn to wisely navigate discourse regarding religion?
Autonomy	Is patient autonomy threatened when a physician engages a patient regarding religion?	Respect	How might a physician engage in discourse which seeks to clarify and promote the patient's flourishing while demonstrating deep respect for the patient?
Neutrality	Is it possible for physicians to dialogue with patients regarding religion while maintaining the neutrality that their professional position requires?	Candor	How should a responsible physician address genuine disagreements regarding religious matters in such a way that he and the patient can respectfully negotiate a mutually acceptable accommodation?

gue that questions about religion are simply a matter of taking the actual person into account, building rapport, and discerning those factors that may be relevant to a patient's experience of illness and medical decision making. Critics counter that spiritual inquiry is misdirected and meddlesome, invading patients' privacy, crossing professional boundaries, and raising the threat of coercion or proselytism.[4-7]

Although they come to different conclusions, proponents and critics of spiritual inquiry share a similar conceptual framework that both defines the relevant moral questions and constrains the possible answers. In that shared framework, dialogue regarding religion is approached as if it were a form of therapeutic technique applied by physicians to patients, who interact clinically as strangers to one another. Alvan Feinstein noted and critiqued the ways that medicine is increasingly practiced and assessed as if it were merely a "technical performance."[8] By this Feinstein meant that medicine is now idealized as a practice that is based on empirical evidence, ordered by practice guidelines and algorithms, refined through techniques of Continuous Quality Improvement, and judged in reference to discrete performance-based indicators.[8] Unfortunately, this technical paradigm also inadvertently devalues the role of relationship in the clinical encounter, a process which has led some to argue that the entire practice of medicine is now "understood and regulated as if it were a practice among strangers."[9] This framework, which emphasizes technique over relationship, gives rise to three particular questions for moral inquiry, summarized in Table 1.

The first question asks, "Are physicians *competent* to engage patients in dialogue regarding religious concerns?" Competency is the first act of kindness, and in our medical tradition, it is demonstrated and governed through accredited certification, but because physicians are unlikely to have any professional training in religious matters, most authors do not consider them competent to address religion.[5, 10-12] Critics note that even if a physician had some religious training, such training would not likely encompass the enormous diversity of religious traditions found among patients.[5, 7] Others have noted that even with training, physicians would still be *relatively* incompetent compared to pastoral care professionals,[3, 11, 13] and they would be much less likely to have the time necessary to adequately address religious concerns.[7] Fearing incompetence, some critics conclude that physicians' attempts to engage patients will lead to erroneous ideas, ill-conceived recommendations,[10] and potentially harmful results.[4] Therefore, the argument goes, physicians should refer religious dialogue to religious professionals.[5-7, 10, 12, 13]

The second question asks, "Is patient autonomy threatened when a physician engages a patient regarding religion?" Physicians' words carry inordinate weight because of the peculiar authority that travels with the profession.[3] Because of this unequal power,[12] it is argued that coercion inheres in any effort that moves beyond "taking note" of a patient's religious concerns toward "taking on" those concerns or the commitments in which they are rooted. Although a physician will not always agree with her patients, some suggest that it would be an unjust "imposition" for the physician to "expound" her own values to an unwitting patient.[11] Patients, it is argued, have a right to "find their own solutions"[11] without the "undue influence"[10, 12] of a physician. Therefore, physicians should neither recommend nor critique religious ideas, unless such ideas conflict with "rational, evidence-based medicine,"[1] in which case a physician may have an obligation to challenge the ideas out of her commitment to beneficence.[3]

The third question asks, "Is it possible for physicians to dialogue with patients regarding religion while maintaining the neutrality that their professional position requires?" Some argue that professional boundaries mitigate against any inquiry into religious matters,[4] but if physicians do inquire, it is agreed that they should not take sides, because patients consult physicians for medical advice — not for dubious and unregulated religious opinions.[13, 14] In addition, it is thought that the languages of religion and science are immiscible,[5, 7] such that trying to add one to the other will only weaken both. For these reasons, Scheurich recently suggested that the medical profession should adopt an approach parallel to the political doctrine of the separation of church and state. To do so physicians would have to remain carefully neutral regarding religious matters.[6]

These three core questions emerge from three moral ideals: competency, autonomy, and neutrality. If these are the right questions, then the only relevant issues involve determining whether and how physicians might engage patients regarding religious concerns in ways that are professionally competent, do not violate patient autonomy, and are carefully neutral regarding religion. However, we contend that a different set of questions, derived from different ideals, will provide a framework better suited for approaching dialogue regarding religion within clinical medicine.

A Critique and a Proposal

Suppose for a moment that dialogue regarding religious concerns is not so much a technique enacted by a powerful stranger upon a weaker one, but rather is a moral discourse governed by an ethic of friendship. By moral discourse we mean a dialogue ordered to clarifying "the good" and negotiating the right ways to pursue that good.[15] By "an ethic of friendship" we are not so much referring to emotional connection as to *moral friendship* whereby a physician would act toward her patient out of desire for the patient's good.[9, 16, 17] Although related to beneficence, moral friendship is a richer concept that aims beyond narrowly defined "goods" toward a more complete sense of human flourishing. To flesh out the ways this new framework would shape interactions between physicians and patients, we will consider again the three questions typically raised about dialogue regarding religion, and then propose alternate questions that follow from the premises of "friendly moral discourse" (Table 1).

Competence Versus Wisdom

Competence is an important aspect of any technique, but when dialogue regarding religion is understood as technique, it is misunderstood. When patients raise religious concerns with their physicians, do we suppose they are looking for professionally certified spiritual therapy? When a patient with newly diagnosed breast cancer says, "Doctor, I think I will just trust God about this and call you in a few months to check in," is the range of appropriate physician responses limited to silence, simple acknowledgement, or referral to trained "religious professionals"? Do we imagine that the patient expects technical competence from her physician's words in the way she will expect competence from the surgeon who will perform her axillary node dissection? No. In such situations a physician appropriately engages in further dialogue with the patient — not because the physician is a certified religious professional nor because his words will be therapeutic, but because the physician must clarify the way his patient comes to her conclusion, and attempt to negotiate a way forward that contributes to the patient's flourishing as the physician understands it.[18, 19]

If the question is not one of competence, then what is it? We suggest it is more a question of, "How might a physician learn to wisely navigate discourse regarding religion?" Aristotle described *phronesis,* or practical wisdom, as the ability to discern which action, among several imperfect options, will best approximate the ultimate good. For Aristotle all choices about how to act are moral choices about which there can be no empirical knowledge.[20] Whereas the intellect allows the physician to learn medical data and the theologian to learn theology, wisdom guides both in discerning when and how such knowledge should be applied in seeking patients' good. Unlike competence, which can be mediated through scientific ways of knowing and technical instruction, wisdom must be developed through experience in a tradition and a way of life.[15, 21] In the medical tradition such wisdom is manifest as "good clinical judgment" in figures such as Sir William Osler. Certainly the wise physician must recognize the limitations of her knowledge, lest in engaging patients' religious concerns she do so badly. Yet, particularly in the case of religious dialogue, it would be naive to assume that a person gains the necessary wisdom solely from professional training. In practice, wise counsel is often given by lay persons who have been shaped and formed by faithful life.

Critics have expressed concern that discourse regarding religion would violate professional boundaries. However, such professional compartmentalization has been challenged by other critics in their search for a more culturally sensitive,[22] patient-centered,[23] integrated,[24] and holistic[25] medicine. These critics note that the divisions of labor that reinforce many professional boundaries can yield an impersonal, technical, fragmented, bureaucratic, and ultimately dehumanizing practice of medicine that undermines genuine interpersonal care and connection. Without doubt, some professional boundaries will always remain essential to medical practice, and forging interpersonal connections will always pose some risk to those boundaries. However, if physicians limit their communication to those areas in which they are professional experts, they will neglect large parts of the human condition including religious and other moral commitments, relationships with family and coworkers, dreams and aspirations, joys and sorrows. It is hard for us to imagine how such sterilization would improve the clinical encounter. It seems, rather, another step down the road toward a sort of medicine that is deeply unsatisfying to patients and clinicians alike.

Autonomy Versus Respect

The second issue concerns the purported threats of religion to patient autonomy. Although the literature carefully notes the dangers of religious coercion, it is easy to forget that physicians engage in moral persuasion on a daily basis. For example, physicians frequently take pains to persuade patients to continue difficult but promising therapies, or to make yet another effort to stop smoking. In these situations, it is apparently appropriate for physicians to use their unequal power judiciously to persuade patients to pursue the goals judged best by the physician. With respect to the principle of patient autonomy, there is a double standard and a secular bias within the current recommendation against engaging religious concerns. On the one hand, discussions regarding religious concerns are considered *prima facie* violations of autonomy, but on the other hand, physicians are encouraged to challenge those religious beliefs that run counter to "evidence-based medicine."[1] Contemporary bioethics often insists that patients have the autonomous right to determine their own values without the meddlesome influence of government, church, family, or friends. However, moral decisions are never made in a vacuum. Whenever a patient says, "I understand the options, Doc, but what do you recommend?" the patient is asking for moral counsel. In such cases, it is the physician's privilege and responsibility to deliberate about the patient's good so as to offer the wisest counsel possible.

If dialogue regarding religious concerns is discourse ordered by an ethic of friendship, the question is not, "Does dialogue threaten autonomy?" but "How might a physician engage in discourse which seeks to clarify and promote the patient's flourishing while demonstrating deep respect for the patient?" Such discourse requires both trust and judgment lest it become patronizing and paternalistic. However, physicians regularly walk this fine line as they persuade patients to follow medical recommendations. Physicians may be less comfortable clarifying the wider goals that contribute to a patient's flourishing, but with practice and care, such discourse is possible. Physicians should never coerce patients to do anything against their will, but neither should they ignore patients' deepest commitments. To take those commitments seriously will at times call for persuasive negotiation, frequently requires an exchange of perspectives, and always requires respect.

Neutrality Versus Candor

Two problematic assumptions are bound up in the final question, "Can physicians engage religious matters with their patients while maintaining the neutrality that their professional position requires?" The first problem is the assumption that physicians can and should be neutral regarding religion. Neutrality is an attractive idea to some,[6, 13, 14] particularly in a secular society which is understandably concerned about tolerance among diverse religious traditions. That concern undergirds the growing preference for addressing "spirituality" rather than "religion," a move which emphasizes commonalities over differences. However, as argued elsewhere, spirituality will not effectively bridge the differences that divide religions because no matter the language used, moral neutrality is not possible.[26] It is *never* possible for individuals to divorce themselves from the specific traditions of knowledge and the moral commitments that shape their lives.[15, 21, 26] Furthermore, feigned neutrality will never be comfortable to the devout person, for whom "setting aside" one's religious commitments would be a form of unfaithfulness.

The second problem is the assumption that religious commitments are private and as such should not influence the professional sphere. Max Weber noted,[27] some say with melancholy,[28] that the modern world fosters the differentiation of distinct social spheres, each of which requires its participants to check their "private" ethics at the door. He concluded that it would therefore be extraordinarily difficult in the modern world for the religious person to live out his commitments publicly.[27] It may indeed be difficult, yet religions such as Christianity, Judaism, and Islam each make totalizing claims, calling the faithful to put God first in every aspect of their lives. Our culture exerts a steady pressure to privatize and relativize religious commitments, but it is a pressure that the faithful are called to resist.[29] We are not suggesting that the profession of medicine give official or unofficial endorsement to a particular religious tradition. We argue rather that neutrality is an ideal that is rooted in secularism and is impossible to achieve.[29] Secularism is not neutral as regards religion.[30]

If the question is not how to maintain professional neutrality, what is it? The wise physician must still ask, "How should a responsible physician address genuine disagreements regarding religious matters in such a way that he and the patient can respectfully negotiate a mutually acceptable accommodation?" Without doubt a generous measure of creativity and good will is necessary to find a way that violates neither the integrity of the physician nor that of the patient. Whatever else it requires, it will certainly require dialogue — the sort of dialogue that is generally unacceptable within the ethical framework that currently prevails. The relevant moral concept is *candor*. A physician need not "tell all to all," but she must seek to be conscious of which judgments are part of professional consensus and which follow from her own moral convictions, and she must take pains to make that distinction clear to patients.[11, 18]

Caveats

The framework we have proposed opens up possibilities that some will find troubling. Some may fear that "Pandora's box" will open and physicians everywhere will persuade, manipulate, or even coerce patients to abandon or change their religious creeds. Although we concede that such is possible, for the moment we would contend that overbearing religious zealots are more populous as specters than as practicing physicians. Others may contend, "I do not want *my* doctor to talk to *me* about religion; my religion is none of his business." Well and good. We do not propose any *obligation* for physicians and patients to engage in dialogue regarding religion. However, research does suggest that a substantial proportion of patients would welcome greater dialogue with their physicians about their religious concerns.[31-33] If so, we might turn an earlier concern on its head and ask, "Why should the preferences of those who do not want discourse be imposed upon those who do?" In addition, some will be troubled by the real possibility that relationships between physicians and patients who have differing religious commitments may at times be undermined by discourse that draws attention to those differences. Although they would likely be uncommon, such occasions would not be surprising. This is where the rubber of diversity meets the road of physician-patient communication. If a patient believes that the difference between his own and his physician's fundamental commitments warrants seeking another physician, such an accommodation, however extreme it may seem, is preferable to a paternalism (secular or religious) which would mask the very difference that the patient finds so important.

Where Do We Go from Here?

Medical education aims to teach the science and art of medicine, but it is not clear that a curriculum for wisdom can be realistically developed. Changes in the economics and practice of medicine are squeezing out the already limited opportunities for senior physicians to mentor medical students and residents in the moral discourse that deliberates about the good and offers wise counsel. In addition, mentorship in practical wisdom depends upon what Aristotle calls *moral virtue:* "Virtue makes us aim at the right target (i.e., the patient's good), and practical wisdom makes us use the right means."[20] Unfortunately, much of medical training still consists of a "hidden curriculum"[34] which does anything but foster the virtue characterized by wisdom, candor, and respect. Given such obstacles, there will be no simple solution or magic bullet. However, we suggest that as medicine endeavors to recover a discipline of moral discourse, such deliberation is likely to be sustained by those communities, both secular and religious, that preserve a vibrant tradition of moral discourse. We remain hopeful that physicians at every level of training might step back from the pressure of daily practice to identify the ways in which wisdom, candor, and respect are fostered, and then make choices to encounter those ways.

Conclusion

In the end we propose a simple approach. Physicians who engage patients in discourse regarding religion should do so in an ethic of friendship, marked by wisdom, candor, and respect. Whether a particular conversation is ethical will depend on the character of those involved and the context of their engagement. In the meantime, the medical profession should exercise restraint in formulating both prescriptions and proscriptions regarding the content of physician-patient discourse. Neutrality is not an option. Physicians must and regularly do make moral choices according to their consciences. To make such choices wisely, physicians will at times need to engage with patients in dialogue regarding religious commitments and concerns.

References

1. Astrow AB, Puchalski CM, Sulmasy DP. Religion, spirituality, and health care: social, ethical, and practical considerations. Am J Med. 2001; 110:283-7.
2. Koenig HG. MSJAMA: Religion, spirituality, and medicine: application to clinical practice. JAMA. 2000; 284:1708.
3. Post SG, Puchalski CM, Larson DB. Physicians and patient spirituality: professional boundaries, competency, and ethics. Ann Intern Med. 2000; 132:578-83.
4. Sloan RP, Bagiella E, Powell T. Religion, spirituality and medicine. Lancet. 1999; 353:664-7.
5. Sloan RP, Bagiella E, VandeCreek L, et al. Should physicians prescribe religious activities? N Engl J Med. 2000; 342: 1913-6.
6. Scheurich N. Reconsidering spirituality and medicine. Acad Med. 2003; 78:356-60.
7. Lawrence RJ. The witches' brew of spirituality and medicine. Ann Behav Med. 2002; 24:74-6.
8. Feinstein AR. Is "quality of care" being mislabeled or mismeasured? Am J Med. 2002; 12:472-8.
9. Childress JF, Siegler M. Metaphors and models of doctor-patient relationships: their implications for autonomy. Theor Med. 1984; 5:17-30.
10. Cohen CB, Wheeler SE, Scott DA. Walking a fine line: physician inquiries into patients' religious and spiritual beliefs. Hastings Cent Rep. 2001; 31:29-39.
11. Lo B, Ruston D, Kates LW, et al. Discussing religious and spiritual issues at the end of life: a practical guide for physicians. JAMA. 2002; 287:749-54.
12. King DE. Spirituality and medicine. In: Mengel MB, Helleman WL, Fields SA, eds. Fundamental of Clinical Practice. New York, NY: Kluwer Academic/Plenum Publishers: 2002; 651-70.
13. Bessinger D, Kuhne T. Medical spirituality: defining domains and boundaries. South Med J. 2002; 95:1385-8.
14. Tarpley JL, Tarpley MJ. Spirituality in surgical practice. J Am Coll Surg. 2002; 194:642-7.
15. MacIntyre A. Whose Justice? Which Rationality? Notre Dame, IN: University of Notre Dame Press; 1988.
16. Aquinas T. Summa Theologica. Second Part of the Second

Part. Section 23. Article 1. Notre Dame, IN: Ave Maria Press; 1981.

17. Wadell PJ. Friendship and the Moral Life. Notre Dame, IN: University of Notre Dame Press; 1989.
18. Cohen CB, Wheeler SE, Scott DA, Edwards BS, Lusk P. Prayer as therapy. A challenge to both religious belief and professional ethics. The Anglican Working Group in Bioethics. Hastings Cent Rep. 2000; 30:40-7.
19. Brett AS, Jersild P. "Inappropriate" treatment near the end of life: conflict between religious convictions and clinical judgment. Arch Intern Med. 2003; 163:1645-9.
20. Aristotle. Nicomachean Ethics. Ostwald M. translator. Book Six. Upper Saddle River, NJ: Prentice Hall; 1999.
21. MacIntyre A. After Virtue: A Study in Moral Theory. 2nd ed. Notre Dame, IN: University of Notre Dame Press; 1984.
22. Carrillo JE, Green AR, Betancourt JR. Cross-cultural primary care: a patient-based approach. Ann Intern Med. 1999; 130:829-34.
23. Laine C, Davidoff F. Patient-centered medicine. A professional evolution. JAMA. 1996; 275:152-6.
24. Snyderman R, Weil AT. Integrative medicine: bringing medicine back to its roots. Arch Intent Med. 2002; 162:395-7.
25. Gordon JS. Holistic medicine; advances and shortcomings. West J Med. 1982; 136:546-51.
26. Hall DE, Koenig HG, Meador XG. Conceptualizing "religion": how language shapes and constrains knowledge in the study of religion and health. Perspect Biol Med. 2004; 47:386-401.
27. Weber M, Mills CW, Gerth HH. From Max Weber: Essays in Sociology. New York, NY: Oxford University Press; 1958.
28. Wolterstorff N. Religion in the University. The Taylor Lectures for 2001. New Haven, CT. Yale Divinity School; 2001: [Unpublished; available on cassette from Yale University Divinity School.].
29. Milbank J. Theology and Social Theory: Beyond Secular Reason. Malden, MA: Blackwell Publishers; 1993.
30. Hall DE, Curlin F. Can physicians' care be neutral regarding religion? Acad Med. 2004; 79:677-9.
31. Ehman M, Ott BB, Short TH, Ciampa RC, Hansen-Flaschen J. Do patients want physicians to inquire about their spiritual or religious beliefs if they become gravely ill? Arch Intern Med. 1999; 159:1803-6.
32. King DE, Buslawick B. Beliefs and attitudes of hospital inpatients about faith healing and prayer. J Fam Pract. 1994; 39:349-52.
33. MacLean CD, Susi B, Phifer N, et al. Patient preference for physician discussion and practice of spirituality. J Gen Intern Med. 2003; 18:38-43.
34. Rafferty FW. Beyond curriculum reform: confronting medicine's hidden curriculum. Acad Med. 1998; 73:403-7.

38 Daniel

Margaret E. Mohrmann

During the time when Sherry's life was dwindling to its close, I was called to the delivery room one afternoon on a semi-urgent basis. The little information I was given over the phone indicated that the obstetrics staff had thought the mother was having a spontaneous abortion — a miscarriage — of a fetus under the age and size of viability. However, the baby, once it appeared, was larger and more mature than they had expected and showed some vigor. A pediatrician was needed after all — but don't rush, they said. They did not expect the baby to survive, but the mother was anxious that everything be done, so they thought it would be politic to have a pediatrician pronounce the child officially "unsalvageable," as the term of art was, and probably still is, as though a human life were analogous to treasure hidden deep on the ocean floor, out of reach of human efforts to snag and retrieve it.

Silently, or maybe not so silently, cursing the bad judgment that had not involved us earlier — easy to do with the clarity of hindsight — I gestured to the medical student to join me, and we strolled the five flights down, two blocks over, five flights up to the delivery room. Along the way, I held forth to my captive student audience on the topic of interdepartmental politics surrounding decision making about fetuses on the cusp of viability.

When we arrived, a nurse pointed us the way to the room where we would find the baby. The room was dimly lit and cool. Over against the far wall, in a line of baby warmers — although this appeared to be a delivery room, it was obviously being used more for storage than for deliveries — stood the obstetrics resident, poking hesitantly with one finger at the chest of a very small baby boy. The warmer was not on; no oxygen was in use. "Oh, good," he said. "You're here. The mother really wants this baby, so I thought maybe we should do what we could."

Well, I thought, you *could* warm him up a bit; you *could* actually *do* something for him. I said, "Fine, here we are," and peered at the baby as I elbowed the obstetrician out of the way. He looked to be close to 1,000 grams and, at first glance, maybe at thirty-two weeks' gestation, which put him well within the limits of viability for premies in 1974. His hair was sparse and fuzzy, his light chocolate skin soft and dry, with some of the wrinkles associated with greater maturity, as opposed to the sleek otter look of the very young premie. Moreover, despite the resident's ineffective care, he was making spontaneous movements and looked like a live baby, not a dead fetus. I jumped into action that by now was rote. Turn on the warmer, check the baby's vital signs. No Apgar score had been given — they did not expect a real baby, after all — and it was now much too long after delivery (twenty minutes? thirty?) to think about that. Nevertheless, the clinical evidence used for Apgar scores was still relevant. Pulse, respiratory effort, muscle tone, color, responsiveness? He was making a weak, desultory effort to breathe, his pulse was slow but steady, and, although he was dusky in color, he did make significant voluntary movements. Not bad, given the circumstances. I placed the ventilating bag over his face and began forcing air into his lungs while I got some information from the resident.

The baby's thirty-five-year-old mother had been trying to get pregnant for many years. This much-desired pregnancy had been free of problems until she had been found on a routine examination to have an "incompetent" cervix and to be at imminent risk of losing the fetus. The obstetricians immediately made an attempt to tighten the cervix, but during the procedure she went into premature labor that could not be stopped. The baby was thought to be of a gestational age (somewhere around twenty-six weeks) and of a weight (estimated to be less than 600 grams) that would not be compatible with extrauterine life then. Therefore no one expected to need a pediatrician. When the baby popped out and cried spontaneously, the mother begged them to do whatever they could to save him: thus the resident's half-hearted attempts at resuscitation in the back room, thus the pro forma call to a pediatrician. It had taken the obstetrics team a while to decide to do any of that. Added to the time it took us to "not rush" over there, it had been more like forty-five minutes since the baby had taken his first breath. Having told me all he knew about the situation, the resident left to attend to the baby's mother.

As I forced oxygen into the baby's lungs, he began moving more, his color improved, and his heart rate climbed into the normal range. What was foremost in my mind, however, was the extended time during which the baby, so I assumed, had been without adequate oxygen. I looked up at the medical student, who was handling his own anxiety by continuous monitoring of the infant's heart rate with his stethoscope. He called out to me each minute the relatively unchanging numbers — 160, 162, 158, 166 — as as though they were a litany of health or of success.

"What are we doing?" I wondered aloud. *Should* we be resuscitating this child? Even if he survived — and I was by no means sure he would — did he not run an enormous risk of being significantly damaged by that long hypoxic period? Were we just "creating," if anything, a baby likely to have severe cerebral palsy? But now the baby was breathing well on his own. What was done was done and could not be undone.

Had my automatic rescue reflexes, assiduously developed over the past couple of years, done something truly immoral here? I was entirely confused. This was not a subject that had ever been discussed in medical school or in my residency thus far. There had been the delivery I had attended the month before when a baby with severe hydrocephalus had been delivered vaginally instead of by Caesarean section. Apparently the diagnosis had been missed, disregarded, or downplayed — I do not know those details — and the enormity of the baby's head had not been recognized until it was inescapably apparent during the delivery. The extraction was difficult, to say the least, requiring a dangerous amount of time and effort to get that large head through the cervix and past the pelvic brim. The dreadful consequence of using the vaginal route was immediately obvious: the baby's huge head had been dramatically compressed, such that cerebral tissue had been squeezed out of the cranial vault, like toothpaste, through the gap at the bony suture lines. I could feel the skull bones, vertical like the sides of an open cereal box top, on either side of the baby's impossibly long narrow head, and then nothing but mushy brain for six inches above where the bones ended. The baby showed no signs of life and we decided not to attempt resuscitation. This was brain damage beyond speculation, this extrusion of cerebrum, squirted away from its anchorage in the all-important brainstem.

That case seemed clear; this one was not, and I had no senior person with me this time nor previous teaching in my head to guide me. I let the baby call the shots. He was breathing, circulating, moving: so be it. Let's take him to the N.I.C.U. On the walk back, the baby in my arms, wrapped in several blankets — there was at this time a certain casualness with premature infants that is well-nigh unbelievable today — I hashed over the problem in my head and came to the conclusion that, from this point on, we should just keep the baby comfortable and attempt to feed him. If he made it, fine; if not, not. But no "heroics": no ventilator, no workup or treatment for sepsis, overwhelming infection. It would be a blessing if some infection took him away quickly and relatively painlessly. We would have given him a chance, and he could either fight his way through or not. That sounded right to me, a good balance that honored the mother's wishes and the baby's theoretical potential but also took seriously the damage done by the long delay before adequate resuscitative measures had been employed. I shared my moral reasoning with the medical student, who managed to look both suitably impressed and dubious and had little to say.

In medical school, we had been told repeatedly that soon we would be in situations in which what we did and did not know about, say, a resuscitation technique or the dose of a medication would determine whether someone lived or died. I was already beginning to realize that this was not quite true, that there were few pieces of medical knowledge or skill whose absence could make such a difference, especially given that residents generally do not practice in solitude. However, I was now also starting to see, with a sort of growing horror that I could not yet let myself examine, that I could, in fact, determine life or death through just the sort of uninformed and insufficiently analyzed moral decision that I was taking upon myself in this situation — a possibility that had never been broached in my education. I am not sure that the addition of instruction in bioethics to medical school curricula in the years since then has done much to alter that discrepancy. It is one thing to teach modes of analyzing and resolving identified bioethical dilemmas; it is quite another to form reflective physicians, able and willing to recognize and address with compassion, humility, and discretion the moral questions that arise continually in the day-to-day care of vulnerable persons.

The baby weighed 930 grams and was assessed to be of thirty-one weeks' gestation. He looked great for the next couple of days. He required no supplemental oxygen, made some attempts to suck a nipple, kept his temperature and heart rate stable and well within the normal range. His mother was overjoyed; she spent as long as she was allowed, sitting in a wheelchair beside her son's incubator, sometimes reaching out a finger for the baby — now named Daniel — to grasp. I was surprised but unmoved in my assessment and continued to be pessimistic in my conversations with his mother, trying not to let her get her hopes up either that Daniel would survive or, if he did, that he would be a normal baby.

On his third day of life, Daniel did not look so good. He was listless and showed some irregularities of temperature and pulse rate. In a premature newborn, this cluster of nonspecific signs is always reason to go looking for and treat on the presumption of sepsis. When the senior resident said as much, my immediate response was to call upon my earlier reasoning about the baby's likely prognosis to pronounce a sepsis workup and treatment ill-advised.

The resident looked at me quizzically. "How long a trial do you intend to give him? He's been fine for almost seventy-two hours. What else does he have to do to prove to you that he's worth treating? Have you looked at *him,* at Daniel, these past few days, or just at your own assumptions about him?"

I stared at him dumbly, and the images of the Daniel I had been examining, checking on, watching with his mother flitted through my mind. He looked and behaved like a real baby, an intact, albeit small and immature, baby. How could I have missed that? My supervisor's words triggered a sort of vision of Daniel's near future: of course, he could grow and mature and be able to go home with his mother. We would see if he had some problems in the future, but he did not appear to be severely damaged, nothing like what I had feared as I resuscitated him in that storage room. Right. Learn something every day. Thank God they don't let me make all the decisions around here.

I did the sepsis workup, which turned out to be negative, and treated him with antibiotics for forty-eight hours, during which time he returned to his previous vigorous state. His recovery of health was unlikely to have been due to the antibiotic treatment. Perhaps he had just been having a bad day, but with premies it may be impossible to know the difference between a bad day and impending doom. I began to talk with his mother about the future, to join in her joy at this unexpected gift of the child she had wanted for so long.

A few weeks later, after Daniel started gaining weight and becoming even more alert, he had another "bad day," another episode of listlessness and decreased appetite, this time accompanied by a slight rise in body temperature, that again signaled the possibility of sepsis — so another sepsis workup was in order. I explained the necessity to his mother and asked her to sit out at the nurses' station while I did the workup. She sat on one side of a tall desk, watching me work. Sitting on the other side of the desk was one of my fellow interns, who had worked in the nursery with me the month before and had returned to complete some paperwork. He and Daniel's mother could not see each other sitting there. He too watched me setting up to do the lumbar puncture and then made one of those collegial, joking remarks that we all used as part of our in-house language with each other. I do not even remember the terms he used now, only that they were disparaging to the patient and suggested that our valuable time and effort were wasted on the likes of him. I winced as he said it, shook my head at him, and said something that I intended to sound professional and serious, to signal to him that this was not the time for such banter. But too late.

Daniel's mother rose up majestically from her chair, peered down at him over the top of the desk, and said, slowly and forcefully, "That is my child you're talking about. What do you mean by saying that?"

The intern turned scarlet and apologized inarticulately, trying vainly to defend the indefensible, and then made a hasty exit from the N.I.C.U. Daniel's mother sat back down with a harrumph and a scowl. I apologized also, without attempting to defend what he had said or that he had said it. All that stuff we were so used to throwing around, all the jokes about our patients that we thought lightened our load but that, more likely, served only to make us feel temporarily impervious to the horror, the grief, the pathos of it all — all of it, indefensible. Once I heard it with her ears, Daniel's mother's ears, I knew, and I was ashamed. I cannot pretend I stopped participating in it from that day; I was much too interested in being part of the professional socialization going on in my residency to exclude myself from the argot. But I never lost the discomfort I learned that day, and I began monitoring myself — not only monitoring the surroundings for listening layfolk, but monitoring myself in order to avoid language that I would not be willing to use to a parent, whether there was a parent around or not.

There is much discussion now of a "dehumanization"

characteristic of today's N.I.C.U.s, full of sophisticated technology that demands as much or more interest and attention than do the babies it is designed to aid. My experience in a pretechnology N.I.C.U., however, suggests that innovative machinery is not necessarily the prime culprit in obscuring the human status of these tiny patients. Dehumanization — blindness to or disregard of the humanity shared by patient, doctor, and family — begins, I believe, with the problem of being an intern: naïve, frightened, thrust into extraordinary situations with insufficient guidance or support, trying hard to be "professional" while having few clear models, the intern's supervisors having learned their professional demeanor in the same dysfunctional way. The pediatrician-in-training is then asked to care for, and about, infants whose prematurity limits significantly their ability to project a fully human identity, a personality. (Many nurses and doctors with long experience working with premies will insist that the babies have distinct personalities. I agree, but I suggest that the assignment of individuality requires a sort of optimistic projection on the part of the observer, a mature and humane decision to recognize a premature infant as fully human, regardless of the baby's ability to evoke that response.) It takes wisdom that many young doctors may not yet have acquired to see the human being in the premature infant, and another kind of wisdom to keep constantly in mind the incalculable value of these babies to their parents. The attainment of this kind of understanding is not inevitable; the defenses learned during one's residency can be a very effective impediment to becoming a wise, humanizing doctor.

Daniel got through that sepsis scare as well as he had the earlier one and had no other interruptions during the rest of his stay in the N.I.C.U. He gained weight steadily and eventually went home with his very happy mother. I followed him, as his primary care pediatrician, for the rest of my residency, another two years and a few months, and he continued to do well, without any signs of damage from those long minutes without adequate oxygen. He was a normal, happy, thriving toddler when I last saw him, developing just as he ought with motor and social skills entirely appropriate for his age. And it is still Daniel I think of when I am tempted to ignore the incorrigible limits to our prognostic skills, no matter how excellent, or to forget the remarkable resilience of even the smallest human beings.

39 AIDS and the Professions of Healing: A Brief Inquiry

Stephen E. Lammers

Introduction

It is not controversial to claim that AIDS has presented the healing professions with a number of challenges, both technical and moral. In this essay I will speak about the particular challenges AIDS has presented to the healing professions, challenges which had as much to do with our societal circumstances as they had to do with the particulars of the disease itself in the late 1980s. What has not been widely celebrated is that there is a consensus within the medical and nursing professions that AIDS patients should be treated even though the patients can be a threat to the caretaker. What I hope to show is how fragile is that consensus, especially fragile because our current moral philosophy is not particularly helpful to us at this point.

This second point is not particularly controversial. Stephen Toulmin pointed up the difficulties of a certain type of philosophy in his essay, "How Medicine Saved the Life of Ethics."[1] In that article Toulmin argues that when philosophers began attending to modern medicine, they moved away from some debates that they had been having and moved towards a more fruitful, in Toulmin's eyes, understanding of human beings, especially human beings in community. Toulmin argues that philosophers had to start attending to the real needs of human beings, instead of worrying about their feelings. In addition, they had to go beyond the discussion of principles to the analysis of cases; thirdly, they had to start thinking about the professional settings within which the particular tasks and duties of so many of us arise, and finally, there was some attention once again to concepts such as equity and reasonableness. Principles alone did not enable persons to talk about professional matters. What Toulmin does not report is that there was a cost of doing medical ethics that way and that much of the cost was borne by the medical professionals, who were being told by the philosophers, and sometimes the theologians, that they had to learn more ethics. Needless to say, this was a message

1. *Perspectives in Biology and Medicine* 25:4 (Summer 1982): 736-50.

This paper was originally prepared for a symposium at Hope College in 1988. I would like to thank the students and faculty at Hope. Their questions led me to correct some of my errors. The rest of them are my own.

that was not often received with a welcome by the healing professions.[2]

At the same time that they were being asked to learn the language of modern ethics, health professionals confronted AIDS. We ought to notice that those persons in the medical profession who are treating AIDS patients are "teaching," and this by example, lessons in ethics which most of us will be unwilling to learn, and, in many cases, to honor. I will return to this later.

I. The Situation of Medicine Today

The healing professions have been under increasing pressure from the larger society. I am going to use the term "the healing professions," although it shall be clear shortly that I am going to focus upon medicine and not upon all of the healing professions. From time to time, I will notice how nursing, for example, might be similar or different from medicine, but nursing is not my main focus of attention. This has more to do with the limitations of time and space and not a lack of inherent interest in the topic.

One pressure comes from members of public interest groups and regulatory agencies who find the costs of health care to be exorbitant and who suggest that members of certain healing professions are greedy and that they are not careful with the public and private monies which they have been given for their work. In addition, there is a concern that medicine has become enamored of expensive technologies. One fairly recent consequence has been the introduction of DRG's, Diagnostic Related Groups, a way of categorizing hospital admissions and trying to give hospitals incentives to hold their costs down. Briefly, what this system does is to limit the amount of reimbursement a hospital can receive for a particular admission, depending upon the diagnosis. Hospitals are given a certain amount, for, say, a gall bladder case. If they can have the patient go home before they spend that money, the hospital can keep the difference. In such a payment plan, hospitals are no longer paid for each and every little thing that they do for and with the patient; they are paid by the case. There are proposals that physicians should receive reimbursement the same way. Obviously, this puts pressures upon hospitals and healers to perform more efficiently. It also should be clear that in their search for efficiency, healers might be tempted to display some biases, preferring younger patients to older ones, for example. These and other problems with DRG's could form the basis of another inquiry; for our purposes it is sufficient to note that the AIDS crisis came upon American medicine at a time when that medicine was under increasing scrutiny about the way in which medicine was practiced, especially the expense of modern medicine.[3]

This has not been the only pressure upon American medicine. At the same time that medicine was being criticized for being wasteful with the public's resources, other persons suggested that healers have been acting immorally, in that they have not permitted patients to exercise their wishes. The term used to describe this phenomenon is medical paternalism. What is argued is that healers assume that they know what is best for persons and they often ignore what patients want. In some forms, this argument asserts that modern medicine, which is often a medicine between strangers, assumed attitudes from the past, when medicine was practiced between friends. We do not have to determine whether such a golden age ever existed. All we know is that what is claimed is that physicians assumed that they knew what was best for their patients and often proceeded to act on what they thought they knew, instead of being guided by their patients. It is argued that this was immoral and should be stopped. Thus the effort to teach ethics to healers so that they will act appropriately.

There are good reasons why people might hold this latter point of view. After all, if the practice of medicine is understood primarily as the application of scientific knowledge, then the knowledge of science is not going to be of much help in resolving ethical questions. Indeed, according to some commentators, it is precisely the assumption that "doctor knows best" that causes many of our current problems in medical ethics. For what has been assumed, so say the critics, is a "generalization of expertise" which is unwarranted.[4]

Thus, healers were undergoing at least two different but not necessarily unrelated crises when AIDS came upon the scene. The first crisis had to do with health care costs and the second with the understanding of the profession. AIDS presented a number of problems, some of which are obvious and others which were not so obvious:

1. AIDS is a wasting disease. The body's immune system, compromised by the disease, cannot fight off ordinary infections. Thus persons with AIDS undergo often a long period where they decline through a number of hospitalizations. Thus far, medical science has been able to do little to reverse this course of events. Among the most devastating effects of AIDS is the diminishing of cognitive capacities in many AIDS patients. It is the case that many AIDS patients are "not themselves" from time to time while they are diseased and this presents difficult problems for physicians who are trying to determine what their wishes are. Further, AIDS is an expensive disease to treat. Often there are many hospitalizations.

2. There is no denying that those persons who were philosophers and theologians and who were invited into the medical setting had to learn the language of medicine.

3. Obviously, American medicine has gone much further in its attempts to control costs since this essay was originally written. Those further developments do not change the claim being made here, that AIDS came upon a medicine newly conscious of its responsibility to control costs.

4. Robert Veatch, "Generalization of Expertise," *Hastings Center Studies* 1:2 (1973): 29-40.

2. Persons with AIDS die, and the persons dying are often in the prime of life. Dying is difficult enough to deal with for healers; we know that beginning medical students are more fearful of death than the general population. When the dying is happening to people who are not old, it is harder on those who care for them.
3. AIDS often occurs in persons who are already stigmatized, if not by one or another member of the healing professions, by some members of the society at large. Thus persons who are homosexual or IV drug users, the two groups thus far most ravaged by this disease in our society, are persons often at the margins of our culture. Here the healing professions sometimes reflect the attitudes of the larger society, in that they join in the stigmatization,[5] and sometimes reflect an older perspective which promised care to anyone, no matter how they contracted their disease. Note that in this case, there are two reasons for the stigmatizing to occur. First, the persons who have AIDS often are engaged in behaviors that many Americans find reprehensible, and second, the disease itself often marks the victim.
4. AIDS threatens the healer. There have been a small number of persons in healthcare who appear to have converted to seropositive status as a result of their occupational exposure to the virus and not as a result of other activities. That is, they show signs of having been exposed to the AIDS virus. The expectation is that they will go on to develop AIDS.

   While the statistical possibility of becoming seropositive is small, the danger to the healthcare worker is perceived by many to be large, precisely because most persons who are seropositive go on to develop AIDS. As a result of this perceived danger, some healers have refused to care for patients either who are seropositive or who in fact have AIDS.
5. But that is only the most dramatic threat. AIDS threatens the healer because of the age of the victim; the young residents who take care of most of the AIDS patients in many public hospitals are closer to AIDS patients in age than their elderly dying patients or the dying infants they may see on the neonatal intensive care wards. This has led to what one author referred to as "AIDS burnout," when the young house officer simply becomes overwhelmed by the psychological toll of the disease.[6] What seems to be especially difficult is to go on in the face of one's own fears and the sense of inevitability that so far is part of the reality of AIDS.
6. Healers are put in a very odd situation, in that they are asked by their own profession to treat persons when such treatment may harm not only the healer but the healer's family. AIDS is passed by contact with body fluids, primarily semen and blood, and if the healer becomes seropositive, so might the spouse. Let me give an example here.

   In one scenario, a pregnant nurse (obviously, it could have been a pregnant physician) was worrying about a recent admission to the ICU because of the nurse's fear that the AIDS patient would suffer a cardiac arrest and she could not find a mouthpiece to create an airway to begin resuscitation while awaiting the crash cart and the team of physicians. In fact the patient suffered the arrest and she gave mouth to mouth resuscitation while awaiting assistance. In this case, not only was the nurse threatened, but also her fetus.
7. When there was a refusal to treat, this refusal to treat has been met with public criticism by the professions of nursing and medicine, although they are not the only ones involved. It is argued that healers have an affirmative obligation to treat persons. There is some tension between this claim and the AMA's statement that physicians have a right to choose their own patients, but the more recent AMA statements have been leaning in the direction of claiming that physicians have a duty to treat that is primary and their freedom of choice is secondary.[7]

While we recognize that some healers continue to give care to AIDS victims, others refuse and they are criticized. This leads me to my central question. On what basis do we ask these men and women to provide this care?

II. Societal Context for the Discussion of Professional Obligations

If we were asked to justify requiring healers to assist the victims of AIDS, what might we say? Most of us, I suspect, would want to make arguments that would lead to the conclusion that physicians have an obligation to treat AIDS patients. We would want to do this because although we may not be at risk for AIDS, or at least we are

5. For an account of how stigmatization can occur, cf. Douglas Shenson, "When Fear Conquers," *The New York Times Magazine*, February 28, 1988, pp. 34ff. Shenson points out the similarities between AIDS and leprosy.

6. Robert Wachter, "Sounding Board: The Impact of the Acquired Immunodeficiency Syndrome on Medical Residency Training," *New England Journal of Medicine* 314 (1986): 177-80.

7. Cf. "American College of Physicians Ethics Manual," *Annals of Internal Medicine* 103 (1984): 129-37, at 131-32. Cf. also American Medical Association Council on Ethical and Judicial Affairs, *Report on Ethical Issues Involved in the Growing AIDS Crisis* (November 1987).

It must be said that the AMA does not demand that each and every practitioner treat AIDS patients but it does insist that the practitioner should not exclude a class of patients from practice because they are HIV positive or have AIDS. In short, it is not something about which the practitioner is totally free; there are obligations which must be fulfilled, even if they do not have to be fulfilled in person. By this standard, those physicians who refuse to treat AIDS patients and who do not make provision for care fail to meet their affirmative duty. I am not claiming that this is an entirely satisfactory resolution of the question. All that should be noted is that the practitioners have lost some of their freedom; they cannot simply walk away from patients.

under the illusion that we are not at risk, we still may become the victim of some disease which is threatening to the healer and would like medical treatment.

It would seem, at first glance, that there are reasons to be fearful that we might not be treated. I want to use the recent work of Robert Bellah and others to make this point.

In their work, *Habits of the Heart,* Bellah and his colleagues attempt first to describe and then to critique some of the assumptions of what they take to be the dominant culture of American society, especially the American middle class.[8] Since it is from that class that the vast majority of physicians come, it would seem fair to look to this work for some indication of what one might think is being thought by the typical physician.

Bellah wants to argue that we have four languages which we might use in America to explain ourselves to one another. The first is the language of biblical religion, the second of the republican tradition, which focused on the good of the state. The third is the language of utilitarian individualism, and the fourth is that of expressive individualism. According to Bellah, the last two languages are the languages that we use to explain ourselves to one another. The languages of republicanism and biblical religion have lost their power in our culture. According to Bellah, most middle-class Americans do not use these languages to explain themselves, either to themselves or to one another. That was not always the case but is the case today. Before we turn to the present, let us take a quick look at the languages of the past.

What is the language of republicanism? This tradition grows out of the classical traditions of Greece and Rome. It assumes that both civic virtue and self-interest are the motivations of citizens. One participates in public life as a way of moral education and one attempts to achieve both justice and public good.

The biblical tradition is carried by Christianity and Judaism. In America, Protestant Christianity is its most influential carrier. One attempts to create a community in which a genuine human life can be lived. One did this under the judgment of a God who cherished you but also held you accountable if your actions led to the destruction of that genuine human life.

But it is the other two traditions which are the focus of much of Bellah's observations and criticism. In the perspective of the topic at hand, we can use the work of Bellah to ask how a health care worker who came at the world using the languages of individualism would understand their situation in terms of the AIDS epidemic.

Bellah starts by describing individualism, since he thinks that all four traditions do agree about one thing with respect to individualism. His claim is that all four traditions believe that the individual has inherent value. The biblical tradition might put this more strongly, claiming that the person was sacred, but there is agreement among all the traditions about the inherent dignity of the individual. There is disagreement, however, about the question, which has priority, the individual or the social order? The republican and biblical traditions claim that the social order is primary, the traditions of utilitarian and expressive individualism claim that the individual is primary.

Utilitarian individualism assumes that there are certain basic appetites, including the desire for power and the fear of sudden death at the hands of others. All of us are assumed to act to maximize our interests relative to those ends. Society arises out of a contract between self-interested individuals. There is a connection between an economic understanding of existence and this tradition.

Expressive individualism arises in reaction to utilitarian individualism. It argues that there is a core of uniqueness at the center of each person, and this core ought to find ways of developing and expressing itself. This core is not necessarily opposed to the center of every other person. Thus, it is possible for persons who hold this view to merge with other persons in their personal journey to express their own uniqueness.

What are the consequences of these views as they appear in our culture? First, argues Bellah, persons holding these views tend to see their lives as encompassed only by their job and their family, if they have one. There is little conception of a public life apart from a social life with like-minded individuals. Nor is one's work related to public goods. Second, one looks at situations in terms of what benefits and risks they represent for the self. In this context, associating with AIDS patients, especially early in the epidemic, was clearly a risky business and should be avoided. The method of transmission was not known for certain, and it appeared even then that the disease was going to be fatal. Our hypothetical utilitarian individualist, for example, would have no reason for associating with AIDS patients, especially when one took into account that the conception of the social world was encompassed by the family. What the rational utilitarian would do in these circumstances would be to avoid AIDS people.

Many physicians wanted to take this route. Yet inevitably, they were subjected to criticism by their peers. We might want to try to explain this criticism by some theory of a social contract, that there is some kind of agreement between a person who will be a physician and the rest of society. In return for the privileges of medicine, there will be some risks.

The social contract is explicitly mentioned in an interesting paper on this topic, and it is rejected as an adequate basis for the discussion of the issue. In a remarkable article in *The Journal of the American Medical Association,* Drs. Abigail Zuger and Steven H. Miles discuss what they call a rights model, a contract model, and a virtue model. Let me give their descriptions of these models and then make some observations about them.[9]

8. Robert Bellah et al., *Habits of the Heart: Individualism and Commitment in American Life* (Berkeley: University of California Press, 1985).

9. Abigail Zuger, MD, Steven H. Miles, MD, "Physicians, AIDS, and Occupational Risk," *JAMA* 258:14 (October 9, 1987): 1924-28.

In the rights model, the patient's right to care creates a duty on the part of healers. The duty is imposed upon the professions but not directly upon the individual healer. It is society which must make arrangements for the provision of medical treatment. This has the consequence that only two classes of physicians have obligations to care for patients who are infectious or who otherwise present a risk to the healer. These would be persons who work in emergency medicine or persons who work in public hospitals. A private practitioner could refuse to treat, under the rights model, on the grounds that he or she is simply exercising a civil liberty which is properly theirs. Thus the rights model gives the person who is ill a right to treatment, but it is a right which must be met by the society only and not the individual physician or nurse. If one is not treated, one has a claim against the larger society for not providing the treatment, but no reason to criticize a particular physician.

There is a second alternative, and here Zuger and Miles examine a version of the contract model. In that model, the assumption is that the contract is between the patient and the physician. The contract imposes a fiduciary obligation on the physician to act in the patient's best interest and to provide competent treatment. Voluntariness is preserved on both sides; the physician can leave after having made alternative provision for medical treatment. Alternatively, the patient may leave the physician at any time. The contract model does protect the infectious patient in that the physician is obligated to provide competent treatment and less than competent care cannot be provided in order to minimize the risk of infection. Note that the physician and patient allow both sides freedom about entering the treatment situation. If the physician does not wish to treat infectious patients, he or she is free to refuse to treat. Zuger and Miles are not content with either of these alternatives. They leave patients vulnerable and, as far as Zuger and Miles are concerned, they do not capture what is at stake in speaking about a physician's responsibility to patients in the face of danger to the physician.

Thus Zuger and Miles proceed to discuss a third alternative, a virtue model. Let me quote directly from the article, in order to give a sense of the flavor of the argument that is being made.

> A virtue-based medical ethic has powerful implications for the care of contagious patients in general, and HIV-infected patients in particular. It recognizes that all HIV-infected persons are in need of the healing art — for counseling and reassurance, if nothing else. It mandates, as well, that because of their prior voluntary commitment to the *professio* of healing, physicians are obliged to undertake the *officia* of caring for these patients. Individual physicians who fail to perform these *officia* are falling short of an excellence in practice implicit in their professional commitment.[10]

10. Ibid., 1927.

Thus Zuger and Miles come to what they call the moral art of medicine. Yet I fear that the moral art of medicine is one which is going to be difficult to sustain in our society.

First, notice the arcane language the authors use in order to explain the obligations of the physician, or in my language, the healers. For example, they speak of the end of medicine as a *professio*. It simply is not part of our vocabulary to speak of these matters in this way. Medicine, in modern parlance, has not one end but many, depending upon what the patient wishes.

Second, notice not simply the language but the implications of the language. The language is a language which involves certain moral commitments, commitments which have costs associated with them, costs in terms of time and materials. The patient's good is to be sought, not some other good or goods. AIDS is not cheap to treat and to ask healers to commit themselves to the treatment of persons with AIDS means that other diseases will go untreated. In an age which wishes to cut the costs of medical treatment, there is something ironic about criticizing healers for refusing to treat AIDS victims and at the same time asking them to cut the costs of medical care in general. If we wish to have AIDS victims treated, then we will have to pay for it. This is what we do not want to have to do. Thus right at the beginning of the process, we can identify difficulties. Indeed, the professional may wish to treat the AIDS victim, but in so doing the professional is making difficulties for another of society's wishes, that the cost of medical care should come down.

But there are further problems. How is a society which uses the language of utilitarian and expressive individualism identified by Robert Bellah going to sustain the vision which has been articulated by Zuger and Miles? The languages of utilitarian and expressive individualism are opposed to the language of virtue. Indeed, one might want to argue that these later languages are set up on the assumption that it would be better if we had a society that did not depend upon virtuous persons in order to be a good society and that we certainly do not go out of our way to produce them.

III. Some Uncomfortable Conclusions

This, of course, leaves us in a paradoxical situation. The behavior of the professional is clearly countercultural. That is to say, what is being maintained is a way of life apart from that of a larger society. We need a vision of what it means to be a healer that is not sustained nor, possibly, sustainable by the moral languages used in the larger society. We are in the odd circumstance of being dependent upon a profession but being unable to articulate the basis of our dependence, and absent that, our sense of what we might have as our responsibilities towards that profession. Further, without any expectation on the part of society, the profession has no conception of when it is or when it is not meeting its responsibilities to the society in which it finds itself. Finally, it should be clear by now that the treatment of AIDS, insofar as it is understood as a duty by the medical profession, has implications for the cost of medicine.

There are two alternatives which one might wish to consider at this point. One alternative would be to declare that if medicine wishes to develop in its practitioners the sense of virtue which is noted above, medicine will have to develop a community of its own to sustain that vision, since that vision is not sustained by the larger society. In this alternative, medicine would have to create its own community to sustain the kind of vision needed to create the kind of persons necessary to care for people with AIDS.

There is another alternative which has been explored by Stanley Hauerwas. Hauerwas would not have medicine create its own community but rely upon a community called church in order to sustain the persons who would practice an appropriate medicine. Hauerwas argues that only in such a community would it be possible to sustain the vision necessary to have these virtues, and to pass that story on to those who would be practitioners of the arts of medicine.[11] Such a vision of the community is an appealing one, in that it involves a willingness to have a medicine which is fallible, which is finite, which is humble in the face of mortality. What Hauerwas suggests, if only by implication, is that the larger society as presently constituted could not sustain such a vision.

Thus far I have been focusing on the responsibilities of the caretakers of the AIDS patient, responsibilities which, if I read the literature aright, we wish to say that the healers have but which we are not easily able to justify. Further, when we find a language which makes that obligation clear, it rings strangely in our ears; we are not quite sure what to do with it. Indeed, it intrigues me that most of the work done in modern ethical theory is not of much help here, since the emphasis upon freedom allows the healer to ignore the cries of the victim on the grounds that the healer is simply exercising his or her freedom. It seems that we are in the curious circumstance of having to learn from behavior that we cannot explain to ourselves, at least not with the languages of the majority culture.[12] We will have to learn, not simply a new set of problems as Toulmin suggested but a new moral philosophy, one learned this time by watching persons who appear to act rightly but who explain to us in languages most of us have difficulty understanding why it is that they do what they do.

But that takes me away from the point that I have been trying to come to for some time. What is at stake is not simply the responsibility of the healer to the victim, but the responsibilities of the larger society both to the victims and to the healers. That issue remains unaddressed in most of the literature. It remains unaddressed because the larger society has been unwilling to look upon the AIDS crisis as one in which it has been implicated. If there is one thing that one could learn by working one's way through Randy Shilts's book *And the Band Played On,* it is precisely this.[13] We are implicated, however, not only insofar as we are at risk for becoming an AIDS victim ourselves but also in the sense that we are being offered a chance to learn something about ourselves and our society and how we respond to difficult human situations. In this sense, we are comfortable in our righteousness criticizing the physician or nurse who refuses to treat AIDS people and at the same time unwilling to either support what they do with our own presence or in some other way that commits us to care for those persons stigmatized by the larger society. Someone else will do it for us, and then we will not have to ask ourselves how we shall deal with it. What is appalling in reading Shilts is to see how the many deaths in the gay community were not thought of as important as deaths in other communities; Shilts's favorite comparison is between the way in which the federal government mobilized for Legionnaire's disease and the way in which it did not mobilize for AIDS victims. While I do not think that Shilts has shown his implicit claim to be true, it is probable that a cure for AIDS could have been found if the United States had been willing to throw enough research dollars at the problem. I am sympathetic to his claim that not enough was done to help AIDS victims. I am also convinced that he is correct when he claims that this was not done because of who the victims were, or, at least, who the vast majority of the victims were.

I am not suggesting that we need to become experts in the care of AIDS patients; that is not the point. The issue is how we support those persons who care for AIDS patients and those patients themselves and what we are willing to commit to treating this particular disease. Most importantly, how we understand who we are as we do this and the reasons that we offer to one another are going to be important.

It is also going to be important that we begin working on what we owe to one another in terms of medical treatment. Whether or not AIDS had come along, the current difficulties in health financing would have developed, and we as a society are having difficulties facing up to them. With AIDS, we have to face up to them, to our responsibilities to victims of a disfiguring disease, and also to our responsibilities, if any, to the professionals that we

11. Stanley Hauerwas, "Salvation and Health: Why Medicine Needs the Church," *Suffering Presence* (Notre Dame: University of Notre Dame Press, 1986), pp. 63-83.

12. I cite only one article. John Arras has written a fine article on the responsibility of physicians to treat AIDS patients. At the end of the day, the most powerful part of the argument is his reference to the history of practice of physicians in the past. All his reference to ethical theory does not do the necessary work of convincing us that, indeed, physicians have duties towards people with AIDS. Cf. John Arras, "The Fragile Web of Responsibility: AIDS and the Duty to Treat," *Hastings Center Report* 18:2 (April/May 1988): 10-20.

13. Randy Shilts, *And the Band Played On: Politics, People, and the AIDS Epidemic* (New York: St. Martin's, 1987).

expect to care for these persons. It may seem odd to include our responsibilities to the healer, but I do this because I fear that we are in a situation in which the patient runs the risk of being excluded from the moral community, and then the healer who treats that patient will be excluded as well. Once you are no longer held to be responsible for your actions, you are excluded from the moral community. William May writes powerfully of how this happens to the elderly in our society, when we no longer hold them responsible for what they do and who they are.[14] I worry that in holding professionals responsible to care for us, even in praising them when they do that at risk to themselves, we might reinforce the notion that we (and by the "we" here I include all of us who will be patients) do not have any moral responsibilities in this area. We are not obligated to challenge one another to aspire to something greater. We do not challenge ourselves to try to find ways of assisting them in their illness, nor do we find ways to express our concern for them. In effect, we have excluded them from our world.

Here, it seems to me, we might appropriate Zuger and Miles's language for our own purposes, to argue for an understanding of the relationship of the self to the larger world which understands the self as having a vocation. To do that would be to ask us to abandon what Bellah calls our dominant languages. That choice is ours. If we do not do it, we will remain in the anomalous situation described above, where we can admire those persons who care for AIDS victims, but find it difficult to honor them. Further, we will set ourselves apart from both them and their patients, forgetting, of course, that one day we will be the patients. The alternative is to join with them and support them as they do their tasks, not in the blind adulation which so often marked the American love affair with medicine in the past, not in awe of medicine's technological skill which marks so much of the discussion of medicine today, but with an attitude of appreciation for what has occurred. Let me be clear, that it is not just the fact that AIDS victims were treated that we should appreciate, but that we learned that it is still possible in this society to envision our world in such a way that victims can be attended to. William May rightly reminds physicians that they must constantly remind themselves of what they owe their patients; without them the physician would not have a practice.[15] It seems to me that it would not be inappropriate for those of us who will be patients to remind ourselves of what we owe our physicians when they treat others, like ourselves, who are possessed by dangerous diseases.

14. William May, "The Aged: Their Virtues and Vices," in *The Patient's Ordeal* (Bloomington: Indiana University Press, 1991), pp. 120-41.

15. William May, *The Physician's Covenant* (Philadelphia: The Westminster Press, 1983).

40 *Exousia:* Healing with Authority in the Christian Tradition

Daniel P. Sulmasy

The contemporary Western world holds tenaciously to a demand for individual liberty which stands radically opposed to an ever increasing need for individuals to be dependent upon the expertise of others. Ironically, the banner of autonomy has been raised high at a moment in history characterized by profound interdependence in a complex, specialized, technological culture. Perhaps this conflict between the demand for independence and the demand for dependence is nowhere more readily apparent than it is in medicine.

It is easy, then, to see why the nature of authority should be such a thorny problem for contemporary society, and particularly for the practice of medicine. The many contemporary meanings of the word "authority" are perhaps reflective of the depth of the doubt about what authority actually is. This confusion is exemplified by the common observation that patients today often go to great lengths to get authoritative opinions regarding their various conditions, only to feel victimized because the very physicians who have rendered such opinions have treated them authoritatively.

Thus, the role of authority in the relationship between doctors and patients is usually understood as a struggle for power between doctors and patients. Power is generally understood as force of knowledge or force of will, and contemporary ethical arguments about authority in the doctor-patient relationship can usually be characterized as advocating either more or less power for either doctors or patients. But the central thesis of this essay is that, from a theological perspective, the whole basis of these arguments is wrongly conceived. The Judeo-Christian notion is best expressed by the Greek word for authority, *exousia.* The *exousia* to heal which Jesus gave his disciples (Mt. 10:1; Mk. 3:15; Lk. 9:1) has nothing to do with a struggle over knowledge and will between doctors and patients. To heal with *exousia* is to heal with an understanding that the only legitimate power (*dynamis*) expressed in the doctor-patient relationship is the *dynamis* of healing itself, and that this *dynamis* has a source which transcends and subsumes that relationship. A medical practice informed by *exousia*

From Gerald P. McKenny and Jonathan Sande, eds., *Theological Analyses of the Clinical Encounter* (Dordrecht: Kluwer Academic Publishers, 1994), pp. 85-104. Used with kind permission from Kluwer Academic Publishers.

might negotiate a new course, avoiding the pitfalls of both unconstrained patient autonomy and physician paternalism. The perspective of *exousia* provides an alternative vision for medicine at a time when the fragmentation of an individualistic medical marketplace and the bureaucratic dehumanization of an unbridled medical technocracy threaten the integrity of the entire medical enterprise.

The Many Meanings of Authority

The meaning of authority is anything but clear. Kierkegaard's complaint about the "confusion involved in the fact that the concept of authority has been entirely forgotten in our confused age" [18] remains valid even today. To help set the many meanings of authority into a framework from which analysis can proceed, I will place these meanings under three basic headings. I will designate an appropriate preposition or article for each of these three uses of the word. Finally, I will define the three senses in which the adjectival form, "authoritative," is most closely associated with each meaning of the noun, "authority."

1. *Authority as Control*

The most typical meaning of authority refers to force of will or the ability of one person to control another's thoughts, words, or deeds. It can refer either to the controlling power that a person actually possesses (e.g. — she is in a position of authority), or it can function as a noun designating the person who is in control, often in the plural (e.g. — she is wanted by the authorities). The typical preposition associated with this usage is "in." To be *in* authority is to have control. Using the word in this sense in a medical context one might say, "Doctors have too much authority." When the adjectival form, "authoritative," is used, it typically refers to an abuse of power or control (e.g. — that surgeon behaves authoritatively).

2. *Authority as Expertise*

The word "authority" is also frequently used when referring to knowledge, skills, precedents, and conclusive statements. It is especially used as a noun to refer to one who has such knowledge or skill. The typical article associated with this usage is "an." To be *an* authority is to possess knowledge and skills superior to others, often rendering the others dependent upon the authority for access to some good or service. Using the word in this sense in a medical context one might say, "Dr. Jones is an authority on ocular melanomas." When the adjective "authoritative" is used in this sense, it means that the opinion or answer is conclusive.

3. *Authority as Warrant*

A less common but by no means archaic use of the word refers either to the freedom granted by one who is in control, or to actions carried out with conviction. The preposition linked to this usage is "with." To act *with* authority is to act in the freedom granted one by someone else or to act with an apparent sense of legitimacy or conviction. In a medical context, using the word this way sounds unfamiliar. But one might say, for example, that "Dr. Smith practices with authority." When the adjective "authoritative" is used in this sense, its meaning can sometimes be approximated by the adjective "legitimate," sometimes by the adjective "genuine," and sometimes by both.

These three clusters seem to capture the families of meaning which come under the broad term "authority." They overlap, of course, and may exclude some marginal meanings of the term, but this classification ought to be sufficient for the purposes of this essay.

Authority, Hobbes, Locke, and Medicine

The use of the word "authority" in political philosophy depends heavily upon the English philosophers Thomas Hobbes and John Locke. This approach has been uncritically accepted by many as the primary means of understanding the role of authority in the doctor-patient relationship, particularly with respect to the concept of informed consent ([6], pp. 76-77; [8], pp. 44-47, 267-68; [10], pp. 13-14, 174-75, 369-73; [44], pp. 190-213). These authors use the word primarily in the first sense (authority as control). The word is also sometimes used in the second sense (authority as expertise), but generally with the assumption that expertise implies control (i.e. — to the extent that the doctor is *an* authority, the doctor is *in* authority). To understand the roots of this conception of authority, one must go to the sources.

For Hobbes, the questions surrounding authority begin with his convictions about human nature. "I put for a general inclination of all mankind a perpetual and restless desire of power after power, that ceaseth only in death" [*Leviathan,* Ch. XI]. Human beings, by nature, seek power, by which Hobbes means control. Liberty, for example, is simply the absence of external control [*Leviathan,* Ch. XIV]. Hobbes' convictions about ownership, coupled with his convictions about an innate human desire to control others and to be free from their control, defines what he means by authority. "He that owneth his words and actions is the AUTHOR: in which case the actor acteth by authority. . . . And as the right of possession is called dominion, so the right of doing any action is called AUTHORITY" [*Leviathan,* Ch. XVI]. Authority, then, is defined negatively: the absence of external control in the disposition of the actions and words one possesses. Finally, Hobbes is convinced that one will give up one's claims to authority only for greater gain, either by individual contract [*Leviathan,* Ch. XVI], or for the sake of self-preservation through participation in the commonwealth [*Leviathan,* Ch. XVIII]. Thus, the Hobbesian conception of authority essentially requires only two things: "effectively uncontested power and the right to rule" [19].

Locke's concept of authority is likewise connected to his concept of political power, which is described in terms of control. "It is impossible that the rules now on earth should make any benefit, or derive any the least shadow of authority from which is held to be the fountain of all power, 'Adam's private dominion and paternal jurisdiction' . . ." [*Second Treatise on Government*, Ch. I]. Closely connected is Locke's concept of negative rights, which limit "the extent of the legislative power." Individuals are not to be interfered with, and others are given "power to make laws but by their own consent and by the authority received from them" [*Second Treatise on Government*, Ch. XI].

The key to understanding authority in contemporary political philosophy is to be aware of its Hobbesian/Lockean roots. Power, considered as the ability to control and be free from control of others, is the implicit assumption which dominates contemporary discussions of authority. Friedman, for instance, suggests that whether one considers authority as the ability to rule or influence (*in* authority), or the ability to inspire belief (*an* authority), it is always control which is at issue. He argues that one must surrender control by surrendering private judgment either in obeying a command or in accepting a premise on authority [14]. Similarly, Raz [36] admits that the contemporary notion of authority comes from a coercive concept of law. However, he suggests that authority be thought of primarily as a moral right to impose a duty, and only secondarily as a right to coerce others into compliance with these duties. But his bottom line is coercion, and the moral right to impose a duty must still be understood as control. Therefore, in contemporary political philosophy, authority is inevitably seen in conflict with autonomy [46].

Both the impetus for the dramatic new role of patient autonomy in medical decision making and the recent evolution of the doctrine of informed consent have depended upon a Hobbesian/Lockean conception of authority in the doctor-patient relationship. Flathman [12], for instance, paints a Hobbesian picture of doctors and patients. He sees two basic models of authority in the relationship:

1. a consensual model in which the physician is authorized to practice only so long as the physician's actions are congruent with the consensually agreed upon values of the community, and
2. a constrained conflict model in which there is no general consensus, and so physicians are placed *in* authority inasmuch as patients will do what physicians say despite their disagreement.

Flathman feels that the latter is more realistic. Patients reluctantly accept dependence upon experts because the price of not doing so is to give up the services the experts provide. Power dominates Flathman's discussion. Knowledge is power. Power is control. Therefore, as experts, physicians exert control through the power of their knowledge. And thus, life in the waiting room is inevitably solitary, poor, nasty, brutish, and short [cf. *Leviathan*, Ch. XIII].

Veatch [43] is also influenced by Locke and Hobbes. He details how physicians do, in fact, act coercively, by controlling access to hospitals and drugs, committing suicidal or psychiatric patients to involuntary admissions, or administering required immunizations. Veatch accepts, however reluctantly, the necessity of giving such control to physicians. Physicians have the expertise to protect the healthy and the sane from the contagious and the psychotic. But while Veatch denies that there are any "value-free facts," he also claims to be able to distinguish facts from values in medical decision making. He insists that the authority of physicians be limited wherever possible to the technical arena, which is more factual than evaluative. He argues that the physicians should be *in* authority only to the extent that the physician is *an* authority. In effect, Veatch argues that patients own not only their bodies, but also the evaluative ideas they have about illness and treatment. Since medical decision making inevitably involves not only the patient's body but also all that the patient values, all medical authority properly belongs to the patient. Even though he thinks it is epistemologically impossible for a real physician to do so, Veatch's ideal physician would dispense "valueless," objective information about the body to patients, who must, regrettably, depend upon physicians for this information. Patients would then be independent in their decision-making. What is at stake in Veatch's theory is, of course, control. The authority of physicians is based on their technical expertise, which defines, for Veatch, the moral limit of their control over patients. He writes, "No one in his right mind would conclude that those who are custodians of a particular value [knowledge of the body] should bear the responsibility for resolving disputes over the relation of that value with other values leading to one's integrated wholeness" [43]. Veatch worries that physicians, like Locke's princes, may overstep their prerogatives. Veatch's solution seems to be equally Lockean. He seems to urge patients, as Locke once urged the prince's subjects, "to get prerogative determined in those points wherein they found disadvantage from it" [*Second Treatise on Government*, Ch. XIV]. That is, Veatch seems to argue that the controlling authority of physicians can be to the disadvantage of patients and hurt them. Therefore, patients should seize control of those liberties traditionally given to doctors which have led to problems for patients. In declaring limitations on the doctor's latitude, Veatch could easily quote Locke and insist that no physician should complain about such a program of transferring control from physicians to patients, "because in so doing they [the patients] have not pulled anything from the prince [physician] that of right belongs to him" [*Second Treatise on Government*, Ch. XIV].[1]

1. It is of interest that while Locke was trained as a physician, he never saw any patients professionally.

The Inadequacies of the Control Model

There are several underlying assumptions in the control model of authority which must be critically examined. These assumptions are foundational. They are so deeply embedded in the ethical theories which flow from them that they often escape attention. But an exposition of these assumptions seems necessary in order to explain some of the difficulties one faces in considering the concept of authority in contemporary medicine, and to look for fruitful alternatives.

Human Nature

First, these Hobbesian and Lockean theories of authority make implicit but striking assumptions about human nature. These assumptions about human nature are certainly not value-free. Notwithstanding Veatch's insistence that physicians be strictly limited to evaluative judgments about the body as such, the theories of both Flathman and Veatch begin with sweeping evaluative assumptions about the nature of the actors in the doctor-patient relationship. First, these theories assume that human beings constitutively seek personal liberty and control over others. Therefore, no one, whether a doctor or a patient or a Native American Chief, is worthy of trust. Second, these theories take the voluntary contract forged between equals to be the paradigmatic human ethical interaction. Therefore, as Hauerwas [16] has observed, these theories presuppose that "all relations that are less than fully 'voluntary' [are] morally suspect."

But such assumptions are largely untrue, particularly in the medical context. First, while acknowledging the reality of sin, it must be argued why one should accept the Hobbesian notion that the primary human drive is to control others and be free of their control. Christian belief, for example, suggests that the primary drive is to love and to be loved. In fact, most persons *can* name other persons that they can trust, and many would place their physicians on their list. Only the most distraught and disheartened say, in their alarm, that no one can be trusted [Ps. 115:2]. Those who cannot count their physicians among the trustworthy generally want another physician, because they understand the critical importance of trust in the doctor-patient relationship.

Second, the most paradigmatic human interactions are not voluntary contract interactions between equals, but involuntary relationships between unequals [4]. The most important human relationships are the ones over which people have no control. No amount of innovation in reproductive technology will ever allow people to choose their own biological parents. Each person enters this world helpless, completely dependent upon others. People have no power to declare themselves immortal or free of the possibility of disease. These conditions are out of human control. And it is precisely in the midst of this absence of control and in relation to the state of dependency which illness engenders that the ministrations of medicine are meted out.

Veatch notes the inadequacies of "raw contracting" as the moral basis of the relationship between doctors and patients, but he unfortunately merely replaces the notion of raw contracting with a boiled down form of contracting [43]. In so doing, he continues to cling to the notion that control is the basis of the doctor-patient relationship. But this view is contradicted by a reality which cannot be otherwise. The doctor-patient relationship is predicated firmly on the fact of illness, which entails the loss of control.

Finally, the increasing interdependence which constitutes our contemporary social relationships, particularly in the medical arena, ought to provide a clue that human beings are not inherently atomistic, but inherently social and interdependent. As Aquinas put it, "man has a natural inclination to know the trust about God and to live in society" [*Summa Theologiae*, I, II, q. 94, art. 2.c]. It would seem obvious this is neither Veatch or Flatham's view of human nature.

Human beings are flawed, of course, and often fail to live out their potential. But a judgment that human beings are naturally selfish and that any behavior which appears to be goodness is really self-interest merely begs the question. Nor is this a matter which can be settled by experience. Experience teaches us only the following: some doctors are mostly good, and some doctors are mostly bad. It will remain an axiomatic choice, a faith assumption, to decide whether the fragile vessel of the physician is a glass half empty or a glass half full. The assumption of the Roman Catholic tradition of Christianity is optimistic: grace can build upon the reasonableness of human nature. Other Christian traditions are not so optimistic about the state of human beings outside of grace, but are at least optimistic to the extent that they believe in the power of grace to fill the fragile human vessel. In contrast to the Hobbesian assumption, Christian belief points to an open possibility that human beings can be better than they are now. Neither physicians nor anyone else will ever be better unless this possibility can be assumed.

An HMO with Only One Member?

The second problem with the control model is that it assumes an intersubjectivist morality for medicine. It assumes that all moral truth in medicine resides in the subjectivity of the autonomous individual. But since individual patients need other individuals called doctors when they seek healing, this poses a problem. More than one subjectivity is involved once a person enters a human relationship. How is one to settle differences if neither has a greater claim to be in the right? The only possible solution under the assumptions of the control model is to construct an *intersubjective* morality, either by contract or consensus. But since such intersubjectivity is never quite objectivity ([22], p. 22), the project is doomed to fail.

Veatch [43] and Engelhardt [8, 9] appear to argue along the following lines. They begin with the assumption that each individual is his or her own moral authority. As Flathman argues [12], when there is complete consensus on what the good is for medicine, there is no need for any external authority in medicine. But Veatch and Engelhardt both agree that such an intersubjective consensus does not exist. Therefore, they conclude that patients and doctors whose views overlap ought to seek each other out, forming voluntary communities of intersubjective agreement in medical morals in which authority can function.

The problems with this view are significant. Taken to its logical conclusion, the theory implies that each person ought to become his or her own personal Health Maintenance Organization (HMO). If there truly is no source of authority (conceived of as control) other than oneself, and conflict is inevitable because human nature implies a need to control others and to be free from their control, then each individual would ideally be his or her own personal health care system, in complete control of his or her own care and free from the control of doctors. Ideally, one supposes, all medical information about one's own body could be processed and analyzed by a computer which would be programmed to provide the treatment one selected from a range of options.

But such a view is far from reality and not ideal for anyone. Medicine is an intrinsically interpersonal enterprise. A purely rational computer medicine could never truly *care* for patients. Care requires persons. Yet Veatch's ideal of value-free information given to completely autonomous patients who are free to decide what to do with that information in light of their own subjective values can only be realized by a machine. No one of right mind would want to be cared for by a health care system which merely objectively provided information about the body and paid no attention to the value of the whole person. There is even emerging evidence that the doctor-patient relationship is itself part of the therapeutic effect [38]. In addition, medicine seems to require (at least in those important cases where people seek out doctors) the presence of another. Self-diagnosis and self-treatment are always dangerous, even for experts. Finally, it seems that medicine is not just an interpersonal interaction between two individuals. It is an inherently communal enterprise. Without a prior commitment of professionals to share knowledge with each other, a system of one-person HMOs, if ever started, would soon grow into an absurd system of isolated, proprietary medical data banks, limited by the narrow experiences of individuals who functioned as their own doctors. The Hobbesian would then face a dilemma. Since medical knowledge is control, and control is what the Hobbesian desires, to share his medical knowledge would be to relinquish precious control over others. In addition, sharing implies accepting information from others, and to do so would be to acknowledge their control over his life, and this too would be unacceptable to the Hobbesian. On the other hand, not to share might lead like-minded persons to be equally stingy, and then he would risk dying from a curable sickness that he would not have the knowledge to treat. Thus he would neither be able to share nor not share. The Hobbesian view cannot be sustained in the limit.

Now a Hobbesian might not concede that there is a problem with his assumptions. Painfully, the Hobbesian might say, the above ideal of private, value-free computer medicine is simply not possible, even though it really *is* what everyone would want. Therefore a Hobbesian patient would reluctantly compromise for the sake of personal interests and accept dependence on medical professionals, but only to the least degree compatible with the patient's interests in pleasure, health, and longevity.

But the counter-argument here is standard. If the real justification for accepting the control of others were the maximization of one's own best interests as one defines them, then the only consistent position would be to lie about one's acceptance of the controlling influence of others in order to gain the benefits offered by contract, but then to do as one pleases in order to escape the control enjoyed by the contract. For example, suppose that a Hobbesian smoker were to join an HMO which forbade smoking in order to eliminate the costs of caring for smoking-related diseases, thereby saving money for everyone in the HMO. The Hobbesian who loves to smoke might promise not to smoke in order to join this HMO and save money. But his actions would be most consistent with the underlying justification of the Hobbesian theory (i.e., self-interest), if he smoked whenever he could do so without getting caught. It is easy to see that once this process became generalized, the very basis for the compromise reached by the social contract would be destroyed. Thus the Hobbesian HMO, whether with one member or many, results in a *reductio ad absurdum*.

Medical Monasticism

As Finnis points out, groups can coordinate action to a common purpose or goal either through unanimity or authority ([11], pp. 231-33). But if there is no unanimity, and if the Hobbesian view is absurd, where can one look for a theory of authority in medicine?

MacIntyre notes that when groups cannot achieve what they must by acting as individuals, practices spring up to achieve those goals. Practices are not forms of political or organizational power, but organized, rule-governed enterprises requiring judgments about how to best understand particular cases or reformulate the rules in the light of particular cases [24]. Medicine, of course, is a practice. And practices are inherently prescriptive. The doctor is said to *prescribe* therapy. To make a prescriptive statements such as, "x ought to be done," is to make "a claim which by the very use of the words implies a greater authority behind it than the expression of feelings or choices" ([24], pp. 51-52). This is true no matter how much one may claim to "own" these feelings or choices.

MacIntyre [24] realistically surveys the contemporary West, in constant rebellion against all forms of tradition and authority, deeply divided and unable to form a consensus about anything, and wonders only why it has taken so long for society to come to the impasse now faced by medicine: the demand for absolute autonomy in the face of its increasing impossibility. In the dissolution of the culture he sees only a profession which has become, "not quite a craftsman's guild, not quite a trade union of skilled workers, not quite anything." He despairs of the possibility of ever achieving enough agreement on the nature and goals of medicine to ever have a true professional practice again. His only positive solution is the possibility of achieving small communities of patients and doctors with a common vision — a vision in which the Western world would be dotted with a series of HMOs operating as medical monasteries in these new Dark Ages. The West only awaits a "new St. Benedict" ([24], p. 263) who will be the founder of these medical communities.

But this view is ultimately also unsatisfactory. MacIntyre is right in calling medicine a practice and right that the institution of medicine is currently threatened by contemporary views of authority. But the practice of medicine still retains enough internal coherence to remain a unified practice. The bodies of atheists and of Christians remain, after all, fundamentally the same. While their ultimate moral views remain radically different, it is hard to see, in the end, how the proposals of Engelhardt ([8], pp. 336-69), Veatch [43], and MacIntyre [24] really differ, except that they vary in the extent to which each thinks that a series of distinct medico-moral communities is a goal to strive for or a state of affairs for which one might reluctantly settle.

Authority, Sociology, and Medicine

Political philosophy is not the only contemporary discipline with important views about authority in the doctor-patient relationship. Sociologists have a view of this relationship as well. The sociological view, however, shares important similarities with the view of political philosophy. The sociological understanding of authority is largely derived from the seminal work of Max Weber, who defined authority as the power to issue commands that will be obeyed ([45], p. 152). As in the work of Hobbes, conflict and control are the essential features for Weber. He did distinguish *Macht,* "the probability that one actor . . . will be in a position to carry out his own will despite resistance," from *Herrschaft,* "the probability that a command with a specific content will be obeyed by a given group of persons." But *Herrschaft* is still conceived of as one will controlling another will. It is simply a less overtly violent imposition of one will upon another. Weber distinguishes three types of justification offered for authority other than simple *Macht:* rational grounds, traditional grounds, and charismatic grounds ([45], pp. 324-52). But it seems, as Hauerwas has noted, that even Weber's typological tryptic "fails to clarify what it means to acknowledge an authority as legitimate" [16].

Talcott Parsons has addressed the issue of authority in the doctor-patient relationship forthrightly ([30], pp. 441-42, 464-65). While not referring to Weber directly in this regard, Parsons also clearly assumes a model of authority based on relationships of power. Parsons suggests a "social control" model based on the advantages to society of giving physicians control over individual patients. This theory results from Parsons' empirical observations. Yet his conclusions are undeniable *interpretations* of his empirical observations and cannot simply be unquestioningly accepted as factual. And even if it is the case that the interpretation of Parsons is true (namely, that doctors really do act as authority figures exerting social control over the ill), it cannot therefore be concluded that this is the way things *ought* to be. This would represent a genuine example of the "Naturalistic Fallacy"; a true violation of the fact/value distinction. The fact/value distinction requires that moral claims not be justified solely on the basis of factual claims ([5], pp. 336-79). On the strength of this principle, even if Parsons were correct in the judgment that physicians used authority to control patients, this would not imply that an interpretation of medical authority based on social control theory is morally correct.

These interpretations of authority as control, based on either sociological theories or the theories of political philosophy or both, are pervasive in the literature of medical ethics. Countless discussions of the conflict between autonomy and beneficence have essentially been based upon this interpretation. It has almost begun to seem as if the fundamental task for medical ethics is to find the proper balance of authority in the power relationship between physicians and patients, with beneficence interpreted to mean authority for doctors, and autonomy interpreted to mean authority for patient. For instance, in their book on informed consent, Faden and Beauchamp acknowledge that "the issue of proper authority for decision making is an implicit theme throughout this volume. In health care, professionals and patients alike see the authority for one decision as properly the professional's and authority for other decisions as properly the patient's" ([10], pp. 13-14). Empirical researchers have used this schema in part, perhaps, because it is amenable to quantification on scales generated by survey instruments and seems to capture at least some of the reality of the interactions between doctors and patients. I myself have fallen into this trap [41], but I am now convinced that the model so constrains the rich reality of the doctor-patient relationship that it is inadequate. A solution is not to be sought by accepting the basic correctness of the model and merely suggesting a shift from "unquestioning acceptance of physician authority, as embodied in the Parsonian model," to a "more egalitarian bargaining" state [20]. The problem lies with the Hobbesian assumptions of the sociological model itself.

Exousia, Dynamis, and Healing

When Jesus sent his disciples out into the world, he gave them "power and authority to overcome all demons and to cure diseases. He sent them forth to proclaim the reign of God and heal the afflicted" [Lk. 9:1-2; cf. Mt. 10:1 and Mk. 3:15]. In this passage, it is important to note that Luke attributes to Jesus a distinction between the power that heals (*dynamis* in the Greek) from the authority (*exousia*) to heal. This is a distinction which is made with remarkable consistency throughout the writings of the New Testament [1, 13, 15, 27]. In making this distinction, it would seem that Scripture is suggesting that neither force of will nor the power of expertise is at issue in a discussion of the authority to heal. This is a perspective which is remarkably different from any account of authority and healing based on Hobbesian/Lockean political philosophy or sociology.

In relation to healing, *dynamis* is the power of healing itself. It was *dynamis* that Jesus felt go out of him when the woman with the hemorrhage touched his cloak and was cured [Mk. 5:30]. *Dynamis* is the pure power to heal. *Dynamis* is power *for,* not power *over* others. In a neo-Platonic sense, *dynamis* is self-diffusive. It has nothing to do with force of will. *Dynamis* goes out from Jesus without his willing it.

Dynamis is also used to characterize expertise. Thus, Simon Magus, the magician, was said to have the *dynamis* to heal [Acts 8:9-25]. But *dynamis* is clearly distinguished from *exousia.* When Simon Magus eventually came to faith, he realized the insufficiency of mere *dynamis.* He also wanted the authority (*exousia*) to impose hands. But the apostles would not grant him that. The very fact that he wanted to buy *exousia* was an indication to them that he was unworthy. And when the Pharisees wanted to know how Jesus had the *dynamis* to forgive sin [Mk. 2:1-12], he avoided the word *dynamis* in his reply. He said, instead, that he had the *exousia* to both heal and forgive sin. He proceeded to demonstrate both.

Exousia presumes *dynamis,* but not vice-versa. In Greek usage *exousia* was an illusion if not backed by real *dynamis* [13]. *Exousia* meant "the warrant or the right to do something" [24]. Thus, *exousia* is really closest in meaning to the third definition of authority set forth at the beginning of this essay. *Exousia* denoted an inner sense, and even a "moral power" in Stoic thought [13]. In the New Testament, *exousia* refers to the rule of God in nature and in the spiritual world, and especially the freedom which is given to Jesus and which he gives to the apostles [13]. While *exousia* is exercised with respect to sickness, the elements, and demons, Jesus specifically rejects any political application of *exousia* [1]. His kingdom, as he tells Pilate, is not of this world [Jn. 18:36]. *Exousia* is intrinsically related to the *Logos.* Nothing takes place apart from the *exousia* of Jesus. It is the freedom given to the community which orients itself to the Word made flesh. Hence, it can never be used arbitrarily [13].

New Testament *exousia* cannot be bestowed or produced. It emerges in practice. It is not more Weberian charismatic authority, which can be used for either good or for evil. *Exousia* rests upon a practical and convincing insight into the Good, the True, and the Beautiful. It springs forth out of tradition. It becomes manifest upon recognition by the community ([15], p. 17). Hence, the magician who already had the *dynamis* to heal cannot buy *exousia* [Acts 8:9-25]. God rebukes those who misuse power as raw *dynamis* and deny the *exousia* of God [cf. Is. 5:8-9]. *Exousia* comes with experience, and is characterized by wisdom, equanimity, talent, charisma, and selflessness ([15], p. 17). William Osler himself could scarcely have done a better job of describing the virtues of a good physician. A physician might have the *dynamis* of actually being *an* authority, but without *exousia,* that physician will never heal *with* authority.

Exousia and Virtue

The Greek terms *dynamis* and *exousia* correspond to the Latin terms *potestas* and *auctoritas,* respectively. The Romans used *potestas* to describe the rule of Nero and Caligula, but *auctoritas* to describe the rule of Caesar and Augustus ([15], p. 52). The Western concept of rights as powers, a concept which strongly influences contemporary discussions of medical ethics, developed around the concept of *potestas* ([9], p. 61). Originally, *auctoritas* or authority had a meaning similar to that of *exousia.* But as discussed above, authority assumed a definition based on the concept of power in the writings of Hobbes and Locke. Since then, it seems that the distinction between power and authority (*potestas* and *auctoritas; dynamis* and *exousia*) has nearly vanished from Western writing. Consequently, contemporary writings about authority in the doctor-patient relationship have been largely oriented either to assert the traditional power of the doctor over the patient or to defend a revolt in which the patient's power is asserted over against the doctor's power.

Exousia represents, to some extent, a *tertium quid* in this examination of the relationship between doctors and patients. In the New Testament understanding, authority does not originate from either the patient or from the doctor. "Like everything human, the measure of excellence in authority is its ordination to God and its success in ordaining its subjects to God" [28].

Exousia is not itself a virtue. It is not an Aristotelian mean in the sense of being the just equilibrium point between the opposed poles of excessive control for either the doctor or the patient. *Exousia* is both an orientation to virtue and the fruit of the vine. *Exousia* results from the recognition by both the doctor and the patient that their relationship is not oriented to one or another of two individual human beings, but to a "third thing" (i.e., to God).

Exousia is an orientation to a *telos*. It is the recognition of the *telos* and the subordination of all related activities to the *telos*. As such, *exousia* is both orientation to virtue and the possibility of virtue. Without a *telos*, there is no virtue. To speak of virtue is to presume the authority of an excellence towards which virtuous activities are oriented. Virtue demands the recognition of authority. And, once one acknowledges an authentic *telos*, one's actions are expected to be virtuous.

Exousia may be likened to grace. One does not earn or own *exousia*. Yet, it can be expressed and it can be recognized. But it cannot emerge unless its divine source has been recognized. And unless it bears fruit in virtuous life and points beyond itself, any claim to *exousia* is disingenuous.

To practice medicine with *exousia* is to ordain one's practice to the good of the patient and to ordain one's practice for the good of the patient to the glory of God. In this way, the *dynamis* to heal, which is already given in nature and in human reason, not only becomes actual but has a context and an ultimate orientation, emerging from God and leading back to God. *Exousia* therefore demands the virtues of practice: wisdom, equanimity, selflessness, trustworthiness, concern, and fidelity. The role of the doctor is defined by an oath to practice in keeping with the virtues demanded by God's free gift of the *exousia* to care for the needs of the sick. A physician practices *with* authority to the extent that this oath is upheld [39].

Virtue is also expected of the patient, but healing is never withheld because a patient does not live up to the perfect fulfillment of these virtues. The patient must also realize that the grace of healing is mediated through flawed and fragile human beings who may not live up to the virtues demanded by *exousia*. The virtues of the patient concern the stewardship of the body, which is given as a gift by God. Patients can be asked to care for their bodies, to avoid what is harmful to their bodies, to be compliant with prescriptions, and to be honest historians. But even the good of the body must be subordinated to the *telos*, which transcends the body itself.

The Wisdom of Ben Sira

The deuterocanonical text of Ben Sira (the Book of Sirach or Ecclesiasticus) is included in the wisdom literature of the Roman Catholic Scriptures and is referred to 82 times in the Jewish Talmud ([37], pp. 17-20). The physician's poem from this text [38:1-15] helps to provide insights into the view of authority in the healing relationship within the Judeo-Christian tradition.

In ancient Hebrew thought, healing was traditionally reserved for God alone. To make a claim to be able to heal, then, was to ascribe to oneself qualities traditionally reserved for God alone, thus making oneself God's equal. This was an abomination. It was among the worst of all sins. It was the practice of magic and darkness associated with the enemies of God: the herbs and spells and incantations of idolaters [40].

But the rational medicine of the Greeks was not only wiser and more efficacious than the medicine of Babylon and Egypt, it made a claim to a rational basis for practice not associated with idolatry. Jews could contemplate availing themselves of the services of these Hippocratic physicians, then, if there were some theological way to reconcile this new rational medicine with the traditional understanding that healing came from the Almighty, not from human beings. Such a theological understanding is expressed in the physician's poem from the Wisdom of Ben Sira (ca. 175 B.C.). This understanding gave Hellenized Jews, for the first time in the history of Israel, an opportunity to practice medicine and ask for the assistance of physicians when sick [40].

While the poem does not use the words for power or authority directly in describing the relationship between doctor and patient, either in the original Hebrew or in the Greek translation written by Ben Sira's grandson, the themes raised by the poem deal quite explicitly with the topic. "From God the doctor has his wisdom," the poem insists. God endows the earth with all the healing herbs the doctor uses. The pure *dynamis* for healing comes originally from God, but it is through the doctor that "God's creative work continues without cease in its efficacy on the surface of the earth." Yet *dynamis* is not enough. The *exousia* to heal must also come from God. The first verse of the poem admonishes the patient to honor the physician not only because his services are "essential" (i.e., that he has *dynamis*), but also because it was God "who established his profession" (i.e., gave him *exousia*).

The orientation of medicine to God is made clear. Both the doctor and the patient are explicitly urged to pray. The physician does not falsely arrogate to himself powers over the patient which properly belong to God. And the patient does not insist on power and rights over and against the physician. Their relationship is a covenant of trust between doctor and patient authorized by the orientation of that covenant to the overarching covenant between God and all of God's people [40]. This view harmonizes with that of contemporary Christian theologians who characterize the doctor-patient relationship as a covenant [26, 35]. Power is not thought of as force of will, but as the actual possibility of healing. Authority is not force of will or the possession of specialized knowledge, but the mutual recognition by both the healer and the healed of the ultimate source of the power to heal and the ultimate source of the warrant to heal. To claim to heal by one's own force of knowledge or will is arrogant. To offer healing as a contract implies ownership of what belongs properly to God, and is thus intolerable. It is only by practicing under both covenants, with the *exousia* which God gives and which demands so much of the doctor, that the *dynamis* of expertise can become an actual act of healing for the patient.

Exousia, Freedom, and Service

The Scriptural perspective which governs the conception of authority covered by the term *exousia* also offers an understanding of the relationship between freedom and authority which differs from contemporary usage. This perspective emphasizes the relationship of loving service to the concept of freedom as well as to the concept of authority. This perspective is highly relevant to discussions of the doctor-patient relationship.

Gunneweg and Schmithals write that the true authority of *exousia* "arises out of freedom and is based upon the possibility of rendering help as a servant" ([15], p. 21). During his final meal with his disciples, a dispute arises among them as to who is the greatest. Jesus admonishes them not to "lord it over" other people, but to fulfill what it means when it is said that those who have *exousia* over people are called their benefactors. Those in positions of true *exousia* must be servants, in imitation of Jesus, who stood among the disciples as one who serves [Lk. 22:24-30]. Similarly, in the Gospel of John, Jesus urges the disciples to follow his example of service and wash each other's feet [Jn. 13:1-17]. Henri Nouwen, implicitly writing with an understanding of authority as *exousia,* asserts that compassion is the substance of legitimate authority ([29], pp. 40-43).

Exousia implies that authority is an assertion of the other in freedom. It is not mere *dynamis,* which is really indifferent to the will of the other, nor is it a coercive use of power, which is the assertion of personal will against the will of the other [28]. *Exousia* is authority which addresses human freedom and human reason. *Exousia* is authority which assumes a mutual orientation towards a *tertium quid. Exousia* is always at the service of others and their freedom. "An earthly authority which does not point beyond itself becomes demonic and will show itself as arbitrary, naked power" [28]. The life of Joseph Mengele provides a chilling example of what can happen when a medical professional distorts the authority of the profession far beyond the legitimacy and genuineness of *exousia.*

The concept of *exousia* captures a sense of human freedom which seems to have been overlooked by the Hobbesian perspective on authority, whether presented in the form of political philosophy or sociology. Hannah Arendt has written that "authority implies an obedience in which men retain their freedom" [3]. Such a statement must seem paradoxical in a culture which considers obedience and freedom as opposites. What kind of freedom is there which does not preclude obedience?

The freedom of *exousia* is the freedom which comes with liberation from self-preoccupation. It is the freedom which only loving service can bring. It is also the free acceptance of human nature with all its inherent limits, including death. It is liberation from the punishment of Sisyphus, condemned to the eternal trial of attempting to make those limits disappear [28]. It is therefore liberation from both the entrepreneurial approach to medicine often assumed by physicians and the consumerist approach to medicine often assumed by patients. Because the doctor does not own the authority to heal, the doctor cannot put healing up for sale on the market. Because the patient cannot purchase immortality, the patient need not expend all his or her human resources on a grandiose, death-denying delusion.

The virtuous doctor, then, will practice with *exousia,* recognizing that healing is authorized by God, who also gives the possibility of healing in the resources of the earth and in the resourcefulness of human reason and imagination. In the covenant which exists between God and the healer, the physician must assume the virtues demanded by *exousia,* placing healing power at the service of others and at the service of their freedom. This means recognizing the dignity and freedom of the patient, and demands, in turn, a covenant between doctor and patient. *Exousia* implies the concept of authority to which Hauerwas referred when he wrote that it is not derived from knowledge or expertise, but from mastery of the practical moral skills involved in the physician's commitment to care for and never abandon the ill and the dying [16]. Likewise, to coerce, manipulate, or ignore the patient is incompatible with the spirit of practicing with *exousia.* Informed consent, then, assumes importance not as the patient's autonomous authorization of the physician's actions, but as the mutual recognition of the gifts of freedom and healing which only God bestows. Authority does not reside with the patient as something to be given to the doctor. Nor is authority something that resides with the doctor as something to be exercised over the patient. Rather, it is the result of the mutual recognition of the dignity of both doctor and patient, each reverencing the life of God in the other.

Exousia, Mystery, and Healing

God is a holy mystery, and the awesome presence of God in the doctor-patient relationship ought never be ignored. But God's mystery ought never be invoked as a stopgap for our knowledge; a mere concept to define the limits of human science. When medical authority is considered only as a control (practicing *in* authority), or when medical authority is considered only as the power of knowledge and expertise (practicing as *an* authority), the fundamental mystery of God's place in the healing relationship is obscured. But when medicine is practiced *with* authority (*exousia*), the holy mystery of God's healing presence opens out before both the doctor and the patient.

Robert Burt has complained that the increasing use of the courts to settle medical cases of ethical concern in advance of any anticipated actions by physicians and patients accepts the false presumptions that medical decision making is certain when it is not, and that direct conversation between the doctor and patient is to be avoided when it ought not. Patients, doctors, and hospitals turn instead "to the last bastion of unquestionable authority in our society: the Judge, the embodiment of the Law" [7]. In going to the courts, they fail to recognize both the ontological and moral ambiguity of those cases which fall at the "edges of life." They seek certitude and security where there is only uncertainty and insecurity. They seek control in situations which are fundamentally out of their control.

But the patient and doctor who recognize *exousia* know that the physician's authority is not called into question when there is no control and there is no knowledge. Those who base their authority on control and knowledge will experience these cases as threats. But *exousia* commits both doctor and patient to a recognition of the fundamental mystery of God's presence in the covenant between them. *Exousia* commits both to a recognition of the mysteries of death and limitation. The foundation of *exousia* is the transcendent, which is revealed in the immanence of sickness and death. In the midst of the powerlessness and confusion wrought by illness and death, faith and reverence replace desperation and delusion. Control slips away from one *in* authority. Expertise slips away from *an* authority. The power and the authority belong to God alone.

Exousia, Medicine, and the Secular City

MacIntyre [24] despairs of the possibility of any kind of moral consensus regarding either what constitutes the good or how various goods ought to be related to one another. He argues that the concept of a profession is inherently linked to the concept of authority. He concludes that the vitality of all professions has been irrevocably destroyed because the concept of authority has lost all meaning in the wake of the loss of moral consensus.

This despair has been challenged by Pellegrino [31]. He notes that the recognition of the legitimacy of the claims of patients to act as moral agents in the doctor-patient relationship is a positive good which ought to be sustained and strengthened. But he also cautions that both patient and physician must be seen as moral agents. Physicians cannot become mere instruments of the patient's autonomous choices.

The view offered here, through the scriptural concept of *exousia,* would seem to obviate these difficulties by transforming the discussion from a debate about power for doctors and patients into a search for that *tertium quid* to which both can point as the source of authority. Paternalism is the mistaken view that authority has to do with knowledge and control which properly belong to the medical profession. "Autonomism" is the mistaken view that authority has to do with control which properly belongs to the patient, but which the patient grants to the physician only because the patient lacks the knowledge. The way of *exousia* is the "third way."

MacIntyre is certainly correct in his assessment that there is no moral consensus, let alone any religious consensus, in the Western world. One might therefore argue that the scriptural notion of *exousia* would be helpful only if one accepted MacIntyre's vision of small communities in which patients and staff shared the Judeo-Christian faith and its conception of the authority to heal. But a great many people would want no part of such communities, either because they have no faith or because their faith does not include the concept of *exousia*.

Does this imply that the concept of *exousia* is irrelevant in a pluralistic society? Does medicine have no unifying goal other than to maximize personal liberty to the extent that others are not harmed? Is total fragmentation of the profession inevitable?

I would suggest that the profession itself will ultimately resist fragmentation into distinct medico-moral practices. Granted, in the wake of intense specialization and subspecialization, it might no longer be possible in a certain sense to talk of a single medical profession. Nonetheless, there seems to be enough unity inherent in the professional activities of contemporary Western physicians to resist fragmentation into little philosophically or religiously distinct professions. The interdependence of medical knowledge, the uniformity of the initial education, the fundamental belief in rational medicine based on scientific evidence, and the oath that physicians take to put this knowledge at the service of patients are critical unifying elements for the profession. Despite the many centrifugal forces which threaten contemporary medical practice, the fact of illness and the act of profession might still form, as Pellegrino points out [32], a secular basis for a *tertium quid* of the sort that could serve as a source of *exousia* for the relationship between doctor and patient. These would constitute integral constituents of the healing relationship, transcending the power concerns of both doctor and the patient. Beneficence and autonomy might cease to be considered antithetical. Pellegrino and Thomasma locate a *telos* intrinsic to the practice of medicine: the good of the patient. This forms the basis, on secular grounds alone, of a new model for the doctor-patient relationship: beneficence in trust [34]. It requires a trusting relationship between doctor and patient not unlike the religious concept of a covenant. It demands virtue of both doctors and patients. Such a model of the healing relationship does not have the power of a truly Judeo-Christian model like the one developed in this paper, but it certainly has secular credibility. And even a secular notion of *exousia* would certainly provide a helpful alternative to the twin vices of physician paternalism and patient "autonomism."

A Clinical Example

To illustrate, in a preliminary and sketchy fashion, how the adoption of a view of medical authority as *exousia* might affect the practice even of secular medicine, I will offer the following example.

Suppose a patient, dying of metastatic lung cancer, is placed on a morphine drip by his doctor to treat his severe pain. Suppose that this patient, quite medically sophisticated, begins to manipulate the drip rate on his own intravenous pump.

A doctor who conceived of authority as power might perceive this patient's behavior as a threat to the authority of the doctors and nurses. If somewhat enlightened, she might interpret this as a manipulative behavior in which the patient was acting out because of fear of death. Her reaction to this behavior would probably be to reassert control by "setting limits" so that the patient would understand the boundaries of proper patient behavior. She might, mercifully, increase the drip rate, but tell the patient that he could only ask for a change in drip rate once per nursing shift, and that he would be carefully watched so that he did not increase the rate on his own. Since he lacked the knowledge (power) to safely adjust the rate, she would insist that control of the morphine dose must be the prerogative of the doctor. If he objected, mutual anger and stalemate might ensue.

On the other hand, if the doctor conceived of authority as *exousia,* she might behave differently. She might ask herself, and the patient, what the *telos* was at this stage of illness and in their doctor-patient relationship. She might ask how they could work towards the overall *telos* of medicine (the good of the patient) in this situation, and how the patient saw his ability to control the rate of the morphine drip fitting into that *telos.* They might agree that the power of the drug (a power which belongs to neither of them) could be better expressed in the service of that *telos* if the patient actually could manipulate the dose of morphine within certain bounds of safety. Thus, the goal both shared could be achieved and the power of medicine more fully expressed in the setting of their mutually trusting relationship.

One can only speculate that it was such an exchange which must have given rise to the wonderful new development of Patient Controlled Analgesia (PCA), in which the patient is given a baseline infusion rate of narcotic but can give additional drug boluses (limited by safety concerns) as necessary to relieve pain not relieved by the baseline infusion. The sum of the boluses required are then used to calculate adjustments in the baseline rate [42].

Some might object that the use of PCA for such a patient merely illustrates an effective redistribution of power and control from doctor to patient, but this interpretation would miss the point. Certainly it is not patient power or doctor power which is at stake here. The things that matter are mutual trust, shared goals, and the expression of a power which belongs not to the doctor or to the patient, but to Humankind or to Nature or to God (or to all three). Certainly it is not control, but loss of control which is the dominant theme in such a situation. To engage in a struggle for control over the rate of morphine infusion as an expression of continued personal control in the face of the overwhelming reality of the patient's imminent, ineluctable death would be absurd for both doctor and patient. The wise physician recognizes the dignity and freedom of her patient even in these final moments, and both doctor and patient ordain their freedom to the common goal of alleviating suffering even in the face of their mutual powerlessness to prevent death. Thus would a wise physician practice *with* authority, in the spirit of *exousia.*

Conclusion

Contemporary discussions of authority in the doctor-patient relationship have largely been based on either sociological or political models. Both of these models assume that authority means control or expertise or both. Under such models, the notion of authority in the doctor-patient relationship has been viewed as a struggle for power between doctors and patients. This perhaps has generated some of the difficulties now confronting medicine, where many physicians continue to exert paternalistic control over patients, while many patients now practice medical consumerism. The New Testament view of authority, *exousia,* provides an alternative view which suggests that the authority to heal is neither a possession of the physician nor of the patient, but a free gift from God. *Exousia* is the warrant to heal. *Exousia* requires virtue from both doctor and patient in a covenant relationship, subsumed under the greater covenant between God and all God's people. The notion of *exousia* also points to a way for secular medicine to move beyond the contradictions of medical authority conceived of as knowledge and control. Perhaps a recovery of the notion of *exousia* can help medicine escape from a spirit of antagonism which is increasingly making the experiences of both going to the doctor and of practicing medicine unsatisfactory for both doctors and patients.

Acknowledgments

I am grateful to Dr. Edmund D. Pellegrino for his thoughtful review of a draft of this manuscript and to the Charles E. Culpepper Foundation for their generous support of my work.

Center for Clinical Bioethics
Georgetown University Medical Center
Washington, D.C., U.S.A.

Bibliography

[1] Amiot, F., and Galopin, P. M.: 1973, 'Authority,' in X. Leon-Dufour (ed.), *Dictionary of Biblical Theology,* 2nd ed., Seabury Press, New York, pp. 36-39.

[2] Aquinas, St. Thomas: 1966, *Summa Theologiae,* vol. 28, Blackfriars edition, T. Gilly, O.P. (ed.), McGraw-Hill, New York.

[3] Arendt, H.: 1968, 'What Is Authority?', in *Between Past and Future,* Penguin Press, Harmondsworth, Middlesex, England, pp. 91-141.

[4] Baier, A. C.: 1987, 'The Need for More Than Justice,' in M. Hanen and K. Nielsen (eds.), 'Science, Ethics, and Feminism', *Canadian Journal of Philosophy* 13 (Suppl.), 41-56.

[5] Beauchamp, T. L.: 1982, *Philosophical Ethics,* New York, McGraw-Hill.

[6] Beauchamp, T. L., and Childress, J. F.: 1989, *Principles of Biomedical Ethics,* Oxford University Press, New York.

[7] Burt, R. A.: 1988, 'Uncertainty and Medical Authority in the World of Jay Katz,' *Law, Medicine, and Health Care* 16, 190-96.

[8] Engelhardt, H. T.: 1986, *The Foundations of Bioethics,* Oxford University Press, New York.

[9] Engelhardt, H. T.: 1991, *Secular Humanism: The Search for a Common Morality,* Trinity Press International, Philadelphia.

[10] Faden, R. R., and Beauchamp, T. L.: 1986, *A History and Theory of Informed Consent,* Oxford University Press, New York.

[11] Finnis, J.: 1980, *Natural Law, Natural Rights,* Clarendon Press, Oxford, England.

[12] Flathman, R.: 1982, 'Power, Authority, and Rights in Medicine,' in G. J. Agich (ed.), *Responsibility in Health Care,* D. Reidel, Dordrecht, the Netherlands, pp. 105-25.

[13] Foerster, W. F.: 1964, 'Exousia,' in G. Kittel and G. Friedrich (eds.), *Theological Dictionary of the New Testament,* vol. II, Eerdmans, Grand Rapids, pp. 562-75.

[14] Friedman, R. B.: 1991, 'On the Concept of Authority in Political Philosophy,' in J. Raz (ed.), *Authority,* New York, University Press, pp. 56-91.

[15] Gunneweg, A. H. J., and Schmithals, W.: 1982, *Authority,* J. E. Steely (trans.), Abingdon Press, Nashville, Tennessee.

[16] Hauerwas, S.: 1982, 'Authority and the Profession of Medicine,' in G. J. Agich (ed.), *Responsibility in Health Care,* D. Reidel, Dordrecht, the Netherlands, pp. 83-104.

[17] Hobbes, T.: 1651 (1946), *Leviathan, or the Matter, Forme, and Power of a Commonwealth, Ecclesiastical and Civil,* M. Oakshott (ed.), Basil Blackwell, Oxford, England.

[18] Kierkegaard, S.: 1955, *On Authority and Revelation: The Book of Adler,* W. Lowrie (trans.), Princeton University Press, Princeton, New Jersey, p. XVI.

[19] Ladenson, R.: 1991, 'In Defense of a Hobbesian Conception of Law,' in J. Raz (ed.), *Authority,* New York, University Press, New York, pp. 32-55.

[20] Lavin, B., Haug, M., Belgrave, L. K., and Breslau, N.: 1987, 'Change in Student Physicians' Views on Authority Relationships with Patients,' *Journal of Health and Social Behavior* 28, 258-72.

[21] Locke, J.: 1690 (1988), 'An Essay Concerning the True Original Extent and End of Civil Government,' in *Two Treatises of Government,* P. Laslett (ed.), Cambridge University Press, New York, pp. 256-428.

[22] Mackie, J. L.: 1977, *Ethics: Inventing Right and Wrong,* Penguin Books, Harmondsworth, Middlesex, England.

[23] MacIntyre, A.: 1967, *Secularization and Moral Change,* Oxford University Press, London, England.

[24] MacIntyre, A.: 1977, 'Patients as Agents,' in S. F. Spicker, and H. T. Englehardt (eds.), *Philosophical Medical Ethics: Its Nature and Significance,* D. Reidel, Dordrecht, the Netherlands, pp. 197-212.

[25] MacIntyre, A.: 1984, *After Virtue,* University of Notre Dame Press, Notre Dame, Indiana.

[26] May, W. F.: 1983, *The Physician's Covenant,* Westminster Press, Philadelphia.

[27] Molinski, W.: 1975, 'Authority,' in K. Rahner (ed.), *The Concise Sacramentum Mundi,* Seabury Press, New York, pp. 60-65.

[28] Myers, A. C. (ed.): 1987, *The Eerdmans Bible Dictionary,* Eerdmans, Grand Rapids, Michigan, pp. 108, 844-45.

[29] Nouwen, H. J.: 1972, *The Wounded Healer,* Doubleday, Garden City, New York.

[30] Parsons, T.: 1951, *The Social System,* The Free Press, Glencoe, Illinois.

[31] Pellegrino, E. D.: 'Moral Agency and Professional Ethics: Some Notes on the Transformation of the Physician-Patient Encounter,' in S. F. Spicker and H. T. Engelhardt (eds.), *Philosophical Medical Ethics: Its Nature and Significance,* D. Reidel, Dordrecht, the Netherlands, pp. 213-20.

[32] Pellegrino, E. D.: 1979, 'Towards a Reconstruction of Medical Morality: The Primacy of Act of Profession and the Fact of Illness,' *Journal of Medicine and Philosophy* 4(1), 32-56.

[33] Pellegrino, E. D., and Thomasma, D. C.: 1981, *A Philosophical Basis of Medical Practice,* Oxford University Press, New York.

[34] Pellegrino, E. D., and Thomasma, D. C.: 1989, *For the Patient's Good: Towards the Restoration of Beneficence in Medical Ethics,* Oxford University Press, New York.

[35] Ramsey, P.: 1970, *The Patient as Person,* Yale University Press, New Haven, pp. xi-xviii.

[36] Raz, J.: 1991, 'Introduction,' in J. Raz (ed.), *Authority,* New York University Press, New York, pp. 1-19.

[37] Skehan, P. A., and DiLella, A. A.: 1987, *The Wisdom of Ben Sira,* Anchor Bible Series, vol. 39, Doubleday, New York.

[38] Suchman, A. L., and Matthews, D. A.: 1988, 'What Makes the Doctor-Patient Relationship Therapeutic? Exploring the Connexional Dimension of Medical Care,' *Annals of Internal Medicine* 108, 125-30.

[39] Sulmasy, D. P.: 1989, 'By Whose Authority: Emerging Issues in Medical Ethics,' *Theological Studies* 50, 95-119.

[40] Sulmasy, D. P.: 1989, 'The Covenant Within the Covenant: Doctors and Patients in Sirach 38:1-15,' *Linacre Quarterly* 55(4), 14-24.

[41] Sulmasy, D. P., Geller, G., Levine, D. M., and Faden, R.: 1990, 'Medical House Officers' Knowledge, Confidence, and Attitudes Regarding Medical Ethics,' *Archives of Internal Medicine* 150, 2509-13.

[42] Tansen, A., Hartvig, P., Fagerlund, C., and Dahlstrom, B.: 1982, 'Patient-controlled Analgesic Therapy: Part II. Individual Analgesic Demand and Plasma Concentrations of Pethidine and Post-operative Pain,' *Clinical Pharmacokinetics* 7, 164-75.

[43] Veatch, R. M.: 1982, 'Medical Authority and Professional Medical Authority: The Nature of Authority in Medicine for Decisions by Lay Persons and Professionals,' in G. J. Agich

(ed.), *Responsibility in Health Care,* D. Reidel, Dordrecht, the Netherlands, pp. 127-37.

[44] Veatch, R.; 1981, *A Theory of Medical Ethics,* Basic Books, New York.

[45] Weber, M.: 1947 (1968), *Theory of Social and Economic Organizations,* A. M. Anderson and T. Parsons (trans.), Free Press, New York.

[46] Wolff, R. P.: 1991, 'The Conflict Between Authority and Autonomy,' in J. Raz (ed.), *Authority,* New York University Press, New York, pp. 20-31.

41 Empowerment in the Clinical Setting

Karen Lebacqz

In *Professional Ethics: Power and Paradox* [17], I proposed that the power of the professional person is morally relevant to determining what should be done in the practice setting and that justice or empowerment of the client becomes a central norm for professional practice.[1] The time has now come to see what justice as empowerment means for the clinical setting. The task is particularly crucial in light of Kapp's recent definition of empowerment as advocating for oneself and participating maximally in one's own significant decisions ([14], p. 5). Under this definition, to choose dependence upon others is to "forego" empowerment ([14], p. 6). I will explore below the adequacy of this definition.

Just as we learn about justice by exploring experiences of injustice [16], so we may learn about empowerment by exploring disempowerment. Disempowerment, and therefore empowerment, within the clinical setting will differ from setting to setting and from population to population. I will examine two populations: those who begin with power and become disempowered in the clinical setting, and those who begin from a position of relative powerlessness and experience the clinical setting from that perspective.

The Disempowerment of the Powerful

Hans Jonas once argued that the ideal research subject is a doctor: the doctor is best positioned to understand the risks and implications of the research, and to give a truly voluntary and informed consent [13]. In short, the doctor as subject is most likely to be empowered in the research setting. Similarly, the doctor as patient is most likely to be empowered in the clinical setting. By looking at the disempowerment experienced by those most likely to retain power in the clinical setting, we begin to develop a sense of what constitutes disempowerment and therefore

1. The definition of justice and dimensions of justice as empowerment are further explored in *Six Theories of Justice* [18] and *Justice in an Unjust World* [16].

From Karen Lebacqz, "Empowerment in the Clinical Setting," in Gerald P. McKenny and Jonathan Sande, eds., *Theological Analysis of the Clinical Encounter* (Dordrecht: Kluwer Academic Publishers, 1994), pp. 133-47. Used with kind permission from Kluwer Academic Publishers.

what would constitute empowerment. So we begin with those who experience no language, cultural, knowledge, or sexual barriers to empowerment.

Yet even white, male, well-educated doctors, when they become patients, experience disempowerment in the clinical setting. The film "The Doctor," based on *A Taste of My Own Medicine* by Ed Rosenbaum [22] and just released at the time of writing this essay, demonstrates precisely this disempowerment. Here is a physician, a surgeon, accustomed to ordering people around in the hospital who must now wait in line, fill out forms by the hour, be told "sorry, the doctor is late today," and undergo any number of forms of indignity experienced routinely by patients.

A similar story is told in Oliver Sacks' delightful treatise *A Leg to Stand On* [24]. Sacks broke his leg in a climbing accident. Not only was the leg broken; Sacks also lost all sense of feeling in his leg, and all ability to move or exercise voluntary control over it. He lost "proprioception," the sense of owning one's own limbs and having command over them. Ironically, proprioception is one of the foci of Sacks' work as a neurologist. Thus, his story is the story of a man who moves not only from the status of physician to the status of patient, but indeed, to the very kind of patient that he himself treats. He thus learned to see from the "inside" what his patients had tried to communicate to him.

Two Miseries, Two Empowerments

To be a patient — at least under critical circumstances — is to live in an altered world. It is almost as though one has entered the "twilight zone." Perceptions are distorted, time and space appear different, even everyday conversation can loom threateningly: "'Execution tomorrow,' said the clerk in Admissions. I knew it must have been, 'Operation tomorrow,' but the feeling of execution overwhelmed what he said" ([24], p. 46).

Illness takes place on two levels. Sacks calls it "two miseries." One is the physical disability, the "organically determined erosion of being and space" ([24], p. 158). The other he calls the "moral" dimension associated with "the reduced stationless status of a patient, and, in particular, conflict with and surrender to 'them' — 'them' being the surgeon, the whole system, the institution . . ." ([24], p. 158).

Illness is not just a matter of physical disability. The clinical setting involves also, and even more importantly, a change in one's structural and sociological status. One becomes a "patient."

Even the most powerful of patients therefore feel disempowered in two ways. First, they have lost some ability previously possessed — in Sacks' case, the ability to walk and even to feel his own leg. Loss of ability is annoying at best, frightening at worst: "I found myself . . . scared and confounded to the roots of my being" ([24], p. 79). This is the first "misery" with which the patient deals, and it is often overwhelming in itself, undermining one's ability to deal normally with the world.

But patients have also lost normal status in the world. For Sacks, and for many others, it is the role of patient as much as physical disability itself that inflicts misery and requires empowerment. "I felt morally helpless, paralyzed, contracted, confined — and not just contracted, but contorted as well, into roles and postures of abjection" ([24], p. 158). For example, Sacks asked for spinal rather than general anesthesia, and his request was denied. He writes, "I felt curiously helpless . . . and I thought, Is *this* what 'being a patient' means?" Sociologists have described the "sick role" or status of patient. From the inside, this status is often a feeling of diminishment. Sacks calls himself a "man reduced, and dependent" ([24], p. 133).

The role of patient is reinforced by institutional structures and practices: "we were set apart, we patients in white nightgowns, and avoided clearly, though unconsciously, like lepers" ([24], p. 163). As Alan Goldman puts it in his examination of professional ethics,

> life in hospitals . . . continues to be filled with needless rituals suggestive of patient passivity, dependence, and impotence. The institutional setting is still structured in such a way as to block the exercise of rights at least partially accepted intellectually. . . . Patients are rarely permitted to see their charts; pills are almost literally shoved into their mouths. . . . Often newly admitted patients perfectly capable of walking are taken to their rooms in wheelchairs, an apt symbol of the helpless pose they are made to assume from the time of their entrance into this alien and authoritarian setting ([10], pp. 224-25).

Ultimately, suggests Sacks, he indeed became an "invalid": in-valid ([24], p. 164). Sacks resisted the patient role at every step. Yet he recognized that both he and the surgeon were, in a sense, "forced to play roles — he the role of the All-knowing Specialist, I the role of the Know-nothing Patient" ([24], p. 105).

If illness is composed of two miseries, then recovery will require two empowerments. "Now we needed a double recovery — a physical recovery, and a spiritual movement *to* health" ([24], p. 164). The patient needs physical healing — in Sacks' case, surgery and physical therapy so that he could once again walk, run, jump, and do things that his body had "forgotten" how to do. But as much as the physical healing, the patient needs recovery from the abject, reduced, dependent status of patient.

Both miseries are disempowering. But it is the "contortion" into roles and postures of abjection that is the core of the power gap between physician and patient. Such contortion need not accompany physical deterioration. Different structures reduce the second "misery."

Nor is such contortion necessarily diminished when physical healing takes place. Too often, we assume that once health is restored, the patient automatically becomes a non-patient and experiences restored moral status. In my experience, this is not true. Effects of dependent status can linger, making future contacts difficult and undermining patients' sense of their own worth and being. While the patient may literally move outside the hospital or clinic and cease being a patient in a technical sense, the psycho-sociological effects of dependent patienthood may remain. Moreover, during the time of clinical care, the dependent status of patient can adversely affect medical treatment.

What can be done to empower patients? The loss of function, the physical disability, is the initial presenting problem. The best the medical team can do in the face of it is to try to heal. But is the loss of status, the diminished sense of personhood that often accompanies being a patient, also necessary? Must there be two miseries? Is there a way to reduce the second misery, to hasten recovery from it, and to empower the patient who experiences it? Using Sacks' experience, we can examine the disempowerment of the powerful and suggest how different structures and responses might empower the patient.

The Central Role of Communication

The clinical context begins with communication. Disempowerment begins with failures of communication. One of the most disempowering things that happens in the clinical context is shutting down the patient's words.

In Sacks' case, this began with his first attempts to share what had happened. "They wanted to know the 'salient facts' and I wanted to tell them everything — the entire story" ([24], p. 47). Something had *happened* to Sacks. It was his story. He wanted to tell it. And he wanted to be heard. So from the first "intake" interview in which Sacks tried to tell the "entire" story and the medical team asked for the "salient facts," things went awry.

Failure to communicate went far beyond this first incident. Sacks knew that something was wrong with his leg because he had lost all feeling in it. He waited (and waited and waited!) for the surgeon to come in order to raise his concerns. The surgeon finally appeared, only to state briskly, "there's nothing to worry about" and disappear before Sacks could say more than "but . . ." Sacks was given no *time* to communicate.

As the days went by and the leg failed to respond to physiotherapy, Sacks became desperate to communicate his concern: "Desperately now, I wanted communication, and reassurance" ([24], p. 88). Above all, he recognized a need to communicate to the surgeon and have the surgeon understand. While he wanted reassurance, he was prepared to accept the truth if no reassurance could be given: "I should respect whatever he said so long as it was frank and showed respect for me, for my dignity as a man" ([24], p. 93).

When the surgeon came, he neither looked at Sacks nor spoke to him, but turned to the nurse and said, "Well, Sister, and how is the patient now?" ([24], p. 104). Rather than being regarded with respect and frankness, Sacks was treated as a nonentity. He was not even addressed by the surgeon, but talked about as if he were not there. Sacks was given no *respect* for himself as a communicator; all the communication was with those around him. Using Kapp's definition of empowerment as advocating for oneself and participating "maximally" in one's own significant decisions, Sacks was clearly disempowered.

Sacks persisted in raising his concern and tried, falteringly, to tell the physician what was wrong:

> It's . . . it's . . . I don't seem to be able to contract the quadriceps . . . and, er . . . the muscle doesn't seem to have any tone. And . . . and . . . I have difficulty locating the position of the leg ([24], p. 104).

I have quoted this speech as Sacks describes it. If it is an accurate representation of what he said, this fact alone is significant. Sacks is a literary man. He writes eloquently, powerfully.[2] It is difficult to imagine him at a loss for words, or stumbling over his words. Yet, confronted with the power of the physician, and in his own dependent state as patient, stumble is apparently what he did. He seems to have stammered, acted hesitant and evidenced confusion.

There may be an important lesson here for empowerment in the clinical context. Few medical people realize how dis-empowering the very context is. Patients generally feel inadequate in their descriptions of what is wrong. They hesitate, stumble, try to find the right words. Nothing seems to come out right. The patient who stumbles over her words is not necessarily stupid, but may simply be experiencing, as Sacks did, a diminishment of her capacity to verbalize.

I went to my physician complaining of pain in my hip joint. He asked me to stand and turn in certain ways, and then declared flatly that it could not be my *joint* which was hurting. It must be the *tendon*, not the joint. To him, this technicality and diagnostic accuracy is very important. To me, only the pain that makes it hard for me to climb stairs is important. I do not care whether the pain originates in the joint, technically speaking, or in the tendon. I care only about what can be done to alleviate it, since I live in a house full of stairs. But his focus on the technicalities made it difficult for me to persist in my query. I had been told that I was *wrong*. I felt inadequate and unable to communicate. I gave up, and no treatment was forthcoming.

Sacks suggests that there is among doctors, "in acute hospitals at least, a presumption of stupidity in their patients" ([24], p. 171). Whether all doctors do in fact consider their patients stupid, in acute or other contexts, failures to communicate often have the subtle effect of giving the patient a sense that she or he is not only stupid but also not worthy of the physician's time and effort.

Failure to hear the patient's story, impatience to get to salient facts, lack of time to listen, failure to address the patient at all, focusing on technicalities or calling the

2. I have also heard him speak publicly and found his address strong.

patient's understanding wrong — all these are disempowering in the clinical context. The patient who has been treated this way often gives up on the effort to communicate.

Many feel keenly their "ex-communication" ([24], p. 110). Not only have they been shut out from the healthy world literally — stuck in the hospital, wrapped in white gowns, and avoided by healthy people — but they are now shut out symbolically by failure to communicate, to listen, to honor their perspective. "As a patient in the hospital I felt both anguish and asphyxia — the anguish of being confronted with dissolution, and asphyxia because I would not be heard" ([24], p. 209). Thus does Sacks describe the life-killing effect of having communication shut off.

Lack of communication is not the only thing that is disempowering in the clinical context. Being denied a legitimate request (e.g. for spinal rather than general anesthesia), being forced to wear unattractive hospital gowns that strip one's individuality, being shunted from department to department like a sack of potatoes — all these and many other routine aspects of clinical care also take power away from patients. But many of these ills would be compensated by careful communication that leaves patients feeling as though they have been treated as persons, as though they can advocate for themselves and participate maximally in decisions. As Sacks puts it, he would have been content with whatever he was told, so long as it was told with respect.

The Liberating Word

If failures of communication are the beginning of disempowerment, then communication can be the beginning of empowerment: "The postures, the passivity of the patient, last as long as the doctor orders. . . ." ([24], p. 133). Sacks points to the importance of the liberating word on several occasions. In order to heal, to regain use of his leg, he had to walk. Rehabilitation is based on action. Yet the action was birthed not just by himself, but by others: "I had to *do* it, give birth to the New Act, but others were needed to deliver me, and *say,* 'Do it!'" ([24], p. 182). He calls this speaking the essential role of the teacher or therapist. It is a form of midwifery. Only as others granted permission could he find the way to do something new.

Once he missed a memorial service that he would have liked to attend, and lamented to the nurse that he was unable to go. "Why not?" she queried. By challenging the limitations he had set for himself, she removed them: "The moment she spoke and said, 'Why not?' a great barrier disappeared. . . . Whatever it was, I was liberated by her words" ([24], p. 184).

Words of support ("do it") and words of challenge ("why can't you?") can both be liberating. Both can set the patient free to take a new step in the healing process and to claim skills and territory that the patient has not been able to claim by herself.

Empathy

But communication goes far beyond words. When Sacks was first injured, a young surgeon danced into his room, and leaped on the bedside table. This surgeon had once had a broken leg, and showed Sacks the scars from surgery. "He didn't talk like a text-book. He scarcely talked at all — he acted. He leapt and danced and showed me his wounds, showing me at the same time his perfect recovery" ([24], p. 44). This visit made Sacks feel "immeasurably better." Here, he encountered someone who had been through it and could demonstrate that there is light at the end of the tunnel. Later, another surgeon came to see Sacks, and Sacks felt that he could communicate with this man. *"I've been through this myself,"* said the surgeon. "I had a broken leg. . . . *I know what it's like"* ([24], p. 183). The empathy that comes from experience communicates and empowers.

Empathy gives authority to speak: "So when Mr. Amundsen said that the time had come to graduate, and give up one crutch, he spoke with authority — the only real authority, that of experience and understanding" ([24], p. 183). Sacks reflects on his own change as a physician because of what he went through as a patient, "Now I *knew,* for I had experienced myself. And now I could truly begin to understand my patients" ([24], p. 202). At the end of the film "The Doctor," the protagonist puts all his physician-in-training through the experience of being a patient in the hospital. Sacks suggests that there is an "absolute and categorical difference" between a doctor who knows and one who does not, and that this difference is because of the personal experience of "descending to the very depths of disease and dissolution" ([24], p. 203).

There is here, then, an important epistemological question that relates to empowerment. One who knows what the patient suffers and can truly hear the patient can empower the patient. But how does one "know" what the patient suffers? Those who have been through a similar experience have readiest access to empathy. This suggests that, where possible, medical care teams should include at least one care-giver who has experienced what the patient suffers. Where this is not possible, groups of patients with similar problems might be assembled. Patients often feel more secure about their position and more enabled to question medical practice when they are with a group that shares their experience.

Art and Religion

Sacks found several other things empowering as well. When he was rebuffed by the surgeon who told him that his concerns were "nothing," he felt as though he had entered a scotoma, "a hole in reality itself" ([24], p. 109). "In this limbo, this dark night," he writes, "I could not turn to science. Faced with a reality, which reason could not solve, I turned to art and religion for comfort . . ." ([24], p. 114). Two additional sources of empowerment, then, are art and religion.

A friend loaned Sacks a tape recorder with only one tape: Mendelssohn's violin concerto. "Something happened" to Sacks from the first playing of the music. The music appeared to reveal the creative and animating principle of the world, his leg. "The sense of hopelessness, of interminable darkness, lifted" ([24], p. 119). When he first tried to walk on crutches, he was unable to do so until suddenly the music began to play in his mind, and then he found that he could move to the rhythm.

In his own medical practice, Sacks finds that music can "center" his patients. It appears to restore a sense of the inner self that has been lost through neurological injury or disease ([24], p. 219). Because healing and empowerment involve both physical rhythms of the body and also the "center" of the self, music might be a powerful tool for empowerment. "Music," writes Sacks, "was a divine message and messenger of life. It was quintessentially quick — the 'quickening art,' as Kant has called it . . ." ([24], p. 148). This makes me wonder what would happen if our hospitals provided not television sets but stereos equipped with the great masterpieces of music from the centuries!

Art is not the only response to realities which reason cannot solve. "Science and reason could not talk of 'nothingness,' of 'hell,' or 'limbo': or of 'spiritual night.' They had no place for 'absence, darkness, death.' Yet these were the overwhelming realities of this time" ([24], p. 114). In order to find a language adequate to describe his experiences, Sacks turned to religion. The patient who faces dissolution of her world needs a language adequate to give voice to that dissolution and to provide a framework within which it can be understood, accepted, and overcome. The language of science and reason is often too sterile for this task. The language of science and reason is often too sterile for this task. The language of religion, precisely because it is often poetic [5] and mysterious, is adequate to the task.

Sacks gives eloquent expression to the power of religious language when he writes, "In a sense my experience had been a religious one — I had certainly thought of the leg as exiled, God-forsaken, when it was 'lost' and, when it was restored, restored in a transcendental way" ([24], p. 190). While he admits that his experience was also a "riveting scientific and cognitive" experience, it had transcended the limits of science and cognition. A language beyond science was needed.

Moreover, it is not only the *language* of religion that is empowering. Sacks went home for a night to see his family. While there, he attended synagogue. Here he experienced "inexpressible joy": "Behind my family I felt embraced by a community and, behind this, by the beauty of old traditions, and, behind this, by the ultimate, eternal joy of the law" ([24], p. 189). Religion is not just a language. It is a community, a set of laws and rituals, a sense of belonging to something larger and more grounding than one's own family or personal universe. All of these things have empowering possibility. They also suggest that Kapp's definition of empowerment is too individualistic and based too much on an autonomy model. Empowerment includes community and connection; it includes strengthening and honoring relationships.

Summary

What Sacks needed was "a leg to stand on." He needed it in two senses: the literal, physical healing of his limb, and the symbolic, "moral" healing of his status in the world. Because there were two miseries, two empowerments — two "legs" — were needed. The second leg is social and spiritual. Although the empowering possibilities of physical healing should not be underestimated, neither should the need for the second leg be neglected. It has to do with the meaning system of the patient, with hope and fear, with anxiety and joy, with community and solidarity. It is a leg composed of the liberating word, the communication that comes from empathy, the centering power of music and art, the adequacy of religious language and the solidity of religious ritual and community.

The Disempowerment of the Powerless

Oliver Sacks was one of the lucky ones. White, male, well-educated, a physician to boot, he was in a position to be as powerful as any patient can be. The mere fact that one so powerful experienced two "miseries" and needed two empowerments gives us many clues as to what happens in the clinical setting. But it does not cover the situation of those who are not powerful at the outset. What about those who suffer language, educational, racial, or sexual barriers when confronting the medical establishment?[3] The experiences of patients who are female, non-white, poor, not well educated, or in some other way less powerful than the white physician suggest some additional dimensions of disempowerment and therefore of empowerment. Those who begin in a more powerless position have many more barriers to empowerment. For them, it will take not only a change in communication, a bit more thoughtfulness, or a little music to give them back their moral status and sense of wholeness. For them, it will take nothing short of a change in the system.

Consent and Rationality

Consider, for example, the case of Maria Diaz, whose doctors recommended tubal ligation while she was in the last stages of a difficult labor. "I told them I would not accept that. I kept saying no and the doctors kept telling me that this was for my own good" ([7], p. 108). Maria Diaz never agreed to be sterilized and signed no consent forms for the procedure; but she was sterilized during caesarian section. Later, she and other Hispanic women

3. Precisely because these patients are already relatively powerless in the system, they are less likely to write books about their experiences than are the more powerful who become patients.

brought a suit against U.S.C.-L.A. medical center where the procedure was performed. In a subsequent study, Dreifus and her colleagues found that nine of 23 physicians interviewed had either witnessed coercion or worked under conditions that border on coercion: "hard-selling, dispensing of misinformation, approaching women during labor, offering sterilization at a time of stress, on-the-job racism" ([7], 1. 116).

Maria Diaz was disempowered in two ways. First, she was treated not simply without her consent but against her explicit will. In spite of her constant advocacy for herself, she did not participate even minimally in a very significant decision. Using Kapp's definition, she was disempowered.

But she was disempowered in another way as well. Sterilization is a life-changing operation with earth-shattering ramifications for women from "machismo" cultures. In "machismo" culture, a man's stature may be measured by the number of children he sires. He may divorce or abandon a woman who cannot bear children. Indeed, this is what happened to Lupe Acosta, whose common-law husband of eight years left her after she was sterilized against her will ([7], p. 107). She ended up on welfare, experiencing not only medical disempowerment, but social and economic disempowerment as well. A decision to refuse sterilization that may not seem "sensible" or "rational" in one culture may be very sensible in another. Empowerment in this context would require sensitivity to such cross-cultural issues, and recognition of the devastating consequences of what might seem a "sensible" decision in white North American culture.

Oliver Sacks may not have been told everything that he wanted to know, and may not have had the kind of communication that he desired. But at no time did he experience the kind of disempowerment that these poor, multiparous women with language and cultural barriers experienced. He was not treated *against* his will, nor was a foreign rationality imposed on him.

Medical Harm

Practices such as forced sterilization would be condemned as unjust by most observers. Harder to uncover are the injustices, the disempowerments, built into ordinary, routine medical practice. Here, there are two levels on which we must look for disempowerment and therefore for empowerment. In Sacks' case, the primary disempowerment came with the social *role* of patient — with losing control, being ignored, and not having social power.[4] But for many women, these social concomitants of the role of patient are only part of the picture. Medical practice historically has contributed not only to this second "misery" for women, but also to the first "misery," the phenomenon of physical disintegration itself.

Feminists and concerned women over the years have exposed a range of obstetrical and gynecological practices that actually *endanger* women's health. Unnecessary hysterectomies [15], use of the Dalkon shield [6], clitoridectomies [4, 23] — any number of practices with serious deleterious impact on women's health have been "routine" or common at one time in our history. For example, a number of studies have documented the movement from childbirth to the "delivery" of children in obstetrical units [11, 29]. Historical evidence suggests that midwifery was safer than obstetrics at the time when the (largely male) medical professionals pushed out the (largely female) midwives. Many women have objected to the health risks presented for both mother and child by routine obstetrical practices. Ethel, who bore 16 children, puts it plainly:

> I had all mine at home except the last six. . . . [I]t was easier to have them at home than to have them at the hospital. . . . They'd take me to the hospital and they'd strap me down. I'd like to never have the baby! When I was home, you know, I'd walk till the pains got so bad that I had to lay down; then I'd lay down and have the baby. Without any anesthetic and never no stitches or nothing, because they waited till time. Now they cut you, you know, and they don't give you time to have it. . . . That's what ruins women's health ([3], p. 229).

That such practices actually are dangerous has been argued by several commentators [21, 25].

In this context, empowerment for women includes having control over one's own body and important medical decisions. The dimension of decision-making that Kapp lifts up remains important. But empowerment also includes better health care practices that do not endanger women or children.

In a study of court cases, Miles and August found that when the patient was a man, the court constructed his preferences for treatment in 75% of cases and allowed those preferences to be determining. But when the patient was a woman, the court constructed her preferences in only 14% of cases, and her preferences were not determinative of treatment decisions. Miles and August conclude that "women are disadvantaged in having their moral agency taken less seriously than that of men" ([20], p. 92). If Sacks had difficulty being heard and treated as a moral agent, imagine what he might have faced had he been a woman instead of a man. Thus, on the level of the second "misery," which Sacks calls the moral level, women are not treated equally with men. Empowerment in such a case means not having a double standard: both male and female patients should be treated with attention to their own expressed preferences as well as to their familial connections.

But it is not only the second level of "misery" on which women are not treated equally. Ayanian and Epstein found that "women who are hospitalized for coronary heart disease undergo fewer major diagnostic and therapeutic procedures than men" ([2], p. 221). Steingart et al.

4. Loss of control and autonomy is a typically male problem; feminist literature suggests that loss of relationship might be more problematic for women.

argue that it is "disturbing" to find that women report more cardiac disability before infraction than do men, but are less likely to receive treatments known (in men) to lessen symptoms and improve functional capacity ([26], p. 230). Just as Miles and August found that women's statements of not wanting to be kept alive were dismissed as "emotional" rather than "rational" desires, so it is possible that women's complaints of chest pain may not be taken as seriously as men's. Empowerment for women in the clinical setting clearly begins with having our voices honored and appropriate interventions utilized.

Empathy and the Non-treatment of Women's Issues

Another subtle form of disempowerment is the non-treatment of or non-focus on women's issues. Coronary artery disease is the leading cause of death in women ([26], p. 226). Yet our common image of "heart attack" is an image of a middle-aged professional man, not an image of a woman. The studies just cited make clear that there is much we do not know about how to treat heart disease in women. We have focused on men's needs, but not on women's.

Similarly, more women die *each year* of breast cancer than men died of AIDS in the first *ten years* of the epidemic [30]. It is estimated that one out of every three women will get cancer during their lifetime, and the breast cancer incidence rate has increased 32% in the last decade [27]. Yet, there is neither the commitment of funds for research and development of new treatments and interventions nor the commitment of public energies and attention to breast cancer that we currently experience for AIDS. Empowerment means *attending* to women's issues, and making them a priority for clinical research and treatment.

The reasons for the relative lack of attention to issues so central to women's lives are complex. Lack of women physicians and researchers may be an important contributing factor. A history of exclusion of women from top ranks of the medical profession leaves its legacy. Walsh concludes her historical study of the discrimination against women in the medical profession with these cautioning words: "There is an interrelationship between discrimination against women as medical students and physicians and against women as patients — resulting in the present lack of research on breast cancer, excessive rates of hysterectomies and surgery on women . . . and generally deficient health care for women" ([28], pp. 281-82).

Lack of women physicians not only influences choices about research and clinical emphasis; it also influences the possibilities for empathy, so important in Sacks' experience of healing. What male physician can truly empathize with the birth pains of a woman patient, or with what it means to a woman to lose a breast to surgery? If empathy is important for empowerment, then women will experience less empowerment than men when they are treated in a system that does not encourage women physicians. Similarly, white care-givers have difficulty empathizing with women and men of color; the well-to-do will not even imagine some problems experienced by those who are economically disadvantaged; and so on. Empowerment in the clinical context will require a change in the system that encourages different care-providers.

Problems of Access

While the focus of this essay is on empowerment *within* the clinical setting, some of the most important empowerment issues for those who are relatively powerless have to do with access *to* the clinical setting. Ectopic pregnancy is now the leading cause of maternal death among African-American women [19]. But in 1982 there were 44,000 women in New York state identified as at "high risk" who became pregnant, had no health insurance, and were not eligible for Medicaid ([19], p. 58). Without health insurance or the means to pay, these women do not get *into* the clinical setting. Their empowerment must begin outside that setting, with changes in political, social, and economic policies, Medicaid eligibility, and access to health care. Similarly, for older women, changes in Medicare to allow access to needed health care is critical.

While problems of access raise larger social and political issues, there are some things that can be done within the clinical setting to address these problems. For instance, would women who are eligible for Medicaid be able to find a physician who accepts Medicaid patients? "The worst medical problems I've had really," says Ethel, a poor mountain woman with 12 living children, "has been since I been on welfare. Trying to see the kinds of doctors that's needed for the children and myself, and they don't take the card — needing to see specialists, and the specialists don't take the card" ([3], p. 231). At the same time that we are experiencing the "feminization of poverty," with women increasingly among the poor who must depend on Medicaid, we are also experiencing a time in which ob-gyns, who specialize in women's diseases and reproductive processes, have the lowest rate of Medicaid participation of all primary care physicians ([19], p. 57). Women who cannot get into the health care system at all are doubly disempowered.

Empowerment in this context means the willingness of clinical care providers to "take the card" and deal with the government red tape, the bureaucratic form-filling, and the loss of income represented by accepting those patients. If more physicians "took the card" and had to deal with these inconveniences, perhaps we would see a faster move toward a more equitable system of access for the poor, many of whom are women.

Alternative Structures

Under these circumstances, it is no wonder that many women and other relatively powerless people have felt that empowerment cannot happen within the system. Empowerment means not only advocating for oneself and participating in significant decisions, but receiving care from a radically re-oriented system.

Some have moved to establishing alternative health care systems. One such organization was called "Jane" [1, 12]. Run by women on a non-hierarchical basis, "Jane" helped women get access to safe abortion during the time that abortions were largely illegal in the United States. "Jane" was part of a larger movement that involved teaching women about their bodies, their sexuality, and their own medical care [8, 9]. Alternative clinics were set up where women were trained to do their own vaginal examinations and to monitor their gynecological health. These organizations were empowering for women because they gave women knowledge, allowed women to help each other in a non-hierarchical structure, and kept control of important bodily processes largely in the hands of women themselves. They strengthened relationships among women patients and providers, and tried to deal with issues that were central from the perspective and rationality of women of different cultures.

But alternative structures outside the system are not the only solution. Recognizing the rise of breast cancer and the crucial place of mammograms in diagnosis and early treatment, the Medical Center of Central Massachusetts set out to discover why women were so reluctant to come in for mammograms and whether something could be done about it. They asked women to talk about what keeps them from having mammograms. Among the factors that keep women away, they found these:

1. lack of child-care;
2. cold and unattractive hospital gowns;
3. lack of privacy;
4. inadequately trained technicians, with resulting pain and discomfort;
5. lengthy waiting time between testing and results.

The mammography unit was redesigned to address these problems: it now provides child-care, privacy, specially trained technicians, attractive and warm clothing, immediate test results, and so on. Such structural changes provide empowerment not just for individual patients, but for the entire class of patients and ultimately for society as a whole.

Summary

The lesson to be learned from those who are relatively powerless is that we need changes in the system, not just changes of attitude in a few care-providers. More thoughtful listening, a willingness to hear the "whole" story and not just the "salient facts," will still be important. But it is the system that must be scrutinized for how it disempowers those who are already powerless, and how it could be made more empowering instead.

Empowerment in the clinical setting will require allowing patients to be their own advocates and to participate in significant decision-making. It will require not treating patients against their will, nor assuming that one culture's "rationality" makes sense for all cultures. It will require honoring those forms of rationality, such as art and religion, that offer a language "beyond" reason and science, a language that may be more appropriate to the patient's needs. It will require recognizing the network of community and relationships that affect patients' lives and decisions. But above all, it will require changing the system so that those who are relatively powerless have access to health care, for without that access, all talk of empowerment within the clinical setting is void.

Pacific School of Religion
Berkeley, California
U.S.A.

Bibliography

[1] Addelson, K. P.: 1986, 'Moral Revolution,' in M. Pearsall (ed.), *Women and Values: Readings in Recent Feminist Philosophy,* Wadsworth, Belmont, CA, pp. 291-309.

[2] Ayanian, J. Z., and Epstein, A. M.: 1991, 'Differences in the Use of Procedures between Women and Men Hospitalized for Coronary Heart Disease,' *New England Journal of Medicine* 325 (4): 221-30 (July 25).

[3] Baker, D.: 1977, 'The Class Factor: Mountain Women Speak Out on Women's Health,' in C. Dreifus (ed.), *Seizing Our Bodies,* Random House, NY, pp. 223-32.

[4] Barker-Benfield, G. J.: 1977, 'Sexual Surgery in Late-Nineteenth Century America,' in C. Dreifus (ed.), *Seizing Our Bodies,* Random House, NY, pp. 13-41.

[5] Brueggemann, W.: 1989, *Finally Comes the Poet: Daring Speech for Proclamation,* Fortress Press, Minneapolis.

[6] Dowie, M., and Johnston, T.: 1977, 'A Case of Corporate Malpractice and the Dalkon Shield,' in C. Dreifus (ed.), *Seizing Our Bodies,* Random House, NY, pp. 86-104.

[7] Dreifus, C.: 1977, 'Sterilizing the Poor,' in C. Dreifus (ed.), *Seizing Our Bodies,* Random House, NY, pp. 105-20.

[8] Frankfort, E.: 1977, 'Vaginal Politics,' in C. Dreifus (ed.), *Seizing Our Bodies,* Random House, NY, pp. 263-70.

[9] Fruchter, R. G., et al.: 1977, 'The Women's Health Movement: Where Are We Now?,' in C. Dreifus (ed.), *Seizing Our Bodies,* Random House, NY, pp. 271-78.

[10] Goldman, A. H.: 1980, *The Moral Foundations of Professional Ethics,* Rowman and Littlefield, Totowa, NJ.

[11] Haire, D.: 1972, *The Cultural Warping of Childbirth,* International Childbirth Education Association, Seattle.

[12] 'Jane': 1990, 'Just Call "Jane",' in M. G. Fried (ed.), *From Abortion to Reproductive Freedom: Transforming a Movement,* South End Press, Boston.

[13] Jonas, H.: 1970, 'Philosophical Reflections on Human Experimentation,' in P. Freund (ed.), *Experimentation with Human Subjects,* George Braziller, NY, pp. 1-31.

[14] Kapp, M. B.: 1989, 'Medical Empowerment of the Elderly,' *Hastings Center Report* 19 (4), (July-August).

[15] Larned, D.: 1977, 'The Epidemic in Unnecessary Hysterectomy,' in C. Dreifus (ed.), *Seizing Our Bodies,* Random House, NY, pp. 195-208.

[16] Lebacqz, K.: 1987: *Justice in an Unjust World: Foundations for a Christian Approach to Justice,* Augsburg Publishing House, Minneapolis, MN.

[17] Lebacqz, K.: 1985, *Professional Ethics: Power and Paradox,* Abingdon Press, Nashville, TN.

[18] Lebacqz, K.: 1986, *Six Theories of Justice: Perspectives from Philosophical and Theological Ethics,* Augsburg Publishing House, Minneapolis, MN.

[19] McBarnette, L.: 1988, 'Women and Poverty: The Effects on Reproductive Status,' in C. A. Perales and L. S. Young (eds.), *Too Little, Too Late: Dealing with the Health Needs of Women in Poverty,* Harrington Park Press, New York.

[20] Miles, S. H., and August, A.: 1990, "Courts, Gender and 'The Right to Die'," *Law, Medicine, and Health Care* 18 (102): 85-95 (Spring/Summer).

[21] Rich, A.: 1986, *Of Woman Born: Motherhood as Experience and Institution,* W. W. Norton, NY.

[22] Rosenbaum, E.: 1988, *A Taste of My Own Medicine;* now published as *The Doctor,* Ivy Books, NY.

[23] Rothman, B. K.: 1979, 'Women, Health and Medicine,' in J. Freeman (ed.), *Women: A Feminist Perspective,* 2nd ed., Mayfield Publishing Co., Palo Alto, CA.

[24] Sacks, O.: 1984, *A Leg to Stand On,* Harper and Row, NY.

[25] Sarah, R.: 1988, 'Power, Certainty, and the Fear of Death,' in E. H. Baruch, A. F. D'Adamo, and J. Seager (eds.), *Embryos, Ethics, and Women's Rights: Exploring the New Reproductive Technologies,* Harrington Park Press, New York.

[26] Steingart, R. M., et al.: 1991, 'Sex Differences in the Management of Coronary Artery Disease,' *New England Journal of Medicine* 325 (4) (July 25), 226-30.

[27] Steingraber, S.: 1991, 'Lifestyles Don't Kill. Carcinogens in Air, Food, and Water Do,' in M. Stocker (ed.), *Cancer as a Woman's Issue: Scratching the Surface,* Third Side Press, Chicago.

[28] Walsh, M. R.: 1977, '*Doctors Wanted: No Women Need Apply': Sexual Barriers in the Medical Profession, 1835-1975,* Yale University Press, New Haven.

[29] Wertz, R. W., and Wertz, D. C.: 1977, *Lying-In: A History of Childbirth in America,* The Free Press, NY.

[30] Winnow, J.: 1991, 'Lesbians' Evolving Health Care: Our Lives Depend on It,' in M. Stocker (ed.), *Cancer as a Woman's Issue: Scratching the Surface,* Third Side Press, Chicago.

42 The Will to Be Healthy

Karl Barth

Let us now raise the question of respect for life in the human sphere. In its form as the will to live, it will also include the will to be healthy. The satisfaction of the needs of the impulses corresponding to man's vegetative and animal nature is one thing, but health, although connected with it, is quite another. Health means capability, vigour and freedom. It is strength for human life. It is the integration of the organs for the exercise of psychophysical functions. . . .

If man may and should will to live, then obviously he may and should also will to be healthy and therefore to be in possession of this strength too. But the concept of this volition is problematical for many reasons and requires elucidation. For somehow it seems to be part of the nature of health that he who possesses it is not conscious of it nor preoccupied with it, but hardly ever thinks about it and cannot therefore be in any position to will it. . . .

If this is so, we must ask whether a special will for health is not a symptom of deficient health which can only magnify the deficiency by confirming it. And a further question which might be raised with reference to this will is whether we can reasonably affirm and seek health independently, or otherwise than in connexion with specific material aims and purposes. . . .

Yet included in the will to live there is a will to be healthy which is not affected by these legitimate questions but which, like the will to live, is demanded by God and is to be seriously achieved in obedience to this demand. By health we are not to think merely of a particular physical or psychical something of great value that can be considered and possessed by itself and therefore can and must be the object of special attention, search and effort. Health is the strength to be as man. It serves human existence in the form of the capacity, vitality and freedom to exercise the psychical and physical functions, just as these themselves are only functions of human existence. We can and should will it as this strength when we will not merely to be healthy in body and soul but to be man at all: man and not animal or plant, man and not wood or stone, man and not a thing or the exponent of an idea, man in the satisfaction of his instinctive needs, man in the use of his reason, in loyalty to his individuality, in the knowledge of its limitations, man in his deter-

From Karl Barth, *Church Dogmatics,* III/4, trans. A. T. Mackay et al. (Edinburgh: T&T Clark, 1961), pp. 357-63. Used by permission.

mination for work and knowledge, and above all in his relation to God and his fellow-men in the proffered act of freedom. We can and should will this, and therefore we can and should will to be healthy. For how can we will, understand or desire the strength for all this unless in willing it we put it into operation in the smaller or greater measure in which we have it? And in willing to be man, how can we put it into operation unless we also will and seek and desire it? We gain it as we practise it. We should therefore will to practise it. This is what is demanded of man in this respect.

Though we cannot deny the antithesis between health and sickness when we view the problem in this way, we must understand it in its relativity. Sickness is obviously negative in relation to health. It is partial impotence to exercise those functions. It hinders man in his exercise of them by burdening, hindering, troubling and threatening him, and causing him pain. But sickness as such is not necessarily impotence to be as man. The strength to be this, so long as one is still alive, can also be the strength and therefore the health of the sick person. And if health is the strength for human existence, even those who are seriously ill can will to be healthy without any optimism or illusions regarding their condition. They, too, are commanded, and it is not too much to ask, that so long as they are alive they should will this, i.e., exercise the power which remains to them, in spite of every obstacle. Hence it seems to be a fundamental demand of the ethics of the sickbed that the sick person should not cease to let himself be addressed, and to address himself, in terms of health and the will which it requires rather than sickness, and above all to see to it that he is in an environment of health. From the same standpoint we cannot count on conditions of absolute and total health, and therefore on the existence of men who are already healthy and do not need the command to will to be so. Even healthy people have great need of the will for health, though perhaps not of the doctor. Conditions of relative and subjectively total ease in relation to the psycho-physical functions of life may well exist. But whether the man who can enjoy such ease is healthy, i.e., a man who lives in the power to be as man, is quite another question which we need only ask, and we must immediately answer that in reality he may be severely handicapped in the exercise of this power, and therefore sick, long before this makes itself felt in the deterioration of his organs or their functional disturbance, so that he perhaps stands in greater need of the summons that he should be healthy than someone who already suffers from such deterioration and disturbance and is therefore regarded as sick in soul or body or perhaps both. And who of us has not constantly to win and possess this strength? A fundamental demand of ethics, even for the man who seems to be and to a large extent really is "healthy in body and soul," is thus that he should not try to evade the summons to be healthy in the true sense of the term.

On the same presupposition it will also be understood that in the question of health we must differentiate between soul and body but not on any account separate the two. The healthy man, and also the sick, is both. He is the soul of his body, the rational soul of his vegetative and animal body, the ruling soul of his serving body. But he is one and the same man in both, and not two. Health and sickness in the two do not constitute two divided realms, but are always a single whole. It is always a matter of the man himself, of his greater or lesser strength, and the more or less serious threat and even increasing impotence. It is he who has been predominantly ill and he who may be predominantly well. Or it is he who must perhaps go the opposite way from predominant health to predominant sickness. It is he who is on the way from the one or the other. Hence he does not have a specific healthy or sick life of the soul with particular dominating or subjugated, unresolved or resolved inclinations, complexes, ties, prohibitions and impulses, and then quite apart from this, in health or sickness, in the antithesis, conflict and balance of the two, an organic vegetative and animal life of the body. On the contrary, he lives the healthy or sick life of his soul in his body and with the life of his body, so that in both, and in their mutual relationship, it is a matter of his life's history, his own history. Again, he does not have a specific physical life in the sound or disordered functions of his somatic organs, his nervous system, his blood circulation, digestion, urination and so on, and then in an upper storey a separate life of the soul. But he lives the healthy or sick life of his body together with that of his soul, and again in both cases, and in their mutual relationship, it is a matter of his life's history, his own history, and therefore himself. And the will for health as the strength to be as man is obviously quite simply, and without duplication in a psychical and physical sphere, the will to continue this history in its unity and totality. A man can, of course, orientate himself seriously, but only secondarily, on this or that psychical or physical element of health in contrast to sickness. But primarily he will always orientate himself in this contrast on his own being as man, on his assertion, preservation and renewal (and all this in the form of activity) as a subject. In all his particular decisions and measures, if they are to be meaningful, he must have a primary concern to confirm his power to be as man and to deny the lack of power to be this. In all stages of that history the question to be answered is: "Wilt thou be made whole?" (Jn. 5[6]), and not: "Wilt thou have healthy limbs or be free of their sickness?" The command which we must always obey is the command to stand upright and not to fall.

From exactly the same standpoint again there can be no indifference to the concrete problems of getting and remaining well. If in the question of health we were concerned with a specific psychical or physical quantity, we might be interested at a distance in the one or the other, and seek health and satisfaction first in psychology and then in a somatic form of health, only to tire no less arbitrarily of one or the other or perhaps both, and to let things take their course. But if on both sides it is a matter of the strength to be as man, on both sides we are free from the anxious or fanatical expectation that real decisions can and must be made, but also free to give to the psychical and physical spheres the attention due to them in this respect because they are the field on which the true decisions of the will for health must be worked out. It is precisely in the continuation of his life of soul and body that the history of man must continue in the strength to be as man. What he *can* do for the continuation and therefore against every restriction of his life of soul and body, he ought to *will* to do if he is to be healthy, if he is to live in this strength, and if his history is to proceed in the strength of his being as man. In order that this strength may not degenerate into a process in which he is only driven as an object and is therefore no longer man, in order that he may remain its subject and therefore man, he must be on the watch and active for the continuation and against the constriction of his psychical and physical life. The fact that he wills to rise up and stand in this power, and not to fall into weakness, is not in the least decided by the various measures which he might adopt to maintain and protect his psychical and physical powers. He could adopt a thousand measures of this kind with full zeal and skill, and yet not possess the will to maintain this strength, thus lacking the will for health and falling in spite of all his efforts. But if he possesses the will to win and maintain this strength, it is natural that he should be incidentally concerned to take the necessary precautions to preserve and protect his psychical and physical powers, and this in a responsible and energetic way in which the smallest thing is not too small for him nor the greatest too great.

At this point, therefore, we may legitimately ask, and must do so in all seriousness, what is good, or not good, or more or less good, for the soul and body. There is a general and above all a particular hygiene of the psychical and physical life concerning the possibilities and limitations of which we must all seek individual clarity by investigation and experience and also by instruction from a third party, and to which we must all keep in questions of what we may or may not do. In such a hygiene God's gifts of sun, air and water will be applied as the most important factors, effective positively in the psychical no less than the physical sphere. Hygiene is the foundation of every prophylactic against possible illness, as it is also the main basis of therapy where illness has already commenced. We have to realise, however, that in all the negative or positive measures which may be taken it is a matter of maintaining, protecting and restoring not merely a strength which is necessary and may be enjoyed in isolation, but the strength even to be at all as man. It is because so much is at stake, because being as man is a history enacted in space and developing in, with and by the exercise of the psychical and physical functions of life, that attention is demanded at this point and definite measures must be incidentally taken by all of us. Sport may also be mentioned in this connexion. But sport has, legitimately, other dimensions, namely, those of play, of the development of physical strength and of competition, so that it may even constitute a threat to health in the true sense of the term as it now concerns us. We shall thus content ourselves with the statement that sport may form a part of hygiene, and therefore ought to do so in specific instances.

The question has often been raised, and will never find a wholly satisfactory answer, whether the measures to be adopted in this whole sphere really demand the consultation of a doctor. The doctor is a man who is distinguished from others by his general knowledge of psychical or physical health or sickness on the basis of tradition, investigation and daily renewed and corrected experience. He is thus in a position to pass an objective verdict on the psychical or physical health or sickness of others. He is capable of assisting them in their necessary efforts to maintain or regain health by his advice or orders or even, if necessary, direct intervention. What objections can there be to consulting a doctor? If we acknowledge the basic fact that we are required to will the strength to be as man, that we are thus required to will psycho-physical forces, and that we are thus commanded to take all possible measures to maintain or preserve this basic power, there seems to be no reason why consultation of a doctor should not find a place among these measures. This is the wise and prudent verdict of Ecclesiasticus in a famous passage (chapter 38): "For of the Most High cometh healing . . . the Lord has created medicines out of the earth, and he that is wise will not abhor them. . . . And he has given men skill that he might be honoured in his marvellous works. With such doth the physician heal men, and taketh away their pains. Of such doth the apothecary make a confection; and of his works there is no end, and from him is peace over all the earth" (vv. 2ff.). Therefore, "give place to the physician, for the Lord has created him; let him not go from thee, for thou hast need of him. There is a time when in their hands there is good success. For they shall also pray unto the Lord, that he would prosper that which they give for ease and remedy to prolong life" (vv. 12ff.).

What do we have against the medical man? Apart from a general and illegitimate passivity in matters of health and sickness, the main point seems to be that there are reasons to suspect the objectivity of the knowledge, diagnosis and therapy of a stranger to whom we are required to give place and confidence at the very heart of our own history, handing over to him far-reaching powers of authority and instruction. The more a man understands the question of health and sickness correctly, i.e., the question of his own strength to be as man and therefore of the continuation of his own life history, the more he will entertain this kind of suspicion in relation to the doctor, not in spite of but just because of his science as general knowledge, and the objectiveness of his verdict, orders and interventions. Is not health or sickness, particularly when it is understood as strength or weakness to be as man, the most subjective thing that there is? What can the stranger with his general science know of this strength or weakness of mine? How can he really help me? How can I surrender into his hands?

Yet this form of argument, and the suspicion based upon it, is quite mistaken, and Ecclesiasticus is in the right against it. For it rests on a misunderstanding in which the doctor himself may share through a presumptuous conception of his position, but which may well exist only on the part of the suspicious patient. Health in the true sense of the term as strength to be as man is not to be expected from any of the measures which can be adopted in the sphere of psychical and physical functions as a defence against sickness or for the preservation or restoration of health. There exists, more perhaps in the imagination of others than on the part of experts, or at any rate of genuine and serious experts, a medical and especially in our own day a psychological totalitarianism and imperialism which would have it that the doctor is the one who really heals. In this form, he must truly be warded off as an unpleasant stranger. There is, in fact, an ancient and in itself interesting connexion between medical and priestly craft. But both doctors and others are urgently asked not to think of the medical man as occupying the position and role of a priest. In all these or similar presumptuous forms, he will probably not be able to help even in the sphere and sense in which he might actually do so. It was probably in some such form that he confronted the woman of whom it is written in Mk. 5[26]: "She had suffered many things of many physicians, and had spent all that she had, and was nothing bettered, but rather grew worse." But in his true form, why should not the doctor be the man who is really able to assist others in his own sphere? And why should he not be looked upon in this way even when he perhaps appears in that perverted form?

In what way can he help? Can he promote the strength to be as man? No, this is something which each can only will, desire and strive for, but not procure nor attain of himself. This is something which even the best doctor can only desire for him. And he will be a better doctor the more consciously he realises his limitations in this respect. For in this way he can draw the attention of others to the fact that the main thing in getting well is something in which neither he nor any human measure can help. If he is a Christian doctor, in certain cases he will explicitly draw attention to this fact. He will then be free to help where he can and should do so, namely, in the sphere of the psychical and physical functions. In relation to these, to their organic, chemical and mechanical presuppositions, to their normal progress and its laws, to their difficulties and degeneracies, to their immediate causes, and to that which can be done in certain circumstances to promote their normal progress and prevent their disturbance, in short, to human life and its health and sickness, there exists more than individual knowledge and opinion. Within the limits of all human knowledge and ability, there are general insights the knowledge of which is based on a history, rich in errors but also in genuine discoveries, of innumerable observations, experiences and experiments, and there are also the general rules to apply this history in the diagnosis and therapy of the individual case. For in this sphere every man, irrespective of his uniqueness before God and among men, is also a specimen, a case among many cases to be classified in the categories of this science, an object to which its rules may be applied. To be sure, each is a new and individual case in which the science and its rules take on a new and specific form. It is the task and business of the doctor to find and apply the new and specific form of the science and its application to the individual case. Hence he is not for any of us an absolute stranger in this sphere. He is a relative newcomer to the extent that each case is necessarily new. But from the standpoint of his science and its practice he is a competent newcomer, and as such he deserves trust rather than suspicion, not an absolute confidence, but a solid relative confidence that in this matter he has better general information than we have, and that for the present we can hopefully submit to his judgment, advice, direction and even intervention in our own particular case. Those who cannot show this confidence ought not to trouble the doctor, nor to be troubled by him. But why should we not show this modest confidence when dealing with a modest doctor?

Ecclesiasticus is quite right to say: "The Lord has created him too." Medical art and science rest like others on a legitimate use of the possibilities given to man. If the history of medicine has been as little free from error, negligence, one-sidedness and exaggeration as any other science, in its main development it has been and still is, to lay eyes at least, as impressive, honourable and promising as, for instance, theology. There is no real reason to ignore its existence or refuse its offer. How can the doctor help? Obviously by giving free play, and removing the obstacles to the will for real health, i.e., the will to exist forcefully as man, which he cannot give to any of us but to which he may supremely exhort us. Psychical and physical illness is naturally a hindrance to this will. It restricts its development. It constitutes an external damaging of it. The doctor's task is to investigate the particular type and form of illness in any given case, to trace its causes in the heredity, constitution, life history and mode of life of the patient, and to study its secondary conditions and consequences, its course thus far, its present position and threatened progress. If humanly speaking everything depends on that will, is it not a great help to be able to learn with some degree of reliability what is really wrong, or more positively what possibilities of movement and action still remain in spite of the present injury, and within what limits one may still will to be healthy? And these limits might, of course, be extended. The doctor goes on to treat the patient with a view to arresting at least the damage, to weakening its power and effect, perhaps even to tackling its causes and thus removing it altogether, so that the patient is well again at least in the medical sphere. And even if the doctor cannot extend the limits of life available, he can at least make the restrictive ailment tolerable, or at worst, if there is no remedy and the limits become progressively narrower, he can do everything possible to make them relatively bearable. All this may be done by the doctor within the limits of his subjective mastery of his medical science and skill. He cannot do more, but at least he cannot do less. And in this way he can assist the will to live in its form as the will to be healthy. In this respect he can encourage man in the strongest sense of the word, and by removing, arresting or palliating the hampering illness he can give him both the incentive to do what he may still do, i.e., to will to be healthy, and also joy and pleasure in doing it. Having done this to the best of his ability, he should withdraw. He has no power in the crucial issue of the strength or weakness of the patient to be as man. He has no control over the will of the patient in this antithesis. Indeed, he has only a very limited power even over the health or sickness of his organs, of the psychical and physical functions in which that strength and the will for it must express themselves in conflict against the weakness. But if he does his best where he can, we must be grateful to him.

Finally, we have to remember that, when seriously posed, the whole question of measures to be adapted for the protection or recovery of the freedom of vital functions necessarily goes beyond the answers given by each of us individually. The basic question of the power to be as man, and therefore of the will for this power and therefore for real health, and the associated question of its expression and exercise, are questions which are not merely to be raised and answered individually but in concert. They are social questions. Hygiene, sport and medicine arrive too late, and cannot be more than rather feeble palliatives, if such general conditions as wages, standards of living, working hours, necessary breaks, and above all housing are so ordered, or rather disordered, that instead of counteracting they promote and perhaps even cause illness, and therefore the external impairing of the will for life and health. Respect for life in the form in which we now particularly envisage it necessarily includes responsibility for the standard of living conditions generally, and particularly so for those to whom they do not constitute a personal problem because they personally need not suffer or fear any threat from this angle, being able to enjoy at least the possibility of health, and to take measures for its protection or recovery, in view of their income, food, working hours, rest and wider interests. The principle *mens sana in corpore sano* can be a highly short-sighted and brutal one if it is only understood individually and not in the wider sense of *in societate sana*. And this extension cannot only mean that we must see to it that the benefits of hygiene, sport and medicine are made available for all, or at least as many as possible. It must mean that the general living conditions of all, or at least of as many as possible, are to be shaped in such a way that they make not just a negative but a positive preventative contribution to their health, as is the case already in varying degrees with the privileged. The will for health of the individual must therefore take also the form of the will to improve, raise and perhaps radically transform the general living conditions of all men. If there is no other way, it must assume the form of the will for a new and quite different order of society, guaranteeing better living conditions for all. Where some are necessarily ill the others cannot with good conscience will to be well. Nor can they really do it at all if they are not concerned about neighbours who are inevitably sick because of their social position. For sooner or later the fact of this illness will in some way threaten them in spite of the measures which they take to isolate themselves and which may be temporarily and partially successful. When one person is ill, the whole society is really ill in all its members. In the battle against sickness the final human word cannot be isolation but only fellowship.

43 Thorn-in-the-Flesh Decision Making: A Christian Overview of the Ethics of Treatment

Richard J. Mouw

The ethical perspectives which get employed in medical ethical discussions often seem rather narrow in scope. Sometimes the methodology seems closely linked to a "values clarification" approach, in which the people involved are encouraged to get clearer about the value commitments with which they operate. Or, ethical issues are introduced within a framework of a kind of "systems analysis," and the questions are put in this way: How can we plug our values into the procedures of medical care? How can we best fit the ethical component into the system of medical decision making?

From a Christian point of view there is something deeply unsatisfactory about these ways of dealing with the issues. This sense of dissatisfaction was expressed to me recently by a medical professional who had been involved in a discussion of ethical issues at a seminar in the hospital where she works. At this seminar she experienced a profound frustration: "I just don't know where to *begin* in bringing my own beliefs to bear on that discussion. I felt like those questions were very important to me, but I also felt that I had to come at those questions in a very different way!"

This experience of frustration is based — or so I judge — on a proper assessment of typical discussions of medical ethics. Very often those discussions move on to casuistry before getting clear about the principles which must inform casuistical deliberation. Nor can the moral principles proper to medical decision making be arrived at merely by explicating our intuitions or by systematizing our hunches. Medical ethical discussion must be rooted in a broad-ranging, self-conscious awareness of the larger moral and more-than-moral contexts in which medical questions arise.

Take, for example, the systems-analysis approach to which I have already alluded. This approach seems to work on the following model. There is a system of medical decision making that encompasses various diagnostic, prognostic, and therapeutic options. This system is taken as a given. The question then is asked whether this system or set of procedures and options is fully adequate without some ethical components being added to it. The view that the system by itself is inadequate seems to be what Ivan Illich has in mind when he complains that in a highly "medicalized" culture "medical ethics have been secreted into a specialized department that brings theory into line with actual practice" (*Medical Nemesis: The Expropriation of Health* [New York: Bantam, 1977], p. 40). Illich's own view calls for an evaluative critique of that system of medical care itself; he is convinced that the basic assumptions of our medicalized society must be called into question. Whatever our own assessment may be of the details of Illich's critique, he does seem to be correct in insisting that we must be sensitive to the basic presuppositions which shape the discussion of medical ethics.

We must recognize the limitations of the medical perspective by looking at the ways in which formulations of that perspective relate to other kinds of concerns, including ethical concerns. But lest that sound like a self-serving statement coming from an ethicist, let me go one step further. We must also recognize the limitations of the ethical perspective by looking at the ways in which formulations of *that* perspective relate to other kinds of concerns, concerns which range more broadly than the issues of ethical rightness and wrongness.

Medical ethics as an area of scholarly and professional inquiry must be tamed — put into its proper place — by the recognition that neither medical nor ethical nor medical ethical discussion is adequate for dealing with the issues which arise in the context of medical decision making. My basic contention here will not be shocking to Calvinists. Medical ethics must itself function within the context of a larger world-and-life view. As Christians we cannot discuss a perplexing medical dilemma for very long without sensing the need to discuss our views of human nature, our perspectives on the society in which we live, and our concepts of health and healing and human well-being and eternal destiny.

For as long as any of us can remember there have been groups around that have reminded us of the role of basic presuppositions in dealing with medical issues. Jehovah's Witnesses have refused blood transfusions; Christian Scientists have rejected conventional definitions of "disease" and "cure"; Seventh Day Adventists have questioned accepted traditions regarding nutrition; the Old Reformed have eschewed preventative medicine. Few of us are convinced by the exegetical and theological cases which these groups offer in defense of their departures from conventional medical wisdom. But, like Ivan Illich's more recent heterodoxies, they do remind us of a *level* of critical concern which we must attempt to maintain — a reminder that has also been reinforced by recent interest in Chinese acupuncture, "indigenous" medicine, the hospice movement, and other phenomena.

Some rather harsh recent criticisms of medical orthodoxy have alleged that there are perverse psychological, social, political and economic forces which have shaped the attitudes and patterns at work in medical decision making. These criticisms have a direct bearing on a consideration of the processes of medical treatment. Elisabeth Kübler-Ross and others have argued that the alleged "objectivity" of medical practitioners is often a cover-up for the insecurity and fear in the presence of suffering and death on the part of those professionals. Others have argued that the medical care professions are tainted by sexism, racism, classism, ageism, and elitism.

As I have said, these latter considerations — which we might think of as having to do with, roughly speaking, the sociology of medicine — bear very directly on the ethics of treatment. It is not necessary here to decide the degree to which these sociological criticisms of medical orthodoxy are correct. But we can allow the sensitivities from which they stem to inform our own discussion. At the very least this means that we ought not construe the treatment process in too narrow a fashion. There is, for example, a distressing tendency in much of the literature dealing with the ethics of treatment to focus almost exclusively on the physician-patient relationship, as if these were the only two roles which have an important place in medical treatment. The fact is that the treatment process encompasses many relationships involving a number of different roles: for example, the relationship between physician and nurse, nurse and patient, physician and family, clergy and patient.

How should we as Christians view these relationships in the context of the treatment process? In a 1956 article published in the A.M.A. *Archives of Internal Medicine,* Thomas Szasz and Marc Hollender distinguished among three basic models of the physician-patient relationship in the hope of showing "that certain philosophical preconceptions associated with the notions of 'disease,' 'treatment,' and 'cure' have a profound bearing on both the theory and practice of medicine." Their first model is that of "Activity-Passivity," which they judge to be the oldest model operating in medical care. Here the physician is viewed as active, the patient as acted upon. "Treatment" takes place irrespective of the patient's contribution and regardless of the outcome. There is a similarity here between the patient and a helpless infant, on the one hand, and between physician and parent, on the other."

The second model is that of "Guidance-Cooperation." Here the patient takes on a more active role than in the previous model. But the decision-making power resides with the physician. The physician "guides"; the patient "cooperates." If the earlier model can be likened to the relationship between parent and helpless infant, this one more closely parallels that between parent and adolescent child.

The third model is given the label of "Mutual Participation," and it is based on "the postulate that equality among human beings is desirable." Patient and physician have roughly equal power, they are mutually interdependent, and they search for decisions which will be satisfactory to both parties.

Several observations are necessary concerning the intentions of Szasz and Hollender in presenting these models. First, they make it clear that no one single model is adequate to all situations involving medical decisions. For example, the Activity-Passivity model may be quite appropriate to a situation where a physician must treat a comatose patient. Second, Szasz and Hollender obviously do think that the third model, Mutual Participation, is the ideal to be strived for. They tell us that "in an evolutionary sense, the pattern of mutual participation is more highly developed than the other two models of doctor-patient relationship." And third, we must highlight the fact that Szasz and Hollender are presenting these models as ways of sorting out different patterns or distributions of power and authority in medical decision making. In the first model, all power resides with the physician; in the second, the patient at least has the right or power to consent to the physician's decision; in the third, power is distributed along egalitarian lines.

I want to comment further on some of these matters. But before doing so, I must briefly observe that Szasz and Hollender themselves manifest the syndrome, which I mentioned earlier, of discussing the treatment process as if it were exclusively an affair between *physician* and patient. I will attempt to remedy that pattern by referring more generally to the relationship between medical professional and patient.

I daresay that many of us in the Christian community would never think of attempting to understand the relationship between medical professional and patient along the lines suggested by the third model proposed by Szasz and Hollender. Nor would we find the first model, that of Activity-Passivity, to be appropriate, except in unusual circumstances. Most of us would take the second model, in which the patient cooperates with the expert guidance of the professional, as quite proper — even the ideal way of viewing medical situations. But of course it is precisely the notion of the "expertise" of the professional which is under attack from the perspective of the egalitarian.

The denial of the expertise of the medical professional comes in two forms today. First, there are those who hold to a pluralistic or relativistic view of medical theory. They reject the notion of a "neutral" or "objective" medical science. Medical theories and technologies are shaped by cultural perspectives, and their formation and formulation are guided by culturally embedded understandings of such things as "health," "disease," and "cure." The Navajo medicine man, the faith healer, the Eastern guru, the shaman, the surgeon from Cincinnati, the practitioner of acupuncture — each is rooted in a different form of social organization embodying a different normative understanding of human nature. To evaluate these perspectives in terms of "primitive" or "modern" or "advanced" is already to be adopting a given cultural archimedian point. There can be no question of whether one system is better than another; each is simply different from the rest. Or, if comparative evaluations *can* be made, they cannot be made superficially; they must be based on an assessment of the larger cultural context from which given perspectives and technologies derive their meaning and effectiveness.

There are important and fascinating issues here — issues which bear directly on questions in the philosophy of science and epistemology. But the second form of the challenge to medical expertise has closer links to medical ethics and the sociology of medicine, so we will look at that version more closely.

The second way in which people challenge the expertise of the medical professional focuses on the role of what are considered to be significant nonmedical factors in medical decision making. Those who issue this kind of challenge may or may not have sympathies with the first form of challenge. Nonetheless they are inclined to view situations of medical decision making in such a way that careful attention is given to various nonmedical features of those situations. The medical professional may be viewed as having some degree of expertise with regard to medical science and technology; but it is argued that the benefits of medical expertise are outweighed by the professional's lack of expertise regarding other, more important, factors at work in situations of medical decision making. Sometimes it is even suggested that medical professionals manifest a systematic bias regarding these nonmedical factors, a bias which distorts and perverts their appeals to medical expertise. For example, a feminist writing under a pseudonym and describing herself as a "fat Radical Therapist" (Aldebaran, "Fat Liberation," in *Love, Therapy and Politics,* ed. Hogie Wyckoff [New York: Grove Press, 1976], pp. 197-212) has argued that the medical establishment and the insurance companies have conspired to suppress and distort accurate information regarding fatness and health. In the course of making her case she refers to "the mystification of medical knowledge which has oppressed fat people for so long," and she alleges that "the hostility of doctors toward fat people is well-documented." This oppression, she suggests, is especially directed toward women: the medical and mental health professions are committed to the ideals of "beauty, poise and health." In foisting these ideals on women in the name of medical "objectivity" they force many people into lives of "anxiety, self-hatred, and, ultimately, more failure."

This line is argument is an extreme case in point for a pattern of thinking which others are inclined to pursue in more modest tones: the medical professions are organized along lines which promote insensitivity to what it means to be a woman, a black, a homosexual, a ghetto-dweller. Yet characteristics of this sort are crucial elements in medical situations. A patient possessing such characteristics is in fact the "expert" regarding the medical situation in which he or she is involved. Prescriptions concerning what is "best" for a person in that situation must be made from the point of view of the patient.

It should be obvious from the little that I have said about this line of criticism of medical professionals that this is an area of discussion where a number of different dynamics are at work. Some critics attribute to medical professionals a systematic bias against certain groups of people; others view medical orthodoxy as a manifestation of a perverse ideology; still others limit themselves to pointing out certain widespread social and psychological insensitivities associated with medical practice.

But underlying some of the criticisms in this area are assumptions which are closely related to the third model described by Szasz and Hollender, the egalitarian model. This does seem to me to be what is going on in Ivan Illich's critique of what he considers our "medicalized society." I offer as evidence the concluding paragraph of his book, *Medical Nemesis:*

> Man's consciously lived fragility, individuality, and relatedness make the experience of pain, of sickness, and of death an integral part of his life. The ability to cope with this trio autonomously is fundamental to his health. As he becomes dependent on the management of his intimacy, he renounces his autonomy and his health *must* decline. The true miracle of modern medicine is diabolical. It consists in making not only individuals but whole populations survive on inhumanly low levels of personal health. Medical nemesis is the negative feedback of a social organization that set out to improve and equalize the opportunity for each man to cope in autonomy and ended by destroying it.

Here we have a clear example of someone who pits human "autonomy" against the "dependency" fostered by medical orthodoxy. According to Illich, the most significant factors at work in a situation of medical decision making are these: as a fragile individual, the questions of how I am going to cope with *my* pain, *my* sickness, *my* death, are an integral part of my life. The autonomous exercise of my ability to cope with these matters is central to my own health. "Health" is not something which can be defined in purely physiological terms, such that a professional intervention on my behalf, an intervention over which I have no control and which brings about a certain state of physiological equilibrium, can make me "healthy." Health *includes* my autonomous coping with my own pain and sickness. Any medical care system which attempts to bypass my active involvement in the decisions which affect these most intimate matters in my life is, as Illich puts it, diabolical: it inevitably reduces my personal health; it makes me dependent on its own alleged expertise. The fact is that the professional is attempting to manage a situation in which I alone may be the true expert; for I alone am qualified to decide how my pain, my sickness, and my death will function in my life plan.

I must confess that my own response to this line of argument is an ambivalent one. Let me first explain the negative side of my reaction. As an orthodox Calvinist I bristle when I hear the word "autonomy." I cut my own theological and philosophical teeth on the writings of Carl Henry, Cornelius Van Til and Herman Dooyeweerd, and I learned my lessons well. "Autonomy" means "self-legislating"; an autonomous agent makes his or her own laws. And from a biblical perspective this simply will not do. People are not their own lawmakers;

they cannot produce their own norms for living. The plea for autonomy is a vain boast, a boast which echoes the arrogance of the serpent in Genesis 3: "when you eat of [the fruit of the tree] your eyes will be opened, and you will be like God."

This is not to say that the word "autonomy," whenever it is used, always means something devilish. Even some orthodox Calvinists have been known to speak of the need for an "autonomous Christian school system" — by which they mean a school system whose direction is not decided by a government or a church but which sets its own course. I do not know whether Illich himself means to use the term in a way that I would consider to be completely perverse. But I do know that sinful autonomy — the prideful desire to set one's own course, thereby refusing to recognize God's sovereign rule — is a very real tendency in the human heart. And it is a tendency which manifests itself in all areas of living and decision making, including those areas having to do with medicine and health. So it is never silly for us to raise the question whether we are hearing echoes from the Garden in contemporary pleas on behalf of autonomous decision making.

But even when we are sure that a given plea for autonomy is diabolical in nature, that does not decide the matter. Even the serpent of Genesis 3 must be given his due. We know that the serpent always lies, that he is always wrong; but we must take pains to discern the nature of his error in a given context. The Bible makes it clear that while the serpent was thoroughly evil, he was not thoroughly stupid. Genesis 3 begins, after all, with the observation that "the serpent was more subtle than any other wild creature that the LORD God had made." The serpent's lie was in fact a perversion of the truth. He was trading on a subtlety. In tempting Eve, the serpent told her that she could become "like God." Now that is not just a simple falsehood — it is a perversion of the truth. In Genesis 1 we learn that Adam and Eve were in fact created in the image and likeness of God. There is a perfectly proper sense in which human beings are "like God." We are God-imagers. The serpent in Genesis 3 was twisting the truth into a falsehood. He was telling a God-imager that she should become a God-pretender; he was encouraging someone who was already made in the image of God to try to *be* a god. In doing so the serpent was trading on a subtlety: he was, as I have already said, twisting the truth.

Now, what does all of this have to do with Ivan Illich's plea for autonomy? I want to suggest that even if we were convinced that Illich was encouraging persons to be autonomous in the straightforwardly sinful sense of Genesis 3, he still might not be *all* wrong. He might be twisting the truth. And then it would be our job to see the truth that might reside in his perversion of the truth.

Let me try to illustrate my contention here by going through a few lines of Illich's paragraph again, but this time substituting references to the image of God for his uses of the concept of autonomy.

> Man's consciously lived fragility, individuality, and relatedness make the experience of pain, of sickness, and death an integral part of his life. The ability to cope with this trio in a God-imaging manner is fundamental to his health. As he becomes dependent on the management of his intimacy, he renounces the divine image and his health *must* decline. . . .

I am of the opinion that this formulation does not sound so off-base to Christian ears. To be healthy in a Christian sense is to be capable of exercising God-given capacities; it is to be able to fulfill one's calling. If conventional medical practice creates the kind of dependency that reduces this capacity in a patient, then it would seem that we must say Christian things about that medical practice which are as harsh as the things being said by Illich and others.

But there is an important "if" in what I just said: "*if* conventional medical practice" reduces God-imaging activity. . . . The important question here is, *Does* it?

A fully adequate answer to this question would, of course, require the sifting of much empirical data. But we can get at the question in a slightly different way by expanding it in this manner: Does it *necessarily?* That is, given the fact that conventional medical practice creates certain kinds of dependencies in patients, are these dependencies necessarily detrimental to God-imaging?

Dependency as such is not a bad thing, viewed from a Christian perspective. Indeed, in a rather basic and crucial way, human beings are radically dependent upon God. Nor is dependency upon the *expertise* of others a bad thing, since the God on whom we are dependent is overwhelmingly expert about everything. Is it, then, that dependency upon the expertise of other *human beings* is something to be avoided? I think not. The notions of individual callings and mutual service suggest that different human beings will develop different kinds of expertise, and that we each must respect the gifts of others and rely on others for guidance in different areas of life. We might put the point this way with reference to medical expertise: dependence on the expert guidance of medical professionals is good and proper if that dependence is an image-promoting dependence. Similarly, expert medical guidance is a good thing for a professional to provide, if that guidance is image promoting.

This way of putting the case is neither trivial nor misleading. The apostle Peter instructs believers to "be subject for the Lord's sake to every human institution" (1 Peter 2:13); and although the immediate context of his remarks seems to be political in nature, I do not think that we violate the spirit of this instruction when we apply it to patterns of authority in other spheres of life. But if this legitimately applies to subjection to medical authority, we must also draw parallels between what the Bible says about the proper exercise of political authority and the proper exercise of authority in the medical sphere. Romans 13 makes it clear that God calls rulers to serve as his ministers, rewarding those who perform good works and punishing evildoers. Similarly, if we extend this pattern of biblical teaching to medical practice, those who would exercise medical authority must minister to those under their care.

If the desire to exercise sinful autonomy is to be condemned in the patient, it must also be condemned in the medical professional. In neither case may a person act like a "self-legislator," pretending that he or she is the sole source or reference point for decision-making norms. Patient and professional alike stand *coram deo,* before the face of God.

But of course the situation is complicated by the fact that not all human beings agree about matters pertaining to the relationship of people to God. Some people, both professionals and patients, do not believe in God. And even among Christians there is much diversity in beliefs concerning what it means to live before the face of God. Even under the best conditions possible in a sinful society, some degree of conflict is to be expected.

The professional-patient relationship can be characterized by four possible distributions of belief and unbelief: Christian professional and Christian patient; Christian professional and non-Christian patient; non-Christian professional and Christian patient; non-Christian professional and non-Christian patient. For our purposes here, let us concentrate on the roles of Christian professional and Christian patient under some of these distributions.

Consider first the role of the Christian patient. I am convinced that the Christian patient ought to have a strong interest in being knowledgeably involved in basic decisions regarding his or her medical treatment. This flies in the face of the attitudes of many professionals, especially in the pre-Kübler-Ross era. For example, in a 1961 study of physicians' attitudes toward "truth telling" in cancer cases (reprinted in *Moral Problems in Medicine,* pp. 109-16), Donald Oken reported that many physicians favored a policy "as little as possible in the most general terms consistent with maintaining cooperation in treatment. . . . Questioning by the patient almost invariably is disregarded and considered a plea for reassurance unless persistent, and intuitively perceived as 'a real wish to know.' Even then it may be ignored. The vast majority of these doctors . . . approach the issue with the view that disclosure should be avoided unless there are positive indications, rather than the reverse."

The language used here is clearly that of power and control. The professional controls information about the patient's condition, dispensing it only when it is judged to be in the "real" interests of the patient to do so. From a biblical point of view, this attitude seems to be clearly unsatisfactory. In almost every case there are prima facie reasonable grounds for thinking that it *is* in the best interests of the Christian patient to struggle knowledgeably with the issues of pain, suffering, and death. In 2 Corinthians 12, the apostle Paul describes his own struggles before the Lord regarding his "thorn in the flesh"; three times he bargained with God in the hope of having the affliction removed. Whether his bargaining process was characterized by emotional maturity and stability is not revealed. But it is obvious that his struggle had an important spiritual outcome, namely, the recognition that God's power could be made perfect in his own weakness. This episode, along with the account of King Hezekiah's negotiations with the Lord regarding the time of his own death, reveals, I think, a biblical pattern for viewing the role of suffering in the life of the believer: we must allow pain, suffering, and the expectation of death — even though these are usually very agonizing factors to confront — to visit us as sanctifying forces in our lives. No medical professional has the unqualified right to deny us these struggles by withholding information from us. Perhaps there are extenuating circumstances in which information may be withheld from a Christian patient, but the bias must clearly be in favor of truth telling, even if such disclosures require educating the patient regarding complex medical analyses. There is, I suggest, a Christian "right to know" about the facts concerning one's physical condition.

But what of the role of the Christian professional in situations in which there is real or potential conflict between professional judgment and the wishes and beliefs of the patient? There is an increasing body of medical and legal literature which argues strongly for the rights of patients to refuse life-saving treatment or even to commit what we might think of as "active suicide." For example, Norman Cantor comes to this conclusion in a 1973 *Rutgers Law Review* article after reviewing a wide variety of medical and legal considerations. He suggests that professional deference to the desires of the patient in refusing treatment must be based on a "sensitivity toward personal interests in bodily integrity and self-determination."

I'm not sure exactly what Cantor means by "bodily integrity," but his appeal to the importance of "self-determination" is clearly related to the "autonomy" theme which we have already discussed. My own hunch is that we as Christians can arrive at a similar conclusion to Cantor's by traveling quite a different route.

It is unfortunate that the phrase "playing God" is often used to describe a pattern whereby professionals override the wishes and desires of a patient in prescribing certain kinds of treatment. This is unfortunate because the biblical God in important respects does not himself "play God" in this manner. The God of the Scriptures is patient with unbelief and sin. He does not override the human will in some tyrannical fashion in order to bring people into conformity with his plans. Even the Canons of the Synod of Dort — which many consider to be the harshest of Calvinist documents — insist that God "does not treat men as senseless stocks and blocks, nor take away their will and its properties, or do violence thereto." The Canons then go on to use the language of "wooing" or courtship to describe God's electing procedures, and they regularly treat the unsaved as being *allowed* by God to remain in the condition of unbelief which they *themselves* have chosen. The biblical God does not "play God" by manipulating people with a disregard to their own choices and convictions.

The Christian professional must imitate God's patience with sinners, refusing to coerce, but choosing instead of invite, to persuade, to educate, and to reason — all of which presupposes a respect for the sincerely held convictions and desires of others. The patient's right to know must be supplemented by the professional's right to attempt to persuade.

In a profoundly Christian sense, medical decision making is a "thorny" business; our decisions must be wrestled with in a world that is presently full of thorns. And our struggles are complicated by the fact that these thorns come in several varieties, from the point of view of theological taxonomy. There are, first of all, the thorns of the curse: "Cursed is the ground because of you; in toil you shall eat of it all the days of your life; thorns and thistles it shall bring forth to you" (Genesis 3:17-18). Surrounded by these thorns, human beings issue forth the groans of their physical suffering, they chafe under the yoke of a host of oppressors, and they are drenched with the sweat of their own labors — sensing in all of this that they are made of dust, and to dust they shall return.

But if we survey the thorn-infested landscape of the fallen world with the eyes of faith, we can also discern the thorns of our redemption. Those thorns, which drew blood when pressed into the Savior's brow, were worn as a crown of victory over the cursedness of the creation: for "he was wounded for our transgressions, he was bruised for our iniquities; upon him was the chastisement that made us whole, and with his stripes we are healed" (Isaiah 53:5). And because of the thorns which were worn on Calvary, we can carry the thorns which become embedded in our own flesh as thorns of sanctification, knowing that in our own weakness, we are made strong in the power of God (2 Corinthians 12:10).

A thorny business indeed. And it is made no easier by the difficulties at times of sorting out the thorns of our cursedness from the thorns of our sanctification. When do I resign myself to suffering and disease and when do I pray confidently for the removal of a thorn lodged in my flesh? In a given encounter with pain, into which garden is the Savior leading me: the Garden of Gethsemane or the garden which surrounds the empty tomb?

The Christian, whether as patient or professional, must face these questions in their complexity and troublesomeness: not in the loneliness of a pretended human autonomy, but with the responsibility of a God-imager, called to share in the exercise of dominion over all that the Lord has placed in the world. In the present age, this necessitates thorn-in-the-flesh decision making. But it is decision making that must take place in the context of the kind of community described so well by Father Henri Nouwen in his excellent little book, *The Wounded Healer* (New York: Doubleday, 1972, p. 96):

> A Christian community is . . . a healing community not because wounds are cured and pains are alleviated, but because wounds and pains become openings or occasions for a new vision. Mutual confession then becomes a mutual deepening of hope, and sharing weakness becomes a reminder to one and all of the coming strength.

CHAPTER SEVEN

Personhood

Medical ethics often talks about "persons." That the language of personhood has currency in medical ethics is unsurprising. After all, this language seems helpful in adjudicating many of the most complicated issues in the field, such as abortion, embryo research, and the termination of life support. The reasoning appears straightforward: if the fetus or embryo or body lying in the bed is a person, then that individual has certain claims on society and medicine. But if it is not a person, then that entity has fewer, if any, claims on us.

There are important disagreements within theological medical ethics about the nature and use of the notion "person." There are debates about what it means to be a person, about the relevance of the human body to being a person, about the criteria of personhood, and about whether we should be developing a list of such criteria at all. Reflecting those disagreements, discussions continue about who counts as a person and about the meaning of the moral requirement of "respect for persons."

The talk about "persons" was initially a language of protest. In reviewing the language of personhood, it is useful to recall these protests, which belong to the beginnings of modern medical ethics. There was a protest against what was frequently called the "depersonalization" of modern medicine. Hospital chaplains and others complained that technological medicine threatened to reduce the patient to a part of nature. To register that protest and to insist that healing not be regarded as simply a matter of curing the body by scientific medicine, hospital chaplains and others called attention to "the whole person."[1]

There was a protest against experiments that made human beings into "guinea pigs." The revelations at Nuremberg of the Nazi experiments — and subsequent revelations of human experimentation in this country as well — provoked outrage and complaint. The resulting protest frequently accused the experimenters of violating the respect due to persons and frequently invoked Kant's second formulation of the categorical imperative: persons must always be treated as ends in themselves and never merely as means to others' ends.

There was also a suspicion of the physicians who performed putatively therapeutic procedures upon patients "for their own good" but without their consent. The suspicion grew into a protest against the power of some people, even benevolent and well-meaning people, over other people. As earlier protests against the unchecked power of kings and priests had insisted on respect for persons, so the protest against the benevolent but despotic physician called for attention to the rights of patients as persons.

Another protest was prompted by the allocation of a scarce medical resource. In 1962, the Admissions and Policies Committee of the Seattle Artificial Kidney Center at Swedish Hospital made decisions about who would have access to the recently developed, but clearly effective, dialysis machine — made decisions, that is, about who would live and who would die — on the basis of *ad hoc* comparisons of the social worth of those who needed it. Shana Alexander, correspondent for *Life* magazine, gave it the name "the Seattle God Committee,"[2] and many protested against reducing the worth of persons to calculations of their respective utilitarian value.

In all of these cases, protests and cries for reform invoked the language of "person." It is therefore little wonder that the ground-breaking works of Joseph Fletcher and Paul Ramsey, *Morals and Medicine* and *The Patient as Person,* respectively, each emphasized the importance of the notion of "person" to moral reflection about medicine. (The preface to the latter is available as selection 46.) Beneath this superficial agreement, however, Ramsey and Fletcher profoundly disagreed about who counted as a person, about the relation of "person" and body, and about what moral requirements were included in the principle of respect for persons.

1. For example, Richard C. Cabot and Russell L. Dicks, *The Art of Ministering to the Sick* (New York: Macmillan, 1936). Another source for the emphasis on "the whole person" was Paul Tournier, *A Doctor's Casebook in the Light of the Bible,* trans. Edwin Hudson (London: SCM, 1954).

2. Shana Alexander, "They Decide Who Lives, Who Dies," *Life* 53 (November 9, 1962): 102-4.

This chapter invites you into the fray about persons. The essays by Joseph Fletcher, Thomas Shannon and Allan Wolter, and Michael Panicola reflect debates about the appropriate criteria for personhood. While those essays assume that there is some such criteria, Oliver O'Donovan, Ian McFarland, Stanley Hauerwas, and Gilbert Meilaender challenge the very idea of developing criteria for personhood. And Keith Meador and Joel Shuman show us that notions of personhood occur within specific communities, with particular histories, practices, and narratives.

What criterion or criteria should be used to delineate who is in or out as a person? The first reading, "Four Indicators of Humanhood — The Enquiry Matures" (selection 45), is a classic piece from Joseph Fletcher. Working from the supposition that rights attach to persons, Fletcher argues that neocortical function — that is, the part of the brain associated with sensory perception, conscious thought, and language — is essential to any plausible understanding of personhood. You cannot be a person without neocortical function, and all other plausible accounts of personhood implicitly presume this function, claims Fletcher.

This specific criterion of personhood is rather different from the approach seen in Thomas Shannon and Allan Wolter's "Reflections on the Moral Status of the Pre-Embryo" (selection 47). Shannon and Wolter do not so much argue for a criterion of personhood as they argue from the presumption that a person is at least an individual. That is, being an individual may not make you a person, but a person is at least an individual. Shannon and Wolter argue that a "pre-embryo" cannot be considered an individual until at least fourteen days, due primarily to the possibility of that "pre-embryo" twinning. In striking contrast, Michael Panicola's "Three Views on the Preimplantation Embryo" (selection 48) worries that lists defining personhood often exclude the most vulnerable members of our community from the protection and respect they deserve. He argues for an understanding of human persons that includes numerous dimensions: physical and material, relational and social, creative and spiritual, morally free and responsible. Panicola contends that "it is not difficult to discern that personal life begins with the completion of fertilization." At that time, we already are dealing with someone who is "participating in the physical and relational dimensions of personal life, and will in time . . . take part in the creative and moral dimensions."

Unlike these debates about criteria for personhood, several essays here dispute the appropriateness of developing such criteria in the first place. For example, in "Again, Who Is a Person?" (selection 49), Oliver O'Donovan believes that efforts to develop criteria for personhood involve a "category mistake" — thinking that the person is simply another kind of constituent or part, like a brain or a heart. Instead, O'Donovan starts from the story of the Good Samaritan to argue that personhood, like "neighbor," is discovered in the midst of personal engagement. We do not know another as person ahead or apart from such engagement. Moreover, much as with infants, the personhood of another must be initially presumed or attributed to him or her as we seek an encounter or begin a relationship.

In similar fashion, Ian McFarland's "Who Is My Neighbor?" (selection 50) starts with the story of the Good Samaritan and the doctrine of the Trinity to challenge the development of criteria for personhood. McFarland notes that the doctrine of the Trinity means that the only true persons are the Father, Son, and Holy Spirit and that the rest of us are persons only because we are treated as such by God. In addition, the doctrine of the Trinity and the story of the Good Samaritan change the focal point: the question is not whether someone else is a person; rather, the question is how do I, as one treated as a person by Jesus Christ, relate to others as the person I have been called to be.

In "Must a Patient Be a Person to Be a Patient?" (selection 51), Stanley Hauerwas challenges the use of "person" language in a slightly different way. Hauerwas suggests that the notion of "person" is being used as a weak substitute for substantive narratives and discerning communities. According to Hauerwas, the language of personhood is functioning as a regulative notion to direct health care, but it is used to disparate ends, sometimes to protect (as was Paul Ramsey's use), sometimes to exclude from protection (as with abortion). Moreover, this regulative use of "personhood" does violence to our everyday language and decision making. "Personhood" is an abstraction; it seldom occurs in the way we typically talk about and make health care decisions. Hauerwas contends that this abstraction simply cannot replace discerning communities and their substantive narratives.

Like Hauerwas, Gilbert Meilaender, "*Terra es animata:* On Having a Life" (selection 52), sees the concept of personhood as increasingly used to limit care or treatment, often by categorizing such treatment as useless or futile. Meilaender challenges the development of personhood criteria by pointing to the importance of the body and the body's history. Meilaender charges that to define personhood according to the presence or absence of certain capacities is to adopt an ahistorical and essentialist view that neglects the natural history of the embodied self, which includes both development and decline. Such an essentialist account of personhood, says Meilaender, pretends that we can abstract ourselves from our own history and precludes viewing ourselves as a whole; it gives privileged status to one moment in one's embodied history, pointing to that moment as the meaning of personhood. But surely our self, our personhood, is more thoroughly tied up with the body's natural history of development and decline, including defect, dependence, and disability.

This chapter's final essay, "Whose We Are: Baptism as Personhood" (selection 53) by Keith Meador and Joel Shuman, draws together reservations about personhood criteria and an emphasis on the importance of a certain kind of discerning community. They argue that there are no historically or morally neutral criteria for designating personhood. All such criteria, including those offered as scientific or rational, depend on historically particular narratives and cultural contexts. The emphasis on minimal mental reflective activity, for example, emerges from modern political philosophy and modern social, political, and economic practices. By contrast, Meador and Shuman argue for an alternative account of personhood found in the practice of infant baptism. "By baptizing infants and others who are unable to speak for themselves into the care and fellowship of the community, the church is acknowledging that they are nothing less than persons. . . . [T]heir identity is not given prior to or apart from their participation in the life of a community in which the members who seem to be weaker are indispensable."

In highlighting baptism, Meador and Shuman underline the importance of the specific community and its practices and convictions for understanding personhood. If they are correct, before developing criteria for personhood, we have to ask about the nature of the community in which that notion is operative. Moreover, certain Christian narratives and practices press toward recognizing the personhood of the seemingly weakest members of the community.

Personhood is a contested notion. Should the determination of personhood center on brain function, individuality, or dynamic traits already evident at conception? Or is the development of such criteria itself a mistake, an abstraction from the body's own history or from specific communities and the difficult work of discernment? And what do we owe a fellow "person"? Or is he or she a "neighbor"?

SUGGESTIONS FOR FURTHER READING

Erickson, Stephen A. "On the Christian in Christian Bioethics." *Christian Bioethics: Non-Ecumenical Studies in Medical Morality* 11, no. 3 (December 2005): 269-79.

Fleischer, Theodore E. "The Personhood Wars." *Theoretical Medicine and Bioethics* 20, no. 3 (June 1, 1999): 309-18.

Garcia, Robert K. "Artificial Intelligence and Personhood." In *Cutting-Edge Bioethics: A Christian Exploration of Technologies and Trends,* ed. John F. Kilner, C. Christopher Hook, and Diann B. Uustal (Grand Rapids: Eerdmans, 2002), pp. 39-51.

Goizueta, Roberto S. "Nosotros: Community as the Birthplace of the Self." In *Caminemos Con Jesus: Toward a Hispanic/Latino Theology of Accompaniment* (Maryknoll: Orbis Books, 1995), pp. 47-76.

Gordijn, Bert. "The Troublesome Concept of the Person." *Theoretical Medicine and Bioethics* 20, no. 4 (1999): 347-59.

Jeeves, Malcolm, ed. *From Cells to Souls — and Beyond: Changing Portraits of Human Nature* (Grand Rapids: Eerdmans, 2004).

Jenson, Robert. "Man as Patient." In *On Moral Medicine: Theological Perspectives in Medical Ethics,* 2nd ed., ed. Stephen E. Lammers and Allen Verhey (Grand Rapids: Eerdmans, 1998), pp. 412-19.

Larson, Edward J. "Personhood: Current Legal Views." *Second Opinion* (Park Ridge, Ill.), no. 14 (July 1990): 40-53.

Meilaender, Gilbert. *Body, Soul, and Bioethics* (Notre Dame: University of Notre Dame Press, 1995), pp. 37-59.

Moreland, J. P., and Scott B. Rae. *Body and Soul: Human Nature and the Crisis in Ethics* (Downers Grove: InterVarsity Press, 2000).

Peters, Ted, Karen Lebacqz, and Gaymon Bennett. *Sacred Cells? Why Christians Should Support Stem Cell Research* (Lanham: Rowman & Littlefield, 2008), pp. 141-52, 207-20.

Ramsey, Paul. *Ethics at the Edges of Life* (New Haven: Yale University Press, 1978), pp. 201-6.

Reinders, Hans S. "Human Dignity in the Absence of Agency." In *God and Human Dignity,* ed. R. Kendall Soulen and Linda Woodhead (Grand Rapids: Eerdmans, 2006), pp. 121-39.

Thomasma, David C., D. N. Weisstub, and Christian Hervé, eds. *Personhood and Health Care* (Dordrecht: Kluwer Academic Publishers, 2001).

Wiredu, Kwasi. "The African Concept of Personhood." In *African-American Perspectives on Biomedical Ethics,* ed. Harley E. Flack and Edmund D. Pellegrino (Washington, D.C.: Georgetown University Press, 1992), pp. 104-17.

44 Luke 10:25-37

The Parable of the Good Samaritan

Just then a lawyer stood up to test Jesus. "Teacher," he said, "what must I do to inherit eternal life?" He said to him, "What is written in the law? What do you read there?" He answered, "You shall love the Lord your God with all your heart, and with all your soul, and with all your strength, and with all your mind; and your neighbor as yourself." And he said to him, "You have given the right answer; do this, and you will live."

But wanting to justify himself, he asked Jesus, "And who is my neighbor?" Jesus replied, "A man was going down from Jerusalem to Jericho, and fell into the hands of robbers, who stripped him, beat him, and went away, leaving him half dead. Now by chance a priest was going down that road; and when he saw him, he passed by on the other side. So likewise a Levite, when he came to the place and saw him, passed by on the other side. But a Samaritan while traveling came near him; and when he saw him, he was moved with pity. He went to him and bandaged his wounds, having poured oil and wine on them. Then he put him on his own animal, brought him to an inn, and took care of him. The next day he took out two denarii, gave them to the innkeeper, and said, 'Take care of him; and when I come back, I will repay you whatever more you spend.' Which of these three, do you think, was a neighbor to the man who fell into the hands of the robbers?" He said, "The one who showed him mercy." Jesus said to him, "Go and do likewise."

45 Four Indicators of Humanhood — The Enquiry Matures

Joseph F. Fletcher

Jean Rostand describes a meeting of French Catholic intellectuals; they spoke of a prosecution for infanticide following the thalidomide disaster of the Sixties.[1] Morvan Lebesque: "After centuries of morality, we still cannot answer questions like those raised by the trial in Liège. Should malformed babies be killed? Where does man begin?" Father Jolif: "No one knows what man is any longer."

That is the situation, exactly. Whether or not we ever knew in the past what man is, in the sense of having a consensus about it, we do not know now. To realize this, make only a quick scan of the wild confusion and variety on the subject gathered together by Eric Fromm and Ramon Xirau in their historical compendium.[2]

First There Was One

Yet it is this question, how we are to define the *humanum,* which lies at the base of all serious talk about the quality of life. We cannot appraise quality or enumerate human values if we cannot first say what a human being is. The *Hastings Center Report* (November 1972) published a shortened version of an essay of mine in which I made a stab at this problem, under the title "Indicators of Humanhood: A Tentative Profile on Man."[3]

In substance I contended that the acute question is what is a *person;* that rights (such as survival) attach only to persons; that out of some twenty criteria one (neocortical function) is the cardinal or hominizing trait upon which all the other human traits hinge; and then I invited those concerned to add or subtract, agree or dis-

1. J. Rostand, *Humanly Possible: A Biologist's Notes on the Future of Mankind,* trans. by L. Blair (New York: Saturday Review Press, 1973), p. 8.

2. E. Fromm and R. Xirau, *The Nature of Man* (New York: Macmillan, 1968).

3. The full text is "Medicine and the Nature of Man," in *The Teaching of Medical Ethics,* ed. by R. M. Veatch, W. Gaylin and C. Morgan (Hastings-on-Hudson, N.Y.: Institute of Society, Ethics and the Life Sciences, 1973), pp. 47-58. It appeared also in *Science, Medicine and Man* I (1973): 93-102.

agree as they may. This was intended to keep the investigation going forward, and it worked; the issue has been vigorously discussed pro and con.

What crystals have precipitated? Without trying to explore them in any detail, as each of them deserves to be, four different traits have been nominated to date as the singular *esse* of humanness; neocortical function, self-consciousness, relational ability, and happiness — the last being included more in a light than a heavy vein. Various additional criteria of the optimal or *bene esse* kind are mentioned in a growing correspondence, but no argument *against* any one of them has been offered: e.g., one correspondent (Robert Morison) wants concern for the meek and dependent stipulated under my eighth trait, "concern for others."

But on the question which one of the optimal traits and capabilities is the *sine qua non,* the essential one without which no combination of the others can add up to humanhood, there are now four contenders in the running. It should be noted at the outset that of the four discrete cardinal criteria thus far entered, none of them is mutually exclusive of any of the others, any more than the optimal indicators are (sense of time, curiosity, ideomorphous identity, obligation, reason-feeling balance, self-control, changeability, etc.). The decisive question therefore appears to be about precondition. Which one of these traits, if any, is required for the presence of the others? To answer this is to find *the* criterion among the criteria.

Now There Are Four

I. Michael Tooley of Stanford contends that the real precondition to "having a serious right to life" or to being the kind of moral entity we call a person, as in the Sixteenth Amendment sense, is subjectivity or self-awareness (no. 2 in my original list). He called it "the self-consciousness requirement."[4] As he points out, fetuses and infants lack that requirement. Machines have no consciousness at all, and therefore may be sacrificed in a competing values situation. Animals are probably not self-conscious, although a few pet lovers claim they are. Once a growing baby's neurological "switchboard" gets hooked up, allowing consciousness of self to emerge, he or she is a person. (Mind is, as Dubos points out, a verb — not a noun; it is not something given but acquired, a process rather than an event.[5] It is what the mind does, not what it is.) So runs Tooley's thesis.

II. Richard McCormick of the Kennedy Center for Bioethics at Georgetown University, on another tack, says "the meaning, substance, and consummation of life is found in human relationships," so that when we try to make quality of life judgments ("and we must"), as in cases of diseased or defective newborns, "life is a value to be preserved only insofar as it contains some potentiality for human relationships."[6] On this basis anencephalics certainly, and idiots probably, lack personal status, with a consequent lack of claim rights. If you lack what he calls "the relational potential" (what I call "the capability to relate to others," no. 7) you cannot be human. "If that potential is simply nonexistent or would be utterly submerged and undeveloped in the mere struggle to survive, that life has achieved its potential" and we need not save it from death's approach.

III. When a pediatrician at the Texas Medical Center (Houston), whose work takes her daily into a service for retarded children, heard me at a grand rounds expound my suggestion that minimal intelligence or cerebral function is the essential factor in being human, she rejected it: "I know a little four-year-old-boy, certainly 20 minus or an idiot on any measurement scale and untrainable, but just the same he is a human being and nobody is going to tell me different. He is happy and that makes him human, as human as you or I." By "human" she meant morally, not only biologically. She described the child's affectionate response to caresses and his constant euphoria. I thought of my neighbor's kitten and recalled the euphoria symptom as happiness without any reason for it, and I remembered Huxley's *Brave New World* where everybody was happy on drugs — except the rebellious intellectuals. I asked her if she really meant to say that euphoria qualifies us for humanhood. I took her silence to be an affirmative answer.

IV. As far as I can yet see, I will stand by my own thesis or hypothesis that neocortical function is the key to humanness, the essential trait, the human *sine qua non.* The point is that without the synthesizing function of the cerebral cortex (without thought or mind), whether before it is present or with its end, the person is nonexistent no matter how much the individual's brain stem and midbrain may continue to provide feelings and regulate autonomic physical functions. To be truly homo sapiens we must be sapient, however minimally. Only this trait or capability is necessary to *all* of the other traits which go into the fullness of humanness. Therefore this indicator, neocortical function, is the first-order requirement and the key to the definition of a human being. As Robert Williams of the University Medical Center (Seattle) puts it, "Without mentation the body is of no significant use."[7]

Discussion Goes On

This search for a *shared* view of humanness, a consensus, may not find a happy ending. James Gustafson's (Univer-

4. M. Tooley, "Abortion and Infanticide," *Philosophy and Public Affairs* 2 (Fall, 1972): 37-65.

5. R. Dubos, *Man Adapting* (New Haven: Yale University Press, 1965), p. 7n.

6. R. A. McCormick, "To Save or Let Die: The Dilemma of Modern Medicine," *Journal of the American Medical Association* 229 (July 8, 1974): 172-76.

7. R. H. Williams, *To Live and To Die* (New York: Springer-Verlag, 1974), p. 18.

The Original Indicators of Humanhood: A Tentative Profile of Man

Positive Human Criteria

1. Minimal intelligence
2. Self-awareness
3. Self-control
4. A sense of time
5. A sense of futurity
6. A sense of the past
7. The capability to relate to others
8. Concern for others
9. Communication
10. Control of existence
11. Curiosity
12. Change and changeability
13. Balance of rationality and feeling
14. Idiosyncrasy
15. Neo-cortical function

Negative Human Criteria

1. Man is not non- or anti-artificial
2. Man is not essentially parental
3. Man is not essentially sexual
4. Man is not a bundle of rights
5. Man is not a worshiper

sity of Chicago Divinity School) skepticism about reaching agreement has now been graduated into skepticism also about applying whatever criterion we might agree to.[8] He thinks now that "intuitive elements, grounded on beliefs and profound feelings," would color our judgments seriously. More sharply, Rostand warns us (p. 66) that looking for a single trait is "a temptation for the fanatics — and there are always fanatics everywhere — to think that his adversary is less human than himself because he lacks some mental or spiritual quality." In scientific and medical circles I find that a *biological* definition is thought to be feasible, but not a list of moral or psychological traits — to say nothing of picking out only one cardinal trait subsumed in all the rest.

One slant on the problem is to deny the problem itself, not as insoluble but as specious (no pun intended). For example, William May of Catholic University, trying to justify the prohibition of abortion, objects to "the thought of Fletcher, Tooley, and those who would agree with them" that membership in a *species* is of no moral significance.[9] He argues that we are human by virtue of what we are (our species), not what we achieve or do. A member of the biological species is, as such, a human being. Thus, we would be human if we have opposable thumbs, are capable of face-to-face coitus and have a brain weighing 1400 grams, whether a particular brain functions cerebrally or not. (I put in the thumbs and coitus to exclude elephants, whales and dolphins, the only other species having brains as big or bigger than man's.) In this reasoning the term "human" slides back and forth between meaning sometimes the biological, sometimes the moral or personal, thus combining the fallacy of ambiguity with the fallacy of ostensive definition. ("He has opposable thumbs, therefore he is a person.")

Tristram Englehardt of the Texas Medical Branch (Galveston) takes a different path: he renounces not the need to define humanhood but the attempt to single out any one crucial or essential indicator.[10] Instead, he is synoptic in the same manner that René Dubos has so superbly shown us in *Man Adapting* and *So Human an Animal.* Englehardt distinguishes the biological from personal life but follows a multifactorial, non-univocal line. Indeed, he points precisely to the traits elected in all three of the major univocal definitions discussed here; together they compose his own — cerebral function, self-consciousness, and relationship or the societal dimension. Yet it is difficult, studying his language, not to believe that he gives cerebral function the determinative place, as when he says that "for a person to be embodied and present in the world he must be conscious in it," but follows that up by adding, "The brain is the singular focus of the embodiment of the mind, and in its absence man as a person is absent" (p. 21).

Being careful in all this is supremely important. Leonard Weber of Detroit urges "caution in adopting a neocortical definition of death" because this is tantamount to a definition of personhood, although he doesn't throw it out of court. He further asks us to make sure "the biological is not being under-valued as a component of human life."[11] On both scores I agree. I take "caution" to mean carefulness, which is always in order, and I certainly want to affirm our physical side, since why even talk of cerebral function apart from a cerebrum? "Mind is meat" may be too crass, but I agree that it contains a vital truth.

Rapprochement?

To Tooley and McCormick I would want to say, "You are on sound ground, so far. Of all the optimal traits of a full and authentic human life, I am inclined with you to give top importance to awareness of self (Tooley's cardinal and my optimal trait no. 2) and to the capacity for interpersonal and social relations (McCormick's cardinal and my optimal traits no. 7 and no. 8)." But I still want to reason that *their* key indicators are only factors at all be-

8. J. M. Gustafson, "Basic Ethical Issues in the Biomedical Fields," *Soundings* 53 (1970): 177; and "Mongolism, Parental Desires, and the Right to Live," *Perspectives in Biology and Medicine* 16 (Summer, 1973): 529-57.

9. W. May, "The Morality of Abortion," *Catholic Medical Quarterly* 26 (1974): 116-28.

10. H. T. Englehardt, Jr. "The Beginnings of Personhood: Philosophical Considerations," *Perkins* (School of Theology) *Journal* 27 (1973): 20-27.

11. L. J. Weber, "Human Death or Neocortical Death: The Ethical Context," *Linacre Quarterly* 41 (May 1974): 106-13.

cause of *my* key criterion — cerebral function. Is this not an issue to be carefully weighted?

Rizzo and Yonder of Canisius College, Buffalo, have argued the case for the neocortical definition.[12] Their conclusion is that "when there is incontrovertible evidence of neocortical death, the human life has ceased." To Professor Tooley and Father McCormick I would say, "Neocortical death means that both self-consciousness and other-orientedness are gone, whereas neither non-self-consciousness nor inability to relate to others means the end of neocortical activity." Just remember amnesia victims when self-consciousness is proposed as the key; just remember radically autistic and schizophrenic patients when the relational key is proposed. The amnesiac has lost his identity, his selfhood, and the psychotic is still *thinking,* no matter how falsely and in what disorder. On these grounds we cannot declare that such individuals are no longer persons, just as we cannot do so at some levels of mental retardation. Only irreversible coma or a decerebrate state is ground for such a serious determination. It seems that possibly the neocortical key is more conservative than some observers of the ethical debate suppose.

The importance of self-awareness is obvious. Abraham Maslow has taught this generation that much. Being able to recognize and respond to others is of the greatest importance to being truly human, as Gordon Allport's interpersonalism made plain. But as Julius Korein, the New York University neurologist, tells us, "Basic to the definition of the death of an individual is identification of the irreversible destruction of that critical component of the system which represents the essence of the person," and that essence, he says, is "cerebral death."[13] The "vegetable" patient, no matter how many spontaneous vital functions may be continuing, is dead, a nonperson, but not at the point he appears to be incapable of self-perception or of relational affect — only when neurologic diagnosis determines that cerebral function has ended permanently.

The non-neocortical theories (or paraneocortical) fail because they do not account for all cases. "Neocortical death," on the other hand, *necessarily* covers all other criteria, because they are by definition impossible criteria when neocortical function is gone. The key trait must be one that covers all cases, no matter how infrequently they are seen clinically. Incidentally but not unimportantly, the neocortical indicator is *medically* determinable, whereas Tooley's and McCormick's are not.

If it proves that very many ethicists feel these issues about a sound hypothesis for the *humanum* are crucial, those whose training has been in the humanities will need the help and advice of psychiatrists, psychologists, and neurologists and brain specialists to teach us the limiting principles involved and expedite our discussion.

12. R. F. Rizzo and J. M. Yonder, "Definition and Criteria of Clinical Death," *Linacre Quarterly* 40 (November 1973): 223-33.

13. J. Korein, "On Cerebral, Brain, and Systemic Death," *Current Concepts of Cerebrovascular Disease* 8 (May-June 1973): 9.

46 Preface to *The Patient as Person*

Paul Ramsey

The problems of medical ethics that are especially urgent in the present day are by no means technical problems on which only the expert (in this case, the physician) can have an opinion. They are rather the problems of human beings in situations in which medical care is needed. Birth and death, illness and injury are not simply events the doctor attends. They are moments in every human life. The doctor makes decisions as an expert but also as a man among men; and his patient is a human being coming to his birth or to his death, or being rescued from illness or injury in between.

Therefore, the doctor who attends *the case* has reason to be attentive to the patient as person. Resonating throughout his professional actions, and crucial in some of them, will be a view of man, an understanding of the meaning of the life at whose first or second exodus he is present, a care for the life he attends in its afflictions. In this respect the doctor is quite like the rest of us, who must yet depend wholly on him to diagnose the options, perhaps the narrow range of options, and to conduct us through the one that is taken.

To take up for scrutiny some of the problems of medical ethics is, therefore, to bring under examination at once a number of crucial human moral problems. These are not narrowly defined issues of medical ethics alone. Thus this volume has — if I may say so — the widest possible audience. It is addressed to patients as persons, to physicians of patients who are persons — in short, to everyone who has had or will have to do with disease or death. The question, What ought the doctor to do? is only a particular form of the question, What should be done?

This, then, is a book *about ethics,* written by a Christian ethicist. I hold that medical ethics is consonant with the ethics of a wider human community. The former is (however special) only a particular case of the latter. The moral requirements governing the relations of physician to patients and researcher to subjects are only a special case of the moral requirements governing any relations between man and man. Canons of loyalty to patients or to joint adventurers in medical research are simply particular manifestations of canons of loyalty of person to person generally. Therefore, in the following chapters I undertake to explore a number of medical covenants among men. These are the covenant between physician and patient, the covenant between research and "subject" in experiments with human beings, the covenant between men and a child in need of care, the covenant between the living and the dying, the covenant between the well and the ill or with those in need of some extraordinary therapy.

We are born within covenants of life with life. By nature, choice, or need we live with our fellow men in roles or relations. Therefore we must ask, What is the meaning of the *faithfulness* of one human being to another in every one of these relations? This is the ethical question.

At crucial points in the analysis of medical ethics, I shall not be embarrassed to use as an interpretative principle the Bible norm of *fidelity to covenant,* with the meaning it gives to *righteousness* between man and man. This is not a very prominent feature in the pages that follow, since it is also necessary for an ethicist to go as far as possible into the technical and other particular aspects of the problems he ventures to take up. Also, in the midst of any of these urgent human problems, an ethicist finds that he has been joined — whether in agreement or with some disagreement — by men of various persuasions, often quite different ones. There is in actuality a community of moral discourse concerning the claims of persons. This is the main appeal in the pages that follow.

Still we should be clear about the moral and religious premises here at the outset. I hold with Karl Barth that covenant-fidelity is the inner meaning and purpose of our creation as human beings, while the whole of creation is the external basis and condition of the possibility of covenant. This means that the conscious acceptance of covenant responsibilities is the inner meaning of even the "natural" or systemic relations into which we are born and of the institutional relations or roles we enter by choice, while this fabric provides the external framework for human fulfillment in explicit covenants among men. The practice of medicine is one such covenant. *Justice, fairness, righteousness, faithfulness, canons of loyalty,* the *sanctity* of life, *hesed, agapē* or *charity* are some of the names given to the moral quality of attitude and of action owed to all men by any man who steps into a covenant with another man — by any man who, so far as he is a religious man, explicitly acknowledges that we are a covenant people on a common pilgrimage.

The chief aim of the chapters to follow is, then, simply to explore the meaning of *care,* to find the actions and abstentions that come from adherence to *covenant,* to ask the meaning of the *sanctity* of life, to articulate the requirements of steadfast *faithfulness* to fellow man. We shall ask, What are the moral claims upon us in crucial medical situations and human relations in which some decision must be made about how to show respect for, protect, preserve, and honor the life of fellow man?

Just as man is a *sacredness in the social, political order,* so he is a *sacredness in the natural, biological order.* He is a sacredness in bodily life. He is a person who within the ambience of the flesh claims our care. He is an embodied soul or ensouled body. He is therefore a sacredness in illness and in his dying. He is a sacredness in the fruits of the generative process. (From some point he is this if he has any sanctity, since it is undeniably the case that men are never more than, from generation to generation, the products of human generation.) The sanctity of human life prevents ultimate trespass upon him even for the sake of treating his bodily life, or for the sake of others who are also only a sacredness in their bodily lives. Only a being who is a sacredness in the social order can withstand complete dominion by "society" for the sake of engineering civilizational goals — withstand, in the sense that the engineering of civilizational goals cannot be accomplished without denying the sacredness of the human being. So also in the use of medical or scientific technics.

It is of first importance that this be understood, since we live in an age in which *hesed* (steadfast love) has become *maybe* and the "sanctity" of human life has been reduced to the ever more reducible notion of the "dignity" of human life. The latter is a sliver of a shield in comparison with the awesome respect required of men in all their dealings with men if man has a touch of sanctity in this his fetal, mortal, bodily, living and dying life.

Today someone is likely to say: "Another 'semanticism' which is somewhat of an argument-stopper has to do with the sacredness or inviolability of the individual."[1] If such a principle is asserted in gatherings of physicians, it is likely to be met with another argument-stopper: It is immoral not to do research (or this experiment must be done despite its necessary deception of human beings). This is then a standoff of contrary moral judgments or intuitions or commitments.

The next step may be for someone to say that medical advancement is hampered because our "society" makes an absolute of the inviolability of the individual. This raises the spectre of a medical and scientific community freed from the shackles of that cultural norm, and proceeding upon the basis of an ethos all its own. Alternatively, the next move may be for someone to say: Our major task is to reconcile the welfare of the individual with the welfare of mankind; both must be served. This, indeed, is the principal task of medical ethics. However, there is no "unseen hand" guaranteeing that, for example, *good* experimental designs will always be morally *justifiable.* It is better not to begin with the laissez-faire assumption that the rights of men and the needs of future progress are always reconcilable. Indeed, the contrary assumption may be more salutary.

Several statements of this viewpoint may well stand as mottos over all that follows in this volume. "In the end we may have to accept the fact that some limits do exist

1. Wolf Wolfenberger, "Ethical Issues in Research with Human Subjects," *Science* 155 (January 6, 1967): 48.

to the search for knowledge."[2] "The end does not always justify the means, and the good things a man does can be made complete only by the things he refuses to do."[3] "There may be valuable scientific knowledge which it is morally impossible to obtain. There may be truths which would be of great and lasting benefit to mankind if they could be discovered, but which cannot be discovered without systematic and sustained violation of legitimate moral imperatives. It may be necessary to choose between knowledge and morality, in opposition to our long-standing prejudice that the two must go together."[4] "To justify whatever practice we think is technically demanded by showing that we are doing it for a good end . . . is both the best defense and the last refuge of a scoundrel."[5] "A[n experimental] study is ethical or not in its inception; it does not become ethical or not because it turned up valuable data."[6] These are salutary warnings precisely because by them we are driven to make the most searching inquiry concerning more basic ethical principles governing medical practice.

Because physicians deal with life and death, health and maiming, they cannot avoid being conscious or deliberate in their ethics to some degree. However, it is important to call attention to the fact that medical ethics cannot remain at the level of surface intuitions or in an impasse of conversation-stoppers. At this point there can be no other resort than to ethical theory — as that elder statesman of medical ethics, Dr. Chauncey D. Leake, Professor of Pharmacology at the University of California Medical Center, San Francisco, so often reminds us. At this point physicians must in greater measure become moral philosophers, asking themselves some quite profound questions about the nature of proper moral reasoning, and how moral dilemmas are rightly to be resolved. If they do not, the existing medical ethics will be eroded more and more by what it is alleged *must* be done and technically *can* be done.

In the medical literature there are many articles on ethics which are greatly to be admired. Yet I know that these are not part of the daily fare of medical students, or of members of the profession when they gather together as professionals or even for purposes of conviviality. I do not believe that either the codes of medical ethics or the physicians who have undertaken to comment on them and to give fresh analysis of the physician's moral decisions will suffice to withstand the omnivorous appetite of scientific research or of a therapeutic technology that has a momentum and a life of its own.

The Nuremberg Code, The Declaration of Helsinki, various "guidelines" of the American Medical Association, and other "codes" governing medical practice constitute a sort of "catechism" in the ethics of the medical profession. These codes exhibit a professional ethics which ministers and theologians and members of other professions can only profoundly respect and admire. Still, a catechism never sufficed. Unless these principles are constantly pondered and enlivened in their application they become dead letters. There is also need that these principles be deepened and sensitized and opened to further humane revision in face of all the ordinary and the newly emerging situations which a doctor confronts — as do we all — in the present day. In this task none of the sources of moral insight, no understanding of the humanity of man or for answering questions of life and death, can rightfully be neglected.

There is, in any case, no way to avoid the moral pluralism of our society. There is no avoiding the fact that today no one can do medical ethics until someone first does so. Due to the uncertainties in Roman Catholic moral theology since Vatican Council II, even the traditional medical ethics courses in schools under Catholic auspices are undergoing vast changes, abandonment, or severe crisis. The medical profession now finds itself without one of the ancient landmarks — or without one opponent. Research and therapies and actionable schemes for the self-creation of our species mount exponentially, while Nuremberg recedes.

The last state of the patient (medical ethics) may be worse than the first. Still there is evidence that this can be a moment of great opportunity. An increasing number of moralists — Catholic, Protestant, Jewish and unlabeled men — are manifesting interest, devoting their trained powers of ethical reasoning to questions of medical practice and technology. This same galloping technology gives all mankind reason to ask how much longer we can go on assuming that what can be done has to be done or should be, without uncovering the ethical principles we mean to abide by. These questions are now completely in the public forum, no longer the province of scientific experts alone.

The day is past when one could write a manual on medical ethics. Such books by Roman Catholic moralists are not to be criticized for being deductive. They were not; rather they were commendable attempts to deal with concrete cases. These manuals were written with the conviction that moral reasoning can encompass hard cases, that ethical deliberation need not remain highfalutin but can "subsume" concrete situations under the illuminating power of human moral reason. However, the manuals can be criticized for seeking finally to "resolve" innumerable cases and to give the once and for all "solution" to them. This attempt left the impression that a rule

2. Paul A. Freund, "Is the Law Ready for Human Experimentation?" *Trial* 2 (October-November, 1966): 49; "Ethical Problems in Human Experimentation," *New England Journal of Medicine* 273, No. 10 (September 10, 1965): 692.

3. Dunlop (1965), quoted in Douglass Hubble, "Medical Science, Society and Human Values," *British Medical Journal* 5485 (February 19, 1966): 476.

4. James P. Scanlan, "The Morality of Deception in Experiments," *Bucknell Review* 13, No. 1 (March, 1965): 26.

5. John E. Smith, "Panel Discussion: Moral Issues in Clinical Research," *Yale Journal of Biology and Medicine* 36 (June, 1964): 463.

6. Henry K. Beecher, *Research and the Individual: Human Studies* (Boston: Little Brown, 1970), p. 25.

book could be written for medical practice. In a sense, this impression was the consequence of a chief virtue of the authors, i.e., that they were resolved to think through a problem, if possible, *to the end* and precisely with relevance and applicability in concrete cases. Past medical moralists can still be profitably read by anyone who wishes to face the challenge of how he would go about prolonging ethical reflection into action.

Medical ethics today must, indeed, be "casuistry"; it must deal as competently and exhaustively as possible with the concrete features of actual moral decisions of life and death and medical care. But we can no longer be so confident that "resolution" or "solution" will be forthcoming.

While no one can do ethics in the medical and technological context until someone first does so, anyone can engage in the undertaking. Anyone can do this who is trained in one field of medicine and willing to specialize for a few years in ethical reasoning about these questions. Anyone can who is trained in ethics and willing to learn enough about the technical problems to locate the decisional issues. This is not a personal plea. It is rather a plea that in order to become an ethicist or a moral theologian doctors have only to quit resisting being one. An ethicist is only an ordinary man, and a moral theologian is only a religious man endeavoring to push out as far as he can the frontier meaning of the practice of a rational or a charitable justice, endeavoring to draw forth all the actions and abstentions that this justice requires of him in his vocation. I am sure that by now there are a number of physicians who have felt rather frustrated as they patiently tried to explain to me some technical medical circumstance I asked about. At the same time, I can also testify to some degree of frustration as I have at times patiently tried to explain some of the things that need to be asked of the science and methods of ethics. Physicians and moralists must go beyond these positions if we are to find the proper moral warrants and learn how to think through moral dilemmas and resolve disagreements in moral judgment concerning medical care.

To this level of inquiry we are driven today. The ordinary citizen in his daily rounds is bound to have an opinion on medical ethical questions, and physicians are bound to look after the good moral reasons for the decisions they make and lead society to agree to. This, then, is a plea for fundamental dialogue about the urgent moral issues arising in medical practice.

No one can alter the fact that not since Socrates posed the question have we learned how to teach virtue. The quandaries of medical ethics are not unlike that question. Still, we can no longer rely upon the ethical assumptions in our culture to be powerful enough or clear enough to instruct the profession in virtue; therefore the medical profession should no longer believe that the personal integrity of physicians alone is enough; neither can anyone count on values being transmitted without thought.

To take up the questions of medical ethics for probing, to try to enter into the heart of these problems with reasonable and compassionate moral reflection, is to engage in the greatest of joint ventures: the moral becoming of man. This is to see in the prism of medical cases the claims of any man to be honored and respected. So might we enter thoughtfully and actively into the moral history of mankind's fidelity to covenants. In this everyone is engaged.

47 Reflections on the Moral Status of the Pre-Embryo

Thomas A. Shannon and Allan B. Wolter

In this paper we wish to review contemporary biological data about the early human embryo in relation to philosophical and theological claims made of it. We are seeking to discover more precisely what degree of moral weight it can reasonably bear. While other ethical conclusions might well be drawn from the results of such a reflective investigation, we limit ourselves to a few moral considerations based on our current knowledge of how human life originates. As Catholics, we too believe that "from the moment of conception, the life of every human being is to be respected in an absolute way because man is the only creature on earth that God 'wished for himself' and the spiritual soul of each man is 'immediately created' by God."[1] But we are also vitally concerned as to when one might reasonably believe such absolute value could be present in a developing organism. We would also like to defuse some of the polar opposition fanned by the rhetoric of both prolife and prochoice advocates that creates a legislative dilemma for morally and religiously responsible politicians. We even hope that a rational analysis of available scientific data might lead to some broad consensus among concerned citizens that the term "human life" is not necessarily a univocal conception.

All life is a many-splendored creation on the part of God; this is especially true of human life at any stage of its development. But we suggest that appropriate protection of the human organism changes with its developmental stages. We wish to present a theory which recognizes the right of every potential mother to a meaningful life and a healthy personality development,[2] but which condemns irresponsible destruction of fetal life.

One of the hallmarks of the Catholic tradition, with certain conspicuous exceptions, has been to be in dialogue with the philosophy and science of its day and to use such insights in articulating the vision of Catholicism. Such efforts have been done better and worse. Many have taken time to evaluate the correctness or usefulness of a particular articulation. But in almost all cases, because of new discoveries in science, changes in scientific theory, and the use of new philosophical frameworks, the insights and articulation of the faith of one generation have differed from those of another. Sometimes such differences have led to severe conflict. One remembers the Copernican revolution, the case of Galileo in the 17th century, and the tensions introduced by the rediscovery of Aristotelian science in the 13th century. Nor can historians of medieval theology forget that certain philosophical views of Aquinas himself were regarded as theologically dangerous by two successive archbishops of Canterbury and condemned by the bishop of Paris in 1277 on the advice of the prestigious university theological faculty, a condemnation that was lifted insofar as it applied to St. Thomas only two years after the saint's canonization in the 14th century.

Anyone who has studied the history of ideas, scientific, philosophical, or theological, knows that there is a usefulness in reviewing the theoretical conceptions of the past, since they have a habit of recurring cyclically in a new and useful scientific garb.[3] The same is true of the theoretic conceptions used by theologians in articulating their faith. We argue that the most recent scientific discoveries fit in more admirably with the epigenetic conception of how a human being originates that was held for centuries by the great theologians and doctors of the Church than does the more recent and now more commonly accepted — though happily not defined — moment of fertilization as coincident with the time of animation. The widespread acceptance of the theory of immediate animation is of post-Tridentine origin,[4] having entered into the tradition only in the early 17th century, and in 1869 the distinction between the formed and unformed fetus was no longer canonically recognized. This assumption about immediate animation still plays a large part in contemporary ecclesiastical documents, as well as do references to the scientific literature purporting to buttress arguments supporting the theory, as we will discuss later.

We would also like to remind our readers, however, that some 40 years ago two learned priests from the University of Louvain,[5] where this theory of immediate ani-

1. Cf. *Donum Vitae,* quoting *Gaudium et Spes,* in Thomas A. Shannon and Lisa Sowle Cahill, *Religion and Artificial Reproduction* (New York: Crossroad, 1988) 147.

2. We are concerned here especially with victims of rape, incest, or sexual abuse.

From Thomas A. Shannon and Allan B. Wolter, "Reflections on the Moral Status of the Pre-Embryo," *Theological Studies* 51.4 (1990): 603-26. Used by permission.

3. Philosophers of science have stressed the important difference between the linear growth of scientific data and theoretic conceptions used to interpret them, for important theories have a life of their own that ensures their perenniality. Or, as Santayana put it, those who forget history are condemned to repeat its mistakes.

4. For theologians at the Council of Trent, in contrasting the virginal conception of Christ with the ordinary course of human nature, asserted that normally no human embryo could be informed by a human soul except after a certain period of time: "cum servato naturae ordine nullum corpus, nisi intra praescriptum temporis spatium, hominis anima informari queat" (*Catechism of the Council of Trent,* Part 1, art. 3, n. 7), cited in E. C. Messenger, *Theology and Evolution* (Westminster, Md.: Newman, 1949) 236.

5. We refer to Dr. Messenger and Canon Henry de Dorlodot.

mation was originally introduced, repudiated its scientific standing and went to some lengths to explain historically how this mistaken interpretation of empirical data was initially accepted. We claim that the most recent scientific evidence concerning fertilization and the development of the very early human embryo does even more to reinforce their view that any theory of immediate animation seems to have become as untenable today as it was commonly held to be for centuries by Catholic thinkers. We think that since scientific observations, now recognized as erroneous, played such a historical role in the development of the position favoring such a theory, new and respected scientific evidence should be utilized by Catholic theologians when they discuss the process of fertilization and conception to determine its moral implications.

We hope our analysis will be welcomed because of our acceptance and use of the methodology of the tradition and because we take seriously the role of science in helping articulate the context of moral problems, as do current ecclesiastical documents. While our conclusions may differ from those of these documents, we think such differences are to be cherished because they help the community understand its beliefs and values at a much deeper level and allow some of the forgotten riches of our Catholic tradition to be expressed to a new audience.

This rearticulation needs careful examination, however, for the fact that something is new does not *ipso facto* make it good or correct. Thus a careful and prayerful process of discernment should also be an important part of the way we rearticulate our tradition, for the community must genuinely receive the reconceptualization of the tradition before it is authentic. This essay is an attempt at such a process of discernment by setting out an account of the process of individuation in the early human embryo in light of modern biology and reflecting on it in the light of some important theological and philosophical insights that seem to have perennial vitality.

The medievals and post-Renaissance theologians articulated their theory of the person, the body, and ensoulment in light of the biology and philosophy of their day. On the basis of this they appropriately drew moral conclusions. We know now that the biology used at any one time, if not out of date, may well need updating. But the philosophy and history of science also make it clear that there is a significant difference as to how our scientific knowledge of the wonder of God's creation grows. We believe that such a moment of review is necessary today if we are to give a reasonable defense of the respect Catholics have traditionally had for human life. For we know that in the male seed there is no homunculus, but it was not until the 1700s that mammalian sperm was discovered, and not until the 1800s that the mammalian egg was found and its role revealed. Modern diagnostic technologies such as ultrasound and fetoscopy have given us a whole new perspective on the development of the human embryo. Thus, while we can correctly say that the biological data of a past era are inadequate in light of the discoveries of modern science, we cannot dispose as easily of the basic philosophical or theological way our scholastic predecessors interpreted those data. And we certainly cannot fault their use of the most advanced scientific knowledge available to them as a necessary condition for articulating any rational philosophico-theological conception of the person, the body, and ensoulment. It is in that spirit that we present this brief review of what embryology has to tell us today.

Contemporary Perspectives on the Human Embryo

1. The Pre-embryo[6]

In mammalian reproduction an egg and sperm unite to produce a new and almost always genetically unique individual. The process, how this occurs, is undergoing tremendous reconceptualization and remodeling in the light of new studies and new diagnostic technologies which allow access to this entity.

A critical discovery of the past two decades is that of capacitation, "the process by which sperm become capable of fertilizing eggs."[7] Human sperm need to be in the female reproductive tract for about seven hours before they are ready to fertilize the egg. This process removes or deactivates "a so-called decapacitating factor that binds to sperm as they pass through the male reproductive tract."[8] This permits the acrosome reaction to occur, which is the means by which lytic enzymes in the sperm "are released so that they can facilitate the passage of the sperm through the egg coverings."[9] Then the sperm are able to penetrate the egg so fertilization can begin.

Fertilization usually occurs in the end of the Fallopian tube nearest the ovary. Sperm usually take about ten hours to reach the egg, and if not "fertilized within 24 hours after ovulation, it dies."[10] Fertilization, however, is

6. This is the term being used to describe this entity from the zygote state to the beginning of the formation of the primitive streak during the third week (see Keith L. Moore, *Essentials of Human Embryology* [Philadelphia: Decker, 1988] 16). The primitive streak gives rise to other structures which continue the physical development of the embryo. The purpose of using this term, as well as other terms such as zygote, embryo, and fetus, is to integrate scientific descriptions into the moral discussion. These terms, as used in this essay, beg no moral questions but help us clearly identify the entity we are discussing. Cf. Clifford Grobstein, *Science and the Unborn: Choosing Human Futures* (New York: Basic Books, 1988) 62. But see *Donum Vitae,* which also uses these terms but attributes "to them an identical ethical relevance, in order to designate the result (whether visible or not) of human generation from the first moment of its existence until birth" (Introduction 1 n.). The text of *Donum Vitae* can be found in Shannon and Cahill, *Religion and Artificial Reproduction* 140ff.; all references will be to this text.

7. Steven B. Oppenheimer and George Lefevre, Jr., *Introduction to Embryonic Development* (2nd ed.; Boston: Allyn and Bacon, 1984) 87.

8. Ibid. 87.

9. Bruce M. Carlson, *Patten's Foundations of Embryology* (5th ed. New York: McGraw-Hill, 1988) 134.

10. Oppenheimer and Lefevre, *Introduction* 175.

not just a simple penetration of the surface of the egg. Rather, it is a complex biochemical process in which a sperm gradually penetrates various layers of the egg. Only after this single sperm has fully penetrated the egg and the haploid female nucleus, one having only one chromosome pair, has developed, do the cytoplasm of the egg and the nuclear contents of the sperm finally merge to give the new entity its diploid set of chromosomes. This process is called syngamy. It takes about 24 hours to complete and the resulting entity is called the zygote. Thus the process of fertilization (and it is important to note that it is a process) generally takes between 12-24 hours to complete,[11] with another 24-hour period required for the two haploid nuclei to fuse.

Fertilization accomplishes four major events: giving the entity the complete set of 46 chromosomes; determination of chromosomal sex; the establishment of genetic variability; and the initiation of cleavage, the cell division of the entity.

Now begins a very complex set of cell divisions as the fertilized egg begins its journey down the Fallopian tube to the uterus. About 30 hours after fertilization, there is a two-cell division; around 40-50 hours there is a division into four cells, and after about 60 hours the eight-stage cell division is reached. "When the embryo approaches the entrance to the uterus, it is in the 12-16 cell stage, the morula. This occurs on the fourth day."[12] Although the cells become compacted here, there is yet no predetermination of any one cell to become a specific entity or part of an entity. On around the sixth or seventh day the organism, now called the blastocyst, reaches the uterine wall and begins the process of its implantation there so that it can continue to develop. Here we have a differentiation into two types of cells: the trophectoderm, which becomes the outer wall of the blastocyst, and the inner cell mass, which becomes the precursor of the embryo proper. This process of implantation is completed by the end of the second week, at which time there is "primitive uteroplacental circulation."[13]

Critical to note is that from the blastocyst state to the completion of implantation the pre-embryo is capable of dividing into multiple entities.[14] In a few documented cases these entities have, after division, recombined into one entity again. Nor must this particular zygote become a human; it can become a hydatidiform mole, a product of an abnormal fertilization which is formed of placental tissue.

Note also that the zygote does not possess sufficient genetic information within its chromosomes to develop into an embryo that will be the precursor of an individual member of the human species. At this stage the zygote is neither self-contained nor self-sufficient for such further development, as was earlier believed. To become a human embryo, further essential and supplementary genetic information to what can be found in the zygote itself is required, namely

> the genetic material from maternal mitochondria, and the maternal or paternal genetic messages in the form of messenger RNA or proteins. In terms of molecular biology, it is incorrect to say that the zygote has all the informing molecules for embryo development; rather, at most, the zygote possesses the molecules that have the potential to acquire informing capacity.[15]

> That potential informing capacity is given in time through interaction with other molecules. . . . This new molecule with its informing capacity was not coded in the genome. Thus, the determination to be or to have particular characteristics is given in time through the information resulting from the interaction between the molecules.[16]

The development of the zygote depends at each moment on several factors: the progressive actualization of its own genetically coded information, the actualization of pieces of information that originate *de novo* during the embryonic process, and exogenous information independent of the control of the zygote.

2. *The Embryo*

The next major stage of development is that of the embryo. This is the beginning of the third week of pregnancy and "coincides with the week that follows the first missed menstrual period."[17] This phase begins with the full implantation of the pre-embryo into the uterine wall and the development of a variety of connective tissues between it and the uterine wall. Eventually the placenta develops and is the medium through which maternal-embryonic exchanges occur.

Two major events now occur. The first is the completion of gastrulation, "profound but well-ordered rearrangements of the cells in the embryo."[18] This process results in the development of various layers which ultimately give rise to the tissues and organs of the entity and is completed by the third week. At this time all expressions of the genes are switched off except those that determine what a particular cell will be. There are now three layers present which are responsible for the development of much of the organism:

> The embryonic ectoderm gives rise to the epidermis; the nervous system; the sensory epithelium of the eye, ear, and nose; and the enamel of the teeth. The embryonic endoderm forms the linings of the digestive and

11. Ibid. 176.
12. Ibid. 175.
13. Moore, *Essentials* 14.
14. Carlson, *Patten's Foundations* 35.
15. Carlos A. Bedate and Robert C. Cegalo, "The Zygote: To Be or Not to Be a Person," *Journal of Medicine and Philosophy* 14 (1989) 642-43.
16. Bedate and Cegalo, "The Zygote" 644.
17. Moore, *Essentials* 16; italics in the original.
18. Carlson, *Patten's Foundations* 186.

respiratory tracts. The embryonic mesoderm becomes muscle, connective tissue, bone and blood vessels.[19]

The second major event, the process of embryogenesis or organogenesis, now begins and is completed by the end of the eighth week. This process results in the development of all major internal and external structures and organs.

By the end of the third week the primitive cardiovascular system has begun to form with the development of blood vessels, blood cells, and a primitive heart. Since the "circulation of blood starts by the end of the third week as the tubular heart begins to beat,"[20] the cardiovascular system reaches a functional state first.

The nervous system progresses from a neural tube to the essential subdivisions of the brain into forebrain, midbrain, and hindbrain.[21] During this time also the upper and lower limb buds begin to appear. The digestive tract begins to form, as do all the external structures such as the head and the eyes and ears. Hands and feet make their appearance, as do, by the end of the eighth week, distinct fingers and toes.

The development of the nervous system is critical because this is the basis for the "generation and coordination of most of the functional activities of the body."[22] The rudimentary brain and spinal cord are present around the third week but are as yet "unspecialized or undifferentiated for neural function."[23] Neuron development begins around the fifth week, and around the sixth week the "first synapses . . . can be recognized."[24] Carlson observes that at about the seventh week "the embryo is capable of making weak twitches in the neck in response to striking the lips or nose with a fine bristle."[28] Grobstein notes "the earliest continuous neuronal circuitry for reflex conduction and behavior could be initiated as early as six weeks."[26] Such a pattern, Carlson says, "signifies that the first functional reflex arcs have been laid down."[27]

In a rather thorough review of the literature Michael Flower describes various embryonic movements and the neural basis necessary for their possibility.[28] Flower notes that the earliest reported elicited reflex response from an embryo occurred at 7.5 weeks. This was a movement away from a stroking stimulus to the mouth. Such movements were typical during this period of the eighth week of development.[29] In the middle of the ninth week the patterns make a transition to whole body responses, and during the 12th week local reflexes dominate. These data indicate a critical level of integration of the nervous system.

This review of embryonic development up to the eighth week shows a dramatic process of development from the initiation of fertilization to the formation of an integrated organism around mid-gestation. The rest of the paper will concentrate on examining what moral implications these data might have. The intent is not to draw a moral ought from a biological is, but to reconsider the compatibility of moral and philosophical claims with what we know of developmental embryology.

Moral Considerations

1. Conception

A critical finding of modern biology is that conception biologically speaking is a process beginning with the penetration of the outer layer of the egg by a sperm and concluding with the formation of the diploid set of chromosomes. This is a process that takes at least a day. This raises a question as to how one ought to understand the term "moment of conception" frequently used in church documents.

One could understand "moment" metaphorically as referring to the process as a whole, or if it is meant to convey an instant of time, then it would seem to refer to either the end of the process of biological conception when the zygote has become an embryo, or to some prior stage of development that has been reached in which this human life form (fertilized egg, zygote, or pre-embryo) has acquired a distinct set of properties. However, it seems that the theologians who framed these carefully crafted documents wished to convey the idea that at the moment of conception (whatever stage of development of human life obtains) everything is present that is required essentially for this human organism to be a person in the philosophical/theological, if not psychological, sense of the term: a rational or immortal soul has been created and infused into the organic body. At the same time, while they wished to set forth guidelines, they declared it was still a theoretically open question and hence they did not want to specify, or define, the moment when such passive conception (as it was called by Catholic theologians for many centuries) took place. Prayerful reflection on what embryology and our Catholic tradition tell us may not yield any direct positive knowledge of when passive conception takes place, but it does seem to throw considerable light on when it has not occurred.

Biologically understood, conception occurs only after a lengthy process has been completed and is more closely identified with implantation than fertilization.[30] The pas-

19. Moore, *Essentials* 18.
20. Ibid. 24.
21. Carlson, *Patten's Foundations* 296.
22. Ibid. 456.
23. Grobstein, *Science* 47.
24. Ibid. 48.
25. Carlson, *Patten's Foundations* 457.
26. Grobstein, *Science* 48.
27. Carlson, *Patten's Foundations* 458.
28. Michael J. Flower, "Neuromaturation of the Human Fetus," *Journal of Medicine and Philosophy* 10 (1985) 237-51.
29. Ibid. 238-39.

30. Norman M. Ford, *When Did I Begin? Conception of the Human Individual in History, Philosophy, and Science* (Cambridge: Cambridge University, 1988) 176-77. This outstanding and comprehensive analysis of the biological data came to our attention af-

toral letter *Human Life in Our Day* speaks of conception "initiating a process whose purpose is the realization of human personality."[31] Such a phrase is biologically correct if applied to implantation and seems to be a reasonable moral description of the typical outcome of conception.

2. *Singleness*

Clearly and without any doubt, once biological conception is completed we have a living entity and one which has the genotype of the human species. As Grobstein nicely phrases it, "conception (fertilization) is the beginning of a new generation in the genetic sense. . . ."[32] This zygote is capable of further divisions and is clearly the precursor of all that follows. But can we say with *Donum Vitae,* quoting the "Declaration on Procured Abortion," "From the time that the ovum is fertilized, a new life is begun which is neither that of the father nor of the mother; it is rather the life of a new human being with his own growth"?[33]

How are we to understand this phraseology in the light of the biology of development? For, while it is correct to say that the life that is present in the newly fertilized egg is distinct from the father and mother and is in fact usually genetically unique, it is not the case that this particular zygote is fully formed and it is not a single human individual, an "ontological individual," as Ford suggests.[34] Because of the possibility of twinning, recombination, and the potency of any cell up to gastrulation to become a complete entity, this particular zygote cannot necessarily be said to be the beginning of a specific, genetically unique individual human being. While the zygote is the beginning of genetically distinct life, it is neither an ontological individual nor necessarily the immediate precursor of one.

Second, the zygote gives rise to further divisions "resulting in an aggregate of cells, each of which remains equivalent to a zygote in the sense that it can become all or any part of an embryo and its extra-embryonic structure."[35] Such cells at this stage are totipotent:

> Within the fertilized ovum lies the capability to form an entire organism. In many vertebrates the individual cells resulting from the first few divisions after fertilization retain this capability. In the jargon of embryology, such cells are described as totipotent. As development continues, the cells gradually lose the ability to form all the types of cells that are found in the adult body. It is as if they were funneled into progressively narrower channels. The reduction of the developmental options permitted to a cell is called restriction. Very little is known about the mechanisms that bring about restriction, and the sequence and time course of restriction vary considerably from one species to another.[36]

Such a process of restriction is completed when the cells have become "committed to a single developmental fate. . . . Thus determination represents the final step in the process of restriction."[37] Such determination begins during gastrulation, three weeks into embryonic development.

Genetic uniqueness and singleness coincide on one level only after the process of implantation has been completed and on another after the restriction process is completed. Thus, if we take implantation as the marker of both conception and human singleness, this does not occur until about a week after the initiation of fertilization. If we use determination and restriction, because of their signaling of the loss of totipotency of the cells, as the markers of human singleness, then individuality does not occur until about three weeks after fertilization. Of critical importance is Ford's observation: *"The teleological system of the blastocyst should not be identified with the ontological unity of the human individual that will develop from it."*[38]

There is, then, a partial answer to the very interesting question[39] *Donum Vitae* asks: "How could a human individual not be a human person?"[40] A Catholic philosopher might well object or reply that this is certainly a very muddled question, for "traditionally speaking" individuality has been considered a necessary, though not sufficient condition for human personhood. The rational soul has never been considered the formal reason why something human is individual. Obviously, "human individual" can have several meanings. If it refers to a fertilized ovum, this is indeed something both human (qua product) and numerically single. Yet, until the process of individuation is completed, the ovum is not an individual, since a determinate and irreversible individuality is a necessary, if not a sufficient, condition for it to be a human person.

Something human and individual is not a human person until he or she is a human individual, that is, not un-

---

ter we had completed much of our own research for this article. We wish to acknowledge how much we have learned from it and to commend it for its exceptionally thorough review of the biological data and philosophical analysis. We also wish to acknowledge the earlier contribution of James J. Diamond, M.D., to this topic: "Abortion, Animation, and Biological Hominization," *TS* 36 (1975) 305-24.

31. *Human Life in Our Day,* par. 84.

32. Grobstein, *Science* 25.

33. *Donum Vitae* I, 2, in Shannon and Cahill, *Religion and Artificial Reproduction* 148.

34. An ontological individual is defined as "a single concrete entity that exists as a distinct being and is not an aggregation of smaller things nor merely a part of a greater whole; hence its unity is said to be intrinsic" (Ford, *When Did I Begin?* 212).

35. Grobstein, "Early Development" 235.

36. Carlson, *Patten's Foundations* 23.

37. Ibid. 26.

38. Ford, *When Did I Begin?* 158; italics ours.

39. Although any conclusions should not be laid at his door, Richard McCormick started Shannon thinking about this problem and was suggestive in phrasing the question.

40. *Donum Vitae* I, 2, in Shannon and Cahill, *Religion and Artificial Reproduction* 149.

til after the process of individuation is completed. Neither the zygote nor the blastocyst is an ontological individual, even though it is genetically unique and distinct from the parents. The potential for twinning remains until the beginning of gastrulation, although it is rare for it to occur this late. Additionally, a zygote that divides can reunite and one individual will emerge. Furthermore, each cell can form a total individual. A human individual, to use the language of the document, cannot be a human person until after individuality is established.

Also, as Grobstein noted, genetic uniqueness does not necessarily imply singleness.[41] That is, when fertilization is complete and the haploid state is reached, the organism has its full complement of genetic information. At this point it is genetically unique. But because of the potentiality for twinning, this uniqueness may be shared by more than one organism. Thus, even though unique, the organism is not necessarily single. Singleness or individuality occurs after the genetically unique organism has implanted and its development is restricted to forming one unified organism.

An individual is not an individual, and therefore not a person, until the process of restriction is complete and determination of particular cells has occurred. Then, and only then, is it clear that another individual cannot come from the cells of this embryo. Then, and only then, is it clear that this particular individual embryo will be only this single embryo.

One can reasonably conclude, then, that if there is no single human entity, there is no person. For the one is the presupposition of the other. Thus, when *Donum Vitae* approvingly refers to the findings of modern science and argues "that in the zygote . . . resulting from fertilization the biological identity of a new human individual is already constituted,"[42] does not this statement of the Congregation fail to make a critical distinction between genetic uniqueness and singleness? In using "individual" rather than "person" in this meticulously worded statement, the Congregation may have sought to sidestep the controversial question of when personhood begins. But if "individual" be taken in its philosophical or technical meaning, scientific data available today hardly justify the claim that a particular zygote is necessarily both genetically unique and an individual.

This is particularly important in assessing the theological intent of the Congregation, particularly since it argues that the "conclusions of science regarding the human embryo provide a valuable indication for discerning by the use of reason a personal presence at the moment of this first appearance of a human life."[43] As the statement stands, three concepts appear to be conflated here: genetic uniqueness, singleness, and personal presence. The argument for the first presence of human and personal life in the zygote relies heavily on scientific claims about the fertilized egg. However, such claims of singleness and personhood cannot be made, the former scientifically and the latter philosophically. We assume that the Congregation would want to adjust its findings in the light of these distinctions.

3. *Ensoulment*[44]

In this section and elsewhere, we will be discussing the principle of immaterial individuality or immaterial selfhood. In the Catholic tradition, and clearly in many of the sources we cite, the usual term for this is "soul." Our practice will be to use the term "soul" when speaking within a clear traditional context. But when we develop our own presentation, we will use the term "immaterial individuality" or "immaterial selfhood," because the term "soul" has many connotations and images connected with it and insofar as possible we wish to avoid problematic usages and confusing images.

a. Issues Although far from being a defined doctrine, there is support in Roman Catholic moral theology for the position that ensoulment is coincident with fertilization or, at least, as early as possible after conception. This position apparently dates from the early-17th-century writings of Thomas Fienus, professor on the faculty of medicine at Louvain.[45] This opinion gradually caught on and became the dominant opinion. This position was complemented by teachings that held that the embryo "possesses all the essential parts of a human body, though very minute in size."[46] This teaching on immediate animation eventually worked its way into the mainstream of Catholic moral theology. If doctors of medicine were Catholics, explains Dorlodot,

> they were told that the theologians of their time held that the soul is created by God immediately after fecundation. The theologians in turn based themselves on the opinion of the doctors, as these did on that of the theologian. In other words, *caecus caeco ducatum praestat.* Finally, the moral theologians, who completely forgot the principles which, according to the great doctors of Catholic morality, render abortion al-

41. Grobstein, *Science* 25.

42. *Donum Vitae* I, 2, in Shannon and Cahill, *Religion and Artificial Reproduction* 149.

43. Ibid. I, 2, in Shannon and Cahill, *Religion and Artificial Reproduction* 149.

44. There is much literature on this, but two interesting articles which are extremely useful for their summaries are Joseph Donceel, S.J., "A Liberal Catholic's View," in *Abortion in a Changing World,* ed. Robert E. Hall (New York: Columbia University, 1970), and Carol Tauer, "The Tradition of Probabilism and the Moral Status of the Early Embryo," *TS* 45 (1984) 3-33. Both articles can be found in *Abortion and U.S. Catholicism: The American Debate,* ed. Patricia B. Jung and Thomas A. Shannon (New York: Crossroad, 1988).

45. Henry de Dorlodot, "A Vindication of the Mediate Animation Theory," in *Theology and Evolution,* ed. E. C. Messenger (Westminster, Md.: Newman, 1959) 271.

46. Dorlodot, "A Vindication" 273.

ways illicit, invoked the danger of favouring abortive or sterilizing practices.[47]

Additionally, the removal from canon law in 1896 of the distinction between the formed and unformed fetus suggests that there is not a time when the body is unformed.[48] The *Ethical and Religious Directives for Catholic Health Facilities* provide another reason when they include in the definition of an abortion the "interval between conception and implantation."[49] Also, we have the 1981 testimony of Cardinal Cooke and Archbishop Roach in support of the Hatch amendment: "We do claim that each human individual comes into existence at conception, and that all subsequent stages of growth and development in which such abilities are acquired are just that — stages of growth and development in the life cycle of an individual already in existence."[50] Finally, in *Donum Vitae* we read: "nevertheless, the conclusions of science regarding the human embryo provide a valuable indication for discerning by the use of reason a personal presence at the moment of this first appearance of a human life."[51]

If this statement is to be accepted as it stands, we suggest that the conclusions of science should be interpreted differently, particularly if we reflect on what we know from science in the light of a centuries-long tradition among Catholic philosophers and theologians. For like them we are struck by both the wonder and sacredness of human life even from its obscure beginnings, as well as to when we could begin to suspect a personal presence might be there. Nor can we forget that for some seventeen centuries the Church indeed condemned abortion, but not on the ground that it might by even the most remote possibility be in all cases a question of murder. Certainly some of the greatest minds and doctors of the Church refused to believe, as many today seem to do, that ensoulment is coincident with fertilization or that we must trace the genesis of each human person back to that moment. Obviously, the Sacred Congregation for the Doctrine of Faith had no intention of definitively settling this question, for it stated pointedly, "This declaration expressly leaves aside the question of the moment when the spiritual soul is infused. There is not a unanimous tradition on this point and authors are as yet in disagreement."[52] It did not believe, however, that such theoretical openness should lead to any rash or precipitous practical action, for it goes on to say: "From a moral point of view this is certain: even if a doubt existed concerning whether the fruit of conception is already a human person, it is objectively a grave sin to dare to risk murder."[53]

Several very critical questions arise here, particularly since abortion was traditionally considered a sin against marriage but not homicide. One of them, concerning the moral possibility of acting on probable knowledge, has already been masterfully treated by Carol Tauer.[54] Others concern practical and philosophical issues relating to the development of the pre-embryo and embryo. It is to these issues that we now turn.

The dominant position of the moral tradition on ensoulment was the acceptance of a time during the pregnancy when the fetus was not informed by the rational soul. Two distinctions were used in discussing this. The first distinction is between active and passive conception and is exemplified in *De Testis* of Benedict XIV, in which the pope comments on the doctrine of the Immaculate Conception.

> Conception can have a twofold meaning, for it is either active, in which the holy parents of the Blessed Virgin, joining each other in a marital role, have accomplished those things which have to do most of all with the formation, organization, and disposition of the body itself for receiving a rational soul to be infused by God; or it is passive, when the rational soul is coupled with the body. This infusion and union of the soul with a duly organized body is commonly called passive conception, namely, that which occurs at that very instant when the rational soul is united with a body consisting of all its members and its organs.[55]

Thus the pope would seem to understand active conception, in our terminology, as the physical union of egg and sperm that will become the embryo, while passive conception would be the moment the rational soul is infused into a suitably organized body, one that results from (begins with) organogenesis.

The second distinction is between mediate and immediate animation by such a soul. The theory of mediate animation is succinctly stated as follows:

47. Ibid.

48. Cf. John Connery, S.J., *Abortion: The Development of the Roman Catholic Perspective* (Chicago: Loyola University, 1977) 212.

49. Washington, D.C.: U.S. Catholic Conference, 1977, 4.

50. Archbishop John Roach and Cardinal Terence Cooke, "Testimony in Support of the Hatch Amendment," *Origins* 11 (1981) 357-72; also in Jung and Shannon, *Abortion* 15.

51. *Donum Vitae* I, 1, in Shannon and Cahill, *Religion and Artificial Reproduction* 149.

52. *Declaration on Abortion* (Washington, D.C.: U.S. Catholic Conference, 1975) 13.

53. Ibid. 6.

54. See n. 44 above. While many have been unhappy with Carol Tauer's article and have dismissed it, Shannon has not yet seen a substantive refutation of her argument that the "application of the probabilist methods would permit some early abortion" (Jung and Shannon, *Abortion* 79).

55. "Conceptio dupliciter accipi potest; vel enim est activa, in qua Sancti B. Virginis parentes opere maritali invicem convenientes, praestiterunt ea quae maxime spectabant ad ipsius corporis formationem, organizationem et dispositionem ad recipiendam animam rationalem a Deo infundendam; vel est passiva, cum rationalis anima cum corpore copulatur. Ipsa animae infusio et unio cum corpore debite organizato vulgo nominator Conceptio passiva, quae scilicet fit illo ipso instanti quo rationalis anima corpori omnibus membris ac suis organis constanti unitur" (Benedict XIV, *De festis,* lib. II, c. 15, n. 1, in *Opera omnia* 9, ed. J. Silvester [Prato: Aldina, 1843] 303a).

> Animation by the intellectual soul is impossible so long as the parts of the brain which are the seat of the imagination and the vis cogitativa (and we might add, the memory) are not suitably organized. But it still is more evident that there cannot be animation by the intellectual soul when the brain is not even outlined, or again, when even the embryo really does not as yet exist. Now that is precisely the case with the ovum, and the morula, and of that which results from its development, so long as there has not appeared, on a particular part of the germ, that which by its ulterior development will become a fetus.[56]

Immediate animation occurs coincidentally with the fusion of egg and sperm, known as the moment of conception. This is the position utilized in the teachings referred to at the beginning of this section. This distinction is also thoroughly discussed by Donceel, as previously noted.[57]

Medieval theologians were particularly interested in clarifying the technical meaning of "conception" in their justification of the celebration of the popular feast of the Bl. Virgin Mary's conception. Henry of Ghent, following common scholastic reasoning, distinguished between the "conception of the seed when fetal life begins" and the conception of the human soul some "35 or 42 days later [when], depending on the sex, a rational soul is created."[58] Such a position echoes St. Anselm's perceptive judgment, "No human intellect accepts the view that an infant has a rational soul from the moment of conception."[59]

Had this saint known of the empirical data on wastage, he would have considered such a claim not only irrational but blasphemous.[60] For only about 45% of eggs that are fertilized actually come to term. The other 55% miscarry for a variety of reasons. Some are related to the biochemistry of the uterus, others are a function of low levels of necessary hormones, while yet other reasons have to do with structural anomalies within the pre-embryo or embryo itself.[61] Such vast embryonic loss intuitively argues against the creation of a principle of immaterial individuality at conception. What meaning is there in the creation of such a principle when there is such a high probability that this entity will not develop to the embryo stage, much less come to term?

Also, given the fact that twinning and recombination is a possibility, what is one to say about the presence of immaterial individuality during that process? If this principle is initiated at fertilization and then a twin is formed, how does one explain the relation of the original principle to the zygote that splits off? And should recombination occur, how does one explain coherently the fate of such a principle of immaterial individuality? Should one freeze the pre-embryo, all organic processes stop for the duration. What is the status of immaterial individuation then? It is genuinely unclear what to think of that in terms of the standard theory of immediate ensoulment. Then there is the issue of whether a soul, in the classic sense of the form of the body, is needed for the fertilized egg to develop into its possible subsequent forms.

b. Commentary The question of the moral significance of the morula and of embryonic wastage has been noted previously in the moral literature. In 1976, for example, Bernard Häring brought together much of the scientific literature and examined its moral significance. His conclusion concurs with one suggestion in our analysis and

56. Dorlodot, "A Vindication" 266. It was here that Messenger and Dorlodot recalled that the only theological attempt to define the role of the rational soul as the substantial form of the body was made by the Council of Vienne (DS 481) and that the fathers and theologians of that council did not subscribe to the immediate-animation theory. Dorlodot uses the definition of the council as the major premise of his argument vindicating the mediate animation theory; see Messenger, *Theology and Evolution* 259.

57. Donceel, "A Liberal Catholic" 48ff.

58. *Quodlibet* 5, q. 13; cited in *John Duns Scotus: Four Questions on Mary*, tr. and intro. by Allan B. Wolter, O.F.M. (Santa Barbara, Calif.: Old Mission, 1988) 6. It is interesting to note that Henry breaks with the tradition and ascribes a longer period of gestation before animation to the male rather than the female as was customary since Aristotle.

59. Anselm of Canterbury, *De conceptu virginali et de originali peccato*, c. 7 in *Anselmi Cantuariensis archiepiscopi opera omnia 2*, ed. F. S. Schmitt (Stuttgart-Bad Cannstatt, 1968) 148 (Anselm of Canterbury 3, ed. and tr. Jasper Hopkins and Herbert Richardson [Toronto: Edwin Mellen, 1976] 152). It is important to keep in mind that the Archbishop of Canterbury is arguing as to when it is possible to contract original sin, something that all theologians in his day agreed required only the existence of a human soul, not any consciousness or voluntary activity on the part of an infant. As he puts it, "Either from the very moment of his conception an infant has a rational soul (without which he cannot have a rational will) or else at the moment of his conception he has no original sin. But no human intellect accepts the view that an infant has a human soul from the moment of his conception. For [from this view] it would follow that whenever — even at the very moment of reception — the human seed perished before attaining a human form, the [alleged] human soul in this seed would be condemned, since it would not be reconciled through Christ — a consequence which is utterly absurd." Today we may have different conceptions as to the nature of original sin and how it is contracted, but we have even less reason than Anselm to believe that there is the remotest possibility of a human will present in what he calls "human seed" at the moment the zygote is formed, or that there is any less rather than a substantially greater amount of "human seed that perishes before attaining a human form."

60. Those who see no insuperable difficulty for the theory of immediate animation in the fact that twins can come from a single fertilized egg should find considerable difficulty in the problem of wastage. To ascribe such bungling of the conceptual process to an all-wise creator would seem almost sacrilegious. One would have to assume that God in His foreknowledge would create souls only for those He foreknew would eventually be born, an argument a pro-choice advocate might well apply to aborted fetuses. On the other hand, Catholics, on the basis of rational argument, can hardly hope to argue for anything more than a suitable level of protection warranted by the development stage of the pre-embryo and its sequelae.

61. C. Grobstein, M. Flower, and J. Mendeloff, "External Human Fertilization: An Evaluation of Policy," *Science* 222 (Oct. 14, 1983) 127-33.

opens the door to other issues: "the argument that the morula cannot yet be a person or an individual with all the rights of the members of the human species seems to me to be convincing as long as we follow our traditional concept of personhood."[62] This conclusion opens up several areas for consideration.

First, we concur with Häring and particularly with the analysis of Ford that, given the biological evidence, there is no reasonable way in which the fertilized egg can be considered a physical individual minimally until after implantation. Maximally, one could argue that full individuality is not achieved until the restriction process is completed and cells have lost their totipotency. Thus the range of time for the achievement of physical individuality is between one and three weeks. One simply cannot speak, therefore, of an individual's being present from the moment of fertilization.

Second, given the standard definition of personhood used in Catholic moral theory — an individual substance of a rational nature — questions are raised about the rational nature. When might one consider such a rational nature to be present? Ford suggests the formation of the primitive streak, which coincides with the time of the formation of the neural tube, as an appropriate criterion.[63] Another criterion would be around eight weeks, when the first elicited responses have been recorded. These are the result of a simple three-neuron circuit. Thus, towards the end of the embryonic period some neural activity is present. A third answer would be the formation of a relatively integrated nervous system, which occurs around the 20th week of fetal development. Of critical importance here is the connection of neural pathways through the thalamus to the neocortex. This allows stimuli to be received, as well as activities to be initiated.

One can speak of a rational nature in a philosophically significant sense only when the biological structures necessary to perform rational actions are present, as opposed to only reflex activities. The biological data suggest that the minimal time of the presence of a rational nature would be around the 20th week, when neural integration of the entire organism has been established. The presence of such a structure does not argue that the fetus is positing rational actions, only that the biological presupposition for such actions is present.

Third, the pre-embryonic form as a system is not totally passive, the recipient only of actions from the outside as it were. It has its own activities arising from the released potencies of the novel combination of its constituent materials. Such potencies are released when these elements form a system, e.g. the embryo. This development of new systems gives rise to new activities and possibilities and serves as the foundation or presupposition for other stages of development. Philosophically speaking, we have every reason to believe that the dynamic properties of the organic matter — the elements of the fully formed zygote — owe their existence to their organizational form or the system. Important to note is that "where there are only material powers — that is, the ability to form material systems — , there is only a material nature or substance."[64] Thus the material system or form of the developing body can explain its own activity. We conclude that there is no cogent reason, either from a philosophical or still less from a theological viewpoint, why we should assert, for instance, that the human soul is either necessary or directly responsible for the architectonic chemical behavior of nucleo-proteins in the human body.

Among the scholastic theologians and doctors of the Church, perhaps St. Bonaventure has given the most helpful model for what we have in mind. For in his interesting Aristotelian interpretation of how St. Augustine's theory of seminal reasons might be explained according to the science of his own day, he argued that if the potencies be understood as active rather than passive, then the Aristotelian formula that the new substantial *form is educed from the potency of matter* made sense. For "the philosopher of nature says that matter first receives the elementary form and by its means it comes to the form of the mineral compound and by means of the latter to the organic form, for he looks to that potency of matter according to which it is progressively actualized by the operation of nature."[65]

If we interpret this in more contemporary terms, it means simply that the new substantial form is nothing more than that of the organic system itself, and that its new and unique dynamic properties stem from the complementary interaction of elements that make up the system. All that is needed is some external agent to bring the elements of that system together, for, as Bonaventure puts it, "in matter itself there is something cocreated with it from which the agent acting in matter educes the form. Not that this something from which the form is educed is such that it becomes some part of the form to be produced, but it is rather that which can be and will become the form, even as a rosebud becomes a rose."[66]

62. Bernard Häring, "New Dimensions of Responsible Parenthood," *TS* 37 (1976) 127. This article is also a good review of the scientific literature of that time period and contains references to other articles which discuss our theme.

63. Ford, *When Did I Begin?* 171ff.

64. Allan B. Wolter, "Chemical Substance," in *Philosophy of Science* (Jamaica, N.Y.: St. John's University, 1960) 108. This citation is an excerpt from a seminal article originally titled "The Problem of Substance." Its primary aim was to present a cosmological account of how mechanical and natural systems differ, why various forms of living substances arise from nonliving matter, and how traditional scholastic philosophical insights and theories such as both the pluriform and uniform hylomorphic conceptions might be helpful as partial insights to a more complex philosophical theory. The psychological role of the rational soul was only discussed peripherally to show how medieval scholastics fitted it into their theories of mediate animation.

65. See J. F. Wippel and A. B. Wolter, *Medieval Philosophy: From St. Augustine to Nicholas of Cusa* (New York/London: Free Press and Collier Macmillan, 1969) 325.

66. Ibid. 320.

These remarks suggest that the principle of immaterial individuality is indeed the ultimate actualization of all the potencies contained within the forms or systems that constitute the organic life of the human being. Thus, finally, we can say that while it is necessary to recognize the distinctions between higher and lower vital functions in the human being, nonetheless there may be "an area where the biochemical theory is the more plausible explanation, and another area where the animistic position seems to be the only tenable view."[67]

The question of when such a principle comes into being is dependent on which level of the system of the human being one is examining and what activities are performed here. The strong implication of these suggestions is that immaterial individuality comes into existence late in the development of the physical individual.

Conclusions

1. Biological Data

a. Physical Individuality Two biological data mandate a revision of our understanding of the beginning of individuality: (1) the possibility of twinning, which lasts up to implantation, which occurs about a week after fertilization begins, and (2) the completion of the restriction process, which prevents individual cells from forming another individual, about three weeks into the pregnancy. While one can speak of genetic uniqueness, in that the fertilized egg has its own genetic code distinct from any other entity (except an identical twin, triplet, etc.), we simply cannot speak of an individual until in fact that individual is present, and the earliest that can be is about two or three weeks after fertilization begins.

b. Neural Development Three markers are significant in neural development: (1) gastrulation, the development of the various layers in the pre-embryo which give rise to the whole organism; (2) organogenesis, the presence of all major systems of the body, occurring around the eighth week; and (3) the development of the thalamus, which permits the full integration of the nervous system, around the 20th week.

Critical here is the necessity of a functioning and probably integrated nervous system for the possibility of rational activity. For if there is no nervous system functioning, it is not clear that the rational part of the definition of a person can be fulfilled, even though the individual part might be. The functioning nervous system is a necessary condition for the possibility of a new stage of development to emerge and is also a sign that the organism is prepared for this. Thus any of the three markers noted immediately above could serve as an indicator of the capacity for rationality, though not necessarily its actuality.

c. Developmental Autonomy Given the philosophical discussion on nature and substance, it is reasonable to argue that the developing body as an organized system is a new substance or nature and has the capacity to elicit the potencies within its own reality. That is, a fully formed zygote is a new nature because it has its own actuality and potentiality. It is in itself a sufficient explanation of its own development and activities. The same is true on each new level of development as the zygote becomes an embryo and, finally, a fetus. On a genetic level, the clearest marker of the presence of self-directing activity which would manifest such a new nature would appear in the zygote after it developed the capacity to manufacture its own messenger RNA and thus be developmentally, though not physically, independent of the mother.

2. Moral Implications

a. Physical Individuality We find it impossible to speak of a true individual, an ontological individual, as present from fertilization. There is a time period of about three weeks during which it is biologically unrealistic to speak of a physical individual. This means that the reality of a person, however one might define that term, is not present at least until individualization has occurred. Individuality is an absolute or necessary condition for personhood.

We conclude that there is no individual and therefore no person present until either restriction or gastrulation is completed, about three weeks after fertilization. To abort at this time would end life and terminate genetic uniqueness, to be sure. But in a moral sense one is certainly not murdering, because there is no individual to be the personal referent of such an action.

Since the zygote is living, has the human genetic code, and indeed possesses genetic uniqueness, this entity is valuable, and its value does not depend on the presence or absence of any or a particular quality or characteristic such as intelligence or capacity for relationships.[68] Thus the zygote and the blastomers derived from it, because they are living, possess ontic value and are in themselves valuable. Thus the general argument made here is not a so-called "quality of life" argument.

Nonetheless, until the completion of restriction or gastrulation, the zygote and its sequelae are in a rather fluid process and are not physical individuals and therefore cannot be persons. The pre-embryo at this state, we conclude, cannot claim absolute protection based on claims to personhood grounded in ontological individuality. Yet, since the pre-embryo is living and possesses genetic uniqueness, some claims to protection are possi-

67. Wolter, "Chemical Substance" 125-26.

68. For a further discussion of this concept, see James J. Walter, "The Meaning and Validity of Quality of Life Judgments in Contemporary Roman Catholic Medical Ethics," *Louvain Studies* 13 (1988) 195-208. Another discussion can be found in Thomas A. Shannon and James J. Walter, "The PVS Patient and the Forgoing/Withdrawing of Medical Nutrition and Hydration," *TS* 49 (1988) 623-47.

ble. But these may not be absolute and, if not, could yield to other moral claims.

b. Immaterial Individuality If one assumes, as we think correct to do, that the potencies actualized in the formation of the new nature of the fertilized egg have the inherent capacity to ground its growth and development, then there is no need to posit a principle of individual immateriality, understood as the Aristotelian *nous* or as the entelechy of the body, in pre-embryonic development.

Since the evidence for such a principle comes from the internal evidence of those who experience it, it is difficult at best to ground any speculation as to when it comes into existence. We would make this argument. On the one hand, the developing pre-embryo as a new nature has within it the potential for future development. On the other hand, if the will as a rational potency is what genuinely distinguishes the person from a nature, then one needs to look to biological presuppositions which enable such a potency to exist. We would argue that the earliest time is around the eighth week of gestation, because then the nervous system is fully integrated.

3. *Summary*

We have reviewed some of the salient biological data about the initial stages of the development of human life, with a view to evaluating the philosophical and theological claims made of them. Reflecting on these from a historico-theological perspective, we have tried to discover whether there exists some rational justification for the absolute value that is attributed to the zygote or pre-embryonic state based on claims to personhood, or whether our earlier long-standing Catholic tradition of mediate animation by a rational soul does not provide a more satisfactory philosophical and theological account. For if we consider judiciously what the great scholastic doctors had to say about the "moment of conception," we seem to have good reason to reintroduce, in interpreting the data of present-day science, the theological distinction between active and passive conception made by Pope Benedict XIV in discussing Mary's immaculate conception.

We thus affirm that any abortion is a premoral evil. That is, it is the ending of life. Consequently we do not want to be understood as proposing or supporting an "abortion on demand" position or assuming that early abortions are amoral. Abortion is a serious issue, because life is involved and one needs always to respect life. We have made one major argument, however, in this essay. Given the findings of modern biology, there is no evidence for the presence of a separate ontological individual until the completion of either restriction or gastrulation, which occurs around three weeks after fertilization. Therefore there is no reasonable basis for arguing that the pre-embryo is morally equivalent to a person or is a person as a basis for prohibiting abortion. That is, there is no biological support for the position that the fertilized egg is from the beginning of the process of fertilization a distinct individual needing no outside agency to develop into a person. Neither is there good philosophical evidence that the principle of immaterial individuality need be present from the beginning to explain the physical development of the pre-embryo.

This position obviously does not support the argument that abortion is to be prohibited because a person is present from the beginning of fertilization. The earliest such an argument could reasonably be made is after the completion of gastrulation. We recognize that this argument will dismay many and comfort others. Our intention in proposing the argument of this essay is to gain a greater coherence between moral theology and modern embryology.

In this sense we are complementing the work of the Roman Congregations and bringing it up to date. We also wish to test the strength of our argument, already subjected to review by several colleagues, in review by a wider and more diverse audience. Additionally, our intention is to develop a position that is reasonable and can be reasonably defended in the public sector.[69] Finally, we think our position on the pre-embryo and embryo can stand rigorous scrutiny, and we propose it as a factor in developing a feasible state and/or national policy on abortion.

One is reminded here of Henry de Dorlodot's evaluation of immediate animation made over 50 years ago in his seminal work *Darwinism and Catholic Thought:* "We are not exaggerating in the least when we regard the fact that this theory [of immediate animation] should still find defenders long after the experimental bases on which it was thought to be founded have been shown definitely to be false, as one of the most shameful things in the history of thought."[70]

69. We suggest that something of the violence between the extreme pro-life or pro-abortionists might be defused, and the political dilemma of Catholic politicians seeking some rational options might be solved, if one were to recognize that the moral status of, and hence the protection appropriate for, a fetus changes with its developmental stages.

70. Quoted by Messenger, *Theology and Evolution* 219.

48 Three Views on the Preimplantation Embryo

Michael R. Panicola

Men pay for the increase of their power with alienation from that over which they exercise their power. Enlightenment behaves toward things as a dictator toward men. He knows them in so far as he can manipulate them. The man of science knows things in so far as he can make them. In this way their potentiality is turned to his own ends.[1]

Max Horkheimer and Theodor Adorno

Advances in reproductive and genetic technologies over the last several decades have generated much public excitement and have expanded the horizon of human possibilities. We now know more about the origin and development of human life than ever before; we can help individuals who were previously unable to have children;[2] we can diagnosis genetic diseases very early in the developmental process; and we are learning how to manipulate the germ-line with the hope of eradicating hereditary diseases.[3] Notwithstanding these benefits, reproductive and genetic technologies have pushed us to the outer moral limits regarding what we can do to human life at its earliest beginnings.[4] These technologies have given rise to public consternation over what will become of the human race and have created difficult ethical and policy issues.

One of the more controversial ethical and policy issues to result from scientific advancement concerns the moral status of the preimplantation embryo.[5] The preimplantation embryo refers to the developing organism that comes into existence after the first cell division of the single-celled zygote and that lasts until the appearance of the primitive streak around the fourteenth day of gestational age.[6] Once hidden in the darkness of the womb and beyond the direct gaze of science, the preimplantation embryo has been nakedly exposed through in vitro fertilization and "examined, probed, and even destroyed, in order to advance human knowledge and ends."[7]

1. Max Horkheimer and Theodor Adorno, *Dialectic of Enlightenment* (New York: Continuum, 1990), 9.

2. For a discussion of in vitro fertilization, see Robert Edwards, *Life Before Birth: Reflections on the Embryo Debate* (New York: Basic Books, 1989); Donald Evans, ed., *Creating the Child: The Ethics, Law and Practice of Assisted Procreation* (London: Martinus Nijhoff Publishers, 1996); and D. A. Valone, "The Changing Moral Landscape of Human Reproduction: Two Moments in the History of In Vitro Fertilization," *Mount Sinai Journal of Medicine* 65 (May 1998): 167-72.

3. For a discussion of preimplantation genetic diagnosis and germ-line gene therapy, see S. J. Fasouliotis and J. G. Schenker, "Preimplantation Genetic Diagnosis: Principles and Ethics," *Human Reproduction* 13 (August 1998): 2238-45; and LeRoy Walters and Julie Gage Palmer, *The Ethics of Human Gene Therapy* (New York: Oxford University Press, 1997).

4. For a discussion of medical technology in general pushing us to the outer moral limits, see several of Daniel Callahan's works, namely: *Setting Limits: Medical Goals in an Aging Society* (New York: Simon and Schuster, 1988); *The Troubled Dream of Life: In Search of a Peaceful Death* (New York: Simon and Schuster, 1993); and *False Hopes: Why America's Quest for Perfect Health Is a Recipe for Failure* (New York: Simon and Schuster, 1998). With particular reference to reproductive and genetic technologies, see Patricia Spallone and Deborah Lynn Steinberg, eds., *Made to Order: The Myth of Reproductive and Genetic Progress* (Oxford: Pergamon, 1987).

5. The moral status of the preimplantation embryo is not a new issue. It has been addressed by a number of ethics boards in past decades. In 1979, the Ethics Advisory Board of the Department of Health, Education, and Welfare decided that "the [preimplantation] embryo is entitled to profound respect; but this respect does not necessarily encompass full legal and moral rights attributed to persons." See Ethics Advisory Board, U.S. Department of Health, Education, and Welfare, "Report and Conclusions: HEW Support Research Involving Human In Vitro Fertilization and Embryo Transfer," *Federal Register* 44 (June 18, 1979): 35033-58, at 35057. In 1984, the Warnock Committee judged that the preimplantation embryo is not accorded the same status as living children or adults but that "the [preimplantation] embryo of the human species ought to have a special status." Mary Warnock, *A Question of Life: The Warnock Report* (London: Basil Blackwell, 1984), 63. In 1986, the Ethics Committee of the American Fertility Society ruled that there is "widespread consensus that the preembryo is not a person but is to be treated with special respect because it is a genetically unique, living human entity that might become a person." See American Fertility Society, Ethics Committee, "Ethical Considerations of the New Reproductive Technologies," *Fertility and Sterility* 46, Supplement 1 (September 1987): 30S. More recently, in 1994, the Human Embryo Research Panel of the National Institutes of Health tackled the issue of the moral status of the preimplantation embryo and concluded that "although the preimplantation embryo warrants serious moral consideration as a developing form of human life, it does not have the same moral status as an infant or child." Human Embryo Research Panel, National Institutes of Health, *Report of the Human Embryo Research Panel* (Bethesda, Md.: National Institutes of Health, 1994), x.

6. Variations of this definition of the preimplantation embryo can be found in the work of several authors. See, for instance, Norman M. Ford, *When Did I Begin? Conception of the Human Individual in History, Philosophy and Science* (New York: Cambridge University Press, 1988); Clifford Grobstein, *Science and the Unborn: Choosing Human Futures* (New York: Basic Books, 1988); and Mary B. Mahowald, "Fetus: Human Development from Fertilization to Birth," in *Encyclopedia of Bioethics*, rev. ed., ed. Warren T. Reich (New York: Simon and Schuster, 1995), 847-57.

7. George Khushf, "Embryo Research: The Ethical Geography of the Debate," *Journal of Medicine and Philosophy* 22 (October 1997): 495-519, at 496.

Originally published in the *National Catholic Bioethics Quarterly* 2.1 (2002): 69-97.

By necessity, rather than choice, we have been charged with the responsibility of deciding whether the preimplantation embryo is a full member of the moral community.[8] How we answer the question of the moral status of the preimplantation embryo will have serious practical implications. Some of these implications include how many preimplantation embryos we allow to be created in vitro for transfer; how we treat preimplantation embryos before transfer; whether we transfer all preimplantation embryos; how we treat those preimplantation embryos not transferred; whether we can remove cells from preimplantation embryos for genetic diagnosis; how we treat genetically defective preimplantation embryos; whether we allow research to be conducted on preimplantation embryos; and given the effects of certain anovulent drugs, how we treat victims of sexual assault who may possibly be pregnant.

The strongest claims concerning the moral status of the preimplantation embryo have been advanced by the moral magisterium of the Catholic Church. In its two most recent statements dealing with the moral status of early human life, the 1974 *Declaration on Abortion*[9] and the 1987 *Instruction on Respect for Human Life in Its Origin and on the Dignity of Procreation,*[10] the magisterium has restated and reinforced its position (hereafter referred to as the *personal position*) that personal life comes into existence at the completion of fertilization and is to be absolutely respected and protected in its inherent dignity.[11] The Declaration specifies that the "tradition of the church has always held that human life must be protected and favored from the beginning, just as at the various stages of its development."[12] Furthermore, the Declaration states:

> In reality, respect for human life is called for from the time that the process of generation begins. From the time that the ovum is fertilized, a life is begun which is neither that of the father nor of the mother; it is rather the life of a new human being with its own growth. It would never be made human if it were not human already.[13]

Following this statement, the Declaration makes two important claims concerning the moral status of early human life. First, the Declaration asserts that "modern genetic science brings valuable confirmation" to its position that a unique human life begins with the completion of fertilization. Science has "demonstrated that from the first instant there is established the program of what this living being will be: a man, this individual man with his characteristic aspects already well determined."[14] Second, the Declaration notes that its conclusion on the moral status of early human life stands "perfectly independent of the discussions on the moment of animation" and that "it is not up to the biological sciences to make a definitive judgment on questions which are properly philosophical and moral, such as the mo-

8. It is important to keep in mind that when discussing the question of the moral status of the preimplantation embryo, the point of issue is not when does human life begin but when does personhood begin. Reasonable people can agree that the preimplantation embryo is human and is living, but what is at issue is when does the preimplantation embryo become a person. As Richard McCormick remarks: "What is present after fertilization is human life. It is *living,* not dead. It is *human;* it will never be canine. So the question 'When does human life begin?' is not really a question: for everyone gives the same answer. The more accurate formulation of the issue is: how should we evaluate human life at the preembryonic stage? Is it a person with potential or a potential person?" "The First 14 Days," *The Tablet* (March 10, 1990): 301-4, at 301. This distinction is important because it focuses the discussion of the moral status of the preimplantation embryo on the question of personhood (not human life) and the respect and protection due to the preimplantation embryo as person or potential person. Albert Moraczewski doubts whether this distinction is necessary because human life and human person "refer to the same objective reality albeit under different formalities." "Personhood: Entry and Exit," in *The Twenty-Fifth Anniversary of Vatican II — A Look Back and A Look Ahead* (Braintree, Mass.: Pope John Center, 1990), 78-101, at 80. Nevertheless, the distinction does clear up some confusion for the public debate as positions are sometimes obscured due to the confusion in terminology.

9. Congregation for the Doctrine of the Faith, "Declaration on Abortion," *Origins* 4 (12 December 1974): 386-91.

10. Congregation for the Doctrine of the Faith, "Instruction on Respect for Human Life in Its Origin and on the Dignity of Procreation," in Thomas A. Shannon and Lisa Sowle Cahill, *Religion and Artificial Reproduction: An Inquiry into the Vatican 'Instruction on Respect for Human Life'* (New York: Crossroad, 1988), 140-77.

11. Several authors have supported the personal position on the moral status of the preimplantation embryo and have contributed arguments to strengthen the position. See, for instance, Benedict M. Ashley, "A Critique of the Theory of Delayed Hominization," in *An Ethical Evaluation of Fetal Experimentation: An Interdisciplinary Study* (St. Louis: Pope John Center, 1976), 113-33; Benedict M. Ashley and Albert S. Moraczewski, "Is the Biological Subject of Human Rights Present from Conception?" in *The Fetal Tissue Issue: Medical and Ethical Aspects,* eds. Peter J. Cataldo and Albert S. Moraczewski (Braintree, Mass.: Pope John Center, 1994), 33-59; Benedict M. Ashley and Kevin D. O'Rourke, *Ethics of Health Care: An Introductory Textbook* (Washington, D.C.: Georgetown University Press, 1994), 149-51; Benedict M. Ashley and Kevin D. O'Rourke, *Health Care Ethics: A Theological Analysis,* 4th ed. (Washington, D.C.: Georgetown University Press, 1997), 227-40; Germain Grisez, "When Do People Begin?" *Proceedings of the American Catholic Philosophical Association* 63 (1989): 27-47; Mark Johnson, "Delayed Hominization: Reflections on Some Recent Catholic Claims for Delayed Hominization," *Theological Studies* 56 (December 1995): 743-63; Jérôme Lejeune, *The Concentration Can* (San Francisco: Ignatius Press, 1992); William E. May, "What Makes a Human Being to Be a Being of Moral Worth?" *Thomist* 40 (July 1976): 416-43; William E. May, "The Sacredness of Life: An Overview of the Beginning," *Linacre Quarterly* 63 (February 1996): 87-96; Moraczewski, "Personhood: Entry and Exit"; Stephen Schwarz, *The Moral Question of Abortion* (Chicago: Loyola University Press, 1990), 67-112; and Robert J. White, "Human Embryo Research," *America* 175 (14 September 1996): 4-5.

12. Congregation for the Doctrine of the Faith, "Declaration on Abortion," 387. It should be pointed out that the Declaration never refers to early human life as the preimplantation embryo. Rather, the Declaration speaks in more generic terms about the developing human organism.

13. Ibid., 388.

14. Ibid., 388-89.

ment when a human person is constituted."[15] Despite not rendering a conclusive assessment on when animation occurs and personhood begins, the Declaration makes an absolute moral judgment about the respect and protection due to early human life: "From a moral point of view this is certain: even if a doubt existed concerning whether the fruit of conception is already a human person, it is objectively a grave sin to dare to risk murder. 'The one who will be a man is already one.'"[16]

The Instruction affirms the teaching of the *Declaration on Abortion* concerning the genetic uniqueness of the human being who comes into existence with the completion of fertilization.[17] The Instruction states that the teaching of the Declaration "remains valid and is further confirmed, if confirmation were needed, by recent findings of human biological science which recognize that in the zygote resulting from fertilization the biological identity of a new human individual is already constituted."[18] Following this statement, the Instruction makes its most pointed comments concerning the moral status of the preimplantation embryo. The Instruction states:

> Certainly no experimental datum can be in itself sufficient to bring us to the recognition of a spiritual soul; nevertheless, the conclusions of science regarding the human [preimplantation] embryo provide a valuable indication for discerning by the use of reason a personal presence at the moment of this first appearance of a human life: How could a human individual not be a human person?[19]

The Instruction continues by expressing that the "magisterium has not expressly committed itself to an affirmation of a philosophical nature [about when animation occurs], but it constantly reaffirms the moral condemnation of any kind of procured abortion." The Instruction concludes its discussion of the moral status of the preimplantation embryo in the following way:

> The fruit of human generation from the first moment of its existence, that is to say, from the moment the zygote has formed, demands the unconditional respect that is morally due to the human being in his bodily and spiritual totality. The human being is to be respected and treated as a person from the moment of conception and therefore from that same moment his rights as a person must be recognized, among which in the first place is the inviolable right of every innocent human being to life.[20]

Thus, the personal position on the moral status of the preimplantation embryo is based on three essential claims.[21] First, human life comes into existence following the process of fertilization (or its physiological equivalent, such as the fusion of genetic material with the ovum, as in cloning). This human life is individual in that it is neither that of the mother nor of the father, and it is unique in that it is endowed with a genetic program that will direct its future growth and development. Second, science alone cannot answer the question of the beginning of personhood, but it does confirm the genetic uniqueness of the developing entity which is a sign for reason's discernment of a personal presence from the very beginning. Finally, even if doubt existed as to the personal status of the developing entity, one is still morally obliged to treat it as if it were a person because it is always a grave sin to terminate or frustrate the biological process of human development once underway.[22]

Though the personal position bases its claims on contemporary scientific data, two other positions have emerged in the ethical and policy discussion of the moral status of the preimplantation embryo that challenge the personal position. The first position (the *pre-personal position*) claims that the preimplantation embryo is in a pre-personal stage of development at least until it attains a certain level of biological stability, which coincides with the formation of the primitive streak, and as such is only entitled to limited respect and protection.[23] This

15. Ibid.

16. Ibid., 389.

17. It should be mentioned that the Instruction makes free use of the terms *zygote, preimplantation embryo, embryo,* and *fetus,* "attributing to them an identical ethical relevance, in order to designate the result (whether visible or not) of human generation, from the first moment of its existence until birth." Congregation for the Doctrine of the Faith, "Instruction on Respect for Human Life in Its Origin and on the Dignity of Procreation," in *Religion and Artificial Reproduction,* 141.

18. Ibid., 148-49.

19. Ibid., 149.

20. Ibid.

21. For a discussion of the personal position on the moral status of the preimplantation embryo, see Michael J. Coughlan, *The Vatican, the Law and the Human Embryo* (Iowa City: University of Iowa Press, 1990); Shannon and Cahill, *Religion and Artificial Reproduction,* 103-32; and William Werpehowski, "Persons, Practices, and the Conception Argument," *Journal of Medicine and Philosophy* 22 (October 1997): 479-94.

22. Benedict Ashley makes the point that the personal position's claims for respect and protection due to early human life are not predicated on its determination of personhood. See his "Delayed Hominization: Catholic Theological Perspective," in *The Interaction of Catholic Bioethics and Secular Society* (Braintree, Mass.: Pope John Center, 1992), 163-80.

23. The pre-personal position has been developed by several authors, namely: Carlos A. Bedate and Robert C. Cefalo, "The Zygote: To Be or Not To Be a Person," *Journal of Medicine and Philosophy* 14 (December 1989): 641-45; Ford, *When Did I Begin?;* Grobstein, *Science and the Unborn;* Bernard Häring, *Medical Ethics,* ed. Gabrielle L. Jean (Notre Dame, Ind.: Fides Publishing, Inc., 1973), 75-85; John S. Mahoney, *Bioethics and Belief* (London: Sheed & Ward, 1984), 52-86; Richard A. McCormick, "Who or What Is the Preembryo?" in *Corrective Vision: Explorations in Moral Theology* (Kansas City: Sheed & Ward, 1994), 176-88; Jean Porter, "Individuality, Personal Identity, and the Moral Status of the Preembryo: A Response to Mark Johnson," *Theological Studies* 56 (December 1995): 763-70; Thomas A. Shannon and Allan B. Wolter, "Reflections on the Moral Status of the Pre-Embryo," in *Bioethics: Basic Writings on the Key Ethical Questions That Surround the Major, Modern Biological Possibilities and Problems,* 4th ed., Thomas A.

first sign of organ differentiation is a morally significant biological marker in that it indicates the developing human organism has become definitively individualized and is no longer capable of being divided through natural twinning or artificial separation in vitro. Since the preimplantation embryo has not achieved this necessary but insufficient criterion for personhood (individuation), the pre-personal position contends that it need not be absolutely respected and protected.[24] The second position (the *nonpersonal position*) claims that the preimplantation embryo is a nonperson and as such is not entitled to any respect or protection.[25] Neither the completion of fertilization nor the appearance of the primitive streak is morally important because the developing human organism still lacks certain fundamental characteristics necessary for claims to consideration, specifically the preimplantation embryo is not even a sentient being capable of experiencing pain or pleasure.

Both the pre-personal position and the nonpersonal positions raise serious questions as to the plausibility of the view that a personal presence is discernible at the completion of fertilization. If either of these positions is accepted in the ethical and policy discussion of the moral status of the preimplantation embryo, severe repercussions for early human life would follow, particularly in the areas of in vitro fertilization and embryo research.[26] Hence, we must determine whether either the pre-personal position or the nonpersonal position stands up under the weight of critical analysis such that it would justify denying the preimplantation embryo the normal standards of moral treatment. Phrasing the issue in such a way admittedly places the burden of proof on these two positions. Some may protest that this is unfair inasmuch as it presupposes the claims made on behalf of the preimplantation embryo by the personal position. Nevertheless, this approach to the issue seems warranted given the fact that incipient human life is at stake. If we are going to exclude the preimplantation embryo from the inner sanctum of the moral community, then we should ensure that we are on solid grounding because a "false step could mean a further erosion of our commitment to defense of the human rights of our most vulnerable fellow human beings."[27]

This paper argues that neither the pre-personal position nor the nonpersonal position on the moral status of the preimplantation embryo has sufficient merit to undermine the personal position and thus justify denying the preimplantation embryo the same degree of respect

---

Shannon, ed. (Mahwah, N.J.: Paulist Press, 1993), 36-60; and Carol Tauer, "The Tradition of Probabilism and the Moral Status of the Early Embryo," *Theological Studies* 45 (1984): 3-33. This position has had quite an impact on the ethical and policy discussion of the moral status of the preimplantation embryo. For instance, in reviewing the reasons why the Human Embryo Research Panel of the National Institutes of Health chose to limit the extent of research on early human life to fourteen days, Carol Tauer, a member of the panel, noted that its position was based largely on the persuasive arguments of those authors who claim that "it is extremely implausible that the [preimplantation] embryo is a human being or a human person before 14 days' gestational age, the usual time of the appearance of the primitive streak." "Embryo Research and Public Policy: A Philosopher's Appraisal," *Journal of Medicine and Philosophy* 22 (October 1997): 423-39, at 429.

24. Thomas A. Shannon, "Issues and Values in Genetic Engineering: A Survey," *Chicago Studies* 33 (1994): 196-204, at 200.

25. The nonpersonal position has been developed by several authors, namely: Stephen Buckle, Karen Dawson, and Peter Singer, "The Syngamy Debate: When Precisely Does Human Life Begin?" *Law, Medicine and Health Care* 17 (Summer 1989): 174-81; H. Tristram Engelhardt, Jr., "Viability, Abortion, and the Difference Between a Fetus and an Infant," *American Journal of Obstetrics and Gynecology* 116 (1 June 1973): 429-34; idem, "The Ontology of Abortion," *Ethics* 84 (April 1974): 217-34; idem, "Some Persons Are Humans, Some Humans Are Persons, and the World Is What We Persons Make of It," in *Philosophical Medical Ethics: Its Nature and Significance,* Stuart C. Spicker and H. Tristram Engelhardt, Jr., eds. (Boston: D. Reidel Publishing Company, 1977), 183-94; idem, "Medicine and the Concept of Person," in *Ethical Issues in Death and Dying,* Tom L. Beauchamp and Seymour Perlin, eds. (Englewood Cliffs, N.J.: Prentice-Hall, 1978), 271-84; idem, "Personhood, Moral Strangers, and the Evil of Abortion: The Painful Experience of Post-Modernity," *Journal of Medicine and Philosophy* 18 (August 1993): 419-21; idem, *The Foundations of Bioethics,* 2nd ed. (New York: Oxford University Press, 1996), 135-54 and 253-77; Helga Kuhse, "An Ethical Approach to IVF and ET: What Ethics Is All About," in *Test-Tube Babies: A Guide to Moral Questions, Present Techniques and Future Possibilities,* William Walters and Peter Singer, eds. (Melbourne: Oxford University Press, 1982), 22-35; Helga Kuhse, "A Report from Australia: When a Human Life Has Not Yet Begun — According to the Law," *Bioethics* 2 (October 1988): 334-42; Helga Kuhse and Peter Singer, "The Moral Status of the Embryo," in *Test-Tube Babies,* 57-64; Helga Kuhse and Peter Singer, "Individuals, Humans and Persons: The Issue of Moral Status," in *Embryo Experimentation: Ethical, Legal and Social Issues,* Peter Singer, Helga Kuhse, Stephen Buckle, Karen Dawson, and Pascal Kasimba, eds. (Cambridge: Cambridge University Press, 1990), 65-75; Peter Singer, "Making Laws on Making Babies," *Hastings Center Report* 15 (August 1985): 5-6; idem, *Practical Ethics,* 2nd ed. (Cambridge University Press, 1993), 83-109 and 135-74; idem, *Rethinking Life and Death: The Collapse of Our Traditional Ethics* (New York: St. Martin's Griffin, 1994), 83-105 and 159-183; Peter Singer and Deane Wells, "*In Vitro* Fertilisation: The Major Issues," *Journal of Medical Ethics* 9 (December 1983): 192-95; Peter Singer and Helga Kuhse, "The Ethics of Embryo Research," *Law, Medicine and Health Care* 14 (September 1986): 133-38; Peter Singer and Karen Dawson, "IVF Technology and the Argument from Potential," *Philosophy and Public Affairs* 17 (Spring 1988): 87-104; Michael Tooley, "Abortion and Infanticide," *Philosophy and Public Affairs* 2 (Fall 1972): 37-65; idem, "A Defense of Abortion and Infanticide," in *The Problem of Abortion,* Joel Feinberg, ed. (Belmont, Calif.: Wadsworth Publishing Company, 1973), 51-91; idem, "Decisions to Terminate Life and the Concept of Person," in *Ethical Issues Relating to Life and Death,* John Ladd, ed. (New York: Oxford University Press, 1979), 62-93; and idem, *Abortion and Infanticide* (New York: Oxford University Press, 1983), 33-305.

26. For a discussion of embryo research, see Gregory Bock and Maeve O'Connor, eds., *Human Embryo Research: Yes or No?* (London: Tavistock, 1986); Anthony Dyson and John Harris, eds., *Experiments on Embryos* (London: Routledge, 1990); and Human Embryo Research Panel, National Institutes of Health, *Report of the Human Embryo Research Panel.*

27. McCormick, "The First 14 Days," 301.

and protection given other human beings. I develop this argument in two major sections. The first reviews and critically evaluates the pre-personal position and the second does the same for the nonpersonal position. An appendix delineating the developmental process of the preimplantation embryo is included below in order to support some of the scientific claims made in the article.

The Preimplantation Embryo as Pre-Personal

The pre-personal position on the moral status of the preimplantation embryo argues that the personal position fails to acknowledge and properly interpret some of the scientific data currently available. The pre-personal position rejects the claim that a personal presence is discernible at the completion of fertilization or its physiological equivalent. Though the pre-personal position admits that the preimplantation embryo is genetically unique, it does not accept that it has become individualized to the point that it warrants absolute respect and protection. This is because genetic uniqueness does not coincide with individuation. Thomas Shannon explains this point:

> The question of individuality is a question different from that of uniqueness. To conflate these questions misreads the biology and leads to unnecessary philosophical complications. One's genome reveals that one is a member of the human species, which is an important part of one's identity but not all of it. Additionally, this genetic profile can be replicated without necessarily harming the entities bearing it. Neither species membership nor an organism's genetic structure says anything about individuality, which is a critical presupposition for personhood.[28]

Individuality is a morally relevant factor because it is only after this has been established that one can speak of an entity that is dedicated to the development of a unified organism incapable of being divided. An individual person cannot be said to exist before a certain biological stability in the organism is present.[29]

While genetic uniqueness is established with the completion of fertilization, the pre-personal position maintains that individuality occurs later in the developmental process. The appearance of the primitive streak at fourteen days' gestation is a significant biological line of demarcation because it indicates that the cells of the preimplantation embryo have lost their ability to differentiate into any type of cell and thus form a new organism or regenerate any part of an organism (totipotency). Until this developmental point has been reached, the preimplantation embryo can divide via natural twinning or artificial separation in vitro and thus cannot be understood to be a single individual. "For by definition, an individual is an entity that cannot be divided or, if it is, becomes two halves neither of which can survive on its own."[30]

Against the personal position that seems to move from the genetic uniqueness of the preimplantation embryo to personal status, the pre-personal position asserts that the manifestation of the human genome does not confer an absolute moral status on the preimplantation embryo.[31] Genetic uniqueness suggests that the preimplantation

---

28. Thomas A. Shannon, "Delayed Hominization: A Response to Mark Johnson," *Theological Studies* 57 (December 1996): 731-34, at 732. Shannon also makes this point in two other articles, namely: "Issues and Values in Genetic Engineering," 200; and "Cloning, Uniqueness, and Individuality," *Louvain Studies* 19 (Winter 1994): 283-306, at 285. See also idem, "Human Embryonic Stem Cell Therapy," *Theological Studies* 62 (December 2001): 811-24.

29. According to some authors who support the pre-personal position, the biological instability of the preimplantation embryo is also evidenced in the relatively high percentage of preimplantation embryos that perish early on in the developmental process (e.g., McCormick, "Who or What Is the Preembryo?" in *Corrective Vision*, 180 and 187; and Shannon and Wolter, "Reflections on the Moral Status of the Pre-Embryo," in *Bioethics*, 49). This phenomenon, known as natural wastage, is said to occur in approximately thirty to fifty percent of all pregnancies. This substantial percentage of natural loss was given considerable weight by Karl Rahner in his reflections on the moral status of the preimplantation embryo. Rahner wondered, "Will [anyone] be able to accept that fifty percent of all 'human beings' — real human beings with 'immortal' souls and an eternal destiny — will never get beyond this first stage of human existence?" "The Problem of Genetic Manipulation," *Theological Investigations* 9 (New York: Seabury, 1972), 236, note 2. While the natural wastage argument may appear to support the pre-personal position, two reasons suggest that this argument is not sufficient to conclude that the preimplantation embryo is not an actual, individual person. First, not all natural losses occur in established pregnancies. Sometimes the process of fertilization is not completed because the gametes fail to unite adequately and the mature oocyte is ill-prepared for further development. See Ashley and O'Rourke, *Health Care Ethics*, 235-36; James J. Diamond, "Abortion, Animation, and Biological Hominization," *Theological Studies* 36 (June 1975): 305-24. Thus, it would be erroneous to state that thirty to fifty percent of all *human beings* never get beyond the pre-embryonic stage of development. Second, a strong argument against the personal status of the preimplantation embryo cannot be made from statistics. It should be remembered that infant mortality throughout history has hovered around 30 to 50 percent, and in some countries at certain times has even exceeded this range. See Ashley, "A Critique of the Theory of Delayed Hominization," in *An Ethical Evaluation of Fetal Experimentation*, 126; Ashley and O'Rourke, *Health Care Ethics*, 235. Even John Mahoney, a proponent of the pre-personal position, rejects the natural wastage argument for denying full personal status to the preimplantation embryo. Mahoney claims that if the matter of personhood can be decided strictly by numbers, "then in principle it does not appear very different, if at all, from arguing from statistics in some countries, or in earlier centuries, of infant or perinatal mortality to the conclusion that the tragically large number of children who die, or have died, at birth could not possibly be all possessed of an immortal soul." In *Bioethics and Belief*, 61.

30. Thomas A. Shannon, "Remaking Ourselves? The Ethics of Stem-Cell Research," *Commonweal* 125 (4 December 1998): 9-10, at 9.

31. Ford, *When Did I Begin?* 117-31; McCormick, "Who or What Is the Preembryo?" in *Corrective Vision*, 182; Shannon, "Delayed Hominization: A Response to Mark Johnson," 734.

embryo is a member of the human species, but *not* that it is a full member of the moral community worthy of absolute respect and protection. The human genome can be passed on successfully to other developing entities and as such is not a sufficient basis for claiming that the preimplantation embryo has passed a critical, albeit not the only, criterion for personhood (individuation). Norman Ford describes this well:

> The genetic code in the zygote does not suffice to constitute or define a human individual in an ontological sense. Identical twins have the same genetic code but they are distinct ontological individuals. Failure to appreciate this significant distinction could lead to a mistake in determining the timing establishing the beginning of a human person.[32]

An individual's established identity requires that it be expressed in the same continuous body. This body cannot be divided without giving rise to two new individuals, each of which is different from the original. Genetic uniqueness neither secures established identity nor protects the existing identity from being split into two separate identities. Furthermore, equating personal status with genetic uniqueness leads to genetic reductionism whereby a person is limited to her or his genetic make-up.[33] While individual genetic structures are vital to personal identity, they do not fully capture the essence of persons.

Thus, the pre-personal position on the moral status of the preimplantation embryo is based on three essential claims. First, human life begins with the completion of fertilization, but personhood does not commence at least until the formation of the primitive streak, which signifies the developing organism has become definitively individualized. Second, genetic uniqueness is not equivalent to individuation and is not sufficient to attribute to the preimplantation embryo personal moral status. Finally, moral doubt regarding the status of the preimplantation embryo does not necessitate that one take the morally safest course and treat the preimplantation embryo as if it were a person. If strong reasons were present that suggested the preimplantation embryo was pre-personal rather than personal, one would be justified in taking a less rigorous course of action toward the preimplantation embryo.[34] The pre-personal position insists that contemporary scientific data provide such strong reasons.

Critical Evaluation of Pre-Personalism

The pre-personal position rejects the view that personal life comes into existence at the completion of fertilization and is to be absolutely respected and protected in its inherent dignity. The pre-personal position's fundamental critique of the personal position is that as long as the cells of the preimplantation embryo remain in a totipotent state, the preimplantation embryo is susceptible to division through natural twinning or artificial separation in vitro and thus cannot be understood to be a single individual. Though the pre-personal position raises serious questions as to the plausibility of the personal position, it ultimately fails in its attempt to refute the personal position for three principal reasons.

First, the pre-personal position places too much emphasis on totipotency, and by association, twinning and individuality. While it is true that the cells that constitute the preimplantation embryo can become the source cells for a separate organism, this only occurs when one of the tightly compacted cells becomes detached from the highly organized cellular mass.[35] Focusing overly on the *possibility* of totipotency "can give rise to the idea that the blastomeres have no real relation to one another" prior to the formation of the primitive streak.[36] However, this would be a misinterpretation of scientific data which confirm that by the eight-cell stage, the originally round and loosely adherent blastomeres begin to change shape and tightly align themselves one with the other through compaction.[37] Hence, as Mark Johnson asserts, "when speaking of the blastomeres as part of the preembryo it is actually, if paradoxically, better to term them 'potentially totipotential,' since their ability to self-regulate and self-develop can occur only on the condition of their being separated from the whole."[38]

Second, the rare phenomenon of twinning does not provide sufficient proof that the preimplantation embryo is not definitively individualized. From the outset of the developmental process the cells of the preimplantation embryo are ordered to the whole and play a role in maintaining life and preparing the developing organism for the process of implantation.[39] These cells are tightly aligned one with the other and operate under the direc-

32. Ford, *When Did I Begin?* 117. Ford's definition of an ontological individual is "a single concrete entity that exists as a distinct being and is not an aggregation of smaller things nor merely a part of a greater whole." Ibid., 212.

33. Shannon, "Issues and Values in Genetic Engineering," 198.

34. For a discussion of the relevance of the tradition of probabilism in the debate on the moral status of the preimplantation embryo, see Mahoney, *Bioethics and Belief,* 79-85; McCormick, "Who or What Is the Preembryo?" in *Corrective Fision,* 185-86; and Tauer, "The Tradition of Probabilism and the Moral Status of the Early Embryo," 3-33. Albert R. Jonsen and Stephen Toulmin offer an excellent presentation on the tradition of probabilism in *The Abuse of Casuistry: A History of Moral Reasoning* (Berkeley: University of California Press, 1988), 164-75.

35. Johnson, "Delayed Hominization," 758. See also Ashley and Moraczewski, "Is the Biological Subject of Human Rights Present from Conception?" 48-49.

36. Johnson, "Delayed Hominization," 758.

37. Ashley and Moraczewski, "Is the Biological Subject of Human Rights Present from Conception?" 40.

38. Johnson, "Delayed Hominization," 759. For a critique of Johnson's understanding of totipotency, see Shannon, "Delayed Hominization: A Response to Mark Johnson," 731-34.

39. Moraczewski, "Personhood: Entry and Exit," 88-94. See also Ashley and Moraczewski, "Is the Biological Subject of Human Rights Present from Conception?" 39-41.

tion of an overarching plan that ordinarily leads to the development of a single organism. Since twinning is more the exception than the rule, "the formation of identical twins should not be the primary basis for deciding the individuality of the zygote and early embryo."[40] Furthermore, identical twinning does not necessarily mean that a single organism has divided. Albert Moraczewski contends that a plausible explanation for this might be that "there never was a single embryo (or person) in the first place. For reasons, unknown at this time, what was thought to be one zygote after fertilization was actually two."[41]

Even if twinning of a single preimplantation embryo does occur, that does not mean it was not an individualized organism. Benedict Ashley and Kevin O'Rourke argue that "the fact that a group of cells is able after separation to develop independently into a second individuated organism in no way refutes the prior existence of an individuated organism, but confirms it."[42] Whenever identical twinning occurs, it is preceded by the development of a single organism. Thus, "if twinning occurred at the first cleavage, then it was preceded immediately by the single-cell zygote. If it took place at some later point in the development of the blastocyst, then it was preceded by the blastocyst," which was a single organism up until this point.[43] The argument that Ashley and O'Rourke are making is that an individualized organism can give rise to another individualized organism.[44] In responding to Thomas Shannon, Sidney Callahan lends support to this line of argumentation: "If the concept of an individual is defined as an 'entity that cannot be divided or, if it is, it becomes two halves neither of which can survive on its own,' then what about the cloning of adult organisms?"[45] This is an intriguing question because cloning of adult organisms involves transferring the nucleus of a somatic cell from an established individual into an enucleated egg, with the possible result being a new individual genetically identical to the individual from whom the nuclear material was taken in the first place.[46] Is this different from a cell of the preimplantation embryo breaking off from the whole and developing into a genetically identical, though distinct organism? Not really, at least not morally. If the pre-personal position is carried forward consistently across the developmental continuum, then no one could be considered an actual, individualized person because in theory everyone today can be cloned. Hence, we may need to start speaking of persons as "pre-persons."

Finally, the pre-personal position states that the preimplantation embryo should be treated with limited (not absolute) respect and protection, but it does not offer legitimate reasons as to why the pre-personal preimplantation embryo should be given any respect and protection.[47] For instance, Richard McCormick insists that the preimplantation embryo should be "treated as a person — that this 'should' is a *prima facie* obligation only, albeit a strong one."[48] Yet, if the preimplantation embryo is not a person, why is it entitled to such profound respect? Why not treat it as other nonpersonal life forms at a similar stage of development? Because, McCormick asserts, the preimplantation embryo is a potential person, even though "its statistical potential for becoming such is greatly reduced."[49] Potential to become a person, however, is not a sufficient basis for conferring a lofty moral status on a being that is not personal. Once the preimplantation embryo is excluded from the inner sanctum of the moral community, it is not clear why it needs to be treated as a person. As John Robertson pointed out in responding to McCormick: "Taking this claim seriously [that the preimplantation embryo is not a person] should permit most of the things that researchers, clinicians, and patients now wish to do with preembryos, including discard, cryopreservation, research, and biopsy."[50] Robertson highlights a major in-

40. Moraczewski, "Personhood: Entry and Exit," 91.

41. Ibid., 89. See also Ashley and O'Rourke, *Ethics of Health Care*, 150.

42. Ashley and O'Rourke, *Health Care Ethics*, 234. See also Ashley and Moraczewski, "Is the Biological Subject of Human Rights Present from Conception?" 50; and Moraczewski, "Personhood: Entry and Exit," 92-93. In discussing the precise time whereby one becomes a person, Jonathan Glover (a noted opponent of the personal position) reinforces this argument. Glover contends that those who claim the preimplantation embryo is not individualized because of the possibility of twinning do not really discredit the view that personhood begins at the completion of fertilization. As Glover remarks: "All the supporters of that view [that personhood begins after fertilization is completed] need do is word their claim carefully: they must say that conception is the point at which at least one person emerges." *Causing Death and Saving Lives* (New York: Penguin Books, 1977), 123.

43. Ashley and O'Rourke, *Health Care Ethics*, 234.

44. We see this all the time in other life forms. For example, a leaf may be taken from a plant and put into another pot so that it may grow and develop. If this leaf does eventually form into a plant, does that mean that the original plant was only a "pre-plant"? Of course not. It means that an individual plant gave rise to another individual plant.

45. Sidney Callahan, "To the Editors: Unique from the Start," *Commonweal* 126 (15 January 1999): 4. For a review of Thomas A. Shannon's response to Callahan, see "To the Editors: The Author Replies," *Commonweal* 126 (15 January 1999): 4, 28.

46. For a discussion of the techniques used in cloning and the ethics of human cloning, see Report and Recommendations of the National Bioethics Advisory Commission, *Cloning Human Beings*, vols. 1-2 (Rockville, Md.: National Bioethics Advisory Commission, 1997).

47. Lisa Sowle Cahill argues that this is a significant pitfall for any position that draws a biological line between personal status and nonpersonal status in "The Embryo and the Fetus: New Moral Contexts," *Theological Studies* 54 (March 1993): 124-42, at 131.

48. McCormick, "Who or What Is the Preembryo?" in *Corrective Vision*, 187. McCormick also makes this point in another article where he states that the prima facie duty to treat the preimplantation embryo as a person is a strong one, "so those who claim exceptions bear the burden of proof" ("The First 14 Days," 302-3).

49. McCormick, "Who or What Is the Preembryo?" 187.

50. John A. Robertson, "What We May Do With Preembryos: A

consistency in the pre-personal position that shows its lack of precision in formulating an adequate response to the personal position. At the least, the pre-personal position should have the tenacity to state its viewpoint (the preimplantation embryo is pre-personal) and carry it through to its logical conclusion (the preimplantation embryo is not entitled to any respect and protection because it is not yet a person).

The Preimplantation Embryo as Nonpersonal

The nonpersonal position on the moral status of the preimplantation embryo claims that the personal position adopts an unsustainable notion of when personhood begins. The nonpersonal position rejects the claim that a personal presence is discernible at the completion of fertilization. Though the nonpersonal position admits that a *human life* comes into existence when a female gamete or oocyte unites with a male gamete or spermatozoon, it does not accept that a *human person* comes into existence at this time. This is because there are two distinct senses of being human. One sense is strictly biological in that it refers to an entity who is a living member of the species *Homo sapiens,* whereas the other sense is strictly personal in that it refers to an entity who now enjoys certain qualities characteristic of human persons.[51] These two distinct senses of what it means to be human are related, but they are not morally equivalent. Peter Singer explains this point:

> These two senses of "human being" overlap but do not coincide. The embryo, the later fetus, the profoundly intellectually disabled child, even the newborn infant — all are indisputably members of the species *Homo sapiens,* but none are self-aware, have a sense of the future, or the capacity to relate to others.[52]

When deciding what respect and protection is due to human beings, the nonpersonal position contends that the main focus should not be on one's membership in the human species, but on one's capacity to take part immediately in the personal dimensions of human life. The demands that human beings place on others, particularly the demands around respecting and protecting life, are contingent upon their being human persons. Tristram Engelhardt describes this well: "That an entity belongs to a particular species is not important in general secular moral terms unless that membership results in that entity's being *in fact* a competent moral agent."[53] It is because members of the species *Homo sapiens* usually possess personal characteristics that being human is morally significant.[54]

The nonpersonal position maintains that to be a full member of the moral community one must be rational, self-conscious, and autonomous.[55] Given the fact that certain human beings lack these personal attributes, it makes no sense to speak of them as beings who have an interest in continued existence because they have no concept of themselves.[56] The preimplantation embryo, the embryo, the fetus, the infant, and the profoundly demented are all examples of human beings who have no understanding of what it means to exist and never have expressed or never will express their desires for continued existence. While all of these beings are members of the human species, they are not persons whose pursuit of life can be thwarted in any real moral sense.[57]

Response to Richard A. McCormick," *Kennedy Institute of Ethics Journal* 1 (1991): 293-302, at 301.

51. Kuhse and Singer, "The Moral Status of the Embryo," 60. A similar distinction has also been made by other authors who support the nonpersonal position on the moral status of the preimplantation embryo. For instance, Tristram Engelhardt distinguishes between human biological life and human personal life. Engelhardt claims that "not all instances of human biological life are instances of human personal life. Brain-dead (but otherwise alive) human beings, human gametes, cells in human cell cultures, all count as instances of human biological life. Further, not only are some humans not persons, there is no reason to hold that all persons are humans, as the possibility of extraterrestrial self-conscious life suggests." "Medicine and the Concept of Person," in *Ethical Issues in Death and Dying,* 273. For a further discussion of this distinction, see Singer, *Practical Ethics,* 85-87 and 150; Tooley, *Abortion and Infanticide,* 50-61; and Mary Ann Warren, "On the Moral and Legal Status of Abortion," in *Today's Moral Problems,* 2nd ed., Richard A. Wasserstrom, ed. (New York: Macmillan, 1979), 35-51, at 43-44.

52. Singer, *Practical Ethics,* 86.

53. Engelhardt, *The Foundations of Bioethics,* 138. Emphasis added.

54. Ibid.

55. This definition of personhood is advanced by both Engelhardt (*The Foundations of Bioethics,* 135-40) and Singer (*Practical Ethics,* 86-87). This more functional notion of what it means to be a human person has clear philosophical precedents. For example, John Locke defines "person" as an "intelligent being, that has reason and reflection, and can consider itself as itself, the same thinking thing, in different times and places; which it does only by that consciousness, which is inseparable from thinking, and, as it seems to me, essential to it: it being impossible for any one to perceive without *perceiving* that he does not perceive." John Locke, *An Essay Concerning Human Understanding* (New York: Dover Publications, 1959), Bk. 2, chap. 27, 448-49.

56. For a contemporary discussion of the moral significance of an individual's concept of self, see Singer, *Practical Ethics,* 96-99; Tooley, "Abortion and Infanticide," *Philosophy and Public Affairs* 2 (Fall 1972): 37-65; and Tooley, "A Defense of Abortion and Infanticide," in *The Problem of Abortion,* 51-91.

57. It should be noted that Engelhardt does not hold to the functional definition of personhood in all cases and apply it across the developmental continuum as do Singer and Tooley. Rather, he develops a twofold concept of personhood that distinguishes between persons in the *strict sense* and persons in the *social sense.* "Some Persons Are Humans," 190-91; and *The Foundations of Bioethics,* 149-51. According to Engelhardt, a person in the strict sense is one who now possesses rationality, self-consciousness, and moral autonomy, whereas a person in the social sense is one who plays a social role but who is not yet (infants and young children), never will be (profoundly demented from birth), or once was but will not again be (permanently comatose) in possession of these distinctive qualities of persons strictly speaking. Engelhardt creates this dual notion of personhood principally so that he does

Singer succinctly captures this point: "It is, other things being equal, a much more serious matter to take the life of a self-conscious being than to take the life of a being without any self-awareness. This is because self-conscious beings have desires for the future that are cut off when they are killed."[58] Since the preimplantation embryo is a human being devoid of the qualities distinctive of human persons, the nonpersonal position holds that it is not entitled to any respect and protection. The preimplantation embryo is not valuable simply because it is a member of the human species. Value may be attributed or imputed to the preimplantation embryo by actual human persons, but it need not be inasmuch as the preimplantation embryo lacks the personal characteristics necessary for making claims to consideration.[59] However, once the developing organism attains some degree of sentience, certain restrictions should apply that limit the extent of research that may cause it pain. The point at which a human organism develops the capacity to feel pain cannot possibly be earlier than six weeks, and even this is a conservative estimate. Therefore, until this point is reached, "the embryo does not have any interests and, like other nonsentient organisms (a human egg, for example), cannot be harmed — in a morally relevant sense — by anything we do."[60]

Thus, the nonpersonal position on the moral status of the preimplantation embryo is based on three essential claims. First, being a member of the human species is not morally equivalent to being a human person. Second, membership in the human species does not secure one's claims to consideration, especially claims to life. Only those beings who are rational, self-conscious, and autonomous have an interest in their continued existence and should be respected and protected. Finally, sentience is morally relevant in that it suggests that a human organism capable of experiencing pain should be treated as "if its pain mattered just as much [as] — or was morally equivalent to — the pain of any other human."[61] Since the preimplantation embryo does not possess the capacity to feel pain, it does not deserve a special moral status that makes it wrong to exploit or destroy it.[62]

Critical Evaluation of Nonpersonalism

The nonpersonal position rejects the view that personal life comes into existence at the completion of fertilization and is to be absolutely respected and protected in its inherent dignity. The nonpersonal position's fundamental critique of the personal position is that it attributes personal moral status to an entity (the preimplantation embryo) that cannot possibly be a person because it does not now enjoy certain qualities characteristic of human persons. Though the nonpersonal position raises serious questions as to the plausibility of the personal position, it ultimately fails in its attempt to undo the personal position for three principal reasons.

First, the nonpersonal position adopts an excessively restrictive view of personhood. Surely, human persons are more than just rational, self-conscious, and autonomous beings.[63] The mystery that we call "person" cannot be summed up in these few characteristics. There is much more to the human person than the nonpersonal position admits. Yet, "What is this 'much more'?" or more precisely, "What does it mean to be a human person?" This is a difficult question to answer because of the complexity of defining personhood.[64] "The human person is one of those common realities which like time — as St. Augustine so aptly noted — everyone knows what it is until asked to define it."[65] Nevertheless, it seems at the most basic level human persons are physical and material, relational and social, creative and spiritual, and morally free and responsible.[66]

not have to accept infanticide as a common practice as do Singer and Tooley. "The Ontology of Abortion," 230; and "Medicine and the Concept of Person," in *Ethical Issues in Death and Dying,* 276. Despite their not being persons in the strict sense, Engelhardt views these beings (listed above) in the social sense who fulfill a social role by being useful to others as objects of pleasure, happiness, and affection. These beings, moreover, are useful and valuable to society in that they represent an illustrative paradigm for the broader social commitments to persons in the strict sense. As Engelhardt remarks: "The social sense of person is a way of treating certain instances of human life in order to secure the life of persons strictly." "Medicine and the Concept of Person," in *Ethical Issues in Death and Dying,* 278.

58. Peter Singer, "Correspondence: *In Vitro* Fertilisation and Moral Equivalence," *Journal of Medical Ethics* 10 (June 1984): 101.

59. Engelhardt, *The Foundations of Bioethics,* 143-44.

60. Kuhse and Singer, "Individuals, Humans and Persons," 73.

61. Singer, "Correspondence: *In Vitro* Fertilisation and Moral Equivalence," 101.

62. Kuhse and Singer, "The Moral Status of the Embryo," 63. While a nonpersonal, sentient being may be entitled to relatively painless treatment, this does not mean, according to the nonpersonal position, that such a being has a claim to life (Singer, "Correspondence: *In Vitro* Fertilisation and Moral Equivalence," 101).

63. Stephen Schwarz persuasively argues against the one-sided or restrictive view of the person as presented by the nonpersonal position in *The Moral Question of Abortion,* 86-112.

64. Ruth Macklin contends that it is fundamentally a futile endeavor to come to a consistent use of the meaning of personhood for bioethics in "Personhood in the Bioethics Literature," *Milbank Memorial Fund Quarterly: Health and Society* 61 (Winter 1983): 35-57. I would agree that it is difficult to define what it means to be a person, but it is nonetheless necessary and possible to make some basic claims about the human person and human life that can guide ethical discussion.

65. Moraczewski, "Personhood: Entry and Exit," 79.

66. These fundamental dimensions of the human person have been discussed in much the same language by a number of authors. See, for instance, Benedict M. Ashley, "Contemporary Understanding of Personhood," in *The Twenty-Fifth Anniversary of Vatican II,* 35-48; Ashley and O'Rourke, *Ethics of Health Care,* 1-12; Ashley and O'Rourke, *Health Care Ethics,* 3-21; Conrad G. Brunk, "In the Image of God," in *Medical Ethics, Human Choices: A Christian Perspective,* John Rogers, ed. (Scottsdale, Penn.: Herald Press, 1988), 29-40; Patrick Derr, "The Historical Development of the Various

Physical and Material Human persons are physical beings who are immersed in the material world.[67] To be a human person means to have a body that exists in a particular time, place, and culture. The pursuit of life's goals and purposes, understood as the material, moral, and spiritual values that transcend physical life, is dependent upon this body as it exists in history.[68] This means in the first place that our bodies are integral aspects of our humanity. We cannot do anything distinctively human without our bodies. We cannot communicate, relate, socialize, love, play, pray, create, or think without first existing physically in the material world. It is in and through our bodies that we express ourselves as human persons. The body is not separate from the human person, but is an indispensable feature of personhood.[69]

Relational and Social Human persons are relational and social beings who are fundamentally directed toward others.[70] To be a human person means to live, grow, and develop within the context of familial and social relationships. Human persons are brought into existence and are continually sustained by way of these relationships.[71] The human relationships that we experience throughout life are essential to our physical survival as well as to our moral and psychological development.[72] The Second Vatican Council makes very much the same point in discussing the dignity of the human person: "For by his innermost nature man is a social being, and unless he relates himself to others he can neither live nor develop his potential."[73]

Creative and Spiritual Human persons are creative and spiritual beings who have the capacity to reason and transcend the material world.[74] To be a human person means to be able to know, to understand, to contemplate, to create, and to move beyond immediate experience. This fundamental dimension of humanity sets human persons apart from other life forms.

The creative and spiritual capacities that human persons possess allow them to connect with themselves and others in more than just physical ways. Through these deeper connections we realize, even if imperfectly, that we are dynamic beings who are open to possibilities beyond ourselves. We also recognize, however, that we are limited beings who can always love more, experience more, and live more.[75] The creative and spiritual capacities of human life also enable us to enter into intimate relationship with the divine. God's self-communication as mediated through human and nonhuman creation is most vividly perceived at this level of human existence.[76]

Morally Free and Responsible Human persons are morally free and responsible beings who must make

---

Concepts of Personhood," in *The Twenty-Fifth Anniversary of Vatican II,* 17-34; Richard M. Gula, *Reason Informed by Faith: Foundations of Catholic Morality* (New York: Paulist Press, 1989), 66-74; Louis Janssens, "Personalist Morals," *Louvain Studies* 3 (Spring 1970): 5-16; idem, "Artificial Insemination: Ethical Considerations," *Louvain Studies* 8 (Spring 1980): 5-13; Timothy E. O'Connell, *Principles for a Catholic Morality,* rev. ed. (San Francisco: HarperSanFrancisco, 1990), 51-76; Kenneth R. Overberg, *Conscience in Conflict: How to Make Moral Choices* (Cincinnati: St. Anthony Messenger Press, 1991), 20-25; James B. Reichmann, *Philosophy of the Human Person* (Chicago: Loyola University Press, 1985), 207-25; and Vincent E. Rush, *The Responsible Christian: A Popular Guide for Moral Decision Making According to Classical Tradition* (Chicago: Loyola University Press, 1984), 25-73.

67. Gula, *Reason Informed by Faith,* 68-70; Janssens, "Artificial Insemination: Ethical Considerations," 5-8; Overberg, *Conscience in Conflict,* 21-22; and Rush, *The Responsible Christian,* 26-29.

68. James Walter provides an excellent reflection on the value and importance of physical life for pursuing life's goals and purposes in "The Meaning and Validity of Quality of Life Judgments in Contemporary Roman Catholic Medical Ethics," in *Quality of Life: The New Medical Dilemma,* James J. Walter and Thomas A. Shannon, eds. (New York: Paulist Press, 1990), 78-88.

69. Congregation for the Doctrine of the Faith, "Instruction on Respect for Human Life in its Origin and on the Dignity of Procreation," in *Religion and Artificial Reproduction,* 144.

70. Brunk, "In the Image of God," 32; Gula, *Reason Informed by Faith,* 67-68; Janssens, "Artificial Insemination: Ethical Considerations," 8-9; Overberg, *Conscience in Conflict,* 23-24; and Reichmann, *Philosophy of the Human Person,* 218-19. In discussing the nature of friendship and happiness, Aristotle also addresses the relational and social dimension of the human person: "No one would choose to have all good things by himself, for man is a social and political being and his natural condition is to live with others." *Nicomachean Ethics,* trans. Martin Ostwald (Englewood Cliffs, N.J.: Prentice Hall, 1962), Bk. 9, chap. 9, 264.

71. Gula makes this point well in claiming: "Human existence does not precede relationship, but is born of relationship and nurtured by it." *Reason Informed by Faith,* 67.

72. Reichmann, *Philosophy of the Human Person,* 219. Rush explores the importance of the physical environment and human relationships for moral and psychological development in *The Responsible Christian,* 32-62.

73. Second Vatican Council, *Gaudium et Spes,* n. 12, in *Proclaiming Justice and Peace: Papal Documents from* Rerum Novarum *to* Centesimus Annus, rev. and exp., Michael Walsh and Brian Davies, eds. (Mystic, Conn.: Twenty-Third Publications, 1994), 167.

74. Ashley and O'Rourke, *Health Care Ethics,* 18; Brunk, "In the Image of God," 31-32; Overberg, *Conscience in Conflict,* 23; and Karl Rahner, *Foundations of Christian Faith: An Introduction to the Idea of Christianity,* trans. William V. Dych (New York: Crossroad, 1994), 31-35. The concept of the human person as a transcendental being is thoroughly developed in another of Rahner's seminal works, namely: *Spirit in the World,* trans. William Dych (New York: Crossroad, 1994).

75. Rahner talks about the human experience of transcendence against the backdrop of limits or human finiteness in *Foundations of Christian Faith,* 31-35, especially 32.

76. For a discussion of God's self-communication through signs and symbols, see Louis-Marie Chauvet, *Symbol and Sacrament: A Sacramental Reinterpretation of Christian Existence,* trans. Patrick Madigan and Madeleine Beaumont (Collegeville, Minn.: Liturgical Press, 1995); Michael G. Lawler, *Symbol and Sacrament: A Contemporary Sacramental Theology* (Omaha, Nebraska: Creighton University Press, 1995); and Edward Schillebeeckx, *Christ the Sacrament of the Encounter with God* (Kansas City: Sheed and Ward, 1963).

moral choices in concrete situations and own those choices as an expression of who they are and want to become in relation to their life's vision.[77] To be a human person means to have *some degree* of self-determination empowered by one's moral conscience in freedom and with knowledge.[78] Yet, the mere fact that we are finite beings limited by our temporal existence implies that we can never act with complete freedom and knowledge. Nevertheless, we are fundamentally free persons at the core of our beings.[79] While our choices may be limited in concrete situations, we are essentially free to choose who we want to become. In his testimony to human freedom and dignity, even amid great hardships, Viktor Frankl provides moving evidence for the fundamental freedom of the human person.

> We who lived in concentration camps can remember the men who walked through the huts comforting others, giving away their last piece of bread. They may have been few in number, but they offer sufficient proof that everything can be taken away from a man but one thing: the last of the human freedoms — to choose one's attitude in any given set of circumstances, to choose one's own way.[80]

In summary, to be a human person means to be physical and material, relational and social, creative and spiritual, and morally free and responsible. While these dimensions of personal life have been considered separately, that does not imply that they are distinct and separate in the human person. Rather, they are interconnected and interwoven to form a complex synthesis that constitutes the human person adequately considered.[81]

The nonpersonal position would have us believe that only those beings who are participating significantly in the creative and moral dimensions count as persons. However, this is too narrow a notion of personhood. If the meaning of personhood is understood more broadly, it is not difficult to discern that personal life begins with the completion of fertilization. At this time, a human person comes into existence who has a material body (physical dimension), and who is growing and developing within the context of an intimate biological relationship with the mother (relational dimension). In time, provided that serious complications do not arise in the developmental process, this human person will actualize the capacities that are already present (though latent) to think and reflect upon itself (creative dimension) and exercise its autonomy as a moral agent (moral dimension).[82]

Second, the nonpersonal position fails to recognize that the nature of a living being is established from the first moment of its existence and unfolds throughout its lifetime. Just because a living being may not appear the same in its more mature form does not mean that it is not the same being who existed from the very beginning. Albert Moraczewski explains this point:

> It should not be overlooked that the most basic and revealing act of what a living thing is, is precisely what it

77. Brunk, "In the Image of God," 31; Gula, *Reason Informed by Faith,* 68-69; Janssens, "Artificial Insemination: Ethical Considerations," 5; O'Connell, *Principles for a Catholic Morality,* 70-72; Overberg, *Conscience in Conflict,* 24-25; Rahner, *Foundations of Christian Faith,* 35-39; and Reichmann, *Philosophy of the Human Person,* 212 and 222-23.

78. Gula, *Reason Informed by Faith,* 68 and 75-88. For a discussion of the theology of the moral conscience, see ibid., 123-62; Richard M. Gula, *Moral Discernment* (New York: Paulist Press, 1997), 11-40; O'Connell, *Principles for a Catholic Morality,* 103-18; and Robert J. Smith, *Conscience and Catholicism: The Nature and Function of Conscience in Contemporary Roman Catholic Moral Theology* (Lanham, Md.: University Press of America, 1998). For a slightly different viewpoint on the moral conscience, see Germain Grisez, with the help of Joseph M. Boyle, Basil Cole, John M. Finnis et al., *The Way of the Lord Jesus,* Vol. 1: *Christian Moral Principles* (Chicago: Franciscan Herald Press, 1983), 73-96.

79. Rahner makes this point in talking about true freedom: "When freedom is really understood, it is not the power to be able to do this or that, but the power to decide about oneself and to actualize oneself. . . . So even when a person would abandon himself into the hands of the empirical anthropologies, he still remains in his own hands. He does not escape from his freedom, and the only question can be how he interprets himself, and freely interprets himself." *Foundations of Christian Faith,* 38-39. Here Rahner is referring to the classical distinction between *liberum arbitrium* (freedom of choice) and *libertas* (freedom to choose God or to create oneself). Interestingly, Rahner parts ways with Saint Augustine, who taught that because of original sin human persons no longer retain *libertas* but only *liberum arbitrium.* For a comparison of Rahner's and Saint Augustine's theological anthropologies, see Stephen J. Duffy, *The Dynamics of Grace: Perspectives in Theological Anthropology* (Collegeville, Minn.: Liturgical Press, 1993); and Roger Haight, *The Experience and Language of Grace* (New York: Paulist Press, 1979).

80. Viktor Frankl, *Man's Search for Meaning,* rev. ed., trans. Ilse Lasch (New York: Simon and Schuster, 1962), 65.

81. Several authors make the claim that the dimensions of the human person must be understood holistically because none of them can be separated from the human person adequately considered. See, for instance, Ashley and O'Rourke, *Health Care Ethics,* 1920; Brunk, "In the Image of God," 33; Gula, *Reason Informed by Faith,* 67; and Janssens, "Artificial Insemination: Ethical Considerations," 4.

82. Ashley and O'Rourke make a similar point in refuting the claim that cerebration marks the beginning of personhood. "Thus, although it is true that the developing fetus first actively exhibits vegetative (physiological) and animal human functions, it possesses from conception the active potentiality to develop all these functional abilities. Only the minimal structure necessary for this active potentiality of self-development (even on the basis of Aristotle's philosophical principles) is required for an organism to be actually a human person, not the brain structures for adult psychological activities." *Health Care Ethics,* 236. The minimal structure necessary for functioning like an adult person can be traced back to the zygote's nucleus, which contains all the "information and active potentiality necessary eventually to develop the brain and bring it to the stage of adult functioning." *Health Care Ethics,* 236. David Wiggins also makes a similar point in outlining his animal attribute view of persons. Wiggins claims that a person is any animal that is part of a species or of a kind that has the *biological capacity* to participate fully in the psychological attributes of persons in more developed stages. *Sameness and Substance* (Cambridge, Mass.: Harvard University Press, 1980), 149-89.

will become in its mature stage. A caterpillar does not fully reveal its nature until it becomes a butterfly or moth. A caterpillar is one developmental stage (larva) of the same creature that later manifests itself as a butterfly or moth. Among living beings the earlier stages of development may, in outward appearance, be very different from the mature stage. Yet it is one and the same individual who has traversed various stages to reach maturity.[83]

Speaking strictly of human persons, a developmental continuum exists between the single-celled zygote, the preimplantation embryo, the embryo, the fetus, the infant, the child, the adolescent, and the adult. There is no clear biological marker that suggests a morally significant dividing line between the nature of a human person in its earlier stages and the nature of a human person in its later stages. The only difference (morally insignificant) is that a human person in its mature form may begin to realize some of the innate capacities of its human nature and may start functioning in more complex ways. This does not, however, mark a radical change in the human person. Stephen Schwarz supports this claim:

> The fact that my capabilities to function as a person have changed and grown does not alter the absolute continuity of my essential being, that of a person. In fact, this variation in capabilities presupposes the continuity of my being as a person. It is *as a person* that I develop my capabilities to function as a person. It is because I am a person that I have these capabilities, to whatever degree.[84]

The marked transformation that the nonpersonal position claims a human being undergoes at some unspecified point in its lifetime seems more consistent with a misguided concept of personhood than with the reality of human experience.

Finally, the definition of personhood that grounds the nonpersonal position is not only excessively restrictive, but also arbitrary. Who says that rationality, self-consciousness, and autonomy are the central properties necessary for being a person? Certainly a broad consensus has not been reached on this matter or else issues such as the one under consideration or abortion would not be so prominent. This indicates that it is an inherently slippery endeavor to define precisely those qualities that constitute full personhood.[85] Formulating any such list is always going to be conditioned by the philosophical commitments one brings to the table and thus is always limited in its applicability. Even if it were determined by a representative body which properties factor into being a human person, the nonpersonal position would still need to resolve two other difficult questions, namely: "To what extent do these qualities need to be developed in a human being for that being to be considered a person?" and "How will these properties or their degree of development be measured?"[86] It should also not go unsaid that by accepting such a narrow and arbitrary definition of personhood, the nonpersonal position tends toward exclusionary practices whereby some members of the human community who do not meet the criteria of personal life are denied the normal standards of moral treatment.[87] As history has repeatedly shown, when most of the important rights due to human beings are predicated on an arbitrary list of what it means to be a human person, some of our most vulnerable fellow human beings are refused the moral respect and protection they deserve.[88]

Conclusion

The question of the moral status of the preimplantation embryo is one of the most controversial ethical and policy issues of the modern day. Previously held views on the value of human life in its earliest beginnings have been called into question, and collectively we have been charged with the responsibility of determining whether the preimplantation embryo is a full member of the moral community. The strongest claims concerning the moral status of the preimplantation embryo have been made by the personal position, which maintains that personal life comes into existence at the completion of fertilization and is to be absolutely respected and protected in its inherent dignity. This position has been challenged on two different fronts. First, the pre-personal position claims that the preimplantation embryo is in a pre-personal stage of development at least until it attains a certain level of biological stability, which coincides with the formation of the primitive streak, and as such is only entitled to limited respect and protection. Second, the nonpersonal position claims that the preimplantation embryo is a nonperson and as such is not entitled to any respect or protection. Both the pre-personal position and the nonpersonal position raise serious questions as to the plausibility of the view that a personal presence is discernible at the completion of fertilization. However, neither position sufficiently refutes the personal position to the point that it would be justifiable to deny the preimplantation embryo the same degree of respect and protection given other human beings.

83. Moraczewski, "Personhood: Entry and Exit," 80.

84. Schwarz, *The Moral Question of Abortion,* 93.

85. Richard McCormick makes a similar claim: "Anyone who would attempt an even tentative personhood inventory is trying to catch, bottle, and display what most men have regarded as ultimately a mystery." *Notes on Moral Theology 1965 through 1980* (Washington, D.C.: University Press of America, 1981), 445.

86. Schwarz, *The Moral Question of Abortion,* 107.

87. Schwarz discusses how the nonpersonal position tends toward discrimination by drawing a fine line between persons and nonpersons. Ibid., 103-105.

88. Reichmann, *Philosophy of the Human Person,* 213. For a discussion of the exclusionary use of personhood, see William Aiken, "The Quality of Life," in *Quality of Life,* 17-25; and Derr, "The Historical Development of the Various Concepts of Personhood," 27-33.

The pre-personal position's fundamental critique of the personal position is that as long as the cells of the preimplantation embryo remain in a totipotent state, the preimplantation embryo is susceptible to division through natural twinning or artificial separation in vitro and thus cannot be understood to be a single individual. One of the problems with this assessment is that it drastically overstates the nature of totipotency, and by association, twinning and individuality. The totipotential capacity that resides within the cells of the preimplantation embryo is rarely actualized for the purposes of developing a separate organism. Identical twinning occurs naturally in approximately one out of 320 births.[89] Since twinning is such a rare phenomenon, it does not provide an adequate basis for deciding the individuality of the preimplantation embryo.[90] Furthermore, twinning does not necessarily mean that the identity of the initial organism is discontinuous. The prospects of cloning adult organisms proves this insofar as a somatic cell from an individualized entity can give rise to another individualized entity with the same genetic composition (the equivalent of twinning). If the pre-personal position was accepted, then we would have to conclude that the adult organism from whom the nuclear material was taken in the first place is not the same individual with the same identity. Surely, this is absurd.

The nonpersonal position's fundamental critique of the personal position is that it attributes personal moral status to an entity (the preimplantation embryo) that cannot possibly be a person because it does not now enjoy certain qualities characteristic of human persons. One of the problems with this assessment is that it narrowly interprets what it means to be a person. The complex and dynamic nature of the human person cannot possibly be limited to a few characteristics such as rationality, self-consciousness, and autonomy. While these qualities must be included in any notion of personhood, they do not constitute the human person adequately considered. At the most basic level, human persons are physical and material, relational and social, creative and spiritual, and morally free and responsible. If the meaning of personhood is understood more broadly, it is not difficult to discern that personal life begins with the completion of fertilization. At this time, a human person comes into existence who is already participating in the physical and relational dimensions of personal life, and who will in time, provided that serious complications do not arise in the developmental process, take part in the creative and moral dimensions of personal life.

While it is *understandable* that some would want to restrict the moral status of the preimplantation embryo to advance human knowledge in the areas of in vitro fertilization and embryo research, it is not *acceptable* to do this in light of the fact that the preimplantation embryo has already embarked on the journey of personal life. The preimplantation embryo is a full member of the moral community and should be treated the same way as other persons in more mature forms. Nothing truly good can come from our attempt to limit the respect and protection due to this defenseless fellow human person. As individuals and as a society, we would be much better off if we just embraced human life in its earliest beginnings and gave up the quest to determine how much value human life has in its more undeveloped stages. Paul Ramsey poignantly expresses this same thought. Though Ramsey speaks of the fetus, his comments apply equally to the preimplantation embryo.

> What life is in and of itself is most clearly to be seen in situations of naked equality of one life with another, and in the situation of congeneric helplessness which is the human condition in the first of life. No one is ever much more than a fellow fetus, and in order not to become confused about life's primary value, it is best not to concentrate on degrees of relative worth we may later acquire.[91]

89. Moraczewski, "Personhood: Entry and Exit," 91.

90. Ibid.

Appendix: Development of the Preimplantation Embryo

Human development begins at fertilization whereby a female gamete or oocyte unites with a male gamete or spermatozoon to form a single-celled zygote. The zygote is a highly specialized, totipotent cell that contains chromosomes and genes from both the mother and father.[92] Once the process of fertilization is completed, the single-celled zygote undergoes a series of divisions and becomes transformed gradually into a dynamic, multicellular organism through cell division, migration, implantation, growth, and differentiation.[93] This complex process of development will be described below.

Fertilization

Every monthly ovarian cycle a secondary oocyte gets expelled from the ovary into the ampulla of the uterine tube. The ampullar region is the longest and widest part of the uterine tube and is the place where fertilization occurs most frequently. Fertilization may take place in other parts of the uterine tube but not in the uterus.[94]

91. Paul Ramsey, "The Morality of Abortion," in *Moral Problems,* James Rachels, ed. (New York: Harper and Row, 1971), 1-27, at 12.

92. In the biological sense, totipotency refers to the cell's ability "to differentiate into any type of cell and thus form a new organism or regenerate any part of an organism." *Stedman's Medical Dictionary,* 26th ed. (1995), s.v. "totipotency."

93. For a description of these developmental processes, see Scott F. Gilbert, *Developmental Biology,* 5th ed. (Sunderland, Mass.: Sinauer, 1997), 121-252.

94. Keith L. Moore and T. V. N. Persaud, *Before We Are Born: Essentials of Embryology and Birth Defects,* 5th ed. (Philadelphia: W. B. Saunders, 1998), 36.

Once in the ampulla of the uterine tube, the secondary oocyte remains viable for as long as twenty-four hours before it loses its capacity to be fertilized.[95] If fertilization does not occur, the oocyte slowly passes through the tube to the uterus, where it eventually degenerates and gets resorbed.

Spermatozoa that get deposited into the vagina pass relatively quickly through the cervix and uterus and into the uterine tube. This ascent through the female reproductive tract by spermatozoa is made possible through the contractions of the musculature of the uterus and the uterine tube.[96] Of the two hundred to three hundred million spermatozoa that get deposited into the vagina by a single ejaculation, approximately three hundred to five hundred make their way to the ampullar region of the uterine tube.[97] Only one of these spermatozoa is needed for fertilization. Once inside the female reproductive tract, spermatozoa retain their capacity to fertilize an oocyte for approximately one to three days.[98]

Fertilization of a secondary oocyte by a spermatozoon occurs in five phases. First, the spermatozoon passes through the outermost layer of the oocyte (corona radiata). Second, the spermatozoon penetrates the glycoprotein shell encompassing the oocyte (zona pellucida). As the head or cap-like structure (acrosome) of the spermatozoon comes into contact with the zona pellucida, it releases certain enzymes that cause the zona pellucida to loosen (lysis), thus enabling the spermatozoon to create a pathway to the oocyte. Third, the head and tail of the spermatozoon enter the cytoplasm of the secondary oocyte, while its plasma membrane is left on the oocyte surface. Immediately after the spermatozoon enters the oocyte, the fertilized egg responds in three important ways, namely: (1) the oocyte membrane becomes impenetrable to other spermatozoa; (2) the zona pellucida changes its composition (zona reaction), precluding the oocyte from being fertilized by more than one spermatozoon (polyspermy); and (3) the oocyte completes the second meiotic division and forms a mature oocyte and a second polar body. Fourth, the nucleus of the mature oocyte becomes the female pronucleus, and the nucleus of the sperm enlarges within the cytoplasm of the oocyte to form the male pronucleus. Both female and male pronuclei have twenty-three chromosomes (haploid) and must replicate their DNA so that each cell of the two-cell stage preimplantation embryo has the normal amount of DNA.[99] Finally, the membranes of the pronuclei break down, the maternal and paternal chromosomes condense and prepare for the mitotic cell division, and a single-celled zygote forms with forty-six chromosomes (diploid).[100]

The complex process of fertilization concludes in twenty-four hours.[101] Fertilization has three main results, namely: (1) creation of a genetically unique human organism, with half the chromosomal complement coming from the mother and the other half from the father; (2) determination of the sex of the human organism, with an X-bearing sperm giving rise to a female and a Y-bearing sperm giving rise to a male; and (3) metabolic activation of the mature oocyte that leads to the initiation of cell division of the zygote (cleavage).[102]

Cleavage

Approximately thirty hours after the completion of fertilization, the single-celled zygote undergoes the first of a series of mitotic divisions, resulting in two smaller daughter cells (blastomeres). With each successive division, the blastomeres become more numerous and progressively smaller as the preimplantation embryo as a whole does not change in size until the surrounding zona pellucida degenerates. By the eight-cell stage, the originally round and loosely adherent blastomeres begin to change shape and tightly align themselves one with the other (compaction).[103] The modification and reorganization that the blastomeres experience via compaction permits greater interaction between the cells and is a prerequisite for the segregation of the inner cells from the outer cells.[104] By the third day, the compacted cells of the preimplantation embryo divide again to form the sixteen-cell morula. At this point, the cells of the morula begin to differentiate, with some moving to the center to form the inner cell mass and others moving to the pe-

95. William J. Larsen, *Human Embryology,* 2nd ed. (New York: Churchill Livingstone, 1997), 16; and T. W. Sadler, *Langman's Medical Embryology,* 7th ed. (Baltimore: Williams and Wilkins, 1995), 29.

96. Sadler, *Langman's Medical Embryology,* 29.

97. Ibid., 29.

98. Larsen, *Human Embryology,* 11. Before a spermatozoon can fertilize an oocyte, it must undergo "a capacitation process, during which a glycoprotein coat and seminal plasma proteins are removed from the spermatozoon head, and the acrosome reaction, during which hyaluronidase and trypsin-like substances are released to penetrate oocyte barriers" (Sadler, *Langman's Medical Embryology,* 39).

99. Moore and Persaud, *Before We Are Born,* 36; and Sadler, *Langman's Medical Embryology,* 31.

100. The various phases of fertilization are treated much the same by Moore and Persaud, *Before We Are Born,* 36-41; Larsen, *Human Embryology,* 11-19; and Sadler, *Langman's Medical Embryology,* 29-33.

101. Moore and Persaud, *Before We Are Born,* 39.

102. Ibid., 39; Sadler, *Langman's Medical Embryology,* 31.

103. Gilbert, *Developmental Biology,* 90; Larsen, *Human Embryology,* 19; Moore and Persaud, *Before We Are Born,* 41; and Sadler, *Langman's Medical Embryology,* 33. This is an important scientific observation because one of the main arguments against the view that a personal presence is discernible at the completion of fertilization is that the blastomeres are loosely held together until implantation and could at any time break off and develop into a unique organism apart from the initial organism (totipotency). While this is theoretically true (as seen in natural twinning or artificially induced blastomere separation), current scientific data suggests that from the eight-cell stage onward, the blastomeres are tightly aligned and dedicated to the development of a single organism.

104. Moore and Persaud, *Before We Are Born,* 41.

riphery to form the outer cell mass. The inner cell mass gives rise to the tissues that constitute the embryo proper, while the outer cell mass develops into the trophoblast, which is the thin outer cellular layer that constitutes the embryonic part of the placenta.[105]

Blastocyst Formation

The morula migrates down the uterine tube to the cavity of the uterus by the end of the third day. Shortly after arriving in the uterine cavity, the morula takes on fluid that passes from the uterine cavity through the zona pellucida into intercellular spaces within the inner cell mass. With the proliferation of fluid in the morula, the intercellular spaces become confluent and the blastocyst cavity is formed.[106] By the fourth day, the morula has developed into a blastocyst. The inner cell mass (now called the embryoblast) extends into the blastocyst cavity and the trophoblast makes up the wall of the blastocyst. On the fifth day, the zona pellucida degenerates and ultimately disappears. The ability to float freely in the uterine cavity and receive nourishment from secretions of the uterine glands without being contained within the zona pellucida enables the blastocyst to grow rapidly. By the sixth day, trophoblastic cells adjacent to the embryoblast begin to implant superficially into the epithelial cells of the uterine mucosa.[107]

Implantation

On the seventh day of development, the trophoblast begins to differentiate into two layers — the cytotrophoblast (inner layer of cells) and the syncytiotrophoblast (outer, multinucleated mass formed by cells with no distinguishable cellular boundaries). By the eighth day, the highly invasive syncytiotrophoblast produces certain enzymes that erode the endometrial connective tissue in the area over the embryoblast and thus allow the blastocyst to penetrate deeply into the endometrium. The embryoblast also begins to differentiate into two layers at this time — the hypoblast (inner layer of cuboidal cells adjacent to the blastocyst cavity) and the epiblast (external layer of columnar cells adjacent to the soon-to-be-formed amniotic cavity).[108] At this point, the embryoblast is referred to as the bilaminar embryonic disc. As implantation of the blastocyst progresses, new cavities develop (amniotic cavity, exocoelomic cavity, and chorionic cavity) and trophoblastic lacunae open within the syncytiotrophoblast establishing primitive utero-placental circulation. On about the tenth day,[109] the blastocyst is completely embedded in the endometrium and the hole in the endometrial connective tissue at the implantation site is filled by the closing plug.[110]

Several days following the completion of implantation (approximately day fourteen), a faint groove appears along the surface of the embryonic disc marking the formation of the primitive streak.[111] This groove runs along the midline of the embryonic disc and eventually becomes the central nervous system of the developing organism. The formation of the primitive streak signifies the commencement of gastrulation, which is when the bilaminar embryonic disc converts into the trilaminar embryonic disc from which all of the organs of the human organism will develop.[112] Once gastrulation has initiated with the appearance of the primitive streak, twinning is no longer possible because the developing organism has sufficiently differentiated and the cells of the organism have lost their totipotency.[113]

105. Ibid.; Larsen, *Human Embryology*, 19; and Sadler, *Langman's Medical Embryology*, 33.

106. Sadler, *Langman's Medical Embryology*, 33.

107. Moore and Persaud, *Before We Are Born*, 41; Larsen, *Human Embryology*, 19; and Sadler, *Langman's Medical Embryology*, 33.

108. Moore and Persaud, *Before We Are Born*, 41; Larsen, *Human Embryology*, 35; and Sadler, *Langman's Medical Embryology*, 41.

109. Moore and Persaud, *Before We Are Born*, 50. There are some disputes as to when exactly implantation is completed. Larsen claims that "between days 6 and 9, the embryo becomes completely implanted in the endometrium." *Human Embryology*, 35. Sadler asserts, however, that "by the 11th or 12th day of development, the blastocyst is completely embedded in the endometrial stroma." *Langman's Medical Embryology*, 43. A recent study of 221 women who had no history of fertility problems showed that implantation occurred eight to ten days after ovulation in most healthy pregnancies. See Allen J. Wilcox, Donna Day Baird, and Clarice R. Weinberg, "Time of Implantation of the Conceptus and Loss of Pregnancy," *New England Journal of Medicine* 340 (June 10, 1999): 1796-99.

110. Sadler offers information that some authors who support the pre-personal position regard as morally relevant to the issue of the moral status of the preimplantation embryo: "Even in selected fertile women under optimal conditions for pregnancy, fifteen percent of oocytes fail to become fertilized, and ten to fifteen percent start cleavage but fail to implant. Of the seventy to seventy-five that implant, only fifty-eight percent will survive until the second week, and sixteen percent of those will be abnormal." *Langman's Medical Embryology*, 51. The moral irrelevance of this information has been discussed above.

111. Moore and Persaud, *Before We Are Born*, 62; Larsen, *Human Embryology*, 51; and Sadler, *Langman's Medical Embryology*, 53.

112. Moore and Persaud, *Before We Are Born*, 41; Larsen, *Human Embryology*, 35; and Sadler, *Langman's Medical Embryology*, 62-65.

113. Gilbert, *Developmental Biology*, 58.

49 Again: Who Is a Person?

Oliver O'Donovan

'And he, desiring to justify himself, said to Jesus, "And who is my neighbour?"' Moral theologians have never tired of pointing out that Jesus did not answer the question in the terms in which it was put. The student of the law knew that he had an obligation to care for a certain class of person, called 'neighbours'; accordingly, he asked for criteria by which he would recognize members of this class. Jesus offered him no criteria, but told a story illustrating how someone discharged the obligation of neighbour-love — someone who might quite plausibly have been held to be outside the category, 'neighbour', because he was not a Jew. 'Which of the three, do you think, proved neighbour to the man who fell among the robbers?' 'The one who showed mercy on him.'

There are at least three ways in which the answer of Jesus defeats the hidden presuppositions of the lawyer's question. In the first place, Jesus' answer clearly implied a 'universalist' doctrine of neighbourhood, whereas the lawyer, we must suppose, had in mind some kind of racial restriction. That is the most obvious, and perhaps least dramatic challenge that Jesus makes to his questioner. In the second place, Jesus' story shows *how* we identify our neighbour; from our active engagement with him in caring for him, sympathizing with him, protecting him. There is, in other words, an epistemology implied in the story; at the *end* of this engagement we can say that the neighbourhood of the two men had become apparent. It would never have become clear *whether* a Samaritan and a Jew could be neighbours, if the Samaritan, like the lawyer, had waited for the question to be answered speculatively before he attended to the Jew at the roadside. The truth of neighbourhood is known in engagement; we act in commitment to someone *as* a neighbour, and thus *prove* the neighbourhood. In the third place, this is a story about how a Jew learned who his neighbour was. He learned it, not by serving him, but by being served by him. And this, perhaps, is the most scandalous element in Jesus' story: that a Jew could *need* a Samaritan as his neighbour, that the natural relation (as he saw it) of patron and client could be reversed, and that he would solve the speculative problem about Samaritans as neighbours not even by caring for a Samaritan in need, but by being cared for, in his need, by a Samaritan.

And who, then, is a person?

The term 'person' is clearly intended to be a universal term, in the way that 'neighbour' is. The question has already taken cognizance of the first challenge that Jesus offered to the lawyer. My case is a very simple one: that the question about 'personhood' has to take notice also of the second and third challenges which Jesus made. That is to say: *(a)* that we can recognize someone as a person only from a stance of *prior moral commitment* to treat him or her as a person, since the question of what constitutes a person can never be answered speculatively; and *(b)* that we know someone as a person as that person is disclosed in his or her personal relations to us, that is, as we know ourselves to be not simply the subject of our own attention to the other, but to be the object of the other's attention to us. On the basis of point *(a)* my account of personhood will be called (and deserves to be called) 'existentialist' — and it is no worse for that, but simply recognizes a fundamental truth about human knowledge which could be found in the New Testament long before anyone declared that it was 'existentialist', namely, that certain kinds of knowledge are given to us only within an active commitment of faith and obedience: 'If any man's will is to do his will, he shall know whether the teaching is from God' (John 7:17). On the basis of point *(b)*, however, we can claim to be safe from the solipsistic tendency into which popular existentialism has too often degenerated. We are not saying that personhood is *conferred* upon the object simply by our willingness to treat him or her as a person. Rather the opposite: we *discover* the personhood of the other by his personal dealings with us. We hold, therefore, to an existentialist *anthropology.* What is required of us is a commitment to be open to the other *as another human agent,* to be open to interaction with him in every form. The term 'person', too, must carry with it this implication of the old term 'neighbour', that we find ourselves with somebody 'next to' us, like us, equal to us, acting upon us as we upon him, as much a subject to whom we become object as he is object to our subject. And this presupposes a doctrine of human nature, and an understanding that we who encounter the equal and opposite other are, with him, mankind.

I

In the first place, then, there are no 'criteria of personhood' by which a person could be recognized independently of, or prior to, *personal engagement.* To say this is to say something about humanity: that members of our species are known (at least to one another) *in a way* that members of other animal species are not known. We may recognize a duck abstractly, by simple observation, and distinguish it from a goose. In the same way, of course, we may distinguish a human being from an elephant; but such observational recognition falls short of the kind of knowledge that it is appropriate for one hu-

From Oliver O'Donovan, "Again, Who Is a Person?" in J. H. Channer, ed., *Abortion and the Sanctity of Human Life* (Exeter: The Paternoster Press), pp. 125-37. Used by permission.

man being to have of another. And, notoriously, it does nothing to answer the moral questions about our fellow human beings which are posed for us by medical technology. When we ask whether someone in an irreversible coma is a 'person' or not, it does no good to answer that he is not an elephant. We want to know whether he still is that same human agent, with whom we have engaged as fellow agents in the business of life, and to whom we therefore owe a brotherly loyalty, or whether he is no longer 'he'. And the point I wish to make is that no conceivable set of purely observational criteria can answer that question positively or negatively for us. It might seem that we could answer it negatively, by adducing certain information about his brain activity (which is not what it was when we used to meet him for lunch and discuss politics). It might seem that we could answer it positively, by showing that the vital functions of respiration and heartbeat are as spontaneously active as they used to be when he tasted wine and drew on his pipe. But both answers would miss the point: it was not his brain that we conversed with about the by-elections. It was he, the agent, the person; and although there would be no possibility of such engagement *without* the functioning brain, respiration and heartbeat, what we met and talked with was not simply the sum of those functions, but another category of subject altogether.

We met *him* — I say 'the person', but it is very important not to think that 'the person' is another *kind* of constituent, like 'the brain' or 'the heart', only different. It would be quite wrong, for example, to say that we met 'the mind'. What we met, simply, was 'Michael', the human being as irreducibly individual, irreplaceable, a member of a species, certainly, but not accounted for simply as 'an instance of kind X', but only as *himself.* To all this the word 'person' points. It is, therefore, from a logical point of view, a category mistake to try to demonstrate the presence or absence of a person by proving that this or that biological or neurological function is present or absent. It is a category mistake to say that a new conceptus cannot be a person until there is brain activity; it is a category mistake to say that it must be a person because there is an individual genetic structure. (I shall be defending a different use of this genetic evidence in a minute; for the moment I merely remark on the impropriety of this use.) For, whatever criteria we take, we end up by reducing the notion of personhood to that one constituent of human functioning.

It has seemed to some that they could evade the implications of this categorical difference by treating personhood as an epiphenomenon supervening upon the presence of biological and neurological functions, and so depending upon them without, nevertheless, being reducible to them. But our thought cannot grasp 'the person', in his unique particularity, by thinking along this route. The most that it can reach is a group of second-order capacities, different in kind from the biological or neurological functions, but no less genetic than they are. It can reach what we call 'personality', which is the cluster of behavioural and relational attributes which characteristically belong to human beings as a kind. It is a common misunderstanding of talk about persons to think that it is interchangeable with talk about personality — as though the difference between the concrete and the abstract meant nothing — or with talk about some aspect of personality, such as the capacity for relationship. But in speaking of the human person we are not speaking of any kind of capacity nor of any kind of attribute. Our argument has not been that we can know persons by *observing* their capacity for relationship. We have said that we know them *in* relationship, which is to say, when we abandon the observer's stance altogether and commit ourselves to treating them *as* persons. Of course, persons are intended for relationship, and will therefore (barring accidents) develop the personal attributes and capacities. But that is a very different thing from taking these attributes as a supposedly objective criterion for determining their status as persons. Personality *discloses* personhood; it does not constitute it. Personal attributes develop, as self-consciousness develops; but persons do not develop, for they are not in the category of quality but of substance.

There is a sermon by Austin Farrer which opens with an account of how he visited a friend who was in an irrecoverable coma; he spoke his name and took his hand, and was profoundly moved to feel the dying man's hand close firmly upon his own in a responsive grasp. But sadly, he reflected, the appearance of relationship was deceptive. The grasp was to be explained as the spontaneous response of the local nerves in the palm of the hand, habituated by years of handshaking; the friend himself was too far gone to know his name or respond to a touch. Now, I put this observation to a neurosurgeon friend of mine, and he was quite uncomprehending. To him it was far from obvious that a deeply comatose person could not hear and respond in some way, and he himself would never discount any such sign, however remote, of awareness. Like many of us when we become fascinated by medical explorations of consciousness, Austin Farrer tried to 'know too much'. Of course, this comatose person's response was not unambiguous; we may well wonder what to make of it, since from an observer's point of view it is quite inconclusive. Farrer's sermon goes on to talk of babies' smiles and wind. Again, what we see is inconclusive; we don't know that a baby is smiling, but we don't know that it is not. Personal presence emerges out of hiddenness, through ambiguous signs, to the point of clear disclosure, and then retreats into ambiguity and hiddenness at the end. There is no sign of behaviour of which we can say, 'There he is present! There he has gone!' — short of death itself, of course, and even there there are ambiguities too obvious to be mentioned. All we can do is *act personally,* as person or as friend.

The importance of this, when applied to the question of human life in its beginnings, the unborn child from conception to birth, is that it allows us to acknowledge the *mysteriousness* of what it is that lives in the womb. No one, I suppose, can have been the parent of a child without experiencing bafflement and amazement at the incomprehensibility of what thought encounters there. It is certainly not what we normally encounter when we engage with some object as a 'person'. Parents have to go *beyond the phenomenon,* and, at first almost playfully, attribute personhood to the living being in the womb — and this playful projection continues in some measure even after birth, as we see in the case of smiles and wind. But it would be quite wrong to imagine that this was simply a sentimental and arbitrary embroidery on some otherwise-specifiable, cold, sober 'facts' about the fetus. Nobody knows any cold, sober facts; they merely observe the ambiguous phenomenon. This commitment of the parents to going beyond the phenomenon, treating the fetus as a baby, and then the newborn baby as a person, is actually *necessary,* if they are to care properly for it and if the baby is ever to develop those 'personal' characteristics which are not themselves personhood but communicate it. Furthermore, it is not arbitrary to think that the fruit of the human womb will, given the right care, develop to the point of evincing personhood through personal characteristics. Parents who do this know what the natural goal of a pregnancy is, and act in expectation of that goal's being reached. In their commitment to that goal, their engagement with the unborn child as their baby, the possibility arises of their knowing their child as a person.

But what is true of the parents in particular has to be true of the whole community. All those who assist in the pregnancy (medically or otherwise) are equally committed to welcoming the new life. And those who have no involvement with *this* pregnancy are nevertheless encouraged to see it sympathetically from the same point of view, and by so doing learn the attitudes which will be important to them when and if they are parents. The commitment of parenting, in other words, is not a private and particular commitment only of *these* parents to *this* fetus, but a generic commitment of a community and its culture to personal care for fetuses in general. This commitment is important for the community's ability to recognize and welcome new members, and will be reflected subsequently in its care for children. Only a very confused culture, such as ours is presently, can arbitrarily treat one fetus in one way and another in another. The confusion must be resolved into a general cultural attitude to the unborn human. And if that attitude does not arise from the practice of parenting, where will it arise from?

I take the practice of *experimenting on embryos* as the clearest indication of what the alternative attitude to the unborn child is. Abortion as such does not express a decisive concept of the fetus; it is the mere *refusal* of parenthood, and can be defended sometimes as the disposal of an impersonal piece of tissue and sometimes as the overruling of one person's rights in favour of another's. Once we confront experiment, however, the philosophy is quite explicit: an embryo is manipulable tissue, which has the double advantage to the researcher of being at one and the same time human tissue, with a high degree of individual organization, and non-personal.

Once again, this philosophy goes beyond the phenomenon, and commits itself in action to a view of the embryo which cannot be demonstrated objectively. Nonpersonhood is every bit as unsusceptible of proof as personhood. The philosophy is demanded not by the phenomena of human beginnings but by the internal requirements of the commitment to scientific experiment itself. Experiment objectifies, assigns its subject to the status of 'thing' — that is the logic of the undertaking. This does not in itself invalidate all experiment on human beings, but it does require a careful structure of symbolic safeguards — requirements of informed consent etc. — which exist to remind us all that the experimenter's perspective on the human subject is an abstraction, and potentially a dangerous one. No comparable safeguards exist in experiment on human embryos, nor could they be introduced without abolishing all useful research. We may therefore regard as purely speculative any suggestions about kinds of research which might be compatible with treating the embryo as a person, and simply say that for practical purposes experiment embodies and requires the decision not to treat it so. And that decision arises from the practice, and not vice versa.

We have to choose, then, between the alternative practices of scientific experiment and parenting as providing rival matrices for the commitment we have to unborn children as a class. This choice cannot be arbitrated existentially, but only on the basis of what is true about the world. In demanding that our common attitude should be formed by the commitment to parenthood, not by the commitment to scientific knowledge (for all the goods of mastery of disease which it promises us), we base ourselves on the truth that those whom we treat as persons when they are yet unborn, become *known* to us as persons when they are children; and that this truth is utterly hidden from us by the alternative practice. The fundamental incompatibility of these two perspectives is ultimately expressed as the decision either to know human beings personally, or not to know them so. The decision to 'play God' — to reidentify the human object — is also, and inescapably, a decision *not* to 'play many', to close ourselves off from the modes of mutual knowledge which essentially belong to the community of mankind.

II

Having said that discerning persons is a matter of commitment to moral engagement, we must add a second point: there are criteria of *appropriateness* for our engaging with other beings as persons in fidelity. It might be thought that the doctrine that we *know* persons only as we *treat* them as persons opened the door to all kinds of fantasy. What do we make, for example, of people who treat their pets or their plants as persons? Certainly the response they get is ambiguous, but that we allowed to be no obstacle; so is the response from the comatose man or the newborn baby ambiguous, but it is appropriate, nevertheless, to commit ourselves to them. Is it equally appropriate to commit ourselves to our plants? No; for, as we made it clear in the beginning, our existential commitment is founded on an anthropology. The commitment to the other is rationally justified because he and we are alike mankind. It is appropriate to commit oneself in engagement with mankind, as it is not with plants; which is not to say that some kind of commitment may not be appropriate also in dealing with plants, but not the kind of commitment that treats them as persons.

'But this,' someone may protest, 'simply begs the whole question. We started off asking whether certain doubtful beings — comatose patients and unborn babies — were really human beings in the full sense of being persons, and you told us that we would discover whether they were only if we assumed that they were and committed ourselves accordingly. Now you tell us that we must, after all, make up our minds *in advance* whether someone is a human being before we know whether to commit ourselves.' The appearance of circularity here is, however, only momentary. For we said also that there was a purely observational level at which we could 'know' human beings and distinguish them from elephants in the same way that we know ducks and distinguish them from geese. This is not knowing 'humanely' — that is as a human being *ought* to know another human being — but it is a form of knowledge, a knowledge of the human *phenomenon* which can render intelligible and appropriate the commitment to treating someone 'as a person'. The question then becomes: what are the criteria for discerning the human *phenomenon?* What is the human 'appearance', or human 'face,' which invites us to commit ourselves to it in expectation and hope of meeting the human 'person'? But this question in turn cannot be answered simply as it stands, for phenomena themselves develop and unfold in time; the more one investigates an object, the more the phenomenon of that object unfolds. Take, for example, a famous shock-scene in Bergman's film *The Seventh Seal.* The hero approaches from behind a figure seated, slightly crouched, upon a rock, and taps him on the shoulder. As he does so, the figure slumps over and his head lurches round at an unnatural angle, to reveal that his eyes have been picked out and that it is nothing but a rotted corpse. The initial phenomenon of a living human being has quickly developed into something quite different. So we might frame the question in this way: how far into the phenomenon do we have to go before we have a sufficient basis for recognizing a human being to whom we may show humane fidelity?

But even in this form the question is misleading. The hero was not *wrong* to think he saw a living human being. That is what makes the shock shocking. It was perfectly appropriate for him to tap this figure on the shoulder, as one might arrest the attention of someone taking a nap. It would not have been appropriate for him to *go on* treating that figure as a living human being; but he had sufficient warrant to *approach* him in that way. It would have been inappropriate, indeed morally wicked, for him to transfix him with an arrow like a beast of prey, for such phenomenal evidence as he had suggested that he had to deal with a living man. So we need to get away from any form of the question which implies that there is a level of proof to be reached before we have warrant to interact with someone as a human being. Rather, the initial appearance of the human form is immediate, and immediately commands a committed humane response. If that appearance then breaks down and turns into something else, then we recognize we have made a mistake and abandon our 'committed' response. But we respond to the 'human face', the immediate self-presentation of humanity, and not to any measure of proof.

Consider the following scenario. The obstetrician cuts the umbilical cord, and the nurse washes the baby, weighs it, takes measures to protect it against infection, wraps it in a blanket to keep it warm; and then, of course, the parents talk to it, call it by its name, try to attract its attention, console its cries. But then the baby shows signs of being in trouble, and in a few minutes dies. It was pointless talking to it, calling it by its name, attracting its attention, for its eyes are sightless, its ears without hearing. But in the first moments it appeared normal. And when we say that the parents were right to *treat* it as a normal child until they knew it was *not* a normal child, we are not merely recommending that one should be on the safe side when in doubt. We are saying that the *only* proper response to the human appearance is the humane response. There could not be any question of *doubt* until the first deviant phenomena occurred; to profess doubt earlier than that would be the purest bad faith. The immediate appearance of a child was a quite sufficient warrant for commitment in those initial moments. (Does this example, perhaps, give us a paradigm for how we may think about natural fetal wastage by spontaneous abortion?)

To say that we respond to the 'immediate appearance' of a human being does not mean that we cannot learn to discern the human appearance more accurately. The first explorers who encountered pigmy peoples may have been in some justifiable doubt as to whether this was the human race or not. Today nobody could be justified in professing doubt on the matter. Many of us might make the mistake of supposing that someone was dead, when the skilled eye of a physician would suspect a coma. We can, in other words, learn to trace the genetic patterns of the human phenomenon and identify some appearances — which lie outside our common experience — as belonging properly to the phenomenon of humanity and others as not doing so. This point is of great importance in assessing the claim on our attention made by the human embryo.

Earlier generations had perfectly legitimate difficulties in recognizing an unborn child (in embryo state) as a human being. The discontinuities of appearance were striking, and, of course, the embryo was never observed alive. Consequently they hypothesized a moment of 'animation' in which this strange body was transformed and brought to life by the coming of the soul. We may compare this kind of thinking to early anthropological speculations about the Bantu races, which tried to show essential discontinuities with the Caucasian races. Subsequent scientific exploration of the phenomena has discredited the impression of such discontinuities. Similarly, scientific study of embryology has laid to rest the notion of a major physiological discontinuity in human development between embryo and fetal stage. Genetic studies have, on the other hand, indicated a major discontinuity at conception, when the parental genotypes re-form into a new genome, the distinct endowment of the new conceptus. (This has meant, not only that the history of the embryo/fetus can no longer be conceived as including a moment of 'animation', but that it can no longer be extended back to include the history of the sperm before conception.)

Our generation cannot avoid the implications of this knowledge. Our recognition of the human face is improved, and we can now see it in the embryo, even in the invisible blastocyst and zygote, where our ancestors could not. This means that pre-modern speculations about the animation of the fetus are now empty of all probative force. (I say this, because there remains among some Anglican Christians a curious belief that this question can be settled simply on the basis of Christian tradition.) This is not to subordinate theology *in principle* to science. Rather, it is to point out that such theological speculations were always *empirical in intent*, lacking only the investigative resources to reach accurate conclusions. And to say that these pre-modern discussions have no probative force is not to say that they have no value for our thinking on the question. They have great *critical* value, in that they expose and refute the philosophical pressures which, then as now, exercise an improper *a priori* influence on what ought to be empirical judgments.

To sum up. The scientific evidence about the development of the unborn child does not prove that the unborn child is a person, because that cannot in principle be proved. We cannot accept any equation of personhood with brain-activity, genotype, implantation, or whatever — for that is to reduce personhood, which is known only in personal engagement, to a function of some observable criteria. However, what the scientific evidence does is to clarify for us the lines of objective continuity and discontinuity, so that we can identify with greater accuracy the 'beginning' of any individual human existence. It is, of course, a purely 'biological' beginning that biology discloses to us; how could it be otherwise? In adopting it as the sufficient ground of respect for the human being, we are not declaring that personhood is merely biological. We are, rather, exploring the presuppositions of personal commitment. The only ground we have for risking commitment in the first encounters with the new human being is biological 'appearance'.

One of the most potent philosophical ingredients from which the giddy modern cocktail of technological materialism is mixed is the idealist distrust of appearances. It has, of course, become almost customary in these days to proclaim emancipation from a 'Cartesian' body-soul dualism, and there can be few intellectual evils which have not been attributed to this source by someone or other. For the most part, however, the emancipation has proved to be an empty boast. The very least that would be implied by it would be a willingness to get a hold on human appearances once again. It would imply that we stopped treating the bodily manifestations of humanity, its genetic and physiological structures, as though we had entirely seen through them and knew that there was nothing there. It would imply that we stopped talking and acting as though we shared some secret knowledge about a real humanity that was disclosed apart from physical appearances. It would imply that we stopped throwing up specious oppositions between 'personalist' and 'biologistic' conceptions of the human being. It is true, as we have emphasized, that the human person resists exhaustive analysis, that it has its root in the mystery of divine vocation whereby God confers our individual existence upon us as he calls us by our names. But to that secret calling there is no public audio-link. We know another person by his unfolding manifestation through appearances, and we know him to be something more than the sum of the appearances only as we attend with seriousness to what the appearances manifest. The Samaritan, who proved to be the Jew's neighbour, was the one traveller upon that road who reckoned that he could trust the evidence of his eyes: 'When he saw him, he had compassion.'

50 Who Is My Neighbor? The Good Samaritan as a Source for Theological Anthropology

Ian A. McFarland

I. The Problem of the Person in Biblical Perspective

Given the degree to which the question of who is to be counted as a person has agitated theologians over the past generation, it is rather disquieting to be reminded of the dearth of biblical reflection on what a person is. To be sure, a search through the concordance of some of the major English translations of Scripture may turn up a hundred or more entries for "person,"[1] but one searches in vain for the kind of technical usage that underlies contemporary debates over the status of the severely retarded, the comatose, unborn, or even certain non-human species. The Greek terms, *hypostasis* and *prosopon,* which were later pressed into service as technical terms for "person," have nothing like this sense in the New Testament.[2] The closest thing to a technical use of the word "person" is probably found in the abstract noun *prosopolempsia* (sometimes rendered "respect of persons") and its variants,[3] but even here the reference is less to a particular quality of human (or other) being than to an individual's social or legal status: to show *prosopolempsia* is less to identify a certain class of beings as persons than to be partial to one class of persons over others.

The reasons for this lack of reference to the problem of personhood in Scripture are not hard to identify. It was only later that the Greek word *prosopon* (along with its Latin equivalent, *persona,* from which the English word is derived) came to be used in a technical sense to describe a particular kind of being. The watershed event in this development was the formulation of the doctrine of the Trinity, in which those whom the Bible names as Father, Son, and Holy Spirit were distinguished as three persons *(hypostaseis* or *prosopa)* within the one divine essence *(ousia).*[4] Interestingly, within this trinitarian framework the term "person" does not name some property common to the Father, Son, and Spirit, but rather identifies their difference from each other.[5]

A crucial juncture in the transition from this specifically theological understanding of "person" to modernity's characteristically anthropological use of the term was Boethius' definition of a person as "the individual substance of a rational nature."[6] Admittedly, Boethius ventured this definition in an effort to explain the theological use of "person" to a general audience, but the effect was to equate personhood with the possession of a particular property or quality, without any necessary reference to a trinitarian framework. Boethius' identification of this crucial property with reason proved enormously influential;[7] but even where some other criterion (relationality, for example) has been proposed, the effect of defining persons as a category of beings has been to cut the term loose from its theological moorings: that which in trinitarian thought identified the Father, Son, and Spirit in their irreducible distinction from one another came to refer anthropologically to some quality or set of qualities that all "persons" were alleged to hold in common.

This latter way of viewing what it means to be a person entails a particular set of presuppositions and practices. First, it presupposes that an individual's identity as a person can be established by viewing that individual in isolation.[8] If personhood is a matter of possessing certain qualities, then an individual's identity as a person is determined by testing for the presence of those qualities.

1. For example, the word "person" occurs 79 times in the RSV, 106 times in the NIV, and 129 times in the NASB. Compare the premodern KJV, in which the word is used only 56 times.

2. *Hypostasis* appears five times: once (Heb. 1:2) it means "essence" or "being" (quite different from the sense it will come to have in the trinitarian theology of the Cappadocians), and the other four (2 Cor. 9:4; 11:17; Heb. 3:14; 11:1) "confidence" or "assurance." *Prosopon* appears many more times (75 in all), but almost exclusively with the meaning of "face" (but cf. Jude 16).

3. *Prosopolempsia* is found in Rom. 2:11; Eph. 6:9; Col. 3:25; Jas. 2:1. Variations found in the New Testament include *aprosopolemptes* (1 Pet. 1:17), *prosopolemptein* (Jas. 2:9), and *prosopolemptes* (Acts 10:34). Note that seven of the nine instances of *persona* in the New Testament Vulgate are translations of these terms.

From Ian A. McFarland, "Who Is My Neighbor? The Good Samaritan as a Source for Theological Anthropology," in *Modern Theology* 17.1 (2001): 57-66. Used by permission of Wiley-Blackwell.

4. See John D. Zizioulas, *Being As Communion: Studies in Personhood and the Church* (Crestwood, NY: St. Vladimir's Seminary Press, 1997), pp. 36-41.

5. This principle takes classic form in the grammatical rule *eadem de Filio quae de Patre dicuntur excepto Patre nomine* — "whatever is said of the Son is said also of the Father, except that the Son is the Father." Bernard Lonergan, *Method in Theology* (New York, NY: Seabury, 1972), p. 307.

6. *"Naturae rationabilis individua substantia."* Boethius, *A Treatise Against Eutyches and Nestorius,* in *The Theological Tractates and The Consolation of Philosophy,* Loeb Classical Library (Cambridge, MA: Harvard University Press, 1973), pp. 84-85.

7. It was endorsed by Thomas Aquinas in the *Summa Theologiae,* Ia, qu. 29, art. 1, and would seem to lie behind Locke's definition of a person as "a thinking intelligent Being, that has reason and reflection, and can consider it self as it self, the same thinking thing in different times and places." John Locke, *An Essay Concerning Human Understanding,* Book II, ch. 27, §9, ed. Peter H. Nidditch (Oxford: Oxford University Press, 1975), p. 335.

8. Note that this is true even if personhood is defined relationally, insofar as within such a relational model personhood is finally inseparable from one's capacity to participate in relationships of a certain type or quality.

Second, to the extent that identity as a person is viewed as something worthwhile — specifically, as something which endows an individual with certain rights withheld from non-persons — it becomes important to identify who is included in the category of persons.

Neither of these presuppositions has any place within a trinitarian context. That the Father, Son, and Spirit are persons is not a fact that can be determined by considering them in isolation: since their personhood refers precisely to that which (unlike the qualities of omnipotence, omniscience, eternity, etc., which pertain to the divine *ousia*) is *not* common to all three, no one of the persons can be identified *as* a person without reference to the other two. This does not mean that divine personhood is in its essence relational, as though the Father, Son, and Spirit's status as persons were the consequence of some capacity, more or less effectively realized, to live in relationship with one another. It is true that the trinitarian persons are *defined* relationally — the Father as the Father of the Son, the Son as the Son of the Father, etc. — but this definition is less reflective of some essence of divine personhood than of our inability to specify any such essence. Because the personal distinctions refer to that which cannot be predicated jointly of the Father, Son, and Spirit, the divine persons' relations to one another do not tell us *what* the Father, Son, and Spirit are, but only provide us a rule for identifying *who* they are. In other words, "person" refers quite specifically to the Father, Son, and Holy Spirit, and is *not* a genus under which individual beings may be subsumed.

II. "Who Is My Neighbor?"

Although one searches Scripture in vain for formal discussion of what constitutes personhood, there is nevertheless a clear biblical analogue to the contemporary question "What is a person?" It comes in Luke 10, in the context of a discussion on the subject of what it is necessary to do in order to inherit eternal life. Under prodding from Jesus, the lawyer who had initially posed the question acknowledges that the requirements are clearly set out in the law as love of God and neighbor (v. 27). The story might well end there (as it does in the Matthean and Markan parallels), but in Luke's version the lawyer asks Jesus a further question: "And who is my neighbor?" (v. 29).

The fact that this question is put into the mouth of a lawyer highlights its parallelism with modern discussions of personhood, which also tend to surface in a legal context. Because persons are understood to have a right to a certain level or quality of treatment — one that would rule out, for example, their being made the objects of medical experimentation without their prior consent — it is necessary to have some criteria for determining who counts as a person. In brief, the fact that I am not allowed to treat persons with the same kind of indifference I might a rock or a tree both confronts me with certain obligations and places definite restrictions on my own freedom of action.

When the matter is put in this way, concern over one's own ethical liability has seemingly eclipsed any genuine interest in the well-being of others. It is therefore not surprising that the lawyer in Luke 10 — who, we are told, asks his question about the identity of his neighbor out of a wish to "vindicate" or "justify" *(dikaiosai)* himself — tends to be viewed in a rather unfavorable light. Yet one need not view his question as prompted purely by the selfish desire to avoid censure or minimize responsibility. If nothing less than eternal life hangs on my love of neighbor, then it is only natural that I should want to determine just who my neighbor is. From this perspective, the lawyer's question to Jesus is a sign of no greater presumption or recalcitrance than the ethically serious efforts of participants in contemporary debates over abortion and euthanasia to find a coherent definition of the person.

Whatever the lawyer's motives in asking his question, Jesus responds by telling the parable of the good Samaritan.[9] The story's plot is straightforward enough: a man (presumably Jewish, inasmuch as his journey begins in Jerusalem) is assaulted on his way to Jericho and left for dead by the roadside. A priest and a Levite, doubtless nervous over the possibility of becoming ritually unclean through contact with a corpse, pass him by. It is a despised Samaritan, evidently unconcerned about any possible effects on his ritual purity,[10] who comes to the victim's aid, tending his wounds, bringing him to a place of shelter, and instructing the innkeeper to spare no expense in his treatment.

Does this story answer the lawyer's question? Considered by itself, the story of the man who fell among thieves might lead the reader (who shares the lawyer's perspective as the one to whom the tale is told) to suppose that the neighbor is the man in need. On this reading, the details of the story are ultimately superfluous, and the parable is only a more or less engaging way of illustrating a fairly straightforward answer to the lawyer's question: your neighbor is anyone who needs your care.

Yet this is not how Jesus himself makes use of the parable. He ends the tale not with a neatly drawn conclusion (e.g., "Count as your neighbor anyone in need"), but with a question of his own: "Which of these three seems to you to have been a neighbor to the one who fell among

9. Joseph Fitzmyer argues that the practical thrust of the passage makes it less a parable than an *exemplum* or extended simile (Joseph A. Fitzmyer, *The Gospel According to Luke (X–XXIV): Introduction, Translation, and Notes* [New York, NY: Doubleday, 1985], p. 883). As the following argument makes clear, I view the story as less straightforwardly "practical" and more parabolic than does Fitzmyer. For another argument against the classification of the parable as *exemplum,* see Robert W. Funk, "The Good Samaritan as Metaphor," in *Semeia* 2 (1974), pp. 75-84.

10. In this context, it is worth pointing out that the Samaritan Pentateuch contained the same injunctions against contact with the dead as the one the priest and the Levite would have consulted.

thieves?" (v. 36). If the parable appears at first glance to accept the terms of the lawyer's question (i.e., the problem of identifying who counts as a neighbor), Jesus' counter-question redirects attention from the status of others to that of the lawyer himself. As it turns out, "neighbor" is not a category that the lawyer is authorized to apply to others; instead, it takes the form of a challenge and recoils back upon him as a moral agent capable either of being or of failing to be a neighbor to someone else.[11] In this way, Jesus asks lawyer and reader alike to consider the possibility that the question of their own status as neighbors might be anthropologically prior to any reflection on the status of other people.

Jesus does not so much answer the lawyer's question as turn it around. His counter-question forces the lawyer to apply the term "neighbor" not to the victim of the assault, but to "the one who showed [literally, 'did'] compassion to him" (Luke 10:37). This is not to suggest that the effect of Jesus' question is merely to replace one possible definition of the neighbor ("someone in need") with another ("one who meets others' needs"). Indeed, it would be hard to imagine a more serious misinterpretation of the parable than the conclusion that the neighbor is the class of those who show mercy to the afflicted, as though one could be justified in refusing to regard anyone who fails to show mercy as a neighbor.

No, a crucial feature of the parable is precisely the fact that Jesus refrains from offering *any* definition of the neighbor.[12] It is true that the one who showed compassion was a neighbor to the man who fell among thieves, but Jesus' final words to the lawyer are in the imperative rather than the indicative mood: "You go and do likewise." The lawyer is not told who his neighbor is.[13] He is simply commanded to imitate the Samaritan's compassion without being given any specific criteria regarding those to whom compassion is owed.[14]

11. Cf. J. M. Creed, *The Gospel according to St. Luke: The Greek Text, with Introduction, Notes, and Indices* (London: Macmillan, 1930), p. 151.

12. Fitzmyer cites the fact that the parable fails to answer the lawyer's question as evidence that it has been joined to the discussion of eternal life only secondarily (Fitzmyer, *The Gospel According to Luke (X–XXIV)*, p. 883). Without venturing to speculate on the pre-history of the Gospel text, the point can nevertheless be made that Jesus' failure to answer the lawyer's question may itself be of important significance for Luke.

13. Fitzmyer is thus right to conclude that "[n]o definition of 'neighbor' emerges from the 'example,' because such a casuistic question is really out of place." His judgment here, however, conflicts rather sharply with his earlier statement (on the same page!) that "[t]he point of the story is . . . that a neighhor is anyone in need with whom one comes into contact and to whom one can show pity and kindness." Fitzmyer, *The Gospel According to Luke (X–XXIV)*, p. 884.

14. In this context, Fitzmyer's judgment that "[t]he point of the story . . . is made without the concluding remark of Jesus" is open to question. See Fitzmyer, *The Gospel According to Luke (X–XXIV)*, p. 883.

III. What Is a Person?

If the lawyer's question as to the identity of his neighbor is in some respects functionally similar to more modern discussions of what makes someone a person, Jesus' response seems equally unhelpful in both contexts. Yet in leaving us without a readily applicable criteriology of personhood, the parable of the good Samaritan arguably honors the trinitarian roots of "person" more effectively than any putative definition of personhood might. As noted above, the term "person" first acquired a technical sense as a means of referring to the Father, Son, and Spirit. Insofar as the term does not identify a common property that these three share, the only possible "definition" of a person that might be derived from the doctrine of the Trinity is "one who participates in the relationships between the Father, Son, and Holy Spirit" — which is really to do no more than to identify the Father, Son, and Spirit as what we mean by persons.

At first glance, it might appear that locating the term "person" in this kind of strictly trinitarian framework simply renders it anthropologically empty. This conclusion, however, is belied by the equally trinitarian confession that one of the three divine persons, the Son, "became incarnate of the virgin Mary, and was made a human being" named Jesus. It follows that at least *this* human being is a person, since he does "participate in the relationships between the Father, Son, and Holy Spirit."[15] Moreover, because the reason for the Son's taking on the human condition was that he might bring the rest of the human family into communion with the triune God, it turns out that the set of human persons is not limited to Jesus alone. On the contrary, as the head of the body into which the rest of us are called (Eph. 1:22-23; 4:15-16; Col. 1:18–2:19), Jesus is the "first-born of many siblings" (Rom. 8:29); and as members of his body, we share in his status as "Son" and are thereby empowered to join with him in calling God "Father" (Rom. 8:15; Gal. 4:5-6; cf. Matt. 6:9; Luke 11:2; Eph. 2:18).

Insofar as all human beings are summoned in and through Christ to participate in the relationships between the three divine persons, they, too, are persons. To be sure, because they are persons only "in" Christ, they have no claim to be persons on their own account, by virtue of some particular capacity or quality they possess. They are persons for the sole reason that they are treated *as* persons by God by being called in Christ to participate in the relationships between the Father, Son, and Spirit.

Correlating the fact of personhood with membership in the body of Christ might appear to suggest that only baptized Christians should be considered persons. Such a conclusion, however, accords ill with Paul's claim that even those who have received Christ's Spirit in baptism still await their adoption as children of God (Rom. 8:23; cf. v. 19). Paul's point here is certainly not to downplay

15. Indeed, it is only by virtue of this incarnation that we are in a position to speak of three persons in God in the first place.

the significance of church membership, but it does serve as a reminder that no human being's final status with respect to the Trinity is known prior to the Last Day. To the extent that the church acknowledges damnation — eternal exclusion from God's presence — as a conceivable destiny for human beings, it remains possible that not all human beings will turn out to be persons; but the identity of such non-persons is not given to us in the here and now.[16]

Here, too, the rule applies that human personhood cannot be correlated with the possession of a given capacity or property, including the "property" of having been baptized.[17] Once again, what counts is how we are treated by the divine persons, and here there are simply no prior limits placed on the range of those called through the Son to live as persons with God. On the contrary, Jesus explicitly commands the gospel to be preached to every nation (Matt. 28:19), and, indeed, to every creature (Mark 16:15; Col. 1:23). From this perspective, the measure of personhood is the fact that we are treated as persons by the Son, who invites us to participate in the communion he shares with the Father and the Spirit.[18]

IV. The Good Samaritan Revisited

Admittedly, the foregoing interpretation of personhood does not seem especially useful for resolving those contemporary ethical dilemmas in which the question of personhood figures prominently. To all appearances, it amounts to a conceptually vacuous latitudinarianism, in which I am obliged to consider every being I encounter as a person until the Last Judgment shows otherwise. In the face of this charge, however, the story of good Samaritan can serve as steadying theological ballast. As argued above, an important feature of that parable is Jesus' refusal to satisfy the lawyer's desire for a readily applicable anthropology. The neighbor is not defined as the one in need, nor as the one who shows compassion to the needy. Instead, Jesus effectively dismisses the lawyer's question and asks the reader to consider that the crucial anthropological issue is not the status of the other whom I face, but rather who I am.

In working out the implications of this latter point, it is worth recalling that throughout most of the church's history, the parable of the good Samaritan has been interpreted christologically. According to this reading, the man who falls among thieves represents humankind, seemingly dead from its sins; the Samaritan is Jesus, who brings us back to life as the persons we were created to be. If the foregoing analysis of the parable is at all accurate, this traditional interpretation may not be as far-fetched as the majority of twentieth-century interpreters suppose.[19] As already noted, the lawyer's question assumes that the status of the other is the crucial theological problem in theological anthropology: love is something he is obliged to show the other — if the other qualifies as a neighbor. But Jesus' counter-question turns things around: it is not the status of the other, but that of the lawyer (and by implication, of the reader) that is at issue.[20]

In this way, the logic of the parable raises the possibility that we first need to be shown compassion by a neighbor as a condition of becoming neighbors ourselves (cf. Eph. 4:32). If "neighbor" is the functional equivalent of "person," it follows that our status as persons can no more be taken for granted than the recovery of the man set upon by thieves. Rather, our life as persons requires a prior act of compassion in which another person treats us as persons. If we adhere to a trinitarian framework in our use of the term "person," then only the divine persons are capable of showing us this kind of compassion. And since only one of those persons has become flesh and dwelt among us, no human being but Jesus can assume the role of the Samaritan for us. The compassion he shows to us by claiming us as sisters and brothers constitutes us as persons sharing his communion with the Father and the Spirit.

Nor is a christological exegesis of the parable lacking in resources for ethical reflection. An unspoken assumption underlying the lawyer's original question to Jesus is that once the identity of my neighbor has been ascertained, the course of action that follows is clear. In other words, the lawyer seems to have no doubts about what love of neighbor entails, only about the range of its application. The same set of assumptions seems to underlie much of the contemporary quest for a criteriology of

16. And, of course, the church has never claimed that baptism constitutes a guarantee of an individual's inclusion or exclusion in the number of the saved.

17. Thus, the church has generally refrained from viewing the fact of baptism as a guarantor of — or its absence as an insuperable obstacle to — salvation.

18. A similar argument is made by Thomas Aquinas in the third part of his *Summa Theologiae*. He first argues that because Christ is properly *(prima et principaliter)* the head only of those united to him in glory (*viz.*, the members of the church triumphant), no human being — Christian or not — is fully incorporated into his body in this life. But he then goes on to argue that Christ is properly considered the head of all human beings insofar as he provides expiation for the sins of the whole world (1 John 2:2) irrespective of present confessional status. It follows that all human beings must be treated as part of his body whether or not they consider themselves to be such. See Thomas Aquinas, *Summa Theologiae,* IIIa, qu. 8, art. 3 (Blackfriars, London: Eyre & Spottiswoode, 1974).

19. Not that modern attempts to affirm a christological interpretation of the parable have been altogether lacking. See, e.g., Jean Daniélou, "Le bon Samaritain," in *Mélanges bibliques rédigés en l'honneur de Andre Robert* (Paris: Bloud et Gay, 1957), pp. 497-465 and B. Gerhardsson, "The Good Samaritan — The Good Shepherd?" in *Coniectanea neotestamentica* 16 (1958), pp. 1-31.

20. "For the question 'Which one was neighbour to the man who was waylaid?' requires that the answer be given from the position of the man in trouble, that the lawyer put himself in the place of the waylaid man." L. P. Trudinger, "Once Again, Now 'Who Is My Neighbour?'" in the *Evangelical Quarterly* 48 (1976), p. 161. Cf. Funk, "The Good Samaritan as Metaphor," p. 79.

personhood. Thus, if the fetus is a person, then I should not abort it; if my comatose aunt is a person, I should not withdraw life support; if monkeys have a claim to personhood, I should not subject them to medical experiments.

Upon further reflection, however, the idea that the range of beings to which love is to be shown is more problematic than the content of love seems a rather odd assumption. Is the status of the other as a person really that crucial to our moral reasoning? After all, though I am quite confident that my wife (for example) is a person, that confidence certainly does not by itself provide me with clear guidelines about how I should behave toward her in any given situation. Indeed, it is precisely in my marriage — arguably the most "personal" relationship I have with another human being (at least as compared with my more formal and routinized relations with the postman, the check-out clerk, or even my colleagues at work) — that I find myself most regularly having to ask myself what love requires.

This is not to deny all moral relevance to reflection on the status of the other. If my wife were to become critically ill and unable to make decisions regarding her own care, my understanding of her condition and prognosis would certainly contribute to any decisions I might be asked to make on her behalf. I suspect, however, that my thinking would not turn on the question of whether or not she still qualified as a person. More importantly, it seems to me that the parable of the good Samaritan provides good theological basis for this suspicion, insofar as this story suggests that the more important ethical question is not whether my wife is a person, but rather how I, as one who is treated as a person by Jesus Christ, relate to my wife (or anyone else) as the person I have been called to be. In other words, the crucial ethical judgment in my behavior toward those I meet on the road is not primarily the determination of the general category under which they fall (however necessary some such judgment may be), but rather the way in which I define my relationship to them in their particularity.[21]

V. Conclusion

Christian doctrine teaches that there are only three persons in the strict sense of the term: the Father, the Son, and the Holy Spirit. It does not presume to say what it means that these three are persons: the term "person" is merely a semantic placeholder that marks this threefold distinction within the Godhead. Strictly speaking, to be a person is simply to be one of these three: the Father, the Son, or the Holy Spirit.

But Christian doctrine also teaches that these three persons have willed to bring others into their fellowship. Those so invited are not persons on their own account, but they are nonetheless persons by virtue of their participation in the life of the Trinity through the Son. They are, so to speak, persons by proxy. Their identity as persons is bound up with their relationship to Jesus, who, as the incarnate Son, is both the model and source of their own personhood.

It follows that Jesus is the proper focus for Christian reflection on what it means to be a person. He assumes this role as the one in whose life is disclosed both the identity of the three divine persons and the form of human personhood they make possible. To know what it means to be a person, one needs to look to Jesus. Because his life is not only the supreme example, but also (and, indeed, primarily) the source of our own identity as persons, it is only on the basis of his prior activity on our behalf that we find ourselves in a position to be challenged by him to "go and do likewise."

21. This last point is beautifully argued by Stanley Hauerwas in his essay, "Must a Patient Be a Person to Be a Patient? Or, My Uncle Charlie Is Not Much of a Person But He Is Still My Uncle Charlie" in *Truthfulness and Tragedy: Further Investigations in Christian Ethics* (Notre Dame, IN: University of Notre Dame Press, 1977), pp. 127-131.

51 Must a Patient Be a Person to Be a Patient? Or, My Uncle Charlie Is Not Much of a Person but He Is Still My Uncle Charlie

Stanley Hauerwas

As a Protestant teaching at a Catholic university, I continue to learn about problems I had no idea even existed. For example, recently I was called down for referring to Catholics as "Roman Catholics." I had been working on the assumption that a Catholic was a Roman Catholic; however, it was pointed out to me that this phrase appeared only with the beginning of the English reformation in order to distinguish a Roman from an Anglo-Catholic. A Catholic is not Roman, as my Irish Catholic friend emphatically reminded me, but is more properly thought of simply as Catholic.

I recount this tale because I think it has something to do with the issue I want to raise for our consideration. For we tend to think that most of our descriptions, the way we individuate action, have a long and honored history that can be tampered with only with great hesitation. Often, however, the supposed tradition is a recent innovation that may be as misleading as it is helpful.

That is what I think may be happening with the emphasis on whether someone is or is not a "person" when this is used to determine whether or what kind of medical care a patient should receive. In the literature of past medical ethics the notion of "person" does not seem to have played a prominent role in deciding how medicine should or should not be used vis-à-vis a particular patient. Why is it then that we suddenly seem so concerned with the question of whether someone is a person? It is my hunch we have much to learn from this phenomenon as it is an indication, not that our philosophy of medicine or medical ethics is in good shape, but rather that it is in deep trouble. For it is my thesis that we are trying to put forward "person" as a regulative notion to direct our health care as substitute for what only a substantive community and story can do.

However, before trying to defend this thesis, let me first illustrate how the notion of "person" is being used in relation to some of the recent issues of medical ethics. Paul Ramsey in his book, *The Patient as Person,*[1] uses the notion of person to protect the individual patient against the temptation, especially in experimental medicine, to use one patient for the good of another or society. According to Ramsey, the major issue of medical ethics is how to reconcile the welfare of the individual with the welfare of mankind when both must be served. Ramsey argues that it is necessary to emphasize the personhood of the patient in order to remind the doctor or the experimenter that his first responsibility is to his immediate patient, not mankind or even the patient's family. Thus Ramsey's emphasis on "person" is an attempt to provide the basis for what he takes to be the central ethical commitment of medicine, namely, that no man will be used as a means for the good of another. Medicine can serve mankind only as it does so through serving the individual patient.

Without the presumption of the inviolability of the "person," Ramsey thinks that we would have no basis for "informed consent" as the controlling criterion for medical therapy and experimentation. Moreover, it is only on this basis that doctors rightly see that their task is not to cure disease, but rather to cure the person who happens to be subject to a disease. Thus, the notion of "person" functions for Ramsey as a Kantian or deontological check on what he suspects is the utilitarian basis of modern medicine.

However, the notion of "person" plays quite a different function in other literature dealing with medical ethics. In these contexts, "person" is not used primarily as a protective notion, but rather as a permissive notion that takes the moral heat off certain quandaries raised by modern medicine. It is felt if we can say with some assuredness that X, Y, or Z is not a person, then our responsibility is not the same as it is to those who bear this august title.

Of course, the issue where this is most prominent is abortion. Is the fetus a human person? Supposedly on that question hang all the law and the prophets of the morality of abortion. For if it can be shown that the fetus is not a person, as indeed I think it can be shown, then the right to the care and protection that modern medicine can provide is not due to the fetus. Indeed, the technological skill of medicine can be used to destroy such life, for its status is of no special human concern since it lacks the attribute of "personhood."

Or, for example, the issue of *when* one is a person is raised to help settle when it is morally appropriate to withdraw care from the dying. If it can be shown, for example, that a patient has moved from the status of being a person to a non-person, then it seems that many of the difficult decisions surrounding what kind and the extent of care that should be given to the dying becomes moot. For the aid that medicine can bring is directed at persons, not at the mere continuation of our bodily life. (Since I will not develop it further, however, it is worth mentioning that this view assumes a rather extreme dualism between being a person and the bodily life necessary to provide the conditions for being a person.)[2]

1. Paul Ramsey, *The Patient as Person* (New Haven: Yale University Press, 1970).

2. For a more extended analysis of this point, see my *Vision and*

Or, finally, there are the issues of what kind of care should be given to defective or deformed infants in order to keep them alive. For example, Joseph Fletcher has argued that any individual who falls below the 40 I.Q. mark in a Stanford-Binet test is "questionably a person," and if you score 20 or below you are not a person.[3] Or Michael Tooley has argued that young infants, indeed, are not "persons" and, therefore, do not bear the rights necessary to make infanticide a morally questionable practice.[4] Whether, or what kind, of medical care should be given to children is determined by whether children are able to meet the demands of being a person. You may give them life-sustaining care, but in doing so you are acting strictly from the motive of charity since nothing obligates you to do so.

As I suggested at the first, I find all this rather odd, not because some of the conclusions reached by such reasoning may be against my own moral opinions, or because they entail practices that seem counter-intuitive (e.g., infanticide), but rather because I think this use of "person" tends to do violence to our language. For example, it is only seldom that we have occasion to think of ourselves as "persons" — when asked to identify myself, I do not think that I am a person, but I am Stanley Hauerwas, teacher, husband, father or, ultimately, a Texan. Nor do I often have the occasion to think of others as persons. I do sometimes say, "Now that Joe is one hell of a fine person," but so used, "person" carries no special status beyond the naming of a role. If I still lived in Texas, I would, as a matter of fact, never use such an expression, but rather say, "Now there is a good old boy."

Moreover, it is interesting to notice how abstract the language of person is in relation to our first-order moral language through which we live our lives and see the kind of issues I have mentioned above. For example, the reason that we do not use one man for another or society's good is not that we violate his "person," but rather because we have learned that it is destructive of the trust between us to do so. (Which is, in fact, Ramsey's real concern, as his case actually rests much more on his emphasis on the "covenant" between doctor and patient than on the status of the patient as a "person.") For example, it would surely make us hesitant to go to a doctor if we thought he might actually care for us only as a means of caring for another. It should be noted, however, that in a different kind of society it might well be intelligible and trustworthy for the doctor rightly to expect that his patient be willing to undergo certain risks for the good of the society itself. I suspect that Ramsey's excessive concern to protect the patient from the demands of society through the agency of the doctor is due to living in an extraordinarily individualistic society where citizens share no good in common.

Even more artificial is the use of "person" to try to determine the moral decision in relation to abortion, death, and the care of the defective newborn. For the issues surrounding whether an abortion should or should not be done seldom turn on the question of the status of the fetus. Rather, they involve why the mother does not want the pregnancy to continue, the conditions under which the pregnancy occurred, the social conditions into which the child would be born. The question of whether the fetus is or is not a person is almost a theoretical nicety in relation to the kind of questions that most abortion decisions actually involve.

Or, for example, when people are dying, we seldom decide to treat or not to treat them because they have or have not yet passed some line that makes them a person or non-person. Rather, we care or do not care for them because they are Uncle Charlie, or my father, or a good friend. In the same manner, we do not care or cease to care for a child born defective because it is or is not a person. Rather, whether or how we decide to care for such a child depends on our attitude toward the having and caring for children, our perception of our role as parents, and how medicine is seen as one form of how care is to be given to children.[5] (For it may well be that we will care for such children, but this does not mean that medicine has some kind of overriding claim on being the form that such care should take.)

It might be felt that these examples assume far too easily that our common notions and stories are the primary ones for giving moral guidance in such cases. The introduction of the notion of "person" as regulatory in such matters might be an attempt to find a firmer basis than these more historically and socially contingent notions can provide. But I am suggesting that is just what the notion of "person" cannot do without seriously distorting the practices, institutions, and notions that underlay how we have learned morally to display our lives. More technically, what advocates of "personhood" have failed to show is how the notion of person works in a way of life with which we wish to identify.

Yet, we feel inextricably drawn to come up with some account that will give direction to our medical practice exactly, because we sense that our more immediate moral notions never were, or are no longer, sufficient to provide such a guide. Put concretely, we are beginning to understand how much medicine depended on the moral ethos of its society to guide how it should care for children, because we are now in a period when some people no longer think simply because a child is born to them

Virtue: Essays in Christian Ethical Reflection (Notre Dame, Ind.: Fides Press, 1974).

3. Joseph Fletcher, "Indicators of Humanhood," *Hastings Center Report,* November, 1972, pp. 1-3; also see my response in "The Retarded and the Criteria of Human," *Linacre Quarterly,* November 1973, pp. 217-22.

4. Michael Tooley, "A Defense of Abortion and Infanticide," in Joel Feinberg (ed.), *The Problem of Abortion* (Belmont: Wadsworth Publishing Co., 1973), pp. 51-91.

5. For an extended analysis of these issues, see my "The Demands and Limits of Care: Ethical Reflections on the Moral Dilemma of Neonatal Intensive Care," *American Journal of Medical Science,* March-April 1975, pp. 269-91.

they need regard it as their child. We will not solve this kind of dilemma by trying to say what the doctor can and cannot do in such circumstances in terms of whether the child can be understood to be a "person" or not.

As Paul Ramsey suggests, we may have arrived at a time when we have achieved an unspeakable thing: a medical profession without a moral philosophy in a society without one either. Medicine, of course, still seems to carry the marks of a profession inasmuch as it seems to be a guardian of certain values — that is, the unconditional commitment to preserve life and health; the responsibility for justifying the patient's trust in the physician; and the autonomy of the physician in making judgments on others in the profession. But, as Alasdair MacIntyre has argued, these assumed virtues can quickly be turned to vices when they lack a scheme, or, in my language, a story that depends on further beliefs about the true nature of man and our true end.[6] But such a scheme is exactly what we lack, and it will not be supplied by trying to determine who is and is not a "person."

The language of "person" seems convenient to us, however, because we wish to assume that our medicine still rests on a consensus of moral beliefs. But I am suggesting that is exactly what is not the case and, in the absence of such a consensus, we will be much better off to simply admit that morally there are many different ways to practice medicine. We should, in other words, be willing to have our medicine as fragmented as our moral lives. I take this to be particularly important for Christians and Jews, as we have been under the illusion that we could morally expect medicine to embody our own standards, or, at least, standards that we could sympathize with. I suspect, however, that this may not be the case, for the story that determines how the virtues of medicine are to be displayed for us is quite different from the one claimed by the language of "person."[7] It may be then, if we are to be honest, that we should again think of the possibility of what it might mean to practice medicine befitting our convictions as Christians or Jews. Yet, there is a heavy price to be paid for the development of such a medical practice, as it may well involve training and going to doctors whose technology is less able to cure and sustain us than current medicine provides. But, then, we must decide what is more valuable, our survival or how we choose to survive.

6. Alasdair MacIntyre, "How Virtues Become Vices: Values, Medicine and Social Context," *Evaluation and Explanation in the Biomedical Services* (Dordrecht: Reidel, 1975), pp. 97-111.

7. For I would not deny that advocates of "person" as the regulatory notion of medical care are right to assume that the notion of person involves the basic libertarian values of our society. It is my claim that such values are not adequate to direct medicine in a humane and/or Christian manner.

52 *Terra es animata:* On Having a Life

Gilbert Meilaender

To live the risen life with God is, presumably, to be what we are meant to be. What can we conclude about our duties to the dying from the medieval belief that we join the hosts of heaven as "animated earth"?

For the past quarter century bioethics has been a booming business in this country. In part that may be because humanists found here a field in which they could compete with scientists for grant money. In larger part, it is surely because medical advance has forced certain problems upon our attention. But, at least in part, it must also be because some of the concerns of bioethics impinge upon everyday life — upon the lives of most people, and at some of the crucial moments of life, in particular birth and death. Bioethics could not have boomed as it has were it not a reflection of some of our central concerns.

I will examine some of the issues that have emerged in bioethical discussions of death, dying, and care for the dying as a way of thinking about what it means to have a life. In particular, I will focus on a concept that has risen to great prominence in our thinking: the concept of a person. Two competing visions of the person — and the relation of person to body — have unfolded as bioethics has developed, and in my view, the wrong one has begun to triumph. We have tried to handle our substantive disagreements on this question by turning to procedural solutions — in particular, advance directives — trusting that they presume no answer to the disputed question. We are, however, beginning to see how problematic such a procedural solution is, how flawed and even contradictory much thinking about advance directives has been. What we need, I will suggest, is to recapture the connection between our person and the natural trajectory of bodily life.

That will be the course of my argument. But, as a way of framing the issues, I begin in what is likely to seem a strange place: with the thought of some of the early Christian Fathers about heaven and the resurrection of the dead. They were attempting to relate the body's history to their concept of the person's optimal develop-

From the *Hastings Center Report* 23, no. 4 (1993): 23-32.

ment. In so doing, they provide a different and illuminating angle from which to see our present concerns.

Patristic Images of the Resurrection of the Body

In his *City of God* Saint Augustine describes the human being as *terra animata,* "animated earth."[1] Such a description, contrary in many ways to trends in bioethics over the last several decades, ought to give pause to anyone inclined to characterize Augustine's thought simply in terms of a Neoplatonic dualism that ignores the personal significance of the body. It may, in fact, be our own constant talk of "personhood" that betrays a more powerful tendency toward dualism of body and self.

This same Augustine, however, found himself puzzled at the thought of the resurrection body. What sort of body will one who dies in childhood have in the resurrection? "As for little children," Augustine wrote, "I can only say that they will not rise again with the tiny bodies they had when they died. By a marvelous and instantaneous act of God they will gain that maturity they would have attained by the slow lapse of time" (22.14). This is, in fact, a question to which a number of the Church Fathers devoted thought.[2]

Origen, for example, understood that throughout life our material bodies are constantly changing. How, then, can the body be raised? He appealed (in good Platonic fashion) to the *eidos,* the unchanging form of the body. Despite the body's material transformations, its *eidos* remains the same as we grow from infancy, through childhood and adulthood, to old age. (For Origen this *eidos* is not the soul; it is the bodily form united with the soul in this life and again in the resurrection. J. N. D. Kelly comments that Origen was charged with having held that resurrected bodies would be spherical; he may have held such a view, in keeping with the Platonic theory that a sphere is the perfect shape.)

From there it is not a long step to suppose that since the *eidos* of each resurrected body will be perfect, it will in every instance be identical in qualities and characteristics. Thus, Gregory of Nyssa, though differing from Origen in some respects, held that in the resurrection our bodies will be freed from all the consequences of sin — including not only death and infirmity, but also deformity and difference of age. This is a view not unlike Augustine's. Bodies may have a (natural) history, but the bodily form is unchanging. That form is the human being at his or her optimal stage of development, the person as he or she is truly meant to be (I write "he or she" not simply to conform to current canons but because Augustine, for example, took trouble to note that the sexual distinction — but not the lust which, in our experience, accompanies it — would remain in the resurrection. All defects would be removed from the resurrected body, but "a woman's sex is not a defect" [*CD* 22.17]. And although intercourse and childbirth will be no more in the resurrection, "the female organs . . . will be part of a new beauty." This is perhaps what C. S. Lewis had in mind when he wrote of the resurrection: "What is no longer needed for biological purposes may be expected to survive for splendour."[3]

Against Origen's notion that the resurrected body would be a purely spiritual *eidos,* Methodius of Olympus held that the body itself — not just its form — would be restored in the resurrection. He based his claim less on a developed philosophical argument than on the resurrection of Jesus, who was raised in the same body that had been crucified (complete, we may recall, with the nail prints in his hands).

Such issues continued to occupy the attention of theologians for centuries to come. For Saint Thomas, the form of the body is the rational soul, and the body reunited with that soul in the resurrection need not reassume all the matter that had ever been its own during temporal life. Rather, as Thomas suggests in the *Summa contra gentiles,* the resurrected man "need assume from that matter only what suffices to complete the quantity due."[4] The "quantity due" is whatever is "consistent with the form and species of humanity." This means that if one had died at an early age "before nature could bring him to the quantity due," or if one had suffered mutilation, "the divine power will supply this from another source" (4.81.12). Saint Thomas is emphatic — against what may have been Origen's view — that our risen bodies will not be purely spiritual. Like Christ's they will have flesh and bones, but in these bodies there will not be "any corruption, any deformity, any deficiency" (4.86.4). Nor, it appears, will there be differences of age; for all will rise "in the age of Christ, which is that of youth [young adulthood], by reason of the perfection of nature which is found in that age alone. For the age of boyhood has not yet achieved the perfection of nature through increase; and by decrease old age has already withdrawn from that perfection" (4.88.5).

Modern Images of the Resurrection

At least to my knowledge, this sort of speculation becomes much rarer after the Reformation — perhaps because Protestants were less inclined to go beyond biblical

1. St. Augustine, *De civitate Dei,* trans. Henry Bettenson (New York: Penguin Books, 1972), 20.20. Future citations will be given by book and chapter number within parentheses in the body of the text.

2. For much of what follows about the early Fathers I draw upon J. N. D. Kelly, *Early Christian Doctrines* (New York: Harper & Row, 1960), pp. 464-79. I am indebted to Robert Wilken for drawing my attention to Kelly's discussion.

3. C. S. Lewis, *Miracles* (New York: Macmillan, 1947), p. 166.

4. Saint Thomas Aquinas, *Summa contra gentiles,* trans. Charles J. O'Neil (Notre Dame: University of Notre Dame Press, 1975), 4.81.12. Future citations will be given by book, chapter, and paragraph number within parentheses in the body of the text.

warrants, even when an intriguing and potentially significant question beckoned. In the fifteenth and last of his charity sermons, Jonathan Edwards does say of heaven: "There shall be none appearing with any defects either natural or moral."[5] And more recently Austin Farrer has approached these questions by asking how it is possible for us to "relate to the mercy of God beings who never enjoy a glimmer of reason."[6] If there never was a speaking and loving person, Farrer asks, where is the creature for God to immortalize? He is less troubled by those who have lost the speaking and loving personhood that once was theirs: God can immortalize them, though Farrer does not tell us whether they are immortalized free of defects or even age differences. But what of those in whom reason never developed? "The baby smiled before it died. Will God bestow immortality on a smile?" Farrer contemplates, without being satisfied by, the possibility that "every human birth, however imperfect, is the germ of a personality, and that God will give it an eternal future" — a speculation not entirely unlike that of some of the early Fathers. And he realizes that there may be some who, though retarded, are not completely without reason — though he never asks, then, what sort of eternal future might be theirs.

If we can overcome both our enlightened bemusement at such speculation and our Protestant refusal to learn from questions that admit of no answer, if instead we enter into the spirit of such questioning, we may find ourselves rather puzzled. Could such a monochromatic heaven really be heavenly? All of us thirty-five-years old, well endowed with (identical?) reasoning capacities? If each of the saints is to see God and to praise the vision of God that is uniquely his or hers, and if the joy of heaven is not only to see God but to be enriched by each other's vision, then why should we not look through the eyes of persons who are very different indeed? Is not the praise of a five-year-old different from that of a thirty-five-year-old, and, again, from that of a seventy-five-year-old? Why should not these distinct and different visions be part of the vast friendship that is heaven? Perhaps it is easier to understand the tendency to eliminate any defects from heaven, but even there, when they closely touch personal identity, we may find ourselves rather puzzled. Edwards was, for example, confident that there would be neither moral nor *natural* defect in heaven. Yet he was willing to grant that friends will know each other there. But if the stump that should have been my leg has shaped the person who I am, the person who has been your friend for forty years, it is hard to know exactly what our heavenly reunion is to be like when the stump is replaced by a perfectly formed leg. "Will God bestow immortality on a smile?" As likely, I should think as that the mother of that child will meet one upon whom God has, in Augustine's words, bestowed in "a marvelous and instantaneous act . . . that maturity they would have attained by the slow lapse of time." We might set against Farrer's view the comment of his fellow Anglican David Smith, who writes that "at the very least it would be hard for Anglicans to hold that a being who might be baptized was lacking in human dignity."[7]

Perhaps I begin to wax too enthusiastic in my own speculations, but the point is worth pondering. To live the risen life with God is, presumably, to be what we are meant to be. It is the fulfillment and completion of one's personal history. To try to think from that vantage point, therefore, is to imagine human life in its full dignity. And to try, however clumsy the speculation, to adopt this vantage point for a moment is to think about what it means to have a life. The questions I have been considering invite us to think about our person, our individual self. Does it have a kind of timeless form? A moment in life to which all prior development leads and from which all future development is decline? A moment, then, in which we are uniquely ourselves? Or is our person simply our personal history, whether long or short, a history inseparable from the growth, development, and decline of our body?

There is some reason to think — or so I shall suggest in what follows — that much contemporary thought in ethics has a great deal in common with Origen. In an age supposedly dominated by modes of thought more natural and historical than metaphysical, we have allowed ourselves to think of personhood in terms quite divorced from our biological nature or the history of our embodied self. In the words of Holmes Rolston, our "humanistic disdain for the organic sector" is "less rational, more anthropocentric, not really *bio*-ethical at all," when compared to a view that takes nature and history into our understanding of the person.[8] Or, put in a more literary vein, the view I will try to explicate is that expressed by Ozy Froats in Robertson Davies's novel, *The Rebel Angels*. Froats, a scientist, is discussing his theories about body types with Simon Darcourt, priest and scholar. Froats believes there is little one can do to alter one's body type, a dismaying verdict for Darcourt, who had hoped by diet and exercise to alter his tendency toward a round, fat body. Froats says of such hopes:

> To some extent. Not without more trouble than it would probably be worth. That's what's wrong with all these diets and body-building courses and so forth. You can go against your type, and probably achieve a good deal as long as you keep at it. . . . You can keep in good shape for what you are, but radical change is impossi-

5. Jonathan Edwards, *Works*, vol. 8, *Ethical Writings*, ed. Paul Ramsey (New Haven: Yale University Press, 1989), p. 371.

6. Austin Farrer, *Love Almighty and Ills Unlimited* (Garden City, N.Y.: Doubleday & Company, 1961), p. 166. For his discussion more generally, see the Appendix, "Imperfect Lives," pp. 166-68.

7. David H. Smith, *Health and Medicine in the Anglican Tradition* (New York: Crossroad, 1986), p. 10.

8. Holmes Rolston III, "The Irreversibly Comatose: Respect for the Subhuman in Human Life," *Journal of Medicine and Philosophy* 7 (1986): 337-54.

ble. Health isn't making everybody into a Greek ideal; it's living out the destiny of the body.[9]

Terra es animata.

Ozy Froats's notion of having a life is not, however, the vision that seems to be triumphing in bioethics. And, to the degree that developments in bioethics both reflect and shape larger currents of thought in our society, those developments merit our attention.

Contra Ozy Froats

The language of personhood has been central to much of the last quarter century's developments in bioethics. It was there at the outset when, in 1972, in the second volume of the *Hastings Center Report,* Joseph Fletcher published his "Indicators of Humanhood: A Tentative Profile of Man." The language had not yet solidified, since Fletcher could still use "human" and "person" interchangeably. But the heart of his view was precisely that which would, in years to come, distinguish clearly between the class of human beings and the (narrower) class of persons.

Among the important indicators (by 1974 Fletcher would declare it fundamental[10]) was "neo-cortical function." Apart from cortical functioning, "the *person* is non-existent." Having a life requires such function, for "to be dead 'humanly' speaking is to be ex-cerebral, no matter how long the body remains alive." And, in fact, being a person has more to do with being in control than with being embodied. Among the indicators Fletcher discusses are self-awareness, self-control (lacking which, one has a life "about on a par with a paramecium"), and control of existence ("to the degree that a man lacks control he is not responsible, and to be irresponsible is to be subpersonal"). Human beings are neither essentially sexual nor parental, but the technological impulse *is* central to their being. ("A baby made artificially, by deliberate and careful contrivance, would be more *human* than one resulting from sexual roulette.")

Even if, in the briskness with which he can set forth his claims, Fletcher makes an easy target, he was not without considerable influence — and it may be that he discerned and articulated where bioethics was heading well before the more fainthearted were prepared to develop the full consequences of their views. Certainly the understanding of personhood that he represents is very different from Augustine's "animated earth" or Ozy Froats's sense that one must live out the destiny of the body. Views of that sort have generally been labeled "vitalism," and their inadequacy assumed.

This is especially evident in our attitude toward death and toward those who are dying. To confront our own mortality or that of those we love is to be compelled to think about our embodiment and about what it means to have a life.[11] How we face death, and how we care for the dying, are not just isolated problems about which decisions must be made. These are also occasions in which we come to terms with who we are, recognizing that we may soon be no more. The approach of death may seem to mock our pretensions to autonomy; at the least, we are invited to wonder whether wisdom really consists in one last effort to assert our autonomy by taking control of the timing of our death. Contemplation of mortality reminds us that our identity has been secured through bodily ties — in nature, with those from whom we are descended; in history, with those whose lives have intertwined with ours. We are forced to ask whether the loss of these ties must necessarily mean the end of the person we are. Such issues, fundamental in most people's lives, have been involved in arguments about how properly to care for the dying, as we can see if we attempt to bring to the surface two contrasting views within bioethics about what it means to have a life.

Having a Life: View 1

For some time the distinction between "ordinary" and "extraordinary" care dominated bioethical discussions of care for the dying. It provided categories by which to think about end-of-life decisions. When this language began to be widely used — and, indeed, it did filter quite often into ordinary, everyday conversation — its chief purpose was a simple one. The perception, in many ways accurate, was that patients needed moral language capable of asserting their independence over against the medical establishment. They needed to be able to have ways of justifying treatment refusals, ways of resisting overly zealous — even if genuinely concerned — medical caregivers. A widespread sense that patients found themselves confronting a runaway medical establishment lay behind arguments that "extraordinary" or "heroic" care could rightly be refused and that no one had a moral obligation to accept such care. Over against a runaway and powerful medical establishment, this language sought to restore a sense of limits and an acceptance of life's natural trajectory. The language proved inadequate, however, meaning too many different things to different people. But it was not simply inadequate; it was also a language that did not, taken by itself, lend stature to the increasingly prominent concept of personhood. And that concept has been used to broaden significantly the meaning of "useless" or "futile" treatment, by divorcing the person from the life of the body.

In recent years we have seen a spate of articles seeking to define futility in medical care. Care that is futile or use-

9. Robertson Davies, *The Rebel Angels* (New York: Penguin Books, 1983), pp. 249ff.

10. Joseph Fletcher, "Four Indicators of Humanhood: The Enquiry Matures," *Hastings Center Report* 4, no. 6 (1974): 4-7.

11. I have discussed this from another angle in chapter 8 of *Faith and Faithfulness* (Notre Dame: University of Notre Dame Press, 1991).

less has in the past been considered "extraordinary" and could be refused or withheld. But what do we mean by futility? Years ago, when I was younger and more carefree, I used to enjoy going out at night in the midst of a hard snowstorm to shovel my driveway. In a sense, this was far from futile, since its psychological benefits were, I thought, considerable. But if the aim was a driveway clear of snow, it was close to futile. Well before I had finished, if the snow was coming hard, the driveway would again be covered. Sometimes I'd do it again before coming in, though aware that those inside were laughing at me. But if the goal was a driveway clear of snow, it just could not be accomplished, no matter how hard I worked while the snow was falling. "In Greek mythology, the daughters of Danaus were condemned in Hades to draw water in leaky sieves. . . . A futile action is one that cannot achieve the goals of the action no matter how often repeated."[12]

This sense of futility we all understand, even if we realize that it may be difficult to apply with precision in some circumstances. Thus, for example, the comatose person (unlike the person in a persistent vegetative state) is reasonably described as "terminally ill." Because the cough, gag, and swallowing reflexes of the comatose patient are impaired, he or she is highly susceptible to respiratory infections and has a life span usually "limited to weeks or months."[13] Because these reflexes are not similarly impaired in the PVS patient, he or she may live years if nourished and cared for. It makes sense, therefore, to describe most medical care for the comatose person as futile, and we understand readily, I think, the language of futility in that context. It is not as obvious, however, that the same language is appropriate in referring to the PVS patient.

Recent discussions make clear that, in light of such problems, "futility" has gradually come to mean something else — and something quite different. If the sense of futility described above is termed "quantitative" (referring to the improbability that treatment could preserve life for long), a rather different sense of futility is now termed "qualitative." Thus, some have argued, treatment that preserves "continued biologic life without conscious autonomy" is qualitatively futile.[14] It is effective in keeping the earth that is the body animated — effective, but, so the argument goes, not beneficial because what is central to being a person cannot be restored.

How ambivalent we remain on these questions becomes evident, however, when we contrast that view with a recent article, "New Directions in Nursing Home Ethics."[15] The authors argue that the standard view of autonomy that has governed so much of our thinking about acute care in the hospital context is not applicable to the nursing home patient. There we need a new notion of "autonomy within community." This may not be the best language to make their point, however, since the authors want to do more than just envision the person within his community of care. They are also concerned to see his medical condition, his chronic needs, his dependence, as internal to the person. Thus, they seek a

> notion of moral personhood that is not abstracted from the individual's social context or state or physical and mental capacity. . . . For now the caring constitutes the fabric of the person's life . . . and the reality of the moral situation is that the person must embrace dependency rather than resisting it as a temporary, external threat.

The aim here is no longer to fend off the threat external to this person and return the patient to an autonomous condition; instead, the aim is to rethink autonomy, to take into it a loss of self-mastery, to accept dependence in order "to give richer meaning to the lives of individuals who can no longer be self-reliant." Perhaps we might even say that the aim is to help the chronically ill person live out the destiny of the body.

How can it be, in essentially the same time and place where this argument is put forward, that we should be moving rapidly away from such an understanding of the person in so many discussions of "futile" medical care? When Dr. Timothy Quill assisted his patient Diane to commit suicide, he did it, he said, to help her "maintain . . . control on her own terms until death." The hands are the hands of Dr. Quill, but the voice is that of Joseph Fletcher, an increasingly powerful voice in our society.

Having a Life: View 2

Around the time that Fletcher was publishing his indicators of humanhood, one of the other great figures in the early years of the bioethics movement, also a theologian, was writing that the human being is "a sacredness in the natural biological order. He is a person who within the ambience of the flesh claims our care. He is an embodied soul or an ensouled body."[16] In those words of Paul Ramsey the vision of the human being as *terra animata* was forcefully articulated. As "embodied souls" we long for a fulfillment never fully given in human history, for the union with God that is qualitatively different from this life — which longing can never, therefore, be satisfied by a great quantity of this life. But as "ensouled bodies" our lives also have a shape, a trajectory, that is the body's. Our identity is marked, first, by the bodily union of our parents, a relationship that then gradually takes on a history. We are a "someone who" — a someone who has a history — and though we may long for that qualita-

12. Lawrence J. Schneiderman, Nancy S. Jecker, and Robert R. Jonsen, "Medical Futility: Its Meaning and Ethical Implications," *Annals of Internal Medicine* 112 (June 1990): 949-54.

13. E. Cranford, "The Persistent Vegetative State: The Medical Reality (Getting the Facts Straight)," *Hastings Center Report* 18, no. 1 (1988): 27-32.

14. Schneiderman et al., "Medical Futility," p. 952.

15. Bart Collopy, Philip Boyle, and Bruce Jennings, "New Directions in Nursing Home Ethics," special supplement, *Hastings Center Report* 21, no. 2 (1991): 1-16.

16. Paul Ramsey, *The Patient as Person* (New Haven: Yale University Press, 1970), p. xiii.

tively different fulfillment, we never fully transcend the body's history in this life. To come to know who we are, therefore, one must enter that history.

It is a history that may be cut short at any time by accident or illness, but in its natural pattern it moves through youth and adulthood toward old age and, finally, decline and death. That is the body's destiny. As Hans Jonas has suggested, we exist as living bodies, as organisms, not simply by perduring but by a constant encounter with the possibility of death.[17] We constantly give up the component parts of our self to renew them, and our continued life always carries within itself the possibility that these exchanges may fail us. Eventually we are worn down, unable any longer to manage the necessary exchanges. The fire goes out, and we are no longer "animated" earth.

To point to some moment in this history as the moment in which we are most truly ourselves, the vantage point from which the rest of our life is to be judged — not just another of the many moments in which we are persons, but a moment at which, presumably, we have personhood — is to suppose that we can somehow extricate ourselves from the body's natural history, can see ourselves whole. It is even, perhaps, to suppose that in such a moment we are rather like God, no longer having our personal presence in the body.

It is not too much to say that two quite different visions of the person — Fletcher's and Ramsey's — have been at war with each other during the three decades or so that bioethics has been a burgeoning movement. But it is equally clear that one view has begun to predominate within the bioethics world and perhaps within our culture more generally. Among the peculiarities of our historicist and purportedly antiessentialist age is the rise to prominence of an ahistorical and essentialist concept of the person. On this view, it is not the natural history of the embodied self but the presence or absence of certain capacities that makes the person. Indeed, we tend to think and speak not of being a person but of having personhood, which becomes a quality added to being. The view gaining ascendancy does not think of dependence or illness as something to be taken into the fabric of the person and lived out as part of one's personal history. It pictures the real person — like Origen's spherical *eidos* — as separate from that history, free to accept or reject it as part of one's person and life. Moreover, to be without the capacity to make such a decision is to fall short of personhood.

This view is not required by any of the standard approaches to bioethical reasoning or any of the basic principles (such as autonomy, beneficence, and justice) so commonly in use. What we do with such principles depends on the background beliefs we bring to them. Those benefits determine how wide will be the circle of our beneficence and whether our notion of autonomy will be able to embrace dependence. The problems we face lie less with the principles than with ourselves. We have lost touch with the natural history of bodily life — a strange upshot for *bio*ethics, as Holmes Rolston noted. How wrong we would be to suppose that ours is a materialistic age, when everything we hold central to our person is separated from the animated earth that is the body.

Embodied Souls sans Competence

It might be, however, that I have overlooked something important. If in some cases we judge care futile when the capacity for independence is gone, and if in other cases of chronic illness we take the need for continual care into the very meaning of personal life, perhaps — one might suggest — the difference lies in what different people want, how they choose to live. One patient chooses to live on; another sees no point in doing so. Hence, the key is autonomous choice, which remains at the heart of personhood. All we need do is get people to state their wishes — enact advance directives — while they are able. Then, if the day comes when others must make decisions for them, we will not have to delve into disputed background beliefs about the meaning of personhood. We will have a procedure in place to deal with such circumstances.

In the wider sweep of history, living wills are a very recent innovation, but the debate about their usefulness or wisdom coincides with the quarter century in which bioethics has grown as a movement.[18] And when we are told that, within a month after the Supreme Court's *Cruzan* decision, 100,000 people sought information about living wills from the Society for the Right to Die, we can understand that this is not an issue for specialized academic disciplines alone. The term "living will" was coined in 1969, and the nation's first living will law (in California) was passed in 1976 — prompted, it seems, by the Karen Quinlan case. By now most states have enacted laws giving legal standing to living wills, and in 1991 the federal Patient Self-Determination Act went into effect, requiring hospitals to advise patients upon admission of their right to enact an advance directive. In a relatively short period of time, therefore, the idea of living wills (and other forms of advance directives, such as the health care power of attorney) seems to have scored an impressive triumph. If we have no substantive agreement on what it means to be a person or have a life, the living will offers a process whereby we can deal with substantive disagreement. Each of us autonomously decides when our life would be so lacking in personal dignity as to be no longer worth preserving, and we pretend that such a process masks no substantive vision of what personhood means.

But it does, of course. Such a procedural approach

17. Hans Jonas, "The Burden and Blessing of Mortality," *Hastings Center Report* 22, no. 1 (1992): 34-40.

18. For the historical information that follows I rely upon George J. Annas, "The Health Care Proxy and the Living Will," *NEJM* 324 (25 April 1991): 1210-13.

brings with it a certain vision of the person: to be a person is to be, or have the capacity to be, an autonomous chooser, to take control over one's personal history, determining its bounds and limits. This substantive view turns out to have a life of its own and — we are beginning to see — can lead in several quite different directions. For a time, perhaps, all choices of once autonomous patients are honored. You choose to die when your ability to live independently and with "dignity" wanes; I choose to live on even when my rational capacities are gone. Each of us is treated as we have stipulated in advance. But then a day comes — and, indeed, is upon us — when the vision of the person hidden in this process comes to the fore.

The Paradox of Autonomy

If the person is essentially an autonomous chooser, then we will not forever be allowed to choose to live on when our personhood (so defined) has been lost. Living wills had, for the most part, been understood as a means by which we could ensure that we were not given care we would no longer have wanted, care that preserved a life regarded as subpersonal and no longer worth having. But in principle, after all, the process could be used to other ends. One could execute a living will directing that everything possible be done to keep oneself alive, even when one's "personal" capacities had been irretrievably lost. What then?

In a case somewhat like this, Helga Wanglie's caregivers answered that question by seeking a court order to stop the respirator and feeding tube that were sustaining her life. Mrs. Wanglie was an eighty-seven-year-old woman who, because of a respiratory attack, lost oxygen to her brain. She did not recover and remained in a persistent vegetative state. Although the costs of her care were covered by the family's insurance policy, the hospital still sought permission to remove life support. In some relatively minor ways, her case does not fit perfectly the hypothetical situation I considered above, for she had no living will. What she had, though, was a husband who was her guardian and who refused to consent to the withdrawal of treatment, believing she would not have wanted him to do so. Also, the medical caregivers went to court challenging her husband's suitability as guardian, rather than directly seeking court approval to terminate treatment.[19] But as Alexander Morgan Capron notes, when the caregivers first announced their intention to go to court, they stated that "they did not 'want to give medical care they described as futile.'"

Thus, in the Wanglie case, at least in the minds of the caregivers, personhood defined in terms of the right autonomously to determine one's future gave way to personhood defined in terms of the present possession of certain capacities.[20] For those who lack such rational capacities, further care is understood as futile — whatever they might previously have stipulated while competent. Similarly, when Schneiderman and his colleagues develop their "qualitative" understanding of futility, they make clear its impact on cases like this one. "The patient has no right to be sustained in a state in which he or she has no purpose other than mere vegetative survival; the physician has no obligation to offer this option or services to achieve it."[21] Ironies abound here. At the heart of the bioethics movement has been an assertion of personal autonomy for patients, which was, of course, ordinarily understood as ensuring their ability to be rid of unwanted treatment. But having built autonomy into the center of our understanding of personhood, having indeed (after *Roe v. Wade)* claimed that such autonomy flows from our right of privacy and may be asserted on our behalf even by others when we are unable to assert our wishes, having used patient autonomy as a hammer to bludgeon into submission paternalistic physicians, we suddenly rediscover the responsibility of physicians to consider what is really best for the patient, to make judgments about when care is futile. We suddenly do an about-face. Against past autonomous patient choice for continued treatment even after "personhood" has been lost, we now assert medical responsibility not to provide present care that is "futile."

Helga Wanglie's caregivers and those who would assert a "qualitative" notion of personhood are both right and wrong — though not in the ways they suppose. They are right in that there is no reason to think that my physicians should forever be bound by what I stipulate (when I am forty-five and in good health) about my future care. That is, they are right in thinking that autonomy alone is far too thin an account of the person and that physicians must concern themselves with patients' best interests, not just their requests or directives. But they are wrong in supposing that care for me becomes futile simply because I have irretrievably lost the higher human capacities for reasoning and self-awareness. They are also confused; for the vision of the person guiding them where they are right is incompatible with the vision of the person at work where they are wrong. In supposing that care for me becomes futile when I have lost my powers of reason (even though I may not be terminally ill), they express a vision of the person that divorces personhood from organic bodily life. They decline to take into their understanding of the person defect, dependence, or disability. But in judging that caregivers need not be bound forever by directions I have stipulated in advance, when my condition was quite different from

19. Alexander Morgan Capron, "In Re Helga Wanglie," *Hastings Center Report* 21, no. 5 (1991): 26-28.

20. My distinction here bears some similarities to James Childress's distinction between autonomy as an end state and autonomy as a side constraint. Cf. his *Who Should Decide? Paternalism in Health Care* (New York: Oxford University Press, 1982), p. 64.

21. Schneiderman et al., "Medical Futility," p. 952.

what it has now become, they accept the need to live out the body's history, and they decline to give privileged status to the person's existence at one earlier moment in time.

Rethinking the *Eidos*

If we could develop an increased sense of irony about the course the bioethics movement has taken, we might be well positioned to think about the important questions for everyday life with which it here deals. The ironies are a clue to our confusions. Is it not striking that just at the moment when the idea of living wills seems to have triumphed, when federal law has required hospitals to make certain we know of our right to execute an advance directive, bioethicists should begin to wonder whether living wills are not themselves problematic? Having gotten what we thought we wanted — a law undergirded by a certain vision of the person — we begin to discern problems.

Thus, for example, John A. Robertson has had "Second Thoughts on Living Wills."[22] There are, he notes, spheres of life in which we do not hold a person to an understanding he or she had previously stated. We do not, for example, hold surrogate mothers to contracts. Yet, we are reluctant to recognize that when Meilaender becomes incompetent — severely demented, let us say — his interests may well shift. We prefer to suppose that his person was complete and perfect at some earlier point in his development — when, say, at age forty-five he executed a living will. We hesitate to consider that what the forty-five-year-old Meilaender thought should be done to and for a demented Meilaender may not be in the latter's best interest. His life circumstances have changed drastically; he has become more simply and completely organism and less neocortex. If we would care for him, we must take that into account. And if we do not take it into our reckoning, if we blindly follow whatever directions the forty-five-year-old Meilaender gave, it is not clear that we can really claim to have the best interests of *this* patient — the Meilaender now before us — at the center of our concern.

Something like that is Robertson's argument, and it makes good sense. For it essentially denies that we should think of the person as a perfect *eidos* captured at a moment in time, and, less directly, it invites us to think of the person as a someone who has a history, as animated earth. But that is not really Robertson's intent. He sees that the living will has become essentially "a device that functions to avoid assessing incompetent patient interests," but his real aim is to encourage us to take up "the difficult task of determining which incompetent states of existence are worth protecting." This can only land him back in the muddle from which he is trying to escape. He is back to thinking of personhood as something added to existence — and well on his way, therefore, to the conception of personhood that gave rise to an emphasis on autonomy, which in turn suggested the living will as a useful way to exercise our autonomy, which — or so he thinks — is a path strewn with "conceptual frailties." He wants us not to live out the destiny of the body but to escape it.

Life as "Someone Who"

To have a life is to be *terra animata,* a living body whose natural history has a trajectory. It is to be someone who has a history, not a someone with certain capacities or characteristics. In our history this understanding of the person was most fully developed when Christians had to make sense of the claim that in Jesus of Nazareth both divine and human natures were joined in one person.[23] Christians did not wish to say that there were really two persons (two sets of personal characteristics) in Christ; hence, they could not formulate his personal identity in terms of capacities or characteristics. They could speak of his person only as an individual with a history, a "someone who." The personal is not just an example of the universal form; rather, the general characteristics exist in and through the individual person. And we can come to know such persons only by entering into their history, by personal engagement and commitment to them, not by measuring them against an ideal of health or personhood.

Perhaps such an understanding of the person is also available to us through reflection upon our life as embodied beings. "Embodiment is a curse only for those who believe they deserve to be gods." If Origen's account of the resurrected body seems to have lost much of what we mean by embodiment, he had at least this excuse: he genuinely believed that God intended to make humankind divine. That bioethics — and our culture more generally — is in danger of losing the body in search of the person is harder to understand, unless in our own way we believe that we deserve to be gods.

James Rachels, arguing that ethics must and can get along quite well without God, has recently distinguished between biological and biographical life, arguing that only the second of these is of any value to us.[24] Biological life has instrumental value, since apart from it there is no possibility of realizing biographical life, but biological life without the possibility of self-consciousness and self-control can be of no value to us. In such a state we no longer have any interest in living, and we cannot be harmed if our life is not preserved.

22. John A. Robertson, "Second Thoughts on Living Wills," *Hastings Center Report* 21, no. 6 (1991): 6-9.

23. I have discussed this point more fully (and acknowledged my indebtedness for it to Oliver O'Donovan) in *Faith and Faithfulness,* pp. 45-47.

24. James Rachels, *Created from Animals: The Moral Implications of Darwinism* (New York: Oxford University Press, 1990), pp. 198ff.

Perhaps, though, such arguments do not take seriously enough the *terra* of which we are made. What Rachels never explains, for example, is why one's period of decline is not part of one's personal history, one's biography. As John Kleinig suggests, "Karen Ann Quinlan's biography did not end in 1975, when she became permanently comatose. It continued for another ten years. That was part of the tragedy of her life."[25] From zygote to irreversible coma, each life is a single personal history. We may, Kleinig notes, distinguish different points in this story, from potentiality to zenith to residuality. But the zenith is not the person. "Human beings are continuants, organisms with a history that extends beyond their immediate present, usually forward and backward. What has come to be seen as 'personhood,' a selected segment of that organismic trajectory, is connected to its earlier and later phases by a complex of factors — physical, social, psychological — that constitutes part of a single history."

Indeed, it is not at all strange to suggest that even the unaware living body has "interests." For the living body takes in nourishment and uses it; the living body struggles against infection and injury. And if we remember "the somatic dimensions of personality, as expressed for instance in face and hands,"[26] we may recognize in the living body the place — the only place — through which the person is present with us. This does not mean that the person is "merely" body; indeed, in such contexts the word "merely" is always a dangerous word. As bodies we are located in time, space, and history; yet, we also transcend that location to some degree. Indeed, from the Christian perspective with which I began, it is right to say that, precisely because we are made for God, we indefinitely transcend our historical location. But it is as embodied creatures that we do so, and our person cannot be divorced from the body and its natural trajectory. This is not vitalism; it is "the wisdom of the body" (p. 358). It is the wisdom to see that every human life is a story and has a narrative quality — a plot to be lived out. That story begins before we are conscious of it, and, for many of us, continues after we have lost consciousness of it. Yet, each narrative is the story of "someone who" — someone who, as a living body, has a history.

Caught as we are within the midst of our own life stories, and unable as we are to grasp anyone else's story as a single whole, we have to admit that only God can see us as the persons we are — can catch the self and hold it still. What exactly we will be like when we are with God is, therefore, always beyond our capacity to say. But it will be the completion of the someone who we were and are, and we should not, therefore, settle for any more truncated vision of the person even here and now.

25. John Kleinig, *Valuing Life* (Princeton: Princeton University Press, 1991), p. 201.

26. Rolston, "Irreversibly Comatose," p. 352.

53 Who/se We Are: Baptism as Personhood

Keith G. Meador and Joel James Shuman

I. The Moral Significance of Personhood

The attempt to arrive at some consensus on precisely what qualifies a human as a person represents one of the more persistently debated and widely significant issues in modern biomedical ethics. The attribution of personhood has been and continues to be a powerful tool in moral discourse, especially at what Paul Ramsey called the "edges" (i.e., the beginning and the end) of life (1978). This is probably because it offers those humans so designated a special, protected moral status. By designating others "persons," we indicate that they are "one of us," by which we typically mean that they are entitled to a particular level of respect and care. Consequently, we believe, there are certain things we may not do to them or allow others to do to them, at least not without their informed consent — a notion about personhood which itself embodies a multitude of assumptions, including autonomy and rationality, which become problematic at some of the above described edges of life.[1]

Biomedical and bioethical debates about personhood seem especially morally significant in late modernity. It is no secret that recent trends in biomedical technology — especially in neonatology, genetic research and organ transplantation — lend these debates a certain urgency. But it is also the case that our attempts to formally articulate universally agreed upon criteria for personhood represent some of the last vestiges of the hope that we can achieve substantial moral agreement in an otherwise morally fragmented world.

At first glance, it appears that in recent years a nearly universal consensus on the issue of personhood has emerged, namely that it exists in an autonomous individual's capacity for a certain level of reflective mental activity. Persons are thinkers, while those humans who for whatever reason cannot think are something other than persons. Yet, as we hope to show in this essay, it is by no means clear that such criteria are so plausible, universally acceptable or morally useful as those who advocate them claim they are.

1. See, for example, Moody (1992).

From Keith G. Meador and Joel James Shuman, "Whose We Are: Baptism as Personhood," *Christian Bioethics* 6.1 (Apr 2000): 71-83. Used by permission.

In what follows we want to argue that, from the perspective of certain strands of the Christian tradition, all bioethics grounded in attempts to develop formal, objective criteria by which we may designate a given individual a person are misguided.[2] Criteria centering on the possession of reflective mental capacity, moreover, are for Christians especially problematic. We suggest that there are no morally neutral ways of designating personhood. All of the criteria we use to designate others persons — including the ostensibly neutral, "scientific" criterion that suggests human personhood consists in minimal reflective mental activity — are historically and morally particular. They are dependent on and emerge from historically contingent narrations of the sorts of things that constitute normal human being and rationality, along with the social practices within which those narrations are embedded.[3] The particularity of these so-called "scientific" accounts, moreover, at least raises the question — which we will address in the second half of this essay — of whether and to what extent they are commensurable with accounts derived from and dependent upon certain strands of the Christian tradition and that tradition's narration of what it means to be a person.

Consider, for example, the work of H. Tristram Engelhardt, Jr. in the second edition of his *Foundations of Bioethics.* The matter of which humans count as persons occupies a central place in Engelhardt's project; he argues that in the public realm of content-less, secular medical ethics, a certain individual, reflective moral *competence* is necessary before a human may rightly be named a person:

> Persons, not humans, are special — at least if all one has is general secular morality. Morally competent humans have a central moral standing not possessed by human fetuses or even young children. It is important to understand the nature of these inequalities in some detail, for physicians and medical scientists intervene in numerous ways in the lives of adult humans, children, infants, fetuses, and laboratory mice. . . . In summary, all persons can envisage *the notion of the peaceable (moral) community.* Insofar as they act in accord with this notion, despite inequalities in intelligence, power, and wealth, they participate with others in *the peaceable (moral) community* (1996, pp. 135 and 137).

Engelhardt's account of personhood is especially helpful from the perspective we want to develop in this essay. It illustrates nicely the ways in which the criteria proposed for personhood by the principals in these various debates are based in particular, historically contingent accounts of human rationality and language that are dependent on and embedded in particular politics, narratives and social practices.[4] For Engelhardt, the politics, narratives and practices in question are those of the procedural liberalism characterizing the modern democratic nation-state, which he sees as a last bastion of universal moral order in an otherwise fragmented and chaotic world. Participation in the procedural state requires that its individual members have the capacity to choose for themselves and to pursue a particular way of life. This capacity to choose a way of life is what makes them persons.

The designation of those with certain reflective mental capacities as persons is thus for Engelhardt one significant step in the establishment of a content-less secular bioethics within which "tolerance, liberality and prudence" are the cardinal virtues (1996, p. 419). Engelhardt makes it clear in the Preface to the second edition of the *Foundations* that as a Christian, he is not satisfied with the sufficiency of such a content-less secular bioethics and its corresponding account of personhood. Nevertheless, he believes it is important to develop a minimalist account of "morality among strangers" (1996, pp. vii-xii). A world such as the contemporary United States, constituted by competing individual self-interests, must be governed by such a morality. For where relationships are understood primarily in contractual terms, the ability to negotiate and to act on one's own behalf and to regard others as so enabled is clearly an advantageous attribute. Apart from the possession of that ability, one is dependent on others in a way that is not conducive to one's flourishing in a world of competing self-interests.

We are more than a little suspicious that Engelhardt's ostensibly content-less secular bioethics is probably not so morally neutral as he supposes. This is especially the case with his account of personhood, which is very much the product of a historically particular understanding of normal human being and rationality that has its origins in the earliest strands of modernity. An implied assumption of self-sufficiency and self-interest and a denial of ongoing mutual interdependence are inherent to this perspective, which is inextricably bound up with particularly modern notions of individual autonomy and competitive political economy (Asad, 1993, pp. 69-70). What is especially problematic about this account, moreover, is the way it denies its own particularity by claiming to be universal and scientifically objective. In so doing, it *de facto* renders implausible other accounts that do not share its assumptions.

2. Quite apart from the Christian account we suggest here, we are inclined to agree with Carl Elliot, who suggests that the "theoretical sensibility" underlying the personhood debates is problematic. Elliot claims that our thinking about personhood is morally significant because we believe that "we can figure out what to do in this case if we can just get straight what a person is. That is, we know how to treat a person so if we decide that this marginal being is a person, . . . then a conclusion about how we should morally treat that marginal being will logically follow" (Elliot, 1999, p. 159).

3. We would stress that this does not necessarily mean that there are not better or worse — or more or less truthful — ways of narrating and accounting for what makes us persons. It means simply that there are no objective (i.e., neutral) criteria for adjudicating between these views.

4. For two quite different defenses of this claim, see Rorty (1979) and MacIntyre (1988).

II. Personhood as Reflective Mentation

The idea that some humans possess a quality or set of qualities called 'personhood' which are properly and exclusively a function of individual reflective mentation has its clearest expression, if not its contemporary origins, in the work of the late Joseph Fletcher. Fletcher's arguments, like those of Engelhardt, seem to be based on the assumptions of certain strands of Enlightenment thought. He presumes first that a human being is essentially and properly mental, and as such is other than and independent of human embodiment. Human reason, moreover, is properly autonomous and cannot rightly be infringed upon. Fletcher argued, beginning in a landmark 1972 essay, that "rights (such as survival) attach only to persons" (Fletcher, 1998, p. 37).[5] Moreover, he said, "out of some twenty criteria one (neocortical function) is the cardinal or hominizing trait upon which all other human traits hinge. . . . To be truly *homo sapiens* we must be sapient, however minimally" (p. 38).[6]

The consequences of this view of personhood are developed (and are altogether consistent with Fletcher's arguments as outlined above) by Mary Anne Warren in her 1973 essay 'On the Moral and Legal Status of Abortion' (Warren, 1998 [1973]). In that article Warren argues that the termination of a pregnancy is morally permissible only if we understand that "a fetus is not a person, and hence not the sort of entity to which it is possible to ascribe full moral rights" (p. 169). She suggests that personhood exists in the possession of a cluster of five traits, each of which is clearly a function of autonomous individual rationality. These include consciousness, reasoning, self-motivated activity, the capacity to communicate, and the presence of self-concepts and self-awareness. It is these traits, she explains, "which are most central to the concept of personhood, or humanity in the moral sense" (p. 178).

III. The Politics and Practices of Personhood as Reflective Mentation

Warren's remarks about the significance of her proposed criteria for personhood offer an especially good insight concerning the politics and practices of such criteria. On the one hand, she appears to deny that her criteria *have* political origins; she asserts that all that is necessary in order to show that a fetus is not a person

> is that any being which satisfies *none* of [the five traits] is certainly not a person. I consider this claim to be so obvious that I think anyone who denied it, and claimed that a being who satisfied none of [the traits] was a person all the same, would thereby demonstrate that he had no notion at all of what a person is — perhaps because he had confused the concept of a person with that of genetic humanity (p. 178).

Thus, Warren contends that the criteria by which we designate others persons are simple matters of fact. She goes on, however, to consider what would happen in the rare instance someone *might* disagree with her account. In such a case, she suggests, "[w]e would probably have to admit that our conceptual schemes were indeed irreconcilably different, and that our dispute could not be settled objectively." Yet, she also claims that such a disagreement is unlikely to occur, "since I think that the concept of a person is one which is very nearly universal" (p. 178).

What is most significant about the closely related accounts of personhood offered by Warren and Fletcher is not simply that they share the fundamental assumptions of modern political philosophy and of the social, political and economic practices with which those assumptions are intertwined. Rather, it is that they assume that the accounts they offer are self-evidently true. By suggesting that there is a human essence that self-evidently and universally consists in an individual's capacity for reflection and inward representation, they deny a very important point, which is that the ascription of personhood is fundamentally social, and as such is dependent upon the practices of some particular society. As Richard Rorty puts it, personhood is "a matter of decision rather than knowledge, an acceptance of another being into fellowship rather than a recognition of a common essence" (1979, p. 38). How this acceptance is mediated and communicated depends upon the particular identity of the community of fellowship and its traditions of membership and acknowledgement of personhood.

IV. The Social and Narrative Nature of Personhood

The criteria we use to ascribe to others the attribute of personhood are in this view as much a function of the way we identify ourselves as the way we identify others. Indeed, suggests Alasdair MacIntyre, these two are largely inextricable. Self-identification is to a significant extent a matter of narration; narrative is in this sense "the basic and essential genre for the characterization of human actions" (1981, p. 208). We make sense of our lives only as we see them situated within one or more of a series of stories we tell about ourselves, our relationships to others, and our place in the world (MacIntyre, 1981, pp. 206-207). Marya Schechtman describes this "reciprocity" inherent in a narrative account of personhood, saying:

5. Fletcher's (1998) essay was first published in the *Hastings Center Report* in December, 1975, and was drawn largely from an earlier essay of his entitled 'Medicine and the nature of man' in the November, 1972 issue of the same periodical.

6. It is interesting to note the circularity inherent in the last sentence of this quotation. Certainly, Fletcher is in some sense correct to claim that *Homo sapiens* are necessarily sapient. A more significant and interesting question, in our minds, is whether *Homo sapiens* is an accurate characterization of the human "essence" or, to put it differently, whether it is even right to suggest that humans have an "essence."

> Personhood, it might be said, is an intrinsically social concept. To enter into the world of persons an individual needs, roughly speaking, to grasp her culture's concept of a person and apply it to herself. It is this recognition which leads to the constraints on an identity-constituting narrative — to be identity defining an individual's self-narrative must conform in certain crucial respects to the narrative others tell of his life (1996, p. 95).

When we understand our lives in this way — as being situated within and made intelligible by various narratives — we discover that while we are both agents in and authors of these narratives, we are neither the sole authors nor the single characters. Both of these are significant factors in the development of our moral agency, for "what the agent is able to do and say intelligibly as an actor is deeply affected by the fact that we are never more (and sometimes less) than the co-authors of our own narratives" (Schechtman, 1996, p. 213). Our lives are often beyond our control; thus, we often may find ourselves in the position of simply telling and retelling, rather than authoring, the stories of our lives (Frank, 1995, p. 176).

Our fellow authors and the other characters in our stories, whether our friends or enemies, are those to whom we are most likely to understand ourselves bound morally. These are the people whom we are most likely to think of as "persons," since "I am forever whatever I have been at any time for others — and I may at any time be called to answer for it — no matter how changed I may be now" (Frank, 1995, p. 217). Consequently, there is never a point in our lives when we can claim to be free from past or present obligations to others. Anthony Thiselton refers to the work of Paul Ricoeur to suggest this interdependence of the narratives that constitute our lives with our accountability to those with whom we share these narratives:

> Whereas for Decartes, for Locke and for Hume, either there are ideas, objects or essences, or there is nothing; for Ricoeur, by contrast, narrative opens up the notion of an entity who acts and suffers within a framework of continuity and change through the changes and continuities of time. Human action seems to carry with it not only initiation of change, which may rebound in changing the self, but also a continuity of accountability as the action of this self. Narratives bring out this feature clearly. We trace the inscribing of actions and events on characters and even of physical appearance and social status (1995, p. 73).

So while it is certainly true that we can narrate our lives and the lives of others as being essentially rational, autonomous, and self interested, it is worth asking whether and to what extent that narration is true or useful. By narrating the world in a way that enumerates our right to existence and the existence of others based on a capacity for mentation, we are creating a world in which persons are essentially isolated from one another. We need to ask ourselves whether that is the world in which we really live and are most likely to flourish. We believe it is not, and in order to show this, we need critically to revisit certain aspects of modern political philosophy.

V. Autonomy or Interdependence?

Characteristic of the intellectual project from which the modern account of personhood is drawn is the assertion that human reason, and hence human identity and agency, are fundamentally and properly autonomous. In this view, our lives are essentially and properly independent of the lives of others, and the practices constituting the ways we live together serve (rightly) to form us in precisely this way. One of the more significant tenets of contemporary liberal political philosophy is that we each need to be left free and unfettered to choose individually the way of life that is best *for each of us.* John Rawls, who is perhaps the best known and most thoughtful defender of the liberal position, argues that since "no general moral conception can provide a publicly recognized basis for a conception of justice," then individuals must "conceive of themselves and one another as having the moral power to have a conception of the good" (1985, pp. 225 and 240). This power tends to be non-discursive, in that for each individual "the good is what is *for him* the most rational long-term plan of life given reasonably favorable circumstances. A man is happy when he is more or less successfully in the way of carrying out this plan. To put it briefly, the good is the satisfaction of rational desire" (1971, pp. 92-93).

Yet the view of human being presumed by this so-called "rational choice theory" is problematic, if not self-deceptive. By suggesting that our relations to one another are freely chosen and have their basis either in the expectation of mutual advantage or in a kind of freely chosen, affective sympathy, rational choice theory ignores the ways in which all humans are at all times fundamentally interdependent (MacIntyre, 1999, pp. 114-115). As Alasdair MacIntyre explains, "What is or would be good or best for me is something on which, apart from the fact that generally and characteristically I know more about myself than others do, I may in many and crucial respects be no more an authority than some others and in other respects a good deal less of an authority than some others" (1999, p. 71).

By asserting the near universality of human interdependence we do not intend to conflate the very real differences in the various ways in and extents to which we require one another's participation in our lives in order to flourish. Certainly there are profound differences in human dependence. Some of these clearly are functions of mental capacity, while others are reflections of developmentally contingent interpersonal patterns (Cushman, 1995). Yet, the simple existence of these differences is not justification in itself for saying that those who are more dependent are less persons. Ascribing personhood to a particular class of human beings based solely on their capacity for autonomous mentation is problematic, in that it is a rather arbitrary denial of the fact that as finite, embodied thinkers whose lives are by nature subject to a wide variety of contingencies, "there is a scale of disability on which we all find ourselves" (MacIntyre, 1995, p. 73).

However, this is an interesting claim only within a society of persons who understand their lives to be constituted in part by goods held in common. In such a society, the interests of those who cannot speak for themselves will be represented by proxies committed to speaking for them in the name *of* the common good (MacIntyre, 1995, pp. 129-130). To suggest that some humans are not persons simply because they are unable to represent themselves is not simply to deny that we are all to greater or lesser degrees dependent. It is also to assert that our personal identities are unable to withstand those fluctuations in our levels of dependence that are inherent in our being embodied social animals (MacIntyre, 1995, pp. 73-74, 94, and 99-100).

VI. Toward a Christian Politics of Personhood

Of course, it is one thing to suggest that an account of personhood as reflective mentation is problematic because it fails to account for normal human interdependence, and it is another thing to envision an alternative account. Standard individualistic accounts of personhood presuppose and arise from a politics that calls attention to and gives priority to individual autonomy. Similarly, any alternative account that is to be viable must describe a politics that calls attention and gives priority to human interdependence. We would suggest that the church possesses in its liturgy the resources for such an account.

We are thinking here especially of the Christian practices of baptism and eucharist. The baptismal liturgy calls Christians to think in a radically different way about themselves, and their obligations to and dependence upon one another. From the perspective of baptism, autonomy and self-interest, rather than dependence, are anomalous. Jean Elshtain suggests that the work of Augustine offers an especially appropriate treatment of these matters by offering a relational, socially contingent understanding of what makes one a person that provides a strong antidote to the modern equation of self with self-interest and self-esteem. "Augustine," she says, "shifts the ontology of the self, relocates the self in a transformed understanding, and moves toward a self that is no longer dominated by a need to dominate, nor bound by the immediacy of desire" (1995, p. 11). The baptized self is a self transformed, a self who no longer has to strive to secure its own existence, a self who is afforded new possibilities for life with God and others (Elshtain, 1995, pp. 124-125).

Baptism transforms the body of the individual, making it a member of the one Body of Christ. This transformation of being subverts the primacy given the individual in contemporary societies. The liturgy helps accomplish this by reminding those participating that their lives are no longer their own, but gifts from God to be received as such. The voice of a community saying to the newly baptized, "We receive you into the household of God. Confess the faith of Christ crucified, proclaim his resurrection, and share with us in his eternal priesthood" (*Book of Common Prayer,* 1979, p. 308), is a call to personhood in its richest form. It embodies a narrative of reception, witness, and sharing with a full acknowledgement of our utter dependence on the other for our present communion as well as our eschatological vision of hope for the future.

The practice of infant baptism and the overtly political language of the baptismal liturgy indicate how this practice might affect the way we tend to think about the moral status of those we typically regard as less than persons, such as embryos, "defective" neonates, mentally retarded children and adults, and the demented elderly. By baptizing infants and others who are unable to "speak for themselves" into the care and fellowship of the community, the church is acknowledging that they are nothing less than persons. Their identity as persons, moreover, because it is based more in the church's practices of baptism and eucharist and what those practices imply than in their capacity for reflective mentation or productivity, exists without respect to who they were or who they might have become apart from their baptism. Their identity is not given prior to or apart from their participation in the life of a community in which "the members who seem to be weaker are indispensable" and in which all "have the same care for one another" (1 Cor. 12:22, 25, NRSV).

Roberta Bondi suggests how baptism may be lived out through eucharistic hospitality to the "weaker members" by speaking about the Christian life as friendship with God and others. She says, "becoming friends of God means we are to love what God loves, we need to bear in mind that God loves people . . . we must also come to yearn for the things God yearns for, including the well-being of the people with whom, left to ourselves, we would rather not share the kingdom" (1991, p. 124). Personhood embodied within a mutually interdependent covenant community necessitates the practice of radical eucharistic hospitality. Inevitably, there are those with whom "we would rather not share the kingdom," but when we understand that we share with them our very being as we claim a shared friendship with God, our understanding of them — and of their undesirability — is transformed. They have become us and we them.

A claim so radical as this — that "they have become us and we them" — is not arbitrary. It flows from the way Christians understand their place in a world created in the image of the triune God. The liturgical imagery suggesting that those who share a baptism and who gather together around the eucharistic table also in some sense share with one another their personhood is simply an expression of the Christian conviction that in baptism human identity has been taken up into and now participates in the identity of the triune God who reveals himself to us as Father, Son, and Holy Spirit. To say that God is Trinity is to say that God exists *as* the continual, mutual interrelationship of the three divine persons. Thus just to the extent we understand ourselves to participate in the life of God, we also understand ourselves to exist in relationship, not simply to God, but to one another as well. For the Christian, "*to be* and *to be in relation* become identical" (Zizioulas, 1985, p. 89).

David Ford depicts this sense of the complementary and reciprocal nature of the life of the Trinity — and hence of the baptismal-eucharistic community — in his imaginative evocation of the ancient comparison of the life of God to a perpetual dance. Dancing, he says, suggests the overflowing and overwhelming dynamic of the love of God. He describes the "internal relationship" and "utter mutuality in dynamic life" of the love expressed through and within the Trinity as an embodiment of the radical hospitality of invitation to personhood found within the baptized community of the Church (1997, p. 194). The invitation to the feast does not stipulate the level of cognitive function and mentation necessary for participation. Rather, it suggests that our "sense of self" derives from our participation in the community of those with whom we share baptism.

We have claimed that the Christian practices of baptism and eucharist constitute individual humans as persons without regard for their capacity for mental reflection or productivity. Such a claim begs for a thick description, such as David Keck provides in his book *Forgetting Whose We Are: Alzheimer's Disease and the Love of God* (1996). There Keck argues that the baptismal communion of saints means, among other things, that the personhood of the cognitively limited and the frail who are no longer productive may in certain instances come to rest almost totally within the community. He suggests that it is possible to understand those who no longer have the individual capacities we typically understand to be necessary for faithful discipleship as being nonetheless faithful and thus still being fully persons. This is possible, he says, because there are others in the community who can be faithful on their behalf. When discussing how a person with Alzheimer's disease might be engaged in Christian practices of preparing for death and of dying well, he says:

> The Christian communities of the patients have to do the dying for them. Just as a person is baptized in the presence of the entire church and just as the congregation may be asked to assume religious responsibilities for the babe, so too may Alzheimer's caregivers rightly ask that a congregation accept responsibility for helping the person die well. As in infant baptism, the powerlessness of babe (or here, the patient) is just as we all are before God. Responsibilities for our families' bodies and persons can be total, and *having responsibility for* is inseparable from *being one with* (1996, p. 139).

The Christian community must remember and tell the stories of baptism and eucharistic hospitality when the cognitively impaired patient can no longer do so for herself. In so doing, the community is *being a person for* the cognitively impaired member, a being-for that extends even to the point of death.

VII. Conclusion

This essay does not constitute anything like a fully alternative account of personhood, nor does it necessarily refute in any definitive way the strengths and the occasional judicious usefulness of the personhood-as-mentation criteria. We have sought merely to draw attention to the fact that these criteria are to a significant extent determined by social and political practices, and that because viable alternative practices exist, so do viable alternative accounts of what makes us persons.

References

Asad, T. (1993). *Genealogies of Religion: Discipline and Reasons of Power in Christianity and Islam,* Johns Hopkins Press, Baltimore.

Book of Common Prayer (1979). Seabury Press, Seabury, Connecticut.

Bondi, R. (1991). *To Pray and to Love,* Fortress Press, Minneapolis.

Cushman, P. (1995). *Constructing the Self: Constructing America: A Cultural History of Psychotherapy,* Addison-Wesley Publishing, Reading, Massachusetts.

Elliot, C. (1999). *A Philosophical Disease,* Routledge, New York.

Elshtain, J. B. (1995). *Augustine and the Limits of Politics,* University of Notre Dame Press, Notre Dame.

Engelhardt, H. T., Jr. (1996). *Foundations of Bioethics,* second edition, Oxford University Press, New York.

Fletcher, J. (1998 [1975]). 'The cognitive criterion of personhood,' in *Classic Cases in Medical Ethics,* G. E. Pence (ed.), McGraw Hill, Boston, pp. 35-41.

Ford, D. (1997). *The Shape of Living,* Baker Books, Grand Rapids.

Frank, A. (1995). *The Wounded Storyteller,* University of Chicago Press, Chicago.

Keck, D. (1996). *Forgetting Whose We Are: Alzheimer's Disease and the Love of God,* Abingdon Press, Nashville.

MacIntyre, A. (1999). *Dependent Rational Animals: Why Humans Need the Virtues,* Open Court, Chicago.

MacIntyre, A. (1988). *Whose Justice? Which Rationality?* University of Notre Dame Press, Notre Dame.

MacIntyre, A. (1981). *After Virtue,* second edition, University of Notre Dame Press, Notre Dame.

Moody, H. (1992). *Ethics in an Aging Society,* Johns Hopkins Press, Baltimore.

Pence, G. E. (ed.). (1998). *Classical Cases in Medical Ethics,* McGraw-Hill, Boston.

Ramsey, P. (1978). *Ethics at the Edges of Life,* Yale University Press, New Haven.

Rawls, J. (1985). 'Justice as fairness: Political not metaphysical,' *Philosophy and Public Affairs* 14 (3), 223-251.

Rawls, J. (1971). *A Theory of Justice,* Harvard University Press, Cambridge.

Rorty, R. (1979). *Philosophy and the Mirror of Nature,* Princeton University Press, Princeton.

Schechtman, M. (1996). *The Constitution of Selves,* Cornell University Press, Ithaca.

Thiselton, A. (1995). *Interpreting God and the Postmodern Self: On Meaning, Manipulation and Promise,* Eerdmans, Grand Rapids.

Warren, M. A. (1998 [1973]). 'On the moral and legal status of abortion,' in *Classic Cases in Medical Ethics,* G. E. Pence (ed.), McGraw Hill, Boston, pp. 169-182.

Zizioulas, J. (1985). *Being as Personhood,* St. Vladimir's Seminary Press, Crestwood, New York.

CHAPTER EIGHT

Embodiment

For millennia, Western culture has toyed with a dualistic view of the self, where the mind or spirit or soul is radically distinct from the body and material reality. Plato's distinction between the sensible, material world and the realm of forms or ideas provides one metaphysical home for this dualism. And much of Hellenistic philosophy associated the mind or soul with that which is pure and immortal but regarded the body as mortal, driven by needs and desires, and dirty or even evil.

While the extent of its influence is debated, Hellenistic dualism is evident in some Christian theology from the Middle Ages onward. It is also evident in some forms of extreme asceticism, which severely deprecate the body, and in the various forms of Gnosticism, which view the immortal soul as trapped in the body. Indeed, this Hellenistic influence is still visible when contemporary Christians too easily talk about the body as destined for the grave but the soul for heaven.

Dualism emerges in more modern forms in the Enlightenment when René Descartes talks about the body as a machine and Immanuel Kant makes a distinction between the realms of phenomena and noumena. And as Lisa Sowle Cahill points out (selection 57) and Gerald McKenny implies (selection 56), some such dualism is likely at work when much of modern science and medicine sees nature or the body simply as raw material for choice and intervention via technology. Dualism also rears its head when advertisers depict our bodies as infinitely malleable to our desires, when media programmers suggest that watching endless hours of violence has no impact on what kind of people we become, and when pornographers suggest that their focus on body parts and sexual acts leaves the people involved untouched.

The biblical material offers a different, more unified view of the self and of the material world. The material world is created good, and the human person *(nephesh, soma, sarx)* is more of a unified whole than a mere composite of body and soul. We are dust into whom the breath of life has been breathed (Genesis 2:7). In Christ, the Word is made flesh (John 1:14). Ultimate redemption is anticipated in the resurrection of the body (Romans 6:5); physical healing is seen as a sign of the kingdom of God (Luke 7:18-23); Paul refers to the church as a body (Romans 12:5) and reminds us that our bodies are temples for the Holy Spirit (1 Corinthians 6:19). What Lisa Sowle Cahill says about the Gospels is true of Christian Scripture as a whole: "one finds, if anything, an anti-dualism about the body."

We are embodied selves. Every aspect of our encounter with the world and with other people is in and through our bodies. We experience the world through our bodies. We express ourselves — our personality, character, beliefs, and so on — in and through our bodies. And when something happens to our bodies, whether it be a kiss or a broken arm, it happens to us.

Yet, we are not "only" or "just" our bodies. The subject or person is not reducible to his or her body. We have a sense of our bodies as "mine." I direct and will "my body" to act in specific ways, to go specific places, to communicate specific things. When something like amputation happens to "my body," I do not stop being me just because my body has been radically altered. Moreover, in situations of illness we can feel betrayed by our bodies; indeed, the body can seem like a foreign "other." And Christians believe that God hangs onto us after death in anticipation of resurrection, a resurrection where our new bodies experience both continuity and discontinuity with our current bodies (1 Corinthians 15:48-58). We are embodied selves, but we are not reducible to our bodies.

Given the nature of medicine, one could argue that nearly every essay in this volume wrestles with the relationship between the self and the body. The works in this section do so explicitly. The opening poem — "Ode on a Plastic Stapes" by Chad Walsh (selection 55) — helpfully raises many issues surrounding embodiment, including the continuity and discontinuity we anticipate in the resurrection. The works by Gerald P. McKenny, Lisa Sowle Cahill, and Wendell Berry (selections 56, 57, and 58) provide historical background and theoretical reflections. Allen D. Verhey and Courtney S. Campbell (selections 59 and 60) then move us to consider the specific issue of organ transplantation.

In "Bioethics, the Body, and the Legacy of Bacon" (selection 56), Gerald McKenny describes what he calls the Baconian project, "the unquestioned commitment to technological control of the body for the sake of eliminating 'misery and necessity.'" According to McKenny, much of contemporary medicine and bioethics subscribes to this project, which began in the Enlightenment. McKenny charges that this project is both theoretical and moral. A mechanistic view of nature and aspirations to the technological control of the body, views that assume the separation of subject from the body, are combined with the modern era's fundamental moral commitments to the relief of suffering and maximization of choice. Lost in this mix is any sense of the role of health, illness, suffering, and finitude within the broader projects of a good moral life and a good society.

By contrast, McKenny suggests that a biblically grounded Christian view would follow St. Paul in refusing to separate subject from body. This view recognizes that embodiment carries the risk of suffering and sin but that it also offers the possibility of redemption and resurrection. From this perspective, suffering, finitude, and bodily imperfection can be part of life's larger moral project, which includes the body as a location of moral and spiritual practices. Moreover, this understanding of embodiment would redirect medical resources: less emphasis on cure, more on comfort care, pain relief, and nursing care; less emphasis on achieving the perfect body, and greater recognition of the moral worth of those who have lost independence or control of body.

Lisa Sowle Cahill's essay, "'Embodiment' and Moral Critique: A Christian Social Perspective" (selection 57), is instructive in several ways. First, she reminds us of the long history of dualism in Western tradition, ranging from the ancient suspicion of the body as the enemy of rational control and unmediated truth to the modern vision of the body as raw material for choice intervention, exercised via technological and instrumental rationality.

Second, she offers examples that show that Christianity is neither intransigently dualistic nor negative about the body but instead offers a positive, integrated approach to the body.

Third, Cahill resists not only a body/soul dualism but also a dualism between self and society. Understanding the self as intrinsically social, Cahill contends that one's self-understanding and social agency always reflect and reinforce social organization. Drawing especially on Michael Foucault and Mary Douglas, Cahill contends that "freedom never exists outside of some social vision; the communal vision which shapes bodily experience also brings the self's embodiment to consciousness, to expression, and to social agency." Since we are embodied, social selves, our experiences and interactions with the world, as well as our understanding of our own bodies, are shaped by society and its vision of the world. But this social process of bodily formation need not be negative, says Cahill. Indeed, a "biblically authentic Christian social vision is characterized by inclusiveness and solidarity, especially toward enemies and toward marginalized and outcast persons and groups." The values and vision of the encompassing social order are often characterized by hierarchy and domination, but Cahill discerns in Christian sources a shaping of the body that functions as a countersign of solidarity and equality.

Interestingly, Cahill claims that an authentic Christian view of the embodied self shifts medical priorities, much as it does for McKenny. Here too there is a vision of inclusive health care that recognizes the inevitability of suffering and death and frames bodily health in relationship to other personal, spiritual, and social goods. Here too is a vision where vulnerability and dependency are partially constitutive of human selfhood and need not be denied or hidden.

In "Health Is Membership" (selection 58), Wendell Berry sees two kinds of dualism at work in modern Western medicine. The first dualism is suggested by the metaphor of the body as machine. Berry suggests that this metaphor is discernible by noting that in the hospital setting it is difficult to rest, the food is often unpleasant, and the costs are extraordinarily high. Rest is important to embodied selves, but not to machines. Food can be something that brings pleasure and healing to an embodied self, but for machines it is simply fuel to be injected. And while cost is surely important if we are concerned about access for everyone, health care is often marketed as another industrial product.

The second dualism is between what Berry calls the "world of efficiency" and the "world of love." This is a dualism between the way we lovingly attend to a specific person in all of his or her history and particularity and the way that medicine (partially of necessity) works from percentages, mechanistic understandings, abstraction, efficiency, and specialization. In the world of efficiency, we can reduce much to percentages — for example, this drug works for 99 percent of people. But the world of love always wants to ask about the 1 percent. In the world of love, people are not reducible to percentages or interchangeable as parts. Intriguingly, Berry suggests with a story that this divide might be partially bridgeable by simple acts of loving attention, such as noticing that what someone might need most is a hug.

Interestingly, the title of Berry's essay is itself a challenge to a kind of dualism — that between self and community. As Berry points out, to be healthy involves being whole, and, as children fortunate enough to be surrounded by love know, "wholeness is not just the sense of completeness in ourselves but also is the sense of belonging to others and to our place; it is an unconscious awareness of community." Thus, a dualism between self and community is a kind of division or dis-ease, and belonging or membership (in the right kind of community) is central to wholeness or health.

Moving to the issue of transplantation, Allen Verhey's "Organ Transplants: Death, Dis-organ-ization, and the Need for Religious Ritual" (selection 59) focuses on the continuity and discontinuity between persons and their mortal remains. Because we are embodied selves, because we are not reducible to minds or disembodied souls or ghosts, there exists a continuity between the person and his or her mortal remains that requires that all due respect be exercised in the retrieval of organs. But because we are not reducible to our bodies, there is also a discontinuity between persons and their mortal remains that allows for transplantation.

Because embodied selves are necessarily social selves, Verhey also calls attention to communal integrity. Much of the ambiguity surrounding transplantation is due to the people left to grieve, due to the relationships that are dis-membered by the loss. The respect owed to the mortal remains is in part owed to those who are grieving. The person who died was a part of relationships, and those relationships should be honored. So too, those who grieve not only need their autonomy respected; they also need people who will stand with them in the loss. They likewise need community and rituals that respect both the continuity between the mortal remains and the person and the discontinuity that death inevitably brings. As communal, embodied events, rituals can acknowledge the hard realities of death and the ambiguities of transplantation; they can provide coping mechanisms and can even help frame the proper context for transplantation.

Courtney Campbell's essay, "Harvesting the Living?" (selection 60), focuses on proposals to address the chronic problem of organ scarcity by modifying the dead donor rule and/or support pre-mortem organ retrieval. Campbell critiques these proposals from several angles, starting with a review of how public surveys on these topics are misused. Campbell's discussion here ultimately forces the question of the extent to which morally normative judgments or public policy should be based on public opinion, itself garnered from surveys.

Campbell also picks out the technological imperative at work in these discussions of transplantation. Campbell charges that the imperative of transplantation technology is so compelling that scholars want society to "change the criteria for the determination of death again, or permit medical professionals to take the lives of those who are not dead by any standard." This charge about the technological imperative resonates with McKenny's and Cahill's claims of the dualism at work in aspirations to the technological control of the body as raw material for choice intervention. Indeed, Campbell specifically views attempts to revise "the dead donor rule to accommodate neocortical criteria for death . . . [as presupposing] an essentialist conception of the person as a disembodied consciousness."

Campbell connects with McKenny and Cahill on another front as well: his final argument about the chronic scarcity of organs for transplantation is that it should prompt us to revise the distribution of medical resources. Rather than a greater focus on life extension technologies, we need a shift to more equitable access to health care and preventative services. The "solution" to organ scarcity is not to give in to the technological imperative; instead, as a matter of justice, we need to refocus on an equitable distribution of health care resources.

Embodiment is at stake in all of medical practice. The essays here put our embodied nature front and center. They ask us to consider the relationship between the self and body. They also challenge us to attend to the various dualisms that are often at work in Western culture and medicine, and they invite a reprioritizing of medical resources.

SUGGESTIONS FOR FURTHER READING

Cahill, Lisa Sowle, and Margaret A. Farley. *Embodiment, Morality, and Medicine* (Dordrecht: Kluwer Academic Publishers, 1995).

Campbell, Alastair V. *The Body in Bioethics* (New York: UCL Press, 2009).

Cherry, Mark J., issue ed. "The Body for Charity, Profit, and Holiness: Commerce in Human Body Parts." *Christian Bioethics* 6, no. 2 (August 2000): Entire Issue (Netherlands: Swets & Zeitlinger).

Davis, Lennard J. *Enforcing Normalcy: Disability, Deafness, and the Body* (New York: Verso, 1995).

Delmonico, Francis L., and Nancy Scheper-Hughes. "Why We Should Not Pay for Human Organs." *Zygon* 38, no. 3 (2003): 689-98.

Frank, Arthur W. *The Wounded Storyteller: Body, Illness, and Ethics* (Chicago: University of Chicago Press, 1997).

Joralemon, Donald, and Phil Cox. "Body Values: The Case Against Compensating for Transplant Organs." *The Hastings Center Report* 33, no. 1 (January-February 2003): 27-33.

Komesaroff, Paul A., ed. *Troubled Bodies: Critical Perspectives on Postmodernism, Medical Ethics, and the Body* (Durham, N.C.: Duke University Press, 1996).

Lysaught, M. Therese. "Vulnerability within the Body of Christ: Anointing of the Sick and Theological Anthropology." In *Health and Human Flourishing: Religion, Medicine, and Moral Anthropology*, ed. Roberto dell'Oro and Carol R. Taylor (Washington, D.C.: Georgetown University Press, 2006), pp. 159-82.

Paris, John J. "Harvesting Organs from Cadavers." *America* 186, no. 14 (April 29, 2002): 9.

Reardon, Patrick Henry, ed. "Forum: Human Harvest. Commerce in Human Body Parts: A Critical Symposium," *Touchstone (U.S.)* 14, no. 5 (June 2001): 28-35.

Toombs, S. Kay. "Taking the Body Seriously." *Hastings Center Report* 27, no. 5 (September 1997): 39.

Toombs, S. Kay. "Vulnerability and the Meaning of Illness: Reflections on Lived Experience." In *Health and Human Flourishing: Religion, Medicine, and Moral Anthropology*, ed. Roberto dell'Oro and Carol R. Taylor (Washington, D.C.: Georgetown University Press, 2006), pp. 119-40.

the modern moral framework is what Taylor calls inwardness (1989, pp. 370-76). Inwardness has deep Augustinian and Cartesian roots, but during the Romantic period it surfaced in the inner conviction of the importance of one's own natural fulfillment. The idea is not only that each individual is unique and original but that this uniqueness and originality determines how he or she ought to live. There is an obligation (more aesthetic than moral) for each person to live up to his or her originality. What follows from this is the importance contemporary moderns place on free self-determination. Together with the ideal of universal benevolence, self-determination also leads to the idea of the subject as bearer of rights of immunity and entitlement. From this follow expectations that the expansion of the reign of technology over the body should be accompanied by, and in fact should make possible, the expansion of the reign of human choice over the body, and that medicine should enable and enhance whatever pattern of life one chooses.

Taylor argues that the Victorian era brought together these Enlightenment and Romanticist trends and bequeathed them to us — along with a view of history as a story of moral progress over our forebears, a progress marked by our greater sensitivity to and eradication of suffering and our greater latitude for human choice (1989, pp. 393-96). This view enabled the Victorians to be convinced of their moral progress over the age of religion even as it enables their successors in this century to be convinced of their moral superiority over the Victorians. As a result, medicine is based on practices and techniques of control over the body rather than on traditions of wisdom about the body. The task of public policy is to negotiate rights of immunity and entitlement rather than to determine the place of health, illness, and medical care in a well-lived and responsible life and in a good community. Traditional moral injunctions that limit or inhibit what medicine can do appear arbitrary, but there is no broader framework to evaluate and criticize the commitments of modern medicine. In the absence of such a framework the commitment to eliminate all suffering combined with an imperative to realize one's uniqueness leads to cultural expectations that medicine should eliminate whatever anyone might consider to be a burden of finitude or to provide whatever anyone might require for one's natural fulfillment. This does not mean that individual conceptions of this burden or this fulfillment are necessarily arbitrary. But it does mean that modern moral discourse provides no vocabulary with which to deliberate about what makes some such conceptions better or worse than others.

This brief sketch of modern moral discourse allows us to identify the major cultural values that standard bioethics draws upon and expresses in its agenda and content. The connection of these values to the Baconian project helps explain the silence of standard bioethics on questions that challenge that project. Moreover, it shows us how this discourse, with its new ways of conceptualizing and objectifying the body and nature, and its new moral valuations, makes it impossible for the moral questions and insights of the discourse of traditional ways of life to gain a hearing. In the modern discourse, moral convictions about the place of illness and health in a morally worthy life are replaced by moral convictions about the relief of suffering and the expansion of choice, concepts of nature as ordered by a telos or governed by providence are replaced by concepts of nature as a neutral instrument that is brought into the realm of human ends by technology, and the body as object of spiritual and moral practices is replaced by the body as object of practices of technological control. From this new perspective the moral and practical concerns of traditional discourses are obfuscated, marginalized, or rejected.

However, four points must be made clear. First, I do not believe that there once was a golden age when medical care was grounded in a robust view of the good or that individual choices now are necessarily arbitrary. Nor do I believe that it is possible or desirable to reverse the technological revolution in medicine and simply return to traditional ways of life. Still less do I believe that publicly enforced consensus about these matters is possible or desirable. On the contrary, efforts to retrieve tradition must take account of the advantages of technology. My argument is the more modest one that modern moral discourse provides no vocabulary with which to deliberate about the meaning of corporeality, what moral purposes the body serves, what goods health should serve, or what limits the control of our bodies by technology should observe. Hence it allows for no discussion of what kinds of suffering should be eliminated, what kinds of choices human beings should make, and what role technology should play in all of this. Second, I do not argue that a commitment to the methods, theories, or principles of standard bioethics entails an explicit endorsement of the Baconian project. But neither is standard bioethics neutral with regard to that project. Negatively, the rejection of all substantive judgments about the moral meaning of bodily life and the ends technological control over the body should serve eliminates any in-principle objection to the Baconian project. Positively, standard bioethics fosters commitments to the elimination of suffering and the expansion of human choice within the moral constraints set by modern moral theories. Third, my account simply identifies some features of the modern moral framework and does not do justice to the rigor with which some bioethicists have articulated and balanced these features. Finally, I do not wish to imply that none of the concerns of standard bioethics are valid or that the alternative I suggest can do without some of these concerns.

Nevertheless my account allows for two conclusions that highlight the obstacles any challenge to standard bioethics must face. First, in regard to technology, it shows how the reign of technology expresses, and is perhaps in part produced by, the deepest moral commitments of modernity: the commitments to eliminate suffering and expand the range of human choices. If I am right about this, modern technology does not render traditional moralities obsolete or call for a new morality so much as it expresses and carries out an existing (modern) morality. Nor does it merely signal a will to dominate nature that levels all moral values and leads to nihilism, as many humanist and existentialist critics of technology charge. Rather, modern technology is surrounded and infused by a certain kind of moral purpose. That this was the case for early prophets of technology is clear to Albert Borgmann in his summary of the projects of Francis Bacon and René Descartes.

> The main goal of these programs seems to be the domination of nature. But we must be more precise. The desire to dominate does not just spring from a lust of power, from sheer human imperialism. It is from the start connected with the aim of liberating humanity from disease, hunger, and toil, and of enriching life with learning, art, and athletics (Borgmann, 1984, p. 36).

Indeed, one of the most characteristic features of technological medicine is the confidence among its practitioners that the elimination of suffering and the expansion of human choice, in short, the relief of human subjection to fate or necessity, are (so long as abuses in implementation are avoided) unambiguous goods whose fulfillment is made possible by technology — a confidence standard bioethics supports and defends. The moral purpose that surrounds technology and the moral confidence it inspires are precisely what make it so difficult to criticize the reign of technology in medicine — a task that would be relatively easy were modern technology simply nihilistic or were the moral purpose it represents unambiguously flawed.

Second, the foregoing account shows why moderns allow medicine to extend its authority over new areas of life. But it offers an additional reason why standard bioethics was able to usurp much of this authority. This reason refers not to the claim of standard bioethics to articulate a common morality in place of a parochial ethic internal to medicine but to its greater success in giving individual persons a sense of control over the powers of medicine. Once again, the challenge to standard bioethics faces a significant obstacle from this perspective. For it is not immediately clear and is difficult to show how standard bioethics has actually failed to give authority and control over technology to individuals rather than to medicine or to society through medicine (as I argue below from a perspective informed by Michel Foucault), or that gaining such control for its own sake is not the ultimate purpose of bioethics.

It is one thing, therefore, to challenge the self-understanding of standard bioethics by pointing out the moral discourse that lends it its agenda, content, and plausibility; it is quite another (and much more difficult) thing to argue that its moral purpose and its understanding of human freedom are inadequate and to argue for an alternative agenda and content for bioethics. Fortunately, as the following section indicates, arguments for such an alternative are as old as the bioethics movement itself.

II. Critics and Alternatives

One set of alternatives to the Baconian project comes from James Gustafson and Hans Jonas, who argue that 1) the Baconian project entails a flawed view of nature and of the relation of humanity to nature, and that 2) modern technology renders the utopian quest for control over nature perilous to humanity and to nature in general. The emphasis on the perils of modern technology in the second point lends a consequentialist flavor to their projects, but their responses to the first point lead them to develop normative conceptions of the human, based on a more adequate understanding of humanity and nature, that extend and qualify the consequentialism and limit technology. Gustafson emphasizes broader and longer-range goods by arguing that both the findings of the sciences and the capacities of modern technology require us to construe human beings as participants in larger human and nonhuman wholes whose well-being is threatened by devotion to human goods pursued in disregard to those larger wholes. Jonas emphasizes an intrinsic good, namely responsibility itself, which arises within and is endorsed by nature itself, and whose possible future existence must be preserved against actions (often supported by ordinary consequentialist calculations) that threaten to turn humanity into a mere product.

Gustafson stands within the ethic of ordinary life which, we have seen, gave rise to the Baconian project. His starting points echo Bacon: humanity is that species which "naturally and properly" extends control over necessity to secure its survival and well-being (Gustafson, 1981, pp. 3-4). Biomedicine, in Baconian fashion, confronts nature as a threat to human survival and well-being that must be overcome (1984, p. 274). However, for Gustafson modern technology requires us to reject the utopian confidence that nature can be reduced to the service of human needs and desires. First, modern technology opens up a huge gap between our technological capacities and our knowledge and control over their far-reaching effects. Second, both science and technology make it clear that the natural world is not ordered only — ultimately nor even primarily — to human survival and well-being. While a Bacon or a John Locke could be confident that God's purposes could be fulfilled by reducing nature to human control and using it, in Locke's terms, "for the Support and Comfort of their being," Gustafson knows that nature does not guarantee such support and comfort, and that if human benefit continues to be the only criterion for intervention the results will likely be catastrophic for human beings and for the rest of nature.

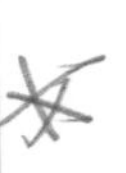

The solution is neither conformity to nature as a fixed order nor control over it for human benefit, but rather participation in the dynamic divine ordering of interdependent wholes (1984, pp. 279-92). Premodern conformity and modern control both yield to a complex determination of the proper ends, scope, and limits of intervention (1984, pp. 298-315). Hence while Gustafson attaches primary moral significance to those points at which interventions into and reorderings of natural, social, and interpersonal processes become possible, this is not because these are the points at which suffering is eliminated and choices are expanded, but because they raise the question of where to draw the fine lines between proper human flourishing and threats to human and other natural wholes. In the case of medicine, this means recognizing the limits to the legitimate needs that can be met by the available resources, taking account in the development and implementation of new kinds of intervention of consequences which affect broader wholes and occur over longer time spans, and accepting the ultimate limits to what medicine can do in the face of death and disease (1984, pp. 272-76).

For Jonas, modern utopianism reverses the ancient priority of *theoria* over *techne:* human perfectibility is no longer found in emulation of a timeless object of contemplation but in human power over the realm of necessity. But modern technology makes this utopianism dangerous. First, the roots of modern technology are in mechanistic science, which by rendering the natural world (ultimately including humanity) both manipulable by human action and neutral with respect to value, made possible control of a nature (including humanity) devoid of any intrinsic norm that would set limits to such control (Jonas, 1974, pp. 45-80). Second, the "dynamics of endless progress" intrinsic to modern technology — its cumulative nature in which each state of progress creates cognitive and material conditions that bring about further progress — ensure that technology will overtake any effort to realize — indeed, even to formulate — any ideal that would direct it (1979; 1984, pp. 126-28). The result is that modern technology is both utopian and nihilistic: it clings to the notion that human perfection is to be realized through progressive control over the realm of necessity while nullifying or surpassing any substantive ideal designed to direct it. In the case of biomedicine it is no longer necessary to spell out, as Bacon and Descartes began to do, the utopia medicine will usher in; it is enough simply to keep pushing the frontiers of life extension, genetic control, forestalling of aging, etc.

This utopianism could radically alter human nature and even turn humanity into a product of our own making. Does human nature demand to be protected against this fate? If so, on what grounds? The task is to identify a certain conception of the human that we have a duty, on the grounds that it is an objective good, to maintain against threats posed to it by our technological power. In a long and complex argument Jonas reconstructs a post-Darwinian, anti-materialist teleology of nature to arrive at the notion of responsibility itself as this good, with the correlative duty (largely but not entirely negative) not to foreclose by technological remaking or by destruction of the natural world the possibility of there being future responsible beings (1984, pp. 25-135).

Gustafson's recognition of intervention into nature as fundamental to human beings and his emphasis on the divine ordering of nature as dynamic entails a more positive stance toward the Baconian project, including a qualified openness to biomedical alterations of human nature, than Jonas, with his concern to preserve humanity as it is and his conviction that nature ratifies this concern, allows. Yet in another sense Gustafson is less Baconian than Jonas, whose chief concern is ultimately anthropocentric. In any case, however powerful their critiques, Gustafson and Jonas share a thin conception of the human which exposes the problem with any effort to oppose the Baconian project by appealing primarily to nature. The problem is that nature itself is too indeterminate a criterion to rule on particular biomedical interventions and, as the alternative paradigms of responsibility and participation indicate, endorses too many versions of the proper stance toward our technological capacities. Gustafson does recognize that it is unreasonable to ask nature alone to provide a conception of the human sufficient to resolve most bioethical issues. But while he rightly points to the need for communities of moral formation and discourse to fill this gap, neither he nor Jonas articulates the convictions and practices that would define such a community and render its moral judgments determinate, nor do they consider that different communities may well have radically different interpretations of nature and its moral significance.

The second set of alternatives to the Baconian Project, those of Stanley Hauerwas and Leon Kass, finds limitations to technological utopianism in the very nature of medicine itself as an inherently moral practice. However, medicine as such a practice is not self-sufficient; it depends either upon a biology and a customary yet reflective morality to determine the kind of human flourishing, with its limitations, at which medicine aims (Kass), or upon a church to sustain by its story-formed virtues the practices of caring that would otherwise, in the face of the inevitable tragedy of human finitude, yield to efforts to eliminate suffering at any cost (Hauerwas).

For both Hauerwas and Kass, medicine is morally committed 1) to the well-functioning of individual patients and 2) to caring for those whom medicine cannot cure or restore. This twofold commitment, moreover, is for both of them derived from the role of medicine in attaining or expressing goods and moral values connected with our embodied life rather than from general moral principles. Hauerwas and Kass differ, however, on which of these two commitments is fundamental, and this difference, I would argue, is grounded in their alternative views of the moral significance of embodiment. For Kass the moral significance of embodiment is found in a life that displays the excellences of embodied life through cultivation of virtues and capacities, and elevates its necessities through custom (as, for example, table etiquette and clothing, respectively, elevate the fundamental dependencies involved in metabolism and the need for protection from the elements) (Kass, 1985, pp. 276-98, 318-45; 1994). Health is either a condition for or is partly constitutive of human flourishing as defined in these terms. Kass therefore begins with health or wholeness as the end of medicine. Given this end, he then recognizes that for individual persons it is realized approximately, under conditions of finitude and vulnerability (1985, pp. 157-246). Hauerwas begins with the opposite point, namely with finitude and vulnerability. Medicine is a tragic profession whose very moral identity, which is found in its commitment to caring for patients when curing is not possible, derives from its limitations. Accordingly, the moral tasks of our embodied life are to determine how our finitude and our subjection to suffering may become part of our moral projects and to care for those whose suffering is pointless and cannot be cured (Hauerwas, 1986, pp. 23-38, 159-81).

From this fundamental difference the key features of their respective accounts follow. For Kass the Baconian project arises from the loss of teleology. Echoing Jonas, Kass argues that the fundamental problem with the Baconian project is its denial of the ethical significance of the natural. The Baconian project is grounded in a modern form of science that seeks to control nature rather than to determine which human aspirations are natural, and in a modern form of ethics that manages our desires and wishes rather than determining which of them represent genuine human aspirations. Modern science and ethics therefore complement each other, and together they remove us from the ordinary understandings of the meaning of embodiment imbedded in our customs and taboos. The results for medicine follow accordingly: the disconnection of our desires and wishes from nature means that medicine is called upon to exert ever greater control over the body in order to fulfill yet more arbitrary wishes and desires. Despite its moral core, medicine is vulnerable to Baconian aims precisely because its knowledge of the meaning of embodiment is only implicit and is thus in need of science and ethics. The antidote to Bacon, then, lies in a biology that articulates the meanings of embodiment and customs that actualize these meanings in institutions and practices.

For Hauerwas the Baconian project follows not so much from the loss of teleology as from the loss of the tragic. The Baconian project denies the tragedy medicine inevitably faces because it deals with beings who are particular, and whose bodies thus do not conform to the relative certainties of a general science, and finite, thus ensuring the ultimate failure of medicine (1977, pp. 184-202). In its denial of the tragic, the Baconian project is for Hauerwas the product of modernity more generally: since moderns have no tradition that enables them to accept tragedy they are unable to find any moral significance in any kind of suffering and therefore call upon medicine to eliminate it all. Bacon and his followers confirm the view that all suffering is pointless and, with their promise to eliminate it by technology, foster illusions about our finitude and subjection to suffering. These illusions about the power of medicine lead to its control over our lives, to the dangerous (because it involves killing those who cannot be cured) and impossible quest for the elimination of disease, and to the abandonment of those whom medicine cannot cure — those who remind us of our own, and medicine's, limitations. In order to resist these forces, medicine is quite radically in need of a particular community (for Hauerwas, the church). First, medicine can restrict itself to the bodily functioning and the care of individual patients only if there are other practices in the community that address the inevitable suffering that accompanies such a restriction. Second, both the demands of care and the pressures to reject and abandon those who remind us of our limitations require a community whose habits embody reconciliation with the suffering other. Third, the role of medicine itself is ultimately determined by a community's understanding of what kinds of suffering fit into its moral projects and how.

There are problems with these projects taken together and separately. First, both overestimate the caring and the contribution to human flourishing that can legitimately be ascribed to medicine. It is both more realistic and ethically more sound, I would argue, to abandon ideals of doctors as gifted with special abilities (or time) to care and special insight into the good, and instead to view medicine as a *techne* which takes its place within a particular community's own forms of caring and is directed to its understanding of the good. (This does not mean, however, that physicians should not be caring people or that they have no role in attainment of the good. Surely physicians should help patients to achieve their goods, determine their capacities for pursuing these goods, and educate them about the likely effects pursuing these goods will have upon their health. In addition, some physicians will, as individuals, also occupy caring roles or be experts in their community's understanding of the good.) Second, Kass seems to think that an adequate account of the proper meaning of embodiment can be found in some entity called "the" western tradition. Hauerwas is right to oppose to this the necessity of a particular community with particular convictions and practices. But, third, Hauerwas tells us very little about the moral projects that at least some kinds of suffering are supposed to serve. A Kassian critique of Hauerwas would rightly insist that a description of these projects requires an articulation of the moral significance of the body that Hauerwas has not yet supplied. In the following section I take a first step toward such an articulation.

The third kind of approach links the Baconian project to a set of discourses and practices regarding the body that, by bringing the body under the seeing eye of clinical-laboratory medical science and the intervening hand of technology, renders it analyzable and manipulable. For these critics, who include Michel Foucault, Drew Leder, and Richard Zaner, the formation of these discourses and practices completed the process initiated by

Bacon and Descartes in which medicine allocates to itself both the problem of human finitude (the subjection of the body to disease, decay, and death) and the task of resolving it. Foucault goes on to show how this same analyzability and manipulability subjects the body to efforts to optimize its capacities and increase its usefulness in accordance with certain interests of modern societies.

Leder and Zaner both begin with the hermeneutical displacement that occurs when the patient's illness narrative is replaced by a disease description. In Zaner's terms, this displacement is grounded in alternative kinds of relation to the body and the substitution of one, the body "in itself" as a material object — a strange body apprehended by and for the Other in a narrative of biological processes — for the other, my lived body which is "for-itself" — my embodied subjectivity narrated in accounts that link illness to various factors in the life-world (Zaner, 1988, pp. 95-97; 1981, pp. 48-50). For Leder and Zaner this hegemony of the body of the Other has dehumanized medicine and rendered it incapable of responding adequately to all but acute conditions, whose causes and cures, unlike those of most conditions, can usually be accounted for in abstraction from the patient's being-in-the-world. Leder and Zaner trace the origin of the body of the Other to Descartes. Zaner argues that Descartes's dualism — not between body and soul but between the ordinary experience of the body (in which the union of body and soul is not problematic) and the body as machine — made possible a scientific basis for anatomy and physiology, which for Descartes require treating the body as an inanimate corpse. He then went on to regard the inanimate corpse as the truth of the body (1988, pp. 115-25). But why privilege the truth of the body as corpse, especially when, according to Zaner, Descartes conceded the superiority for clinical purposes of the body of ordinary experience? The reason, Leder argues, is Descartes's quest for a solution to the existential threats of disease, decay, and death, which he hoped could be met by relegating them to a sphere of objectification and quantification where medical science and technology would eventually eliminate them from humanity (Leder, 1990, pp. 138-41). Hence the result I referred to above, in which medicine gains the authority to formulate and resolve the problem of finitude. In Foucault's terms "health replaces salvation": in place of the spiritual techniques and practices one engaged in when suffering or death was unavoidable, the techniques and practices of medicine aim at eliminating or postponing disease and death (cf. Rose, 1994).

Foucault argues that the body as machine also makes it possible to optimize the capacities of bodies and increase their usefulness, both of individuals and of the society as a whole. Through a wide range of interacting forces — the sciences of medicine and public health, dissemination of health information and advertising, forms of screening and monitoring, etc. — bodies of individuals and populations are now measured against norms related to utility, amenability to profitable investment, capacity for being usefully trained, and prospects of survival, death, and illness (Foucault, 1980, pp. 121-23, 172). By internalizing and acting according to these norms, we come to desire, for ourselves and others, bodies that approximate the norms (1983, p. 208; 1987, pp. 10-11). As a result, modern societies can accomplish through our own choices and desires what they could never have accomplished by force. Eugenics is a case in point. Where eugenic goals once required suppression of the desire of some to procreate, they now operate through stimulation (by health information, advertising, prenatal and neonatal monitoring and screening, and the fear of having an imperfect child in a society that values and constantly measures persons with reference to their usefulness) of the desire for a perfect child.

Leder and Zaner are quite right to draw attention to the role of the body of the Other in the constitution of the subject through the experience of illness and our responses to it. They also help break the hold of the Baconian project by emphasizing that the body of the Other, as that which escapes and thwarts my intentionality, is not merely a product of objectifying science and technology but one way in which the body reveals (often by concealing) itself in experience, thus overcoming the effort to isolate the body of the Other from the subject. But Leder and Zaner are mistaken in believing that the Baconian project can be overcome by reincorporating the body of the Other into the lived body. This belief assumes that the lived body is a genuine expression of embodied selfhood, so that by reorienting medicine to the lived body we recover an essential, nonalienated self as the basis of medical practice in contrast to the alienation of self and the dehumanization of medicine that, they argue, results from the primacy of the body of the Other in Baconian medicine. The problem, as many observers have pointed out, is that the lived body is also marked by the attitudes and practices of one's society or particular way of life. The lived body too is in part a social body, and not a pure expression of self. Medicine oriented to the lived body will still involve techniques of monitoring the body, disciplines, and even the formation of desires and choices — all of which not only express but also form our subjectivity.

This, of course, brings us to Foucault, who seeks to show how technological control of the body is connected with the production of certain kinds of bodies and the formation of certain kinds of subjects. And if this is always the case with any way of interpreting and acting upon the body (as ascetics have always realized), then it also forces us to realize that the task is not to recover an essential humanity behind these attitudes and practices but to determine what kinds of bodies and subjects we should cultivate. From this perspective, the most significant point about the Baconian project is not the alienation it involves or the "dehumanized" medicine it causes. Rather, the significant points are, first, that the body of the Other — the body in its susceptibility to disease, suffering, and death — is construed through attitudes and practices that reduce it to an object of technological control rather than attitudes and practices that find moral and spiritual significance precisely in the otherness of the body, and second, that this reduction of the body of the Other to technological control is connected with a vast range of norms, institutions, forms of knowledge, techniques of monitoring, etc. which increasingly form our bodies, in large part by already having formed (and been formed by) our desires to eliminate suffering and our choices for what we have now come to regard as a good body. In short, as I argued in the first section, a set of attitudes and practices grounded in one discourse of the body has been substituted for another, and the task of bioethics is to determine what set of attitudes and practices should form our bodies and ourselves as subjects, whether those of the Baconian project or some other. But this requires a move from the genealogical (in Foucault's sense) task of pointing out how various attitudes and practices form us to the ethical task of determining which ones *should* form us.

III. The Moral Significance of the Body in Christianity

The problem is that if the genealogist of Baconian medicine is right, we have already been formed by the Baconian project in a way that determines our answer to the ethical question in its favor. The challenge to the Baconian project must come from a set of interpretations and practices regarding the body that constitutes an alternative to Baconian medicine. I will now try to show how certain Christian convictions would, if fully developed, make it possible to understand how Baconian medicine has formed us as subjects and to answer Plato's questions regarding the attention or vigilance we should exercise over our bodies, the control we should give medicine over our bodies, the ends that should determine what counts as a sufficiently healthy body, and the limits we should observe in improving our bodies and eliminating suffering. Underlying this alternative is a fundamental conviction that the attempt to render our bodies free from suffering and wholly subject to our choices is morally impoverishing — that the kind of vigilance over the body it entails produces subjects who are incapable of understanding the nature and meaning of embodiment, of recognizing and accepting the limits of medicine, of caring adequately for those who embody those limits and who fall victim to our efforts to deny them, and of rightly ordering the goods of the body (including those made possible by technology). The remainder of this section spells out this conviction.

The Christian discourse that subjugates medicine to the moral uses of suffering is connected with a subject formed by certain attitudes and practices regarding the body. What distinguishes these attitudes and practices from their modern counterparts is their refusal to separate the body of the Other from the subject. Rather, they recognize that the body of the Other is inextricable from the subject, so that the subject is separated from and within itself. This understanding of the body can be traced to Paul, for whom, as Rudolf Bultmann and a succession of later scholars have concluded, "the *soma* [body] is not a something that outwardly clings to a man's real *self* (to his soul, for instance), but belongs to its very essence, so that we can say man does not *have* a *soma;* he *is soma* . . ." (Bultmann, 1951, p. 194). In phenomenological terms, the body for Paul is a lived body; it is oneself as related to the external world. But according to Bultmann, the body for Paul is also that in which one experiences oneself as "subjected to an occurrence that springs from a will other than [one's] own" (1951, p. 196). The body, then, is oneself as separated from oneself. Phenomenologically speaking, this is the body of the Other: oneself as subject to powers external to one's own willing or intentionality. And it brings with it the temptation to allow the separation within the subject to become a separation in which, as in Gnosticism, the body becomes alien and foreign to the subject (1951, p. 199). The refusal of Paul — in contrast to Plato as well as the Gnostics — to resolve the problem of alterity by separating the body from the true subject as alien to the latter is highly significant. For it means that for him the alterity recognized by all of these ancient writers does not occur between the subject and something external to it, but within the subject itself. Hence a Christian view of the body will understand the body of the Other as integral to the subject and will therefore interpret alterity — the body as it escapes the dominion of will and intentionality — as the separation of the subject from and within itself.

But for Paul, in contrast to some phenomenological accounts, the body of the Other is not altogether negative. While it poses the threat of wresting one from oneself (i.e. sin), it also harbors the promise, fulfilled in the resurrection of the body, of redemption, which is itself the work of a power that escapes one's will and intentionality (Bultmann, pp. 198, 201). In short, the body of the Other is for the Christian inseparable from the determination of the subject by sin and grace, so that the body of the Other is the key to the Christian meaning of embodiment and to the attitudes and practices that carry that meaning. Since illness and bodily imperfection are primary occasions in which the body of the Other breaks through the body as expression of will and intentionality — the state of being at one with oneself — it is appropriate for Christians to view illness and healing in analogy (though not in a causal relationship) to sin and redemption (cf. Khushf, 1995). Hence one way in which illness or bodily imperfection has served the moral projects of Christians is as an occasion for meditation on sin and the need for grace, and the disciplines and ways of monitoring the body Christians have developed have sought to form subjects accordingly.

From this perspective Descartes's effort to separate himself as a subject from his body prone to disease, decay, and death, or more generally, the quest to make the body perfect and perfectly subject to our choices, can only be understood as a denial of the moral and spiritual significance of the body. And the disciplines and ways of monitoring of the body and its processes that carry out this quest produce subjects constituted by their denial of the body of the Other. This denial prompts the use of medicine to eliminate all traces of the body of the Other in their own bodies. Medicine is accordingly called upon to postpone death, stall or reverse biochemical aging processes, restore youthful anatomical features, and in general eliminate or alter anything that is unwanted. Just as significantly, this denial of the Other equates the meaning of embodiment with control over the body. When the body of the Other is denied, the end of life may become a desperate quest for control through physician-assisted death.

From a Christian perspective, therefore, when one monitors and acts upon one's body in a way that denies the body of the Other, one becomes incapable of the use of illness and bodily imperfection to form oneself in an awareness of sin and grace. One wrongly supposes that medicine can resolve the crisis of alterity and overcome the separation of the subject by rendering the body the full expression of one's will and intentionality. But this denies the limits of medicine, which does not expel the Other but only delays his inevitable appearance, and which cannot dispel the deeper question of sin and redemption. Moreover, those who deny the body of the Other end up affirming it in a most ironic way, since efforts to perfect the body and bring it under the realm of choice do not restore the body to the willing and choosing subject but instead place it under the hegemony of a society that produces the subjects whose desires and choices enable it to accomplish its normalizing ambitions.

Acceptance of the body of the Other that separates the subject from and within itself is the condition for receptivity to the body of the Other in a second sense, as the suffering of the Other. The Baconian project fails from this perspective because it does not address and in fact contributes to this kind of suffering. Just as the Baconian-Cartesian subject is formed by monitoring and acting upon himself in accordance with societal standards for the body, so he internalizes his society's concern with producing other bodies that approximate these standards. His compassion for the suffering of others is thus formed by and expressed in these normalizing processes. The suffering of the other is elicited and responded to in terms of utility, efficiency, prospects of healthy survival, etc. Medicine exercises compassion by measuring individuals against these norms and helping them to approximate them to the highest degree possible. But as Edith Wyschogrod has argued (with respect to postmodern, not Christian, ethics), such a subject is incapable of responding to the pain of the Other because it never allows the Other to break through the codes (such as those of normalization) that inscribe the body in the text of society (Wyschogrod, 1990, pp. 98-99, 103-4; 1995, pp. 26-27). It is not surprising, therefore, that as Hauerwas argues, compassion for the suffering results in elimination of the sufferer who will never approximate the standards. It is also not surprising that as Baconian medicine keeps increasing the standards for a "normal" body in a society that measures and calculates bodies according to these standards, the marginalization of those whose bodies cannot meet the standards is increased and their worth in the eyes of society is diminished. On the other hand, acceptance of the vulnerability of the body that separates the subject from itself opens up a receptivity to the Other that resists reducing the Other to social codes (Wyschogrod, 1990, p. 99). In Hauerwasian terms, a subject for whom the susceptibility of the body to suffering and death is integral to interpretations of and actions upon the body may welcome the other who reminds us of the limits of medicine or whose body refuses to conform to the normalizing demands of society.

This understanding of the body has direct and thoroughgoing implications for the practice of medicine and the care for the ill more generally in a community formed according to this understanding. First, such a community is prepared to recognize and accept the limits of medicine and to reorganize health care around this recognition. It is becoming clear to many observers that the quest of medicine to find a "magic bullet" cure for every disease or unwanted condition has been founded on an exaggeration of certain accomplishments of medicine in this century (Golub, 1994). The prevalence and persistence of chronic diseases, the yawning gap between genetic diagnosis and effective therapy, the growing resistance of bacterial strains to antibiotics — these and many other similar factors assure us that the Baconian quest to eliminate suffering is not only being delayed but is an illusion. This is not to deny the many accomplishments of technological medicine — to the contrary, my point is that once we accept the limits of medicine in elimination suffering, we will be in a better position to use technology, as part of a more general commitment to caring, in ways that help more and more people to live better with conditions that cannot be eliminated. But if chronic conditions, the gap between diagnosis and therapy, and the like will characterize medicine for the foreseeable future, then from a Christian perspective Baconian medicine has done those who suffer from these factors a double disservice. By defining all suffering as pointless and holding out the false promise of eventually being able to eliminate it all, it has discouraged them from coming to understand what for Christians is the truth of the body (namely, one's place in the drama of sin and redemption) while also failing to provide adequate resources and other support for those who, due to the limitations of medicine in general or for a particular patient, cannot be cured. Because the Christian approach to the body and to bodily suffering as I have described it is committed to the transformation of suffering into the moral and spiritual projects I have identified, it is in a position not only to recognize and accept the limits of medicine in eliminating suffering but to form a practice of health care that assigns a much higher place to the forms of care and support that enable people to live with their conditions in such a way that they can accomplish the transformation.

Second, because a community formed according to this understanding of the body denies that all incurable suffering is pointless or that the worth of one's life is determined by how closely one conforms to societal standards of bodily perfection, it will see no "need" to eliminate those who suffer in order to spare them a life of suffering. It is necessary at this point to understand Baconian medicine in relation to the larger society that it makes possible but that also supports it. The Baconian project is bound up with an entire social and economic system that virtually demands that we be independent of the need to care for others or be cared for by them. Those who cannot or can no longer maintain their independence or control over their bodies are therefore abandoned to specialized forms of care which, due to the devaluation of this kind of care and support in view of the priorities of Baconian medicine criticized in the previous paragraph, are unable to meet their needs. In these circumstances we are taught to value independence and control over our bodies and to fear their loss far more, I surmise, than our predecessors were. To the same extent we are inclined to deny the moral worth of those who cannot or can no longer exercise independence or control their bodies, including ourselves. In this context it is clear why many would kill others to spare them a life of suffering or call for assistance in dying as a way to regain control and independence. But for a subject constituted by the body of the Other, loss of control over the body may signal an occasion for oneself and others to grasp the truth of the body: the need for grace and the experience of it through the care of families and communities who recognize their duty to care in such circumstances. This is not to idealize or romanticize the loss of control; it can be a deeply troubling experience for everyone involved. Nor does it by itself resolve the status of those who are irreversibly incapable of responding to the care of others or whose incurable pain or tragic sense of abandonment at the end of life precludes accomplishment of any moral or spiritual transformation of suffering. My point is only that from a Christian perspective one does not lose one's moral worth or one's moral task in life simply because one has lost independence or control of one's body. A community committed to this perspective would form its institutions and order its health care priorities accordingly. In the case of the dying, this would involve a rather thoroughgoing redirection of resources from efforts to extend life to efforts to develop more effective comfort care, including pain relief, high quality nursing care, and support of family caregivers.

Third, members of a community formed by this approach to the body would no longer measure themselves or others by the norms of a society bent on producing bodies designed for optimal levels of productivity, beauty, and success. Because the body is no longer measured, calculated, and valued according to such norms, the need to reorder it in accordance with these norms disappears. In such a community, the uses of medicine to eliminate all traces of the body of the Other, some of which I referred to above, would simply disappear. This does not mean that all uses of medicine to enhance bodily functioning would disappear, but it does involve two implications. The first is that members of such a community will find the place of the pursuit of health and bodily excellence within the space opened up by the body of the Other and the moral and spiritual tasks and duties it entails for oneself and for others. The second is that it is clear how little is contributed to this task by efforts to draw lines between, say, treatment of a disease and enhancement of a trait. Rather, the process of discernment requires determination of how one's own body, with its capacities and limitations, best carries out the tasks and duties just mentioned and orders the rest of life in accordance with them.

In his study of sexual renunciation in early Christianity Peter Brown shows how "Christian attitudes to sexuality delivered the death-blow to the ancient notion of the city as the arbiter of the body" (Brown, 1988, p. 437). A subject formed by the body of the Other in the twofold sense I have described possesses both the self-regarding and other-regarding moral commitments to frame a way of practicing health care that is capable of rejecting as arbiters of the body Baconian medicine and the society that underwrites it. But this interpretation of the body is, of course, only the beginning. It indicate the attitudes and practices Christians should bring to occasions of suffering but does not tell us specifically what kinds of suffering should be eliminated or what choices should be made with regard to the capacities of technology. It tells us in general what priorities a health care system organized around these moral convictions should have but does not tell us in detail how to order the goods of the body. It shows how the twofold imperative of Baconian medicine fails on its own terms insofar as it delivers the body over to society rather than to human freedom and increases certain kinds of suffering in its effort to eliminate other kinds. But it does not offer a detailed alternative to the Baconian project. And if contemporary Christians are to reject Baconian medicine as arbiter of the body in the same way that their ancient predecessors rejected the Roman city, there is a final and much more important deficiency. That is the need for a concrete community (including health care institutions) to form subjects according to these attitudes and practices regarding the body as fully as the broader society forms subjects by the attitudes and practices of the Baconian project.

Sources

Bacon, Francis, 1894, *Works of Lord Bacon*, edited by Joseph Devey, London: George Bell and Sons.

Bacon, Francis, 1960, *The New Organon and Related Writings*, edited by Fulton H. Anderson, New York: Liberal Arts Press.

Borgmann, Albert, 1984, *Technology and the Character of Ev-*

eryday Life: A Philosophical Inquiry, Chicago: University of Chicago Press.

Brown, Peter, 1988, *The Body and Society: Men, Women, and Sexual Renunciation in Early Christianity*, New York: Columbia University Press.

Bultmann, Rudolf, 1951, *Theology of the New Testament*, vol. 1, New York: Scribner's.

Edelstein, Ludwig, 1967, *Ancient Medicine: Selected Papers of Ludwig Edelstein*, edited by Owesei Temkin and C. Lillian Temkin, Baltimore: Johns Hopkins University Press.

Foucault, Michel, 1980, *Power/Knowledge: Selected Interviews and Other Writings, 1972-1977*, edited by Colin Gordon, New York: Pantheon Books.

Foucault, Michel, 1983b, "The Subject and Power," Afterword to Hubert L. Dreyfus and Paul Rabinow, *Michel Foucault: Beyond Structuralism and Hermeneutics*, Chicago: University of Chicago Press, pp. 208-26.

Foucault, Michel, 1987, "The Ethic of Care for the Self as a Practice of Freedom," in James Bernauer and David Rasmussen, eds., *The Final Foucault*, Cambridge, Mass.: Massachusetts Institute of Technology Press, pp. 1-120.

Golub, Edward S., 1994, *The Limits of Medicine*, New York: Times Books.

Gustafson, James M., 1981, *Ethics from a Theocentric Perspective*, vol. 1: *Theology and Ethics*, Chicago: University of Chicago Press.

Gustafson, James M., 1984, *Ethics from a Theocentric Perspective*, vol. 2: *Ethics and Theology*, Chicago: University of Chicago Press.

Hauerwas, Stanley, 1977, *Truthfulness and Tragedy: Further Investigations into Christian Ethics*, Notre Dame, Ind.: University of Notre Dame Press.

Hauerwas, Stanley, 1986, *Suffering Presence: Theological Reflections on Medicine, the Mentally Handicapped, and the Church*, Notre Dame, Ind.: University of Notre Dame Press.

Jonas, Hans, 1974, *Philosophical Essays: From Ancient Creed to Technological Man*, Chicago: University of Chicago Press.

Jonas, Hans, 1979, "Toward a Philosophy of Technology," *Hastings Center Report* 9, no. 1 (February), pp. 34-43.

Jonas, Hans, 1984, *The Imperative of Responsibility: In Search of an Ethics for the Technological Age*, Chicago: University of Chicago Press.

Kass, Leon R., 1985, *Toward a More Natural Science: Biology and Human Affairs*, New York: The Free Press.

Kass, Leon R., 1994, *The Hungry Soul: Eating and the Perfection of Our Nature*, New York: The Free Press.

Khushf, George, 1995, "Illness, the Problem of Evil and the Analogical Structure of Healing: The Difference Christianity Makes in Bioethics," *Christian Bioethics* 1, pp. 102-20.

Leder, Drew, 1990, *The Absent Body*, Chicago: University of Chicago Press.

MacIntyre, Alasdair, 1984, *After Virtue*, 2nd edition, Notre Dame, Ind.: University of Notre Dame Press.

Plato, *The Republic*.

Rose, Nikolas. "Medicine, History and the Present," in Colin Jones and Roy Porter, eds., *Reassessing Foucault: Power, Medicine and the Body*. New York: Routledge, 1994, pp. 48-72.

Taylor, Charles, 1989, *Sources of the Self: The Making of the Modern Identity*, Harvard University Press.

Wyschogrod, Edith, 1990, *Saints and Postmodernism: Revisioning Moral Philosophy*, Chicago: University of Chicago Press.

Zaner, Richard M., 1981, *The Context of Self: A Phenomenological Inquiry Using Medicine as a Clue*, Athens, Ohio: Ohio University Press.

Zaner, Richard M., 1988, *Ethics and the Clinical Encounter*, Englewood Cliffs, N.J.: Prentice-Hall.

57 "Embodiment" and Moral Critique: A Christian Social Perspective

Lisa Sowle Cahill

"Embodiment" is frequently lifted up as central in critiques of the Western moral tradition on both sex and medicine. Yet the prominence of this theme is in some respects puzzling. After all, talk and practice in these two areas could hardly be more explicit about having the "body" as a key concern. Indeed, ethics as discourse about human relations and practices is always at some level about the body. . . .

What, then, could be intended by current appeals to recover the significance of the body for moral discourse? Most ethicists use the theme of embodiment to counteract a dualism about body and mind in which the body tends to come off as the inferior partner in an uneasy relationship. Contemporary ethicists, both religious and philosophical, see the integration of body and mind or spirit as a value and goal. Yet, somewhat paradoxically, choice, consent, and autonomy can be so central in (Western) moral and policy discussions that protection of freedom serves to justify almost any medical or technological manipulation of his or her body that an informed moral agent elects. Moreover, liberal moral theory about choice rarely succeeds in integrating the body and the embodied agent or self with their social context. Integration needs to occur not only between body and mind, but also among body, mind, and society. The body is always central in defining the self, while in all cultures, the meaning of the body reflects and augments social relationships. To understand the significance of embodiment for bioethics, it will be useful to set references to the body in sexual and medical ethics against broader discussions of body and society in philosophical, anthropological, and religious discourse. In so doing, it must be noted that society influences and shapes the bodily experience of the self not only in negative, repressive ways, but also in positive, expressive ways.

A thesis I want to develop is that a positive, integral view of the self as embodied and as intrinsically social does not require the rejection of control of the body in relation to the values of an encompassing social order. To advance this thesis, I will review dualism in the Western tradition, including modern versions of it which focus on autonomy; will examine recent critiques of mind-body dualism; and will examine the proposal, differently elaborated by Michel Foucault and Mary Douglas, that the self-understanding and social agency of the embodied self reflect and reinforce social organization. Drawing on their work as well as that of Peter Brown, I will use Christian sources to show that the disciplined body can and has functioned as a countersign to hierarchy and domination, and as an inaugural sign of a new social order characterized by solidarity and equality. Consequences for the practice of medicine follow from changed relationships in general, and in particular from Christian symbolization of the new order through the experiences of bodily illness, pain, healing, and death.[1]

From L. Sowle Cahill and M. A. Farley, *Embodiment, Morality, and Medicine* (Dordrecht: Kluwer Academic Publishers, 1995), 199-214. Slightly abridged and edited from the original. Used with kind permission from Kluwer Academic Publishers.

Dualism and Western Tradition

A matter of concern for many ethicists is a body-spirit dualism which pervades Western (North Atlantic) culture, and which was expressed in Christian tradition by a negative view of the body as unruly and in need of control. In contemporary medical practice, we find a different but not unrelated objectification of the body as the site of technical intervention, and as the material or even property regarding which autonomous persons exercise free consent.

This dualism about the body's relation to the mind or spirit has not been a problem to the same degree in many other cultures and religions. Islam and Judaism assume a strong integration of body and spirit, even though those traditions, like others, are occasionally beset by dualistic strands and the denigration of women's bodies ([5], pp. 23-55). African religious traditions see the body as so essential to the person that the physical integrity of the body is crucial to the individual's successful passage into the afterlife ([5], pp. 141-53). Similarly, in many Asian philosophical traditions (for instance, those of India, China, Japan), the mind-body relation might be better described as a symbiotic "polarity" within an integrated whole, than as a "duality" ([1], p. 159). Moreover, the relation of mind to body becomes in these traditions not a philosophical or epistemological problem of the reconciliation of two diverse elements, but a practical matter of improved integration of the self through ritual and self-cultivation or training.

> The process may proceed by the mind's training the body or the body's training the mind. In the former case, the mind sets a pattern for the body to follow; in the latter the body leads the mind (through controlled breathing, for example) to a state of tranquility or creativity. . . . The unity of mind and body is not to be discovered, but achieved ([10], p. xviii).

1. Thanks to Francis Elvey, S.J., Margaret Farley, Karen Lebacqz, Therese Lysaught, and James Nelson for very helpful critical comments on a first version of this essay.

June O'Connor's account of abortion in Japan shows precisely that it is through a *ritual practice* of recognizing the aborted fetus that issues of women's choice to abort, the social circumstances of the abortion, women's and men's emotions about the event and their physical parenthood, and the physical-spiritual existence of the unborn child are brought into conjunction and addressed, if not resolved ([5], pp. 93-111).

In much of the Western tradition, however, mind and body have often been seen as discrete entities whose conjunction is uncertain, posing a philosophical problem. Modern science builds a strictly material body, and locates the causes of its illness and health in material causes, tending thereby to erode both the interdependence of spiritual and physiological states, and the connectedness of the embodied self with other elements and presences in the cosmos ([18], p. 133). Many place the blame on Descartes and his metaphor of the body as "machine" (e.g., [5], pp. 169-83). By philosophically privileging thought over physical existence as constitutive of the person, Descartes laid the way for later disembodiments and dehistoricizations of subjectivity, and for the body's deprivation of its role in knowledge and in moral valuation.

But Western dualism did not originate in the seventeenth century. While Aristotle cultivated virtue through practical wisdom in daily, bodily, social life, other ancient Greek philosophers deliberated on the distance between the world of lived experience and the world of unmediated truth and goodness. The heights of spiritual and intellectual accomplishment seemed to require escape from the exigencies and tensions of physical function and survival. The Platonists, and to a lesser extent the Stoics, armed their approach to the body with asceticism and rational direction, an approach attractive to many later Christian authors. On the one hand, the problematic body is subject to an impressive number of "contingencies," such as the need for food and shelter, and the liability to torture and imprisonment. On the other, when the drive to fulfill its own needs becomes stronger than the rational purposes by which one tries to channel or restrain them, the body seems to have a "mind of its own" ([13], pp. 130-31). In dualistic views of the body and mind or spirit, body still defines self insofar as the virtues of rationality and asceticism move to center stage precisely in reaction to bodily realities.

Body and Self in Christianity

One finds, if anything, an anti-dualism about the body in the gospels. God's reign is realized in the life and ministry of a man formed bodily in the womb of a woman, a man who in his very walking, sleeping, eating, drinking, talking, touching, fasting, night-watching, pain, and death makes present the compassion of God for human suffering. Human persons are drawn into God's own love and life through the resurrection of their bodies. In earthly existence, the healing of illness is linked to faith, and human beings are called to alleviate the physical hunger, nakedness, and pain of neighbors and enemies alike.

St. Paul may reflect some of the anxieties of the philosophers when he laments that "I delight in the law of God, in my inmost self, but I see in my members another law at war with the law of my mind and making me captive to the law of sin which dwells in my members" (Rom 7:22-23). But despite his appreciation of the recalcitrance of the body in conforming to spiritual aims, Paul more generally understands "flesh" in terms of any sinful turning from God or captivity to the world and its powers. "Spirit" as flesh's opposite transforms not only the mind but the whole person to a life of righteousness through the indwelling Spirit of God. Certainly, notwithstanding its potentially hierarchical uses, Paul's master metaphor of the Christian community as "Body of Christ" depends on the literal incorporation of disciples in all their physical reality. In his reaction against prostitution, he insists, "The body is not meant for immorality, but for the Lord, and the Lord for the body. . . . Do you not know that your bodies are members of Christ? . . . Do you not know that your body is a temple of the Holy Spirit within you . . . ? So glorify God in your body" (1 Cor 6:13-20).

Ambivalence toward the body assumed a higher profile in the tradition, however, as Christians battled, and were in the process influenced by, gnostic and other dualistic worldviews. An early example is Origen, who, like Plato, saw the differences among creatures as marks of their deviation from an original unity of being, and who was reputed at least to have had himself castrated by a doctor in order to avoid either sexual incontinence or the appearance of immorality in his spiritual relationships with women ([2], p. 168). Augustine is another great thinker whose dualistic inclinations were eventually reconciled to but never eliminated from his defense of the body against Manichean assaults on marriage and childbearing. Though Augustine defined procreation of offspring as a "good" of marriage (*On the Good of Marriage,* 6-7, trans. Deferrari), he was nevertheless able to speculate that in the Garden of Eden conception might have been accomplished by a passionless act of the will (*City of God,* XIV, trans. Dods).

Despite the ultimate victory of the orthodox Christian view that the body is not only essential to the person, but is good as created and redeemed, the uncertainty of much of the tradition's investment in that view led not only to now-incredible theological proposals, but also to much agony of human spirit and body alike. "The very matter-of-fact manner in which monastic sources report bloody, botched attempts at self-castration by desperate monks shocks us by its lack of surprise" ([2], p. xviii).

Dualism in Contemporary Views

The "old" dualism of Western culture, reinforced historically by Christianity, saw the body (especially the sexual body) as the enemy of rational control and requiring subjugation. A "new" dualism, which sees the body as raw material for choice and intervention, is exercised via the technical and instrumental rationality guiding much of modern science. . . . Defining instrumental reason as the calculation of maximum efficiency in pursuing means to a given end, Charles Taylor notes its evidence "in the prestige and aura that surround technology," making us believe that "we should seek technological solutions even when something very different is called for" ([19], pp. 5-6).

The reign of informed consent in bioethics today is a symptom of technical rationality operating within a lingering body-mind dualism. The self is defined as an autonomous, private, and self-constituting will. After Nuremberg, we may hardly forget that the principle of consent is important to maintain the dignity and inviolability of persons. However, the near absoluteness and self-sufficiency of this criterion in moral decisions about medical care and research reveals a modern version of the idea that the body is inferior and essentially alien to personal freedom. The rhetoric of choice promoting a legal right to physician-assisted suicide or euthanasia is a glaring example, as is the array of "new reproductive technologies" designed to take advantage of all available means to force the realization of the self's chosen aims. The body relates to the self's freedom primarily as matter to be manipulated, matter which, when resistant to the self's elected projects, may and must be overcome or circumvented.

It would be foolish to repudiate all forms of medical resistance to bodily limitations or failures, or to conform the identity of the self to physiological capacities (as do patriarchal definitions of women's roles). The issue is not a choice between bodiliness and freedom, but the appropriate integration of the self *as* body, mind, will, and spirit. The moral exclusions and permissions a wise and practicable integration would entail are no simple matter to define, and no doubt cannot be defined finally or abstractly. Suffice it to say that a naturalist morality of the body, a libertarian morality of the will, a rationalist morality of the intellect, and a fundamentalist morality of divine command all fail to meet the standard of a nuanced and experientially true approach to moral agency. All the constitutive dimensions of the self should be mutually engaged and allowed to carry some normative moral force.

One dangerous consequence of holding informed consent not only as necessary but as the sufficient principle of bioethics is that to do so keeps out of our range of vision broader social relations which impinge on the identity of the self and its "free" choices, including relations and practices focused on the body. Obvious examples are gender, race, and class expectations that make choices less than free, or that create blindnesses and injustices which cannot be redressed by focusing narrowly on providing information and eliciting a decision. . . . The informed consent criterion also tends to neglect positive moral experiences and values which may be important to moral identity but which are not captured by the simple ideal of well-informed choice. . . .

Embodiment as a Critical Theme in Sexual and Medical Ethics

It is in sexual ethics that the appeal to embodiment has been most visible. This appeal typically supports a claim that traditional moral norms have been defined in the abstract (with authority attributed to God or to nature), and with inadequate attention to the normative value of the actual, embodied experience of sex. For example, to define procreation as the principal purpose of sexual intercourse is to neglect if not ignore other aspects of sexual experience, such as pleasure, intimacy, and homoeroticism. These aspects might also define goods and values whose claim should be recognized in moral choices. No doubt it *is* actual experience in precisely such dimensions that the experientially incommensurate norms are intended to control. In this sense, they do address sexual reality, even if only to assert a norm over against it. But this fact only verifies the critique: received sexual norms themselves do not build constructively on the embodied experience of the persons they are aimed to address. As far as sex is concerned, then, the corrective advanced via "embodiment" is the counteraction of repressive attitudes toward the body with a more positive attitude toward the fullness of its capacities, an important feature of which is the potential of the sexual body for intimacy and pleasure as well as for procreation.

Because it is derived from biological sex as its social interpretation, gender also enters into the positive reconstrual of the body. Specifically, women's bodies are affirmed as constituting selves who are equal to men in moral agency and moral value. Women's reproductive capacities in no way signal lesser rational or volitional abilities, nor should women's roles be constrained or accorded lesser value on account of women's distinctive reproductive contributions. Women's bodies are a source of moral knowledge equal to, if somewhat different from, that yielded by the male embodied experience.

In medicine, the point commonly advanced by means of the theme of embodiment is that the "patient" whose body is manipulated is also a "person" who is embodied. The self is constituted by the person's materiality as much as by his or her intellectual, spiritual, and psychological dimensions. The body enters into the subjectivity of the person, mediates that subjectivity to the world, and is a medium through which the world and other persons interact with the subject as embodied self. In the words of Merleau-Ponty, "the body expresses total existence, not because it is an external accomplishment to that existence, but because existence comes into its own in the body" ([14], p. 166). Bodies are not just living organisms which as such become the objects of scientific, technical interventions. Bodies are the spatiality and temporality of selves, and it is to persons — not only to bodies — that medical professionals must respond. In medicine, the corrective which "embodiment" brings is a holistic view of the person. In addition to the unity of self and body, this holism extends to a unity of all the physical parts and processes of the body in their personal and social meanings.

It is just this emphasis on holism that often brings sexual discourse into conjunction with biomedical talk of the significance of body, especially in the case of the medical relevance of biological sex socially mediated as gender. The self as embodied is quite strongly constituted by the social significance of gender as an elaboration of maleness or femaleness. Medical practice can become oppressive to women to the extent that it incorporates patriarchal gender models in its approach to women's health. A revealing treatment of the practical interpenetration of sexual and medical discourses is Emily Martin's *The Woman in the Body* ([12]). In the medicalization of women's reproductive processes, the female body is often objectified in a way reflecting cultural views of women's passivity and inferiority. The obstetrician, for instance, often assumes the role of "supervisor or foreman" of a labor process in which two images compete: "the uterus as a machine that produces the baby and the woman as laborer who produces the baby" ([12], p. 63). If Gerda Lerner is right that patriarchy is the first and paradigm case of oppression ([11]), then we will not be surprised to see further objectification of the bodies of those in "lower" racial, ethnic, and class groups, all of which are compounded when the medical subject/object is a woman.

In overview, Western authors writing today . . . are almost unanimously inclined to see dualism as bad and integration as a value, and to affirm that the body's contribution to selfhood is not only essential but is a component of the highest levels of human value and accomplishment, such as love, friendship, moral insight, and art. Contemporary Western affirmations of embodiment as a value may be seen to address three axes along which the body is understood, each structured by an internal polarity. Affirmations of embodiment are generally intended to move perception and practice away from the first pole in each set, and toward the second. These axes are *dualism — integration* (of body and mind, reason, or spirit); *denigration — affirmation* (of the body as part of the person); and *control — freedom* (presence or absence of a definite social ordering of the parts and processes of one's own body, as well as of one's own person in relation to the bodies of others). The third move in combination with the first two has a somewhat paradoxical effect at the level of moral practice and public policy. There we find a cultural and philosophical insistence on the freedom to control, reshape, or even kill the body as a prerequisite of genuine moral agency and as a form of resistance to the heteronomous control of social institutions which serve the vested interests of some groups of individuals in control over the bodies of others.

We find examples in the phrasing of the morality of avoiding or undertaking parenthood as a matter of reproductive choice, and when sexual morality is phrased as a matter of creating or constructing one's own sexual identity. The merits of both agendas lie in their unmasking definitions of the body's moral significance which employ a rhetoric of the biologically natural to disguise social power relationships. However, such critiques would be strengthened by the development of positive alternative ways to bring freedom back into interdependence with the body, and with the other material and social conditions of freedom. Charles Taylor instructs us that any nontrivial "choice" reflects a set of value priorities which at the very least highlight the realms of moral conduct which are of highest importance, and which reflect a dialogical community of other moral agents ([19], p. 39).[2] Freedom as a moral value makes no sense without a material and social context.

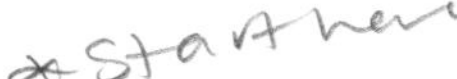

The Body as Symbol of Social Organization

A lesson that we learn in different ways from Mary Douglas and Michel Foucault is that the individual body is always interpreted and ordered to reflect social relationships. It is both a symbol of those relations and a medium through which they are realized, realigned, or replaced. Conceptions of the individual body and of the social body are interdependent. Interestingly, writers who explore the social history behind the early Christian religious world often draw on Mary Douglas and, less centrally, on Foucault. (Peter Brown [2] cites both in his bibliography; see John Dominic Crossan [6], p. 77 for a discussion of Mary Douglas.)[3] A counterpoint to the social interpretation of the body is the fact that the body is to some extent a biological given. Presumed "universals" of human embodiment include need for food and shelter, sexuality and reproduction, pain and pleasure, health and disease, aging and death. At the same time many commentators on embodiment focus on the variety of ways in which such embodied experiences as these have been understood and on how religious understandings of embodiment have changed or remain in need of change.

Foucault writes precisely to resist the "universals" of reason and nature by showing that experience and knowledge are thoroughly historical. He argues that our

2. Taylor perceptively explains why "authenticity" as "self-determining freedom" has to depend on "the understanding that independent of my will there is something noble, courageous, and hence significant in giving shape to my own life." Within the horizon of values against which moral authenticity takes place, some issues and values are more important than others, or "the very idea of self-choice falls into triviality and hence incoherence" ([19], p. 39).

3. I am grateful to Francis Elvey, S.J., for sharing with me his work in progress on the relevance of Foucault and Douglas to Christian conceptions of the body, which he applies to Thomas Aquinas's use of the body as a metaphor for society.

self-consciousness, our freedom, our values, and our very construal of what is central in our own experience are created by social practices which represent and perpetuate power relationships. Part of the originality of his contribution lies in his demonstration that in order to shape the self at its deepest levels, power does not need to coerce consciousness or behavior directly. Power determines consciousness through a comprehensive set of strategies which focus on the body (whether through hospitals, prisons, insane asylums, education, theories of sex, and — across all of these — modern medicine), and which determine the parameters within which we imagine our identity and our options. Foucault convincingly displays the ways in which power "controls" bodies as a positive and constructive force, not just by repression and constraint. He writes of "deployment" of discourses or "regimes" of knowledge and power which induce people to construct reality on their terms. He regards the whole notion of "sexuality" as such a discourse ([9]). He illustrates how Christian confessional practice and medical-psychiatric discourses about sex, supposedly responsible for repression, have actually resulted in endlessly proliferating talk about sex and in our conviction that the secret and truth of our very being lie in our sexual identity and behavior.[4] Our present quest for sexual "liberation" is no more than the ultimate victory of a discourse of sexuality which procures our consent to our own domination by means of a discipline of the body which we all too readily embrace ([9], pp. 151-59). While Foucault resists describing power as the "power of" any distinct social group by which it is consciously and purposively exercised, he often portrays medical science as facilitating the control both of individuals and of whole populations by its socially aggressive definitions of the body's significance.

Mary Douglas also sees the meaning of the body as culturally determined to a large extent. She finds in all cultures a human "drive to achieve consonance between social and physical and emotional experience" which finds expression in the use of the body as a natural symbol of the social order. The symbolic potentials of the body are in some ways culturally constant. To present the front rather than the back of one's body signifies respect; physical closeness signifies intimacy; the casting off of physical waste products (spitting, urinating) is incompatible with formal discourse and may be used to interrupt it; and the more strongly classified and controlled is the social hierarchy, the more controlled the individual's bodily movements will be, even to the point of "etherealization" or the relative disembodiment of personal interactions ([7], pp. 100-101).

In cultures in which there is a strongly defined structuring of the roles of individuals and groups, controlled and formal behavior will also be highly valued ([7], p. 99). Conversely, in societies in which individuality and freedom are prized over and above social expectations, freedom of physical movement and expression — the individual's "control" over his or her own body — will also be accepted and valued. It is important to make explicit the implication, however, that even in ostensibly unrestricted societies, the significance of the body and its movements still follow social norms, are still ordered and even in a sense controlled by the social ethos.

Douglas discerns a movement in Western societies away from systems characterized by a high respect for social roles and structures, and the duties they present for individuals, to systems in which the sincerity and authenticity of the subject become more important than structures, and in which personal success eventually overrides respect for roles and duties ([7], p. 50). The latter sort of society, to which Douglas says "we" now belong, sees a demise of ritualism in public and private ("the celebration of Sunday dinner"), and a great informality of social and family life (the disappearance of rank according to age and sex, as reflected in the arrangement of living room chairs) ([7], p. 55). Children are educated to be interested in their own internal states and the feelings of others. But the "seeds of alienation" ([7], p. 190) are contained in the relocation of control to the personal system, and the lack of integration of the individual with the social body. We may infer that alienation from the social significance of one's own body will also result, so that individuals neither realize the social shaping of their embodied behavior nor take into account the social effects of their choices to execute their sincere and "autonomous" life-plans by means of embodied relationships. They may even see the body as, in Douglas's phrase, an "alien husk" from which to escape ([7], p. 191).

Despite a common emphasis on socialization of the body, Douglas and Foucault obviously differ in significant ways. First, Douglas sees the body in its physicality as in some sense a universal which is socially interpreted ([7], p. ivx), while Foucault edges toward the claim that the body is itself a social construction. Second, Douglas avoids Foucault's heavy, even cynical, association of social control with domination, leaving open in her cross-cultural studies the possibility that the body and its parts can be ordered to reinforce social relationships which are not necessarily repressive, or which are at least characterized by a solidarity in which the embodied individual immediately participates.

In her study of trance states ([7], pp. 104-10), Mary Douglas also paves the way to a recognition, fully achieved for instance in the work of Caroline Walker

4. As Michael Foucault shows so well, a "controlling" discourse about sex all the better serves to accentuate it, to elevate sex as the secret of the self's identity, so that the long-run effect is guilty fascination or confessional self-display, rather than repression. Perhaps a Christian dualism about sex has ensured the repetition of social situations in which a normative discourse of strict sexual control has been accompanied by or broken out into anarchic practices of sexual perversion, especially by those in power — including the age-old rape and prostitution of women and sexual exploitation of children, the Victorian "double standard," and sexual abuse by clergy.

Bynum ([4], [3]), that Christianity, along with most or all other societies, sees the body (not only the spirit) as an avenue of transcendence and even of union with the divine. "Control, discipline, even torture of the flesh is, in medieval devotion, not so much the rejection of physicality as the elevation of it — a horrible yet delicious elevation — into a means of access to the divine" ([3], p. 182). Among the most universal bodily routes to the divinity are sex, food, and death, along with death's foretastes, pain and illness. Christianity has used all three.

The Body and Christian Society

While positive construals of the religious significance of sexual activity may have been scarce in Christian culture until the modern period,[5] permanent virginity as a religiously dedicated and ideal sexual identity was a distinctive contribution of early Christianity (1 Cor 7:8; this is Peter Brown's thesis [2]). Moreover, Bynum illustrates that the self-expressions of many mystics have strongly physical and indirectly sexual overtones ([4], p. 248; [3], p. 133). Food becomes a physical sharing in the divine life in the eucharistic meal ([4], pp. 252-53); in the sharing of food with the poor in imitation of God's mercy (Lk 6:36; Acts 6:1-6); in mystical and symbolic experiences of giving and receiving nurturance through feeding, even nursing ([4], pp. 269-76; [3], p. 133); and in the renunciation of food by fasting, complemented by the feast in celebration of divine grace and presence ([4], p. 250).

Likewise, Christianity is hardly alone among the world's religions in seeing death as a point of entry into a transcendent realm and of approach to God. Christians elaborate the religious significance of death in terms of last rites for the dying, funerary and burial practices, veneration of the dead and of their relics, martyrdom, resurrection, eternal life, eternal reward and punishment, and God's sharing in human death through the Cross of Christ. Anticipations of death in this life, often called "mortifications" of the body, include ascetic deprivation of the body and deliberate infliction of pain on it (including fasting); religious interpretations of illness as a trial, a gift, or a sign of sanctity; healing of illness, including the New Testament healing miracles and the religious ministries of healing which have existed throughout Christian tradition; and the actual bodily manifestation of the wounds which caused Christ's death (stigmata). Mystical experience also can include sensations of pain and of dying or of being near death or of passing through it. . . .

These examples serve to demonstrate that Christianity has been neither intransigently dualistic nor negative about the body. They also indicate that a positive, integrated approach to the body and soul, or body and mind, need not exclude — indeed, may depend upon — an ordering of the body in relation to a social vision. But where Foucault tends to portray social forces which determine the significance of the body as discourses of power-knowledge which serve regimes of domination, Douglas permits us to see that the background of social conditions within which we are embodied provides us with a framework for channeling, shaping, and disciplining our embodied experiences. Freedom never exists outside of some social vision; the communal vision which shapes bodily experience also brings the self's embodiment to consciousness, to expression, and to social agency.

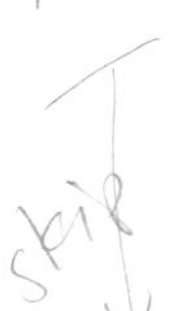

Like other societies, Christianity both channels a social vision through the body, and defines community partly in terms of bodily experiences and roles. As current scholarship attests, the biblically authentic Christian social vision is characterized by inclusiveness and solidarity, especially toward enemies and toward marginalized and outcast persons and groups. The solidarity of the New Testament communities challenged social relations built on status, power, and economic dependency, even if it did not completely overturn them.[6] Inclusive solidarity as a defining feature of Jesus' kingdom preaching is familiar in the Sermon on the Mount's Beatitudes (Matt 5:1-12) and in Jesus' instruction to "love your enemies, do good to those who hate you" (Lk 6:27); in the parable of the Good Samaritan (Lk 10:30-37); in Jesus' association with sinners and outcasts; in his approach to women; in his sacrificial death. A representative restatement of the cultural challenge presented by Jesus and his first followers is offered by John Dominic Crossan. In Jesus' teaching, life, and death,

> the Kingdom of God is a community of radical or unbrokered equality in which individuals are in direct contact with one another and with God, unmediated by any established brokers or fixed locations ([6], p. 101).

Crossan uses Mary Douglas on the body as a microcosm of the social order to show how Jesus manifested social equality through practices of table fellowship, itinerancy, healing, the raising of Lazarus, and exorcisms. Jesus' healing miracles are of special relevance to medical practice. For Crossan, their significance does not consist in any intervention into the natural, physical order of "disease" but into the social world of "illness," in which disease often meant ritual uncleanness and social ostracization. Jesus' violation of the purity code by contact with a leper challenged both the body politic and the priestly authorities, impugning "the rights and prerogatives of society's boundary keepers and controllers"([6], p. 82). Jesus' healing miracles are important for their so-

5. Take possibly Ephesians 5:23-32 on husbands and wives, and recall the sacramental status of marriage in at least some Christian communities, e.g., the Roman Catholic.

6. Several authors have recently made this argument, based on a social history approach to the distribution of power and status in the communities in which Christianity first arose. An example is Halvor Moxnes ([15]). This literature commonly draws on Moses Finley's description of client-patron relationships in first-century society ([18]).

cial significance, for their relevance to the new kingdom which includes the "marginalized and disenfranchised" ([6], p. 83), and refuses the traditional boundaries of order and exclusion symbolized in the disordered and thus excluded body of the sick. The Christian transformation of the social significance of the diseased body both symbolizes and advances at the practical level an inclusive community in which traditional hierarchies are overturned. A particularly good example is Jesus' healing of the woman who had had a "flow of blood" for twelve years (Mark 5:25-34), since she was not only sick but female. She would have been especially stigmatized if the hemorrhage from which she suffered involved menstrual blood, making her ritually impure.

Peter Brown illumines ways in which the early churches shaped the sexual body to advance this same vision. Especially in its implications for gender relations and for social relations of unequal power in general, this reshaping too is relevant to medical practice. Brown contrasts the hierarchical household of the ancient world with egalitarian Christian communities which threatened the social order. Celibacy was sometimes practiced in the ancient world, but it never replaced marriage as the general ideal and cornerstone of the social welfare. When undertaken, it was often temporary (as in the case of the Vestal Virgins). In Roman society, the sexual act, the relation of human and wife, their marriage, the hierarchy of the household, and the government of the state were not only analogous as concentric circles of order, but were dependent upon one another for their existence.

Although conservation of seed was thought to enhance the vitality and strength of a man, "eugenic sex," in which man and woman united their seed with full concentration and proper decorum, was a social duty and would have positive effects on the health, character, and even sex of the resulting child ([2], pp. 20-210). The concord of the couple in marriage elaborated their sexual cooperation, and was the foundation of the properly ordered household. While the early Roman ideal was unity in body and mind of the spouses, the married couple was seen by the beginning of the late antique period "less as a pair of equal lovers than as a reassuring microcosm of the social order" ([2], p. 17). This order was clearly not only hierarchical but patriarchal. It encompassed first of all the household and estate, where the husband cultivated the traits of active virility in his own body and deportment, and administered the bodies of wife, children, and slaves. The household mirrored the public order maintained by the governing classes.

Against this environment, Christian sexual renunciation may be seen, not as a mere repression of the body under the influence of dualistic philosophical and religious currents, but as a form of resistance to the hierarchical social order maintained through the reality and the symbolism of sex, marriage, and family. Perpetual virginity transformed the bodies of both men and women in their social significance, and enabled Christians (perhaps most especially women) "to break with the discreet discipline of the ancient city" ([2], p. 31). And beyond transforming the orders of personal relationships taken for granted in the ethos of the age, continence also broke with the continuity of history and of generations, announcing the eschatological advent of the Kingdom of God, and a "new creation" ([2], pp. 32, 64, 435).

Paul had a distinctive way of refracting Christian social cohesiveness through the body. The body is sanctified and an inauguration of the new age insofar as it is a "temple of the Holy Spirit" (1 Cor 6:19). The community of disciples as a whole is the material and historical presence of the body of Christ. The body of the believer participates in this communal identity to so great an extent that an act of sexual immorality will contaminate the very body of Christ (1 Cor 7:15). Corinth was a place where division based on status had fractured the community and introduced disorder into this transformed community. Some at Corinth apparently had taken the solution of embracing celibacy and totally dissolving the household. Paul himself recognized the radical effects of Christian baptism as an induction into a new social order (Gal 3:28). However, he resisted complete separatism from the pagan world, and emphasized the continuing validity of social bonds, including marriage and slavery.

While Paul's preference for celibacy may reflect a Stoic dualism of reason and passion to some extent, it also signifies a radical critique of the social order in which hierarchy reigned. His stated reasons for the preference are a suspicion neither of women (for he addresses both the wife and the husband) nor of the body, nor of sex itself.[7] Marriage should be avoided specifically to avoid "anxiety about worldly affairs" — the business and ordering of the household. Paul desires "to promote good order" but instead, that is, "to secure your undivided devotion to the Lord" (1 Cor 7:32-35). In other words, celibacy is for the sake of the transformed and transforming social order of the eschatological community, of which the body is a symbol.

Even in preferring celibacy ("I wish that all were as I myself am" (1 Cor 7:7), Paul does not make this sign of the new order into an entrance requirement ("But each has his own special gift from God, one of one kind and one of another" (1 Cor 7:7). The egalitarian solidarity of discipleship can also be at least partially reflected in marriage, even though Paul anticipates that it will in that state be more difficult to maintain. For instance, wife and husband "rule" equally over one another's bodies (1 Cor 7:4); neither partner is to divorce an unbelieving spouse who is willing to continue the relationship, though either may do so if the spouse is not (1 Cor 7:12-16); and Christians are exhorted to enact the transforma-

7. Scholars widely agree that 1 Cor 7:1 ("It is well for a man not to touch a woman") is Paul's restatement of his opponents' position, to which he is about to reply.

tive effects of mutual love even within the hierarchical household (Eph 5:21-6:9).[8]

Yet, as we have seen, Paul specifically contrasts the social ordering celibacy symbolizes to the social order of that household. In later Christianity, celibacy became an instrument of hierarchical control over believers, especially clergy and religious. Yet, following Brown's lead, we may say that permanent virginity for early Christians signals, not merely or simply the evils of the sexual body, but the solidarity of the kingdom, which is radical and total. Involvement with sex, even sex "well-ordered" from a cultural point of view, will involve the disciple with a set of social relationships (organized around sex, gender, procreation, and family) in which it will be difficult to live out fully the equality, solidarity, compassion, and mercy among men and women, slave and free, and finally Jew and gentile (Gal 3:28) in which the kingdom of God is present.

Paul's representation of the sexual body as not fundamentally compliant with the norms of the social order is carried out in the early Christians' presentation of the body and its functions as in other ways subversive of power and hierarchy. Many disciplines of the Christian body have to do with eating or feeding in a way which symbolizes the unity of the community. For instance, Paul accuses those who maintain distinctions among rich and poor at the eucharistic table, by providing sumptuously for themselves while others go hungry, of "profaning the body and blood of the Lord" (1 Cor 11:27). Ministers to the needy were appointed in the community, and were charged with such duties as distribution of food to widows. Whether Jewish or Greek, the widows should be treated similarly (Acts 6:1-6). Concerning whether Christians should partake of meat that has been offered to idols, Paul acknowledges that idols have no real existence (1 Cor 8:4), and that food in and of itself does not establish one's relationship with God (1 Cor 8:8). Nonetheless, each should be concerned for the consciences of others in the community, and should not cause scandal to "weaker" members who may not yet have reached the same freeing knowledge (1 Cor 8:7; 10:28-29). "'Knowledge' puffs up, but love builds up" (1 Cor 8:1). Love as solidarity in community is symbolized by a control of the body which denies that the knowledgeable are "superior."

Symbolizations of the new order by means of bodily suffering and death pervade the gospels and epistles, and center on the death and resurrection of Jesus. We may add just a few examples of the appropriation of this unifying death in the Christian life. Paul, whom later historical sources attest was eventually martyred, sees his own imprisonments as a confirmation of his defense of the gospel and as a means of strengthening other members of Christ's body in their commitment to the faith (Phil 1:7, 14; see also Col 4:10; Eph 3:1; 4:1; 6:20). In his own name as "a prisoner for the Lord," Paul implores the church at Ephesus "to lead a life worthy of the calling to which you have been called, with all lowliness and meekness, with patience, forebearing one another in love, eager to maintain the unity of the Spirit in the bond of peace" (Eph 4:1-3). Paul rejects the bodily mark of circumcision because it is used to distinguish higher religious status, to set off the "glory" of those who belong from those who do not (Gal 6:12-15). Instead, he says, he bears on his own body "the marks of Jesus," possibly a reference to his having been beaten (Gal 6:7). Although Paul's death is not recounted in the New Testament, the Acts of the Apostles tells of other martyrdoms, including the stoning of Stephen (Acts 7:57-60) and the death of James at the hands of Herod (Acts 12:1-2). Stephen, like Jesus, dies praying for the forgiveness of his persecutors (Acts 7:60).

8. The critical question is whether a transformation which still leaves the essential hierarchical structure intact is an adequate social adaptation or a betrayal of kingdom solidarity ([16]).

Overview and Recommendations

Certainly in the tradition, perhaps most of all in Augustine's writings, Christian control of the sexual body has come into alignment with dualistic and negative currents, leading Christians to see the body preeminently as a temptation to sin. This negativity is not only not required by, but is inconsistent with, New Testament symbolization of the body, especially the presence of God's reign in Jesus' birth, life, death, and resurrection; the Christian community as inclusive Body of Christ; the resurrection of the body as the full incorporation of the whole person into God's kingdom.

As we bring Christian views of the body toward medical practice, what perhaps is most in need of emphasis is the positive *social* significance of those views. A first significance of embodiment for a Christian ethics of medicine and healing is the importance of a stance of compassion toward the sick on the part of the care-givers. The point is not pity, but an empathic identification with the suffering of the other, which, to the extent humanly possible, reaches through boundaries of race, gender, class, and economic status. Only then can one serve, as did the Good Samaritan, as a "neighbor" to those who are injured and vulnerable.

A second significance proceeds partly from that identification; it is the realization that we too suffer and die, whether pain and mortality mark us already in profound ways or in temporarily subtle ones. With that realization comes the recognition of the vulnerability of every human being, and the need of everyone for redemptive inclusion in the unity of all being which the Christian eucharist signifies and of which the mystics of all religions have had a premonition. Doctors and patients are but provisionally set apart by the pain and supplication of the latter. A third significance proceeds both from compassion and from the universality of disease and death. That is the moral importance of a genuinely inclusive social practice of health care, which alleviates suffering, even while acknowledging the inevitability of death and the interdependence of health and bodily life with other social, personal, and spiritual goods.

The social significance of embodiment for a Christian bioethics is neither a knowing priesthood of the medical professions, nor a resignation to human suffering as "God's will," nor an absolutization of the individual's "right to life," nor even the cultivation of altruistic virtues by members of care-giving professions. It is the challenge to create a community of solidarity in which suffering and death are healed and avoided when possible, and are recognized as constitutive of human selfhood even after they are not. In such a community, the suffering and dying self would not experience dependency as defilement, but as an extenuation and deepening of the self's social destiny. All persons in such a community might learn to take their own bodily vulnerability as an occasion for self-transcendence through compassion for the vulnerability of others and in openness to the sustaining communion of being which Christians symbolize as "resurrection life."

Bibliography

[1] Ames, R. T.: 1993, "The Meaning of the Body in Classic Chinese Philosophy," in T. P. Kasulis et al. (eds.), *Self as Body in Asian Theory and Practice,* State University of New York Press, Albany, pp. 157-77.

[2] Brown, P.: 1988, *The Body and Society: Men, Women, and Sexual Renunciation in Early Christianity,* Columbia University Press, New York.

[3] Bynum, C. W.: 1991, *Fragmentation and Redemption: Essays on Gender and the Human Body in Medieval Religion,* Zone Books, New York.

[4] Bynum, C. W.: 1987, *Holy Feast and Holy Fast: The Religious Significance of Food to Medieval Women,* University of California Press, Berkeley, Los Angeles and London.

[5] Cahill, L. S., and Farley, M. A. (eds.): 1995, *Embodiment, Morality, and Medicine,* Kluwer Academic Publishers, Dordrecht.

[6] Crossan, J. D.: 1993, *Jesus: A Revolutionary Biography,* HarperCollins Publishers, New York.

[7] Douglas, M.: 1973, *Natural Symbols: Explorations in Cosmology,* Barrie & Jenkins, London.

[8] Finley, M. I.: 1973, *The Ancient Economy,* University of California Press, Berkeley and Los Angeles.

[9] Foucault, M.: 1978, *The History of Sexuality,* Vol. 1: *An Introduction,* R. Hurley (trans.), Random House, New York.

[10] Kasulis, T. P.: 1993, 'Introduction', in T. P. Kasulis et al. (eds.), *Self as Body in Asian Theory and Practice,* State University of New York Press, Albany, pp. ix-xx.

[11] Lerner, G.: 1986, *The Creation of Patriarchy,* Oxford University Press, New York and Oxford.

[12] Martin, E.: 1987, *The Woman in the Body: A Cultural Analysis of Reproduction,* Beacon Press, Boston.

[13] Meeks, W. A.: 1993, *The Origins of Christian Morality: The First Two Centuries,* Yale University Press, New Haven and London.

[14] Merleau-Ponty, M.: 1962, *Phenomenology of Perception,* C. Smith (trans.), Routledge and Kegan Paul, London and Henley, N.J.

[15] Moxnes, H.: 1988, *The Economy of the Kingdom: Social Conflict and Economic Relations in Luke's Gospel,* Fortress Press, Philadelphia.

[16] Schüssler Fiorenza, E.: 1983, *In Memory of Her: A Feminist Theological Reconstruction of Christian Origins,* Crossroad Publishing Company, New York.

[17] Sheets-Johnstone, M. (ed.): 1993, *Giving the Body Its Due,* State University of New York Press, Albany.

[18] Sheets-Johnstone, M.: 1993, "The Materialization of the Body: A History of Western Medicine, A History in Progress," in M. Sheets-Johnstone (ed.): 1993, *Giving the Body Its Due,* State University of New York Press, Albany, pp. 132-58.

[19] Taylor, C.: 1991, *The Ethics of Authenticity,* Harvard University Press, Cambridge, Mass., and London.

[20] Turner, B. S.: 1984, *The Body and Society: Explorations in Social Theory,* Basil Blackwell, Oxford and New York.

58 Health Is Membership

Wendell Berry

I

From our constant and increasing concerns about health, you can tell how seriously diseased we are. Health, as we may remember from at least some of the days of our youth, is at once wholeness and a kind of unconsciousness. Disease (dis-ease), on the contrary, makes us conscious not only of the state of our health but of the division of our bodies and our world into parts.

The word "health," in fact, comes from the same Indo-European root as "heal," "whole," and "holy." To be healthy is literally to be whole, to heal is to make whole. I don't think mortal healers should be credited with the power to make holy. But I have no doubt that such healers are properly obliged to acknowledge and respect the holiness embodied in all creatures, or that our healing involves the preservation in us of the spirit and the breath of God.

If we were lucky enough as children to be surrounded by grown-ups who loved us, then our sense of wholeness is not just the sense of completeness in ourselves but also is the sense of belonging to others and to our place; it is an unconscious awareness of community, of having in common. It may be that this double sense of singular integrity and of communal belonging is our personal standard of health for as long as we live. Anyhow, we seem to know instinctively that health is not divided.

Of course, growing up and growing older as fallen creatures in a fallen world can only instruct us painfully in division and disintegration. This is the stuff of consciousness and experience. But if our culture works in us as it should, then we do not age merely into disintegration and division, but that very experience begins our education, leading us into knowledge of wholeness and of holiness. I am describing here the story of Job, of Lazarus, of the lame man at the pool of Bethesda, of Milton's Samson, of King Lear. If our culture works in us as it should, our experience is balanced by education; we are led out of our lonely suffering and are made whole.

In the present age of the world, disintegration and division, isolation and suffering seem to have overwhelmed us. The balance between experience and education has been overthrown; we are lost in experience, and so-called education is leading us nowhere. We have diseases aplenty. As if that were not enough, we are suffering an almost universal hypochondria. Half the energy of the medical industry, one suspects, may now be devoted to "examinations" or "tests" — to see if, though apparently well, we may not be latently or insidiously diseased.

If you are going to deal with the issue of health in the modern world, you are going to have to deal with much absurdity. It is not clear, for example, why death should increasingly be looked upon as a curable disease, an abnormality, by a society that increasingly looks upon life as insupportably painful and/or meaningless. Even more startling is the realization that the modern medical industry faithfully imitates disease in the way that it isolates us and parcels us out. If, for example, intense and persistent pain causes you to pay attention only to your stomach, then you must leave home, community, and family and go to a sometimes distant clinic or hospital, where you will be cared for by a specialist who will pay attention only to your stomach.

Or consider the announcement by the Associated Press on February 9, 1994, that "the incidence of cancer is up among all ages, and researchers speculated that environmental exposure to cancer-causing substances other than cigarettes may be partly to blame." This bit of news is offered as a surprise, never mind that the environment (so called) has been known to be polluted and toxic for many years. The blame obviously falls on that idiotic term "the environment," which refers to a world that surrounds us but is presumably different from us and distant from us. Our laboratories have proved long ago that cigarette smoke gets inside us, but if "the environment" surrounds us, how does *it* wind up inside us? So much for division as a working principle of health.

This, plainly, is a view of health that is severely reductive. It is, to begin with, almost fanatically individualistic. The body is seen as a defective or potentially defective machine, singular, solitary, and displaced, without love, solace, or pleasure. Its health excludes unhealthy cigarettes but does not exclude unhealthy food, water, and air. One may presumably be healthy in a disintegrated family or community or in a destroyed or poisoned ecosystem.

So far, I have been implying my beliefs at every turn. Now I had better state them openly.

I take literally the statement in the Gospel of John that God loves the world. I believe that the world was created and approved by love, that it subsists, coheres, and endures by love, and that, insofar as it is redeemable, it can be redeemed only by love. I believe that divine love, incarnate and indwelling in the world, summons the world always toward wholeness, which ultimately is reconciliation and atonement with God.

I believe that health is wholeness. For many years I have returned again and again to the work of the English

From Wendell Berry, "Health Is Membership," in *Another Turn of the Crank* (Washington, D.C.: Counterpoint, 1996), 86-109.

agriculturist Sir Albert Howard, who said, in *The Soil and Health,* that "the whole problem of health in soil, plant, animal, and man [is] one great subject."

I am moreover a Luddite, in what I take to be the true and appropriate sense. I am not "against technology" so much as I am for community. When the choice is between the health of a community and technological innovation, I choose the health of the community. I would unhesitatingly destroy a machine before I would allow the machine to destroy my community.

I believe that the community — in the fullest sense: a place and all its creatures — is the smallest unit of health and that to speak of the health of an isolated individual is a contradiction in terms.

We speak now of "spirituality and healing" as if the only way to render a proper religious respect to the body is somehow to treat it "spiritually." It could be argued just as appropriately (and perhaps less dangerously) that the way to respect the body fully is to honor fully its materiality. In saying this, I intend no reduction. I do not doubt the reality of the experience and knowledge we call "spiritual" anymore than I doubt the reality of so-called physical experience and knowledge; I recognize the rough utility of these terms. But I strongly doubt the advantage, and even the possibility, of separating these two realities.

What I'm arguing against here is not complexity or mystery but dualism. I would like to purge my own mind and language of such terms as "spiritual," "physical," "metaphysical," and "transcendental" — all of which imply that the Creation is divided into "levels" that can readily be peeled apart and judged by human beings. I believe that the Creation is one continuous fabric comprehending simultaneously what we mean by "spirit" and what we mean by "matter."

Our bodies are involved in the world. Their needs and desires and pleasures are physical. Our bodies hunger and thirst, yearn toward other bodies, grow tired and seek rest, rise up rested, eager to exert themselves. All these desires may be satisfied with honor to the body and its maker, but only if much else besides the individual body is brought into consideration. We have long known that individual desires must not be made the standard of their own satisfaction. We must consider the body's manifold connections to other bodies and to the world. The body, "fearfully and wonderfully made," is ultimately mysterious both in itself and in its dependences. Our bodies live, the Bible says, by the spirit and the breath of God, but it does not say how this is so. We are not going to *know* about this.

The distinction between the physical and the spiritual is, I believe, false. A much more valid distinction, and one that we need urgently to learn to make, is that between the organic and the mechanical. To argue this — as I am going to do — puts me in the minority, I know, but it does not make me unique. In *The Idea of a Christian Society,* T. S. Eliot wrote, "We may say that religion, as distinguished from modern paganism, implies a life in conformity with nature. It may be observed that the natural life and the supernatural life have a conformity to each other which neither has with the mechanistic life."

Still, I wonder if our persistent wish to deal spiritually with physical things does not come either from the feeling that physical things are "low" and unworthy or from the fear, especially when speaking of affection, that "physical" will be taken to mean "sexual."

The *New York Review of Books* of February 3, 1994, for example, carried a review of the correspondence of William and Henry James along with a photograph of the two brothers standing together with William's arm around Henry's shoulders. Apropos of this picture, the reviewer, John Bayley, wrote that "their closeness of affection was undoubted and even took on occasion a quasi-physical form." It is Mr. Bayley's qualifier, "quasi-physical," that sticks in one's mind. What can he have meant by it? Is this prurience masquerading as squeamishness, or vice versa? Does Mr. Bayley feel a need to assure his psychologically sophisticated readers that even though these brothers touched one another familiarly, they were not homosexual lovers?

The phrase involves at least some version of the old dualism of spirit and body or mind and body that has caused us so much suffering and trouble and that raises such troubling questions for anybody who is interested in health. If you love your brother and if you and your brother are living creatures, how could your love for him not be physical? Not spiritual or mental only, not "quasi-physical," but physical. How could you not take a simple pleasure in putting your arm around him?

Out of the same dualism comes our confusion about the body's proper involvement in the world. People seriously interested in health will finally have to question our society's long-standing goals of convenience and effortlessness. What is the point of "labor saving" if by making work effortless we make it poor, and if by doing poor work we weaken our bodies and lose conviviality and health?

We are now pretty clearly involved in a crisis of health, one of the wonders of which is its immense profitability both to those who cause it and to those who propose to cure it. That the illness may prove incurable, except by catastrophe, is suggested by our economic dependence on it. Think, for example, of how readily our solutions become problems and our cures pollutants. To cure one disease, we need another. The causes, of course, are numerous and complicated, but all of them, I think, can be traced back to the old idea that our bodies are not very important except when they give us pleasure (usually, now, to somebody's profit) or when they hurt (now, almost invariably, to somebody's profit).

This dualism inevitably reduces physical reality, and it does so by removing its mystery from it, by dividing it absolutely from what dualistic thinkers have understood as spiritual or mental reality.

A reduction that is merely theoretical might be harmless enough, I suppose, but theories find ways of getting into action. The theory of the relative unimportance of physical reality has put itself into action by means of a metaphor by which the body (along with the world itself) is understood as a machine. According to this metaphor — which is now in constant general use — the human heart, for example, is no longer understood as the center of our emotional life or even as an organ that pumps; it is understood as "a pump," having somewhat the same function as a fuel pump in an automobile.

If the body is a machine for living and working, then it must follow that the mind is a machine for thinking. The "progress" here is the reduction of mind to brain and then of brain to computer. This reduction implies and requires the reduction of knowledge to "information." It requires, in fact, the reduction of everything to numbers and mathematical operations.

This metaphor of the machine bears heavily upon the question of what we mean by health and by healing. The problem is that, like any metaphor, it is accurate only in some respects. A girl is only in some respects like a red rose; a heart is only in some respects like a pump. This means that a metaphor must be controlled by a sort of humorous intelligence, always mindful of the exact limits within which the comparison is meaningful. When a metaphor begins to control intelligence, as this one of the machine has done for a long time, then we must look for costly distortions and absurdities.

Of course, the body in most ways is not at all like a machine. Like all living creatures and unlike a machine, the body is not formally self-contained; its boundaries and outlines are not so exactly fixed. The body alone is not, properly speaking, a body. Divided from its sources of air, food, drink, clothing, shelter, and companionship, a body is, properly speaking, a cadaver, whereas a machine by itself, shut down or out of fuel, is still a machine. Merely as an organism (leaving aside issues of mind and spirit) the body lives and moves and has its being, minute by minute, by an interinvolvement with other bodies and other creatures, living and unliving, that is too complex to diagram or describe. It is, moreover, under the influence of thought and feeling. It does not live by "fuel" alone.

A mind, probably, is even less like a computer than a body is like a machine. As far as I am able to understand it, a mind is not even much like a brain. Insofar as it is usable for thought, for the association of thought with feeling, for the association of thoughts and feelings with words, for the connections between words and things, words and acts, thought and memory, a mind seems to be in constant need of reminding. A mind unreminded would be no mind at all. This phenomenon of reminding shows the extensiveness of mind — how intricately it is involved with sensation, emotion, memory, tradition, communal life, known landscapes, and so on. How you could locate a mind within its full extent, among all its subjects and necessities, I don't know, but obviously it cannot be located within a brain or a computer.

To see better what a mind is (or is not), we might consider the difference between what we mean by knowledge and what the computer now requires us to mean by "information." Knowledge refers to the ability to do or say the right thing at the right time; we would not speak of somebody who does the wrong thing at the wrong time as "knowledgeable." People who perform well as musicians, athletes, teachers, or farmers are people of knowledge. And such examples tell us much about the nature of knowledge. Knowledge is formal, and it informs speech and action. It is instantaneous; it is present and available when and where it is needed.

"Information," which once meant that which forms or fashions from within, now means merely "data." However organized this data may be, it is not shapely or formal or in the true sense in-forming. It is not present where it is needed; if you have to "access" it, you don't have it. Whereas knowledge moves and forms acts, information is inert. You cannot imagine a debater or a quarterback or a musician performing by "accessing information." A computer chock full of such information is no more admirable than a head or a book chock full of it.

The difference, then, between information and knowledge is something like the difference between a dictionary and somebody's language.

Where the art and science of healing are concerned, the machine metaphor works to enforce a division that falsifies the process of healing because it falsifies the nature of the creature needing to be healed. If the body is a machine, then its diseases can be healed by a sort of mechanical tinkering, without reference to anything outside the body itself. This applies, with obvious differences, to the mind; people are assumed to be individually sane or insane. And so we return to the utter anomaly of a creature that is healthy within itself.

THE MODERN HOSPITAL, where most of us receive our strictest lessons in the nature of industrial medicine, undoubtedly does well at surgery and other procedures that permit the body and its parts to be treated as separate things. But when you try to think of it as a place of healing — of reconnecting and making whole — then the hospital reveals the disarray of the medical industry's thinking about health.

In healing, the body is restored to itself. It begins to live again by its own powers and instincts, to the extent that it can do so. To the extent that it can do so, it goes free of drugs and mechanical helps. Its appetites return. It relishes food and rest. The patient is restored to family and friends, home and community and work.

This process has a certain naturalness and inevitability, like that by which a child grows up, but industrial medicine seems to grasp it only tentatively and awkwardly. For example, any ordinary person would assume that a place of healing would put a premium upon rest, but hospitals are notoriously difficult to sleep in. They are noisy all night, and the routine interventions go on relentlessly. The body is treated as a machine that does not need to rest.

You would think also that a place dedicated to healing and health would make much of food. But here is where the disconnections of the industrial system and the displacement of industrial humanity are most radical. Sir Albert Howard saw accurately that the issue of human health is inseparable from the health of the soil, and he saw too that we humans must responsibly occupy our place in the cycle of birth, growth, maturity, death, and decay, which is the health of the world. Aside from our own mortal involvement, food is our fundamental connection to that cycle. But probably most of the complaints you hear about hospitals have to do with the food, which, according to the testimony I have heard, tends to range from unappetizing to sickening. Food is treated as another unpleasant substance to inject. And this is a shame. For in addition to the obvious nutritional link between food and health, food can be a pleasure. People who are sick are often troubled or depressed, and mealtimes offer three opportunities a day when patients could easily be offered something to look forward to. Nothing is more pleasing or heartening than a plate of nourishing, tasty, beautiful food artfully and lovingly prepared. Anything less is unhealthy, as well as a desecration.

Why should rest and food and ecological health not be the basic principles of our art and science of healing? Is it because the basic principles already are technology and drugs? Are we confronting some fundamental incompatibility between mechanical efficiency and organic health? I don't know. I only know that sleeping in a hospital is like sleeping in a factory and that the medical industry makes only the most tenuous connection between health and food and no connection between health and the soil. Industrial medicine is as little interested in ecological health as is industrial agriculture.

A further problem, and an equally serious one, is that illness, in addition to being a bodily disaster, is now also an economic disaster. This is so whether or not the patient is insured. It is a disaster for us all, all the time, because we all know that, personally or collectively, we cannot continue to pay for cures that continue to get more expensive. The economic disturbance that now inundates the problem of illness may turn out to be the profoundest illness of all. How can we get well if we are worried sick about money?

I WISH IT WERE not the fate of this essay to be filled with questions, but questions now seem the inescapable end of any line of thought about health and healing. Here are several more:

1. Can our present medical industry produce an adequate definition of health? My own guess is that it cannot do so. Like industrial agriculture, industrial medicine has depended increasingly on specialist methodology, mechanical technology, and chemicals; thus, its point of reference has become more and more its own technical prowess and less and less the health of creatures and habitats. I don't expect this problem to be solved in the universities, which have never addressed, much less solved, the problem of health in agriculture. And I don't expect it to be solved by the government.

2. How can cheapness be included in the criteria of medical experimentation and performance? And why has it not been included before now? I believe that the problem here is again that of the medical industry's fixation on specialization, technology, and chemistry. As a result, the modern "health care system" has become a way of marketing industrial products, exactly like modern agriculture, impoverishing those who pay and enriching those who are paid. It is, in other words, an industry such as industries have always been.

3. Why is it that medical strictures and recommendations so often work in favor of food processors and against food producers? Why, for example, do we so strongly favor the pasteurization of milk to health and cleanliness in milk production? (Gene Logsdon correctly says that the motive here "is monopoly, not consumer health.")

4. Why do we so strongly prefer a fat-free or a germfree diet to a chemical-free diet? Why does the medical industry strenuously oppose the use of tobacco, yet complacently accept the massive use of antibiotics and other drugs in meat animals and of poisons on food crops? How much longer can it cling to the superstition of bodily health in a polluted world?

5. How can adequate medical and health care, including disease prevention, be included in the structure and economy of a community? How, for example, can a community and its doctors be included in the same culture, the same knowledge, and the same fate, so that they will live as fellow citizens, sharers in a common wealth, members of one another?

II

It is clear by now that this essay cannot hope to be complete; the problems are too large and my knowledge too small. What I have to offer is an association of thoughts and questions wandering somewhat at random and somewhat lost within the experience of modern diseases and the often bewildering industry that undertakes to cure them. In my ignorance and bewilderment, I am fairly representative of those who go, or go with loved ones, to doctors' offices and hospitals. What I have written so far comes from my various efforts to make as much sense as I can of that experience. But now I had better turn to the experience itself.

On January 3, 1994, my brother John had a severe heart attack while he was out by himself on his farm, moving a feed trough. He managed to get to the house and telephone a friend, who sent the emergency rescue squad.

The rescue squad and the emergency room staff at a local hospital certainly saved my brother's life. He was later moved to a hospital in Louisville, where a surgeon performed a double-bypass operation on his heart. After three weeks John returned home. He still has a life to live and work to do. He has been restored to himself and to the world.

He and those who love him have a considerable debt to the medical industry, as represented by two hospitals, several doctors and nurses, many drugs and many machines. This is a debt that I cheerfully acknowledge. But I am obliged to say also that my experience of the hospital during John's stay was troubled by much conflict of feeling and a good many unresolved questions, and I know that I am not alone in this.

In the hospital what I will call the world of love meets the world of efficiency — the world, that is, of specialization, machinery, and abstract procedure. Or, rather, I should say that these two worlds come together in the hospital but do not meet. During those weeks when John was in the hospital, it seemed to me that he had come from the world of love and that the family members, neighbors, and friends who at various times were there with him came there to represent that world and to preserve his connection with it. It seemed to me that the hospital was another kind of world altogether.

When I said early in this essay that we live in a world that was created and exists and is redeemable by love, I did not mean to sentimentalize it. For this is also a fallen world. It involves error and disease, ignorance and partiality, sin and death. If this world is a place where we may learn of our involvement in immortal love, as I believe it is, still such learning is only possible here because that love involves us so inescapably in the limits, sufferings, and sorrows of mortality.

LIKE DIVINE LOVE, earthly love seeks plenitude; it longs for the full membership to be present and to be joined. Unlike divine love, earthly love does not have the power, the knowledge, or the will to achieve what it longs for. The story of human love on this earth is a story by which this love reveals and even validates itself by its failures to be complete and comprehensive and effective enough. When this love enters a hospital, it brings with it a terrifying history of defeat, but it comes nevertheless confident of itself, for its existence and the power of its longing have been proved over and over again even by its defeat. In the face of illness, the threat of death, and death itself, it insists unabashedly on its own presence, understanding by its persistence through defeat that it is superior to whatever happens.

The world of efficiency ignores both loves, earthly and divine, because by definition it must reduce experience to computation, particularity to abstraction, and mystery to a small comprehensibility. Efficiency, in our present sense of the word, allies itself inevitably with machinery, as Neil Postman demonstrates in his useful book, *Technopoly*. "Machines," he says, "eliminate complexity, doubt, and ambiguity. They work swiftly, they are standardized, and they provide us with numbers that you can see and calculate with." To reason, the advantages are obvious, and probably no reasonable person would wish to reject them out of hand.

And yet love obstinately answers that no loved one is standardized. A body, love insists, is neither a spirit nor a machine; it is not a picture, a diagram, a chart, a graph, an anatomy; it is not an explanation; it is not a law. It is precisely and uniquely what it is. It belongs to the world of love, which is a world of living creatures, natural orders and cycles, many small, fragile lights in the dark.

In dealing with problems of agriculture, I had thought much about the difference between creatures and machines. But I had never so clearly understood and felt that difference as when John was in recovery after his heart surgery, when he was attached to many machines and was dependent for breath on a respirator. It was impossible then not to see that the breathing of a machine, like all machine work, is unvarying, an oblivious regularity, whereas the breathing of a creature is ever changing, exquisitely responsive to events both inside and outside the body, to thoughts and emotions. A machine makes breaths as a machine makes buttons, all the same, but every breath of a creature is itself a creature, like no other, inestimably precious.

LOGICALLY, in plenitude some things ought to be expendable. Industrial economics has always believed this: abundance justifies waste. This is one of the dominant superstitions of American history — and of the history of colonialism everywhere. Expendability is also an assumption of the world of efficiency, which is why that world deals so compulsively in percentages of efficacy and safety.

But this sort of logic is absolutely alien to the world of love. To the claim that a certain drug or procedure would save 99 percent of all cancer patients or that a certain pollutant would be safe for 99 percent of a population, love, unembarrassed, would respond, "What about the one percent?"

There is nothing rational or perhaps even defensible about this, but it is nonetheless one of the strongest strands of our religious tradition — it is probably the most essential strand — according to which a shepherd, owning a hundred sheep and having lost one, does not say, "I have saved 99 percent of my sheep," but rather, "I have lost one," and he goes and searches for the one. And if the sheep in that parable may seem to be only a metaphor, then go on to the Gospel of Luke, where the principle is flatly set forth again and where the sparrows stand not for human beings but for all creatures: "Are not five sparrows sold for two farthings, and not one of them is forgotten before God?" And John Donne had in mind a sort of equation and not a mere metaphor when he wrote, "If a clod be washed away by the sea, Europe is the less, as well as if a promontory were, as well as if a manor of thy friend's or of thine own were. Any man's death diminishes me."

It is reassuring to see ecology moving toward a similar idea of the order of things. If an ecosystem loses one of its native species, we now know that we cannot speak of it as itself minus one species. An ecosystem minus one specics is a different ecosystem. Just so, each of us is made by — or, one might better say, made as — a set of unique associations with unique persons, places, and things. The world of love does not admit the principle of the interchangeability of parts.

When John was in intensive care after his surgery, his wife, Carol, was standing by his bed, grieving and afraid. Wanting to reassure her, the nurse said, "Nothing is happening to him that doesn't happen to everybody."

And Carol replied, "I'm not everybody's wife."

In the world of love, things separated by efficiency and specialization strive to come back together. And yet love must confront death, and accept it, and learn from it. Only in confronting death can earthly love learn its true extent, its immortality. Any definition of health that is not silly must include death. The world of love includes death, suffers it, and triumphs over it. The world of efficiency is defeated by death; at death, all its instruments and procedures stop. The world of love continues, and of this grief is the proof.

In the hospital, love cannot forget death. But like love, death is in the hospital but not of it. Like love, fear and grief feel out of place in the hospital. How could they be included in its efficient procedures and mechanisms? Where a clear, small order is fervently maintained, fear and grief bring the threat of large disorder.

And so these two incompatible worlds might also be designated by the terms "amateur" and "professional" — amateur, in the literal sense of lover, one who participates for love; and professional in the modern sense of one who performs highly specialized or technical procedures for pay. The amateur is excluded from the professional "field."

For the amateur, in the hospital or in almost any other encounter with the medical industry, the overriding experience is that of being excluded from knowledge — of being unable, in other words, to make or participate in anything resembling an "informed decision." Of course, whether doctors make informed decisions in the hospital is a matter of debate. For in the hospital even the professionals are involved in experience; experimentation has been left far behind. Experience, as all amateurs know, is not predictable, and in experience there are no replications or "controls"; there is nothing with which to compare the result. Once one decision has been made, we have destroyed the opportunity to know what would have happened if another decision had been made. That is to say that medicine is an exact science until applied; application involves intuition, a sense of probability, "gut feeling," guesswork, and error.

In medicine, as in many modern disciplines, the amateur is divided from the professional by perhaps unbridgeable differences of knowledge and of language. An "informed decision" is really not even imaginable for most medical patients and their families, who have no competent understanding of either the patient's illness or the recommended medical or surgical procedure. Moreover, patients and their families are not likely to know the doctor, the surgeon, or any of the other people on whom the patient's life will depend. In the hospital, amateurs are more than likely to be proceeding entirely upon faith — and this is a peculiar and scary faith, for it must be placed not in a god but in mere people, mere procedures, mere chemicals, and mere machines.

It was only after my brother had been taken in to surgery, I think, that the family understood the extremity of this deed of faith. We had decided — or John had decided and we had concurred — on the basis of the best advice available. But once he was separated from us, we felt the burden of our ignorance. We had not known what we were doing, and one of our difficulties now was the feeling that we had utterly given him up to what he did not know. John himself spoke out of this sense of abandonment and helplessness in the intensive care unit, when he said, "I don't know what they're going to do to me or for me or with me."

As we waited and reports came at long intervals from the operating room, other realizations followed. We realized that under the circumstances, we could not be told the truth. We would not know, ever, the worries and surprises that came to the surgeon during his work. We would not know the critical moments or the fears. If the surgeon did any part of his work ineptly or made a mistake, we would not know it. We realized, moreover, that if we were told the truth, we would have no way of knowing that the truth was what it was.

We realized that when the emissaries from the operating room assured us that everything was "normal" or "routine," they were referring to the procedure and not the patient. Even as amateurs — perhaps *because* we were amateurs — we knew that what was happening was not normal or routine for John or for us.

That these two worlds are so radically divided does not mean that people cannot cross between them. I do not know how an amateur can cross over into the professional world; that does not seem very probable. But that professional people can cross back into the amateur world, I know from much evidence. During John's stay in the hospital there were many moments in which doctors and nurses — especially nurses! — allowed or caused the professional relationship to become a meeting between two human beings, and these moments were invariably moving.

The most moving, to me, happened in the waiting room during John's surgery. From time to time a nurse from the operating room would come in to tell Carol what was happening. Carol, from politeness or bravery or both, always stood to receive the news, which always left us somewhat encouraged and somewhat doubtful. Carol's difficulty was that she had to suffer the ordeal not only as a wife but as one who had been a trained nurse. She knew, from her own education and experience, in how limited a sense open-heart surgery could be said to be normal or routine.

Finally, toward the end of our wait, two nurses came in. The operation, they said, had been a success. They explained again what had been done. And then they said that after the completion of the bypasses, the surgeon had found it necessary to insert a "balloon pump" into the aorta to assist the heart. This possibility had never been mentioned, nobody was prepared for it, and Carol was sorely disappointed and upset. The two young women attempted to reassure her, mainly by repeating things they had already said. And then there was a long moment when they just looked at her. It was such a look as parents sometimes give to a sick or suffering child, when they themselves have begun to need the comfort they are trying to give.

And then one of the nurses said, "Do you need a hug?"

"Yes," Carol said. And the nurse gave her a hug.

Which brings us to a starting place.

59 Organ Transplants: Death, Dis-organ-ization, and the Need for Religious Ritual

Allen D. Verhey

"'Brain-dead,' said the doctor." It's the first line in Richard Selzer's story of Hannah in "Whither Thou Goest."[1] It's the first line, but it is hardly the last word.

Hannah and Sam, her husband, had celebrated his thirty-third birthday by spending a weekend at the beach together. On the trip home Sam had stopped their pickup to help a stranded motorist change a tire. Good Samaritan Sam was himself assaulted, shot in the head, and left in the road with a halo of blood. Three weeks later, as preface to his request that Hannah donate her husband's organs for transplantation, the doctor announced that Sam was brain-dead. It seemed reasonable enough, supported by an electroencephalograph that the doctor unrolled to display a tidy flat line. In an effort to reassure Hannah, however, the doctor added, "The only thing keeping him alive is the respirator." That remark, hard on the heels of the doctor's confident announcement that Sam was brain-dead, confused Hannah — and revealed a messy ambiguity that no flat line on a graph could hide.

"Let him go," the doctor said, evidently unable to comprehend the implication of his own diagnosis that he was already gone. The doctor pressed on toward the request. "We would like your permission to harvest Sam's organs for transplantation," he said. And, as if to make it easier for Hannah, he added, "That way your husband will live on. He will not really have died. . . ."[2] This statement confused Hannah still more, and in an effort to restore some sense to this conversation she responded, "Dead is dead."

In spite of her confusion — or perhaps because of it — Hannah allowed the hospital to "harvest" Sam's organs. A week later she received a thank-you letter from the doctor. It informed her that, thanks to her generous gift (and "to the miracle of modern science"), Sam's organs were benefiting seven people. There was a little list of organs and recipients, including information that Sam's heart had been given to "a man just your husband's age

1. Richard Selzer, *Imagine a Woman and Other Tales* (New York: Random House, 1990), 3-28.

2. Ibid., 4.

in a little town near Arkansas."[3] This information, too, confused Hannah. She was baffled by this situation. She found getting on with her life difficult. "'Dead is dead,' she had told that doctor. But now . . . she wasn't so sure."[4] "Maybe, she thought, it was a matter of percentage — if more than 50 percent of your husband was dead, you were a widow."[5] She even stopped going to the Evangelical Baptist Church cemetery to visit Sam's grave. "It wasn't Sam in that cemetery, not by a long shot. It was only parts of Sam, the parts that nobody needed. The rest of him was scattered all over Texas. And, unless she had been misinformed, very much alive."[6]

Along with the doubts came resentment. She resented the doctors for covering up their dismembering of people by "soft words of husbandry and the soil" like "harvest" and "transplant." Worse than that, she began to resent Samuel, who "was participating in not one but seven lives, none of which had anything to do with her."[7] And she resented the radio preacher's talk about resurrection of the flesh. "It's a big lie," she said to her born-again cousin Ivy Lou. "There is no such thing. . . . What about Samuel Owens on your resurrection day? . . . They going to put him back together again when the day comes, or is it that to the recipients belong the spoils? Tell me that."[8]

Hannah remembered a story Sam had told her of his own bewilderment with loss. Sam's father had died suddenly of a heart attack when Sam was twelve years old. For a long time afterward, he would think that he had seen his father on the street and would run after the man, calling out, "Daddy." When he caught up with the man, of course, he always discovered that he had been mistaken. His behavior got him into some trouble with strangers and with his mother. When it finally stopped happening, Sam had said, he had felt a mixture of relief and disappointment. Hannah remembered how she had wept for the little boy "who couldn't let go of his father" when Sam had told her that story.[9]

In her own bewilderment Hannah decided to seek out the man with Sam's heart in that little town near Arkansas and to plead with him to permit her to listen to Sam's heart for a little while. Then "she would be healed," she was confident.[10] After she succeeded in identifying the man, she wrote to him, requesting permission to listen to Sam's heart. After the man replied with a polite refusal, she wrote again. After the man reported that his doctor doesn't think it would be a good idea, she wrote to tell him that doctors "haven't the least idea about the human heart except to move it from place to place."[11] The man still refused, but he admitted that he felt bad about it, "like ungrateful or something."[12] Hannah's next letters reminded him of the gift, assured him that she doesn't want it back, and promised that, if he would permit her to listen to Sam's heart, "you will have repaid me in full."[13]

The man's replies grew increasingly impatient and attempted to put an end to the correspondence. In what she promised would be her last letter Hannah asked the man for the gift of a photograph of him. When he sent a picture in reply, Hannah was sure that "that heart is working," and wrote to thank him.[14] The thank-you note evidently succeeded where the request for repayment had failed, for a little while later the man sent Hannah an invitation to come to that little town near the Arkansas border and to listen to Sam's heart for an hour.

She accepted the invitation. The preliminaries were a little awkward, and when she finally lowered her ear to his left nipple, she could feel the man wince. But she could hear the heart plainly. "Oh, it was Sam's heart, all right. She knew the minute she heard it. She could have picked it out of a thousand."[15] After an hour of listening and remembering, there was a change in both the man and Hannah. He was tender and gentle, even wondering whether Hannah would want to come to listen again. But Hannah said, "There will be no need," confident that her life had been retrieved from the shadows and grateful for the man whose chest, it seemed to her, "was a field of golden wheat in which, for this time, it had been given to her to go gleaning."[16] She was ready to get on with her life, and she was glad for the gift she gave and for the gift she was given.

It is an outrageous story in a way, but it artfully displays certain ambiguities in transplantation procedures. First is the ambiguity that attends the determination of death; the tidy and reasonable criteria for determining that a person is "brain-dead" do not eliminate (and cannot hide) this ambiguity. There is an ambiguity in the responsibilities of care; the needs of the grieving may conflict with the needs of a prospective recipient. These ambiguities can conspire to undercut confidence in physicians. The gift relationship between donor and recipient is itself ambiguous. And religious traditions have had an ambiguous relationship with transplantation. The experience (and the language) of both caregivers and survivors is frequently messy. The task undertaken here is not to eliminate the messiness but to understand it, to appreciate why it cannot be altogether eliminated, and to suggest the potential of religious ritual for pointing a way through the mess in ways that honor both the dead and their gifts.

"'Brain-dead,' said the doctor." Consider first the development of tidy and reasonable criteria for the deter-

3. Ibid.
4. Ibid., 6.
5. Ibid., 7.
6. Ibid.
7. Ibid., 7-8.
8. Ibid., 8-9.
9. Ibid., 10.
10. Ibid.
11. Ibid., 19.

12. Ibid.
13. Ibid, 20.
14. Ibid., 23.
15. Ibid., 27.
16. Ibid., 28.

mination of death. It was, of course, the ambiguities that attended the first heart transplant that made it important and necessary to develop some tidy and reasonable criteria for the determination of death. The criteria for the determination of brain death, however, as necessary as they may be, do not eliminate the ambiguities.

I am old enough to remember billboards urging motorists to drive safely by joining a picture of Dr. Christian Barnard in scrubs to the message, "Slow down! Dr. Barnard wants your heart!" When I saw that billboard (sometime close to 1968, I presume), I slowed down a little and, muttering something about the fact that I was still using mine, I wondered how Dr. Barnard could take a living heart from a person without killing that person. One wanted to assume, of course, that the person from whom the heart was taken was already dead, but how can you know that someone with a beating heart is dead? The question was unavoidable, and the first moral challenge for heart transplantation procedures was to answer that unavoidable question.

The challenge was met with the development of a remarkable consensus that one could determine death by the irreversible cessation of whole brain function, which could be made independently on either cardiac or respiratory arrest. Already in 1968, a Harvard ad hoc committee recommended criteria by which such a determination of death could be made. In 1972, an influential study group from the Hastings Center endorsed these criteria, and in 1981 the President's Commission gave their approval and drafted a Uniform Determination of Death Act. That model law was endorsed by both the American Medical Association and the American Bar Association and eventually adopted by all fifty states.

The unavoidable question had an answer. There is a way to determine that someone with a beating heart is dead, a way to determine that a person is dead independently of heart and lung function, which can be mechanically supported. The answer, the consensus that supports it, and the legislation that gives it effect are of obvious importance to transplantation procedures; indeed, they are morally necessary to certain transplantation procedures. Even so, Hannah's story reminds us that the reasonable and tidy criteria meet the challenge only in part. They do not eliminate the messiness of the situation, or the ambiguity of death, or the kind of confusion that Hannah experienced.

Her confusion is not difficult to understand. The "neomort" appears very much alive, and every reasonable effort is made to "keep it alive" for the sake of the transplant. Brain-dead and ready for surgery, the cadaver is warm, has a good color, and continues to digest and eliminate. Moreover, monitoring continues, along with interventions designed to preserve the cadaver's "health." Even our language almost inevitably expresses this confusing situation. A "healthy cadaver" is an oxymoron. But for the sake of it, we have "brain-dead" bodies on "life-support" systems. After the transplant, the "brain dead" are removed from the ventilator and "allowed to die" or "allowed to die all the way" or "really die." The point is not to call into question the rightness of the criteria, but to suggest why they are insufficient.

The criteria are tidy, but the experience is confusing and sometimes disconcerting even for those who are practiced in it. The doctors and nurses who work in transplantation are no strangers to this confusion. In a fascinating study of nearly two hundred physicians and nurses likely to be involved in organ procurement, Stuart Youngner and his colleagues demonstrated the dissonance between the intellectual understanding of criteria for the determination of brain death and the experience of those who care for brain-dead organ donors. In one part of the study, the doctors and nurses were presented with two cases and asked both whether the patients were legally dead and whether, aside from legalities, they themselves regarded the patients as really dead and why. Only about a third of the total number of respondents and about two-thirds of the physicians were able to identify the criteria for determining death correctly, and "the personal concepts of death varied widely."[17] The "conceptual disarray" that Youngner and his colleagues demonstrated did not suggest that death was being misdiagnosed or that patients were being prematurely declared dead and their organs removed. But the study did conclude that "[t]hough clinicians can tell which patients have permanent loss of all brain function there is no consensus over whether, and especially why, this means they have died."[18] If the professionals find this experience confusing and sometimes disconcerting, then one can imagine how much more difficult it must be for families. For families, of course, the "neomort" is not just a cadaver, but Mom or Son or Sam.

Even without the complicating factor of organ transplantation, the tidy criteria are insufficient. Joseph Fins tells the story of a seventy-seven-year-old Chinese woman who was assessed for brain death. The patient, a widow with a history of poorly controlled hypertension, had come to New York to visit her youngest son and his wife. The daughter-in-law, who had been trained as a physician in China, had urged the patient to see a physician, but the patient had refused. Then she suffered a severe anoxic brain injury after a large intracranial hemorrhage and subsequent cardiac arrest. The son and daughter-in-law were distraught, of course, and when they were informed that the patient would be assessed for brain death, they objected. (Under New York law clinicians are required to make "reasonable accommodation" for religious and moral objections to brain-death criteria.) The daughter-in-law was feeling guilty that she had not been able to convince the woman to have her

17. S. J. Youngner, S. Landefeld, C. J. Coupon et al., "'Brain Death' and Organ Retrieval: A Cross-sectional Survey of Knowledge and Concepts among Health Professionals," *Journal of the American Medical Association* 261 (21 April 1989): 2205-2210.

18. D. Wikler and A. J. Weisbard, "Appropriate Confusion over 'Brain Death,'" *Journal of the American Medical Association* 261 (21 April 1989): 2246.

blood pressure monitored, and she worried that the family in China might blame them for the woman's death. The son felt "marooned between life and loss."

Because his mother was "alive," he could not bring himself to grieve. The tidy criteria for brain death were not what this family needed to clarify their situation and to recognize the death of their mother. The doctors withheld their determination of death while the daughter-in-law and son went through rituals appropriate to dying in their culture.

The daughter-in-law read a large Chinese placard to the patient. With tears in her eyes, she read plaintively rocking back and forth in a trance-like state as she held the bed rail for support. The message, dictated by relatives back home, was one of wishes and blessing, "saying goodbye and asking for forgiveness."

The assessment for brain death was done after the rituals were complete and the family had left the room. The neurologist who performed the test dismissed the concerns of the family about the application of the brain-death criteria by saying, "You are your brain." Others in the room, Fins reported, "were not so sure" anymore.

> After the patient did not breathe on her own, the endotracheal tube was removed. She looked quite peaceful. Her coloring remained good. She remained in a normal sinus rhythm on the monitor. After about eight minutes, she flexed her arms and brought them to the midline in what appeared to be a purposeful movement, only to let them fall slowly to her side. . . . After this, she became dusky. Though it was almost certainly a physiologic response, the change struck me as a profound moment of transition. One resident in the room commented that the patient now "looked dead." One colleague later described it as the patient's true passage. And that certainly was the intuitive sense that many of us had in spite of our training in biomedical science. Even as the neurologist reassured us that what we had witnessed was just a cervical reflex often described as a "Lazarus sign," the intensivist quickly reached for his stethoscope to listen to the patient's heart and lungs. Reflexively, he had to confirm that the patient was truly dead by conventional means, notwithstanding the declaration of brain death that had been made moments earlier. At that moment, science only took us so far.[19]

The story not only displays the insufficiency of the tidy brain-death criteria to eliminate the confusion about the determination of death; it also identifies why the criteria are insufficient: "science only took us so far." Death is a human event. It may not simply be reduced to simple scientific criteria. When the criteria are not acknowledged as insufficient, we risk the sort of reductionism to which the neurologist gave voice. Human rituals are as important to the recognition of death as the scientific criteria that are used to determine brain death. We will return to the importance of ritual, but first it will be useful to summarize the ambiguity surrounding brain death and to attend to certain other ambiguities in transplant.

There may be no better way to summarize the problem than to remember one of the initial challenges to the brain-death criteria. In spite of the developing consensus in 1974, Hans Jonas wrote an essay, "Against the Stream." The worries and suspicions he voiced in that essay did not stem the stream, but they seem remarkably prescient after twenty-five years. Jonas criticized the position of the Harvard ad hoc committee for its effort to provide a sharp line between life and death when, in fact, according to Jonas, life often shades imperceptibly into death. "Giving intrinsic vagueness its due is not being vague," he said. "Aristotle observed that it is the mark of a well-educated man not to insist on greater precision in knowledge than the subject admits. . . . Reality of certain kinds — of which the life-death spectrum is perhaps one — may be imprecise in itself, or the knowledge obtainable of it may be. To acknowledge such a state of affairs is more adequate to it than a precise definition, which does violence to it."[20]

Even if we admit the necessity of some precise criteria, Jonas reminds us of the inevitable ambiguity and warns us against pretending that any tidy criteria can eliminate that ambiguity. Such pretense violates the human experience of both caregivers and survivors.

In addition to this claim about the intrinsic vagueness of the borderline between life and death, Jonas also complained about the consequences and about the sources of the tidy new definition. Concerning the consequences, he worried that the new definition would substitute a diagnostic question for the axiological one and that the body would be commodified: "[T]he question is not: has the patient died? but: how should he — still a patient — be dealt with? Now this question must be settled, surely not by a definition of death, but by a definition of man and of what life is human. That is to say, the question cannot be answered by decreeing that death has already occurred and the body is therefore in the domain of things. . . ."[21]

Jonas may have been wrong when he attempted simply to set aside the question, "Has the patient died?" That question, I think, is morally unavoidable. He was right, however, in insisting that a definition of death not be allowed to substitute for the question "How should he — still a patient — be dealt with?" Both questions are morally important. The danger comes when we assume that we resolve the moral ambiguities surrounding the death of a patient when we can answer the first question. Then

19. Joseph Fins, "When Brain Death Pulls at the Heart Strings," in *Personal Narratives on Caring for the Dying,* 2d ed. (American Board of Internal Medicine, forthcoming), 21-22.

20. Hans Jonas, "Against the Stream: Comments on the Definition and Redefinition of Death," in *Philosophical Essays: From Ancient Creed to Technological Man* (Englewood Cliffs, N.J.: Prentice-Hall, 1974). Reprinted in *Contemporary Issues in Bioethics,* ed. Tom L. Beauchamp and LeRoy Walters (Encino, Calif.: Dickenson Publishing Co., 1978), 263.

21. Ibid., 264.

we risk thinking that the situation can be adequately handled "by decreeing that death has already occurred and the body is therefore in the domain of things."

Concerning the sources of the new definition, Jonas identified them as "the ruling pragmatism of our time" and "the old body-soul dualism." And he was suspicious of both. It was pragmatism, he said, that motivated a definition of death that served the interests of the expanding powers of transplantation. His suspicion of pragmatism is captured in his characterization of it as "the relentless expanding of the realm of sheer thinghood and unrestricted utility."[22] And it was body-soul dualism, he said, even if in its "new apparition" as "the dualism of brain and body," that allowed us to hold "that the true human person rests in the brain, of which the rest of the body is a mere subservient tool."[23] Against such dualism he insisted, "My identity is the identity of the whole organism, even if the higher functions of personhood are seated in the brain. How else could a man love a woman and not merely her brains?"[24] Hannah would have understood. The neurologist in Fins's story evidently did not.

"They haven't the least idea about the human heart except to move it from place to place." Perhaps it is inevitable that Hannah would be suspicious of doctors like the neurologist in Fins's story. It is not that Hannah, or people like her, sees the doctor as a villain, although, of course, there is the old suspicion of greed. Rather, I think, they see the doctor as a hero but as a tragic hero; as a hero with a tragic flaw of character, as a hero so committed to a certain good end that he ignores the evil, the injustice, or the indignity of certain means to accomplish it. They see those skilled in transplant surgery as crusaders, as powerful do-gooders who are prepared to overlook (or undercut) the vulnerable in order to achieve the good they can do and long to do for other patients.[25]

The public polls concerning transplantation suggest such a view of physicians. On the one hand, the public supports transplantation and celebrates the good it can sometimes do. According to the 1985 Gallup poll commissioned by the American Council on Transplantation, three-quarters of those polled approved of organ donation.[26] And in a 1993 Gallup survey, 85 percent of those polled approved of organ donation.[27] People are evidently glad that we are not quite so helpless and so hopeless in the face of diseased and damaged organs; they are grateful that the powers of medicine can intervene in these sad stories and sometimes give them a happy ending after all, and they are ready to regard the doctors as heroes.

On the other hand, the same polls testify to the public's suspicions. Even those who approve of transplantation are evidently reticent to donate their organs. According to that 1985 Gallup poll, although three-quarters of those polled approved of organ donation, only one-quarter said they would be "very likely" to donate their own organs at death, and only 17 percent said they had completed donor cards.[28] And in the 1993 survey, although 85 percent approved of organ donation, only 37 percent said they would be "very likely" to donate their organs, and only 28 percent reported that they had granted permission for organ donation on a driver's license or donor card.[29] The reasons for this reticence, however, are more interesting than the statistics. In that 1985 Gallup poll those who said they would not donate their own organs gave a variety of reasons: "They might do something to me before I'm really dead." "Doctors might hasten my death." "I don't like to think about dying." "I don't like someone cutting me up after I die." "I never thought about it." "I want my body intact for the afterlife." "My family might object." "It's against my religion." "It's complicated to give permission."[30] Only some of these reasons testify to the public suspicion of doctors, of course. Nevertheless, it is noteworthy that in 1985, some years after the consensus on the criteria for brain death had been formed, 23 percent of the people polled by Gallup said, "They might do something to me before I die," and 21 percent said, "Doctors might hasten my death." (Moreover, those numbers were up significantly from a 1983 poll by Gallup.)

The explanation is not, I think, simply that the public was unaware of the developing consensus concerning brain death. Rather, they were suspicious of it because, as we have already observed, there is evidently some dis-

22. Ibid., 266.

23. Ibid.

24. Ibid.

25. The image of physician as crusader helps to clarify, I think, why so much of medical ethics and public discourse about medical ethics focuses on the "rights" of patients. It also helps us to understand what is good and what is bad about that focus. It is good because the language of "rights" is the most powerful language we have to constrain and restrain the powerful do-gooder. It is bad because it is essentially adversarial — it will not (cannot) nurture or sustain the loyalty and trust that are essential not only to healing but to the effort to procure organs for transplant. Adversarial relationships and distrust are serious barriers to procuring organs for transplant. Legalistic attention to the "rights" of patients and their families will not nurture the necessary trust, and any actions that are seen as compromising the loyalty physicians owe patients and their families will threaten that trust. Medical ethics could contribute to alleviating suspicion by developing alternative ways to talk about these issues. And religious communities have access to other ways of talking about professional obligations, like the image of "covenant" that William F. May has used so compellingly.

26. Task Force on Organ Transplantation, *Organ Transplantation: Issues and Recommendations* (Washington, D.C.: U.S. Department of Health and Hunan Services, 1986), 31.

27. The Partnership for Organ Donation, *The American Public's Attitudes toward Organ Donation and Transplantation: Summary Results of a Gallup Survey Prepared for The Partnership for Organ Donation* (Boston: The Partnership for Organ Donation, 1993), 3, 6.

28. Task Force on Organ Transplantation, *Organ Transplantation,* 31.

29. Partnership for Organ Donation, *American Public's Attitudes,* 3, 6.

30. Task Force on Organ Transplantation, *Organ Transplantation,* 31.

tance between the acceptance of tidy, scientific, and eminently reasonable criteria for the determination of death and the messy, human, and emotional reality of a "neomort." But they also were suspicious of those who sponsored the developing consensus; they were suspicious that it was the work of crusaders.

It is not hard to understand the public's suspicion of the new criteria. When the Harvard ad hoc committee issued its landmark report in 1968, it reported that one reason for updating the definition of death was to make it easier to obtain organs for transplant. That was unfortunate, and it was more unfortunate that that justification for the new criteria was frequently repeated in public discussion of the developing consensus. People got the idea that the reason for the new definition of death was to make organ transplantation possible. The consensus sounded, frankly, opportunistic. Those who did not want doctors to hasten their deaths for the sake of their organs also did not want doctors calling them dead prematurely for the sake of their organs. The public may have regarded doctors as heroes, but they also suspected that they were flawed by their very commitment to care for their patients, ready to hasten the moment at which other patients would be regarded as dead in order to obtain their organs.

That particular suspicion may have been unjustified. The consensus concerning whole brain death may not have been formed in quite so opportunistic a fashion. Indeed, many of those who urged the acceptance of the new criteria, including the influential Hastings Center task force, quite deliberately rejected the need for organs as a reason to adopt the criteria. The need for organs was part of the occasion for the reconsideration of the determination of death, along with the development of life-support technology, but it was not regarded as a justification of the new criteria.[31] Rather, the consensus was formed in the recognition that traditionally death meant not the death of the whole organism but the death of the organism as a whole. It was (and is) an essentially conservative concept of death, even if the criteria for determining the death of the organism as a whole now involved technical assessment of brainstem activity.

If the public was (unfairly) suspicious of the new consensus, that suspicion hints at the public's suspicion of the medical profession itself, and especially of transplant physicians, as tragic heroes equipped with powers to do good but flawed by their hubris. That suspicion of transplantation medicine was shared and expressed in the book by medical anthropologists Renee Fox and Judith Swazey, *Spare Parts: Organ Replacement in American Society*. Their decision to "leave the field" after thirty years of work was a public complaint, not only of inequities but also of the hubris of the transplantation industry. Their complaint about hubris is a description of crusaders who, in their desire to cure organ failure, are unmindful of the evil they sometimes do, ready to trample the embodied integrity of their patients and to neglect their suffering. Such hubris can be traced to a mechanistic dualism that reduces the body either to the battlefield where the war against disease and death is waged or to "spare parts." Hannah's complaint, "They haven't the least idea about the human heart except to move it from place to place," found an echo in the work of these medical anthropologists.

If the public suspicion of the new criteria for brain death was unfair, it is less clear that suspicion of the doctors who supported it was unfair. Indeed, that suspicion has been reinforced by other behaviors. For example, if the transplantation community looked a little like crusaders when they advocated whole-brain-death criteria on the grounds that such criteria would increase the supply of organs for transplant, it reinforced that image when suggestions were made to utilize anencephalic babies for the sake of the great good of making infant organs available. The effort to redefine death or to create a special category of the "brain absent" in order to increase the supply of badly needed organs was understandable enough, but it was troubling. Gilbert Meilaender made the moral point eloquently. "Our obligation," he said, "is not to achieve all the good we can, as if our responsibilities were godlike. It is, rather, to effect all the good that we can within the limits morality places upon us. Not only what we accomplish but what we do counts."[32] Alexander Capron said clearly that what we must not do is kill the living, even if — or especially if — they are among the most vulnerable of the living (or the dying). And he warned the transplant community that to yield to this crusader temptation would lead to the sort of public suspicion and distrust that would, in the long run, be counterproductive to the supply of organs.[33]

To be sure, the public continues to celebrate the good that medicine does and can do, but it regards physicians as ambiguous heroes, tempted by their power. Consequently, the relationship of physician and patient has become increasingly distrustful.

"Hannah . . . cried for the young boy who couldn't let go of his father." The tidy and eminently reasonable criteria for the determination of death do not quite fit with the messy and not altogether manageable experience of death. Death brings a sense of loss and grief. And when transplantation takes place in the context of death, it takes place also in the context of a grief that finds no remedy in tidy criteria. To be sure, those invited to consider donating a loved one's organs need information. They need to be told about the criteria for brain death and why these criteria justify treating a patient not only as dying but also as dead. And they need procedures to

31. May, *The Patient's Ordeal*, 176-77.

32. Gilbert Meilaender, "Case Studies: The Anencephalic Newborn as Donor," *Hastings Center Report* 16 (April 1986): 23.

33. Alexander Capron, "Anencephalic Donors: Separate the Dead from the Dying," *Hastings Center Report* 17 (February 1987); see also Arthur Caplan, "Fragile Trust," in *Pediatrics, Brain Death, and Organ Transplantation*, ed. H. Kaufman (New York: Plenum Press, 1989), 299-307.

protect their rights. But because we are dealing with death, it should not surprise us that they need more than tidy criteria and rational moral principles. Death involves us and repels us more deeply than that. It is not so easily managed and domesticated. Death requires more than just rational criteria and just impartial calculation of self-interested individuals. It is always a religious event; it invokes consideration of — and attention to — the powers that bear down on us and sustain us (or do not). And it is always a communal event; it involves the dis-member-ment of some community, the dis-organization of our relationships. When death is the context for transplantation, it is little wonder that the "soft words of husbandry and the soil"[34] seem deceptive. The event of death is a dis-member-ment, and transplantation in the context of death can seem the epitome of this dis-member-ment. In this light, one can understand why even those who support the idea of transplantation in the context of health sometimes find consent difficult in the context of death. If, for example, the potential donor is a suicide, the family will be understandably anxious about any action toward the mortal remains that could be interpreted as mistreatment of the person. If the potential donor is an accident victim, the family will desperately hold to the continuity between mortal remains and the person they have lost. And if the efforts to save a person's life had justified treating him or her like manipulable nature, like an object, then it is not surprising if the family insists that the person's death ought to put an end to such treatment, not justify continuing it.

The old body-soul dualism of which Jonas complained is surely operative in the reduction of the body to "spare parts." Surely doctors must sometimes "objectify" the body in an effort to heal a person; surely sometimes they must treat the body as manipulable; but the risks are both familiar and great. Human beings are not to be reduced to their bodies, but neither are their bodies to be consigned to the realm of mere things. We are not in our bodies the way Descartes's ghost was presumably in the machine. We are embodied selves, and communal selves as embodied. People do not live or die or suffer as ghostly minds nor as mere bodies but as embodied and communal selves.

To be sure, because persons may not be reduced to their bodies, there is a discontinuity between persons and their mortal remains. But because persons may not be reduced to minds or ghosts or disembodied souls, there is also continuity between persons and their mortal remains. The continuity helps us to understand why some who refuse to make organ donations give as their reason "I don't want someone cutting me up after I die." It helps us to understand why the first experience of medical students in the gross anatomy lab is frequently repulsive to them[35] and why some family members are reticent to consider the dis-member-ing of their beloved son or daughter or parent. The discontinuity helps us to understand how medical students can settle down to the tasks of learning anatomical parts, their places, their relations, and their functions, and also how family and friends experience in the presence of mortal remains that the one they loved is somehow gone.

What the grieving need is not simply a tidy definition of death or procedures that protect their individual autonomy. They need to acknowledge the reality and the sadness of death. They need people to stand with them in acknowledging the loss, the disorganization of their communal selves. They need people who will discipline the human tendencies to deny death and to flee from it, who will stand with the grieving, attentive to the mortal remains, once — and still — identified with the person who has died, once — and still — the medium by which family and friends displayed the affection and loyalty of various relationships. They need people who will respect not only their autonomy but their communal integrity, who will respect both the continuing connections of the mortal remains with the person and the community and the hard reality of the discontinuity that death inevitably brings. They need, that is, something like a funeral ritual.[36] The person is dead; relationships are broken; communities are dismembered. Family and friends need to surrender the person and the mortal remains; they need to "let go." But neither they nor doctors can by decree or fiat reduce the body to "spare parts." It is appropriate to remind those sickened medical students of the discontinuity. However, students who treat their cadavers cavalierly need to be reminded of the continuity, need to be reminded that the cadavers remain the mortal remains of someone who experienced the sights and sounds and smells of the world in it, someone who loved and blushed in it. Similarly, it is appropriate to remind those who refuse to consider organ donation of the discontinuity. And it is necessary to remind all that reduce the newly dead to "manipulable nature" or to exchangeable parts of the continuity. While the discontinuity makes dissection morally possible, the continuity requires that the retrieval of organs be undertaken with all due respect not only for the recently deceased but also for those who are dis-membered by the loss and need to grieve.

"[Y]ou will have repaid me in full." If the first challenge for transplant surgery was the proper diagnosis of death, the second surely was — and remains — appropriate consideration for the recently dead and for the grieving. And if there are possibilities for being mistaken for a crusader in response to the first challenge, the second challenge contains even more such possibilities.

One part of the solution here was provided by the language of "gift." Transplantation has been described from the very beginning as a "gift of life." The Uniform Anatomical Gift Act was an effort to make such gifts easy and routine. The language and the legislation recognized that

34. Selzer, *Imagine a Woman,* 7.

35. Leon Kass, *Toward a More Natural Science* (New York: Free Press, 1985), 277-78.

36. May, *The Patient's Ordeal,* 182-87.

although Dr. Barnard might want my heart, it was not his to take; it could only be given — and only by those with the authority to make such a gift, that is to say, by the person whose body it is while alive and/or by the family whose responsibility it is to dispose of the body appropriately when the person dies.

The recognition of organ transfer as "gift" is to be affirmed and commended, and the gift relationship is to be protected from the crusaders who would simply take. However, the language of "gift" meets this challenge only in part. Relationships established by "gift" are themselves more ambiguous than we sometimes think. And, in spite of the best efforts of those who would encourage voluntary gifts, death — and thus a gift in the midst of death — can hardly be made routine.

First, then, let it be affirmed that the intuitions that accompanied the Uniform Anatomical Gift Act were sound. Organ donation is gift, and organ recipients receive a gift. The donative aspects of transplantation should not be ignored, and it is perilous to deny them. And to deny them for the sake of increasing the supply of organs looks like the work of a crusader. The continuity of the mortal remains with the person whose body it was (and is) requires that we respect the dead person by treating his or her corpse in ways that reflect the reality of the union between persons and their bodies. It is impossible altogether to separate the way we treat a person and the way we treat that person's body. Indeed, the way we treat a corpse is often the final display of respect or contempt. To requisition the body or its parts would discredit the dignity that should be accorded to the person while alive. It would treat the person, and not just the corpse, with negligible dignity. The gift character of organ exchange protects against the indignity.

The Uniform Anatomical Gift Act affirmed that organs for transplant were gifts; indeed, it capitalized on the characterization of donation as a "gift of life." Although it wanted to make such gifts in the context of death routine, however, neither death nor donation has been routinized.

The transplant community reminds us that donation, or what Arthur Caplan has called the policy of "encouraged voluntarism," has not kept up with the demand for organs. It is appropriate to be reminded of the sad story that many patients "die waiting" for organs. And the response to that sad story must, of course, be compassion and sympathy and an effort to increase the supply of organs for transplant. Compassion, however, needs to be joined not only with artifice, with technology, but also with wisdom and piety. It ought to be a motive not just to "do something," which can mean anything, but to act in ways that are fitting to human experience and appropriate to the human condition. Otherwise, compassion can be the motive of crusaders.

Caplan has effectively advocated an alternative to the policy of "encouraged voluntarism": the policy of "required request." The latter attempts to increase the supply of organs while continuing to acknowledge the normative significance of donation and consent. The idea is simply to ensure that the families of potential donors will be informed of the transplantation option and asked to make a donation. It was quickly drafted into law and adopted by most state legislatures and mandated for all institutions that receive Medicare or Medicaid funds.

Caplan's own telephone survey of ten states where the legislation had been in effect for at least six months revealed two trends. First, there were some small gains in the number of organs available for transplant, but second, there was quite a remarkable rate of noncompliance with the new legislation among doctors and nurses involved in organ procurement, more than 50 percent in many states. Before one joins Caplan in attributing this noncompliance to "professional arrogance,"[37] one might consider the following: the emotional investment in the "neomort" in spite of reasonable (and accepted) criteria for the legal determination of death; the clinical difficulty of attending to a patient both as a patient and as a potential organ donor; or the professional difficulty of both supporting the family in their grief and being the advocate of unknown potential recipients of the organs of their recently dead relative. One might consider, in short, whether the "discretion and sensitivity" the law itself commands are not exercised in at least some noncompliance.[38] What Caplan celebrates as the "routinization of requests"[39] does not make death or grief routine. To be sure, potential donors must be identified and inquiries must be made, but to refuse to allow a physician's "discretion and sensitivity" to override the requirement of a request looks like the decision of a crusader. Death and gifts in the context of death cannot be made routine.

The other proposals to increase the number of organs available for transplant include "presumed consent" and creating a market for organs. A policy of "presumed consent" would allow the routine harvesting of needed organs from any potential donor. It is called "presumed consent" because of the important qualification that a donor or a family would have the option of opting out. That qualification acknowledges that organ donation remains — and must remain — a gift. Moreover, since procrastination and aversion presumably would continue to play a role in these decisions (or in avoiding them), donors and their families would need to be informed of the practice of routinely harvesting organs and of their right to opt out. And presumably a physician's "discretion and sensitivity" would still sometimes override providing that information and making that request (now whether they want to opt out). That is to say, in spite of the policy differences between "required request" and "presumed consent," the practices might not be so different.

37. Arthur Caplan, "Professional Arrogance and Public Misunderstanding," *Hastings Center Report* 18 (April-May 1988): 34-37.

38. Susan Martyn, Richard Wright, and Leo Clark, "Required Request for Organ Donation: Moral, Clinical, and Legal Problems," *Hastings Center Report* 18 (April-May 1988): 27-33.

39. Caplan, "Professional Arrogance," 36.

James Childress, however, has expressed concern that in some of the places where this policy is in force donors and their families have not been informed of the policy or of their right to opt out.[40] Other critics find it hard to understand on what basis in an individualistic society consent could be presumed and organs taken. Although such a policy favors the language of voluntary gifts and consent even while it licenses the routine salvaging of organs, it acknowledges the importance of the gift relationship too much the way a lie acknowledges that the truth ought to he told. It looks suspiciously like "taking" organs rather than receiving them as gifts. To conscript donors unless they apply for the status of conscientious objectors risks violating the communal integrity of those who are "members one of another" before they are members of the state as well as the embodied integrity of persons by reducing their bodies to "parts" for social use. Transplantation does involve gifts, however much crusaders would prefer it if they could reduce organs to waste to be retrieved to serve a human good.

What "presumed consent" puts at risk, creating a market in organs simply violates. The commercialization of transplantation, the selling and buying of organs as commodities, alienates us both from our communities and from our bodies, rendering us individual choice makers tied to others only by the contracts of a marketplace and rendering our bodies (our selves) commodities. Such a marketplace policy was advanced in 1983 by Dr. H. Barry Jacobs, of International Kidney Exchange, Incorporated. He wrote to thousands of hospitals to inquire whether they would be interested in his plan to purchase kidneys from persons living in poverty here and abroad as cheaply as possible and sell them to sick Americans who could afford to buy them. The reaction was appropriately outrage both in Congress and among transplant surgeons. In 1984, the National Organ Transplantation Act expressly outlawed commercial markets in organ procurement and distribution, and in 1985 The Transplantation Society adopted a special resolution: "No transplant surgeon/team shall be involved directly or indirectly in the buying or selling of organs/tissues or in any transplant activity aimed at commercial gain to himself/herself or an associated hospital or institute," and made violation a cause for expulsion from the society.

Preserving the gift relationship offers donors and their families the best protection against exploitation by a crusader and against the mechanistic dualism that would reduce the body and its members to spare parts. Moreover, gifts are wonderful tokens of a way of life that religious thinkers have regularly commended. It is good to give of ourselves to others, to be generous with others in ways that surpass any claim they may have on us, and graciously to include strangers as well as friends and family in the range of our generosity. Gifts establish or cement relationships. And, to be sure, both donor and recipient celebrate "the gift of life." A bond may be created between donors, recipients, and their families because a part of the donor remains and functions within the recipient, and that bond is often experienced as an enriching and ennobling thing.

The act of giving is a glorious thing, but let it also be recognized that the glorious act of giving can be ambiguous. That point was made eloquently by Renee Fox and Judith Swazey. They point out the ambiguity just below the surface in the mechanisms to protect relatives whose psychological tests suggest that they are not appropriate donors by telling them that they are not compatible.[41] They point out the recognition of ambiguity in the policy of anonymity surrounding cadaver organs, whereas formerly transplant teams were disposed to reveal not only identities but also details about the lives of donors, recipients, and their families. But the ambiguities surface most visibly in what Fox and Swazey call "the tyranny of the gift," the psychic and social effects of being bound to another by a gift that it is impossible adequately to repay, of being trapped either as benefactor or recipient into a creditor-debtor relationship. That ambiguity surfaced in Hannah's effort to manipulate the consent of the man with her husband's heart by reminding him of the gift and of his obligation somehow to repay it. Ironically, it seems not to have been the tyranny of the gift that wins Hannah an audience with Sam's heart but her own gratitude for a simple act of kindness that the donor had shown.

To insist that organs are gifts is not wrong, but it is insufficient. It does not, and cannot, remove the ambiguities surrounding transplantation.

"What about Sam Owens on your resurrection day?" Religious convictions and communities do not provide an easy transcendence over the ambiguities in transplantation. The story of Hannah, for example, reminds us that transplantation has sometimes been seen as inconsistent with Christian conviction about resurrection. Hannah resented the radio preacher's talk of the resurrection of the flesh. "It's a big lie," she said, and used Sam Owens's flesh, now part of the flesh of seven others, as her evidence.[42] Others, convinced of the truth of resurrection, have resented the request that they should be donors. On their "great getting-up morning," they figure, they will need their organs. Cheryl Sanders reports that this conviction (along with distrust of physicians and fears that donors will be declared dead prematurely) contributes to the reluctance of African Americans to donate organs. But she also reports that the effort of certain members of the transplantation community to respond to this conviction by dismissing it as "superstitious," mythological, and nonscientific looks like the act

40. James Childress, "Ethical Criteria for Procuring and Distributing Organs for Transplantation," *Journal of Health Policies, Policy and Law* 14 (1989): 87-113.

41. Renee C. Fox and Judith A. Swazey, *Spare Parts: Organ Replacement in American Society* (New York: Oxford University Press, 1992), 40.

42. Selzer, *Imagine a Woman*, 8-9.

of the crusader. Sanders calls for theological inquiry and conversation, not dismissive ridicule.[43]

Theological inquiry and instruction are obviously important when religious communities confront issues like transplantation. Theological conversations could be instructive both to those who could donate their organs and to those who would harvest them. Theological inquiry, however, should be conducted in the service of particular religious communities, tested by the wisdom of their respective traditions, not conducted in the service of the transplantation community or tested by whether it increases the number of organ donors.

The Christian conviction concerning the resurrection of the body, for example, does not make resurrection depend on the intact condition of the body when it is buried. Rather, resurrection depends on the power of God to make "all things new." The conviction of the resurrection, therefore, is not inconsistent with the donation of organs. At the same time, however, by reminding Christians of the significance of embodiment, the conviction of resurrection of the body should challenge the old dualism of body and soul (and its "new apparition" in "the dualism of brain and body") that renders us immortal souls in a disposable body. And by reminding Christians that the victory over death is finally a divine victory rather than a technological one, it should challenge the hubris of crusaders.

Most religious people are ready to celebrate the good that transplantation sometimes does. Because developments in transplant surgery enable a more effective human response to the sad stories of diseased and damaged organs and the premature deaths they sometimes cause, religious people give thanks to God and celebrate human service to the cause of God. And modest celebration is certainly appropriate. Many religious groups have adopted resolutions approving and encouraging organ donation. Moreover, many religious groups have overcome initial reservations about whole brain death and have explicitly accepted such criteria for the determination of death. (See Appendix.)

Such resolutions may provide a significant reply to some religious persons who refuse to consider organ donations because "It's against my religion." They may contribute to alleviating suspicion of the new consensus concerning brain death. They do not, however, provide a remedy for the ambiguities of transplantation. Moreover, the merely formal acceptance of brain-death criteria in the context of affirming the good transplantation can achieve will probably be seen as insufficient and might be regarded as suspiciously like an ecclesiastical blessing on the crusaders, which has happened before, of course.

Religious communities have provided theological position papers, resolutions encouraging organ donation, and official acceptance of brain-death criteria. Communities that have advocated organ donation as a worthy response in death to the giver of life have an opportunity and a responsibility to develop religious rituals for transplantation, which would acknowledge the reality and the sadness of the deaths of potential organ donors and would honor their gifts. More than once in the course of this paper's account of the ambiguities of transplant we have encountered something of the need for ritual. Ritual actions do not eliminate ambiguities, but they can acknowledge them and provide a way to cope with them. They can recognize tragedy and help the grieving find their way through it. They can provide order in the context of the dis-organ-ization wrought by death. They can nurture community in the context of the dis-memberment death brings. They can recognize and deal with the human experience of continuity and discontinuity with mortal remains. Death and a gift in the midst of death can hardly be made routine, but they can be made a matter of ritual and liturgy.

In her fine book on ritual, Catherine Bell defines "ritualization" as a way of acting that is designed and orchestrated to distinguish and privilege what is being done in comparison to other, usually more quotidian, activities. As such, ritualization is a matter of various culturally specific strategies for setting some activities off from others, for creating and privileging a qualitative distinction between the "sacred" and the "profane," and for ascribing such distinctions to realities thought to transcend the powers of human actors.[44]

Stuart Youngner, whose study of "conceptual disarray" among transplant teams was cited earlier, has also called for the "ritualization" of transplant procedures. He has suggested that new nursing rituals should be developed for transplantation as a way of meeting the challenge of ambiguity against which the tidy definition of death seems powerless. Such rituals, he said, should "symbolically distinguish caring for the cadaver donor from that of patients and . . . infuse the macabre nature of what is involved with 'gift of life' meaning."[45] There is wisdom there. "Specific strategies for setting some activities off from others" would be helpful to distinguish care for the newly dead from patients in critical condition and to remind all parties that the "life support system" is not supporting a life. These strategies could involve little things, perhaps drapes that look more like shrouds than sheets, perhaps black sheets. Little things ritually performed can powerfully reinforce the fact of death and the professional commitment to honor both patients' mortal remains and their gifts. Even so, to give control over the rituals surrounding transplantation to medical professionals would be to surrender control over the appropriate way to act to the medical community. Patients and their families should be able to draw on their own reli-

43. Cheryl J. Sanders, "African Americans and Organ Donation: Reflections on Religion, Ethics and Embodiment," in *Embodiment, Morality, and Medicine,* ed. L. Sowle Cahill and M. A. Farley (Dordrecht: Kluwer, 1995), 141-53.

44. Catherine Bell, *Ritual Theory, Ritual Practice* (New York: Oxford University Press, 1992), 74.

45. Cited in Fox and Swazey, *Spare Parts,* 63.

gious and cultural traditions to deal with death and with the questions of giving organs in the context of death. No "generic" ritual will do, and no purely private ritual will do. To avoid the suspicion that "ritualization," too, can be the work of crusaders, the ritual must privilege death as a human event that inevitably invokes attention to God and to community, and not just as an opportunity for transplant. Religious traditions that have issued resolutions in approval of transplant bear some responsibility for the construction of rituals for such occasions. All traditions have rituals for death;[46] all of them recognize and deal with the human experience of continuity and discontinuity; and many of them have elements that could be used in the context of transplantation. The Park Ridge Center has begun a project investigating ritual as a resource for responding to the needs of patients, families, and caregivers.[47]

There is liturgical work, as well as theological work, to be done. Only so will the horror of death be acknowledged and our aversion to death be disciplined by commitments to a continuing community and to some transcendent cause. The Christian tradition offers resources for that liturgical work. It might be as simple as selecting parts of the funeral liturgy for use in the hospital when organs are to be harvested from deceased members of the Christian community. Other resources include the dirge and the psalms of lament in scripture.

The most complete and powerful dirge in scripture is David's dirge at the death of Saul and Jonathan (2 Sam. 1:19-27). It is a remarkable song. God is not addressed or even mentioned. The dead are eulogized, but the decisive feature of this and every dirge is the contrast between past glories and present misery. In its refrain and conclusion, "How the mighty have fallen," there is a sharp and total contrast to the remembered glories of Saul and Jonathan. Once they were "beloved and lovely"; once "they were swifter than eagles, . . . stronger than lions"; now "how the mighty have fallen." The contrast so important to the form of the dirge has been called "the tragic reversal." It acknowledges the reality and horror of death and gives the grieving voice.

Grief also finds voice in the psalms of lament, but now a voice addressed to God. They are not funeral liturgies, but Hermann Gunkel has identified the individual psalms of lament as "the place where the religion of the psalms comes into conflict with death." The laments reverse the tragic reversal. By their attention to God they move from distress to renewal, from powerlessness to confidence, from anger to assurance, from grief to gift. The invocation of God allows the pattern of the dirge to change, but it does not disallow the sorrow. Laments acknowledge the real experiences of life and the honest emotional reactions that those experiences evoke. There is no pretense, no denial, and no withdrawal to some otherworldly realities. There is no romantic effort to reduce the hurt to some domesticated account of nature, and no technical effort to accomplish a surrogate immortality. Lament calls the faithful to deal with real life and real death. Lament gives the suffering voice, but it also holds them to a meaning and a covenant that promise that the tragic reversal is not the last word. Lament gives form and limits to the venting of emotions and thus helps to give direction to the sufferer, helps to encompass the hurt within a faithful identity. In the psalms of confidence (for example, Ps. 22), the lament reaches past the certainty of a hearing to the gifts of thanksgiving. The psalmist pledges a gift as a token of gratitude; it is gift answering to gift. Resources are available here for ritualizing both death and gift, for the construction of a liturgical acknowledgment of the horror of death and a liturgical pledging of the gift of organs. In the very presence of death, such gifts can be celebrated as a response to the one who gives mortal life and rules even death so that we can rise above our fear and horror in order to serve God's cause and some other's good.

A ritual could signify and express both the continuity and the discontinuity between persons and their mortal remains. The liturgies would not create the simultaneous continuity and discontinuity, but they could help us and force us to acknowledge it. Rituals will not make suicide or accident or any death less sad, but they may provide a way to acknowledge the sadness and to honor the gift, to free families both for grief and for generosity.

Religious rituals could also be helpful in minimizing the "tyranny of the gift," for the gift would be seen as response to God, as response to the one before whom we are all recipients and debtors, as gift answering to gift. Then organ donors and organ recipients are not trapped as benefactors or recipients into a creditor-debtor relationship; they are recipients, bound together by their common indebtedness to God, and giving and sharing are mere tokens of community. If, for example, some lustration or sprinkling with water were a part of a Christian ritual for such occasions, participants could remember the baptism of the person whose corpse they attend, could acknowledge that baptism and this death as sharing in the death of Christ, and could celebrate both the gift of grace and the gift of this person's life. And in response to the gift of grace and in anticipation of the resurrection, they could not only surrender this member of their body to death but also surrender in death the members, the organs, of this member of their body in the service of others. Such a ritual would also serve, I think, to lower the rhetoric of a surrogate immortality.

In baptism Christians are instructed that "if we have died with Christ, we . . . will also live with him" (Rom. 6:8). The hope is not that our Sams will continue to survive in the breast of another, but that God's cosmic sovereignty will be unchallenged. The hope is not in technol-

46. For a brief summary of several rituals, see Kenneth Kramer, *The Sacred Art of Dying: How World Religions Understand Death* (New York: Paulist Press, 1988).

47. Laurence J. O'Connell, "Ritual Practice and End-of-Life Care," *The Park Ridge Center Bulletin* 5 (August/September 1988): 14.

ogy, but in the power of God that makes things new, the same power that raised Jesus and will raise Sam from the dead. Death cannot be made routine, but it can be an occasion for liturgy. Part of preparation for this liturgy could be the request for donation. We would have the functional equivalent of "required request" within particular communities. Indeed, the point could be made more strongly than that. In the Christian tradition, for example, the preparation for this liturgy could remind Christians that, while they recognize life and health as good gifts of God, they also recognize that faithfulness to God does not permit them to make their own ease and survival the law of their being. They may expect physicians to be committed to their ease and survival, but they recognize more important obligations for themselves. And among those obligations are duties to help a neighbor in need, duties to answer the primordial giver with little tokens of their gratitude and generosity. This legitimate expectation of consent would still require "discretion and sensitivity." As death cannot be made routine, neither can gifts in the context of death. Rituals will not eliminate the ambiguities of death and grief and gift in transplantation, but they can help us to acknowledge those ambiguities and to journey through them in ways that nurture both respect for the one now recently dead and the readiness to give the organs that others may live.

Oh, one thing more: Drive carefully!

Appendix: Statements within Religious Traditions

Jewish

Definition of death: The Chief Rabbinate of Israel, on November 3, 1986, accepted "verification" of death by means of "proving that the brain, including the brainstem . . . , has been totally and irreversibly functionally destroyed." A Halakically acceptable variation of "whole brain death" has been found in the concept of "physiological decapitation." Contemporary rabbis continue to express dissenting opinions.[48]

Transplantation: "The following issues are of Halakic concern: the prohibition of desecrating or mutilating the dead, the prohibition of deriving benefit from the dead, the prohibition of delaying the burial of the dead, and the positive commandment of burying the dead. All these concerns and prohibitions are set aside if necessary in order to eliminate a danger to the life of a human being."[49]

Roman Catholic

Definition of death: "wide agreement among Catholic bishops, physicians and theologians that whole brain death . . . is sufficient to constitute death, and that there are available clinical tests which . . . show when this state of affairs obtains."[50]

From "Holy Living and Holy Dying — A United Methodist/Roman Catholic Common Statement," 1989: "The gift of life in organ donation allows survivors to experience positive meaning in the midst of their grief and is an important expression of love in community. [Transplantation is supported] . . . as long as death is not hastened and is determined by reliable criteria."[51]

Anglican-Episcopalian

According to Resolution A-097, adopted by the 1991 General Convention of the Episcopal Church in the U.S.A., the church "recommends and urges" members to consider the opportunity to donate organs after death so that others may live.[52]

Latter-day Saints

There is no official policy encouraging or discouraging donation; the decision to "will" organs for transplant is left to individual consciences. Reports of counsel not to will organs because of the doctrine of the literal resurrection of the physical body are counterbalanced by enthusiastic endorsement of transplantation by individual Mormons (Sen. Jake Garn, Barney Clark, William DeVries). Strong encouragement to donate organs was given in an article by Cecil Samuelson in *Ensign,* the official LDS monthly periodical.[53]

Lutheran

In 1984, the Lutheran Church in America adopted a resolution that observed that "the donation of renewable tissue and live organs can be an expression of sacrificial love for a neighbor in need," encouraged the use of donor cards, and urged those wishing to donate to communicate such wishes to families, physicians, pastors, and hospitals. It urged pastors and church agencies to facilitate donation and governments to encourage voluntary donation, to discourage "coercive donation," to disallow a market in organs, and to assure equitable distribution of organs. The Lutheran Church Missouri Synod adopted a resolution in 1981 that called the church to implement programs to promote donation.[54]

Methodist

A 1988 United Methodist resolution, observing that "selfless consideration for the health and welfare of oth-

48. Andrew Lustig, ed., *Bioethics Yearbook,* Vol. 1: *Theological Developments in Bioethics, 1988-1990* (Dordrecht: Kluwer, 1991), 193.

49. Ibid., 194.

50. Andrew Lustig, ed., *Bioethies Yearbook,* Vol. 3: *Theological Developments in Bioethics, 1990-92* (Dordrecht: Kluwer, 1995).

51. Cited in Lustig, *Bioethics Yearbook,* Vol. 1, 158.

52. Lustig, *Bioethics Yearbook,* Vol. 3.

53. Lustig, *Bioethics Yearbook,* Vol. 1, 36-38.

54. Ibid., 139.

ers is at the heart of the Christian ethic," affirmed organ donation as "life-giving" and a source of comfort to surviving loved ones, and urged members to become organ and tissue donors by signing donor cards.[55]

Eastern Orthodox

Evangelos Mantzouneas, "Organ Donations in the Orthodox Church in Greece," concludes that organ donations "do not violate" a Greek Orthodox account of Christian ethics but "every form of payment is prohibited." Organ donation has been approved by the Holy Synod of the Church of Greece. Serapheim, Archbishop of Athens, stated in 1985 that "to put words into practice" he had willed his kidneys and eyes for donation at his death.[56]

Islamic

Definition of death: A 1989 study sponsored by the Islamic Organization for Medical Sciences, after a thorough discussion, recommended that the diagnosis of brainstem death should be regarded as a sufficient indication of death.

Transplantation: The Islamic Code of Medical Ethics (endorsed by the First International Conference on Islamic Medicine, 1981) reads in part: "If the living are able to donate, then the dead are even more so, and no harm will afflict the cadaver if heart, kidneys, eyes or arteries are taken to be put to good use in a living person. This is indeed a charity . . . and directly fulfills God's words: 'And whosoever saves a human life it is as though he has saved all mankind.' A word of caution, however, is necessary. Donation should be voluntary. . . . In the society of the faithful, donation should be in generous supply and should be the fruit of faith and love of God and His subjects."[57]

Buddhist

It is possible to interpret Buddhist ideals to support the donation of organs, since one ought to help people who are in need. But Buddhist ideals require that the recipient not desire the donor's death "nor desire to prolong his own life." Moreover, "[b]rain death, in contrast to organ transplantation, seems unequivocally opposed to Buddhist ideals."[58]

55. Ibid., 158.
56. Ibid., 89-90.
57. Ibid., 114-16.
58. Ibid., 66-67.

60 Harvesting the Living? Separating "Brain Death" and Organ Transplantation

Courtney S. Campbell

The chronic shortage of solid organ donors has reached critical proportions with no obvious resolution in sight. The case of Horacio Alberto Reyes-Camarena, in the spring of 2003, is illustrative. Reyes-Camarena's otherwise obscure social status as an inmate on death row in Oregon drew national attention when the state considered providing him with a kidney transplant. The state anticipated savings of $40,000 per year if Reyes-Camarena received a kidney transplant rather than the continuation of dialysis; at the time of this controversy, 203 persons in Oregon (and nearly 55,000 nationwide) were on the kidney transplant waiting list. Reyes-Camarena eventually was denied a transplant on grounds that he failed to meet medical criteria for transplant eligibility, but his case revived debates over the priority of transplants within a healthcare system that does not provide equitable access to basic care, the economic tradeoffs of transplants, methods of fairness in allocating scarce resources, and the rights of inmates to medical care (Spencer 2003).

A further illustration of the crisis is the recent solicitation of virtually every person on bioethics list-serves from an organization called the "LifeSharers." Describing their proposal as a "simple and obvious solution" to the deaths of 6,000 Americans annually due to organ shortages, LifeSharers is comprised of members who have agreed to donate their organs when they die on condition that fellow members will have first access to the organs. The expectation of the organization is that being assured a reasonable chance to have access to an organ will expand the pool of donors to the point that the organ shortage eventually will diminish altogether (LifeSharers 2003). However, this seems excessively optimistic; since relatively few people upon death are eligible to become organ donors, a substantial proportion of the national population would need to be enrolled in such a program for it to have an impact on organ scarcity (personal communication with Laura Siminoff, Case Western Reserve University School of Medicine, Cleveland, OH, 29 August 2003).

The Reyes-Camarena case illustrates the microalloca-

From Courtney S. Campbell, "Harvesting the Living? Separating 'Brain Death' and Organ Transplantation," *Kennedy Institute of Ethics Journal* 14.3 (2004): 301-18.

tion problem of organ transplantation: there are not enough scarce resources to provide for everyone in need. The LifeSharers proposal exemplifies the macroallocation dilemma: what methods can be used to increase the scarce resource without violating important social and ethical values. In the past decade, arguments for commerce in organs have been debated with some frequency (Richards 1996). Other proposals have included variations on what has been termed "rewarded gifting," that is, offering potential donors and families certain financial incentives, such as compensation for funeral costs, to permit greater recovery of organs.

Still another alternative for increasing the supply of donor organs is through a reconceptualization of the understanding of "donor" and of "death." Some proposals advocate modifying or abandoning altogether the so-called "dead donor rule" (cf. Robertson 1999), permitting organ retrieval from persons who have not yet met the legal standards for death. In its more dramatic version, this reconceptualization approach would increase the number of prospective donors through revision of the standards or criteria by which death is determined. In particular, leading ethicists have argued for an expanded concept of death, such that current whole-brain standards of death would be supplemented with higher-brain or neocortical criteria of death (Youngner, Arnold, and Schapiro 1999) or even displaced in favor of pre-mortem organ retrieval.

The data collected by Laura Siminoff, Christopher Burant, and Stuart Youngner (2004) furnishes valuable insights for the bioethics community and policymakers into public attitudes about the occurrence of death and assessments of the various options for remedying the organ shortage problem. This information can help bridge the conceptual and practical gaps between professionals, providers, and the general public. Still, I am concerned that data gathered from the public, and incorporated by bioethicists in service of an agenda to bring coherence to the definition of death debate, or to resolve the crisis in scarce organs, can be misread, or selectively used, leading to bad policy and bad ethics. I argue here that the "bridging" work the data do will not provide sufficient grounds for either revising the criteria of death or for modifying the dead donor rule; indeed, either approach will violate important social values upon which the integrity of the transplant process rests. Moreover, I contend that the chronic problem of organ scarcity should prompt bioethicists to revisit the question of the priority of organ transplants in the overall package of healthcare benefits provided to most, but not all, citizens.

Public Precautions

Virtually every scholar who writes on the subject of organ donation contends that the public is very supportive of the practice, and indeed views it as a paradigm illustration of what is meant when one refers to the "miracles" of modern medicine. In many instances, a transplant literally does rescue a person from the jaws of death. At the same time, the public is held to be somewhat confused and mystified by the process undertaken by transplant teams to recover an organ from a donor whose vital respiratory and circulatory functions are maintained by machines.

Indeed, when the recovery process is publicized, intellectual advocacy and moral commendations for donation can meet the resistance of emotional revulsion; this intellectual-emotional conflict was thoughtfully described by Willard Gaylin (1974) in his classic article, "Harvesting the Dead," published in the beginnings of the transplantation era. As Gaylin (1974, p. 30) put it, "After all the benefits are outlined, with the lifesaving potential clear, the humanitarian purposes obvious, the technology ready, the motives pure, and the material costs justified — how are we to reconcile our emotions?" It fell to moral philosophers, Gaylin suggested, to be attentive to these conflicts and to work out proposals to enable the use of life-saving technologies, including transplantation technologies, without simultaneously eroding our humanity and the qualities for which life is worth saving.

In the three decades since, I think it likely that the routinization of organ transplants within the medical field has provided an aura of the familiar that has diminished the revulsion. Transplants on their own seldom make it into the headline-grabbing attention of public consciousness; some other possibly scandalous association — a death-row inmate receiving a transplant, a child denied a transplant, racial stratification, or celebrity priorities — seems required for transplant policy to be deemed newsworthy. Philosophical argumentation and institutional implementation also may have had a role in resolving the moral conflict on the side of the rationality of beneficence rather than revulsion. What these influences seem not to have succeeded in doing is to eliminate the confusion over the relationship of death and organ retrieval; indeed, such confusion persists among members of the medical community who are much closer to the actual process than the public. Hence, it is entirely possible that public attitudes about transplantation are not fully clear and coherent, or at least as coherent as is assumed by bioethicists who want to appropriate public perspectives and survey responses in service of policy reform or "progress."

There is an academic or professional culture of bioethics that is somewhat disconnected from the experiences and decisions of a public that is responding to survey questions or having to face such choices as part of their personal or familial healthcare experience. As observed by Stuart Youngner, Robert Arnold, and Renie Schapiro (1999, p. xv):

> Debates about the definition and determination of death have occurred almost solely among academics. By all appearances, the public has little understanding

or even interest in the issue. . . . What is probably true, based on the evidence we have, is that the public cares a great deal about the actual determination of death but conceptualizes or frames the issues in a very different manner from that of academic physicians, philosophers, lawyers, and social scientists.

Moreover, the disciplinary training of bioethicists requires assuming certain canons of argumentative articulation: clarity, consistency, coherence, completeness, and comprehensiveness, among others. Matters are simply messier for persons whose daily dilemmas are not about the standards for determining death, but about choices for living a quality life, including adequate nutrition, assisting with public education, ensuring the children get to soccer practice, or overseeing the completion of homework.

This simply means that analysis of public attitudes on organ transplants and brain death requires substantial caution. How might bioethicists apprehend the information revealed by empirical surveys and draw out its normative implications? With no pretension to comprehensiveness, let me suggest several recurrent patterns.

(1) One alternative is to support what might be called a *democratic* approach to data. Survey data may show a majority of popular preference for a particular policy, for example, the legalization of physician-assisted suicide. Arguments then can be generated to reform, or to maintain, policy in the direction preferred by the public. This approach should be inadequate for bioethicists, who will need to enquire in greater detail about not simply the conclusions, but also the rationales and values behind the public views. In addition, although the democratic approach has been influential in several venues on bioethics issues (Campbell, C. 1995), bioethicists are likely to be skeptical about deriving a moral imperative or policy "ought" from an empirical fact.

(2) A second approach reflects a form of intellectual *authoritarianism*. Bioethicists can be tempted to render an interpretation of public preferences that presumes reliance on their disciplinary canons of rational argumentation. In this circumstance, the professional may be advancing a claim about what the respondents ought to have said if they were thinking clearly and coherently, that is, as a professional bioethicist is supposed to have thought. This can generate moral arguments or proposals that are paternalistic even as they are cast in the guise of promoting the public interest.

(3) A third method reflects what I think of as bioethical *hermeneutics*. It involves the selective use or appropriation of data to confirm or buttress a position that is already held on other grounds. The method is analogous to "proof-texting" in theological discussions, in which a particular passage of sacred text is extracted from its narrative and historical context and used to advance a position on an issue like abortion or homosexuality. In both cases, the previously accepted conclusion directs selective (and arbitrary) interpretation of the data.

(4) A fourth approach reflects a *pragmatist* understanding. Even though a moral position or policy might be considered not only ethically defensible, but also ethically preferable, it may be deemed impractical or unfeasible when institutional practices are examined through empirical research on public attitudes. This disparity may lead to abandonment or substantial modification of the position or policy. An illustration of this is displayed in the response of some in the bioethics community to the results of the SUPPORT study, which showed that advance directives, patient education, and caregiver communication appears to have minimal impact on the manner of dying (SUPPORT 1995). In light of these and related findings, leading scholars in bioethics seemed to abandon the use of advance directives as a feasible way to promote patient autonomy. As Arthur Caplan (1998, p. 202) asserted: "It is time to head back to the drawing board to seek new approaches to death in a technological age." Similarly, in the context of the controversy over organ procurement and the standards of death, bioethicists may mull over the chronic crisis of organ scarcity, consider public attitudes to death, and answer Robert Truog's (1997) question, "Is it time to abandon brain death?" in the affirmative.

These recurrent patterns in the bioethics literature regarding interpretation of the *vox populi* warrant both caution and a greater engagement of bioethics with the social sciences, an issue I return to in the concluding section of this essay. Bioethicists need to see data about public views as illuminating, as setting the questions of bioethics in a new light. Research on public preferences provide a context for understanding how a moral problem can arise or is experienced, but the moral context does not dictate moral content: Public perceptions should not be taken to require prescriptive patterns or normative generalizations.

At the very least, there is a methodological issue to which bioethicists need to be attentive, namely, the strong possibility of differences between what the public will *say* when confronted in the abstract with a scenario laden with ethical choice, and what such individuals actually will *do* when experiencing such a dilemma in "real" life. It is entirely possible that the general attitudes expressed by the public in responding to the abstract dilemma — which is the grist for bioethical reflection — will show greater support for certain policy options deemed as more progressive than will the donating public confronted with actual decisions about the determination of death or the disposition of the organs of their (nearly) deceased relative.

The prospects of disciplinary disconnection, selective interpretation of data, or data appropriation to advance a policy proposal lead me to contend that we should avoid recommending dramatic shifts in existing policies *if* the primary rationale for such a policy shift is that of "public support." My caveat here includes proposals that address defining concepts for humanity such as the idea of "death," as well as the implications of such a shift in this boundary concept for a practice like organ transplantation. There may be other grounds, and legitimate reasons, for adoption of neocortical criteria to determine death or for modification of the dead donor rule, such as philosophical coherence or social utility, but I am not convinced such changes can be grounded in a claim that the public is "on board" with the proposals.

I think moral wisdom lies in requiring the burden of proof to be on those who advocate change from current policies to new criteria for death or for being a donor to show real and tangible, nonspeculative benefits from the changes *and* to show that the anticipated benefits occur in greater proportion than the certain harms; the burden should not be on those who defend current policy to demonstrate the harms of forgoing the changes. Some exemplifications of this precautionary approach follow below.

The Public Stake in "Brain Death"

The professional stake in getting the issue of "brain death" "right" was articulated long ago by Henry Beecher and the Ad Hoc Committee of the Harvard Medical School: first, avoiding the burdens — physical, emotional, financial — to patients, families, and displaced patients of maintaining the biological functions of persons who but for the mechanical interventions would be considered "dead," and second, avoiding controversy in obtaining organs for transplantation (Harvard Medical School Ad Hoc Committee 1968). In subsequent years, needs for practical implementation, policy formulation (President's Commission 1981), and philosophical justification of a "brain death" standard became additional interests of professionals involved in the definition-of-death discussion.

I suspect, by contrast, that the principal reason the concept of "brain death" has garnered public attention is due to confusion, perpetuated through media misstatements about whether a "brain-dead" person is "really dead." Clearly, the public, no less than professionals, has an important stake in a clear and comprehensible understanding of the definition of death. Yet, the insistent need for transplantable organs is ultimately of greater interest for the public than are the discussion and potential resolution of the interesting philosophical puzzles or policy perplexities. Public interest in the "brain death" question is present because it mediates a greater interest in increasing organ procurement, or put another way, we care about the standards of death because of the hope of offering continued life to recipients.

This context is important because some scholars (Truog 1997, p. 34) have argued that whole-brain criteria for death are an obstacle to increased organ procurement and some of the data presented in the study by Siminoff and colleagues can be read as supporting such a position. With variations depending on the specific scenario, a meaningful proportion of the respondents indicated that even when the hypothetical patient is alive, they were willing to donate the patient's organs. That is, they seemed to support pre-mortem organ retrieval. Certainly interpretive caveats are warranted here: donating hypothetical organs and those of an actual (nearly) deceased relative are likely to be two quite different endeavors. Nonetheless, in principle at least, numerous respondents seem to indicate that an *act* of organ donation is more important to them than ensuring that the patient is actually dead prior to organ retrieval.

Supportive attitudes for pre-mortem organ retrieval seem to imply that, subject to obvious limits, the "dead donor rule" may be more a construct of policymakers and academic bioethicists than an actual guiding norm for the public. Alternatively, the data might suggest that the dead donor rule could be reconstructed such that patients in a persistent vegetative condition would now be considered dead.

The approval of some respondents to allow organ procurement from a nearly-deceased individual in a hypothetical context is an important finding. It deserves careful study and comment, but I have three reservations about its significance as a basis for changing public policy or supporting philosophical positions. First, as John Rawls (1955) argued, it is important to distinguish between *acts* and *practices*. We may be able to justify an act in a particular circumstance as coherent with a world view and as morally permissible. The justification of a practice (or policy) is not, however, contained within the justification of a particular act. The practice or policy must be justified on its own grounds or principles. Hence, from the support of some respondents for pre-mortem organ retrieval in a limited circumstance, it does not follow that we are warranted in concluding there is significant support for a policy instantiated in a practice in which increasing organ supplies takes preeminence over satisfying current criteria for a determination of brain death.

This leads to a second reservation. The interest in "brain death," I have claimed, resides in its door-opening role to increasing organ procurement. In the broader study conducted by Siminoff and colleagues, pre-mortem organ retrieval from the nearly-deceased was the *least* supported option of the procurement alternatives presented to the respondents (Siminoff 2002). Respondents also were asked in general about their attitudes toward what bioethicists conventionally have termed "presumed consent" approaches as well as about "rewarded gifting." In their responses, the public was much more supportive of both of these procurement proposals than of recovering organs from persons still considered alive. Thus, if the public interest in "brain death" really does rest on its ramifications for organ transplantation, then I think the responsibility of the bioethics community is first to explore, advocate, and argue about alternatives that involve re-envisioning notions of "consent" and "donation" rather than to engage in a reconstruction of the concept of "death."

There is a third reason to approach the apparent willingness to approve pre-mortem organ retrieval with great caution. It is one thing to contend that the public is confused in its understanding of, or inconsistent in its application of, current "brain death" criteria and that the dead donor rule replicates, and perpetuates, this confusion at the policy level. It is quite another to say that this confusion can be exploited to the point that the dead donor rule must be modified to encompass PVS patients or abandoned. It is unlikely that public confusion over "whole-brain death" can be supplanted readily by enlightened clarity regarding "neocortical death."

There may be legitimate reasons for reconstructing the dead donor rule so it expands the definition of deceased persons from whom organs can be recovered. However, those arguments already have been developed and would be advocated regardless of what the public survey data reveal or conceal. Perhaps the true test of the adequacy of such philosophical argumentation is not whether it draws upon the data from Siminoff and colleagues to confirm positions that have been arrived at independently, but rather whether it is susceptible to revisions and modifications by a preponderance of data to the contrary.

Rule or Maxim?

Another interpretation of the finding of some public support for pre-mortem organ recovery is possible. Perhaps the attitude reflects neither confusion over "whole-brain death" nor dissatisfaction with an inadequate rule. Moreover, the view may not represent an uninformed public that is "lagging behind" the policy and ethical discussions. On the contrary, this finding could be interpreted as populist progressivism, a public view about the priority of organ transplants as a life-saving technology that is "ahead" of even the cutting edge of both medicine and its academic commentators. This would not be without precedent: In other contexts of bioethics, such as physician-assisted suicide, public opinion has driven changes both in medical practice and in public policy (Campbell, C. 1995). In this interpretation, the dead donor rule possesses no binding or prescriptive force, but functions as a moral maxim. A maxim is a summation and generalization of received wisdom from the past. It can provide guidance, of course, but it also can be discarded as the circumstances arise, particularly circumstances of social utility.

Treating the dead donor rule as a maxim would allow both the law and medicine to dispense with various imposed requirements that are tantamount to fictions and ritualistic charades performed for the sake of compliance with the rule. Norman Fost, among others, has long argued that these impositions impede the prospect for medical treatment and social gains from donation after "cardiac-death" protocols. It should be possible, he maintains, to retrieve organs from nearly deceased persons with their consent and comply with a (to-be-developed) statute that furnishes the transplant team with immunity from homicide charges (Fost 1999, pp. 172-74).

Since first hearing Fost advocate his proposal several years ago, I have included it as an option for my class in biomedical ethics in our deliberations about methods to increase the supply of organs, along with others such as presumed consent, rewarded gifting, organ commerce, expropriation, and xenotransplantation (organ cloning from embryonic stem cells is too distant to consider it an option for patients dying right now). Although, in general, most students, dying patients and waiting lists notwithstanding, are content with the status quo, perhaps because they are distanced from the medical reality and urgency of need, I continue to be surprised that, when forced to choose, the option of pre-mortem organ retrieval is the option to which a plurality of my students give their primary support. I take this constant support as a sign of a reasonably sound proposal or of remarkably bad teaching on my part.

I do not find the pre-mortem organ retrieval proposal compelling because it does not deal adequately with the very real fact of public distrust of institutions and systems, including distrust of the medical transplant system. In the mid-1980s, the two primary reasons cited for public unwillingness to sign organ donor cards were fears that physicians might take action prematurely to obtain organs or that physicians might hasten death (Childress 1997, p. 269). The image of physician as devourer of the patient, rather than rescuer of the recipient, seemed quite prominent. Given the various economic and bureaucratic incentives that have permeated medicine the last two decades, and the concomitant emergence of a *caveat emptor* ethos in medicine, as well as the general decline of trust in public institutions, I am very dubious that the level of distrust in medicine as a system has diminished.

It may be countered, however, that generalized distrust in medicine is one thing and that the particularities of transplant medicine has or can escape this diminished trust. In particular, an element of what might be called the "constituency" factor can work to mitigate the distrust. The constituency factor in medicine appears similar to that in politics: as a citizen, one can be distrustful, even contemptuous, toward "the government," but nonetheless be strongly and trustingly supportive of one's own representative. Similarly, it is possible to imagine a nearly-deceased patient and his or her family who are generally distrustful of the "system" or institution of medicine. However, when approached by their personal physician about pre-mortem organ retrieval, they may be very cooperative and compliant because of their familiarity with the physician and their long history of a professionally respectful and caring relationship.

Still, transplant medicine traditionally has been marked by a separation of roles to provide procedural checks and balances against abuse and because of the latent potential for conflict of interest and for poor and even unethical judgments. The personal physician is not, after all, an isolated actor: The practices of declaring death, requesting organs, retrieving and transporting the organs, and transplanting the organs into a recipient involve both an institution and a system, ones that are heavily regulated. Thus, the constituency argument as a rationale for why transplantation may be exempt from the endemic distrust fails to be compelling and is somewhat disingenuous.

There may be legitimate medical, political, and philosophical reasons for abandoning the dead donor rule, or at most giving it a status equivalent to a maxim rather than a rule. But, as illustrated in Post and others, such arguments have been articulated previously irrespective of a finding of limited public support. Will that public support be retained when the public is informed that in order to enact these preferences the laws regarding homicide will need to undergo revision? My position here reflects my concern about trying to generalize from apparently compassionate acts to institutionalized and legal practices, particularly when the fragility of trust in medicine is given full consideration. I am persuaded that it is morally preferable to seek to increase organ supplies through alternative methods that accommodate the institutionalized nature of transplant medicine and that endeavor to ensure public trust. The extent to which other alternatives are incorporated into and inform the case for abandoning the dead donor rule, or the case for an exemption to homicide, is in my view, a test of the adequacy and integrity of the argument for pre-mortem retrieval.

Resisting the Technological Imperative

There are few better examples of the technological imperative at work in contemporary medicine than in the incessant demand to increase organ procurement. There is little question that the technology is available to provide life-extension, or that it is becoming increasingly proficient. Yet, the number of persons on waiting lists for organs increases by several thousand every year, and those who die while on waiting lists by several hundred. The principal impediment in this social enterprise has been, and continues to be, the limited number of transplantable organs.

In order to comply with the technological imperative, the bioethics community is now giving serious consideration to proposals that modify the dead donor rule and/or support pre-mortem organ retrieval. That is, so compelling is the imperative of transplantation technology that leading scholars are willing to argue that society change the criteria for the determination of death again, or permit medical professionals to take the lives of those who are not dead by any standard.

Increasing organ supplies through such measures seems to me to indicate a good we want too much. The reservations of theological ethicist William F. May (1991, p. 183) seem relevant: "a tinge of the inhuman marks the humanitarianism of those who believe that social need [for organs] overrides all other considerations. . . ." I contend that the moral and social costs embedded in these procurement proposals are excessive. A revision of the dead donor rule to accommodate neocortical criteria for death presupposes an essentialist conception of the person as a disembodied consciousness. The advocacy of pre-mortem organ retrieval necessitates carving out a new exception in homicide law to the prohibition of killing in medicine. These are hardly existentially or ethically innocuous considerations, but they are morally minimized by the relentless insistence on "more" from transplantation's technology imperative.

Moreover, there is no guarantee that such proposals will solve the problem of organ scarcity, and precedent for thinking they will exacerbate that problem. In the last two decades, the expectations that a few thousand more organs would become available each year via public educational programs and adoption of routine-inquiry protocols have not materialized, nor have these measures, as was anticipated, alleviated the problem of organ scarcity. Instead, continued refinements and successes in transplantation medicine have so increased patient expectations that the waiting list has increased fourfold from the 1980s.

The debate over the current proposals to increase organ procurement presents important challenges for the identity and integrity of the bioethics community. First, the empirical data reveal a pressing need for a more engaged and constructive dialogue between bioethics and the social sciences. As Robert Zussman (2000, p. 8) has noted, "whether we are reading about informed consent, or reproductive rights, or managed care, suddenly [bioethics] arguments turn out to hinge in large part . . . on empirical propositions." This seems especially significant in the realm of bioethics under scrutiny here, namely, normative bioethics arguments that recommend changes in public or institutional policies in order to obtain certain socially desired outcomes. Zussman (2000, pp. 9-10) further observes:

> If an ethical claim is based on an assertion that a practice or arrangement is ethically questionable because it results in a particular outcome, then that claim is empirically testable. Philosophical medical ethicists rarely mount those tests themselves. . . . There is a sufficient body of social science research, bearing on informed consent, organ transplantation, end of life treatment, and any number of issues as well as managed care, to suggest that some of the consequentialist claims will be confirmed, that others will not, and that confirmation of some will modify others.

This contention seems especially salient for the kinds of studies, such as that conducted by Siminoff and colleagues, that seek to provide a fuller understanding of public attitudes and beliefs and for the outcomes-oriented policy implications that are drawn from them. Bioethics's early self-understanding, after all, was that of giving credibility and voice for a populist movement against the paternalistic authoritarianism of traditional medicine. This helped to establish the primacy of the principle of respect for autonomy in the bioethics lexicon and supported the incorporation of public interests in policy deliberations, at least as a countervailing presence to the technical views of institutionalized and bureaucratic power elites.

Although normative ethics cannot, on my view, be reduced to eliciting the preferences of individual persons or of the broader public, attentiveness and incorporation of such public views is one criterion of adequacy of a normative ethic. Moreover, bioethical theory needs to be open to revision and modification when studies provide empirical evidence of public views that run contrary to what the theory had assumed as a given. Indeed, as James Lindemann Nelson (2000, p. 15) suggests, a critical engagement with the social sciences by bioethics may involve a re-evaluation of the primacy of autonomy: "The social sciences might make a contribution to bioethics by helping the field's practitioners understand better what's behind its deeply installed respect for individual autonomy and whether it has assumed more the character of an ideology than a moral philosophy."

A second challenge for the bioethics community consists in examining whether the criteria for determining death are entirely socially constructed and thereby subject to ongoing evolution and manipulation in accordance with social needs. The irreversible cessation of certain biological functioning in the human organism is an occurrence that we mark by the term "death." This also signifies a shift in ontological status; the corpse of the deceased is open to medical manipulations, from organ retrieval to autopsy, that are precluded by law and ethics from being conducted on the living person, and the community engages in various rituals surrounding the disposition of the body to memorialize the person.

As noted previously, there are important social interests embedded in this question, including avoiding both premature determination of death as well as post-death assaults on the body, and in making decisions about when technologies of life extension legitimately can be terminated as well as initiated. Yet, it is also clear that social constructions of death cannot be disconnected from the underlying biological phenomenon. The dispute centers on which biological venue is socially and ontologically significant. However, the concern that either whole-brain or neocortical standards are arbitrary criteria deployed for social utility has led some authors recently to advocate non-brain-based, biologically validated standards (Potts, Byrne, and Nilges 2000). In short, the bioethics community continues to have work to do to articulate criteria for the determination of death that meet standards of philosophical defensibility, biological adequacy, and public intelligibility (Campbell 2001).

A third challenge concerns the degree of continuity or extent of separation between the medical and philosophical debates about the standards for determining death and the social policy interest in increasing organ procurement. Clearly, the former has implications for the latter; a non-brain-based standard will preclude most organ retrieval and subsequent transplantation and a higher-brain standard will expand both practices substantially. What raises legitimate concern, I believe, is when the relationship is reversed and the goal of organ procurement, or its lower than desired recovery ratio, directs the standard of death that society adopts.

It is a momentous undertaking to render and reform understandings of the defining boundaries — "life" and "death" — of human existence. Reconstructing these understandings to accommodate needs for transplantable organs will permeate the transplantation process with distrust and suspicion — were these organs recovered from the living or the dead? — and infuses the philosophic discussion with arbitrariness — does it really matter how we answer the preceding question?

My contention is that the discussion of the criteria used in the determination of death needs to proceed according to its own scientific and philosophic logic, and not be driven by the pragmatic interest in procurement. There are, moreover, numerous possible alternatives to increase transplantable organs short of revising the current standard of death or of resorting to harvesting from the living. If bioethics is to be taken seriously about its rhetoric of self-determination as a critical factor in social policy, it must examine these other alternatives, seek to implement them, and evaluate their efficacy, prior to meaningful consideration of an alternative, such as premortem organ retrieval, that receives the least support among the sampled public.

Finally, in concluding this essay, I return to an issue highlighted at the outset and challenge the bioethics community to have the courage to take seriously the question of the priority of organ transplants relative to other modes of healthcare. The Oregon Health Plan, now in its second decade, displays qualified acceptance by a large public constituency of a policy priority to forgo technologies of life extension, including some transplant technologies, so that more equitable access to preventive care services can be provided. Some priorities reflect a willingness to say an anguished "no" to present, identifiable patients on some matters of great expense that benefit one person in order to secure a better health future for the collective interests of the rising generation.

There are numerous philosophical arguments that contend that current healthcare priorities, which emphasize rescue medicine — for which transplantation is the paradigm example — are badly misplaced (Callahan 1990; Daniels 1988). Although these accounts are intellectually compelling, I find those positions rooted in religious and theological language inspiring and motivating. The Abrahamic faith traditions — Judaism, Christianity, and Islam — offer repeated prophetic critiques of institutions and cultures whose economic well-being betrays an ethical superficiality, as revealed in its neglect of those on the social margins. Alastair V. Campbell (1995) has eloquently articulated these concerns of the faith traditions in the context of healthcare prioritization in his book *Health as Liberation.* Campbell contends that "the fundamental injustices in the delivery of health care in modern society [are] forms of oppression, the taking away of the freedom of weaker members of society by those who hold power." Moreover, "unless we confront these issues of freedom, oppression, and liberation, we will have missed the central problem of modern health care ethics" (Campbell, A. 1995, pp. 1-2).

This is an important rejoinder to the view, voiced by some in the theological community as well as by professional bioethicists, that justice in the realm of healthcare allocation is politicized to the point that it is morally intractable. Hence, this position runs, the bioethics community ought to devote its attention to those matters, such as institutional policy on end-of-life care or transplantation procedures, in which it can have some meaningful influence, rather than try to tilt at the windmills of substantive healthcare reform. It is my position, by contrast, that the moral integrity of bioethics turns on its commitment to social justice in healthcare access, and that bioethicists first need to speak the truth of equal dignity to the corporate, industry, and institutional brokers of power in healthcare.

Campbell similarly rejects this compartmentalization between the ethical ideal and the political feasible. He affirms "a hope based on a refusal to accept that we have no power to change things" (Campbell, A. 1995, p. 122), which is generated through a focus on the experience of the poor, the marginalized, and the oppressed. "Thus, the substance of any hope for change can come only from some 'community of faith' which has the perseverance to return constantly to the places where suffering is to be found and to bring that suffering to the awareness of the whole society" (Campbell, A. 1995, p. 123).

This is the social justice challenge that the bioethics community needs to take up with a vigor equal to that displayed in debates over "whole-brain death" and increasing organ procurement. A dialogue over healthcare priorities can be informed by philosophical and religious traditions both about sharing of self and about meaningful death that can give point and purpose to the practice of organ transplantation. Ultimately, the commitment to justice is a distinctive mark and sign of the ethical seriousness of bioethics.

References

Callahan, Daniel. 1990. *What Kind of Life: The Limits of Medical Progress.* New York: Simon & Schuster.

Campbell, Alastair V. 1995. *Health as Liberation: Medicine, Theology, and the Quest for Justice.* Cleveland, OH: Pilgrim Press.

Campbell, Courtney S. 1995. When Medicine Lost Its Moral Conscience: Oregon Measure 16. In *Arguing Euthanasia,* ed. Jonathan Moreno, pp. 140-67. New York: Simon & Schuster.

———. 2001. A No-Brainer: Criticisms of Brain-Based Standards of Death. *Journal of Medicine and Philosophy* 26: 539-51.

Caplan, Arthur. 1998. *Due Consideration: Controversy in the Age of Medical Miracles.* New York: John Wiley & Sons.

Childress, James F. 1997. *Practical Reasoning in Bioethics.* Bloomington: Indiana University Press.

Daniels, Norman. 1988. *Am I My Parents' Keeper?* New York: Oxford University Press.

Fost, Norman. 1999. The Unimportance of Death. In *The Definition of Death: Contemporary Controversies,* ed. Stuart J. Youngner, Robert M. Arnold, and Renie Schapiro, pp. 161-178. Baltimore, MD: Johns Hopkins University Press.

Gaylin, Willard. 1974. Harvesting the Dead. *Harpers* (September): 23-30.

Harvard Medical School Ad Hoc Committee. 1968. A Definition of Irreversible Coma. Report of the Ad Hoc Committee of the Harvard Medical School to Examine the Definition of Brain Death. *JAMA* 205: 337-40.

LifeSharers. 2003. Solicitation received from David J. Undis, Executive Director, June 5. Available at www.lifesharers.com. Accessed 9 July 2004.

May, William F. 1991. *The Patient's Ordeal.* Bloomington: Indiana University Press.

Nelson, James Lindemann. 2000. Moral Teachings from Unexpected Quarters. *Hastings Center Report* 30 (1): 12-17.

Potts, Michael; Byrne, Paul A.; and Nilges, Richard G., eds. 2000. *Beyond Brain Death: The Case Against Brain Based Criteria for Human Death.* Dordrecht, The Netherlands: Kluwer Academic Publishers.

President's Commission for the Study of Ethical Problems in Medicine and Biomedical and Behavioral Research. 1981. *Defining Death.* Washington, DC: U.S. Government Printing Office.

Rawls, John. 1995. Two Concepts of Rules. *Philosophical Review* 64: 3-32.

Richards, Janet R. 1996. Nephrarious Goings On: Kidney Sales and Moral Arguments. *Journal of Medicine and Philosophy* 21: 375-416.

Robertson, John. 1999. The Dead Donor Rule. *Hastings Center Report* 29 (6): 6-14.

Siminoff, Laura A. 2002. Presentation at conference on Brain Death and Organ Transplantation. Case Western Reserve University, 15 November.

———; Burant, Christopher; and Youngner, Stuart J. 2004. Death and Organ Procurement: Public Beliefs and Attitudes. *Social Science & Medicine,* in press. Available to subscribers online at http://www.sciencedirect.com.science/journal/02779536. Reprinted without conclusions in *Kennedy Institute of Ethics Journal* 14: 217-34.

Spencer, Camille. 2003. Panel Denies Transplant for Inmate on Death Row, but Issue Persists. *The Oregonian* (11 June): B1, 8.

SUPPORT. 1995. A Controlled Trial to Improve Care for Seriously Ill Hospitalized Patients. *JAMA* 274: 1591-98.

Truog, Robert D. 1997. Is It Time to Abandon Brain Death? *Hastings Center Report* 27 (1): 29-37.

Youngner, Stuart J.; Arnold, Robert M.; and Schapiro, Renie, eds. 1999. *The Definition of Death: Contemporary Controversies.* Baltimore, MD: Johns Hopkins University Press,

Zussman, Robert. 2000. The Contributions of Sociology to Medical Ethics. *Hastings Center Report* 30 (1): 7-11.

CHAPTER NINE

Care of Patients and Their Suffering

Medical personnel confront suffering on a daily basis. How does a medicine shaped by Christian convictions understand suffering? What stance does it take toward suffering? One of the perennial temptations is to deny the seriousness of suffering, and Christians are, perhaps, especially tempted to negate suffering as a mere external and "earthly" reality in the enthusiastic flight to a better and other world. If we can deny the reality of suffering, we feel more comfortable ourselves. But this sort of "Gnostic" dualism was called a heresy early in the church's history.

If the first temptation is avoided, a second awaits us. It is easy and comfortable to think of suffering as constituted solely by physical pain. If Bradley Hanson is to be believed (selection 62), that is not the experience of the sufferer; and if the Christian tradition is to be believed, the external person, the body, is never quite so neatly separated from the inner person. But while the Christian tradition of an embodied soul or ensouled body may keep us from either denying suffering or reducing it to physical pain, what does it contribute positively to our understanding of suffering and to our response to it? "Well," you say, "it teaches us to be compassionate toward the sufferer." But what is it to be compassionate? Compassion is a visceral response to the suffering of another — so far, so good. It moves us to want to do something in response to another's suffering — a little further, and still unobjectionable. We see suffering, and we want to do something, anything, to put a stop to it. With this small step a divide has suddenly opened up between what may be called a "modern" compassion and an ancient virtue. The ancient virtue fit the story of one who, God with us, made the human cry of lament his or her own cry; "modern" compassion wants to stop the crying. The ancient virtue was the strength to suffer with others; "modern" compassion wants to put an end to the suffering, and by whatever means necessary. When we celebrate the "modern" compassion, the ancient virtue sounds suspiciously like an invitation to masochism and a license for sadism; suffering should be eliminated, after all, not shared.

But perhaps there are reasons to be suspicious of the "modern" compassion, too. Perhaps the "modern" compassion is a failure — or at least a temptation — of the Baconian project described by Gerald McKenny in the previous chapter. One should be grateful, of course, for the successes of medical technology in response to human suffering, thankful for any little token of God's good future. The ancient virtue itself, after all, does not delight in suffering but in God's cause and in the neighbor's good. It was surely compassion that prompted the gradual development of a medical science and technology that no longer leave us quite so helpless and hopeless in the face of the sad stories of human suffering and premature dying. But the suspicion of more than one of the essays in this chapter is that modern medicine is tempted to neglect an ancient virtue and to distort compassion into its "modern" counterfeit.

Compassion tells us, in view of suffering, to do something, but it does not tell us what thing to do. Given our confidence in the Baconian project, it is not surprising that the thing to do is to use the tool at hand. "Modern" compassion simply (and blindly) arms itself with superior technique, relying not on wisdom but on artifice against suffering. This modern counterfeit moves those unskilled in medical technology to assign the sufferer to the care of those armed with artifice, to abandon the sufferer to medicine, and so to remove the suffering. And then it moves those skilled with such tools, those armed with artifice, to attempt to give the story a happy ending by their technology; and if and when they fail, it licenses their withdrawal since they cannot do the patient any "good" anymore — as if the only good were the elimination of mortality or suffering. Meanwhile, such patients, abandoned by both friends and experts, and surrounded by technology rather than by a community that knows and shares their suffering, suffer alone and pointlessly.

This chapter asks you to consider the meaning of care. It invites you to consider the shape of a compassion armed not only with artifice but also with wisdom, and not only with wisdom but also with faith. To equip compassion with wisdom, it is necessary first to attend to the suffering, and it is there that the chapter begins.

W. H. Auden gives us a tour of a surgical ward and an initiation into the world of the suffering in selection 61. His observations, confirmed by the testimony of sufferers, call attention to at least three marks of the suffering of the sick. There is a marginalization, or "isolation," of the sufferer; "we stand elsewhere." There is a simultaneous identification with and alienation from the body; "who when healthy can become a foot?" And there is a loss of voice; the "groans they smother."

Bradley Hanson's description of his suffering (selection 62) corroborates Auden's analysis, especially the marginalization of the sufferer, but he writes as one who has recovered his voice and as one who interprets his suffering as a divine pedagogy. He has learned, he says, to share the suffering of others and to share the suffering of Christ. He has learned the ancient virtues of compassion and patience.

The essay by M. Therese Lysaught (selection 65) identifies those same three marks of the suffering of patients, but she shows that medicine can sometimes ironically reinforce a patient's suffering rather than relieving it. A patient can suffer not only from a disease but also from the treatment for it. Margaret Mohrmann, too (selection 64), is attentive to the ways in which medicine can further isolate the patient, can silence (or neglect) the patient's voice, and can identify the patient with the patient's body (or disorder) while reinforcing the experience of the body as the enemy. The challenge of medicine as a "ministry" to the suffering is not just to "feel compassion," nor simply to master a technique. The first challenge is to get to know the patient so that one can recognize his or her suffering. One context for this would presumably be the practice of taking a patient's history; Mohrmann's complaint that this practice is "significantly flawed" and her proposal to nurture a practice of listening to the patient's story are worth pausing over. It may be hard to "listen," of course, to one struck dumb by suffering; a compassion armed with wisdom will be prepared to practice a silent and empathetic presence that can break the desolating isolation of suffering and nurture the readiness of a patient both to tell his or her story and to begin to write "the next chapter."

The other selections in this chapter focus on the resources of the Christian tradition for both sufferers and those who would care for them. Together with some of the other essays they attempt to arm compassion not only with artifice but with faith. Lysaught (selection 65) sets suffering and care in the context of the liturgical tradition of the Rite of the Anointing of the Sick. She argues that the ritual offers "an alternative vision of the world" and of our suffering; it offers community to the otherwise marginalized, an appreciation of the embodied life of a mortal self when we feel both reduced to body and alienated from it, and a voice, a witness, not only *to* the suffering but also *of* the suffering.

Earl Shelp and Ronald Sunderland (selection 63) retrieve New Testament materials on suffering, especially the stories of the healing ministry of Jesus, in order to provide a model for a Christian response to people with AIDS. The stories present Jesus as compassionate and "as a combatant"; Jesus' compassion moves him not to judge but to heal, to oppose with his power the power of death and sickness. They contrast the New Testament materials with later theological efforts that train us to respond to suffering, they suggest, by trying to figure out what wrong had been done or what lesson was to be learned.

One might usefully compare the suspicion of suffering as pedagogical in the essay by Shelp and Sunderland with the account by Hanson of his suffering as a school. And one might contrast the importance of appeals to "sharing in Christ's suffering" or "sharing in the cross" in some of the other essays with the effort of Shelp and Sunderland to make "a clear distinction" between suffering "for Christ's sake" and suffering due to disease or disability. That same "clear distinction" allows them to focus on Jesus as "combatant" in his healing ministry as the model for Christian compassion and discipleship in response to the suffering caused by disease and disability. One might ask whether they are at risk of underwriting the "modern" compassion with their distinction and emphasis. Conversely, one must ask whether a Christian account of compassion may neglect the stories of Jesus' healing ministry. Without such stories to guide our response to suffering, what we called the ancient virtue may be at risk of complacent acceptance of suffering.

Stanley Hauerwas and Charles Pinches (selection 66) revisit the descriptions of patience in Cyprian, Tertullian, Augustine, and Aquinas. They find in that ancient Christian virtue and in those commentaries on it a strength to recognize the sadness of our lives and of our world and to endure it without giving up hope. Without the strength to acknowledge truthfully the brokenness of our world and the limits of our power, caretakers are tempted to remove all traces of pain and suffering, even if that finally requires the removal of the sufferers. Without the readiness to bear evils without inflicting them, we will not learn to care for those we cannot cure. Patience is not Stoic fatalism, not complacent indifference to suffering; but Hauerwas and Pinches also contrast patience not only to Stoicism but also to the restless impatience and limitless desires of modern patients, who demand the medical miracle that will eliminate their mortality and vulnerability to suffering. They contrast patience, if you will, to a "modern" compassion. And they retrieve patience as a resource for equipping compassion both with wisdom and with faith in the patient care of God, as a resource for restoring this other ancient virtue.

SUGGESTIONS FOR FURTHER READING

Cassell, Eric J. *The Nature of Suffering and the Goals of Medicine* (New York: Oxford University Press, 1991).

Dougherty, Flavian, C.P. *The Meaning of Human Suffering* (New York: Human Sciences Press, 1982).

Dyck, Arthur J. *On Human Care* (New York: Abingdon, 1977).

Farrar, Austin. *Love Almighty and Ills Unlimited* (New York: Doubleday, 1961).

Fichter, Joseph Henry. *Religion and Pain: The Spiritual Dimensions of Health Care* (New York: Crossroad, 1981).

Hauerwas, Stanley. *God, Medicine, and Suffering* (Grand Rapids: Eerdmans, 1994).

Kliever, Lonnie D., ed. *Dax's Case: Essays in Medical Ethics and Human Meaning* (Dallas: Southern Methodist University Press, 1989).

May, William F. *The Patient's Ordeal* (Bloomington: Indiana University Press, 1991).

McGill, Arthur C. *Suffering: A Test of Theological Method* (Philadelphia: Westminster, 1982).

McKenny, Gerald P., and Jonathan R. Sande. *Theological Analysis of the Clinical Encounter* (Dordrecht: Kluwer Academic Publishers, 1994).

Nouwen, Henri. *The Wounded Healer* (Garden City, N.Y.: Doubleday, 1972).

Ricoeur, Paul. *The Symbolism of Evil* (Boston: Beacon Press, 1967).

Sabatino, Frank G. "AIDS as a Spiritual Journey." *Second Opinion* 18, no. 1 (July 1992): 94-99.

Sölle, Dorothee. *Suffering*, trans. Everett Kalin (Philadelphia: Fortress, 1975).

Taylor, Rodney L., and Jean Watson, eds. *They Shall Not Hurt: Human Suffering and Human Caring* (Boulder: Colorado Associated University Press, 1989).

61 Surgical Ward

W. H. Auden

They are and suffer; that is all they do;
A bandage hides the place where each is living,
His knowledge of the world restricted to
The treatment that the instruments are giving

And lie apart like epochs from each other
— Truth in their sense is how much they can bear;
It is not like ours, but groans they smother —
And are remote as planets; we stand elsewhere.

For who when healthy can become a foot?
Even a scratch we can't recall when cured,
But are boist'rous in a moment and believe

In the common world of the uninjured, and cannot
Imagine isolation. Only happiness is shared,
And anger, and the idea of love.

62 School of Suffering

Bradley Hanson

The School of Suffering has a demanding curriculum that includes practical experience as well as thinking and reading. The practical requirements make this school different from any humanly designed institution of higher learning, for most of its students have not requested entrance. Admission usually happens to one rather than is sought. Yet once one becomes a student in the School of Suffering, one finds that it has a distinguished faculty.

My own recent illness thrust me into the school and, although I am not a biblical scholar, I was impelled to seek out one of its greatest teachers, the apostle Paul, and to especially ponder his Second Epistle to the Corinthians. I found that Paul has four major lessons on suffering. His first two lessons cast light on my experience of suffering and in turn were confirmed and illuminated by that experience. His third lesson is rather advanced for me, and I have only begun to comprehend it. The fourth is well beyond me, and I can do little more than identify it.

I

Paul's first lesson is that the sufferer is not forgotten, because God cares and often expresses his caring through the comfort given by other people. I learned this the hard way over a period of about four months when I endured increasing pain. I learned to distinguish between levels of pain. At the lowest level is an ache. While it is a bother, if one becomes engaged in something the ache is forgotten. The next level is a mild pain, sharper and more noticeable than an ache. Yet again if one becomes fully involved in some activity or conversation, the mild pain is forgotten. As the level of pain increases, the pain occupies more and more of one's consciousness. At the upper limit pain crowds out awareness of anything else; this is excruciating pain. A notch below is what I came to call intense pain, in which pain occupies nearly all of one's awareness; other things are noticed only as peripheral and subordinate to the pain. One cannot forget about intense pain. As the weeks passed the visits of intense pain came more often and lasted longer.

One result of the pain was that I was pushed to the margins of life. Many things that I enjoyed had to be given up — playing football with my sons, attending a concert or a play, spending an evening in conversation with friends, and the enjoyable activities that remained — became clouded by pain. Life became dull and uninteresting as it took all available energy just to get through the day's minimum duties.

Not only is existence on the margins of life flat, it tends to be lonely. My friends and associates were at the center, and I felt increasingly like a crippled child left on the sidelines while other children play a game. Adding to the sense of loneliness was a certain privacy about my experience of physical pain. Much suffering has a communal character. When a family member dies, the survivors share their common grief. When a minority endures discrimination, they have many common elements in their experience. But few of the people around me know first hand what it was to endure chronic intense pain. There are many who suffer like this, with no one near who fully understands their plight. Whatever the particular circumstances, being pushed to the margins of life in some form or other is nevertheless a universal feature of human suffering.

It is precisely because all genuine suffering includes psychological and social dimensions as well as the physical, that comfort from others is so terribly important. The sufferer longs to be assured that others care, and that others are striving to relieve the suffering. To feel abandoned, alone in one's suffering, would crush the sufferer with an unbearable burden.

The powerful need for this assurance was brought home to me late one night in September. I awoke as usual about 2 a.m. with intense pain. Usually it had lasted 30-45 minutes, but this night it kept on and on. After about two hours I began to cry, not a gentle weeping but great gasps. I felt unable to stand up to the pain any longer, and I cried out in anguish at being overwhelmed. My cries were also a call to my wife that I needed her. She awoke and held and stroked me. The pain did not cease for some time, but her presence made it more tolerable.

A few days later Paul's words caught my eye, "But God, who comforts the downcast, comforted us by the coming of Titus . . ." (II Cor. 7:6 RSV). When Paul speaks of comfort, he uses it against the Old Testament background in which comfort includes deliverance as well as tender stroking (e.g. Isaiah 40:1, 2). The news that the Corinthian church had taken Paul's severe letter well delivered him from his anxiety; but first he mentions that the mere arrival of his friend and associate Titus was a comfort.

Paul sees this ordinary series of events in theological perspective. The arrival of his friend with good news encourages Paul, who has been afflicted with anxieties and conflicts in his work; but it is ultimately God who has comforted him through Titus. "But God, who comforts the downcast, comforted us by the coming of Titus." Thus for Paul the aid that one human being gives to another is a human transaction grounded in and manifesting the character of God, "The Father of mercies and God of all comforts" (II Cor. 1:3).

From *Dialog* 20 (Winter 1981): 39-45. Used by permission.

When strong and privileged socially concerned Christians hear that God comforts sufferers through other people, they are likely to hear only a call to be active in relieving the suffering of others, but that is not what *sufferers* need to hear. To issue such an ethical challenge to those who suffer is to increase their trouble by laying another burden on them. The strong and privileged are able to give; the sufferer needs first of all to receive. So Paul's first word to those Corinthian Christians who endure sufferings with him is to bless "The God and Father of our Lord Jesus Christ, the Father of mercies and God of all comfort, who comforts us in all our afflictions . . . " (II Cor. 1:3, 4). If those who suffer are to interpret the meaning of their suffering within the Christian perspective, they need to know they are not abandoned in their suffering. Others care, and God cares. This word of comfort, rather than a word of moral challenge, is the first lesson in learning the Pauline meaning of suffering.

II

Paul's second lesson is that those who have received comfort from God in their suffering are called to give comfort to other sufferers, for God "comforts us in all our affliction, so that we may be able to comfort those who are in any affliction . . ." (II Cor. 1:3,4). Paul's "so that" expresses purpose.

Of course, Paul's audience and his own situation shape what he says. Paul speaks as a man who has endured much affliction yet has lived through it all; and his audience are Christians in Corinth and the province of Achaia who also were no strangers to suffering. Paul does not consider those whose suffering is such that they do not live through it or fail to receive comfort in their suffering. He considers only those cases in which people are able to learn something from their suffering. He also is not speaking to non-sufferers, even though they might be eager to help those less fortunate. The admission fee to this particular lesson on suffering is high — it requires suffering, for comfort is received only in suffering. It is sufferers who are given comfort "so that" they may comfort others.

It is true that Paul's "we" in II Cor. 1:3-11 refers primarily to himself, but the plural "we" likely indicates that the pattern of affliction and comfort so dramatically exemplified in the apostle's existence has wider application. He certainly does not set himself totally apart from the Corinthians, whom he also recognizes as sharing in comfort and suffering.

So Christians who have been comforted in their suffering may affirm as part of its meaning that their experience of suffering and comfort includes God's call to comfort others and that the experience itself equips them to do it. There is a psychological aspect to this, because someone who has experienced a certain kind of affliction is peculiarly equipped to help others with that affliction. Having known poverty first hand can enable one to more fully understand the plight of the poor and to bring genuine comfort. To be sure, deliverance from suffering often requires also the technical knowledge of a physician or economic changes on a broad front. Still, direct experience of suffering and comfort gives a depth and sensitivity to compassion which is irreplaceable in the total effort to comfort the afflicted.

The truth of this lesson began to dawn on me one night shortly before entering the hospital. My wife was helping me use a heat lamp, and we began to talk about the meaning of my suffering. I had to admit that the most prominent feature of the suffering up to this point had been its emptiness of purpose. There had been no goal which I could affirm and strive for, except to fight against the pain and seek healing. The suffering itself was an experience of passivity, of being acted upon by negative forces beyond my control. The pain was a harsh reminder of the blind physical roots of life, an irrational reminder without purpose. I felt kinship with the insect accustomed to living in the supportive environment of black soil suddenly turned on its back in the sun, legs moving helplessly. The brute physical reality of pain was devoid of meaning. The only glimmer of meaning I could own at this time was that I now felt much greater sympathy for others who had to suffer, especially those who had to endure chronic pain without hope of relief.

Upon further reflection after my suffering was over, I came to see that the scope of "suffering with others" should not be unduly extended by overdramatized portrayals of the Christian life which picture the concerned Christian as suffering with the afflicted. There are tendencies toward this sort of rhetoric in Dorothee Sölle's book *Suffering*.

There are at least three distinct ways for Christians to bring comfort through sharing in the suffering of others. One way is to have concern and sympathy for those who suffer and to express it in some concrete way. Such active compassion is an expression of love for neighbor. Paul's collection for the needy in Jerusalem appealed to this sort of compassion.

Another way to bring comfort by sharing in the sufferings of others is by enduring the same suffering they do (e.g. to starve with the starving). Very infrequently would one choose to suffer with others in this way and only when it would serve some constructive end.

A third way to share in the suffering of others is through profound identification with them. Paul does not define suffering for us; but a good definition is that a person is suffering when being acted upon in such a way that the person wishes strongly that his or her state were different.[1] If the sun is shining on one during a hot summer's day walk, one is uncomfortable but not suffering. If one were forced to walk 20 miles in scorching heat, one would suffer. The wish that one's state were otherwise would be very powerful indeed. Using this definition to

1. Cf. David R. Mason, "Some Abstract, Yet Crucial, Thoughts About Suffering," *Dialog* 16 (Spring 1977): 94-96.

suffer with another would mean that the other's suffering would have such a deep impact on a person that one would fervently wish that the other's state (and one's own) would be changed. Parents who agonize over the serious illness of their child genuinely suffer; their anxiety causes them to lose sleep, to weep, etc. To suffer with another in this way requires a profound identification with that other person; the other's welfare is intimately linked with one's own.

While Christians frequently exhibit active concern for others in affliction, they seldom actually suffer with them. This should be honestly recognized. When there was mass starvation recently in Cambodia, I prayed for them and sent contributions through Oxfam and church. This and other manifestations of compassion are good, but it is not suffering.

A final comment about receiving comfort in order to comfort others. It would be reading too much into Paul to infer from this lesson that God *sends* suffering in order to build character. That pedagogical view of suffering may or may not be true, but Paul does not consider such a question of justification for suffering. He begins with the fact of suffering and comfort, and says that God sends *comfort* at least in part so that those who are comforted may be able to comfort others.

Paul also sees this principle of "comforting as one has been comforted" in theological depth, for Christians are to comfort others "with the comfort with which we ourselves are comforted by God" (II Cor. 1:4). This brings us back to the foundation of Paul's first lesson — the ultimate source of comfort is not our own skill or personality but God's compassion for His creatures.

III

The third Pauline lesson is that suffering Christians share in the suffering of Christ. I found this to be the most difficult lesson to understand and appropriate. Two obstacles stood in the way.

I encountered the first obstacle when I read Second Corinthians while in the hospital. When I first read Paul's list of his own sufferings in II Cor. 11:23-29, I felt that my own affliction from pain did not qualify as suffering that shares in the suffering of Christ. Paul mentions sufferings from persecution as a Christian missionary — he was imprisoned, beaten, lashed, and stoned. He also speaks of hardships that came with being a traveling missionary — the dangers of first-century travel, hunger, and cold. On top of all that was the anxiety he felt as an apostle for all the churches.

My suffering found no place among those listed by Paul. I was not persecuted for the faith. About the only hazard I faced in carrying out my vocation as a professor of religion was a loss of muscle tone from sedentary work. And while some Christians can confess anxiety over the church, I could not recall losing any sleep for that reason. If only persecution, hardship, and anxiety for the faith could count as sharing in the sufferings of Christ, then I, and by far most American Christians, were left out.

Later, after serious study of Paul's thought, two things led me to include myself as having shared in Christ's suffering. One is that Paul refers to two personal afflictions which were very likely physical. In II Cor. 1:8 he mentions "the affliction we experienced in Asia" which brought him very near death. And in II Cor. 12:7 he alludes to his "thorn." Although Paul never tells us exactly what either of these were, the bulk of commentators think that the indications make physical afflictions the best guess.

The second reason is that Paul does not set himself totally apart from other Christians, for he says that they are comforted when they "patiently endure the same sufferings that we suffer" (II Cor. 1:6). It could hardly be literally true that they experienced the same sufferings as the well-traveled apostle. It is likely that other Christians at Corinth underwent some persecution, especially the Jewish Christians, but such opposition most likely focused on Paul as the instigator of changes (Acts 18:12-17). While the disciplic pattern of suffering/death and resurrection is most vividly evident in the apostle's life, still he recognizes its presence in the more ordinary lives of other Christians as well.

It is very doubtful that Paul meant to set strict boundaries to what sort of sufferings share in the sufferings of Christ. The specific afflictions he cites from his own experience are merely examples, and even these examples are varied, including anxiety, illness, and physical disability. It seems likely that Paul would agree with I Peter 4:12-19 that suffering as a murderer or wrongdoer would not count, but he opens the circle beyond the persecution cited by Peter to include any innocent suffering. Thus those Christians whose more settled circumstances do not expose them to persecution and hardship for the faith will still at times have sufferings which bring them to share in the sufferings of Christ.

Having surmounted the first obstacle, another still loomed ahead: What does it *mean* to share in Christ's sufferings? A number of commentators think that at least part of what Paul means is connected with his beliefs about the end times. C. K. Barrett points out that there was a Jewish notion of the "sufferings of the Messiah" which did not mean that the Messiah himself would suffer but that the age of the Messiah would be a time of tribulation prior to eternal bliss. Paul probably believed that Jesus had taken most of this end-time tribulation upon himself, yet in the brief time remaining before the end some of this messianic suffering had "overflowed to" Jesus' followers. "For as we share abundantly in Christ's sufferings" (II Cor. 1:5) is perhaps better rendered ". . . as the sufferings of Christ overflow to us."[2]

If these commentators are correct, there is the question what this can mean for us today. When Paul believed that the Christians of his time were living in the

2. C. K. Barrett, *A Commentary on the Second Epistle to the Corinthians* (New York: Harper & Row, 1973), pp. 61-62.

last days, the idea of sharing in the end-time woes with Christ lent drama and rich meaning to their suffering. It might have given a sense of high privilege to be among this chosen band. But what happens after 1900 years have elapsed and belief in the imminent end has waned? Most of the power in this interpretation of suffering is lost.

Of course, it is not impossible to view the course of human history in Paul's framework if one lengthens the end time considerably, but it is difficult not to lose the vibrancy of that belief unless one believes this nearly 2000-year end-time era is about to close. Jehovah's Witnesses, Seventh-Day Adventists, and dispensationalist-minded Christians can resonate to this interpretation of sharing in Christ's suffering, but it leaves me unmoved. For me, and I suspect for most mainline church-goers, its power has been dissipated by the passage of time and numerous failed prophecies of when the end would come. We simply do not approach each day thinking this might be the day when Christ returns.

The more important and durable meaning of sharing in Christ's suffering depends on Paul's conception of the relationship between Christ and believers as expressed in the terms "Body of Christ" and "in Christ." Considerable historical study is required to grasp what Paul might have meant with these expressions, for they are many-leveled metaphors. Eduard Schweizer's discussions of these terms are a happy contrast to numerous murky treatments of Paul's mysticism. Much of what Schweizer says can be grouped under three heads.

First, Schweizer says that when Paul speaks of the body of Christ and being in Christ, he is following the Jewish way of thinking in terms of spheres, in which there are certain places or spheres where God's lordship is experienced more directly than in other places, e.g. the temple. Such a sphere of life could bear the stamp of a man such as Abraham, Jacob, or Moses. When Paul speaks of the church as the body of Christ, he is speaking of the place or sphere bearing the stamp of Christ.[3]

Secondly, "body of Christ" has several rich overtones which make it especially suitable as a metaphor for the community/sphere in which Christ's stamp is manifest. One level of its meaning is always the historical body of Christ sacrificed on the cross. In Paul's day this reminder that God expressed His love for people supremely in that physical realm counteracted common Hellenistic tendencies to escape from the physical world into some pure spiritual realm. For Christians the body is the appropriate place and means for meeting and serving others. By extension the Christian community is also appropriately called the body of Christ, because in this down-to-earth sphere people are accepted by God on the basis of Christ's bodily sacrifice and are called to obedient service. Life in this community bears the stamp of Christ. "Life in the body of Christ is identical with life 'in Christ.'"[4]

Thirdly, Schweizer says that the expressions "body of Christ" and "in Christ" are also part of Paul's translation of Jesus' call to discipleship for a Hellenistic audience. When Jesus called Matthew and others to be his disciples, it meant to come with him as he traveled from place to place, but after the resurrection that sort of accompaniment was no longer possible. Discipleship to Christ needed reinterpretation. Paul translated Jesus' call to discipleship into spatial images readily understandable to the Hellenistic mind already accustomed to calling a social group a "body" and to thinking in Platonic and Stoic fashion of the world as the body in which God dwells as its soul. It was not a great step for them to think of the Christian community as the body in which Christ dwells.[5]

What had special appeal to the Hellenistic audience was to say that following Christ would mean being glorified with him and elevated above the trials of this physical world; but to say only this would have falsified the account of Christian discipleship. Paul had to say that following Christ also means obedience to Him in daily life with its defeats as well as its victories. Indeed, following the crucified Christ means that his disciples cannot expect to be delivered from the ills of life; their way will also include suffering and death.

I think the idea of discipleship is the key to a contemporary interpretation of how Christians share in Christ's suffering. My own experience of suffering suggests how the relationship of lord and disciple can be understood to involve participation in the Lord's suffering. There were a few people who shared by suffering to the extent that they suffered with me; above all it was my wife, to a lesser extent my children and parents. There were friends and other relatives who were concerned and sympathetic to my situation, yet could hardly be said to suffer with me. What seems to account for the difference between the sympathizers and the fellow sufferers is that those who suffered with me were so closely identified with me that I was included in their sense of self; their own identity as persons was closely intertwined with me as husband, father, or son.

There is a useful analogy here to the believer's participation in the sufferings of Christ, although the basis of the participation is the relationship of disciple to lord rather than husband and wife, father and children, son and parents. The identity of the disciple is inseparably linked with the lord, and the identity of the lord with his disciples ("Saul, Saul, why do you persecute me?" Acts 9:4). Christ's relationship with his disciples belongs to his very being as Christ; he cannot be Christ all by himself. The relationship of disciples with Christ is also constitutive of their being; they cannot be Christians apart from identifying with Christ as their lord.

The relationship of Christ with his disciples is asymmetrical, for the relationship rests on his choosing them while it is their secondary place to respond to the lord's

3. Eduard Schweizer, *Jesus* (Richmond: John Knox, 1971), p. 110.

4. Ibid., p. 113.

5. Eduard Schweizer, *Lordship and Discipleship* (London: SCM, 1960), pp. 104-13.

call. Therefore the sufferings of Christians are also Christ's sufferings fundamentally because Christ identifies himself so closely with his church. If a concerned parent hurts when the child hurts, how much more does Christ share in the suffering of his people. So our sufferings are his primarily because he makes them his. He wills to include us in his own being as Christ the lord.

Secondarily, disciples of Christ are called to recognize that suffering is an integral part of Christian discipleship. If they hope to be glorified with Christ, they should also expect to share in his suffering by following the way that includes suffering. To identify with the crucified one as lord is to include in one's own self-definition the expectation of suffering. When the son of a Nigerian territorial ruler came to medical school in the United States, he refused to do some dirty work expected of beginning medical students in the hospital. That lay outside his self-definition, and he was prepared to drop out of the university rather than do that menial work. Suffering does not lie outside the self-definition of Christians.

Because the disciple's identity is dependent upon that of the lord, the disciple's sufferings are not just his or her own but are a sharing in the lord's suffering. That is to say, the disciple's identity is patterned after the lord's identity. So when the disciple of Christ suffers, it is not simply sharing in a common human experience as it is when one laughs or plays; it is more importantly a sharing in the specific way of Jesus Christ.

Not every path of discipleship follows that way. Suffering cannot be ignored, but one after another religious leaders point a way out of it, and suffering is usually regarded as a sign that disciples are failing to follow their leader. Jesus Christ leads his disciples more deeply into suffering, for he himself went into the depths of suffering before the resurrection. Thus while suffering comes to every human being, Christians can believe that their suffering is not alien to their relationship to Christ, but an integral part of it. Even as Christ shares in their suffering by virtue of his identification with his church, so also Christians share in his suffering by following his way.

I have found that this Pauline lesson is not as easily appropriated as the first two. To be sure, I take comfort in the thought that Christ has so closely identified himself with the community of believers that he makes their suffering his own. That is a reassuring expression of God's love for me. But the idea that suffering is an integral part of Christian discipleship is contradictory to human inclinations. I am very much like that African medical student who refused to do menial work. I shy away from including suffering in my self-definition.

My tendency is to assume that it is my *right* to be healthy, to be able to run, to have good eyesight and hearing, to have the normal functioning of all my limbs and organs. I believe it is my right to be happy, and I become enraged at any violation of these rights. Thus I deny my creatureliness, for I assume that God (or "life") owes me happiness as though the cosmic order were established by some grand social compact like a club or nation. I do not want to admit that, as a creature, whatever I have has been given to me. Certainly health and happiness are goods which I should seek, but there is no cosmic bill of rights which guarantees that I should have them.

Just as Paul's lesson goes against our denial of creaturely limits, so it also goes against our tendency to deny being disciples of Christ. I definitely think of myself as a "Christian" or a "believer in Jesus Christ." I realize that when those terms are properly understood, they include discipleship, but my inclination is not to understand myself as one who is called to obediently follow the way of Christ, a characteristic basic to discipleship. I am more interested in what comfort Christ can give to me than in the summons to follow him. So I tend to ignore the call to take up my cross and follow him even when the cross has knocked me flat on my back. The resistance to being a disciple is strong.

Christ did not claim any right to a happy normal life (not even equality with God was a thing to be grasped). He accepted God's call to service and followed it through suffering and death. "A disciple is not above his teacher." So Christians need to include suffering in their self-definition. Not that they should welcome affliction or go looking for it, but there should be a recognition that suffering is both an inevitable risk for human creatures and an integral element in Christian discipleship.

Because my resistance to discipleship is so strong, I have barely opened the book on this lesson. Yet in an elementary way I have found that suffering brings lord and disciple into closer fellowship. I am drawn closer to Christ as I more fully appreciate the nature of the sufferings that he endured. The sheer physical pain must have been excruciating and prolonged. Scholars often downplay this because it is not unique to Jesus, but having known extended intense pain myself, I marvel at anyone voluntarily undergoing great pain. Adding to Jesus' suffering was the sense of abandonment by most disciples. And depending on the interpretation of Jesus' words, "My God, my God, why hast thou forsaken me?" most terrifying of all may have been abandonment by God and apparently meaningless suffering. Since my illness, I have felt a bond with anyone who suffers pain or illness. I am even drawn closer to Christ, for in some sense he suffered for me.

Being drawn closer to the suffering Christ has revealed that discipleship is a fulfilling relationship of deeper fellowship between lord and disciple. In this relationship the disciple finds fulfillment in surprising ways. There has been a glimpse of the truth that through following the lord's way of suffering, my own true identity is being fashioned, for it is mysteriously intertwined with Christ.

IV

Yet another lesson that Paul teaches about suffering is that it has the potential for being a means through which

God's power can be revealed to others. Paul accepted his thorn in the flesh when told, "My grace is sufficient for you, for my power is made perfect in weakness" (II Cor. 12:9). Besides whatever else it means that God's power is made perfect in weakness, it means that the divine power is especially evident when the human vessel is weak (II Cor. 4:7). God's power is more apparent when his will is accomplished in and through one who lacks the human power of strength, beauty, wealth, etc. So Paul gladly boasts of the weaknesses evident in his own sufferings, because through them God's power is plainly revealed to others.

This too is a teaching difficult to appropriate, and it may be that it does not have as wide an application as the previous lessons. It seems presumptuous to regard one's own affliction as a vehicle for God's revelation except when circumstances clearly warrant it. I know of nothing in my own suffering that made it a means for divine revelation to others. One cannot assume that one's suffering is automatically being used in this way, but one can certainly pray that God will so use it and one can seek to be open to the grace that will make that possible. If it turns out that one's suffering becomes a medium of revelation to others, that is grounds for seeing yet another profound meaning in one's suffering.

V

Very likely Paul has other lessons on suffering, but these are enough for one term. Learning Paul's lessons is not easy, because the required involvement in suffering is a very high tuition to pay for the School of Suffering. Yet more than enough suffering will come to every Christian over a lifetime even without choosing it, so it is good that Christians can draw upon Paul's insights. When we can affirm for ourselves some of his rich meaning in suffering, then we too can paradoxically rejoice in our suffering at the same time that we long for deliverance.

63 AIDS and the Church

Earl E. Shelp and Ronald H. Sunderland

Illness in Christian Perspective

The question of how to account for the existence of illness, suffering, and tragedy as integral parts of daily life has preoccupied the human psyche throughout history. In particular, the Christian church has struggled with the relationship of illness to faith. The Gospels provide little insight regarding the role of illness and suffering in creation. Issues of how to justify the ways of God seem to have been unimportant to Jesus, who clearly gave priority to the urgency of proclaiming the gospel. We seemingly cannot forgo our human preoccupation with attempts to explain illness and suffering, but apparently Jesus did not join these discussions. He was too busy going about healing the sick, casting out demons, and, in so doing, manifesting God's compassion and love toward the afflicted. The church attempts to keep a balance between these two functions, engaging in acts of compassion and support to people in need and reflecting theologically on the relationship of this ministry to the church's confession and mission. If the New Testament is a guide, ministry must remain in the forefront of the church's activity. But theology as critical reflection on the work of ministry is not a secondary function. Rather, each function informs and corrects the other; each fulfills a servant role, so that the church's work may be done.[1]

It is important to pursue this interrelationship with respect to the AIDS epidemic. The dimensions of this crisis, the needs of people with AIDS, and societal reactions to people with AIDS demand a response from the church. We must discover the appropriate form such a response must take, as to both the nature of compassionate ministry and the theological imperatives by which care and concern are shaped and corrected. In the course of exploring these issues, we will discover that the scriptures do not offer simple answers to questions related to the existence of illness and suffering. Rather, they call the people of God to serve their neighbors. At this moment, that includes people with AIDS.

1. For an elaboration of this theme, see *The Pastor as Theologian*, Earl E. Shelp and Ronald H. Sunderland, eds. (New York: Pilgrim Press, in press).

New Testament Perceptions of Suffering

The New Testament recognizes suffering as a part of daily living that must be accepted and endured with fortitude. The troubles to be borne in this earthly existence are of little consequence compared to the life that is "hidden with Christ in God" (Col. 3:3). The New Testament, however, addresses sufferings at three levels. First, some afflictions clearly were the consequences of imprisonment and persecution because of the believer's witness to faith in Jesus Christ as Lord. Thus was Stephen stoned to death. Second, suffering may be the result of oppression by one person or group of another person or group. The most frequently cited biblical example is the oppression of the weak and helpless by the wealthy and powerful. Third, pain and suffering may be due to disease or physical or mental disability.

Suffering "For Christ's Sake"

Peter refers to suffering "for Christ's sake," for example, when he warns his readers that they may suffer "trials of many kinds." These trials come so that their faith "may prove itself worthy of all praise, glory, and honour when Jesus Christ is revealed" (1 Peter 1:6-7). Paul expresses the same thought frequently. Writing to the Corinthians, he offers the example of his faithful witness:

> As God's servants, we try to recommend ourselves in all circumstances by our steadfast endurance: in distress, hardships, and dire straits; flogged, imprisoned, mobbed; overworked, sleepless, starving. . . . Dying we still live on; disciplined by suffering, we are not done to death; in our sorrows we have always cause for joy; poor ourselves, we bring wealth to many; penniless, we own the world." (2 Corinthians 6:4-5, 9-10)

One of the richest sources of this image is in the eleventh chapter of the same letter:

> Five times the Jews have given me the thirty-nine strokes; three times I have been beaten with rods; once I was stoned; three times I have been shipwrecked, and for twenty-four hours I was adrift on the open sea. I have been constantly on the road; I have met dangers from my fellow-countrymen, dangers from foreigners, dangers in towns, dangers in the country, dangers at sea, dangers from false friends.
>
> (2 Corinthians 11:23-26; see also, for example, Romans 8:19, 21-23; 1 Corinthians 4:9-13; 2 Corinthians 1:8-11; 4:8-12, 16-18)

These "trials of many kinds" were anticipated in phrases attributed to Jesus in the Beatitudes: "How blest you are, when you suffer insults and persecution and every kind of calumny for my sake. Accept it with gladness and exultation, for you have a rich reward in heaven; in the same way they persecuted the prophets before you" (Matt. 5:11-12). Suffering "for Christ's sake" on the part of his followers is thus incorporated into the suffering for the sake of righteousness that characterizes both Old and New Testaments. In the Old Testament, it is linked to the concept of the Suffering Servant. In the New Testament, Peter recognizes that such human suffering participates in the suffering of Christ:

> My dear friends, do not be bewildered by the fiery ordeal that is upon you, as though it were something extraordinary. It gives you a share in Christ's sufferings, and that is cause for joy; and when his glory is revealed, your joy will be triumphant. . . . If anyone suffers as a Christian, he should feel it no disgrace, but confess that name to the honour of God. (1 Peter 4:12-13, 16)

Such passages often seem to be advanced in support of the claim that when suffering in the form of physical illness is experienced, it ought to be accepted and endured as an ordeal in the sense intended by Peter: that is, a trial sent to test the believer's faith. A clear distinction, however, should be made as to the source of the suffering before physical hardship and illness are so linked, as will be noted.

Suffering as a Result of Oppression

The Gospels note a second source of suffering against which Jesus cried out in protest, and which is to be opposed at every point: suffering that results from human injustice and oppression of the poor. Luke begins his record of Jesus' ministry with the account of the visit to Nazareth. The words from Isaiah 61 are applied to the ministry of Jesus: "[The Lord] has sent me to announce good news to the poor" (Luke 4:18). The announcement is clearly intended to address the concerns that so roused the prophets: the need to proclaim liberation to broken victims and release to the captives. It is usual to link with these phrases the complementary passages from Isaiah. Thus, the Gospel calls for the loosing of the fetters of injustice, untying the knots of the yoke, snapping every yoke, and setting free those who have been crushed. To the cry for compassion toward the crushed is added the call to proclaim recovery of sight to the blind and to clothe the naked, provide hospitality to the homeless poor, feed the hungry, and satisfy the needs of the wretched (Isa. 58:6-10). In denouncing the religious authorities, Jesus pointed to their greed: "Beware of the doctors of the law. . . . These are the men who eat up the property of widows, while they say long prayers for appearance' sake; and they will receive the severest sentence" (Luke 20:45-47).

Luke is not alone among the Evangelists in identifying Jesus as championing the cause of the poor and oppressed, but his gospel is noteworthy for this emphasis. With Matthew, Luke cites Jesus' reply to John's disciples, who sought confirmation that Jesus was really "the coming one." Jesus' ministries of healing and liberation were explicit signs of the reign of God — for those who had eyes of faith to see. The fact that, in the liberating actions of Jesus, John possessed all the evidence he needed to satisfy his uncertainty leads to only one conclusion: the power of God is present in Jesus. In its presence, evil — in the form of oppression of the innocent, injustice levied against those too weak to speak for themselves, or exclusion of the humble from the community's concern and care — is being overturned. The message is clear. Evil cannot continue to exist in the presence of God's love.

The hospitality of the Kingdom is extended without hesitation to those whom society has oppressed or ignored: the poor, the crippled, the lame, and the blind (Luke 14:21), those whose homes are the city's streets and alleys (v. 21) or the roads and hedges of the countryside (vs. 23-24). Such gracious acts are extended to people who, because of their very weakness, even their failure to thrive, are unable to return the gift of hospitality. That they cannot is the best reason for inviting them. The inability of the poor to return the kindness is the measure of their need of it. The words and actions of Jesus are those of confrontation: the causes and consequences of poverty, injustice, and exclusion from the community are to be opposed. Not only will those who oppress the poor not inherit the kingdom; even those who fail to minister to the least of the Lord's brothers and sisters will go away to eternal punishment, "to the eternal fire that is ready for the devil and his angels" (Matt. 25:41). Jesus accused the Pharisees of having no care for justice and love of God, and the lawyers of loading men with intolerable burdens (Luke 11:42, 46). The scene in the temple in which the money-changers' tables were overthrown and the pigeons freed from their cages expresses the same sense of outrage at the afflictions imposed on the poor. For the robbery being practiced involved not only the fraudulent activities of the money-changers against worshipers, but the stealing of this house from God. "Moreover, the thefts from me were not limited to the Temple precincts, as Jeremiah knew, but included the dog-eat-dog practices outside the Temple by men who then took part in the worship (Jer. 7:8-15)."[2]

Jesus' work in the temple was a prophetic sign of God's wrath, in accordance with God's desire to make God's house a place of worship for all nations. God had promised to bring foreigners and gather the outcasts to rejoice in the benefits of the temple (Isa. 56:6-8). "It was this promise which Jesus fulfilled and which the priests repudiated, so that this episode becomes an epitome of the Messiah's whole career."[3] As a result, Christians are not urged to accept or tolerate such affliction with passive resignation; they are bidden to lift the yoke of oppression and to fill the role of champions of the downtrodden. The followers of Jesus walk in his footsteps only if they are filled with a like concern for the poor (we discuss this theme more comprehensively in chapter 4).

2. Paul S. Minear, *The Gospel According to Mark,* vol. 17 of the Layman's Bible Commentary, Balmer H. Kelly, ed. (Atlanta: John Knox Press, 1960), p. 109.

3. Ibid.

Suffering Due to Disease or Disability

Just as injustice cannot exist in the presence of the Lord's anointed, neither can sickness endure against God's power. The citing of the Isaianic passages (Luke 4:18-19) signals Luke's emphasis on Jesus' ministry to the poor and oppressed, included among whom, true to the Old Testament passages, are the sick and disabled in body and mind. This aspect of the discussion should be set in the context of the attribution of causality for sickness and affliction, and the perceived relationship between illness or disability and ritual defilement, that has characterized Judeo-Christian thought. Judaism struggled with the notion that sickness was a consequence of sin and therefore a punishment. Acts of healing were acknowledged by proving to a priest that the symptoms of disease or disability had vanished, whereupon the priest declared that the defilement was lifted and the formerly disabled person was restored to the community and to the full benefits of the law. Ritual defilement resulted from any affliction, since it was axiomatic that the disease would not have occurred if the victim's relationship with God was not disordered.[4]

It is in this context that the ministry of Jesus to the sick should be set. Jesus was at pains to discard the ancient attribution of illness or disability as punishment for some act of disobedience of God's law: that is, as God's retribution for human sin. The tradition was long and deep. Sirach, or ben Sira, the author of Ecclesiasticus, declared in the second century B.C. that

> From the beginning good things were created for
> the good,
> and evils for sinners.
> The chief necessities of human life
> are water, fire, iron, and salt,
> flour, honey, and milk,
> the juice of the grape, oil, and clothing.
> All these are good for the god-fearing,
> but turn to evil for sinners.
>
> There are winds created to be agents of retribution,
> with great whips to give play to their fury;

4. This was the case, for example, with respect to leprosy. In this respect, it is important to recognize that the term to which reference is made in the Jewish scriptures and in the New Testament carried a different connotation from that of the disease known commonly as leprosy in the twentieth century. The leprosy of the ancient Near East actually encompassed a range of dermatological disorders that seldom approached the seriousness or evoked the level of fear with which today's leprosy (Hansen's disease) is associated. Such common skin diseases as psoriasis, eczema, and other common rashes and lesions were probably included under the general heading of "leprosy."

The real suffering of lepers was not so much due to physical discomfort as to the isolation and ostracism that sufferers met in the general community. It is a similar isolation and ostracism experienced by people with AIDS that links the two. More important, given this association, the response of Jesus to people with leprosy suggests the model for the response of God's people to people with AIDS.

on the day of reckoning, they exert their force
and give full vent to the anger of their Maker.
Fire and hail, famine and *deadly disease,*
all these were created for retribution;
beasts of prey, scorpions and vipers,
and the avenging sword that destroys the wicked.
They delight in carrying out his orders,
always standing ready for his service on the earth;
and when their time comes, they never disobey.
(Ecclesiasticus 39:25-31; emphasis added)

Sirach clearly reflected a popularly held perception against which Jesus protested. John records the disciples' questioning of Jesus regarding a blind man: "Rabbi, who sinned, this man or his parents? Why was he born blind?" Jesus responded: "It is not that this man or his parents sinned; he was born blind so that God's power might be displayed in curing him" (John 9:2-3). Jesus rejected the notion that God had deliberately disabled this man — and, conceivably, others — on account of sin, or merely to provide an opportunity to demonstrate God's power. Indeed, Mark presents Jesus as requiring the disciples to keep silent concerning such acts lest they be regarded by the populace as merely displays of power designed to coerce a positive response to the gospel — and thus be misunderstood. Luke records that Jesus was challenged to explain the sufferings of the innocent: for example, the Galileans slaughtered by Pilate and the eighteen upon whom the tower of Siloam fell (Luke 13:1-9). An easy solution would be to say, echoing Job's friends, that the fate of the Galileans overtook them in the providence of God, a just punishment for some iniquity of which they were doubtless guilty. While it is precisely this theory that Jesus rejects, he does not advance any alternative explanation at this point.[5] The question of the problem of suffering is unanswered, for Jesus treats the story, and another that he raises, as parables. And the whole issue of the parables is the urgency of the gospel. It is this urgency which is offered as the basis for the Johannine statement: "While daylight lasts we must carry on the work of him who sent me; night comes, when no one can work. While I am in the world I am the light of the world" (John 9:4-5).

The issue for Jesus is the primacy of the gospel. He had come into Galilee "proclaiming the Gospel of God" (Mark 1:14). What followed, whether teaching, confronting, ministering compassionately, or healing, was the manifestation of the power of God at work: "If it is by the finger of God that I drive out the devils, then be sure the kingdom of God has already come upon you" (Luke 11:20). The healing acts were entailed by the message he proclaimed. Nothing, including disease and devils, could impede the progress of the kingdom's unveiling or withstand its power. Hence, the Markan "secret": the healing acts would only be correctly perceived when people recognized them as outbreaks of the kingdom's presence. In any other context, they would appear as mere "signs and wonders," which Jesus refused the Pharisees.

When one turns to examine how Jesus acted when confronted by human distress arising from disease and disability, the evidence is overwhelming: Jesus responded at every opportunity to relieve such affliction. Healing was often performed in a manner indicative of confrontation with illness. The Gospels identify Jesus as engaged in two types of healing activity: the driving out of demons and the healing of the sick and physically disabled. The twelve disciples were sent out with instructions to heal the sick, raise the dead, cleanse lepers, and cast out devils (Matt. 10:8). In Capernaum, the crowds brought to him all who were ill or possessed by devils (Mark 1:3). To Pharisees who urged him to escape from Herod, he replied, "Go and tell that fox, 'Listen: today and tomorrow I shall be casting out devils and working cures'" (Luke 13:32). The separate identification of the two activities suggests two functions. In the case of demon possession, the confrontation with evil is emphasized, but such actions are viewed in the context of the struggle between the power of the evil one and the power of God. Edward Schillebeeckx notes, "As Jesus pursues his ministry and manifests himself, this in itself is regarded by the evil powers as an act of aggression (Mk. 1:23-24 and parallels; 5:7ff. and parallels; 9:20-25). Against the evil and hurtful results produced by these powers Jesus sets only good actions, deeds of beneficence."[6]

The exorcisms are presented to show that God's eschatological kingdom is now present. Illness in general, however, was a sign of disorder in God's creation that ends with physical death. While sickness and death are customarily assumed to be evidence of the activity of evil, the healing of the sick is set in the context of the announcement of the kingdom and of Jesus' compassion for those who, because of their illness, are unable to live life to its fullest. Again and again, he is represented as reaching out to people at their points of need. Acts 10:38 states that witnesses can bear testimony to all that he did in the Jewish countryside and in Jerusalem: he went about doing good and healing all who were oppressed by the devil, "actively showing pity for the sick and those who by the standards of that time were held to be possessed by 'the demon' or by 'demons,' 'the prisoners' whom the eschatological prophet was to set free (Isa. 61:1-2)."[7] The commitment of Jesus on behalf of people in distress became the basis for the early church's emphasis on the preaching of the "glad tidings of Jesus Christ" (Mark 1:1). The Gospels report that the response of Jesus to those whose lives were disordered was one of tenderness and compassion. Nothing aroused his anger more spontaneously than unfeeling and uncaring legalists who saw not the distress of a person crippled in mind or body but an opportunity to moralize on the basis of some fine

5. T. W. Manson, *The Sayings of Jesus* (London: SCM Press, 1954), p. 273.

6. Edward Schillebeeckx, *Jesus: An Experiment in Christology* (New York: Crossroad Publishing Co., 1985), p. 184.

7. Ibid., p. 180.

point of the Torah (Mark 3:1-6; see also Matt. 23:23: "You pay tithes of mint and dill and cummin; but you have overlooked the weightier demands of the Law, justice, mercy, and good faith. . . . Blind guides! You strain off a midge, yet gulp down a camel!").

The intensity of Jesus' response to human suffering is illustrated in the story of the healing of a man with a crippled hand (Mark 3:1-6). The healing is necessary on the Sabbath, since in Hebrew thought not to heal the man would leave him nearer to death — for sickness is proximity to death.[8] That is, the struggle against sickness is a struggle to save the sufferer from the power of death and the threat it poses. Since sickness opposes the Creator God's saving power, it must be righted and the creation restored. Jesus is the Redeemer in whom the mercy of God is present. What is new in his ministry is that the beneficiaries of God's mercy are not the religious authorities and legal scholars but those considered outsiders: the poor, the disabled, the sick, and the bereaved. Jesus made himself accessible to those who needed him, ignoring conventional limitations and thus according proper recognition to those who were cast out of society for whatever reason. Consistently, he met people at their particular points of need and addressed those needs. Jesus is presented as a combatant, constantly opposing with his power those forces that kept people in subjugation. Whatever held people back from experiencing the fullness of the gospel must be confronted and its power to do so destroyed. Thus, the sick were healed, the disabled returned to full activity, and the oppressed freed.

When Jesus welcomed the sick and disabled with open arms, he presented a potent model to his followers. The manner in which churches and their members respond to people with AIDS is an indication of the degree of seriousness with which they follow the example of Jesus. A response of love and compassion — an open-arms response — is demanded of God's people. It is a mandate expressly given by Jesus, as, for example, in the parable of the Judgment (Matt. 25:31-46). Further, such a response is a sign of God's gracious love, not only to people with AIDS and to their loved ones but to the wider community. It announces for all to see and hear that the kingdom is being realized, that it is taking shape in the world. If AIDS, in fact, means that the sick person has fallen into death's realm of power, loving acceptance of people with AIDS announces that God's saving power takes the field against death's destructive power.

During a recent hospitalization, a young man who knew that his struggle with numerous infections occasioned by AIDS was reaching its inevitable end drew comfort from the knowledge that his membership in a local church had led to the development of a support group for AIDS patients in the congregation. During the final days of his struggle he was visited by members of the group. His family gathered to support him. He was distressed that his family, in particular, would remember him racked with pain and broken by disease. With a supreme effort, he spent some time with each family member, leaving each with a message of how important was their support and love and how strong his love was for them. The ministry of the religious community was one of the undergirding forces in the hospital room, both for the patient and for his family. It symbolized God's gracious and reconciling love. Such compassion is a first call upon God's people in the crisis created by the AIDS epidemic.

The "Problem of Suffering"

In marked contrast to the fact that Jesus was concerned to show compassion to the afflicted rather than to establish the causes of disease and disability, Western scholars have tended to be preoccupied with the latter concern, connecting their response to issues of morality. The church's response to sickness and disability has been influenced by both emphases, which have existed side by side in Western culture. The ministry of compassion, so integral to the ministry of Jesus, is manifested, for example, in the establishment of an infirmary in Rome as early as the late fourth century, a logical development of Christian charity. The commandment to love the neighbor (Matt. 19:19; 22:39; Mark 12:31-33) was not simply a piece of advice, it was a categorical imperative. Love for the neighbor can be manifested in a variety of ways, but spiritual concern must never take precedence over immediate material or physical help for those in need, as the Letter of James bluntly states: "Religion that is pure and undefiled before God and the Father is this: to visit orphans and widows in their affliction" (1:27, RSV).

The visitation, care, and comfort of the afflicted became an obligation incumbent upon all Christians and was repeatedly stressed in early Christian literature. This duty to attend the sick and the poor conferred on them a preferential position that has lasted until now. The example of Christ was followed in the mid-third century when, during an outbreak of plague, Christians ministered to plague victims. In a letter by Dionysius written in A.D. 263, he describes how "our brethren were unsparing in their exceeding love and brotherly kindness. They held fast to each other and visited the sick fearlessly and ministered to them continually, serving them in Christ. . . . And many who cared for the sick and gave strength to others died themselves . . . so that this form of death, through the great piety and strong faith it exhibited, seemed to lack nothing of martyrdom."[9] The com-

8. For a development of the concept that illness and affliction place the sick person "nearer to death," see Klaus Seybold and Ulrich B. Mueller, *Sickness and Healing* (Nashville: Abingdon Press, 1981). They state, "The sick person as such has fallen into death's realm of power, not only because sickness possibly brings death . . . but because sickness *eo ipso* belongs to death's domain" (p. 123).

9. *Nicene and Post-Nicene Fathers,* Series 2, Philip Schaff and Henry Wace, eds., vol. 1, *Eusebius* (Grand Rapids: Wm. B. Eerdmans Publishing Co., 1979), p. 307.

mitment to the outcast sick is evident in the nineteenth century, exemplified by Fr. Damien on the island of Molokai, and into the twentieth century, with Mother Teresa and countless nameless people for whom the needs of the sick and dying become a call to ministry.

Yet this often sacrificial gesture of compassionate response has been accompanied by efforts to explain the existence of pain and suffering in terms of retribution. For example, Calvin identified two purposes served by suffering caused by such events as pestilence, disease, poverty, or any other suffering in body or mind. First, suffering is punishment for high crimes and misdemeanors against God, a punishment justly deserved. Calvin prayed that God's chastisements — the affliction of disease or poverty, for example — would be effective for the reformation of the sufferer's life. In this sense, suffering has an expiatory force which imparts the assurance to the believer that guilt is thereby atoned, reflecting the Talmudic statement that the one who has suffered in this life is thereby assured of rewards in the life to come. Second, suffering is perceived to have an educational purpose. Calvin directed ordained pastors who visit those afflicted by disease or "other evils" to

> console them by the word of the Lord, showing them that all which they suffer and endure comes from the hand of God, and from his good providence, who sends nothing to believers except for their good and salvation. . . . Moreover, if he sees the sickness to be dangerous, he will give them consolation, which reaches farther, according as he sees them touched by their affliction; that is to say, if he sees them overwhelmed by the fear of death, he will show them that it is no cause for dismay to believers, who, having Jesus Christ for their guide and protector, will, by their affliction, be conducted to the life on which he has entered. By similar considerations he will remove the fear and terror which they may have of the judgment of God.[10]

This manner of presenting poverty and disease — and, in fact, misfortune generally — has endured into modern Western usage and remains a powerful influence on contemporary attitudes to disease and disability. During a morning TV news presentation late in 1986, the parents of a promising college athlete who had died during 1986 were interviewed. Asked what meaning they attached to their son's death, his mother responded that God had made their son an example to other youth "so that millions might live." The same attribution of suffering is evident in the tracts left in hospital waiting areas or placed on bedside tables that carry such messages as: *Sickness is an opportunity to mature inwardly; The Lord does not place burdens upon us that are more than we can bear; Affliction is God's test of our faith; We must pray for strength.*

It seems that either the experience of personal affliction or the awareness of suffering in another person inevitably drives humanity back to the question asked poignantly by the psalmists: Why do righteous people suffer? Attempts to answer that question seem endless. The Hebraic perception of God, which attributed all phenomena to a divine purpose, was carried over into early Christendom and remains a pervasive influence in much "folk religion." As the Renaissance paved the way ultimately for the enhancement of the sciences, however, larger and larger areas of human life were explained on the basis of a growing body of scientific data. Included in this explosion of knowledge was the matter of illness. A small group of British scientists was convened in the late 1950s to review the relationship between religion and science. The group recalled that in the Middle Ages people crowded into churches to seek deliverance from plagues, whereas twentieth-century societies dig drains and educate the public concerning matters of hygiene. Whereas primitive societies prayed for rain and abundant harvests, we invest resources in water conservation and teach third world countries the benefits of fertilizers and crop rotation. When humans were forced to account for phenomena they could not understand, the tendency was to fall back upon the age-old measure of attributing causality to some unfathomed divine purpose.

The problem arose, however, that as rational explanations emerged to account for more and more areas of human experience, the extent of experience ascribed to a purposive God began to shrink. Now that science can explain in intricate detail the manner in which viruses enter and affect the human body, and how the body's immune system defends itself against such attacks, it is tempting to divide human experience into two (or more) parts, granting science control over one while retaining the control of religion over the other. This is a mistake. To assert that some sort of hedge can be planted in the country of the mind to mark the boundary where a transfer of authority takes place is a twofold error. First, it presupposes an intolerable dichotomy of existence. Second, it invites "science" to discover new things and thence gradually take possession of that which "religion" once held.[11] Soon, God becomes no longer necessary because the gap between the explained and the unexplained is closed. If this image is applied to the science of medicine, any attempt to remove disease from the arena of medicine to that of religion assumes the same dichotomization, an untenable position. God does not reserve certain areas of life in which to dabble. In particular, AIDS was not "sent" on some divine intention to communicate a message; for example, to remind humans that God retains some areas in which to manifest initiative.

There is a second and more disturbing objection to the notion that the answer to suffering is to be found in some divine purpose. Dorothee Sölle put the issue forcefully when she objected to what she termed "theological

10. John Calvin, *Tracts and Treatises on the Doctrine and Worship of the Church,* vol. 2 (Grand Rapids: Wm. B. Eerdmans Publishing Co., 1958), p. 127.

11. Charles A. Coulson, *Science and Christian Belief* (Chapel Hill, N.C.: University of North Carolina Press, 1955), p. 19.

sadism." For her, "Christian masochism" had "so many features that merit criticism: the low value it places on human strength; its veneration of one who is neither good nor logical but only extremely powerful; its viewing of suffering exclusively from the perspective of endurance; and its consequent lack of sensitivity for the suffering of others." But what bothered Sölle was not the well-meaning attempts of onlookers to comfort a disabled person; such attempts may be genuine efforts to speak in comfort and compassion. Her greatest discomfort and anger arose because "the picture changes as soon as theologians, in a kind of overly rigorous application of the masochistic approach, sketch in as a companion piece a sadistic God." Her concern was that such a God who causes affliction and suffering is presented as one who demands the impossible and then tortures people.[12]

As this chapter was being written, a father sat for three weeks at the bedside of his dying twenty-eight-year-old son. He dealt with his grief out of images derived from the Middle Ages. He stated simply that what was happening was God's will, which he had no alternative but to accept. When the chaplain asked how he would feel if he were to discover that his son's imminent death was not "willed" by God but that instead God "grieved" over the death of one of God's children, he dismissed the image without consideration. The chaplain did not return to the theological issue; at that moment such a discussion was not appropriate. The father's conviction that his son's death was at God's behest was his only source of comfort. It might have been easier to accept his perception if his consolation had been deep and genuine. But it was as if he were engaged in a never-ending struggle to hold back the waters of bitterness behind a narrow dike, with his finger plunged into a fissure through which the waters seeped, constantly threatening to become a surge that would overwhelm him. Similarly, a hospital chaplain recounted a ten-year-old patient's struggle to come to terms with his diagnosis of AIDS. Who knows the source of the child's images? Had some well-meaning relative, friend, or pastor sought to comfort him by suggesting gently that God had "chosen" him? He sat up in bed and cried out, "Why did God choose me? I did not want to be chosen!"

These images of God are derived from perceptions of God's transcendence that leave little room for immanence such as manifested in the life of Jesus of Nazareth, who sat beside a woman alienated from her community, or who crouched in a dusty village street alongside another threatened woman. These biblical pictures contrast sharply with the image of a transcendent God, far removed from human concerns except to use them as teaching opportunities. It is right to criticize radically all attempts to reconcile God with misery or, worse, to represent God as sanctioning misery. Such a God, who uses affliction merely or primarily to reprove, correct, or educate, cannot be separated from the accusation of injustice. If God "comes to a sufferer only with pedagogical intent,"[13] then God seems deaf to the anguished protest of a ten-year-old child or any other person with AIDS, on whose behalf all must cry out for justice and compassion.

To attribute suffering to an all-powerful God who uses such power to inflict pain and misery upon humanity flies in the face of the incarnation of God's love in Jesus Christ. Such love is expressed in an active goodwill toward people, moved by a genuine sensitivity to their deepest needs. This type of love includes, but is not limited to, compassionate sympathy. Sympathy indeed has received a bad press, with the contemporary emphasis by social scientists on terms such as "empathy." Sympathy involves being present with a person — weeping with the sad, rejoicing when there is cause for celebration. It is comforting for one who is sick to know that he or she is not alone and that others care. "Empathy," on the other hand, is a construct that more fully expresses a human attempt to speak of God's love. The term involves a relationship between the helper and the afflicted person in which the helper knows, or can imagine, the depth of the pain and struggle the other is experiencing. It is a relationship that opens the possibility of change or, if that is not possible, assures the struggler that the helping person has the ability to enter into the feeling of helplessness or even despair and know what it means. If these images may be applied validly to God's love, they suggest that God is in touch with our pain, that God "feels" our anguish and is affected by it. This conception is in stark contrast to the Greek notion of divine impassibility that has permeated traditional theism, a notion that sharply restricts the biblical perception of divine love that is responsive to human suffering.

The idea that God's knowledge of the world is complete and unchanging implies that God has determined every aspect of the world, down to the last detail. Nothing can happen that is not immutably known. There is little provision for creaturely freedom in such a fixed system. Process theology, on the other hand, sees God's creative activity as based upon responsiveness to the world. Since the very meaning of actuality involves internal relatedness, God as an actuality is essentially related to the world. Since actuality as such is partially self-creative, future events are not determined. Even perfect knowledge, process theologians argue, cannot know the future. Thus, God does not wholly control the world. God's power, even creative power, is persuasive, not coercive.[14]

Process thought has three immediate consequences for this inquiry. First, it provides a theological basis for the assertion that God does not select specific diseases to punish certain human behaviors. If God's power is persuasive, not controlling, finite actualities can fail to con-

12. Dorothee Sölle, *Suffering* (Philadelphia: Fortress Press, 1975), p. 22.

13. Ibid., p. 26.

14. John B. Cobb, Jr., and David Ray Griffin, *Process Theology: An Introductory Exposition* (Philadelphia: Westminster Press, 1976), pp. 51-52.

form to the divine aims for them. Deviations from divine aims may give rise to evil. Since deviation is possible, though not necessary, evil is not necessary. It is the *possibility* of deviation that is necessary, and that makes the *possibility* of evil necessary. The risk in all this for humanity is that a new actuality may develop which introduces a novel element into creation. It may add to the variety of existence, and so to the value that can be enjoyed. But the new reality may be a strain of virus which leads not to enjoyment but to discord.[15] Human immunodeficiency virus (HIV) surely falls into this category. If the intention had been to exclude the possibility of all discord, God would simply have abstained from creating a world altogether, and so have guaranteed the absence of all suffering. Risk is part of the created order, a price paid for freedom, God's trump card. Thus, God does not "send" AIDS for some retributive purpose (such a thought flies in the face of the New Testament witness to a loving God). Rather, God "risked" creating a world in which HIV could develop.

The second consequence of process thought centers around the question of persuasiveness vs. control. It is on just this issue that conservative Christians oppose radically any stance to the left of their own positions. "Fundamentalist" and "liberal" Christians may fight over matters of ecclesiology and biblical and historical theology, but what is at stake is the political issue of management styles and measures of control and freedom. This battle has certainly invaded areas of ethics and theology in accounting for human suffering, but it also plays a key role in the form that pastoral care takes — for example, in shaping attitudes toward people with AIDS. Care and compassion can be offered to people in need without attempting to coerce them into adopting the caregiver's religious commitments. It is appropriate for ministries to reflect religious and moral values; it is not appropriate, however, to expect the other person to adopt those values as the *conditions* for the relationship and the care.[16]

Both the Hebrew scriptures and the New Testament characterize God as choosing to deal freely with humanity. God offers humanity choices. The question then is whether the choices made are trivially or morally evil or are genuine attempts at responsible living. This matter of choice is always unambiguous. It is the choice expressed by Joshua to the Israelites: "Hold the LORD in awe then, and worship him in loyalty and truth. Banish the gods whom your fathers worshipped beside the Euphrates and in Egypt, and worship the LORD. But if it does not please you to worship the LORD, choose here and now whom you will worship. . . . I and my family, we will serve the LORD" (Josh. 24:14-15). The choice is presented as sharply by Jesus to the rich young ruler: "Jesus said to him, 'If you wish to go the whole way, go, sell your possessions, and give to the poor . . . and come, follow me'" (Matt. 19:21).

The fact of freedom places the responsibility for decision and choice on the only one who can assume such responsibility, the person who must decide. The attempt to control the choices of others is a constant temptation for caregivers. One of the temptations is to reject a person who has made a decision with which one disagrees or, more pointedly, which is offensive to one's own moral judgment. It is also tempting to use the power implicit in the role of the caregiver to overwhelm the person who needs help and to make help contingent upon the adoption of an "acceptable" lifestyle.[17]

This raises the third consequence of process thought for this inquiry. It is logical to argue that if God's relationship with humanity is persuasive, that characteristic should be the model for our own interpersonal relationships. It should apply particularly to the role of caregiver. If persuasion, rather than control, is the divine mode of relation, this manner of doing things is expected of believers. These images of relationship — offer, freedom, and persuasion — are true to the gospel. The object of preaching the gospel is "full life" (John 10:10). That invitation is offered, but in large measure it is up to each of us how that full life will be appropriated. God's creative purpose for humanity is loving because God is always a completely *gracious* God. God's aim for people is existence that they experience as intrinsically good. But God is not in complete control. We are in part responsible for who we are and what we shall become. We are certainly responsible for the choices we make and for their consequences. The freedom God offers humanity is therefore risky, but it is a necessary risk if there is to be the chance for greatness. Thus the question as to whether God is indictable for evil reduces to the question of whether the positive values enjoyed by the higher forms of life and experience are worth the risk of the negative values; namely, the sufferings. Should humans, therefore, risk possible suffering in order to have at least the possibility of intense enjoyment? Process theologians Cobb and Griffin respond affirmatively, explaining that the divine reality is an Adventurer who not only enjoys humanity's experience of the pitch of enjoyment but who also experiences sufferings.[18] God knows what it is like to taste the bitter waters of our valleys of Marah (Ex. 15:23).

The desert plains across which lie our paths, as we press forward looking for Canaan, that land flowing with

15. The philosopher Alfred North Whitehead suggests that, to the extent that conformity to the divine aims is incomplete, there is evil in the world. New actualities or realities (such as AIDS) may lead not to enjoyment but to discord, a term Whitehead uses to refer to physical or mental suffering which is simply evil in itself, whenever it occurs. See Alfred North Whitehead, *Religion in the Making* (New York: Macmillan Co., 1926), p. 60, and *Adventures of Ideas* (New York: Macmillan Co., 1933), pp. 329-30, 342.

16. See James A. Wharton, "Theology and Ministry in the Hebrew Scriptures," in Earl E. Shelp and Ronald Sunderland, eds., *A Biblical Basis for Ministry* (Philadelphia: Westminster Press, 1981), pp. 62-69.

17. See Alan Keith-Lucas, *Giving and Taking Help* (Chapel Hill, N.C.: University of North Carolina Press, 1972), p. 9.

18. Cobb and Griffin, p. 74.

milk and honey, are broken by more than one valley of Marah. The ancient pilgrimage of the children of Israel remains a prototype for all. AIDS is but the latest tragedy to evoke from humanity the age-old question, "Why, Lord? Why me?"

It has been suggested that from the most primitive of ancient cultures to the more highly developed religious forms, humanity has always struggled with the tragedy of affliction, resolving the paradox of life pockmarked by suffering by attributing disease and disability to the gods' anger at human failure and sin. Primitive Hebrew thought incorporated this concept, and much of contemporary Christian "folk religion" reflects it. Yet the biblical response is one of affirmation. It does not answer the question, "Why me?" other than to remind us, through metaphor, that we are called to be children of our Father in heaven, who makes the sun rise on good and bad alike and sends the rain on the honest and dishonest (Matt. 5:45). We are assured that God makes those whom society denigrates God's people. It is salutary to remember that the first epistle of Peter was addressed to just such people: domestics, street sweepers, laborers, and Gentiles. The writer's joy is in seeing people who once were "no people" becoming "God's people." Those who had not previously received mercy were now recipients of God's mercy. Nobodies were receiving the dignity and the joy of being God's children. Is there any comfort for a patient in the theological notion that his or her God, who has rejoiced in human achievements and enjoyments, now shares in the pain and physical discomfort of his or her dying?

There is no formula for erasing the pain and anguish of people with AIDS and of their loved ones. Moreover, as sick and disabled people constantly remind those who just stand around, one who has not experienced catastrophic crisis cannot know the feelings it evokes in the sufferer. But in the face of such pain, the witness of scripture is plainly and simply stated: God is a God of unfathomable love who tends people like a shepherd tends the flock. The human analogy is of a loving parent who loves to the uttermost. This affirmation moves Paul to reassure his readers that nothing can separate people from the love of God revealed in the Christ. Not persecution, hunger, nakedness, peril, or sword; not illness, disability, or AIDS. But our thoughts are not God's thoughts; neither are our ways God's ways. We do not rise to Paul's level of maturity but continue to judge from our human point of view. We cannot say, with the apostle, that "worldly standards have ceased to count in our estimate of any man" (2 Cor. 5:16). So we continue to place people in categories, creating new groups of "the poor" from whom, because they do not fit our stereotypes, we distance ourselves.

64 Stories and Suffering

Margaret E. Mohrmann

Paying Attention

We should not read the Bible for lists or rules or for direct answers to most of our specific moral questions. Nevertheless, scripture is a unique and inescapable authority for Christian ethics, although not an absolute judge (only God is absolute).[1] Therefore, let us consider what can be found in our reading of scripture.

There is a long tradition in Christian thought, dating back to at least Augustine (in *De doctrina Christiana*, for example), that teaches us that understanding scripture requires that we come to it prepared to be changed by it.[2] From the standpoint of theological ethics, it is for that change, rather than for any rules or answers, that we go to scripture. Christian ethics, as Richard McCormick has written, is not norms and principles but transformation.[3]

> Do not be conformed to this world, but be transformed by the renewing of your mind, so that you may discern what is the will of God — what is good and acceptable and perfect. (Rom. 12:2)

The crux of biblically informed ethics is that the story of God's love for us is transformative. It has the power to shape us into the sorts of persons who want and are able to discern what is good, and who then can and will act morally. That story also has the power to shape the church into the sort of community that enables and encourages both the transformation and the empowered action of its members.

To what end is this transformation? There is only one encompassing purpose: to love God with all our being and to love our neighbors as ourselves. The scripture that transforms us comes to us as story, and thereby teaches us to see that our lives and the lives of those we love and serve are also stories and not random collections of disconnected episodes. The transforming story is one that

1. James M. Gustafson, introduction to *The Responsible Self,* by H. Richard Niebuhr (New York: Harper and Row, 1963), p. 22.

2. Charles M. Wood's *Formation of Christian Understanding* (Valley Forge, Pa.: Trinity Press, 1981) teaches much the same lesson as Augustine.

3. Richard A. McCormick, "Theology and Bioethics: Christian Foundations," in *Theology and Bioethics,* ed. E. Shelp (Dordrecht, Netherlands: D. Reidel Publishing Company, 1985).

From Margaret E. Mohrmann, M.D., *Medicine as Ministry* (Cleveland, Ohio: The Pilgrim Press, 1995), pp. 62-88. Edited slightly from the original. Used by permission.

both reveals and compels love. The narrative form of scripture and the agape command that is at the heart of the ethics of the Bible are inseparably intertwined. The story makes no sense without its meaning of love; the love it compels has no content without the narrative that shows us what love is and how love acts.

The metaphor of ever-expanding, ever-clearer vision has long been used in Christian thought to describe this process of transformation, the process of moral and spiritual growth toward the mind of Christ. The more our minds are renewed by the transforming power of God, the more clearly we can see: see what loving God and our neighbor means; see the injured person by the side of the road; see the Samaritan who comes with healing for us; see all the pain, all the suffering that perhaps we would rather not see; see both the infinitely precious object and the incalculably high cost of love. To be transformed is to live and love with open eyes.

In her powerful and painful book on suffering, Dorothee Sölle tells us that, just as freedom from pain is nothing but death, so freedom from suffering is only a blindness that fails to perceive suffering.[4] The truth we must hear, as ministers of medicine, is that we must first see the suffering if we are to help relieve it, and that we cannot see it without in some sense experiencing it. To be transformed, to love with open eyes, is to join in the suffering of the world, as Jesus did.

The story of Jesus' suffering is the basis for the belief that it was his very participation in our pain that makes our salvation possible. Likewise, it is our willingness to see, and thereby to partake of, the suffering of those we wish to serve that makes our service effective.

In love's service there is no substitute for seeing, recognizing, hearing (to use another metaphor) those who are suffering. To acknowledge a sufferer in all her anguish is to begin the process of restoring her to full personhood.[5] In Arthur Miller's play *Death of a Salesman,* Willy Loman's wife seems to understand the crucial role of recognition, for she pleads the case of her desperate husband this way: "He's a human being, and a terrible thing is happening to him. So attention must be paid. He's not to be allowed to fall into his grave like an old dog. Attention, attention must be finally paid to such a person."[6]

Paying attention to those who suffer — hearing their pain, seeing their damaged selves as damaged selves and not just as vehicles for interesting diagnoses — means, more than anything, listening to the stories they have to tell us. In 1985, Richard Baron wrote a thought-provoking essay in the *Annals of Internal Medicine* titled "I Can't Hear You While I'm Listening." He makes the essential point that we need to take human experience as seriously as we do anatomy and pathology.[7] To do this, we must hear what our patients have to tell us about their experiences.

The more than twenty years I have spent being a doctor have taught me two things that constitute, I believe, the heart of medical practice. One is the importance of the physician's silent presence with those whose lives she or he has changed forever by information and intervention, a presence that allows a true sharing of the burdens of knowledge and fear that pass between healer and sufferer. I shall say more about this silent presence in the final chapter [of *Medicine as Ministry*] when I speak of the importance of being with the patient through the suffering.

The other thing I have learned is how to take a history — or, rather, how to hear a story. I believe that much of what we teach medical students about taking medical histories from their patients is significantly flawed. We teach them, in effect, how not to listen, how not to hear the human experiences that have brought the patients to seek their help. We accomplish this by teaching the student to force the patient's experience into a prefabricated structure that sorts and separates information in ways foreign to the patient's story as it has been lived.

Anyone who teaches clinical medicine will have observed that hospitalized patients in medical centers often love the green third-year medical students assigned to them, and look upon them as their primary doctors during their hospital stay. I am sure there are many reasons for this phenomenon, but one in particular, I am convinced, is that the students have not yet "mastered" history taking as it is taught to them.

Students are given an enormous list of questions to ask and, usually, some method of selecting the appropriate questions for particular complaints. However, they cannot remember all the questions, and they get nervous, playing doctor for the first time. When they go in to take a history, they often end up just listening to the patient's flow of words, hoping that somehow the answers will appear by chance or that something in the monologue will jog from their memory some question to ask. They do not yet know enough to direct the story into the structured lines that they are taught to use. Consequently, their patients feel that they have finally been heard by someone.

If I were now teaching medical students about taking histories from patients, the first thing I would tell them is that all the lists of questions are to be used, but only to flesh out the story. The questions may clarify details, or stimulate further revelations, or recall a rambling storyteller to the main plot, but they are never a substitute for the story itself. There is much to be learned from the way patients tell their own tales of suffering: what they emphasize, the chronology as they have experienced it, the

4. Dorothee Sölle, *Suffering* (Philadelphia: Fortress Press, 1975), pp. 37-39.

5. Howard Brody, *Stories of Sickness* (New Haven, Conn.: Yale University Press, 1987), p. 125.

6. Arthur Miller, *Death of a Salesman,* in *The Portable Arthur Miller,* ed. Harold Clurman (New York: Viking Press, 1971), p. 50.

7. Richard J. Baron, "An Introduction to Medical Phenomenology: I Can't Hear You While I'm Listening," *Annals of Internal Medicine* 103 (1985): 606-11.

side events that sound unrelated to us but clearly are not to them, what they fear it all means. Only when we hear all of this can we dare to insert our own questions — about whether a certain symptom is also present, or whether the pain has this or that character — so that the answers fit into the patient's story. Otherwise, the answers create simply our own story: a description of a patient whom we have not heard, a human experience we have not touched.

Understanding illness is mostly a matter of getting the description right, and the description involves far more than just a diagnosis. Diagnosis is one of the extraordinary powers given to physicians, the power of naming. I know, however, that more often than not we get the name wrong, or at least dramatically incomplete. We often get the diagnosis right, but diagnostic labels primarily serve as shorthand tags that physicians find useful for encompassing a theory of pathophysiology and related treatment. A diagnosis is not always a helpful or meaningful label for the illness as experienced by the patient. The following examples illustrate this point.

In Flannery O'Connor's letters, she occasionally spoke of the lupus that was her constant companion and that eventually killed her at the age of thirty-nine. However, when she was very anemic, she did not speak of anemia — much less of bone marrow suppression — as her problem; she spoke of fatigue. When, only a month before her death, she referred to her illness, she did not mention circulating immune complexes, or even nephritis and renal failure. She said simply, "The wolf, I'm afraid, is inside tearing up the place."[8] Her experience was not systemic lupus erythematosus. It was, rather, her awareness of the chaotic, destructive, wolflike gnawing inside that she knew was gradually but inexorably disassembling, "tearing up" her self.

John Updike's story "From the Journal of a Leper" is told by a man who suffers from psoriasis. Although we have learned to laugh at the phrase "the heartbreak of psoriasis," how he describes the disease makes it clear that heartbreak may be a truer name for the illness than the term psoriasis, which he calls "a twisty Greek name it pains me to write." Here is his description.

> I am silvery, scaly. Puddles of flakes form wherever I rest my flesh. Each morning, I vacuum my bed. My torture is skin deep: there is no pain, not even itching; we lepers live a long time, and are ironically healthy in other respects. Lusty, though we are loathsome to love. Keensighted, though we hate to look upon ourselves. The name of the disease, spiritually speaking, is Humiliation.[9]

It is important to get diagnoses right: to recognize psoriasis and lupus, cancer and schizophrenia, AIDS and alcoholism. However, it is no less important to get the name of the illness right. It is no less important to recognize that for the sufferer the name of the disease, spiritually speaking, is humiliation or fear or malaise or endless pain or loneliness or despair or the end of a career or the end of a life. It is no less important to recognize that this is a human being to whom a terrible thing is happening and, whatever other name this terrible thing bears, its name is tragedy. There is nothing harder or less sentimental than Christian realism. Christian realism knows how to call a tragedy a tragedy, and not some other "twisty Greek name."

Tragedies come in all shapes and sizes, minor and major, but they all have three things in common: they are sad stories; they have flawed heroes; and they represent conflicts of good intentions or, more often, gatherings of evil possibilities.[10]

I have said enough about the importance of stories, and of recognizing our patients' lives and histories as stories; I shall not belabor the definition of tragedy as a story. However, I want to emphasize the adjective "sad." Being Christian does not spare us from the sorrow evoked by all that our open eyes see. On the contrary, the concentrated gaze of Christian realism allows us to experience true Christian sorrow[11] with and for those who suffer. This sorrow is not the sentimental, effortless tears we shed for distant starving children on the evening news. It is rather a deep, aching, compelling sorrow that breaks our hearts even while it motivates and empowers our resolve to understand and to love. It is a sorrow that binds us to those we serve as surely as Jesus' tears bound him to Lazarus, Martha, and Mary.

Our sorrow is for the flawed heroes of the sad story, the ones who suffer the action of the tale. "Flawed," in this context, has at least two meanings. Medically, it implies the defect of disease: the disintegration or unwholeness caused by the attack on self-identity that illness inflicts. In a Christian sense, it also implies the imperfection of sinfulness we all bear: sick and well alike, we are all flawed heroes in our own stories.

The word "hero" is at least as interesting. It seems somewhat out of place in the midst of discussion of sad stories and tragic suffering. However, I suggest that identifying sufferers as the heroes within their own stories is a healing move,[12] similar to the healing power evoked by recognition of the complex stories of our patients' lives.

A sometimes difficult corollary of seeing the patient as hero is that the physician is *not* the hero; this adjustment of perspective is probably salutary. We often hear and speak of the heroism of modern medicine, with the term invariably referring to "heroic" actions by members

8. Flannery O'Connor, *The Habit of Being*, ed. Sally Fitzgerald (New York: Random House, 1980), p. 591.

9. John Updike, "From the Journal of a Leper," in *Problems and Other Stories* (New York: Alfred A. Knopf, 1979), p. 181.

10. Hessel Bouma et al., *Christian Faith, Health, and Medical Practice* (Grand Rapids, Mich.: Eerdmans, 1989), pp. 124-32.

11. Arthur C. McGill, *Suffering: A Test of Theological Method* (Philadelphia: Westminster Press, 1968).

12. Rita Charon, "Doctor-Patient/Reader-Writer: Learning to Find the Text," *Soundings* 72 (1989): 147.

of the medical professions — the desperate fight to save a life with resuscitation techniques, the gallant flight of a transplant team to retrieve a life-saving organ, the dedicated twenty-four-hour efforts of intensive care nurses and doctors. All these people seem heroic; they certainly may be of critical importance to their patients. But they are not the true heroes in these stories.

To do one's job well and thoroughly is an excellent accomplishment, but it is not heroic. To bear the suffering that disease and its remedies bring can be heroic. As William May puts it, "the heavy burden of heroism in medicine falls not on the physician but on the patient and the patient's family."[13] The label of hero belongs only to those who bear the burden of the heroism.

Recognizing the patient as hero should make us think twice about imposing the burden of our own heroics on one who might not choose that particular form of courage. More important, it should add considerably to the reempowering of a person otherwise trapped in the impotence of illness. Such reempowering requires the patient's reintegration, the restoration of his wholeness. It begins with our enabling the patient to regain her voice by our paying attention to her and her story. The process continues with our unwavering recognition of who the hero truly is in this tragedy.

The perception of the true owner and protagonist of the story evokes a much richer sense of patient autonomy than most discussions of medical ethics allow. With our transformed, open eyes we can see the one who suffers as a person in all his wholeness — a person with self-creating relationships and with an intact and meaningful life story into which the present suffering can be incorporated and, therefore, comprehended.

Beyond any minimalist notion of respecting a patient's right to determine his or her own fate, we can now see this burdened hero as the only one who knows all the threads of the story well enough to weave them into the next panel of the tapestry. That panel's colors and textures and design can be congruent with all that has gone before only if the hero who lives within the tapestry, and those who have been allowed to share it, can direct the weaving. Somewhat less metaphorically, it has been said of the patient's autonomy that "the freedom we must honor is not the arbitrary freedom to will one thing one moment and another the next, but the freedom to establish an identity and to maintain integrity."[14]

I speak of "empowering" the patient, but this may have become too glib a catchword. It requires clarification if it is to fit into a specifically Christian ethical proposition. The power I speak of is the gleaming, grueling power that streams through these words of Paul to the Christians at Rome:

> We also boast in our sufferings, knowing that suffering produces endurance, and endurance produces character, and character produces hope, and hope does not disappoint us, because God's love has been poured into our hearts through the Holy Spirit that has been given to us. (Rom. 5:3-5).

"We also boast in our sufferings." This is not a frivolous notion of enjoyment, no masochistic reveling in pain. There is too much in scripture and theology to warn us against choosing suffering for its own sake. The solemn "joy" of suffering is only in knowing where it can lead: to endurance, to character, to hope, to the love of God.

"Suffering produces endurance." In the rolling Latin of the Vulgate, this statement is *tribulatio patientiam operatur,* which can also be translated "tribulation produces patience." To be a patient is to be one who is patient, one who endures. To be a patient is to be one who suffers not only in the sense of feeling pain but also in the sense of allowing the pain, of acknowledging and incorporating it as a true thing that is actually happening and that must be dealt with as such. The power of acknowledgment and incorporation — the power to exercise the freedom to establish an identity and to maintain integrity — is the power available to and essential for the suffering ones we wish to serve. It is the power that our recognition of their suffering can evoke and enhance.

It should be clear, then, that in speaking of patience, of endurance, I am not talking about a "stiff upper lip." I am not talking about a foolish, isolating, and fundamentally impotent refusal to admit the presence of pain and to seek its elimination. The stolid, stoical "patience on a monument" that denies its need for healing is not the Christian virtue of patience.

The first known moral essay in Christian history, written around the year 200 C.E. by Tertullian, was entitled *De patientia,* "On Patience." Tertullian makes the pivotal point that the Stoic ideal of patience is designed to result in resignation. In contrast, Christian endurance produces hope. The difference is crucial.

The Christian virtue of patience is the power that looks suffering square in the face, sees it for what it is, and then decides what is to be done about it. It is in this process of clear vision, open acknowledgment, and careful decision that endurance produces character, the sort of character that is full of the hope that neither suffering nor anything else in all creation will ever be able to separate us from the love of God (Rom. 9:35, 39).

Writing the Next Chapter

We who minister to the ill in the name of the faithful community are transformed by the Word of God to be persons who can see. We can now perceive the tragedy that befalls "the patient one" as a sad story centered around a flawed hero. Our perception helps empower in the sufferer a hopeful and virtuous endurance so that she or he also may look upon the tragedy with open eyes and

13. William F. May, *The Patient's Ordeal* (Bloomington: Indiana University Press, 1991), p. 3.

14. Bouma et al., *Christian Faith,* p. 15.

work with us to discern what is to be done, what is, in Paul's words, "good and acceptable and perfect."

It sounds as though we may finally have arrived at the point where we shall have to talk about more traditional medical ethics — about problem solving, about what is to be done. Maybe.

William May, in *The Patient's Ordeal,* makes a distinction, which he attributes to T. S. Eliot, between two sorts of problems. One type of problem raises the question "What are we going to do about it?"; the other asks, "How are we going to behave toward it?" May proposes that many, if not most, of the problems we seek to solve in responding to the suffering of our neighbors are those of the latter sort.[15] For example, if I am coping with the news of a disease likely to be fatal to me, there are things I must do: I must make decisions about therapy, get my affairs in order, and the like. However, these sorts of decisions surely take a back seat to, and in fact depend on, my response to the second question about how I shall behave toward this news. I must first ponder how I choose to conduct the rest of my life in the light of the new, self-shattering information. I must consider how to complete my life in a way that is congruent with who I am and congruent with the way I have lived my life thus far.

The metaphor that leads us to seek "solutions" to our problems may reveal more than we have realized about the intricate process of problem solving. In their book about the largely unnoticed prevalence of metaphorical language in our everyday speech, Lakoff and Johnson tell the story of a young man who was learning to speak English. When he encountered the phrase "the solution of a problem," he adopted with enthusiasm the chemical metaphor that no longer stands out for native speakers familiar with it.[16] His explanation of the image is worth considering as an alternative to the usual notion that to solve a problem is to eliminate it.

When the young man heard "the solution of a problem," he pictured a huge vat of solvent in which problems of various types are suspended. In order to get any particular problem into solution, it is necessary to alter the chemical nature of the solvent. The problem will then become dissolved and seem to disappear. However, if the solvent is altered again, perhaps to handle another problem, the first problem may precipitate; it may come out of solution and, once again, cloud its fluid environment.

Reclaiming the chemical basis of the metaphor of problem solving reminds us that the solution of a problem may at times depend not on its removal but on a change in its environment. "Solutions" may require alterations in the other aspects of one's life that now have to adjust to this new problem in order to fit it in, and thus solve it by assimilating it. It is also worth remembering that later adaptations to newer dilemmas may make old problems reappear, an experience likely to be familiar to most of us.

Some problems, like strep throat or a broken arm, can be eliminated sooner or later. In contrast, many others, like chronic arthritis, alcoholism, cancer, grief — indeed, virtually all the afflictions that entail the kinds of suffering that call for virtuous and hopeful endurance — can find their "solutions" only by being acknowledged and incorporated into the embracing whole of a lifetime's narrative. "Incorporate" is the Latin-based equivalent of the Anglo-Saxon word "embody." What some problems need is embodiment: they need to be given bodies that allow them to fit into the story, forms that are compatible with the story. The rich nuances of the forgotten metaphor embedded in the notion of problem solving can, therefore, lead us toward the adoption of a different metaphor to explain our task. I suggest that we can offer more to those we serve by consciously adopting the metaphor of *story,* so that we can see the process of healing as a process not of solving problems, but of giving narrative form to the events. It is the process of "writing the next chapter."

The stories of all our lives have always been under joint authorship. I may rightly consider myself to be the chief author of my own tale (although, at times, "editor" seems to be the better word, because my life typically happens to me while I am making other plans, and much of my task seems to be to correct the spelling and the punctuation). However, I am well aware that there has been no time when I have been the sole contributor to this work. Parents and siblings, school friends and teachers, children and colleagues, all the people we love and those to whom we commit ourselves — all these people participate in varying degrees in writing the chapters of our life stories. In addition, when a time of medical crisis arrives, the members of the healing community — the pastor and the physician, the comforter and the therapist — will also be part of the composition that solves the problem by continuing the narrative. Together with the family and friends who are old hands at this particular manuscript, they will help the flawed hero embody this newest sad episode within the story of his or her life.

There are several criteria for the writing of that next chapter. First, it has to be part of the hero's story and no one else's. It is undeniably true that our contributions to the stories of those we serve are themselves important parts of our own narratives. However, it is essential that we remember whose crises we are involved in and that we ensure that the paragraphs we add are crafted to fit those persons' tales and not our own.

Second, the next chapter has to make sense. It has to fit the story as it has unfolded to that point. There is no sense in trying to tack the last chapter of *Anna Karenina* onto the first half of *Gone with the Wind.* Scarlett would never have thrown herself in front of a train, even if there had been any railroad tracks left in Georgia, and there is no point in considering such an incongruous outcome.

15. May, *Patient's Ordeal,* pp. 3-4.

16. George Lakoff and Mark Johnson, *Metaphors We Live By* (Chicago: University of Chicago Press, 1980), pp. 143-44.

The meaning of the next chapter must include and somehow continue the themes that have defined the hero's life. This requirement may entail a strenuous examination of previous parts of the story in order for the significance of past activities to be understood, so that the content can be continued even if the activities themselves cannot, because of changes wrought by illness or injury. The process of ensuring continuity may call for an expansion or an altered comprehension of the meanings that animate the story, but such rethinking characterizes healing and growth in their most basic forms.

The work of finding new interpretations and new expressions for the essential meanings of one's life satisfies the third criterion of a good chapter: the new chapter should be able to lead the story on to the other chapters that are to follow. It must be not only continuous with what has gone before but also generative of what is to come: the re-formed, reintegrated life of a whole person.

Sometimes, when the next chapter is actually the final chapter in the story, it leads to the continuation of important threads of the hero's tale in the lives of those who have shared the story. Sometimes the succeeding chapters can be read only in the lives of those left behind to remember and to sustain the meaning of that memory.

The next chapter in the hero's story may be the last chapter, or it may be a chapter so shattering that finding strands of continuous meaning and creative hope seems scarcely possible. To acknowledge this is to recognize once again that the part of the story we are concerned with is indeed a tragedy. Beyond all poetic talk of the tragedy as a sad story about a flawed hero, the fact remains that tragedy is dark confusion and chaos swirling around a conflict of good intentions and, most painfully, a gathering of evil possibilities.

The conflict that characterizes tragedy is perhaps most evident in situations that ask for impossible decisions, situations that seem to need ethics consultants. A good example is the case of Debbie, . . . in which the good of preserving life comes into uncompromising conflict with the good of relieving suffering, and the evil of failing to respond to pain confronts head-on the evil of ending a life. However, the multiple evils and conflicting goods that create and intensify suffering appear long before that final decision point is reached. It is characteristic of the tragedy of human suffering that it is always a compound insult; the attack is always on more than one front.

Many authors have correctly described illness as an assault on the identity of the patient, or have explained it in terms of damage to the person's wholeness. Others have spoken of a fundamental internal division, a violent separation of the parts of the self that were created to live an integrated life. William May's way of putting it — which I find particularly applicable to an understanding of the communal nature of healing — is that our human identity is best understood in three dimensions: that of the body, our physical presence in the world; that of the community, our relations with each other; and that of the ultimate, our perception of transcendent reality, our connection to God.[17]

With this compound notion of identity, illness can be understood as a simultaneous assault at all three levels, physical, communal, and religious. One conclusion to be drawn from such a perspective is that, to be fully restorative, healing must attend to all three levels. Such an approach affirms the point made in the Introduction that healing involves all segments of the healing community — medical, lay, and clerical. Medicine is a ministry in which doctors are not the only ordinands.

I shall analyze briefly each of these dimensions of healing, and the response to each by the part of the community most closely related to it. However, I wish to make it clear from the start that such a pairing off of the three levels of suffering and the three categories of healers, while it may create neat rhetorical parallels, belies the actual interplay of real patients and real ministers. There is and there should be considerable overlap among these three areas; I do not want my assignment of apparently separate tasks to obscure the complexity of our interactions with those we serve.

Having made this disclaimer, I can say that the physical dimension of illness, which involves a disruption of the patient's unique embodied state in some fashion, is preeminently the domain of the medical professional. It is the obligation of the physician, nurse, or therapist to witness materially to the will of the community to relieve suffering and to reestablish the patient's physical participation in the world of sense, activity, and communication.

Specifically, much can be said about the primacy of the physician's obligation to relieve suffering: to do everything possible to alleviate the illness, to remove the impediment to health, to attend to the patient's physical well-being. One can find innumerable warrants for the doctor's task in scripture, especially in the healing work of Jesus. Although Jesus asked some interesting questions of his patients, he never suggested to them that they would be better off just bearing their pain. Jesus' consistent willingness to relieve physical suffering adds a necessary qualifier and counterbalance to any discussion of the glorious endurance that suffering can produce.

The sort of suffering of which Paul speaks in Romans, the "tribulation that produces patience," must satisfy at least two criteria in order to be productive of the endurance that strengthens character and engenders hope. First, the suffering must be unavoidable. This ineluctability can mean either that the suffering cannot be eliminated — the pain is intractable, the loss irretrievable, the prognosis undeniable — or that what is required for its elimination is unacceptable — a loss of consciousness, say, or a renunciation of deeply held principles.

Second, it must be possible for the suffering in question to produce those goods of endurance and character and hope. There is no point in talking about character building when the torture is so intense and shattering

17. May, *Patient's Ordeal*, pp. 9-12.

that there may be virtually no self left to be strengthened or to comprehend the idea of hope. Moreover, there is no point in talking about the productivity of suffering when the one who suffers has no discernible capacity to learn from the experience — a person in irreversible coma, for example, or perhaps a newborn infant. As William May writes, "suffering does not always ennoble."[18] It can crush rather than strengthen its bearer.

Therefore, while we recognize and understand the creative potential in suffering, we also know that we are not asked to bear unnecessary suffering. We know that there is some pain that cannot lead to more abundant life. Our Christian hope is built partly upon the assurance that God does not test us beyond our power to endure, but always provides means of escape (1 Cor. 10:13). Such avenues of escape are often under our control. We may not test God's children more rigorously than God would by blocking access to the escape routes God provides.

The suffering that a serious illness inflicts results not only from the assault on the person's physical well-being and sense of embodiment,[19] but also from the threat to that person's relations with those who comprise his or her community. For example, the physician may fully be able to relieve the devastating physical pain of a severe burn, but the psychic pain of permanent disfigurement and its inevitable alteration of relationships does not respond to analgesics. The damage done to a person's self-identification as part of a community can be healed only by the ministrations of that community.

Just as it is the doctor's task to witness to the will to relieve physical suffering and restore the patient's damaged embodiment, so it is the task of the community to witness to the will to sustain relationship with the injured one. In so doing, the community confirms the patient's continued identity as a whole and treasured member. By our refusal to allow suffering to separate the patient from us, we repeat the truth that nothing can separate us from the love of God. We also proclaim an essential fact about human existence, theologically understood: none of the negative aspects of life — sickness and crime and grief and meanness and pain — is absolute in this world. Their elimination is not required for us to be able to live a fully human existence.[20] What is required for a truly human life is not the absence of pain but the presence of others, the maintenance of living bonds with other human beings. It is these relations that are threatened during any self-assaulting illness. As part of their healing, those who suffer require from us assurance that our relationships with them endure.

Sickness is isolating; one of the pains that any serious illness inflicts is the pain of loneliness. The loneliness cannot be completely overcome, because illness is, ultimately, an intensely personal experience. However, the loneliness that accompanies suffering, though it may still be present, can be stripped of much of its ability to destroy if it is transformed into a sign of the patient's unique and central position within a community that focuses its healing love on him or her.

Flannery O'Connor wrote, "I have never been anywhere but sick. In a sense sickness is a place, more instructive than a long trip to Europe, and it's always a place where there's no company, where nobody can follow."[21] She would probably be quick to acknowledge that she wrote this in a letter to a close friend whose weekly correspondence and frequent visits were part of a network of relationships that kept O'Connor unshakable in her identity and capable of stunningly creative work through all her years of living in that lonely place called sickness. She would also be quick to remind us — and it is important that we not forget — that, despite that supportive network, she could still write this kind of statement and know it to be true.

The third dimension of illness is its assault on one's relation to God. This is the level of suffering to which ordained clergy especially are called to respond. Serious illness shatters our understanding of the way the world works by bringing into question God's power to protect us and even God's love for us.

I considered briefly the possibility of devoting part of this book [*Medicine as Ministry*] to questions of theodicy, to the problem we have in reconciling a belief in both God's goodness and God's omnipotence with the obvious presence of evil and suffering in the world. I have chosen, however, not to linger on theodicy, not only because there has already been much written on the subject, most of which focuses appropriately on our misunderstanding of power as an attribute of God, but also because I do not think that it is a particularly helpful emphasis for those who wish to minister to the suffering. None of us wants to be in the role of Job's comforters; we want to be real comforters, real healers. That task requires attention not to the fine points of theological doctrine but to the reality of the patient's experience of pain and to our certainty of God's love.

The theological witness needed to reestablish and reaffirm the patient's relationship to God is the witness of the cross and its double message that evil is real and God is good. It is a message that both validates the reality of the suffering and denies that the pain is absolute. Suffering is real (we cannot accept the stance of Christian Science); suffering may not always be explainable (we are not God, but creatures bound in time); but suffering is not the ultimate reality (we are not lost out here in the stars). And nothing can separate us from the love of God.

Suffering produces hope, "because God's love has been poured into our hearts through the Holy Spirit that has been given to us" (Rom. 5:5). It is, finally, that truth

18. Ibid., p. 50.

19. "Embodiment" here is not intended to signal the varied philosophical and experiential nuances that the term carries in, for example, feminist thought. In the context of this book, embodiment refers simply to the fact of human physicality, especially as it seizes our attention in situations of pain and disease.

20. Ibid., p. 153.

21. O'Connor, *Habit of Being*, p. 163.

— the truth of God's love in our hearts — that we bring to those who suffer when we treat their bodies, when we sustain our relationships with them, when we assure them that the pain working at them is being vanquished by the love working for them. From these overlapping responses to the several dimensions of illness we can enable in those we serve and in ourselves the transformation of vision that we need, not only to see the suffering itself, but also to see the meaning of the pain.

65 Patient Suffering and the Anointing of the Sick

M. Therese Lysaught

A physician, reflecting on the early days of his medical training, recounts a relationship with a patient suffering from a rare form of bone cancer. He recalls the following:

> In the hospital, it was the habit [of this patient] to roam the halls late at night after his wife and small children had gone to their lodging. I never asked him whether it was pain that kept him moving or perhaps loneliness and a simple desire for conversation. One night, having completed my work for the day, feeling too tired to read on my own, and facing no other prospect but to give in to sleep, I felt like talking.
>
> On that night, and on other nights following, we discussed nothing in particular. Our conversation might turn to his aspirations at work . . . or to my thoughts about medicine. For a time he would talk about his plans for the future as though they were still foremost in his mind, but before long he would lapse into the past tense and grow sullen. I think that a part of him was looking for encouragement, but what little I knew of his condition made medical reassurance nearly impossible. I hid from his pain by focusing on the bright side of things. It was a kind of dishonesty, though at that early point in my medical training I did not recognize it as such. What we had was better than silence, but we never really talked.
>
> One night, after I had been away for several days, I met him again in the semidark hallway near the nurses' station. He was asking a nurse to bring something to his room. . . . For some reason, she proceeded to introduce the two of us — a rare event by hospital standards. Equally strange, neither he nor I spoke up to say that we already knew one another. I put out my hand to shake his, and he started to do the same; then it hit me: his arm was missing. It had been amputated as part of his treatment. I should have anticipated the amputation . . . but it came as a surprise to me. In the instant before my hand withdrew and I looked down, at a loss for what to say or do, I caught in his eyes a look of sorrow, perhaps even shame. I begged his pardon, but we did not speak further. . . . We never met again. (Gunderman 15-16)

From M. Therese Lysaught, "Patient Suffering and the Anointing of the Sick," *The Cresset*, February 1992, pp. 15-21. Used by permission.

A week or so later, the patient dies, and the rapidity of the deterioration and the injustice of the illness creates a crisis for the physician. He feels that he has failed this patient, though not medically as this was not his patient. He senses that he has failed morally, although according to the principles and canons of biomedical ethics, he has done nothing 'wrong.' The physician is disturbed that nothing in his medical training or in his medical ethics prepared him, guided him, instructed him in how to attend to this man's pain and suffering.

As it did with this physician, suffering confronts us, compels us, and condemns us. It confronts us with shock that can upheave our unified, positive, progressive vision of our world, our lives, and our selves. It compels us to act — to alleviate it or to flee from it — in order to restore our sense of unity shattered by its eruption into our present. It condemns us — our fictions of unity, peace, and invulnerability, our factual self-centeredness and complicity in its creation and sustenance, our paralysis in its face and our evasion of responsibility.

Suffering similarly confronts theological theory, accusing it of being ephemeral and inadequate, assuming the role of a problematic, a contradiction, a paradox. It compels us to speak words that comfort and justify. It condemns all theorizing that posits a metastructure more important than the real and everyday or that posits a God who could cause or allow suffering, convicting it of complicity and generativity of conditions, of privileging an airtight image of God that we have created over the chaos of those who suffer.

Suffering similarly convicts biomedical ethical theory. In confronting biomedical ethics, the physical and social suffering of patients rarely finds itself addressed adequately. The reality of this suffering condemns a biomedical ethics that privileges the construction of clean and clear formulaic principles aimed primarily at facilitating the decision-making of medical practitioners and that allies itself with a theoretical structure which cannot account for the suffering of patients — a suffering which is the *raison d'être* for medicine and the locus for much of the moral significance of medicine. As for this physician, the sufferings of patients compel us to look beyond biomedical ethics.

This essay, then, undertakes three tasks. Part one offers a construction of some of the philosophical commitments of biomedical ethics, arguing that these prevent it from adequately conceptualizing two crucial characteristics of patients: (1) the fact that they are suffering and (2) religious/moral interpretations patients give to their own suffering. In order to highlight this problem, part two describes some of the dynamics of suffering as drawn from narratives of patients and phenomenological analyses of suffering. Finally, part three reflects on one way in which the Christian tradition has incorporated these dimensions of sickness and suffering into its corporate life, namely the Rite of the Anointing of the Sick.

Biomedical Ethics and Its Theoretical Alliances

Biomedical ethics failed this physician, failed to give him the conceptual or moral tools with which to act or to understand his lack of actions. It failed to convict his actions as wrong, although he profoundly knew that he had behaved badly. What do we mean by 'biomedical ethics' in this context, and why do they often fail to provide the necessary guidance or illumination?

Biomedical ethics might profitably be understood as a 'discourse' in the Foucauldian sense. Arthur Frank defines discourses as "cognitive mappings of the body's possibilities and limitations, which bodies experience as already there for their self understanding. . . . These mappings form the normative parameters of how the body can understand itself" (Frank 48). By situating themselves at the intersection of a number of discourses offered by societies, individuals formulate what Frank calls a 'code' by which we understand, and hence navigate, both the world and our identities. Biomedical ethics, then, insofar as it offers societal expectations of normative ideals of individual performance, might be understood to function in part as an agent of social regulation.

This might seem a strange categorization for those of us familiar with a biomedical ethic that speaks the language of principles, rights, autonomy, and decision-making. But the power of this description is evident in H. Tristram Englehardt's *Foundations of Bioethics.* Englehardt is the most articulate and forthright spokesperson for the majority position in biomedical ethics, namely 'pluralist biomedical ethics.'[1] Pluralist biomedical ethics see themselves as a "general attempt at secular ethics," derived from the "logic of pluralism," a logic which seeks to describe a neutral framework for the peaceable resolution of controversies (Englehardt 6, 11, 39).

To create this framework, pluralist biomedical ethics utilize normative anthropological and sociological dualisms that structure the liberal philosophy of pluralist society. The taken-for-granted dichotomies of mind/body, reason/desire, public/private, lead Englehardt to make some bold claims. First of all, he posits the moral landscape as bifurcated into "two tiers" mirroring traditional distinctions between public and private. These "two tiers" of the moral life he names the "peaceable secular community" and "particular moral communities" (54). The "peaceable secular community" functions as a conceptual space in which public disputes are resolved by 'rational' (i.e., impartial, unprejudiced, anonymous, universal) arguments made by rational beings "anywhere in the cosmos" who have transcended the boundaries of their particular communities (10, 81, 105); ethical reason-

1. I would assert the case for three approaches to biomedical ethics: (1) pluralist — represented by Engelhardt, and the work of Beauchamp and Childress in *Principles;* (2) an ethics of medicine — represented by Leon Kass, as well as Pellegrino and Thomasma in *A Philosophical Basis;* and (3) Roman Catholic biomedical ethics — represented by Richard A. McCormick, S. J., Lisa Sowle Cahill, and Charles E. Curran.

ing and moral judgments derive authority through correlations with procedures of this general standpoint and not from any particular content.

While the second tier, particular moral communities, is the locus of moral content and meaning, these communities rely on premises that, because of their particularity, "cannot be secured by [rational] argument," so that judgments of these communities cannot be validated as "rationally" authoritative (54). Particularities and affectivities, commitments nurtured within particular moral communities, which for our purposes means especially *religious* commitments and convictions, therefore, cannot be admitted as premises in rational moral arguments. While moral agents live their lives within particular, substantial, concrete communities, for moral purposes they must disembed themselves from these attachments if they wish to function in the public, moral domain.

Englehardt also provides criteria for membership in the "peaceable secular community," criteria that are necessary insofar as "not all humans are equal . . . [as he says] persons, not humans, are special" (104). The criteria, namely, rationality, self-consciousness, and a sense of worthiness of blame and praise, define a being as an autonomous moral agent. A body — a human body — does not qualify one to be a moral agent; correlatively, bodies are not theoretically required for moral agency. Bodies tend to be practical correlatives of moral agents, but they have no moral or rational value or content.

This distinction between 'persons' and 'humans' greatly simplifies the task of biomedical ethics. Englehardt argues that there are only two methods by which to resolve an ethical controversy: agreed-to-procedures or force. The autonomy of the members of the 'peaceable secular community' constrains society and other persons from using 'unconsented-to' force against them. But 'non-persons,' who can make no claim to autonomy, are not protected from such force.

Thus, a contradiction becomes apparent. On the one hand, a primary object of pluralist biomedical ethics is 'bodies,' and the task is to authorize legitimate use of force against bodies — for example, who decides what is to be done with a particular (now incompetent) body; when do we stop sustaining a body; when do we let newborn but malformed bodies expire; should we kill bodies; whose body will have access to health care? But this same human body does not count as a legitimate epistemological or even anthropological moral resource. Moral subjectivity is equated with rational mind, and 'knowledge' is available only of those things predicated as accessible to all minds; human embodiment, the locus of human illness and suffering and the site of the practice of medicine, are overlooked.[2]

2. It is important to emphasize here that I am distinguishing between medical ethics and medicine. Clearly medicine attends to bodies and the bodily in a significant manner, both conceptually and practically. My remarks are directed solely at medical ethics at this point.

The Sufferings of Patients

The patient's suffering and pain convict the physician of moral failing.[3] If biomedical ethics were to attend to the embodied sufferings of patients, what might they discover?

If nothing else, they would discover that the sufferings of the sick differ widely. This fact alone renders suffering inaccessible to biomedical ethics (see Smith 261). Not only are different kinds of sufferings associated with different kinds of illnesses — emergency traumatic injury vs. chronic illness vs. terminal illness that moves rapidly vs. a life-threatening condition that persists for twenty years vs. illness that has intense social stigmas — but each individual body will be inscribed differently by the intersection of the cultural discourses of class, race, gender, age, religion, science, and politics with the individual's personal history. The matrix comprised of these intersections of discourses, relationships, and histories provides our ongoing identity, the code by which each individual deciphers and negotiates the world. In instances of suffering, this 'code' is broken.

In spite of this irreducible particularity, phenomenological and autobiographical accounts of suffering note three consistent dynamics. In the first dynamic, experiences of illness or pain often re-situate patients *vis-à-vis* their bodies, re-ordering taken-for-granted relationships between "self" and "body." Experiences of illness serve as a reminder that "selves" depend on the integrity of bodies, that health and lives are radically contingent. In illness the body often moves from the background to the forefront of perception, and patients increasingly identify their selves with their bodies, a move which also unfortunately often encourages medical professionals to do the same. Some describe this aspect of patients' experiences as "essentially on ontological assault" in which the body becomes the enemy, interposing itself between "us and reality," standing "opposite the self" (Pellegrino/Thomasma 207-8), challenging a culturally instilled sense of the transcendence of self over body.

While this reorientation can be illuminating, more likely it can be alienating. Pain and illness can first effect alienation by counteracting "the human being's capacity to move out beyond the boundaries of his or her own body into the external, sharable world" (Scarry 13). Restrictive and dissociative, pain "chains down our thoughts," breaks connections between "body" and "world." In addition to impeding motion beyond personal boundaries, pain also alters the nature of these boundaries: "It is the intense pain that destroys a per-

3. On the other hand, I do not distinguish too clearly between the notions of 'suffering' and 'pain.' The distinction, which is commonly employed, relates suffering to one's self and identity, while pain is understood primarily in bodily terms. Although it is now rather standard to make this distinction, and the distinction can be helpful within certain arguments, I would resist making it too clear-cut, as I am concerned that it might buy into a mind/body dualism that will only exacerbate the problems I am trying to address.

son's self and world, a destruction experienced spatially as either the contraction of the universe down to the immediate vicinity of the body or as the body swelling to fill the entire universe" (Scarry 35). The body can become one's "world" as pain occupies more and more of one's consciousness and crowds out awareness of anything else. Alienation can also be effected by experiencing the body as the "enemy," the "agent of the agony."

Secondly, patients often experience a loss or usurpation of their "voice." Voice may literally be "lost" as a function of pain, or legitimate "voice" may be denied or repressed because it does not fit with normative medical or moral language. As Elaine Scarry notes, one characteristic of physical pain is that, for the most part, it is "inexpressible." While I can *tell you* of my pain, for example, there is no way for you to truly grasp its reality — either *that* it is real, or how real, how intense it is; your doubt of my pain cannot be decisively dispelled (4). This inexpressibility, this unsharability, can isolate patients from those close to them and prevent them from effectively communicating their distress to medical practitioners. Moreover, Scarry continues, "pain does not simply resist language, but [can] actively destroy it, bringing about an immediate reversion to a state anterior to language, to the sounds and cries a human being makes before language is learned" (Scarry 4). (An alternative suggestion is that these sounds actually *are* the language of pain.) It can achieve this effect because physical pain resists objectification. Undoubtedly, this characteristic of pain underlies medicine's tendency to identify patients with their bodies: this identification is a first step in trying to "objectify" the pain, to give it the referent, the object, that it lacks. As Arthur Frank notes, illness can also result in "the loss of capacity to express through the body" (Frank 85).

But in many ways, the medical establishment furthers the patient's experience of loss of voice. As many have noted, when it comes to medicine, the patient is a "stranger in a strange land" (Engelhardt 256); medicine is foreign country filled with unfamiliar languages and customs. Kleinman, for example, perceptively comments on how medical facilities seem designed to be navigated only by those who are familiar with them. Often, patients' lack of knowledge of the language of medicine can intimidate them, leaving them speechless. When patients do "find" their voice, they often speak of the "lived experience" of their illness in non-scientific and often subjective "common-sense ways accessible to all lay persons in their social group" (Kleinman 4). But, all too often, in order to participate in the medical cure, patients must conform themselves to the world of medicine rather than vice versa, learning its language; their accounts of their own illness are translated into the language of the profession.

Kleinman notes that practitioners "have been taught to regard with *suspicion* patients' illness narratives and causal beliefs" (17). Physicians often feel they have to sift out meaning from confused and messy narratives of patients, listening selectively "so that some aspects are carefully listened for and heard (sometimes when they are not spoken), while other things that are said — and even repeated — are literally not heard" (Kleinman 52, 16; Scarry 6-7). 'Subjective' experiences of patients' illnesses become 'objective' categorized diseases. Moreover, not only are patients' narratives at times suspect, but at times, as a result of the "inexpressibility" of their pain, patients' claims of illness or pain are doubted, if not explicitly denied, especially in the cases of chronically ill patients or in cases where the "explanatory framework" of medicine has not yet shifted to allow an illness into "reality." (Contemporary examples of this might include early sufferers of AIDS and chronic fatigue syndrome.) Alternatively, patients who reject a diagnosis of disease, or who do not conform to acceptable modes of dealing with a diagnosis, may be labelled as "in denial"; the physiological "interpretation" is given higher epistemic status than the patient's lived experiential interpretations. Patients, along with their voices, can be rendered inadequate, unhelpful, wrong, inactive, silenced.

But, just as a crucial characteristic of suffering is its ability to dissolve and destroy language, a first step toward dissolving and destroying suffering, then, is linguistic. As pain and suffering "resist objectification in language" and de-objectify the world, they can be overcome only by "forcing [them] into avenues of objectification," an objectification correlated with the body in which they reside (Scarry 5, 6, 17; see also Sölle 70-72). We find this same notion of "objectification" in descriptions of "work." Work, an inextricably social process, is the vehicle through which we "objectify" ourselves, a multi-directional process through which the "self" is constituted and through which the self constitutes the "world." Dorothee Soelle employs this concept to suggest that "working on" suffering is best understood as "transforming the act of suffering into purposeful activity. . . . nothing [she maintains] can be learned from suffering unless it is worked through" (126).

A fundamental shape that this work takes in the lives of the ill and suffering is that of creation of 'narratives.' As Kleinman notes, "the illness narrative is a story the patient tells, and significant others retell, to give coherence to the distinctive events and long-term course of the suffering" (49). Kleinman further affirms that not only does the story reflect the experience of illness, "but rather it contributes to the experience of symptoms and suffering" (49). Arthur Frank confirms this process, noting that "in illness, the body finds itself progressively unable to express itself in conventional codes. Sometimes, with the right kind of support, it creates a new code" (85).

It is noteworthy that Frank remarks, "with the right kind of support." The dynamics of suffering in illness all contribute to a sense of isolation and marginalization voiced by many who have been ill. Consequently, this process of narrative creation depends on the resources, options, and opportunities offered to the individual by the social situation. Often these prove insufficient. But importantly, those who initiate this narrative process need not be the victims of suffering themselves; in fact, often they cannot be. Thus Kleinman includes as a "core clinical task" what he calls "empathetic witnessing. That is the existential commitment to be with the sick person and to facilitate his or her building of an illness narrative that will make sense of and give value to the experience" (54; see also Scarry 6). This corporate dimension is indispensable in the dissolution of suffering, for the sufferer to move from the state of isolation caused by the destruction of her world, through expression and communication to solidarity through which change is possible. Thus, potential for deriving meaning from suffering lies not in some inherent quality suffering possesses, nor in the abilities of its victims. It lies rather in the resources offered by society and in the willingness of individuals to participate in this process, to enter into solidarity, to pay "attention" to those who suffer.

Suffering and Illness in a Liturgical Framework

Given the secular commitments of pluralist biomedical ethics described in section one, the Christian community might seem an unlikely place to turn to find resources to aid and inform our physician. But Christian tradition has, from its earliest beginnings, been significantly committed to attending those who suffer. This commitment has led to the development of practices which in their contemporary forms attend to many of the dynamics of suffering outlined above and thereby shape contemporary Christian relationships to suffering, both individual and communal. In this third section, I would like to focus on one practice in particular — liturgical rites of anointing and healing. For our purposes, I will draw on the Roman Catholic tradition's Sacrament of the Anointing of the Sick.

Before turning to the Rite, it is important to highlight the centrality of suffering and healing in Christian practice. Healing of the sick was one of three primary activities associated by the Evangelists with Jesus' ministry, inextricably linked with his preaching and teaching. John Dominic Crossan, in a recent article, attends to this fact and suggests that Jesus' particular bodily practices (i.e., eating and healing) embodied his message and had radical religiopolitical ramifications. Crossan locates his argument within the matrix of anthropological claims that correlate regulation of bodily boundaries with regulation of social boundaries. Drawing on Mary Douglas, Peter Farb, and George Armelagos, as well as Pierre Bourdieu and Caroline Walker Bynum, Crossan begins with the position that in Jesus' Jewish culture, who one ate with defined and identified one's location in the social matrix: "those decisions about what we eat, where we eat, when we eat, and above all, with whom we eat . . . form a miniature map of our social distinctions and hierarchies" (1195). It probably would have been rare, we can imagine, to find a Jew eating with a Samaritan or a Pharisee with a tax collector. Furthermore, bodies who were sick, menstruating or dead were denoted as ritually "unclean" and would have been categorized as those one ought not touch, let alone eat with. Thus, food customs and illness customs provided clear social divisions, with some designations excluding people entirely.

Within this matrix, Crossan argues, Jesus' proclamation of the advent of the Kingdom of God contained a radical social challenge. Crossan maintains that Jesus' practices and message championed a radically egalitarian "reciprocity of open eating and open healing" (Crossan 1195). Thus we find Jesus scandalizing onlookers by those he chooses to eat with (tax collectors and sinners, taking water from a Samaritan woman). Parables tell of the kinds of people he healed — lepers, the blind, the lame, a woman "with a flow of blood" — those understood within the culture to be blemished or unclean. And importantly, in these parables it is clear that Jesus often healed by touch, as Crossan notes:

> [Jesus] healed the illness by refusing to accept the official quarantine, by refusing to stay separate from the sick person, by touching him [or her], and thereby confronting others with a challenge and a choice. By so doing, of course, he was making extremely subversive claims about who defined the community, who patrolled its boundaries, who controlled its entries and exits, who, in other words, was in charge. (1197)

Crossan implies that these two practices — open eating and open healing — were identifiable marks of what he calls the "Jesus movement." Those who had been healed were enjoined only to carry the message, and those who carried the message were charged to carry with them no other provisions but to trust that message and miracle would open the homes and hearths of those they healed. These two practices are embodied in the contemporary Church in the Eucharist and in the practice of ministry to the sick. While this is not the place to argue for a stronger liturgical and ecclesial understanding of the constitutive nature of the latter practice, I would like to suggest that Christian liturgies of healing, at least as represented in the Roman Catholic Rite, are both responsive to the existential situation of those who suffer and continue to embody the meaning that Jesus' healing practices suggest.

As can be seen from the text of its Introduction, the *Rite of Anointing and Pastoral Care of the Sick* responds to a number of the dynamics of the sufferings of patients noted in part two above. First of all, the Rite is fundamentally liturgical, reconfigured from its earlier privatized forms in light of the Second Vatican Council call to liturgical renewal. Properly liturgical actions embody and intend the Church as a whole, and the Introduction to the Rite stresses this corporate dimension:

> Like the other sacraments, these too have a communal aspect, which should be brought out as much as possible when they are celebrated. . . . The faithful should clearly understand the meaning of the anointing of the sick so that these sacraments may nourish, strengthen,

and express faith. It is most important for the faithful in general, and above all for the sick, to be aided by participating in it, especially if it is to be carried out communally. ("Rite of Anointing" 191)

The communal context of the action emphasizes that, over against the social and cultural realities of isolation and marginalization that attend illness, the sick are not alone. The ecclesial community continues to understand them as included, and in fact, to be an integral part of the community: "If one member suffers in the body of Christ, which is the Church, all the members suffer with him" (I Corinthians 12:26) ("Rite of Anointing" 190). This bond is reinforced in the ritual actions of touch — the laying on of hands and the anointing.

In addition to communal support being integral to ameliorating the burdens of suffering, in part two Scarry, Kleinman, Sölle and others further suggested the importance of "working on" or "transforming the suffering into purposeful activity." The Rite of Anointing of the Sick as a liturgical act can be understood as 'work' in precisely this sense. On the one hand this dimension can be seen etymologically, as the Greek term 'leitourgia' is derived from the two terms 'laos' (people) and 'ergon' (work). 'Liturgy' is precisely 'work' done by all the people in the Body of Christ. Equally importantly, in the Rite, it is 'work' done by the sick person. The sick are not understood as passive and, in fact, are enjoined special duties and activities which give meaning to their suffering.

> The sick in return offer a sign to the community: In the celebration of the sacrament they give witness to their promises at baptism to die and be buried with Christ. They tell the community that in their present suffering they are prepared to fill up in their flesh what is lacking in Christ's sufferings for the salvation of the world. . . . And the sick are *believed* to be and seen as productive members of the community, contributing to the welfare of all by associating themselves freely with Christ's passion and death. . . . In the sacrament, the faith of the sick person gives us, the healthy, a sign — an embodiment — of the words of Paul to Timothy: 'You can depend on this: If we have died with him, we shall also live with him. If we hold out to the end, we shall also reign with him' (2 Tim. 2:12). (*Study Text,* 20-21.)
>
> The sick are challenged not to isolate themselves from the community, not to withdraw in embarrassment or fear. They are called to continue acting as a part of the body of Christ, called to forge ahead in the face of their difficulties, modelling discipleship and so serving as "ministers to the whole church in their illness" (*Study Text,* 41). In this way, "meaningless" suffering — of which suffering associated with illness is especially a case — is given a use, purpose, meaning.

Finally, we noted in part two that illness inflicts suffering partly by breaking apart a person's "code" — that set of discourses, relationships, and histories by which one understands and interprets one's world and identity. The Rite addresses this in two ways. On the one hand, most of those to whom this Rite reaches inhabit a 'code' derived partly from Christian formation and partly from secular culture. In instances of illness, especially in contemporary Western culture, part of the crisis of illness is created by presuppositions supplied by secular culture. For example, illness can pose a grave threat not only to psychological identity but also to physical security in a culture that values to the point of ideology the idea of individual autonomy. By preaching and living the gospel of a God who is essentially dependent and self-giving, the sacramental rite informs those who practice it with an alternative vision of the world.

On the other hand, as we noted above, Kleinman and others advocate that those involved with the sick encourage the creation of 'narratives.' While this is important, the Church, especially through the practice of the Rite of Anointing of the Sick, invites those who suffer to locate their narratives in an ongoing story, to learn anew the stories of others who have suffered and the interpretations they give their experiences, to truly hear — possibly for the first time — what it means to worship a God whose relationship to humanity was revealed on a cross.

Sacraments and Medical Ethics?

It might be objected that all this is well and good, but it doesn't really aid us in the difficult task of making day-to-day decisions about which technologies to use, and when, and for how long. But the power of the simple dynamic involved in these liturgical rites is easy to underestimate when compared to the power exercised by biomedical technologies and interventions. Like Jesus' practices of open eating and open healing, Christian understandings of suffering, illness, and healing embodied in the rites and liturgies of common worship challenge contemporary cultural understandings. The Church's 'discourses' challenge those of secular society. They refuse to locate a creature's value solely in its rationality, refusing to accept the designation 'enemy' for the realities of suffering and death, refusing to validate a posture that is closed to the world and fearful and ostracizing of those who are 'other.'

Those physicians and patients formed by ecclesial practices of Christian communities will find themselves navigating the world of medicine and biomedical ethics along a different path, for what they see as 'persons,' 'threats,' 'dilemmas,' and even 'the world' may differ significantly from their colleagues. For the physician whose story opened these reflections, the Sacrament of the Anointing of the Sick might have supplied him with alternative understandings of sufferings and a disposition toward openness and vulnerability that would have enabled him to reach out to the patient with a touch that healed. As importantly, it might have opened him to the touch of the patient that would have left him with the hopeful memory of shared community in addition to the empty sorrow of aloneness.

WORKS CITED

Beauchamp, Tom and James Childress. *Principles of Biomedical Ethics,* 2nd edition. New York: Oxford University Press, 1983.

Bourdieu, Pierre. *An Outline of a Theory of Practice.* New York: Cambridge University Press, 1977.

Bynum, Caroline Walker. *Holy Feast and Holy Fast: The Religious Significance of Food to Medieval Women.* Berkeley: The University of California Press, 1987.

Cahill, Lisa Sowle. "Can Theology Have a Role in 'Public' Bioethical Discourse?" *Hastings Center Report 20.4.* A Special Supplement, July/August: 1-14, 1990.

Campbell, Courtney. "Religion and Moral Meaning in Bioethics." *Hastings Center Report 20.4.* A Special Supplement, July/August: 4-10, 1990.

Cassell, Eric. "Recognizing Suffering." *Hastings Center Report 21,* May-June 1991: 24-31.

Crossan, John Dominic. "The Life of a Mediterranean Jewish Peasant." *The Christian Century* 108, December 18-25, 1991: 1194-1200.

Elshtain, Jean-Bethke. *Public Man, Private Woman.* Princeton, N.J.: Princeton University Press, 1981.

Engelhardt, H. Tristram, Jr. *The Foundation of Bioethics.* New York: Oxford, 1986.

Frank, Arthur. "For a Sociology of the Body: An Analytical Review," in *The Body,* Mike Featherstone, Mike Hepworth, and Bryan Turner, eds. London: Sage Publications, Ltd., 1991.

Finkelstein, Joanne L. "Biomedicine and Technocratic Power." *Hastings Center Report 20.4,* July/August: 13-16, 1990.

Gunderman, Richard B. "Medicine and the Question of Suffering." *Second Opinion* 14: 15-25, 1990.

1979. "Rite of Anointing and Pastoral Care of the Sick." *Instruction on the Revised Roman Rites.* London: Collins.

Heller, Agnes. *Everyday Life.* Trans. G. L. Campbell. New York: Routledge and Kegan Paul, 1984.

Kleinman, Arthur, M.D. *The Illness Narratives: Suffering, Healing and the Human Condition.* New York: Basic Books, Inc., 1988.

McGill, Arthur C. *Suffering: A Test of Theological Method.* Philadelphia, Pa.: Westminster Press, 1982.

Musser, Donald M., 1987. "On the Edge of Uncertainty: Twenty Years with Cancer." *Second Opinion* 5: 121-27, 1982.

National Council of Catholic Bishops. *Study Text 2: Pastoral Care of the Sick and Dying.* Washington, D.C.: Office of Publishing Services, United States Catholic Conference, 1984.

Pellegrino, Edmund and David Thomasma. *A Philosophical Basis of Medical Practice: Toward a Philosophy and Ethic of the Healing Profession.* New York: Oxford University Press, 1981.

Scarry, Elaine. *The Body in Pain: The Making and Unmaking of the World.* New York: Oxford University Press, 1984.

Smith, David H. "Suffering, Medicine and Christian Theology," in *On Moral Medicine: Theological Perspectives in Medical Ethics.* Stephen E. Lammers and Allen Verhey, eds. Grand Rapids: William B. Eerdmans Publishing Company, 1987.

Sölle, Dorothee. *Suffering.* Trans. Everett R. Kalin. Philadelphia: Fortress Press, 1975.

Springstead, Eric. *Simone Weil and the Suffering of Love.* Cambridge, Mass: Cowley Publications, 1986.

Turner, Bryan. *The Body and Society: Explorations in Social Theory.* Oxford: Basil Blackwell, 1984.

Weil, Simone. *Waiting on God.*

Wendell, Susan. "Toward a Feminist Theory of Disability." *Hypatia* 4.2 (Summer): 104-24, 1989.

Wind, James P. "What Can Religion Offer Bioethics?" *Hastings Center Report 20.4.* A Special Supplement, July/August: 18-20, 1990.

66 Practicing Patience: How Christians Should Be Sick

Stanley Hauerwas and Charles Pinches

1. The Terms of Our Professions

In our current setting there is something of a rush to call any and every line of work a profession. A number of interesting consequences have followed from this, including that the term "professional" has broken free of older ties in our language to the originating idea of a calling for a special service to the common good. This is not to say, however, that the term "professional" has lost its moral power. If anything it has gained more, albeit of a different kind. For there is now no more stinging charge against an aspiring inductee into any one of a legion of careers we call professions than that he or she has acted "unprofessionally."

What counts as unprofessional varies, of course, but in all cases it has some connection with how the professional has treated his "client." Indeed, it is this term that has seized the day, becoming a virtual pair with the ubiquitous "professional." Their intertwining is not, however, entirely complete, a fact that gives us our subject for this essay. For in the practice of medicine, even though some physicians may treat their patients as clients, or, worse, customers, they yet call them "patients." Indeed, as we shall attempt to show, the retention of "patients" in medicine and the continued practice of patience by patients is key to the good practice of medicine.

When we fix on the connection between patience and patients we cannot but feel some discomfort. It is an empirical fact that often patients are extremely impatient. As a society, nothing upsets us more than having to wait for our bodies. Indeed, our bodies are like our cars: they are to serve as we direct without calling attention to themselves (although we may use them to call attention to us). If they do call for our attention, we are quick to anger, with both our bodies and cars, and with those whose job it is to repair them. This impatience is of interest to us. At the least, and as we shall briefly try to show, it dooms the practice of medicine. More important, however, is the shape of the patience it lacks. Christians are called to be a patient people, in health and in sickness. Indeed, impatience is a crucial sin that carries us into other sins. The shape of Christian patience, then, will be our chief concern in this chapter, although we mean to describe it concretely as it relates to the practice of medicine. If Christians are faithful, they will be, we think, the most patient of patients. As such they will embody the skills necessary for the sustenance of the practice of medicine.

From Stanley Hauerwas and Charles Pinches, *Christians among the Virtues: Theological Conversations with Ancient and Modern Ethics* (Notre Dame: University of Notre Dame Press, 1997). Reprinted by permission.

2. The God That Failed: The Pathos of Medicine in Modernity

The title *The God That Failed* originally was used for a book of essays by former communists describing how they became communists and why and how they lost their faith in communism.[1] Arthur Koestler, one of the essayists, notes that communism, like all true faiths, "involves a revolt against the believer's social environment, and the projection into the futures of an ideal derived from the remote past. All utopias are fed from the sources of mythology; the social engineer's blueprints are merely revised editions of the ancient text."[2] For many today, medicine is to be viewed analogously. As they suggest, modern medicine is fueled by the utopian presumption that illness can be cured or tamed by skill and science. As such, medicine represents another utopia, another god that has failed.

According to its critics, as a failed god medicine is not the mode of liberation it professes to be but rather a legitimating ideology that allows some people to control others in the name of liberation. Moreover, like most effective forms of control, the power that medicine exercises is covert, since it stems from and is secured by its invisibility. As such, medicine is but another of the supervisory strategies so prevalent in modern political regimes.[3] Insofar as we desire what medicine teaches us to desire, we willingly shape our lives to become pliant medical subjects. The very understanding of our bodies, our "biology," produces and reproduces us to be good servants of the medical regime.[4]

1. *The God That Failed,* ed. with an introduction by Richard Crossman (New York: Harper and Row, 1963). The book was first published in 1949. It contains essays by Arthur Koestler, Ignazio Silone, Richard Wright, Andre Gide, Louis Fisher, and Stephen Spender.

2. Ibid., 16.

3. See Michel Foucault, *The Birth of the Clinic* (New York: Vintage Books, 1973).

4. For a wonderful set of essays that question the understanding of the body prevalent in modern medicine, see Paul Komersaroff, ed., *Troubled Bodies: Critical Perspective on Postmodernism, Medical Ethics, and the Body* (Durham, NC: Duke University Press, 1995). In his introduction Komersaroff observes, "The infiltration of the categories of medicine into the way we think about pregnancy and childbirth, the menopause, sexual relationships and caring for a sick relative, for example — or, for that matter, merely eating, exercising or just lying in the sun — may profoundly transform the quality of these experiences. In these cases, medical modes of thought introduce into previously unproblematic life experiences evaluative criteria that are formulated in purposive-rational terms. That is, they are presented as purely technical values" (3).

As for the rise of medical ethics in the past twenty-five years, say the critics, it is but icing on the ideological cake. Just as princes once surrounded themselves with priests whose function it was to legitimate their power to rule, so physicians now employ "ethicists" for structurally similar purposes. A strange creature that only modernity could produce, the "ethicist" may imagine himself to be the patient's advocate against the power of the physician when he champions — as he is doing with increasing frequency — the "autonomy" of the patient. Ironically, however, the stress on autonomy turns out to produce just the kind of ahistorical account of moral agency that so effectively disguises medicine's power over us. Indeed, it is the job of the "ethicist" to devise rules and guidelines that, while ostensively helping us to resolve hard decisions about life and death, in the end convince us that our lives are nothing without such "decisions."[5]

One device we have found effective in teaching students something of the power the church once held over people's lives is to ask them to reflect on how it feels to experience the amazingly technical, administrative, and bureaucratic complexity of a major medical center. Those of us unfortunate enough to have found ourselves patients in such centers recognize deep feelings of powerlessness in the fact of such a faceless giant, feelings that more often than not are followed by an overwhelming sense that we must please those "caring" for us or else they will hurt us. Indeed, the hierarchical politics of such medical centers are enough to make the description "Byzantine" inadequate. Medicine, in fact, has become more powerful and pervasive in our lives than the church ever was and surely far more powerful than it is today. This may explain why the current attack against medicine appears ready to exceed the furor of the revolt against the church. It is perhaps the only sort of revolt that makes sense in modernity now that the church is far too weak as an institution to make revolt against it worthwhile.

Despite our deep sympathies with the shape of this revolt against medicine, however, we cannot entirely credit its story. Those currently in revolt against medicine in our society overestimate the intensity of public antipathy toward medicine and its servant, medical ethics. In fact, the revolt has had to this point very little effect, since the questions it has raised can easily be dismissed as extreme moralistic nonsense.

That the revolt is so effortlessly deflated, absorbed, or repudiated may be, as the rebels allege, another sign of medicine's iron grip on our minds. We think, however, that it is a sign of the insufficiency of the moral resources the rebels have brought to bear on medicine as an institution. Modern medicine is not quite a god that failed. It is, rather, a failed substitute for God when God was failed by us. For *modern* medicine was formed by a modern culture that forced upon medicine the impossible role of bandaging the wounds of societies that are built upon the premise that God does not matter.[6] Such social orders,

5. For an extraordinary account of how "ethics" has served to legitimate the presumptions of modern medicine, see Gerald McKenny, *To Relieve the Human Condition: Bioethic and the Technological Utopianism of Modern Medicine* (Albany: State University of New York Press, 1996). McKenny observes, "A moral discourse which related the health of the body as well as its mortality and its susceptibility to illness and suffering to broader conceptions of a morally worthy life was succeeded by a moral discourse characterized by efforts to eliminate suffering and expand human choice and thereby overcome the human subjections to natural necessity or fate. The result is that standard bioethics moves within the orbit of the technological utopianism of what I call the Baconian project, and its agenda and content are designed to resolve certain issues and problems that arise within that project." McKenny identifies the "Baconian project" with the attempt to eliminate suffering and to expand the realm of human choice through technology.

6. Colin Gunton is to be commended for his attempt to read modernity in this fashion. See his *The One, the Three, and the Many: God, Creation, and the Culture of Modernity* (Cambridge, England: Cambridge University Press, 1993). We are sympathetic to Gunton's account, though we may have a different reading of who have been and currently are friends and enemies. John Milbank's *Theology and Social Theory,* which we have drawn on extensively in "The Renewal of Virtue and the Peace of Christ" (1997) in [*Christians among the Virtues*], provides an important contrast to Gunton. Gunton suggests that Milbank is insufficiently trinitarian and, as a result, fails to see that "modernity" did not begin with nominalism and the Reformation but is rooted earlier (p. 55).

We lack the learning to enter into such debates, but it is clear to us that the hard problem with which both Gunton and Milbank are struggling is how to narrate the "secular" theologically. Secular modes of discourse are now so powerful that theological claims no longer seem to do any work; thus we fail to supply what MacIntyre says we must, that is, a *theological* critique of secular culture and morality.

Few have accomplished this task better than Cardinal John Henry Newman. According to Robert Pattison, Newman regarded what most people take as the character of liberalism — that is, a movement for individual rights, free markets, and material progress — as only the trappings of liberalism. For Newman, liberalism's political program was but a symptom of the heretical belief that shaped its basic principles. Liberalism was only a modern version of the Socinianism of the Reformation and that was but a version of the Arian heresy of the fourth century. According to Newman, what offended the Arians about Nicaea and Constantinople was not that the church declared the Son to be "the same in nature" as the Father, but that anything at all was declared about God. The Arians denied our knowledge of God in Christ and as a result became the first liberals.

In the face of the limits of language and our inability to express the truth fully within its parameters, truth must finally be constructed as a contest of wills. Pattison, a liberal, admires Newman because "he was the last good mind in which the dogmatic principle still excited all the ideological excitement of seventeenth-century controversy. As a result, he denominated ancient theological errors and modern social theories indifferently by the interchangeable names Arianism, Socinianism, Hoadlyism, and liberalism. Newman is the missing link between the belief of the old world and the ideology of the new. As he seemed absurd to his brother, so must he to us; his absurdity is inseparable from his message, which is that those things that the worldly mind of the modern era considers ridiculous — namely the orthodox assertion that belief has a real object, that truth is abiding, and that words can dogmatically state truth — are in fact sublime realities" (Pattison, *The Great Dissent: John Henry Newman and the Liberal Heresy* [Oxford: Oxford University Press, 1991], p. 143).

which we rightly call liberal, take as their central problem how to secure cooperation among self-interested individuals who have nothing in common other than their desire to survive. Cooperation is secured by bargains being struck that will presumably secure the best outcomes possible for each individual.[7]

"Liberalism" names those societies wherein it is presupposed that the only thing people have in common is their fear of death, despite that fact that they share no common understanding of death. So liberalism is that cluster of theories about society that are based on the presumption that we must finally each die alone. Our fear of such a death becomes the resource for cooperation as we conspire to create social practices that embody the presumption that holds so many moderns in its grip, namely, that there is nothing quite important enough in our lives to risk dying for.[8] Yet, at the same time, we all know we must die. Even more telling, we know that the way we die is the result of the very forms of cooperation (often taking the form of competition) that are created to hide our own deaths from ourselves and from one another. In such social orders, medicine becomes an insurance policy to give us a sense that none of us will have to come to terms with the reality of our death.

Nowhere is this better seen than in the abandonment of the traditional medical imperative "Do no harm" in its correlating form: "When in doubt do not act." If there is a cardinal rule now in medicine, it is that in any and every state of uncertainty, physicians must nonetheless find something to do. If a physician does not act, her patient will quickly either lose hope in medicine, or, more likely, come to believe her incompetent. Moreover, the imperative to act has driven medical research to discover ever newer and more fantastic modes of intervention, which, while temporarily increasing confidence in a medicine of technological miracles, may in the long run undercut it more deeply. For the risk of error is all the greater and the fall to death all the more jolting since the technological miracles have schooled us in the false hope that death might be avoided altogether. To avoid error, physicians have become increasingly specialized, hoping that by knowing more and more about less and less they will be prone to fewer mistakes, a strategy that ironically results in more mistakes, since, as a matter of fact, the patient happens to be more than the sum of his parts. Unfortunately, he is increasingly cared for by a medicine that is something less than the sum of its specializations.

To position ourselves clearly, we are not distant from the rebels against modern medicine in our diagnosis of its problems. Where we differ profoundly, however, is in the ascription of blame to the institution of medicine for our present state of ill health. No one can or should be blamed. The simple fact is that we are getting precisely the kind of medicine we deserve. Modern medicine exemplifies a secular social order shaped by mechanistic economic and political arrangements, arrangements that are in turn shaped by the metaphysical presumption that our existence has no purpose other than what we arbitrarily create.

In such a world it makes perfect sense to call physicians "health professionals" and patients "clients." Nevertheless, modern medicine has stuck with the anachronisms — which we think demonstrates the true pathos of medicine. For in fact the practice of medicine was formed under a quite different set of presumptions than those now so widely held. This is why at least some physicians still presume that they are to care for a patient even though they cannot cure, or even alleviate to any significant extent, the patient's malady.[9] This kind of behavior makes little sense if physicians are there for the sole purpose of repairing our bodies when they don't serve us as we like. Medical care, moreover, is still governed by the presumption that patients are to be cared for in a manner independent of and preceding all other considerations concerning their worth to wider society.

This pathos — whereby physicians and patients yet engage in practices that are unintelligible within our predominant modern self-descriptions — is one of the reasons that medicine has seemed such a fertile ground for theological reflection. At the least, some of the practices of medicine continue to form a space where theological claims retain a semblance of intelligibility and persuasiveness. Ironically, however, theologians, propelled by the worry of their increasing irrelevancy to the newer trends

7. Obviously the account of such bargains varies from Hobbes to Locke to Rousseau, and in our own day, to Rawls and Nozick. Such differences matter, but we are concerned with how to articulate how medicine works in social orders so conceived. The current enthusiasm for rational choice methodologies in the social sciences is a wonderful confirmation of bargaining as the central metaphor for social organization today. For a good critique of the inability of rational choice methods to deliver what they promise, at least in political science, see Donald P. Green and Ian Shapiro, *The Pathologies of Rational Choice Theory: A Critique of Applications in Political Science* (New Haven: Yale University Press, 1994).

8. This paragraph is a slight rewording of a footnote from Hauerwas's *Naming the Silences: God, Medicine, and Suffering,* p. 123. I (Hauerwas) think it the heart of the argument of that book, though few have recognized the importance I attribute to this point. That is, of course, not the fault of my readers, since I was in truth trying to disguise the main argument of that book. *Naming the Silences* is allegedly a book about the suffering and death of children, and I hope it is at least that. But I also wanted to make the case that medicine has become the theodical project of modernity, part of whose task is to save liberalism. That is why I claimed that the book was really an exercise in political theory. We are here simply trying to articulate in a straightforward fashion what I attempted to do indirectly in that book. *Naming the Silences* has recently been reprinted by Eerdmans under the title *God, Medicine, and Suffering.* Eerdmans thought my original title was hurting the sales of the book. So much for being subtle.

9. We are acutely aware that this puts the issue too simply, since part of the power of modern medicine is constituted by its ability to name the "illnesses" that then become subject to medical intervention. For a more extended (but hardly exhaustive) discussion of these issues, see Hauerwas's *Suffering Presence: Theological Reflections on Medicine, the Mentally Handicapped, and the Church* (Notre Dame: University of Notre Dame Press, 1986).

in medicine and elsewhere, have been quick to shed their theological garments and join the ranks of the philosophical ethicists.[10] In this rush next to nothing has been said about the peculiar fact that medicine still calls its patients "patients." But what could it mean to be called "patient" given the impatience that so imbues the modern practice of medicine and the social order it serves?

3. The Christian Virtue of Patience

The recent retrieval of the virtues in modern ethics has even more recently begun to affect thinking in medical ethics.[11] However, it is not clear that medicine provides the kind of soil in which the virtues can take firm root. For while medicine usually gives us birth and surrounds us as we die, it does not form or mold us in the time in between. Indeed, when we meet medicine full in the face it comes to us as we or those we love are sick or dying. If, therefore, medicine attempts to form us into virtuous people on its own turf it will inevitably fail, for it will be too little too late. Indeed, if the first time we are called on to exercise patience is as patients, we will surely be unable, for there is no worse time to learn patience than when one is sick. So, if we are to understand the vital importance of patience as a virtue, we cannot begin by considering it in the context of medicine. For us, this will mean that before we can say much about being patient patients we will need to take the time to look at how and why patience is integral to the Christian life.

As a strategy this has its liabilities. For if the virtues in general have been ignored in modern Christian ethics, the virtue of patience has especially been ignored.[12] Happily, however, patience played a prominent role in much earlier Christian accounts of the moral life. It is to these we now turn for needed help in considering the shape of Christian patience.

Saint Cyprian begins his "On the Good of Patience" by observing that philosophers also claim to pursue the virtue of patience, but "their patience is as false as is their wisdom." How can anyone be either wise or patient unless he knows the wisdom and patience of God? In contrast, Christians "are philosophers not in words but in deeds; we exhibit our wisdom not by our dress, but by truth; we know virtues by their practice rather than through boasting of them; we do not speak great things but we live them. Therefore, as servants and worshipers of God, let us show by spiritual homage the patience that we learn from heavenly teachings. For that virtue we have in common with God. In Him patience has its beginning, and from Him as its source it takes its splendor and dignity. The origin and greatness of patience proceed from God its Author. The quality that is dear to God ought to be loved by man."[13]

10. In an article in a special issue of the *Journal of Medicine and Philosophy* on theology and medicine edited by Hauerwas and James Gustafson, Alasdair MacIntyre issues the following challenge: "What we ought to expect from contemporary theologians in the area of medical ethics: First — and without this everything else is uninteresting — we ought to expect a clear statement of what difference it makes to be a Jew or a Christian or a Moslem, rather than a secular thinker, in morality generally. Second . . . we need to hear a theological critique of secular morality and culture. Third, we want to be told what bearing what has been said under the two headings has on the specific problems which arise for modern medicine" ("Theology, Ethics, and the Ethics of Medicine and Health Care: Comments on Papers by Novak, Mouw, Roach, Cahill, and Hartt," *Journal of Medicine and Philosophy* 4 [1979]: 435). That challenge was issued in 1979. Subsequent developments have made it clear that that issue did little to convince anyone that theology had or has anything distinctively important to say about these matters. MacIntyre challenges theologians to accent their differences, but in this time called modernity most theologians have attempted to downplay them. Their task has been to suggest that Christians believe pretty much what anyone would believe on reflection. For example, the call for theology to be a "public" discourse seems carried by the urge to show that theological convictions do in fact measure up to standards of truthfulness generally recognized in liberal democratic societies. Only if theology meets these standards can Christians enter into the public arena without apology. (For a succinct chronicle of these developments as well as some interesting comments about the rise of recent promising dissent, see Scott Giles and Jeffrey Greenmen, "Recent Work on Religion and Bioethics: A Review Article," *Biolaw: A Legal and Ethical Reporter on Medicine, Health Care, and Bioengineering* 2, nos. 7-8 [July-August 1994]: 151-60.)

11. See, for example, *Virtue and Medicine: Explorations in the Character of Medicine,* ed. Earl E. Shelp (Dordrecht: D. Reidel, 1985). Karen Lebacqz's essay, "The Virtuous Patient" (275-88), is particularly relevant for what we are trying to do here. Lebacqz argues that three virtues — fortitude, prudence, and hope — are central to the task of being a patient. Our only difficulty with her account is knowing from whence such virtues come. William May has also developed the importance of the virtues in "The Virtues in a Professional Setting," in *Medicine and Moral Reasoning,* ed. K. W. M. Tulford, Grant Gillet, and Janet Martin Soskice (Cambridge, England: Cambridge University Press, 1994), 75-90. For an overview of recent work in medical ethics on the importance of virtue, see Hauerwas's "Virtue and Character" in *Encyclopedia of Bioethics,* rev. ed. Warren Thomas Reich, editor in chief (New York: Macmillan, 1995), 5:2525-532.

12. Typically out of step with his contemporaries, over twenty years ago John Howard Yoder observed that apparent complicity with evil, which the nonresistant stance allegedly involves, has always been a stumbling block to nonpacifists. In response, Yoder points out that "this attitude, leaving evil to be evil, leaving the sinner free to separate himself from God and sin against man, is part of the nature of *agape* itself, as revealed already in creation. If the cutting phrase of Peguy, *'complice, c'est pire que coupable,'* were true, then God Himself must needs be the guilty one for making man free and again for letting his innocent Son be killed. The modern tendency to equate involvement with guilt should have to apply *par excellence,* if it were valid at all, to the implication of the all-powerful God in the sin of His creatures. God's love for men begins right at the point where he permits sin against Himself and against man, without crushing the rebel under his own rebellion. The word for this is divine *patience,* not complicity." *The Original Revolution* (Scottdale, PA: Herald Press, 1971), pp. 64-65. Drawing on Yoder, Hauerwas argued in [*The Peaceable Kingdom*] that hope and patience are central Christian virtues. See especially pp. 102-6.

13. Cyprian, *De Bono Patientia: A Translation with an Introduction and Commentary,* by Sister M. George Edward Conway,

According to Cyprian, God's patience is clearly shown by the way he endures profane temples, replete with earthly images and idolatrous rites meant to insult God's majesty and honor. Yet nowhere is God's patience more clearly exemplified than in the life of Christ. Tertullian likewise observes that the patience of God made it possible for him to be conceived in a mother's womb, await a time for birth, gradually grow up, and even when grown be less than eager to receive recognition, having himself baptized by his own servant. Throughout his ministry he cared for the ungrateful and even refrained from pointing out the betrayer who was part of his own company. "Moreover, while He is being betrayed, while He is being led up 'as a sheep for a victim' (for 'so He no more opens His mouth than a lamb under the power of the shearer'), He to whom, had He willed it, legions of angels would at one word have presented themselves from the heavens, approved not the avenging sword of even one disciple."[14]

Tertullian and Cyprian alike make much of Matthew 5:43-48, where the refusal to return evil for evil is highlighted as in the very character of God, and, through imitation, the way the sons and daughters of God are made perfect. As Tertullian says, "In this principal precept the universal discipline of patience is succinctly comprised, since evil-doing is not conceded even when it is deserved."[15] Such patience is not only in the mind, according to Tertullian, but in the body, for "just as Christ exhibited it in his body, so do we. By the affliction of the flesh, a victim is able to appease the Lord by means of the sacrifice of humiliation. By making a libation to the Lord of sordid raiment, together with scantiness of food, content with simple diet and the pure drink of water in conjoining fasts to all this; this *bodily* patience adds a grace to our prayers for good, a strength of our prayers against evil; this opens the ears of Christ our God, dissipates severity, elicits clemency."[16] Thus, that which springs from a virtue of the minds is perfected in the flesh, and finally, by the patience of the flesh, does battle under persecution.[17]

For the fathers of the church, bodily patience puts suicide out of the question. Job is the great exemplar in this regard as he resists his wife's suggestion that he should curse God and die. Augustine calls upon those who would kill themselves under persecution to look to "this man," meaning both Job and Christ. Like true martyrs who neither seek death nor invite it prematurely, we ought to bear all patiently rather than "to dare death impatiently." According to Augustine, all that can be said to those who have killed themselves under persecution is "Woe unto them which have lost patience!"[18]

Following Tertullian and Cyprian, Augustine maintains that only patience shaped by Christ is true patience. As he says, "Properly speaking those are patient who would rather bear evils without inflicting them, than inflict them without bearing them. As for those who bear evils that they may inflict evil, their patience is neither marvelous nor praiseworthy, for it is not patience at all; we may marvel at their hardness of heart, but we must refuse to call them patient."[19] Such patience cannot come from "the strength of the human will,"[20] but rather must come from the Holy Spirit. Behind it, of course, is the greatest of all the Spirit's gifts, namely, charity. "Without [love] in us there cannot be true patience, because in good men it is the love of God which endureth all things, in bad men the lust of the world. But this love is in us by the Holy Spirit which was given us. Whence, of Whom cometh in us love, of Him cometh patience. But the lust of the world, when it patiently bears the burdens of any manner of calamity, boasts of the strength of its own will, like as of the stupor of disease, not robustness of health. This boasting is insane: it is not the language of patience, but of dotage. A will like this in that degree seems more patient of bitter ills, in which it is more greedy of temporal good things, because more empty of eternal."[21]

S.S.J. (Washington, DC: Catholic University Press of America, 1957), p. 65. Cyprian's account of patience closely parallels Tertullian's earlier treatise "On Patience." The latter can be found in volume 3 of *The Ante-Nicene Fathers* (Grand Rapids, MI: Eerdmans, 1989), pp. 707-17. Augustine drew on both Tertullian and Cyprian for his "On Patience," which can be found in *A Library of Fathers of the Holy Catholic Church, Anterior to the Division of the East and West,* trans. Members of the English Church (Oxford: John Henry Parker Press, 1937), pp. 542-62. Sister Conway provides a very helpful comparison of these three treatments of patience. Augustine is careful to explain that just as God is jealous without any darkening of spirit, so He is patient without "thought of passion," p. 544.

14. Tertullian, p. 708.

15. Ibid., p. 711. Cyprian's reflections on Matthew are found on pages 68-69.

16. Ibid., p. 715.

17. Cyprian observes that the Christian should not hasten to revenge the pain of persecution, since vengeance is the Lord's. "Therefore, even the martyrs as they cry out and as they hasten to their punishment in the intensity of their suffering are still ordered to wait and to show patience until the appointed time is fulfilled and the number of martyrs is complete," p. 89.

18. Augustine, pp. 550-51.

19. Ibid., p. 544. Aquinas uses this quote to counter the claim that patience is not a virtue, since it can sometimes be found in wicked men. See *Summa Theologica* (New York: Benziger Bros., 1947), II-II, 136, 1.

20. Augustine, p. 551.

21. Ibid., pp. 557-58. Augustine, like all the Christian fathers, makes constant appeals to Scripture in support of this argument — I Corinthians 13:4 being, of course, the central text. Charity must form patience, but it is equally the case that charity needs patience. In a remarkable passage Cyprian says, "Charity is the bond of brotherhood, the foundation of peace, the steadfastness and firmness of unity; it is greater than both hope and faith; it excels both good works and suffering for faith; and, as an eternal virtue, it will abide with us forever in the kingdom of heaven. Take patience away from it, and thus forsaken, it will not last; take away the substance of enduring and tolerating, and it attempts to last with no roots or strength. Accordingly, the apostle when he was speaking about charity joined forbearance and patience to it, saying: Charity is magnanimous, charity is kind, charity does not envy, is not puffed up, is not provoked, thinks no evil, loves all things, believes all things, hopes all things, endures all things. By this he showed that charity can persevere steadfastly because it has learned how to

Following the fathers before him, Aquinas maintained that true patience comes from God. Like them, he was aware that many people display the semblance of patience without the gift of the Spirit. Yet patience taken as a "natural virtue" cannot be shaped by the appropriate sadness and joy constitutive of Christian patience. For Aquinas a true understanding of our place as creatures must include an insuperable sadness and dejection about our condition. Christ's suffering on the cross exemplifies the sorrow that must be present in every Christian's life.[22] Christians must "be saddened by their own frailty, by the suffering present in the world, and by their inability to change either fundamentally."[23]

From Aquinas's perspective, the problem is how to prevent the sadness, which we appropriately feel, from becoming depression, despair, or apathy. And this falls to patience. "Patience is to ensure that we do not abandon Virtue's good through dejection of this kind."[24] It makes us capable of being rightly saddened without succumbing to the temptation to give up hope. A patience-formed sadness can be held together with joy, because each is the effect of charity. Holding such a joy, we rightly "grieve over what opposes this participation in the divine good in ourselves, or in our neighbors, whom we love as ourselves."[25]

Lee Yearley suggests that Aquinas's account of patience combines two different, even apparently paradoxical attitudes. Christians must judge their earthly life according to the standard evident in God's goodness, yet they must also adhere to the future good of possible union with God and the present good evident in God's manifestations in the world and in people's lives. Neither side of

endure all things. And in another place he says: bearing with one another in love, taking every care to preserve the unity of the Spirit in the union of peace. He proved that neither unity nor peace can be preserved unless brothers cherish one another with mutual forbearance and preserve the bond of unity with patience as intermediary" (p. 81).

22. We are indebted once again to Lee Yearley's wonderful *Mencius and Aquinas: Theories of Virtue and Conceptions of Courage* (New York: State University of New York Press, 1990), particularly pp. 136-43. Crucial for understanding Aquinas's views is the significance of his account of the passions and, in particular, sadness as a passion. See *Summa Theologica* I-II, 35-39. Yearley rightly observes that Aquinas thinks his understanding of the place of sadness in the Christian life is the crucial difference between Stoicism and Christianity. The Christian cannot seek to be free of sadness, for without the appropriate sadness we lack the ability to be joyful.

The Stoics' understanding of the passions was much more complex than they are usually given credit for. See, for example, Martha Nussbaum's treatment of Stoicism in *The Therapy of Desire: Theory and Practice in Hellenistic Ethics* (Princeton, NJ: Princeton University Press, 1994), pp. 359-438. Nussbaum, quoting Seneca, observes, "'Where you take greatest joy you will also have the greatest fear.' Just as there is unity among the virtues, all being forms of correct apprehension of the self-sufficient good, just so there is a unity to the passions — and also to their underlying dispositional states. But this means, too, that there is a unity to the cure of the passions. 'You will cease to fear, if you cease to hope. . . . Both belong to a soul that is hanging in suspense, to a soul that is made anxious by concern with the future.' The world's vulnerable gifts, cherished, give rise to the passionate life; despised, to a life of calm. 'What fortune does not give, she does take away'" (pp. 388-89). Against such a background the importance of Aquinas's insistence that Christians are the most passionate of people can be understood not only as a claim about what we must be as Christians, but also as a claim about the way the world is. If God, at least the God that Christians worship, does not exist, then our joy and our sadness, schooled by our hope, is a lie.

23. Yearley, p. 137. This point should be qualified with the insistence that Thomas's account of patience does not entail passivity. Patience is a necessary component of fortitude, which, as Josef Pieper observes, seems incongruous for many people because for them patience "has come to mean an indiscriminate, self-immolating, crabbed, joyless, and spineless submission to whatever evil is met with or, worse, deliberately sought out. Patience, however, is something quite other than indiscriminate acceptance of any and every evil: "The patient man is not the one who does not flee from evil, but the one who does not allow himself to be made inordinately sorrowful thereby." To be patient means to preserve cheerfulness and serenity of mind in spite of injuries that result from the realization of the good. Patience does not imply the exclusion of energetic, forceful activity, but simply, explicitly and solely the exclusion of sadness and confusion of heart. Patience keeps man from the anger that his spirit may be broken by grief and lose its greatness. Patience, therefore, is not the tear-veiled mirror of a 'broken' life (as one might easily assume in the face of what is frequently presented and praised under this name), but the radiant embodiment of ultimate integrity. In the words of Hildegard of Bingen, patience is 'the pillar which nothing can soften.' And Thomas, following Holy Scripture (Luke 21:19), summarizes with superb precision: 'Through patience man possesses his soul.'" *The Four Cardinal Virtues* (South Bend, IN: University of Notre Dame Press, 1966), p. 129.

24. Aquinas, *Summa Theologica* II-II, 136, 4, 2. Yearley highlights this wonderful passage.

25. Aquinas, *Summa Theologica* II-II, 28, 2. (This is Yearley's translation of this passage.) Crucial for sustaining such joy in the midst of sadness is the kind of materialism required in the Christian belief in the Incarnation and Resurrection. Our belief in the bodily Resurrection — that is, that the resurrection is not so much a throwing off of our human flesh but rather an exchanging of our present body for a new body so that we may dwell in a new heaven and a new earth — means that Christians' hope that "all manner of things shall be well" can never be a facile optimism that evades the reality of pain. As James Fodor observed to one of us (Hauerwas), "simply to encourage people to see things differently, while leaving things as they are, is to reinforce their slavery, the reinforcement of which is all the more insidious precisely because it is disguised as a proclamation of the truth to set us free. Christianity, in other words, is not merely a way of 'regarding,' 'looking at,' or 'interpreting' reality. Christianity is not a 'theory' but a way of life, a way of discipleship. And discipleship is concrete, specific; it occurs — or fails to occur — in particular practices and patterns of engagements, relations, suffering, and worship. Thus the importance of the practice of 'bodily patience' for guarding against the tendency, all too common among many modern Christians, to affirm 'the primacy of the spiritual' to the neglect of the material conditions of redemption. The practical, material display of Christian virtue necessary for patience is in finding a gift from God and not something we cultivate willfully or from our own strength, apart from God's help. In fact, patience is often something we reluctantly accept, if at all, and then only after a long and painful struggle to acknowledge our creaturely limits and the sense in which most things in our life remain out of our control."

such an attitude can be lost. We must persist in sadness, yet it must not be allowed to overwhelm the pursuit of the good, the accurate recognition of its forms, and a correct belief about the world's ultimate character. "This attitude is distinctive enough that it can arise, Aquinas thinks, only from the theological virtues. Charity's friendship with God is most crucial, but the attitude manifest in patience also rests on faith and displays the mean between presumption and despair that appears in hope."[26]

Like all the virtues that come from charity, Christian patience is a gift. As we noted earlier with courage [see "Courage Exemplified," essay 14 in Yearley's *Mencius and Aquinas*], there are always semblances of the virtues produced apart from charity; patience in particular is frequently confused with its semblances. For example, there is a kind of tempered optimism in which people "either rest too confidently on their past experiences of overcoming dejection or manifest a phlegmatic or unreflective disposition at inappropriate times. Their optimism, then, reflects a flawed hope that is close to dullness or presumption. It displays an intemperate attitude that expresses itself in the naive belief that all will turn out for the best."[27] Christians have no such wan hope, sustained as we are by a patience that looks to our misfortunes, even the misfortune of our illness and death, as part of our service to one another as God's people.

4. Christian Patience and Patients

The matter of whether true patience can be had without God is particularly relevant to our own time and especially to the medicine practiced within it. We suspect that those committed to living in the world without God will find no time for the patience described by the likes of Cyprian, Tertullian, Augustine, and Aquinas. Indeed, we moderns fill our lives with what Albert Borgmann characterizes as a kind of addiction to hyperactivity. Believing that we live in a world of infinite possibilities, we find ourselves constantly striving, restless for what, we are not sure.[28] We call our restlessness freedom, but more often than not our freedom seems more like fate, especially when we get what we have strived for only to discover that it does not satisfy — thus the peculiar combination in modern life of an attitude of metaphysical indeterminism with Stoic fatalism.

All this is what Christians might call impatience; we should not be surprised to discover it, for we live in a world governed by sin. Indeed, Tertullian went so far as to attribute the creation of impatience to the devil, since he could not ensure the patience God exemplified in creation. According to Tertullian, the devil passed to Eve that same impatience when, through his speech, he "breathed on her a spirit infected with impatience: so certain is it that she would have never sinned at all, if she had honored the divine edict by maintaining her patience to the end."[29] She passed her impatience on to

26. Yearley, p. 139.

27. Ibid. Yearley notes that Aquinas did not examine the semblances of patience in the systematic manner in which he explored the semblances of courage. Yet, given patience's close relation to endurance, the crucial aspect of courage, Yearley rightly uses the semblances of courage to suggest analogies for how Aquinas might have understood the semblances of patience. Though the comparisons of the semblances of patience with true patience (or the semblances of courage with true courage, or the semblances of prudence with true prudence) are usually negative, it is a mistake to assume that positive comparisons are not also a possibility. Since we are God's good creatures we should expect to find in those who are not Christians indications of God's patience. The problem, then, is not that non-Christians fail to exhibit any of the virtues, but that they do and because they do they are just as likely to display them in ways that may be destructive rather than constructive. The Christian advantage is to be part of God's people, which makes us vulnerable to the judgments of others who have acquired the wisdom necessary to understand the interrelation of the virtues.

28. Albert Borgmann, *Crossing the Postmodern Divide* (Chicago: The University of Chicago Press, 1992), pp. 97-102.

29. Tertullian, p. 710. Gerald J. Schiffhorst in a similar fashion argues that in *Paradise Lost* Milton "relies on patience to express the Christian's proper response to the divine will while ironically revealing the anti-heroism of Satan, whose blind impatience reverses what Milton called the 'better fortitude' of patience. Satan's struggle to fight God is undercut by the 'pleasing sorcery' of a false heroism whereas Adam learns to arm himself with patience 'to overcome by suffering' what God will unfold. The centrality of 'patience as the truest fortitude' (*Samson Agonistes*, 654) in revealing this fundamental contrast demonstrates the importance of the virtue in the poem." "Satan's False Heroism in *Paradise Lost* as a Perversion of Patience," *Christianity and Literature* 38, no. 2 (winter 1984), p. 13.

Schiffhorst provides a very helpful contrast of Christian patience with Stoic indifference by noting the difference between the Christian understanding of providence and the Stoic idea of fortune. He notes that "this basic Christian-pagan distinction helps us recall that Christ's victory over death was a victory over Fortune, and so the virtuous Christian can have everlasting life by imitating Christ's perfect patience. As Miles Coverdale says in his important Elizabethan treatise on patience, 'the impatient man complains against God and ascribes prosperity to his own wisdom, blaming blind Fortune for adversity.' Without ascribing dispassionate Stoic virtues to Satan, we can nevertheless say that his false heroism is rooted in a stubborn pride and that he exhibits all the passions of the impatient man: wrath, despair, grief, and envy," pp. 14-15.

For a wonderful collection of essays on patience, see Gerald J. Schiffhorst, ed., *The Triumph of Patience: Medieval and Renaissance Studies* (Orlando: University Presses of Florida, 1978). Particularly interesting is Elizabeth Kirk's essay entitled "'Who Suffreth More Than God?': Narrative Redefinition of Patience in *Patience* and *Piers Plowman*," ibid., pp. 88-105. She not only provides a wonderful commentary on the medieval poet of the Pearl, but ends with a delightful quote from Chaucer's Parson that she thinks contains everything written large in *Patience and Piers Plowman*: "Patience that is another remedie agayns Ire, is a vewru that suffreth sweetly every mannes goodness, and is not wroth for noon harm that is doon to hym. . . . This vertu maketh a man lyk to God, and maketh hym Goddes owene deere child, as seith Crist. This vertu disconfiteth thyn enemy. And therefore seith the wise man, If thow wolt vengukysse thyn enemy, lerne to suffer. . . . And understond wel that obedience is parfit whan that a man dooth gladly and hastily, with good herte entirely, al that he should do," p. 102.

Adam, which in turn produced impatient sons. The very impatience that "had immersed Adam and Eve in death, taught their son, too, to begin with murder."[30] That murder was the fruit of impatience, as Cain impatiently refused his God-given obligation to his brother.

Surely medical care is one of God's gifts that it is our prerogative to use as a hedge against the impatience of the world. To care for one another when we cannot cure is one of the many ways we serve one another patiently. To be committed to alleviating the other's pain in a manner that makes all other considerations irrelevant makes no sense if we have not been made to be patient people. Yet, as we tried earlier to display, the powers of impatience have breathed heavily on the practice of modern medicine, leading it to promise more than it can or should deliver. Indeed, in the frustration of being unable to meet impatient expectations, we are threatened with a medicine that, in the name of relieving suffering, kills.

We Christians are, of course, as implicated in this strange reversal as our non-Christian neighbors. But these issues are far too serious to play "Who is to blame?" The challenge is rather whether Christians have any contribution to make that would help us discover the proper limits of our care of one another through the office of medicine. It is not the unique task of Christians to suggest new and better theories about medical care, though some Christians engaged in that care undoubtedly have contributions to make. Rather, if Christians have anything to offer, it is to be patients who embody the virtue of Christian patience.[31]

To be patient when we are sick requires first that we learn how to practice patience when we are not sick. God has given us ample resources for recovering the practice of patience. First and foremost, we have been given our bodies, which will not let us do whatever we think we should be able to do.[32]

We are our bodies and, as such, we are creatures destined to die. The trick is to learn to love the great good things our bodies make possible without hating our bodies, if for no other reason than that the death of our bodies is our own death. To practice the patience of the body is to be put on the way to holiness as we learn that we are not our own creations.

Second, we have been given one another. To learn to live with the unavoidability of the other is to learn to be patient. Such patience comes not just from our inability to have the other do our will; more profoundly, it arises with the love that the presence of the other can and does create in us. Our loves, like our bodies, signal our deaths. And such love — if it is not to be fearful of its loss, a very difficult thing — must be patient. Moreover, patience sustains and strengthens love, for it opens to us the time we need to tell our own story with another's story intertwined and to tell it together with that other. So told, the story in fact constitutes our love.

Third, we have been given time and space for the acquisition of habits that come from worthy activities such as growing food, building shelters, spinning cloth, writing poems, playing baseball, and having children. Such activities not only take time but they create it by forcing us to take first one step and then another. These activities will outlive us, so long as we take the time to pass them on to future generations through shared activities and stories. So too, patience gives us the ability to engage in these activities with our children, to teach by doing, and to tell them worthy stories worthily so that we and they may be rightly entertained.[33]

These resources, these practices of patience, are not simply "there" but arise within the narrative of God's patient care of the world, which is but another way of insisting, with Aquinas, that it is impossible to have pa-

30. Tertullian, 710. As pacifists we find Tertullian's suggestion that our violence lies in our impatience as intriguing as it is persuasive.

31. Our emphasis on patience as the virtue essential to the doctor-patient relationship may appear particularly perverse because it seems to make the patient even more powerless. There is rightly an asymmetry between the doctor and patient inasmuch as the physician has authority that the patient does not or should not have. However, once it is understood that medicine names an activity in which doctor and patient are jointly involved, patience can work in such a relationship to decrease rather than increase the abuse of power. Crucially, both Christian patience and obedience require the church for display. Without the kind of friendship, dependency, trust, and mutual nurturing imbedded in the worship of God, patience and obedience always risk the possibility of becoming malformed. That is why Hauerwas suggested in *Suffering Presence* that institutionalized medicine requires a church for sustaining the kind of presence that physicians, nurses, and others in medical settings provide. The hospital is the best exemplification of the kind of care the church should make possible and sustain, although, as we suggested earlier, "the hospital," increasingly detached from the practices of the church which gave it birth, may be on its way to an entirely new sort of existence.

32. We are acutely aware, as anyone must be after the work of Foucault, that appeals to the "body" are anything but unproblematic. Recent historical work helps us better understand why Paul could say that nothing was more "spiritual" than the body. Moreover, understanding the body as peculiarly "spiritual" we think has great potential for helping us reexamine the relation of Christian practices and the practice of medicine. See, for example, Peter Brown's *The Body and Society: Men, Women and Sexual Renunciation in Early Christianity* (Boston: Faber, 1988), and Dale Martin's *The Corinthian Body* (New Haven: Yale University Press, 1995).

Particularly important is a better understanding of the "therapy of desire" characteristic of Christian practice in contrast to the assumptions of Galen and the other Hellenistic philosophical schools. For example, we need a Christian account parallel to Nussbaum's *The Therapy of Desire.* Brown's book is obviously a good beginning, but one has the feeling that we are just beginning to understand what Augustine and Aquinas grasped far better than we do about the nature of the passions. We are indebted to Thomas Harvey, a graduate student at Duke, for a paper in which he explored how Augustine provided an alternative to Galen's understanding of the body.

33. For a fuller development of how our practices not only take but also create time, see "Taking Time for Peace: The Ethical Significance of the Trivial," in *Christian Existence Today: Essays on Church, World, and Living in Between* (Durham: Labyrinth Press, 1988), pp. 253-66.

tience without charity — that is, without friendship with God. Put simply, our ability to take the time to enjoy God's world, when we are well as when we are sick, depends on our recognition that it is indeed God's world.

When we are sick, reminders of joy may seem to be the gestures of a false courage. Indeed, the Christian is charged with the responsibility of speaking truthfully about the sadness that riffles our lives. As Aquinas maintained, sadness must be recognized and lived with. But the acknowledgment of such sadness, upheld by patience, becomes integral to the Christian gift for sustaining the ill and those who care for them. Hence, those formed by the virtue of patience can be patients who do not believe that life is an end in itself. The patient patient knows — and can teach others, including physicians — that the enemy is neither the illness nor the death it intimates, but rather the fatalism these tempt us to as we meet our "bad luck"[34] with impatience.

If Christians could be such patient patients — and there is every reason to think that we can — we might well stand as witnesses to our non-Christian neighbor of the truth of the story of God's patient care of God's creatures. We might find we have something to say, not only about how illness and death can be met with grace and courage, but also about how those called to be physicians and nurses might care patiently for their patients, and perhaps even about the kind of training they will need to become capable of this high calling. To do this Christians will need to risk being different, but that should not be beyond a people who, having learned the patience of God, can find the time, even in the midst of a frenzied world, to give themselves over to such worthy work.

34. We put quotes around this phrase to indicate its everyday usage but also to mark our unease. As we implied earlier, luck is a Stoic, not a Christian, notion that implies fortune, which is blind. Christians do not believe the world is ruled by fortune but rather by God's providential care.

IV. Vulnerable Persons

CHAPTER TEN

Persons with Mental Illness

Few topics remain as taboo in contemporary culture as major mental illness. The terrain has shifted somewhat over the past two decades with the development and marketing of selective serotonin reuptake inhibitors (SSRIs). Since the first SSRI, Prozac, was introduced by the pharmaceutical company Eli Lilly in 1987, the use of SSRIs and other psychoactive medications (including Paxil, Zoloft, Luvox, Celexa, Elavil, Anafranil, Norpramin, Tofranil, Pamelor, Nardil, Parnate, Ascendin, Wellbutrin, Serzone, Effexor, Buspar, Valium, Ativan, Klonapin, and Xanax, in addition to the antipsychotics Haldol, Risperdol, Zyprexa, Lamictal, Geodon, Lithium, Tegretol, and Depakote, to name only some) has skyrocketed. It is estimated that 65 million prescriptions are written in the U.S. every year for antidepressants, for conditions ranging from major depression to obsessive-compulsive disorder, panic disorder, and social anxiety disorder; off-label prescriptions are written for premenstrual syndrome, bulimia, premature ejaculation, insomnia, borderline personality disorder, hypochondria, and fibromyalgia.

Reports estimate that approximately one in five adults suffers from a personality disorder, a number that has remained relatively stable from 1993 (when it was first reported by the National Institute of Mental Health) through 2008. Some of the taboo surrounding mental illness has been breached by the willingness of celebrities and public figures to share their own stories and by the growth in the relatively new literary genre of psychobiography. The prevalence of the above psychoactive medications has contributed to the mainstreaming of mental illness as well.

Yet the theological literature remains relatively quiet on the subject of mental illness. Few theologians have ventured to comment upon the way in which the advent of psychopharmaceuticals has changed the landscape of psychiatry as well as understandings of the self, identity, and health. Few have followed psychiatrist Peter Kramer's landmark book *Listening to Prozac* (1993) and the concerns he raised about the psychopharmacologization of American culture. Much has been written on the positive role religion can play in sustaining mental health, but thick theological engagement with issues surrounding mental illness remains wanting.

Kathryn Greene-McCreight concurs. We open this chapter with a selection from her book *Darkness Is My Only Companion*.[1] Greene-McCreight, a theologian and Episcopal priest, writes of her own experience with bipolar disorder. She writes in large part because, as a person with a major mental illness, she found little that could address her theological concerns. Greene-McCreight's "Darkness" (selection 67) provides an important contextualization for the rest of the essays in this chapter. It tells the story of mental illness from one patient's perspective; it situates mental illness in the context of a "normal," everyday life; it suggests some of the ramifications of such illness; and it points to one woman's theological wrestlings and resources.

However, most of the "religion and mental health" literature is written not from the perspective of the patient or those involved in "religion," but from the perspective of mental health professionals, particularly psychiatrists, psychiatric social workers, counselors of various kinds, family therapists, pastoral counselors, and still others. Harking back to the first chapter of this anthology, the very terms that shape this field raise again the relation of religion to medicine. Psychiatry is formed of two Greek words, *psyche* (breath, spirit, soul) and *iatreia* (healing); its sister discipline psychology is rooted in *psyche* (breath, spirit, soul) and *logia* (study of). Thus, the fields of psychiatry and psychology claim, in their etymology, to be about the study and healing of the soul or spirit.

Until the late nineteenth century, however, the care, study, and healing of souls was considered primarily the domain of a different institution, namely, the church. Clergy long regarded "the care of souls" as part of their task.[2] The term "curate," long used to refer to clergy, captures the centrality of this work. Traditional practices of the care or cure of souls entailed the (sometimes) sacramental practices of confession, penance, and reconcilia-

1. Kathryn Greene-McCreight, *Darkness Is My Only Companion* (Grand Rapids: Brazos, 2006).

2. John T. McNeill, *A History of the Cure of Souls* (New York: Harper & Row, 1977).

tion, as well as spiritual direction, preaching, and other forms of pastoral care.[3]

Thus, behind much of the literature on religion and mental health lies a contest over jurisdiction and turf: Who are the proper practitioners of "soul healing"? What are the proper methods? Where, institutionally, ought this work be located? And on what authority? Sigmund Freud, one of the Masters of Suspicion of religion (along with Karl Marx and Friedrich Nietzsche), sets the tone for much of contemporary psychiatry and psychology, seeing religiosity itself as a form of mental illness — an "obsessional neurosis" and "a system of wishful illusions."[4] Carl Jung, on the other hand, regarded religion as necessary for mental health, because "it is the role of religion to give a meaning to the life of man."[5] There remain differences of opinion among therapists about whether religion is pathological or therapeutic.[6]

Yet regardless of where psychiatry eventually lands on the question of religion, some would argue that religion has effectively conceded the field to psychiatry, jettisoning traditional theological language and religious practices in favor of psychological jargon and techniques. Eminent child psychiatrist Robert Coles, for example, takes issue both with his own profession and with Christianity. In his essay "Psychology as Faith" (selection 68), he not only protests against the "secular idolatry" of psychology and psychiatry as they usurp the role previously played by clergy. He also launches an equally scathing critique against clergy, those who are properly charged with the "cure of souls" but who have surrendered the traditional practices of believing communities and adopted instead the tools of the therapist, the ends-and-means language of psychology. Why do we hear, Coles might lament, of Jung and stages of faith development in our sermons and spiritual direction rather than of the cross or Christian practices? Similar critiques of pastors and chaplains were raised in some of the essays in Chapter Five of this anthology.

An interesting embodiment of Coles's critique of psychiatry can be found in Ian S. Evison's essay "Between the Priestly Doctor and the Myth of Mental Illness" (selection 69). Evison provides a helpful historical account of the development of the field of psychology and uses two eminent psychiatrists, Robert J. Lifton and Thomas Szasz, to display contrasting accounts of the relation of psychiatry to ethics. Evison traces the philosophical roots of their different perspectives (Lifton's to Romanticism and communitarianism and Szasz's to the Enlightenment and laissez-faire individualism), but he goes beyond this polarity to call psychiatry and its practitioners to pursue "the admittedly ethical but limited goal of basic human functioning." Evison regards his position as a form of "public theology," one that brackets the larger, richer, and more particular visions of individual and social good while not succumbing to the pretense of value-neutrality.

But whence, we might ask, will Evison construct his standard of "adequate functioning"? Will such a thin "public theology" be able to guide and to limit the powers of psychiatric medicine? Lifton might respond that such a psychiatry would inevitably become co-opted by the "forces of death" in a culture like Nazi Germany[7] — or in our own — especially if the standard of "adequate functioning" would seem to presume some account of what a person is "for." We know what a watch is for, of course, and so we have reasonable standards for judging whether a watch is functioning adequately, and particular theologies have some ideas about what human beings are "for," but can a psychiatric "public theology" judge whether a person is functioning adequately?

To illustrate this point, one needs only passing familiarity with the controversies surrounding the periodic revisions of the *Diagnostic and Statistical Manual of Mental Disorders* (DSM), which was first issued in 1952. The past sixty years have seen certain conditions (e.g., homosexuality) liberated from the category of deviation or disorder and others (e.g., ADHD, pre-menstrual dysphoric disorder) created. This history certainly reflects changes in biological and sociological data, but it has equally been driven by political advocacy, changes in U.S. culture, changes in the practical infrastructure of everyday life, and the burgeoning growth of the pharmaceutical industry since 1980. Thus, one must ask: To what extent does psychiatry's vision of basic or adequate human functioning simply reflect its cultural context?

These questions regarding the normative power of psychiatry to define basic or adequate functioning, or what human persons are for, take on renewed urgency in light of the increased use of psychopharmaceuticals in the U.S. over the past twenty years, particularly by children, young adults, and those not generally understood to have a *major* mental illness. But that story is but a part of a longer history of psychoactive medications in the U.S., the first chapter of which is deeply intertwined with

3. Annemarie Kidder, *Making Confession, Hearing Confession: A History of the Cure of Souls* (Collegeville: Liturgical Press, 2010).

4. Sigmund Freud, *The Future of an Illusion* (Garden City, N.Y.: Doubleday, 1961; first published in 1927), pp. 71-72.

5. Carl Jung, ed., *Man and His Symbols* (London: Aldus Books, 1964), p. 89. Like Jung, Gordon Allport considered religion a potentially important contributor to mental health; see, for example, *The Individual and His Religion* (New York: Macmillan, 1950).

6. See, for example, the debate between Allen Bergin and Albert Ellis in *Journal of Consulting and Clinical Psychology* 48 (1980): Allen E. Bergen, "Psychotherapy and Religious Values," pp. 95-100; Albert Ellis, "Psychotherapy and Atheistic Values: A Response to A. E. Bergin's 'Psychotherapy and Atheistic Values,'" pp. 635-39; Bergin, "Religious and Humanistic Values: A Reply to Ellis and Walls," pp. 642-45. See also David B. Larson and Susan S. Larson, "Religious Commitment and Health: Valuing the Relationship," *Second Opinion* 17, no. 1 (July 1991): 27-40, which combines an autobiographical account of David Larson's confrontation with a prejudice against religion in his psychiatric training with a survey of the empirical research on the contribution of religion to mental health.

7. Besides the books mentioned in Evison's bibliography, Robert J. Lifton is also the author of *The Nazi Doctors* (New York: Basic Books, 1985).

the history of deinstitutionalization. Paul S. Appelbaum narrates this history in his essay "Crazy in the Streets" (selection 70). In this story of triumph and tragedy, it is clear that the goal of at least some who advocated a policy of deinstitutionalization, which psychopharmaceuticals made plausible, was the reduction of the population (and the costs) of state mental institutions rather than a concern about the mental health of the residents.

Since Appelbaum and others call for some reversal in the policy of deinstitutionalization, it is worth considering again some of the issues prompted by "total institutions," and the selection by William F. May "Afflicting the Afflicted: Total Institutions" (selection 71) does that splendidly. The history of institutionalization — whether of the mentally ill or of any other population — is generally not a pretty story. Beyond May, those interested in this topic are encouraged to read Michel Foucault's *Madness and Civilization: A History of Insanity.*[8] Foucault provides a broader account of the development of totalizing institutions, and he also shows how contemporary constructs of "madness" and "insanity" emerged in the late seventeenth century, in concert with the Age of Reason and the development of market capitalism. May's essay is important not only for the subject of mental illness but, clearly, for consideration of other vulnerable groups within our culture, especially the elderly (see Chapter Eleven, below), as well as for health care generally, insofar as the major location of health care delivery remains the hospital.

The Christian response to deinstitutionalization includes not only contributions to the public discussion about state institutions but also reflections about the Christian community's responsibility to be hospitable and supportive to mentally ill persons. In this task, many churches have not behaved in an exemplary fashion. John Swinton, in "Community and Friendship: The Church as a Liberating Community" (selection 72), calls on the church as an institution to become a site of care for persons with mental illness in a whole new way. As a registered mental health nurse who has worked with persons with severe mental health issues, Swinton understands the important role played in such care by psychiatric medicine and psychopharmaceuticals. But, such value notwithstanding, Swinton questions whether "the medicopsychiatric definitions, understandings, and strategies . . . [are] the most appropriate way of defining" and responding to mental health problems. Swinton asks Greene-McCreight's question: "what does it mean to live with a mental health problem?" And he argues that the socio-relational dimension — which is fundamental to the oppression attending such illnesses — is far more critical than the strictly biomedical.

Swinton, as a theologian, calls the church to reclaim its responsibility for the "cure of souls" and to be a social institution that practices and embodies "radical messianic friendship" toward those with mental illness. Such a notion of friendship is, of course, markedly different from the way we normally understand the term, and so Swinton's vision of such friendship occurring within the context of religious congregations presents challenges to the way we normally think about the church. Yet, for Swinton, "caring for the needs of people living with mental health problems is not an option for the church. Rather it is a primary mark of its identity and faithfulness."

What a contrast of visions — from sequestering people with severe mental health issues in May's totalizing institution to caring for them in an institution shaped by radical messianic friendship. With Swinton the chapter comes full circle from Kathryn Greene-McCreight's opening reflection. Neither rejects psychiatric medicine or pharmaceuticals, but nor do they believe such interventions are sufficient. Both challenge and qualify certain assumptions about mental health care and the goals and means of particular therapies, while resituating the care and cure of souls within its original institutional context — the church — and its practices. In doing so, they point toward new ways to better care for the mentally ill among us, paths Robert Coles would undoubtedly applaud.

8. Michel Foucault, *Madness and Civilization: A History of Insanity* (New York: Vintage, 1988).

SUGGESTIONS FOR FURTHER READING

Elliott, Carl. *Prozac as a Way of Life* (Chapel Hill: University of North Carolina Press, 2004).

Elliott, Carl. "Pursued by Happiness and Beaten Senseless." *Hastings Center Report* 30, no. 2 (March/April 2000): 7-12.

Swinton, John. *From Bedlam to Shalom: Towards a Practical Theology of Human Nature, Interpersonal Relationships, and Mental Health Care.* Pastoral Theology, vol. 1 (New York: Peter Lang, 2000).

Swinton, John. *Resurrecting the Person: Friendship and the Care of People with Mental Health Problems* (Nashville: Abingdon, 2000).

67 Darkness

Kathryn Greene-McCreight

Affliction is the best book in my library.

Martin Luther (1483-1546)

My thirtieth birthday found me as content as the next person, as happy as I had always been, in fact quite unremarkably normal. I was well adjusted, highly productive, married to the man of my dreams, with an active and healthy toddler, beginning to earn recognition in my chosen field of study. I understood myself to be mentally quite healthy. I had had a stable and happy childhood, blessed with the benefits too often lacking from many other childhoods. The only exception to the streams-of-mercy-never-ceasing was a somewhat unusual series of tragedies that had struck like waves throughout my youth and young adult years. But even these I had weathered well, or so I had always thought.

When I became a mother for the second time, however, the hem of my mental health began to fray. Motherhood by nature challenges the mental, emotional, spiritual, and physical endurance of any woman. It is a highly overromanticized and underestimated pressure cooker, matched in potential not only for the creation of a new family but also for the destruction of both mother and child. Think — with horror — of the Susan Smiths and Amanda Yateses of the world. Smith drowned her two children in a pond by seatbelting them into the car and pushing the car into the water. Yates killed all six of her children, the youngest a newborn, by drowning them in the family bathtub. Of course, not all postpartum sufferers are this detached from reality.

I cannot speak, of course, from experience of the role of the father. I do not mean to discredit his difficulties. I am not aware of the role of the fathers in the Smith and Yates cases. I do know that without the father of my own children, I simply would not have survived thus far. His support and care took the edge off most of my symptoms, especially at this early stage. Without my husband's staunch faithfulness and belief that I would see light beyond this, I simply would not have made it through.

Motherhood, I believe, was only the precipitant for an internal agony that I had been holding back for years. Maybe God had postponed my storm at sea until I could be buoyed by the hopefulness and joy that I derived from my children and husband. The experience as a whole and the experiences that constituted the eventual illness were at the least bewildering and at most terrifying. The blue sky, which normally fills my heart, stung my soul. Beautiful things like oriental rugs and good food like bean soup absolutely exhausted me. Noise was amplified in my ears, and I fled sound and conversation in search of silence. Small tasks became existential problems: how and why to fold the laundry, empty the dishwasher, do the grocery shopping. My memory failed me. I was unable to read or write (except for sermons, by the Holy Spirit's providence, I believe). And it went downhill from there. A back and forth in and out of darkness lasted for years.

There are many psalms of lament, but Psalm 88 seemed to fit me. It ends in the Book of Common Prayer and in the King James Version with "Darkness is my only companion." Yes, even some of my friends deserted me, except ones who are now the dearest and truest of friends. I was no fun to be with whatsoever, so why not desert me? "What has got her? Why is she in such a bad mood? She can't even remember my name!"

I have a chronic disease, a brain disorder that used to be called manic depression and is now, less offensively, called bipolar disorder. However one tries to soften the blow of the diagnosis, the fact remains that bipolar disorder is a subset of the larger category unhappily called "major mental illness." By the latter part of my thirties, I had sought help from several psychiatrists, social workers, and mental health professionals, one a Christian but mostly non-Christians. I had been in active therapy with a succession of therapists over several years and had been introduced to many psychiatric medications, most of which brought quite unpleasant side effects and only a few of which relieved my symptoms to some degree. Those medications that have in fact been helpful, I must say despite my own disinclination toward drugs, have been a strand in the cord that God has woven for me as the lifeline cast out in my free fall. The medications have helped me to rebuild some of "myself," so that I can continue to be the kind of mother, priest, and writer that I believe God wants me to be. "A threefold cord is not quickly broken" (Ecclesiastes 4:12). The three cords to my rope were the religious (worship and prayer), the psychological (psychotherapy), and the medical (medication, electroconvulsive therapy, and hospitalization).

Yet while therapists and counselors, psychiatrists and medications abound, I found no one to help me make sense of my pain with regard to my life before the triune God. I write this book, then, by way of an offering, as what I wish someone had written to help me make sense of the pain and the apparent incongruity of that agony with the Christian life. Those Christians who have not faced the ravages of mental illness should not be quick with advice to those who do suffer. Platitudes such as "Pray harder," "Let Jesus in," even "Cast your anxiety on

From Kathryn Greene-McCreight, "Darkness," in *Darkness Is My Only Companion: A Christian Response to Mental Illness* (Grand Rapids: Brazos Press, 2006).

him, because he cares for you" (1 Peter 5:7), which of course are all valid pieces of advice in and of themselves, may only make the depressive person hurt more.

This is because depression is not just sadness or sorrow. Depression is not just negative thinking. Depression is not just being "down." It is being cast to the very end of your tether and, quite frankly, being dropped. Likewise, mania is more than speeding mentally, more than euphoria, more than creative genius at work. The sick individual cannot simply shrug it off, or pull out of it. While God certainly can pick up the pieces and put them together in a new way, this can happen only if the depressed brain makes it through to see again life among the living. At the time of free fall such a possibility seems absolutely unimaginable. Christians who have not experienced either pole — the high of mania or the low of depression — must try to accept that this is the case, even if they cannot understand it.

> I loathe my life;
>   I will give free utterance to my complaint;
>   I will speak in the bitterness of my soul.
> I will say to God, Do not condemn me;
>   let me know why you contend against me.
> Does it seem good to you to oppress,
>   to despise the work of your hands
>   and favor the schemes of the wicked?
>
> Job 10:1-3

Job is, of course, the quintessential sufferer in the Bible. He suffers immensely and yet always brings his complaint before God. Even when God seems to have abandoned him, Job continues to pray "Do not condemn me . . ." Even though he speaks "in the bitterness" of his soul, he recognizes that he is a soul, and that soul, despite the suffering, is related to God. "Does it seem good to you to oppress, to despise the work of your hands and favor the schemes of the wicked?" Even though God seems to favor the wicked, to whom does Job utter his complaint? God.

> Again I saw that under the sun the race is not to the swift, nor the battle to the strong, nor bread to the wise, nor riches to the intelligent, nor favor to the skillful; but time and chance happen to them all.
>
> Ecclesiastes 9:11

When I asked God why this happened, Ecclesiastes answered: Why not? Time and chance happen to all. Why not this time, this chance, and me?

* * *

Chopping vegetables for a stir-fry. Baby fussing in the background, three-year-old running his toy truck between my feet. Suddenly I see on the cutting board, in place of celery, the severed fingers of my baby daughter. Neat, clean, bloodless. I blink. They are gone now, the celery has returned, the baby is still fussing, her fingers still attached to her hands where they should be, the truck still rumbling along the kitchen floor. I turn back to fixing dinner as though nothing had happened.

An effective coping mechanism: pretending everything is all right, pretending nothing upsetting has happened. It had served me well for some thirty years. Now the storage area in my soul for all the hurts that had been pretended away is overflowing. I need help. Before what I sloughed off was just psychological pain; now my brain is playing tricks on me. Darkness is my closest companion. I need something, but I don't know what. I don't even know how to tell if or when I need help. I don't know what it means to let myself be helped. I never ask for help, even on the odd occasion when I recognize my need for help. That is the definition of me: strong. But now I don't sleep well, can't eat, can't read (a problem for a graduate student), draw no pleasure from the little things anymore.

Physical symptoms bother me. I see my general practitioner: must be a sinus infection or the flu, or . . . he runs test after test and concludes from the exam and blood work that there is nothing physically wrong with me. He suggests that I be seen in Mental Hygiene upstairs. I am appalled at the thought, but he convinces me.

* * *

"Kathryn, from all of the symptoms you have mentioned and from your answers to my questions, I would say that you are in a major depression and that . . ."

I don't hear the rest. A close friend has just been unsuccessfully treated for depression with electroconvulsive therapy. My father and brother had suffered bouts of depression. But I was the cheery one, the well-adjusted one, the happy face of the family. I try to listen to the doctor above the roaring din of my thoughts scrambling to understand, to piece together the meaning of the incidents I had just recounted to him. How could this be and yet I had not even guessed? What does this mean? My head wails, I cannot hear.

* * *

Kay Jamison's book *An Unquiet Mind* is the story of her lifelong struggle with manic-depressive illness and of her career as a psychiatrist specializing in the treatment of mood disorders. Beyond the narrative framework, though, the book does have a thesis (rather unlike William Styron's *Darkness Visible* or Kathy Crosby's *At the Edge of Darkness*). Her thesis is that love pulls one through the suffering. Sounds sweet, almost trite. The kindnesses of strangers and friends, the acceptance of her disease by those who were able, the love of several men who serially played major roles in her healing: love heals.

Why should this seem trite to me? Shouldn't I see this as an authentic, powerful, and appropriate explanation of what pulls us through? Is it just because I am depressed, or naturally cynical, or a theologian? Maybe all those things. But when one looks at the problem of mental illness from a completely secular perspective, her statement (clearly meant to be hopeful and hope-filling) in fact can fill me with more despair than ever. After all, human love can seem particularly unreliable and fleeting. At times it is unattainable, at others inexpressible, and usually for the depressed, human love is unsensed, and indeed nonsense. Of course, for the depressed individual, divine love can be unsensed and nonsense as well. But at least it never fails! "Love bears all things, believes all things, hopes all things, endures all things" (1 Corinthians 13:7). This is true of divine love, and only thereby derivatively of human loves. So "love pulls you through," when it is not tied to the love of God in Christ but to the random kindnesses of people who happen at the moment to be in a better humor than I, is flat. Yet human loves, such as that of my husband, can certainly be a conduit for divine love, even for those who do not recognize love's true source. If it is the love of God that we see in the face of Christ Jesus that is promised to pull us through, a love that bears out to the edge of doom even for the ugly and unlovable such as we, then the statement that love heals depression is in fact the only light that exists in the dark tunnel.

This leads me to wonder how people who are depressed and do not have the conviction of God's unconditional love to hold them steady (even when they cannot feel or sense that conviction) can survive depression. Maybe they do not have such a pessimistic (or what I would prefer to call realistic) understanding of human love. But anyhow, I am a Christian, and how will I survive my depression? God, please enable me to survive. I must allow God to touch me through those people who by God's grace are enabled to love beyond mere human capacity. And maybe it is this sort of love to which Jamison refers after all, although she never says so explicitly. Again, the love of my husband is like this, a grace-filled love. I suppose, though, that we should not fail to recognize God's love extended toward us even in the seemingly trite kindnesses of the otherwise potentially unkind. Even in the listening and patient ear of a psychotherapist, yes, even though I am financing the relationship. I must allow for the possibility for God to work through that relationship. I suppose we have to allow for the possibility for God to be active even among those who are not aware of his presence. It doesn't matter whether they know it or not; God is big enough to handle their potential ignorance.

> Help me, O Lord, to make a true use of all disappointments and calamities in this life, in such a way that they may unite my heart more closely with you. Cause them to separate my affections from worldly things and inspire my soul with more vigor in the pursuit of true happiness.
>
> Susanna Wesley (1669-1742)
> mother of John and Charles Wesley,
> and seventeen other children

Why, with my religious convictions about the love and mercy of God, with my belief in the unconditional and free grace of God poured out in Jesus even in spite of my basest longings and actions, why would I not be filled with joy at every moment, eager to greet the day with the love of the Lord? Especially with a new, perfect baby, a little girl, our Grace, born healthy after some twenty weeks of preterm contractions. I had had, from the outside, a happy and comfortable, indeed privileged, childhood: a two-parent family, a stable home, a good education. I was never neglected by my parents, was always given material blessings that most of the world's children do not have. Amazing that someone even in that cushioned atmosphere should end up in my position, struggling on the edge of sanity sometimes. One of my psychiatrists once suggested that my symptoms as a twelve-year-old sounded like a depression arising from post-traumatic stress syndrome. This syndrome is frequently experienced by soldiers who were traumatized by the atrocities they witnessed and committed in war. How could I have had post-traumatic stress syndrome? As a child and young person I did know many people who committed suicide or died in accidents. The symptoms of post-traumatic stress syndrome can look somewhat like those of depression. But still, I read about the woman who, as a child, was the subject of the famous photo of the naked girl engulfed in napalm flames as she ran through the Vietnamese jungle. Now an adult, disfigured and disabled from the burns, she was able to embrace with her remaining arm the weeping, repentant man who had dropped the bomb that killed her family and maimed her for life. She forgave him. *Forgave him.* She leads a productive life. I lead a productive life too, some of the time, but I never faced the atrocities she did. She does not appear to have post-traumatic stress syndrome. How then could I?

I have been challenged by tragedy, but it was always witnessing the tragedy of others, and even now it is witnessing the tragedy of others that I find absolutely unbearable. It sends me into a complete tailspin. One day recently I saw an old man get hit by an oncoming car as he was walking across the street — the thud of his body against the car, the sight of him dropping to the ground, then trying pitifully to rise. I was the first to reach him, the one to drag him back to his car as he attempted to walk away, the one to take his keys and sit with him until the ambulance came. I was shaky for the next few days. Witnessing the tragedy of others is very difficult for me.

I remember the first time I was confronted with death. Other than hearing of grandparents and uncles dying, the first time I was struck with the reality of my own mortality was the week I turned twelve years old. One of my church choir buddies was killed when a tree fell on her in her backyard. She lingered for about a day, but it was clear that she would not pull out of the coma. I don't remember how I felt, but I do remember adopting the habit of crossing off the days on my bedside calendar with a perfect black *X* after that. I was crossing off the days I had that Cindy would no longer have. A strange undiagnosed illness kept me in bed for about a month sometime after that. I suffered head-splitting pain that made me scream out in the middle of the night. I could not keep food down. I remember being quite content to listen to my purple transistor radio in bed all day. My doctor suggested that may have been my first episode of depression, but at the time no one ever considered that.

Between middle school and college, more tragedies rolled over me. My science lab partner in eighth grade, André, shot himself with his father's hunting rifle one night in a fit of despair. That same year, one of my classmate's older brothers, Tim, killed himself, leaving a note indicating that he had reached his potential in life and had nothing more to "do," as though life were a board game that he had prematurely won. When I was sixteen, my first "real" date, Matthew, was in a motorcycle accident. He lingered for a few days, but his head injuries claimed his life. Then there was Gary, the brother of our church youth group leader, killed in a drunk driving accident; Sandy, my gymnastics teammate, killed herself by diving into an empty pool; Brent, a friend from church youth group, shot himself with his own hunting rifle; Glenn, my co-counselor from church camp, threw himself off a cliff in Hawaii; and Sean, a former student, took an overdose. Later, during my fifth hospitalization in Yale Psychiatric Institute, now Yale New Haven Psychiatric Hospital, another childhood friend hung herself while on suicide watch in another mental hospital in the state. This is not even a complete roster, but by this point I was used to it, if such a thing can be said.

But one thing truly terrified me, and that was witnessing my brother's depression. Of course I knew where it could lead. Once when he and I were both home from college one summer, I begged him never to do that, never to kill himself. He refused to promise. He said he just could not make that promise. That meant that every time he became depressed, would be awake knocking about the house at 3:00 a.m., I would be terrified that he would hurt himself. I found myself wanting to scream out, "Just do it, just get it over with and kill yourself if you are not willing to fight! Don't prolong our agony and yours if that is how this will end anyway!" I felt terrible for having such thoughts and feelings.

Yet I did gain some insight from my brother's and father's depressions. They helped me learn how to protect others from my own depression years later. I would come to refuse the self-pity and blaming of others. I learned to remind myself of my belief that life is a gift. No matter how I felt about my own life, I refused to give in to suicidal thoughts and acts, even though I often ruminated wildly about them. Still, my compassion for my brother was matched only by this anger toward him. He was clearly suffering, and there was nothing I could do about it. Or at least that is the way I thought about it then.

I think that people who have not dealt with such grief, either first or second hand, simply do not know what happiness is, what joy is, because they do not know what the depths of pain can be. It is like this: you cannot know the import of the cross and resurrection unless you have grasped the weight of sin. All those smiley people out there who are always on an even keel have no idea what joy can be seen from the underside, because they have no idea of the really awful pain life can bring. As Augustine said, the hills drive back the water, but the valleys are filled by it (Sermon 27). In the valleys of depression, one can find a "well-watered garden" if one is so blessed. That is, sometimes depression can be a blessing, because one can learn about God through his hiding. That usually only comes afterward, because during depression, as during the flood, the waters of death cover the face of the earth. As with Noah, it is only afterward that the dove can return with the olive leaf in its beak, a sign of blessing. Only after the storm can God set his bow in the clouds as a sign of the covenant.

> Truly, you are a God who hides himself,
> O God of Israel, the Savior.
>
> Isaiah 45:15

Even here, Isaiah does not say, "Truly he is a God that hides himself." Isaiah addresses God directly, even in God's apparent absence. He acknowledges that this absent God is still his own God and the God of his people. And Isaiah acknowledges that God is Savior, even in hiding. *Truly, you are a God who hides himself, O God of Israel, the Savior.*

During a depression, as during Noah's flood, the good providence of God is hidden from view. All I can see is the storm, all I can smell is the dung of my own ark, and all I can perceive is the very wrath of God. And worse than Noah, I have no companions in my ark, just stinky, contentious inner beasts. Darkness is my only companion.

> O blessed Jesus, you know the impurity of our affection, the narrowness of our sympathy, and the coldness of our love; take possession of our souls and fill our minds with the image of yourself; break the stubbornness of our selfish wills and mold us in the likeness of your unchanging love, O you who alone can do this, our Savior, our Lord and our God.
>
> William Temple (1881-1944)

Certainly, mental illness manifests itself differently from person to person. Symptoms can differ. Some can get out of bed, some sleep too much, some can't sleep, some eat too much, some can't bring themselves to eat. So the diseases are not the symptoms. It is not like cancer, where one can cut out the afflicted sections of the body. The symptoms plague the whole body and mind.

I am not necessarily sad when I am depressed. I am not necessarily "down." Sometimes I just have a gnawing, overwhelming sense of grief, with no identifiable cause. I grieve my loved ones as though they were dead and contemplate what their funerals would be like. I feel completely alone; darkness is my only companion. I feel as if I am walking barefoot on broken glass. When one steps on broken glass, the weight of one's body grinds the glass in further with every movement. The weight of my very existing grinds the shards of grief deeper into my soul. When I am depressed, every thought, every breath, every conscious moment hurts.

So what do I do? I try to distract myself. Enduring episodes of depression requires that I expend huge amounts of energy just to distract myself. My work, when I can by sheer force of will overcome the depression enough to engage in work, is solace. Prayer, when I can climb out of the hole depression throws me into, helps momentarily. Of course, theologically speaking, I know it helps more than just momentarily, but that is not the way it feels. Sleeping, while I am sleeping, if I can sleep, helps as an escape. Tasks, busyness, gardening, tidying up: distractions. Mustn't think, mustn't be conscious, mustn't reflect. This escape from consciousness is at the heart of suicidal energy. It is *not* wanting to hurt the self. It is simply wanting *not to hurt.* When I am depressed, it seems that the only way not to hurt is to cease being a center of consciousness.

Distracting myself, though, is itself depressing, to use the term loosely, because I end up feeling that my every action and thought is a futile flight from pain that will ease up. Of course, I am not always depressed; in fact usually I am no longer depressed at all. But when I am, there is no "other side," no perspective, no reminding myself that this will pass . . . yes, of course I remind myself of this, but it only enters the top of my brain and then flits right out again. It is never a sure and certain knowledge.

Other than my childhood episode with what now has been suggested to have been depression, my first real head-on toss into the pit as an adult was, as I have said, after my daughter Grace was born in 1992. Postpartum depression is not pretty. It is tragic. Every instinct in the mother pushes toward preserving the life of the child. Most mothers would give their own life to protect their babies. But in a postpartum depression, reality is so bent that that instinct is blocked. Lack of sleep could alone make anyone depressed and hallucinatory, but on top of that the new mother has a rush of hormones playing havoc with body and brain. Perfectly good mothers have their confidence shaken by the thoughts and feelings they endure in postpartum depression.

I realize now that after my son Noah was born in 1989 I also was not well, but at the time I was under so much stress that I just did not attribute my ill health to anything except to having entered a doctoral program with a two-and-a-half-month preemie slung across my front. Two months of bed rest for preterm labor prior to Noah's birth, and hospitalizations afterward because of complications with his health, had left me exhausted and dazed. Looking back further, I can remember times in college that I couldn't get out of bed, was incredibly irritable for weeks at a time, when my friends were strained beyond their capacity to bend with my brain chemistry.

Now, by the grace of God and help from psychotherapy and medicine, I have learned how to protect those around me from my depressive episodes and to prevent the shadows from damaging my relationships with family and friends. Some mentally ill folk use the illness as an excuse to lash out at loved ones. Some disown family and friends, either by running away or by severing relationships. Divorce is a ready exit from either side of the marriage when one partner is mentally ill. Especially in the case of bipolar sufferers, manic episodes with their impetuous affairs and drastic overspending can ruin marriages. Some abuse their family verbally and/or physically, blaming them for the sufferings of the self. Thanks be to God that I never was subject to any of this. When I was manic, my therapist kept a tight rein on me, seeing me every day if needed. The same was true when I was suicidally depressed. She even accepted phone calls in her off hours and figuratively held my hand through many a rough time.

My method of dealing with bipolar energies was to dance with my daughter, who would look at me with unbelieving delight, expecting a depressed mommy. I would garden. I would play the piano and sing at the top of my lungs all the show tunes I knew. This got rather loud and annoyed the children. I would avoid stores and thus the temptation to overspend. But being disciplined with oneself during this stage is very difficult; mania is almost defined by lack of discipline.

My method of dealing with depression was not to lash out but to retreat. When I was depressed I would curl up on our bed and sleep. I could sleep at any time of the day or night, and sleep soundly for hours. I would avoid the family, in part because the noise was so painful to me that I could not stand it and in part because I did not want to make others miserable by my presence. I did not understand at that time that my family and friends truly missed me. I later came to realize this and moved my nest from our bed to the living room as I improved. I was silent and still unable to move, but at least I was there, with the children and my husband.

This leads me to a warning about the children of the mentally ill. Children are often very sensitive and perceptive; they understand much more than we give them credit for. Parents must explain to their children what the nature of the problem is, or the children may create scenarios in their minds that are worse than the realities of the situation. They may even blame themselves. My children pretended they were comfortable with Mommy's spiritual, psychological, and physical absences behind the door of the bedroom, but they became absolutely unhinged when I went into the hospital. Grades slipped, moods dropped. My son became more aggressive, and my daughter withdrew. My husband and I were so embarrassed at the hospitalization that we did not even tell teachers at the children's schools. This was a big mistake that at the time we did not recognize.

We had not prepared the children well enough for my first hospital stay and did not share the details with them. Children need communication at times even as horrible as these, but it must be judicious communication. Do not mention suicidal thoughts or gestures. Just something simple. "Mommy is sick. She is very sad. She needs to go to the hospital. She will get better and be home soon. The doctors will take good care of her." Even telling children that "Mommy has a brain disorder" is better than saying nothing, or than saying that her heart hurts. Children have heard about heart attacks and know how serious they are. Don't bring in half-truths for the sake of protecting the children. Speak matter-of-factly, quietly, calmly. Stress that the hospital is a good place for those who are sick.

When the children did come for a visit to the hospital, they became entirely unglued. They didn't like seeing people catatonic, jumpy, uncontrollable, nor did they like seeing me in such a pale state. My son decided deep in his eight-year-old brain that germs had caused these maladies, and he took to washing his hands obsessively for some time after that. He refused to return to visit me in the hospital. Of course I thoroughly understood. If I had been well, I wouldn't have wanted to be there either. Even though my husband had tried to make the whole situation positive by promising Happy Meals afterward, that first visit was not much of a success. However, the children and I did get to cuddle on the couch, which was very reassuring for all of us. Once again I could be Mommy, even at such a low energy point, and they could be children who weren't expected to suck it up for the sake of the outside world.

So family is very important. The support of a loving spouse is very comforting. My husband was the most loving and most patient partner I could ever imagine. I could never have asked for more. I would question how he was putting up with this blob of a me, or with the zippy version, with no in-betweens. The chores of the household fell on him: laundry, cooking, shopping, child minding. And he still had a full-time job, which he had to cut back. He is a helpmate given by the grace of God. What I would have done without his support and encouragement I shudder to think. Maybe my suicidal urges would have become reality: in many ways I owe my life to him.

My mother came to stay with the children and to help run the household while I was in the hospital. I don't remember how long she was with us, but it was not a short stint. She bore the yeoman's burden while I was in the hospital, cooking and cleaning and taking the children to school. This allowed Matthew to get his own work done and kept the children on a fairly even keel. I don't even remember any more than this, because that time is still fuzzy in my memory and according to my psychiatrist it will always be. Some things I remember quite clearly, and others I cannot recall at all.

Not only family but friendship is so important for the mentally ill. I think I might not have crashed so hard after Grace's birth if a particular close friendship had remained an important support in my life. A host of factors, including my symptoms of depression, which ironically she did not recognize even though her father too has bipolar disorder, tested my friend beyond the point of her ability to love me. Having that support knocked out from under me was a blow that I could not absorb at the time. In depression, it is as though you lack shock absorbers for the potholes, so that these make you bottom out easily. Friendship is very important for those with poor mental health, but it is *very* hard to be a true friend to someone in such a condition. It is just too difficult for some people, for some relationships.

> Even my best friend, whom I trusted,
> who broke bread with me,
> has lifted up her heel and turned against me.
>
> Psalm 41:9

One way to help your friends understand is, as with children, to explain calmly and objectively your diagnosis. I told my friend of my illness only years later. How could she want to be associated with such a groaning blob as I was? If I had told her why I was in such a state, I imagine now that she would not have been so impatient with me, but at the time I felt so alone I could not even reach out. I am not advocating telling everyone you know that you are ill; this is a challenge to handle as you see fit. But those who are closest to you should be warned that your behavior is different from usual and will be for a while, until the medicines get sorted out. They may even be able to help you with feedback. Tell your friends when you are on a new medicine and ask them to let you know how you seem after a few weeks. Do you seem outwardly peppier, with more energy, less grumpy?

Being on the receiving side of friendship is another matter, and sometimes a mentally ill person is capable only of the receiving end. Yet it can for this reason be extremely difficult to be the friend of someone with a mental illness. Often they are not very fun to be with, or they are so much fun that it makes you worry. It is hard to stick with a person who has no conversation to make, no desire to go out with you, eat with you, talk to you.

How can friends of mentally ill patients show their support? Personally, I hated having people ask me how I felt, because I was trying very hard to be OK and didn't want anyone noticing that I was not well. This is, however, not the case for everyone. Reaching out to the mentally ill will least be appreciated as a token of friendship and concern. One suggestion is simply to ask the patient how you can help. What can you do? The most helpful things for me were the meals, the offers to do a load of laundry or take care of the children for the afternoon. Even though I often did not accept these offers because of a misplaced sense of pride, which depression can foster, knowing that someone cared enough to offer was a source of encouragement.

The friends who were present in their concern but did not demand anything of me were helpful. This meant sometimes not communicating for weeks or months, when I was incapable of conversation. During my hospitalizations, I generally asked friends not to visit. I was too embarrassed. I think I would approach this differently were I to be hospitalized again. It might have lessened the monotony for me and also might have helped my friends not to worry so much.

But frankly, I wondered throughout the time whether

I had any friends at all. This was not because of my friends but because of the nature of my illness. While in mania, I felt that everyone loved me and found me scintillating; indeed I found myself scintillating. However, in depression you cannot imagine that anyone would really love you, want to be there for you, find you still worthy of friendship and love. Truly darkness seemed my only companion. Of this I was quite convinced.

One very important way to help your friends who suffer from mental illness is to pray for them. The assurance that people were praying for me, since I had so much trouble praying for myself, was a salve. My true friends during this time were the ones I knew were praying for me. It can be very difficult to pray for someone day in and day out, over and over again, especially when you see little improvement, when you feel like a scratched CD uttering the same phrases over and over, like the woman who pounded and pounded on the door of the judge: "Grant me justice against my opponent" (Luke 18:3). Even so, this was so vital for me. I do not mean to say that the *idea* of people praying for me was a great comfort, although I do suppose this is true to an extent. I mean the *fact* that people were praying for me was key in my dealing with my illness. In other words, it is not just that I was touched that people would think of me. Prayer is more than merely thinking of someone, even though it does involve thought. My point here is that I believe in the efficacy of prayer, in God's pleasure at hearing our desires and needs and providing for that which we seek in prayer. That many people were knocking on God's door for me strengthened me in putting up with the disease and sped the healing, even though the full healing was years in coming. Maybe it would never have come if people had not been praying.

68 Psychology as Faith

Robert Coles

At various moments in these columns I have made snide references to the secular idolatry which it has been the fate of psychology and psychiatry to become for so many of us. My wife and our sons have suggested I spell out some of my thoughts on this subject, hence this essay. I must say that I speak as one of the gullible, the susceptible, the all too readily devotional — having put in years of teaching in medicine and pediatrics, in psychiatry and child psychiatry, in psychoanalysis, and done so with an eagerness and zeal and self-assurance, if not self-importance, I have yet to shake off, no matter these words, and others I'll write before I go to meet my Maker. "Once smitten, for life smitten," as a teacher of mine in high school used to say, and how we mocked his arrogant determinism, we who were so sure that no one or nothing would get its teeth into us unless we rationally and with utterly independent judgment had decided that such be the case.

In fact, I think we need to know why that teacher's observation does so commonly turn out to be true — the intellectual and psychological, and not least, social and economic "investment," so to speak, we make in what amounts to a way of thinking, as well as a career. The issue, as always, is pride, the sin of sins. To be a psychiatrist in America today, one says with all the risks of even more pride, of narcissism, is to take a substantial risk with one's spiritual future, as Anna Freud obliquely declared in one of her books (*Normality and Pathology in Childhood*). There she rendered a chronicle of the unblinking credulity accorded any and every psychoanalytic assumption, however tentatively posited; and as she said more bluntly to a few of us at Yale Medical School in a meeting both instructive and unsettling during the mid-1970s: "I do not understand why so many people want us to tell them the answers to everything that happens in life! We have enough trouble figuring out the few riddles we are equipped to investigate!"

Well, of course, she *did* understand only too well what has happened, especially in America: the mind as a constant preoccupation for many people who are basically agnostic, and who regard themselves as the ultimate, if passing, reality — which preoccupation constitutes a socially and historically conditioned boost to the egoism or

---

From Robert Coles, *Harvard Diary: Reflections on the Sacred and the Secular* (New York: Crossroad, 1984), pp. 92-94. Used with permission of the Crossroad Publishing Company.

narcissism we all must confront in ourselves. The result is everywhere apparent: parents who don't dare bring up their children, from infancy on, without recourse to one expert's book, then another's; students who are mesmerized by talk of psychological "stages" and "phases" and "behavioral patterns" and "complexes"; grown-up people who constantly talk of an "identity crisis" or a "mid-life crisis"; elderly men and women who worry about "the emotional aspects of old age," and those attending them at home or in the hospital who aim at becoming versed in steering the "dying" through *their* "stages" or "phases"; newspaper columnists, if not gurus, and their counterparts on television who have something to say about every single human predicament — the bottom line being, always, a consultation with a "therapist"; and worst of all, the everyday language of our given culture, saturated with psychological expressions, if not banalities, to the point that a Woody Allen movie strikes one not as exaggeration, caricature, or satire, but as documentary realism.

Especially sad and disedifying is the preoccupation of all too many clergy with the dubious blandishments of contemporary psychology and psychiatry. I do not mean to say there is no value in understanding what psychoanalytic studies, and others done in this century by medical and psychological investigators, have to offer any of us who spend time with our fellow human beings — in the home, in school, at work, and certainly, in the various places visited by ministers and priests. The issue is the further step not a few of today's clergy have taken — whereby "pastoral counseling," for instance, becomes their major ideological absorption and the use of the language of psychology their major source of self-satisfaction. Surely we are in danger of losing our religious faith when the chief satisfaction of our lives consists of an endless attribution of psychological nomenclature to all who happen to come our way.

I am tired, for instance, of the unwarranted, undeserved acquiescence some ministers (and alas, recently, priests as well) show to various "experts" who tell them about important "relationships" (talking about psychological jargon) and about "mental health" (whatever *that* is) and about the supposed "value" of religion (the height of condescension) in a person's so-called "psychic economy." I am tired of watching ministers or priests mouth psychiatric pieties, when "hard praying" (as I used to hear it put in the rural South) is what the particular human being may want, and yes, urgently require. I am tired of all the "value-free" declarations in the name of what is called "social science"; tired, too, of the complexities, ambiguities, and paradoxes of our moral life being swept into yet another "developmental scheme," with "stages" geared to ages.

As Walker Percy reminded us, and we ought to keep reminding ourselves, one can "get all A's and flunk life" — meaning one can answer some psychological theorist's hypothetical moral scenarios brilliantly in a given office or research setting, and then go into this world of sin and drive a car like an arrogant murderer, or push ahead in dozens of other ways that any moment may provide.

Back in the 1930s a host of brilliant people, including psychiatrists, psychologists, physicians, and alas, philosophers, ministers, and priests made their various accommodations, if not scandalous agreements of support, with the Nazis. Those highly educated ones might have scored well in some psychological theorist's "scale" of moral development; might have obtained good results in a Rorschach test, in a TAT test; might have mastered the Minnesota Multi-Phasic examinations; might have gotten top scores in our SAT tests given prospective college students; might have been pronounced in possession of "stable personalities" by an examining psychiatrist — all too "stable," they were, all too in resonance with that much touted "reality principle," namely Hitler's murderous authority.

Dietrich Bonhoeffer was a singular person indeed, and when he blasted psychology and psychiatry, as he did in his prison letters, we ought to take sharp notice. (We ought to take sharp notice, too, of efforts to stifle criticism of aspects of psychology or psychiatry. When such criticism gets called "resistance," or a mark of a "problem" — then an ideology is at work; agree with us or be banished!) Bonhoeffer, it seems, was prophetic not only with respect to his nation's tragedy in the 1930s and early 1940s, but also with respect to the continuing threats which certain aspects of 20th-century Western thinking pose to people of religious faith.

69 Between the Priestly Doctor and the Myth of Mental Illness

Ian S. Evison

What should be the relationship of psychiatry to social ethics? Should psychiatry seek to be value neutral, to base its judgments wholly on scientific criteria? Or should psychiatry — must psychiatry inevitably — seek to promote a determinate view of the good person and the good society? Psychiatry has struggled with this problem since the beginnings of the profession in North America in the nineteenth century. Psychiatry has found itself involved in each great social conflict in the past century and a half. Before the Civil War, psychiatrists discussed whether *drapetomania,* slaves running away from their masters, was a mental disease (Cartwright 1851, 707). During the suffragette campaigns of the late nineteenth century psychiatrists discussed whether the discontent of women was a form of "nervousness" that might be remedied by a "rest cure" (Gilman [1892] 1980). During the Vietnam war, psychiatrists discussed how to cure the "inappropriate" reluctance of soldiers to go into battle (Bloch 1969). And during recent revisions in the standard diagnostic manual, the DSM-III psychiatrists have classified smoking as an illness and no longer refer to homosexuality as an illness.

During some periods, psychiatry has been confident that it finally has disentangled itself from social ethics, yet retrospectively it is hard to say that this was so. What is notable is the correlation between periods when psychiatry has been confident about its ethical neutrality, and periods when the nation has been complacent about the ethical virtue of existing social arrangements. Since every movement from abortion to women's liberation has turned up new insights about the ethical presuppositions of psychiatric diagnosis, the conclusion is unavoidable that the entanglement of psychiatry with ethics is permanent.

Yet it is an empty victory simply to force upon psychiatry the realization that judgments concerning mental illness have an ethical core. For psychiatry has at the same time a need to establish itself as independent of ethical entanglement. Nor is this drive based simply on Cartesian anxiety concerning relativism inherited from Western philosophic traditions (Bernstein 1983, 16-17). It also arises from the concrete exigencies of practice. Reliable and responsible ways to make difficult decisions need to be found.

Is there a third option beyond both the improbable claim to be ethically neutral and the impractical suggestion that psychiatry resign itself to relativism? Will psychiatry drown in indeterminacy if it lets go of the claim to be purely scientific? My aim in this paper is to describe such a "third option." To establish it, I propose to use practical theology and its reflection on the affirmations of ultimate concern of a community in terms of their implications for the goals, norms, and means of practice. In particular, I hope to show that, although the basic orienting goals of psychiatric practice cannot be determined by empirical technical reasoning, this does not mean that the ends must remain indeterminate: our choices concerning ultimate ends (*theo*) can be informed, if not determined, by reasoned discussion (*logy*). In this reasoned discussion, theological ethics plays a central role (Tracy 1977, 88).

A way to balance the ethical dependence and independence of psychiatry — I will argue — is to see the orienting goal of psychiatry as a minimum one of promoting "basic human functioning." A psychiatry that understood itself as in service of such a basic goal would be free from broader agendas of personal and social reform, and yet would have a solid base from which to develop limited self-critical and social-critical roles.

This paper is organized in three sections. In each I will bring into conversation representatives of the two tendencies in psychiatry that I have identified: Robert Lifton and Thomas Szasz, as representatives of activism and value-neutrality respectively. In the first section, I will sketch out an interpretation of the history of psychiatry broad enough to show how the historical arguments made by Lifton and Szasz are not simply contradictory, but rather are part of a larger whole. In the second, I will use the conversation between Lifton and Szasz to bring out the orienting world views of each. And in the third, I will add my own voice to the conversation as a mediation, arguing that each is partly right and that the profession of psychiatry should understand itself as serving the limited ethical end of *basic human functioning.*

The Social and Historical Context

The history of psychiatry has most often been written as an account of developing technologies of treatment; however, this view does not do justice to the complexity of the relationship of the professions to culture. The issues at stake are not narrowly technical. Lifton and Szasz each see part of this. The first task is to place their differing insights within a single larger history of the professions.

The psychiatrist who will serve in this paper as an example of activist psychiatry, Robert Lifton, found precedence for his ethically committed vision in the derivation of the word *professional.* Speaking of the struggle be-

From Don S. Browning et al., eds., *Religious and Ethical Factors in Psychiatric Practice* (Chicago: Nelson-Hall, 1990), pp. 131-57.

tween ethically committed and ethically neutral visions of the professions, Lifton commented:

> One source of perspective on that struggle was a return to the root idea of profession, the idea of what it means to profess. Indeed, an examination of the evolution of these two words could provide something close to a cultural history of the West. The prefix "pro" means forward, toward the front, forth, out, or into a public position. "Fess" derives from the Latin *fateri* or *fass,* meaning to confess, own, acknowledge. To profess (or be professed), then, originally meant a personal form of out-front public acknowledgment. And that which was acknowledged or "confessed" always (until the sixteenth century) had to do with religion: with taking the vows of a religious order or declaring one's religious faith. But as society became secularized, the word came to mean "to make claim to have knowledge of an art or science" or "to declare oneself expert or proficient in" an enterprise of any kind. (Lifton 1976, 165-66)

There is truth in Lifton's observation of the religious origins of the professions. Law and medicine arose in the twelfth and thirteenth centuries as specialties among the clergy (Ullman 1975; Berman 1985). We can still see the faint religious imprint in the fact that the word *professional* carries connotations of responsibility and seriousness as well as technical competence, and in the respect that people in the professions, especially in the "learned professions" of ministry, medicine, and law, command in areas far beyond their technical competencies.

Yet one must be careful. Lifton concluded that the idea of ethical neutrality is a later addition and a by-product of secularization. This is not so. The independence of the professions, if not their ethical neutrality in the modern sense, is as old as the dependence of the professions on the religious substance of the culture. The independence of the profession is rooted in the relationships of independence and dependence implicit in the covenanting between Yahweh and the people of Israel and in the covenanting of feudal lords and vassals in which suzerainty relationships were reaffirmed — relationships in which the vassals provided services to the lords in return for privileges. The professions by analogy were in service of God and society but had independent domains in which they were entitled to exercise stewardship.

This heritage has been mediated to us through the figures of the Protestant Reformation who translated the substance of the medieval understanding of the relationships of the professions to society by the concepts of *calling* and *vocation.* In the call is the origin of both a special dependence upon God of the one called and the legitimation of certain independent actions. The pervasive influence of these ideas has become well-known through Weber's *The Protestant Ethic and the Spirit of Capitalism.* Calvin's own summary in the *Institutes* captures the essentials:

> The Lord bids each one of us in all life's actions to look to his calling. For he knows with what great restlessness human nature flames, with what fickleness it is born hither and thither, how its ambition longs to embrace various things at once. Therefore, lest through our stupidity and rashness everything be turned topsy-turvy, he has named these various kinds of living "callings." Therefore each individual has his own post so that he may not heedlessly wander about throughout life. Now, so necessary is this distinction that all our actions are judged by it, often indeed far otherwise than in the judgment of human and philosophical reason. No deed is considered more noble, even among philosophers, than to free one's country from tyranny. Yet a private citizen who lays his hand upon a tyrant is openly condemned by the heavenly judge. (Bk. 3, ch. 10, sec. 6)

Secular occupations are "from God," and they imply a responsibility to society as a whole, yet not — as Calvin took pains to explain — an unlimited license to political activity. Also, contrary to the thesis that ethical neutrality is a by-product of secularization, it should be noted that Calvin gave solidly theological reasons for the independence from politics of people in secular callings.

In fact, so strong are Calvin's theological arguments against political involvement that one might ask whether he was condemning it completely. Within the concept of a "vocation" or a "profession" there is always a dialectic between involvement and detachment, and while Calvin stressed the detachment side of the dialectic, he did not destroy the dialectic itself. Calvin's statements against political involvement must be seen against the background of the debacle of the peasant's revolt in Münster in 1535, which raised the fear that the Reformation might lead to complete anarchy (Williams 1975, 378-81). When Calvin said cautionary things about political involvement by Christians, he was concerned that if involvement could be structured and limited, the possibility for both religious and political reform would be destroyed. He did not proscribe all political activity but only the questioning of the ultimate grounding or political organization of society.

The religious substance of the concept of calling in the professions dissipated with the rise of professional schools associated with universities in Paris, Berlin, and Bologna, and the general secularization of European culture in the seventeenth and eighteenth centuries. This resulted not in the loss of the wider responsibility of the professions, but rather in a transformation of it. For example, the privilege of wearing an academic robe implied a responsibility to the wider cultural heritage, transmitting, transforming, and applying the ethos of the culture in an evolving situation (Adams 1986, 269).

The rise of the professional associate in Anglo-Saxon cultures caused an important development in the dialectic of professional involvement in and independence from the wider culture. Thomas Hobbes called voluntary associations of all sorts "worms in the entrails of the sovereign": they made possible organized dissent by providing independent centers of legitimation and authority.

Yet the ultimate decision of our political system has been to allow and encourage such associations. They have been important vehicles for mediation and for making politically effective the involved yet detached nature of groups in society (Adams 1986, 276). The professional association is a further development in which voluntary associations representing professions receive quasi-governmental powers within certain spheres. In its special status, the professional association repeats the same dual identity: it is a private group, yet corresponding with its special privileges it has a special responsibility to society as a whole.

Although to be "professional" has always meant to have special technical knowledge (as the priest knowing the liturgy), this knowledge did not become what we think of as technical knowledge — empirically based and supported by massive technology — until comparatively recently. Nor was it seen as the exclusive source of legitimacy. A number of factors, including the explosive growth of science and technology in the later nineteenth and early twentieth centuries, contributed to an expanded understanding of a profession as a group of people defined by their technical ability to perform a task or provide a service. In fact this definition eclipsed the understanding of the broader cultural involvement of professions.

In Germany, the consolidation of the unified state and the concomitant development of a rationalized bureaucracy led to the understanding of the professions as serving particular limited duties in a larger structure. In England, development of laissez-faire mercantilism gave rise to an understanding of professionals as independent business people who dealt with clients on the basis of freely negotiated contracts. Thomas Szasz finds precedence for his views of value-neutrality in this era:

> Doctors and patients have come a long way since the nineteenth century, but we had better think twice before we conclude it has all been progress. It is of more than passing interest to note, in this connection, one of the definitions of the word *profession* in the *Oxford English Dictionary*. "A profession in our country," wrote a British gentleman named Maurice in 1829, "is expressly that kind of business which deals with men as men, and is thus distinguished from a Trade, which deals primarily for the external wants or occasions of men." Until recently, this criterion applied particularly to the practice of medicine and law, the relations between practitioners and their clients being based on mutual respect and trust and, of course, the studied avoidance of coercion. (Szasz 1987, 129)

While there are problems with this interpretation, Szasz is correct to turn to the era of the rise of British mercantilism for the antecedents to his views, including his opinion that the professional has no social roles aside from the services to individuals rendered in fulfillment of contracts (all other activities being without contract and hence, in his view, coercive).

The American professions were massively influenced by their German and British counterparts in the latter nineteenth and early twentieth centuries. The foreign impulses toward functionalism combined with domestic impulses, most notably the increasing pluralization of society that was occurring with massive immigration. Paul Starr has noted that the multiplication of nonstandard medical practitioners and the protection to incompetence provided by the anonymity of urban life led the medical establishment to assert a right to a monopoly on care (Starr 1982, 18). Further, in the increasingly pluralistic environment, ways were needed to serve people that were not dependent on commonality of culture or even language between professional and client. In medicine the triumph of the functional view was marketed by the publishing of the Flexner report in 1910, *Medical Education in the United States and Canada,* and the reorganization of the AMA in 1901.

The history of psychiatry in the later nineteenth and early twentieth centuries is both an example of these developments and a reaction against them. James Luther Adams, speaking from an acquaintance with Erikson and Fromm, said that "the appearance of the psychiatrist is itself a sign of the demand for professional men who are capable of a wider competence than is suggested by the term 'specialty of function.'" Yet Adams immediately questioned whether "the average psychiatrist has the professional training that fits him for his dealing with the basic questions of ethos having to do with the very meaning of life" (Adams 1986, 273). While the development of psychiatry can be interpreted as a reaction against the functionalization of medicine, it is also an example of it. The development of psychiatry testifies to the continued concern of the medical profession for something more than the narrowly functional, and it is also an extension of the functional view into new areas.

While it is tempting to interpret the history of the professions as one of inexorable increase in technical competence and functionalism, and to project this inexorable increase into the future (Ramsey 1970, xvi), this view is simplistic. It suggests that the only ethical challenge of the professions is to decide how to use new technologies. The complexity of the ethical challenge was highlighted at a recent conference in honor of the Flexner report ("Flexner and the 1990's: Medical Education in the 20th Century," University of Illinois at Chicago, June 10-11, 1986). The picture of medicine that emerged was one in which the technology of medicine would continue to develop, but in which the development of medicine as a whole would not be technology driven. It was pointed out that, in spite of popular views to the contrary, no "cures" to major diseases have been discovered since the polio vaccine in the 1950s and that researchers on the major "killer diseases" of cancer and heart disease hardly speak in terms of discovering "cures."

Psychiatrists have realized that the high hopes for "cures" to the major mental illnesses that accompanied the introduction of antipsychotic drugs and the resulting sharp reductions in population of mental institutions in the late fifties were inflated (Freedom et al. 1975, 1921). The mentally ill homeless today on the nation's streets are a guilty reminder that deinstitutionalization was not cure, and even has led some to question whether it is correct to speak of "cures" to mental illnesses at all.

The impulses towards functionalism in medicine that characterized the "Flexner Era" seem to be spent. If they are, it will mean that economic and social factors will drive medicine as much as technological ones. Social and preventive medicine will attain new prominence. It will mean also a new rapprochement between technical reasoning about means of accomplishing specific ends, and practical moral reasoning about how it is good to live.

Works that search out the historical conditioning and the ethical presuppositions of science have multiplied in recent decades (e.g., Kuhn 1970). While these works perform the hermeneutical task of showing the ethical and religious components of "scientific" ideas, few take the additional step of critically showing how the ethical or religious ideas can be evaluated. This is a crucial omission, since one of the reasons that professions in the late nineteenth century began to claim to be "value-free" was that they despaired of the possibility of ethical discussion in a pluralistic society. The insight that our ideas must depend on ethical presuppositions without the demonstration that our practices can depend on them is a counsel of despair. It leaves only the options of fideism and nihilism.

Having provided a broad cultural interpretation of the changing fortunes of the ethical dimension of the professions, I must immediately point out that one cannot go directly from an undertaking of the ethical dimension to practical decisions about what is to be done. The cultural situation is only one factor impinging on practice. The institutional roles of psychiatrists are evolving. Patient populations and the economics of psychiatric practice are changing. The technological base is developing. Yet, it is perhaps in such a complex situation that higher-level orienting perspectives for this profession become the most important.

The Contemporary Debate between Activist and Value-Neutral Psychiatry: Robert Lifton vs. Thomas Szasz

Two contrasting visions for psychiatry have in recent years fought for dominance: ethical commitment and ethical neutrality. To explore these positions and to help develop a mediating option I will bring representatives of these two tendencies into conversation in this section: Robert Lifton on the side of activist psychiatry and ethical commitments, and Thomas Szasz on the side of value neutrality. Although these two figures are alienated from much of contemporary psychiatry, they represent ideal types who embody significant tendencies in the profession.

Within psychiatry there is a significant undercurrent of belief that tends toward the view that "neuroses of society" produce individual neuroses and therefore psychiatrists must to some extent take responsibility for "treating" society as well as the individual. The implications of this activist view would enlarge psychiatry to almost priestly dimensions, giving the profession a role in writing ethical prescriptions for the good society. On the other hand, some believe that social problems will be generated as long as individuals are unregenerated. Taken to its extreme, this view implies that the only route to changing society is through changing individuals, and further, that one should only work to change individuals in the sense of seeking to restore or promote an ethically neutral quality of health. Most psychiatrists avoid both these extremes and claim that their concern is with something much less grandiose than whether ultimately society causes individual problems or individuals cause social problems. Yet, in order to explore the issues that exist between the activist and the value-neutral positions, I have not chosen people who represent this middle view. Like the doctor who waited for her patients to get sicker so that diagnosis would be easier, I have chosen, rather, two extreme cases. Although my purpose in this section is to point out the philosophical issues between the different prescriptions for change in the psychiatric profession, I do not mean to imply that the position of either Lifton or Szasz is without empirical grounding or that the existence of a philosophic dimension to their thought ipso facto brings into question its validity.

Robert Lifton

Robert Lifton has become known as a psychohistorian. Many of his books have been studies of individuals caught up in the dynamics of history. If one looks at how he interprets the actions of a specific person, it is easy to see the connection between the judgments he makes and his much broader views about human action and responsibility. His broader philosophical and ethical commitments and his related thoughts about the role of psychiatry are exemplified in his involvement in the defense of Patty Hearst.

Patty Hearst appeared to Lifton as a bland wisp of a woman caught up in terrorism. For him the analogy to the victims of Chinese brainwashing during the Korean war was clear. The *New York Times* reported his testimony:

> Prisoners of the Chinese, he said, were cut off from their past to make them reliant on their captors. Dr. Lifton said that in Miss Hearst's case the bank robberies cut her ties to the past. But he also said that "there was no ideological conversion" although her compliance with orders was "absolute."
>
> Finally, the prisoners returning to Hong Kong seemed to be confused and to want to indicate some remaining tie to the behavior and thought pattern set by their treatment, Dr. Lifton said.

> It was in that connection that he sought to explain another thing that has been a problem for Miss Hearst's defense: the clenched fist salute she repeatedly gave immediately after her arrest.
>
> "That is the sort of thing that I described as the last act of compliance among those coming back from China." (February 28, 1976, p. 32)

Lifton clearly believes that his ideas about people caught up in the dynamics of history could lead to insights of more general applicability:

> In my work . . . I found that studying an extreme situation such as that facing the survivors of the atomic bomb can lead to insights about everyday death, about ordinary people facing what Kurt Vonnegut has called "plain old death." Our psychological ideas about death have become so stereotyped, so limited and impoverished, that exposure to a holocaust like Hiroshima, or My Lai, or the entire American involvement in Indochina, forces us to develop new ideas and hypotheses that begin to account for some reactions we observe. (Lifton 1976, 29)

At the furthest reaches of generality these "new ideas and hypotheses" imply that the best way to understand human action generally is *as caught up in history.* As Lifton expressed it, the theme of death and the continuity of life became in his later work his controlling image (Lifton 1976, 61). This image became a "new paradigm" for understanding life (Lifton, 1976, 60).

Lifton asserted that, whereas in Freud's day the major psychological dynamics were repression and release of sexual energy, today the major dynamics are better understood in terms of the struggle of life against the forces of death (Lifton 1973, 20). He quoted Camus's character, the plague doctor, Dr. Rieux: "The task of life is to construct an art of living in times of catastrophe in order to be reborn by fighting openly against the death instinct at work in our history" (Lifton 1976, 116). Yet in stark contrast to the view of Camus, the struggle against the death instinct was not for Lifton a struggle of will, but of impersonal forces of life and death. The forces of life arise out of a mythic zone, which, quoting Eliade, he described as "the zone of the sacred, the zone of the absolute reality" (Lifton 1976, 145). The true principle of life is a principle of Protean transformation (Lifton 1961, 316). If Lifton thought the individual will has any significance, he did not discuss it. When he described the My Lai massacre there were no actors present, only embodiments of social forces. There was no massacre, only an "atrocity-producing situation," a combination of elements that were "inevitably genocidal" (Lifton 1973, 109).

> In all, it is not too much to say that the illusions surrounding an aberrant American quest for immortalizing glory, virtue, power, control, influence, and know-how are directly responsible for the more focused My Lai illusion. (Lifton 1973, 66)

Likewise, Patty Hearst is a tragic figure because "given who she was and what had happened to her, there was really no other path she could have taken" (Lifton as quoted by Szasz 1976a, 11).

In this understanding, the task of the doctor and of the good person generally becomes more the cure of a sick society than the cure of individuals:

> As a giver of forms the insurgent survivor must perforce become a leader. Dr. Rieux, the central figure of *The Plague,* is called upon to provide both medical and spiritual therapy. His antagonist is not only the plague itself, but the more general evil the plague stands for — "the feeling of suffocation from which we all suffered and the atmosphere of dread and exile in which we lived." (Lifton 1976, 120)

The role of a professional is to pro-fess. Doctors who claimed to be ethically neutral but provide "curative" treatment for soldiers who refuse to fight in an unjust war were for Lifton paradigmatic examples of those who would use the forces of life for the purposes of death.

Psychotherapy must be more than a means of curing the individual. When Lifton led group therapy sessions for Vietnam veterans, their aim was not so much to help individuals as to create new social arrangements and rejuvenate old ones.

> The rap groups have been one small expression . . . of a much larger cultural struggle . . . toward creating animating institutions. Whether these emerge from existing institutions significantly modified or as "alternative institutions," they can serve the important function of providing new ways of being a professional and of working with professionals. (Lifton 1976, 161)

Like the stone the builders discarded, the Vietnam veterans became the cornerstone of the new society. "I want to raise the question of the significance of an important change undergone by a relatively small group of men for a larger change in human consciousness now sought from many sides" (Lifton 1976, 21).

Is this psychology or social philosophy? It is hard to say at what point this line is crossed, but it is also hard to avoid the resonances of this with such clear exemplars of social philosophy as John Winthrop's "City on a Hill." The Massachusetts Bay Colony, like the veterans' rap groups, was created as an "animating institution." It was created to regenerate Europe "weighted down with the weight of death." Both Lifton and Winthrop assumed that in a regenerated society individuals would be regenerated. Both ran into problems when this did not happen.

Looked at in historical perspective, Lifton's rap groups continue the communitarian theme in American social philosophy, which has been renewed in a myriad of forms from Brook Farm through the Owenite communities, the social settlement movement, the Pullman Community, the Great Society programs, and the communes of the sixties. In each there was the assumption that in the society was the salvation of the individual, and that the way to rejuvenate society was to create model institutions. All of these experiments ran into trouble over the fact that even in the most regenerate of social arrangements some people remained stubbornly unregenerate.

It is intriguing how Lifton, like many American communitarians, shares features with romanticism and its responses to Enlightenment rationalism. His reference to the Middle Ages as a time before rationalism (for Lifton before professional*ism*) had vitiated ability of the will to act with conviction, is reminiscent of romantic nostalgia for that era exemplified by Novalis's *Christianity and Europe* of 1799. Yet like Balzac in *The Quest for the Absolute,* Lifton does not denigrate the scientists but rather enlarges their role to almost priestly dimensions. The way Lifton emphasizes reason as symbol-making in the mythic realm, in contrast to discursive reason, also closely parallels the distinction Kant made and Coleridge developed between Understanding and Reason (*Verstand* and *Vernunft*). Further in common with romanticism, Lifton is deeply conscious that there is a dark and destructive side to what lies beyond consciousness (as shown in Schopenhauer's *The World as Will and Idea,* 1818). Patty Hearst is a tragic figure, not because of the terrible consequences of her choices but because she is helpless before forces greater than herself. Most basically, there is the affinity at the level of anthropology: for the romantics, the Enlightenment had made people the masters of their own fates at the price of emphasizing what Wordsworth termed the "inferior faculties" of reason, and at the price of cutting them off from access to the dimension of truth itself, the "principles of truth" (Baumer 1973, 203). Like Schopenhauer and Coleridge in their rebellions against Lockean and Humean empiricism, Lifton breaks out of rationalism at the price of reducing the function of the will to that of receptivity to the forces of the universe, thus losing a conceptual place for choice in his thought.

Thomas Szasz

Thomas Szasz is a perceptive critic of Lifton because his basic affinities of thought are precisely opposite. He agrees with Lifton that psychiatry hides its dependence on ethical presuppositions, but his view of what should be done about the problem is precisely opposite. Whereas Lifton proposes that psychiatry should become explicit about its ethical commitments, Szasz believes that any hope for psychiatry — and on the question of whether there is hope he has become ever more doubtful — rests in reestablishing psychiatry on a value-neutral basis. This opposition between Lifton and Szasz arises from diverse sources, starting with the fact that each takes different practical problems in professional practice as symptomatic of the problems of psychiatry in general, and ending with the fact that each draws upon a different stream of social thought and a different philosophic tradition. Whereas Lifton's orientation was towards the communitarian tradition of American social thought, and to romanticism, Szasz's orientation is towards individuals and the Enlightenment.

The task of sketching out the philosophic dimensions of Szasz's thought is both easier and harder than it was for Lifton. It is easier in that, while Lifton is rarely explicit or even conscious of how he draws on wider cultural resources, Szasz is both conscious and explicit. There is no need to conjecture about which philosophers he is indebted to. He tells us: Locke, Hume, and Mill (Szasz 1987, 354-55). However, the philosophic dimensions of Szasz's thought are also harder to trace than those of Lifton because, in spite of his voluminous writings, he rarely elaborates his own constructive proposals. Never an optimist, in recent years he has become bleakly cynical about the possibilities for change in psychiatry or society.

It is thus necessary to review the thinking of Szasz in two stages, first, to summarize his criticism of our representative of activist psychiatry, Lifton, and, second, to review Szasz's constructive position from such hints of it as can be found in the nooks and crannies of his work.

Whereas Lifton developed his position by reflecting on the role of psychiatrists in such world-transforming dynamics as war, Szasz began to develop his position by reflecting on the role of psychiatrists in involuntary hospitalization of mental patients and, slightly later on, what he decided was the mirror problem, the role of psychiatrists as court witnesses. His observation was that involuntary hospitalization had become a means by which society or a person's family could control behavior that was bothersome but not illegal. Likewise, the insanity defense became a means whereby a person could be excused for actions that were illegal. Both practices make end runs around fundamental principles of democratic government — that a person can be deprived of liberty only by a finding of criminal guilt in a public trial, and that a person who performs a criminal act will be held accountable.

Especially at the time he wrote his original work on the myth of mental illness, Szasz was making observations on which there was broad, if not universal, accord both in the psychiatric profession and in the general public. What was controversial about Szasz's position was his generalizations of his more limited observations.

He arrived at his sweeping conclusion that mental illness is a "myth" by roughly this chain of reasoning: hospitalization for mental diseases has been subject to abuse, whereas hospitalization for physical diseases has not. Hence is it logical to look for the cause of the abuse in the distinction between mental and bodily diseases. What is the distinction? Szasz noticed that there is a fundamental difference between saying that someone has mental disease and saying she has liver disease. This distinction is revealed in the nuance of language. When it is said that a person's liver is diseased, the presumption is that an examination of the liver could be made and some physical anomaly found; the same cannot be said concerning a mental disease. It might be possible to perform an operation on a person's brain and find a physical anomaly there, but then it would not be mental disease but brain disease. In fact, it is in the space between mind disease and brain disease that Szasz located the possibilities for abuse. To say that a person has a "diseased mind" is, he argued, like saying there is a disease in the body politic. It is a metaphor expressing disapproval of actions that we judge to be wrong.

> Illnesses of the body reflect a general consensus on the definition of health. However, the behavior which people come to criticize and view as mental illness is simply a disagreement on whether or not such a behavior should be permitted. (Szasz 1983, 218)

Nor does it change the metaphorical nature of the judgment that a relationship can at times be established between mental diseases and physical diseases.

When a psychiatrist says that someone is mentally "ill," she is making a value judgment. Yet psychiatrists claim to make purely empirical judgments:

> [I hold] that contemporary psychotherapists deal with problems of living, rather than mental illnesses, and their cures stand in opposition to a currently prevalent claim according to which mental illness is just as "real" and "objective" as bodily illness. This is a confusing claim since it is never known exactly what is meant by such words as "real" or "objective." I suspect, however, that what is intended by the proponents of this view is to create the idea in the popular mind that mental illness is some sort of disease entity, like an infection or a malignancy. . . . In my opinion, there is not a shred of evidence to support this idea. (Szasz 1960, 116)

For psychiatrists and their patients to act as though mental disease is real disease is a double impersonation in which a patient pretends to be sick and a psychiatrist pretends to give treatment.

Szasz pointed out that belief in mental illness, or at least acting as if one believed in mental illness, can function as belief in myth — hence his well-known claim that mental illness is mythical. From this follow his radical normative claims about the practices of psychiatry: since they are based on claims concerning "mythical" illnesses, neither involuntary hospitalization nor the insanity defense is ever legitimate, and psychiatry can be made legitimate, if at all, only by reestablishing it on a value-free foundation.

In saying this, Szasz does not intend to argue that the phenomena referred to as mental illness do not exist. "While I have argued that mental illnesses do not exist, I obviously do not imply that the social and psychological occurrences to which this label is currently attached also do not exist" (Szasz 1960, 11). His point rather is anthropological (Szasz 1983, 207, 227). He wishes to "criticize and counter a contemporary tendency to deny the moral aspects of psychiatry (and psychotherapy) and to substitute for them allegedly value-free medical considerations" (Szasz 1960, 116). "The problem with the medical model is that it disguises moral matters as medical" (Szasz 1983, 221).

How is morality disguised as medicine? Supposedly mental disease causes a person to lose the capacity of moral responsibility, much as multiple sclerosis causes loss of muscle control. In actuality the direction of the logic is precisely the reverse:

> Critical consideration of the connections between mental illness and responsibility thus points to a relationship of profound negation: as death negates life, insanity negates responsibility. It is not so much, as is commonly believed, that insanity diminishes or annuls the mentally ill person's capacity for responsibility; instead it is rather that our idea of insanity itself negates our concept of responsibility. Although it appears as if nonresponsibility were a condition separate from insanity but sometimes caused by it . . . in fact nonresponsibility and insanity are essentially synonymous. (Szasz 1983, 269)

The problem caused by the negation of responsibility is not only, or even primarily, injustice to individuals; at a more profound level the harm is that all are diminished as human beings.

The logic of determinism does not — Szasz argues — admit of distinctions. If one chooses to view life according to the logic of determinism, all free will becomes an illusion. Szasz quotes Freud:

> Many people, as is well known, contest the assumption of complete psychical determinism by appealing to a special feeling of conviction that there is free will. This feeling of conviction exists; and it does not give way before a belief of determinism. (However) . . . what is left free by one side receives its motivation from the other side, from the unconscious; and in this way determinism in the physical sphere is still carried out without a gap. (Szasz 1987, 243)

While psychiatrists may often think, like Freud, that they free people to love and to work, they instead promote a view of the human as determined. While claiming to extend the sphere of reason in human life, psychiatry extinguishes it in a revived doctrine of predestination.

Thomas Szasz's response to Lifton's testimony in the Hearst case began with this broadside:

> Dr. Robert Jay Lifton, professor of psychiatry at Yale University, testified (as he was quoted as saying in the *New York Times*) that Patty Hearst "came under the category that I wrote about in my book of the obviously confused about what had happened to her." In the style characteristic of the courtroom psychiatrist, he thus makes Hearst into a "case" about whose conduct he, the brainwashing expert, knows more than does the "patient" herself. Such psychiatric self-flattery is acquired at the expense of the patient's self-esteem, not to mention, in this case, her father's money. (Szasz 1976a, 11)

Lifton discussed a metaphorical disease, brain-washing, as if it were a literal disease and so transformed a discussion of whether what Hearst did was right or wrong into a discussion of whether she was sick or healthy. Szasz commented:

> The crucial question becomes: What is "brainwashing"? Are there, as the term implies, two kinds of brains: washed and unwashed? How do we know which is which?
>
> Actually, it's all quite simple. Like many dramatic terms, "brainwashing" is a metaphor. A person can no more wash another's brain with coercion or conversation than he can make him bleed with a cutting remark.
>
> If there is no such thing as brainwashing, what does this metaphor stand for? It stands for one of the most universal human experiences and events, namely for one person influencing another. However, we do not call all types of personal or psychological influences "brainwashing." We reserve this term for influences of which we disapprove. (Szasz 1976, 11)

In spite of this pointed criticism, Szasz was less concerned with the specifics of Lifton's testimony than with the principle that psychiatrists have no role in the courtroom. Such a role subverts the political system. This same criticism applied equally to Lifton's conclusion that My Lai was "an atrocity-producing situation," and to any conclusion that a person's actions are caused by social forces. Lifton was able to uncover the "fact" that actions are determined because he had assumed it.

However, Szasz's position was not simply a psychiatric version of law-and-order politics. His point was more fundamental: it is dangerous to excuse someone on the basis of lack of moral responsibility. This danger is evident if we note the affinity between how Lifton excused Patty Hearst's actions and how her father dismissed them — just as he dismissed the views of Patty's mother and of women in general as childlike (Weed 1976).

Another plausible psychological interpretation of Patty's "conversion" to that of her captors was that she wanted to force her father to take her seriously. If this was so, Lifton's "defense" that she was not responsible for her action was a cruel extension of her father's and society's sexism. As Szasz has said:

> That this psychiatric-psychoanalytic view on responsibility encourages lay people to be irresponsible and physicians to be paternalistic is obvious and requires no further comment. Perhaps because it is less obvious, people often do not realize that relieving a person of his responsibility is tantamount to relieving him, partly or entirely, of his humanity as well. The person who claims that he, not his brother, is responsible for his brother's welfare and happiness, stabs at the very heart of his brother as a person. (Szasz 1987, 245)

The insight has not been lost on oppressed groups that it is a short step from being excused on the basis of not being responsible for one's actions, to being dismissed as not fully human.

What has Szasz accomplished with his critique? Although he has not proven that action is free, he has refuted the opposing position advocated by Lifton. Thus, he has made two important contributions. First, he has shown, from a different, less sympathetic angle, what was said in my earlier discussion of Lifton's position: that in building his position Lifton must have drawn from sources other than empirical observation. I would not say that this fact invalidates Lifton's position, but I do agree heartily that Lifton did something other than deduce conclusions from evidence. However, I would put the case more positively, saying that in Lifton's position there is an interplay between empirical and philosophical perspectives. This does not mean that the involvement of psychiatrists in the judicial process, which Lifton advocates, is completely illegitimate, but we do need a discussion of whether such hybrid practical moral conclusions have grounds for legitimacy.

The second way in which Szasz's critique advances the discussion is to suggest the need for a second look at Szasz's own position. If he has not proven that actions are free on the basis of deductions from empirical evidence, then what is the source of this conclusion? It emerges that there is just as much of a dialectic between empirical observations and world view for Szasz as there is for Lifton. Whereas the communitarian stream of social thought and romanticism inform Lifton's work, individualism and Enlightenment rationalism mediated through laissez-faire perspectives inform Szasz.

It remains to investigate Szasz's own constructive position. Although this position appears only infrequently in his work, and hardly at all in his most recent publications, it is decisively important if we are to understand the commitments which lie behind his critiques. He presents himself as wanting simply to establish the truth by exposing falsehood, yet he is guided in decisive ways in his pursuit of these goals by broader visions of the good person and the good society.

Szasz's observation that specific actions are not determined shades into a more general conclusion: the world is a place in which actions are free.

> Man's actions represent free choices for which he is responsible, but for which he may rhetorically seek to avoid responsibility, most prominently through attributing behavior to literal and/or figurative gods. The traditional Judeo-Christian monotheistic god would be an example of the former, while physicians might be classified as the latter.
>
> The crucial moral characteristic of the human condition is the dual experience of freedom of the will and personal responsibility. (Szasz 1983, 23-24)

Szasz seems blind to the fact that the *will* is "mythical" in the same sense he argued *mind* or *mental illness* to be. Luckily for him this does not mean that *free will* is necessarily an illegitimate concept, but only that it is philosophically rather than empirically based, and is connected with a broader philosophical point of view.

Szasz's understanding of action as free is connected with his understanding of the struggle of reason against irrationalism.

> Man's awareness of himself and of the world about him seems to be a steadily expanding one, bringing in its wake an ever larger burden of understanding. . . . This burden, then, is to be expected and must not be misinterpreted. Our only rational means of lightening it is more understanding, and appropriate action based on such understanding. The main alternative lies in action as though the burden were not what in fact we perceive it to be and taking refuge in an outmoded theological view of man. (Szasz 1960, 177)

The hero of this world view is the person who takes on the burden of understanding, aware of her limits, content with the slow gains of reason, and steadfastly refusing blandishment of the "theological view of man" and its successors. For Lifton, the paradigmatic examples of human wrongdoing are the psychiatrists who use the forces of life to promote war. But for Szasz, the chief examples are the psychiatrists who are the successors to the historic opponents of free will: the theologians and priests.

Recently Szasz has become so cynical about the alliance of psychiatry and medicine with the forces of determinism and irrationalism that he rarely mentions his ideals for psychiatry. However, he did indicate his vision for the profession in his early works. In *The Ethics of Psychoanalysis* Szasz proposed a vision of psychiatry that he called "autonomous psychotherapy."

> I chose this expression [autonomous psychotherapy] to indicate the paramount aim of this procedure: preservation and expansion of the client's autonomy. To emphasize the nature of the therapeutic method, rather than its aim, the procedure could also be called "contractual psychotherapy"; the analyst-analysand relationship is determined neither by the patient's "therapeutic needs" nor by the analyst's "therapeutic ambition," but rather by an explicit and mutually accepted set of promises and expectations, which I call "the contract." (Szasz 1965, 7)

The contract for Szasz was not one feature of therapy, but rather its essence. The ability to keep a contract became for him both the goal of therapy and the definition of health:

> In large part, the analysis of the analytic situation is the analysis of the contract. A contractual agreement, by its very nature, may be broken in one of two ways: by underfulfilling or by overfulfilling one's obligations. These two types of contract violation correspond, roughly, to the characterological postures of the person who exploits and the one who allows himself to be exploited. To an extent, the former is typical of the so-called oral-demanding, or greedy, individual or of the sadist, and the latter, of the so-called mature, or generous person or of the masochist. (Szasz 1965, 191)

The ability to give fair measure — the ultimate commercial virtue — is the norm of health. Self-sacrifice — except as it is required to precisely fulfill contractual obligations — is not only a questionable good; it is positively a vice. By this extension of his logic, Szasz revealed that "ethically neutral" is not ethical neutrality. If Szasz wants psychiatrists to stand above the fray of moral disagreements, and above the efforts to improve society, it is so as to be more visible as a beacon pointing beyond them:

> Perhaps the relationship between the modern psychotherapist and his patient is a beacon that ever-increasing numbers of men will find themselves forced to follow, lest they become spiritually enslaved or physically destroyed. (Szasz 1961, 310)

"Autonomous" psychotherapy produces the prototype of the good person and the psychotherapeutic relationship is the norm of all relationships.

Szasz's image of the good person was also an image of the good society, since he presumed, as all advocates of *laissez-faire* must to remain consistent, that there is a preestablished harmony of interests:

> In a modern society, based more on contract than on status, the autonomous personality will be socially more competent and useful than his heteronomous counterpart. Moreover, and very significantly, autonomy is the only positive freedom whose realization does not injure others. (Szasz 1965, 22)

If only each person would act autonomously, the best result would be achieved for all. To accept the notion that one person can hurt another by pursuit of self-interest is, Szasz concluded, like accepting the notion that "a sadist is one who refuses to hurt a masochist" (Szasz 165, 23).

This is the Enlightenment as it filtered through Locke, Hume, and Mill, and even more directly into the American experience through Emerson. The standard of good becomes the good inside, and doing anything other than realizing this is betrayal:

> Nothing is at last sacred but the integrity of our own mind. . . . On my saying, "What have I to do with the sacredness of traditions, if I live wholly from within?" my friend suggested — "But these impulses may be from below, not from above." I replied, "They do not seem to me to be such, but if I am the devil's child, I will live then from the devil." No law can be sacred to me but that of my nature. (Emerson 1899, 47-48)

When developed to this point, autonomy is more than a good. It has swallowed up the good.

The social ideal of *laissez-faire* individualism has traveled a crooked course from the eighteenth century, when it was the battle cry of the middle class against aristocratic privilege, to the nineteenth century, when it reversed its meaning to become the battle cry of the robber barons against social legislation. The dictum that each is entitled to the fruits of his labors came to mean whoever has got it must deserve it. Emerson's "Self-Reliance" became William Graham Sumner's succinct answer to the question of what social classes owe to each other: nothing (Sumner [1883] 1986). Not only is social activism not morally obligatory, it is a disruption of social laws, what Szasz called "coercion," and what Sumner called "social meddling." Whereas Lifton's ideal of the professional was someone who pro-fesses, Szasz's ideal is of a professional who at all costs avoids doing so.

Lifton's and Szasz's views of the relation of professionalism to ethics are two parts of an earlier dual concept. Robert Lifton's understanding of the professions, as committed to sustaining and transforming the ethical vision of culture, is a distant relative of the view that callings are from God and of the understanding expressed in such customs as the wearing of academic robes by professionals. Thomas Szasz's understanding of the professions as independent from ethics is similarly related to theological understandings of the independence of those who practice a calling within an appointed domain of stewardship. There is a family resemblance between Calvin's view that we each serve God best by sticking to our individual callings, and Szasz's view that society profits most when each person sticks to a policy of noninterference.

Furthermore, these differing views of the professions are rooted in differences in basic anthropology. In *The Nature and Destiny of Man,* Reinhold Niebuhr has shown how romantic understandings of the human as determined and rationalist understandings of the human as free are by-products of the breakup of classic theological understandings of the human as self-transcending. This basic theological understanding originates in an Augustinian concept of the human as made in the image of God. Paul Tillich, also drawing heavily on this Augustinian heritage, described determinism and free will as a basic polar opposition in the ontological structure of the human. As Tillich described it, free will and determinism, or freedom and destiny, exist in dialectical relationship. Destiny is a structured aspect of myself and my environment that makes me who I am. It is the concreteness out of which decisions arise. Freedom, on the other hand, is the structure of destiny made real (Tillich 1951, 182-86).

Yet this view contains a danger. To say that two divergent tendencies in the understanding of the relationship of ethics to the professions are the "broken halves" of a classic theological understanding of calling or vocation points prematurely to a normative solution. Even if the two tendencies were once held together in classical theological formulations, this does not mean that they can be, or should be, again. It still needs to be argued that those theological concepts meet contemporary demands, particularly the demand that they be compatible with radical pluralism.

The reasons for this go beyond the fact that arguments based on the authority of a particular religious tradition are unlikely to succeed in a public forum. There are theological objections to any proposal that replaces the present with the past. History moves forward, not only chronologically but also theologically. Lifton and Szasz have done more than move away from theological understandings of vocation; they have advanced those understandings — and have done so for compelling reasons. Given this, can classic traditions of reflection still serve as guides?

Solution

Can a theological concept help guide our understanding of the relationship between ethics and the professions? In the 1820s, de Tocqueville observed that in America a distinguishing feature of public life was the way theological, and explicitly Christian, presuppositions guided public discourse: "Christianity reigns without obstacles, by universal consent; consequently, everything in the moral field is certain and fixed, although the world of politics is given over to argument and experiment" (*Democracy in America* [1835, 1840] 1969, 292, as quoted in Bellah 1986, 80).

Yet, in spite of what de Tocqueville said, the question of the proper role of such concepts is perennial. A generation ago John Dewey, John Courtney Murray, and Walter Lippmann all argued the need for a public philosophy which, if it were not quite a public theology, would be at least informed by particular cultural traditions. As Bruce Kuklick has argued, neither Lippmann nor Dewey quite managed to do public philosophy without doing public theology (Bellah 1986, 82), and, of course, Murray did not argue that one should try. Although Lippmann, Dewey, and Murray disagreed on the substance of a public theology, Murray's statement of the need for one speaks for all three.

> And if this country is to be overthrown from within or from without, I would suggest that it will not be overthrown by Communism. It will be overthrown because it will have made an impossible experiment. It will have undertaken to establish a technological order of most marvelous intricacy, which will have been constructed and will operate without relations to true political ends; and this technological order will hang, as it were, suspended over a moral confusion; and this moral confusion will itself be suspended over a spiritual vacuum. This would be the real danger resulting from a type of fallacious, fictitious, fragile unity that could be created among us. ("Return to Tribalism," *Catholic Mind,* January 1962, as cited in Neuhaus 1984, 84)

The issue has surfaced again recently, first in Solzhenitsyn's Harvard speech, and then in Richard Neuhaus's *The Naked Public Square.* Yet there remains the suspicion that those who have been most strident in their criticisms have not understood fully the legitimate claims of pluralism. This is certainly true for Solzhenitsyn, whose own view of public life is both theocentric and Christocentric.

There is a group who would argue that "public theology" is an oxymoron. Or, rather, there are two groups who have historically opposed the concept of a public theology. Channing first observed that the extreme secularists and the extreme religionists come together to support the notion that if an issue is not resolvable by narrowly empirical means, then it is not amenable to rational discussion at all (Channing 1849, vol. 3, 66). William James similarly observed the affinities between narrow empiricists and supernaturalists (James [1902] 1925, 19).

Does theology have a place in public discussion? Szasz stressed the human capacity for choice; Lifton stressed what lies outside the human choice. Each criticized religion for including in its understanding of the human that part of the dual understanding that he excluded. Tillich commented that in the contradiction between free will and determinism, reason looks into its abyss. Whether to view the human as a creature of reason or as a creature of vitality cannot be decided by theoretical reason or reduced to narrowly empirical terms.

A characteristic of classic theological understandings of the human is that they have held together free and determined aspects of the human spirit. Even when the human capacity for choice has been emphasized least, voluntaristic elements have been retained in theological discussion. There has rarely, if ever, been a time without general agreement that human beings must be recognized as responsible. This has not been simply a political necessity of a ruling power. It has also been an insight held most tenaciously when the church was most oppressed. The reason for this is one that Szasz accurately recognized: to be "understood" in the sense of being held to be not responsible is also to be dismissed, or regarded as not fully human.

In affinity with Lifton, an appreciation of the limitations of the will has also been part of classic theological understandings. The human capacity for choice is limited first by physical limitations and by habit, but more profoundly we are limited by internal divisions of the will that the apostle Paul referred to when he said, "what I would, that I do not; but what I hate, that I do" (Romans 7:15).

Whatever the ultimate foundations of religious truth, a proximate norm for it must be that it accord with common human experience. The further limits of religious truth may be beyond rational discussion; yet there exists an arena of discourse that is authentically theological, but about which broadly empirical public discussions and evaluations are possible.

While no imposition of the understandings of a particular religious tradition can or should be made, it may be possible for the concept of the professions to be renewed by allowing itself to be instructed by both tendencies of the classic theological concept of calling. Such an understanding of the professions would borrow its form from the theological concept; yet its content would be independently justifiable as a mediation between such poles of thinking as are represented by Lifton and Szasz.

Psychiatry should not seek either to "base itself wholly on science" or to serve expansive visions of individual and social good, but should rather serve the admittedly ethical but limited goal of *basic human functioning.* Basic functioning is a basement concept on which can be built the more expansive ideas of virtue. It contains a rudimentary view of what it is to be a good person, but only in the minimal sense of a person whose actions could be discussed as good or bad. It is a goal defined formally as that norm which, when violated, brings into question the humanness of an action, not its morality, and materially as the community consensus refined by reflection and critique.

A psychiatry which served the goal of basic human functioning would not claim to be based purely on science, but it would still be scientific in a number of respects. It would include reasoning about how to achieve the end of adequate functioning, and about whether a person corresponds to the minimum concept of adequate functioning. Furthermore, it would retain the asceticism often characteristic of science in that it would hold itself back from direct participation in debates about more complete understandings of the nature of the good person and the good society. Psychiatry has been accused of a poverty of ends. In the understanding I am proposing, psychiatry would make this fault a virtue, taking a "vow of poverty" concerning ends, practicing an ascetic attitude concerning larger visions of individual and social good, and making use of only that which is necessary for practicing its own vocation.

Yet this understanding of psychiatry could also be instructed by Lifton's side of the concept of calling. It could say, when asked to treat a soldier who would not fight, that it could serve the larger end of combat effectiveness of the unit only by serving the narrower end of basic functioning. To the extent that soldiers who were capable of basic functioning still chose not to fight, psychiatry would have no role in convincing them to change their minds. Likewise, psychiatry could not say anything about the metaphysical validity of religious beliefs, but would be able to say that particular religious practices undermined the capacity for basic functioning. Thus, although such a psychiatry could not follow Lifton in his larger demand that psychiatry help build the good society, it could contribute to a social good greater than the sum of its contribution to the adequate functioning of individuals.

Such an understanding of the role of psychiatry as serving a limited but authentically moral end, is in keeping with its position as a profession. A profession organizing itself into a voluntary association, such as the American Psychiatric Association, occupies a mediating function in society (Adams 1986, 268). Unlike a political party or a religious denomination, a professional association has a fiduciary responsibility to society as whole. Because of the fact that it is a private organization, not directly regulated by the government, and yet has a larger public role, one could argue that it rightfully should be conservative in the ends it chooses to serve. Such an end as adequate functioning is one that would allow psychiatry to serve both its narrower and its larger roles in society.

In the specific case of Patty Hearst, psychiatry would be able to testify concerning how her actions corresponded to a norm of adequate functioning. However, it could not make the kinds of global claims that Lifton made at the trial. It would need to recognize that in entering the courtroom it had entered an area beyond its fiduciary responsibility. Such a position in fact corresponds to the emerging self-understanding of the profession. The American Psychiatric Association has endorsed the position that psychiatrists should not be allowed to testify about "'ultimate issues' such as whether or not the defendant was, in their judgment, 'sane' or 'insane,' 'responsible' or not. . . ." (American Psychiatric Association 1982, 13). Even Szasz has suggested that within such bounds there may be a place for psychiatric testimony (Szasz 1983, 146).

The suggestion I make that adequate functioning become the governing norm of mental health has precedent in the American context. Richard Cabot, in a 1908 article entitled "An American Type of Psychotherapy," proposed a moral component to psychiatry that could be established on the basis of a broad social consensus; this is not altogether different from the concept of adequate functioning I propose (Cabot 1908, 7). His proposal did not win the day then, but may bear reconsidering now.

References

Adams, James L. 1986. *Voluntary Associations: Socio-cultural Analyses and Theological Interpretation.* Chicago: Exploration Press.

American Medical Association. 1983. "The Insanity Defense in Criminal Trials and Limitations of Psychiatric Testimony." Report G of the Board of Trustees.

American Psychiatrist Association. 1982. *American Psychiatric Association Statement on the Insanity Defense.*

Baumer, Franklin L. 1973. "Romanticism." In *Dictionary of the History of Ideas,* pp. 198-204. New York: Scribner's.

Bellah, Robert N. 1986. "Public Philosophy and Public Theology in America Today." In *Civil Religion and Political Theology,* ed. Leroy S. Rouner. Notre Dame: University of Notre Dame Press.

Berman, Harold. 1985. *Law and Revolution: The Formation of the Western Legal Tradition.* Cambridge, Mass.: Harvard University Press.

Bernstein, Richard J. 1983. *Beyond Objectivism and Relativism.* Philadelphia: University of Pennsylvania Press.

Bloch, H. Spencer. 1969. "Army Clinical Psychiatry in the Combat Zone — 1967-1968." *American Journal of Psychiatry* 126, 3 (September): 289-98.

Cabot, Richard C. 1908. "The American Type of Psychotherapy." *Psychotherapy* 1, 1:5-13.

Calvin, John. 1966. *The Institutes of the Christian Religion* (1559). Volume 1. Philadelphia: Westminster Press.

Cartwright, Samuel A. 1851. "Report on the Diseases and Physical Peculiarities of the Negro Race." *New Orleans Medical and Surgical Journal,* May, pp. 691-715.

Channing, William E. 1849. *The Works of William E. Channing.* Boston: George G. Channing.

Emerson, Ralph Waldo. 1899. *Essays: First Series.* Philadelphia: Henry Alemus.

Flexner, Abraham. 1910. *Medical Education in the United States and Canada.* Bulletin no. 4. New York: Carnegie Foundation for the Advancement of Teaching.

Freedman, Alfred M., Harold I. Kaplan, and Benjamin J. Sadock, eds. 1975. *Comprehensive Textbook of Psychiatry.* Second edition. Baltimore: Williams and Wilkins.

Gamwell, Franklin I. "Religion and Reason in American Politics." *Journal of Law and Religion* 2:325-42.

Gilman, Charlotte Perkins. 1892. "The Yellow Wallpaper." *New England Magazine,* January, pp. 3-20.

———. 1980. *The Charlotte Perkins Gilman Reader.* New York: Pantheon Books.

Ingleby, David, ed. 1980. *Critical Psychiatry: The Politics of Mental Health.* New York: Pantheon.

James, William. 1922. *Pragmatism: A New Name for Some Old Ways of Thinking.* London: Longmans, Green and Co.

———. 1925. *The Varieties of Religious Experience* (1902). New York: Longmans, Green and Co.

Kuhn, Thomas. 1970. *The Structure of Scientific Revolutions.* Chicago: University of Chicago Press.

Kuklick, Bruce. 1977. *The Rise of American Philosophy.* New Haven: Yale University Press.

Laor, Nathaniel. 1982. "Szasz, Feuchtersleben, and the History of Psychiatry." *Psychiatry* (November): 316-24.

———. 1984. "The Autonomy of the Mentally Ill: A Case Study in Individualistic Ethics." *Philosophy of Social Science* 14:331-49.

Lifton, Robert Jay. 1961. *Thought Reform and the Psychology of Totalism: A Study of Brainwashing in China.* New York: Norton.

———. 1961. *History and Human Survival.* New York: Random House.

———. 1967. *Boundaries: Psychological Man in Revolution.* New York: Random House.

———. 1973. *Home from the War: Vietnam Veterans, Neither Victims nor Executioners.* New York: Simon and Schuster.

———. 1976. *The Life of the Self: Toward a New Psychology.* New York: Simon and Schuster.

———. 1979. *The Broken Connection: On Death and the Continuity of Life.* New York: Simon and Schuster.

Maxim, Jerrold S. 1986. *The New Psychiatry.* New York: Mentor.

Neuhaus, Richard. 1984. *The Naked Public Square: Religion and Democracy in America.* Grand Rapids: Eerdmans.

Niebuhr, Reinhold. 1941. *The Nature and Destiny of Man: A Christian Interpretation,* Volumes 1 and 2. New York: Scribner's.

Ramsey, Paul. 1970. *The Patient as Person.* New Haven: Yale University Press.

Rouner, Leroy, ed. 1986. *Civil Religion and Political Theology.* Notre Dame: University of Notre Dame Press.

Schleiermacher, Friedrich. 1966. *Brief Outline on the Study of Theology.* Richmond, VA: John Knox Press.

Starr, Paul. 1982. *The Social Transformation of American Medicine.* New York: Basic Books.

Sumner, William Graham. 1986. *What Social Classes Owe to Each Other* (1883). Caldwell, ID: Caxton Printers.

Szasz, Thomas. 1957. "Commitment of the Mentally Ill: Treatment or Social Restraint?" *Journal of Nervous and Mental Diseases* 125:293-307.

———. 1960. "The Myth of Mental Illness." *American Psychologist* 115:113-18.

———. 1961. *The Myth of Mental Illness: Foundations of a Theory of Personal Conduct.* New York: Harper and Row.

———. 1963. *Law, Liberty, and Psychiatry: An Inquiry into the Social Uses of Mental Health Practices.* New York: Macmillan.

———. 1965. *The Ethics of Psychoanalysis: The Theory and Method of Autonomous Psychotherapy.* New York and London: Basic Books.

———. 1973. *The Manufacture of Madness: A Comparative Study of the Inquisition and the Mental Health Movement.* Frogmore, St. Albans: Granada Publishing Ltd.

———. 1976a. "Mercenary Psychiatry." *New Republic,* March 13, pp. 10-12.

———. 1976b. "Some Call It Brainwashing." *New Republic,* March 6, pp. 10-13.

———. 1977. *The Theology of Medicine: The Political-Philosophical Foundations of Medical Ethics.* Baton Rouge: Louisiana State University Press.

———. 1978. *The Myth of Psychotherapy. Mental Healing as Religion, Rhetoric, and Repression.* Garden City, NY: Anchor Press.

———. 1983. *Thomas Szasz: Primary Values and Major Contentions,* ed. Richard E. Vatz and Lee S. Weinberg. Buffalo: Prometheus Books.

———. 1987. *Insanity: The Idea and Its Consequences.* New York: Wiley.

Tillich, Paul. 1951. *Systematic Theology: Volume I.* Chicago: University of Chicago Press.

Tocqueville, Alexis de. 1969. *Democracy in America.* 1835, 1840. New York: Doubleday Anchor.

Tracy, David. 1977. "Revisionist Practical Theology and the Meaning of Public Discourse." *Pastoral Psychology* 26, 2 (Winter): 83-94.

Ullman, Walter. 1975. *Law and Politics in the Middle Ages.* Ithaca, NY: Cornell University Press.

Weed, Steven. 1976. *My Search for Patty Hearst.* New York: Crown.

Williams, George. 1975. *The Radical Reformation.* Philadelphia: Westminster Press.

70 Crazy in the Streets

Paul S. Appelbaum

I

They are an inescapable presence in urban America. In New York City they live in subway tunnels and on steam grates, and die in cardboard boxes on windswept street corners. The Los Angeles City Council has opened its chambers to them, allowing them to seek refuge from the Southern California winter on its hard marble floors. Pioneer Square in Seattle, Lafayette Park in Washington, the old downtown in Atlanta have all become places of refuge for these pitiable figures, so hard to tell apart: clothes tattered, skins stained by the streets, backs bent in a perpetual search for something edible, smokable, or tradable that may have found its way to the pavement below.

Riddled by psychotic illnesses, abandoned by the systems that once pledged to care for them as long as they needed care, they are the deinstitutionalized mentally ill, the detritus of the latest fashion in mental-health policy. The lucky ones live in board-and-care homes where they can be assured of their next meal; perhaps they have a place to go a few hours a week for support, coffee, even an effort at restoring their productive capacity. Those less fortunate live in our public places, existing on the beneficence of their fellow men and God. It is extraordinary how quickly we have become immune to their presence. Where we might once have felt compassion, revulsion, or fear, now we feel almost nothing at all.

There are times, of course, when the reality of the deinstitutionalized breaks through our defenses. Three days after the Statue of Liberty extravaganza in the New York harbor last July, in the shadow of the icon of huddled masses, a psychotic man ran amok on the Staten Island ferry, slashing at enemies in a war entirely of his own imagining. Two victims died. Investigations ensued. For a moment we became aware of the world of shelters and emergency rooms, a world where even those willing to accept help and clearly in need of it are turned away because the state has deliberately dismantled the system where they might once have received care. Briefly, the curious wondered, how did this come to be?

Like its victims, the policy of deinstitutionalization has been taken for granted. It is difficult to recall that mentally ill persons ever were treated differently. Yet the process that came to be called deinstitutionalization (no one knows when the term was coined) only began in the mid-1950's, and did not move into high gear until a decade later. Although the term itself suggests a unitary policy, deinstitutionalization has had complex roots, and at different times has sought diverse goals. Its failure, however, was all but preordained by several of the forces that gave it birth. Any attempt to correct the debacle that has attended the contraction — some might say implosion — of our public mental-health systems will require an understanding of those forces.

II

The idea that the states bear some responsibility for the care of the mentally ill was not immediately obvious to the founders of this country. Through the colonial and federalist periods, care of psychotic and other dependent persons was the responsibility of local communities. They responded then as many of them do today. Almshouses and jails were overrun with the mentally ill, who, though thrown together with the criminal, tubercular, and mendicant, were often treated with a cruelty visited on none of the others.

Change came in the second quarter of the 19th century. New interest was stimulated among a small number of physicians in a system of treatment of the mentally ill begun in a Quaker hospital in England and called "moral" care. The name — with its ironic allusion to the immorality that had governed most other efforts to deal with the mentally ill — denoted a therapeutic system based on the radical idea that the mentally ill were more like us than unlike. If they were treated with kindness, encouraged to establish order in their lives, given the opportunity to work at productive trades, and provided with models of behavior, their mental illnesses might dissipate.

The belief that the mentally ill could be treated, and thus need not be relegated to the cellars of local jails, was championed by Dorothea Dix, a spinster Sunday-school teacher from Massachusetts, who traversed the country, cataloguing the barbarities inflicted on mentally ill persons and petitioning legislatures to establish facilities where moral treatment might be applied. Her efforts and those of others resulted in the creation of a network of state-operated hospitals. As the states assumed ever wider responsibility for the mentally ill, the hospitals grew in size, absorbing the denizens of the jails and poorhouses.

In the wake of the Civil War, as the burdens created by waves of immigration stood unrelieved by increases in funding, the public hospitals surrendered the goal of active treatment. They continued to expand, but changed into enormous holding units, to which the mentally ill were sent and from which many never emerged. Once again sliding to the bottom of the list of social priorities, the mentally ill were often treated with brutality. At best, they suffered from benign indifference to anything more than their needs for shelter and food.

Such had been the condition of public mental hospitals for nearly eighty years as World War II came to a close. Periodic efforts at reform had left them largely untouched. Over one-half million patients languished in their wards, accounting for half of the occupants of hospital beds in the country. The state hospitals had swelled to bloated proportions. Pilgrim State Hospital on Long Island, New York's largest, held nearly 20,000 patients. St. Elizabeth's in Washington, D.C., the only mental hospital operated directly by the federal government, had its own railroad and post office. Most facilities, located away from major population centers, used patients to work large farms on their grounds, thus defraying a good part of the costs of running the institution.

A new generation of psychiatrists, returning from the war, began to express their disquiet with the system as it was. They had seen how rapid-treatment models in hospitals close to the front and the introduction of group therapy had drastically cut the morbidity of psychiatric conditions evident earlier in World War I. With the belief that patients need not spend their lives sitting idly in smoky, locked wards, they determined to tackle a situation which Albert Deutsch had described as the "shame of the states."

These psychiatrists and their disciples, emphasizing the desirability of preparing patients for return to the community, began to introduce reforms into the state systems. Wards that had been locked for nearly a century were opened; male and female patients were allowed to mix. Active treatment programs were begun, and many patients, particularly elderly ones, were screened prior to admission, with efforts made to divert them where possible to more appropriate settings. The effects soon became evident. More than a century of inexorable growth in state-hospital populations began to reverse itself in 1955, when the number of residents peaked at just over 558,000. The first phase of deinstitutionalization was under way.

A second factor was introduced at this point. In 1952, French scientists searching for a better antihistamine discovered chlorpromazine, the first medication with the power to mute and even reverse the symptoms of psychosis. Introduced in this country in 1954 under the trade name Thorazine (elsewhere the medication was called Largactil, a name that better conveys the enormous hope that accompanied its debut), the drug rapidly and permanently altered the treatment of severe mental illness. The ineffective treatments of the past, from bleedings and purgings, cold baths and whirling chairs, to barbiturates and lobotomies, were supplanted by a genuinely effective medication. Thorazine's limitations and side-effects would become better known in the future; for now the emphasis was on its ability to suppress the most flagrant symptoms of psychosis.

Patients bedeviled by hallucinatory voices and ridden by irrational fears, who previously could have been managed only in inpatient units, now became tractable. They still suffered from schizophrenia, still manifested the blunted emotions, confused thinking, odd postures that the disease inflicts. But the symptoms which had made it impossible for them to live outside the hospital could, in many cases, be controlled.

Psychiatrists still argue over whether the new ideas of hospital and community treatment or the introduction of Thorazine provided the initial push that lowered state-hospital censuses. The truth is that both factors probably played a role, with the medications allowing the new psychiatric enthusiasm for community-based care to be applied to a larger group of patients than might otherwise have been the case. The effects of the first stage of deinstitutionalization can be seen in the figures for patients resident in state psychiatric facilities. By 1965 that number had decreased gradually but steadily to 475,000.

III

Until the mid-1960's, deinstitutionalization had been a pragmatic innovation; its driving force was the conviction that some patients could be treated and maintained in the community. Although large-scale studies supporting this belief were lacking, psychiatrists' everyday experiences confirmed its validity. Further, control of the process of discharging patients was solidly in the hands of mental-health professionals. By the end of the first decade of deinstitutionalization, however, the process was in the midst of being transformed.

What had begun as an empirical venture was now about to become a movement. Deinstitutionalization was captured by the proponents of a variety of ideologists, who sensed its value for their causes. Although their underlying philosophies were often at odds, they agreed on what seemed a simple statement of mission: all patients should be treated in the community or in short-term facilities. The state hospitals should be closed.

Some of the earliest advocates of this position were themselves psychiatrists. Unlike their predecessors, who first let light and air into the back wards, these practitioners were not content to whittle away at the number of patients in state hospitals. They sought systemic changes. The pragmatism of the psychiatrists, persuaded on their return from the war that many patients could be treated without long-term hospitalization, was transmuted into a rigid credo. No patient should be confined in a massive state facility, it was now declared. All treatment should take place in the community.

These advocates, who saw themselves as part of a new subspecialty of community psychiatry, were heavily influenced by the sociologists of institutional life, notably Erving Goffman, the author of *Asylums*. The book, based on a year of observing patients and staff at St. Elizabeth's Hospital in Washington, D.C., catalogued the ways, subtle and blatant, in which patients were forced by the demands of a large institution into an unthinking conformity of behavior and thought. The rules that constrained their behavior, Goffman wrote, derived not from a consideration of therapeutic needs, but from the desires of hospital staff members to simplify their own tasks. From Goffman's work a new syndrome was defined — "institutionalism": the progressive loss of functional abilities caused by the denial of opportunities to make choices for oneself, leading to a state of chronic dependency. Robbed of their ability to function on their own, state-hospital patients had no alternative but to remain in an environment in which their lives were directed by others.

Community psychiatry embellished Goffman's charges. Articles in professional journals began to allege that the chronic disability accompanying psychiatric illnesses, particularly schizophrenia, was not a result of the disease process itself, but an effect of archaic treatment methods in which patients were uprooted from their own communities. With the attachments of a lifetime severed, often irretrievably, patients lost the incentive and then the will to maintain their abilities to relate to others and function in social environments. Thus, state hospitals, in addition to subjecting patients to abominable physical conditions — the stuff of exposés since the 1860's — were exacerbating and embedding the very symptoms they purported to treat. The only way to prevent the development of a new generation of dysfunctional chronic patients was to close the hospitals.

Of course, alternative places of treatment would have to be created. In 1963, the new community psychiatrists persuaded a President already interested in mental-health issues and a receptive Congress that, with a new approach, chronicity could be averted. The consensus that emerged was embodied in the Community Mental Health Center Act of 1963. With seed money from the federal government, the law encouraged the development of outpatient clinics in every area of the country. Ultimately, it was hoped, no citizen would live outside one of the 2,000 designated "catchment areas" in which community-based treatment could be provided.

Psychiatric proponents of closing the state hospitals found unlikely allies in a group of civil-libertarian attorneys who were now turning their attention to the mentally ill. Fresh from victories in the civil-rights movement, and armed with potent new constitutional interpretations that restricted the power of the state to infringe personal liberties, these lawyers sought the dismantling of state hospitals as the first step in eliminating all coercive treatment of the mentally ill. They sought this end not simply because they believed that encouraging autonomy reduced chronicity, as the community psychiatrists claimed, but because in their own hierarchy of values individual autonomy was paramount.

Mentally ill persons seemed particularly appropriate targets for a crusade against governmental power, for the state was depriving them of liberty — with ostensibly benevolent aims, yet in conditions that belied the goal of treatment. It appeared to these critics that ultimately the state was concerned most with maintaining imbalances of power that favored the privileged classes and with suppressing dissent. By confining and discrediting the more obstreperous members of the lower classes, the mental-health system served as a pillar of the ruling elite.

Critiques of this sort were not rare in the late 1960's, when skepticism of established power was, for many, a prerequisite of intellectual discourse. Its application to psychiatry was encouraged, however, by the writings of iconoclastic psychiatrists like Thomas Szasz, who maintained that mental illness was a "myth," perpetuated only as a mechanism for social control, and R. D. Laing, whose books touted the value of the psychotic experience for elevating one's perceptions of the meaning of life. Additional academic support for Szasz's views came from sociologists known as labeling theorists, who believed that deviance was a creation of the person with the power so to name it.

Whereas the community psychiatrists initially sought to achieve their ends through a legislative reconstruction of the mental-health system, the civil-libertarian attorneys favored the judicial route. They attacked the major mechanism for entry into the public mental-health system, the statutes governing involuntary commitment. These laws, they charged, were unconstitutionally broad in allowing any mentally ill person in need of treatment to be hospitalized against his will. Surely individual liberty could not legitimately be abridged in the absence of a substantial threat to a person's life or to the life of others. In addition, they alleged that the wording of the statutes, many little changed for one hundred years, was impermissibly vague; particularly problematic for the civil libertarians were the definitions of mental illness and the circumstances that rendered one committable.

In an era of judicial activism, many courts, both federal and state, agreed. Involuntary commitment came to be limited to persons exhibiting danger to themselves or others; strict, criminal-law-style procedures came to be required, including judicial hearings with legal representation. As the trend in the courts became apparent, many legislatures altered their statutes in anticipation of decisions in their own jurisdictions, or in emulation of California, where civil libertarians won legislative approval of a tightened statute even without the threat of court action.

The final common pathway of this complex set of interests led through the state legislatures. Although concerns about better treatment for chronic patients and the enhancement of individual liberty were not foreign here, more mundane concerns made themselves felt as well. The old state mental hospitals took up a significant proportion of most state budgets, in some jurisdictions the largest single allocation. Advocates of closing the old facilities were not reticent in claiming enormous cost savings if patients were transferred to community-based care. And even if real costs remained constant, the availability of new federal entitlement programs such as Supplemental Security Income and Medicaid, to which outpatients but not inpatients would have access, promised a shift in the cost of supporting these people from the states to the federal government.

In many states, this was the final straw. The possibility that patients could be cared for in the community at less expense, perhaps with better results, and certainly with greater liberty, was an irresistible attraction. Deinstitutionalization was too valuable a tool of social policy to remain a discretionary option of state-hospital psychiatrists. It now became an avowed goal of the states. Quotas were set for reductions in state-hospital populations; timetables were drawn up for the closure of facilities. Individual discretion in the release of patients was overridden by legislative and administrative fiat. Patients were to be released at all costs. New admissions were to be discouraged, in some cases prohibited. In the words of Joseph Morrissey, if the first phase of deinstitutionalization reflected an opening of the back door, the second phase was marked by a closing of the front door.

Thus did deinstitutionalization assume the form in which we know it today.

IV

If a decrease in patient population is the sole measure for gauging the outcome of deinstitutionalization, the success of the policy is unquestionable. From 1965 to 1975, in-patient populations in state hospitals fell from 475,000 to 193,000. By 1980, the figure was 137,000, and today all indications are that the number is even smaller. Relatively few of the state hospitals closed. The majority shrank from bustling colonies with thousands of patients to enclaves of a few hundred patients, clustered in a few buildings in largely abandoned campuses.

Yet by the mid-1970's professionals in the field and policy analysts had begun to ask whether the underlying goals espoused by the advocates of deinstitutionalization were really being met. Are the majority of the mentally ill, by whatever measure one chooses to apply, better off now than before the depopulation of the state hospitals? The inescapable answer is that they are not.

A large part of the reason for the movement's failure stems from its overly optimistic belief in the ability of many mentally ill persons to function on their own, without the much-maligned structure of state-hospital care. Rather than liberating patients from the constraints of institutional life, the movement to reduce the role of state hospitals merely shifted the locus of their regimented existence. Indeed, *trans*institutionalization may be a better term to describe the process that occurred. It is estimated that 750,000 chronic mentally ill persons now live in nursing homes, a figure nearly 50 percent higher than the state-hospital population as its 1955 apogee. Additional hundreds of thousands live in board-and-care homes or other group residences. Many of these facilities, particularly the nursing homes, have locked wards nearly indistinguishable from the old state hospitals. They are, in psychiatrist H. Richard Lamb's evocative phrase, the asylums in the community.

Many of the mentally ill, of course, have drifted away

entirely from any form of care. Given the freedom to choose, they have chosen to live on the streets; according to various estimates they comprise between 40 and 60 percent of homeless persons. They filter into overcrowded shelters — as Juan Gonzalez did before becoming the agent of his fantasies on the Staten Island ferry — where they may experience fleeting contact with mental-health personnel. The lack of external structure is reflected in their internal disorganization. Whatever chance they had to wire together their shattered egos has been lost.

What of the hopes of the community psychiatrists that liberating patients from state hospitals would prevent the development of the chronic dependency which stigmatizes the mentally ill and inhibits their reintegration into the community? They learned a sad lesson suspected by many of their colleagues all along. The withdrawal, apathy, bizarre thinking, and oddities of behavior which Goffman and his students attributed to "institutionalism" appear even in the populations maintained outside of institutions. They are the effects of the underlying psychiatric illnesses, usually schizophrenia, not of the efforts to treat those conditions. And contrary to the claims of the labeling theorists, it is the peculiar behavior of severely psychotic persons, not the fact that they were once hospitalized and "labeled" ill, that stigmatizes and isolates them in the community. Studies of discharged patients demonstrate that those who continue to display the signs of their illnesses and disrupt the lives of others are the ones who suffer social discrimination.

To some extent, the community psychiatrists never had a chance to test their theories. The community mental-health centers in which they envisioned care taking place were, for the most part, never built. Fewer than half of the projected 2,000 centers reached operation. Of those that did, many turned from the severely ill to more desirable patients, less disturbed, easier to treat, more gratifying, and, above all, as federal subsidies were phased out, able to pay for their own care. A few model programs, working with a selected group of cooperative patients, are all the community psychiatrists have to show for their dreams. But the evidence suggests that even optimal levels of community care cannot enable many mentally ill persons to live on their own.

The goals of the civil libertarians, except in the narrowest sense, have fared little better. If one conceives that liberty is enhanced merely by the release of patients from the hospitals to the streets, then perhaps one might glean satisfaction from the course of deinstitutionalization to date. But if individual autonomy implies the ability to make reasoned choices in the context of a coherent plan for one's life, then one must conclude that few of the deinstitutionalized have achieved autonomy. One study found fewer than half the residents of a large board-and-care home with a desire to change anything at all about their lives, no matter how unrealistic their objectives might be. If the facade of autonomy has been expanded, the reality has suffered.

Finally, and with fitting irony, not even the hope that deinstitutionalization would save money has been realized. It was originally anticipated that the closing of state hospitals would allow the transfer of their budgetary allocations to community facilities. But state hospitals proved difficult to close. As many hospitals existed in 1980 as in 1955, despite a fourfold reduction in patients. Even with current, broad definitions of who can survive in the community, tens of thousands of patients nationwide continue to require institutional care, often long-term. They are so regressed, self-destructive, violent, or otherwise disruptive that no community can tolerate them in its midst. Moreover, the communities that derive jobs from the facilities have fought hard to preserve them. As censuses have fallen, per-capita costs of care have increased, pushed up even further by pressure to improve the level of care for those who remain. Many costs for the treatment of out-patients have been redistributed, with the federal and local governments bearing heavier burdens; but no one has ever demonstrated overall savings. Even as the quality of life for many mentally ill persons has fallen, state mental-health budgets have continued to expand.

V

Both the failure of deinstitutionalization and our seeming paralysis in correcting it stem from the same source: the transformation of deinstitutionalization from a pragmatic enterprise to an ideological crusade. The goal of the first phase of the process — to treat in the community all mentally ill persons who did not require full-time supervision and might do equally well or better in alternate settings — was hardly objectionable. Had state-hospital populations been reduced in a deliberate manner, with patients released no faster than treatment, housing, and rehabilitative facilities became available in the community, the visions of psychiatry's Young Turks of the 1950's might well have been realized.

Once the release of state-hospital patients became a matter of faith, however, this individualized approach was thrown to the winds. In the Manichaean view that soon predominated, confinement in state hospitals came to be seen as invariably bad. Freedom was always preferred, both for its own sake and because it had a desirable, albeit mysterious therapeutic value. Further, we came to doubt our own benevolent impulses, yielding to those who claimed that any effort to act for the welfare of others was illegitimate and doomed to end with their oppression. Thus, although we may now recognize the failure of deinstitutionalization, we as a society have been unable to reverse course; these same ideologies continue to dominate our policies not by the power of logic but by the force of habit.

It is time to rethink these presuppositions. That freedom *per se* will not cure mental illness is evident from the abject condition of so many of the deinstitutionalized. More difficult to deal with is the belief that even if the lives of hundreds of thousands of mentally ill persons have been made objectively more miserable by the emptying of our state hospitals, we have no right to deprive people of liberty, even for their own benefit. In the currently fashionable jargon of bioethics, the value of autonomy always trumps the value of beneficence.

Interestingly, this position is now being challenged by a number of our leading public philosophers, who have called attention to its neglected costs. Robert Burt of the Yale Law School and Daniel Callahan of the Hastings Center, for example, have taken aim at the belief that the freedom to do as we please should be our primary societal value. This emphasis on individual autonomy, they point out, has come to mean that in making our choices, as long as we do not actively infringe on the prerogatives of others, we face no obligation to consider them and their needs. The result has been the creation of an atomistic community in which, relieved of the duty to care for others, we pursue our goals in disregard of the suffering that surrounds us. This lack of an obligation to care for others has been transmuted in some cases into an actual duty to ignore their suffering, lest we act in such a way as to limit their autonomy.

Although Burt and Callahan have not addressed themselves to mental-health policy *per se,* there is no better illustration of their thesis. The right to liberty has become an excuse for failing to address, even failing to recognize, the needs of the thousands of abandoned men and women we sweep by in our streets, in our parks, and in the train and bus stations where they gather for warmth. We have persuaded ourselves that it is better to ignore them — that we have an obligation to ignore them — because their autonomy would be endangered by our concern.

But the impulse to act for the benefit of others is the adhesive substance that binds human communities together. A value system that loosens those bonds by glorifying individual autonomy threatens the cohesion of the polity. Nobody wants to live in a society characterized by unrestrained intervention (even with benevolent intent), but that does not mean we must reject altogether the notion that doing good for others, despite their reluctance, is morally appropriate under some conditions.

Meaningful autonomy does not consist merely in the ability to make choices for oneself. Witness the psychotic ex-patients on the streets, who withdraw into rarely used doorways, rigidly still for hours at a time, hoping, like chameleons on the forest floor, that immobility will help them fade into the grimy urban background, bringing safety and temporary peace from the world which they envision as a terrifying series of threats. Can the choices they make, limited as they are to the selection of a doorway for the day, be called a significant embodiment of human autonomy? Or is the behavior rather to be understood on the level of a simple reflex — autonomous only in a strictly formal sense?

Far from impinging on their autonomy, treatment of such psychotics, even coercive treatment, would not only hold out some hope of mitigating their condition but might simultaneously increase their capacity for more sophisticated autonomous choices. To adopt the typological scheme of the philosopher Bruce Miller, patients might thereby be enabled to move from mere freedom of action to choices that reflect congruence with personal values, effective rational deliberation, and moral reflection. Our intervention, though depriving them of the right to autonomy in the short term, may enhance that quality in the long run. In such circumstances, benevolence and autonomy are no longer antagonistic principles.

VI

Deinstitutionalization is a remnant of a different era in our political life, one in which we sought broadly-framed solutions to human problems that have defied man's creativity for millennia. In the 1960's and 70's we declared war on poverty, and we determined to wipe out injustice and bigotry; government, we believed, had the tools and resources to accomplish these ends; all that was needed was the will.

This set of beliefs, applied to the mentally ill, allowed us to ignore the failure of a century-and-a-half of mental-health reform in this country, in the conviction that this time we had the answer. The problem, as it was defined, was the system of large state hospitals. Like a cancer, it could be easily excised. And the will was there.

Unfortunately, the analysis was wrong. The problems of severe mental illness have proved resistant to unitary solutions. For some patients, discharge from the state hospitals was a blessing. For all too many others, it was the ultimate curse. Far from a panacea, the policy created as many problems as it solved, perhaps more. To be sure, it is never easy to admit that massive social initiatives have been misconceived. The time has come, however, to lay deinstitutionalization to rest.

It would not be difficult to outline a reasonable program to restore some sense to the care of the mentally ill; moderate expansion of beds in state facilities, especially for the most severely ill patients; good community-based services for those patients — and their number is not small — who could prosper outside of an institution with proper supports; and greater authority for the state to detain and treat the severely mentally ill for their own benefit, even if they pose no immediate threat to their lives or those of others.

Deinstitutionalization has been a tragedy, but it need not be an irreversible one.

71 Afflicting the Afflicted: Total Institutions

William F. May

This chapter will examine institutions as symbols of death, not those institutions and movements that obviously traffic in killing — war, concentration camps, revolutionary terrorism — but rather our health care institutions, which, though devoted to the fight against death, often become its instrument and symbol. Our total institutions reflect primordial images for sickness and death, images of hiding and devouring prominent in folklore, literature, dream life, and ritual behavior.[1]

Traditional societies interpreted sickness as the soul's departure from the body; and death as the soul's irreversible journey to a hidden realm. The enfeebled condition of the sick man or woman suggested that the animating principle, that is, the soul, had obviously vacated the body and retired to an invisible place, inaccessible to ordinary folk. Only the shaman could heal by tracking after and retrieving the soul, a feat which the healer accomplished by going into an ecstatic trance. He left his own body to fetch back the soul of the afflicted.

On death, when, at length, the soul departed for good, the body of the deceased turned into a shroud, a mask; that is, it now hid rather than revealed the soul that once animated it. Fittingly, funeral rites must shroud the shroud, that is, wrap up the body, and hide it away permanently in the ground. This final ritual of hiding carried the weight of a religious duty with which none could interfere. Thus Sophocles' King Creon horrified Antigone by refusing to let her bury her traitorous brother's body. No crime could place a man's body beyond the dignity of burial. Polyneices' corpse should not remain exposed to view where men could stare at it. Antigone had an indefectible duty to hide it from sight.

Sickness and death additionally suggest the image of devouring. To this day, we associate some diseases with eating. We call tuberculosis "consumption"; the malignant tumor feeds off its host; high fever burns and consumes. "Eating, devouring, hunger, death, and maw go together," writes Erich Neumann, "and we still speak, just like the primitive, of 'death's maw,' a 'devouring war,' a 'consuming disease.'"[2]

Total Institutions and the Temptation to Hide the Sick, the Aged, the Imprisoned, and the Mentally Ill

Increasingly, in the modern world, we have placed the sick, the aged, the criminal, and the mentally impaired and disturbed in total institutions, thereby segregating them from the society at large. Some 80 percent of Americans will eventually die not in the home, but in a total institution. The nursing home industry has expanded rapidly in recent decades, and special regions of the country have turned into huge territorial nursing homes where we hide the aged and they hide from us. It used to be said that children should be seen but not heard. Now we imply to many of the aged that they should be neither seen nor heard. Long before their death, we bury them in the folds of the total institution, hidden, out of sight and out of mind, until we are called upon, finally, to bury them again.

Similarly, mental hospitals and penal institutions subliminally associate with the oblivion of death. "'The prisoner,' a Sing Sing chaplain observed, 'was taught to consider himself dead to all without the prison walls."[3] A warden in 1826 prohibited contacts with the outside world, saying, "while confined here . . . you are to be literally buried from the world."[4] Such strictures on communication with the outside world have lessened today, but, still, prisoners call themselves the forgotten men. Our society has insisted on the thick walls of prisons and other institutions not only to keep inmates in but also to keep the world out. The walls say two things to an inmate: do not expect to *escape* from here, but also do not really expect others to visit you here. The society preaches the same message to many of the mentally disturbed and the chronically ill when it consigns them to institutional bins where they sometimes receive minimal, custodial care until their final disappearance.

This colonization of the distressed occurs for all the understandable reasons that obtain in a highly differentiated society with its specialized functions and services. The seriously distressed or disabled often overload the already burdened nuclear family. American society has

1. For a discussion of death as a "Hider-Goddess," see Edgar Herzog, *Psyche and Death, Archaic Myths and Modern Dreams in Analytical Psychology* (London: Hodder and Stoughton, 1966). Hermann Güntert's language studies of the Indo-Germanic (and pre-Indo-Germanic) period lead Herzog to state (p. 39) that a "mysterious hiding and shrouding has been experienced as the first essential character-trait of the numinous, hidden power of death in early times."

From William May, *The Patient's Ordeal* (Bloomington: Indiana University Press, 1994), pp. 142-55. Used by permission.

2. Erich Neumann, *The Origins and History of Consciousness* (Princeton, NJ: Princeton University Press, First Princeton/Bollingen Paperback Printing, 1970). For further explorations of death as devourer, see Richard and Eva Blum, *Health and Healing in Rural Greece* (Stanford, CA: Stanford University Press, 1965), p. 129, and Herzog, *Psyche and Death*, Ch. 4, "The Death Demon as Dog and Wolf."

3. David J. Rothman, *The Discovery of the Asylum* (Boston: Little, Brown and Co., 1971), p. 95.

4. Ibid.

not offered enough assists to family caregivers to provide them with some respite and relief. Institutions, moreover, can deliver important technical services that only mobilized professional resources can offer. I am not a Luddite who would urge that we smash the bureaucracies, that we "total" the total institutions or recklessly "deinstitutionalize" their residents. When we cast out the mentally disturbed from the huge custodial institutions where they were formerly incarcerated and recolonize them in third-rate hotels unattended, they go off their medication and end up in the streets. The heartless 1980s made that clear.

Yet we need to acknowledge candidly the suffering that our efforts to heal impose, the ordeals which the residents of our institutions face, partly gratuitous and eliminable, partly ineradicable, if we would offer what we can compassionately and effectively.

Some nursing homes have provided particularly cynical, even scandalous care; the mentally disturbed often receive notoriously poor treatment of their physical ailments. One harassed hospital administrator in New York City spoke with particular bitterness: apparently, he said, the emotionally disturbed are miraculously endowed with immunity to disease once committed to a mental hospital. For, in the New York City hospitals with which he is familiar, the insane never seem to come down with cancer, gall bladder trouble, or pulmonary or heart conditions serious enough to treat.

Although such neglect is remediable, institutionalization, whether good or bad, often tends to afflict the afflicted more subtly, by depriving them of community. The existentialists used to define being human as "being present" to others and letting others be present to oneself. Institutionalization often not only deprives the inmate of the opportunity to be present to the community but also relieves the larger society of the need to be present to the aged and distressed.

Although one would not want to do without the technical services that our health bureaucracies offer, they can exact a high price by imposing upon residents a kind of premature burial. The institution forces upon them a loss of name, identity, companionship, and acclaim — an extremity of deprivation of which the ordinary citizen has a foretaste in his complaints about the anonymous and impersonal conditions of modern life. To this degree, the nursing home for the poor, the prison, and the chronic care hospital serve as destination and symbol for a society at large that already operates to deprive its citizens of significance. Many people have suffered a loss of community long before their institutionalization. Indeed, the institution may in fact provide them with more community than they have enjoyed for years.

The Hospital and Death as Devourer

While disease wracks his body, the acutely ill patient often has a more general sense of being exhausted and consumed by a world that has depleted all his personal resources. In the recent Western past, when a member of the middle class suffered a breakdown in health he sought respite in the sanctuary of the home, where the doctor visited him. This pattern of care prevailed for the middle and upper classes through the nineteenth and early twentieth centuries. Treatment for the poor differed. The poor went to the teaching hospitals, where, in exchange for medical services, they sometimes signed over to the staff their cadavers for research purposes. Thus the hospital acquired, especially for the poor, associations as an institution that not only serves, but consumes the body.

Today, care for the seriously ill among the middle and upper classes has moved to the hospitals, thus giving other members of society a taste of the earlier plight of the indigent. Despite its indisputable technological advantages over the home, the hospital exacts a high price both psychologically and financially. Psychologically, it gnaws — with its alien machines, rhythms, language, and routines — at that identity which a person previously maintained in the outside world. The patient must surrender his customary *control* of his world not only to the disease but to those who fight against it. His capacity for *savoring* his world is also numbed by the disease and by those procedures imposed upon him in the fight against it — diet, drugs, X-rays, surgery, nausea-inducing therapy, and sleeping potions. Finally, his capacity for *communicating* with his world erodes as he loses his social role. Just as disease rips him out of his usual place in the community and makes him feel less secure in his dealings with fellows, the procedures of the hospital remind him acutely of this loss by placing him in the hands of professionals — the nurse and the doctor — precisely those who seem unassailably secure in their own identities.

The financial trauma patients face makes it difficult to think of the hospital as sanctuary. Not only disease but medical expenses devour the patient, and if not the patient, the patient's family. Current systems of national health care, while distributing costs somewhat, have caused the total social expense of medicine to rocket to nearly 12 percent of the gross national product without increasing commensurately, as compared with other developed nations, the quality of health care. Nothing quite matches inflation for producing a sense that one's world is a devouring world; and no item has matched health care in the inventory of rising costs.

Chronic, even more than acute, care centers have acquired associations with death as devourer. Erving Goffman has worked out this theme in his long essay on asylums, a term which covers prisons, mental hospitals, monasteries, and the like, places where "a large number of like-situated individuals, cut off from the wider society for an appreciable period of time, together lead an enclosed, formally administered round of life."[5] Such an

5. Erving Goffman, *Asylums* (Garden City, NY: Anchor Books, 1961), p. xiii.

institution devours in the sense that it can deprive systematically the sick, the deviant, and the aged of their former identities.

> The recruit comes into the establishment with a conception of himself made possible by certain stable social arrangements in his home world. Upon entrance, he is immediately stripped of the support provided by these arrangements. In the accurate language of some of our oldest institutions, he begins a series of abasements, degradations, humiliations, and profanations of self. His self is systematically, if often unintentionally, mortified. . . .[6]

Goffman particularly attends to admission rites and procedures. The act of taking off one's old clothes and donning new garments impresses symbolically upon the inmate the price he must pay for entering into the total institution: the surrender of his old personal identity and autonomy and the acquisition of a new identity oriented to the authority of the professional staff and to the aims and purposes and the smooth operation of the institution. (The metaphor of changing clothes, of course, dates all the way back to the Benedictine Rule, and behind that to the letters of the Apostle Paul, and, still earlier, to rites of passage in primitive societies. It tells the prospective candidate that his new life demands devouring of the old, though in the case of the asylum inmate the new identity itself often leads eventually to the oblivion of death.)

The word "total" refers not simply to the comprehensive way in which the institution organizes all activities — eating, sleeping, working, leisure, and therapy sessions — but also to the strategies by which the institution invades the interior life of its inmates. In civilian life, Goffman observes, institutions usually claim the resident's overt behavior alone, releasing to the individual the question of his private attitude toward the organization. But in total institutions, the staff can legitimately busy itself with the resident's interior reactions to authority through a process that Goffman calls "looping." The resident finds to his dismay that his protective response to an assault upon his dignity itself collapses back into the situation and provides the staff with reasons for yet further controls; ". . . he cannot defend himself in the usual way by establishing distance between the mortifying situation and himself."[7] The all-monitoring eye of the supervisor surveys both his inner and his outer life and organizes the prison of his therapy.

The Motives for Institutionalization

However sensitively run, total institutions can exact from their residents a price, as they impose upon the segregated the ordeals of banishment and deprivation. What explanations can we offer for their attraction, above and beyond the original philanthropic impulses that founded them and the technical services they orchestrate? (I set aside in answer to this question the motives for entering the handsomely designed and expensive three-tier retirement centers to which the affluent elderly often move themselves.)

Philip Slater, a sociologist, offers the rawest explanation of their appeal in America. He argues that Americans are tempted to solve their problems by resorting to what he calls "the toilet assumption." We behave as though the most efficient and sanitary way of solving a problem is to avoid it by voiding it. To argue the depth of this tendency in the American character, Slater offered a revisionist view (in the *Pursuit of Loneliness*) on the motives of immigrants who settled this country. Our celebratory histories to the contrary, Americans were not the most heroic of Europe's millions. Rather, they were self-selectively those most inclined to solve the problems of an ancient continent and aging relatives by escaping from them. Americans have endlessly repeated this strategy of abandonment: as an immigrant people became a migratory people, moving from the East across the plains to the West; then, as a migratory people became a mobile people, leaving small towns in order to "make it" in the city; and then, after making our cities uninhabitable, fleeing from the city to the suburbs; and, finally, retreating from the tedium of the suburbs to the weekend retreat in the country. Slater sees in this ruthlessness the work of the toilet assumption — the American tendency to dispose of problems by flushing them.[8]

But why are we so drawn to the toilet assumption? Slater's attempt to explain it as a special character defect of those who migrated to America is historically dubious. Most immigrants did not come to the United States in order to flush the problems of their native countries. Certainly not the blacks, and probably not most of the whites. In his essay *Going to America,* Terry Colman notes that English absentee landlords in the late 1840s sought to get rid of huge numbers of Irish peasants on their estates by shipping them off to America. The practice was commonly known as "shoveling out."[9] It would appear that some of our forebears were not the flushers as much as the flushed.

Furthermore, if Michel Foucault's *Madness and Civilization* can be credited, Europeans in the Classical period of the seventeenth and eighteenth centuries already exhibited the tendency to solve problems by banishing a defiled population to a special institution. In this respect, the Age of Reason differed from the earlier medieval and renaissance worlds. Medieval society, according to Foucault, except for its treatment of lepers (and religious minorities), incarcerated its own members for reasons of deviancy much less often than did the reputedly more

6. Ibid., p. 14.
7. Ibid., p. 36.

8. Philip Elliot Slater, *The Pursuit of Loneliness* (Boston: Beacon Press, 1976), pp. 21-23.
9. Terry Colman, *Going to America* (New York: Random House, 1972), p. 216.

tolerant Age of Reason. Renaissance society let the mad and the indigent mingle in the society at large. But by the seventeenth and eighteenth centuries, rulers incarcerated the idle, the poor, the insane, and the criminal without distinction in lazar houses.

The religious ritual of confession, Foucault believes, helped shape and reflected the more generous, earlier medieval attitude toward deviancy. Confession concedes the fact of human imperfection, but also implies some confidence that evil can be let out into the open without engulfing those who pray. But classical Europe, with its proud celebration of human reason, "felt a shame in the presence of the inhuman"[10] that the earlier ages did not experience. After the seventeenth century, Western society increasingly assumed that one can handle evil only by banishing it. Put another way: an age that aspires to total autonomy admits with more difficulty the dependent, the defective, and the irrational into its life. These imperfect members of society represent a negativity so threatening and absolute that a society pretending to autonomy can only put them out of sight.

Foucault knew that this impulse to banish did not spring from crude brutality. He recognized the philanthropic element in the move to sequester: "Interest in cure and expulsion coincide."[11] But it took David Rothman's *The Discovery of the Asylum* to show the intimate historical connection between the impulse to rehabilitate and the compulsion to segregate. The American historian documented the drastic change that occurred in the 1820s and afterward in the United States in the handling of crime, madness, and indigency. Until the early nineteenth century, Americans either whipped, pilloried, drove out of town, or hanged their criminals. Jails served as little more than temporary lockups until the penal system decided on the appropriate punishment. Not until the 1820s did this country adopt the strategy of building, and isolating criminals in, huge penitentiaries.

Similar changes occurred about the same time in the handling of the indigent and the insane. Until the 1820s, welfare funds largely supported families or surrogate families to take care of the poor. But increasingly in the nineteenth century, America constructed, and incarcerated the poor in, its great workhouses. Similarly, the country moved the mad from the attic and the hovel at the edge of town to the insane asylum.

Reformers made these changes for the philanthropic purpose of removing stricken populations from the evil influences of the society at large to the protected environment of the penitentiary or the asylum, where, under carefully controlled conditions (including isolation, work, discipline, and obedience under the authority of professionals), the distressed had a chance to recover. By the end of the Civil War, however, these massive, standardized facilities deteriorated into institutional bins, manned by professionals and subprofessional staff and filled with racial minorities.

In the medieval church, as a priest and his assistants dragged a leper out of the church with backward step and committed him to the lazar house, they would say to him: "And howsoever thou mayest be apart from the church and the company of the Sound, yet art thou not apart from the grace of God."[12] In the last one hundred years, our implied ritual address to the mad, the aged, and the criminal has been: "And howsoever thou mayest be apart from the community and the company of the Sound, yet art thou not apart from the ministrations of the Professional."

Thus rationalism, philanthropy, and professionalism intertwine with banishment and deprivation.

In my judgment, however, both Slater's attempt to locate the toilet assumption uniquely in the American immigrant experience and Foucault's effort to blame the impulse to banish exclusively on classical rationalism fail to persuade. Solving problems by dodging them dates back at least to the parable of the Good Samaritan. "Passing by on the other side" tempted ancient priests and levites as well as the modern middle class as a way of achieving some distance from the distressed. The impulses both to sequester and to devour spring from within humankind and not just idiosyncratically from careerist Americans or eighteenth-century rationalists.

We underestimate, moreover, the real power of these impulses within us in adopting too moralistic a view of their origin — in assuming that they issue from a gratuitous ruthlessness or complacency. Our neglect of the indigent does not result solely from the fact that we are too smug or too engrossed in our own riches to bother with them. If we examine our excuses for neglect,[13] including our reasons for institutionalization, we discover not so much smugness but anxiety, not self-assurance but a sense of harassment, not riches but a feeling of bankruptcy. The statement "I am too busy to care for her now" often betrays a free-floating anxiety: "I am riddled with concern about my own affairs. I can't break free from the grip of my own needs. They hold me in a vise. Maybe next year will be different. But this year is impossible."

Or again, the question "What can I do?" often blurts out no more than one's own despair: "I have nothing for the real needs of another because what I have doesn't satisfy my own. What help could I possibly offer him? It is better to avoid him. To face him would be too depressing. He would remind me of the emptiness of my own fate." Many a man avoids a visit to the bed of a dying friend for reason of the latter dread. He knows he has nothing to say that will help. He feels resourceless before his friend's imminent death and his own. He himself is in

10. Michel Foucault, *Madness and Civilization* (New York: Random House, Vintage Books, 1973), p. 68.

11. Ibid., p. 7.

12. Ibid., p. 6.

13. See William F. May, *A Catalogue of Sins* (New York: Holt, Rinehart, and Winston, 1967), Ch. 6, for a fuller treatment of the sin of neglect.

need, and a face-to-face meeting with his friend would remind him of his own exigency.

Not all expediency in our treatment of the distressed springs from gross callousness; rather, we are busily engaged in obscuring from view our own poverty: both hiding from ourselves and hiding our selves. We consign to oblivion the maimed, the disfigured, and the decrepit, because we have already condemned to oblivion a portion of ourselves. To address them in their needs would require us to permit ourselves to be addressed in our needs. But we recoil from accepting the depths of our own neediness. The hidden away threaten us with what we have already hidden away from ourselves. For some such reason, we prefer, even at great expense, to remove them from sight. And what better way to place them in the shadows and to obscure our own neediness, than to hand them over to professionals whose métier it is to make a show of strength, experience, and competence in handling a given subdivision of the distressed? Thus the exigent provide an opportunity for the community to exhibit its precedence and power over them.

A Concluding Comment

Three major and differing political reactions have emerged in interpreting the problems raised in this essay — conservative, reformist, and revolutionary. These reactions require comment in the light of the religious tradition that engages me as a theologian.

The modern, pragmatic, libertarian conservative would find in David Rothman's account of the emergence and decline of the asylum vindication for his skepticism about reform. The degeneration of the asylum provides but another sad tale of reform gone to seed. In the brief period of forty years, institutions with utopian aspirations deteriorated into dumping grounds for the desperate. Why bother, Mr. Reformer? Spare me your plans and save me some change.

Hobbes and his latter-day descendants among conservatives would darken this particular historical lesson into a comprehensive pessimism. Our institutions can do little more than keep human misery in check because of the murderous appetites to which human beings are subject. The impulses to sequester and devour derive from human nature; they are not just a cultural accident. Hobbes provided the anthropological foundations for this claim by observing: animals hunger only with the hunger of the moment, but man, like Satan, hungers and thirsts *infinitely.* His boundless, devouring hunger makes man "the most predatory, the most cunning, the strongest, and the most dangerous animal."[14] Moreover, Hobbes linked, by implication, this activity of devouring with the further impulse to sequester when he argued that men characteristically differ from animals in their "striving after honor and positions of honor, after precedence over others and recognition of this precedence by others, ambition, pride, and the passion for fame."[15] One man's glory demands another man's eclipse. When we aspire to step forward into the light, we betray the underside of this aspiration in our readiness to see others overshadowed by our illumination. Man's boundless craving, and specifically his appetite for honor and precedence, generates that enmity among humankind which justifies, in Hobbes's estimate, his characterization of the state of nature as "solitary, poor, nasty, brutish, and short." Thus, devouring and overshadowing connect, and our fears that others will devour and surpass us reinforce these murderous impulses. Hobbes resolved our sorry plight by arguing that we must accept our irrevocable duties of obedience to the state and its agencies, which, albeit oppressive, exercise a monopoly over the power of death and thereby keep terror within limits.

In their differing ways, both conservative skepticism and Hobbesian pessimism justify the *status quo* or the *status quo ante* for those institutions that consume, consign to oblivion, or oppress. Hobbes warns, in effect, leave well enough alone. Things are bad, but could be worse. Neither the skeptic nor the Hobbesian conservative appreciates the very real differences institutions (and public institutions) can make, not just in maintaining order, but in aspiring to the good. Without some sense of the distinctions between better and worse and the ineliminable and the reformable, one leaves very little room for improving the lot of the needy, ourselves included.

At the opposite end of the political spectrum, utopian reformers and revolutionaries tend to locate death in our institutional life alone. They see individuals and groups as relatively innocent victims of an oppressive social order. The reformer does battle with social evils, discrete and episodic, in the hope of making things better. But the revolutionary views the specter of overtaxed clinics in ghetto neighborhoods, rotting vegetables in wards, infected blood in banks, and foul overcrowding in jails as symptoms of a generally discredited social and political structure. The system serves the excellors and the devourers rather than the failed and the deprived. Since, however, individuals and groups are relatively innocent victims of the system, reformers and revolutionaries believe that humankind possesses the moral resources either for the piecemeal improvement of the system (the reformer's aim) or for the total displacement of the current system by one superior to it (the revolutionary's hope).

The positions of Hobbesian conservatives and of revolutionaries, like many other opposites, ultimately resemble one another. Both parties think too globally. The conservative wholly justifies and the revolutionary wholly repudiates institutions as they are. As such, they fail to distinguish sufficiently between varied total institutions, better and worse, and to discriminate among varied proposals for their discrete improvement. The

14. Leo Strauss, *The Political Philosophy of Hobbes* (Oxford: The Clarendon Press, 1936), p. 9.

15. Ibid., p. 11.

chapters in this volume [*The Patient's Ordeal*] on the institutionalized retarded and on the aged attempt to show some of those qualities of total institutions that make them both indispensable and praiseworthy and the workers and residents within them deserving of our admiration. Thus, while I have emphasized in this chapter the ordeals which institutionalization imposes, I have not done so with the intent of repudiating the institutions. They impose some ordeals intrinsically and inevitably and others gratuitously. Wise reforms will eliminate the gratuitous, reduce to a minimum the inevitable, improve the necessary, and reserve institutionalization to as small a population as possible.

What response can one make theologically to these contending general assessments of institutions in our time? Reinhold Niebuhr offered the most influential theological response during the period under review. Niebuhr faulted the Hobbesian pessimists for locating destructiveness exclusively within the murderous impulses of humankind and for dealing too kindly with its institutional manifestations. However, Niebuhr also criticized the reformers and the revolutionary optimists for locating oppression exclusively in the social system and for exculpating individuals and groups as its relatively innocent victims. Niebuhr urged, instead, a more complex anthropology that sought to do justice both to the human and institutional capacity for good and to the individual and social capacity for destructiveness.

While salutary, Niebuhr's theological response did not address the more metaphysical question that underlies the social debates of our time. Both parties to the political debate, despite their differences, share in common a somewhat gloomy metaphysical vision. They both tend to define their politics by the experience of death and destruction alone. Conservatives justify institutions and revolutionaries justify their overthrowal in reaction to a negativity rather than to the experience of some positive, nurturant power which may offer hope of rebirth and thus authorizes their action. The fear of death and destruction keeps the conservative defensive about institutions; the hatred of death often provokes the revolutionary to attack them.

Fear supplies the hydraulic fluid and pressure that make the system work for the Hobbesian conservative. Inasmuch as institutions derive their power from the fear of death, we cannot expect them to dispense with this fear. Leviathan — and all its attendant institutions — deserves a monopoly over the power of death for fear of that even more murderous state of affairs that afflicts us in a state of nature without its ministrations.

Correspondingly, the hatred of death usually provides revolutionaries and often reformers with their life's meaning and vocation. Such activists may rightly see the evils of the system, but wrongly define their vocation by that perception alone. Evil serves them as that absolute which authorizes their activities and shapes their plans for a new or better society. They seek relentlessly to eliminate the negative from human life as their passion and calling.

Perhaps the eighteenth-century European and nineteenth-century American experiments with total institutions teach a somewhat different lesson. They emphasize that an ethic defined by resistance alone usually imposes on others what it seeks to depose. The total institution failed partly because it operated reflexively against negativities, the absolute negativities of madness, crime, dependency, and decrepitude. Society assumed that the negative absolutely must be eliminated (through the ministrations of the professional) and, when it cannot be eliminated, it must be sequestered or eliminated by being sequestered.

It may be less pernicious to assume that the negative is not absolute and therefore that its elimination is not the precondition of a truly human existence. Once conservatives, reformers, and revolutionaries no longer treat negativities as absolutes, then the conservative may be less tempted to justify institutional repression and reformers less tempted to lay upon professionals the fatal charge to eliminate negativity or to banish ruthlessly its host. This deflation of evil, moreover, need not lead to quietism or complacency. Action against evil does not require that we inflate it absolutely.

Where, however, does one find theological warrant for this alternative vision of the metaphysical setting in which social action takes place? In my own efforts to puzzle over this problem as a Christian theologian, I have found myself drawn to the passages about the "suffering servant" in Isaiah. Remarkably enough, the text locates God's servant in the very arena of death that we have been exploring. He exposed himself to deprivation and oblivion. "He was despised and rejected by men; a man of sorrows and acquainted with grief, and as one from whom men hide their faces, he was despised, and we esteemed him not" (Isaiah 53:3). The passage furthermore does not suggest that this move into the site of deprivation and death engulfs him. Though "he was cut off from the land of the living" and though he "poured out his soul to death," his resources do not thereby deplete or thin out. Quite the contrary: in and through his outpouring of service, the will of the Lord actually prospers in his hand. God's servant "suffers" — not simply as tortured, but as determinedly subject to the will of God. God may will him to places where he must endure. But his suffering resembles more "suffer the little children to come unto me" than "look what suffering I have endured for your sake, ungrateful woman!" He suffers but also suffers as an attending to, a following, a tracking after the powerful will that creates, preserves, and upholds in love. Therefore, the passage suggests a peculiarly intimate connection between love's flourishing and his own dying.[16]

The assertion of any such link between dying and

16. The now-deceased Professor Arthur C. McGill of Harvard Divinity School offered the best examination of this topic in an as yet unpublished paper on "Identity and Death," in the care of the literary executor of his estate, Professor David Cain, Mary Washington College.

prospering contrasts starkly with our ordinary conception of social action. In traditional social action, we assume some kind of dualistic battle in which either we gradually prevail over death (in which case death diminishes) or we find our resources gradually thinned out by death (in which case we diminish). But this passage suggests that the suffering servant makes his own dying, that is, his own laying down of his life, an essential ingredient in that life which he shares with the community. "By his stripes we are healed."

Christians have traditionally drawn a moral implication from this passage. A community that professes such a servant as savior cannot avoid going into places marked by rejection, pain, and oblivion. In failing to do so, the community would defect from its own mission in the God from whom no secret places are hid.

Concretely, such a savior demands of the churches that they not leave health care exclusively in the hands of the bureaucracies and their professional staffs which serve as the current chief instruments of a society's sequestering. The churches must find ways to open themselves up to loving the institutionalized needy: (1) to provide supplemental services above and beyond those that the bureaucracies can provide; (2) to criticize bureaucracies for their failure to provide what they ought to provide and thereby to assist in their improvement; (3) to encourage the development of alternative delivery systems where appropriate; and (4) to provide the community at large with sufficient contact with the plight of the deprived and the forlorn so as to effect a more favorable ethos in the society toward them and the ordeals that beset them.

But a moralistic reading of the passage from Isaiah does not cut through to the nerve of the problem. The problem we face consists not simply of other people's suffering but of our own. We avoid the failures of others because we cannot bear to see our own failures reflected in their faces; we deprive the needy because we absorbingly attempt to overcome our own limitless sense of deprivation; and rarely are we so tempted to impose pain on others as when we are hellbent on relieving it, convinced of the absolute righteousness of our cause and the indispensability of our contribution in promoting that cause.

Thus the final word spoken in Isaiah 53 must address our own metaphysical plight.

If the anointed of God has exposed himself to deprivation and oblivion, then men and women need fear no longer that the death and failure that they know in themselves can separate them from God. Those powers they fear as absolute have been rendered of no account, either as they appear in them or as they beset their fellow creatures.

This position of metaphysical optimism differs from the vision of the conservative who elevates the powers of darkness and disorder into a divine figure of chaos which institutions must grimly contain; and it differs from the pessimism of the revolutionary whose cause derives its inspiration from the repressive institutional negativity that he seeks to overcome. The act of dying for others penetrates, rather than sidesteps or merely reacts to, the negative. Death looms as one of the principalities and powers, to be sure, but a creature for all of that, incapable of separating human beings from the substance of self-expending love. As this love takes hold of men and women, they suffer rebirth, perhaps in blood and fire, perhaps in water, but, in any event, reconnected to creative, nurturant, and donative love.

This vision of the human plight should not undercut the motive for works of mercy and relief among people and the reformation of defective institutions. Quite the contrary, it should enable them, for it deprives the negative of its ultimacy and therefore its power to paralyze, dominate, and distort. It relieves men and women of the burden of messianism. They need no longer repress the negative in themselves, or impose it on others, or obsess on it in their enemies, or protect themselves from it through the shield of the professional. They can freely perform whatever acts of kindness they can and even receive such acts from others, as a limited sign of a huge mercy which their own works have not produced.

72 Community and Friendship: The Church as a Liberating Community

John Swinton

Why Bother with Friendship?

The central theme of this book [*Resurrecting the Person*] is *friendship.* At first glance, the suggestion that friendship should take center stage in the church's care of people with severe mental health problems may appear to be a rather unusual proposition. In a medicopsychiatric world that places a strong emphasis on therapy, pharmacology, and medical technology, it is difficult to conceive of something as apparently basic as friendship as a serious form of pastoral care for people encountering such difficulties. One might justifiably suggest that this was one area of care that should remain firmly within the domain of the mental health professions. Is it not rather simplistic, one might ask, and perhaps even dangerously naive, to suggest that such a basic relationship as friendship could be central to the mental health care of people living with severe forms of mental health problems? At one level this is a fair question. Few would want to discard the need for specialist interventions designed to understand and help control the worst manifestations of psychological disorder. As we shall see, mental health professionals can contribute to the enabling of people with severe mental health problems to deal constructively with their conditions and to live lives appropriate to their status as human beings, made in the image of a relational God.

The object of this book, rather than to develop an alternative model of care, is to explore ways in which the church can enter into critical prophetic *dialogue* with current strategies for caring, with a view to constructive collaboration that will enable liberation for all. The concept of dialogue is highly significant theologically, as will become clear as the book moves on. For now it is important to highlight that the art of dialogue depends on the honesty and integrity of the two partners. It is not about developing theologies and practices that simply support caring strategies as they are at the moment. Rather, critical prophetic dialogue involves respecting the position of the other, while at the same time adopting a stance that challenges implicit or explicit biases or injustices. Accepting that conventional strategies may be necessary (although always open to critique), this book argues that they are certainly not sufficient. Medicopsychiatric definitions, understandings, and strategies can be helpful when accepted discerningly. However, they only go so far. It is true that such approaches can help identify particular difficulties and suggest strategies and interventions that can significantly improve the lives of people living with long-term mental health problems. Difficulties arise if we begin to assume that such a way of defining mental health problems is the *only,* or even the most appropriate, way of defining them. The issue is one of power, specifically the power that the perspective of psychiatry has to define the "true" nature of a condition and what the most appropriate strategies are for effective intervention. The important conspirational critiques of psychiatry offered by antipsychiatrists such as Szasz[1] and Laing,[2] though open to serious critique themselves, have offered some challenging insights into the potential that the mental health professions have, implicitly or explicitly, to abuse the power that society invests in them. While this is *not* in any way an antipsychiatry book, it is nonetheless important to bear in mind the level of psychological and social power that the medicopsychiatric community has to define how those with and those without mental health problems perceive psychological distress and react to it.

We in the West belong to a culture that has been profoundly influenced by the medical model of care.

> The medical model assumes that a disorder has a specific aetiology, a predictable course, manifests describable signs and symptoms, and has a predictable outcome modifiable by certain technical manoeuvres. In this model, the illness or problem is understood as an isolated "bad spot" which it is the task of the health professional to excise or control using whatever means are at her disposal. The objective is to return the individual to their previously healthy state and to enable them to retake their former position within society. Within this model, health is defined primarily as the absence of disease or infirmity. Ill health is understood in terms of specific pathology that needs to be identified, categorised and eradicated. To be deemed healthy is to be freed from pathology and to experience life as closely to the expected social norm as possible.[3]

It is, therefore, not insignificant that mental health research has increasingly moved toward a focus on science and biology as an explanatory framework within which

From John Swinton, "Community and Friendship: The Church as Liberating Community," in John Swinton, *Resurrecting the Person: Friendship and Care of People with Mental Health Problems* (Nashville: Abingdon Press, 2000).

1. Thomas Szasz, *The Myth of Mental Illness* (London: Penguin Books, 1973).
2. R. D. Laing, *The Divided Self* (London: Penguin Books, 1990).
3. John Swinton, *Building a Church for Strangers,* Contact Pastoral Monographs, No. 9, 1999, pp. 16-17.

mental health problems should be understood. Under the influence of the medical model, which the public and mental health professions conceptualize mental health problems primarily in terms of the biomedical model. Current research agendas, for example, predominantly focus on issues of pathology and specific etiology. The objective is to discover the biological roots of each mental health problem and do all that can be done, (a) to normalize and destigmatize it and (b) to seek more effective ways to eradicate the worst manifestations of it.

Of course, these are good aims to have. As will be discussed later, it is proper that we explore the biological roots of mental health problems in order that we may increase public awareness of them and educate the public on how people with these problems should be perceived and treated. Such an approach does much to destigmatize mental health problems and to free people from oppressive attitudes and exclusionary practices. However, the medical model's approach, while perhaps necessary, is certainly not sufficient. Though biology tells us some things about the mechanics of human beings and the technicalities of mental health problems, it tells us nothing of what it means to be human and to live humanly even in the midst of our particular difficulties. The danger with oversomaticizing mental health problems is that it tends to individualize the problem, thus drawing attention away from the critical sociorelational dimension that this book argues is fundamental to the process of oppression in the lives of people with various forms of psychological distress. If the problem is perceived as purely biological, then presumably it belongs to the individual quite apart from the particular social context within which the individual experiences it. This is an error based on the assumptions of the medical model, an error that enables society to abrogate responsibility for the oppression and disablement of people with mental health problems. As such, it requires a liberating counter-understanding.

At best, approaches based on the medical model reveal only a part, and perhaps not even the most significant part, of what it means to live with a mental health problem. Mental health problems are much more than biological defects that require being fixed or controlled by specialist interventions. They are human experiences that happen to unique individuals within particular circumstances. More than that, they are *social* experiences. Whereas the medical model's approach locates the difficulty within the genes or the neurobiology of the individual, this book argues that a major part of the individual's difficulty lies in the society within which a person experiences his or her difficulties. While the medical model's approach may drive us to focus on the eradication and control of pathology, the specific mental health problem may well *not* be of ultimate concern to the individual experiencing it. Frequently one finds that the primary concern of individuals experiencing mental health problems lies with issues of personhood and personal relationships, which, while not unconnected with their particular difficulties, cannot be fully understood by focusing on psychopathology alone.

Yale University professor of psychiatry John S. Strauss in "The Person — Key to Understanding Mental Illness" observes:

> . . . In the process of doing research interviews, conducting rounds and seeing patients in other contexts, it is increasingly striking to me how little I recognise in these people many of the key concepts that dominate the ways we as mental health professionals work. The things patients talk about and the way they talk do not seem to reflect our concepts, or at the very least, our concepts seem to reflect only such a very narrow range of what is going on in these people.[4]

As an illustration he offers the following story:

> This 28-year-old man had had the first onset of his schizophrenia ten years previously. He had spent three years in the hospital, and then from the period between seven and five years before my interview had been able to manage outside the hospital. However, five years before my interview he had been readmitted to the hospital and had remained there since. As part of our interviews, we try to delineate the various general levels of illness, at several times in the past. We then determine levels of social relations and work functioning, symptoms and hospitalisation during those times and plot a time line of course of disorder. This line is generated by rating scales of established reliability. In this particular study, we also enquire about the worst year the person has had since becoming ill. I expected that when I asked that question of this young man he would say that it was one of the times when his functioning scores were lowest, his symptoms highest, and when he was in the hospital. He said the worst year was about six years ago, a time when by our scores he was doing fairly well and was not in the hospital. He said that he had been living with his mother and then finally had been kicked out of her house and was living in an apartment. About two weeks after leaving her house he called home. She answered the telephone. He started talking, but when she heard his voice, she said "You have the wrong number" and hung up. He said that was the worst year of his life. My heart sank as he told his story. It was not difficult to understand what he meant, but the worst year according to him and the worst year according to our rating scales were very different. Who was right?[5]

What one has here is a clash of interpretations and priorities and a fundamental difference in situational definition — two narratives revolving around the same situation, one focusing on the person-as-illness, the other focusing on the person-as-person, and both coming to signifi-

4. John S. Strauss, "The Person — Key to Understanding Mental Illness: Toward a New Dynamic Psychiatry, III," *British Journal of Psychiatry,* Vol. 161 (Supplement 18) 1992, pp. 19-26, 109.

5. Ibid., p. 104.

cantly different conclusions as to priorities and life expectations. To the clinicians, from their medicopsychiatric perspective the "natural" assumption was that the "schizophrenic's" (as opposed to person's) worst time was when his illness was at its peak, that is, when his clinical symptomatology was most obvious (when the objects of the researcher's particular area of interest were most obvious). In other words, their position as medical researchers offered them a perspective whereby they defined him, his emotions, his expectations, and his hopes according to their perception of his problem and its implications, that is, as if his illness were inevitably the most important thing in his life. The reality was that what took priority, what had the greatest impact on him was the nature of his personal experiences, in particular his relationship with his mother.

Strauss's final question "Who was right?" is highly significant. In a sense both narratives are correct from the standpoint of the individuals involved. However, as will become apparent, people with mental health problems are seriously disempowered. When it comes to the question of whose voice will be listened to within such a process of narrative negotiation, the chances are that it will be the voice of the professional who comes through loud and clear. Though Strauss's central interest is in recentering the person within the process of mental health care, he is not in the majority within the mental health professions. In a medicocentric culture, the narrative of the health professions will almost inevitably tend to take priority over the other narratives. It is vital that we bear these thoughts and propositions in mind as we move on to explore contemporary interpretations of schizophrenia. While acknowledging the importance of the medicopsychiatric view, we must be careful not to allow the power of its voice to prevent us from hearing the voices of those who may be victims of an overly medicalized definition of what mental health problems are and what appropriate responses should be.

Focusing on Friendship

Strauss's vignette suggests that even in the midst of the most profound forms of mental health problems there is a vital relational dimension that is frequently *more* significant, from the perspective of the sufferers, than other factors within their illness. It also suggests that this dimension is often not given adequate priority within standard professional understandings of what psychological disorders are and what they might mean to the people who have them. It is here, within the area of personal relationships, that the Christian community has a vital contribution to make to the care of people with mental health problems. The role of the Christian community lies not only in creating a context that will nurture relational development and enable people to find wholeness in the midst of their brokenness, but also in actively countering the wider interpersonal and social forces that act to stigmatize, alienate, oppress, and exclude many people with mental health problems from full social inclusion.

The primary conduit through which such a task can be fulfilled is the relationship of *friendship*. Christian friendships based on the friendships of Jesus can be a powerful force for the reclamation of the centrality of the *person* in the process of mental health care. It is within the relationship of friendship that we discover a critical tool of liberation and healing. This can enable the church to fulfill its task of rehumanizing those whom society has dehumanized through its attitudes and its refusal to relate with them in a way that is meaningful and life enhancing. To understand the significance of this proposition, we begin by exploring the relationship of friendship, drawing out precisely why it offers distinctive and unique opportunities for the mental health ministry of the Christian community.

Friendship is a deeply intimate and committed relationship that encompasses people in all their fullness. It is not bounded or dictated by stereotypical presumptions of biological malfunctioning. *The priority of friends is the personhood of the other and not the illness.* As such, a focus on the role of friendship as a primary mode of caring offers a vital counterbalance to the types of positivistic, medicalized approaches highlighted above. It allows us to move beyond pathology, and begin to explore those aspects of *people* with mental health problems that fall outside the boundaries of the medical model. A focus on friendship enables us to ask critical questions that are often not on the agenda of those whose horizons are bounded by the medical gaze of psychiatry and whose focus lies primarily within pathology. A concentration on friendship releases us from an overdependence on technology and allows us to explore issues of human relationships, personhood, spirituality, value, and community, all of which can easily be overlooked or seen as of secondary importance within standard definitions and treatment models of mental health care.

Friendship as a Gift of the Community

Unlike specialist/professional relationships, friendship is a form of human affection that is potentially available to and from the *whole* of the Christian community and from the whole of society. A focus on friendship opens up the possibility that the care of people with severe mental health problems is a communal, lay-oriented enterprise rather than an exclusively individualized specialist task, and suggests that the church community may have a specific responsibility within this area. Such a focus on friendship enables the church to offer a *distinctive* contribution to the process of care. Nancy Eiesland suggests that friendship is the distinctively Christian gift that the church offers to marginalized people:

> Whereas we [the church] might like to imagine ourselves as part of the mainstream or "normal" popula-

> tion — Christians have accepted a mission that perpetuates a marginal position. Thus we call to other marginalized individuals for friendship not from the center of society — where we are not either demographically or in terms of political/social power — but at the periphery, where we are because of Christ's radical call to be for the other. Thus the contention is that friendship is the Christian call to all who are on the periphery by virtue of [our] decisions to follow the model of friendship of Jesus; thus we are in no position to worry whether [others], such as people with AIDS, people with physical disabilities, people with learning disabilities, etc., are going to be a "burden" to us.[6]

When the church is truly being the church, it does not sit at the center of power and politics, seeking to establish God's reign through the exercise of power, violence, and exclusion. The task of the church is not to reestablish the reign of Constantine,[7] but rather to live out the rule of Christ, the one who sat on the margins of society with those whom the world deemed to be unlovable. Caring for "strangers" is not an act of charity, but a revelation of the true nature of the church and the true character of the God whom we worship and seek to image. Friendship is necessary, not simply for effective mental health care, but in order for the church to be the church in any kind of meaningful sense. Friendship enables us to take seriously the personhood and social context of marginalized people and seeks to actualize the proposition that all people are made in the image of a relational God, and as such, created for loving relationships with God and with one another.

What Is Different about Christian Friendship?

One of the reasons we underplay the healing potential of friendship is that we take for granted that we know what it is. The type of friendship this book will focus on differs from the assumed norm of everyday Western friendship. The form of friendship here is *radical* in that it transcends the relational boundaries that are constructed by contemporary tendencies to associate with others on the basis of likeness, utility, or social exchange. It is radical also in that its primary dynamic is toward the outcast and the stranger, those whom society rejects and marginalizes. It is a profoundly humanizing relationship that reveals something of the coming kingdom of God as revealed in the person of Christ in whom the possibility of reconciliation and shalom becomes a reality; the enmity between human beings finds resolution and healing and the fragmentation of the human family is swept up and mended by the power of the coming Kingdom. In Christ, servants are transformed into friends, boundaries of prejudice and difference are torn down and the wholeness of the human family is revealed as a genuine possibility.

Such radical friendship is perhaps best described as *messianic friendship* in that, inspired by the power of the Spirit, it takes its shape from the relationships of Jesus the Messiah, and seeks to embody and act out something of his life and purpose. In order to understand and justify such a position, it is necessary to begin by exploring the nature and purpose of the church. In clarifying precisely what the church community is (or at least should be in its ideal form) the shape of the model of friendship that forms the heart of this book will begin to emerge.

Imaging the Messiah: The Church as Sign and Sacrament

Avery Dulles in his book *Models of the Church* identifies five major ecclesial types. He suggests that the church can be viewed as: an institution, as the mystical Body of Christ, as a sacrament, as a herald, or as a servant.[8] For current purposes it will be useful to examine some aspects of Dulles's propositions concerning the sacramental nature of the church. The model of church-as-sacrament emphasizes the present reality of the grace of Christ in the world, with the church being seen as the sign of that reality. "If Christ is the sacrament of God, the Church is for us the sacrament of Christ; she represents him, in the full and ancient meaning of the term, she really makes him present. She not only carries on his work, but she is his very continuation, in a sense far more real than that in which it can be said that any human institution is its founder's continuation."[9] Thus the Christian community as the Body of Christ is seen to be the living continuation of the earthly and messianic ministry of Christ. The church is founded on the historical Christ, sustained and guided by the power of the Holy Spirit,[10] and gathered around and shaped by the biblical narrative.[11]

John Calvin describes sacraments as "effectual signs; the means whereby God leads us to Himself via earthly elements."[12] In like manner, Dulles defines a sacrament as "a sign of grace."[13] By "sign," Dulles means not a mere pointer to something that is absent, but a sign of something really present. "Beyond this a sacrament is an efficacious sign; the sign itself produces or intensifies that of

6. Nancy L. Eiesland, personal correspondence. Used with Dr. Eiesland's permission.

7. Stanley Hauerwas, *Resident Aliens* (Nashville: Abingdon Press, 1989).

8. Avery S. J. Dulles, *Models of the Church* (London: Gill and Macmillan, 1976).

9. Henri Lubac in Dulles's *Models of the Church,* p. 59.

10. Jürgen Moltmann, *The Church in the Power of the Spirit* (London: SCM Press, 1992).

11. Stanley Hauerwas, *The Peaceable Kingdom: A Primer in Christian Ethics* (Notre Dame, Ind.: University of Notre Dame Press, 1983).

12. Brian Easter, "Sacraments and MH People," in *Liturgy,* Vol. 9, No. 5, June/July, 1985, p. 193. He is discussing John Calvin's definition of sacraments.

13. Dulles, *Models of Church,* p. 61.

which it is a sign. Thanks to the sign, the reality signified achieves an existential depth; it emerges into solid, tangible existence."[14] The church understood as a sign of grace does not simply point toward an ideal, but actually reveals something of that ideal in its life and ministry. In this sense the church might legitimately be understood as the physical manifestation of God's redemptive love. Thus, the task of the church is to signify the redeeming grace of Christ in a historically tangible form.

> It stands under a divine imperative to make itself a convincing sign. It appears most convincingly when its members are evidently united to one another and to God through holiness and mutual love, and when they visibly gather to confess their faith in Christ and to celebrate what God has done for them in Christ. . . . The church never fully achieves itself as church. It is true church to the extent that it is tending to become more truly church.[15]

The church is not a perfect institution.[16] It works out its ministry within the continuing eschatological dialectic between the cross and the Resurrection; what is and what will be. Although it cannot reveal the coming kingdom in all of its fullness, it is charged with the task of revealing signs of how that kingdom will be in the fulfillment of the eschaton. Hodgson explains the paradoxical dialectic that marks the ongoing life of the church in terms of the difference between *basileia* and *ecclesia,* that is, between the kingdom of God and the church.[17] He argues that *basileia* is "an image of a new way of being human in the world in relation to God and neighbour — new community, communion of love, liberation, a new and radical family based not on blood relationships but on human and ethical ones."[18] The church then, as Moltmann correctly observes, is the "anticipation of the kingdom of God under the conditions of history, the vanguard of the new humanity."[19] It is that body which reveals something of the new humanity that has been given to us in Christ (2 Corinthians 4:4). Inevitably the church becomes an institution, an *ecclesia,* that has to maintain itself within history. However, this ecclesia is also "an image, sign, sacrament, and foretaste of the *basileia,* embodied in the diversity of historical churches. As such it discloses the *basileia* vision unambiguously but actualizes it only fragmentarily."[20] Thus while the church community is called to reveal the coming kingdom in its actions and thinking, it is not an ideal community. It is flawed and struggles to live up to its own identity. Nevertheless, it does contain the messianic vision for the future and reveals something of the coming kingdom if imperfectly.

The Centrality of Christ

Central to the identity of the church is the figure of Jesus. Dulles sees the church as fundamentally centered on the person of Jesus Christ: "God's grace is for all people, but the church is the place where it appears most clearly that the love that reconciles men to God and to one another is a participation in what God communicates most fully in Christ. Christians are those who see and confess Jesus Christ. As the supreme efficacious symbol — the primordial sacrament of God's saving love stretched out to all."[21]

Such a Christocentric view of the church has important implications for the character of the church's caring ministry. Hoekendijk presents a powerful argument for the church to understand itself as a "Messianic community" by following Jesus' example of self-emptying servanthood.[22] He argues that the life of the church must be imitated from the Messiah, which means living the self-emptying life of the suffering servant. Hoekendijk states that the church received her "charter" thus: "Let the same mind be in you that was in Christ Jesus, who, though he was in the form of God, did not regard equality with God as something to be exploited, but emptied himself, taking the form of a slave, being born in human likeness. And being found in human form, he humbled himself and became obedient to the point of death — even death on a cross!" (Philippians 2:5-8).

Hoekendijk applies this model, then, to the role of the church: "If someone asks where the church is, then we ought to be able to answer; there, where people are emptying themselves, making themselves as nothing. There where people serve, not just a little, but in total service, which has been imitated from the messiah servant, and in which the cross comes into view. And there, where the solidarity with the fellow man is not merely preached, but is actually demonstrated."[23]

The church is called to embody God's passion for the world that was revealed in the life of Jesus, and to adopt the ethical priorities that were so clearly revealed in his life and death. The truth of the gospel can only be understood when it is manifested in the lives of a people who have experienced and been transformed by the love of Christ. The authenticity of the gospel is always judged by the ability of Christians to live their lives in ways that reflect the truth of the message. The message that in Christ

14. Ibid.

15. Ibid., p. 6.

16. The use of the term "institution" is not meant to limit conceptualizations of the church to the institutional church. The term "institution" indicates the whole church in all its variegated forms as it works out its historical existence.

17. John Patton, *Pastoral Care in Context: An Introduction to Pastoral Care* (Louisville: Westminster/John Knox Press, 1993), p. 25. Quoting Peter Hodgson, *Revisioning the Church: Ecclesial Freedom in the New Paradigm* (Philadelphia: Fortress, 1988), p. 52.

18. Ibid.

19. Moltmann, *Church in the Power of the Spirit,* p. 196.

20. Hodgson, *Revisioning the Church,* pp. 58-63. (Quoted in Pattison).

21. Dulles, *Models of Church,* p. 66.

22. J. C. Hoekendijk, *The Church Inside Out* (London: SCM Press, 1967), pp. 71-72.

23. Ibid., p. 71.

God was reconciling himself to the world (2 Corinthians 5:19) only becomes truth as it is embodied within a people whose primary desire is to love and to reach out in compassion to the needy.

The messianic church cares for the world with the passion of Christ and strives to reflect that care in its life and attitudes. This being so, the nature of Jesus' ministry and mission, which is fundamental in forming the character of the church, will inevitably be reflected in the forms of care that the church deems it legitimate to adopt, and the priorities and goals that guide the practice of that care.

Friendship and Liberating Discipleship

As we reflect on the life of Jesus, it becomes clear that the types of relationships he entered into were of a special quality and frequently had a specific focus. His relationships were marked by such things as unconditional acceptance (John 4:5), solidarity with the poor and the marginalized (Matthew 9:10), and total commitment to others, even unto death. The name that he and the other gospel writers gave to this form of committed relationship was *friendship.* It would not be unreasonable to define discipleship as friendship with Jesus: "No one has greater love than this, to lay down one's life for one's friends. You are my friends if you do what I command you. I do not call you servants any longer . . . but I have called you friends" (John 15:13-15).

Sacrificial friendship is the definition of love. Sacrificial friendship, which works itself out as solidarity with the poor, reveals the true meaning of discipleship and faithful living that images the messiah. Bearing in mind what has already been suggested concerning Christ as the pattern for ministry, mission, and the church, we see the importance of such reflections on the centrality of friendship for our understanding of discipleship. By laying down friendship as a pattern for discipleship and a way of being that embodies the coming kingdom, Jesus outlines the specific shape and form that the church's ministry of care should take. Christians are called to be disciples: *friends of the poor.*

Redefining Friendship

Of course, the type of friendship that is revealed in the life and mission of Jesus differs quite markedly from normal Western understandings of friendship. For most of us, friendship is a common relationship of which everyone assumes they know the meaning. Mary Hunt comments:

> Friendship is available to everyone, at least potentially. The tiny baby who is befriended by her mother is learning friendship. The elderly person around whom a community gathers when she is dying is capable of teaching friendship. Friendship, by its nature, assumes that persons live in relationships, and that relationships are good.[24]

At one level, then, friendships, along with kinships, are the essence of the relational fabric within which all human beings work out their lives. At this level friendship is the most common relationship, available to all and special only in its importance for general human flourishing. Irrespective of its implications for mental health care, friendship is a fundamental and vital form of human relationship. Such an observation should come as no real surprise. For many people, the essence of life, that which makes it worthwhile, is the presence of friends. The prevalence of friendship is a natural extension of the image of God in human beings. Human beings are social creatures, made in the image of a social God who is trinity; a God who *is* love and relationship in essence. God is a community of Father, Son, and Holy Spirit, eternally indwelling one another in a community of love. It is only natural that creatures made in God's image should seek after relationships in all of their various forms.

For most of us, our friendships are based on the principle that like attracts like. We normally assume that making friends depends on sharing common interests and activities and having a shared frame of reference within which we communicate and share our experiences. When we reflect on our own relational networks, we find that the majority, if not all, of our friends are very much like ourselves. This cultural presumption reflects the thinking of Aristotle, whose writings have provided the major philosophic source in Western Christian tradition for dealing with friends and for making sense of most relationships.[25] This way of approaching human relationships has been deeply influential within Western culture and, by implication, on the church that is embedded within that culture. Aristotle distinguished between three kinds of friendships: friendships of *utility,* friendships of *pleasure,* and friendships of *goodness.* A friendship of *utility* is a friendship based on usefulness. The friends are friends only insofar as they are useful to each other. They are useful to each other as long as they can provide the goods the other person needs. This category of friendship would include work mates, those with whom we do business, and so forth. Such people are "a necessary part of our relational landscapes. They provide what is useful to the common good."[26] Friendships of *pleasure* are based on the amount of pleasure the participants get from the relationship. They are friends primarily for the enjoyment they bring to one another. The third kind of friendship, the highest according to Aristotle, is the friendship of *virtue* or *goodness.* This kind of friendship is exclusive, in the sense that it can only be between two people, both of whom are able to actualize the virtue of goodness. "One or two

24. Ibid., p. 105.
25. Ibid.
26. Ibid., p. 93.

persons in a lifetime come along who are 'most completely friends, since each one loves the other for what the other is in himself and not for something he has about him which he need not have.' Those friendships are based on mutual goodness and the desire to respond in kind to that goodness."[27]

Unlike friendships of utility and pleasure, where there can be a circle of friends, the friendship of goodness is an exclusive and deeply intimate relationship that takes place between two people, both of whom *must* share the virtue of goodness. The intensity of this relationship means that the friends have no love to spare for other less virtuous friendships.

There are a number of difficulties with such an understanding of friendship. I will highlight two here. First, for Aristotle, friendship could occur only between *equals,* that is, two good people serving to actualize the virtue of goodness within their friendship relationship. In this model, as Sallie McFague correctly observes, "friendship is finally not love of another but of oneself. One needs a friend, says Aristotle, in order to exercise one's virtue; one needs someone to be good in order to be good."[28]

Such an understanding is the antithesis of the types of friendship revealed in the life and death of Christ.

> In the incarnation, one finds God willingly entering into friendship with his creatures who could never be his equal. In the earthly life and ministry of Jesus one finds a continuing picture of a man entering into friendships not with social equals, but with those whom society had downgraded and considered unworthy of friendship. In the death of Jesus one discovers a man committed to these same friends even unto death.[29]

People with severe mental health problems such as schizophrenia are at times radically different in their outlook, behavior, and attitudes. Friendships based on the principle that like attracts like will inevitably exclude those who for whatever reason are different. Thus, a faithful Christ-centered church cannot accept the premise of "like attracts like" as an adequate foundation for its caring practices.

Second, Aristotle focused primarily on *quality* as opposed to *quantity.* He considered friendship something that decreased in quality as it increased in quantity. However, as we reflect on the friendships of Jesus, we see that the quality of his relationships remained the same, not just for intimates but for all the people he encountered. Certainly the level of intensity of his relationships varied. Jesus had close friends and friends for whom his love was openly expressed in a way that it was not in other relationships (John 19:26). However, though the intensity may have fluctuated, the quality and texture of his friendships always remained the same. While Aristotle retains a hierarchy among friends, Jesus offers a radically new understanding of friendship.

> When "respectable society" calls Jesus a "friend of sinners and tax collectors," it wants only to denounce and compromise him. In keeping with the law according to which its ranks are organised, respectable society identifies people with their failings and speaks of sinners; it identifies people with their profession and speaks of tax collectors; it identifies people with their diseases and calls them lepers and the handicapped. From this society speaks the law, which defines people always with their failings. Jesus, however, as the Son of man without this inhuman law, becomes the friend of the sinful and sick persons. By forgiving their sins he restores to them their respect as men and women; by accepting lepers he makes them well. And thus he becomes their friend in the true sense of the word. The denunciatory, contemptuous name "friend of sinners and tax collectors," unintentionally expresses the deep truth of Jesus. As friend he reveals God's friendship to the unlikable, to those who have been treated in such unfriendly fashion. As the Son of Man, he sets their oppressed humanity free.[30]

In befriending those who were cast out by society, and claiming that this is the way of the emerging kingdom of God, Jesus presents us with a model of liberation, an "inescapable moment of radical change" in our perceptions of friendship. In this moment of liberation and revelation, Jesus flattens the relational hierarchy of the Aristotelian model of friendship and presents a new and radically open understanding of friendship — a friendship that is open to those who are, in the perception of society, "not good" — the outsiders, the tax collectors, and sinners, those who are in many respects radically unlike himself. More than that, by moving the status of his disciples from servants to friends, and by suggesting that true friendship demands commitment even unto death, Jesus presents a model of committed friendship that more than transcends the boundaries of utility and pleasure.

Thus, in the friendships of Jesus we find a model of friendship, not as a closed relationship with a single like-minded individual, but as an open relationship focused on "the outsider," a form of relating that should form the template and the core of any church that seeks to follow and to image him faithfully.

> If one takes the friendship of Jesus as paradigmatic of the friendships that are expected of the church, then it becomes clear that the quality of the church's friendships *must* reflect the God whom they image and the messiah they claim to follow. The church community will find its true identity when it comes to understand itself as a community of friends, wholly and selflessly committed to God, one another, and the world.[31]

27. Ibid.

28. Sallie McFague, *Models of God: Theology for an Ecological, Nuclear Age* (London: SCM Press, 1988), p. 161.

29. John Swinton, *From Bedlam to Shalom* (In press).

30. Jürgen Moltmann, *The Open Church — Invitation to a Messianic Lifestyle* (London: SCM Press, 1978), p. 56.

31. Swinton, *From Bedlam to Shalom* (in press).

The church then is a "fellowship of the friends of Jesus,"[32] called to live in the world in a manner that is appropriate to such a status.

Agape and an Ethic of Solicitude

Such a model of friendship is based on a radical ethic of *solicitude.* Stephen Post in *The Moral Challenge of Alzheimer's Disease* argues that the ethical principle of *solicitude* — the anxiety over the good of another — is fundamental for all moral behavior. Drawing on the thinking of Soble, Post suggests that solicitude can take three forms. The first of these is property based, in the sense of being dependent on a person's having certain properties that make him or her attractive or worthy of care in the eyes of another person. In the first model, "the caregiver looks for some comprehensible and explanatory source of his or her solicitude." Such solicitude is property based, that is, "When x loves y, this can be explained as the result of y's having, or x's perceiving that y has, some set (S) of attractive, admirable, or valuable properties; x loves y because y has S or because x perceives or believes that y has S."[33]

A second form solicitude can take is memory based. Faced with a loved one's severe neurological damage and profound loss of memory, caregivers remain solicitous "because that person was near and dear and, no matter how dismantled, continues to be honored in reciprocation." Such a form of solicitude is still property based, but retrospectively so.

While both of these models of solicitude have their place within this study, it is Post's third model that is of particular relevance here. The third is based on a very different principle: the radical *agape* love of God for human beings. This view of solicitude is very much in line with the Christian understanding of *agape* love. Quoting Soble,[34] Post suggests that it "denies the need to be grounded in y's attractive properties (S) or in x's belief or perception that y has S." Such solicitude is not property based, not is it explicable or easily comprehensible. Such solicitude is a matter of bestowal rather than appraisal, it is unconditional rather than conditional on certain properties in its object, and it is therefore not extinguished by unattractive properties. This solicitude "is its own reason and love is taken as a metaphysical primitive. Such is the structure of agapic personal love."[35]

There is a real danger that property-based solicitude, by definition, is dependent on the continuity of certain properties within the individual. If these are no longer present, then the maintenance of solicitude can be troublesome. Even with memory-based solicitude, there is an implicit assumption that there is a radical discontinuity between the person remembered and the person experienced in the present. If solicitude is based solely on memory, then one is faced with some serious questions as to the nature of the personhood of the person one is attempting to relate with in the present. However, the type of non–property-based solicitude presented in Post's third definition offers a model of solicitude that is grounded in the reality of God's unending and unconditional love for the individual — a love that bestows worth and dignity upon the individual irrespective of context, situation, or any radical change that may occur within particular properties. This kind of solicitude offers a "non-appraisive attitude of radical equality" underpinned by an ethic and an attitude that adopts a position of moral solidarity with the other, irrespective of circumstance. Such a stance is very much in line with the ethical and social position adopted by Jesus — the one who came to reveal God's agapic love in all of its fullness. As such, it offers a powerful ethical underpinning to the model of friendship that has been developed thus far.

Friendship and Virtue

It is, of course, vital to bear in mind that while solicitude may find its ultimate exposition in the life of Christ, it should not be understood as something that is solely the heroic achievement of outstanding individuals. The attainment and maintenance of such an attitude of solicitude-in-friendship requires a community that understands and seeks to live out the implications of taking such a way of being seriously. While there may be legitimate criticism directed at certain aspects of Aristotle's model of friendship, there are dimensions of his thinking that are important to retain. If what has been presented thus far is correct, then Christian friendship is considerably more than simply "another human relationship." Rather it is both a virtue and, as Paul Waddell suggests, "a moral enterprise."[36] It is a way of living that ensures that human beings can be enabled to live their lives humanly. It is a form of praxis (embodied theology) through which we acquire the wisdom necessary and in particular the self-knowledge we require to be people of virtue.

Understanding friendship as a virtue is an important emphasis for the purposes of this book. In *The Nichomachean Ethics,* Aristotle describes virtue as a state of excellence *(arete)* or disposition whose aim is the highest Good *(eudaimonia).*[37] In essence, for Aristotle the term *virtue* meant "that which causes a thing to perform its function well." *Arete* was an excellence of any kind that

32. Moltmann, *The Open Church,* p. 60.

33. Stephen G. Post, *The Moral Challenge of Alzheimer's Disease* (Baltimore: Johns Hopkins University Press, 1995), p. 37.

34. A. Soble, *The Structure of Love* (New Haven: Yale University Press, 1990), pp. 5, 6.

35. Stephen G. Post, *The Moral Challenge of Alzheimer's Disease,* p. 38.

36. In Stanley Hauerwas, *Sanctify Them in the Truth: Holiness Exemplified* (Edinburgh: T&T Clark, 1998), p. 111.

37. Aristotle, *The Nichomachean Ethics,* David Ross, tr. and intro. (New York: Oxford World's Classics Set, Oxford University Press, 1998).

denotes the power of anything to fulfill its function. Thus the virtue of the eye is seeing, the virtue of a knife is its cutting edge, the virtue of a horse is running, and so forth.[38] Human virtue is that which causes us to fulfill our function in a way that is appropriate to our status as human beings.[39] Understood in this way, the activity of friendship is that which trains us to be virtuous in the art of being Christlike and, by implication, being fully human.

The suggestion that friendship is an *activity* is significant. Friendship is not a social status or a static human relationship. Rather it is a dynamic activity within which we seek to live virtuous lives worthy of being called truly human. Such a way of living is based on the life of Christ in whom we discover the ultimate definition of what it means to be human (2 Corinthians 4:4), The process of friendship and the process of community development are deeply interlinked. Friendship is not something that we embark upon on our own. Friendship is a skill that is learned in community and in turn contributes to the formation of a specific type of community. Thus we develop the skill of friendship as we encounter one another in friendship and experience the friendship of Christ as he works out his purposes in and through those who seek to follow him. "Friendship is not just a necessity for living well, but necessary if we are to be people of practical wisdom. Through character-friendship we actually acquire the wisdom necessary, and in particular the self-knowledge, to be people of virtue."[40]

From our discussion thus far it has become clear that friendship, like all the virtues, is context dependent — that is, the word "friendship" does not have a universal meaning. The meaning and praxis of friendship can be understood only within the context of the particular community within which it is being practiced, and the specific moral tradition within which it is rooted.[41] The model of friendship presented previously offered roots itself within the Christian tradition in general and the Gospel narratives in particular, and takes the figure of Christ as the primary exemplar of this form of relational praxis. Virtue-friendships that reflect the friendships of Jesus, the one true image of God, give us a means and a form of self-knowledge that allows us to live life humanly and to begin to move toward the actualization of our status as creatures made in the image of God.

If we contextualize this understanding of friendship within the realm of mental health care, we find that friendship is that virtue which enables us to care with the compassion, humanity, and vision of Christ. The activity of Christlike friendship moves us beyond our socially bound expectations, and opens up new horizons and possibilities for human relationships, community, and mental health care. Christ-centered friendship demands that the church become a community that is deeply committed to those who are, in some senses, "least like us." It demands that we sit with the poor, commune with the marginalized, and sojourn with those whom society despises. In the virtue of friendship as defined by the tradition of the Gospels and the example of Christ, we discover the continuation of the incarnation and the possibility of a radical new vision of both society and church.

Radical Friendship

Reflecting on the discussion thus far, it becomes clear why one might legitimately refer to Christian friendship as *radical* friendship. The *Collins English Dictionary* defines the word "radical" as "favoring or tending to produce extreme or fundamental changes in political, economic, or social conditions, institutions, habits of mind." On reflection, it is clear that one of the goals of the type of friendship described above, rooted in a new way of being human revealed to us in the life of Christ, is to produce just such radical changes within individuals, the church, and the wider community. Such friendships axe both *centripetal* and *centrifugal,* reaching inward to contribute to the building of a loving and inclusive community, and outward to embrace and stand with the "outsiders," those who are oppressed and forced to stand on the margins of acceptable society. As such, *messianic* friends are always necessarily pushing against the boundaries of oppressive political and economic systems, ideologies, social conditions, and false epistemologies that might cause the suppression of the *imago Dei* in portions of the community. When Christian friends come together in solidarity and loving commitment, they encounter the world at a different level and see it from a different perspective. It is this radical edge to the friendship relationship that images the friendships of Jesus and enables friends to "see the world differently," and in seeing differently, move toward the initiation of liberation.

As the following chapters will show, people living with severe mental health problems are often defined as essentially "other," and marginalized, discriminated against, and excluded accordingly. Due to the nature of their condition and its psychological and social consequences, they are among the poorest and most marginalized within society. This being so, and in the light of the argument of this chapter, it becomes clear that *caring for the needs of people living with mental health problems is not an option for the church. Rather, it is a primary mark of its identity and faithfulness.* The church community cannot simply choose whether it should or should not minister to people with severe mental health problems. Quite the opposite. In order to *be* the church in any kind

38. Andrew Mackie and John Swinton, "Community and Culture: The Place of the Virtues in Psychiatric Nursing," *Journal of Psychiatric and Mental Health Nursing,* January, 2000, p. 36.

39. Stanley Hauerwas, *A Community of Character* (Notre Dame, Ind.: University of Notre Dame Press, 1981), p. 116.

40. Stanley Hauerwas, *Sanctify Them in the Truth,* p. 111.

41. For a development of this point, see Alasdair MacIntyre, *After Virtue: A Study in Moral Theology* (Lubbock, Texas: Duckworth, 1996).

of meaningful sense, it *has* to seek to minister to people living with mental health problems in all of their diversity. To minister within this area is a confirmation of the church's faithfulness to its calling. If God does have a "bias toward the poor," and if the church truly wishes to image Christ in his ministry of liberation and rehumanization, then the church must take the needs of this group of people most seriously. It is out of a desire to enable the church truly to be the church by developing a new and transformative form of ecclesial praxis that images the relationships and attitudes of Jesus, that this book finds its rationale and its goal.

CHAPTER ELEVEN

Aging and the Elderly

Every day we grow older — individually and as a society. In 1900, one out of twenty-five Americans (or 4 percent of the population) was over the age of 65. By 2003, that number had risen to 12 percent. These increases will continue dramatically. The "baby boomer" generation in the U.S. is beginning to turn 65 in 2011; by 2030, 20 percent of the U.S. population will be over the age of 65. By 2050, 5 percent of all Americans will find themselves in the category of the "old old" or "the third age" — those over the age of 85.[1] These trends are not unique to the United States.[2]

With aging comes greater likelihood of health problems or disability and therefore greater utilization of health care services, both high tech and low. Yet while our population is aging, particular cultural trends over the past fifty years — such as greater geographic mobility, dual-career households, a greater focus on nuclear rather than extended families — have eroded traditional networks that helped families care for their elderly members. Thus, in addition to the greater need for an array of health and support services, the shifting demographics signal a greater need over the next thirty years for viable options for long-term care.

But such care is costly, and poverty rates rise with advancing age. Why? In part because the elderly population is largely female. Women, on average, live longer than men. In 2000, women comprised almost 60 percent of the over-65 age group and 71 percent of those over the age of 85. Consequently, elderly women are more likely than their male counterparts to live alone, decreasing both their household income and their in-home support. Women, traditionally, have also entered occupations less well-compensated than those held by men, have received lower wages for similar work, or have spent more years outside the world of paid employment caring for children, parents, or spouses.

Conventional wisdom extrapolates from this data and concludes that the aging of our population is one of the major causes of the annual growth of health care spending in the U.S. Economist Uwe E. Reinhardt effectively debunks this myth and provides a more nuanced understanding of how health care costs for the elderly factor into overall health spending.[3] Reinhardt notes that when the data is analyzed carefully, "the per-capita health spending of nations is virtually independent of the age structure of its population," and that "the process of the aging of the population by itself adds only a very small part — usually about half a percentage point — to the annual growth in per-capita health spending in industrialized societies. . . . The bulk of annual spending growth can be explained by overall population growth (about 1.1 percent per year), increases in the prices of health care goods and services, and the availability of ever more new, often high-cost medical products and treatments used by all age groups." Nonetheless, the question of how to think about the use of health care resources in relation to elderly persons remains a central question in U.S. bioethics.

Before turning to these questions, we open with what we believe is a prior question: the nature of aging itself. Is it a natural part of the life course, a reality with its own unique gifts and resources? Or rather ought we to understand aging as a "disease" for which we should seek a "cure"? Should it be postponed, reversed, or even, perhaps, overcome? What if we could extend life — a relatively youthful form of life — indefinitely, to live to be as old as Methuselah or at least as old as many of the matriarchs and patriarchs of the Old Testament? Aubrey D. N. J de Grey takes up this question in his article "The Urgency Dilemma: Is Life Extension Research a Temptation or a Test?" (selection 73). De Grey notes how anti-aging medi-

1. U.S. Census Bureau, "65+ in the United States: 2005" (December 2005), http://www.census.gov/prod/2006pubs/p23-209.pdf. Last updated October 2006. See also: The UNC Institute on Aging, "United States Aging Demographics" (October 2006), http://www.aging.unc.edu/infocenter/slides/usaging.ppt.

2. K. Steel, "Research on Aging: An Agenda for All Nations Individually and Collectively," *Journal of the American Medical Association* (1997): 278, 1374-75.

3. Uwe E. Reinhardt, "Why Does U.S. Health Care Cost So Much? (Part III: An Aging Population Isn't the Reason)" (December 5, 2008), http://economix.blogs.nytimes.com/2008/12/05/why-does-us-health-care-cost-so-much-part-iii-an-aging-population-isnt-the-reason/. Anyone interested in a succinct and clear account of the economics of health care in the U.S. would benefit greatly from reading through the related series of articles by Reinhardt posted on the Economix site.

cine — and allied products available from pharmacies to boutiques — has become a huge business. In 2009, it was estimated that the market for what are now known as "cosmeceuticals," as well as memory-enhancers, sexual dysfunction treatments, and other interventions, would top $20 billion. De Grey, a scientist who works in anti-aging research, believes that it is imperative that we do all we can to postpone aging, and that the imperative is even more profound for Christians than for those who do not believe in eternal life. Aging, according to de Grey, is ghastly, causing unnecessary suffering. Christians are called to overcome this suffering, and to extend the abilities of others or oneself to continue to do God's work in the world.

While de Grey's assumptions might square well with broader Western culture, one might ask: How consistent are his assumptions with the Christian tradition? Is aging just ghastly, to be avoided at all costs? Is there more to "aging" than just physical and mental decline? And how does this factor into how we think about the relationship between health care and the elderly? Dennis Sansom in his essay "Why Do We Want to Be Healthy? Medicine, Autonomous Individualism, and the Community of Faith" (selection 75) challenges de Grey's claim. He raises the important question of the *telos* of American society, the *telos* that shapes health care. He identifies it as "autonomous individualism." He shows how this *telos* particularly shapes how we think about health care *vis-à-vis* the elderly. Drawing on the important yet controversial work of Daniel Callahan, Sansom raises the question of how we might understand mortality and aging as part of our destiny.

As mentioned earlier, while many are spending lots of money in pursuit of eternal — or at least a few more decades of — youth, many other people who have reached "the third age" (85 or older) find themselves increasingly constrained *vis-à-vis* health care resources to care for the sorts of issues that attend aging. John Kilner, in his essay "Age-Based Rationing of Life-Sustaining Health Care" (selection 74), harkens back to the conversation in Part II and our discussion of how to think theologically and ethically about questions of the allocation of health care resources, especially the notion of rationing (see Lustig in Chapter Four, selection 25) and how these questions can translate into disparities of care that ultimately cost lives. Kilner challenges the usual warrants typically invoked to limit the use of health care for the elderly. He notes the fundamental utilitarian bias of American culture and its focus on productivity and social contribution. He also assesses seemingly just criteria, such as equal opportunity, the notion of a natural life span, and even the virtue of prudence, to show how these criteria continue to think of elderly persons in quantitative rather than qualitative terms and to subtly mask discrimination. He argues that thinking about the use of health care with the elderly should be shaped by an approach informed by biblical, cross-cultural, and medical criteria.

When, we might ask, is the proper time to start thinking about aging, about being elderly, about the physical challenges that will come, and even about our own death? D. Stephen Long turns the conversation in this direction. Looking forward to Christopher Vogt's essay in Chapter Twenty-one, Long raises the question of what it means to "die well," a question that was central to Christian practice until the dawn of modern medicine. As he notes, learning to die well begins not when we are 82 or when we receive the diagnosis of a terminal illness, but right now — whether you (fair reader) are 18 or 48 years old. Long also picks up on Kilner's opening observation about the way the elderly are assessed in terms of "productivity" and takes this observation much deeper. In his essay, "The Language of Death: Theology and Economics in Conflict" (selection 76), Long demonstrates, step-by-step, how deeply the ways in which we now think and speak about aging and death are imbued with economic assumptions. He puts contemporary "givens" and debates in historical context, showing how many of our current practices involving "the elderly" are the result of certain economic assumptions and arrangements. He then shows how radically our picture of aging, burden, and care change when aging and economics are situated within a larger, overarching theological perspective — and how radically our practices might change as well. He particularly challenges the notion of the biological family as the place where this care takes place.

Long's focus on the church as the site of the creation of alternative practices of care for the elderly and Kilner's closing observation that current arguments for age-based rationing might subtly mask other forms of discrimination — like gender discrimination — come together in Amy Laura Hall's essay "Ruth's Resolve: What Jesus' Great-Grandmother May Teach about Bioethics and Care" (selection 77). It is probably not accidental, theologically, that "the widow" plays such a prominent role in the scriptural narrative, in both the Testaments. Hall leads the reader to dwell deeply in one of these narratives — the story of Ruth and her widowed mother-in-law Naomi. Hall dismantles thin, romanticized, and disempowering notions of women as innately caring and shows how the story of Ruth is one of resolute, courageous, arduous fidelity and is a model for contemporary Christians — women and men — faced with the call to care for the elderly in their midst. Hall challenges individual Christians and the contemporary church to ask themselves: Do we turn away from or walk with Naomi? Hall's essay appeared in an issue of *Christian Bioethics* devoted to aging and women, in conversation with two other essays of note.[4]

We close with one of the most difficult questions in medicine with relation to aging and the elderly — the question of dementia and Alzheimer's Disease. We in-

4. Two additional essays from this issue of *Christian Bioethics* (11 [April 2005]) engage and expand the question of women, aging, and bioethics: M. Cathleen Kaveney's "The Order of Widows: What the Early Church Can Teach Us about Older Women and Health Care," pp. 11-34; and M. Therese Lysaught's "Practicing the Order of Widows: A New Call for an Old Vocation," pp. 51-68.

clude the second chapter from David Keck's profound reflection on what he calls "the Theological Disease" in his book *Forgetting Whose We Are: Alzheimer's Disease and the Love of God.*[5] Keck's theological reflections on Alzheimer's are rooted in his family's experience of his mother's affliction with this disease. Keck's book is difficult to excerpt. Each of the eight chapters treats a different theological locus from the perspective of Alzheimer's, and each chapter is theologically rich and existentially profound. The selection offered, "Memory and Canonicity" (selection 78), engages the question of memory: How do we think about the "self" or the "personhood" of the patient with Alzheimer's when what is attacked is a central component of the "self" — our very ability to remember? Keck sets the Alzheimer's patient's loss of memory within a scriptural account of memory, both human and divine.

In the end, we hope readers leave this chapter convinced of three things: (1) that the primary question with regard to aging and the elderly is not one of resource allocation; (2) that more fundamental questions pertain to how we think about aging and how we think about the elderly among us; and (3) that through critical analysis of the assumptions of contemporary culture, wedded with a more thickly theological and scriptural understanding of aging and the elderly, we will be able to craft more adequate practices of caring for those who have reached the second or third age of life.

SUGGESTIONS FOR FURTHER READING

Hauerwas, Stanley, Carole Bailey Stoneking, Keith G. Meador, and David Cloutier, eds. *Growing Old in Christ* (Grand Rapids: Eerdmans, 2003).

Huebner, Chris K. "Curing the Body of Christ: Memory, Identity, and Alzheimer's Disease by Way of Two Mennonite Grandmothers." In *A Precarious Peace: Yoderian Explorations on Theology, Knowledge, and Identity* (Waterloo and Scottdale: Herald Press, 2006), pp. 163-75.

McFadden, Susan H., and John T. McFadden. *Aging Together: Dementia, Friendship, and Flourishing Communities* (Baltimore: Johns Hopkins University Press, 2011).

Mitchell, C. Ben, Robert D. Orr, and Susan A. Salladay, eds. *Aging, Death, and the Quest for Immortality* (Grand Rapids: Eerdmans, 2004).

Post, Stephen G. *The Moral Challenge of Alzheimer Disease,* 2nd ed. (Baltimore: Johns Hopkins University Press, 2000).

5. David Keck, *Forgetting Whose We Are: Alzheimer's Disease and the Love of God* (Nashville: Abingdon Press, 2006).

73 The Urgency Dilemma: Is Life Extension Research a Temptation or a Test?

Aubrey D. N. J. de Grey

The prospect of greatly postponing, or even reversing, the aging process has in recent years moved emphatically from the realms of science fiction to being science foreseeable. While many differences of opinion between experts remain concerning likely timeframes, an increasing number of specialists in the biology of aging (including the author) now take the view that we (a) know enough about the molecular and cellular basis of aging, and (b) possess versatile enough tools for modifying cells and molecules, that aging may well come within range of effective medical intervention within the lifetimes of many people alive today. In this essay I will explore some of the issues this raises for people in general and Christians in particular. I will focus especially on what I feel the Christian ethical framework says about the rights and wrongs of developing life-extension medicine and thereby postponing death.

The Pro-aging Trance

Anti-aging medicine is big business, despite being a blatant misnomer. Why is this, and does it matter?

The above questions will not form the basis for the bulk of this essay, but they are key aspects of the background information on which I will build. The fact that so many people choose to spend so much money on products that do not do what they are superficially advertised to do is a sociological phenomenon that we should understand, or at least explore, if we are to do justice to the issues that will be raised in the future by products and therapies that will more accurately be described as anti-aging medicine. Therefore, it is also key to any discussion of what we — Christians and/or non-Christians — should do today to influence the pace of development of those future therapies.

The quest for a "cure" to aging long predates Christianity — and so does our ambivalence concerning that

From Aubrey D. N. J. de Grey, "The Urgency Dilemma: Is Life Extension Research a Temptation or a Test?" *Update (Loma Linda University Center for Christian Bioethics)* 21.1 (June 2006): 6-10. Used by permission of Loma Linda University Center for Christian Bioethics.

quest. The tale of Gilgamesh is an obvious example. More instructive, perhaps, is the myth of Tithonus, the warrior who won the heart of the goddess Eos. Eos, who was of course immortal already, asked Zeus to make Tithonus immortal, and Zeus obliged — but Eos forgot to ask Zeus to make Tithonus eternally youthful, so he became frailer and frailer as time went on and eventually Eos turned him into a grasshopper. The relevance of this myth to the present discussion is the fact that it was invented at all (and has survived so well, even finding its way into popular culture such as "The X-Files"). The idea that if we extend life span we will necessarily do so by keeping frail people alive, rather than by keeping youthful people youthful, is of course ridiculous in principle and could never be introduced in rational debate, yet here it is introduced by the back door through a story. The message being surreptitiously conveyed is that postponing aging is tempting but ultimately a bad idea, even though we can't quite put our finger on what's bad about it. Evidently this is a message that we subconsciously like to hear, or else the myth would have been forgotten long ago.

The anti-aging industry has many of the same features. The actual, specific claims made for products that form the anti-aging industry are modest — as they must be, given the lack of evidence to support anything more robust. But the slipperier language that is given prominence on packaging and advertising is another matter entirely, including phrases such as "grow younger." This is possible mainly because aging is very hard to measure, and vendors know that advertising language is only illegal if it can be proved to be false, rather than if it cannot be proved to be true. But as with the "Tithonus error" (as it has come to be known), this ambiguity seems to be a positive attraction to the general public, who seem to like to suspend disbelief enough to engage in cosmetic efforts to combat aging, possibly comforted by the back-of-the-mind knowledge that they are indeed merely cosmetic. The alternative interpretation that most purchasers of "anti-aging" products truly believe they will live much longer as a result is, I feel, too harsh an estimation of the typical consumer's acumen.

In summary, my answer to the first question I posed above — why is anti-aging medicine big business? — is that society is deeply conflicted concerning aging, on the one hand recognizing that it is a curse to be combated, but at the same time shying away from all-out determination to combat it, for reasons that it cannot adequately crystallize. So to my second question: Does this matter?

If we take the view that modest postponement of aging is all that humanity will ever achieve by medical means, there is a good case that this incongruous attitude does not matter — indeed, that it is positively rational. Quite apart from the point that adults are entitled to spend their money on whatever they like so long as they are not palpably misled into doing so, and that the anti-aging industry is hardly alone in rose-tinting the efficacy of its wares, we must acknowledge that when faced with a fate that is both ghastly and unavoidable, there is a certain logic to putting it out of one's mind so as to make the most of what time one has left. Once this is accepted, we can go further and note that since such people are in the business of psychological self-management, it does not actually matter how irrational are the lines of reasoning that they may resort to in order to achieve that objective. In short, humanity's tendency to cling to the Tithonus error and its friends is a perfectly reasonable, rational response to the inevitability of aging. I have termed it the "pro-aging trance."

However, as soon as the inevitability of aging begins to look a little less certain, the above logic collapses. Worse, the depth of the pro-aging trance means that what was once a valid psychological strategy is transformed into an immense barrier to reasoned, objective debate concerning the desirability of postponing aging. This is why, as a fairly high-profile member of the life extension research community, I currently spend as much of my time on the social context of this field as on the science. Thus, the answer to my question "does the anti-aging industry matter?" is, in a nutshell: "It used not to matter, but now it matters a great deal."

Thus far I have discussed the attitudes of society in general and have not addressed issues that might relate specifically to Christians. The latter will be the focus of the remainder of this essay. As will be seen, I feel that Christians face a particularly formidable challenge to reasoning objectively about the merits of life extension. Paradoxically, however, when that challenge is overcome, it can be seen (or so I shall argue) that the imperative to do all one can to postpone aging is even more profound for Christians than for those who do not look forward to the prospect of God-given immortality.

Indefinite Life Extension and Immortality: An Unfortunate Confusion

Aging is a side-effect of living. The immensely complex network of biochemical processes that maintain our bodies in a fully functional state until middle age has side-effects, some of which build up throughout life. This molecular and cellular "damage" is initially harmless because our metabolism is able to work around it, but eventually it becomes abundant enough that metabolism is impaired and physical and mental decline ensue. There are seven main types of damage, encompassing cell loss, mutations, indigestible molecules, and stiffening of elastic tissues.

My work focuses on the development of therapies that will repair the various types of damage just mentioned. Others in the life extension research field are focusing on therapies that do not seek to repair pre-existing damage but instead to slow its subsequent accumulation. Repairing damage may sound harder than pre-empting it — after all, prevention is usually better than cure — but in this case it turns out, in my view at least, that while preventive measures are ideal in principle, truly effective ones are not in sight, simply because our understanding of the immense complexity of metabolism is still so superficial that we have no foreseeable prospect of designing interventions that do not do more harm than good. Additionally, of course, repair therapies can in principle rejuvenate those who are already suffering the effects of aging, whereas retardation therapies cannot. This is not in any way to say that retardation therapies are useless, but it does mean that they should be pursued mainly as potential adjuncts to rejuvenation therapies.

There is another difference between repair and retardation that must be emphasized at this point. Just like all other pioneering technologies, life extension technologies will be highly imperfect when they first arrive and will be progressively improved thereafter. For both repair therapies and retardation therapies, this means that the benefits someone can expect to obtain from access to the latest advances will exceed what they would get from the first therapies they receive. But this disparity is much more pronounced for repair therapies. In fact, it is highly likely that, once repair therapies exist that can confer 30 or so extra years of youthful life on those who are in their 50s or younger when the therapies arrive, the rate of improvement of the therapies will outpace the rate at which the types of damage that are not yet reparable are accumulating. In other words, even though aging will still be happening in the sense that damage is being laid down, and even though the problem of eliminating more damage is getting more difficult (because the easy types of damage have yielded to the already-developed therapies), the overall amount of damage in these people's bodies will be declining: they will be getting progressively more youthful and further from the prospect of dying of old age. This therefore constitutes indefinite life extension — indefinite maintenance of the probability of dying in the next year at a level typical of young adults.

I have called this situation "longevity escape velocity." I think that is quite a pithy, evocative phrase — it captures the idea that there is a threshold rate of progress beyond which a qualitatively different end result occurs, and the use of "escape" (from aging) seems apposite. However, despite my best efforts, the media predictably describe my work as an attempt to engineer "immortality."

Let me, therefore, be quite clear: That description is erroneous. Immortality is not what I'm engineering. Aging is one cause of death — a very common one, to be sure, killing roughly twice as many people worldwide as all other causes of death combined, but still just one cause. If aging was eliminated, we would in many ways be restoring our lives to the state they were in a few thousand years ago, when death from infections, starvation, and violence were each considerably more common than death from aging: Death would still occur, but the likelihood that you would die in the coming year would not be strongly influenced by your age.

The above answers the first key question that arises whenever the concept of indefinite life extension is discussed — that such work constitutes "playing God," depriving God of His right to decide when we should die. It quite clearly does nothing of the kind. Whether you die of aging at 80 or of being hit by a truck at age 800, God's influence over that event is the same. So when you see my work and similar efforts being described as engineering immortality, I hope you will count to 10, remind yourself that that is simply journalistic hype, and read on in the knowledge that what I actually seek to engineer is the elimination of one major cause of death.

Aging Doesn't Just Kill People, It Kills Them Horribly

Having disposed of an issue that is terminologically problematic but logically (and thus ethically and theologically) simple, I now turn to issues that are of more substance. In this short section I will discuss the pros and cons of various causes of death from the point of view of the suffering associated with them, and in the next section I will discuss some aspects of life extension research that I feel are wrongly thought by some to be relevant to the ethical (whether Christian or otherwise) status of that endeavor. That will conclude the groundwork for my discussion in the final section of the "urgency dilemma" to which the title of this essay refers — a dilemma that applies specifically to those who believe in an afterlife.

Death before the age of 60 is now relatively rare in the developed world — rare enough that when a friend dies that young we typically consider it a great loss (whether to us, to their family, or to the world in general). Conversely, when someone dies in their 80s, people tend to take the view that he or she had a "good innings" — there is a sense that the loss is somehow less. Is this rational?

I would like to suggest that it is not rational, because it neglects the fact that death at an advanced age invariably follows an extended period of physical decline, and usually mental decline too. That decline varies greatly in its severity and duration, to be sure, and the stated aspirations of many biogerontologists are centered on minimizing both those variables. But as compared to the severity and duration of the decline associated with death from age-independent causes, it is immense in almost everybody. And decline means suffering — for the individual concerned, for their loved ones, and even (in a more low-grade way) for society in general, which allocates resources to modestly alleviating that suffering and thus increases the suffering of others through lack of those resources. The suffering caused by the shock of losing a loved one in a fatal accident is meaningful, certainly, but it cannot and must not be considered to outweigh the aging-derived suffering just described — it does not compare.

A hasty perusal of the preceding paragraph might lead you to believe that I favor the banning of seat belts and crash helmets and, more generally, the compulsory adoption of highly risky lifestyles in order to minimize aging-related suffering. Of course I favor no such thing. I favor the bringing about of a shift in the causes of death, so that fewer people die of old age and more die of accidents, but I favor doing this by enabling people to stay biologically young and thereby avoid dying of old age, not by raising the risk of having a fatal accident in any given year. In this way, the suffering of aging will be eliminated. There will be a modest side-effect, however . . . we can expect to live at least 10 times as long as we do today.

Action, Inaction, and Urgency

I hope by this point to have reminded you that aging is rather a pity. What I will discuss next is where it objectively ranks in the canon of things that are undesirable and against which we have reason to expend our effort. As noted, I will not yet move to arguments that apply specifically to Christians.

One aspect of this issue that is often raised is whether action and inaction are morally equivalent. The logical position here is blindingly clear: If you're not doing something, you're doing something else, so there's no such thing as inaction, only choices between actions. Hence, if it's wrong to cause suffering by an action that directly inflicts it, it's also (and equally) wrong to cause that same suffering by an action that you do instead of an action that alleviates it. But there is a good reason why this question comes up so much: However clear it may be that action and inaction are logically identical, they are very far from identical psychologically. It's emotionally easier to pass by on the other side and put someone's suffering out of your mind than it is to cause the same result by actually doing something. Or conversely, it's easier to find the strength to refuse to do something that causes suffering (but which has some upside for you) than to find the strength to "act" to alleviate the suffering when "doing nothing" would have that upside. But being easier doesn't change the ethics of the situation.

Another way in which some influences on suffering might appear to differ importantly from others is the time that elapses between the action (or "inaction") that alters the suffering and the actual outcome (the occurrence or otherwise of the suffering). Intuitively, one may feel that priority should be given to alleviation of more imminent suffering, because there will be time to work on the more delayed potential suffering afterwards. But this is only correct if the opportunity to alleviate the more delayed suffering will still exist at that later time, and it may not: Events may be beyond one's control unless one acts now, even if those events will take time to unfold. In many real-world situations this is not a particularly important argument, because events that are a long way in the future almost always can still be influenced even if one attends to more urgent matters first. But there are exceptions.

The exception I'm thinking of — one to which my action/inaction point also sharply applies — is, of course, postponement of aging. On both counts, even once we appreciate that aging is the cause of immense suffering and thus should be combated, we are in danger of deprioritizing the postponement of aging in favor of other good deeds, either because those good deeds are not deeds so much as the avoidance of bad deeds, or because the suffering that we can alleviate in other ways is imminent, whereas any attempt (however concerted) to postpone aging will certainly not achieve its objective for at least a decade or two and probably longer. It is thus imperative to understand that, as I have just explained, these apparent justifications for leaving aging unchallenged are not ethically sound.

The Urgency Dilemma

The urgency that I discussed in the last section, i.e., the importance (or not) of prioritizing the alleviation of imminent suffering — is not the urgency to which I refer in the title of this essay. The urgency in the title concerns the afterlife.

For all those who believe in heaven, or that the soul survives after the body is gone, or that God will in due course make his chosen people immortal, or any other variant on this theme, death is the beginning of a new life that is incomparably more, well, heavenly than this life ever was. Thus, from a selfish point of view, the sooner death comes, the better. The fact that it's from a selfish point of view is the stumbling block, of course: Selfishness is a sin, so engineering one's own premature death might not have the desired effect.

But what does a belief in a better life to come mean for one's desire to postpone aging? For some devout Christians with whom I have discussed this issue, it means rather a lot — but for very poor reasons. Specifically, it causes them to view the postponement of aging as a double-edged sword: They accept that it would alleviate suffering but they note that it would also postpone bliss, so they see it even less as a priority than others do. Added to this is that the action/inaction argument often features in these discussions, despite the clear relevance of the parable of the Good Samaritan.

So I come, at the end of this essay, to the question in its title. Is life extension research a temptation for those of faith — something that would be sinful, taking control of a matter that should be God's prerogative — or is it a test, something that we should energetically embrace even though it will postpone our entry into the kingdom of heaven? It seems incontrovertible to me that the latter is the case — that by treating the prospect of the afterlife as a reason not to strive to combat aging, we are making a decision ethically no different from the person who commits suicide in order to reach God sooner. In some ways it is a more problematic decision even than that, because by committing suicide one turns down the opportunity to continue doing good in the world, but by not participating in the "war on aging" one is not only acquiescing in others' possibly avoidable suffering but also helping to deprive them of a longer life of doing good. These do not seem to me to be outcomes of which we are taught God would approve.

Conclusion

In this essay I have attempted to show that the popular belief that working to postpone aging would be "playing God" and thus sinful is in fact the exact opposite of the correct interpretation of Christian doctrine: In fact, it is a sin not to work to postpone aging. I have dwelt at length on issues that are not specific to Christians, such as the relationship between lack of aging and immortality or between action and inaction, for two reasons. First, without these underpinnings the argument that life extension research is imperative is weakened, whether or not one believes in the afterlife. Second, Christians are just as susceptible as others to the psychological traps that can make sinning easy; as such, it is vital to remind Christians that they are indeed traps, in order to give the inevitable conclusion that we have a duty to combat aging with our full force. By this essay I hope to have opened a few eyes to the horror of a phenomenon that humanity has always been so determined to ignore, and to the duty that I feel we all have to consider what we can contribute to the war on aging.

74 Age-Based Rationing of Life-Sustaining Health Care

John F. Kilner

Thousands of people die annually — even in developed countries like the United States — for lack of access to widely available high-tech treatments such as organ transplantation. Vastly greater numbers die worldwide for lack of access to immunizations, antibiotics, and prenatal care.[1] The inescapable question echoes around the world: When there is not enough for everyone, who gets it and who does not? Who lives and who dies?[2]

Sometimes the problem is that health care becomes very expensive, or that the resources allocated to it become limited by other priorities — perhaps misplaced priorities. So it may be a question of tight money;[3] or it may be a question of other scare resources, such as organs for transplant.[4]

Valiant efforts have been made to save the lives of those who cannot get transplants. The artificial kidney — hemodialysis — was developed to save the lives of those who could not have kidney transplants. That development created a new allocation problem: who would get the available dialysis machines? In 1962, *Life* magazine ran a now infamous exposé about how hospitals were deciding who would live and who would be left to die. People who were socially attractive were the winners.[5]

1. UNICEF, *The State of the World's Children 2002* (New York: UNICEF, 2002).

2. Victor R. Fuchs, *Who Shall Live? Health, Economics, and Social Choice,* expanded edition (River Edge, N.J.: World Scientific, 1998); William D. Frazier, "Rationing of Health Care — Who Determines Who Gets the Cure, When, Where, and Why?" *Annals of Health Law* 2 (1993): 95-99; John F. Kilner, *Who Lives? Who Dies?* (New Haven, Conn.: Yale University Press, 1990).

3. Paul Menzel et al., "Toward a Broader View of Values in Cost-Effectiveness Analysis of Health," *Hastings Center Report* 29 (May-June, 1999): 7-15; Jack W. Snyder, "Making Medical Spending Decisions: The Law, Ethics, and Economics of Rationing Mechanisms," *Journal of Legal Medicine* 19 (March 1998): 143-50.

4. Volker H. Schmidt, "Selection of Recipients for Donor Organs in Transplant Medicine," *Journal of Medicine and Philosophy* 23 (February 1998): 50-74; Thomas Gutmann and Walter Land, "The Ethics of Organ Allocation: The State of the Debate," *Transplantation Reviews* 11 (October 1997): 191-207.

5. Shana Alexander, "They Decide Who Lives, Who Dies," *Life*

From John F. Kilner, "Age-Based Rationing of Life-Sustaining Healthcare," in *Aging, Death, and the Quest for Immortality,* ed. Ben C. Mitchell, Robert D. Orr, and Susan A. Salladay (Grand Rapids: Wm. B. Eerdmans, 2004), pp. 58-74.

The matter went to the floor of the United States Congress. Congress understandably was not eager to tackle the issue of how to decide who should live and who should die. No Congressional hearings were held on the matter. Less than thirty minutes of debate took place on the Senate floor. Congress was able to escape developing ethical criteria by deciding to fund dialysis for everyone.[6] What was projected to cost a few hundred million dollars at the time skyrocketed to two billion dollars in the first decade, and then well beyond that.[7] Everyone realized then that the next time a major artificial organ developed, it could not simply be given to everyone.[8] Ethical criteria would be unavoidable.

We have now witnessed the use of a totally implantable artificial heart in humans, and huge demand is predictable.[9] Other lifesaving technologies will not be far behind. The pressure to develop ethical allocation criteria will only be escalating in the days ahead.[10]

One approach to this challenge is to bar older people from receiving life-sustaining health care such as organ transplants and implants[11] — or possibly even allowing them only limited intensive care space.[12] There is evidence that similar age considerations affect treatment decisions in many other areas of health care as well.[13] Prominent bioethicists such as Daniel Callahan, Robert Veatch, and Norman Daniels have all expressed support for some form of age-based rationing, as will be discussed shortly. Why this mushrooming interest in age-

---

53 (November 9, 1962): 102-25. See also David Sanders and Jesse Dukeminier Jr., "Medical Advance and Legal Lag: Hemodialysis and Kidney Transplantation," *UCLA Law Review* 15 (February 1968): 366-80; "Scarce Medical Resources," *Columbia Law Review* 9 (April 1969): 620-92. For additional sources, see Kilner, *Who Lives? Who Dies?* p. 28.

6. The arguments voiced by a majority of the senators during the brief floor debate confirm this interpretation: United States Congress, *Congressional Report* 118 (September 30, 1972): 33007. See also Leonard M. Fleck, "DRGs: Justice and the Invisible Rationing of Health Care Resources," *Journal of Medicine and Philosophy* 12 (May 1987): 184; James F. Childress, "The Gift of Life: Ethical Problems and Policies in Obtaining and Distributing Organs for Transplantation," *Critical Care Clinics* 2 (January 1986): 144-45; George J. Annas, "The Prostitute, the Playboy, and the Poet: Rationing Schemes for Organ Transplantation," *American Journal of Public Health* 75 (February 1985): 187; Lorraine R. Adams, "Medical Coverage for Chronic Renal Disease: Policy Implications," *Health and Social Work* 3 (1978): 42.

7. Eugene L. Meyer, "Tax Money for Transplant Operations: Who Pays?" *Washington Post* (September 12, 1984): 18; Glenn Richards, "Technology Costs and Rationing Issues," *Hospitals* 58 (June 1, 1984): 81; *National Heart Transplantation Study* (Seattle: Battelle Human Affairs Research Centers, 1984): ch. 44:41; R. W. Schmidt et al., "The Dilemmas of Patient Treatment for End-Stage Renal Disease," *American Journal of Kidney Diseases* 3 (July 1983).

8. Ruth Macklin, *Mortal Choices* (New York: Pantheon, 1987), p. 160; Drummond Rennie et al., "Limited Resources in the Treatment of End-stage Renal Failure in Britain and the United States," *Quarterly Journal of Medicine*, n.s., 56 (July 1985): 227; Glenn C. Graber et al., *Ethical Analysis of Clinical Medicine* (Baltimore: Urban and Schwarzenberg, 1985), p. 208; Minnesota Coalition on Health Care Costs, *The Price of Life: Ethics and Economics* (Minneapolis: M.C.H.C.C., 1984), p. 33; Institute of Medicine, *Disease by Disease Toward National Health Insurance? Implications of a Categorical Catastrophic Disease Approach to National Health Insurance* (Washington, D.C.: National Academy of Sciences, 1973), pp. 8-9.

9. For a discussion of the development of the artificial heart, including the latest trials regarding the totally implantable artificial heart and the 100,000 or so lives that might be saved annually by it in the United States alone, see www.heartpioneers.com. Cf. Dale Jamieson, "The Artificial Heart: Reevaluating the Investment," in *Organ Substitution Technology*, ed. Deborah Mathieu (Boulder, Colo.: Westview, 1988).

10. Even the provision of dialysis for everyone in the United States — not to mention elsewhere — has come under huge pressure, because of the great costs involved. See John K. McKenzie et al., "Dialysis Decision Making in Canada, the United Kingdom and the United States," *American Journal of Kidney Diseases* 31 (January 1998): 12-18; Gregory W. Rutecki and John F. Kilner, "Dialysis As a Resource Allocation Paradigm: Confronting Tragic Choices Once Again?" *Seminars in Dialysis* 12 (January-February 1999): 38-43; Shahid M. Chanda et al., "Is There a Rationale for Rationing Chronic Dialysis? A Hospital Based Cohort Study of Factors Affecting Survival and Morbidity," *British Medical Journal* 318 (January 23, 1999): 217-23.

11. Schmidt, "Selection of Recipients"; James Neuberger et al., "Assessing Priorities for Allocation of Donor Liver Grafts: Survey of Public and Clinicians," *British Medical Journal* 317 (July 18, 1998): 172-75; Peter A. Ubel and George Loewenstein, "Distributing Scarce Livers: The Moral Reasoning of the General Public," *Social Science and Medicine* 42 (April 1996): 1049-55; Mary C. Corley and Gilda Sneed, "Criteria in the Selection of Organ Transplant Recipients," *Heart and Lung* 23 (November-December 1994): 446-57.

12. John D. Lantos et al., "Resource Allocation in Neonatal and Medical ICUs: Epidemiology and Rationing at the Extremes of Life," *American Journal of Respiratory and Critical Care Medicine* 156 (July 1997): 185-89; William Meadow et al., "Distributive Justice across Generations: Epidemiology of ICU Care for the Very Young and the Very Old," *Clinics in Perinatology* 23 (September 23, 1996): 597-608; Janet Baltz and Judith L. Wilson, "Age-Based Limitation for ICU Care: Is It Ethical?" *Critical Care Nurse* 15 (December 1995): 65-73; P. Frisho-Lima et al., "Rationing Critical Care: What Happens to Patients Who Are Not Admitted," *Theoretical Surgery* 9 (December 1994): 208-11; Society of Critical Care Medicine Ethics Committee, "Attitudes of Critical Care Medicine Professionals Concerning Distribution of Intensive Care Resources," *Critical Care Medicine* 22 (February 1994): 358-62.

13. N. J. Turner et al., "Cancer in Old Age: Is It Inadequately Investigated and Treated?" *British Medical Journal* 319 (July 31, 1999): 309-12; Marshall B. Kapp, "*De Facto* Health-Care Rationing by Age: The Law Has No Remedy," *Journal of Legal Medicine* 19 (September 1998): 223-49; Robert P. Giugliano et al., "Elderly Patients Receive Less Aggressive Medical and Invasive Management of Unstable Angina: Potential Impact of Practice Guidelines," *Archives of Internal Medicine* 158 (May 25, 1998): 1113-20; Mary Hamel et al., "Seriously Ill Hospitalized Adults: Do We Spend Less on Older Patients?" *Journal of the American Geriatrics Society* 44 (September 1996): 1043-48. For a large number of additional sources describing age-based rationing criteria in organ transplantation, intensive care, and a wide range of other health-care settings, see John F. Kilner, "Why Now? The Growing Interest in Limiting the Lifesaving Health Care Resources Available to Elderly People," in *Choosing Who's to Live: Ethics and Aging*, ed. James W. Walters (Urbana, Ill.: University of Illinois Press, 1996), pp. 144-47.

based rationing of health care? Are the reasons ethically legitimate? What insights does a Christian perspective give us into the present debate?

The Influence of Economy and Utility

The most commonly cited reason for limiting the lifesaving resources available to older people in the United States is the economic impact of the rapidly growing number of elderly persons.[14] The percentage of the American population over age sixty-five has grown from less than 2 percent in 1790 to nearly 12.5 percent in 2000. Particularly fast-growing are the ranks of the oldest persons — those eighty-five years or older. By 2000, their number in the United States had topped 4.2 million, representing 1.5 percent of the population; moreover, this number is projected to increase considerably in the future.[15]

These escalating numbers, particularly of the oldest persons, signal a rapidly growing need for assistance. Those eighty and older have substantially higher rates of illness and disability even when compared only with persons in their seventies and sixties. Moreover, elderly persons who have severe disabilities are more likely to experience chronic disease, to be older and poorer, and to be more dependent than other elderly persons.[16]

The association of age and cost is an understandable one. As the reasoning goes, health care for elderly persons is costing more and more money, so in order to cut costs it will be necessary to cut back on the health-care resources that will be available to them. Nevertheless, three observations challenge this simple economic rationale for age-based allocation of health care.

First, health-care costs are increasing as a result of a variety of factors, many of which have no special connection to elderly persons. Why are older people as a group singled out to bear the brunt of cutbacks in lifesaving care?[17]

Second, resource constraints are (for the most part) due to the fact that the sum total of individuals' various desires exceeds the total of available resources. In a country that can justify spending $3 billion annually on potato chips, for example, why would people consider preventing a certain group of patients from obtaining lifesaving health care to be one of the best ways to pursue cost savings?[18]

Third, when it is claimed, economically speaking, that elderly persons are receiving a "disproportionate share" of health-care resources, the question must be raised, "disproportionate to what?" They are not receiving disproportionately to their medical need (assuming that medical criteria are being applied equitably to all). Why do those concerned about disproportionate shares so readily assume that the appropriate frame of reference for "proportion" is age?

These three observations suggest that a more complicated economic trend is at work in the United States than merely a concern to reduce health care or other expenditures. There appear to be other reasons for targeting elderly persons in particular for cutbacks. That lifesaving care is an issue even raises the possibility that there is something undesirable about elderly persons *per se*.[19]

The view that health care ought to be rationed for the elderly is attributable, at least in part, to the utilitarian orientation of American culture. Utilitarianism is an outlook that identifies right actions as those producing the greatest good for the greatest number of people. When employed consciously or unconsciously as a means of determining who should receive limited resources, it predisposes one to view people in terms of whatever contributions are valued most highly by the society, with a bias toward contributions most readily quantifiable and thus comparable.

In a market-driven society like the United States, economic productivity is at the top of the list. So it is no surprise that older people, who are less likely to be viewed as economically productive, are not highly valued. They are "retired" — or even more succinctly put, "retirees" — no longer productive in the ways that matter most in contemporary society. Efforts to defend elderly persons by promoting the image of old age as a time of new possibilities and productivity (the slogan "I'm retreaded, not retired," for example) only reinforce this utilitarian perspective. What matters is productivity.[20]

14. For a fuller discussion of this economic justification for age-based rationing of health care, see Kilner, "Why Now? The Growing Interest," pp. 122-26.

15. United States Census Bureau, "Profiles of General Demographic Characteristics," *2000 Census of Population and Housing* (Washington, D.C.: U.S. Dept. of Commerce, May 2000); American Medical Association, "Ethical Implications of Age-Based Rationing of Health Care," downloaded from www.ama-assn.org/ama1/upload/mm/369/15b.pdf on July 10, 2001; Jane A. Boyajian, "Sacrificing the Old and Other Health Care Goals," in *Aging and Ethics*, ed. Nancy S. Jecker (Clifton, N.J.: Humana, 1991), p. 320.

16. Robert H. Binstock and Stephen G. Post, "Old Age and the Rationing of Health Care," in *Too Old for Health Care?* ed. Binstock and Post (Baltimore: Johns Hopkins University Press, 1991), pp. 7-8; Boyajian, "Sacrificing the Old," p. 320.

17. For further probing of this question, see Robert H. Binstock, "Another Form of Elderly Bashing," *Journal of Health Politics, Policy, and Law* 17 (summer 1992): 271.

18. This matter is discussed further in Christine K. Cassel, "The Limits of Setting Limits," in *A Good Old Age?* ed. Paul Homer and Martha Holstein (New York: Simon and Schuster, 1990), p. 200.

19. Needless to say, there are a host of other reasons given by proponents of age-based allocation for limiting lifesaving care. The point here is not that the "real reason" is something different, but that there are forces at work in the culture that may well make the reasons offered more intuitively attractive (or less offensive) than they would otherwise seem on their own merits.

20. For further discussion on this point, see p. 83 of Christine K. Cassel and Bernice L. Neugarten, "The Goals of Medicine in an Aging Society," and pp. 165 and 171 of Thomas H. Murray, "Meaning, Aging, and Public Policy," both in *Too Old for Health Care?* ed. Binstock and Post. See also Henry C. Simmons, "Countering Cultural Metaphors of Aging," *Journal of Religious Gerontology* 7 (1990): 156.

This emphasis on productivity helps explain American society's preoccupation with youth. Youth is the time of greatest productivity and thus possibility — a time most worthy of society's attention and protection. Accordingly, elderly people are commonly referred to in terms of either their distance from youth (e.g., "over the hill") or their decline from youth (e.g., their "sunset years").

The utilitarian way of thinking that sustains the emphasis on youth and productivity in the United States has been criticized harshly. For instance, comparing everyone's social contribution is extremely difficult, since everything potentially of benefit to anyone in society must be considered. Utilitarian thinking has also been castigated for its lack of inherent protections against how badly a person or group can be treated if society finds such treatment to be economically beneficial. Even if, however, a utilitarian way of thinking were workable and theoretically sound, the question of what should count as a "contribution to society" remains. The tendency to focus on economic contributions in the United States is rather different from the perspective of some other societies around the world.

While European and Asian examples could be cited, a particularly good example of an alternative outlook may be found among the Akamba people of Kenya.[21] The great respect accorded to older people there is intimately bound up with their view of the relationship between the individual and the community. Whereas the utilitarian view conceives of the social good atomistically in terms of individual (mainly job-related) contributions summed over the breadth of society, the Akamba view presupposes a social network of interpersonal relations of which one becomes more and more an essential part the older one becomes. The more interwoven a person becomes with others through time, the greater the damage done to the social fabric when that person is torn away by death.

When we look at the economic, especially utilitarian, context of health-care resource allocation in countries like the United States today, it is no wonder that age criteria have such a strong, albeit often unconscious, appeal. But as we have seen, there are indeed viable alternatives to the economic, individualistic, youth-oriented outlook so influential in the United States.

A Biblical Alternative

The utilitarian outlook is not the only major cultural consideration underlying the contemporary openness to age-based rationing of health care in the United States and elsewhere. In recent decades, Americans have witnessed an increasing reluctance to include biblical-Christian perspectives and arguments in public policy discussions, as a result of concerns over "separation of church and state." What difference has that made in how society has come to view its elderly members? To put the same question differently, if one were open to considering the wisdom that a biblical outlook on life offers, what would that outlook tell us about elderly people and how elderly people should be treated? Regarding the distinctive characteristics of older people, two characteristics stand out at various points in the biblical writings: their wisdom and their weakness.[22]

First, older people are generally wise. "Is not wisdom found among the aged?" Job asks rhetorically, and "Does not long life bring understanding?" (Job 12:12 NIV; cf. 15:10; 32:7). The elders (normally elderly) are, therefore, in the best position to give good counsel (e.g., Deut. 32:7); and a family that has lost all of its elderly has been severely punished (1 Sam. 2:31). In fact, a city with men and women of "ripe old age" is considered blessed (Zech. 8:4).

The difference that the wisdom of elderly counsel can make is nowhere more dramatically illustrated than in 1 Kings 12 (cf. 2 Chron. 10). There, a large assembly of God's people ask King Rehoboam to lighten their harsh workload. The king consults with two groups of counselors — one of old men and one of young men. His failure to heed the wise counsel of the old men leads to the dramatic break-up of God's kingdom into the two antagonistic kingdoms of Israel and Judah! Wisdom, then, is generally presented as a function of the life experience that only elderly persons have. Because, however, it is also the product of righteousness and God's Spirit, it is possible occasionally for young people to have wisdom (Job 32:8-9; Eccles. 4:13) and older people to lack it (Job 12:20).

A second characteristic of many elderly persons — at least at some point — is that they are weak. Old age is acknowledged in the Scriptures as a time of suffering and vulnerability (Eccles. 12:2-5; 2 Sam. 19:35). It is a time of failing eyes (e.g., Gen. 27:1; 48:10; 1 Sam. 4:15; 1 Kings 14:4), failing feet (e.g., 1 Kings 15:23), and declining overall bodily health (e.g., 1 Sam. 4:18; 1 Kings 1:1). Knowing that insensitive people take advantage of the weakness of older people, the psalmist prays, "Do not cast me away when I am old; do not forsake me when my strength is gone" (Ps. 71:9; cf. v. 18).

Such weakness may be a general characteristic but not an absolute characteristic. Elderly people, therefore, should not automatically be written off as mentally or physically incapable simply because of their age. God often breaks through stereotypes. Who would have thought that Sarah and Abraham would have a child in

21. John F. Kilner, "Who Shall Be Saved? An African Answer," in *Choices and Conflict*, ed. Emily Friedman (Chicago: American Hospital Association, 1992), pp. 22-27.

22. An earlier version of portions of the biblical-Christian discussion in this chapter may be found in John F. Kilner, *Life on the Line: Ethics, Aging, Ending Patients' Lives, and Allocating Vital Resources* (Grand Rapids: Eerdmans, 1992), and in John F. Kilner, "The Ethical Legitimacy of Excluding the Elderly When Medical Resources Are Limited," *The Annual of the Society of Christian Ethics* (1988): 179-203.

their very old age (Gen. 18:11-14; 21:5-7); or that the Shunammite woman would have a baby with her elderly husband (2 Kings 4:14ff.); or that the elderly Elizabeth, relative to Jesus' mother Mary, would bear a child (Luke 1:36-37)? Who would have expected Jacob to father Joseph at such an old age that Joseph became special for that reason (Gen. 37:3)? While weakness is often present in older people, it must be discovered and documented — never assumed.

Both the wisdom and weakness of elderly people call for appropriate responses, namely, respecting and protecting. We respond appropriately to wisdom by respecting it and those who possess it. Evil peoples are sometimes characterized by their lack of respect for those who are older (Deut. 28:50; 2 Chron. 36:17; Isa. 47:6). It is an evil day when "the young will rise up against the old" (Isa. 3:5 NIV), when elders are shown no respect (Lam. 5:12). The young are to resist the temptation to despise the old (e.g., Prov. 23:22), and instead are to recognize gray hair — i.e., old age — as a crown of splendor (Prov. 20:29). People are to "rise in the presence of the aged," says the Lord. They are to "show respect for the elderly" (Lev. 19:32). This particular command is one of seven commands in Leviticus 19 that ends with something like the words "I am the Lord," thereby underlining their importance by emphasizing God's authority. This command regarding elderly people adds — before those closing words — the call to "revere your God."

It appears here that the connection between God and older people is special. God is not simply saying that this, like all other commands, should be obeyed. The point, instead, is that obedience to this command in particular expresses a special reverence for God. By showing respect for the elderly, we are revering God.

If we rightly respond to wisdom by respecting those who possess it, we appropriately respond to the relative weakness of the elderly by protecting them. God is frequently portrayed in biblical writings as the protector of the weak (Exod. 22:22-27; Ps. 10:14; 35:10; 140:12; Acts 20:35; 1 Cor. 8:9-12; 2 Cor. 12:9-10), and God's people are challenged to be the same (Prov. 31:8-9; 1 Thess. 5:14). So it is not at all surprising to find God affirming that "Even to your old age and gray hairs I am he, I am he who will sustain you" (Isa. 46:4 NIV).

That God says "even" in old age emphasizes that, from a human perspective, it is easy to find reasons to support younger people, and that, in this utilitarian world, it is all too easy to neglect older people. King David observed this phenomenon in his day, which is why he implores God to sustain him, as he puts it, "even when I am old and gray" (Ps. 71:18 NIV). Because God is a sustainer of elderly people, it is natural to expect that godly people will do the same (e.g., Ruth 4:15).

Elderly people are as worthy of staying alive and even receiving lifesaving care as anyone else. In fact, whether a particular society values the wisdom of the elderly or not is ultimately beside the point. All persons are God's creation in God's own image (Gen. 1:27) and are the objects of God's sacrificial love in Christ (John 3:16). God pours out the Spirit on the old as well as on the young (Joel 2:28; Acts 2:17). The equal worth of all persons demands that all be respected and that the weak accordingly receive special protection.

What are the implications of all this for age-based rationing of life-sustaining health care? First and foremost, a straightforward utilitarian exclusion of older people, because they are less productive in some sense, is just as straightforwardly unethical. It misunderstands what is important about a person and it rests on a philosophy that undergirds some of the most oppressive attitudes and episodes in the history of humanity.

Non-Utilitarian Justifications

There are, however, other justifications for age criteria that do not overtly appeal to utilitarian values. What about them? First of all, that the intuitive appeal of such justifications is greatly strengthened by a utilitarian social context is unavoidable. Against such a backdrop, we should be highly skeptical of arguments for age-based rationing of life-sustaining health care, no matter how philosophically pure they may appear. We also need to address such justifications on their own terms.

Medical Benefit

Perhaps the most commonly invoked non-utilitarian justification of age-based rationing criteria in health care involves an appeal to medical benefit: "This patient is elderly, and elderly patients don't live as long or as well as other patients, and treatment is less likely to be successful in elderly patients — so this patient shouldn't receive treatment."[23] If the real concern here is medical, then the medical criteria involved should be invoked as such. Age *per se* is not the issue. We have to be careful how we use language. We should take care to identify as "medical" only those qualities and criteria that are, in fact, medical.

Age *per se* is not a medically relevant factor in determinations about individual patients, since medical problems that make one elderly person a bad candidate for a given treatment may not affect another. We generally cannot even assume that a particular elderly person has a short life expectancy. It is certainly true that many elderly patients are so physically weakened that they make poor candidates for organ transplantation or intensive care; but others bear up fairly well in these circumstances. Similarly, although elderly patients have often been excluded from dialysis treatment, many of those who have received it have done well.

Accordingly, age is best not identified as a separate ra-

23. For a more in-depth discussion of the ethical issues involved here, see Kilner, *Life on the Line,* chap. 8; and John F. Kilner, "Age Criteria in Medicine: Are the Medical Justifications Ethical?" *Archives of Internal Medicine* 149 (October 1989): 2343-46.

tioning criterion at all. Rather, its most appropriate role is probably as one of many "symptoms" to be assessed by the physician making the medical assessment required for any treatment decision. Like any observed symptom, age can be an indicator of a possible medical problem. Age serves best as a tool the physician uses in applying a medical criterion, not as a criterion in its own right. From this perspective it is inappropriate to identify age during a discussion of rationing criteria in a way that implies that it is more than just one among many symptoms considered in a medical assessment.

Even in this more restricted role, however, age considerations must be handled carefully to ensure that they are not accorded more influence than is warranted medically. It is easy enough to underestimate the ability of some elderly patients to endure treatment when life is at stake; and technological developments consistently make treatments more endurable. In the end, the only way to know with confidence how elderly people will bear up under a given treatment may well be to treat them in large numbers, as was done during the early days of dialysis in Italy.[24] Whenever possible, a therapeutic trial can be employed to facilitate more individualized assessments.

Three other non-utilitarian justifications for age-based rationing have also been put forward by contemporary bioethicists such as Robert Veatch, Daniel Callahan, and Norman Daniels. They are based on ethical appeals to equal opportunity, natural life span, and prudence.[25] The appeal to equal opportunity contends that the most important equality at issue here is the equal opportunity to live to the same age as others. Some notion of a *prima facie* right to a minimum number of life-years may be involved.[26] The life span justification holds that there is a natural life span (perhaps seventy, perhaps eighty years) — a span which is normative rather than merely a statistical average at the present moment in history. Once people have reached this age, medicine should generally no longer be concerned with extending their lives.[27] The appeal to prudence maintains that people should be treated equally not so much in the present moment as over a lifetime. Health care should be provided in the way that enables all people to live as long as possible. To achieve this end, the resources available must be prudentially distributed throughout each person's lifetime in a way that will protect against early death. Expensive life-sustaining resources, then, might be made available only to young persons, with personal care services enhanced for those who are older.[28] Each of these three justifications warrants a closer look.

Equal Opportunity

Equal-opportunity justifications for age-based rationing support giving people an equal opportunity to live a long time, thereby maximizing the life-years saved. The most dubious aspect of this justification is the way that it values *life-years* rather than *lives* (i.e., persons). People are more than sums of life-years that are accumulated like nickels. Accordingly, murderers are typically not punished less for killing sixty-five-year-olds than for killing twenty-five-year-olds. Life is equally precious at any age. Although it is indeed better, where possible, to preserve someone's life for a longer rather than a shorter time, it is another thing to suggest that we should seek to preserve one person's life for a long time at the price of denying any chance of living to another.

Two problems unrelated to maximizing life-years are also involved in attempting, by means of an age criterion, to equalize the opportunity people have to live a long life. The first of these involves the manner in which we calculate the patient's opportunity to experience life. Say two women need the same scarce lifesaving resource. One of them is thirty-five years old; the other is thirty-six years old but has recently emerged from more than a year spent in a coma. If we are making decisions on the basis of an age criterion, whom do we choose? Usually the younger woman would be the preferable candidate on the grounds that her shorter life has given her less opportunity to experience life. In this case, however, the older woman has had the lesser opportunity. If we concede that it is valid to consider issues like these in making a decision in the matter, we open the door to any number of imprecise qualitative considerations in the assessment of who has had the least opportunity to experience life.

One proponent of this approach admits that such as-

24. Terrie Wetle, "Age As a Risk Factor for Inadequate Treatment," *Journal of the American Medical Association* 258 (July 24/31, 1987): 516; G. D'Amico, "Treating End-Stage Renal Disease: An Age Equivalence Index," *Annals of Internal Medicine* 96 (April 1982): 417-23.

25. For a more in-depth discussion of the ethical issues involved in these approaches, see Kilner, *Life on the Line,* chap. 9; and John F. Kilner, "Age As a Basis for Allocating Lifesaving Medical Resources: An Ethical Analysis," *Journal of Health Politics, Policy, and Law* 13 (fall 1988): 405-23.

26. This ethical appeal can be traced back to classical formulations put forward by Robert M. Veatch in two settings, among others: "Justice and Valuing Lives," in *Life Span,* ed. Robert M. Veatch (San Francisco: Harper and Row, 1979), p. 218; and "Ethical Foundations for Valuing Lives: Implications for Life-Extending Technologies," in *A Technology Assessment of Life-Extending Technologies,* Supplementary Report, vol. 6 (Glastonbury, Conn.: Futures Group, 1977), p. 232. Cf. Paul T. Menzel, *Medical Costs, Moral Choices* (New Haven, Conn.: Yale University Press, 1983), p. 191.

27. This ethical appeal can be traced back to classical formulations put forward by Daniel Callahan in two settings, among others: *Setting Limits: Medical Goals in an Aging Society* (New York: Simon and Schuster, 1987), pp. 137ff.; and "Aging and the Ends of Medicine," *Annals of the New York Academy of Sciences* 530 (1988): 128-29.

28. This ethical appeal can be traced back to classical formulations put forward by Norman Daniels in two settings, among others: *Just Health Care* (London: Cambridge University Press, 1985), pp. 96-97; and *Am I My Parents' Keeper?* (New York: Oxford University Press, 1988), pp. 8-9, chap. 5.

sessments would be "an overwhelmingly complicated task," calling it "procedurally and administratively a nightmare."[29] Yet, how would we justify excluding such factors? A patient's socioeconomic or spiritual condition may have much more to do with her or his lifetime experience of well-being than does age. Age provides too rough an approximation of lifetime well-being (or present physical health for that matter) to be determinative when something as important as life is at stake.

The other problem related to equalizing the opportunity to live long concerns past access of patients to resources. Should a younger person who has already received years of life-extending medical care be automatically preferred to an older person who has received very little? A strictly employed age criterion would say so, although it seems less than accurate to suggest that the younger person has not been given as great an opportunity to live as the older person.

Life Span

No less problematic is a variation of the equal-opportunity justification that limits lifesaving care to those who have not yet reached their natural life span. The very notion of a normative life span requires more critical attention. Even if a theoretical biological limit to the human life span is granted, the actual life span has grown through the years as life-extending care for the elderly has improved. An age criterion of the sort envisioned here would hinder medicine from extending even good-quality years at the end of life.

Furthermore, such an age criterion would demean those living beyond the natural life span. One supporter candidly admits this problem, given the world as it presently exists.[30] However, the problem is also intrinsic to the justification. Those who support this justification assume that extending medical care to those beyond the natural life span is not warranted because these people have already "accomplished" and "achieved" everything of significance that they can.[31] An implicit productivity orientation is revealed here: what matters is what one succeeds in doing. The significance of life, though, is to be found as much in "being" as in "doing" — as much in relating to others as in completing tasks. Moreover, our life goals change as we grow older. We have different values at different ages. Those who argue that elderly people no longer have any goals left to reach may be thinking only in terms of their own largely productivity-oriented life goals.

While those who support the life-span justification may not be explicit about their productivity bias, they do typically acknowledge a commitment to maximizing quality of life. In fact, this commitment may in the end provide more support for a quality-of-life criterion than for an age criterion. One supporter candidly admits that an age criterion excluding elderly patients from care is not warranted unless their quality of life is low.[32]

Whether either a quality-of-life or age criterion is really in view here, both are riddled with practical difficulties. It is no easier to assess another person's quality of life precisely than it is to determine if people have essentially completed their life goals — at least without relying on the statements of the patients themselves. There is little reason to assume that all older persons will value their continued life less than younger persons value theirs. Moreover, neither group is likely to be forthright about the degree to which they no longer value their lives if what they say could cost them their lives. The alternative is to withhold resources only from those who voluntarily forgo treatment — but that is to impose neither an age nor a quality-of-life criterion.

Prudence

The final justification of an age-based rationing, prudence, is also problematic for multiple reasons. First of all, it is unjust. While it might not be as thoroughly discriminatory as racism or sexism, it is discriminatory nonetheless. It assumes that all persons move through all age categories and will receive the different types of services provided for each age group. The fact is that many people are born with congenital, genetic, or environmental handicaps that will prevent them from living as long as others. What they give up when young, in order to receive when old, may well never be accessible to them. In fact, defenses of this justification suggest that the real concern here is precisely what is most needed by older people: personal care services. If that is their primary need, then an age criterion for acute care is not necessary in order to meet their need. Instead, a greater priority could be placed on personal care services when the larger allocation decisions are being made.

What ultimately makes this justification inadequate, however, is that it is hopelessly idealistic. In an ideal world this proposal might be appealing, but even proponents admit that it would be wrong to introduce age criteria in one health-care setting and not in another. They also admit that age criteria may be politically unacceptable in any setting.[33] The potential strength of the proposal lies in its vision of distributing vital resources equitably throughout an individual's lifetime, but in the end

29. Robert M. Veatch, "Distributive Justice and the Allocation of Technological Resources to the Elderly," Contract Report prepared for the U.S. Congress Office of Technology Assessment, Washington, D.C. (1985), p. 43; Robert M. Veatch, *The Foundations of Justice* (New York: Oxford University Press, 1986), p. 146.

30. Daniel Callahan, *Setting Limits,* pp. 184-85.

31. See, e.g., Daniel Callahan, *Setting Limits,* pp. 16, 172. Accordingly, Callahan does not consider elderly people to be as worthy of attention as younger people; "the primary orientation" of older people, he suggests, "should be to the young" ("Aging and the Ends of Medicine," p. 128).

32. Daniel Callahan, *Setting Limits,* pp. 184-85.

33. Norman Daniels, *Am I My Parents' Keeper?* pp. 96-97; *Just Health Care,* p. 111.

elderly people will likely experience the reality of exclusion from treatment more keenly than they will appreciate the theory that lies behind it. The politics of the issue centers on which groups will gain greatest access to the most resources. Moreover, were the proposal applied throughout a nation such as the United States, existing social and economic injustices could cause the application of an age criterion to make things worse. The potential injustice of an age criterion is so compelling that even those who in theory support age-based rationing may be forced to admit, as one of them has frankly acknowledged, that their proposal "is in no way a recommendation for the introduction of such practices in our present world."[34] That is quite a disclaimer, since that's the world we are talking about in the debate over age-based rationing of health care.

A Christian Perspective

While this critique of particular secular justifications for age-based rationing has rarely appealed explicitly to biblical or theological arguments, such a critique is not irrelevant from a Christian perspective. It exposes the internal problems of the justifications themselves. It demonstrates the weaknesses of these justifications on the basis of widely acknowledged human concerns. A Christian perspective also gives us a larger frame of reference from which to evaluate such justifications by giving us a clearer view of what is at stake. Four elements of a Christian perspective will close this chapter.

First, as we have already seen, a Christian perspective reminds us that elderly people tend to be wise and weak, relative to others. So we should be inclined to respect and protect those who are older. This outlook fosters an appropriate skepticism about any approach to health-care resource allocation that singles out older people, as a group, to receive less access.

Second, a Christian perspective reminds us of the importance of cross-cultural understanding, so that our views are not shaped unconsciously by the worst values in our own culture. One of the most striking teachings of Christianity is that there is neither Jew nor Greek, barbarian nor Scythian; but all are one in Christ and all peoples are loved and sought by God (see, for example, Col. 3:11; 2 Pet. 3:9). If that is the case, then those of us steeped in the cultural values of North America need to be challenged by alternative values in other cultures such as that of the Akamba of Kenya. We cannot assume that our culture is normative.

A third Christian insight that has important bearing upon age-based rationing is the sinfulness of the world. People as well as the policies and institutions they establish are less than God intends them to be because people are fundamentally self-oriented rather than God-and-other-oriented (Ps. 14:2-3; Jer. 17:9; Rom. 3:10-12, 23). While it is possible to turn from self-centeredness to God and others, experience and the biblical materials alike testify that the majority of people will never truly do so (see Matt. 7:13-14; Luke 13:23-24).

Accordingly, there is a pressing need for social strategies that take this reality into account and seek to promote the best possible policies in light of it. Good intentions and commitment to laudable concerns such as equal opportunity, a natural life span, and prudence are not enough. It is misleading and perhaps even dangerous to propose age criteria that would be immoral if implemented "in our present world."

Lastly, a Christian perspective sensitizes us to make sure that there are not other hidden injustices built into age-based rationing — that other groups besides older people are not victimized by this approach. What we find is that women, in fact, would bear the brunt of age-based allocation. While the ratio of elderly women to elderly men in 1960 was four to five, older women now outnumber older men three to two. More specifically, of those sixty-five to seventy-four, 55 percent are women; of those seventy-five to eighty-four, 61 percent are women; of those eighty-five and over, 71 percent are women. For those ninety and over, the figure rises to 76 percent.[35] So particularly if very elderly people are to be barred from lifesaving health care, it is predominantly women who are in view. A specific age cut-off for receiving lifesaving health care, then, will likely be set high enough to ensure a "full life" as life is typically experienced by men — implicitly devaluing the years beyond that point, which are primarily years of women's lives.

Age-based victimization, as with the victimization of other vulnerable groups, is contrary to the spirit and teaching of Christianity. The biblical materials identify the female/male distinction with slave/free and racial distinctions as inappropriate categories used by one group to assert superiority over another (e.g., Gal. 3:28). Biblical writings exhort the community to provide special protection and care to older women in particular, who are frequently widows (e.g., Isa. 1:17; James 1:27). If we are really concerned about such matters as equal opportunity and full life span, we will not support age-based rationing of life-sustaining health care.[36]

34. Margaret P. Battin, "Age Rationing and the Just Distribution of Health Care: Is There a Duty to Die?" *Ethics* 97 (January 1987): 340. Cf. Norman Daniels, *Am I My Parents' Keeper?* p. 96; *Just Health Care*, p. 113.

35. United States Census Bureau, *Census 2000*, Summary File 1, Matrices P13 and PCT12.

36. For further discussion of age-based rationing, see David C. Thomasma, "Stewardship of the Aged: Meeting the Ethical Challenge of Ageism," *Cambridge Quarterly of Healthcare Ethics* 8 (spring 1999): 148-59; Kenneth Boyd, "Old Age, Something to Look Forward To," in *The Goals of Medicine*, ed. Mark Hanson and Daniel Callahan (Washington, D.C.: Georgetown University Press, 1999), pp. 152-61; Mary Beth Hamel et al., "Patient Age and Decisions to Withhold Life-Sustaining Treatments from Seriously Ill, Hospitalized Adults," *Annals of Internal Medicine* 130 (January 19, 1999): 116-25; Norman G. Levinsky, "Can We Afford Medical Care

Conclusion

A Christian perspective, then, can help us to gain a better insight into the current debate over age-based rationing of life-sustaining health care. Utilitarian intuitions, combined with a predisposition against Christian influences in public policy, make openness to age-based rationing quite understandable. Nevertheless, this form of rationing is objectionable on broadly accepted ethical grounds, as well as on Christian theological grounds.

Our elderly and aged deserve our respect and our protection. Rationing their health care because of their age is to treat them with disdain rather than with dignity.

for Alice C?" *Lancet* 352 (December 5, 1998): 1849-51; Sara T. Fry, "The Ethics of Health Care Reform: Should Rationing Strategies Target the Elderly?" in *Current Issues in Nursing,* ed. Joanne Comi and Helen Grace, fifth ed. (St. Louis: Mosby, 1997), pp. 626-31; Alan Williams and J. Grimley Evans, "Rationing Health Care by Age: The Case for and the Case Against," *British Medical Journal* 314 (March 15, 1997): 820-25; Eric Rakowski and Stephen G. Post, "Should Health Care Be Rationed by Age? Yes and No," in *Controversial Issues in Aging,* ed. Andrew Scharlach and Lenard Kaye (Boston: Allyn and Bacon, 1997), pp. 103-13.

75 Why Do We Want to Be Healthy? Medicine, Autonomous Individualism, and the Community of Faith

Dennis Sansom

Eric J. Cassell, in *The Nature of Suffering and the Goals of Medicine,* observes that the medical profession is now realizing that an exclusive interest in the patient's "physical biology" does the patient an injustice. "[I]llness is a biopsychosocial phenomenon and cannot be completely described in any lesser terms. It is not that patients with diseases also have psychological or social problems, the sick are sick in all dimensions simultaneously."[1] Suffering due to pain attacks the whole person, not just a particular body part, because it debilitates the person's relationships to family, others, work, recreation, future goals, and assumed obligations. This is why, when we lose our health because of suffering from pain, we feel attacked. We value health because it is a condition by which we have enough strength (whether physical, psychological, interpersonal, and/or spiritual) to live as humans, having a personal center from which we hope to organize our lives into a meaningful whole.

The loss of health challenges our personal integrity. It disrupts our ability to be centered in the world, because it makes us too feeble to continue with the ways we have been ourselves up to that point. On a simple level we expect health care and medicine to restore our health, but actually the expectations are greater than merely removing pain from our bodies. We expect health care and medicine to help secure our integrity as humans when suffering due to pain overwhelms us.

In a sense we look to health care and medicine to empower us when we become weak due to suffering from pain. We want empowerment because we value our integrity, and we know we need health to fulfill our goals in life. Health requires power. Karl Barth notes, in *Ethics,* that the concept of health implies power as well. "[Our life] wills to be lived also in the maintaining and achieving of its possibilities, in *power.* To be healthy is to be in possession of one's physical and intellectual powers. It is to will what is necessary to achieve and assert these pow-

1. Eric J. Cassell, *The Nature of Suffering and the Goals of Medicine* (Oxford: Oxford University Press, 1991), p. 206.

From Dennis Sansom, *Christian Scholar's Review* 23 (March 3, 1994): 300-306. Used by permission.

ers."[2] Since power must be included in an understanding of health, then it is easy to see why we expect empowerment from health care agencies and medicine. With the loss of health, we need power to regain it.

Yet it's not enough just to link health and power, and ill-health and the need for empowerment. If power is understood as the ability to accomplish certain ends, goals, or purposes (i.e., *telos*), then the *telos* determines what kind and amount of power are necessary for us. The *telos* which guides a person informs her of the means by which she lives meaningfully within society. It also defines the nature and use of power. Therefore, if we are to understand why we want to be healthy, we not only need to understand personhood, power, and the value of the health care industry, but we also need to understand our society's *telos*. Hospitals, medicine, and health care in general manifest our societal moral commitments, and it is in observing these manifestations that we see the large differences between the effects of what I shall call the "autonomous individualism of the Enlightenment" and "the community of faith of Christianity" upon our expectations for health care.

Since our society is complex, it is always risky to generalize about it, but I will venture to say that to a great extent our society's *telos* is shaped by one aspect of the Enlightenment's moral agenda — autonomous individualism. Of course that period of intellectual growth and religious tolerance had many good effects (e.g., ending the sectarian wars, promoting personal responsibility in moral matters, and encouraging intellectual rigor and creativity), but we have funneled the Enlightenment's legacy into the single value of personal autonomy, which has become the moral *telos* of our liberal democracy.

The autonomous adult who freely chooses her own moral principles and who produces effectively in our free market economy is the pinnacle of our society. We are committed to removing as many obstacles as possible to achieving this autonomous, self-made personhood. We accept only those restrictions of our own choosing. Ill-health is obviously a restriction, and if in our society we are primarily committed to establishing conditions in which we can live, move, and work according to our own choosing, then we pressure the health industry to restore our autonomy. We expect the industry to take away health obstacles, and the greatest of these obstacles is death. Certainly, no one thinks that medical science can make us immortal, but nonetheless we act in a practical sense as though medical science can keep extending our lives indefinitely. We insist that medical science keep finding cures for all fatal diseases and genetic maladies, and we keep utilizing as many life-prolonging technologies as possible until the only time we choose to die is when we artificially are kept alive beyond our own sense of dignity.

In August, 1987, Daniel Callahan wrote the controversial article "Limiting Health Care for the Old?" and in it he maintained that our inability to know when to die has put undue pressures upon health care in our society. Callahan is bothered primarily by three urgent issues.[3] First, "an increasing large share of health care is going to the elderly." Second, "the elderly, in dying, consume a disproportionate share of health care costs." And third, the elderly use most of the medical technology primarily to prolong their lives. According to Callahan, we have these pressing concerns in health care because we assume that we can extend middle age with medicine's accomplishments. Because we assume that health care can keep us middle-aged, and we do not want to grow old and suffer the restrictions of aging, we conclude we do not have to grow old.

However, this attitude is the problem, according to Callahan. "By pretending that old age can be turned into a kind of endless middle age, we rob it of meaning and significance for the elderly."[4] In trying to push back the experience of death and dying, we forget our mortality and become ignorant and incapable of learning how to grow old.

We are mortal, no doubt about it, and we need to consider our mortality as part of our destiny and not deny it. However, we keep demanding that medical science invent new life-prolonging technology so that we can be resuscitated one more time to prevent death. What is missing in our modern moral vocabulary is what Callahan is urging us to revive — "a fresh vision of what it means to live a decently long and adequate life, what might be called a 'natural life span.'"[5] We need to recognize that we have physical and temporal limitations, and that knowing when to die is one of the most important attitudes to cultivate in our personal pilgrimages. The desire to stay autonomous without restrictions eventually compels us either to forget a practical sense of our mortality or to deny it.

To remedy this attitude, Callahan proposes three principles for public policy.[6] First, due to our sense of a collective social obligation, the government should help people to live out their natural life span. Second, what life-extending technology is used should be restricted to the application of the first principle. And third, beyond a patient's natural life span, the government should provide only for the relief of suffering.

Not everyone agrees with Callahan's article. Amitai Etzioni is typical of negative criticism against it.[7] Etzioni believes that Callahan's argument starts down a slippery slope with no place to stop. The argument is built on too

2. Karl Barth, *Ethics*, edited by Dietrich Braun, translated by Geoffrey W. Bromiley (Edinburgh: T&T Clark, 1981), pp. 129-30.

3. Daniel Callahan, "Limiting Health Care for the Old," in *Taking Sides: Clashing Views on Controversial Bioethical Issues*, third edition, edited by Carol Levine (Guilford, Connecticut: Dushkin Publishing Group, 1989), pp. 328-29.

4. Callahan, p. 331.

5. Callahan, p. 330.

6. Callahan, pp. 331-32.

7. Amitai Etzioni, "Spare the Old, Save the Young," Levine, ed., in *Taking Sides*, pp. 333-37.

many ambiguous ideas whose meanings would have to be changed only slightly for Callahan not to want to live with the consequences. For instance, the term "elderly" fluctuates according to death rates, general health trends, and size of population. It is conceivable that population pressures and environmental deterioration could make fifty-five-year-old people "elderly" and subject to the denial of some health care under Callahan's limitations.

Etzioni is also afraid that Callahan's policy would cause intergenerational strife between the young and old, making the old inferior. According to Etzioni, discrimination against the elderly is contrary to democracy and undermines our society. Furthermore, Etzioni thinks Callahan would probably not want to impose draconian restrictions on cigarette smokers who disproportionately tax society's medical budget, even though he wants to impose draconian restrictions on the elderly because they do disproportionately burden society.

In Etzioni's eyes, Callahan oversteps the bounds of democracy. Yet Callahan does find a sympathic reader in Stanley Hauerwas, of Duke University. Like Callahan, Hauerwas sees one of the major issues in health care to be society's moral assumptions. In the book *Naming the Silences: God, Medicine, and the Problem of Suffering,* Hauerwas criticizes in his typical fashion the Enlightenment's legacy of autonomous individualism.

> In a way, modern medicine exemplifies the predicament of the Enlightenment project, which hopes to make society a collection of individuals free from the bonds of necessity other than those we choose. In many ways that project has been accomplished, only now we have discovered that the very freedom we sought has, ironically, become a kind of bondage.[8]

Autonomous individualism is crippling society, and one way we suffer by it is in health care. As a liberal society, we want fewer and fewer inhibitions, and obviously illness and death are major restraints which prevent us from realizing the goals we choose for ourselves. We thus demand that medical science cure our illnesses and prolong our lives. We create technologies to help keep death farther from us and to give us more control of our lives.

Of course, to admit our finitude we do not need to eliminate health care or life-prolonging technology. Yet medicine should help us fulfill our creaturely limitations, not be a symptom of our practical denial of them.

Hauerwas does criticize Callahan for not being more precise about the meaning of "natural life span" and "tolerable death."

> The problem with Callahan's recommendation for a recovery of these notions is that such concepts remain far too formal. He talks, for example, about having "one's life possibilities accomplished," but what precisely does that mean? I should like to live long enough to have read all of Trollope's novels twice — but even if I accomplished that, I suspect I would want to try it three times. . . . But in the end the crucial issue is not whether one's death seems offensive to others, rather the kind of expectations we ought to have so that death, perhaps even an untimely death, is an event to be accepted — accepted with sorrow, but accepted nevertheless.[9]

According to Hauerwas, Callahan does not go far enough in rejecting autonomous individualism, because he still assumes that our lives are our own making, but in fact, according to Hauerwas, it is truer to admit that "we more nearly discover rather than create our lives."[10]

Callahan's ideas of "natural life span" and "tolerable death" lack coherence outside of a moral tradition which enables a person to integrate her life from birth to death under what Hauerwas calls a narrative unity. The concept of narrative unity is a key notion for Hauerwas. It refers to the way a community defines the meaning of life from birth to death according to that community's moral and spiritual traditions. Such a tradition enables us to realize that illness and death need not be alien to us but can be events, as painful and as sad as they are, which do not necessarily destroy our lives' integrity and meaning.

> Interestingly, a life experienced as a narrative unit is one in which events are not experienced or remembered as foreign. A kind of fatalism in which one's life is seen as fundamentally out of control, in which one is a victim of time, is rendered impotent by a narrative construal, which allows one to integrate one's misfortunes into an ongoing framework.[11]

The Christian affirmations that our lives with all their blemishes and illnesses are not alien to God and that God promises to live with us and empower us even in our death provide a narrative unity in which sickness and dying do not rob one of a *telos.*

Theology becomes a way of telling ourselves that in the midst of our tragedies and sufferings we have a unity which cannot be taken away because the unity is given by God, and because of this theological narration about our lives in God we do not need to exhaust our lives and natural resources by trying to prevent the inevitability of illness and death. We expect medicine to give us enough power when needed to fulfill our places within the community which has given us our destinies through its moral and spiritual traditions.

Yet from the Enlightenment's legacy we expect medicine to empower us to overcome our restrictions, and this is a different justification for health care. According to Hauerwas, medicine in the Enlightenment tradition becomes a secular theodicy in which we try to justify our lives by trying to deny our creaturely finitude and the natural consequences of being mortal. With our fixation upon life-prolonging technologies we even think medi-

8. Stanley Hauerwas, *Naming the Silences: God, Medicine, and the Problem of Suffering* (Grand Rapids: William B. Eerdmans, 1990), p. 108.

9. Hauerwas, pp. 108-9.

10. Hauerwas, p. 111.

11. Hauerwas, p. 119.

cine can control our greatest foe — death. Instead of religious faith providing a hope by which we believe evil and death will not destroy our *telos,* medicine usurps the role of faith by saying that we do not need to appeal to God or a transcendent hope to integrate our lives but through science and technology we can obtain our *telos.*

If it is true, as Hauerwas implies, that underneath our appreciation and expectations for modern medicine lies a theodicy, then we ask a lot of it. We ask it to change reality. There are different kinds of theodicies. The one undergirding the Enlightenment's rationale for medicine is an "ontological theodicy," by which we desire to alter our creaturely limitations and thereby show that we can change reality to conform to our desires.

One of the consequences of the Enlightenment's *telos* of autonomous individualism is that we are exhausting our resources to pay for a health care system in which we hope that our mortality can be checked. But we can look at medicine in another way. Instead of seeing medicine as an "ontological theodicy," we can see it as a "soul-making theodicy" (to borrow a phrase from John Hick's interpretation of Irenaeus' theodicy). That is, medicine can help us mature our souls, our identity as moral and spiritual beings, by providing us with enough power when we are ill so that we can continue to live virtuously towards others and God. In this sense our *telos* in life is not autonomous individualism but living virtuously within a community of people in whom we find our purpose. If living virtuously before God within a community is our goal in life, then what we expect out of medicine is to help us have enough physical power to exhibit those virtues which build up the community in which we find our narrative unity. There comes the time in which we need to exhibit how a virtuous person dies, affirming in our dying the moral and spiritual commitments by which we discovered our own unity within the community's stories of faith. Medicine does its greatest service when it assists us in this *telos.*

We learn what is a "natural life span" and a "tolerable death" by living in a community in which we see and learn from others who have discovered their own narrative unity through their faith in God. By living in a community of faithful people who are shaped by the life, teachings, death, and resurrection of Jesus Christ, we see how people integrate their lives, how they deal with sickness and dying. The model of these relationships equips us to integrate our lives and to accept our limitations, even illness and dying. In knowing that our meaning as humans is found in what we derive and contribute to the legacy of the community of faithful people, we expect of medicine to help us bear witness to the Gospel of Jesus Christ.

Of course, in the community of faith we want just as much as in the Enlightenment's tradition to alleviate excruciating pain, to save the lives of our children, to cure diseases, and to keep ourselves healthy, but the primary difference is the goal for medicine. As long as we think our *telos* is autonomous individualism, then we will pressure medicine to empower us to overcome more and more of our physical limitations, to change our finite nature. In a sense what happens in a society shaped by the ethos of autonomous individualism is that the very plausible and common sense desire to stay healthy is distorted into the desire to live without illness and dying, a form of practical immortality.

But if our *telos* is to live faithfully within a community of people who treasure its particular spiritual and moral tradition, then we ask medicine to restore our health to us so that we may fulfill our role within the community of faith. We don't ask of medicine to do the impossible, i.e., help us to pretend we are immortal, but we ask of it to help us be healthy enough to act in ways indicative of a person who knows that the *telos* of life is not dominating over the restrictions of our natural finitude but living faithfully towards God within the community of faith.

Certainly, this justification for medical care does not prohibit further research or life-prolonging treatments. When illness or injury obviates our natural life span, then we need medical science to help us to live. But the question is — what is our natural life span? We find an answer within a community of people who understand that life's purpose is in being faithful to our spiritual and moral legacy, our families, our community of faith, and to the continuation of this tradition of believers in God. The best that we can determine within our own finitude and *telos* is that our natural life span is the amount and level of health it takes to fulfill this level of faithfulness. It may come early or it may come late. It may come with grief or it may come with peace. But all along the ultimate focus of our life becomes not how much of life we can enjoy or how much we get out of it, but how we can live and die as a faithful person. We value medical care because it can help us fulfill that *telos.*

76 The Language of Death: Theology and Economics in Conflict

D. Stephen Long

How shall we assist our elders in dying well? When we answer this question we will also know how to live well because living a good life includes learning to die well. Such an art has become a neglected and forgotten theme in Christian theology. This was not always the case. Works such as Jeremy Taylor's *Holy Dying* recall a time when theologians put forth obligations to prepare the faithful for death. The "art" of "dying well," suggested the Anglican divine, required daily practices of general preparation. For Taylor, this general preparation was based on three precepts: First, the person who would die well "must always look for death every day knocking at the gates of the grave; and then the gates of the grave shall never prevail upon him to do him mischief." Second, "he that would die well must all the days of his life, lay up against the day of his death." The necessary provisions, stated Taylor, were "faith and patience." Third, to die well required a life that eschewed "softness, delicacy and voluptuousness" in favor of "a life severe, holy and under the discipline of the cross." Taylor then suggested daily activities that would assist us in this general preparation for death such as examination of conscience and the exercise of charity.[1]

Jeremy Taylor put forward these duties in the mid-seventeenth century,[2] and they provide a context within which we think about not only our own deaths but also the deaths of our elders. To honor one's elders would be to help them complete life with a holy death. But more than two centuries later, Taylor's general precepts seem alien, if not morbid, to us. We focus our attention not on death itself, but on that period prior to death known as "retirement" or the "third age."[3] We speak of "aging" rather than of "dying." We still possess preparatory duties for death, but these duties take as their primary purpose a comfortable retirement before death so that we will be the least burdensome on our relatives, friends, and enemies. Such duties can easily conflict with previously practiced theological duties to prepare daily for death at all ages through a severe and holy discipline. The language of dying is no longer cloaked in garments such as fasting, prayer, and preparation for suffering. Instead, it is dressed up with retirement, pensions, and security.

This change in dress has some distinct advantages and reflects positive social changes since Taylor's time: we bury our children less, our parents and grandparents live longer and healthier lives, we physically suffer less from diseases and poor health.[4] These changes have resulted in a new language. We now speak of a "third age," or a third stage in life where we must learn to adjust to the process of aging — adjustments our forebears had little opportunity or necessity to make. Only a masochist could find in these new developments something to bemoan, for no one should seek suffering and an early death for their own sake. Yet the difficulty with acknowledging the positive gains of these changes is the social and political narrative that is often given credit for them. That narrative suggests that these gains were realized primarily by the creation of the free market as a neutral technical instrument that allocates scarce resources in the most efficient way possible, diminishing pain and suffering and furthering life and prosperity.

This narrative creates two problems. First, by viewing the market as a neutral technical instrument, it abstracts it from any analysis or consideration of the social, political, and theological conditions that make such a market possible and that such a market produces.[5] Second, once this narrative is conceded as the source of this best of all possible worlds we now live in, then the dominant language available to think and speak about aging and death is the language of the economists. That language will always find preparatory duties such as Taylor's alien. It will also produce false contexts within which people of faith can easily be misled in their good intentions to fulfill religious obligations such as honoring one's elders.

1. Jeremy Taylor, *Holy Living and Dying; With Prayers Containing the Complete Duty of a Christian* (New York: D. Appleton, 1859), pp. 42-57.

2. Taylor himself was no stranger to death and suffering, having faced imprisonment, poverty, and the burial of two sons.

3. See Peter Laslett's *A Fresh Map of Life: The Emergence of the Third Age* (London: Widenfeld and Nicolson, 1989).

4. Who constitutes the "we" in these sentences is intended in a limited sense. It applies to those who might read this essay — educated, middle- or upper-class people. These changes are not uniform throughout all places and among all people. It is still the case that one's socioeconomic status while working basically determines one's socioeconomic status in retirement.

5. Another problem with this interpretation is that it seems to be false. Sociological interpretations of statistics do not show direct correlations between increased life expectancy and modernization and industrialization. Laslett notes, "The developing countries today have already been described as beginning to age in the sense of the lengthening of life, well before industrialization has been achieved. If present trends and politics continue, it could be that aging in the further sense of having large proportions of old will also supervene in those countries, especially China, before industrialization and 'modernization' have made much progress" (*Fresh Map of Life*, p. 83).

From D. Stephen Long, "The Language of Death: Theology and Economics in Conflict," in *Growing Old in Christ*. Ed. Stanley Hauerwas, Carol Bailey Stoneking, Keith G. Meador, and David Cloutier (Grand Rapids: Wm. B. Eerdmans Publishing Company, 2003), 129-50.

Perhaps the reason we find terms such as "fasting, severe discipline and preparation for suffering" strange and yet are comfortable with the language of "retirement, pensions, and security" is precisely that our dying is defined more by considerations of "economics" than by moral, political, and theological considerations. Our language of aging and dying has implicitly and explicitly become defined by the "burden of dependency," which is given definition by economists:

> From an economic point of view, a person who has retired from the labor market is a "burden" on society in the specific sense that his current consumption expenditure outweighs his current contribution to the total marketable output.[6]

This technical definition of retired persons is not intended to imply a value judgment; it supposedly reflects nothing but a necessary presupposition for the economic analysis of intergenerational resource distribution. Nevertheless, such language does produce different moral considerations for the process of aging and dying than did language such as Taylor's or obligations to honor one's elders. It prompts us to secure our future aging so that we will be the least burdensome on others. Our preparatory duties for death include securing our future not only against want but also against any dependence on the charity of others. But these preparatory duties are not the result of some natural desire for autonomy; they arise from the demands of a particular sociopolitical order, one that was given shape by the marginalist revolution.

Speaking of Death as the Optimal Allocation of Scarce Resources: The Language of Economics

Economists describe the relationship between the elderly and the young in terms of the marginalist rationality (also known as neo-classical liberalism) that revolutionized economics in the latter part of the nineteenth century.[7] This rationality assumes that the starting point for economic analysis is individuals who must make choices concerning exchanges in conditions of scarcity.[8] The market is a neutral, value-free technical instrument to effect these exchanges in the most efficient and rational way possible. Such reasoning abstracts both from the social conditions within which these individuals are situated and from conditions of accumulation by assuming that "the initial allocation of goods is taken as given historically and so is no matter for the economist to investigate."[9] The task of the economist is to optimize efficiency with the social and political conditions assumed as given.

Marginalist Rationality: Natural or a Political Abstraction?

Marginalist rationality does not describe something which is natural, i.e., just the way things are; rather, it assumes the normativity of a social order — capitalist society — which it seldom acknowledges, because economics presents itself as something of a natural science. This is important for intergenerational economic analyses because marginalist rationality also assumes a "natural" conflict of interest between the generations. In fact, some economists believe we will face an economic crisis because of our aging population. We shall examine this possible crisis below; however, whether such a crisis exists or not, intergenerational economic analyses assume conflict. As one economics textbook puts it,

> Is a $20,000 hip replacement for a ninety-year-old with a life expectancy of a few years the most valuable use of society's resources? These are difficult and unpleasant questions but as long as society as a whole bears the brunt of these costs, through its Medicare and Medicaid programs, there is no way of avoiding them.[10]

The economist's question seems "natural" enough. We have a straightforward and stark choice, and we are told there is no way to avoid it. Either we expend "society's resources" on a ninety-year-old individual's hip replacement or we expend these resources on something else more valuable. The mathematics is simple. We have X amount of resources. Y equals the value of a ninety-year-old individual's hip replacement. Z equals other "more valuable uses of society's resources." The result is an obvious equation: $X = Y + Z$. If we increase expenditures on Y then we decrease possible expenditures for Z. But a little reflection and this apparently natural choice disappears, and we see how misleading and abstract it is

6. See Richard Disney, *Can We Afford to Grow Older?* (Cambridge, Mass.: MIT Press, 1996), p. 17. Such "conventional approaches to the 'economics of aging'" then give rise to discussions of aging in a "burden of dependency" model, which uses "static . . . measures of the burden, calculated with varying degrees of sophistication" (p. 12). It should be noted that Disney's work develops a different model than this burden of dependency model, although he does assume that the retired are a "burden" in this putatively neutral technical sense.

7. For a good analysis of the marginalist revolution see Simon Clarke's *Marx, Marginalism and Modern Sociology: From Adam Smith to Max Weber* (London: Macmillan, 1982), particularly pp. 145-85.

8. This language is not only prevalent in economics; it is also the language within which sociologists work. For example, Ronald and Jacqueline Angel begin their sociological analysis of care for the elderly by stating, "In the United States today, programs for the old and for the young compete for the same limited resources. If real economic growth remains relatively low, increased outlays for the elderly can only come at the expense of other social goods, including programs for children" (Ronald L. Angel and Jacqueline L. Angel, *Who Will Care for Us? Aging and Long-Term Care in Multicultural America* [New York: New York University Press, 1997], p. xxi).

9. Clarke, *Marx, Marginalism, and Modern Sociology*, p. 153.

10. Joseph E. Stiglitz, *Economics*, 2nd ed. (New York: W. W. Norton, 1997), p. 920. Stiglitz has served as President Clinton's chairman of the council of economic advisers as well as chief economist at the World Bank.

because it hides its politics behind a putatively "natural" choice.

The first abstraction we encounter is in the terms of the comparison itself. We find a "ninety-year-old individual's hip replacements" compared with "more valuable uses of resources." But the comparison assumes that all ninety-year-old people in need of hip replacements share a similar socioeconomic status. This is simply false. Some ninety-year-olds will have access to resources other than federal expenditures for health care. All such people should be exempted from the comparison. Then we realize that the comparison works only between those who depend on federal expenditures for their health care and other "more valuable uses of resources"; the comparison is between the poor and "more valuable uses of resources." Yet what are these "more valuable uses of resources"? What does "Z" represent? Nuclear armaments? Tobacco subsidies? Bicycle trails? Enterprise zones for inner cities? Expenditures for special prosecutors? Until we know what we are comparing, we simply are incapable of exercising any practical judgment.

This brings us to the second abstraction with which we meet. Who is the "we" that is assumed to make these practical determinations about the allocation of "society's resources"? We are asked which use of "society's resources" is more advantageous as if "we" had some direct political mechanism to make this determination. But of course "we" do not, and marginalism works on the assumption that we should not. No political mechanism should exist other than the choices of individual consumers. Choice is exercised by individuals, each of whom determines for herself what she wants, and the market merely acts as a neutral instrument to index those preferences by matching wants with products and services. Thus if either the elderly or those concerned about them find it useful to employ their resources for hip replacements, then the market will provide. The market will provide such services until the marginal utility of such an employment of resources is no longer viable; that is to say, until individual consumers determine that the employment of their limited resources for other services or products is of more use to them than hip replacements for ninety-year-olds.

These collected and indexed preferences are all that the marginalist economists can mean by "society's resources." Politically, the logic of their position entails that institutions refrain from social constraints on the market; otherwise, the "rationality" of marginal utility would be adversely affected. If the government, or some other institution, subsidizes hip replacements, then I as a consumer might be able to employ my resources for both my grandmother's hip replacement and my son's college education, not recognizing that this is an "irrational" employment of resources because the costs are hidden in such a way that I am not forced to allocate my own resources in the most efficient way possible. So to use the expression "society as a whole bears" is within a marginalist analysis both an abstraction and misleading. Few, if any, "social resources" exist, and "we" have no political mechanism to make judgments about the control of such resources other than as individual consumers.[11]

Of course, in the equation above, X (the amount of resources available at a given time) is not indefinitely fixed. It may be fixed momentarily at the point where I must choose between utilizing my resources on hip replacements or on a child's education, but it is not fixed over time. The only possible alternative to difficult decisions between competing values is to increase X as much as possible. So the best possible answer to our social problems will always be increased economic growth. But here we see a contradiction, because the very same economists who argue that in the long term we must increase growth and that the advantage of capitalist society is that it is the most efficient form of wealth production also tell us that the means to achieve this most efficient form of production is by recognizing that we must choose in the present between our elders' hip replacements and our children's education or other "more valuable uses of resources."

So we are confronted with the economist's abstract logic: "These are difficult and unpleasant questions, but as long as society as a whole bears the brunt of these costs . . . there is no way of avoiding them." But of course what we have discovered is that we do not have a society that bears the brunt of these costs and that economics works to prevent us from any concrete discernment about uses of resources other than as individual consumers. It permits us the privilege of avoiding social and political questions about the allocation of scarce resources. The purpose of the economist's question is not to exercise practical judgment about the expenditures of social resources; the question functions merely as a way to legitimate the economist's social and political starting point — we are all individuals who must make choices about scarce resources, and the most efficient way to do this is to leave it to the "neutral" working of the market.

The market decides, and we must realize that the market is the most rational form of life available to us. We have no politics available to us that would allow us to live otherwise, for such a politics would require that questions such as "What is a good use of our resources?" could be answered. We would need some common conception of a good life for which people should aim. But this is precisely what our democratic process protects against.[12] Thus, the market is our only politics.

Once the market has become our politics, then we should not be surprised that we begin to speak of the el-

11. The one exception would be through taxation, but what impacts us directly is the amount we will be taxed. We have little recourse as to how those taxes will be utilized, for all the political options present accept the basis of marginalist rationality.

12. For a fuller explanation of this point, see Michael Sandel's *Democracy's Discontent: America in Search of a Public Philosophy* (Cambridge, Mass.: Belknap Press of Harvard University Press, 1996), particularly his first chapter, "The Public Philosophy of Contemporary Liberalism," pp. 3-24.

derly, aging, and death in terms intelligible within the market. To honor our elders is to submit them to the logic of the economist's rationality. We must now think of our elders as economic burdens whose care should be subject to the conditions of marginal utility. This is not because health care is "by nature" a scarce resource whereby choices must inevitably be made between hip replacements and children's education. This is a feature of our particular social order.

The Impending Social Security Crisis

Even those programs which could potentially be "social resources," such as Social Security, Medicare, and Medicaid, do not function within social and political arrangements whereby people can exercise practical judgments about what constitutes a good expenditure of society's resources. The debates around all social security programs occur within the logic of marginalism. Economists tell us that federal expenditures for the elderly are currently $16,000, while they are only $1,200 for children under the age of eighteen.[13] Such figures raise questions about the optimal use of resources by an aging population. Of course, these figures are also abstractions that overlook the social and political context within which the elderly and children live. These federal expenditures to the elderly are the entitlements granted by Social Security and Medicare. The extent to which the economy can continue to provide these kinds of entitlements to the elderly is a question beguiling economic prognosticators.

We are told that the Social Security system in the United States faces an impending crisis. A number of factors account for this. First is the increase in life expectancy. In 1935 the expectation for those who had lived to sixty-five was that they would live another twelve years. In 1995 that expectation had increased to seventeen years and it is estimated that by 2040 it might climb as high as nineteen to twenty-one more years.[14] Such increased life expectancy places an added burden on Social Security, which has been a mixture between a "pay-as-you-go" model and a trust fund. The pay-as-you-go model works on the basis of economic transfers between current working generations and those who are retired. Increased life expectancy places burdens on the revenues that will need to be redistributed from the current working generation to those in retirement as well as on the funds available for the elderly.

Second, the numbers within, and the age of, the working generation have been decreasing at the same time that the numbers of the retired generation have been increasing. The past century's declining fertility rates have led to fewer persons available to support the elderly and thus restrict the potential for the pay-as-you-go system, creating more of a demand for a trust system.[15] That declining fertility rates pose serious intergenerational economic problems contains a curious irony, since both the classical liberal economists and the marginalists told us that population control (especially among the poor) was essential for a healthy economy. Fertility rates in the United States reflect the very measures economists urged on society. Now we are told that the success of this population control could place the ability to care for the elderly in jeopardy.

A third reason for the possible impending crisis is that the trust system has been primarily placed in government bonds, which are used to finance the debt; thus the rate of return is not as high as it could be.

A fourth reason for the crisis is public opposition to increased taxation. To fix the system, some economists suggest, would require a 3 percent increase in taxes. But the suggestion of a tax increase in the current cultural climate is simply not possible.

A fifth reason for the crisis stems from changes in family and community structures and in the nature of work. As Angel and Angel state, "For most of human history, as is still the case for a large fraction of the world today, people worked until they could no longer participate in paid or domestic labor, and then they survived on the charity of family and community until they died."[16] This social practice, however, has now been replaced by a relatively new one known as "retirement" in which we hope to age free from charity doled out by family or community.[17]

The current practice of retirement has developed within the last fifty years and was brought on by changes in the family structure that resulted from capitalism. From 1947 to 1976 the "labor-force participation rate of men over 65 fell from 47.8% to 20.0%."[18] This declining participation ratio is not only for workers sixty-five and older; it is also found among workers between the ages of forty-five and sixty-five. As a social practice, retirement has been both forced and voluntary. Insofar as it has occurred through lay-offs, plant closings, and shifts in labor employment resulting in changes from industrial production to a service economy, such retirements were forced. Insofar as it has occurred from choices made available because of private pension funds and Social Se-

13. Stiglitz, *Economics,* p. 918.

14. Stiglitz, *Economics,* p. 916.

15. See P. A. Samuelson's "The Optimum Growth Rate for Population," in *International Economic Review* 16 (October 1975): 531-38.

16. Angel and Angel, *Who Will Care for Us?* p. 2.

17. One of the reasons for this loss of family structure is mobility, which works against the perseverance of family and community structures and is central to the logic of capitalism. Within capitalist society, people, like commodities, must be mobile. Without mobility, strains are placed on the most efficient allocation of scarce resources, including labor. We all must go where the jobs are. While some of the technological achievements of the past few decades make it easier to maintain contact with family, these achievements have not allowed us to sustain a bodily presence to our elders. Current efforts underway to provide "elder care" long-distance are certainly one way the market allows some of us to address this issue, but such care remains a contractual arrangement between producers and consumers.

18. Disney, *Can We Afford to Grow Older?* p. 193. Most of my reflections on retirement are indebted to Disney's chapter, "Retirement: The Labor Supply of Older Workers in an Aging Society."

curity, it is viewed as voluntary. Even if retirement is a function of choice, suggest the economists, it may still not be "utility maximizing," for many of these retirees are still capable of "productive" services. Thus, incentives may be needed to entice the elderly to remain in the workforce.[19]

Social Security and private pension funds have made those who cease working less dependent on family and community structures. Sociologist Peter Laslett, however, views the decline of the family structure not as a loss but as a gain for the elderly. He suggests that the diminishment of the extended, residential family structure was necessary for the development of retirement because "the co-residential family group is very difficult to adapt to all the eventualities of the individual life course, and providing for old age seems to be beyond its capacities."[20] Co-residential families, he argues, produce dependency and intergenerational hostility. For the elderly to be free from such dependence they must first have sufficient means to sustain themselves separate from familial means. Intimacy at a distance, he suggests, is more conducive to healthy third-age living. Thus his "theory of the third age" suggests that retirement reflects a natural desire of the elderly to be independent from familial constraints, a state now made possible by capitalist society.[21]

Should those in the "third age" expect a comfortable, independent existence free from the burdens of family, work, and the needs of community life? What moral resources could we draw upon to answer such a question? Would provisions for such a life fulfill the religious obligation to honor one's elders? If this is a morally valid expectation, can the economy continue to support an elderly generation marked by increased longevity, higher medical bills, early retirement age, and fewer family and communal networks, by a declining number of workers? Economists suggest that it can, that we face no economic crisis of aging;[22] but the economy will not be able to provide for the practice of retirement through the current re-distributive practices of Social Security. Only through increased private pensions will the economy continue to work for the elderly. But this of course raises the possibility of increased relative disparities between the poor and the rich. We face no economic crisis of aging, but we continue to suffer deep divisions between rich and poor, and these categories cannot be equated with working and retired.

Increased utilization of private pension plans is many economists' remedy for the problems brought to the economy by an aging population. Another possible remedy is to increase the power of the state. This seems to be a remedy more favorable to sociologists. "All of these changes mean that in the future the elderly will have little alternative but to turn to the state when they become dependent," write Angel and Angel.[23] But, of course, turning to the state will also entail turning away from family and other community structures. Either the state or the market will give us the language to speak about preparing our elders to die. In the face of such a reality, preserving a theological language for aging is itself politically significant, for if it gives us nothing else, it can give us the moral resources by which our expectations of aging and dying should be formed.

Dying as a Participation in Charity: The Language of Theology

How can we relate theology to this socioeconomic analysis? The question is improperly stated. It assumes that economics is a technical science like auto mechanics, gall bladder surgery, or housing construction. Because these are neutral, technical disciplines, we need not relate theology to them; nor should they encroach upon theological language. While this may be the case with carburetor adjustments, economics constantly surpasses its proper limits and imposes its logic on all aspects of human life; and theology must refuse to concede any intellectual space free from its own intrinsic logic. This is a necessary feature of Christian theology because it is a "metadiscourse" that positions all other discourses within its own narrative order of creation and redemption. Any Christian theology which refuses to do this will cease to express adequately its own internal logic

19. "An alternative view [to that of involuntary early retirement] is that the secular decline in labor-force participation rates, especially among elderly men, is an outcome of choice. For these individuals, the prospect of higher retirement income, stemming from (e.g.) the growth of private pensions and the ability to liquidate other assets such as housing equity, exceeds the utility derived from continued employment at an age when they might expect to live for another 25 years. Then the decision to retire is optimal for the individual. . . . In a 'forward-looking' (lifetime) model, the individual will evaluate the expected streams of earnings and nonwork income and the marginal utility of leisure per remaining period. This could lead still productive individuals to choose to forgo paid work. In such circumstances, it is hard to think of a social regime under which it would be desirable to force such individuals to work beyond their chosen retirement age. What is then needed, if the decline in the participation rates of the elderly is to be curtailed, is a structure of economic incentives that persuades the potential worker to continue working" (Disney, *Can We Afford to Grow Older?* p. 199).

20. Laslett, *Fresh Map of Life*, p. 125. For a historical analysis of retirement see his chapter, "Retirement and Its Social History," pp. 122-39.

21. Laslett writes, "In disposing of the myth that the English elderly in the past always lived and died surrounded by bevies of their relatives, we need not accept the belief that it would always and necessarily have been better for them if these had been the circumstances" (*Fresh Map of Life*, p. 126).

22. See Angel and Angel, *Who Will Care for Us?* pp. 150-53.

23. Angel and Angel, *Who Will Care for Us?* pp. 17-19. In fact, without federal intervention such as Social Security, "retirement" is not possible for many persons who were gainfully employed throughout their life. In 1990, 41 percent of retirees had nothing but Social Security to live on.

and become dependent upon other discourses for its intelligibility.[24] Theologians on both the political left and right have denied this claim by making space for economics or social analysis as an autonomous sphere. But such concessions inevitably reduce theology to the status of the irrational, cultural, or valuational over against the factual.

All Things Fulfilled in Christ and Subject to His Authority

Christian theology cannot concede space to other intellectual disciplines because the logic of theology arises from a universal meta-claim (always mediated historically) that Christ is Lord and that such lordship cannot be superseded. The strength of a theological analysis of aging is that it explicitly gives us what economics conceals — a common conception of a good life for which people should aim and to which judgments about good uses of resources can and should be subordinate. This is because no higher authority exists than Christ's. Thus no intellectual discourse can position theology within some authoritative structure other than the logic of Christ's sacrifice. As Karl Barth put it,

> His sacrifice meant the closing of the time of the divine holding back, the time of the mere passing over of human sins endlessly repeating themselves, the time of the alternation of divine grace and divine judgment, in which human priests had their function and the offerings made by men had a meaning. His sacrifice means that the time of being has dawned in place of that of signifying — of the being of man as a faithful partner in covenant with God, and therefore of his being at peace with God and therefore of the being of the man reconciled with Him and converted to Him. We are told in John 19:28 concerning the crucified Jesus that He knew "that now all things were finished *(tetelestai)*." And His last word when He died was "it is finished *(tetelestai)*" (John 19:30). Jesus knew what God knew in the taking place of His sacrifice. And Jesus said what God said: that what took place was not something provisional, but that which suffices to fulfill the divine will, that which is entire and perfect, that which cannot and need not be continued or repeated or added to or superseded, the new thing which was the end of the old but which will itself never become old, which can only be there and continue and shine out and have force and power as that which is new and eternal.[25]

In the all-sufficient, unsurpassable sacrifice of Christ, Christian theology suggests, *all things* are completed. Nothing escapes the force of the "all things" here, all things have received their proper end. Christ's sacrifice is the "perfect redemption."[26] The logic of this perfect redemption is such that all other intellectual discourses must be positioned in terms of its truth and never vice versa.

While theological engagement with other intellectual discourses must position all other discourses within its own internal logic, it must also reflect the nature of its own logic, which is Christ's sacrifice, and not become a form of tyranny. As Milbank reminds us, "There is a continuity between Jesus' refusal of any seizure of power and the early church's refusal to overthrow existing structures, in favor of the attempt to create alternative ones, as local areas of relative peace, charity and justice."[27] This continuity should exist not only between Jesus and the early church; it must be a permanent feature of the church's life, for it is intrinsic to the logic of the gospel. The task of relating theology to economics is not then to overthrow the existing structures in some cataclysmic revolutionary act. We are not waiting for the proletariat to rise up and control the means of production through a violent seizure of power any more than we are waiting for the free market to work its miracle and provide its always-not-yet-achieved wealth of nations. Neither are we waiting for the imposition of some "righteous" theocracy. Instead, the theological task is to create space for faithful Christian practice wherever that space can be found and whatever the consequences entailed in the production of such a space. For this reason, a theology of aging need not begin by responding to the economists' and sociologists' analysis. They should seek to be relevant to theology and never vice versa.

Christian theological reflection does not begin with the allocation of scarce resources among individuals; it begins with the appropriate distribution of the fullness of life Christ offers in his cross and resurrection. This claim must be something more than pious sentiment if theology is to matter substantively. By beginning with the fullness of life Christ offers I am not denying the possibility of tragic conflicts; we still might need to tell ninety-year-olds that hip replacements are not the appropriate use of our resources. Such judgments, however, will be based on an understanding of an ecclesial mission subject to Christ's authority and not simply on the abstract calcula-

24. I recognize that many theologians would find this claim objectionable, but I find John Milbank's argument in *Theology and Social Theory: Beyond Secular Reason* (Cambridge, Mass.: Basil Blackwell, 1991) convincing on this point. Milbank writes, "The pathos of modern theology is its false humility. For theology, this must be a fatal disease, because once theology surrenders its claim to be a meta-discourse, it cannot any longer articulate the word of the creator God, but is bound to turn into the oracular voice of some finite idol. . . . If theology no longer seeks to position, qualify or criticize other discourses, then it is inevitable that these discourses will position theology: for the necessity of an ultimate organizing logic cannot be wished away" (p. 1).

25. Karl Barth, *Church Dogmatics* IV.I.

26. The language comes from the Anglican and the United Methodist Articles of Religion. The expression is ecumenical. I do not intend to eclipse the "not-yet" character of this eschatological claim into a fully realized eschatology. The very effort to subordinate an economic analysis of aging to theological considerations is a sign of the "not-yet" character present in these claims.

27. Milbank, *Theology and Social Theory,* p. 116.

tions of marginal utility, which always hide politics behind "usefulness."

Jesus' fullness of life breaks the boundaries of race, class, family, and nation to produce a new form of social reproduction which we call "church." The church is the visible inauguration of God's reign, which is both founded by Jesus in his teachings, death, and resurrection and endowed with certain sacramental structures by which all people are called to Jesus' ongoing mission through participation in his life. Jesus' actions reveal to us the role our elders have within the new community he has established. They provide the context within which we can faithfully honor our elders. Jesus provides this by fulfilling the law revealed to Moses on Mount Sinai.

When Jesus tells us that the entirety of the law is fulfilled in the commandment to love God and our neighbor, he is directing us to the realization of the Torah revealed at Sinai to Moses and now fulfilled in him.[28] This does not constitute a decisive break with Israel, but retells the story from the perspective of Christ as the one who decisively brings and enacts God's reign.[29] All social, political, and economic institutions are now subjected to the authority of Christ. We can begin to see how this works for the family, and the care of the elderly, by observing the odd way Christ fulfills the fourth commandment — honor your father and mother.

Honoring Our Elders

Law is never an end in itself; if it were, obedience would be arbitrary, it would mean merely observing commandments. Law directs human actions to virtuous ends; it assumes a virtuous life as the context for its intelligibility. Law without virtue is capricious; virtue without law lacks direction. Jesus presents to Christians the social and political life that directs our actions toward virtuous ends. When we examine the fourth commandment, however, the social life Jesus presents to us seems to contradict rather than complete the commandment. His treatment of his elders appears dishonorable.

Luke tells the story of Jesus' disappearance from his parents' care for three days to spend time in the temple. When Mary finds him and says, "Son, why have you treated us so? Behold your father and I have been looking for you anxiously," Jesus' response is, "How is it that you sought me? Did you not know that I must be in my Father's house?" (Luke 2:48-49). Jesus dismisses his parents' anxiety as unwarranted, and this is not the only occasion on which Jesus seems dismissive of his family. Mark records Jesus' response to the announcement that his mother and brothers are waiting for him as "Who are my mother and my brothers? . . . Here are my mother and my brothers! Whoever does the will of God is my brother, and sister, and mother" (Mark 3:31-35). In their narration both Matthew and Luke seem to soften this encounter by retaining Jesus' words but not juxtaposing them to his mother's search quite so severely (Matt. 12:46-50; Luke 8:19-21); yet both Matthew and Luke record a statement of Jesus against the family that Mark does not have. Luke puts it in its starkest form: "If anyone comes to me and does not hate his own father and mother and wife and children and brothers and sisters, yes, and even his own life, he cannot be my disciple" (Luke 14:26; see also Matt. 10:37-39).

Both Matthew and Luke record one of Jesus' harshest sayings against the family, when he turns to a disciple who wants to bury his father and says, "Follow me, and leave the dead to bury their own dead" (Matt. 8:22; Luke 9:60). Such statements do not seem to hold forth much promise for any attempt to develop a theology of aging and dying. John's Gospel likewise recounts a shocking statement of Jesus to his mother when she tells him that the wine has run out at a marriage at Cana in Galilee: Jesus says, "O woman, what have you to do with me? My hour has not yet come" (John 2:4). So we find in Scripture multiple attestations from diverse sources that Jesus acted almost dishonorably toward his own elders. The urgency of his mission seems to leave little room for a theology focused on the needs and concerns of the elderly, including the needs of his own parents.

Jesus' harsh actions toward his elders, however, need to be supplemented with the poignant scene in John's Gospel when Jesus, suffering on the cross, saw his mother and John "standing near" and said to Mary, "Woman, behold, your son!" and to John, "Behold your mother!" (John 19:26-27). This agonizing scene does not contradict the harsh ones mentioned earlier. Rather, it sets them in an appropriate order. In fact, this scene occurs right before Jesus remarks, "It is finished" *(tetelestai).* The bequeathment of his mother to the disciple is part of Jesus' completion of all things. From this we learn that the family has been restructured and brought into submission to the authority of Christ. Beneath the suffer-

28. See Thomas Aquinas, *Summa Theologiae* I-II.108.

29. Oliver O'Donovan has persuasively narrated the political implications of Christ's victory in his *The Desire of the Nations: Rediscovering the Roots of Political Theology* (Cambridge: Cambridge University Press, 1997). He notes that "The kingly rule of Christ is God's own rule exercised over the whole world. It is visible in the life of the church, but not only there. St. Paul declared that God has 'disarmed the principalities and powers and made a public show of them in Christ's triumphal procession' (Col. 2:15). That must be the primary eschatological assertion about the authorities, political and demonic, which govern the world: they have been made subject to God's sovereignty in the Exaltation of Christ. The second qualifying assertion is that this awaits a final universal presence of Christ to become fully apparent. Within the framework of these two assertions there opens up an account of secular authority which presumes neither that the Christ-event occurred nor that the sovereignty of Christ is now transparent and uncontested" (p. 146). O'Donovan then narrates how secular authority both submits to and contests Christ's rule. Something like O'Donovan's argument must also be made with respect to the family. As Christ subjects, and will subject, all nations to his authority, so also does he, and will he, subject the family. To understand how he subjects the family to his authority we must be attentive to the scriptural narratives that characterize the subordination of the family to Christ's mission.

ing of the cross, John receives Jesus' mother and provides a space for her in his own home.

This scene can serve us well in our efforts to think about an appropriate theology of aging and death. Raniero Cantalamessa explains its significance well: "Beneath the cross, Mary therefore appears as the daughter of Zion, who after the death and loss of her sons received a new and more numerous family from God, but by the Spirit and not the flesh."[30] The fourth commandment is fulfilled not by dishonoring the family, but by restructuring it. Just as there is no longer male nor female, Jew nor Gentile, slave nor free in the community of faith, so there is also neither parent nor child. As Jesus commanded, all the faithful are to be brothers, sisters, and mothers to one another. This commandment assumes the virtues of charity and hope. Charity is present because we must take others into our homes, and provide for them out of our resources, as John did for Mary. Hope is present because death will not leave the widowed and orphaned abandoned. Within the church, they are to find new homes. Our use of resources must bear witness to this new reality that is made present beneath the cross.

That we are to be brothers and sisters to one another is easily explained, but that we are to be mothers is certainly surprising. This surprised St. Augustine such that he wrote, "I understand that we are Christ's brethren and that the holy and faithful women are Christ's sisters. But how can we be mothers of Christ?" Augustine did not let his puzzlement prevent him from using the expression, and he explained it ecclesiologically.

> Who gave you birth? I hear the voice of your hearts answering "Mother Church!" This holy and honored mother, like Mary, gave birth and is virgin. . . . The members of Christ give birth, therefore, in the Spirit, just as the Virgin Mary gave birth to Christ in her womb: in this way you will be mothers of Christ. This is not something that is out of your reach; it is not beyond you, it is not incompatible with you; you have become children, be mothers as well.[31]

St. Augustine also finds in Jesus' bequeathment of John and Mary to each other evidence of his humanity and divinity. The harsh sayings of Jesus toward his elders represent for Augustine Jesus' divinity; they reveal that Jesus is not bound by biological ties to the family. Jesus' bequeathment, on the other hand, evidences his humanity. "Then it was, as a man on the cross, that He acknowledged His human mother and commended her in a most human fashion to the Apostle he loved most."[32] The love for his mother was natural and more; it was also supernatural. And thus it was grounded in grace, in his freedom to love through and beyond the biological ties of family. It was not necessary; it was gift.

The bequeathment of Mary and John to one another occurs prior to Jesus' proclamation, "It is finished." The all-sufficient sacrifice on the cross includes Christ's restructuring of the family so that our duties toward the elderly are no longer merely obligations to biological family. Instead, the family is expanded. To honor one's parents is for John to take Mary into his home now that she has lost her son. To honor one's parents is also to honor those who are parents to us in the faith. Our obligations to our parents include not only that we be children to them but parents as well. Vice versa, parents' obligation to their children includes not only the role of parenting but also a readiness to allow our children to be mothers to us, to birth in us faith. This does not imply any disrespect for our own parents, for as Jesus made preparations for his mother on the cross, so he teaches us that disciples are to prepare such a place for their own parents within the community of faith.[33] Nor does this imply that "Mary" stands as some symbol for the "elderly" per se. Mary is,

> as St. Ambrose taught, . . . a type of the church in the order of faith, charity, and perfect union with Christ. For in the mystery of the Church, which is itself rightly called mother and virgin, the Blessed Virgin stands out in eminent and singular fashion as exemplar both of virgin and mother. Through her faith and obedience she gave birth on earth to the very Son of the Father, not through the knowledge of man but by the overshadowing of the Holy Spirit, in the manner of a new Eve who placed her faith, not in the serpent of old but in God's messenger without wavering in doubt. The Son whom she brought forth is he whom God placed as the first born among many brethren (Rom. 8:29), that is, the faithful, in whose generation and formation she cooperates with a mother's love.
>
> The Church indeed contemplating her hidden sanctity, imitating her charity, and faithfully fulfilling the Father's will, by receiving the word of God in faith becomes herself a mother.[34]

By her faithfulness, Mary is mother to us all. She is the symbol of the church and a symbol of the restructuring of family bonds.

30. Raniero Cantalamessa, *Mary: Mirror of the Church,* trans. Frances Lonergan Villa (Collegeville, Minn.: Liturgical Press, 1992), p. 121.

31. St. Augustine, *Sermons* 72A; quoted in Cantalamessa, *Mary: Mirror,* p. 69.

32. Augustine, *Faith and the Creed,* p. 325. St. Augustine also finds in the relationship between Jesus and his mother evidence for God's love and redemption of both sexes. "We must likewise repudiate those who deny that the Lord Jesus Christ had Mary for His mother on earth, since His temporal plan ennobled each sex, both male and female. By possessing a male nature and being born of woman He further showed by this plan that God has concern not only for the sex He represented but also for the one through which He took upon Himself our nature."

33. That the disciple took Jesus' bequeathment seriously can be seen in the Acts of the Apostles where Luke tells us that Mary was with the disciples when they returned to Jerusalem after the Ascension (Acts 1:12-14).

34. *Lumen Gentium,* in *Vatican Council II: The Conciliar and Post Conciliar Documents,* ed. Austin Flannery (Collegeville, Minn.: Liturgical Press, 1981), para. 63-64.

The way we think, speak, and act concerning our aging, and the aging of our elders as well, should reflect that the family has now been restructured and subordinated to the authority of Christ as have "all things." The well-known description of Mary as the "daughter of her son" reflects the completed ordering of the family. This restructuring of the family should become our politics and provide us with the language we use in speaking of preparing our elders, and ourselves, to die.

Languages in Conflict

Once we begin not with the abstract calculations of marginalism but with a theological politics where all things are, and shall be, subordinated to the authority of Christ, we do not then have ready-made answers to perceived economic problems of aging. Instead, what we have is a different context within which arguments and concrete determinations could take place.

1. An alternative space must be created.

The first theological task in preparing our elders to die is to create some alternative space where the elderly can be cared for within the context of the ecclesial community. Only such a space allows for theology to circumscribe the language of aging and dying with its own logic. Such a space will include subordinating all our needs to the authority of Christ and the ecclesial mission. It involves duties and habits of preparation which recognize our sufferings and those of our parents as purposive; they fulfill what is lacking in the all-sufficient sacrifice of Christ (Col. 1:24).

Theology must not accommodate the analysis of aging to either the economists or the sociologists. Instead, it should show the abstract nature of their arguments as well as their hidden political and social valuations. Aging cannot be adequately assessed solely on the basis of marginal utility, for usefulness per se does not give us sufficient resources to exercise concrete determinations necessary for the sake of our ecclesial mission. As St. Thomas stated, an action is useful because it is directed to an end.[35] Until we know that end we cannot properly speak of the useful. To speak of the useful without knowledge of any end is foundational to marginalism. This is why it always reduces politics to market considerations. Christians should not countenance such a political reductionism. Our politics must bear witness to the end of all creation present in Christ. This entails that economic considerations find their purpose in the ecclesial mission, which is to be a sign and foretaste of the subordination of all things to Christ. Such a mission does not give us a priori principles about whether we as the elderly, or the elderly entrusted to our care in hospitals, nursing homes, and families, should be given hip replacements. But it could provide a political context within which such a debate could take shape. We can begin to ask questions such as, "Must we practice medicine in such a way that it is viewed as a scarce natural resource?"

The "we" here takes on some definitiveness in its reference to people of faith bound together into a catholic unity serving a common mission. We can now ask in a concrete way, "What 'other valuable resources' could serve our mission better?" Free medical clinics in the inner city? Perhaps we could ask our suburban elderly to forego such operations for the sake of some greater mission, thus extending the life of charity.

2. The healing power of the resurrection is essential.

At the same time that subjection to the authority of Christ recognizes a place for suffering, and recognizes that suffering does not diminish the life of charity, it also must bear witness to the healing power brought by the resurrection. Suffering is not the only enemy we know, but it remains an enemy. As Mary always had a place among the disciples, should we not expect that our parents will also receive a place where sons and daughters will tend to them? Such "tending" will seek to diminish the pain associated with aging and dying as much as possible. Death and its entourage is no friend; it remains an enemy, and one that was vanquished in the cross and resurrection even if it is not yet fully vanquished. For this reason we must not sacrifice our elderly to the idols of a false security. When a ninety-year-old foregoes a hip replacement and endures suffering for her last few years, and the Pentagon is granted more money than it requested, then we can be sure we have denied the healing power of the resurrection.

3. No solution can be found in the biological family (or the state or the market).

The church should never rest content with a care for the elderly situated in the biological family, the market, or the state. There may be some truth to Laslett's contention that co-residential families create intergenerational hostility rather than structures for virtuous living; yet Christians need not fear such revelations about the family since it has been restructured, and we need not hold romantic illusions about it. Nevertheless, Laslett's replacement of charity by earned assets and autonomy is problematic, for the community of faith has as part of its task the charitable redistribution of its resources to care for those who no longer have them. A system of care such as Social Security, insofar as it redistributes wealth across biological family lines, reflects more an appropriate subjection to Christ's authority over the family than does either leaving such care to the family alone or leaving such care to individual earnings. Nevertheless, not even the state is entrusted with the charisma to restructure the family along the lines of God's reign. That is the task of

35. Aquinas, *Summa Theologiae* I-II.7.2 ad 1.

the church alone, a task it accomplishes through the sacrament of baptism. The church must assist in the practice of redistribution so that needs are met rather than wants satiated. This has been an ancient teaching of the church,[36] and it implies that families within the church should recognize Christ's authority over their resources. By providing for those who cannot provide for themselves, the church fulfills the pentecostal mission.

4. The threat to God's rule is not the division between the elderly and the young but between the rich and the poor.

The serious threat to God's rule is not the disparity that exists between young and old in our churches but that between poor and rich. Only insofar as the elderly are found among the broader category known as the poor should they be entitled to charitable provisions. While our Social Security system may be facing a crisis, this does not necessarily translate into any "crisis of aging" per se.[37] The crisis is between the increasing relative distance between rich and poor, both culturally and economically. The church cannot begin to address the problems of the elderly poor only during their "third age"; such problems must be addressed from birth. The crisis for the church is that this economic disparity is insufficiently challenged; instead, it is reflected in the church's increasing divisions based on class interests.

5. The elderly are not individuals in a calculation of burden.

The elderly must not be treated as individuals in a calculation of burden of dependency — even in a technical sense. They are persons who by virtue of their baptism were granted gifts for the upbuilding of the church. Baptism, like ordination, brings with it lifelong tasks. The goal of the Christian life is not leisure, forced or voluntary, at the end of life, but faithful service. This must be demanded from the faithful even when we rejoice with them in their cessation of work as daily toil.

6. We must think again about the creation of an alternative practice.

But all of this requires the creation of an alternative space where Christians would practice medicine and care for the elderly in ways that we do not yet see prevalent in contemporary church life. Such alternative arrangements are present both within the church's ministries and outside of them. The church could learn from community-based health care such as the On Lok program in San Francisco's Chinatown, where medical and social services are provided to the elderly so that they can remain in their own homes and community.[38] Insofar as the church has a financial interest in the proliferation of nursing homes for the well-to-do elderly it will be hampered in its ability to subject even our family relationships to the authority of Christ. This poses a serious problem for any theological analysis of the economics of aging, for the conflict between theology and economics occurs not at some abstract level of linguistic differences; it must be a conflict of languages made necessary by ecclesial practice. If such concrete practice is not forthcoming, we will have no alternative but to use the dominant language of the market; our dying will be described in terms of the burden of dependency.

36. See Acts 2-5. A similar sentiment is found in Catholic teaching on the church: "in accordance with the venerable example of former times, bishops should gladly extend their fraternal assistance, in the fellowship of an all-pervading charity, to other Churches, especially to neighboring ones and to those most in need of help" (*Lumen Gentium,* para. 23).

37. See Disney, "Some Salient Conclusions" (chap. 11 in *Can We Afford to Grow Older?*), where he argues, "There is not a crisis of aging." He suggests, "It is common to blame 'aging' for the budget deficits and payroll-tax increases associated with social security programs in the 1980's. But the sources of these (correctly perceived) crises have little to do with aging per se. In pay-as-you-go social insurance, financing crises have far more to do with the chain-letter or Ponzi-scheme nature of such programs as practiced by governments and voters, which pre-commit future generations to excessive forced transfers" (pp. 307-8). While he reassures us that aging itself is not the problem we face, his prediction that increased private pension plans will increasingly replace Social Security is not so reassuring, for this will only exacerbate the class divisions between the poor and others.

38. See Angel and Angel, *Who Will Care for Us?* pp. 150-53.

77 Ruth's Resolve: What Jesus' Great-Grandmother May Teach about Bioethics and Care

Amy Laura Hall

I. Introduction

So Naomi returned together with Ruth the Moabite, her daughter-in-law, who came back with her from the country of Moab. They came to Bethlehem at the beginning of the barley harvest. (Ruth 1:22, NRSV)[1]

M. Cathleen Kaveny prophetically beckons Christians to remember "the Order of Widows" and the church's historic calling to bring "the *almanah* into its center rather than pushing her to its margins" (see [*Christian Bioethics* 11.1], pp. 11-34). Kaveny calls on the church again to enable and encourage the hard work of caring for the often forgotten and ignored women at the margins of society. When thinking about the intersection of care and Christian bioethics, it may also be helpful to read about the young Moabite widow who chose to turn away from security to walk alongside her grieving mother-in-law to Bethlehem. Remembering Ruth's story may, I hope, further encourage readers to heed Professor Kaveny's summons. As Kaveny well explains toward the end of her essay, the particular bioethical "case-study" questions about euthanasia and physician-assisted suicide may lead to a larger interrogation of the context in which these procedures appear necessary. She argues that one route to current, bioethical quandaries has much to do with neglect of the vulnerable in general and women in particular. Disabled, elderly, and terminally ill people are seen and even see themselves as expendable in part due to individual and corporate disregard. Hearing the scriptural account of a tenacious great-grandmother in the canon, readers may recall another way. Ruth's care for Naomi is a powerfully prophetic act.

This foreign convert to the faith of Israel is appropriately a mentor for works of Christian faith. In Matthew's genealogy (1:1-6), Jesus Christ is the son of Tamar and of Rahab and of Ruth, three women remembered for their unconventional acts of courage on behalf of God's people.[2] Rather than recalling these matriarchs with fond sentimentality, as Christians are known to do, readers may attend to their particular narratives and consider the contours of a life lived similarly. By hearing specifically the account of Jesus' grandmother Ruth, those who profess Christ may be prompted further to hear the truth about faithful care of widows and others on the margin. In bioethical discussions about death and its options, Christians may ask more probing questions about the distribution and details of faithful care for the vulnerable.

Those acquainted with Ruth often overhear merely a portion of the story. Her words of determined love to Naomi have been snipped neatly in order to embellish many a wedding ceremony. I will here seek to stitch them back into Ruth's actual narrative in order to display the Christian calling to difficult service.

When discussing an ethic of care, Christians are too often tempted to employ a vague assessment of women's ways of serving, assuming that women have some innate capacity to care effectively for others.[3] Reading Ruth may be of use for resistance to this unreflective and unscriptural notion. When Ruth vows "may the Lord do thus and so to me, and more as well, if even death parts me from you" (1:17b), she is not merely tapping into her compassionate, feminine self. The narrative resists such a (suspiciously convenient) reading. This foreign woman inextricably links her future with that of her justifiably cynical mother-in-law through a vow that is more than an example of sororal camaraderie. Ruth's vow is one of resolute, courageous fidelity. Those who hear the narrative may note that this prompt — faithful care is not a gender trait. Faithful care in this story is saliently arduous work. I will here consider Ruth's testimony as a storied guide for those who attempt or are ineluctably called to similar tasks.

Ruth's story also implies that care is dependent upon the fidelity of the God of Israel. True patience and fidelity to another may involve an active turn from Moab to face Bethlehem. In her decision to care for Naomi, Ruth directs her adopted mother toward her ultimate home. Their destination informs their journey, as it will inform the journey of those who follow them. The scriptural account may encourage Christians of both genders to seek, in faith, to follow this young matriarch. Rather than the default, feminine *modus operandi,* care in this story is a matter of tenacious fidelity, a practice that is prayerfully possible for women and men who receive God's grace and live expectantly.

These promptings from Ruth have many concrete implications for Christians called by Jesus to care for oth-

1. All Scripture references are to the New Revised Standard Version, copyright 1989 by the Division of Christian Education of the National Council of the Churches of Christ in the United States of America.

Amy Laura Hall, "Ruth's Resolve: What Jesus' Great-Grandmother May Teach about Bioethics and Care," *Christian Bioethics* 11.1 (2005): 35-50. Used by permission.

2. See the stories of Tamar, who poses as a prostitute in order to trick her negligent father-in-law into impregnating her (Genesis 38), and of Rahab, an actual prostitute who protected Joshua's spies and confessed the Lord's name, thereby saving her family from the destruction of Jericho (Joshua 2 and 6:22-27).

3. Feminists, both Christian and secular, have resisted and spoken against this tendency to view the capacity to care as a physiological trait. See, for example, Margaret Farley (1991).

ers. If women are not by sheer anatomy suited to tend to the young, old, and vulnerable, if care is a virtue cultivated and encouraged through faith, then readers would do well to ask why so few men in the United States are performing the difficult tasks of hearing those who cry, of wiping noses, of wrapping wounds, and of changing Pampers or Depends undergarments. Those who hear and read Ruth may stand against the temptation to understand women as uniquely fitted for such work and instead ask why so few men envision and act on the faith narrated in Ruth's story. This interrogation may depend on a faith sufficient to enable the courage and patience required to stay engaged rather than opting to turn away, as does Orpah. A close reading may also prompt a renewal of Christian commitment. Ruth the Moabite accepts Israel's trust in God's goodness, and she is thus able to refuse her mother-in-law the last word. Their circumstances, as Naomi perceives them, do not ultimately define their future; Naomi's hopelessness does not preclude Ruth's faith on behalf of them both. Christians may glean from Ruth an important cue: those who would care for others faithfully may daily turn towards Bethlehem and receive the only sustenance sufficient for the task. This sustenance is, for Christians as for Ruth, to be found in the bread given by God.

I will follow closely the first few acts in Ruth's drama, paying particular attention to the narration of her resolve to remain alongside her mother-in-law. I will then move from the text to consider what a bioethic of care modeled after Ruth would look like, and suggest how such an ethic may inform general conversations on women, men, and embodied service. Finally, I will propose several ways that Ruth's story may shape Christian, bioethical conversations regarding end-of-life care.

II. Ruth's Resolve

Naomi had much reason to be, as she defines herself, "bitter." To be a widow was to be vulnerable. To be a widow without a male child was significantly worse. Naomi finds herself with neither a husband nor a son, and she is in a foreign land. The skillful storyteller who tells us of Naomi's plight moves quickly from abundance to apparent desolation with terse Hebrew prose. This is the calamity that begins the real story. Naomi is initially blessed with a husband, fertile fields in a foreign land, and two eligible sons. Her husband dies. Her sons marry, and with marriage comes hope for fertility. Yet, in the immediately subsequent verse, her sons die as well. And, significantly, they leave their wives childless. This first section ends with a blunt summary of Naomi's fate: "so that the woman was left without her two sons and her husband" (1:5). This alien woman with no men has every reason to be angry, for all obvious sources of protection and selfhood are gone. As Phyllis Trible puts it, "From wife to widow, from mother to no-mother, this female is stripped of all identity" (1978, p. 167).

The first real scene in this drama comes as Naomi decides to return to Judah. When Naomi hears that God has "visited his people to give them bread," this old, foreign widow who is, effectively, no one, herself recalls, however tenuously, that she is one of God's people. This line about an infertile widow is, itself, pregnant with meaning. An echo of God's prior deeds on behalf of his people and a poetic allusion to God's future work mark this line as significant. As "God looked upon the Israelites, and God took notice of them" in their time of slavery in Egypt (Exodus 2:24), so Naomi hears that God has "considered his people and given them food" (1:6). The echo serves as a reminder, for Naomi and for those who hear the story, of God's prior acts of mercy toward Naomi's people. The Hebrew is also beautifully alliterative. The phrase "give to them bread" is *latet lahem lachem,* and the poetic repetition is to accentuate Naomi and Ruth's eventual destination. They are, in time, to reach *bêt lechem,* Bethlehem, or, literally, house of bread. God gives to his people bread, and this hungry widow resolves to return to the house of bread. The storyteller thus gives us the first, albeit fragile, signs that Naomi will not perish. Those who hear this story may anticipate the possibility that Naomi will not remain an unidentified foreigner. She may instead reach the land of her own people, God's people, and the source of nourishment that is *bêt lechem.*

But at this point, Naomi's perspective is merely one notch above grim. Leaving Moab for Judah, Naomi turns to the two young, childless widows before her and insists that they turn away from Judah, back to Moab. If these two women are to flourish, they had best leave her (infertile) side and take up their much better chances with another deity. Naomi's speech to them begins and ends by speaking with warranted pessimism about her own circumstances and with cynicism about the *chesed* of God. The Lord may "deal kindly" with these young, Moabite women, but, she concludes, "the hand of the Lord has turned against" his own daughter, Naomi. She builds toward this conclusion by juxtaposing their fertile wombs to her own barrenness. They may return to Moab and find "security" with new husbands. She herself will return, childless, to the supposedly promised land. With brittle sarcasm about God's infidelity and their own prospects, she responds to her daughters' gestures of affection: "So God gives me a husband this very night, and I conceive two more sons, would you foolishly wait for them to become men? No, that is ridiculous, go home to your own mothers." Life, she concludes, "has been far more bitter" for Naomi, one of the Lord's own, than for these two Moabite women (1:14).

With this apparently irrefutable estimation of their circumstances, Orpah leaves Naomi's side. Accepting Naomi's perspective as true and her command as incontrovertible, Orpah chooses to turn back towards her own home. Phyllis Trible writes of Orpah: "Her decision is sound, sensible, and secure . . . [and] ironically, [Orpah's] alliance with Naomi means separation from that mother-in-law" (1978, p. 173). Her daughter-in-law's departure returns the story to the trajectory of loss and bereavement narrated in the first section. Having lived in Moab as a family of six, Naomi is now down to a family of two. Life has met her morose expectations. Naomi's next statement to Ruth echoes the religious despair of her previous speech to both young women. "See," she says to Ruth, "your sister-in-law has [prudently] gone back to her people and to her [more reliable] gods" (1:15, bracketed additions mine). Naomi tells her one remaining family member that if she has any sense, she will, like Orpah, put her trust elsewhere.

According to the Septuagintal tradition, the book of Ruth immediately follows Judges. The narrative of her heroic faith begins just after the ominous closing line of judges, "In those days there was no king in Israel; all the people did what was right in their own eyes" (21:25). The placement of Ruth's story is potent. At this crucial juncture in the canon, a young, foreign woman does what is right in the eyes of the Lord. Ruth refuses and carefully refutes Naomi's realistically pessimistic vision. Instead of accepting her mother-in-law's perspective, as does Orpah, Ruth adamantly embraces Naomi and indirectly exhorts her to remember her own identity as a daughter of Abraham:

> Do not press me to leave you or to turn back from following you! Where you go, I will go; where you lodge, I will lodge; your people shall be my people, and your God my God. Where you die, I will die — there I will be buried. May the Lord do thus and so to me, and more as well, if even death parts me from you! (1:16-17)

Ruth insists that she will stay with Naomi, and at the center of her insistence is the claim that, by her act of fidelity, she is one of the people of God. Naomi, one of the daughters of Abraham, cannot presently trust in God. Her foreign daughter's testimony stands in contrast. Ruth attests to a radical faith of which Naomi is, for ample reason, incapable. She vows before Naomi and before God that, while the decision may be ludicrous, she will remain with Naomi beyond death. In so doing, she seeks to adjust Naomi's perspective, she takes on a perfected hope, and, in effect, she carries her adopted mother-in-law toward Bethlehem.[4]

Naomi sees that Ruth is "determined," as the NRSV translates the word *mit 'ammetset.* It is helpful to dust off the *Brown-Driver-Briggs* and dwell on the wording here. This Hebrew word is the reflexive form of the verb *'amets,* to be "strong or bold," and in this form the verb means more specifically to "strengthen oneself" or to "confirm oneself in a purpose" (Brown, 1979, p. 54). This is significant for the purpose of understanding faithful care. The Hebrew does not suggest that Ruth found her inchoate desire felicitously coincident with what was right in the eyes of the Lord. Rather, those who hear are told that Ruth strengthens herself to the purpose of fidelity to God and to Naomi. The wording explicitly connotes the mustering of strength and thus of moral exertion on Ruth's part. It would have made much more sense for Ruth to leave this widow, to return to her own kin, to food, to a new husband, and to the promise of future children. It is not possible to parse precisely the set of factors separating Ruth's intrepid faith and Orpah's compliance. Perhaps only through the lens of subsequent interpretation may Christians name the difference grace. What readers do know from the text itself is that one woman turned to walk back to Moab and another resolved herself, strengthened herself, to stay bound with an old woman who had faith insufficient for the journey back to Bethlehem.

Ruth's resolution carries over into the next line, "So the two of them went on until they came to Bethlehem" (1:19). Ruth's commitment to Naomi alters the previous trajectory of loss. The momentum of her courageous decision propels the narrative beyond Naomi's next, angry announcement to the women gathered at the entrance to Bethlehem. Naomi's long, heated greeting to these women stands as a threatening parallel to Ruth's prior declaration of fidelity, but there is reason to hope that Naomi's resentment will not overshadow her daughter's words. Naomi insists to the women that she returns "empty," that "the Lord has dealt harshly" with her, that "the Almighty has brought calamity" on her (1:21). Her language is even stronger than her previous witness against God. But the women must observe that Naomi has not returned empty. She has returned with an outrageously loyal new daughter. And those who overhear her story of anguish know how this daughter dealt with Naomi's previous speech. Here and throughout the remaining story, Ruth will not allow Naomi to rename herself "Mara," literally "bitter," just as she did not allow Naomi's case against God to stand uncorrected. Her tenacious, courageous presence with this woman testifies to God's power more effectively than Naomi's case against God's goodness. The storyteller then closes this first scene in Bethlehem with a displacement of the last lines in Moab. "So that the woman was left without her sons and her husband," is overturned by the statement, "So Naomi returned together with Ruth the Moabite, her daughter-in-law, who came back with her from the country of Moab" (1:22). Ruth's presence stands as evidence of a faith that surpasses even great pain and loss.

III. Following Ruth

Moving from the text to particular lives, it is helpful to avoid gutting the narrative with allegory. Naomi cannot easily "stand for" the danger of despair in the face of suffering, nor does Ruth serviceably "represent" determined

4. Trible writes, Ruth "has disavowed the solidarity of family; she has abandoned national identity; and she has renounced religious affiliation. In the entire epic of Israel, only Abraham matches this radicality, but then he had a call from God" (1978, p. 173).

fidelity. Much of the narrative's power derives from its capacity to catch the hearer up in the story, to involve the reader's imagination as one considers what it might look like to choose a life shaped by these women's words and decisions. Watching and listening, one's moral imagination may quicken in a way that one may, with grace, follow Ruth. To put an ecclesial spin on this power, those who are bound to Jesus also hear that this woman is a great-grandmother for the Church. Reading the story of this, an ancestor, Christians may think about the shape of a life true to her memory. If her grandchildren were to live out the family resemblance, how might the patterns of compassion and attention change? What might it look like to be with another as Ruth remains with and for Naomi? The lived answers to these questions will be as particular and varied as the characters of this and other scriptural narratives. Those who suffer loss respond in many different ways, and the contours of individual responses will necessarily vary. But perhaps I may, with reasonable assurance, name some salient features of faithful bioethical care modeled after Ruth. I will now seek to describe the considerable work of caring for the bitter, refuting the trajectory of loss, having faith sufficient for two, and moving toward Bethlehem.

However one translates the Hebrew word for Ruth's "determination" (to use the NRSV), one may recognize from the onset of this section that serving similarly demands a kind of movement akin to resolve. I will try to intimate further on the source of resolve, but scripture and sobriety call for the reader first to consider the difficulty involved. While there may be some blessed people who are capable of binding themselves to the needy with no inner resistance, most find caring for others (any others) to be quite often exhausting, frustrating, and tedious. As is the case with Ruth, caring faithfully for another implies effort. Perhaps one example will serve helpfully here. One of the most compelling and common portrayals of immediate, natural, almost effortless attention to another person in art and poetry is the love of a new mother for an infant. Most who have tended to an infant know that this characterization is an oversimplification, to put it mildly. Many new mothers will attest that such nurture is indescribably rewarding, even blissful, and most would not trade the experience for any price. Yet caring for a baby is also exhausting, frustrating, and tedious. Mothers will attest with equal passion that it is by sheer force of will (enabled by the sustaining grace of God) that one crawls out of bed for feedings in the wee hours. Now, to take another step back, this maternal scene is easily marketable — it is a cultural "best-case scenario," so to speak. Remaining with someone who is resentfully hopeless, helplessly despondent, or sarcastically angry — each a difficult task this culture does little to champion, beautify, or reward — arguably calls forth a different order altogether of "strengthening oneself for the purpose" of fidelity to God and neighbor. The work of caring for the perpetually vulnerable and the dying may be more difficult for some than for others, but it is undeniably *work*, regardless.

In Ruth's case, the task of care involves binding herself to another woman, not her kin, whose sarcasm is brittle to the point of breaking. Following Ruth, one needs to be prepared to receive and critically engage others whose loss has rendered them almost unrecognizable. Naomi tells the women in Bethlehem to call her Mara, an explicit acknowledgement that her loss has made her, in effect, a different person. Old age and loss threaten to redefine Naomi to the point where her identity is bitterness itself. Naomi is not Ruth's kin. Ruth does not have childhood memories or blood ties binding her to Naomi. This facet of the story will be significant for many. But it is perhaps even more difficult to commit to remain with someone known well, when that person becomes someone else. Memories of a child or of an elder ineluctably carry expectations for the future. When illness, loss, age, grief, or anger form that beloved person into someone not known, it is all the more tempting to turn back to the safely familiar, as Orpah turned back to Moab.[5] Remaining to tend to the bitter necessitates a kind of theological recollection, to know from whence this unrecognizable person came. Ruth's declaration of love for Naomi is linked with her declaration of love for Naomi's people and for the God of Israel. She is capable of binding herself to Naomi in part because her fidelity is not only to this, her mother-in-law. Ruth remains with Naomi perhaps due to the truth that the narrative of Naomi, as a daughter of Abraham, began long before Ruth married Chilion and will continue long after these two widows return to Bethlehem. Ruth's refutation of Naomi's new name says, in effect, "You are not, dear Naomi, Mara. You are one of God's chosen." Even if Naomi is not able to name this truth, Ruth's own knowledge allows her to walk with Naomi toward Judah.

By refusing to leave Naomi, as Naomi compels her to, Ruth blocks and diverts the story's trajectory, turning it from one of loss to one of hope. In so doing, Ruth does not blithely deny that Naomi is justifiably angry with her circumstances or with God, nor does she perkily tell Naomi to be of good cheer regarding their future. In her oath to Naomi, Ruth instead faces head-on the prospect of death. These two childless widows may indeed die soon, but Ruth vows that Naomi will not die alone. The hope Ruth offers Naomi is thus not equivalent to plucky optimism. Intrinsic to the care Ruth offers is an acknowledgement of suffering and a refusal nonetheless to remain. Caring in like manner does not necessitate a blithe ignorance of circumstances. Ruth fully turns toward the possibility of further grief, refusing to break and splinter off. What Ruth does refute, in her words and in her actions, is Naomi's testimony against God. The sheer act of *staying with* people who decide, as does Naomi, that "the Lord has brought calamity" upon them, stands as counter-

5. Here I am indebted to David Keck's powerful book *Forgetting Whose We Are: Alzheimer's Disease and the Love of God* (1996).

evidence.[6] By her sheer presence, Ruth testifies that, to the contrary, God provides. The Lord has not "brought" Naomi "back empty," as she proclaims. Ruth is with her. The sign of hope in this story is a strange one: a young Moabite widow. Mere humans are often strangely inadequate but effective signs of hope for those who are grieving. Through grace one may, by one's presence, remind people whose they are.

Ruth's hope is tied up with her conviction that binding herself to Naomi's seemingly unreliable God is not an act of sheer lunacy. Her story implies that, in order to attend faithfully in such circumstances, one needs to remember who God is, serving with such memory to remind the person currently incapable of faith. This is a perilous task, and many are likely to falter and fail in the attempt. Some err on the side of downplaying the grieving or suffering person's pain, deeming it easier to remain in proximity if indeed the circumstances seem less than dire. Yet, Naomi's acrid cynicism is a portion of the truth, and a memory of Ruth's work will also take in that portion. The storyteller could have written a humorous tale painting Naomi with broad strokes as an unreasonably bitter old woman, contrasting her to the stalwart young Ruth, but that story would have avoided the truth of Naomi's chaos. In the course of a mere ten years, Naomi's husband and her two children die. She has ample reason to estimate a grim future. Naomi turns back to Judah after hearing that God "had considered his people and given them food," but she cannot help but contrast God's seeming abandonment of her with God's generous visitation on his people. When Naomi decides to return to Judah, she is acting on her belief that, in some way, she is God's own and that God is, in some sense, good. But her trust in God is shaken at the root. Faithfully caring for one who suffers will involve not so much changing her, but standing as firm as possible herself. It is here that Ruth is able to witness to God's grace, by her own faith. In a sense, Ruth is able to have faith enough to keep them both moving toward Bethlehem.

Christians read this story knowing that the same young widow who reminds Naomi of God's goodness became the grandmother of the savior. As these two women turn toward Bethlehem in hope of bread, Christian readers will, with anticipation, hear of the Messiah later to be born there. The reader hears that in Bethlehem God sustains Naomi and Ruth, and Christian readers may recognize that in Bethlehem God provides Christ for the salvation of all Israel. Those who receive the bread, Christ's body, at the Eucharist may hear in Ruth's story a call to return to the table, continually, for sustenance. It is there that those who follow Ruth's grandson recall the deeds of God on behalf of his people. It is there that Christians physically and spiritually receive the one whose power infuses every effort to tend faithfully to another. As Ruth cannot be for Naomi a faithful presence without turning away from Moab, toward Bethlehem, so perhaps must others take on the constant, daily and lifelong tasks of caring for others with consistent recourse to the Eucharist. For Christians, perhaps this is the prescription that underlies the story. Those who follow Jesus may best live a life approximating Ruth's resolve by turning, as does she, toward *bêt lechem,* toward the bread of heaven.

This prescription may have individual and corporate implications. When speaking about Holy Communion, some Christian traditions emphasize the gathering of the Christian community, for others the emphasis falls on the actual work of the sacramental elements on the individual believer. According to my own Wesleyan tradition, the bread and wine are themselves efficacious for the one who receives, but we also recognize that the people gathered around the Eucharist become Christ's body — that through the Holy Spirit the Church sustains believers and brings about "the redemption of the world."[7] As it seems impossible to parse scrupulously the inner workings of Ruth's resolve, so Christians may not meticulously delineate the specific workings of the Eucharist as a means of grace; both Ruth's resolve and the Lord's Supper may best be named as matters of God's mysterious work. Yet, by turning one's focus from the reception of the elements to the community gathered at the table, one may sense another facet of incarnate fidelity modeled after Ruth. Care for the dying may necessarily call upon the entire community of faith. As Ruth and Naomi journey towards Bethlehem and begin hoping for a future there, Ruth stands as a reminder that Naomi belongs to a particular people. Ruth, the Moabite, brings Naomi back to these particular people and, in the following days, reminds these people of their commitment to Naomi. Ruth's arrival in Bethlehem with Naomi is a provocative act. Boaz, Naomi's kinsman, says to Ruth, "you left your father and mother and your native land and came to a people that you did not know before" (2:11). What's more, she has done this in order to care for a woman to whom she was not bound by blood. Implicit in Boaz's praise of Ruth's fidelity is the question: How much more is he, who *is* bound by blood, called to care for Naomi? His implied question may become a question for others who now hear the scriptural account of Ruth. If this foreign woman stays with Naomi, how much more are those bound together by Christ's blood called to pray and work alongside those who would name themselves bitter? Ruth's relationship to Naomi is a prophetic act. To live a life that approximates Ruth's involves becoming for one another the living Body of Christ, particularly for the sake of those who would otherwise be deemed, and deem themselves, extraneous.

6. See Stanley Hauerwas (1986).

7. My own tradition, as stated in the Doctrinal Standards of the United Methodist Church, in the United Methodist *Book of Discipline,* explains that through the "partaking of the blood" and "the body of Christ," God works our salvation. See Part II, Section III, Article XVI "Of the Sacraments" in *The Book of Discipline of The United Methodist Church* (1996).

IV. Speaking of Boaz . . .

This is perhaps a good point to ask again a crucial question. If care is a hard-won, grace-filled commitment rather than a gender trait, then why is the church not explicitly calling more men to this ethic of care? It is plausible that some Christians do not think that men are called to tend to the daily needs of others, or believe that men are called to care, but in a different, less hands-on way, than are women. Even conceding this last point, we may ask whether men can attend to others in any truly meaningful way if they reside at such a distance. It is difficult to attend when one is simply not there. One recent study revealed that men in the United States spend on average a mere twelve minutes a day with the children in their own households.[8] Whether attending to the difference between a newborn's cry of hunger or of fear, dressing the wounds of an elderly woman suffering from bed sores, or reading the daily news to a man homebound with cerebral palsy, women disproportionately do the work.[9] One might again cheaply attribute this to the "fact" that women are naturally suited to such tasks. Yet to fail to call men to such embodied endeavors is to ignore not only Ruth's story but also the particular life of her great-grandson. Even if one were to strike Ruth out of the running as a mentor for Christian men, there is still the story of a savior who prophetically sat with and healed old paralytics and young coma victims, who sought out unsociable demoniacs, and who, much to the chagrin of his disciples, sat visiting with small children. Those who follow Jesus Christ and who learn from Ruth may rightly ask why men in the United States are significantly less likely to be dancing a baby in the crying room, playing with the toddlers in the church nursery, teaching children's Sunday School, taking care of their elderly mother, or volunteering at the nursing home. One provocative way to name Christian feminism is "the radical notion that men are called to be servants." Those who methodically or unquestioningly sidestep the tasks of embodied service may be evading a constitutive practice of faith.

To deny that men are also called by Christ to do this hard work of caring for the vulnerable is to become involved in exegetical gymnastics. Why then is this kind of work so disproportionately women's work? Perhaps a clue as to why so few men actually tend to the bodies and hopes of the vulnerable and/or bitter can be found in Ruth's story itself. Most who hope to follow Ruth must strengthen themselves to commit to women like Naomi because an ethic of care involves tedious work. Those with power, money, prestige and cultural capital will more often than not opt out of such grueling, "demeaning" tasks as wiping noses and bottoms. This seems exponentially true when one adds to the scene the bitter tone understandably common to those who suffer. This may go some way toward explaining why male immigrants from the two-thirds world, compared to white men, disproportionately participate in what are called the "helping" professions, and why white women have, as we have gained power, paid less powerful women or men to perform the tasks supposedly "beneath" us.[10] The Church may speak prophetically about this inequality of service labor, not only as an injustice, which it surely is, but also as an implicit refusal of God's own power to be found in Bethlehem. Even the faithful often act for the sake of the power to be gained from higher salaries, prestige with colleagues, and the envy of neighbors. Ruth's presence with her suffering mother-in-law is a countertestimony to Naomi's invective against God's goodness. The absence of Christians may stand as evidence against the faithful. If Ruth is able to leave the security and worldly promise of Moab behind in order to bind herself to her angry, widowed mother-in-law, traveling to a place she knows only by faith, then those who hope to be true to her memory may, by grace, find the strength to care for children and even bitter, aging relatives.

V. Ruth and End of Life Care

Much of the North American Church currently stands with Orpah, facing Moab. As the dominant economy becomes one ever more intent on speed and innovation — with a superstructure built on and around the Internet and a substructure consisting of the "dirty work" of the service industry — able-bodied adults will have many incentives likewise to turn away from Naomi and face Moab. Those who are privy to dominant American culture hear every day that Moab is, in fact, a sure thing. There, in the "new economy" one may invest one's money, one's time, one's hope. At the beginning of the technological upsurge, advertisers claimed that technology would grant more time to spend with loved ones. Working at home would grant the flexibility needed to be with young children and aging parents. Companies have now shed these claims, aiming with precision at the young and unencumbered viewer. Advertisers further recognize that many of the not so young and unencumbered (who do have children and/or aging parents) would prefer not be reminded of such obligations.[11] The consumer of the new economy can, with only a trace of guilt, turn toward Moab and away from Bethlehem, traveling

8. See Arlie Hochschild (1989). There she narrates with detail the lived reality of a society wherein women who work outside the home spend an average of three hours per day on housework to men's seventeen minutes and who spend fifty minutes per day exclusively with their children in comparison to men's twelve minutes. How can someone care faithfully if present for only twelve minutes a day?

9. I write all of this while my husband takes care of my daughter, my brother takes care of my parents, and my father takes care of my grandmother. There are men faithfully doing this work, witnessing to what is possible.

10. See Ehrenreich and Hochschild (2003).

11. See Hochschild (2001).

toward the more reliable sources of financial gain and domestic security. A decision to spend quantity time with either children or the elderly may thus seem as imprudent as was Ruth's choice to remain with Naomi. Given serious economic incentives, those who wish to succeed are constantly encouraged to make Orpah's choice.

The Church and the academy are subject to the same critique. As if caught in a rapidly moving current, even Christian professionals swim desperately to keep up, throwing off those who might weigh one down. This is particularly the case when the weights are elderly people or those with chronic or terminal illness. While currently "well" children carry with them the promise of future "success," the elderly and chronically or terminally ill persistently carry with them the promise of death. Their photographs cannot prettily adorn offices. They do not look like *Baby Gap* or *Limited Too* ads, cute with just the right touch of perky persistence needed in the new millennium. Instead, by their mere existence they stand as testimony against dreams of immortality and perpetual productivity. Even more, the young, ill, and elderly involve slow, hands-on, patient care. One cannot swim in the fast lane or keep jogging the track while carrying a woman with multiple sclerosis. Choosing to remain present with an overtly needy person, to walk toward Bethlehem with only one's faith, is an arguably reliable roadmap for worldly failure when the needy one is an aging and/or incurably ill person. (Again, at least when taking time off for an otherwise well child one is caring for a future participant in the new economy and a potential sustainer of our retirement.) The incentives for neglecting the elderly dangerously now slip into incentives for justifying their death.

As M. Cathleen Kaveny reports, "the vast majority of Jack Kevorkian's clients have been female" (see [*Christian Bioethics* 11.1], pp. 11-34). Many of these women, she continues, were not on the verge of death but rather suffered from conditions that made them a burden to others. The testimony of these women may serve as a deafening wake-up call. Perhaps they found themselves in Naomi's position and, perhaps, either ignored, or simply were not offered any, refutation. Perhaps their rising perspective against life and God remained undisputed. Kaveny explains:

> [A]n inadequate appreciation for their own dignity and worth may lead elderly and chronically ill women to request assisted suicide or euthanasia to avoid becoming a burden to others. Their families and physicians might very well agree with them. Victims of the enduring sin of sexism, such women will misperceive the choice of their own deaths as the last, best gift they can give to their own aging daughters.

This parallels Naomi's plight, as she insists to her younger daughters-in-law that they must turn away from her and seek new husbands. She will only be a burden to them, she insists, and their prospects will be better if they will only separate their future from hers. In her command for them to leave her side, Naomi further witnesses against God's fidelity, suggesting that the Moabite pantheon is more reliable. Those who are currently able-bodied may recognize through this story that many are currently obeying Naomi's morose command by neglect. Many are by default accepting Naomi's estimation of God's fidelity. How might those around the ill and suffering currently hasten their death by leaving their testimony unchallenged?

The prospect of spending one's last days painfully connected to feeding, breathing, and waste-removal tubes while tactically disconnected from home and family leads many aging Christians to sign documents prohibiting the use of such potentially "heroic" measures when they approach death. While Christians disagree about the proper delineation of ordinary and extraordinary care, most agree that advance directives are in a different moral category from active euthanasia or physician-assisted suicide.[12] I believe that Christians should, for many reasons both contextual and deontological, prohibit active euthanasia in whatever way it might be administered. Yet, as the ill become increasingly a burden on a fast-paced economy, those who are not ill or yet elderly may need to question *each* effort to preclude life and "accept" death. With the increasing incentives for families to let the ill, disabled, and elderly stumble along toward death alone, even advance directives may carry with them a taint of despair. Supposedly licit "do not resuscitate" orders may still elicit scrutiny when so many aging and ill adults daily find no one beside them. When bed-bound people spend more time each week with technologically administered sisters like Oprah or Ellen DeGeneres than they do with real neighbors and loved ones, it may be little surprise that they ask under no condition to be revived. In such a context, Christians may need to consider such requests for death a witness against imposed solitude.

One way to read Ruth alongside such questions in bioethics is to find that, alas, individual Christians and the corporate church face the choice of turning away from or walking with Naomi. The next generation of Christians in the U.S. is neglecting its elders (to an arguably unprecedented extent) not only out of forced economic mobility, but also out of familial infidelity. Leaving Christian care up to the few women who still tenaciously enjoy the work or to the women and men desperate for whatever service job they may find is a morally untenable solution. Many more in the Church must, like Ruth, receive strength for the purpose of walking with the ill and aging toward God's sustenance. Ruth acknowledges in her vow to Naomi that they may die in the endeavor. She harbors no illusions about the risks involved. To turn back to Moab, with its promise, would be more "prudent." Leaving that world behind will be difficult. A faithful bioethic of care may thus entail salient sacrifices of prestige and material comfort. But the burden need

12. Margaret Farley has a characteristically wise take on the relevant distinctions. See Farley (1995).

not be debilitating. Those who follow in Ruth's footsteps may know themselves walking towards Bethlehem, towards the body of Christ, toward the Church. As Kaveny compellingly suggests, the church needs to *corporately* take up the task of supporting and assisting caregivers in their work, lest the faithful merely contribute to the currently vicious cycle of sexism and ageism. Those who faithfully choose to do this work of attention and tending can act as prophetic witnesses and in so doing enrich and direct a Christian ethics of care, in particular, a Christian bioethics of care, calling those still unable so to choose to receive frequently the bread of heaven. For, in a potent way, Christians need not merely anticipate the arrival in Bethlehem. Through Eucharist, many among the faithful arrive there each week. With God's grace, may more Christians bring Naomi along.

References

Brown, F. (1979). *The new Brown, Driver, Briggs, Gesenius Hebrew and English lexicon: With an appendix containing the Biblical Aramaic.* Peabody: Hendrickson Publishers.

Ehrenreich, B., and Hochschild, A. R. (Eds.). (2003). *Global woman: Nannies, maids, and sex workers in the new economy.* New York: Metropolitan Books.

Farley, M. (1991). Love, justice and discernment: An interview, *Second Opinion,* 17 (2), 80-91.

Farley, M. (1995), *Issues in contemporary Christian ethics, The choice of death in a medical context.* Santa Clara: Santa Clara University Department of Religious Studies.

General Conferences of the United Methodist Church. (1996). *The Book of Discipline of the United Methodist Church.* H. J. Olson (Ed.). Nashville: The United Methodist Publishing House.

Hauerwas, S. (1986). *Suffering presence.* Notre Dame: University of Notre Dame Press.

Hochschild, A. (1989). *The second shift.* New York: Viking Penguin.

Hochschild, A. (2001). *The time bind: When work becomes home and home becomes work.* New York: H. Holt.

Kaveny, M. C. (2005). The Order of Widows: What the early Church can teach us about older women and health care. *Christian Bioethics,* 11, 11-34.

Keck, D. (1996). *Forgetting whose we are: Alzheimer's disease and the love of God.* Nashville: Abingdon.

Trible, P. (1978). *God and the rhetoric of sexuality.* Philadelphia: Fortress.

78 Memory and Canonicity

David Keck

And he said, "Jesus, remember me when you come into your kingdom."

Luke 23:42

It is impossible for us to distinguish between ourselves and our memories. Even the act of reading this sentence (let alone this paragraph) presupposes a memory of what the first words of the sentence are. We are our memories, and without them we have but a physical resemblance to that person we each suppose ourselves to be. Memories function canonically, telling us authoritatively who we are, giving us resources for who we will become. It should be obvious, then, that the apparent dissolution of the mnemonic capacities experienced by Alzheimer's disease patients raises most serious and profound questions about human existence.

But we are not simply what we remember. We are also what others remember of us, especially what God remembers. The Old Testament witness clearly identifies human existence with being remembered. In his *Memory and Tradition in Israel,* Brevard Childs observes that idiomatically "not to be remembered" is "not to exist."[1] God's very presence, grace, and mercy are expressed through the divine memory. The blinded Samson's strength is reborn when God answers his prayer to be remembered (Judg. 17:28), and Rachel is able to conceive because "God remembered Rachel" (Gen. 30:22). By contrast, in Psalm 88, the person whom God has forgotten, has no strength, is already in the grave, already in "the regions dark and deep." Although God's remembering of a person is crucial, the role of human memory is also underscored, especially in the case of the unrighteous. In Job 24:20, the names of the wicked are forgotten in the towns, and so "wickedness is broken like a tree."

The task of this chapter is to arrive at a theological appreciation of memory, an appreciation that is faithful to the Christian tradition and takes account of the modern world's contributions and contexts. This description of memory helps delineate the most important ways in

1. Brevard Childs, *Memory and Tradition in Israel* (London: SCM Press, 1962). I will make frequent reference to this important study.

which memory shapes who we are, how we should live our lives, and even whose we are. My concern will be, above all, to examine the witnesses of the two Testaments and the Christian tradition concerning the role of memory in the lives of persons and the church. How have prophets, psalmists, apostles, theologians, and others understood memory? Is it a purely cognitive element of human life? What does it mean when a narrative begins, "He forgot the Lord God and . . ."? How can it be said, in the case of an Alzheimer's patient, that family and friends (and ultimately God) remember *for* someone? As we shall see, there are important affinities between human memory and the church's canonical witnesses. Each is constitutive for self-understanding; each serves as a *kanon,* a "rule" or "measuring rod" for life. What will emerge from this examination of our heritage is a clear sense that the problem of Alzheimer's, the problem of memory loss, is no stranger to the Biblical and Christian traditions.

Because everything pertaining to human existence passes through the memory, this chapter risks employing "memory" equivocally. Just as horses yoked together to a chariot always run side by side, a consideration of memory brings along with it the topics of imagination (which draws on memories for all its work) and historical criticism and narrative (which, like memory, appreciate the fundamentally temporal nature of human existence). And as a perusal of Plato, Aquinas, Freud, and countless others would demonstrate, terms such as memory, habit, imagination, reason, consciousness, and repression are employed in quite different senses in different epistemologies. One person's "memory" may be another's "habit" or "imagination." Hence, we will need to distinguish carefully between memory itself and each of these topics.

The first sections of this chapter examine Christian beliefs concerning God's memory, human memory, and the relationship between faith and memory. Building on Brevard Child's analysis of the Hebrew root for memory, *zkr,* we unfold the many rich meanings and uses of memory in the lives of Israel, individual persons, and the church. The next section examines the phenomena of forgetting both as a perennial problem and as a condition peculiarly affecting the modern world. The final section discusses the impact of the twentieth-century revolution concerning the study of memory and highlights the Bergsonian concept of *durée* as an important element for this study. This chapter concludes with a theological appreciation of memory. In particular, it contrasts imagination with memory and draws together the many links between canonicity and memory evoked by previous sections.

God's Memory, the Foundation of Our Hope

God remembers. Despite humanity's regrettable habit of forgetting God, and despite the dissolution of human memories, the encouraging witness of both Testaments is that God does remember. When confronted by the phenomena of Alzheimer's (or when we remember all those millions who died suffering), it is ultimately God's memory, not ours, which must be, in the language of 1 Peter 3:15, the reason for the hope that is within us. Truly, our cry is the cry of the thief in Luke 23:42, "Jesus, remember me when you come into your kingdom."

Although speaking of God's "memory" may seem to be an anthropomorphism, the prophets, apostles, psalmists, and even Jesus himself all invoke God's memory, for to speak of this is to speak of God's fidelity. In this sense, it is a "parabolic" expression of the workings of the divine mind, rendered in such a fashion as to make such a mystery comprehensible.[2] Augustine in his *On the Trinity* located in memory, understanding, and will a Trinitarian image of God in humanity. Memory, he argued, was particularly to be associated with the Father, and memory and omniscience become inseparable. Moreover, we cannot forget that when the Logos became man, he possessed human knowledge, and hence human memory. When we speak of God's memory, we may be speaking of one of several aspects of God's faithfulness, creative knowledge, and redemptive work.

The first four chapters of Deuteronomy encapsulate many of the themes suggesting that God's memory is the key to our memory. The great emphasis on memory and remembering has led commentators to observe that Deuteronomy offers a "theology of remembering."[3] After the great work of liberation wrought by God in the Exodus, itself a manifestation of God's faithful memory, it is Israel's duty to remember these deeds and to employ this communal memory as a spur to the fulfillment of the law. Hence, it is not with Job or Lamentations that a study of the theological dimensions of Alzheimer's begins. Rather, it commences with Deuteronomy — with the earliest cultic formation of Israel. For the community, its worship and God's own memory all precede and shape the experience of individual suffering, not vice versa.

These chapters comprise the beginning of Moses' final address to the people he has led out of Egypt and through the wilderness for four decades. He first recapitulates the history of the tribes' wanderings, a history of God's faithful memory and Israel's recurrent rebellion, and then enjoins the people of Israel to be faithful to God and God's work and law. What is suggested by Moses' address in Deuteronomy 4:1-10 is that that which is to be learned is prior to the community and the communal narrative itself. In other words, divine pedagogy precedes human epistemology. We do not discover God in order to remember; rather, we remember what has been done in order that we may discover God.

Moses — and as far as Israel and the early church were concerned the author is Moses — well aware of the frag-

2. On the figurative, parabolic sense of Scripture, see Aquinas, *Summa Theologiae,* §1.1.10.

3. Childs, *Memory and Tradition,* 77-79.

ile nature of human memory, prophesies that the people of Israel, despite all they have received, will continue to grow forgetful of God's works. The particular form of forgetfulness which Moses identifies is idolatry, choosing to worship creatures such as fishes, stars, beasts, and even humans. "Take heed to yourselves, lest you forget the covenant of the LORD your God, which he made with you, and make a graven image in the form of anything which the LORD has forbidden you" (Deut. 4:23). Idolatry, in its ancient or modern guises, is a form of forgetfulness to which every generation seems to be susceptible.

Deuteronomy 4:30-31 serves as a coda to Moses' prophecies, a coda which transforms a warning of human wretchedness and misery into a proclamation of God's greatness:

> When you are in tribulation, and all these things come upon you in the latter days, you will return to the LORD your God and obey his voice, for the LORD your God is a merciful God; he will not fail you or destroy you or forget the covenant with your fathers which he swore to them.

God's mercies and God's memory are inseparable. The theme of the covenant which Moses stresses underscores the importance of the prevenience of God's memory. It serves as the basis for many invocations of God in many diverse situations in the history of Israel, and prophets or psalmists frequently invoke the covenant in the context of a confession of infidelity and forgetfulness.[4] As with the phenomena of Alzheimer's disease, because of its forgetfulness, Israel seems constantly to be in danger of complete dissolution, and only God's memory prevents total destruction.

God's remembering is not a purely mental operation; it also implies providential, salvific activity. In the Old Testament, the use of the root word for memory, *zkr*, with God as the subject, frequently employed the directional preposition *le*. Lexicographically, when God remembers, God brings something into the divine mind simultaneously with an implied divine motion towards the object. For God, remembering is thus never the same as acting, but at the same time it is never separated from action either.[5] To confess that God remembers is to affirm that God is faithful to the covenant he established with Abraham. To confess God's fidelity is to confess his sustaining love.

In the context of Alzheimer's, families, especially those families who have entrusted one of their own to anonymous professionals, frequently beseech God to remember those who no longer seem capable of remembering. The proclamation of God's memory of those in distress occurs several times in the Old Testament (cf. the barren Rachel in Gen. 30:22 or the blind Samson in Judg. 16:28). As Jeremiah 15:15 underscores, not only is God's memory invoked, but also his divine presence: "O LORD, thou knowest; remember me and visit me." As anyone in a nursing home will tell us, not only is it important to be remembered, it is also crucial to be visited.

But God's memory, especially God's faithful visitation with the suffering, as witnessed in the Old Testament, assumes a rather different meaning in light of the New Testament, in light of Christ and Christ's suffering. God's memory of the covenant was frequently seen as vicarious. God extends mercy to the faithless for the sake of the patriarchs (cf. Exod. 32:11-14 and Lev. 26:45). Now we recognize that God remembers not only Abraham but also himself. Luke explicitly links the Incarnation to God's memory of the covenant. Mary declares, "He has helped his servant Israel, in remembrance of his mercy," and Zechariah, "filled with the Holy Spirit," proclaims that God will "remember his holy covenant" (Luke 1:54 and 72). In some sense, the Incarnation, death, and resurrection can be seen as God's great act of memory. Because of Christ, the new covenant, God forgives, and forgiveness is phrased as the forgetting of sins. Hebrews 8:12, reinterpreting — re-remembering or re-canonizing — Jeremiah 31:34 in light of the Gospel, presents God's declaration: "For I will be merciful toward their iniquities, and I will remember their sins no more." God's forgetting is a sign of love and power, our forgetfulness is a reminder of our solipsism and weakness.

In Isaiah 44:21, divine and human memory become interwoven, but in the union of the two natures, God's divine memory and Jesus' human memory become one. Human nature, made in the image of God, partakes of the depths of divine memory (omniscience), and the divine memory assumes into itself the weakness of the human. More specifically, God divinizes human memory. Jesus' cry, "My God, my God, why have you forsaken me?" is the lament of a man who possesses the fullness of divine memory — yet who himself simultaneously experiences being forgotten. His soul at once encompasses all of history and more, yet he himself is cast outside of it completely. This seems to be a horrible mental counterpart to the physical pains of the nails and thorns. When God remembers us, then, he also remembers being forgotten himself, a terrifying abandonment for which we sinners all share responsibility. We may wonder, perhaps, if his own experience on the Cross facilitates his remembering of Alzheimer's patients in nursing homes.

Human Memory, Faith, and Apostolicity in Israel and the Church

"This is my body, which is given for you. Do this in remembrance of me" (Luke 22:19). The central act of the Christian community is an act of remembering God's saving work. The acceptance of the canon, Christ's Supper, and his Lordship by a person is the acceptance of an authoritative shared memory and the basis of the

4. See, for example, Exod. 32:13, Lev. 26:45, Jer. 14:21, and Ezek. 16:60.

5. See Childs, *Memory and Tradition*, 31-33.

church's apostolic communion.[6] As we shall see in this section's exploration of the many roles of memory in Israel and the church, this shared memory stands at the heart of Christian faith and is the basis of our relationship with God. Consequently, memory plays a crucial role in the dynamics of morality, sin, and forgiveness.

To remember God seems at times synonymous with belief; that a person remembers God and behaves accordingly resembles an experience of faith. It would seem contradictory to say that an agnostic or atheist can remember God — for such a memory implies a commitment to the reality of that which is remembered. And Christians often call this commitment faith. Remembering the divine is not a neutral, dispassionate epistemological process — indeed, we should expect nothing less when we use phrases such as "Do this in remembrance of me." Whether faith is understood primarily as a series of truth-claims, a fundamental disposition in a person, or a sense of trust, whether it is viewed in terms of Barth's "truth as self-involving" or seen in scholastic terms of faith formed by love, Christian faith and memory combine both cognitive and affective elements. Remembering theologically not only entails recalling certain facts or propositions about God and humanity but also presumes a soteriological, ethical, and existential disposition in the rememberer.

Lexicographically, *zkr,* memory, and faith became related during the unfolding of Israel's history. As Brevard Childs has demonstrated, the identification of the Hebrew root for memory with not only cognitive processes but also existential claims was the result of three distinct historical crises in the cultic life of Israel.[7] The "theology of memory" produced by the Deuteronomist was in response to the need to make the Exodus experience a reality for those generations who had not been in Israel. Responding to another gulf between the experiences of the exiles and the professed history of the covenant and Exodus, Deutero-Isaiah uses the Israelite's remembering of God as a bridge spanning present experience and the history of God's salvific activity. Similarly, Ezekiel's use of memory provides a way for those of subsequent generations to identify themselves directly with the covenant.

In each case, Israel's remembering of God and God's work provides existential "memories" for those who could neither have experienced the events nor even seen the land which had been promised. Childs employs the term "actualization" to describe this process for the Israelites. The rememberer "entered the same redemptive reality of the Exodus generation." The event transmitted to another's memory becomes as real as the original experience.[8] Thus, at Passover, Jews eat bitter herbs to remind themselves, to actualize for themselves, what Jews have experienced before. Memory is thus efficacious. Childs stresses that this use of *zkr* exhibits a distinct appreciation for the dynamic, existential qualities of salvation history and human memory. For the Israelites in the exile, memory was not mythical but historical. Memories did not re-create or manifest a mythical understanding of origins; rather, they linked the rememberers to God as God works in history.

For several reasons, the historical contexts for the New Testament understanding of memory and its relationship to faith are in important respects quite different from those of Israel. First, the Gospel narratives' concerns for the past are overwhelmed by the present reality of God in the person of Jesus Christ. Hence the Gospels speak little *per se* of memory (though the Lukan Magnificat and Benedictus, Luke 1:46-55 and 67-79, link the conceiving of Jesus and the birth of John to God's remembering of the covenant). Prophecies may be remembered, but they are remembered insofar as they point to the present manifestation of God. There is no doubt that the Pharisees remember the Exodus; the issue is whether they believe that the man before them is the Messiah. Nevertheless, Christ's words of institution for the Eucharist remind us in the central act of the church of the importance of remembering him.

Second, whereas the Hebrew term for memory was undifferentiated from responsibilities, affections, and ultimately action, the Greek understanding of memory by the time of Christ had experienced the rigorous epistemological analyses of Plato and Aristotle.[9] In the hand of philosophers, terms for mental processes became distinguished and separated. Whereas many Homeric Greek mnemonic terms semantically resemble the Hebrew *zkr,* Greek terms after Plato and Aristotle exhibit differentiated memories such that remembering can be understood as a purely epistemological, completely neutral action in the mind. These memories do not entail any particular responsibilities, duties, attitudes, or personal struggles. Aristotle's *On Memory and Reminiscence* appears to be a treatise on data processing.

Third, and reinforcing this distinction between cognitive recalling and acts of the entire person, the New Testament emphasis on belief and conversion suggests that the process of "entering sacred reality" cannot be expressed adequately by memory. Rather, the self-conscious will becomes more important. Whereas Israelites are born into a genetic community with specific historical memories which define its existence, gentiles may choose to join a community which professes certain truths. Thus, confessions and creeds begin with "I believe" not "I remember."

Finally, the understanding of the Holy Spirit's role as Paraclete also changed the theological understanding of

6. For a good discussion of the church's communion described through the shared liturgical memory of Christ, see David S. Yeago, "Memory and Communion: Ecumenical Theology and the Search for a Generous Orthodoxy," in Ephraim Radner and George R. Sumner, eds., *Reclaiming Faith: Essays on Orthodoxy in the Episcopal Church and the Baltimore Declaration* (Grand Rapids: Eerdmans, 1993), 247-71.

7. This is one of the central theses of Childs, *Memory and Tradition.*

8. Ibid., 85-89.

9. Ibid., 25-27.

memory. The Spirit remains present in each generation, even though the narrative of Jesus is received through the memories and witnesses of others. As Paraclete, the Spirit comforts directly; Christians have more than memories of the covenant in times of duress. Consequently, instead of enjoining Timothy to remember the truths of Christ, pseudo-Paul states, "Guard the truth that has been entrusted to you by the Holy Spirit who dwells within us" (2 Tim. 1:14). Nevertheless, despite these historical changes in the manifest reality of God, important links between memory and faith remain; Hebrews 11:22 makes it explicit — by faith Joseph remembered the Exodus. And through our faith, we remember Joseph and the author of this epistle.

It should not be surprising that memory becomes more important in the pastoral epistles, letters written for readers several generations after the Resurrection. First, as with Deuteronomy, the author must bring those who have heard into the realm of those who were present. The same problem of "actualization" remains. Second, both Deuteronomy and the Pastorals seem to expect that sin will cause people to forget who God is and what God has done (cf. 2 Tim. 3:1ff). But because false Christs were being preached at this time, the issue became not only *whether* Christ is remembered but *how* Christ is remembered. Consequently, in these epistles which testify to the development of the church, authoritative teaching assumes a position of paramount importance (cf. 1 Tim. 4:13 and 2 Tim. 4:2). Timothy is not only to remember Christ but to remember Christ "as preached in my [Paul's] gospel" (2 Tim. 2:8). Memory is inseparable from the crucial ideas of apostolicity and canonicity.

The great emphasis on apostolicity in the writings of the Fathers emerges from this context of preserving the accurate, faithful memory of who Jesus was and why he became man. As much as we might like to, we should not choose to remember any Jesus we please. Nineteenth- and twentieth-century liberal, often Marcionite, attempts to separate Jesus from his Jewishness are, to put it most charitably, a failure of memory. Significantly, it was in part through the challenge of Marcion that the early church had to establish formally what constituted the canon of Scripture. Both in the life of a person and the life of a church, challenges to faithful memory produce a need for canonicity, a need for authoritative self-description.

Finally, the Christian experience of conversion and the willful assumption of the church's memories into one's own memories — the process of growing strong in faith — may also entail a very important transformation of memories. The Resurrection, for example, changed the memories of the disciples (John 2:22 and 12:16). The fresh insights brought by Augustine's new faith as he presented them in his *Confessions* provide a clear example of how conversion completely alters old memories. He is able to recall his former life in the context of his new realization of God's work in his own life. The "once . . . but now" of the hymn *Amazing Grace* similarly expresses this important transformation of memory by faith. We look back on our lives with the fresh knowledge of God's love and work for us — our experiences are transformed and we are filled with hope for the future. For the convert as for the Israelite, faith actualizes and transubstantiates human memories. A conversion experience resembles receiving a diagnosis of Alzheimer's disease because this medical revelation compels us to re-remember the previous months of strange behavior and forgetfulness. Unfortunately, this re-remembering entails a new sense of dread, not a sense of hope.

The link between faith and memory underscores the importance of the narrative context in which we remember.[10] The discussion of Psalm 25:6-7 in the first section highlighted the importance of how God remembers. God remembers according to his "steadfast love." Similarly, human memory does not occur in a vacuum. Rather, memories interact dialectically with our own sense of who we are and how we are to live. This sense expresses itself as our life's story or narrative, and in consciously or unconsciously remembering, we bring the past into the present moments of this ongoing narrative. Similarly, past memories assert themselves by shaping this narrative in ways which we may not perceive. Accurately or not, we see ourselves as a certain type of character or characters (say, a certain type of spouse, parent, or professional), and we remember our pasts accordingly, sometimes with regret, sometimes with satisfaction. The questions become, then, What are the canonical events, principles, and habits for our remembering? Do we remember as Christians according to faith, hope, and love? With pride, despair, or anger in our hearts? Have our lives been sufficiently shaped by the church's traditions that our remembering may be guided by service to Christ's lordship?

Because of this strong identity between faith and memory, memory becomes interwoven with all aspects of our relationship with God. One of the central elements of this relationship is praise; as my father's *The Church Confident* reminds us, the act of praise ought to be the defining characteristic of the church and its worship.[11] As many passages suggest, to remember the covenant with Abraham or the liberation of Israel — to remember God's work — is also to be compelled to praise. The link between memory and praise is, in part, a feature of Hebrew. Especially in some later passages of the Old Testament, the hiphil of *zkr* can also be translated as "extol,"

10. The link between memory and our personal narratives is important in John Kotre, *White Gloves: How We Create Ourselves Through Memory* (New York: The Free Press, 1995), and Theodore Plantinga, *How Memory Shapes Narratives: A Philosophical Essay on Redeeming the Past* (Lewiston, NY: The Edwin Mellen Press, 1992). As their subtitles might suggest, Alzheimer's disease renders their notions of memory's creative and redemptive powers ultimately suspect.

11. See Leander E. Keck, *The Church Confident* (Nashville: Abingdon Press, 1993), chapter 1.

"proclaim," "praise," or "confess."[12] Psalm 105, a great psalm of praise and memory, links praise of God with the recalling of God's works. Similarly, the rememberings in 2 Timothy 1–2 evoke praise from the author. Theologically speaking, memory is doxological, and the culture of the church is a culture of praise.

At the same time, memories can also be painful, and perhaps the most disturbing memories are the memories of sin. Ezekiel prophesies Israel's future remembering of her sins — this remembering, quite naturally, will produce lamentations and shame (Ezek. 16:61; 20:43; 36:31).[13] Yet in some elements of the tradition, there is also a clear sense that painful memories, purgation, and reconciliation are linked. In Ezekiel, the future remembering of sins appears to be part of the process of the recovery of Israel, a recovery possible only because God does not forget (16:59-63). In the medieval drama *Everyman,* the eponymous hero's recollection of the scourging of Christ is "penance strong that [he] must endure."[14] In his *Lament for a Son,* Nicholas Wolterstorff intimates that we need an afterlife to confess our sins to our loved ones, to purge our memories of all of the shortcomings, failures, and iniquities which we know all too well.[15] His son's unexpected death, as with the loss of cognitive presence in Alzheimer's, deprived him of the chance to apologize, to rectify, and to forgive and be forgiven. As we shall see in chapter 6, the burdens of sin in the memory lead us to consider the importance of eschatology.

A comparison with Greek traditions underscores the strangeness of the Jewish and Christian understandings of human memories, especially painful ones. Mnemosthene, Memory, was mother of the Muses because Memory is the source of the arts. But, according to Hesiod, the nature of these daughters "is forgetfulness of evil and rest from cares. . . . The gifts of these goddesses instantly divert the mind."[16] In Aristophanes' account of Eros in Plato's *Symposium,* sexual pleasure becomes a vehicle for forgetting the wretched state of a deeply wounded humanity. And in the underworld, the departed soul is to receive the gift of a sip of the waters of Lethe, of forgetfulness. In the *Odyssey,* the souls of the dead must drink blood for vitality and memory. Ultimately, in the Greek world — at bottom a world circumscribed by tragedy — human memories are to be forgotten.

By contrast, Zophar, one of Job's interlocutors, seeks to comfort the afflicted man by telling him that one day he will forget his miseries (11:16). Job soundly rejects this idea, for to do so would be to deny both himself and God. Liturgically, we express the importance of grievous memories when we confess, "The burden of our sins is intolerable." Christians are to remember even their sins. As patristic scholars have shown, Job's notion of his own personhood would have been impossible for the ancient Greeks. Indeed, for the Greeks, "person" could mean but a mask, a mask devoid of distinct, ontological content.[17] The unique human person as a being with a special set of historical memories, however painful or joyous, was not an idea available to most Greeks, whose doctrines of reincarnation or of Lethean forgetfulness precluded such personhood.

Dante's Christianization of Lethe suggests the special dimensions of the Christian constructions of memory. In canto XXXI of the *Purgatorio,* the poet's own cleansing in this river is a purging only of his self-confessed, woeful memories which impede his progress into heaven. After he emerges from the water he partakes symbolically of the Eucharist. He drinks a blood which is quite different from the blood which the shade of Achilles drank in the *Odyssey.* Through Christ, the poet retains his memories, his personhood, and is prepared for beholding the divine. Not all experiences of sorrow can so smoothly lead, as they do in Psalm 77, to memories of God and God's work and the concomitant evocation of praise and joy. But in the Christian world, the sufferer can hear God say, "But remember, I made all this, and raised my Son from the dead, so. . . ."[18]

It is precisely this dimension of grace, this dimension of God's activity, and our ability to cooperate with it, which marks the peculiar dimensions of memory in the Jewish and Christian worldviews. Because God created humans in his own image, for example, it is possible for Augustine to argue that by remembering with the aid of the Spirit, the *imago Dei* in humans becomes more like the divine.[19] By contrast, for Polybius, ultimately, human memories of the past are embedded in a rather bleak present. He states that he feels compelled to write history because "the only method of learning how to beat with dignity the vicissitudes of Fortune is to be reminded of the disasters of others."[20]

As Polybius suggests, memory is crucial not only for our emotional and spiritual experiences but also for our behavior. At the most basic level, ethical reflection and moral growth seem impossible without memory, for without knowledge of past events there is no ability to learn for the future. Thus, Polybius declares that "certainly mankind possesses no better guide to conduct

12. Article on *"zakhar"* by H. Eising in G. Johannes Botterweck and Helmer Ringgren, eds., *Theological Dictionary of the Old Testament,* 7 vols. (Grand Rapids: Eerdmans, 1973-1974), 4:74. The list provided here includes Exod. 20:24; Isa. 26:13; 48:1; and Ps. 45:18 (17). See also Childs, *Memory and Tradition,* 14.

13. See Childs, *Memory and Tradition,* 59-60.

14. A. C. Cawley, ed., *Everyman and Medieval Miracle Plays* (New York: Dutton, 1958), 223.

15. Nicholas Wolterstorff, *Lament for a Son* (Grand Rapids: Eerdmans, 1987), 65.

16. Hesiod, *Theogony,* trans. Norman O. Brown (New York: The Liberal Arts Press, 1953), section 1, 54-56.

17. See, for example, J. D. Zizioulas, *Being as Communion: Studies in Personhood and the Church* (Crestwood, NY: St. Vladimir's Seminary Press, 1985), chapter 1.

18. Wolterstorff, *Lament for a Son,* 102.

19. Augustine, *On the Trinity,* §14.12.15.

20. Polybius, *The Rise of the Roman Empire,* trans. Ian Scott-Kilvert (New York: Penguin Books, 1982), Introduction, 41.

than the knowledge of the past."[21] But whereas the Greek historians provided useful lessons and character studies, Moses also revealed binding commandments. And Moses sought to strengthen Israel's ability to fulfill the law by strengthening its memory of God. In Deuteronomy, the instruction in the law is inseparable from the Israelites' memory of the Exodus. Without the latter, the former is ineffectual and meaningless.[22]

Further, the actualizing of other peoples' suffering is to strengthen the person in her faithfulness to the community: "You shall remember that you were a slave in Egypt; and you shall be careful to observe these statutes" (Deut. 16:12), here concerning the proper treatment of slaves. The Israelite is not to imagine what it would be like to be a slave, nor is he or she to recall that previous generations were enslaved in Egypt. Rather, there is a clear existential link in the memory of subsequent generations. Through the covenant, memories are handed down, like the land, from generation to generation. To remember God is a commandment, but likewise so is remembering human beings. "Remember those who are prison" (Heb. 13:3) and "remember the poor" (Gal. 2:10). The implication is clear, and the history of this century underscores it all too well — it is all too convenient for humans, especially those removed from normal society (as in a nursing home), to be forgotten. Quite appropriately, John Patton's *Pastoral Care in Context: An Introduction to Pastoral Care* places a great emphasis on memory, and remembering in pastoral care.

Memory strengthens us not only through reminding us of our duties. An important theme in some Stoic writings is the deep joy which we experience when we recall our own virtuous deeds. Conversely, Christ says in *The Imitation of Christ,* "Remember your sins with deep sorrow and displeasure."[23] By regret, we become better prepared to avoid sin. By recalling both pleasures and pains, then, we strengthen our capacity to live a life pleasing to God. To say that a person has a clean conscience is to say that the person's memories do not contain the knowledge of her own willful evil. The Thomistic conception of cooperating with grace and the infusion of virtuous habits reminds us that habit, like memory, makes past deeds active in the present ethical contexts. For good and for ill, we develop mnemonic habits which shape our conduct.

Forgetting, Sin, and Modernity

Despite the importance of memories for all aspects of our existence, human beings seem to be the most forgetful of creatures. Things "slip our mind" frequently, and we are often looking for car keys. As anyone who has attempted to present an autobiography will recognize, even the memories of many central events in our lives seem uncertain. Rousseau's *Confessions* contain many apologies for his weak memory. Given the sheer amount of sensory impressions we receive at any moment and the data we gather through reading, watching, or listening, it is not surprising that we are unable to recall everything. According to Henri Bergson, we should be glad that one of the functions of the brain is to sort and discard unnecessary data.

More importantly, perhaps, human memory is not only inherently forgetful, it is also fallible.[24] Contemporary studies in the legal profession have demonstrated that memories of witnesses are highly susceptible to alteration and emendation. Interrogators may be able to change a witness' memories by introducing false data concerning a crime scene unobtrusively in early questions and eliciting these bits of information from the witness in subsequent questions: "So, you were standing near the blue Ford when . . . What was the color of the Ford?" The car may have been white, but the witness may now remember it as blue. Moreover, memories can be altered by emotions and personal biases. John Dean's famous detailed Watergate testimony about conversations he had was substantially correct, but later comparisons with the actual tape recordings of the talks reveal that he magnified his own role in his memories. We remember in specific situations, and our egos, emotions, prejudices, and personal narratives greatly affect a supposedly neutral memory of events.

Neurologists describe these problems in terms of the physiological complexity of memory. Impressions from the different senses are stored in different parts of the brain, while the brain's limbic system has the responsibility of integrating such data into a whole. Age is important, too; children's brains are immature and do not retain memories well, and some brain deterioration is normal in old age. Scientists speak of the brain's encoding new data over old bits, and so it becomes possible to imagine how a seemingly simple memory can be altered, lost, or made meaningless as it loses connectedness to the rest of a person. (Many readers' own experiences with fickle computer files and hard drives may illustrate this problem of memory, too.)

More dramatically, the recent cases of "repressed memories" and the alleged recovery of memories of crimes (such as the one involving Cardinal Bernardin of Chicago) complicate our understanding of memory. They plant seeds of uncertainty about our own past. Are memories supposedly recovered through hypnosis and/or the use of the hypnotic drug sodium amytal genuinely

21. Ibid.

22. See Childs, *Memory and Tradition,* 50-52.

23. Thomas à Kempis, *The Imitation of Christ,* §3.4. Quoted from the translation by Leo Sherly-Price (New York: Penguin Books, 1984).

24. The information in this paragraph comes from the good introduction to the problem of forgetting to be found in Alan Baddeley's "The Psychology of Remembering and Forgetting" in Thomas Butler, ed., *Memory: History, Culture, and the Mind* (Oxford: Basil Blackwell, 1989).

a part of who we are? Or are they false memories implanted by quack therapists in violation of a person (or of a whole family, since many of the legal cases involve incest or rape)? Apparently, it is disturbingly easy to plant a false memory which will appear so real as to be indistinguishable from the subject's true memories. The literature on this topic has become enormous; within the last several years many major publishers have come out with major books on the subject. Given the importance of memory in general, and given the legal, professional, and personal issues at stake, we should not be surprised that those who argue both for and against the authenticity of these "memories" become quite passionate.

With Alzheimer's patients who still retain lucidity, memory seems fickle indeed. Sometimes your wife recognizes you, sometimes she does not. Sometimes a caregiver may feel like Socrates the midwife. By asking the right questions diligently, the caregiver helps the patient give birth to the knowledge she already has. The patient crying out to her father may come to remember that he died many years ago. But at the same time, caregivers themselves risk dangers similar to those of therapists recovering repressed memories. When you repeatedly rephrase a question in order to get a patient to answer, are you inadvertently eliciting a true or a false memory? Will the patient suddenly expect her father to enter the room as he did yesterday?

Therapists in the repressed memory debate have been following Freud's lead in believing that traumatic experiences early in life would be repressed only to produce neuroses or hysteria later as the repressed events continued to assert themselves unconsciously. According to Freudian theories of repression, the memory is still there buried somewhere in the unconscious. With Alzheimer's disease, by contrast, damage to the brain may suggest that the memories no longer exist. Human memories may be like computer files — once you destroy the computer's "memory" the data simply no longer exist. (When we consider the soul in chapter 4 [of *Forgetting Whose We Are*], we will return to the material or metaphysical basis for human memories.) Regardless of how court cases and psychoanalytical procedures resolve the legitimacy of these practices, the issues raised do highlight the potentially fragile nature of memory. We do forget, repress, or deny parts of our past experiences.

A theological appreciation of memory requires that we consider the forgetfulness and fallibility of memory as it pertains to our religious existence, and such a consideration is most concerned with the relationship between sin and memory. Although academics of all disciplines are holding conferences on memory, rarely do such investigations touch on this crucial relationship. Neurology, in particular, does not seem well suited to investigating how character and memory intersect, since such a linkage presupposes something neurology does not address adequately: the quality and existential significance of our memories. Any attempt to construct a psychology of remembering and forgetting without reference to the effects of "man's first disobedience" (in Milton's phrase) will inevitably fail to do justice to the human condition *coram Deo*.

According to diverse Biblical witnesses, sin is both a cause and effect of forgetting. Despite the Deuteronomist's warning to the Israelites to take heed lest they forget the Lord and sin (Deut. 8:11), the Israelites were quite proficient at not remembering. Israel's idolatry and ingratitude towards the late Gideon's family is interwoven with the fact that "the people of Israel did not remember the LORD their God" (Judg. 8:34). Similar tapestries of forgetfulness and sin are found throughout the prophets (e.g. Neh. 9:17). Likewise, the testimonies of our own forgetfulness are legion. The adulterer forgets the spouse, the rich forget the poor, the friend forgets the friend. We forget the simplest acts of writing thank you and birthday cards. Perhaps we are too busy to remember. Remembering, after all, takes time, and if we follow the rich connotations of the Hebrew *zkr,* remembering also entails distinct responsibilities.

But the psychology of sin and memory is more complicated, as Augustine's penetrating *Confessions* reveals. He describes the way he initially coped with his sins: "I had noticed my iniquity, but I had dissembled it, and contained it, and forgotten it."[25] Our capacity to forget God is exceeded, perhaps, only by our ability to manipulate our own memories so that we can discard our sins mentally. Only God's ability to justify us exceeds our ability to legitimate ourselves. Thus, as we have seen, the *Imitation of Christ,* like Augustine's *Confessions* a perceptive study of spiritual psychology, recommends that we be certain to remember the weakness of our sinful nature, for unless we recall this unfortunate condition we are all too likely to forget the many resolutions we make against sin.[26] Memory *of* sin can be transformed into memory *against* sin. For this reason, it is all the more important that we train ourselves through the church's traditions to strengthen those memories which do contribute to a life of love and virtue, a life pleasing to God.

Because humans seem predisposed to forgetting, Israel and the church have been given a great variety of means for remembering. The Israelites are to wear tassels on the corners of their garments for the sake of remembering the commandments of the Lord (Num. 15:39). As we have already discussed, the pastoral epistles emphasize the importance of regular preaching, and the central act of the church itself, the Eucharist, is an act done in memory. Orthodox liturgies perhaps do a greater service to worshippers as prayers are repeated; such repetition strengthens memory and tempers the soul. The liturgical calendar itself serves as a mnemonic guide for the diversity of religious celebrations and days of remembrance. Our burial practices — tombstones, brass rubbings, sarcophagi, memorial bequests to universities — all express our desire to remember and to be remembered. But the

25. Augustine, *Confessions,* §8.7.

26. Thomas à Kempis, *The Imitation of Christ,* §1.22.

sad reality is that in most cases people are forgotten within a few decades or even years after their death.

That God helps human beings remember (through commanding the Israelites to wear tassels, through sending prophets, or through the institution of the Eucharist) is also one of the central elements of the Biblical witness. Jesus' pedagogical practices — his use of parables, hyperbole, rhetorical questions, etc. — seem designed specifically to promote the remembering of his teachings.[27] In the New Testament, the divine assistance for memory is attributed to, in part, the Holy Spirit. In John 14:25-26, Jesus states, "These things I have spoken to you, while I am still with you. But the Counselor, the Holy Spirit, whom the Father will send in my name, he will teach you all things, and bring to your remembrance all that I have said to you." Throughout the New Testament and Christian tradition, the Paraclete has helped to actualize the past, has aided humans as they seek to remember the divine mercies which have been given in time. Because of the Paraclete, we can have hope for human memory and human faith. We may ask the same rhetorical question asked in the *Imitation of Christ,* "How can I forget You, who have deigned to remember me, even after I was corrupted and lost?"[28]

Emphasizing the divine roles in the process of human memory seems to be needed now more than ever. Although the history of sin from the Old Testament on reveals that humans have been forgetting God for millennia, for many reasons modern Christians seem to have more difficulty in remembering than previous generations. Contemporary Christian understandings of memory do not have the same dense meanings — existential, cognitive, ethical, historical, communal — which were associated with the Hebrew root *zkr.* We would do well to remind ourselves about our modern obstacles to memory and why we need to take great care to appreciate memory theologically. If we are to recover some of the richness of *zkr* — a recovery I believe Alzheimer's provokes us to attempt — then we will need to consider some of the peculiar problems of our age.

In large part, the contemporary problem of memory and faith is the problem of history, or rather, of our time and place in history. Writing his *Democracy in America* over a century and one half ago, Alexis de Tocqueville, at once the herald and critic of the new age of democracy, suggested that democratic peoples would not be as interested in history as previous generations had been. Earlier societies, which he termed aristocratic, were more closely tied to their histories, in part because the aristocratic rulers derived their authority from the past. By contrast, democratic peoples would have their eyes fixed on the present and the future, ever eager to put their pasts behind them, ever desiring to generate new lives and new opportunities for themselves. The past could be a source of knowledge, but rarely of inspiration or authority. Tocqueville was a Frenchman describing America in the 1830s, and for a man who could see the monuments and art produced by centuries of Europeans, America was bound to seem curious and ahistorical. Hannibal, Caesars, Holy Roman Emperors, Napoleon — these men had already crossed the Alps, but what great names had ever crossed the Appalachians or the Rockies at the head of an army to change history?

The peculiar aspects of the American experience led R. W. B. Lewis, in *The American Adam,* to interpret American history, and especially American literature, in terms of the Genesis typology. Each generation of Americans is a new Adam, boundlessly free to make of the American garden what he will, living without a past, capable of choosing afresh between good and evil. This American predisposition has been strengthened by the seductive idea of Progress which we have inherited. Despite the horrors of this most progressive century, our assumptions about progress and the constant improvement of the human condition make us look condescendingly, not devotionally, towards the past. In this regard, Americans are far more Greek (Athenian) than Hebrew. We are democratic, predisposed to shorter historical memories, and ever seeking to be rational and pragmatic. Of the Titans, Americans are Promethean, great makers, and Protean, always capable of change; we are less intimate with another of the Titans, Mnemosyne (memory).

The new American spirit of democracy was, in part, the result of the Enlightenment, an age that combined radically historical and anti-historical elements. Or rather, it placed history in the service of critical reason, detaching the historian from the past as it sought to liberate all humanity from the intellectual and political chains of history, tradition, and authority. This period has weakened the capacity of modern Christians to remember faithfully in four related ways.

Hans Frei's *The Eclipse of the Biblical Narrative* has identified one of the central changes in Christianity in this period which have transformed our ability to *zkr* (if I may refashion a verb). Whereas pre-Enlightenment Christians understood their own worlds through the world of Scripture, theologians and scholars of this era began to locate the meaning of Scripture in terms of their own contemporary worlds. To reformulate the problem in light of this study, whereas to *zkr* could be a logical result of pre-modern exegesis and preaching, there has developed a tendency away from "remembering" the past and making it active in the present. In its place has arisen a habit of locating the present in the past. The Bible is relevant to the extent that it depicts something we already can recognize. Now, human epistemology precedes divine pedagogy.

Along with this transformation strides the most important feature of the Enlightenment for modern Christian memory — the rise, development, and ascendancy of the historical-critical method. This method, despite its apparent historicity, has in fact made the church less his-

27. See Robert H. Stein, *The Method and Message of Jesus' Teaching* (Philadelphia: Westminster Press, 1978), 32.

28. Thomas à Kempis, *The Imitation of Christ,* §3.10.

torical; over the past two to three centuries, church people have grown less and less confident about their own past. That the historical-critical method has made it harder to remember the past can be seen in one of its greatest exponents, Adolph von Harnack. His antidogmatic agenda led him to use history as a tool for distinguishing between the genuine life and teachings of Jesus and ecclesiastical, historical, Christianity. It is hardly surprising that Harnack himself came to espouse Marcionite views about the Old Testament.

The third important Enlightenment legacy for Christian self-understanding which bears directly on the problem of our memories is the emphasis on reason. The quest for an intelligible understanding of the life of the mind, a quest which emphasizes rationality, scientific certainty, and consciousness, enervated the narrative aspects of theology. (This, too, was an important theme for Frei.) But memory and narrative are interwoven, and consequently the memorial elements of theology are enervated as well. Moreover, with the Enlightenment's distrust of received authority and its emphasis on the individual's own rational thinking, the communal aspects of memory — so powerful in Deuteronomy — become diminished as well. In more recent decades in America, the ability to appropriate the story of Israel, the story of a people, has become even weaker in a culture which emphasizes religion as a private matter. (This loss of communal memories is one of the concerns of Robert N. Bellah and other communitarians.)

Finally, human pain and distress, another inextricable part of the Biblical discussions of memory, was not something the Enlightenment could be comfortable with. Memories of human suffering constitute a great threat to the abstract reasonings of philosophers.[29] Enlightenment optimism does not know how to address this since the Enlightenment, informed by the idea of Progress, proceeds from the assumption that suffering is not endemic to the human condition. Presumably, suffering, like superstition, is susceptible to elimination.

Romanticism, another modern strand, one that runs counter to the Enlightenment (while also drawing from its energy), has likewise enervated the modern church's ability to remember. Rousseau's emphasis on feelings and the imagination and Schleiermacher's regrounding religious faith in the experiences and feelings of the believer distanced and separated Christians from their ancestors. The new code words of Romantic discourse — feeling, experience, imagination, spontaneity — are not the code words which easily lend themselves to the memorial apprehension of the past. Rousseau privileges the authenticity of his feelings over the rest of his memories in the *Confessions* — a move which seems akin to privileging general intent over actual deed (we intend the good, whether we act upon that is not so important). Although Romantics frequently turned to the past for their inspiration, histories written under this muse often tell us far more about the author's age than about the historical subjects themselves. The emphasis on the individual, one of the glories of some strains of Romanticism, likewise makes it difficult for modern Christians to appropriate communal memories as their own.

The existential appropriation of the Incarnation which began with Kierkegaard also reduced and circumscribed the God of history (especially when combined with the sophisticated techniques of de-mythologization). God is not remembered from the past, but the report of this God is confronted in this present. In its more extreme forms, it almost seems as if we no longer need the historical events themselves. The existential reading of the New Testament at times has a rather unknowable God who appeared briefly on the field of human history only to recede again. God becomes a blip in time. Love, it would seem to me if I read 1 Corinthians 1:13 correctly, would endure, not disappear. Love would stick around through sorrows and sufferings. If God loves, God permeates history. If we love, we should remember.

None of these modern traditions, Enlightenment, Romantic, existential, can make the same memorial appropriation of the past as can the psalmist of Psalm 105 who can remember *all* of the history of Israel as part of God's providential, merciful redemptive plan. We need to recover our memories — we need to recover the full memories of God's never-failing presence in the world.

Dynamism and Durée: Modern Contributions to Memory

We have as of yet refrained from attempting to define precisely what the cognitive or epistemological functions of memory might be. This is in part because certain intellectual, cultural, and neurological transformations of the modern period have dramatically altered contemporary understandings of memory. Another obstacle to a working definition of memory is that defining memory requires certain commitments to related concepts such as — habit, idea, sensation, feeling, thought, imagination, consciousness, and, in the case of theology, sin. As Jacques Le Goff observes, "The idea of memory is an intersection."[30] Hence, a review of the issues and directions taken by some modern thinkers may help to clarify the difficult task of describing memory. In particular, a theological description of memory will benefit from a concept associated with the work of Henri Bergson: *durée*. As we shall see, his idea of the dynamism of memory and its powerful, often uncontrollable influences on the pres-

29. On this point, see Johann Baptist Metz, "A Short Apology of Narrative," in Stanley Hauerwas and L. Gregory Jones, eds., *Why Narrative? Readings in Narrative Theology* (Grand Rapids: Eerdmans, 1989), 251-62.

30. Jacques Le Goff, *History and Memory*, trans. Steven Kendall and Elizabeth Claman (New York: Columbia University Press, 1992), 51. This text contains a useful review of how problems of memory have become important for modern historians.

ent will provide us with an important way of thinking about memory theologically.

Before turning to the modern world and its uses of cognitive memory, it will be useful to consider some of the major views prior to the nineteenth century. Christian reflections on the epistemological aspects of memory have tended to follow philosophical or medical leads on what memory actually is. Augustine's reflections on memory in Book X of the *Confessions,* for example, follow Platonic traditions. And Aquinas' *Summa Theologiae* draws heavily for its interpretation of memory on Aristotle. What is perhaps most striking in the writings of both philosophers and theologians before the twentieth century is the relative simplicity of memory. Plato and Aristotle speak of memory as a wax tablet, something which merely records sensory impressions. Augustine describes memory as a great cave, and Locke chooses the metaphor of a storehouse.[31] Regardless of the actual image, the functioning of memory appears, by modern standards, straightforward. The dynamics and cognitive processes of memory appear relatively uncomplicated.

Moreover, the memory in the process of receiving stimuli remains passive — it is a tablet onto which impressions are put. Consequently, remembering itself seems relatively simple. We can imagine Plato searching through his tablets, Augustine rummaging around in his cave, or Locke scanning the shelves of his storehouse in order to find the information concerning what each had for breakfast. Today, perhaps, we would use computer metaphors, and we would be inserting various disks into our mind's computer. Both Aristotle and Aquinas, as might be expected, pay some attention to the problem of organic dysfunctions and the concomitant loss of mnemonic function, but for both men these are merely diversions.

By contrast, philosophers, psychologists, artists, and doctors of the last century have viewed memory as highly problematic, confusing, and not nearly so simple as first imagined. Students of memory now readily distinguish between many different types of remembering as well as of several distinct stages in the process. Semantic memory, for example, refers to factual memory (how many nickels are in a quarter), and it is a type of memory often retained by amnesiac patients. By contrast, episodic or autobiographical memory denotes one's own particular experiences and the capacity to reflect upon them. Generally we think of amnesiac patients as having lost this. Others speak of instrumental memory, the process whereby the elderly enhance their sense of self by recalling past successes.[32] Although I sometimes describe Alzheimer's families' experiences in light of these different categories, I have not thought that these distinctions about types of memory are crucial for a theological discussion of Alzheimer's disease. Eventually a patient comes to lose all of his memories and mnemonic capacities. Hence, it is the nature of memory as a whole which needs theological elucidation.

The dramatic shift in modern thinking about memory occurred in large part because of changes in fundamental categories of existence. In *The Culture of Time and Space,* Stephen Kern examined the transformations wrought by various modern trends on our views of time, space, speed, duration, and memory. The key revolutions for memory were changes in perceptions about time itself. So dramatic was the metamorphosis in thinking that it became possible to identify Bergson as "the first philosopher to take time seriously."[33] Quite naturally, a change in human thinking about temporality makes for alterations in human thinking about memory.

Beginning with the end of the last century, innovations and events such as electric clocks, time cards, the cinema, the development of geology, the standardization of world time by the acceptance of Greenwich Mean Time, even the profound spatial and temporal dislocations of trench warfare — all these and more led to a new awareness of the pervasive problematic character of time. Scholars of various disciplines and artists of all sorts responded with a flurry of new views about time, memory, and the nature of human existence. Examining differing religious calendars, for example, Durkheim argued that time itself was a social construction, that it was qualitative rather than quantitative. Jaspers, too, argued against a universal, abstract, mechanical time, believing that time is primarily subjective (he was especially concerned with the case of the mentally ill).

In their own ways, these moderns were drawing on Kant's rejection of ordered, Newtonian, absolute time in his *Critique of Pure Reason.* Given our biological nature — a nature which admits of problematic perceptual dimensions as well as passions, hopes, and fears — time simply cannot be experienced as the Englishman had conceived of it. Consequently, Kant argues that the human memory is active when it receives sensory impressions. It cannot be understood as a simple, regularly-ordered storehouse or any such passive metaphor. Both the time card and the simple wax tablet appear to be gross distortions. Any child who, while waiting for the bell to ring, looks at the school clock repeatedly in the last five minutes of the school day, will confirm the fact that mechanical concepts of minutes and seconds are inadequate descriptions of the human experience of time.

Consequently, the number of different theories of memory and time increased dramatically in the decades before and after the turn of the century. William James,

31. Specific references to the *loci classici* on memory and a good introduction to the problem can be found in the article "Memory" in *The New Catholic Encyclopedia* (New York: McGraw-Hill, 1967).

32. A good introduction to modern ways of thinking about memory can be found in Baddeley's "The Psychology of Remembering and Forgetting," in Butler, ed., *Memory.* On instrumental memory and for another discussion of memory see Kotre's *White Gloves.*

33. This remark by a British philosopher, Samuel Alexander, in 1890, is quoted in Stephen Kern, *The Culture of Time and Space, 1880-1918* (Cambridge: Harvard University Press, 1983), 33.

Freud, Bergson, Joyce, Proust, Kafka, Nietzsche — all of these and many more offered new visions of what memory is and how it relates to human existence. As the now-common phrase "stream of consciousness" suggests, the rather neatly arranged filing space of the ancients gave way to a construal of memory which was fluid, dynamic, and, like a river, potentially raging and chaotic. As one cannot dissect a stream in the way one can separate a set of shelves, so we cannot distinguish neatly between moments in the flow of consciousness. What comes to the fore in modern discourse is not the way we control the remembering of specific events but the way in which our minds often spontaneously and unpredictably are capable of splashing from one memory to the next — from a baseball game to a library to a poem to a love affair to a snowy evening to a pair of boots. A river seems to have flooded the storehouse and scattered the memories all about.

A consequence of this fluvial construction of memory is a concentration on the dynamism of past and present, wherein memories can well up, flood, or pour into consciousness. For Proust, many memories of the protagonists in *Remembrances of Things Past* were spontaneous intrusions into consciousness. The French title of this work is even more suggestive for Alzheimer's patients and their families: *A la recherche du temps perdu* — or "In Search of Times Lost." Freud's idea of repression and the suppression of events too horrible to think about can also be seen in such watery terms; the pressure from the dammed or repressed memories creates a pounding and stress on the conscious. Memories thus are not always easily compartmentalized. Rather, they impinge on the present, assuming a vitality, almost a life of their own.

For Freud and Proust especially, memories were private. But the work of sociologists, especially Maurice Halbwachs, suggests that human memories have important social dimensions. He spoke of the "social framework of memory" and stressed the social aspects of our recollection and transmission of the past. We retain the past not only individually but also communally. Whereas Proust's and Joyce's protagonists often experience their memories in isolation, most of us share our memories at school reunions, with families, or at any number of different gatherings. That we recall and retell our pasts, often with people who shared the same experiences, suggests that we cannot consider memory as a phenomenon of individuals. Following Stanley Fish's use of the term "interpretive communities" to describe the way groups of people share certain assumptions about how to read a text, Peter Burke understands the collective apprehension of the past through "memory communities."[34] This view of memory would not have seemed new to the Deuteronomist.

Precisely because of the social dimension of human memory, our personal remembrances are subject to distortion, political use, and manipulation. Recent vehement debates about a Smithsonian exhibition on the atomic bomb and about the nature of Polish, Jewish, Soviet, and/or gay memorials at Nazi concentration camps illustrate the significant implications of public remembering. Foucault and his followers proceeded from the assumption that items from the past represent the attempts of those in power to legitimate their power and dominate the memories of the future. While this may well be an over-generalization for much of humanity's past, certainly this seems to hold true for much of the former Eastern bloc, wherein the State assumed the formal role of historian, or memory-keeper, of the people. Since the eighties, especially with the increasing popularity of works such as Milan Kundera's *The Book of Laughter and Forgetting,* we in the West have become increasingly aware of the precarious attempts of many ordinary people to have their own memories. It is hardly surprising that some Russians, seeking to create space not only for discourse but also for their persons, founded a journal called *Pamyat',* or *Memory.* Freedom and memory are inseparable. There is a powerful political potential for the manipulation of memories. The first task of a Revolution is to rewrite the past.

There has been, thus, a revolution in memory, but these modern views are sometimes quite different construals of memory from the associations that the root *zkr* exhibits. Indeed, some of these interpretations, one might say obsessions, appear to point in an opposite direction from *zkr.* Joyce, Proust, Nietzsche, and Freud, in particular, emphasize the personal (often self-indulgent), the aesthetic, the free. By contrast the Hebrew uses of *zkr* and the Christian tradition's own understanding of memory have stressed the communal, the historical, and the ethically responsive.

One aspect of this modern discussion, however, holds great promise for a theological appreciation of memory — Bergson's rich descriptions of *durée,* a term simplified in its translation as "duration." In *Matter and Memory, Time and Free Will* and in *Creative Evolution,* his discussions of memory and *durée* become interwoven with a number of other central Bergsonian concepts: intuition and intellect, space/time, the life-force, and creativity.[35] Although we do not need to accept all of Bergson's premises and categories, *durée* does seem to be an accurate description of how God's work both in the past and in the present bears on our lives each moment. Thus, Bergson's ideas of time and memory were highly influential for H. Richard Niebuhr's *The Meaning of Revelation.*[36] In

34. Peter Burke, "History as Social Memory," in Butler, ed., *Memory,* 107. This essay is a very good introduction to modern discussions of the social aspect of memory.

35. For a scathing, if idiosyncratic, evaluation and critique of Bergson's thought, see Bertrand Russell, *A History of Western Philosophy* (New York: Simon and Schuster, 1972), 791-810. Bergson is discussed extensively and compared with other modern thinkers in the first four chapters of Kern, *Culture of Time and Space.*

36. Some passages from Niebuhr's *The Meaning of Revelation* read as if they were straight from Bergson. For a discussion of the particular influence of Bergson's understanding of faith and reli-

this light, I want to underscore some key points which will be important for the rest of this study.

As already noted, the past for Bergson flows into the present and comes to interpenetrate it. He speaks of "osmosis" as a way of describing how the past endures. The "past" as we commonly understand it, he argues, never really ceases to exist. Moreover, the past has power. To say that something has *durée* is to say that it gnaws and impinges on the present, often without our being aware of it. We do not control our memories as much as we interact with them. Often the sight of something associated with a person or event evokes a powerful response from our memories. Sometimes we enjoy such a serendipitous recollection, at other times, as with Peter and the cock's crowing, the memory is simply too painful. Denial may be possible, but not always.

As a consequence of this understanding of *durée,* Bergson argues, the free person is one who is able to act within the totality of her memories. She acts in continuity with who she is, not in discontinuity or randomness. The dancer becomes more free by being able to utilize the total repertoire of movements she has learned throughout her life. For the Christian, freedom must be considered in the context of God's grace. Hence, this linking of freedom and memory suggests that we can understand the freedom of a Christian as being able to live within the total memory of God's work in Israel and the church. To participate in the communion of the saints is to be able to actualize their memories in one's own life. This total memory includes, of course, memories both of faithfulness and failures.

Following Bergson's notion of *durée,* we can see how memories both of sin and of Christ impinge upon our thought processes without our control, the former sometimes driving us to guilt and the latter shaming us as well as giving hope. Our need for forgiveness is so strong precisely because of the powerful *durée* of sin. At the same time, some memories have increased *durée* because of sin. Human weakness, an integral part of our temporal or narrative existence, creates openings for sinful memories or imaginings. In part because of sin, we do not control all of our conscious thought processes, and the imagination and memory conspire to insert unlawful ideas into our heads. I recall (or imagine) the sin, but I do not regret it; indeed, I recall it with some pleasure. Because we do not know how to remember properly — because we do not always interpret these memories or notions in the context of Christ's work — we entertain these thoughts and empower them. We can legitimate ourselves by yielding unfaithfully to *durée.*

At the same time, the grace given through the Holy Spirit enters into our souls through a similar process. It may be that the Spirit helps evoke, in the words of the gospel song, the "Precious memories [which] flood my soul." Why is it that at some times we suddenly find ourselves remembering something Christ said or did? Why is it that Jeremiah discovers that, despite his attempts to forget and deny God, "there is in [his] heart . . . a burning fire" (20:9)? It may be because habit and mnemonic associations assert themselves. It may also be that the Spirit is at work, prodding and eliciting through the memory, strengthening the *durée* of some of our memories.

The need to cooperate with this *durée* — to confess our sins, to discern the Holy Spirit, and to proclaim and obey Christ's lordship — suggests that we need to learn how to remember properly. For this, we need the church and its memories. The conclusion of this chapter now considers how this understanding of *durée* complements a theological appreciation of memory, canonicity and the church.

gious institutions on Niebuhr, see Jaroslav Pelikan, "Bergson Among the Theologians," in Thomas Hanna, ed., *The Bergsonian Heritage* (New York: Columbia University Press, 1962), 54-73. For Bergson's influence on Maritain, see Maritain's *Bergsonian Philosophy and Thomism,* trans. Mabelle L. Andison and J. Gordon Andison (New York: The Philosophical Library, 1955).

A Theological Appreciation of Memory: Memory as Canon

Building upon some basic lexicographical and historical observations concerning the Hebrew root *zkr,* we have sought to appreciate the complexity and centrality of memory for our existence as religious persons. We have tried to describe the facets of memory — to discern its density and consider how normative or canonical it should be for theological reflection.

I began this chapter with Deuteronomy and God's memory of the covenant as the foundation for our theological memories. A modern historical-critical discussion surrounding the covenant illustrates the similarities between memory and canonicity. Old Testament scholars have debated the role of the covenant in Israel's theology and religion because it appears to be the work largely of the Deuteronomic school.[37] This theme, which is so important for seeing the unity of Old and New Testaments, may be a later interpolation into earlier texts. Similarly, just as we re-remember older events in light of newer ones (Oedipus horribly re-remembers his marriage to Jocasta when he learns whose son he is), so too does canonical acceptance lead to re-remembering the past relations between God and Israel. It is possible for later Israelites to re-remember Abraham in light of their own developing ideas of the covenant. Similarly, Christians remembering Abraham are re-remembering the Old in light of the New. Some memories provide the dominant contexts for reinterpreting other memories of the past. These central memories are, in effect, our canonical memories, the ones which give the primary energy to our identities.

37. For a review of this problem, see Brevard Childs, *Biblical Theology of the Old and New Testaments: Theological Reflection on the Christian Bible* (Minneapolis: Fortress Press, 1992), 413-21.

In concluding this chapter it is important to distinguish between memory and imagination; such a distinction further clarifies how we form canonical memories. Memory, in some senses of the word, may seem to be grounded in the imaginative, ordering, synthesizing faculties of the mind.[38] Epistemologically, imagination is inseparable from memory, and in the pre-nineteenth-century understanding of mental processes, the relationship was quite clear. In essence, memory stored sensory data, and the imagination was able to use this data for its own free synthesizing and creations. But as memory became more fluvial and assumed its own powers, the memory became more active, and distinguishing between the active imagination and the passive memory of old no longer made much sense. Given the interwoven character of memory and imagination, it may be that the distinction between memory and imagination is a distinction of connotation more than anything else. Still, the different connotations are crucial to the theological implications of the two terms.

The modern affection for the imagination stems from Rousseau, for he imbued the term with all sorts of delightful qualities. Indeed, in *Emile,* the imagination is what bridges the great gap between human beings, linking us all together in sympathy and compassion. "Imagination" currently means different mental processes to different theologians, and it now encompasses many features of what used to go by reason, contemplation, and memory. Imagination as some employ the term is the vehicle for self-understanding, a capacity for employing paradigms to order the world. It thus allows for an aesthetic unifying of life's experiences. It can serve as the basis for the formation of the Christian character, and it can provide directions for the lived life. As discussed by some theologians, the imaginative faculty shares with *zkr* its appropriative, existential functions. The imagination is seen as "an activity of the psyche as a whole."[39] That is, whereas Deuteronomy might say, "Remember that you were in Egypt," to a generation many decades removed from that experience, we might today say, "Imagine that you, too, were in Egypt."

But a comparison of the two sentences reveals crucial differences. While it may appear that imagination as the appropriation of images and events is the same as *zkr,* to say that "one remembers" suggests that something actually happened and that one submits oneself to the reality of that event and accepts it. To say that "one imagines" leaves so much room for the question of reality. Indeed, for the imagination, the functions of history could be as adequately served by the stage as by the past. The Greek tragedies are not historical, but they do fire the imagination.

Compare likewise these two sentences: Remember that God in Jesus Christ died on the Cross so that human beings might enjoy eternal life. Imagine that God in Jesus Christ died on the Cross so that human beings might enjoy eternal life. The first is open to *durée.* That is, it accepts the fact that this act of remembering inherently will impinge upon the present. It will drive us in certain directions, and we willfully surrender to it. We accept the narrative of the Cross as canonical. The second seems to leave open the question of whether one should accept this reality or not. The imagination, which is derived from the freedom of the creative subject, here remains free. Because Alzheimer's disease exposes this creative subject as vulnerable to dissolution, we learn that what God does for us is crucial. While how we imagine God is important, our salvation lies in remembering, not in imagining. Because memory acknowledges and accepts God's prevenience, it is more open to God's present reality than the imagination. Again, this discussion is describing how "memory" and "imagination" connote fundamentally different attitudes, not what each necessarily is.[40] But these connotations are important because they affect our devotional fervor and the energy we bring to loving God and neighbor.

Faith and memory are linked in ways more profound than faith and imagination. Imaginative efforts may provide genuine depth and content to a person's faith. But memory is linked to history, to a belief that certain events did transpire in very specific ways and for specific purposes. We may follow Loyola's injunctions to imagine the details of the nativity of Christ, but when we do so, we give priority to the limits of what we have in the historical narrative. In viewing different paintings of the nativity, we acknowledge the artist's imagination, but we use the Gospel account to set limits for our ability to accept the artist's imaginative construction. Memory considers itself to be relentlessly accurate, relentlessly faithful to God and to the past, especially the past we share with others. By contrast, the imagination entertains its own creativity. Memory accepts God's activity and God's role in history in ways more dramatic than the imagination. Memory, in a way, accepts the irresistibility of God's grace. By contrast, as Hume observed, "Nothing is more free than the imagination of man."[41]

While our imaginations are socially informed, they remain personal in a way that our memories do not. With good reason we speak more readily of shared memories than of shared imaginings (small utopian communities might be the exception that proves the rule). Hence, while

38. See, for example, Plantinga, *How Memory Shapes Narrative,* 45-47.

39. Stephen Crites, as quoted by Julian Hartt in Hauerwas and Jones, eds., *Why Narrative,* 281. For a discussion of different views of the imagination as they pertain particularly to the problem of narrative, see the essays by both Crites and Hartt in [*Why Narrative*].

40. Harold Bloom's discussion of how the imaginative and creative powers of great writers emerge from a struggle with the impinging literary memory of the canon illustrates both how memory is canonical (here, in a literary sense) and how imagination and memory may interact. See his *The Western Canon: The Books and Schools of the Ages* (New York: Harcourt Brace, and Company, 1994).

41. David Hume, *An Inquiry Concerning Human Understanding,* §5.2.

the term imagination can adumbrate a number of epistemological functions, it remains more individual than communal. Ecclesiologically, we should prefer memory to imagination. Shared authoritative memories provide a canonical description of our shared identities.

Some who advocate theology as a fundamentally imaginative enterprise openly accept the fabricative connotations of imagination, for above all they intend to underscore the tentative and non-reified nature of theology. Such an approach to theology does little good to those families that have to experience the phenomena of Alzheimer's. If only these events were imaginative. Caregivers come to fear the imaginations of the patients — especially those who become paranoid. Similarly, having to acknowledge the fact that your parent now imagines you to be someone else, perhaps even her parent, is a terrible moment. Consequently, caregivers do not want to dwell upon what goes on in the imaginations of victims, for such contemplation produces only sorrow. Moreover, what caregivers need so desperately to see in patients is some sign that memories do remain. Particularly in the most ambiguous phases of the disease, when a patient requires complete care but is still able to communicate, indications of memory are desperately sought after. No one wants to know that they are forgotten.

It is precisely in the area of pastoral care that theology as primarily an imaginative enterprise seems weakest. It is here that memory and being faithful to memory become crucial. Ultimately, the lonely and the sick are to be remembered, not imagined. Even if one grants the imagination to be a "complete act of the psyche" and imbues it with all sorts of rich connotations, it still falls flat. And as *zkr* means to remember with responsibility, so too does remembering the dying prompt us to act, to become faithful caregivers or better friends. Sins and forgetfulness are quite closely linked, and hence cultivating faithful memories becomes necessary.

Perhaps the most important difference between memory and imagination emerges from a consideration of God. We use the phrase "God remembers" as a way of expressing God's omnipotence. How might we use the phrase "God imagines"? Moreover, what would its significance be? God might imagine a way of life pleasing to the divine or might imagine the kingdom of God, but it remains unclear how that might relate to human existence. Some proponents of imagination, such as Gordon Kaufman, have no problem with this issue since for them God is active in human affairs only to the extent that an imaginative construct of human minds can affect human behavior.

Imagination maximizes human freedom, but theology seeks, above all, to maximize human fidelity. And for that task, we need to return to *zkr* as a departure point. As the subsequent chapter [in *Forgetting Whose We Are*] will make clear, there are important roles for the imagination. But these creative faculties need to be exercised within the canonical framework which the church's memory provides.

ogy of Disability: Disabling Society, Enabling Theology (Binghampton, N.Y.: Haworth Pastoral Press, 2004).

Vanier, Jean. *From Brokenness to Community* (New York: Paulist Press, 1992).

Wendell, Susan. *The Rejected Body: Feminist Philosophical Reflections on Disability* (New York: Routledge, 1996).

Yong, Amos. *Theology and Down Syndrome: Reimagining Disability in Late Modernity* (Waco: Baylor University Press, 2007).

79 Encountering the Disabled God

Nancy L. Eiesland

I recently read an article entitled "Disability for the Religious" in *The Disability Rag* — an American magazine primarily for disability rights activists. The article implied that religion offers no relevant answers to the query, "What is disability?" According to the author the following answers are available: disability is (a) a punishment; (b) a test of faith; (c) the sins of the fathers visited upon the children; (d) an act of God; or (e) all of the above. If these were the only choices, I would have to agree that religion has no relevant answers.

Christianity has often been cited as the source of destructive stereotypes about people with disabilities.[1] In countering these views, the challenge for people of faith is (i) to acknowledge our complicity with the inhumane views and treatment related to people with disabilities, and (ii) to uncover this hidden history and to make it available for contemporary reflection.

As a person with a disability, I could not accept the traditional answers given to my query, "What is disability?" Since I have a congenital disability, I have had opportunities to hear and experience many of these so-called answers. They included: "You are special in God's eyes, that's why you were given this painful disability," which didn't seem logical. Or "Don't worry about your pain and suffering now, in heaven you will be made whole." Again, having been disabled from birth, I came to believe that in heaven I would be absolutely unknown to myself and perhaps to God. My disability has taught me who I am and who God is. What would it mean to be without this knowledge? I was told that God gave me a disability to develop my character. But at age six or seven, I was convinced that I had enough character now to last a lifetime. My family visited faith healers with me in tow. I was never healed. People asked about my hidden sins, but they must have been so well hidden that even I misplaced them. The theology that I heard was inadequate to my experience.

However, in my teen years, I became actively involved

1. For example, the introduction to a collection of essays by mostly Canadian women with disabilities includes this statement: "Many people, including the disabled, still believe the traditional myths about the disabled. Some of these negative attitudes have their origins in ancient religious beliefs that regarded the disabled as devil possessed, or as corporeal manifestations of family guilt."

Taken from the article "Encountering the Disabled God," by Nancy L. Eiesland, published in *Bible in TransMission*, Spring 2004, and is reproduced here with the permission of Bible Society.

in the disability rights movement — the worldwide movement that has sought basic human rights for the now approximately 650-million persons with disabilities worldwide. Within the movement I came to understand why we people with disabilities have such depreciated views of ourselves and why so many of us are lacking in genuine convictions of personal worth. I began to see the "problem" not within my body, but with the societies that have made us outcasts, and viewed and treated us in demeaning and exclusionary ways. In America, I was among those who organised sit-ins to achieve access to public transport, to seek access to public facilities, and to promote human and civil rights legislation. I became passionately committed to the view that society must be changed in order for our full value as human beings to be acknowledged.

While the disability rights movement and activism addressed my experience, it didn't always respond to my more spiritual and theological questions about the meaning of my disability. For a long time, I experienced a significant rift between my participation in the movement and my Christian faith. The movement offered me opportunities to work for change that I thought were unavailable in Christianity, but my faith gave a spiritual fulfilment that I found elusive elsewhere. Within the Church, other people with disabilities were often uninterested in political and activist matters. In the rights movement, fellow participants saw religion as damaging or at least irrelevant to their work.

Although I began to answer my own question of the meaning of my disability by articulating God's call for justice for the marginalised, thus including people with disabilities, I felt spiritually estranged from God. However, the return path towards intimacy with God began to be cleared as I read a passage from the Gospel of Luke, after an encounter with several other people with disabilities. The setting was the Shepard Centre, the local rehabilitation hospital for people with spinal cord and traumatic brain injuries. I had been asked by the facility's chaplain to lead a Bible study with several residents. One afternoon, after a long and frustrating day, I shared with the group my own doubts about God's care for me. I asked them if they could tell me how they would know if God was with them and understood their experience. There was a long silence, then an African-American young man said, "If God was in a sip/puff maybe he would understand."[2] We talked about the image for a while and concluded.

Several weeks later, I was reading Luke 24.36-39. It is set within the account of Jesus' death and resurrection, but the focus of this passage is really on his followers who are anxious and depressed. The passage reads: "While they were talking about this, Jesus himself stood among them. . . . They were startled and terrified, and thought that they were seeing a ghost. He said to them, 'Why are you frightened, and why do doubts arise in your hearts? Look at my hands and my feet; see that it is I myself. Touch me and see.'" It wasn't God in a sip/puff, but here was the resurrected Christ making good on the promise that God would be with us, embodied, as we are — disabled and divine. Reading this passage, I came to realise that here was a part of my hidden history as a Christian. The foundation of Christian theology is the resurrection of Jesus Christ. Yet seldom is the resurrected Christ recognised as a deity whose hands, feet, and side bear the marks of profound physical impairment. The resurrected Christ of Christian tradition is a disabled God. This disabled God understood the experience of those in my Shepard Centre Bible study, as well as my own, and called for justice not from the distant reaches of principle but by virtue of God's incarnation and ultimate knowledge of human contingency. Christian theology, insofar as it is an incarnational theology, has a calling to stand by contingency, mortality and the concreteness of creation and suffering.

This encounter with the disabled God was the source of the liberatory theology of disability that I have written about in *The Disabled God,*[3] which calls both for justice and the recovery of vital Christian symbols and rituals. In promoting this vision, we also counter the prevailing sentiment that the religious practices and history of the able-bodied constitute the only relevant spiritual pulse and narrative, and that whatever is outside this ambit is of little, if any, significance.

What is the outcome of a life-changing encounter with the disabled God? Such an encounter highlights the need for justice for people with disabilities and the temporarily able-bodied. What is justice? Justice and just action are primarily virtues and practices of full participation, of persons deliberating about particular visions of human flourishing and working together to remove barriers in their institutions and relations so that they embody reciprocity and mutual appreciation of difference.

Justice is first about just listening, listening for the claims for justice made in the process of everyday life. This means attending to the ways in which everyday talk (and sometimes commonly accepted silence) makes claims about justice. They are not theories to be explicated or fully developed agendas to be followed; they are instead calls, pleas, or claims upon some people by others. Personal and social reflection on the demands of justice begins in heeding a call rather than in asserting and mastering a state of affairs. The call to be just is always situated in concrete social and congregational practices. Encounter must begin with listening, hearing the calls for justice expressed by people with disabilities who are among us.

Encountering the disabled God then makes possible thoroughgoing re-analysis of the connection between the myth of bodily perfection and the theological lengths to

2. A sip/puff is a head mounted accessory used to actuate a two position switch by a simple sip or puff.

3. Nancy Eiesland, *The Disabled God: Toward a Liberation Theology of Disability* (Nashville: Abingdon Press, 1994).

which we are willing to go in order to protect it. If Christ resurrected still participated fully in the experience of human life — including mysteriously the experience of impairment — we must be scandalised by our theological tendencies to perpetuate the myth of bodily perfection in our defence of heavenly (or, indeed, earthly) perfection. The disabled God nails the lie in our belief in a paradise in which we are "released" from the truth of worldly and bodily existence. That which God has called good, and in which God has participated through the incarnation, cannot be simply viewed as a temporary "evil" which we repudiate in order to participate in the promised fullness of life.

Furthermore, a theology that examines our own complicity in the theological justification of the myth of bodily perfection allows us to interrogate our own rage at mortality. The truth of mortality is threaded in our bones and genes and yet we, who are categorised as "unhealthy," find it hard to love God and ourselves. We would be a god. We rage within at God or at ourselves. We constantly kick against the limits of being human. We devise inhuman schedules, inhumane expectations of others and ourselves, and inhumane needs of wealth and success. Stress-induced impairment will soon be among the leading causes of disability in the Western world, as we work our bodies beyond God-given limits. Affecting men and women in their thirties to fifties, stress-induced disabilities, like repetitive strain injury, stroke, and heart attack, teach us that we have yet to hear God's call to be fully human, which means accepting our mortal limits. It is worth noting that our limits are neither constant nor uniform. Yet in the practice of ordinary faithfulness to our call to be human and to be for the others, we must learn to love our mortality as God does.

Finally, we must develop a risky imagination as a result of encountering the disabled God. Being at risk is the fundamental experience of human life. It is our birthright. The theological use we make of this is up to us. We can cultivate a risky imagination which understands that as we seek to address the meaning of disability and chronic illness we may find new ways of being in the world. Moving towards change is risky. But staying where we have been is deadly. Hopelessness takes no risk; it's what we have been taught. The will to practice hope in the context of our own lives, our spiritual homes and in the world is risky. We have no assurance that our efforts will be repaid, our lamentations heard, our joys celebrated, our pain reverenced. We do not know that justice will be done and yet we must practice hope and work for justice. This is hope as a spiritual discipline.

Theologically, people with disabilities have tried most, if not all, of the well-trodden theological paths in responding to our queries about the meaning of disability. We have found most treacherous and inaccessible. We are unsatisfied and willing to risk new imaginings, new symbols and renewed efforts to uncover our hidden history. We put the question to others who care: Are you willing to risk understanding God more fully as you move toward full participation of people with disabilities and the chronically ill in your midst and beyond? Will we together develop a risky theological imagination that asks what is God's vision of human flourishing not just for some but for all, not just for able-bodied but for the disabled, not just for those in the Western world but for the whole world?

People with disabilities can enable Christian communities to rethink the meaning of difference in our midst. Our presence reminds everyone that the boundaries of group difference are ambiguous and shifting, without clear borders. Individuals who are currently able-bodied have a greater than 50 per cent chance of becoming physically disabled, either temporarily or permanently. Ours is a minority you can join involuntarily, without warning, at any time. This risk can produce creativity and openness to what God will do.

For some, simply encountering the disabled God is risky. But, I believe that this encounter can open the possibility for conceiving the ways that God is already acting in the world, and for developing new and better imaginings. The Church needs to take risks to see justice enacted. I am convinced that if we look carefully and critically at our Christian tradition, we can uncover bits of a hidden history and perhaps more importantly find guide markers that can take us to a further place along the path towards human flourishing. If we risk encountering the disabled God, we may apprehend with greater clarity the fullness of God in the distinctiveness and diversity we see around us.

The time is now for justice and vision for the faith that includes just listening with people with disabilities and with chronic illness. We are called forth to risk the bread of life and eschew the crumbs. Only then can we articulate the implications of a theology of full participation.

80 Human Dignity in the Absence of Agency

Hans S. Reinders

Introduction

Let me introduce you to Kelly, a young girl whom I encountered a number of years ago in an institution for people with mental disabilities. Kelly is endowed with very little mental capacity to live her life as a human being. At birth she was diagnosed as micro-encephalic, meaning that a significant part of the normal brain was missing. Kelly is what some people prefer to call a "vegetable."

The first time I visited the group where Kelly lives, I found a twelve-year-old-girl with beautiful red hair and big brown eyes, sitting in a wheelchair, "staring without seeing," as was my first reaction. I asked the staff a few things about her and was invited to stay for the afternoon in order to get an impression of how she lived. So I stayed. I noticed that the nurses around her never spoke of Kelly as if she were a "vegetable." For them Kelly was simply Kelly, who could be just as "happy" or "sad" as any other human being. The view that leads others to speak of human beings in her condition as "vegetables" was not completely alien to the institution where she lives, however. This I inferred from what the director of this institution told me about her condition when she was a little baby:

> When Kelly was still a baby, the only thing she seemed capable of doing was taking a deep breath now and then. In her case we did not think of "sighing" as if she were lamenting her condition, but assumed her taking a deep breath was only a respiratory reflex. We thought this until somebody noticed that it depended on who spoke to her. When she was spoken to by particular voices, the changing respiration pattern stopped. Once the voice stopped, she started again. Thank heavens! At last she could do something, even if it was only "sighing." Our Kelly turned out to be human.

The guiding idea in assessing Kelly's condition was, presumably, that in order to be truly human one has to be capable of at least *doing* something, even if it is only as little as responding to a voice by taking a deep breath. The relief that the director testified in this connection is very significant, I think, because it indicates a sense of awkwardness. It is the sense of awkwardness that reflective people in our society feel in thinking about human beings such as Kelly. Suppose that Kelly had not been capable of something as minimal as "sighing," how could she then be called "human" other than in a vegetative sense?

Given the sensibilities of our secular moral culture, the question of what it means to be human raises all kinds of vexing questions in the face of profoundly disabled people like Kelly. This is especially true when the disabling condition is such that we doubt to ascribe "being a self" to the person. If we follow the moral presuppositions of our culture, the notion of a person does not even seem to apply. That notion presupposes the capacity of being aware of ourselves, even if only in a limited sense. Human lives, in our culture, are lives of subjects with a potential for being meaningful to them. Human lives are lived "from the inside."

These reflections suggest that, given the presuppositions of our moral culture, only lives that meet the conditions of self-referentiality and subjectivity can be properly called "human."[1] Within this culture, the point of being a subject is that one has at least a conception of what it is to be "oneself." That conception being absent, one's humanity is questionable — not in the biological sense, of course, but in the moral sense. Once one's *humanity* is questionable in the moral sense, however, so is one's dignity, because dignity is ascribed to human persons, not merely to human beings.

This essay addresses the question how to think theologically about human beings like Kelly. If human beings like her are to be dignified, then the ground of this dignity cannot be found in human agency, unless one wants to accept a "different" kind of human dignity for a "different" kind of human being. The theological task, then, is to think about human dignity in the face of people like Kelly in a way that avoids the implication of an anthropological "minor league." This requires that the presuppositions of our moral culture are overturned to the extent that they deny Kelly a share in our humanity. From a Christian point of view this denial cannot but mean that she is denied as a creature of God. While for many Christians the denial will be intuitively objectionable, as it should be, it is by no means clear what to say positively about Kelly's humanity.

A Theological Approach to the Question

How do we speak theologically about human dignity with regard to someone like Kelly? The question forces

From Hans S. Reinders, "Human Dignity in the Absence of Agency," in *God and Human Dignity,* edited by R. Kendall Soulen and Linda Woodhead (Grand Rapids, MI: Eerdmans, 2006), pp. 121-39.

1. See Hans S. Reinders, "Mental Retardation and the Quest for Meaning: Philosophical Remarks on 'The Meaning of Life' in Modern Society," in *Meaningful Care: A Multidisciplinary Approach to the Meaning of Care for People with Mental Retardation,* ed. Joop Stolk, Theo A. Boer, and R. Seldenrijk (Dordrecht: Kluwer, 2000), pp. 65-84.

us to think about the characteristically human that is implied in that notion. For whatever human dignity may mean, it must have something to do with what we consider to be special about humans. So what is it?

Initially the answer to that question may appear to be quite simple. "Being human" is defined by the fact that one is born out of human beings, as the Roman Catholic Church teaches. To define the characteristically human solely in terms of biological origin, however, is not sufficient for a theological anthropology. This requires a more demanding answer, one that includes not only the origin but also the destiny of human beings. After all, Christians do not simply believe in God; they believe in God the Father, and the Son, and the Holy Spirit. The Trinitarian understanding of God entails both the beginning and the end, Alpha and Omega, protology and eschatology. To speak of the former is to speak of the latter. To be a creature is to be created, and to be created is to be created with a purpose. That is why our destiny as humans is not a *donum superadditum* — something that is added to a subsistent being.[2] This implies that theological anthropology cannot explain what it is that dignifies human beings without referring to both their origin and their destiny. What the Christian faith tells us about our final destiny, that we will be resurrected with Christ, is intended in the beginning. And what it tells us about our origin, that we are created in the image of God, is consummated in the end.[3] All of which is to say that theological anthropology, as it is understood here, must be grounded in the Christian narrative as it is found in Scripture.

But even on its own account the biological answer is not sufficient to answer our question. This is clear when we ask what it is that makes human beings special. From classical antiquity the biological answer to that question has been that the human being is a "rational animal." As a matter of fact it is quite obvious that from the point of view of biology human beings such as Kelly cannot but be characterized as "defective" because they do not fit the description of the *Homo sapiens*. Whatever one may want to say about Kelly, she is not a "rational animal."

Can a theological account succeed in avoiding such qualifications? It occurs to me that in order to succeed, theological explanation cannot proceed from the presuppositions of our contemporary moral culture. It cannot proceed, that is to say, from a description of the necessary conditions of what distinguishes human beings from other beings in order to declare these conditions to be the ground for human dignity.

A theological anthropology that is grounded in Scripture should follow none of these steps. Giving the preferred set of necessary conditions for being "human" espoused by our moral culture — the conditions that constitute moral selves — that culture has no grounds left to reject the view that people who fail to be "moral selves" can be considered human only in a marginal sense. The problem is revealed by its spatial metaphor of "marginal cases," which implies that some human beings are more human than others, and some may even be considered not human at all. Since this strategy dominates most of modern moral philosophy, it will have a hard time recognizing the humanity of people such as Kelly.

Theological anthropology, in my view, does not proceed this way because it has a different point of reference. Its point of reference is the belief that we are God's children because he is our loving Father. From the point of view of Christianity — a viewpoint shared with Judaism and Islam — our humanity is given, not in the sense of *data* but as *donum*.

Nor is there any need for theological anthropology to proceed in this way, we should add. Theologically speaking, our humanity is received as a gift before it is anything else, which is something human beings like Kelly share with the rest of us. This is what theology has to explain, which it cannot do if it also starts with defining the human by means of biological, psychological, or philosophical description. Christians believe — again, together with Jews and Muslims — that all human beings are created in the divine image. They do not believe that God created only some human beings in his image. To put it briefly, but not inaccurately, Christians claim that in the loving eyes of God the Father there are no marginal cases of being "human."

But theology, as I understand it, does not need to refute philosophical understanding. It has its own logic, depending on the story of the God of Israel who came to be acclaimed by Jesus as his Father. Theological understanding is couched in narrative, not in philosophical conceptualization or classification.

Defending a distinctive theological approach to the question of what it means to be human, however, one must expect an objection, namely, that the truth about human nature cannot be claimed for a particular religious tradition. What is true about human nature should at least be accessible to all human beings. That rules out any reference to particular sources of knowledge to understand the meaning of "being human."

I am not inclined to take this objection very seriously. First of all, answering the question of what constitutes our human dignity from the perspective of biblical faith in no way rules out that what is claimed holds true for all human beings. It does rule out, however, the possibility of establishing this truth independently from that faith. Second, the fact that many people do not believe the basic tenets of the Christian religion to be true does not imply that they cannot be adequately explained to them. There is a distinction between explanation and justification. People may see what you mean without accepting

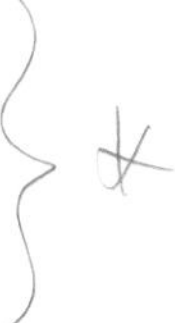

2. Cf. Martien E. Brinkman, *The Tragedy of Human Freedom: The Failure and Promise of the Christian Concept of Freedom in Western Culture* (Amsterdam: Rodopi, 2003), p. 32.

3. Here I am referring implicitly to Karl Barth's famous dictum of how the covenant between God and man is the inner ground of creation, whereas creation is the external ground of the covenant. Karl Barth, *The Doctrine of Creation*, vol. 3 of *Church Dogmatics*, trans. G. Bromiley (Edinburgh: T&T Clark, 1958), part 1, §41.

that what you mean is true. Third, this epistemic condition holds for any other approach to our question as well. To answer the question about human nature from the perspective of, say, evolutionary biology in no way rules out that what is claimed in that regard holds true for all human beings. It also does not rule out that its tenets can be adequately explained to those who doubt the truth of evolutionary biology. But it does rule out that this truth can be established independently from the philosophical presuppositions of evolutionary biology.

The Image of God in the History of Western Theology

Keeping these preliminary thoughts in mind, where to start? The answer to this question is fairly obvious. If there is a single notion in Christian theology that resists deferring particular human beings to an anthropological "minor league," it surely must be the notion that all human beings are created in the image of God. As the history of this doctrine shows, however, theological reflection has always been tempted to explain the divine image in terms of individual human capacities and faculties.[4] Unsurprisingly, the powers of reason and the will have frequently served as the prime candidates for the "seat" of the image.[5] It is not at all clear, therefore, that the theological tradition on the meaning of *imago Dei* is helpful with regard to our question.

Contrary to what some might expect, this verdict holds true also for the Protestant tradition, despite the fact that it is known for its insistence on a "relational" rather than a "substantial" view of the image. The issue between Protestantism and Roman Catholicism has been, of course, the question of how "nature" relates to "grace." One way to pose that question is this: are our human capacities to be valued because they allow us to receive the gift of grace, or does the gift of grace expose the esteem for our human capacities as the source of our sinfulness? On this issue the Roman Catholic tradition defined its position by saying that grace does not eliminate human nature but makes it more perfect: *gratia non tollit naturam sed perficit.* Human capacities obviously deserve to be kept in high esteem, a view that returns in Roman Catholic thought in the knowledge of God as the ultimate end of human beings.[6]

In contrast, the Protestant tradition has by and large always understood the question of "nature" and "grace" in terms of opposition rather than continuity. There is nothing in fallen human beings that qualifies them for receiving the grace of God, because only God overcomes human sinfulness. Consequently, our human capacities cannot be the mark of our worth before God. As it is often put: the coordinates of Protestant theology are "sin" and "grace" rather than "nature" and "grace."

Outside the context of human salvation, however, matters often appeared to be different. Regarding the powers of reason and the will, classical Protestant sources spoke of *reliquiae,* "remnants" or "vestiges," particularly with regard to morality.[7] In spite of the claim that, soteriologically speaking, the elevation of human capacities was the mark of sinfulness, these capacities often reappeared on the stage in a more positive tone as soon as the possibility of ethics was considered.[8] While the doctrine of salvation invoked the possibility that the divine image had been lost in the fall, that very possibility was regarded as implausible with regard to the moral life. Accordingly, the notion of "remnants" provided the ground for distancing anthropology and ethics from soteriology. The argument was that the fall had robbed human beings of their relation with God but had not eliminated their humanity. After the fall, the capacity for taking moral responsibility remains intact.[9]

Whatever the correct explanation of this theological state of affairs may be, the point to be kept in mind here is simply that with regard to theological anthropology

4. Berkhof claims that the tradition has by and large explained the image in terms of a "static-idealistic-individualistic conception of man." Hendrikus Berkhof, *Christian Faith: An Introduction to the Study of the Faith,* trans. Sierd Woudstra (Grand Rapids: Eerdmans, 1979), p. 180.

5. Fletcher, for example, understood the divine image to refer to the capacities for "intelligent causal action." See Joseph Fletcher, *Morals and Medicine* (Boston: Beacon, 1954), p. 218. That Fletcher stood in a long tradition in this respect is shown in D. J. Hall, *Imaging God: Dominion As Stewardship* (Grand Rapids: Eerdmans, 1986), pp. 89-98.

6. For a recent specimen of this thought see Josef Pieper, *Happiness and Contemplation,* introduction by Ralph McInerny (South Bend, Ind.: St. Augustine's Press, 1998).

7. See Gerrit C. Berkouwer, *Man: The Image of God* (Grand Rapids: Eerdmans, 1962), pp. 117-47. Berkouwer shows how the Protestant confessions maintained the notion of "remnants" in relation to the knowledge of good and evil in civil life. See also E. Brunner, *Der Mensch im Widerspruch* (Zürich: Zwingli Verlag, 1937), pp. 94-98, 154. According to Brunner, not only Luther himself but also Melanchthon and Calvin spoke of *reliquiae* in connection with the *lex naturalis.* Further, see Hall, *Imaging God,* p. 22a, fn. 34.

8. The exception to this rule is Karl Barth, who developed his conception of Christian ethics as obedience to God's word ("das Gebot der Stunde"), which presupposes an actual relationship with him. Barth's conception never gained much support in Protestant ethics. The same is true for Barth's interpretation of the *locus classicus* for the divine image — Genesis 1:26-27 — in terms of an analogy of the relation between God and man on the one hand and the relation between men and women on the other. See Hans S. Reinders, "Imago Dei As a Basic Concept in Christian Ethics," in *Holy Scriptures in Judaism, Christianity and Islam: Hermeneutics, Values and Society,* ed. Hendrik M. Vroom and Jerald D. Gort (Grand Rapids: Eerdmans, 1995), pp. 187-204.

9. Hall, *Imaging God,* p. 100 (especially fns. 33 and 34). The notion of *vestigia* in fact continued the theological tradition that since Irenaeus of Lyon had distinguished between "similitudo" and "imago" — the Latin translation of the Hebrew phrase *tselem wa demut* of Genesis 1:26-27 — saying that in the fall we lost the former but not the latter. In this way the Western tradition created anthropological space to talk about human nature independently from the work of Christ.

the Christian tradition has by and large adhered to an anthropology of individual capacities and faculties.[10] Since that anthropology does not have much to say for those human beings who are lacking in individual capacities and faculties, the question is how this tradition can repair its own inadequacy at this point.[11]

That it needs to be repaired can hardly be a matter of dispute, in my view. Given the presuppositions of our moral culture, many of our contemporaries doubt the humanity of human beings like Kelly. But for Christians, I take it, the decisive question is how we are seen in the loving eyes of God, regardless of what our moral culture tells us about ourselves. Consequently, any view implying that only some but not all human beings have been created in God's image must for that very reason rest on a theological mistake. To accept any such view would be to accept that the existence of mentally disabled human beings is a creational error. To my knowledge the Christian tradition has never endorsed this possibility, which means that there is reason to look for a theological conception that neither entails nor allows it.[12]

The possibility of repair will be explored by looking at recent accounts of Trinitarian theology that rethink the classical doctrine not as a piece of theological metaphysics but as part of the biblical narrative. The outstanding feature of these attempts is that they ground the Christian understanding of personhood in the story of the Father, Son, and Holy Spirit. I will explore what this development in Trinitarian thought implies for our understanding of human dignity.[13]

10. Cf. Hall, *Imaging God,* p. 89, where he writes: "A long and influential tradition of Christian thought looks upon the *imago dei* as referring to something inherent in *homo sapiens.* Humankind in God's image, according to this view, means that as it is created by God, the human species possesses certain characteristics or qualities that render it similar to the divine being." The underlying concept was that of human nature as a particular kind of substance. Hence the notion of a "substantialistic concept of *imago Dei*" (p. 89).

11. Cf. Brinkman, *The Tragedy of Human Freedom,* p. 31, who brings out the implication: "Thus both the Protestant and the Roman Catholic tradition recognize a central continuity with respect to fallen human beings remaining human. The fallen human person has not become an animal." From the perspective of the *animal rationale,* Kelly is merely an animal. This conclusion is inevitable when the individual capacities of reason and freedom are identified as the *continuum* of the human.

12. In this connection Martin Luther is frequently mentioned as the proverbial exception to this rule, because he once suggested to the prince of Sachsen Anhalt that an apparently mentally disabled youngster be drowned because he was nothing more than a *massa carnis* — a heap of flesh — without a soul. Martin Luther, *Tischreden* (Stuttgart: Reclam, 1987).

13. This exploration will take us far away from Kelly and the people in her group home, but it is their existence that we will have in mind all the way. A theological account of their existence has to take the burden of asking what its own history contributed to the cultural marginalization of these people's lives. Looking at that history will make us realize that the task ahead is quite formidable indeed.

The Turn to Inwardness[14]

The elevation of the powers of reason and the will as the characteristically human has been the hallmark of Western thought since its inception in ancient Greece. But there is a peculiar twist to this tradition that identified the powers of reason and the will as constituting the individual self. Consequently, the tradition of the West embarked on a course that located the characteristically human in an inner space. This development was inspired by Augustine's psychological doctrine of the Trinity. In Augustine's view, divine personhood was understood in terms of relation, but the distinguishing feature of Augustinian persons turned out to be that they have a relationship *with themselves.*

Augustine's mature view on anthropology is found in his treatise on the Trinity. There he reasons that if human beings are created in the image of God, and if this God is a triune God, then the Christian doctrine of man must somehow reflect the Trinity. Hence the fact that Augustine's psychological doctrine of the Trinity is mirrored in a psychological doctrine of man. The crucial step in this connection has been what Charles Taylor has coined as Augustine's turn to radical reflexivity.[15] "Radical reflexivity" in Augustinian sense means that the understanding of the subject as itself is a reflective act. The "I" as the source of its own existence is a model that Augustine draws from his understanding of God as "Being itself." For the theologian in the fourth century that he was, this implied the understanding of the relations between God as the Father, Son, and Holy Spirit. According to Augustine, the relationships between the three could not be relations of difference. They had to be relations of identity. Accordingly, he argued that divine personhood was predicated of the Father with respect to the Father himself. God the Father is called a person not in relation to the Son or the Spirit, but in respect to himself, just as he is called "good," "great," "just" in respect to himself.[16] Thus "Father" refers to God's being, "not insofar as He is Father," as Augustine puts it, "but insofar as He is."[17] In conceptual terms, the three are God because they equally possess

14. The theological move that follows is dependent upon recent developments in Trinitarian theology in which "relationality" is a key concept. My approach to the discussion owes a great deal to Catherine Mowry LaCugna, *God for Us: The Trinity and Christian Life* ([San Francisco]: HarperSanFrancisco, 1991). For a brief overview covering much of the literature, see David S. Cunningham, *These Three Are One: The Practice of Trinitarian Theology* (Malden, Mass.: Blackwell, 1998).

15. See Charles Taylor's *Sources of the Self: The Making of Modern Identity* (Cambridge: Cambridge University Press, 1989), pp. 117-41.

16. Augustine, *De Trinitate* VII.6.11: Quocirca ut substantia patris ipse pater est, non quo pater est sed quo est; ita est persona patris non aliud quam ipse pater est. Ad se quippe dicitur persona, non ad filium vel spiritum sanctum; sicut ad se dicitur deus et magnus et bonus et iustus et si quid aliud huiusmodi.

17. Augustine, *De Trinitate* VII.6.11.

the divine *ousia* but not because of the differentiating relations between them.

Augustinian explanation of divine personhood has stirred much debate in recent times because it fails to recognize the crucial importance of relationships for Christian theology. Accordingly, Robert W. Jenson has commented that in Augustine's view the differentiating relations between the three are irrelevant to their being God.[18] For a relational understanding of personhood, Augustine's conclusions are fatal, because when he says that "person" does not refer to a relation between the Father and the Son, but to the Father *with respect to himself,* he in fact inaugurates the concept of a self-enclosed relationality.[19]

Grounded in this model of Trinitarian thought, the Western conception of human personhood in terms of a relational interiority emerged. Just as Augustine's conception refers to God the Father in respect of himself, so the Western conception of human personhood refers to the human individual in respect of itself.[20]

The seeds of the latter conception are already apparent in Augustine's *De Trinitate.* There he argues that the "trinity in man" cannot be found in love, because this involves a three-term relationship: the one who loves, that which is loved, and the love that brings them together *(amans, amatum,* and *amor).*[21] Since this three-term relation locates one of its terms outside man — the object of his love — it does not satisfy the condition of being like the Trinity in God, because that Trinity is a relation of three equal hypostases within one being or essence. Consequently, not love but self-love provides the solution. Self-love allows for the conceptual possibility of a relation within the soul between the self as both the one loving and the one loved, and the love of self as the middle term between these two. In this manner "we discern a trinity, not yet indeed God, but now at least an image of God."[22]

I want to suggest that the notion of the human person grounded in this psychological introspection has deeply influenced Western anthropology and ethics. Augustine can be held only partially responsible for this development because for him the inward road is the road to God.[23] The step that severed this connection was made by Descartes. It is a huge leap from Augustine to the seventeenth century, of course, but even then it does not seem to be inappropriate for Charles Taylor to speak about Augustine as a "Proto-Cartesian."[24] Without ignoring that Augustine's view was radically distinct from what Descartes believed, the conclusion must be that relational personhood in *De Trinitate* is located in the domain of interiority.[25] In other words, the concept of personhood as a relation of the self with the self was not what Augustine intended, but he opened up a possibility that eventually would lead to the elevation of interiority and self-referentiality as the defining characteristics of the human.

18. Robert W. Jenson, *Systematic Theology,* 2 vols. (New York: Oxford University Press, 1997-1999), vol. 1, p. 112. The conclusion seems correct in that Augustine explains "person" as equivalent of "great," "good," and "just," each of which cannot be relative terms with regard to God. The deity is not both God and great, because God *is* greatness in the absolute sense.

19. Schmaus concludes from this argument that "Ist 'Person' kein relativer Begriff dann ist er ein absoluter. Der Schriftsteller [sc. Augustine] betont die vollständige Identität von Wesen und Person. . . . Person sein, gut sein, gross sein, und Wesen liegen alle auf der gleichen Linie. Wohl behauptet Augustinus so die Substanzialität der Personen, spannt aber zugleich die Identität von Person und Substanz so hoch, dass die Relativität der Person verloren geht und auch für subsistente Relationen kein Platz mehr bleibt." Michael Schmaus, *Die psychologische Trinitätslehre des Heiligen Augustinus* (Münster, Westf.: Aschendorf, 1967), p. 149. See for a similar conclusion LaCugna, *God for Us,* p. 103.

20. This is not to suggest, of course, that Augustine shared the modern conception of the individual, but it is to suggest that in Augustine's *De Trinitate* there is a clear correspondence between the "inner life" of God and the inner life of man. Cunningham (*These Three Are One,* pp. 229-30) has defended Augustine against criticisms that make him responsible for the development of "modern forms of individualism" by arguing that Augustine's was a "communal," not an individual, understanding of the human faculties. His argument fails to address the point at stake, however, which is not whether in Augustine's view the faculties of the mind were "communally shaped," but whether the relations of the self are constituted by interiority. See also David S. Cunningham, "Trinitarian Theology Since 1900," *Reviews in Religion and Theology* (1995): 4, 8-16, where the author makes the same point: "Augustine was well aware that an individual cannot reflect the inner life of God, because it is not an *individual* who is created in the image of God." But, as we will see shortly, Augustine in *De Trinitate* says that the *vestigia trinitatis* in man cannot be touted in an exterior relation between one human being and another. He explicitly denies that the concept of love can provide us with a proper understanding of the Trinity in man.

21. Augustine, *De Trinitate,* IX.2.

22. Augustine, *De Trinitate,* XIV.8.

23. Moltmann states that Augustine's view contains the first theological traces of the notion of the "absolute personhood" of God. He explains: "Every human being finds in himself the mirror in which he can perceive God. The knowledge of God in his image is surer that the knowledge of God from his works. So the foundation of true self-knowledge is to be found in God." Jürgen Moltmann, *The Trinity and the Kingdom* (Minneapolis: Fortress, 1993), pp. 14-16.

24. Taylor, *Sources of the Self,* pp. 132-33. Taylor points out the difference between Augustine and Descartes by saying that in Augustinian introspection the soul discovers its ultimate ground in God, who is closer to the self "than my own eye," while Cartesian introspection results in the sure inference by my own intellectual powers. Whereas Augustine is in search of an encounter with God "within," in Descartes the soul finds itself.

25. *Pace* Cunningham I do not see that Augustine's *De Trinitate* can be regarded a key source of Trinitarian thinking against "the modern cult of the individual" (see Cunningham, *These Three Are One,* pp. 229-30). Brian L. Horne has argued that in the *Confessions* Augustine develops a quite different and much more convincing view on personhood. Brian L. Horne, "Person As Confession: Augustine of Hippo," in *Persons, Divine and Human,* ed. Christoph Schwöbel and Colin E. Gunton (Edinburgh: T&T Clark, 1991), pp. 65-73.

Interlude: A Moral Point about Language

The analysis of Augustinian theology shows how the possibility of an anthropological "minor league" is opened up by the turn to inwardness. Without a relationship "within," no inner life; without an inner life, no "self"; and without a self, no person in the modern sense. Doubts about people's selfhood must lead to doubts about their dignity as humans. It is only with regard to human beings lacking a self in this sense that people may venture to argue that in taking their lives we cannot take anything that is valuable to them.[26]

At this point, I want to go back to Kelly, the severely disabled girl introduced in the opening section of this essay. The afternoon when I first visited the place where she lives, I noticed a nurse coming in for the late afternoon shift. Having entered the room she approached Kelly with a spontaneous, "you are looking cheerful today." On subsequent visits to Kelly's home, I noticed that such ascriptions of mental states were frequently made. It might be that somebody said that she looked sad, or that she loved to be bathed. Apparently Kelly was included in the language we use to speak to and about one another.

I realized that from the perspective of individual selfhood this language raises serious questions when used to refer to people like Kelly. Each of the phrases in question — "looking cheerful," "being sad," "love to be bathed" — imply intentionality on her part. They presuppose a capability of having mental states and of engaging the world in certain ways. Since this is highly questionable with regard to Kelly, we are forced to conclude that the things said about Kelly are in fact said metaphorically. To use intentional language in her case is to turn that language into metaphor. People speak to and about Kelly *as if* she were happy, or *as if* she were sad.

The problem arising from these considerations, it occurred to me, is that from the perspective of individual selfhood one cannot in good faith talk about Kelly as a human being. That is to say, one cannot talk that way when one knows that the language that implicates her as a human being is used metaphorically. In other words, people speak about Kelly *as if* she were a human being. If correct, what to say then to the skeptic who argues that using this language with regard to Kelly is a form of self-delusion?[27]

Pondering these thoughts made me very uneasy. Suppose that the people who work with Kelly and her friends[28] also believe that having the mental states of inwardness is what makes us human. Suppose they then realize that they cannot in good faith speak to and about Kelly as a human being without fooling themselves. What would be the effect of that belief on their practice of caring? To take the possibility seriously is in fact quite chilling, What is the point of treating something as if she were a human being when one knows for a fact that she is not a human being? The question is inevitable, it occurred to me, once one has accepted the perspective of selfhood as the originating source of our humanity. From that perspective, it is difficult to see how one could regard Kelly otherwise than as a "vegetable," which is, indeed, to regard her as a "something."

I then asked myself what the staff in Kelly's group home would say to all this. Supposedly many of them *do* believe something like modernity's claim that being human is being in the possession of a self. But somehow it does not seem to hold them back from engaging themselves in the practice of caring for Kelly and her friends. For them Kelly is just Kelly, as I said before. They include Kelly in the language that constitutes and shapes the meaning of what is going on in her home. To give an account of that language, I take it, they have no use for the philosophical beliefs of modernity, regardless of whether these beliefs may in fact coincide with their own. This does not mean, of course, that they don't have the responsibility to think critically about what they are doing within their practice of caring. But it does mean that their critical reflection will not proceed from presuppositions that invite them to question Kelly's humanity.

The point of these reflections is to open our eyes to what the preoccupation with selfhood in our contemporary moral culture may do to our understanding of the practice of caring for dependent human beings such as the severely disabled. The language of that culture cannot but make the practice appear as an oddity remaining from a religious past that is in rapid decline. This does not necessarily mean that the practice of caring for the disabled is as such in danger, but it does mean that the moral grounds that once served to support and inspire it are exposed to cultural erosion. Among the more important of these grounds was the view that they too are children of God. Now that our society has the technological means to enhance selective procreation, many of our contemporaries have ceased to look upon their children in this light. Instead they believe that it is our duty to make "responsible reproductive decisions."

Notwithstanding the fact that many of our contemporaries hold this view, the task for Christian theology, I want to suggest, is to sustain the practices of caring for disabled human beings such as Kelly and her friends. This is not to say that, subjectively, these practices are dependent upon a theological meta-discourse. That is obviously not the case. Usually the professionals involved in it do not have much use for meta-discourse of any kind because they are too busy running the place. I do mean to say, however, that *objectively* the practices of

26. Cf. Peter Singer and Helga Kuhse, *Should the Baby Live?* (Oxford: Oxford University Press, 1985).

27. I vividly remember a scene when the director of an institution introduced me in a group home similar to Kelly's. We watched a nurse who said she was playing a game with a severely disabled man. Upon leaving the scene, the director apologized to me for the nurse: "Of course the man has no clue what is going on, but I greatly admire these nurses. I could not do it." That remark indicated a skeptical mind.

28. Note how skeptical doubts about the language immediately start to multiply: can one work "with" someone like Kelly? Can she have "friends"?

caring for the mentally disabled — in particular the severely disabled — cannot be accounted for from the perspective of modernity and its beliefs about selfhood as the originating source of our human dignity.

"Ecstatic Personhood": The Greek Orthodox Alternative

Therefore, a theological alternative to the moral discourse of modernity is called for. Given the problem resulting from the turn to inwardness, the question before us is how to think about the human in a way that is not premised by a psychology of the human faculties. Regarding this question I believe Augustine was right in thinking that theology's conception of humanity is grounded in its understanding of God. But unlike the tradition following Augustinian inwardness, I think that the relations constituting divine and human beings are relations *between* persons, rather than *within* an absolute personhood.

Recent Trinitarian accounts to support this claim have been developed in close conversation with the Greek Orthodox tradition. It is well known that compared with the West, the tradition of Greek Orthodoxy has approached the doctrine of the Trinity in a distinctively different key.[29] By and large the West has followed Augustine's neo-Platonism by emphasizing God's simplicity. "Being itself" — *Ipsum esse* — is considered the first ontological principle. In contrast, Greek Orthodoxy, particularly in the Cappadocian Fathers, proceeded from the "monarchy" of the Father. In their view God's fatherhood is ontologically prior.

The Greek Orthodox theologian who has defended this tradition consistently is John D. Zizioulas.[30] His work in this connection has been recognized as an influential contribution to contemporary Trinitarian thought.[31] As Zizioulas shows, the Cappadocian replaced the neo-Platonic "Being" as the ultimate principle of reality by God the Father from whom everything else proceeds.[32] This procession is not a matter of ontological necessity. Instead, Zizioulas argues, the procession is an act of communion by which the Father brings forth the Son and the Spirit. The act of communion that constitutes the Holy Trinity is a free act of love. Accordingly, Greek Orthodoxy regards divine personhood as constituted by an *ecstatic* act of communion. It is ecstatic in the sense that God's very being is identified in an act of communion. That is how God exists.[33]

What follows, according to Zizioulas, is that human personhood necessarily depends on divine personhood. The reason is that the main characteristic of personhood is freedom. Personhood breaks the chain of ontological necessity. This is what the phrase "being as communion" is intended to convey. To be free as a person is to be free for another in an ecstatic movement. Now the question arises how humans can be free from the necessity of their temporal being. We find ourselves inevitably determined by all sorts of conditions that make us the concrete beings we are. Zizioulas responds that the movement of "ecstatic being" can never be complete in the case of natural beings. The only person who can absolutely affirm its own existence as *freedom* is God the Father. Only his is true freedom because freedom cannot plausibly be derived from necessity.

According to Zizioulas, this means that as a "biological hypostasis" man is intrinsically a tragic figure. Unlike the persons of the Trinity that exist as communion, human persons are characterized by the *separateness* of their being in the natural world. Humans cannot per se exist freely on the ontological level. Therefore, Zizioulas argues, the possibility of ontological freedom is only realized in our union with God that is realized in Christ. Hence the "locus" of true human freedom is the ecclesial community where we anticipate what we will be in the "final outcome of our existence." This eschatological reality is mediated, according to Zizioulas, by the sacraments and the liturgy of the church. Only it can defeat the separation between individuals caused by natural necessity.

Going back to the question that we are pursuing in this essay — the question about the dignity of those that have no conception of themselves as humans — it is clear that the notion of ecstatic personhood looks like a promising move in Trinitarian thinking. It does not presuppose any notion of the human person as an individually subsistent being. Participation in ecclesial personhood is not premised by what we as individuals can or cannot do, but in what God does for us. It is grounded in God's act of communion that is mediated in the Eucharist.

Here the question arises of whether God's act of com-

29. See Walter Kasper, *Der Gott Jesu Christi* (Mainz: Matthias Grünewald, 1982), p. 361, who argues that "the Greeks" proceeded from the three persons to establish the unity, whereas "the Latins" proceeded the other way around. See also Jenson, *Systematic Theology*, vol. 1, pp. 115-16.

30. See in particular John D. Zizioulas, *Being As Communion: Studies in Personhood and the Church* (Crestwood, N.Y.: St. Vladimir's Seminary Press, 1985).

31. See Jenson, *Systematic Theology*, vol. 1, p. 116. See also Miroslav Volf, *After Our Likeness: The Church As the Image of the Trinity* (Grand Rapids: Eerdmans, 1998).

32. Zizioulas, *Being as Communion*, pp. 36-37, 40f.

33. See Jenson, *Systematic Theology*, vol. 1, p. 103. Jenson argues along similar lines that engaging himself in relation with the Son, and, thereby, with human history, is how God exists: against the timeless and immutable deity of the surrounding Hellenistic culture that saved human beings from the contingencies of their existence, "the gospel proclaims a God who is not in fact distant, whose deity is identified with a person of our history; antiquity's struggle to overcome a supposed gulf between deity and time is discovered to be moot in light of the gospel." In Jenson's thought "overcoming a supposed gulf between deity and time" is exactly why the relation that identifies the Father with the Son is crucial in the biblical narrative. Consequently, God "himself" cannot be abstracted from this person, nor from his death, nor from his career, nor from anything else that characterizes the Son's mission into the world.

munion is connected to human acts of communion. The question arises because Zizioulas does not seem to have any use for other acts of communion in his account. As acts of natural beings, such acts cannot be truly free, which presumably means that they cannot be true acts of communion either. The reason is that on the ontological level natural human beings cannot exist as persons. The fallenness of human beings means that we are indeed separated individuals. This points to the conclusion that Zizioulas inadvertently reinforces the traditional Western view of the individual as a self-enclosed being. In his view, openness for the other is realized in the Eucharist as the act of God's love that draws us into the triune existence. But somehow this act, as Zizioulas explains it, does not inform our understanding of how we in reality exist as human beings.

Robert Jenson's Account of Personhood

It is with regard to this question that I finally turn to Robert Jenson's account of Trinitarian personhood. Jenson shares much of the criticism I directed against Augustine, most notably the fact that Augustine regards Trinitarian personhood as predication of God's being. This results in the view that when the triune God acts he acts singly, which eliminates the differentiation between the agency of the Father, the Son, and the Spirit that is attested by the biblical narrative. Notwithstanding the objections to Augustine's Trinitarian theology, however, Jenson also wants to criticize the one-sidedness of the Cappadocian view, which he sees as precisely located in their limited account of the ontology of Trinitarian personhood.

Jenson points to the fact that the Cappadocians recognized three ontological questions — "Is it?" "What is it?" and "How is it?" — and taught that only the third question applies to the Trinitarian *hypostasis.* Their explanation of the divine persons was about their "way of having being," not about the two other questions. What they wanted to say is that only the question "How is it?" differentiates the persons, not "Is it?" or "What is it?" Consequently, what kind of being the *hypostasis* were implied to be remained obscure.

For this reason, Jenson argues for an ontological definition of the concept of the person as a relation in the mode of substance. The divine person is a relation that itself subsists and is not merely a connection between subsistent entities. This definition gives the concept of personhood a clearly distinctive ontological status. It states that the Trinitarian persons are, in Jenson's language, "relational identities." He credits Tertullian for having seen — long before the Eastern tradition — that *persona* signifies a subsistent social relation. With his understanding, Tertullian specified an identity "that is constituted in a particular set of social relations of address and response." Moreover, this view enabled Tertullian to remain faithful to the mutual exchanges in the biblical dramatic narrative in which the Father, the Son, and the Spirit have different agencies that shape their different parts as *dramatis Dei personae.* Consequently, Tertullian ruled out the view that regarded "Being" as somehow the "real" God of which the three persons were the concrete manifestations. The triune God is no other than the Father who exists in relation to the Son from which relation proceeds the Spirit.[34]

The conceptual space created by the notion of personhood as relational identity is further developed when Jenson makes his second move, which is to consider the possibility of different ways of "being personal."[35] It is customary in the Western tradition to think of a person as the focus of consciousness, that is, as an "I" which is the originating source of its own self. From the act of identifying the transcendental "I" with the self springs the possibility of freedom. But this freedom must then be "a relation internal to a fundamentally closed single entity," which results in the view of selfhood as self-enclosure. Jenson wants to break away from this "conceptual straightjacket" by considering the possibility that personality and identity are not necessarily correlated one-to-one: "There may be *more than one way to be personal,* even to be 'a' person, so that indeed, . . . I may in one way be one person with Adam and Christ and in another way distinct from them not only by identity but also personally."[36] Accordingly, there can be more identities related within one person, as when we speak of a corporate person, which is said of Israel standing before God and addressed as one person, but also of the human race as Adam's descendants, or of the Christian community that is one person with Christ. The person as a subsistent social relation is not necessarily limited to the relatedness of one being to another, but it is conceivable as the complex relatedness of beings with different identities in communion. This, I think, is in fact what Zizioulas's notion of "being as communion" is intended to express. The freedom that for Zizioulas and Jenson is the hallmark of personhood is not necessarily a "relation internal to a single entity" as modernity believes it to be. Instead it is a relation grounded in an act of communion between beings with different identities. In this sense it can be said, as does Zizioulas, that to be free as a person is to be free for another in an ecstatic movement. Our freedom is received from God the Father who created us with and for another in the name of the Son and the Spirit.

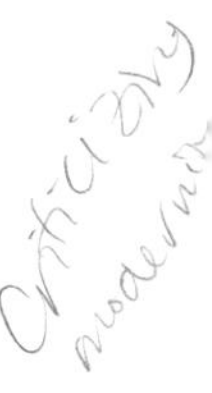

34. Augustine explicitly denied the explanation of the relational being if that implied that "neither is the Father God without the Son nor the Son without the Father, but only both mutually are God." See Jenson, *Systematic Theology,* vol. 1, p. 112.

35. The problem Jenson addresses in this connection is that of interpreting the Trinity itself as personal without introducing a fourth person in it. This problem will not be my concern, but only its anthropological implication for understanding human personhood.

36. Jenson, *Systematic Theology,* vol. 1, p. 120; emphasis added.

Conclusion: Kelly's Dignity

If the theological tour de force undertaken here is to be helpful with regard to our initial question, it must give substance to the phrase written above this final section. Given what I explained about Kelly's existence, what does it mean to speak of her dignity? First of all, the notion of dignity cannot refer to any subjective condition as it is implied in the notion of the person as a self-reflective agent. Human dignity does not have individual action as its originating source. But then, this is no shortcoming, because the argument in its entirety was conceived precisely to avoid grounding dignity on such notions. Kelly's dignity does not depend on what she is or is not capable of doing. It is a dignity she possesses as a human person with a relational identity. It is a dignity that is communicated to her in the acts of people caring about her and about her well-being. If the chaotic force of her natural condition would have had its way, Kelly would have been dead years ago. Her dignity is that she has been accepted as God's creature, which is what she shares with all of us. For others to accept her and include her in their relationships *is* a genuine act of communion.

The theological warrant for this view is that human beings are dignified, regardless of their state or condition, by a divine act of communion. In the resurrection of Christ, God the Father draws human beings into his own relationship with the Son and the Spirit and saves them from the bonds of natural necessity. This does not mean, as Zizioulas seems to imply, that personhood is the prerogative of ecclesial beings participating in the sacramental life of the church. But it does mean that in participating in that sacramental life, we learn to see what and how God intended us to be from the beginning. We learn to see that including Kelly in our relationships is a genuine act of communion that glorifies God the Father.

Having explained our dignity as originating from the act of communion by which God has first created us, and then has re-created us, we have shown that our humanity is a gift from the beginning to the end. We have received it, before we did anything, and we are promised the fullness of this gift in the end. This indicates why divine agency — not human agency — is the primary concept of theological anthropology. Because of what God does, we can see Kelly as a child of God who is lovable in his eyes just like any other of his children. When seen in that light, Kelly fits Jenson's description of personal being, according to which "a person is one whom other persons may address in hope of response."[37] The hope of response in her case must be eschatological hope, the hope for what she and we will be in the final state of our existence, as Zizioulas did put it. Given that Christian hope, we may regard the acts of communion that include her in personal being as acts that prefigure the future of God.

37. Jenson, *Systematic Theology,* vol. 1, p. 121.

81 Unremitting Compassion: The Moral Psychology of Parenting Children with Genetic Disorders

Richard B. Steele

Interrupted Sleep

About a year ago, one of my younger colleagues, fresh out of graduate school, announced that he and his wife were expecting their first child. I responded by doing what any seasoned, middle-aged father of three would do: I gave him some unsolicited advice. "Get as much sleep as you can before the baby is born," I told him. "You'll want to remember afterwards how good it used to feel." Gamely playing his part in this obligatory ritual of male bonding, my friend groaned in mock agony at the thought of all those midnight diaper changes and 2:00 A.M. bottle feedings to come — as if this thought had not yet occurred to him. Of course, both of us had been through such rituals countless times, and understood that the giving of dour "advice" is the masculine way of offering heartfelt congratulations. Joking about the troubles of parenthood is how we share its exquisite joys without lapsing into maudlin sentimentality. Both of us knew — and each of us knew that the other knew — that having to endure a few months of wakeful nights goes with the territory, and also that these months pass quickly as the child learns to sleep the whole night through.

What I did not tell him, at least just then, is that not every child does learn to sleep the whole night through, and that for the parents of those who do not, the memory of how good eight hours of unbroken shut-eye feels is just that — a fond but distant memory. My wife Marilyn and I are among those for whom interrupted sleep, as well as many other forms of daily and nightly unpleasantness, is a way of life. Our oldest daughter, Sarah, now thirteen, gets us up two or three times every night. Whenever she needs to use the toilet, shift position, have an itch scratched, a pillow fluffed, or finds that she has dropped any of the three items she always takes to bed with her (a luminescent wristwatch, her crook-shaped plastic "reacher," and an old headband she uses to screen the morning light from her eyes) she calls out, "Maaaaaaahhhm" or "Daaaaaaaaaad." And one or both

From Richard B. Steele, "Unremitting Compassion: The Moral Psychology of Parenting Children with Genetic Disorders," *Theology Today* 57.2 (July 2000): 161-74. Used by permission.

of us run, or stumble, to her bedside. Often we know from the sound of her voice which of these various things she needs even before we get there. Sarah has developed — though she may not be aware of this — a distinct "call" for each need, with its specific tone quality, volume level, and note of urgency.

Sarah cannot do these simple things for herself because she suffers from two catastrophically debilitating physical disorders. I am not going to explain these disorders in full detail, but I will say enough about them to indicate the kind of unremitting, round-the-clock care she requires. This will help to illustrate the issues that I discuss here, namely the moral responsibilities and psychological effects upon parents of raising children with severe, incurable, untreatable genetic disorders. Thus, my focus will not be on suffering children, but on the parents who must suffer with and for them.

The first of Sarah's two conditions is a rare genetic disease called Fibrodysplasia Ossificans Progressiva (FOP).[1] As its name implies, this condition involves the gradual calcification of her exoskeletal muscles. Put simply, her body is not content with one skeleton, the one she was born with, so it is growing a second. It does so by turning most of her muscles first into masses of cartilage, and then into bones. These are perfectly healthy bones, complete with perfectly healthy marrow, but they grow where bones do not belong — some jutting out at odd angles from normal bones, some crossing joints, some even penetrating the skin from the inside out. As the years go by, this second skeleton gradually rigidifies the human body, turning it into a kind of living statue. Sarah's case has progressed much faster than most. She still has some movement of her hands, forearms, and legs — enough to feed herself, do certain handicrafts, and (with the aid of sticks) type on a computer, but not enough to walk, or dress herself, or use the toilet, or put on her own glasses or hearing aids, or bathe, or turn her head, or roll over in bed.

1. For a more extensive discussion of FOP, and of Sarah's case in particular, see my "Accessibility or Hospitality? Reflections and Experiences of a Father and Theologian," *Journal of Religion in Disability and Rehabilitation* 1 (1994), 11-26 and the literature cited in notes 6, 8, and 9. Great strides in understanding the disease have been made since that time by Frederick Kaplan, M.D. and Eileen Shore, Ph.D. and their collaborators at the FOP Laboratory of the University of Pennsylvania School of Medicine in Philadelphia, and several promising treatments are currently being developed. This research is summarized in J. Michael Connor, "Fibrodysplasia Ossificans Progressiva — Lessons from Rare Maladies," *The New England Journal of Medicine* 335/8 (August 22, 1996): 591-93 and in Wade Roush, "Protein Builds Second Skeleton," *Science* 273/5279 (August 30, 1996): 1170. A longer and less technical description of the disease and recent research is Thomas Maeder, "A Few Hundred People Turned to Bone," *The Atlantic Monthly* 281/2 (February 1998): 81-89. Unfortunately, there is little likelihood that the debilitating effects of the disease in its advanced state can be fully reversed, and thus the recent research has little bearing on the present article, which describes the effects upon the parents of having to give day-to-day care to children with severe and permanent disabilities.

As if FOP were not enough, Sarah was also born with a craniopharyngioma, a kind of brain tumor. Although "benign" (not cancerous), it would have blinded her, and eventually killed her, had it gone untreated. We first learned of its existence when she was eight years old and began having vision problems. It was successfully resected, and five years later there is no evidence of recurrence. But her pituitary gland had to be removed, so she has endocrine deficiencies and diabetes insipidus. She takes numerous hormones orally, and her diet is limited to eight hundred calories a day.

FOP occurs in about one in two million births, and craniopharyngioma in about one in fifty thousand. So the chances that anyone would have both conditions are about one in one hundred billion — a number larger than the total number of human beings who have ever been alive. And because her case is medically unique, no one can say for sure how best to care for her. Marilyn and I must figure that out as we go along. Of course, we have a phalanx of doctors, nurses, pharmacists, physical therapists, genetic counselors, respite care workers, insurance agents, wheelchair technicians, adaptive equipment vendors, teachers, teacher's aides, lawyers, financial consultants, and sympathetic friends and relatives who provide all sorts of valuable information, advice, assistance, and medical care. God bless them all! We could not manage without them, and over the years we have been exceedingly fortunate in finding competent and compassionate people to help us. But — and this brings me to the main topic of this paper — there are distinct differences between the sort of compassion displayed by even the best professional caregiver or well-meaning friend and that required of a parent of a sick child.

The Double-Sidedness of Compassion

It will help to begin by giving a general account of this emotion. Or should we call it, rather, a virtue?[2] Indeed, part of what makes compassion such a remarkable human quality — and part of what makes those who possess this quality such remarkable human beings — is what I shall call its "double-sidedness."[3]

2. The following account of compassion depends heavily on three sources: Lawrence Blum, "Compassion," in Amélie Oksenberg Rory, ed., *Explaining Emotions* (Berkeley: University of California Press, 1980), 507-17; Simon G. Harak, *Virtuous Passions: The Formation of Christian Character* (New York: Paulist, 1993); and Milton Mayeroff, *On Caring* (San Francisco: Harper & Row, 1971).

3. Although neither Blum nor Harak specifically describes compassion as "double-sided," both have observed this characteristic. The second and third sections of Blum's article, for example, are titled "The Emotional Attitude of Compassion" and "Compassion and Beneficent Action," respectively. And Harak's expression, "virtuous passion," in its quite intentional paradoxicality, is meant to point out something that modern psychology often overlooks or denies, namely the moral appraisability of the emotions. I have borrowed the term "double-sidedness" from Gustaf Aulén, *Christus Victor* (New York: Macmillan, 1931), 31, 35, 56-60, 67. But

On the one hand, it is clearly an emotion. That is, it is something we experience, something we feel, something that happens in us. And it can be an agonizing experience, although, as we shall see, it can also be a very joyful one. Yet, curiously, it is a secondary, indirect, and vicarious experience. That is, it is *my* experience of someone else's suffering, my identification with the misery I observe in another. And this identification is usually spontaneous and uncontrived (though we would not say "automatic"). It arises in me unbidden, and is thus a mark of my own vulnerability to another person's distress. Indeed, genuine compassion seems to be something that is almost torn out of us by the grievous circumstances under which someone else lives.[4] Any attempt to induce this emotion (or any other emotion) in ourselves by a sheer act of willpower, under an onerous sense of duty, will only result in a simulacrum of the real thing.

And yet there *is* a sense in which compassion is voluntary. Or at least it is a trait of character that we must intentionally cultivate and that typically grows in scope and intensity as we mature morally. For although we do not exactly "choose" to be compassionate (in quite the same way that we might choose, say, to perform one specific action instead of another), nevertheless we can, over time, train ourselves to be open to the needs of others. Indeed, compassion can become so deeply embedded in our character, and so forceful in its regulation of our conduct, that it might better be called a "disposition." That does not imply that it is less intensely felt than other emotions, but only that it is less vicissitudinous. Some emotions, such as anger, come and go rather quickly, as circumstances dictate. But dispositions are notable for their constancy and for the way they shape large areas of our life. Compassion is that way. It gentles our character as a whole, rendering us more patient and respectful toward others, more attentive to and interested in people's thoughts and feelings, even when they are not suffering.

Compassion is also distinguished from many other emotions because it must be *learned.* We do not ordinarily have to learn how to "feel" emotions: they seem almost to be "hard-wired" into our nature (although what we feel emotional *about,* and how we express our emotions, will change as we grow). But compassion is an acquired trait of character, which we must foster and develop by putting ourselves in situations where we can practice it. Certainly it would be a mistake to suppose that some people simply have a taste or a knack for it. Nobody "enjoys" being compassionate (though, again, we may "take joy" in helping others), and it does not come naturally to us. Indeed, those who do acquire this trait often come by it the hard way, that is, by undergoing some intense suffering of their own, and perhaps also by receiving the generous care of others in their time of need. It often takes a tragedy to activate our human capacity for self-transcendence. We might even say that learning compassion takes a kind of "conversion," a transformation in our fundamental orientation toward life, away from our endemic self-preoccupation and toward an open-hearted concern for the well-being of others.

The fact that compassion is both voluntary and learned differentiates it from other kinds of suffering, which are involuntary and connate. Thus, a starving man does not need to "let" himself experience the pain in his empty belly. But a well-fed man who reads a newspaper account of an African famine must, in a sense, "let" himself feel the agony of the victims. For he could, of course, shrug off such grim tidings and move on to the sports page. This is why our various ways of responding to other people's sufferings are morally appraisable. Those who willingly open themselves to the sufferings of others are to be admired for their courage and sensitivity. Those who are unwilling to do so, or who, from long habit of indifference, have grown quite incapable of entering imaginatively and caringly into other people's situations, are deemed psychologically and/or morally defective.[5]

At the same time, the number of suffering people for whom I can reasonably be expected to feel compassion is rather limited. For I am not God, who alone is both willing and able to bear the sorrows of the whole world. People who have not learned to differentiate between those to whom they owe compassion and those whose sufferings are none of their business are prey to a refined, self-deceived, and self-destructive grandiosity.

This brings us to the other side of compassion. Precisely because it is voluntary and learned, we can call it a

Aulén's use of the term has nothing directly to do with moral psychology.

4. This emotion is sometimes so intense that it produces somatic effects, such as a flood of tears or a "pit in the stomach." Such manifestations are suggested by the word for compassion used in the Greek New Testament, namely *splanchna.* The literal meaning of this term is "bowels" (cf. Acts 1:18, where it is used with reference to Judas Iscariot's gruesome death). But in several places it refers to the "gut feelings" of personal affection among Christians (e.g., Phil 1:8, 2:1, Phlm 7, 12, 20) or, what is more apropos of the present argument, of intense commiseration with the sufferings of others (e.g., Matt 9:36, Luke 10:29-37, 2 Cor 7:15, Col 3:12, 1 John 3:17).

5. Lawrence Blum writes: "My neighbor suffers; in 'suffering with' him there is a sense in which I suffer too, but my suffering is much less than his" ("Compassion," 513). There is a certain *prima facie* truth to this statement: The starving orphan suffers more than the compassionate newspaper reader. Yet, I would prefer to locate the difference between suffering and compassion, not in the intensity of the agony endured, but in the fact that the latter contains an element of intentionality and vicariousness that the former lacks. And might there not be cases in which that very intentionality actually heightens the suffering of the compassionate person to a degree greater than that of the primary sufferer? As a Christian, for example, I believe that Christ experiences my sufferings to an infinitely greater degree than I experience my own. Moreover, as I shall argue later, the parent of an infant who has just been diagnosed with a genetic disorder may suffer, at least for a time, far more acutely than the child. For the parent can foresee, or at least imagine, what is to come for the child, even though the child may not yet exhibit painful or debilitating symptoms.

moral virtue and the lack of it a vice. To possess a virtue (or a vice) is to be in the habit of acting in a certain way. And the actions that spring from compassion are those aimed at alleviating the sufferings of others — perhaps even at great cost to oneself. This is what differentiates genuine compassion from condescending pity on the one hand and phony moral outrage on the other. Some will react to the news of the famine by shedding a few alligator tears for the "poor unfortunates." Others will indulge in a bit of armchair speechifying about how awful "the System" is. But the truly compassionate person will avoid both bathos and bluster, and quietly figure out something constructive to do to put food in the mouths of the hungry. Genuine compassion involves the capacity to focus one's attention on those in need, and a corresponding indifference to one's own reputation for being "compassionate." The conversion that compassion works in a person renders her immune to the desire to think of herself, or to be thought of by others, as "sensitive" or "well-informed about the world's problems." True self-sacrifice is truly self-forgetful.

Of course, just as I cannot feel everybody else's sufferings, I cannot help every sufferer. I must target my efforts or waste them. For again, I am not God, but at best only one of God's instruments. And it sometimes happens that those whom I most wish to help cannot be helped very much. Or rather, the help I can give them does not consist in alleviating their suffering, but in refusing to abandon them to it. For people whose pain is irremediable or whose grief is too deep for words, the most I may be able to do is to sit in silent vigil with them or to pray for them. But in such cases, what may appear to be a purely "useless" ministry of quiet presence will really be a far more compassionate thing than a flurry of pointless activity or a barrage of distracting chatter.[6] The value of the "active" element in compassion is measured not by the amount of sheer energy expended on the sufferer's behalf, but by the suitableness and sincerity of what is done.

Thus the double-sidedness of compassion: As an emotion, it is something we feel, something elicited from us at the sight of another's distress. But as a virtue, it is something we must labor to develop, a disposition of responsiveness to human need, a certain alertness to situations that call for our intervention, as well as a sensitivity to the types of intervention that are suitable to given circumstances. And these two elements thoroughly interpenetrate, so that a compassionate person always displays both. She will have that capacity for self-transcendence that allows her to suffer *with* others, and that capacity for self-sacrifice that allows her to suffer *for* others. She will have that limpid emotional vulnerability that only comes when a person begins to shed her fear of being hurt and her need of being in control. Conversely, she will have that robust practical availability for others that only comes when a person begins to see her time, energy, and resources as gifts to be shared, rather than property to be hoarded.

6. On "Presence" as a Christian virtue, see James Wm. McClendon Jr., *Ethics: Systematic Theology, Volume I* (Nashville: Abingdon, 1986), 106-9.

Parental Compassion for Suffering Children

Having offered this general description of compassion, I now want to describe the specific character of this "virtuous passion" as it manifests itself in parents who must exercise it toward children with serious genetic or congenital disorders. For although I believe that genuine compassion always involves both suffering with and suffering for another, it seems obvious that the precise way in which it is displayed in any given case depends in large measure on the nature of the social relationship between the sufferer and the person of compassion. Thus, the character of a parent's compassion for an ill child differs from that of a doctor's compassion for a patient, and again, from a conscientious suburbanite's compassion for a starving orphan. Both the degree of emotional involvement felt and the nature of the merciful actions performed differ substantially among these cases. Moreover, it would be a mistake to regard any of these cases, however exemplary in itself, as morally superior to the others. For the authenticity of someone's compassion is at least partly a function of the social appropriateness of her conduct vis-à-vis the sufferer.[7] My aim, then, is not to recommend the way in which a parent exercises compassion upon a child with birth defects over other ways, but simply to *describe* the oddities and special demands of the case.

Based on my own experience (which, admittedly, is a perilously small sample from which to draw conclusions), there seem to be three peculiar features of parental compassion for special-needs children. The first of these is the sheer *horror* that one feels upon learning that one's child suffers from a genetic disorder or congenital defect. Now, horror is an exceedingly complex emotion, an amalgam of at least four other emotions: *fear, guilt, eeriness,* and *grief.* Let me say a word about each of these in turn.

Take fear. When any child falls ill, her parents get worried. In most cases, the child eventually recovers from or outgrows the condition, and her parents' anxiety subsides. Of course, children get sick often, and so their parents are often anxious. Yet the very frequency of childhood illness can serve to reduce the intensity of parental anxiety over time. The first time your child gets sick is terrifying; but after going through a few dozen "bugs," fevers, and infections with her, you come to ex-

7. This is why an excess of compassion is just as blameworthy as a deficiency of it. Hence we rightly condemn both the parent who is too "distant" from her children and the nurse who is too "involved" with her patients. Of course, as Aristotle taught us, virtues that are practiced in ways disproportionate to what the circumstances call for are really vices, in this case indifference and overprotectiveness, respectively.

pect recovery and learn to handle each bout as it comes with a certain businesslike calm. But when your child begins to manifest strange, painful and/or debilitating symptoms that the doctor cannot at first explain, and when, after she undergoes the usual battery of tests and procedures, you finally get a positive diagnosis and learn that she has an untreatable, incurable genetic condition, your fear becomes "fixed," and at a rather high level.

But fear is soon joined by three other emotions. One is guilt, which arises when you realize that, biologically, you are the cause of your child's condition. Of course, at an intellectual level you may understand that no one is really "to blame" for this catastrophe. Nevertheless, you feel viscerally that you have committed some kind of outrage against your child, and that in the very act of giving her life you have condemned her to a great deal of agony.[8]

Another component of horror is a sense of eeriness. You find yourself gazing at your child and thinking, "She's different. She's abnormal. My God, she's a . . . freak!" This sense that you are in the presence of something monstrous may cause you to feel emotionally alienated from your child, from your family and friends, and even from yourself. The eeriness of the child's condition itself is compounded by the fact that caring for her places many new and onerous demands on your schedule, disrupts your familiar routines, and sends you at times to strange, distant, and forbidding places, such as radiology labs and wheelchair showrooms. It is as if you had been teleported to a different world.

Finally, the situation produces grief. You find yourself suffering the death, not of the child, but of all your cherished expectations for her life. You find yourself thinking that parenthood will not be a joyous task of helping your child to thrive, but a grim business of simply keeping her alive — which is to say, of keeping her in a state of constant discomfort, unpleasantness, pain, and social stigmatization.[9]

These four emotions blend with and feed back upon each other in bizarre ways to generate what I am calling "horror." For example, feeling that there is something eerie about your own daughter can itself be the cause of yet more guilt. Moreover, these emotions can produce still other ones, as when you begin to feel resentment toward the person who is the occasion of all your fear and grief . . . only to feel yet more guilt for resenting someone who has done nothing wrong.

Now the question arises: How is it possible, in the midst of such overwhelming emotions, to suffer with and for your child in appropriate and helpful ways? For as we have seen, compassion presupposes a certain detachment from the victim of suffering, even as it entails identification with her. This is what we meant by saying that compassion is a kind of "secondary" or "vicarious" suffering. But the parent of a child with a severe genetic disorder does not have the luxury of detaching herself from the victim's sufferings and limitations: They impose constant burdens and responsibilities that become, in time, a form of suffering in its own right. Suffering with and suffering for the child seem to shade into suffering from the child.

The second feature that affects, or distorts, the way in which parents express compassion toward children with genetic disorders is the chronic *fatigue* that eventually sets in. People who visit our home are astounded by the sheer number of times that Sarah asks for things. Her wants and needs are those of a highly intelligent and psychologically healthy teenager; but her capacity to fulfill these for herself is more like that of an infant. Of course, unlike an infant, Sarah can express herself verbally. Indeed, that is her sole means of controlling her environment, and she has become a master of self-expression and assertiveness. For this we are very glad, but we are painfully aware of its shadow side. She is prone to treat other people simply as instruments of her will, without bothering to observe the proper social conventions that indicate respect and gratitude: "Find my book, fetch my craft, turn on the TV, turn off the light, take me to the bathroom, reposition me in the chair, serve me dessert, set up a game, scratch my itch, get me a washcloth, do this, do that, run here, run there." On and on and on, all day, every day, forever. It seems absurd to make her say "Please" and "Thank you" every time. Indeed, it would be cruel, for it would only underscore her dependency in the most humiliating fashion. On the other hand, it is infuriating for those who love her and want to help her to be bossed around and manipulated.[10] Put sharply, paren-

8. It may, of course, be your spouse's genes, not your own, that caused the defect. In that case, you may feel resentment toward your spouse rather than personal guilt. These are certainly very different emotions, and they will have significantly different effects on your self-concept and on your relationship to your spouse. I suspect, however, that as alternative ingredients in the complex emotion of horror, resentment, and guilt (that is, blame and self-blame, respectively) function in more or less the same way. The same goes even if the doctors cannot determine which parent is the donor of the "bad" gene, for then one experiences both blame and self-blame by turns.

9. Upon receiving the crushing news that one's child has a genetic disorder or birth defect, parents may suppose that the future has suddenly grown unrelievedly bleak. They realize that many of the wonderful things they dreamed of for their child will never come true, and that many ghastly things they never imagined before may be in store for their child and for themselves. I suspect, however, that most parents soon discover that special needs children, like all other children, have an irrepressible capacity to bring their parents joy. Indeed, I have come to believe that one of the chief moral responsibilities that parents of special needs children bear is to show the wider community that human flourishing does not depend nearly as much as we tend to think on "perfect health" and body beautiful.

10. I shall bypass the question of how parents should provide moral and spiritual training for children whose capacity to *sin*, just like their capacity to do everything else, is affected by their impairments. This is a topic for another article. But to give the reader a sense of the peculiarities and subtleties of the problem, I might simply ask him or her to ponder the following question: How does one instill the virtues in a person who is physically incapable of practicing most of the vices?

tal compassion bids us do what we can to make her life as pleasant and normal as possible. But doing so turns our lives into an endless string of errands, favors, and interruptions. One is reminded of the ancient Greek myth of Sisyphus. He was sentenced to push a huge rock up a steep hill, but whenever he got it to the top, it would roll down again. In our case, however it is not a single boulder that we must push; it is ten thousand pebbles. This is why, at least in my own case, decisionist ethics is so unsatisfactory, and narrative ethics so attractive. As the parent of a child with so many little demands and requests, I need a sense that my life is not some kind of Sartrian "bad infinite," just one damned thing after another, but an integrated whole. I do not "decide" to take Sarah to the toilet each time she has to go: I simply do it. The question is, can I do it in a manner that will not make Sarah feel guilty or ashamed for having to ask me to do it? Only if I can feel, so deeply that I am hardly "conscious" of feeling, that such tasks are all of a piece, parts of the "storied" whole that is my life . . . and hers.

This brings us to the third distinctive feature of parental compassion for the child with severe disabilities: its apparent *futility*. The net result of carrying out the routines of good care sometimes seems to be nothing more than buying ourselves one more day of hassles. Milton Mayeroff has argued that one of the marks of genuine caring is its willingness to adjust itself to the condition of the "other," so that the other will grow:

> If caring is to take place, not only are certain actions and attitudes on my part necessary, but there must also be developmental change in the other as a result of what I do; I must actually help the other grow. To determine whether I am caring, I must not only observe what I do, feel, and intend, but I must also observe whether the other is growing as a result of what I do.[11]

Mayeroff is surely right that caring for someone means paying attention to her concrete and ever-changing needs and interests, and to the ways in which one's actions on her behalf actually touch and affect her. You think more about the other than about yourself, more about whether your conduct is helpful to her than about the fact that you are trying to help her. All of that certainly applies to the parent who must care for a child with severe disabilities. But is it true that the child "grows as a result" of what the parent does? The child's observable growth may be negligible. Indeed, when a child has a progressive disease, the care she needs simply to stay alive may have the grimly ironic effect of buying her the time for her symptoms to get worse. And surely *that* is not the kind of "developmental change" Mayeroff wants the caring person to promote. True, Sarah is growing in many other ways. She is a straight-A student, and is very gifted in vocal music, poetry, and some handicrafts. We have good reason to hope that she will go to college and find a career suitable to her capacities. So perhaps our parental efforts on her behalf would satisfy Mayeroff's requirements. But it is hard to imagine that Sarah will ever become "independent" or "self-determining," as Mayeroff believes that caring people should help the objects of their care become. And to the extent that Marilyn and I devote ourselves to enabling all three of our children to grow toward such goals, our labors for Sarah will always seem unavailing in comparison to those for the other two. Or at least the results will be meager in proportion to our investment of time, energy, and money. For me, the hardest thing about being Sarah's father is not the horror I feel at her sufferings and limitations, or the fatigue I feel in caring for her, but the aggravation I feel at the fact that it takes so much to accomplish so little. I want to see results . . . and so often I do not.

Thus, like all kinds of compassion, the compassion of the parent for a special-needs child is "double-sided." It reveals the characteristics of emotional identification with the victim's suffering and of concrete action ordered toward promoting the victim's well-being. But so overwhelming is the parent's emotional and physiological reaction to the sufferings of the child ("his own flesh and blood"), and so constant and arduous is the work that raising the child requires, that parental compassion may be said to differ significantly from, say, the doctor's compassion for her patients or the suburbanite's compassion for famine victims. The parent is constantly reminded of the child's needs, limits, and pains — and hence of his own responsibilities and inadequacies. Again, I am not suggesting that this constitutes some kind of special moral heroism. I only mean that the sheer uninterruptedness and interminability of the attention that the parent must give to the child, coupled with the extreme anguish he feels, turn parental compassion into a primary and direct, not merely a secondary and vicarious, form of human suffering.

The Peace That Passes Understanding

Parents must either learn to live with this, or they will eventually collapse. In the concluding section of this article, I discuss how I, for one, have learned to live with the horror, fatigue, and sense of futility arising from the task of raising Sarah.

Before doing so, I wish to make two things quite clear about the following argument: First, it is not meant as a "theodicy."[12] I have no interest in "justifying the ways of God," if that turns out to mean (as it usually does) giving a rationale for the evil that God "permits" in the world, and thereby giving some kind of cosmic legitimation for the suffering of little children . . . and their parents. Second, it is not meant as an implicit censure of those par-

11. Mayeroff, *On Caring*, 39.

12. For my views on theodicy, see "All or Nothing: Reflections on the Suffering of Children, Prompted by Albert Camus' *The Plague*," *Stauros Notebook* 18 (Winter 1998).

ents of special needs children who *have* "collapsed." I am no more interested in criticizing the coping abilities of other people than I am in justifying the ways of God. In particular, I am profoundly contemptuous of those who appeal to Scripture (for example, "God . . . will not let you be tempted beyond your strength, but with the temptation will also provide the way of escape . . ." [1 Cor 10:13]) in order to argue that those who buckle under the pressures of parenting a child with special needs must lack faith. I do believe in divine providence, but I do not believe that the causal weave of creation is so tight that God has specifically chosen just *these* parents to raise just *these* children, and has guaranteed these parents all the resources necessary for the job — if only *they* are willing. That is, nothing I am about to say should be used as a stick for beating those parents who simply cannot manage to hold themselves, their marriage, and/or their family together. Those who are defeated by the extraordinary demands that parental compassion imposes are themselves deserving of compassion, not reproach! My aim here is very modest and, in keeping with the autobiographical and introspective approach I have used throughout this essay, I simply will catalog some of the things I have learned from my situation that have immeasurably enriched my life. Whether I might have learned these lessons in some other way, I do not know. That God expressly caused Sarah's illnesses in order to teach me these lessons, I certainly do not believe. Here I shall content myself with stating the good that God has wrought for me, or rather, the conversion that God has wrought in me, through my situation.

Put quite simply, I have come to believe that you can live with suffering only if you learn how to grow from it.[13] You must construe your misfortunes as opportunities, convert your "fate" into "destiny," and search out what might be called the "surplus of meaning" implicit in every calamity. There is, of course, nothing especially novel about this belief. It is a central theme in the Bible and in much Jewish and Christian literature. The God in whom Jews and Christians believe is mysterious, and one of the most mysterious things about this God is that instead of rescuing us *from* our troubles (as we would like), God redeems us *through* them, and that instead of *reducing* our sufferings (as we would prefer), God uses them to *increase* our wisdom (see for example, Ps 37, Ps 73, and Job 42:1-6). Each person must apply this belief to his or her own situation.

How, then, have I grown from the horror of seeing my daughter's body turn into a statue? Certainly I will never "outgrow" the horror itself — or if I do, it will be I who have become monstrous! But I have nevertheless grown from this horrible spectacle by learning that human flourishing is possible in spite of it. When Sarah was first diagnosed with FOP, my hope was for a cure that would enable her to live a "normal" life. When that hope died, I was forced to ask whether it was still possible for her to live a "happy" life. And the answer was "Yes," provided that her happiness did not depend on attaining the ideals of physical beauty dictated by Madison Avenue and the ideals of economic productivity dictated by Wall Street. But then it dawned on me how thoroughly I had internalized those ideals and how I myself was imposing them on Sarah — and in so doing, helping to condemn her to a life of frustration and disappointment. But in refusing to be the servant of the powers and principalities that are hell-bent on adding emotional insult to my daughter's physical injuries, I was thrown back upon the Christian gospel, which offers a quite different view of human well-being, and one that does not assume that disabled people are disqualified from attaining it. For the gospel says that happiness is the result of standing in a right relationship to God and neighbor, and it is only sin, not suffering, that can prevent that. Thus, the horror of my daughter's condition exposed the demonic illusion under which I, for all my theological training, was still unwittingly laboring, namely that happiness is a function of our fame, fortune, or photogeneity. It brought home to me the liberating truth that faith, hope, and love are finally what make life worth living. Sarah can have these . . . and so can I.

And how have I grown from the fatigue caused by the constant care of someone with serious disabilities? Certainly the fatigue never goes away. Indeed, it gets worse and worse as I age, for all my efforts to keep healthy and fit, to furnish our home with adaptive equipment, and to make use of the available resources for respite care. The Scriptures admonish us not to "grow weary in well-doing" (Gal 6:9; 2 Thess 3:13), but even if one manages not to grow weary *of* well-doing, one eventually grows weary *from* well-doing. Lifting a delicate eighty-pound body twenty times a day, running countless errands, getting called in the night — all of these things have forced me to realize how far short my abilities and resources fall of the demands of our situation. This realization has been profoundly humiliating to me, being thoroughly steeped in the American myth of self-reliance and arrogant enough to believe that I can manage on my own. But it has also taught me why the Scriptures regard self-reliance as folly and insist that the experience of humiliation is an opportunity to learn the virtue of humility. Thus, my fatigue has exposed both my limits and my illusion of limitlessness. For this I am grateful. For I have become more able to accept help and advice from others without reluctance, resentment, or shame, and to depend less on my own strength and ingenuity. In other words, it has made me more open to the grace of God and more receptive to the kindness of others.

Finally, how have I grown from the sense of futility that dawns on you when all your labors on behalf of a child with a severe, incurable, untreatable, and progressive disorder produce such limited and ever-diminishing results? By now it will be obvious that, for me at least, the

13. See Viktor E. Frankl, *Man's Search for Meaning: An Introduction to Logotherapy*, rev. ed. (New York: Washington Square Press, 1963).

answer is to reframe the question, and to ask myself why I suppose that my "labor" must yield "results." Are there not certain activities (such as prayer) whose value is intrinsic to the doing of them and not dependent on any extrinsic outcomes that may accrue? Is not our tendency to estimate the value of an activity by its outcomes an example of the modern worship of the idols of production and consumption, hard work and competitive play? Does not our furious quest for greater profits, higher scores, faster times, better mousetraps, and bigger monuments to ourselves plunge us into a frantic state of perpetual dissatisfaction, rob us of the present moment, and force us to fixate on what we *will* do, *will* get, *will* make, or *will* have — tomorrow? Our need to see "results" for everything we do thereby renders any activity that is performed for its own sake, because of its inherent worth, suspect in our eyes. But that is precisely why caring for a child who will never be "cured" or "healed" or "rehabilitated" is so morally salutary. It *must* be done, regardless of the fact that it does not seem to accomplish anything, simply because it is *right,* simply because one cannot do otherwise without grave sin. The sheer immediacy of the child's needs, the sheer inescapability of the child's claim on our attention, can teach us to be fully *present* where we are, and not always rushing off to somewhere else.[14] Sarah has become for me a kind of anchor to the here and now, and caring for her a kind of sacrament, an outward and visible sign of the inward and spiritual grace that meets us *where we are* and *as we are.* And I am not only the minister of this sacrament, but, perhaps even more than Sarah, its beneficiary.

St. Paul urges us to "rejoice in the Lord always" (Phil 4:4), even in suffering, and even in the suffering that comes from suffering with and for others. And he promises that if we can manage to rejoice in all circumstances, we will experience the "peace of God, which surpasses all understanding" (4:7). I certainly do not rejoice *that* Sarah must suffer as she does, or that Marilyn and I must undergo the collateral sufferings associated with caring for her. But I am slowly learning how to rejoice *in* our sufferings, because it is there, more than anywhere else, that I have felt the inexpressible peace that comes when God begins to strip us of our selfishness and our illusions.

14. This, I suspect, is one reason that we are so obsessed with medical research in our day. It is not just that it promises to "relieve human suffering," but also that it purports to "give hope" to those who suffer; it allows them to live where modern people are most comfortable living: in the future. Moreover, I suspect this is why we are increasingly tempted to kill people whose sufferings are unrelievable (a practice we call, euphemistically, "euthanasia" or "physician-assisted suicide"), namely, that we cannot bear the presence of people whose sufferings are a standing reproach to the present limits of medical science, and who probably will not live long enough to benefit from the results of tomorrow's experiments. Their suffering thus becomes an embarrassment, even to themselves.

82 Love without Boundaries: Theological Reflections on Parenting a Child with Disabilities

Thomas E. Reynolds

In Dostoevsky's classic novel *The Brothers Karamazov,* the most morose and cynical of the three Karamazov brothers, Ivan, makes a confession to his brother Alyosha that is at once amazingly perceptive and disturbing. He states, "I never could understand how it's possible to love one's neighbors. In my opinion, it is precisely one's neighbors that one cannot possibly love. . . . It's still possible to love one's neighbor abstractly, and even occasionally from a distance, but hardly ever up close." While Ivan admits that selfless acts "up close" do occur, he claims they are for the most part disingenuous, stemming more from what he calls "the strain of a lie, out of love enforced by duty, out of self-imposed penance," than from genuine kindness or care. He goes on, "If we're to come to love a man, the man himself should stay hidden, because as soon as he shows his face — love vanishes."[1] Yes, people may *seem* altruistic, but they are either living in a dream world, loving humanity in some vague and general sense, or else repudiating themselves in an act of prescribed self-hatred. And for Ivan, neither option has integrity.

When I first read *The Brothers Karamazov,* I must admit that my initial reaction to the conversation between the two brothers favored the viewpoint of the tender and good-hearted Alyosha, who believes in the redemptive possibility of Christ-like love for one's neighbor in everyday life. Ivan's appraisal of humanity seemed hopelessly pessimistic. But now, upon further reflection, I have reconsidered my initial inclination. There is a hard truth to Ivan's perspective. Indeed, compassionate regard and self-giving care do seem easier and more alluring as general ideals rather than as particular realities. For, once we encounter other human beings and acknowledge their genuine difference from us, recognizing the peculiar ways they call us to respond to and affirm their uniqueness apart from our own agendas or expectations, it is difficult to love. At close range, face-to-face, the little details get in the way. But it is only at close range that love becomes active and real.

1. Fyodor Dostoevsky, *The Brothers Karamazov* (New York: Vintage, 1991), 236-7.

From Thomas E. Reynolds, "Love without Boundaries: Theological Reflections on Parenting a Child with Disabilities," *Theology Today* 62.2 (2005): 193-209. Used by permission.

Love is life-giving generosity, a compassionate regard that draws near and attends to the beloved for its own sake and with its good in mind. And such generous concern requires that we adjust or even give up our hold on reality as we see it and open ourselves to the unfamiliar, strange, perhaps threatening presence of another without imposing conditions that restrict or exclude their own particular capacities and ways of being. Genuine love signifies being summoned into a relational space of giving that happens outside the order of predetermined calculations and expectations, beyond the boundaries of "tit-for-tat" systems of exchange, beyond universal concepts of right and obligation. This is what makes love so difficult, indeed traumatic: Its gesture of giving hinges around letting go of those things by which we domesticate and manage reality so as to feel ourselves secure and in control.

The difficulty of which I speak here has been brought home to me with particular power in my own family life. I am now more sympathetic with Ivan's viewpoint because of the challenges my wife and I have faced in raising a child with chronic disabilities. My son Chris, who is fourteen years old, is diagnosed with Tourette syndrome, bipolar disorder, and Asperger's syndrome.[2] Abstract love from a distance is not an option here. It would be absurd to speak of loving my son in some disinterested or general sense. Indeed, it is hard to think of a more concrete example of love "up close" than familial love. And here lies the rub.

Chris's temperament, needs, and difficulties have challenged our family to the core, overturning conventional expectations about what home life might be. Attending to him has meant "letting go" of our own preconceived ideals and comfortable ways of showing care and loving kindness, and instead learning to listen — and listen deeply — to the ways his own human individuality requires affirmation, attending, and empowerment. This has been disconcerting and painful at times, and has demanded patient and persistent practice. But Chris's particular beauty radiates outward and serves something other than satisfying the needs of his parents. It is its own good, precious in its own right. Therefore, loving him as a parent — seeking to enable his future potential for fulfillment and happiness — is not merely something my wife, Mary, and I do *in order that* we receive some benefit in return, performed essentially for ourselves and with our own ends in mind. Rather, such love struggles and suffers, but in the process begins to cultivate a relation that rises above any economy of exchange or tit-for-tat policy of equivalency. In this way, acting with life-giving generosity toward Chris has meant moving beyond the boundaries of customary presumptions and anticipations about parenting. And the discoveries have surprised us, deepening our experience of love in unexpected and marvelous ways.

In this essay, then, I wish to explore the boundary-transgressive power of love through my own life experience as a parent of a child struggling with disabilities. There is truth to Ivan's view of human love, but I believe that there is a much richer tapestry woven into human relations than Ivan recognizes. I affirm the possibility of genuine love at close range, the possibility that love is more than an imposed duty or superficial feeling of benevolence for humanity in general, more than stoic self-sacrifice or a state of emotional elation that is a mile wide but an inch deep and all too easily manipulated to cloak self-serving agendas. Love is something already at work at the deepest level of existence, a creative and expansive relational power *into which* we enter as the ultimate source and consummation of our lives. I make such an assertion not simply because I am a theologian by trade, but because of the daily and unrelenting reality of caring for my son. Learning to attend to Chris with compassionate regard has been a life-transforming process that might best be expressed in religious terms as a kind of redemptive healing. Learning *from him* what it means to let go and genuinely attend to a life at once inseparably joined with yet distinct from my own, I have been persuaded that concrete love — up close — opens to a surplus of grace that can only be called divine. Present in the concrete, relational experience of love is a universal dynamism at work. Indeed, love is at the heart of the universe.

In a kind of reflective-autobiographical style that aims to be more suggestive than definitive, I shall describe how this is true in essentially two ways.[3] First, letting go

2. Tourette syndrome is a neurological disorder of the brain that causes involuntary movements (motor tics) or vocalizations (verbal tics), in many cases involving obsessive-compulsive and attention-deficit disorders. Bipolar disorder is psychiatry's name for manic-depression, which entails extreme mood cycling that, in children, often appears in symptoms like prolonged raging, separation anxiety, precociousness, night terrors, fear of death, oppositional behavior, sensitivity to stimuli, problems with peers, and so on. Asperger's syndrome is a high-functioning form of autism, in many cases associated with Tourette syndrome or bipolar disorder. For more information, consult Tracy Haerle, ed., *Children with Tourette Syndrome: A Parent's Guide* (Rockville, MD: Woodbine House, 1992); Ruth Dowling Bruun and Dertel Bruun, *A Mind of Its Own: Tourette's Syndrome: A Story and Guide* (Oxford: Oxford University Press, 1994); Mitzi Waltz, *Bipolar Disorders: A Guide to Helping Children and Adolescents* (Sebastopol, CA: O'Reilly, 2000); Demild Papolos and Janice Papolos, *The Bipolar Child* (New York: Broadway, 1999); George T. Lynn, *Survival Strategies for Parenting Children with Bipolar Disorder* (Philadelphia: Jessica Kingsley, 2000); and Tony Attwood, *Asperger's Syndrome: A Guide for Parents and Professionals* (Philadelphia: Jessica Kingsley, 1998).

3. I do not intend to moralize on the basis of my own experience. Neither do I seek to "use" my son merely as a theological example. My particular area of research is the philosophy of religion and global theology; so this essay draws me outside the box somewhat. While I do make ethical and theological claims, I seek more fundamentally to explore my localized experience in a way that draws upon theological and philosophical resources and begins — albeit tentatively — to formulate a vision that, for me, not only makes sense but offers constructive possibilities for fruitful living and humanizing relationships. To this end, I walk a tenuous line

and becoming open to another in love entails the traumatic but ultimately fulfilling experience of being released from self-enclosure, from the gravitational pull of ego-centeredness, toward a relation of mutual belonging that transgresses all boundaries and conditions. In this, secondly, love trades on and harnesses a relational power that encompasses the whole of reality, marking what philosopher Paul Ricoeur calls a "logic of superabundance"[4] that ripples through all things and is itself, I believe, the transformative presence of God. Love is at once a conversion to others and to God.

Love as a Conversion to an Other

Love is not something I do to someone, a skill I possess in myself. Rather, it is the nature of a certain correlation between myself and another, a certain way that we belong together. I am drawn into love by the proximity of an *other* who stands before me and lures me outward, summoning me to respond and attend to something otherwise than myself. I am thus caught up in an event that is larger than I, that occurs between me and someone else, a Thou with personal force of presence. And this in-between zone is the dynamic, expansive space of relation.[5] What is it that calls me outward? A particular presence reveals itself "up close" as precious in its own right, inviting me to pay attention to it, leading me beyond the orbit of myself. A concrete *other* calls out to me, "Love me." The Jewish philosopher Emmanuel Levinas calls this an experience of the "face," a confrontation with that distinct feature of personal presence that is irreducible to any condition or horizon of expectation.[6] Encountering another human being in this way means that I have been touched by a singular value that cannot be measured according to standards of exchange or absorbed into my own agendas or desires. This sets it at a distance from me, even as it entices me into relationship with it and makes me answerable to it. I am invited to recognize, show regard for, and celebrate an *other* for its own sake, to reveal to it its own value. Here lies the fundamental source of generosity. Love is born in the space of relation.[7]

The relational dimension that is established here, however, is not one of easy bliss. It can be quite disturbing and painful. For an *other* is by nature different, set apart from me. An other resists being grasped and treated like an object or possession, thereby putting me into question, disrupting my world — my way of seeing things and mapping out what should or should not be the case. For Ivan, it is precisely this disruption that human beings cannot handle, at least if they are honest, for the price is too high, causing too much discomfort, even anguish. The temptation is to turn away, to refuse relational connection.

When I think of my son in this regard, however, difficult questions arise. By all standard assumptions, it might seem that loving one's own child is a much easier task than loving a complete stranger, for there is a basic biological tie that stimulates instinctive family bonding. After all, is not a child an extension of oneself? And does this fact not assuage the temptation to turn away? The reality, however, is more complicated. Yes, Chris is my child. Yes, in ways too mysterious to fathom he reflects dimensions of me, a mirror of me genetically, emotionally, environmentally. But precisely this is also a source of difficulty: His own distinctiveness and the struggles that accompany it have made my own limitations, expectations, and ideals painfully obvious. We may ride waves on the same body of water, but we do not ride the same waves. Chris does not "fit the mold"; his peculiar difference sets him at a distance from the way I have set up parameters and calculated conditions that (often falsely) measure what counts for a "normal" family life, for the way my son "should" be if he is truly *my* son. Indeed, every child is born into a symbolic household upheld by many taken-for-granted assumptions about who he or she will be.[8] And Chris has challenged our "household"

between the "personal" and the "academic," between sharing my own struggles and being reserved for the sake of grappling with concepts and issues that transcend the scope of my own life alone. Theology cannot help but be personal and localized; but it is also public in a way that speaks to a community of human beings sharing common concerns and struggles. I offer these reflections in the midst of an ongoing struggle to love, hoping that readers may find in them something of value — regardless of whether they are parents or caregivers of a child in similar circumstances.

4. See Paul Ricoeur, *Figuring the Sacred* (Minneapolis: Fortress, 1995), chs. 11, 16, 19, 21.

5. The in-between space of relation is a central theme in the influential works of Gabriel Marcel and Martin Buber. For Marcel, see "On the Ontological Mystery," in *The Philosophy of Existentialism* (New York: Citadel, 1984), 9-46, and "The Ego and Its Relation to Others," in *Homo Viator: Introduction to a Metaphysics of Hope* (Gloucester, MA: Peter Smith, 1978), 13-28. For Buber, see *I and Thou* (New York: Charles Scribner, 1958) and "Elements of the Interhuman," in *The Knowledge of Man: Selected Essays*, ed. Maurice Friedman (Atlantic Highlands, NJ: Humanities, 1988), 62-78.

6. On the theme of the "face" see Levinas, "Signification and Meaning," in *Philosophical Papers* (Dordrecht: Kluwer, 1987) and *Totality and Infinity: An Essay on Exteriority* (Pittsburgh: Duquesne University Press, 1969). For a good introduction to Levinas, see the collection of interviews in *Ethics and Infinity* (Pittsburgh: Duquesne University Press, 1985).

7. Those familiar with Levinas will note that I am softening his language here in a way that places more stress on love as a correlative relation between me and an other. For Levinas, the relation to the other is tied principally to the ethical call of responsibility (see *Ethics and Infinity*, chs. 7-8). Levinas, in this regard, sees relation in ethical terms as a unilateral act of giving myself over to another, a gesture of service and self-sacrifice. In my view, this tends to overlook the celebrative, joyful, compassionate, and even playful elements in love as a mutually life-enhancing endeavor.

8. One need only attend a "Little League" baseball game to see this phenomenon in action — parents yelling at their kids to cajole them into performing "up to expectations." Parents also often seek, with great subtlety, to suppress in their children those visible signs of inadequacy that they find so uncomfortable to see in themselves.

to the core, rather pointedly forcing me to recognize the ways I have set up boundaries that close me in on myself and constrict my ability to be open to his unique way of being, indeed tempting me to turn away.

It is true that human beings need a predictable and safe world — a place to belong that orients us in life — and they often go to drastic extremes to insure its security against perceived threats. We are not ready-made for surviving and thriving in the world. Indeed, we are instinct-deprived and require anchoring in social relationships that create and preserve our needed sense of belonging and orientation. To this end, we cultivate cultural practices and establish social orders that organize relationships according to economies of utility and exchange. And these economies function by placing value on those things that benefit a corporate way of dwelling together. We thus learn from early in our youth what it means to be recognized as of worth, to have something to offer, to be a "somebody." Our sense of ourselves depends upon being included in a group, upon how we "fit" into its taken-for-granted framework of assumptions and values.[9]

It seems only too natural, then, that we make judgments and behave in ways that serve to place under surveillance or exclude those persons who do not "fit" within the boundaries of the system, who cannot be assimilated or integrated and are in effect "nobodies" because they do not present what is normative and esteemed as "of value." In fact, we come to fear such people. Why? Because their difference puts the economy of exchange into question. Their strangeness disrupts the predictable world and so disorients us.[10]

In the name of charity, special provisions may be made to accommodate the nobody, the outsider. We might establish care-facilities and offer aid. And, on the surface, this is well and good. But a deeper problem exists, for such acts of charity keep those who do not naturally "fit in" at a distance. Charity, as it is commonly understood, tends to favor the ideal of donation, giving those values we have in abundance and condescending to the "needy," who by our standards have been judged as lacking.[11] This, however, trades on and nourishes a disingenuous sense of privilege, presuming that those who receive aid are of no use and have nothing to offer in return. That the nobody is often institutionalized and isolated from mainstream society exemplifies the point.[12]

The problem here is compounded by the fact that love has so often been regarded as a disinterested and unilateral act of self-denial. According to such a view, genuine love can be only indiscriminate and general. I give to the *other* not out of an experience of the other's own value, but because of some external criterion of measurement by which value is conferred upon the other and by which I am directed to forget myself and attend to it. By this logic, however, love entails no real relation, no zone of mutual encounter. It is directionless. For the unique difference of another person — that which makes someone alluring and special — is disregarded and overlooked. Indiscriminate and disinterested love renders a person essentially anonymous, of no particular value at all. This is ironic, given that love is prized as an ideal form of relation. The motivation to love in this manner can be only out of a general sense of duty enforced by an authority (perhaps even God), or out of a self-centered desire to see oneself recognized by others (perhaps even God) as loving. In either case, the concrete *other* is not loved "up close." Indeed, it becomes easy to see how, in the name of charity, we may even resort to violence. Ivan's cynicism comes to the fore yet again, haunting us: An economy of exchange is still at work in disinterested self-giving, albeit it in a more subtle and difficult-to-recognize form than its utilitarian counterpart.

Hence, learning to love my son has meant putting aside presumptions about what love is, what is of value in a person, what being human entails. And it has been difficult to avoid falling into patterns of resentment and bitterness. Try as my wife and I might to change things, Chris's uniqueness resists conforming to our calculations of what family life should be. When we struggle, I must confess my first impulse is to feel disappointed, cheated, even betrayed by life. Chris's presence ruptures my planned and predictable world. Somehow things have gone awry, the pieces scattered in disarray, hopes deferred. Because of this, it is also easy to feel a sense of failure — as if I am flawed in some basic way, have done something horrible to traumatize Chris, or have not yet done enough to oblige Chris to accommodate to my vision of how a "normal" child should be, essentially fashioning him in my own ideal image. But after going through behavior modification programs, attending parent skill-building workshops, reading the disability literature, getting family therapy, and talking individually with psychologists and psychiatrists, I realize that Chris is neither simply an inconvenient burden nor an example of how I have failed.[13] There is something more basic and more powerful at work.

9. On this need for value orientation, see Charles Taylor, *Sources of the Self: The Making of Modern Identity* (Cambridge, MA: Harvard University Press, 1989), chs. 1-2.

10. Charles Taylor develops the multicultural implications of this point with great subtlety. See "The Politics of Recognition," in *Multiculturalism,* ed. Amy Gutmann (Princeton, NJ: Princeton University Press, 1994), 25-73.

11. This criticism of charity is made forcefully by Ada Maria Isasi-Diaz in "Solidarity: Love of Neighbor in the 21st Century," in *Lift Every Voice,* ed. Susan Brooks Thistlethwaite and Mary Potter Engel (Maryknoll, NY: Orbis, 1998), 30-9.

12. This point has been well established by Michel Foucault. See *Madness and Civilization: A History of Insanity in the Age of Reason* (New York: Vintage/Random House, 1973) and *Discipline and Punish: The Birth of the Prison* (New York: Vintage/Random House, 1979).

13. A resourceful book that has helped in this regard is Harold S. Koplewicz, *It's Nobody's Fault: New Hope and Help for Difficult Children* (New York: Times, 1996).

Chris's genuine otherness continually breaks through my self-pity and astonishes me as something surprisingly precious in its own right. His is a young life seeking to affirm itself, thwarted by conditions that he did not ask for and for which he is not responsible. This vulnerability and beauty rouse me to attend to him in ways that lure me outward beyond self-preoccupation. The first taste of this conjures something akin to repentance. Confronted by Chris's vulnerability, I am humbled and brought to recognize how my own needs, expectations, and ideals have closed me in on myself and set up boundaries that condition and thereby limit my capacity to be open toward him, to be there with and for him in *his* struggle. On occasions too numerous to mention, parenting has highlighted my own shortcomings, my own poverty and brokenness as a human being. And it has been difficult, in turn, not to despise myself for feeling resentful, for not being that ideal parent whose love is unconditional and untiring. Given Chris's needs, I could be more than I am. But these feelings of shame and guilt, natural as they are, often serve to further exacerbate a logic of self-enclosure, leaving Chris standing on the outside. I have asked myself more than once, "Is it possible to let go and step beyond this cycle of ego-centered paralysis?"

My relationship with Chris has helped me come to believe that it is possible, even if only gradually and in a finite sense. By honestly confronting and accepting my own vulnerability and limitations, I have grown in the capacity to let go of my need for control and to risk moving beyond my own fears and self-accusations, affirming Chris for who he is. There is, oddly enough, a strength in weakness, a "usefulness" in being of no use. Embracing our own weakness allows us to welcome weakness in an other. And it is by encountering weakness in an other that we come to discover it in ourselves. Jean Vanier, the founder of L'Arche, a network of communities that house people with intellectual disabilities, writes on this theme with particular poignancy. He states: "Weakness carries with it a secret power. The cry and trust that flow from weakness can open up hearts."[14] Why? Because we all at the core are vulnerable and receive our existence from one another.

We are frightened by those who do not fit in, who are different, because they threaten the existing order and bring us to confront our own vulnerability in the possibility of failure or rejection.[15] Accordingly, Vanier suggests that those who embody weakness and are considered "nobodies" in society's economy of exchange — that is, people with disabilities — "have profound lessons to teach us."[16] They invite us to move out from behind closed walls of false security and exclusion to acknowledge and accept our common human vulnerability. Jürgen Moltmann corroborates the point: "A person with disabilities gives others the precious insight into the woundedness and weakness of human life."[17] Disability is a profound symbol of universal human brokenness.[18] Of course, we can suppress or deny our human weakness, fleeing from it by pushing away those others whose difference more overtly exhibits it as something we deem ugly or dirty, flawed or deficient. But by doing this, we shun what is perhaps most human about all of us — the need to belong and to be recognized as of value by others.

Learning to embrace ourselves and others as we are in our weakness releases us from self-enclosure and empowers us to risk the openness of genuine relationship out of which love is born.[19] In this way, through time, I can learn to accept my common limitations as a human being and to forgive myself for those shortcomings — characterological or otherwise — that inhibit and condition my regard for Chris.[20] Even more, I can tell him "I am sorry" during times when I lose patience or misunderstand him, acknowledging my weakness openly. Time and again, Chris's forgiveness and patience with me have become a sustaining grace. His humor and sense of irony about things help lighten my often overwrought solemnity and seriousness (we often joke together about our shortcomings). The paradox here is that, far from inhibiting my ability to attend to Chris, such openness actually works to establish a more profound mutuality that cultivates compassionate regard. After all, compassion literally means to undergo, feel, or suffer with an other. The "with" is key. Compassion signifies a relation of involvement, of empathetic attunement.[21] Certainly this is a far cry from disinterested charity. It is, I suggest, nothing less than *communion*.

Communion is connection, solidarity, and reciprocal belonging, a way of living in the "between" zone of gen-

14. Jean Vanier, *Becoming Human* (Mahwah, NJ: Paulist, 1998), 40.

15. Ibid., 71.

16. Ibid., 45.

17. Jürgen Moltmann, "Liberate Yourselves by Accepting One Another," in *Human Disability and the Service of God*, ed. Nancy L. Eisland and Don E. Saliers (Nashville: Abingdon, 1998), 105-22, 121.

18. See Stuart Govig, *Strong at the Broken Places: Persons with Disabilities and the Church* (Louisville: Westminster/John Knox, 1989).

19. I should add here that Chris has a younger brother, Evan, who has learned this lesson in his own way. Evan is remarkably compassionate for a child of eleven years. He struggles with Chris but is open to his brother in ways that show his mother and father a thing or two about familial bonding and love.

20. That is to say, I can forgive myself for what I am and for what I am not. Indeed, Chris mirrors back to me certain things about myself that are sometimes unattractive and painful to acknowledge. And, even more, he has many positive features that I often fail to acknowledge for all my preoccupation with the difficulties.

21. The nature of compassion is beautifully portrayed in an article by Richard B. Steele, "Unremitting Compassion: The Moral Psychology of Parenting Children with Genetic Disorders," *Theology Today* 57 (2000): 161-74. Steele, a parent of a chronically ill daughter, suggests that compassion is both an emotion and a virtue, a spontaneous affective response to the suffering of another as well as an acquired trail of character that grows in its concern for the well-being of others.

uine relation.[22] In communion, I share myself with another person and together we begin to form a bond of mutuality by which we each become more than ourselves alone. Indeed, each "I" is now enlarged, becoming a "we" through identifying with and belonging to something larger than both of us. This does not mean that selfhood loses its integrity by being assimilated into the world of an other or a collective unity. Neither does it mean self-sacrifice. To the contrary, communion actually enriches and expands the integrity of the self. Communion establishes a relation that transgresses self-enclosure and its debilitating paralysis, enticing the self beyond the gravitational pull of its own orbit, thus serving as the fertile ground from which love can blossom in acts of life-giving generosity. Love leads us to become "larger" and more fully alive. In this way, communion involves self-transcendence, a liberating release from the deadness of fear-based individual isolation into a life-giving mutuality of vulnerability and empowerment. The result is a conversion of self to an other in relationship. Chris has taught me how to love him. And, in this, he also has grown.

All this happens, however, outside of the economy of exchange that dominates our social order. For the process begins neither because love is socially useful or expedient, nor because it is a general ethical duty or obligation owed universally to everyone, but because a particular, unique *other* bids me to attend to it as an exception, precious in its own right, apart from the standard rule. I do not love simply "in order to" fulfill a social prescription or become richer as a human being; these are byproducts of love that are misplaced if given priority as ends in themselves. I love because of the revelation to me of an other's intrinsic value.[23] Ethical codes originate in the deep fullness and joy of this experience, not in puritanical acts of self-effacement and asceticism. But it is also paradoxically true that such fullness and joy do come from love — as a surprise, an unsought bonus rather than a fulfilled objective. Why? Because another's vulnerability and singular beauty invite me to let go of conditions that reflect my need for security and control and to risk a relation beyond foreseeable calculations and expectations, so becoming response-able to that person's peculiar way of being.

There is an odd logic at work here: The *other* discloses itself as having a worth and value inborn, not parceled out according to predetermined conventions. From this fact, a question arises. If not according to external conventions, wherein does lie the value of this *other* whom I encounter, especially in its weakness? Where does such preciousness — in its singular instance — originate? In light of this question, I suggest, we enter into a distinctly religious space of orientation.

22. Vanier, 29.

23. Vanier makes the point that love begins with the revelation of value (22-3).

Love as a Conversion to God

In all of what is described above, a *fundamental affirmation* is at work that exceeds estimation and escapes containment within any finite framework of value-orientation.[24] I suggest that this is nothing other than a declaration of gratitude for the gift of existence, and it rises to the surfaces of our lives in a tenacious posture of hope. Thus, the particular presence of another person holds out before us a gift — the promise of mutual relation as an empowering grace. Because of this, we continually push past the apparent finality of senselessness and failure, destruction and violence, and risk-affirming life amidst and in spite of the reality of death. Such a gesture cannot help but transgress the limits of finitude, invoking a sense of the divine. Let us examine this in more detail.

Recognizing an *other* as vulnerable and precious means welcoming a gift, an empowering value. I am confronted suddenly, unexpectedly, by a beauty that is more than I arranged for or expected, that surprises me by its very appearance in weakness and fragility, in its capacity to be denied and broken. Astonished, I am awakened and lured into another way of being that suspends the laws of production and distribution so characteristic of the typical economy of exchange. Another, more primary, economy is at work here, one in which the other offers me nothing useful, nothing at all according to standard conventions — nothing, that is, but its own being. Here there are no calculable "reasons" that bid me to enter into a contractual relation with it in order that I may gain something in return, for it shows itself as a value precisely in its weakness, its inability to offer "anything" in return. Apart from all external conditions and utilitarian appraisals of worth, a human being stands before me in sheer givenness. And from this surprising, incalculable occurrence rises in me a profound acknowledgement: *To exist is good, a grace received.*

In its uniqueness and difference, an *other* is precious merely because it is. What is more, this *other* is a gift set before me, with whom I am invited into relation. This astonishing fact testifies to the sheer gratuity, as well, of my own existence. This is why another person's weakness has such extraordinary power: It contains not only the ability to bring me to acknowledge and accept my own weakness, luring me into the between-space of mutual relation, but also the ability to elicit in me the affirmation of existence itself as an inestimable value. Being is good simply because it *is* (compare the Augustinian formula, *esse que esse bonum est*).[25] All living creatures desire to be, to discover their value, and, in turn, to see their value

24. With some modifications, I am drawing the idea of an original affirmation from Paul Ricoeur. See *The Conflict of Interpretations,* ed. Don Ihde (Evanston, IL: Northwestern University Press, 1974), 341, 452.

25. In a rich and evocative way, Erazim Kohák testifies to this affirmation in his book, *The Embers and the Stars: A Philosophical Inquiry into the Moral Sense of Nature* (Chicago: University of Chicago Press, 1984).

reflected back to them through the recognition of others.[26] Seeing my son struggle to affirm life and wrestle with his condition has brought this truth home to me with particular poignancy.

Such an affirmation yields what Paul Ricoeur calls a "logic of superabundance," a surplus of value that exceeds quantification and control.[27] The fact of existence is a given, a grace received. I did not do anything to deserve to be, to justify the essential worth of being. My being at all is a mysterious gift handed over to me, for which I can take no credit. And its intrinsic goodness implies an extravagant generosity at work in the universe, a superabundance of grace that spills over and endows my life and all things with inestimable individual value. In all its concreteness and multiplicity, the universe is a horizon of excessive plentitude, a fathomless mystery given over continually and creatively in each moment of finite existence.

The recognition of this transcendent prodigality yields nothing less than *gratitude,* a gesture of thanksgiving by which we concede to the fact that we are radically dependent, not our own possession. As individuals, we are only part of a complex network of relationships that is itself contingent and gratuitous. After all, the universe might not ever have been. It is a wonder that there is something at all and not nothing. To be is to express value, and, accordingly, to sound an inescapable and original "thank you."[28]

Such gratitude, however, is no easy panacea or superficial optimism. It is tenacious and realistic. It affirms the gift of existence amidst those things that would deny or suppress it, giving cause for despair. It is not blind to tragedy; rather, it is an exigency that refuses to let failure and tragedy become the final word. This determination fuels the posture of *hope* — what Ricoeur calls a "passion for the possible" — that asserts the surplus of meaning and value over bland repetition, chaos, and destruction.[29] Hope refuses and pushes past all closures and finalities, even death. It is as if the fact of existence held out a promise that is now only partially and fragmentarily realized, opened up toward a future of possibility. Hope anticipates.

Caring for Chris is such a gesture of anticipation — holding out for his good, working toward a future of possibility for him even as limiting conditions impose themselves daily. Is this gesture in vain? Perhaps. But I cannot be in communion with Chris and believe so. When he cries out to me in anguish after a day of struggle, and I hold him gently, saying, "It will be all right, tomorrow is another day," what am I doing? Am I just placating him with verbal anesthetics? Am I perpetuating a delusion? At the core of my being, however, I believe that I am, instead, reflecting an acknowledgement that his existence is value-laden and full of promise despite its imperilment. Despite evidence that might lead to a contrary stance, I hope. And more, I seek to validate and cultivate in him the disposition of hope, reflecting back to him the giftedness of existence in his own being.

Hope survives, then, not by denying despair through some naive utopian vision, but precisely amidst the very real temptations to despair. Hope arises only with a felt sense of lack or deprivation, and in terms of an acknowledgement of vulnerability. Existence is tragic in its gratuity; it is fragile, conditioned by situations of interdependency that limit the scope of well-being and invariably cause discontent and suffering.[30] In this fragility, hope overcomes the possibility of despair by stretching forward, imagining concrete fulfillment that actualizes the fundamental affirmation of value underlying gratitude. But because such value is an inestimable and irreducible surplus, hope can never be brought to complete fruition in this life.[31] There are no guarantees, only finite and fallible approximations. Despair remains ever an option. Yet, beyond all probability, beyond all conditioned expectations, hope asserts that the heart of existence is not anonymous and indifferent, that the world is not merely a collection of interchangeable quantities reducible simply to their function in the whole. Hope asserts that the mysterious depth at the heart of things wills my being, Chris's being, all beings. Existence is trustworthy, holding out an eschatological promise: "It will be all right." In this, hope extends ever forward toward a fullness of life — indeed, a salvation — an exigency animated by gratitude.[32]

Precisely this tenacious sense of gratitude leads toward the religious sense of God. For the logic of superabundance trespasses all finite categories. Attending to an other as precious in its own right breaks the hold of all conventions and boundaries, signaling the trace of a horizon of excess value giving itself over in things, bestowing a grace to which we are indebted. This sense of giftedness rises from an inbuilt proclivity not merely to give thanks in some vacuous and inchoate sense, but as directed toward an unconditioned reference-point that symbolically houses superabundant value. As Mary Jo Leddy puts it, "In the awareness of having received something for free, there is a movement to wanting to acknowledge the giver."[33] Who is this giver? Ultimately, the gift we receive points to a plentitude that can only be called divine, a transcendent power of generosity from which existence originates and toward which hope is directed. Perhaps, then, it is not altogether outlandish to say that humans are disposed to something akin to

26. Ricoeur, *The Conflict of Interpretations,* 329, 452.

27. Ricoeur, *Figuring the Sacred,* 206-7, 279, 300.

28. On this sense of gratitude, see Mary Jo Leddy's insightful book, *Radical Gratitude* (Maryknoll, NY: Orbis, 2002).

29. Ricoeur, *Figuring the Sacred,* 207.

30. For an excellent discussion of the tragic structure of existence, see Edward Farley, *Good and Evil: Interpreting a Human Condition* (Minneapolis: Fortress, 1990), 29, 121-4.

31. Ricoeur, *Figuring the Sacred,* 211.

32. I am indebted here to Gabriel Marcel's articulation of hope in "On the Ontological Mystery" and "Sketch of a Phenomenology and a Metaphysic of Hope," in *Homo Viator,* 29-67.

33. Leddy, 51.

"praise," seeking out a higher power or object to worship that is personal, in some sense a life-giving will. The symbol "God" functions in precisely this way in Abrahamic and other monotheistic traditions.

Thus, the affirmation of being is simultaneously an affirmation of God. Genesis 1 expresses this in calling the world a "creation," fashioned with purpose and value by a God who declares that it is "good." We are created by God, endowed with integrity and value simply in the fact that we exist. And, as creatures with inherent worth, we are loved. This evident love underlying our pure giftedness enables us to profess that God not only is agential and personal, but also is loving, the ultimate life-giving generosity out of which we have our being. Love is thus at the heart of existence, not simply spread out in some homogeneous way, but rather taking on a particular, incalculable form with each created thing.[34] Each created thing is loved into being, fashioned to depend upon and be part of a larger, interconnected whole, the fabric of which is relational through and through. Because it is gratuitous, this whole — as a creation — is rooted in something much more significant than a distributive economy of exchange: It is rooted in an economy of grace.[35] No reason exists that could justify or account for the fact that we are loved into being by God; God's love is freely given. All things are good; nothing is taken for granted. Each depends upon the other, vulnerable and beautiful, attended to infinitely as unique by God. God is the life-giving relational power of the whole of reality.

Given this created interrelation of all existence, with its roots in God's own gratuitous love, finite human gestures of compassionate regard for others are themselves sacred invocations that participate in the infinite, life-giving generosity of the divine. Loving creatures is another way of loving God. When I affirm the goodness of an *other* and attend to it for its own sake, recognizing the unique value that inheres in its being, I am simultaneously affirming God, riding the wave of an excessive power rolling through all creation. This is what the New Testament writer expresses by stating: "Beloved, let us love one another; for love is of God, and the one who loves is born of God and knows God" (1 John 4:7). Human love for God may begin with a sense of gratitude to the divine, but ultimately it spills out toward creation, attending to the particular value of concrete *others,* up close and personal. Giving thanks to God entails giving recognition to the inherent worth of others — accepting the generosity that God has already given and letting it run over into the between-space of human relations. Because existence has been given to me, I give to others.[36] Existence is a gift overflowing with generosity. My given life is a gift to be life-giving for others, to be there for and with them. In this way, my love for God becomes manifest concretely in communion with others, and vice versa.

At this point, it is fitting that we note that, in *The Brothers Karamazov,* Dostoevsky offers us a counter to Ivan's despair-prone vision of love in the beautifully narrated story of a holy man, Father Zossima (Alyosha's teacher), and his encounter with a woman who doubts her faith. The woman asks him how we can prove the existence of God and the reality of life after death. Father Zossima replies that there is no proof available, though we can be convinced by "the experience of active love." He proposes that she strive to love her neighbor, suggesting that to the degree she perfects this task she will grow surer of the presence of God and her immortal soul.[37] But Father Zossima recognizes that this is no easy task. He goes on to say that active love is hard labor and requires fortitude, a "harsh and fearful thing compared with love in dreams" — that is, with love at a distance.[38] Up close, love is difficult, and thus Father Zossima exhorts the woman to be patient and forgiving of herself. In this, contrary to Ivan, Father Zossima preaches that love is not only possible; it is a window into the divine.

In terms of my relationship with my son, this truth has become apparent in two basic ways. First, my own religious sense of gratitude has been amplified by daily encounters with Chris's uniqueness. This is not to say, of course, that I am thankful for the privilege of not having to struggle in the way that he does. Rather, I have learned through his distinctive presence that each and every person, created and loved by God, has something wonderful to give the world. Consequently, because my life is itself a gift, I am more aware that it is not its own possession, but is meant to be given back, given in life-giving generosity.[39] The experience of sheer gratuity opens my world up to the fact that creation is not simply "there for me," something to be taken for granted or exploited for my own interests. Creation exists by, with, and for love. Specifically, Chris is not "there" to meet my expectations; rather, my wife and I have been given one who helps us see that our lives are meant to be invested in something outside the boundaries of all our expectations, something more humanizing — what Father Zossima calls "active love." Loving is a way of thankful celebration. And this has opened up the reality of God to me in radically new ways.[40]

Second, the nature of Chris's suffering has made the tenacity of hope something quite real. Hope keeps alive the possibility of his unique fulfillment as an individual

34. Ibid., 57. This is also one of the key points in Jonathan Sacks' book, *The Dignity of Difference: How to Avoid the Clash of Civilizations* (New York: Continuum, 2002).

35. See Ricoeur, *Figuring the Sacred,* 324-29.

36. Ibid., 325.

37. Dostoyevsky, 56. See also Leddy, 66-7.

38. Ibid.

39. See Ricoeur, *Figuring the Sacred,* 324-26.

40. Before his death, Henri Nouwen wrote a beautiful book depicting his experience of caring for a disabled person at Daybreak, a L'Arche community in Toronto. He writes that his sense of God's radical love was deeply enhanced, in fact pulling him out of a prolonged period of depression. See *Adam: God's Beloved* (Maryknoll, NY: Orbis, 1997).

— even if there is no "cure" available. And such hope has made the difficulties we have faced seem like stepping stones to his greater good, a good undetermined, yet palpably real. I cannot guarantee the future for Chris, but I do trust the grammar of the universe in a way that faith in God upholds and deepens. When he cries out to me in frustration, I can say to him without false pretense, "It will be all right." But God is no easy answer, an opiate for covering up Chris's pain and ignoring the pain of human suffering in general. If we are to be realistic, we must admit that, even as it is a gift, existence is also vulnerable and tragic. God is rather a way of naming the element of trustworthiness in the fragility of things, a way of persistently living out the affirmation that "it is good." My hope is that such hope blossoms in Chris, and that he will see his own giftedness as a child of God, loved into being by God.

Conclusion

In this essay I have pushed the logic of love to a certain extreme, with the intent of uncovering dynamics and assumptions at work in the character of my relationship with my son. While Chris's disabilities make our family situation somewhat unique, the essential ideas I have tried to express — tentative and exploratory as they may be — apply broadly not only to family life but to the human situation in general. To love without boundaries, to be open to an *other* and attuned to the other's singular worth outside standardized systems of economic exchange or utility, means to love without conditions, unconditionally. On the one hand, this is truly an impossible feat given the limitations of human life. The cultures and societies on which we depend rest upon conventional values, norms, and frameworks of orientation that govern reciprocity and provide for group accord. It is a fact that our relationships are unavoidably conditioned by "tit-for-tat" forms of value-exchange. Yet, on the other hand, there is also already operative in all economics of exchange an economy of grace, an economy of the gift that underlies and is presumed by all human acts of reciprocity, even if they are distorted by violence. The revelation of the *other* as precious in its own right is fundamental. Love, therefore, exists as a possibility within human relations — indeed, within reality itself — as a gratuitous gift. Communion is the inborn potential of human life.

Paul Ricoeur pushes this point further. He notes that the economy of grace, based as it is in a logic of superabundance, acts as a balancing corrective to the ideals of distribution and equality inherent in the notion of justice. Justice is grounded in a logic of equivalency that gives each its due. While this serves the social order well, legal forms of insuring "fairness" can be value-neutralizing, reducing all to exchange-equivalency. Rather than preserving society, this equalization homogenizes the concrete, singular value of differences. True, justice is an ideal measured according to the "golden rule." But "giving unto others as you would have them give unto you" can easily be perverted and drawn into a utilitarian mode of "I give *in order that* you will give." What protects against this perverse interpretation? Ricoeur suggests it is the commandment to love one's neighbor, to give as it has already been given unto you, even to the point of loving one's enemies. This "hyper-ethical" injunction runs counter to the utilitarian economy of exchange, not because it entails self-sacrifice, but because it is based in an economy of grace, an awareness of preexisting gratuity built into the nature of human relations from the beginning.[41] Neighbor-love stems from the revelation of value in another person that is basic to the way we find ourselves with others in the world. It points toward the always already possible reality of love, of mutual relation in communion, of compassionate regard and life-giving generosity.

Love is at the heart of existence. This is no sentimental assertion. It is a hard truth. And it is why caring for a child with disabilities has been a vehicle of redemption for me. Chris is teaching me how to love, to become more open to the revelation of his own particular value and, in turn, to become more able to attend to him in a way that reflects back to him his own particular value. As Jean Vanier proclaims, "To love is not just to do something for [others] but to reveal to them their own uniqueness, to tell them that they are special and worthy of attention. We can express this revelation through our open and gentle presence."[42] For me, this has been difficult and exhausting, but ultimately healing. Seeing Chris's own life-giving potential, his own distinctive way of loving, come into its own has been and continues to be a source of great joy. Chris is a creative, intelligent, funny, and deeply caring person with much to "offer" the world. The gift of my son has opened me to the unique differences of the many people and things that surround me, to which I would otherwise have been dead, and has allowed me to sense the power of God in a radically new way. Such deep satisfaction and joy are the fruits of a love that I could never have planned for or arranged on my own terms. And I am thankful.

41. Ricoeur, "Love and Justice," in *Figuring the Sacred,* 315-29.
42. Vanier, 22.

83 Welcoming Unexpected Guests to the Banquet

Brett Webb-Mitchell

The focus of this article is the challenge of discovering the place of people with disabilities in the life of a congregation or parish. The article's message is appropriate for such occasions of the church's life as Christian Family Sunday in May, or Access Sunday, or Ability Awareness Sunday, in which the gifts of all people, including those with disabilities, are emphasized. The names are fictitious due to confidentiality.

It is a cool summer morning in the hills surrounding Montreat, North Carolina, as parents gather together to share something they have in common: a child with a disabling condition. The topic of discussion for this gathering has to do with how their individual congregations first responded to the presence of their child with a disability. The parents' responses echoed one another as they told of congregations who, though scared at first, learned to at least accept that the couple had a child with a disabling condition. Most of the parents learned how to work with their churches so that their child had a place in Sunday school, youth groups, and worship. Karen, whose two children have cerebral palsy and developmental problems, shared that her congregation has grown to accept her children and involve them in the life of the church. But Joy, whose son has Down's syndrome, said that the support was fragile at best. She handles the fragile support by no longer expecting much from the church but expecting much from God to care for her and her family.

Other parents of children with disability and adults with disabilities have experienced the church's fragile support. Many people with disabling conditions are angry at their church for what feels like a lack of caring support, a feeling that carries over to their relationship with God. Some people with disabilities feel that "if a healthy child is a perfect miracle of God, who created the imperfect child?"[1] For the writer Bern Ikeler, the whole family questioned and cried to the Creator: "What is happening to us?" Born with cerebral palsy, Bern's birth was the death of the family's dream child. Unlike a child's physical death, a disability is a death that happens hundreds of times each day, as the child is unable to do what "normal" children could do.[2]

It isn't only those intimately connected with a person's disabling conditions who have felt the fragility of support. Church leaders have also admitted that their support is fragile. Many say they don't know what to say or do for the family of the person with a disability. Continually afraid of saying something offensive at the wrong time, offering help not needed, some choose to say and do nothing at all. Practical signs of support are absent, the comforting words of care needing to be expressed are rarely heard, and the gift of being present in the challenging times in a disabled person's life is withheld.

This reaction is not isolated to churches. We live in a society which has created a mistaken belief that shapes our collective perception, or misperception, of disabled people. We have been lured to believe that having a disabling condition means one is less than fully human, regardless of what combination of gifts and talents a person might have; people focus on one's physical, mental, or sensory limitations. The person with a disabling condition is a provocative, painful sign of our own mortal condition and something that we'd rather deny than accept.[3] As the theologian Stanley Hauerwas writes, the natural response to the misperceived stereotype that people with a disabling condition are in pain is to get away from the person as quickly as possible.[4] Such pain, or illusion of pain, is a threat to our communities.

Misperception of people with disabling conditions in congregations is not an individual problem, but is a dark, knotted disturbing thread that runs throughout the richly textured fabric of congregational life. The challenge for the church is to rightly perceive that some people have physical, mental, or sensory conditions that naturally impose real limitations in terms of what some can and cannot do in life. Members of Christ's community are to look *through* and *beyond* one's abilities or disabilities into the heart of the other person as we come to be with another person, whether in times of exuberant celebration or righteous anger. We are called to live with one another as a sign of God's grace.

The gospel message affirms this message of grace in Jesus' call to love God with our whole being, and to love our neighbor as ourselves (Matt. 22:39). Overt exclusion of another person in God's family, regardless of one's abilities or limitations, hurts and offends everyone in the body of Christ. Jesus emphasized that Christians share a spiritual bond of loving care with one another that transcends our own previous, natural kinship network. Jesus points to the existence of a spiritually ordered commu-

1. Helen Featherstone, *There's a Difference in the Family* (New York: Penguin Books, 1980).

From Brett Webb-Mitchell, "Welcoming Unexpected Guests to the Banquet," *Journal for Preachers* 16, no. 3 (1993): 15-19. Used by permission.

2. Bernard Ikeler, *Parenting Your Disabled Child* (Philadelphia: Westminster Press, 1986).

3. Ernest Becker, *The Denial of Death* (New York: Free Press, 1973).

4. Stanley Hauerwas, *Naming the Silences* (Grand Rapids: Wm. B. Eerdmans Publishing Co., 1990).

nity of neighbors, where we view ourselves as selves-embedded-in-community rather than disconnected individuals living in the selfish and unjust order of the scarcity paradigm.

The anthropologist Richard Katz wrote that the scarcity paradigm assumes we live in a world of scarce, nonrenewable resources, and only those who are rich or powerful enough may accumulate and control the distribution of these resources. Such resources include items like oil, water, and health care provisions for people with disabilities.[5] Whatever truth there may be in a scarcity of natural resources, the paradigm can be used to distort important elements of human life. Some, for example, perceive love as a scarce resource, fearful that they may squander it in the wrong places, thus using it all with no love left in reserve for an emergency. They are not aware that this is backward thinking as, in reality, the more we share love with one another, the more we have of it.[6] The scarcity paradigm is a justified description of our contemporary American culture, and from such cultural pressures none of us are exempt, including those of us who consider ourselves members of Christ's body.

Juxtaposed with the scarcity paradigm as applied to culture is the alternative spiritually ordered community of caring love found in Jesus' vivid description of God's kingdom. Throughout the gospel accounts, Jesus keeps pointing his disciples to the powerful reality of God's kingdom, the embodiment of a paradigm of abundance. The theologian Lesslie Newbigin suggests that the church on earth, called into existence by God in Christ, is a signpost on the arduous journey of faith, pointing the faithful followers of Jesus to the eventual, glorious destination.[7] Yet Jesus' vision of God's kingdom is more than our final destination. Instead, it is a different lens on reality, a new spiritually ordered lifestyle that we should be committed to living out in this time and place. The Church is called by God in Christ to live life on earth with an eye on this kingdom whenever we pray the Lord's Prayer: "Thy kingdom come, Thy will be done, on earth as it is in heaven" (Matt. 6:10, RSV).

In telling his followers about God's kingdom, Jesus used many parables, metaphors, and analogies. One powerful parable that reveals the inclusive nature of God's kingdom is found in the parable of the "Great Banquet Feast" (Luke 14:15-24, NIV). In this parable, Jesus takes the Old Testament image of the messianic banquet, which is prepared and hosted by Yahweh, surrounded by the leaders and prophets of the children of Israel, and uses this banquet as metaphor for God's kingdom, with God as the host and Jesus as the servant.

To summarize the story, the host has invited three prominent, wealthy men, and probably their families, to come to a large banquet he has prepared, but they all refuse him: they are all too busy with their ordinary lives to take time to accept the gracious invitation of the host to this most delicious love feast. The claim of God, the host, upon their lives was crowded out by things of this world. The host, angry at such a response, tells the servant, "Go out at once into the streets and lanes of the town and bring in the poor and maimed and blind and lame" (vs. 21). This most likely included the outcasts of Jewish society, like those people from the leper colonies, those who sat at the city gates and begged for money, and those who stole from others along the dark alleyways of Jerusalem to support themselves. At first, many probably stalled because they did not feel worthy and, in feeling unworthy, declined the invitation. The host then tells the servant to *compel* the people to come "that my house may be filled" (vs. 23).

In verse 24, the host is telling the servant the theological point of the story: None of those who were first invited will taste my dinner. But this isn't by God's choice to exclude them, for the invited guests excluded themselves from the banquet. Instead, these vacancies have been filled by those seen as the most unlikely, unworthy, unexpecting guests at this feast: the poor, disabled outcasts of Jewish society. By turning to these rejected, disabled citizens, those who hid along the highways and the hedges, God transforms them from unwanted social outcasts to wanted, honored, though unexpected guests in God's kingdom.

Are those who are disabled in this story symbolic of only those who are obviously disabled in our time and place? I think not. Those who are disabled in this story represent all humankind. The people who are disabled represent all who come before God every Sunday, all too aware of wounds and brokenness, filled with the painful knowledge that God knows the sinful condition of their lives, aware of their human limitations and inadequacies, yet who still dare to come and share in the love feast presented before us by the Creator, our all-forgiving host.

This simple yet profound parable of God's kingdom has important theological implications that may enable congregations to learn how to invite, welcome, and accept all who wish to enter the church, regardless of their abilities or limitations. To begin with, we need to remember that the good news of this story is that the invitation to God's banquet table is not based upon our human good works, nor dependent upon our money or fame. Instead, the invitation to this banquet is the gift of salvation extended through God's gift of grace. We are invited because God first loved us. The only way one can remain outside and away from the banquet is by consciously turning down the invitation. The New Testament theologian Joseph Fitzmyer writes, while we cannot save ourselves, we can very well damn ourselves.[8]

5. Richard Katz, "Empowerment and Synergy: Expanding the Community's Healing Resources." Unpublished manuscript (Cambridge, Mass.: Harvard University, 1984), p. 1.

6. This perception of love came from conversation with Stanley Hauerwas.

7. Lesslie Newbigin, *Sign of the Kingdom* (Grand Rapids: Wm. B. Eerdmans Publishing Co., 1980).

8. Joseph Fitzmyer, *The Gospel According to Luke X-XXIV*, Anchor Bible Commentary (New York: Doubleday, 1985).

This idea of grace runs contrary to the implied message of the scarcity paradigm that suggests that such love and attention are limited resources. The scarcity paradigm is overtly and covertly communicated to many people with disabling conditions and their families. Many leaders in congregations determine whether disabled persons may attend worship or other activities by asking the narrow question, "What can they *do* in worship?" as if God values us only for what we can do, not for who we are.

Nowhere in Scripture is it written that one has to be able to *do* certain things in order to worship God, or that one must have a specific I.Q., or behave in a socially appropriate fashion. It has been said by many who worship with those who have been labeled severely or profoundly mentally retarded that the greatest gift they give is the understanding that God valued and enjoys *who* we are, as children of God's, rather than what we *do*. What one finally gets out of worship is, most likely, between the "invited guest" and the "host" of the banquet.

Another important lesson is the realization that God's banquet table is big enough for all who are invited to sit at it and enjoy the meal. There is no sense in the parable that the banquet room was not big enough or overly crowded. There was so much space left over at one point that the servant was sent out a second time to bring in more people. Each person has a special place at God's table at this love feast. No one is shunted away from the feast.

This lesson from God's banquet table runs contrary to some congregations which may resemble a family reunion. When I grew up, dinners at the family reunions were in two different rooms. In the dining room was the adult table, with china, crystal, the best silver on an Irish linen tablecloth, with a floral bouquet, and candles in the center. Meanwhile, the kitchen was the room for the children with a rickety card table, folding chairs, plasticware, and no flowers. This room was child proof.

Many churches have opted for this family reunion paradigm for worship. Some churches have set aside a separate chapel, sometimes called the "Weeping Chapel," located off the main sanctuary for those with disabilities to sit in along with nursing mothers and their crying, babbling babies. Others, like those with hearing impairment, are tired of feeling closed out of the hearing-centered parish during worship and have established their own churches for the "deaf community" in their denominations. This parable raises a question for our churches: Is this banquet table symbolic of our gathering, willing to welcome all who wish to enter?

The final lesson is remembering that each person who was invited and came to the banquet had this one, essential characteristic in common: they probably had never seen themselves as members of a community of love. Each person had seen themselves as disconnected individuals, with long-forgotten family connections, isolated from the Jewish community. They were hiding in the alleyways because they were lonely outcasts.

Being brought together through the host's gracious invitation, gathered around a common table, they began to see that they were more or less like the other invited guests: they saw other poor strangers transformed, unexpectedly, into invited honored guests. Who would have thought that the one with leprosy, the outlaw, the disenfranchised, the undervalued, would be God's welcomed guests? All it took was accepting the invitation to come to God's feast.

What is moving in this story is that not one of these people could ever repay the host in kind, for none of these individuals had ever tasted or seen such splendor as was found at this feast. They simply accepted God's invitation to "taste my banquet." And in accepting this invitation, their lives were forever changed.

The challenge for the church is to break away from the dominant culture's misperceptions, which keep those who have a disabling condition on the disenfranchised, undervalued margins of our society. Jesus' parable establishes a vision of God's kingdom that gives those who are disabled a place not only close to God's heart in God's kingdom, but more importantly, the realization that the one with a disabling condition has an invaluable place in the living body of Christ. But Jesus' parable calls for nothing less than a conversion of the church's collective heart in inviting and welcoming all who wish to worship God. To God, people with disabling conditions are not just another special-interest social-action task force and project for our churches. This is more than social posturing; this is kingdom of God ethics ruling.[9] People who, by the way, have some real limitations and unique gifts, have been invited to have a seat at the finest meal at God's love feast.

The reason that Jesus told the parable is so that we have a practical, concrete vision of the loving nature of God's kingdom in our churches. Such love, writes social critic Wendell Berry, is never abstract: "It does not adhere to the universe of the planet or the nation or the institution or the profession, but to the singular sparrows of the street, the lilies of the field, 'the least of these my brothers and sisters.' "[10]

Jesus is calling the church to live its life according to this alternative vision of God's kingdom. We are to move over on the pews and discover that God wants all who wish to enter our sanctuaries to worship God to be free to do so. Christ's body is made of those who think they are able and those whom we have labeled "disabled," who appear less fortunate, broken, and wounded. We need these "unexpected guests" to be invited in order to be reminded that it is God in Christ alone who can heal the wounds deep within, and mend the broken hearts, because we are God's children. God's banquet table is a place for all Christians, upholding the common good of all members of Christ's body, on earth as it is in heaven.

9. John Howard Yoder, *The Priestly Kingdom* (Notre Dame: University of Notre Dame Press, 1984).

10. Wendell Berry, *Home Economics* (San Francisco: North Point Press, 1987).

84 The Body of Christ Has Down's Syndrome: Theological Reflections on Vulnerability, Disability, and Graceful Communities

John Swinton

Over the past year it has been my pleasure to manage a major research project within the United Kingdom that has sought to explore the spiritual lives of people with developmental disabilities and those who offer care and support to them. The project will last for two years and is funded by the Foundation for People with Developmental Disabilities, which is a London-based charitable organisation. We are right at the halfway stage at the moment, and some fascinating findings are beginning to emerge. The more we explore this area and take time to listen to and reflect on the experiences of people with developmental disabilities and their carers, the more apparent it becomes that this is an area of tremendous theological importance for the church. In this paper I want to share some of our initial findings and to give you a feel for the importance of the research and its implications for the ways in which we understand God, human beings, and what it might mean for the church to live as a graceful community.

I also want to begin to reflect on what practical theology actually is as a theological and a practical discipline. Many people still have an image of practical theology as simply providing "handy household hints for ministers." Within this understanding, practical theology is a parasitic discipline that simply takes data from the other theological disciplines and attempts to apply them to particular areas of ministry. While practical theology is certainly focused on enhancing the ministry and practice of the church, it is not simply a pragmatic discipline in the sense of merely applying theory. Practical theology is a deeply theological discipline which seeks to utilize the Kingdom of God as a critical hermeneutic, which can be used to test and determine the authenticity and faithfulness of the practices of the church. A basic definition would be that *practical theology is theological reflection on the praxis of the church as it strives to remain faithful to the continuing mission of the Triune God in, to, and for the world.* Practical theology seeks to guide and critique ecclesial praxis as the church strives to fulfil its role as "the hermeneutic of the gospel" (Newbigin 1989 pp. 222-223), which is that place where the gospel is lived out and interpreted to the world through the actions and character of its participants.

L'Arche as a Revelation of the Way That God Loves

Let me begin by clarifying what I mean by the term *profound developmental disability.* Within the United Kingdom the terminology used for this group of people is *learning disabilities;* elsewhere terms such as intellectual disability and mental retardation are common currency. The constant debate about the appropriateness and inappropriateness of terminology indicates the difficulties society has in conceptualizing and understanding this group of human beings. For current purposes I will use the term *developmental disability,* a term which has a degree of international recognition and acceptance. Developmental disability refers to a group of human beings who are deemed by the majority within society to have limited communication skills, restricted or no self care skills, significant intellectual and/or cognitive difficulties and who essentially will be dependent upon others for even their most basic needs throughout their lives. The important thing to bear in mind is that within a society that uses the criteria of independence, productivity, intellectual prowess and social position to judge the value of human beings, there will always be questions relating to the value of people with this profound type of disability.

As we have spent time with carers and support workers, one of the things that has struck us is the way in which people's lives and worldviews have been radically transformed through their encounters with people who have profound developmental disabilities. In encountering people with profound developmental disabilities in friendship, people's lives are changed, their priorities are reshaped and their vision of God and humanness are altered at their very core. What we are discovering is the occurrence of a process of *transvaluation* (Young 1990 p. 144) within which personal encounter with people with profound developmental disabilities initiates a movement towards a radically new system of valuing. In this paper I want us to think about this process of transvaluation and to reflect on the potential impact it may have for our theology and practice.

One of the contexts we have explored that has had a particular impact on us is the way of life manifested within the L'Arche communities. These communities provide a very powerful exemplar of Christian community. A focus on the L'Arche communities will enable us to understand this process of *transvaluation* and its implications for Christian theology and, in so doing, point us towards revised understandings and forms of practice which will enable each of us to live more faithfully as individuals and communities.

From John Swinton, "The Body of Christ Has Down's Syndrome: Theological Reflections on Vulnerability, Disability, and Graceful Communities," *The Journal of Pastoral Theology* 13.2 (Fall 2003): 66-78. Used by permission of *The Journal of Pastoral Theology.*

L'Arche: A Sign of Hope

The L'Arche communities are an international network of inclusive communities within which people with developmental disabilities live together with people who do not have such disabilities. L'Arche is founded on the Beatitudes, and in particular Jesus' teaching that the person who is poor in what society generally values is, in fact, blessed and has deep gifts to offer. L'Arche began in 1964 when Jean Vanier and his spiritual director, Father Thomas Philippe, invited two men with profound developmental disabilities, Raphael Simi and Philippe Seux, to come and share their life in the spirit of the gospel and of the Beatitudes. From this first community born in France and rooted in the Roman Catholic tradition, communities have been developed across the globe, the ethos being to share in the lives of people with developmental disabilities in the spirit of the Beatitudes.

L'Arche is a place where disabilities exist, but don't really matter. In other words, within L'Arche the meaning of disability is very different from the cultural norm. Within the philosophy and theology of L'Arche disabilities are not viewed as problems to be solved, but rather as particular ways of being human which need to be understood, valued and supported. The focus is on discovering ways of loving and living together that recognize the naturalness and beauty of difference and the theological significance of weakness and vulnerability. The L'Arche communities "seek to offer not a *solution,* but a *sign* — a sign that a society, to be truly human, must be founded on welcome and respect for the weak and the downtrodden" (L'Arche Charter in Young 1997 p. xv). In a divided world, L'Arche wants to be a sign of hope (L'Arche International 1999 p. 3). It wants to manifest in its life and practices that the way society is may not be the way of life within the Kingdom of God.

Loving for the Sake of the Other

At the heart of L'Arche lies the act of *welcoming* and *accepting.* Within the L'Arche communities people with developmental disabilities are accepted and welcomed not for what they can or cannot do, but simply for what they are. In like manner to the way in which Augustine claimed that we do not choose our friends but that they are brought to us by God, so the L'Arche communities welcome all people as *gifts* which have divine dignity, meaning and purpose. A gift is something to be received with thankfulness and love for what it is, not for what it might become or for what it is not. A gift is loved because it is a gift. Offering care and support to people with profound developmental disabilities is thus not an act of charity, but rather it is an act of *faithfulness* within which people respond in love to those whom God has given to them.

If those with whom we seek to have communion are understood as gifts, this opens up the possibility of loving people *simply for what they are.* While the suggestion that we should love people simply for what they are is not particularly revolutionary, it is! Societies such as our own thrive on meritocracy and processes of valuing that are contingent on the exchange of particular social, psychological or material goods. If we are honest with ourselves, most of our relationships are contingent on some kind of benefit that they will bring to ourselves. If our relationships no longer yield this benefit, we have a tendency to move on to forms of relationship that give us what we want. More significantly, this principle often transfers into our spiritual lives. Our relationship with God is often contingent on what God can do for us, rather than on what God is as God. And yet we expect God to love us simply for what we are. This is an important point. David Ford suggests that "the greatest mystery relates to God's love for us *for our own sake* and the possibility of loving God *for God's own sake*" (Ford 2002). What might it mean simply to love someone for their own sake; not for what they can do for us, but simply for what they are? What might it mean simply to love God for God's own sake, not for what God can do for us but simply for what God is? When we begin to think in this way it takes us to the heart of the contemplative vocation within which one turns one's whole being towards God, not because of what one can get out of God, but *for God's sake* (Ford 2002). Only when we can begin to love God for God's sake and to recognize that we are loved simply for our own sake, can we begin to understand what it means to *care for the other simply for their sake.*

Reclaiming this contemplative dimension of the pastoral task is vital for authentic pastoral praxis. The apparently simple practice of loving people for what they are, on a deeper reflection turns out to be a profound spiritual exercise which is vital for effective Christian pastoral care. Pastoral care with people who have profound developmental disabilities or indeed of any other human being does not begin with theories of psychology, rehabilitation or human development. *Pastoral care that is genuinely Christian begins with the development of forms of practice that will enable people to grow into the discipline of loving God for God's sake and loving others for their own sake.* To do this is much harder than learning an idea or a set of theories. To grow into loving God demands an approach that involves the whole person to be committed to love in every dimension of their being. To grow into loving God demands that as we think about training pastors and pastoral carers, we must expand our standard models of pastoral care and begin to reflect on the role of such things as hospitality (welcoming the stranger as a gift), spiritual direction, contemplation, and spiritual exercises. To grow into loving God demands a community that can support such practices. The L'Arche communities in their practice and liturgical exercises offer a model of such a community and an indication that it might be possible.

L'Arche: A Community of Gentleness

Within the theology of L'Arche, people with developmental disabilities represent the poor. This poverty is manifested most clearly in the relational isolation and the cultural marginalization which marks the life experience of many people with this and other forms of disability (Swinton 2002; 2001; Vanier 1992). As Vanier puts it,

> The greatest pain is rejection, the feeling that nobody really wants you "like that." The feeling that you are seen as ugly, dirty, a burden, of no value. That is the pain I have discovered in the heart of our people. (Vanier 1998 p. 8)

Couple this marginalization and rejection with the very real spiritual, and material poverty which people experience and it quickly becomes clear that the label of "poor and oppressed," is not altogether inappropriate (Curtice 2001). The L'Arche communities recognize this poverty and seek to begin their theology from and shape their practices according to the perspective of "the poor." However, the theology that underpins L'Arche is not a theology of liberation. While L'Arche would wish to emphasise that God is in some sense "on the side of the poor," the form of practice which emerges from this assumption by that is significantly different from the perspective of liberation theology.

The Weakness of God

At the heart of the theology of L'Arche lies a particular image and understanding of God. Within the L'Arche communities God is perceived to be with the poor not as a revolutionary political presence, but as a fellow sufferer who comes into the midst of the poor in weakness and in vulnerability. As Vanier puts it:

> It is true that at times Jesus became powerful, he worked great miracles but he feared that people would see in him the Powerful One who does great things instead of the One who seeks to give Communion. So Jesus becomes little, he is humble and this because we admire the powerful, but we love the little ones, the child, the person who is weak, fragile. So for me Jesus is the One who becomes little, he is God who becomes little, who hides in the poor, the humble, the weak, the dying, the sick; because all these people who are particularly fragile are longing for love and I see this as the mystery of Jesus and that Jesus is love. Just as God is Love. Jesus is Love. (Vanier 1997)

It is in the immanence of Christ that the presence of God is experienced and revealed within the L'Arche communities. In this sense there are significant similarities between the theology of L'Arche and Bonhoeffer's theology of the suffering God as he sketches it in *Letters and Papers from Prison*. For Bonhoeffer, the power of God is revealed in the suffering of Christ.

> God is weak and powerless in the world, and that is exactly the way, the only way in which he can be with us and help us. Matthew 8:17 makes it crystal clear that it is not by his omnipotence that Christ helps us, but by his weakness and his suffering . . . only a suffering God can help. (Bonhoeffer 1953 p. 164)

Bonhoeffer's point is not that the suffering God is helpless but rather that recognizing this dimension of God enables us to see new strands of a providential understanding of life. Within L'Arche, these new strands of providential understanding are actualized and worked out within the day-to-day practices of the community. God is with the poor, not in triumphalistic revolution, but in the weakness and vulnerability that is experienced in the everyday tasks of living together in community. Importantly, within this theological frame, the weakness and vulnerability of people with profound developmental disability is not indicative of lives that are incompatible with being fully in God's image. Quite the opposite, the experiences of people with profound developmental disabilities remind us of dimensions of God which have been hidden by our culture's preference for such things as power, strength and intellectual prowess.

Idolizing Jesus and the Practice of Gentleness

Francis Young suggests that perhaps one of the most significant dangers for the church today is the idolization of Jesus (Young 2002). To idolize Jesus is to create Jesus in our own image and according to our own desires. It is to turn Jesus into a kind of superman who is available and willing to grant our every desire, extrapolate us from every unpleasant situation and protect us from the pain, suffering and sickness which is a mark of life in a fallen world. When this happens, we remove the scandal of the cross, the theological significance of Jesus' littleness and the strength of his weakness and vulnerability that reveals the wisdom of God. When we confuse earthly with divine power we miss dimensions of God that are vital. When power is equated with might, strength and force, we forget the significance of tenderness, gentleness and weakness, dimensions of the incarnated Son which are crucial for a balanced understanding of the Trinitarian God.

The communal life of L'Arche and its daily encounters with the weak, the poor and the voiceless, and its ability to see God in the midst of these encounters, moves us away from idolization and the flight from suffering, and forces us to consider the possibility that the nature, character and actions of God may be radically different from our socially constructed norms. When such a reframe occurs, we are freed to explore "hidden" dimensions of God that open up new possibilities for more faithful pastoral practices.

If we take one particular attribute that is often overlooked this will help make the point. David Ford, in reflecting on the Beatitudes and the life of Christ, suggests that the life of the L'Arche communities calls forth the theological significance of *gentleness*. Ford, reflecting on the Beatitudes and Jesus' statement "I am gentle" (Matt 11.29), makes an important point:

> Gentleness is usually practiced, if at all, as an optional extra, as something peripheral and secondary. It is nothing short of a revolution to imagine it at the heart not only of individuals but of groups and institutions. But might that be part of the implication of Jesus' beatitude? Is it conceivable? (Ford in Young 1997 pp. 82-83)

To conceive of our political institutions being governed by the liberatory principle of gentleness, is indeed unthinkable. To think of our churches governed in ways that are gentle and kind may, sadly, be equally as unthinkable. Yet, Jesus says, "I am gentle." He does not say that he acts gently, or that gentleness is a good thing to practice. Jesus says that he *is* gentle; Jesus who *is* God who *is* love and in whom the image of God is revealed *is* gentle in his very being. Gentleness is not an option; it is an aspect of the Divine.

Gentleness sits at the heart of the gospel. Jesus who is God enters the world in weakness and vulnerability, dependent on the gentleness of his parents for his very survival. Gentleness was a mark of Jesus' ministry: gentleness as he gathered children to himself; gentleness as he dealt with the weakness and faithlessness of his disciples; gentleness as he moved his disciples from "discipleship to friendship," a movement which is very much part of the dynamic of L'Arche; gentleness towards women, the outcast, the marginalized. And gentleness was a mark of his death and resurrection. The gentleness of the women who held and washed his broken, lifeless body, the gentleness of his words towards Thomas in spite of all his doubting. What would our churches be like if we began to develop the virtue of gentleness? How would we lead, how would we teach, how would we relate to one another, what would be the shape of our friendships?

This might sound idealistic, impractical, and unworkable. Yet it is precisely this dynamic life of gentleness that is modelled and indeed is a fundamental mark of the way of life within the L'Arche communities. It is clearly this eschatological sign of hope that L'Arche offers to church and world. By living gently,

> in the everydayness of attending to bodily functions, feeding and defecating, in the gentle gestures of washing and dressing . . . the sanctity of bodies [is] acknowledged, but in a context in which their transformation is not through miracles, but through the recognition of God's love and power in mutual need. (Young 2002)

What develops within L'Arche is a *theology of gentle presence* "in communion and community, a kind of contemplative mode of waiting on God with one another, which is far removed from political activism or patronising charity" (Young 2002). God is the one who comes amongst the poor, who suffers with and for the poor, and in so doing transforms their poverty and brokenness into gentle humanness. Within L'Arche, liberation comes when people begin to let go of their individuality and to recognize the strength that comes from gentleness, mutuality, weakness and brokenness. In this way, those who accompany people in L'Arche find themselves, who they are, what they are, why they are, in the mutuality of life with others.

The Body of Christ Has Down's Syndrome?

This idea of finding oneself in the mutuality of life together with others is important, not least because it reflects something of the dynamic of the Triune God. As John Zizioulas has helpfully highlighted in his reflections on the trinity, God in God's self is a community within which each person is constituted by the other. Each receives their existence in and through their relationship with the other. God does not exist in *what* God is for others, but rather in *who* God is for the particular other (Zizioulas 1989).

Scottish philosopher John Macmurray (1961/1995) has pointed towards a similar relational dynamic within the development of human personhood. For Macmurray, it is a person's *relationships* that constitute who they are as persons. "I exist as an individual only in personal relation to other individuals. Formally stated, I am one term in the relation 'You and I' which constitutes my existence" (1995 p. 28). We become who and what we are according to the types of relationships that we experience within our lives. In a very real sense we are responsible for the construction of the personhood of those whom we choose to relate with. This, of course, is a distinctively counter-cultural position. In Neo-Liberal capitalism, one is offered a picture of human beings as fundamentally individual beings who choose to get together to form societies, the primary purpose of which is to attain the greatest benefits for the largest number of individuals. In other words, the individual *precedes* the community. In contradistinction, Macmurray's formulation proposes that the individual is the *product* of a community.

For most of us this process of becoming persons-in-relation occurs through interaction with a very limited range of people. For the most part, those whom we become persons-in-relation with are pretty similar to ourselves. We develop our sense of self, our personal constructs, and we shape our interpretative universes in dialogue with our partners, pastors, friends, our academic colleagues, and so forth, all of whom, for the most part, are people who are not particularly different from ourselves. We then assume that the theology and practices which emerge from such interactions are both real and universal. Most people rarely get the opportunity to become persons-in-relation with people whose life experience and existential perspectives are significantly different from their own.

This begs the question of what it would be like if individuals and communities were to become persons-in-relation, with people who have profound developmental disabilities, in other words, to genuinely allow their perspective on the world to become part of their own inner space. How would we approach the task of theology, ministry and being the church, if our theology was constructed in dialogue with people who have profound developmental disabilities; if their "worlds" were brought into dialogue with that which the majority perceive to be the "real" or "normal" world, what would we see? What kind of persons would we become, and how would that fresh perspective affect our understandings?

Friendship-in-community

The primary emphasis within L'Arche is on friendship and mutuality-in-community. Within the L'Arche communities it is in and through the relationship of friendship that people are transformed, "reconstructed," and taught how to be persons-in-relation with those whose life experiences are very different from the perceived norm. It is the relationship of friendship that brings about the type of transvaluation I mentioned earlier. When they meet together in mutually constructive relationships of friendship with people who have profound developmental disabilities, assistants are changed and transformed in significant ways. When this happens, disability is transformed from pathology into mere difference and a genuine mutuality is initiated within which assistants learn not only to respect difference, but actually to incorporate dimensions of the experience of disability into their own lives and worldviews. As the assistants encounter people with developmental disabilities in friendship and community, and as they internalize the radically different experience and perspective that is offered to them, they begin to reconstruct who they are as persons-in-relation both with God and with other human beings. In so doing, their sense of what it means to be human and to live humanly is expanded to include what might be described as the "normality of difference," that is, the recognition that difference need not be pathological and indeed may be a source of blessing and revelation.

The Scandal of the Incarnation

This provides assistants with the type of theological perspective that has been explored thus far. It also gives them the freedom to reflect on dimensions of God using concepts that initially appear distinctly odd, to those who have not had this "conversion experience," but on reflection are deeply challenging. In closing, let me give you an example. One Roman Catholic woman, who is an assistant in a L'Arche community in Belfast in Northern Ireland, told me how difficult it was to live in what remains in many senses a war zone. As a Catholic woman, she is terrified to go out on the streets of Belfast. If she went out alone, she would be in genuine danger. However, if she goes out with the people from the L'Arche communities, she knows that she is always safe. Indeed, when she has people with developmental disabilities with her, she, a Catholic woman, has even been allowed to speak in Protestant churches, which is extremely unusual. As we chatted, she made a quite startling statement. "*When I am with people with profound developmental disabilities I can go anywhere and say anything. The barriers come down on both sides of the divide, Protestant and Catholic. Wherever they go, they seem to bring peace and reconciliation, and if I am with them I can share in that peace. You know, I sometimes wonder if Jesus had Down's syndrome.*" She wasn't joking. She wasn't using metaphorical language; her question was wistful but genuine. Her encounters with people with profound developmental disability had changed the way she saw the world and the ways in which she understood God to be at work in the world. Gone were images of God as the bringer of liberation and peace through God's great power and might. Instead the possibility of God being very different from assumed norms, incarnating God's self within the body of a person with Down's syndrome, opened up new vistas of hope, reconciliation and revelation. Because she had entered into relationships with people who have profound developmental disability, and allowed those relationships to challenge the way in which she viewed herself, God and the world, the suggestion that Jesus with Down's syndrome was neither shocking nor outrageous. Why should it be? Nowhere in scripture are we told what Jesus looked like, what his IQ was, why people ridiculed him. We simply assume that Jesus looked "something like us." Why do we construct an image of Jesus that is able-bodied and able-minded? Why do we explicitly or implicitly assume that Down's syndrome is inequitable with the divine image? Think for a moment on the implications of Stanley Hauerwas' reflections on the relationship of disability to the Body of Christ:

> God's face is the face of the retarded; God's body is the body of the retarded; God's being is that of the retarded. For the God we Christians must learn to worship is not a God of self-sufficient power, a God who in self-possession needs no one; rather ours is a God who needs a people, who needs a Son. The Absoluteness of being or power is not a work of the God we have come to know through the cross. (Hauerwas 1986 p. 178)

Within the L'Arche communities, such an image of God springs naturally from deep relationships of friendship with people whose life experiences challenge us to think and to re-think the nature of God and the glory of Christ, who is the image of God.

At this point, some readers may be wrestling with the dissonance between such an image and our personal image of God as all-knowing, all-powerful and so forth. But the challenge is to wrestle with *why* such an image may be disturbing; and if it is disturbing, what that might mean for how we *really* feel about people with developmental disabilities who are made fully in the image of the triune God who is love. If this image is incompatible, then how does that affect the way in which we view and act towards people with developmental disabilities? If the image is compatible, what does that say to our understanding of what it means to be human and to live humanly in community and fellowship with people with profound developmental disabilities?

Conclusion

In conclusion, what I have tried to do in this paper is to illustrate and work through some of the dynamics of practical theology as a reflective, theological discipline. By reflecting on the lives of people with developmental disabilities as they are conceptualized and worked out within the communities of L'Arche, we have been offered a number of significant theological challenges which call for significant changes in pastoral practice. We have learned the significance of such practices as spiritual direction, contemplation, friendship, hospitality and gentleness for a balanced, trinity-centred model of pastoral care which is applicable not only to the care of people with profound developmental disabilities, but to all people. This of course is exactly as it should be. In the end, people with profound developmental disabilities are no different from anyone else. They have the same needs, desires, hopes, and dreams, and they are foundational to the shape and texture of the Body of Christ. Indeed, if we take seriously Paul's metaphor of the Body of Christ, it is clear that their disabilities are our disabilities and our disabilities are their disabilities. *The Body of Christ has profound developmental disability.* What we all need to do is to begin to learn what it means to live gracefully and faithfully within that Body within which there is "neither Jew nor Greek, slave nor free, male nor female . . . black nor white, able bodied nor handicapped" (Young 1991 p. 192), only friends working out the meaning of friendship-in-community.

References

Bonhoeffer, Dietrich. (1953) *Letters and Papers From Prison.* London: SCM Press Ltd.

Curtice, L. (2001) The social and spiritual inclusion of people with learning disabilities: a liberating challenge? *Contact* 136 pp. 115-23.

Ford, David. (2002) What is the Wisdom of L'Arche? Unpublished paper presented at a conference for theologians held at 'La Ferme' in the community of L'Arche in Trosly-Breuil, France, in December of 2002. (Quoted with permission from the author)

Hauerwas, Stanley. (1985) *Suffering Presence: Theological reflections on medicine, the mentally handicapped, and the church.* Edinburgh: T&T Clark Ltd.

L'Arche International. (1999) *A Covenant in L'Arche: An expression of our spiritual journey.* Paris: L'Arche International.

Macmurray, John. (1961) *Persons in Relation.* London: Faber and Faber.

Macmurray, John. (1995) *Persons in Relation* London: Faber.

Newbigin, Lesslie. (1989) *The Gospel in a Pluralist Society.* Grand Rapids: Eerdmans.

Swinton, John. (2002) *Resurrecting the Person: Friendship and the care of people with severe mental health problems.* Nashville: Abingdon Press.

Swinton, John. (2001) *A Space to Listen: Meeting the spiritual needs of people with learning disabilities.* London: The Foundation for People With Learning Disabilities.

Vanier, Jean. (1992) *From Brokenness to Community* (The Wit Lectures). New York: Paulist Press.

Vanier, Jean. (1997) Jesus Christ, humble and poor, all-powerful. *Tertium Millennium* N.3/July 1997 http://www.vatican.va/jubilee_2000/magazine/documents/ju_mag01071997_vol-iii-index_en.html.

Vanier, Jean. (1998) The need to be loved. *Shepherds of Christ: A spirituality newsletter for priests.* A publication of Shepherds of Christ Ministries.

Vanier, Jean. (1999) *Becoming Human.* New York: Paulist Press.

Young, Francis. (2002) The Contribution of L'Arche to Theology. Unpublished paper presented at a conference for theologians held at 'La Ferme' in the community of L'Arche in Trosly-Breuil, France, in December of 2002. (Quoted with permission from the author)

Young, Francis (Ed.). (1997) *Encounters with Mystery: Reflections on L'Arche and living with disability.* London: Darton, Longman and Todd.

Young, Francis. (1990) *Face to Face: A narrative essay in the theology of suffering.* Edinburgh: T&T Clark.

Zizioulas, John. (1985) *Being as Communion: Studies in personhood and the church.* London: DLT.

CHAPTER THIRTEEN

Research Ethics and Experimental Subjects

Abuses of human subjects by researchers, especially researchers who were also physicians, constituted a main catalyst of the emergence of the field of bioethics. After the Second World War, the world was horrified to learn that Nazi physicians had conducted experiments upon human beings against their will. Jews, gypsies, and others were subjected to painful and often lethal experiments, ostensibly for the sake of information useful to the war effort. People were especially outraged that physicians had taken part in these experiments. The Nuremberg Tribunal condemned the behavior of these physicians, and in authoring the Nuremberg Code — the first international guidelines for the conduct of research with human subjects — it set as the first principle of research that the voluntary consent of participants is absolutely required before they may be made subject to a scientific experiment.[1]

Issued in 1947, the Nuremberg Code did not have an immediate effect upon the practice of research in the U.S. Perhaps it was easy enough to believe that only Nazis and fascists would compromise the well-being of humans in scientific experiments, that only those without a moral conscience needed such guidelines. But the 1960s and 1970s proved otherwise, as story after story of research abuses in the U.S. emerged. The first to come to light was the hepatitis study at the Willowbrook State School, an institution for children with mental disabilities. In the 1950s and 1960s, researchers infected healthy children with profound mental disabilities between the ages of 3 and 11 with various strains of the hepatitis virus, to study the natural history of the disease and later to test the effectiveness of gamma globulin against the disease. Then in 1966, Henry K. Beecher, an eminent physician and researcher at Harvard, published a study in the *New England Journal of Medicine* criticizing twenty-two specific medical experiments involving human subjects, all of which had been published in medical journals.[2] Two years later, Henry Pappworth published a book similarly criticizing five hundred studies.[3]

In 1972, the story of the Tuskegee Syphilis Experiment broke.[4] Beginning in 1932 and continuing for forty years (or twenty-five years after the Nuremberg Code was published), the U.S. Public Health Service sponsored a study of the natural history of syphilis in untreated black men in Tuskegee, Alabama. The men involved in this study were not told the purposes of the study; they were not given a truthful diagnosis; and after an easy and effective treatment for the disease — penicillin — was discovered in 1945, they were not offered that treatment. All along, articles from the study were published in reputable scientific journals — seventeen articles in all between 1936 and 1972.

A major outcome of the public outrage over these scandals was the development of federal guidelines for human subjects research in the U.S. In 1972, the U.S. government mandated that all proposed experiments receiving federal funding be reviewed by an Institutional Review Board (IRB), a group comprised of professionals (sometimes also community representatives) to evaluate the scientific merit and ethical compliance of proposed research using human subjects. Over the next nine years, a series of panels and government agencies crafted the federal regulations governing human subjects research, referred to as 45 CFR 46.[5] Finally promulgated in 1981, the

1. The Nuremberg Code, http://ohsr.od.nih.gov/guidelines/nuremberg.html (accessed February 20, 2009).

2. H. Beecher, "Ethics and Clinical Research," *New England Journal of Medicine* 274 (1966): 1354-60.

3. H. Pappworth, *Human Guinea Pigs* (Boston: Beacon Press, 1968).

4. For the definitive study of the Tuskegee case see James Jones, *Bad Blood: The Tuskegee Syphilis Experiment* (New York: Free Press, 1981). See also Emilie M. Townes's chapter on the Tuskegee study in her book *Breaking the Fine Rain of Death: African American Health Issues and a Womanist Ethic of Care* (Eugene: Wipf & Stock Publishers, 2006; previously published by Continuum Publishers, 1998), pp. 81-106.

5. Code of Federal Regulations, Title 45, Public Welfare, Department of Health and Human Services, Part 46, Protection of Human Subjects, Revised and Effective June 23, 2005. Available at: http://www.hhs.gov/ohrp/humansubjects/guidance/45cfr46.htm (accessed February 20, 2009).

federal regulations are periodically updated to reflect changes in the nature of scientific interventions and contemporary understandings of human subjects.

The federal guidelines reflect the two foundational principles that came to shape medical ethics through the 1970s and 1980s: autonomy and utility. Following Nuremberg, autonomy — now cast as the principle of informed consent — remains the first and foremost principle of human subjects research. All persons participating in an experimental protocol must be fully informed as to the nature of the research and their participation in it, and must freely and voluntarily consent to such participation. Yet autonomy alone is not sufficient. For an experiment to be ethical, it must also have a positive ratio of benefits to costs or risks or harms. In all cases, experiments must be scientifically well designed, so as to produce useful information. Previous laboratory and animal studies must provide support for the hypothesis in question. And in seeking to demonstrate that the intervention is beneficial, risks of harm to the human subjects must be as minimal as possible. Even if a human subject agrees to let a researcher cut off her hand in a badly designed experiment, that consent alone will not render the experiment ethically justifiable. Or, even if the potential benefit to scientific knowledge and even humanity is certain and profound, one cannot enroll a subject in an experiment that will surely kill him, even if he consents. That, too, would be unethical.

Most conversations on research ethics from 1968 forward have been shaped by these basic parameters. Yet any study of this literature quickly reveals how ill is the fit between the practice of research and these principles. For example, they provide little help on the question of animal research, apart from the ideal of inflicting minimal harm. Our opening selection by C. S. Lewis on "vivisection" offers at least one perspective on this question (selection 85).

Nor do they provide needed guidance on a critical question: the identity of the participants. When shaping their guidelines for experimentation, Nuremberg and various other national and international bodies presume a specific scenario: that of a researcher (a pure scientist) and a human subject (a healthy volunteer) who meet as equals for the common reason of altruistic commitment to the common good through the advancement of knowledge. This scenario forms the backdrop for the profound essay by the Jewish philosopher Hans Jonas, "Philosophical Reflections on Experimenting with Human Subjects" (selection 86). This classic piece on experimentation raises still pertinent issues. It introduces into the conversation the inconvenient third party always operative in the question of human experimentation, but whom the category of autonomy has a hard time conceptualizing, namely "society" (as in "research is necessary for the good of society"). Jonas also raises the important question of obligation — might persons, healthy or sick, have an *obligation* to participate in scientific or clinical research? This was a live question in the early days of research ethics, one that has somewhat fallen by the wayside in recent decades. In addition, Jonas addresses the important notion of the "conscription" of consent; it is worth reading through his essay to get a thick understanding of the meaning and sufficiency of "free and informed consent."

Jonas closes his essay by raising a question that seems odd in retrospect: Should patients be research subjects? For Jonas, fundamental moral wisdom tells us patients are the "last and least" group who ought to be conscripted into research; yet he acknowledges that some must participate in research if it is to achieve its goal. Are patients able to understand the research and be fully informed? Might their disease, its physiological burden, the pain it brings, not to mention the effects of medication, hamper their ability to understand? Might their fear of pain and death compromise their freedom? Most patients who participate in experimental protocols do so because proven treatments have failed and they feel they have "no other options" — in other words, they feel they "have no other choice." How does this change the ethics of the situation?

Many patients agree to participate in experimental research protocols because they think (hope, pray) that the experimental agent might help them. The purpose of research, however, is to prove whether or not an intervention might work.[6] Many clinical trials are not even designed to prove effectiveness. Phase I trials — the first step that all trials using human subjects are required to complete — are designed solely to test toxicity. If the intervention does not harm the subject, then the protocol is permitted to advance to a Phase II trial, where researchers continue to test safety but also begin to gather preliminary data on effectiveness. Only Phase III trials — a phase that the vast majority of research protocols never reach — are designed to test effectiveness. Yet today, with the diagnosis of a serious illness, many patients will scour the Internet, looking for research protocols in which they might enroll, seeing them as their "last hope."

In spite of Jonas's reservations, by the mid-1970s, the literature on human experimentation evidences an important shift, a transition from speaking of researchers and subjects to speaking of physicians and patients. Undoubtedly, one reason for this shift was a change in the pool of available research subjects that occurred in the early 1970s. As Adriana Petryna notes in her contribution to this chapter (selection 87), until the 1970s the primary population to which researchers turned in search of subjects was prisoners; at that time, 90 percent of pharmaceutical testing being carried out in the U.S. involved prisoners. In light of the scandals in the late 1960s and early 1970s, this practice came under severe criticism and was heavily curtailed — for, can prisoners really give "informed consent"? Can their participation be fully "volun-

6. See M. Therese Lysaught, "Reconstruing Genetic Research as Research," *Journal of Law, Medicine, and Ethics* 26 (1998): 48-54.

tary," given that their autonomy is constrained in just about every other way?

And if this is the case with prisoners, what about other potential subject populations with compromised ability to understand or to give complete and voluntary consent — those with mental disabilities (as in the Willowbrook experiment), those with mental illness, children, pregnant women, the comatose, the newly dead, fetuses, embryos? Students of human subjects research will note that much of the literature from the 1970s through the 1990s seeks to adjudicate the propriety of involving various potential subject populations in research. It seems obvious that such persons should not participate in medical research. Yet critics of such a strict application of the Nuremberg standard have argued that such experimentation is necessary to test the safety and effectiveness of treatments for children (and persons with mental disabilities or mentally ill patients) — whether the treatments are traditional, innovative, or investigational. Unless some of them are involved in controlled tests, whole classes of persons (the mentally ill), persons with rare diseases, or persons with child-onset diseases risk becoming what are called "therapeutic orphans."[7]

And what of the "physician-researcher"? Does such a hyphenated identity, which is now very commonplace, introduce an intrinsic conflict-of-interest? We expect physicians to be committed to the "benefit of the sick," as the Hippocratic Oath put it long ago. Certainly to benefit the sick, we expect the field of scientific-clinical medicine to acquire knowledge that physicians can use. But ought physicians be the primary agents working to gain this knowledge, with their own patients . . . or with others' patients? This question was mainly a philosophical question in the late 1960s, when Hans Jonas penned his essay. But the changing economics of clinical research — when physicians can make an average of $7,000 for each patient they enroll in a clinical trial (at least in 2001) — makes the question more pressing. Might such economic incentives, or even the incentives that come with being the principal investigator on a major industry-funded trial, introduce irreducible conflict-of-interest? In the end, to whom or to what is the physician-researcher finally loyal?

Moreover, how might these incentives, by which physicians are encouraged to enroll their own patients in clinical trials, affect patient informed consent? We noted in Chapter Six that because of the very nature of illness, combined with the structure of the contemporary hospital or clinical setting, a significant imbalance of power exists between physicians and patients, even with patients who are high-powered elsewhere in life. Patients frequently depend upon their physicians; sometimes they acquiesce to a physician's request out of fear of losing care or because they trust the physician's commitment to their well-being. And sometimes, to be sure, they urge their physicians to try "the latest" thing, before it has been proven safe or effective. The issue is only exacerbated by the fragmentation of medical care, when a particular patient — especially one with a serious condition — will be seen by specialist after specialist, many of whom will not understand the patient to be her or his primary responsibility.

The nature of human subjects research has changed so radically over the past twenty years that some background information on the scope, structure, and nature of international biomedical research is necessary for beginning to understand the contemporary questions. No longer is biomedical research about university-based scientists or indefatigable physicians working in their labs, interacting occasionally with individual patients. Biomedical research has become an enormous international, multi-national industry in its own right. Several legislative and policy changes in the early 1980s laid the groundwork for this transformation. Among these, two are landmarks. First, the Bayh-Dole Act enabled universities and small businesses to patent discoveries derived from taxpayer funded research sponsored by the National Institutes of Health (NIH) and then to grant exclusive licenses to drug companies. Second, the Hatch-Waxman Act (1984) extended monopoly rights for brand-name drugs.[8]

Marcia Angell, M.D., who spent twenty years on the editorial staff of the *New England Journal of Medicine,* closing her career there as Editor-in-Chief, outlines a series of significant concerns about the pharmaceutical industry in her book *The Truth About Drug Companies: How They Deceive Us and What To Do About It.* Here she explains, in lay person's terms, how clinical, scientific research works in the U.S. She cites the nature of Contract Research Organizations (CROs), the size of pharmaceutical research alone (a $7 billion industry in 2001), and the number of Americans enrolled in clinical trials — some 2.3 million people in 2001! Given these new industrial and economic realities, considerations of questions in research ethics must move beyond an oversimplified picture of a conversation between a physician and patient.

Adriana Petryna, in her essay "Globalizing Human Subjects Research" (selection 87), continues Angell's argument, but steps back to look at the industry involving human subjects on a global scale. Petryna focuses primarily on pharmaceutical research, but her findings are pertinent to research in other areas as well. How do we think about "outsourcing" (formerly known as "offshoring") something like human subjects research? What constraints are placed on the "informed" part of informed consent when working across significant cultural differences? How free, voluntary, and autonomous can consent truly be in impoverished populations who usually lack access to the most basic medical care, let alone in-

7. See, e.g., Richard A. McCormick, "Proxy Consent in the Experimental Situation," *Perspectives in Biology and Medicine* 18, no. 1 (1974): 2-20.

8. For more on this history see Marcia Angell, *The Truth about Drug Companies: How They Deceive Us and What To Do about It* (New York: Random House, 2004), pp. 3-20.

come, voting rights, or any other human rights? Which issues of justice are raised when researchers and pharmaceutical countries turn to "overseas" populations for the testing of drugs and medical interventions that will be distributed primarily in contexts where people have the means to pay for them? Who, in other words, bears the burdens of medical research, and who reaps the benefits? Given the massive number of people now involved in clinical trials here and especially abroad — in contexts where regulations and guidelines may be much less stringent than ours or even non-existent — how can oversight be orchestrated and abuses of subjects — of real persons — be avoided?

The closing chapter by Thomas Nairn, "The Use of Zairian Children in HIV Vaccine Experimentation: A Cross-Cultural Study in Medical Ethics" (selection 88), provides a case-study for the issues raised by Angell and Petryna. Nairn provides helpful background on the question of enrolling children in medical experimentation and shows how these difficult questions become far more complicated by issues of international politics, industrial economics, research pressures toward discovery and publication, and more. Nairn's study makes clear that it is largely the poor who bear the risks of experimentation while the middle and upper classes will benefit from the research. What used to be the case on a local scale — when it was the poor in the wards and clinics of teaching hospitals that bore the risks of experimentation — is now also occurring on a global scale. The sort of "preferential option for the poor" documented by Petryna and Nairn is not quite what Christian social teaching means by that principle.

This chapter, we hope, will leave you with more questions than answers, but they are critical questions, precisely the questions that Christians and bioethics must turn to in the near-term. For as we come to the end of this introduction and turn to what attentive readers will note is a very short chapter, a lacuna must be recognized. Christian and Jewish theologians and philosophers such as Hans Jonas, Paul Ramsey, Richard McCormick, Al Jonsen, and Karen Lebacqz were key figures in shaping the normative principles for human subjects research, both through their contributions to the literature of the nascent field of bioethics as well as through their participation in national commissions.[9] Yet since the publishing of the federal regulations in 1981, human subjects research *per se* has received little if any attention from scholars situated in theology or religious studies. Much theological ink has been spilt on particular issues — e.g., stem cell research or embryo research — but apart from an occasional essay,[10] the basic philosophical and institutional parameters for human subjects research have been largely ignored by the religious academy, in spite of the dramatic changes in human subjects research outlined above. The time has come for the theological academy to again turn its attention to questions regarding human subjects research. Informed by our tradition's advocacy for the poor, its attention to embodiment and the material reality of human life, its critique of structural injustices, its greater ability to recognize and name idolatry, and three decades of scholarship in political economy,[11] theologians may well be able to again find themselves at the forefront of charting new directions in the ethics of human subjects research, directions that move past principles that have come to mask more operative dynamics toward a framework that fully respects human persons and advances healing without sacrificing human bodies on the altar of profit.

SUGGESTIONS FOR FURTHER READING

Childress, James F., Eric M. Meslin, and Harold T. Shapiro, eds. *Belmont Revisited: Ethical Principles for Research with Human Subjects* (Washington, D.C.: Georgetown University Press, 2005).

Elliott, Carl. "Guinea Pigging," *The New Yorker* (January 7, 2008).

Elliott, Carl. "Not-So-Public Relations: How the Drug Industry Is Branding Itself with Bioethics," *Slate* (December 15, 2003).

Final Report of the Advisory Committee on Human Radiation Experiments. *The Human Radiation Experiments* (New York: Oxford University Press, 1996).

Fisher, Jill. *Medical Research for Hire: The Political Economy of Pharmaceutical Clinical Trials* (New Brunswick, NJ: Rutgers, 2009).

Lysaught, M. Therese. "Docile Bodies: Transnational Research as Biopolitics," *Journal of Medicine and Philosophy* 34 (2009): 384-408.

Mirowski, Philip, and Robert Van Horn. "The Contract Research Organization and the Commercialization of Scientific Research," *Social Studies of Science* 35 (2005): 504-48.

9. John H. Evans, *Playing God? Human Genetic Engineering and the Rationalization of Public Bioethical Debate* (Chicago: University of Chicago Press, 2002).

10. See, e.g., M. Therese Lysaught, "Respect: or How Respect for Persons Became Respect for Autonomy," *Journal of Medicine and Philosophy* 29 (2004): 665-80; and M. Therese Lysaught, "Gene Therapy: A Test Case for Research with Children," in *Genetics and Ethics: An Interdisciplinary Study*, ed. Gerald McGill, 216-52. St. Louis: St. Louis University Press, 2004.

11. Cross-over resources — those that see the connections between theological claims and socio-economic realities — abound for such analysis. Clearly the resources of liberation theology, not as readily available in the mid-1970s, would inform such a new framework. The economic analyses produced by advocates of global health, particularly the Institute for Health and Social Justice at Harvard University, are informed by just such a perspective. Interestingly, it is this putatively secular institute that is not afraid to use the word "idolatry" to refer to the relentless pursuit of profit at the expense of the health and well-being of the poor (see the penultimate subhead in Ch. 1, "The Idolatry of Growth," in Jim Yong Kim et al., eds., *Dying for Growth: Global Inequality and the Health of the Poor* [Monroe, ME: Common Courage Press, 2004], p. 44). John Paul II in his encyclical on globalization entitled *Sollicitudo Rei Socialis* also invokes the role of idolatry in neoliberal economics (§ 31 and 37). That "idolatry" may not translate well into secular, public dialogue does not mean that it might not be an accurate analytical category.

Petryna, Adriana. *When Experiments Travel: Clinical Trials and the Global Search for Human Subjects* (Princeton: Princeton University Press, 2009).

Washington, Harriet. *Medical Apartheid: The Dark History of Medical Experimentation on Black Americans from Colonial Times to the Present* (New York: Doubleday, 2006).

85 Vivisection

C. S. Lewis

It is the rarest thing in the world to hear a rational discussion of vivisection. Those who disapprove of it are commonly accused of 'sentimentality', and very often their arguments justify the accusation. They paint pictures of pretty little dogs on dissection tables. But the other side lies open to exactly the same charge. They also often defend the practice by drawing pictures of suffering women and children whose pain can be relieved (we are assured) only by the fruits of vivisection. The one appeal, quite as clearly as the other, is addressed to emotion, to the particular emotion we call pity. And neither appeal proves anything. If the thing is right — and if right at all, it is a duty — then pity for the animal is one of the temptations we must resist in order to perform that duty. If the thing is wrong, then pity for human suffering is precisely the temptation which will most probably lure us into doing that wrong thing. But the real question — whether it is right or wrong — remains meanwhile just where it was.

A rational discussion of this subject begins by inquiring whether pain is, or is not, an evil. If it is not, then the case against vivisection falls. But then so does the case for vivisection. If it is not defended on the ground that it reduces human suffering, on what ground can it be defended? And if pain is not an evil, why should human suffering be reduced? We must therefore assume as a basis for the whole discussion that pain is an evil, otherwise there is nothing to be discussed.

Now if pain is an evil then the infliction of pain, considered in itself, must clearly be an evil act. But there are such things as necessary evils. Some acts which would be bad, simply in themselves, may be excusable and even laudable when they are necessary means to a greater good. In saying that the infliction of pain, simply in itself, is bad, we are not saying that pain ought never to be inflicted. Most of us think that it can rightly be inflicted for a good purpose — as in dentistry or just and reformatory punishment. The point is that it always requires justification. On the man whom we find inflicting pain rests the burden of showing why an act which in itself would be simply bad is, in those particular circumstances, good. If we find a man giving pleasure it is for us to prove (if we criticise him) that his action is wrong. But if we find a man inflicting pain it is for him to prove that his action is right. If he cannot, he is a wicked man.

Now vivisection can only be defended by showing it to be right that one species should suffer in order that another species should be happier. And here we come to the parting of the ways. The Christian defender and the ordinary 'scientific' (i.e., naturalistic) defender of vivisection have to take quite different lines.

The Christian defender, especially in the Latin countries, is very apt to say that we are entitled to do anything we please to animals because they 'have no souls'. But what does this mean? If it means that animals have no consciousness, then how is this known? They certainly behave as if they had, or at least the higher animals do. I myself am inclined to think that far fewer animals than is supposed have what we should recognise as consciousness. But that is only an opinion. Unless we know on other grounds that vivisection is right we must not take the moral risk of tormenting them on a mere opinion. On the other hand, the statement that they 'have no souls' may mean that they have no moral responsibilities and are not immortal. But the absence of 'soul' in that sense makes the infliction of pain upon them not easier but harder to justify. For it means that animals cannot deserve pain, nor profit morally by the discipline of pain, nor be recompensed by happiness in another life for suffering in this. Thus all the factors which render pain more tolerable or make it less totally evil in the case of human beings will be lacking in the beasts. 'Soullessness', in so far as it is relevant to the question at all, is an argument against vivisection.

The only rational line for the Christian vivisectionist to take is to say that the superiority of man over beast is a real objective fact, guaranteed by Revelation, and that the propriety of sacrificing beast to man is a logical consequence. We are 'worth more than many sparrows',[1] and in saying this we are not merely expressing a natural preference for our own species simply because it is our own but conforming to a hierarchical order created by God and really present in the universe whether anyone acknowledges it or not. The position may not be satisfactory. We may fail to see how a benevolent Deity could wish us to draw such conclusions from the hierarchical order He has created. We may find it difficult to formulate a human right of tormenting beasts in terms which would not equally imply an angelic right of tormenting men. And we may feel that though objective superiority is rightly claimed by man, yet that very superiority ought partly to *consist in* not behaving like a vivisector: that we ought to prove ourselves better than the beasts precisely by the fact of acknowledging duties to them which they do not acknowledge to us. But on all these questions different opinions can be honestly held. If on grounds of our real, divinely ordained, superiority a Christian pathologist thinks it right to vivisect, and does so with scrupulous care to avoid the least dram or scruple of unnecessary pain, in a trembling awe at the responsibility which he assumes, and with a vivid sense of the high mode in which human life must be lived if it is to justify the sacrifices made for it, then (whether we agree with him or not) we can respect his point of view.

But of course the vast majority of vivisectors have no such theological background. They are most of them naturalistic and Darwinian. Now here, surely, we come up against a very alarming fact. The very same people who will most contemptuously brush aside any consideration of animal suffering if it stands in the way of 'research' will also, in another context, most vehemently deny that there is any radical difference between man and the other animals. On the naturalistic view the beasts are at bottom just the same *sort* of thing as ourselves. Man is simply the cleverest of the anthropoids. All the grounds on which a Christian might defend vivisection are thus cut from under our feet. We sacrifice other species to our own not because our own has any objective metaphysical privilege over others, but simply because it is ours. It may be very natural to have this loyalty to our own species, but let us hear no more from the naturalists about the 'sentimentality' of anti-vivisectionists. If loyalty to our own species, preference for man simply because we are men, is not a sentiment, then what is? It may be a good sentiment or a bad one. But a sentiment it certainly is. Try to base it on logic and see what happens!

But the most sinister thing about modern vivisection is this. If a mere sentiment justifies cruelty, why stop at a sentiment for the whole human race? There is also a sentiment for the white man against the black, for a *Herrenvolk* against the non-Aryans, for 'civilized' or 'progressive' peoples against 'savage' or 'backward' peoples. Finally, for our own country, party, or class against others. Once the old Christian idea of a total difference in kind between man and beast has been abandoned, then no argument for experiments on animals can be found which is not also an argument for experiments on inferior men. If we cut up beasts simply because they cannot prevent us and because we are backing our own side in the struggle for existence, it is only logical to cut up imbeciles, criminals, enemies, or capitalists for the same reason. Indeed, experiments on men have already begun. We all hear that Nazi scientists have done them. We all suspect that our own scientists may begin to do so, in secret, at any moment.

The alarming thing is that the vivisectors have won the first round. In the nineteenth and eighteenth century a man was not stamped as a 'crank' for protesting against vivisection. Lewis Carroll protests, if I remember his famous letter correctly, on the very same ground which I have just used.[2] Dr. Johnson — a man whose mind had as much *iron* in it as any man's — protested in a note on

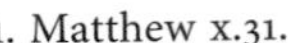

1. Matthew x.31.

2. 'Vivisection as a Sign of the Times', *The Works of Lewis Carroll*, ed. Roger Lancelyn Green (London, 1965), pp. 1089-92. See also 'Some Popular Fallacies about Vivisection', *ibid.*, pp. 1092-1100.

Cymbeline which is worth quoting in full. In Act I, scene v, the Queen explains to the Doctor that she wants poisons to experiment on 'such creatures as We count not worth the hanging, — but none human.'[3] The Doctor replies: 'Your Highness / Shall from this practice but make hard your heart.'[4] Johnson comments: 'The thought would probably have been more amplified, had our author lived to be shocked with such experiments as have been published in later times, by a race of men that have practised tortures without pity, and related them without shame, and are yet suffered to erect their heads among human beings.'[5]

The words are his, not mine, and in truth we hardly dare in these days to use such calmly stern language. The reason why we do not dare is that the other side has in fact won. And though cruelty even to beasts is an important matter, their victory is symptomatic of matters more important still. The victory of vivisection marks a great advance in the triumph of ruthless, non-moral utilitarianism over the old world of ethical law; a triumph in which we, as well as animals, are already the victims, and of which Dachau and Hiroshima mark the more recent achievements. In justifying cruelty to animals we put ourselves also on the animal level. We choose the jungle and must abide by our choice.

You will notice I have spent no time in discussing what actually goes on in the laboratories. We shall be told, of course, that there is surprisingly little cruelty. That is a question with which, at present, I have nothing to do. We must first decide what should be allowed; after that it is for the police to discover what is already being done.

3. Shakespeare, *Cymbeline*, I, v. 19-20.

4. Ibid., 23.

5. *Johnson on Shakespeare: Essays and Notes Selected and Set Forth with an Introduction by Sir Walter Raleigh* (London, 1908), p. 181.

86 Philosophical Reflections on Experimenting with Human Subjects

Hans Jonas

Experimenting with human subjects is going on in many fields of scientific and technological progress. It is designed to replace the over-all instruction by natural, occasional experience with the selective information from artificial, systematic experiment which physical science has found so effective in dealing with inanimate nature. Of the new experimentation with man, medical is surely the most legitimate; psychological, the most dubious; biological (still to come), the most dangerous. I have chosen here to deal with the first only, where the case *for* it is strongest and the task of adjudicating conflicting claims hardest. . . .

I. The Peculiarity of Human Experimentation

Experimentation was originally sanctioned by natural science. There it is performed on inanimate objects, and this raises no moral problems. But as soon as animate, feeling beings become the subjects of experiment, as they do in the life sciences and especially in medical research, this innocence of the search for knowledge is lost and questions of conscience arise. The depth of which moral and religious sensibilities can become aroused over these questions is shown by the vivisection issue. Human experimentation must sharpen the issue as it involves ultimate questions of personal dignity and sacrosanctity. One profound difference between the human experiment and the physical (beside that between animate and inanimate, feeling and unfeeling nature) is this: The physical experiment employs small-scale, artificially devised substitutes for that about which knowledge is to be obtained, and the experimenter extrapolates from these models and simulated conditions to nature at large. Something deputizes for the "real thing" — balls, rolling down an inclined plane for sun and planets, electric discharges from a condenser for real lightning, and so on. For the most part, no such substitution is possible in the biological sphere. We must operate on the original itself,

Reprinted by permission of *Daedalus,* Journal of the American Academy of the Arts and Sciences, from the issue entitled "Ethical Aspects of Experimentation with Human Subjects," Spring 1969, Vol. 98, No. 2.

the real thing in the fullest sense, and perhaps affect it irreversibly. No simulacrum can take its place. Especially in the human sphere, experimentation loses entirely the advantage of the clear division between vicarious model and true object. Up to a point, animals may fulfill the proxy role of the classical physical experiment. But in the end man himself must furnish knowledge about himself, and the comfortable separation of noncommittal experiment and definitive action vanishes. An experiment in education affects the lives of its subjects, perhaps a whole generation of schoolchildren. Human experimentation for whatever purpose is always *also* a responsible, nonexperimental, definitive dealing with the subject himself. And not even the noblest purpose abrogates the obligations this involves.

This is the root of the problem with which we are faced: Can both that purpose and this obligation be satisfied? If not, what would be a just compromise? Which side should give way to the other? The question is inherently philosophical as it concerns not merely pragmatic difficulties and their arbitration, but a genuine conflict of values involving principles of a high order. May I put the conflict in these terms? On principle, it is felt, human beings *ought not* to be dealt with in that way (the "guinea pig" protest); on the other hand, such dealings are increasingly urged on us by considerations, in turn appealing to principle, that claim to override those objections. Such a claim must be carefully assessed, especially when it is swept along by a mighty tide. Putting the matter thus, we have already made one important assumption rooted in our "Western" cultural tradition: The prohibitive rule is, to that way of thinking, the primary and axiomatic one; the permissive counter-rule, as qualifying the first, is secondary and stands in need of justification. We must justify the infringement of a primary inviolability, which needs no justification itself; and the justification of its infringement must be by values and needs of a dignity commensurate with those to be sacrificed. . . .

II. "Individual Versus Society" as the Conceptual Framework

The setting for the conflict most consistently invoked in the literature is the polarity of individual versus society — the possible tension between the individual good and the common good, between private and public welfare. . . . I have grave doubts about the adequacy of this frame of reference, but I will go along with it part of the way. It does apply to some extent, and it has the advantage of being familiar. We concede, as a matter of course, to the common good some pragmatically determined measure of precedence over the individual good. In terms of rights, we let some of the basic rights of the individual be overruled by the acknowledged rights of society — as a matter of right and moral justness and not of mere force or dire necessity (much as such necessity may be adduced in defense of that right). But in making that concession, we require a careful clarification of what the needs, interests, and rights of society are, for society — as distinct from any plurality of individuals — is an abstraction and, as such, is subject to our definition, while the individual is the primary concrete, prior to all definition, and his basic good is more or less known. Thus the unknown in our problem is the so-called common or public good and its potentially superior claims, to which the individual good must or might sometimes be sacrificed, in circumstances that in turn must also be counted among the unknowns of our question. Note that in putting the matter in this way — that is, in asking about the right of society to individual sacrifice — the consent of the sacrificial subject is no necessary part of the *basic* question.

"Consent," however, is the other most consistently emphasized and examined concept in discussions of this issue. This attention betrays a feeling that the "social" angle is not fully satisfactory. If society has a right, its exercise is not contingent on volunteering. On the other hand, if volunteering is fully genuine, no public right to the volunteered act need be construed. There is a difference between the moral or emotional appeal of a cause that elicits volunteering and a right that demands compliance — for example, with particular reference to the social sphere, between the *moral claim* of a common good and society's *right* to that good and to the means of its realization. A moral claim cannot be met without consent; a right can do without it. Where consent is present anyway, the distinction may become immaterial. But the awareness of the many ambiguities besetting the "consent" actually available and used in medical research[1] prompts recourse to the idea of a public right conceived independently of (and valid prior to) consent; and, vice versa, the awareness of the problematic nature of such a right makes even its advocates still insist on the idea of consent with all its ambiguities: an uneasy situation either way.

Nor does it help much to replace the language of "rights" by that of "interests" and then argue the sheer cumulative weight of the interest of the many over against those of the few or the single individual. "Interests" range all the way from the most marginal and optional to the most vital and imperative, and only those sanctioned by particular importance and merit will be admitted to court in such a calculus — which simply brings us back to the question of right or moral claim. Moreover, the appeal to numbers is dangerous. Is the number of those afflicted with a particular disease great enough to warrant violating the interests of the nonafflicted? Since the number of the latter is usually so much greater, the argument can actually turn around to the contention that the cumulative weight of interest is on *their* side. Finally, it may well be the case that the individual's interest in his own inviolability is itself a public

1. Cf. M. H. Pappworth, "Ethical Issues in Experimental Medicine" in D. R. Cutler (editor), *Updating Life and Death* (Boston, 1969), pp. 64-69.

interest, such that its publicly condoned violation, irrespective of numbers, violates the interest of all. In that case, its protection in *each* instance would be a paramount interest, and the comparison of numbers will not avail.

These are some of the difficulties hidden in the conceptual framework indicated by the terms "society-individual," "interest," and "rights." But we also spoke of a moral call, and this points to another dimension — not indeed divorced from the social sphere, but transcending it. And there is something even beyond that: true sacrifice from highest devotion, for which there are no laws or rules except that it must be absolutely free. "No one has the right to choose martyrs for science" was a statement repeatedly quoted in the November, 1967, *Daedalus* conference. But no scientist can be prevented from making himself a martyr for his science. At all times, dedicated explorers, thinkers, and artists have immolated themselves on the altar of their vocation, and creative genius most often pays the price of happiness, health, and life for its own consummation. But no one, not even society, has the shred of a right to expect and ask these things in the normal course of events. They come to the rest of us as a *gratia gratis data.*

III. The Sacrificial Theme

Yet we must face the somber truth that the *ultima ratio* of communal life is and has always been the compulsory, vicarious sacrifice of individual lives. The primordial sacrificial situation is that of outright human sacrifices in early communities. These were not acts of blood-lust or gleeful savagery; they were the solemn execution of a supreme, sacral necessity. One of the fellowship of men had to die so that all could live, the earth be fertile, the cycle of nature renewed. The victim often was not a captured enemy, but a select member of the group: "The king must die." If there was cruelty here, it was not that of men, but that of the gods, or rather of the stern order of things, which was believed to exact that price for the bounty of life. To assure it for the community, and to assure it ever again, the awesome *quid pro quo* had to be paid over again.

Far should it be from us to belittle, from the height of our enlightened knowledge, the majesty of the underlying conception. The particular *causal* views that prompted our ancestors have long since been relegated to the realm of superstition. But in moments of national danger we still send the flower of our young manhood to offer their lives for the continued life of the community, and if it is a just war, we see them go forth as consecrated and strangely ennobled by a sacrificial role. Nor do we make their going forth depend on their own will and consent, much as we may desire and foster these. We conscript them according to law. We conscript the best and feel morally disturbed if the draft, either by design or in effect, works so that mainly the disadvantaged, socially less useful, more expendable, make up those whose lives are to buy ours. No rational persuasion of the pragmatic necessity here at work can do away with the feeling, a mixture of gratitude and guilt, that the sphere of the sacred is touched with the vicarious offering of life for life. Quite apart from these dramatic occasions, there is, it appears, a persistent and constitutive aspect of human immolation to the very being and prospering of human society — an immolation in terms of life and happiness, imposed or voluntary, of few for many. What Goethe has said of the rise of Christianity may well apply to the nature of civilization in general: "*Opfer fallen hier, / Weder Lamm noch Stier, / Aber Menschenopfer unerhoert.*"[2] We can never rest comfortably in the belief that the soil from which our satisfactions sprout is not watered with the blood of martyrs. But a troubled conscience compels us, the undeserving beneficiaries, to ask: Who is to be martyred? In the service of what cause and by whose choice?

Not for a moment do I wish to suggest that medical experimentation on human subjects, sick or healthy, is to be likened to primeval human sacrifices. Yet something sacrificial is involved in the selective abrogation of personal inviolability and the ritualized exposure to gratuitous risk of health and life, justified by a presumed greater, social good. My examples from the sphere of stark sacrifice were intended to sharpen the issues implied in that context and to set them off clearly from the kinds of obligations and constraints imposed on the citizen in the normal course of things or generally demanded of the individual in exchange for the advantages of civil society.

IV. The "Social Contract" Theme

The first thing to say in such a setting-off is that the sacrificial area is not covered by what is called the "social contract." This fiction of political theory, premised on the primacy of the individual, was designed to supply a rationale for the *limitation* of individual freedom and power required for the existence of the body politic, whose existence in turn is for the benefit of the individuals. The principle of these limitations is that their *general* observance profits all, and that therefore the individual observer, assuring this general observance for his part, profits by it himself. I observe property rights because their general observance assures my own; I observe traffic rules because their general observance assures my own safety; and so on. The obligations here are mutual and general; no one is singled out for special sacrifice. Moreover, for the most part, *qua* limitations of my liberty, the laws thus deducible from the hypothetical "social contract" enjoin me from certain actions rather than obligate me to positive actions (as did the laws of feudal

2. *Die Braut von Korinth:* "Victims do fall here, / Neither lamb nor steer, / Nay, but human offerings untold."

society). Even where the latter is the case, as in the duty to pay taxes, the rationale is that I am myself a beneficiary of the services financed through these payments. Even the contributions levied by the welfare state, though not originally contemplated in the liberal version of the social contract theory, can be interpreted as a personal insurance policy of one sort or another — be it against the contingency of my own indigence, be it against the dangers of disaffection from the laws in consequence of widespread unrelieved destitution, be it even against the disadvantages of a diminished consumer market. Thus, by some stretch, such contributions can still be subsumed under the principle of enlightened self-interest. But no complete abrogation of self-interest at any time is in the terms of the social contract, and so pure sacrifice falls outside it. Under the putative terms of the contract alone, I cannot be required to die for the public good. . . .

But in time of war our society itself supersedes the nice balance of the social contract with an almost absolute precedence of public necessities over individual rights. In this and similar emergencies, the sacrosanctity of the individual is abrogated, and what for all practical purposes amounts to a near-totalitarian, quasi-communist state of affairs is *temporarily* permitted to prevail. In such situations, the community is conceded the right to make calls on its members, or certain of its members, entirely different in magnitude and kind from the calls normally allowed. It is deemed right that a part of the population bears a disproportionate burden of risk of a disproportionate gravity; and it is deemed right that the rest of the community accepts this sacrifice, whether voluntary or enforced, and reaps its benefits — difficult as we find it to justify this acceptance and this benefit by any normal ethical categories. We justify it transethically, as it were, by the supreme collective emergency, formalized, for example, by the declaration of a state of war.

Medical experimentation on human subjects falls somewhere between this overpowering case and the normal transactions of the social contract. On the one hand, no comparable extreme issue of social survival is (by and large) at stake. And no comparable extreme sacrifice or foreseeable risk is (by and large) asked. On the other hand, what is asked goes decidedly beyond, even runs counter to, what it is otherwise deemed fair to let the individual sign over of his person to the benefit of the "common good." Indeed, our sensitivity to the kind of intrusion and use involved is such that only an end of transcendent value or overriding urgency can make it arguable and possibly acceptable in our eyes.

V. Health as a Public Good

The cause invoked is health and, in its more critical aspect, life itself — clearly superlative goods that the physician serves directly by curing and the researcher indirectly by the knowledge gained through his experiments. There is no question about the good served nor about the evil fought — disease and premature death. But a good to whom and an evil to whom? Here the issue tends to become somewhat clouded. In the attempt to give experimentation the proper dignity (on the problematic view that a value becomes greater by being "social" instead of merely individual), the health in question or the disease in question is somehow predicated on the social whole, as if it were society that, in the persons of its members, enjoyed the one and suffered the other. For the purposes of our problem, public interest can then be pitted against private interest, the common good against the individual good. Indeed, I have found health called a national resource, which of course it is, but surely not in the first place.

In trying to resolve some of the complexities and ambiguities lurking in these conceptualizations, I have pondered a particular statement, made in the form of a question, which I found in the *Proceedings* of the earlier *Daedalus* conference: "Can society afford to discard the tissues and organs of the hopelessly unconscious patient when they could be used to restore the otherwise hopelessly ill, but still salvageable individual?" And somewhat later: "A strong case can be made that society can ill afford to discard the tissues and organs of the hopelessly unconscious patient; they are greatly needed for study and experimental trial to help those who can be salvaged."[3] I hasten to add that any suspicion of callousness that the "commodity" language these statements may suggest is immediately dispelled by the name of the speaker, Dr. Henry K. Beecher, for whose humanity and moral sensibility there can be nothing but admiration. But the use, in all innocence, of this language gives food for thought. Let me, for a moment, take the question literally. "Discarding" implies proprietary rights — nobody can discard what does not belong to him in the first place. Does society then own my body? "Salvaging" implies the same and, moreover, a use-value to the owner. Is the life-extension of certain individuals then a public interest? "Affording" implies a critically vital level of such an interest — that is, of the loss or gain involved. And "society" itself — what is it? When does a need, an aim, an obligation become social? Let us reflect on some of these terms.

VI. What Society Can Afford

"Can Society afford . . . ?" Afford what? To let people die intact, thereby withholding something from other people who desperately need it, who in consequence will have to die too? These other, unfortunate people indeed cannot afford not to have a kidney, heart, or other organ of the dying patient, on which they depend for an extension of

3. *Proceedings of the Conference on the Ethical Aspects of Experimentation on Human Subjects,* November 3-4, 1967 (Boston, Mass.), pp. 50-51.

their lease on life; but does that give them a right to it? And does it oblige society to procure it for them? What is it that *society* can or cannot afford — leaving aside for the moment the question of what it has a *right* to? It surely can afford to lose members through death; more than that, it is built on the balance of death and birth decreed by the order of life. This is too general, of course, for our question, but perhaps it is well to remember. The specific question seems to be whether society can afford to let some people die whose death might be deferred by particular means if these were authorized by society. Again, if it is merely a question of what society can or cannot afford, rather than of what it ought or ought not to do, the answer must be: Of course, it can. If cancer, heart disease, and other organic, noncontagious ills, especially those tending to strike the old more than the young, continue to exact their toll at the normal rate of incidence (including the toll of private anguish and misery), society can go on flourishing in every way.

Here, by contrast, are some examples of what, in sober truth, society cannot afford. It cannot afford to let an epidemic rage unchecked; a persistent excess of deaths over births, but neither — we might add — too great an excess of births over deaths; too low an average life expectancy even if demographically balanced by fertility, but neither too great a longevity with the necessitated correlative dearth of youth in the social body; a debilitating state of general health; and things of this kind. These are plain cases where the whole condition of society is critically affected, and the public interest can make its imperative claims. The Black Death of the Middle Ages was a *public* calamity of the acute kind; the life-sapping ravages of endemic malaria or sleeping sickness in certain areas are a public calamity of the chronic kind. Such situations a society as a whole can truly not "afford," and they may call for extraordinary remedies, including, perhaps, the invasion of private sacrosanctities.

This is not entirely a matter of numbers and numerical ratios. Society, in a subtler sense, cannot "afford" a single miscarriage of justice, a single inequity in the dispensation of its laws, the violation of the rights of even the tiniest minority, because these undermine the moral basis on which society's existence rests. Nor can it, for a similar reason, afford the absence or atrophy in its midst of compassion and of the effort to alleviate suffering — be it widespread or rare — one form of which is the effort to conquer disease of any kind, whether "socially" significant (by reason of number) or not. And in short, society cannot afford the absence among its members of *virtue* with its readiness for sacrifice beyond defined duty. Since its presence — that is to say, that of personal idealism — is a matter of grace and not of decree, we have the paradox that society depends for its existence on intangibles of nothing less than a religious order, for which it can hope, but which it cannot enforce. All the more must it protect this most precious capital from abuse.

For what objectives connected with the mediobiological sphere should this reserve be drawn upon — for example, in the form of accepting, soliciting, perhaps even imposing the submission of human subjects to experimentation? We postulate that this must be not just a worthy cause, as any promotion of the health of anybody doubtlessly is, but a cause qualifying for transcendent social sanction. Here one thinks first of those cases critically affecting the whole condition, present and future, of the community we have illustrated. Something equivalent to what in the political sphere is called "clear and present danger" may be invoked and a state of emergency proclaimed, thereby suspending certain otherwise inviolable prohibitions and taboos. We may observe that averting a disaster always carries greater weight than promoting a good. Extraordinary danger excuses extraordinary means. This covers human experimentation, which we would like to count, as far as possible, among the extraordinary rather than the ordinary means of serving the common good under public auspices. Naturally, since foresight and responsibility for the future are of the essence of institutional society, averting disaster extends into long-term prevention, although the lesser urgency will warrant less sweeping licenses.

VII. Society and the Cause of Progress

Much weaker is the case where it is a matter not of saving but of improving society. Much of medical research falls into this category. As stated before, a permanent death rate from heart failure or cancer does not threaten society. So long as certain statistical ratios are maintained, the incidence of disease and of disease-induced mortality is not (in the strict sense) a "social" misfortune. I hasten to add that it is not therefore less of a human misfortune, and the call for relief issuing with silent eloquence from each victim and all potential victims is of no lesser dignity. But it is misleading to equate the fundamentally human response to it with what is owed to society: it is owed by man to man — and it is thereby owed by society to the individuals as soon as the adequate ministering to these concerns outgrows (as it progressively does) the scope of private spontaneity and is made a public mandate. It is thus that society assumes responsibility for medical care, research, old age, and innumerable other things not originally of the public realm (in the original "social contract"), and they become duties toward "society" (rather than directly toward one's fellow man) by the fact that they are socially operated.

Indeed, we expect from organized society no longer mere protection against harm and the securing of the conditions of our preservation, but active and constant improvement in all the domains of life: the waging of the battle against nature, the enhancement of the human estate — in short, the promotion of progress. This is an expansive goal, one far surpassing the disaster norm of our previous reflections. It lacks the urgency of the latter, but has the nobility of the free, forward thrust. It surely is worth sacrifices. It is not at all a question of what society can afford, but of what it is committed to, beyond all necessity, by our mandate. Its trusteeship has become an established, ongoing, institutionalized business of the body politic. As eager beneficiaries of its gains, we now owe to "society," as its chief agent, our individual contributions toward its *continued pursuit.* I emphasize "continued pursuit." Maintaining the existing level requires no more than the orthodox means of taxation and enforcement of professional standards that raise no problems. The more optional goal of pushing forward is also more exacting. We have this syndrome: Progress is by our choosing an acknowledged interest of society, in which we have a stake in various degrees; science is a necessary instrument of progress; research is a necessary instrument of science; and in medical science experimentation on human subjects is a necessary instrument of research. Therefore, human experimentation has come to be a societal interest.

The destination of research is essentially melioristic. It does not serve the preservation of the existing good from which I profit myself and to which I am obligated. Unless the present state is intolerable, the melioristic goal is in a sense gratuitous, and this not only from the vantage point of the present. Our descendants have a right to be left an unplundered planet; they do not have a right to new miracle cures. We have sinned against them, if by our doing we have destroyed their inheritance — which we are doing at full blast; we have not sinned against them, if by the time they come around arthritis has not yet been conquered (unless by sheer neglect). And generally, in the matter of progress, as humanity had no claim on a Newton, a Michelangelo, or a St. Francis to appear, and no right to the blessings of their unscheduled deeds, so progress, with all our methodical labor for it, cannot be budgeted in advance and its fruits received as a due. Its coming-about at all and its turning out for good (of which we can never be sure) must rather be regarded as something akin to grace.

VIII. The Melioristic Goal, Medical Research, and Individual Duty

Nowhere is the melioristic goal more inherent than in medicine. To the physician, it is not gratuitous. He is committed to curing and thus to improving the power to cure. Gratuitous we called it (outside disaster conditions) as a *social* goal, but noble at the same time. Both the nobility and the gratuitousness must influence the manner in which self-sacrifice for it is elicited, and even its free offer accepted. Freedom is certainly the first condition to be observed here. The surrender of one's body to medical experimentation is entirely outside the enforceable "social contract."

Or can it be construed to fall within its terms — namely, as repayment for benefits from past experimentation that I have enjoyed myself? But I am indebted for these benefits not to society, but to the past "martyrs," to whom society is indebted itself, and society has no right to call in my personal debt by way of adding new to its own. Moreover, gratitude is not an enforceable social obligation; it anyway does not mean that I must emulate the deed. Most of all, if it was wrong to exact such sacrifice in the first place, it does not become right to exact it again with the plea of the profit it has brought me. If, however, it was not exacted, but entirely free, as it ought to have been, then it should remain so, and its precedence must not be used as a social pressure on others for doing the same under the sign of duty.

Indeed, we must look outside the sphere of the social contract, outside the whole realm of public rights and duties, for the motivations and norms by which we can expect ever again the upwelling of a will to give what nobody — neither society, nor fellow man, nor posterity — is entitled to. There are such dimensions in man with trans-social wellsprings of conduct, and I have already pointed to the paradox, or mystery, that society cannot prosper without them, that it must draw on them, but cannot command them.

What about the moral law as such a transcendent motivation of conduct? It goes considerably beyond the public law of the social contract. The latter, we saw, is founded on the rule of enlightened self-interest: *Do ut des* — I give so that I be given to. The law of individual conscience asks more. Under the Golden Rule, for example, I am required to give as I wish to be given to under like circumstances, but not in order that I be given to and not in expectation of return. Reciprocity, essential to the social law, is not a condition of the moral law. One subtle "expectation" and "self-interest," but of the moral order itself, may even then be in my mind: I prefer the environment of a moral society and can expect to contribute to the general morality by my own example. But even if I should always be the dupe, the Golden Rule holds. (If the social law breaks faith with me, I am released from its claim.)

IX. Moral Law and Transmoral Dedication

Can I, then, be called upon to offer myself for medical experimentation in the name of the moral law? *Prima facie,* the Golden Rule seems to apply. I should wish, were I dying of a disease, that enough volunteers in the past had provided enough knowledge through the gift of their bodies that I could now be saved. I should wish, were I desperately in need of a transplant, that the dying patient next door had agreed to a definition of death by which his organs would become available to me in the freshest possible condition. I surely should also wish, were I drowning, that somebody would risk his life, even sacrifice his life, for mine.

But the last example reminds us that only the negative form of the Golden Rule ("Do not do unto others what you do not want done unto yourself") is fully prescriptive. The positive form ("Do unto others as you would wish them to do unto you"), in whose compass our issue falls, points to an infinite, open horizon where prescriptive force soon ceases. We may well say of somebody that he ought to have come to the succor of B, to have shared with him in his need, and the like. But we may not say that he ought to have given his life for him. To have done so would be praiseworthy; not to have done so is not blameworthy. It cannot be asked of him; if he fails to do so, he reneges on no duty. But *he* may say of himself, and only he, that he ought to have given his life. *This* "ought" is strictly between him and himself, or between him and God; no outside party — fellow man or society — can appropriate its voice. It can humbly receive the supererogatory gifts from the free enactment of it.

We must, in other words, distinguish between moral obligation and the much larger sphere of moral value. (This, incidentally, shows up the error in the widely held view of value theory that the higher a value, the stronger its claim and the greater the duty to realize it. The highest are in the region beyond duty and claim.) The ethical dimension far exceeds that of the moral law and reaches into the sublime solitude of dedication and ultimate commitment, away from all reckoning and rule — in short, into the sphere of the *holy*. From there alone can the offer of self-sacrifice genuinely spring, and this — its source — must be honored religiously. How? The first duty here falling on the research community, when it enlists and uses this source, is the safeguarding of true authenticity and spontaneity.

X. The "Conscription" of Consent

But here we must realize that the mere issuing of the appeal, the calling for volunteers, with the moral and social pressures it inevitably generates, amounts even under the most meticulous rules of consent to a sort of *conscripting*. And some soliciting is necessarily involved. This was in part meant by the earlier remark that in this area sin and guilt can perhaps not be wholly avoided. And this is why "consent," surely a non-negotiable minimum requirement, is not the full answer to the problem. Granting then that soliciting and therefore some degree of conscripting are part of the situation, who may conscript and who may be conscripted? Or less harshly expressed: Who should issue appeals and to whom?

The naturally qualified issuer of the appeal is the research scientist himself, collectively the main carrier of the impulse and the one with the technical competence to judge. But his being very much an interested party (with vested interests, indeed, not purely in the public good, but in the scientific enterprise as such, in "his" project, and even in his career) makes him also suspect. The ineradicable dialectic of this situation — a delicate incompatibility problem — calls for particular controls by the research community and by public authority that we need not discuss. They can mitigate, but not eliminate the problem. We have to live with the ambiguity, the treacherous impurity of everything human.

XI. Self-Recruitment of the Community

To whom should the appeal be addressed? The natural issuer of the call is also the first natural addressee: the physician-researcher himself and the scientific confraternity at large. With such a coincidence — indeed, the noble tradition with which the whole business of human experimentation started — almost all of the associated legal, ethical, and metaphysical problems vanish. If it is full, autonomous identification of the subject with the purpose that is required for the dignifying of his serving as a subject — here it is; if strongest motivation — here it is; if fullest understanding — here it is; if freest decision — here it is; if greatest integration with the person's total, chosen pursuit — here it is. With the fact of self-solicitation the issue of consent in all its insoluble equivocality is bypassed *per se*. Not even the condition that the particular purpose be truly important and the project reasonably promising, which must hold in any solicitation of others, need be satisfied here. By himself, the scientist is free to obey his obsession, to play his hunch, to wager on chance, to follow the lure of ambition. It is all part of the "divine madness" that somehow animates the ceaseless pressing against frontiers. For the rest of society, which has a deep-seated disposition to look with reverence and awe upon the guardians of the mysteries of life, the profession assumes with this proof of its devotion the role of a self-chosen, consecrated fraternity, not unlike the monastic orders of the past, and this would come nearest to the actual, religious origins of the art of healing. . . .

XII. "Identification" as the Principle of Recruitment in General

If the properties we adduced as the particular qualifications of the members of the scientific fraternity itself are taken as general criteria of selection, then one should look for additional subjects where a maximum of identification, understanding, and spontaneity can be expected — that is, among the most highly motivated, the most highly educated, and the least "captive" members of the community. From this naturally scarce resource, a descending order of permissibility leads to greater abundance and ease of supply, whose use should become proportionately more hesitant as the exculpating criteria are relaxed. An inversion of normal "market" behavior is demanded here — namely, to accept the lowest quotation last (and excused only by the greatest pressure of need); to pay the highest price first.

The ruling principle in our considerations is that the "wrong" of reification can only be made "right" by such authentic identification with the cause that it is the subject's as well as the researcher's cause — whereby his role in its service is not just permitted by him, but *willed.* That sovereign will of his which embraces the end as his own restores his personhood to the otherwise depersonalizing context. To be valid it must be autonomous and informed. The latter condition can, outside the research community, only be fulfilled by degrees; but the higher the degree of the understanding regarding the purpose and the technique, the more valid becomes the endorsement of the will. A margin of mere trust inevitably remains. Ultimately, the appeal for volunteers should seek this free and generous endorsement, the appropriation of the research purpose into the person's own scheme of ends. Thus, the appeal is in truth addressed to the one, mysterious, and sacred source of any such generosity of the will — "devotion," whose forms and objects of commitment are various and may invest different motivations in different individuals. The following, for instance, may be responsive to the "call" we are discussing: compassion with human suffering, zeal for humanity, reverence for the Golden Rule, enthusiasm for progress, homage to the cause of knowledge, even longing for sacrificial justification (do not call that "masochism," please). On all these, I say, it is defensible and right to draw when the research objective is worthy enough; and it is a prime duty of the research community (especially in view of what we called the "margin of trust") to see that this sacred source is never abused for frivolous ends. For a less than adequate cause, not even the freest, unsolicited offer should be accepted.

XIII. The Rule of the "Descending Order" and Its Counter-Utility Sense

We have laid down what must seem to be a forbidding rule to the number-hungry research industry. Having faith in the transcendent potential of man, I do not fear that the "source" will ever fail a society that does not destroy it — and only such a one is worthy of the blessings of progress. But "elitistic" the rule is (as is the enterprise of progress itself), and elites are by nature small. The combined attribute of motivation and information, plus the absence of external pressures, tends to be socially so circumscribed that strict adherence to the rule might numerically starve the research process. This is why I spoke of a descending order of permissibility, which is itself permissive, but where the realization that it is a *descending* order is not without pragmatic import. Departing from the august norm, the appeal must needs shift from idealism to docility, from high-mindedness to compliance, from judgment to trust. Consent spreads over the whole spectrum. I will not go into the casuistics of this penumbral area. I merely indicate the principle of the order of preference: The poorer in knowledge, motivation, and freedom of decision (and that, alas, means the more readily available in terms of numbers and possible manipulation), the more sparingly and indeed reluctantly should the reservoir be used, and the more compelling must therefore become the countervailing justification.

Let us note that this is the opposite of a social utility standard, the reverse of the order by "availability and expendability": The most valuable and scarcest, the least expendable elements of the social organism, are to be the first candidates for risk and sacrifice. It is the standard of *noblesse oblige;* and with all its counterutility and seeming "wastefulness," we feel a rightness about it and perhaps even a higher "utility," for the soul of the community lives by this spirit.[4] It is also the opposite of what the day-to-day interests of research clamor for, and for the scientific community to honor it will mean that it will have to fight a strong temptation to go by routine to the readiest sources of supply — the suggestible, the ignorant, the dependent, the "captive" in various senses.[5] I do not believe that heightened resistance here must cripple research, which cannot be permitted; but it may indeed slow it down by the smaller numbers fed into experimentation in consequence. This price — a possibly slower rate of progress — may have to be paid for the preservation of the most precious capital of higher communal life.

XIV. Experimentation on Patients

So far we have been speaking on the tacit assumption that the subjects of experimentation are recruited from among the healthy. To the question "Who is conscriptable?" the spontaneous answer is: Least and last of all the sick — the most available of all as they are under treatment and observation anyway. That the afflicted should not be called upon to bear additional burden and risk, that they are society's special trust and the physician's trust in particular — these are elementary responses of our moral sense. Yet the very destination of medical research, the conquest of disease, requires at the crucial stage trial and verification on precisely the sufferers from the disease, and their total exemption would defeat the purpose itself. In acknowledging this inescapable necessity, we enter the most sensitive area of the whole complex, the one most keenly felt and most searchingly discussed by the practitioners themselves. No wonder it touches the heart of the doctor-patient relation, putting its most solemn obligations to the test. There is nothing new in what I have to say about the ethics of the doctor-

4. Socially, everyone is expendable relatively — that is, in different degrees; religiously, no one is expendable absolutely: The "image of God" is in all. If it can be enhanced, then not by anyone being expended, but by someone expending himself.

5. This refers to captives of circumstances, not of justice. Prison inmates are, with respect to our problem, in a special class. If we hold to some idea of guilt, and to the supposition that our judicial system is not entirely at fault, they may be held to stand in a special debt to society, and their offer to serve — from whatever motive — may be accepted with a minimum of qualms as a means of reparation.

patient relation, but for the purpose of confronting it with the issue of experimentation some of the oldest verities must be recalled.

A. *The Fundamental Privilege of the Sick*

In the course of treatment, the physician is obligated to the patient and to no one else. He is not the agent of society, nor of the interests of medical science, nor of the patient's family, nor of his co-sufferers, or future sufferers from the same disease. The patient alone counts when he is under the physician's care. By the simple law of bilateral contract (analogous, for example, to the relation of lawyer to client and its "conflict of interest" rule), the physician is bound not to let any other interest interfere with that of the patient in being cured. But manifestly more sublime norms than contractual ones are involved. We may speak of a sacred trust; strictly by its terms, the doctor is, as it were, alone with his patient and God.

There is one normal exception to this — that is, to the doctor's not being the agent of society vis-à-vis the patient, but the trustee of his interests alone: the quarantining of the contagious sick. This is plainly not for the patient's interest, but for that of others threatened by him. (In vaccination, we have a combination of both: protection of the individual and others.) But preventing the patient from causing harm to others is not the same as exploiting him for the advantage of others. And there is, of course, the abnormal exception of collective catastrophe, the analogue to a state of war. The physician who desperately battles a raging epidemic is under a unique dispensation that suspends in a nonspecifiable way some of the strictures of normal practice, including possibly those against experimental liberties with his patients. No rules can be devised for the waiving of rules in extremities. And as with the famous shipwreck examples of ethical theory, the less said about it the better. But what is allowable there and may later be passed over in forgiving silence cannot serve as a precedent. We are concerned with non-extreme, non-emergency conditions where the voice of principle can be heard and claims can be adjudicated free from duress. We have conceded that there are such claims, and that if there is to be medical advance at all, not even the superlative privilege of the suffering and the sick can be kept wholly intact from the intrusion of its needs. About this least palatable, most disquieting part of our subject, I have to offer only groping, inconclusive remarks.

B. *The Principle of "Identification" Applied to Patients*

On the whole, the same principles would seem to hold here as are found to hold with "normal subjects": motivation, identification, understanding on the part of the subject. But it is clear that these conditions are peculiarly difficult to satisfy with regard to a patient. His physical state, psychic preoccupation, dependent relation to the doctor, the submissive attitude induced by treatment — everything connected with his condition and situation makes the sick person inherently less of a sovereign person than the healthy one. Spontaneity of self-offering has almost to be ruled out; consent is marred by lower resistance or captive circumstance, and so on. In fact, all the factors that make the patient, as a category, particularly accessible and welcome for experimentation at the same time compromise the quality of the responding affirmation that must morally redeem the making use of them. This, in addition to the primacy of the physician's duty, puts a heightened onus on the physician-researcher to limit his undue power to the most important and defensible research objectives and, of course, to keep persuasion at a minimum.

Still, with all the disabilities noted, there is scope among patients for observing the rule of the "descending order of permissibility" that we have laid down for normal subjects, in vexing inversion of the utility order of quantitative abundance and qualitative "expendability." By the principle of this order, those patients who most identify with and are cognizant of the cause of research — members of the medical profession (who after all are sometimes patients themselves) — come first; the highly motivated and educated, also least dependent, among the lay patients come next; and so on down the line. An added consideration here is seriousness of condition, which again operates in inverse proportion. Here the profession must fight the tempting sophistry that the hopeless case is expendable (because in prospect already expended) and therefore especially usable; and generally the attitude that the poorer the chances of the patient the more justifiable his recruitment for experimentation (other than for his own benefit). The opposite is true.

C. *Nondisclosure as a Borderline Case*

Then there is the case where ignorance of the subject, sometimes even of the experiment, is of the essence of the experiment (the "double blind"-control group-placebo syndrome). It is said to be a necessary element of the scientific process. Whatever may be said about its ethics in regard to normal subjects, especially volunteers, it is an outright betrayal of trust in regard to the patient who believes that he is receiving treatment. Only the supreme importance of the objective can exonerate it, without making it less of a transgression. The patient is definitely wronged even when not harmed. And ethics apart, the practice of such deception holds the danger of undermining the faith in the *bona fides* of treatment, the beneficial intent of the physician — the very basis of the doctor-patient relationship. In every respect, it follows that concealed experiment on patients — that is, experiment under the guise of treatment — should be the rarest exception, at best, if it cannot be wholly avoided.

This has still the merit of a borderline problem. The same is not true of the other case of necessary ignorance of the subject — that of the unconscious patient. Drafting him for nontherapeutic experiments is simply and unqualifiedly impermissible; progress or not, he must never be used, on the inflexible principle that utter helplessness demands utter protection.

When preparing this paper, I filled pages with a casuistics of this harrowing field, but then scrapped most of it, realizing my dilettante status. The shadings are endless, and only the physician-researcher can discern them properly as the cases arise. Into his lap the decision is thrown. The philosophical rule, once it has admitted into itself the idea of a sliding scale, cannot really specify its own application. It can only impress on the practitioner a general maxim or attitude for the exercise of his judgment and conscience in the concrete occasions of his work. In our case, I am afraid, it means making life more difficult for him.

It will also be noted that, somewhat at variance with the emphasis in the literature, I have not dwelt on the element of "risk" and very little on that of "consent." Discussion of the first is beyond the layman's competence; the emphasis on the second has been lessened because of its equivocal character. It is a truism to say that one should strive to minimize the risk and to maximize the consent. The more demanding concept of "identification," which I have used, includes "consent" in its maximal or authentic form, and the assumption of risk is its privilege.

XV. No Experiments on Patients Unrelated to Their Own Disease

Although my ponderings have, on the whole, yielded points of view rather than definite prescriptions, premises rather than conclusions, they have led me to a few unequivocal yeses and noes. The first is the emphatic rule that patients should be experimented upon, if at all, *only* with reference to *their disease.* Never should there be added to the gratuitousness of the experiment as such the gratuitousness of service to an unrelated cause. This follows simply from what we have found to be the *only* excuse for infracting the special exemption of the sick at all — namely, that the scientific war on disease cannot accomplish its goal without drawing the sufferers from disease into the investigative process. If under this excuse they become subjects of experiment, they do so *because,* and only because, of *their* disease.

This is the fundamental and self-sufficient consideration. That the patient cannot possibly benefit from the unrelated experiment therapeutically, while he might from experiment related to his condition, is also true, but lies beyond the problem area of pure experiment. I am in any case discussing nontherapeutic experimentation only, where *ex hypothesi* the patient does not benefit. Experiment as part of therapy — that is, directed toward helping the subject himself — is a different matter altogether and raises its own problems, but hardly philosophical ones. As long as a doctor can say, even if only in his own thought: "There is no known cure for your condition (or: You have responded to none); but there is promise in a new treatment still under investigation, not quite tested yet as to effectiveness and safety; you will be taking a chance, but all things considered, I judge it in your best interest to let me try it on you" — as long as he can speak thus, he speaks as the patient's physician and may err, but does not transform the patient into a subject of experimentation. Introduction of an untried therapy into treatment where the tried ones have failed is not "experimentation on the patient."

Generally, and almost needless to say, with all the rules of the book, there is something "experimental" (because tentative) about every individual treatment, beginning with the diagnosis itself; and he would be a poor doctor who would not learn from every case for the benefit of future cases, and a poor member of the profession who would not make any new insights gained from his treatments available to the profession at large. Thus, knowledge may be advanced in the treatment of any patient, and the interest of the medical art and all sufferers from the same affliction as well as the patient himself may be served if something happens to be learned from his case. But this gain to knowledge and future therapy is incidental to the *bona fide* service to the present patient. He has the right to expect that the doctor does nothing to him just in order to learn.

In that case, the doctor's imaginary speech would run, for instance, like this: "There is nothing more I can do for you. But you can do something for me. Speaking no longer as your physician but on behalf of medical science, we could learn a great deal about future cases of this kind if you would permit me to perform certain experiments on you. It is understood that you yourself would not benefit from any knowledge we might gain; but future patients would." This statement would express the purely experimental situation, assumedly here with the subject's concurrence and with all cards on the table. In Alexander Bickel's words: "It is a different situation when the doctor is no longer trying to make [the patient] well, but is trying to find out how to make others well in the future."[6]

6. *Proceedings,* p. 33. To spell out the difference between the two cases: In the first case, the patient himself is meant to be the beneficiary of the experiment, and directly so; the "subject" of the experiment is at the same time its object, its end. It is performed not for gaining knowledge, but for helping him — and helping him in the *act* of performing it, even if by its results it also contributes to a broader testing process currently under way. It is in fact part of the treatment itself and an "experiment" only in the loose sense of being untried and highly tentative. But whatever the degree of uncertainty, the motivating anticipation (the wage, if you like) is for success, and success here means the subject's own good. To a pure experiment, by contrast, undertaken to gain knowledge, the difference of success and failure is not germane, only that of conclusiveness and inconclusiveness. The "negative" result has as much to teach as the "positive." Also, the true experiment is an act distinct from the uses later made of the findings. And, most important, the subject experimented on is distinct from the eventual beneficiaries

But even in the second case, that of the nontherapeutic experiment where the patient does not benefit, at least the patient's own disease is enlisted in the cause of fighting that disease, even if only in others. It is yet another thing to say or think: "Since you are here — in the hospital with its facilities — anyway, under our care and observation anyway, away from your job (or, perhaps, doomed) anyway, we wish to profit from your being available for some other research of great interest we are presently engaged in." From the standpoint of merely medical ethics, which has only to consider risk, consent, and the worth of the objective, there may be no cardinal difference between this case and the last one. I hope that the medical reader will not think I am making too fine a point when I say that from the standpoint of the subject and his dignity there is a cardinal difference that crosses the line between the permissible and the impermissible, and this by the same principle of "identification" I have been invoking all along. Whatever the rights and wrongs of any experimentation on any patient — in the one case, at least that residue of identification is left him that it is his own affliction by which he can contribute to the conquest of that affliction, his own kind of suffering which he helps to alleviate in others; and so in a sense it is his own cause. It is totally indefensible to rob the unfortunate of this intimacy with the purpose and make his misfortune a convenience for the furtherance of alien concerns. The observance of this rule is essential, I think, to at least attenuate the wrong that nontherapeutic experimenting on patients commits in any case.

XVI. Conclusion

There would now have to be said something about nonmedical experiments on human subjects, notably psychological and genetic, of which I have not lost sight. But I must leave this for another occasion. I wish only to say in conclusion that if some of the practical implications of my reasonings are felt to work out toward a slower rate of progress, this should not cause too great dismay. Let us not forget that progress is an optional goal, not an unconditional commitment, and that its tempo in particular, compulsive as it may become, has nothing sacred about it. Let us also remember that a slower progress in the conquest of disease would not threaten society, grievous as it is to those who have to deplore that their particular disease be not yet conquered, but that society would indeed be threatened by the erosion of those moral values whose loss, possibly caused by too ruthless a pursuit of scientific progress, would make its most dazzling triumphs not worth having. Let us finally remember that it cannot be the aim of progress to abolish the lot of mortality. Of some ill or other, each of us will die. Our mortal condition is upon us with its harshness but also its wisdom — because without it there would not be the eternally renewed promise of the freshness, immediacy, and eagerness of youth; nor would there be for any of us the incentive to number our days and make them count. With all our striving to wrest from our mortality what we can, we should bear its burden with patience and dignity.

---

of those findings: He lets himself be used as a means toward an end external to himself (even if he should at some later time happen to be among the beneficiaries himself). With respect to his own present needs and his own good, the act is gratuitous.

87 Globalizing Human Subjects Research

Adriana Petryna

The number of people participating in and required for pharmaceutical clinical trials has grown enormously since the early 1990s. The number of clinical trial investigators conducting multinational drug research in low-income settings increased sixteenfold, and the average annual growth rate of privately funded U.S. clinical trials recruiting subjects is projected to double by 2007.[1] This essay considers the evolution of commercialized clinical trials and ethical and regulatory environments as they contribute to a dramatic growth of human subjects' involvement in research. It focuses on the operations of U.S.-based contract research organizations and on the ways in which drug trials are being outsourced and expedited. Many of these new trials are being performed in areas of political and economic instability and unprecedented healthcare crises. Drug companies' accessibility to such areas raises questions about the unequal social contexts in which research is being performed and about how conditions of inequality remake a global geography of human experimentation.[2]

Pragmatic issues have overwhelmed ethics in terms of who controls international guidelines for ethical research and their capacity to protect the rights, interests, and well-being of human subjects globally.[3] Social scientists have critiqued bioethicists for focusing discussions about new global experimental orders almost exclusively on procedural questions of informed consent and clinical conduct, narrowing the view of the complexity of emergent ethical dilemmas in the arena of global human subjects research. Such a focus has led to a disconnect between bioethics — an abstract philosophical discourse grounding a set of codified norms for medical practice and research — and empirical reality.[4] Arthur Kleinman (1999), for example, points to a "dangerous break" between bioethics and the realities of local moral worlds that poses a danger to persons and their bodily integrity. Veena Das (1999) links international immunization programs and the manner of their implementation with the reemergence of local epidemics in India. Her work raises questions about the relation between bioethics and accountability in democratic societies and about the forms such ethics takes and to whom it is accountable.

Other anthropological work on the ethics of biotechnology and new medical technologies has shifted attention away from issues of individual autonomy and has deepened the analysis of new biomedical technologies as they affect new patterns of civic, medical, and commercial organization.[5] This work examines an important dimension of ethics beyond its universal and regulatory (or normative) frameworks. New technologies raise new contexts of decision making over doing what is right; thus, beyond defining instances of moral certainty, ethics also involves a set of tactics that can generate new human conditions and events (Rabinow 1996a, 2003; Fischer 2001, 2003).

In my ethnographic work with various professionals within the contract research organization (CRO) community (including company founders, CEOs, clinical trial managers, and health economists), the nurses and physicians with whom CROs contract, and pharmaceutical consultants and regulators in various countries, I came to

1. Business Communication Co., Inc. 2003. This figure is derived from industry surveys, the U.S. General Accounting Office, and the annual reports of seven major philanthropic organizations.

2. The Office of Inspector General, Department of Health and Human Services, states that "among the countries that have experienced the largest growth in clinical investigators [for commercially sponsored trials] are Russia and countries in Eastern Europe and Latin America" (2001:i). Clinical trials typically have been conducted on patients living in major pharmaceutical markets, the United States and Western Europe (and to a lesser extent Canada, Australia, and Japan). These regions comprise the leading global pharmaceutical markets. By the early 90s, this picture of commercialized drug research began to change. The outmigration of clinical research to so-called non-traditional research areas — countries undergoing demographic shifts or holding a relatively small market share — signals a sea change in a fundamental assumption in clinical trial participation. In the new clinical trials "markets," citizens are not long-term beneficiaries of new drugs. The reciprocal cycle of test subjects typically conceived of as end users/consumers of drugs is being broken.

3. Benatar and Singer 2000; Rothman 2000; Schuklenk and Ashcroft 2000; Benatar 2001; Lurie and Wolfe 2001; Office of the Inspector General, Department of Health and Human Services 2001; Farmer 2002a.

4. For earlier warnings on the dangers of ethics becoming disassociated from the empirical realities it claims to know, see Jonas 1969 and Toulmin 1987. Histories of bioethics and medical humanities approaches speak of the loss of intimacy in medical care as codes and norms (related to informed consent, for example) transform the patient-doctor relationship so that it is "no longer the intimate affair that it once was" (Rothman 1991:4). Intimacy, as anthropologists and historians of colonial and postcolonial settings suggest, is rarely a part of medicine in these settings, where it is the control of populations, rather than of individuals, that becomes the focal point of medicine (see Lindenbaum 1978; Comaroff and Comaroff 1992; Scheper-Hughes 1992; Vaughan 1992; Arnold 1993; Prakash 1999; Misra 2000; Anderson 2003; Briggs and Mantini-Briggs 2003; Biehl 2005; among others).

5. Strathern 1992; Franklin 1995; Cohen 1999; Rapp 1999; Dumit 2000; Biehl 2001; DelVecchio Good 2001; Lock 2001; Petryna 2002; Scheper-Hughes 2004.

From Adriana Petryna, "Globalizing Human Subjects Research," in *Global Pharmaceuticals*, pp. 33-60.

see that the global dynamics of drug production plays an important role in shaping contexts in which ethical norms and delineations of human subjects are changing. As violations of individual bodily integrity in human research continue to be exposed in the media, social scientists are also challenged to chart and consider how whole populations are brought into experimental orders and why the available discourses and protective mechanisms are unable to intervene to assist these groups.

I also discovered an ethical variability at work in the globalization of trials, one of several modes helping pharmaceutical sponsors to mobilize much larger populations of human subjects much more quickly. Ethical variability refers to how international ethical guidelines (informed by principles and guidelines for research involving human subjects) are being recast as trials for global research subjects are organized.[6] The international standardized ethics has starkly failed to account for local contexts and lived experience (Cohen 1999; Das 1999; Kleinman 1999). In an industrial pharmaceutical context, ethical variability evolves as a tactic informing the regulation and organization of commercial clinical trials. It takes the specificities of local context and lived experience as a given and as a basis on which to consolidate a cost-effective variability in ethical standards in human research.

Variability, however, is not meant to evoke the notion of "cultural relativism," although it has been interpreted in such terms (Christakis 1992). Reliance on culture to explain differences in global health practices has been central to the field of medical anthropology for decades. Knowledge of such cultural differences, as translated into the healthcare arena, tends to focus on "unbridgeable" moral divides between Western and non-Western groups. In the ethical imperialism versus relativism debate (Macklin 1999), anthropologists working in healthcare arenas and elsewhere have been faulted for blindly defending local cultural tradition, making them susceptible, as Clifford Geertz says, to the "moral and intellectual consequences that are commonly supposed to flow from relativism-subjectivism, nihilism, incoherence, Machiavellianism, ethical idiocy, esthetic blindness, and so on" (Geertz 2000:42).

Medical anthropologists, by contrast, have recently contended that a focus on cultural and moral difference in healthcare has become dangerous to the very people and practices anthropologists have sought to understand, particularly in the contexts of massive epidemics and debates over treatment access. As Paul Farmer (1999), Jim Yong Kim et al. (2003), and others point out, culture understood as difference has been used to explain "why" the poor are somehow less responsible regarding treatment regimes. The absence of an anti-HIV drug market in Africa, for example, has been blamed on the allegedly undependable medical and economic behaviors of that continent's desperately poor HIV sufferers. Farmer and Kim et al. have addressed the way moral assumptions in international health can further entrench inequality, warranting some interventions while preventing others.

Other anthropologists have moved beyond emphasis on difference and have shown, via careful ethnography, how courses of local epidemics are influenced by international policy and its technical forms (Cohen 1999; Das 1999; Biehl 2001). Differences in how institutions assigned to administer health problems (state governments, welfare agencies, insurance companies, medical bureaucracies, and religious and humanitarian groups) are arranged produce programs and actions that can shape different courses of health and sickness and affect the outcomes of both.

These works point to the kind of empirical precision that is required to address the moral, ethical, and cultural realities of emergent global drug markets. In this essay, I explore how ethical variability works, particularly in the conjuncture of accelerated drug development and the realities of global public health crises. I specify the effects of this variability on how research that uses human subjects is governed across various political and economic spheres, particularly in the absence of clear legislation in the United States and of transnational regulatory policy.[7] Ethical variability has become central to the development and global testing of pharmaceutical drugs, and it provides the means through which pharmaceutical sponsors and their third-party CROs achieve recruitment successes.

More Human Subjects

What drives the demand for larger pools of human subjects? First, it is the sheer number of trials being run. One

6. Rules and regulations for conducting human subjects research have been evolving since the Nuremberg Code was established in 1947. The World Medical Association's Declaration of Helsinki states ethical principles that should guide investigators and participants in medical research. The U.S. Food and Drug Administration (FDA) and other government and professional organizations also issue guidelines. The Office of Human Research Protection of the Department of Health and Human Services (DHHS) and the Declaration of Helsinki follow the ethical principles outlined in the Belmont Report (National Commission for the Protection of Human Subjects of Biomedical and Behavioral Research 1974). Yet these guidelines apply only to companies and institutions receiving DHHS funding. In the United States as well as in other countries, clinical trials are monitored by institutional review boards (IRBs). The number of commercial IRBs is growing.

7. By "government" of human subjects research I mean its ethical codes, the mechanisms of its growth, and its regulation. One goal of my research is to understand how wider ethnographic contexts inform the design and operation of clinical trials. Harry Marks's (1997) work is particularly illuminating in showing how ethics was incorporated into the design of the controlled, randomized trial in the United States in the interwar period. Elsewhere (Petryna forthcoming) I address the many forms and functions that human subjects research assumes at local and national levels and how the terms of commercialized human subjects research are being challenged so as to redirect economic, moral, and scientific investments in particular contexts.

market research company estimates that as of 2000, about 7,500 new clinical projects were being designed for research and development worldwide. By 2001 that number had purportedly grown to 10,000 (Brescia 2002).[8] Second, to satisfy U.S. regulatory demands, increasingly large numbers of patients must be included in clinical trials to prove products' long-term safety, especially for drugs intended to be widely prescribed. Third, some therapeutic categories — such as hypertension — are being overwhelmed by new drugs. Competition to get these drugs approved and to bring them to market intensifies the search for subjects. Fourth, there is a "drug pipeline explosion": patent applications are flooding the U.S. Patent Office for new compounds that have yet to be clinically tested.

Shifts in the very science of drug development also influence the decision to increase subject recruitment. As a vast amount of potential molecular therapeutics is generated, making right decisions regarding which molecules to test becomes more difficult. Consider antisense, a technology made up of genetic snippets that pass through cells and prevent the expression of certain harmful proteins. Wall Street investors learned that when the technology showed signs of failure in a late-phase clinical trial for patients with skin cancer, researchers recruited more research subjects in an attempt to find a statistically significant positive result.

Finally, the available pool of human subjects in the United States is shrinking. The relatively affluent U.S. population is using too many drugs (Gorman 2004). "Treatment saturation" is making Americans increasingly unusable from a drug-testing standpoint, as our pharmaceuticalized bodies produce too many drug-drug interactions providing less and less capacity to show drug effectiveness and making test results less statistically valid.

Indeed, whatever an American is ready to provide as a human subject, owing to a belief in scientific progress, altruism, or therapeutic need, will never be enough to satisfy the current level of demand for human subjects in commercial science. And that fact is pushing the human subjects research imperative to other shores. In this section, I examine historical aspects and operations of North American CROs, members of a specialized industry that began listing and selling securities on public exchanges in the early 1990s and that focuses on efficient and cost-effective human subjects research and recruitment.

The demand for human subjects in developing countries is directly related to the dynamics of industry-sponsored pharmaceutical drug testing in the United States. The roots of the expanding drug-testing regime are traceable to the post–World War II pharmaceutical boom in the United States, when a fee-for-service industry evolved in response to a demand for more safety testing in animals. Another point of origin for the expansion of human subject recruitment efforts dates back to the early 1970s, when the use of prisoner subjects in the United States was exposed and severely limited. According to one prominent executive, widely regarded as the founder of the CRO industry, pharmaceutical companies in the United States began internationalizing their human subject recruitment efforts as a response to regulatory limitations on prison research. (He directed the internationalization effort for one company in the mid-1970s.)[9] The scale of U.S. prison research was impressive: An estimated 90 percent of the drugs licensed prior to the 1970s were first tested on prison populations (Harkness 1996). When use of prisoners was banned (for particular phases of testing), pharmaceutical companies lost almost an entire base of human volunteers. In response, they shifted a good deal of their research elsewhere, primarily to Europe (and countries with regulatory-friendly environments), but also to other areas with large subject pools whose access could be guaranteed because of centralized health systems and the closed nature of referral systems.

By the early to mid-1980s, pharmaceutical companies were routinely outsourcing laboratory and clinical services — including preclinical bioassays, in which the activity of a chemical is assessed (mainly in animal models) — and the monitoring of investigational sites and clinical data. By the early 1990s, drug development had become a globalized endeavor, in part under the aegis of the International Conference on Harmonisation, or ICH (in which the U.S. FDA played a key developmental role).[10] The ICH created international standards for ensuring and assessing the safety and quality of testing procedures for experimental compounds, including the Good Clinical Practice guidelines for investigators and the implementation of institutional review boards (IRBs). Most important, it eased the acceptability and transference of clinical data from foreign investigational sites to the FDA for regulatory approval of new drugs.[11]

Today, CROs are highly competitive transnational

8. Estimates for the current number of clinical trials range from twenty-five thousand to eighty thousand (see, e.g., CenterWatch 2002). Such ambiguity suggests a global field of experimental activity whose true scope is largely unknown and prone to guesswork and that requires ethnographic attention. Dickersin and Rennie suggest that major barriers to a comprehensive repository of clinical trials include "industry resistance, the lack of a funding appropriation for a serious and sustained effort, lack of a mechanism for enforcement of policies, and lack of awareness of the importance of the problem" (2003:516). I thank Nicole Luce-Rizzo for her insights and generous research assistance here and elsewhere.

9. I interviewed this individual in June 2003.

10. The full name of this initiative is the International Conference on Harmonisation of Technical Requirements for Registration of Pharmaceuticals for Human Use.

11. Testing requirements are typically established by national regulatory agencies and can differ from country to country; duplicate testing threatened to delay foreign market access and affect the global trade in pharmaceuticals. Japan, perceived to be a potential large consumer market for U.S. pharmaceuticals, is famous for its intransigent regulatory system. See the chapter by Applbaum in [*Global Pharmaceuticals*].

businesses that run clinical trials for pharmaceutical, biotechnology, and medical device industries. They offer expertise in submission of clinical trial data to regulatory bodies and in conducting market analyses of existing and prospective drugs. Their main source of revenue comes from conducting clinical trials in an efficient and cost-effective manner, particularly the second and third phases of clinical trials, and they are paid to know the constraints and opportunities afforded by country and regional regulations related to drug testing.[12] CROs are rapidly expanding into the Third World and the former Second World of Eastern Europe, statistically and innovatively carving out new populations for larger and more complicated trials to assess the drug safety and efficacy demanded by U.S. regulators and consumers.

CROs claim to recruit patients quickly and more cheaply than academic medical centers. Most firms are involved in locating research sites, recruiting patients, and in some cases drawing up the study design and performing analyses. Elements considered in situating a cost-effective trial include local levels of unemployment, population disease profiles, morbidity and mortality rates, per-patient trial costs, and potential for future marketing of the approved drug. CROs investigate the host country's regulatory environment. They ask whether universal access to health is in place. They assess regulatory priorities and capacities of host countries (e.g., efficacy of local ethical review boards outlooks and regulations on placebo use).

In managing clinical trial sites CROs sometimes work with site management organizations, which may include primary healthcare facilities, general practitioner networks, hospitals, or consortia of specialists focusing on a particular therapeutic area. U.S.-based CROs have alliances with site management organizations in countries in Eastern Europe, Latin America, the Middle East, and Africa. Some even have their own centralized IRBs for single-investigator trials or for multicenter trials that can involve studies of up to ten thousand people in ten to twenty countries.[13] IRBs are, ideally, independent boards composed of scientific and nonscientific members whose duty is to ensure the safety of patients in a trial. Their purpose is to review and approve the trial protocol and methods to be used in obtaining and documenting the informed consent trial subjects. The ethics committee model for monitoring the conduct of research, as sociologists and anthropologists of bioethics have noted, turns the ethical universe in which researchers operate into an essentially procedural one (Guillemin 1998; Bosk 1999, 2002, 2005; Bosk and de Vries 2004; de Vries 2004) and deflects attention from structural circumstances that can contribute to increase risk and injustice (Chambliss 1996; Marshall and Koenig 2004). Do clinical researchers have the patient's informed consent? Does the local investigator agree to accept all responsibility in case of an adverse reaction or death? In the international context of drug development, the IRB model avoids the challenge of variability across distinct political and economic contexts. At stake is the construction of an airtight documentary environment ensuring the portability of clinical data from anywhere in the world to U.S. regulatory settings, even if those data were derived in the middle of an epidemic or in a war zone.[14]

Treatment Naiveté

This work evolved out of my research and writing on the Chernobyl nuclear disaster in the former Soviet Union (Petryna 2002). Working in government-operated research clinics and hospitals in the mid to late 1990s, I observed a rapid growth of pharmaceutical and clinical trial markets in Ukraine and its neighboring countries. Physicians who tended to Chernobyl sufferers routinely expressed eagerness to learn how to conduct clinical trials and to attract clinical trial contracts from multinational pharmaceutical sponsors because of the abundance of various untreated diseases.[15] They were also eager because the scientific infrastructures on which they were dependent were quickly deteriorating in the absence of state funding. The combination of local public health crises and commercial and scientific interest led to the sudden revaluing of patients who themselves had lost state protection in the form of guaranteed healthcare. It was not quite the dream "of Neel, Chagnon, and their gold-rush, tourist-hunting allies 'to turn the Yanomami's homeland into the world's largest private reserve,' a six-thousand-square-mile research station and 'biosphere' administered by themselves," described by Geertz (2001:21).[16] But scientists' rush to reconceptualize their

12. Drug development is broken down into four phases (preclinical, clinical, marketing, and postmarketing). Forty billion of the estimated $55 billion that is being invested in drug research and development goes to development. The CEO of one major contract research organization told me, "Probably 60 percent of that $40 billion is spent on phase two and three trials. So big money is there." Hundreds of CROs operate worldwide and employ a labor force of nearly 100,000 professionals (Rettig 2000). The move toward outsourcing increased dramatically in the 1990s. By 2004, nearly 42 percent of all pharmaceutical drug development expenditures had been committed to outsourcing (compared with only 4 percent in the early 1990s). The pharmaceutical industry is outsourcing an increasing number of operations ranging from discovery research to clinical trials operations to manufacturing, final packaging, and distribution as well as sales and marketing activities.

13. For an assessment of the commercialization of ethical review boards, see Lemmens and Freedman 2000.

14. See Jonathan Moreno's analysis of the ethics of human experiments for national security purposes. The focus on standards of consent in a time of international crisis can be read as a means through which a "postwar national security state protects itself from critics of expanded governmental power" (Moreno 2004:198).

15. Post-Soviet scientists were new to the randomization aspect of modern controlled clinical trials.

16. Geertz's quote continues: "The problem was that the anthros (and the médicos), reductionist to the core, conceived the object of their study not as a people but as a population. The Yanomami,

object of study "not as a people but as a population" to be brokered as valued research subjects on the pharmaceutical world scene was certainly there.

Currently a turf war is raging among pharmaceutical sponsors for human subjects. The competition is not only about the number of subjects a given company can recruit, it is also about recruiting subjects quickly. As one veteran recruiter told me, "It's really a problem. I don't know anybody who has really cracked the code. Sometimes you get lucky and you fill the study quickly, but for the most part, patients are really difficult to find, and they are difficult to find because everybody is looking for them." CROs see Eastern Europe as a particularly good recruitment site due to the collapse of basic healthcare there. Postsocialist healthcare systems are conducive to running efficient trials because they remain centralized. High literacy rates in this region mean that subjects offer more "meaningful" informed consent, thus smoothing potential regulatory problems in the future. Large Latin American cities such as Lima and São Paulo are also considered premium because, as one CRO-based recruiter told me, "Populations are massive. It's a question of how many patients I can get within a limited area, which reduces travel cost." CROs, he said, battle over "who gets those patients, who I can sign up to be in my alliance so that when I do attract a sponsor, I can say, 'I can line up 500 cancer patients for you tomorrow morning.' You are seeing that happening a lot because recruitment is one of the most time-consuming and expensive portions of the plan." Eastern Europe and Latin America are particularly attractive because of the extent of so-called treatment naiveté, the widespread absence of treatment for common and uncommon diseases. Treatment-naive populations are considered "incredibly valuable" because they do not have any background medication (medications present in the patient's body at the time of the trial), or any medication, for that matter, that might confuse the results of the trial. CROs make themselves competitive by locating the treatment-naive. One researcher told me that these populations "offer a more likely prospect of minimizing the number of variables affecting results and a better chance of showing drug effectiveness."[17]

On the one hand, pharmaceutical markets are growing. On the other hand, drug developers are now focusing on the biology of populations experiencing acute healthcare crises — populations whose life expectancies increased and whose incidence of infectious disease and mortality rates decreased under the demographic health transition, but whose lives are now shorter, more chronically diseased, and less socially protected.[18] The public health practice of demarcating disease to prevent disease (involving epidemiology, prevention, and medical access) is now used to carve out new catchment areas of human subjects who are targeted precisely because of their treatment naiveté. This move may appear exploitative, but the pharmaceutical industry argues that it is positive because in these regions clinical trials have become social goods in themselves.[19] And they may well be: they provide healthcare where there is none (see the chapter by Whyte et al.) and medical relief for participants' specific ailments for the duration of the trial.

Although industry and U.S. regulators would not dare codify such justifications for promoting clinical trials in poor areas, in many ways such justifications have already become an industry norm. Yet the question of precisely what made the move of the human subjects research enterprise to resource-poor settings both ethical and opportune remains unaddressed. In the next section I consider some key moments in the recent ethical and regulatory discussion of globalizing research in contexts of crisis, which have implications for how experimental groups are being defined and pursued globally today.

Ethical Variability: Constructing Global Subjects

The controversy over placebo use in Africa in 1994 during trials of short-course AZT treatment to halt perinatal transmission of HIV was a watershed in the debate over ethical standards in global clinical research (Angell 1988, 1997, 2000; Bayer 1998; Crouch and Arras 1998; Lurie and Wolfe 1998, 2000; Botbol-Baum 2000; de Zulueta 2001). Here I consider it as a watershed of another kind: for understanding how a cost-effective consolidation of variability in ethical standards overtook efforts to make a universal ethics (as codified in key ethical guidelines for human subjects research) applicable and enforceable worldwide. Underpinning this process is a more general

who indeed had the requisite sorts of brains, eyes, and fingers, were a control group in an inquiry centered elsewhere" (2000:21).

17. This short genealogy points out some reasons why subjects in health resources–poor areas became desirable for recruitment. Not only are they "desperate" and willing to participate in trials (Rothman 2000), they also fit a regulatory framework backed by a particular vision of appropriate scientific evidence promulgated by the FDA.

18. *Health transition* refers to the role that the cultural, social, and behavioral factors of health play in the rising life expectancy at birth (the mortality transition) and the decreasing proportion of all deaths caused by infectious diseases (the epidemiological transition). "Studies of the health transition focus on the institutional aspects that promote such change including public health interventions that control disease and promote modern healthcare" (Johansson 1991:39).

19. The fall of Communism in Poland, for example, marked the beginning of revolutionary changes in the field of cardiology and cardiac intervention. Poland, as the rest of Eastern and Central Europe, was plagued by inordinately high rates of cardiovascular deaths or a "cardiovascular disaster," as the former director of Poland's top cardiology institute (ANIN) called it. Clinicians and epidemiologists in this field were among the first Polish medical workers to participate in multi-nationally sponsored trials. One Polish CRO executive told me in 2005 that by the late 1990s ANIN became a major clinical trial site, "awash in thrombolytics for experimental use, so much so that the Institute had no need to buy them."

anthropological problem of how new subject populations are forged at the intersection of regulatory deliberation, corporate interests, and crises (upon crises) of health. My specific inquiry here centers on how the ability of the pharmaceutical industry to recruit treatment-naive subjects was solidified.

In this well-known case, some American researchers argued that giving less than standard care to those on the placebo arm of the study was ethically responsible, even if in the United States the standard of care medication was already known (a placebo is an inactive treatment made to appear like real treatment; it amounts to no treatment).[20] Critics viewed the use of a placebo arm in this case as highly unethical. They charged that research carried out in developing countries was being held to a standard different from those in effect in developed countries. Marcia Angell (2000), for example, noted patterns of conduct reminiscent of the Tuskegee experiment; that is, low-income communities were providing standing reserves of exploitable research subjects. Harold Varmus of the National Institutes of Health and David Satcher of the Centers for Disease Control, among the U.S. government institutions that authorized and funded the trial, claimed the trial was ethically sound (Varmus and Satcher 1996). They cited local cultural variables and deteriorated health infrastructures as making the delivery of the best standard of care infeasible. It would be a paternalistic imposition, they argued, for critics in the United States to determine the appropriate design of medical research in a region undergoing a massive health crisis when deciding the appropriate conduct of research and treatment distribution was within the jurisdiction of local and national authorities.

Ethical imperialism or ethical relativism? The debate, as it stands, is unresolved. Yet these catchphrases represent current responses to the ethics of the trial. The first position builds on well-known cases of marginalized communities acting as human subjects, and those cases, as medical historian Harry Marks (2002) suggests, may obscure more than they reveal about the contexts of experimental communities today. The second position relativizes ethical decision making as a matter of sound science, but it fails to consider the uptake of this relativizing move in corporate research contexts. The African AZT trial — and the ethical debates that followed it — highlight the role of crisis in the consideration of differences in ethical standards in the area of human research; indeed, that crisis conditions legitimate variability in ethical standards. Historically, some crises have led perhaps inescapably to experimentation (Smith 1990; Petryna 2002). But one can also ask, are crises exceptions or are they the norm? To what extent does the language of crisis become instrumental, granting legitimacy to experimentation that otherwise might not have any?

The debate over the ethics of the AZT trial prompted the sixth revision of the Helsinki Declaration, first issued in 1964. The declaration deals with all dimensions of human biomedical research, furnishing guidelines for investigator conduct in research involving human subjects.[21] The 2000 revision reiterated a position against placebo use when standards of treatment are known: "The benefits, risks, burdens, and effectiveness of a new method should be tested against those of the best current prophylactic, diagnostic, and therapeutic methods. This does not exclude the use of placebo, or no treatment, in studies where no proven prophylactic, diagnostic, or therapeutic method exists" (World Medical Association 2000:3044).[22] Although the ethics was unambiguous, the regulatory weight of the declaration was not. In this latter domain the winners and losers of the placebo debate would be named.[23] Pharmaceutical companies, already eagerly expanding operations abroad and calculating the economic advantages of placebo use (placebos lower costs, and, many argue, placebo trials produce unambiguous evidence of efficacy), were scrambling to learn from regulators about the legal enforceability of the declaration and were finding ways to continue using the placebo arm.

Haziness brought clarification of the rules of the game. Dr. Robert Temple, associate director of medical policy of the Center for Drug Evaluation of the FDA, undercut the regulatory significance of the declaration and threw his support behind placebo advocates, stating, "We'll have to see if the Declaration of Helsinki remains the ethical standard for the world" (Vastag 2000:2983). He cited the International Conference on Harmonisation (ICH-E10 2001) as the more authoritative guideline on the ethics of placebo use. This guideline states, "Whether a particular placebo controlled trial of a new agent will be acceptable to subjects and investigators when there is a known effective therapy is a matter of patient, investigator, and IRB judgement, and acceptability may differ among ICH regions. Acceptability could depend on the specific trial design and *population chosen*" (Temple 2002:213, emphasis added). In other words, the ethical standard for the world was claimed to be variability.

Temple's support for the placebo trial was ostensibly guided by his desire for high-quality scientific data. His reaction is also indicative of how regulatory regimes can influence the definition of experimental groups. Let me

20. The placebo control trial typically consists of a placebo arm and a treatment arm; its alternative, the active control trial, consists of an arm of treatment with known efficacy (active control) and an experimental arm.

21. The Declaration of Helsinki has been modified five times since its first edition in 1964.

22. This statement, of course, does not pertain to instances in which risk from withholding a proven therapy is lacking — as, for example, in the case of analgesics and antihistamines.

23. At stake in the placebo debate was something more than the issue of standard of care and patients' right of access to it. The regulatory weight of the Helsinki Declaration, the ability of IRBs to enforce proper research conduct globally, and the definition of just redistribution (particularly in resource-poor areas of the world) remained unaddressed.

briefly trace the logic of this relation. The alternative to the placebo control is the active control trial. Its purpose is to compare a new drug with a standard one, to show the superiority of the new drug to the active control or to at least show a difference. (Many patients and clinicians consider the comparative effectiveness of a new drug in relation to a standard therapy to be the most relevant information.) But showing difference or superiority is not enough because "many kinds of study defects decrease the likelihood of showing a difference between treatments" (Temple 2002:222) and make data on difference less reliable. Study defects arise from external factors like poor patient compliance, poor diagnostic criteria, and the use of concomitant medication that can obscure the effect. Other defects can include inconsistencies in how the disease is defined, the use of insensitive or inappropriate measures of drug effectiveness, and the chance of spontaneous recovery in a study population. These factors can be "fatal to a trial designed to show a difference," Temple claimed (2002:222; also see Pocock 2002:244-245). They can decrease difference or increase the chances of finding no difference, such that, in the end, in Temple's words, "you don't know if either of them worked" (Vastag 2000:2984). By contrast, a placebo control trial is capable of showing difference, and, much more important, makes it possible to distinguish between effective and ineffective treatments. That ability is considered a key marker of reliable evidence of the effectiveness of a new drug. Active control trials fail to make such a distinction and are therefore not preferable from a regulatory standpoint.

A certain kind of global human subject is at stake in Temple's description of the failure of active control trials. Most people in low-income countries, where many clinical trials are being or will be performed, are subject to the external factors that are said to lead to the study defects cited above. They may have medical histories that are patchy at best, thus making cross-cultural interpretation of the meaning of drug effectiveness less reliable. Their diagnoses can be inconsistent, also confusing evidence on drug effectiveness. Not only is quality of data in doubt with active control trials, so is the "quality" of the research subjects. Researchers must standardize medical histories if they are to ensure their comparability, and this is a time-consuming, costly, and all but impossible task.

Temple's invalidation of the active control trial is anthropologically and economically significant — the treatment-naive become preferable from a regulatory standpoint that emphasizes the importance of an efficient (and foolproof) global research subject. Precisely because they are often poor and lack a treatment history and treatment itself, the treatment-naive are the more foolproof and valuable research subjects!

Ethics as a Workable Document

In responding to the Helsinki Declaration revision, American regulators conveyed the value of research efficiency to industrial clinical researchers. And the murky ethics of the placebo could be bypassed by providing for what is known as equivalent medication — not necessarily the best or standard treatment, but whatever is available as the best local equivalent. "Do I give them a sugar pill or vitamin C?" one researcher cynically asked me. In the meantime, the study will be ethical, the data will have integrity, and, sadly, the patients will remain treatment-naive.

Another researcher echoed this shift from concerns about redistribution to efficiency-based standards in global research when he told me that ethics has come to be seen as a "workable document." "Equivalent medication in Eastern Europe is not the same as equivalent medication in Western Europe, so you could work the Helsinki Declaration," he said. In the name of efficiency, pharmaceutical companies and CROs intensified their search for treatment-naive populations worldwide.

In tracing the relation between regulation and the making of ethics in human research, Marks notes, "it is as if ethical discourse and the regulations governing research exist in two parallel universes which share some common elements but do not connect" (2000:14). But I would argue that the aftermath of the 1994 AZT trials shows how linked those universes are. Regulatory response in the context of debates over the Helsinki Declaration's revision (itself a response to controversial uses of human subjects) is now instantiating new populations of human subjects — the treatment-naive.

The story told here is about how regulatory decision making at the transnational level encourages the evolution of "local" experimental terrains whose ethics are workable and whose subjects can be (justifiably) variably protected under current international ethical codes such as the Helsinki Declaration. I say variably because some national governments faced with a sudden growth of human subjects research have minimal bureaucracies to cope with structures of liability in cases of adverse or catastrophic events.[24] Nor do all have the bargaining power

24. CROs and pharmaceutical sponsors tell me that their greatest concern is liability. In Europe, for example, governments require CROs, pharmaceutical sponsors, or both to purchase insurance. As one lawyer who arranges research contracts told me, "What if something goes wrong? What if the patient dies? What if there is some horrible side effect? Who is going to pay? That is big dollars. In the United States we have a legal system that we all understand, and the liability will be divided based upon negligence. . . . But in all of these other countries you really have to think about who is going to be responsible. At one recent conference that brought together representatives of the human subjects research industry from all over the world, I watched as pharmaceutical industry representatives lobbied some developing country officials to avoid "the insurance path" and to rely on systems of universal health coverage to cover costs. Legislation is pending in Brazil that would require CROs to register with the state's national health surveillance agency (ANVISA). According to one Brazilian official, this legislation is being put into place "because often what happens is that big pharmaceutical companies work through third parties. The CRO comes in and, let's say there is an adverse event, someone

or the desire to press for fairer procedures and access to drugs during and after the trial. Thus, a distinction is to be made between ethical codes (in which the definition of what constitutes biomedical harm is fairly unambiguous) and ethical regulation (in which deliberation of those definitions is balanced against economic, scientific, and regulatory constraints and demands). Ethical regulation entails minimally enforceable procedures governing human research as inscribed in public policy and law. It is also a realm of contingent practice where the allocation of protection for human subjects research is far from settled.

The ethical arrangements that have grown up around populations and their diseases can be elucidated by examining the spatial and temporal complexities associated with global pharmaceutical development and by analyzing the practices of the CROs that fill this demand.

Starting in the early 1990s, just four years before the controversial AZT trials, the FDA began to actively promote the globalization of clinical trials, declaring "the search for sites and sources of data" to be "part of its mandate to determine the safety and efficacy" (Office of the Inspector General, Department of Health and Human Services 2001:42) through the establishment of the ICH. Participation in American-sponsored research began to swell among clinical investigators in countries that had voluntarily agreed to harmonizing standards in the field of commercial drug testing: Argentina, Brazil, Hungary, Mexico, Poland, Russia, and Thailand, among others. As a result, the number of international human subjects involved in clinical trials grew dramatically between 1995 and 1999 (in 1995, 4,000; in 1999, 400,000; these are only partial estimates; see Office of the Inspector General, Department of Health and Human Services 2001).[25]

This global growth of research brought with it a new set of unknowns related to the circumstances of research as well as concerns about possible exploitation of foreign subjects. Currently, no U.S. legislation or international regulatory policy is aimed at controlling or monitoring the conduct of these globalizing clinical trials, although many proposals have been made for improving the monitoring system. In 1999, the Office of the Inspector General (OIG), a body that carries out periodic reviews of the FDA, told that agency after careful review that "in spite of its active promotion of the search for sites and subjects elsewhere," the FDA is not able to protect human subjects in research elsewhere.[26] The OIG recommended that the FDA support and in some cases help to construct local ethical review boards.

The regulatory preference for the expansion of the IRB model is reflected in a recent National Bioethics Advisory Commission (2000) report recommending that studies submitted to the FDA receive ethical committee review both in the United States and in the country in which the research is being carried out (as opposed to the present situation, in which only foreign ethical review and approval are mandated). The report supported the idea of dual review but stated that if host countries have working ethical review committees, then only their approval is required.

These approaches involve monitoring, data collection, and more local ethics committees and lean heavily toward what Iris Young (2004) calls the "liability model" of accountability: Let regulators name the responsible local parties (in some cases, set them up first), and surely those parties can gather information and make the right decisions; surely they can stop inappropriate research from taking place. Much is also assumed about who is and is not the agent of abuse, typically defined as the individual investigator.

What about instances in which risks arise in the structure of the research itself? These instances tend not to find proper nouns in ethical discussions, beyond designation as "interesting" or "scandalous" cases. The fact is that certain conditions have to be met for liability to work: States themselves need to act as protectors and not abusers; transnational corporations need to respect the rights and dignity of all research subjects and recognize that different situations elicit different kinds of coercion; and international ethics codes must be enforceable in cases of clear violation.

None of this occurred, unfortunately, in Nigeria in 1996 during industry-sponsored research involving Trovan, a drug manufactured by Pfizer, Inc. Trovan was once one of the most widely prescribed antibiotics in the United States, but it was taken off the market because it was found to produce liver-damaging side effects. In an effort to gain FDA approval for a new use of Trovan to treat bacterial meningitis a team of Pfizer researchers traveled to the city of Kano during a bacterial meningitis

needs surgery, and the CRO is not held liable, even though the pharmaceutical company guarantees liability coverage." This official put it very succinctly: "The patient-subject signs the informed consent form but the protection is a fiction. They are not insured."

25. These numbers refer to new drug applications only. In Brazil, for example, the number of clinical investigators grew from 16 in 1991 to 187 in 1999. In Russia, the number grew from 0 in 1991 to 170 in 1999. These countries and others experiencing growth have seen political upheavals during democratic transition and are currently competing to consolidate their clinical trials markets in a neoliberalizing context. In collaboration with the ICH, a harmonizing initiative is under way in the Americas called the "Pan American Network for Drug Regulatory Harmonization." The European Union recently implemented the EU Clinical Trials Directive for EU countries and accession states.

26. The OIG's mission statement is as follows: "The mission of the Office of Inspector General, as mandated by Public Law 95-452 (as amended), is to protect the integrity of Department of Health and Human Services (HHS) programs, as well as the health and welfare of the beneficiaries of those programs. The OIG has a responsibility to report both to the Secretary and to the Congress program and management problems and recommendations to correct them. The OIG's duties are carried out through a nationwide network of audits, investigations, inspections and other mission-related functions performed by OIG components" (Office of Inspector General, Department of Health and Human Services n.d.).

outbreak (which they found out about on the Internet). They were in search of pediatric victims of this disease who were most likely treatment-naive. Doctors Without Borders was already distributing a cheaper antibiotic, proven effective for treating bacterial meningitis, at a main local hospital.

The trial protocol for testing a new use of Trovan was not approved by an American ethics committee and received a grossly inadequate, perhaps nonexistent, review in the host country, which was suffering civil unrest under the Abacha military dictatorship. Legal documents show that the informed consent forms used in Pfizer's defense are backdated.[27] The Pfizer team went to the hospital where the cheaper drug was being distributed and selected one hundred children who were waiting in line to receive treatment. Researchers are alleged not to have explained the experimental nature of Trovan to the subjects; parents believed their children were receiving a proven treatment.[28] Some of these children were given Trovan in a form never before tested on humans; others were given a lower dose of the standard of care for meningitis (ceftriaxone) that, according to the complaint filed by the New York law firm representing the parents, allowed Pfizer researchers to show that Trovan was more efficacious (Lewin 2001). This low dosing, the parents claim, resulted in the deaths of eleven children.

This is the first case brought by foreign citizens against a U.S.-based multinational pharmaceutical company. The plaintiffs' lawyers suggested that a chain of complicity in making the children available for research included Nigeria's military rulers and state officials, Ministry of Health officials, and local hospital administrators; U.S. FDA regulators who authorized an unapproved drug's export to Nigeria for "humanitarian" purposes; and the Pfizer researchers who selected subjects for an industry-sponsored clinical trial. All were involved, lawyers claimed, in violating principles of the Nuremberg Code and other codes of human subjects protection, referred to in plaintiffs' court documents as "customary laws" that are "made up of fundamental principles of a civil society that are so widely held that they constitute binding norms on the community of nations" (*Rabi Abdullahi et al. v. Pfizer Inc.*, 01 Civ. 8118 (WHP) [2000]).[29]

The defendant's lawyers downplayed the authority of the code and stated that it and other such guidelines "are not treaties." (In some domestic cases, federal judges have ruled that internationally accepted codes of human subjects protection, in this case the Nuremberg Code and the Helsinki Declaration, cannot be relied on as the basis of civil suits in U.S. courts.) The defense situated Pfizer researchers' activities in the context of a "massive epidemic killing more than 11,000 people," whose outbreak they attributed to "woefully inadequate" sanitary conditions. By suggesting that their experimental treatment could only do good in such a desperate context, the defense obscured the criteria by which to judge the difference between experimental and standard-of-care treatment. Pfizer's defense further stated that it would be "paternalistic" for an American court to adjudicate the appropriate conduct of medical research in a country undergoing a public health crisis, and echoed the ethically relativizing stance already familiar in the African AZT case *(Rabi Abdullahi et al. v. Pfizer Inc.)*.

One aspect of this legal parrying is worth stressing. As much as one would like to see the Kano case as an instance of the "dubious" or the "para" (paralegal, pararegulatory, paraethical), an interlocking set of regulatory, commercial, and state interests is at play in such situations that can potentially introduce uncertainty with respect to the observability of international ethics codes in local contexts, or even suspend the relevance of such ethics altogether.[30] In this case, a functional ethical review of U.S. industry-sponsored research might have prevented this tragedy. But from the Nigerian side of things, interests were not on the side of protection but overwhelmingly on the side of making populations accessible to research.

The Trovan case is still being adjudicated, but deliberations so far suggest that knowledge of wrongdoing does not necessarily translate into the ability to regulate or prosecute wrongdoers. The case exemplifies how contextual factors (crisis and its humanitarianisms) and defenses fold into and construct new experimental scenarios and groups. Ethical positions, particularly those revealed by the AZT case, that relativize decision making over appropriate conduct of research to local context inform a legal defense strategy to make acts of experimentation — particularly those enacted in public health crises — either reachable or unreachable by international ethics codes.[31] What appears as scandalous activity with respect to global human subjects research may in fact be seen as legitimate under evolving ethical and legal notions of fair play.

As I noted above, this "expedient" experimentality first caught my attention in the context of the scientific

27. I am grateful to Elaine Kusel for providing relevant legal documents, and to Michael Oldani for referring me to this case.

28. Pfizer contracted a CRO, European based at the time, to organize the transfer of blood samples to its laboratory in Geneva to conduct assays on children's spinal fluid samples. The Trovan story illustrates how the political economy of drug development links seemingly disconnected worlds and jurisdictions. At the same time, the legal viability of existing international codes of human subjects protection is being thrown into doubt.

29. The Nuremberg Code was established in response to Nazi medical experiments on prisoners in concentration camps. The code instituted norms of protection for subjects of scientific research experiments in the form of informed and voluntary consent and human rights guarantees.

30. For another instance of lawyers attempting to eliminate ethical limitations, rather than to assert them, see Alden 2004.

31. The domain of international law in remunerating human subjects violations is beyond the scope of this essay. See Das's (1995b) consideration of the Bhopal Union Carbide case.

management of the Chernobyl nuclear crisis. Here, too, the language of crisis became instrumental, granting legitimacy to what might be considered questionable experimentation. A public health disaster combined with the state's incapacity to protect the life of citizens, and this combination of circumstances justified a commercially sponsored clinical trial that would have been impossible to conduct elsewhere at the time. Human research whose exploitativeness might have been hard to judge was justified under the rubric of humanitarianism; and this process in itself may lie outside the bounds of what ethical discourse about human subjects research and even legal codes can capture.[32]

Occurring at a time when research priorities in the world of international science were shifting toward biotechnology, Chernobyl afforded a venue for biotechnological research.[33] The Soviet state's response to the crisis is widely documented as having been grossly inadequate, particularly in the first days after the disaster.[34] Under strong pressure to restore the credibility lost by the state's initial inadequate response, General-Secretary Gorbachev agreed to cooperate in an unprecedented Soviet-U.S. scientific venture. He personally invited a team of American oncologists and radiation scientists to conduct experimental bone marrow transplants on workers from the "Zone" (an area thirty kilometers in diameter circumscribing the destroyed nuclear reactor site) whose exposures were beyond the lethal limit and for whom no treatment was available.

In exchange for the credibility garnered from this move, Soviet medical authorities gave in to the American research team's demands to conduct human testing of a genetically engineered hematopoetic growth factor molecule (rhGM-CSF, thought to regenerate stem cell growth and to be useful for treating leukemia). Some animal testing had been under way in the United States using highly irradiated chimpanzees and dogs, but human testing of the molecule had not been approved by the FDA. The humanitarian ethics to treat in a crisis where there was no other treatment legitimated the transfer and use of unapproved experimental drugs.

The lead scientist on this trial told me that he had no clinical trial protocol but that he had acted consistently "with what was legal."[35] He did not know the exact number of individuals on whom the molecule was tested (he guessed it was over four hundred). During our 1996 interview he described his interests in the Chernobyl cohort as short term. In his view, the accident offered his team a ready-made set of experimental conditions: "The Chernobyl accident for the firemen at the power plant was exactly what we do at the clinic every day. Potentially, there were patients with [leukemic] cancer exposed to acute whole body irradiation." This scientist, who has gained fame and admiration for his humanitarianism, spoke to me about these unregulated trials in a surprisingly confident fashion, suggesting that political arrangements gave him adequate refuge from ethical sanctions. "No one was going to believe what Gorbachev had to say about Chernobyl," he told me. "I convinced them of that [in my negotiations]. They had no credibility."

This scientist's confidence illuminates a political, regulatory, legal, and ethical milieu that lay beyond the procedures governing relations between researchers and their human subjects. Disaster reframed as humanitarian crisis presented a unique scientific and political opportunity. Politically, normal rules of conduct were suspended. Scientifically, the disaster offered a set of negative health circumstances that, because of codes of ethics prohibiting human experimentation, would have been impossible to simulate in normal clinical trial circumstances in the United States. In other words, the crisis provided a ready-made scenario for bioscientific research: it gave researchers liberal access to a pool of highly endangered people. This pool became attractive precisely when a nonhuman model showing the effects of a particular molecule was lacking. Although the results of this trial were deemed largely unsuccessful, both sides gained significantly from their short-term arrangement. The American scientist's team and its major pharmaceutical backer got a valuable jump-start on the emerging biotechnological market in growth-factor molecules, and Soviet officials got a rare opportunity to shore up the state's credibility locally and internationally.

Biological Citizenship

As the Trovan and Chernobyl cases show, a humanitarian crisis can create a space that appears to be "ethics free" precisely because it is disastrous, beyond the reach of regulation. With the sudden suspension of normalcy, whole groups of people actually or potentially become experimental subjects.[36] Both cases also demonstrate to a

32. The literature and practice on human rights versus humanitarianism have highlighted this state of affairs over the past decade (see, e.g., Ignatieff 2001 and Rieff 2003). Also see Rabinow 2003.

33. For evidence of the view of Chernobyl as a kind of "experiment" allowing scientists to corroborate or refute biomedical data concerning the long-term health consequences of nuclear exposure, see "Chernobyl's Legacy to Science."

34. Because of government inaction, tens of thousands of people were either knowingly or unknowingly exposed to radioactive iodine-131 — which is absorbed rapidly in the thyroid — resulting, among other things, in a sudden and massive onset of thyroid cancers in children and adults as soon as four years later. This disaster could have been curtailed had the government distributed non-radioactive iodine pills within the first week.

35. He said he had approval from the FDA.

36. While the rhGM-CSF trials were taking place in a clinic in Moscow, Soviet, European, and U.S. nuclear industry officials met in Vienna to decide how to portray the scope of the disaster to the world. In their press release they announced that thirty-one cleanup workers had died in the course of work in the Zone. As the officials were negotiating over this number, hundreds of thousands of workers were being sent into the Zone in a massive, ongoing effort to contain the flames and radioactivity of a burning reactor. Humanitarianism in the form of scientific cooperation provided

greater or lesser extent a breakdown in consent processes and in citizens' ability to trust and rely on state systems of public health and protection. Ethics is used variably and tactically by all actors in a chain of interests involved in human subjects research. Such chains now function in states where lives of citizens are not adequately protected by traditional health or welfare systems. The biological indicators of whole groups, however formed or damaged by social and economic context, are enfolded into regimes of international and local forms of protection in which ethics becomes a "workable document." The issue of human subjects protection thus moves beyond scripted procedural issues of informed consent and into questions of legal capacities and the aggregate human conditions of which they are generative (Marks 2000).

What alternatives are there to counteract abuse and inadequate protection of research subjects? What work can be done locally, scientifically, and administratively to link biology back to regimes of protection? In the Chernobyl context, I documented how, in the newly independent Ukrainian state, radiation research clinics and nongovernmental organizations mediated an informal economy of illness and claims to "biological citizenship" — a massive demand for but selective access to a form of social welfare based on scientific and legal criteria that both acknowledge injury and compensate for it. Such struggles over biological citizenship took place in a context of fundamental losses related to employment and state protections against inflation, widespread corruption, and the corrosion of legal and political categories.[37] Assaults on health became the coin sufferers paid for biomedical resources, social equity, and human rights.

This type of biosocial fabric, in which the very idea of citizenship becomes charged with the superadded burden of survival (also see the chapter by Biehl [in *Global Pharmaceuticals*]), is one of many being converted into a model of cost-effective ethical variability in globalized human research. Commercial sponsors argue that clinical trials provide social and material goods to treatment-naive populations where those goods otherwise might not be available; if these populations do not want the goods, sponsors can always go somewhere else. "There are so many places that we can work that we just bypass it altogether," one CRO executive told me. In other words, sponsors are free to bargain down the price and "work the ethics" (in terms of equivalent medications) of any trial.[38]

The circulation of such experimental goods and the relative absence of public scandal over how they circulate do not make the task of gathering more information on the sites and sources of clinical research data any less urgent — particularly while the FDA actively promotes the "search for sites and sources of data" around the world to fulfill its "mandate to determine the safety and efficacy" of new drugs (Office of Inspector General, Department of Health and Human Services 2001:42). In the early 1970s, when the scandal over the use of prison subjects broke, the FDA claimed it had little documentation, citing its duty to protect intellectual property. Today the FDA resists gathering data on the out-migration of human research on the basis that location of testing is proprietary information. One might want to rethink whether anonymity of the sources of clinical research data is a defensible idea anymore.

Conclusion

In this chapter I have sketched an ethnographic approach to human subjects research — examining its practices and strategies across a variety of international, state, and economic spheres — in the context of an emerging industry of such research. The overriding empirical problem centers on the apparent ease of access to new treatment-poor populations. In the pharmaceutical industry's pursuit of these new global subjects one can observe how deliberations over the ethics of research in crisis-ridden areas are set against — and even eclipsed by — the market ethics of industry scientists and regulators. Rather than leveling the starting conditions in which global human subjects research is conducted, ethical variability itself has become the industry norm, to the point of being consciously deployed in pharmaceutical development. Ethics should protect people from harm. Case-based observation and analysis suggest that the procedural issues researchers rely on in realizing human subjects protection are insulating researchers from the contexts of inequality in which they work.

In contrast, current bioethical commentary on the movement of human trials to developing countries centers on the need to produce better ways of deriving informed consent from human subjects and exporting the IRB model at a quicker pace. The purpose here is to ensure that the autonomy of individuals takes precedence over the demands of science or the interests of society, with the idea that such autonomy can counteract coercion in research wherever it takes place. An exclusive focus on informed consent narrows one's vision of the

---

the Soviet state some protection in organizing this massive labor recruitment. The number of deaths is not known because of lax monitoring and medical follow-up (Petryna 2002).

37. Social protections include cash subsidies, family allowances, free medical care and education, and pension benefits for sufferers and the disabled. Affected persons, legally designated *poterpili* (sufferers), number 3.5 million and constitute a full 7 percent of the Ukrainian population.

38. In the language of bargaining theory, individual threat points vary globally. A threat point is the level of well-being that could be achieved if bargaining fails. Thanks to Joe Harrington for clarifying this point. Once again, variability seems to be the norm rather than the exception, as access to clinical trial subjects in contexts of minimal or no care becomes easier. And this variability includes a biological component because in some environments states can no longer protect the lives of their citizens.

broad array of factors that are overwhelming ethics. The incursion of procedural norms has not (at least not yet) evidenced itself in the exercise of free will by autonomous agents in human research. Rather, population-wide processes that support reification (and in some cases capitalization) of social and biological difference continue to operate.

This ethnographic assessment of the human subjects research industry brings into focus emergent ethical arrangements around disease and populations where states have collapsed and where the creation of new poverty is a chronic process. Rather than focusing on normative theory of ethics and ideal conditions, I maintain the importance of apprehending the norms that are being propagated and how they are being reconstructed in actual and diverse conditions. Understanding the existing variability in the regulation of ethics and the coinages through which consent, autonomy, and drug markets evolve helps build an ethnographic context that may ultimately provide the basis for a critique of market-driven human research.

References

Alden, Edward. 2004. US interrogation debate: Dismay at attempt to find legal justification for torture. *Financial Times,* 10 June.

Anderson, Warwick. 2003. *The Cultivation of Whiteness: Science, Health, and Racial Destiny in Australia.* New York: Basic Books.

Angell, Marcia. 1988. Ethical imperialism? Ethics in international collaborative clinical research. *New England Journal of Medicine* 319 (16): 1081-1083.

Angell, Marcia. 1997. The ethics of clinical research in the Third World. *New England Journal of Medicine* 337 (12): 847-849.

Angell, Marcia. 2000. Is academic medicine for sale? *New England Journal of Medicine* 342 (20): 1516-1518.

Arnold, David. 1993. *Colonizing the Body: State Medicine and Epidemic Disease in Nineteenth-Century India.* Berkeley: University of California Press.

Bayer, R. 1998. The debate over maternal-fetal HIV transmission prevention trials in Africa, Asia, and Caribbean: Racist exploitation or exploitation of racism? *American Journal of Public Health* 88 (4): 567-570.

Benatar, Solomon. 2001. Distributive justice and clinical trials in the Third World. *Theoretical Medicine and Bioethics* 22 (3): 169-176.

Benatar, Solomon, and Peter A. Singer. 2000. A new look at international research ethics. *British Medical Journal* 321 (7264): 824-826.

Biehl, João. 2001a. Vita: Life in a zone of social abandonment. *Social Text* 19 (3): 131-149.

Biehl, João, with Denise Coutinho e Ana Luzia Outeiro. 2001b. Technology and affect: HIV/AIDS testing in Brazil. *Culture, Medicine, and Psychiatry* 25:87-129.

Biehl, João. 2005. *Vita: Life in a Zone of Social Abandonment.* Berkeley: University of California Press.

Bosk, Charles. 1999. Professional ethicist available: Logical, secular, friendly. *Daedalus* 128 (fall): 47-68.

Bosk, Charles. 2002. Now that we have the data, what was the question? *American Journal of Bioethics* 2 (4): 21-23.

Bosk, Charles. 2005. *What Would You Do? The Collision of Ethnography and Ethics.* Chicago: University of Chicago Press.

Bosk, Charles, and Raymond de Vries. 2004. Bureaucracies of mass deception: Institutional review boards and the ethics of ethnographic research. *Annals of the American Academy of Political and Social Science* 595 (1): 249-263.

Botbol-Baum, Mylène. 2000. The shrinking of human rights: The controversial revision of the Helsinki Declaration. *HIV Medicine* 1 (4): 238-245.

Brescia, Bonnie. 2002. Better budgeting for patient recruitment. *Pharmaceutical Executive.* Electronic document, http://www.pharmexec.com. Accessed 10 September 2004.

Briggs, Charles, and Clara Mantini-Briggs. 2003. *Stories in the Time of Cholera: Racial Profiling During a Medical Nightmare.* Berkeley: University of California Press.

Business Communication Company. 2003. *The Clinical Trials Business.* Report B-171. Norwalk, Conn.: Business Communication Company.

CenterWatch. 2002. CenterWatch launches first-of-its-kind consumer guide to the risks and benefits of volunteering for clinical trials. Electronic document, http://www.centerwatch.com/newsreleases/4-1-2002. Accessed 1 September 2004.

Chambliss, Daniel F. 1996. *Beyond Caring: Hospitals, Nurses, and the Social Organization of Ethics.* Chicago: University of Chicago Press.

Christakis, Nicholas. 1992. Ethics are local: Engaging cross-cultural variation in the ethics for clinical research. *Social Science and Medicine* 35 (9): 1079-1091.

Cohen, Lawrence. 1999. Where it hurts: Indian material for an ethics of organ transplantation. *Daedalus* 128 (fall): 135-165.

Comaroff, John, and Jean Comaroff. 1992. Medicine, colonialism, and the black body. In John Comaroff and Jean Comaroff, *Ethnography and the Historical Imagination,* 215-235. Boulder, Colo.: Westview Press.

Crouch, Robert A., and John D. Arras. 1998. AZT trials and tribulations. *Hastings Center Report* 28 (6): 26-34.

Das, Veena. 1995b. Suffering, legitimacy, and healing: The Bhopal case. In Veena Das, *Critical Events: An Anthropological Perspective on Contemporary India,* 137-174. Delhi: Oxford University Press.

Das, Veena. 1999. Public good, ethics, and everyday life: Beyond the boundaries of bioethics. *Daedalus* 128 (4): 99-133.

de Vries, Raymond. 2004. How can we help? From "sociology in" to "sociology of" bioethics. *Journal of Law, Medicine, and Ethics* 32 (2): 279-293.

de Zulueta, P. 2001. Randomised placebo-controlled trials and HIV-infected pregnant women in developing countries: Ethical imperialism or unethical exploitation? *Bioethics* 15 (4): 289-311.

Dickersin, Kay, and Drummond Rennie. 2003. Registering clinical trials. *JAMA* 290 (4): 516.

Dumit, Joseph. 2000. When explanations rest: "Good enough" brain science and the new biomental disorders. In Margaret Lock, Alan Young, and Alberto Cambrosio, eds., *Living and Working with the New Medical Technologies: Intersections of Inquiry,* 209-232. Cambridge: Cambridge University Press.

Farmer, Paul. 1999. The consumption of the poor: Tuberculosis in the late twentieth century. In *Infections and Inequalities: The Modern Plagues,* 184-211. Berkeley: University of California Press.

Farmer, Paul. 2002a. Can transnational research be ethical in the developing world? *Lancet* 360 (9342): 1301-1302.

Fischer, Michael M. J. 2001. Ethnographic critique and technoscientific narratives: The old mole, ethical plateaux, and the governance of emergent biosocial polities. *Culture, Medicine and Psychiatry* 25 (4): 355-393.

Fischer, Michael M. J. 2003. *Emergent Forms of Life and the Anthropological Voice.* Durham, N.C.: Duke University Press.

Franklin, Sarah. 1995. Science as culture, cultures of science. *Annual Review of Anthropology* 24:163-185.

Geertz, Clifford. 2000 [1984]. Anti anti-relativism. In Geertz, *Available Light: Anthropological Reflections on Philosophical Topics,* 42-67. Princeton: Princeton University Press.

Geertz, Clifford. 2001. Life among the anthros. *New York Review of Books* 48 (2): 18-22.

Good, Mary-Jo DelVecchio. 2001. The biotechnical embrace. *Culture, Medicine and Psychiatry* 25 (4): 395-410.

Gorman, James. 2004. The altered human is already here. *New York Times,* 6 April.

Guillemin, Jeanne. 1998. Bioethics and the coming of the corporation to medicine. In Raymond de Vries and Janardan Subedi, eds., *Bioethics and Society: Constructing the Ethical Enterprise,* 60-77. Upper Saddle River, N.J.: Prentice-Hall.

Harkness, Jon M. 1996. Research behind bars: A history of nontherapeutic research on American prisoners. PhD diss., University of Wisconsin, Madison.

Ignatieff, Michael. 2001. *Human Rights as Politics and Idolatry.* Princeton: Princeton University Press.

Johansson, S. Ryan. 1991. Health transition: The cultural inflation of morbidity during the decline of mortality. *Health Transition Review* 1 (1): 39-68.

Jonas, Hans. 1969. Philosophical reflections on human experimentation. *Daedalus* 98 (spring): 219-247.

Kim, Jim Yong, Joia S. Mukherjee, Michael L. Rich, Kedar Mate, Jaime Bayona, and Mercedes C. Becerra. 2003. From multidrug-resistant tuberculosis to DOTS expansion and beyond: Making the most of a paradigm shift. *Tuberculosis* 83 (1-3): 59-65.

Kleinman, Arthur. 1999. Moral experience and ethical reflection: Can ethnography reconcile them? A quandary for "the new bioethics." *Daedalus* 128 (fall) 69-99.

Lemmens, Trudo, and Benjamin Freedman. 2000. Ethics review for sale? Conflict of interest and commercial research ethics review. *Milbank Quarterly* 78 (4): 547-584.

Lewin, Tamar. 2001. Families sue Pfizer on test of antibiotic. *New York Times,* 30 August.

Lindenbaum, Shirley. 1978. *Kuru Sorcery: Disease and Danger in the New Guinea Highlands.* New York: McGraw-Hill.

Lock, Margaret. 2001. *Twice Dead: Organ Transplants and the Reinvention of Death.* Berkeley: University of California Press.

Lurie, Peter, and Sidney M. Wolfe. 1998. Unethical trials of interventions to reduce perinatal transmission of the human immunodeficiency virus in developing countries. *New England Journal of Medicine* 337 (12): 853-855.

Lurie, Peter, and Sidney M. Wolfe. 2000. Letter to the National Bioethics Advisory Commission regarding their report on the challenges of conducting research in developing countries. HRG Publication no. 1545. Electronic document, http://www.citizen.org/publications. Accessed 12 December 2003.

Lurie, Peter, and Sidney M. Wolfe. 2001. Comments on the draft health and human services inspector general's report: The globalization of clinical trials (OEI-01-00-00190). HRG Publication no. 1591. Public Citizen's Research Group, 5 July 2001. Electronic document, http://www.citizen.org/publications. Accessed 12 December 2003.

Macklin, Ruth. 1999. *Against Relativism: Cultural Diversity and the Search for Ethical Universals in Medicine.* Oxford: Oxford University Press.

Marks, Harry. 1997. *The Progress of Experiment: Science and Therapeutic Reform in the United States, 1900-1990.* Cambridge: Cambridge University Press.

Marks, Harry. 2000. Where do ethics come from? The role of disciplines and institutions. Paper prepared for Conference on Ethical Issues in Clinical Trials. University of Alabama, Birmingham, 25 February.

Marks, Harry. 2002. Commentary. Third Annual W. H. R. Rivers Workshop: Global Pharmaceuticals: Ethics, Markets, Practices. Harvard University, 19-21 May.

Marshall, Patricia, and Barbara Koenig. 2004. Accounting for culture in a globalized ethics. *Journal of Law, Medicine, and Ethics* 32 (2): 252-266.

Misra, Kavita. 2000. Productivity of crises: Disease, scientific knowledge and state in India. *Economic and Political Weekly* 35 (43-44): 3885-3897.

Moreno, Jonathan D. 2004. Bioethics and the national security state. *Journal of Law, Medicine, and Ethics* 32 (2): 198-208.

National Bioethics Advisory Commission. 2000. *Ethical and Policy Issues in International Research: Clinical Trials in Developing Countries.* Bethesda, Md.: National Bioethics Advisory Commission.

National Commission for the Protection of Human Subjects of Biomedical and Behavioral Research. 1974. *Protection of Human Subjects: Ethical Principles and Guidelines for the Protection of Human Subjects of Research* [Belmont Report]. Washington: Department of Health, Education, and Welfare.

Office of the Inspector General, Department of Health and Human Services. 2001. *The Globalization of Clinical Trials: A Growing Challenge in Protecting Human Subjects.* Boston: Office of Evaluation and Inspections.

Office of the Inspector General, Department of Health and Human Services. n.d. OIG Mission. Electronic document, http://oig.hhs.gov. Accessed 22 September 2004.

Petryna, Adriana. 2002. *Life Exposed: Biological Citizens after Chernobyl.* Princeton: Princeton University Press.

Petryna, Adriana. Forthcoming. The human subjects research enterprise. Princeton: Princeton University Press.

Pocock, Stuart. 2002. The pro's and con's of non-inferiority (equivalence) trials. In Harry A. Guess, Arthur Kleinman, John W. Kusek, and Linda W. Engel, eds., *The Science of the Placebo: Toward an Interdisciplinary Research Agenda,* 236-248. London: BMJ Books.

Prakash, Gyan. 1999. *Another Reason: Science and the Imagination of Modern India.* Princeton: Princeton University Press.

Rabinow, Paul. 1996a. *Essays on the Anthropology of Reason.* Princeton: Princeton University Press.

Rabinow, Paul. 1996b. *French Modern: Norms and Forms of the Social Environment.* Chicago: University of Chicago Press.

Rabinow, Paul. 2003. *Anthropos Today: Reflections on Modern Equipment.* Princeton: Princeton University Press.

Rapp, Rayna. 1999. *Testing Women, Testing the Fetus: The Social Impact of Amniocentesis in America.* New York: Routledge.

Rettig, Richard. 2000. The industrialization of clinical research. *Health Affairs* (March-April): 129-146.

Rieff, David. 2003. *A Bed for the Night: Humanitarianism in Crisis.* New York: Simon and Schuster.

Rothman, David J. 1991. *Strangers at the Bedside: A History of How Law and Bioethics Transformed Medical Decision Making.* New York: Basic Books.

Rothman, David J. 2000. The shame of medical research. *New York Review of Books* 47 (19): 60-64.

Scheper-Hughes, Nancy. 1992. *Death Without Weeping: The Violence of Everyday Life in Brazil.* Berkeley: University of California Press.

Scheper-Hughes, Nancy. 2004. Parts unknown. *Ethnography* 5 (1): 29-74.

Schuklenk, U., and R. Ashcroft. 2000. International research ethics. *Bioethics* 14 (2): 158-172.

Smith, Jane. 1990. *Patenting the Sun: Polio and the Salk Vaccine.* New York: William Morrow.

Strathern, Marilyn. 1992. *After Nature: English Kinship in the Late Twentieth Century.* Cambridge: Cambridge University Press.

Temple, Robert. 2002. Placebo-controlled trials and active controlled trials: Ethics and inference. In Harry A. Guess, Arthur Kleinman, John W. Kusek, and Linda W. Engel, eds., *The Science of the Placebo: Toward an Interdisciplinary Research Agenda,* 209-226. London: BMJ Books.

Toulmin, Stephen. 1987. National Commission on Human Experimentation: Procedures and outcomes. In Tristam Engelhardt Jr. and Arthur L. Caplan, eds., *Scientific Controversies: Case Studies in the Resolution and Closure of Disputes in Science and Technology,* 599-613. Cambridge: Cambridge University Press.

Varmus, Harold, and David Satcher. 1996. Ethical complexities of conducting research in developing countries. *New England Journal of Medicine* 337 (14): 1003-1005.

Vastag, Brian. 2000. Helsinki discord? A controversial declaration. *JAMA* 284 (23): 2983-2985.

Vaughan, Megan. 1992. *Curing Their Ills: Colonial Power and African Illness.* Stanford: Stanford University Press.

Whyte, S. R., S. Van der Geest, and A. Hardon. 2002. *Social Lives of Medicines.* Cambridge: Cambridge University Press.

World Medical Association. 2000. Ethical principles for medical research involving human subjects [Declaration of Helsinki]. *Journal of the American Medical Association* 284:3043-3045.

Young, Iris. 2004. Responsibility and historic injustice. Paper presented at the Institute for Advanced Study, School of Social Science, Princeton, N.J., 19 February.

88 The Use of Zairian Children in HIV Vaccine Experimentation: A Cross-Cultural Study in Medical Ethics

Thomas A. Nairn

I. The Situation

In April of 1991, John Crewdson, a reporter for the *Chicago Tribune,* began a series of articles about three deaths which had occurred in Paris as a result of an AIDS vaccine experiment conducted by Dr. Daniel Zagury, a immunologist of the Institut Jean Godinot of the Université Pierre et Marie Curie.[1] Although all three of the victims had been infected with the HIV virus prior to the experimentation, the deaths resulted from acute necrosis, a vaccinia disease.

The articles tell of an investigation by the National Institutes of Health (NIH) and its Office for Protection from Research Risks (OPRR) into the research of Dr. Zagury. The NIH was concerned with the work of a French researcher because Zagury had been a collaborator with Robert Gallo of the National Cancer Institute (NIC) since 1984 when a Materials Transfer Agreement was executed between the NCI and Dr. Zagury.[2] Even more problematical was the transfer to Dr. Zagury by Dr. Bernard Moss of the National Institute of Allergy and Infectious Diseases of a recombinant vaccinia strain into which Moss had inserted HIV envelope proteins.[3] It was

1. John Crewdson, "Three Deaths in AIDS Vaccine Tests," *Chicago Tribune,* 14 April 1991, pp. 1, 16-17; "U.S. Health Agency Will Probe 3 Deaths from AIDS Vaccine Tests," *Chicago Tribune,* 26 April 1991, p. 14; "After 3 Die in Tests, France Bans AIDS Vaccine," *Chicago Tribune,* 16 June 1991, pp. 1, 10; "Secret AIDS Tests on African Kids Detailed," *Chicago Tribune,* 17 July 1991, pp. 1-2.

2. Saul Rosen and Alison Wichman, memorandum to F. William Dommel, Jr., Director, Division of Human Subjects Protections, OPRR, 5 October 1990, p. 2. The memoranda and letters cited in this essay are on file with the author.

3. William C. Eby, memorandum to F. William Dommel, 14 March 1991, p. 2. Crewdson explains: "Moss's idea was to use the vaccina virus as a delivery system for the AIDS virus gene. Since his vaccinia recombinant contained only a part of the AIDS virus, recipients were in no danger of getting AIDS. But their immune systems might generate antibodies to the protein produced by the inserted gene that would protect them against the later infection with AIDS." Crewdson, "Secret AIDS tests on African Kids Detailed,"

From *The Annual of the Society of Christian Ethics* (Baltimore: Georgetown University Press, 1993). Used by permission.

apparent that this was the vaccinia strain that had been used in the experiments that occasioned the three deaths. Thus the NIH investigation was into possible noncompliance with the Department of Health and Human Service's regulations for the Protection of Human Research Subjects.

The investigation extended into several of Zagury's research projects. In addition to the phase I trial with 28 seropositive patients at the Hôpital Saint Antoine in Paris, these experiments included several studies which occurred in Zaire: immunotherapy on two Zairian subjects with advanced AIDS, a phase I vaccinia study on nine HIV-seronegative Zairian children, a similar study on 45 HIV-seronegative volunteers from Zaire's military with some civilians, and a fourth study (taking 4-5 years) analyzing blood samples from HIV seropositive members of the Zairian military.[4] These experiments were in addition to a variety of *in vitro* and animal experiments that Zagury had previously conducted.

For the purposes of this paper, I will concentrate on the phase I vaccinia study on Zairian children in order to address some of the biomedical issues involved when one conducts research in a cross-cultural setting. Although I will touch upon a variety of questions that this experimental protocol raises,[5] I will concentrate on (1) the understanding of informed consent in the use of *children* in such a phase I study and (2) the use of children *of a different culture* in such a study. Rather than being two different questions, they might be better understood as two foci of the same ethical question.

Beginning in November of 1986, Dr. Zagury conducted a phase I vaccine trial involving ten seronegative individuals. One of the ten was Zagury himself, but the other nine experimental subjects were Zairian children ranging in age from two to twelve. All the children's fathers had already died of AIDS, and all of their mothers had tested positive for the HIV virus. The children themselves, however, were all seronegative and had no additional risk for contracting the virus than others living in sub-Saharan Africa.[6] The experimental protocol was reviewed by an ethics committee in Zaire[7] but none in France. In his series of articles, Crewdson maintains that there were eleven children in this group, including a six-year-old girl, a five-year-old boy and two three-year-old girls. He also contends that a month later, another eleven Zairian children were inoculated, including a twenty-two-month-old baby.[8]

Although some of the OPRR reports question the ethical justification for enrolling children in such a phase I trial,[9] Zagury himself defended this decision. In a letter to Charles McCarthy, the Director of the OPRR, Zagury stated that the use of children was in accord with French (if not American) law, as long as there was the written consent of the parents. He quoted specifically from the Huriet law.[10] He steadfastly maintained that the mothers of all the children had signed consent forms.

In the same letter, he maintained that his motivation for these tests was compassion. He stated:

> I should stress that in our action we profited by compassionately allowing for the participation of the children. Their fathers had died of AIDS; and their mothers, wasting away because of the same disease, begged us to do something for their children. This inoculation, evidently good, did not bring them either clinical or human harm. All the children came through the experiment well. Rather than harm, our action proved to be a source of comfort and hope for their families.[11]

In this letter and elsewhere[12] he continued to emphasize that all children developed no immediate or later complications from the immunization. He concluded his report by suggesting that the NIH itself had resorted to a sort of ethical imperialism, narrowly focusing on the supposed moral superiority of its own policies and procedures and not being sensitive to the importance of the work which had been done:

> We deplore the entire action of the OPRR arising from the allegations, which it did not attempt to substantiate, made by the journalist John Crewdson, whose motives, which are very often alien to this profession, . . . were not examined by the OPRR.
>
> We regard it as deplorable that in a matter like AIDS we should mire ourselves in procedures that have nothing to do with the disease and are fraught with errors that are serious and dangerous for everyone, which hinder and destabilize the researchers who are entirely

pp. 1-2. Dr. Moss maintains that the vaccine was intended for use only in animals and that "he gave no authorization for administration to humans." See Rosen/Wichman memorandum, p. 4.

4. Eby memorandum, pp. 1-4.

5. It is interesting to note that several reports to the OPRR cite possible violations of ethical principles but do not necessarily include the use of children among them. The violations most often mentioned were the use of Moss's recombinant vaccinia strain on humans, though it was only to be used for *in vitro* or animal experimentation and enrolling subjects at the Hôpital Saint Antoine who were already receiving AZT, thus deviating from the approved protocol. See, for example, the Eby memorandum, p. 6; Priscilla A. Campbell, Report to the OPRR, 15 March 1991, pp. 2-3. I will not deal with these questions in this paper.

6. Rosen/Wichman memorandum, p. 4.

7. This committee was organized at the request of Dr. Zagury, who had been advised to do so by Dr. Robert Gallo. See Rosen/Wichman memorandum, pp. 4-5.

8. "Secret AIDS Tests on African Kids Detailed," p. 2. Furthermore, there is an unconfirmed report that at least three of these children have already died in Kinshasa, Zaire. See *Africa Faith and Justice Network Update,* 13 February 1992.

9. See, for example, the Rosen/Wichman memorandum, p. 4.

10. "La loi Huriet en précise les modalités: 'le consentement signé des parents à cette vaccination.' " Daniel Zagury and Odie Picard, letter to Charles McCarthy, 21 June 1991, p. 5. Zagury also emphasized that the first person in the world to be vaccinated by Louis Pasteur was an eight-year-old French child.

11. Zagury/Picard letter to McCarthy, p. 5.

12. Daniel Zagury, reply to the OPRR's Interim Report, delivered through his attorney, Bernard Dartevelle, 15 July 1991, p. 14.

committed to their work, and above all, the sufferers, who should not be forgotten.[13]

II. Background

As noted above, Zagury defended his work by maintaining the general ethical appropriateness of his experimental protocol and by noting that the motivation for his inclusion of Zairian children was compassion, thereby providing "a source of comfort and hope." One must therefore begin this study by asking about the nature of Zagury's research itself.

A. The Development of an AIDS Vaccine

Since the discovery of the HIV virus, there have been many attempts to develop a vaccine against infection, reprsenting an entire spectrum of approaches: the use of killed-virus preparations, nonpathogenic variants of the virus, virus subunits, anti-idiotypes, and a variety of genetically engineered recombinant viruses utilizing subunits of the HIV virus.[14] The genetic engineering approach "appears to be a major choice to be considered seriously."[15] This is precisely the sort of vaccine developed by Moss and tested by Zagury.

Yet, there have also been obvious problems with the development of any vaccine. Animal studies are almost impossible. Only members of the great ape family, that group most closely related to humans, have been reported to be susceptible to infection from the HIV virus.[16] Most of these species are endangered or threatened, and the chimpanzee remains the most suitable model by means of which to study the disease. Yet even this animal model is problematic. Aside from the high cost of using and keeping these animals, no chimpanzee has yet developed the clinical syndrome of AIDS even though infected.[17] One can therefore question their ultimate benefit in such studies.

Human research has also been hampered by multiple problems. These include the nature of the spread of the disease, the prolonged period from infection to display of symptoms, the fact that the virus frequently mutates even within the same individual, and the current reality that the very "definition of protective immunity against initial infection with HIV remains unknown."[18]

13. Ibid., p. 19.

14. Peter J. Fischinger, et al., "Toward a Vaccine Against AIDS: Rationale and Current Progress," *The Mount Sinai Journal of Medicine* 53, 8 (December 1986): 639-40.

15. Ibid., 640.

16. Robert H. Purcell, "Animal Models for the Development of a Vaccine for the Acquired Immunodeficiency Syndrome," in Anthony Fauci, moderator, "Development and Evaluation of a Vaccine for Human Immunodeficiency Virus (HIV) Infection," *Annals of Internal Medicine* 10, 5 (March 1989): 382.

17. Ibid.

18. Anthony S. Fauci, "Vaccine for Human Immunodeficiency Virus Infection," in ibid., 373-74.

One needs to understand these facts in evaluating the study of Dr. Zagury, both as regards its possibilities and also as regards its limits. There is no downplaying the importance of developing the vaccine. Yet one must investigate Zagury's understanding of the purpose of his experiments as opposed to what his African subjects might have understood. Finally, one must ascertain the ethical implications not only of the use of Africans in such experimentation but especially that of African children.

B. The Nature of a Phase I Vaccine Study

Traditionally, experimental trials occur in three phases:

> A phase I trial involves testing a small group of subjects (members of AIDS risk groups or others) to evaluate the short-term safety and immunogenicity of the vaccine;
>
> a phase II trial determines the ideal dose and spacing of the vaccine through larger safety and immunogenicity trials; and
>
> a phase III trial determines the actual protection against HIV infection through large scale efficacy trials involving as many as 1,000 to 2,000 subjects. A phase III trial would be randomized, double-blind, and controlled.[19]

Thus, phase I trials are typically conducted at the beginning of a study, utilize small numbers of subjects, and evaluate the effects, including possible toxic side effects, of given experimental agents upon the subjects.[20] The purpose of a phase I study is therefore not to test the success of a drug's long-range immunogenic activity on a class of subjects. In a report on his study of the children, Zagury himself concluded:

> We suggest that this approach be considered as a prototype candidate vaccine against AIDS. However, whether the above described immune state against HIV confers protection against AIDS has to be established. Indeed, an estimation of the efficacy of a vaccine for protection against AIDS can only be achieved after a large scale clinical trial in a group of volunteers with a high risk of natural infection and followed for an adequate period of time.[21]

It is difficult to maintain that those taking part in such a phase I trial are not exposed to risks. The very fact that three patients died in the Saint Antoine experiment from a reaction to the vaccinia attests to this point. In addition

19. See Nicholas A. Cristakis, "The Ethical Design of an AIDS Vaccine Trial in Africa," *Hastings Center Report* 18, 3 (June/July 1988): 32.

20. See David Byar, "Design Considerations for AIDS Trials," *New England Journal of Medicine* 323, 19 (8 November 1990): 1343.

21. Daniel Zagury, et al., "A Group Specific Anamnestic Immune Reaction Against HIV-1 Induced by a Candidate Vaccine Against AIDS," *Nature* 332, 21 (April 1988): 730. It is interesting to note that nowhere in this article does Zagury mention that the subjects of this study were children.

to the possible risks inherent to the initial administration of any viral vaccine preparation, there is also the possibility that because of a partial tolerance developed in the phase I study, a subject may not be able effectively to use a possible AIDS vaccine developed in the future.[22]

Given these considerations, there are certain ethical limits within which these studies ought to be undertaken. While some maintain that phase I studies should utilize only animal subjects, most admit that such a principle is too restrictive. This may be especially true in dealing with the HIV virus. Nevertheless, having acknowledged that the participation of human subjects in phase I vaccine studies can be ethical, can one justify the use of Africans in such tests? For many, this raises the specter of racism such as that associated with the Tuskegee Syphilis Study.[23] Thus, it has been stated that "when a new vaccine is first given trial in a primitive African tribe, one needs to go no further. The investigator feels insecure and unsafe with the material and wants to get his quick answer from a group in whom consent is impossible, information is totally lacking, and the backlash is insignificant."[24] Consequently, according to a statement issued by the Consultation on Criteria for International Testing of Candidate HIV Vaccines sponsored by the World Health Organization's Global Programme on AIDS in 1989: "In general, initial Phase I trials should be conducted in the country of origin of the vaccine. Phase I results, including those that indicate toxicity which prevents further trials of the vaccine, should be made public."[25]

Yet, this analysis seems too simplistic. There can be reasons for such testing of African adults. Among the reasons are the high incidence of the infection on the continent,[26] its probable benefit for Africans in general, and — more controversial — because of the reduction of high-risk behaviors among high-risk groups in countries such as the U.S., the incidence of HIV infection is declining in these countries. Researchers are facing the possibility "that longer phase III trials of AIDS vaccine may have to be done in groups in the United States who are traditionally less compliant or in populations of certain foreign countries where the incidence of infection is still high."[27] Accordingly, the use of Africans may likely lead to speedier and more accurate trials.

Acknowledging the potential ethical difficulties inherent in a French researcher using African subjects in a phase I vaccine study, I would like to bracket these questions for the sake of the present study. One can potentially justify the use of human subjects for phase I vaccine studies, as opposed to animal or *in vitro* studies. One might even justify, though with greater hesitancy, the use of adults from another nation or culture in such studies. I will now concentrate on the use of children, especially children of a different culture and race, in such a phase I study.

III. Anthropology and the Ethics of Experimentation on Zairian Children

In the case described above, a French experimenter is being investigated by a U.S. government agency for research conducted on Zairian children. Such a case demands some sort of cross-cultural analysis. Yet, when one enters such an international and multicultural arena, ambiguities multiply.

There has been an ongoing debate among both experimenters and ethicists when faced with the situation of experimenting on subjects from a different culture. One way of formulating the central question of this debate has been: "Should ethical standards be substantially the same everywhere, or is it inevitable that they differ from region to region, reflecting local beliefs and custom? . . . Underlying these concerns is the fundamental issue of whether ethical standards are relative, to be weighed against competing claims and modified accordingly, or whether, like scientific standards, they are absolute?"[28] Much ink has been spilt over this question, defending a spectrum of points of view.

While this question is important, one does not necessarily have to answer it in order to acknowledge the ambiguities present when dealing with ethical issues involving persons from a different culture. Still less does acknowledging the insights of anthropology detract from the ethical nature of such an investigation. Both anthropology and ethics can become tools in analyzing the mo-

22. See Joan P. Porter, et al., "Ethical Considerations in AIDS Vaccine Testing," *IRB: A Review of Human Subjects Research* (May/June 1989): 2. This essay was quoted in Carol Levine, Report to the Office for Protection from Research Risks, 14 March 1991, p. 5.

23. See, for example, James Jones, *Bad Blood: The Tuskegee Syphillis Experiment* (New York: The Free Press, 1981). See also Patricia A. King, "The Dangers of Difference," *Hastings Center Report* 22, 6 (November-December 1992): 35-38.

24. Francis D. Moore, "Therapeutic Innovation: Ethical Boundaries in the Initial Clinical Trials of New Drugs and Surgical Procedures," *Daedalus* 98, 2 (Spring 1969): 520. While this is undoubtedly an overstatement regarding the study I am investigating, it is of interest that an unidentified source close to Zagury claimed that they conducted the trial there because "[i]t was easier to get official permission [in Zaire] than in France." See Cristakis, "The Ethical Design of an AIDS Vaccine Trial," 31.

25. Quoted in Levine, Report to the Office for Protection from Research Risks, p. 2.

26. Of the 10 million people who have been infected with the HIV virus world-wide, 6.5 million live in Sub-Saharan Africa. In many African cities, more than 10% of all young adults are infected. Between 20 and 30% of pregnant women are infected, and 40% of the children born to these women will have developed AIDS perinatally. See Roy M. Anderson and Robert M. May, "Understanding the AIDS Pandemic," *Scientific American* 266, 5 (May 1992): 59. See also Erik Eckholm, "AIDS, Fatally Steady in the U.S., Accelerates Worldwide," *New York Times*, 28 June 1992, E5.

27. Fauci, "Vaccine for Human Immunodeficiency Virus Infection," 374.

28. Marcia Angell, "Ethical Imperialism? Ethics in International Collaborative Clinical Research," *New England Journal of Medicine* 319, 16 (20 October 1988): 1081.

rality of the experiment described above. In making this move, one acknowledges that anthropology does have something to say, in either a broad or limited manner, to the ethicists evaluating a situation such as this phase I vaccine experiment. For example, reading the account given by Dr. Zagury, even in the most positive light, one might properly ask the anthropologist whether what Zagury claimed he understood as occurring between him and the mothers would be at all similar to what mothers of these children understood as occurring.

One insight of anthropology, which can assist the ethicist here, is that of the notion of a health care system. As articulated by Arthur Kleinman:

> Patients and healers are basic components of such systems and thus are embedded in specific configurations of cultural means and social relationships. They cannot be understood apart from this context. Illness and healing also are part of the system of health care. Within that system, they are articulated as culturally constituted experiences and activities, respectively. In the context of culture, the study of patients and healers, and illness and healing, must, therefore, start with an analysis of health care systems.[29]

The interaction between Dr. Zagury and the Zairian mothers and their children represents the interplay between two different and possibly antagonistic health care systems. One system constructs reality by means of symbols dependent upon the scientific method and "professionalism,"[30] a system which would also be at home with a Western philosophical understanding of concepts such as autonomy, informed consent, and substituted judgment. The other might be understood more in terms of a "folk system."[31] If this is correct, one confronts two questions: (1) whether and how the notion of experiment, and especially "phase I experiment," easily understood within the scientific-professional health care system, might be understood within a "folk" health care system, especially when Dr. Zagury himself seemed to have spoken to the mothers in terms of "comfort and hope"; and (2) how the related concepts of informed consent and proxy consent for those without capacity to competently make their own judgments can be understood once these concepts are separated from the broad Western tradition that has given them meaning.

In attempting to answer these questions, I will first analyze the traditionally Western concepts of informed consent and substituted judgment in order to question the morality of Zagury's experiment from a broadly European/North American perspective. I will then attempt to ask these questions from an African perspective in order to investigate the issues involved when confronting culturally different health care systems.

IV. Experimentation with Children: Western Style

From its beginnings in the last century, the discipline of experimental medicine has acknowledged the tension between the experimenter as scientist and the experimenter as physician dedicated to the health of the subject.[32] Recent decades have witnessed the development of a variety of codes of ethics regarding human experimentation, most importantly the Nuremberg Code of 1947 and, more recently, the Declaration of Helsinki of 1964 (amended in 1975, 1983, and 1989). These codes, and others like them, recognize that experiments on human subjects must be undertaken within a certain ethical and legal context. They have stressed the dignity and rights of the individual, and derived from this, the necessity of informed and voluntary nature of any consent to becoming a subject of experimentation. This area of informed and voluntary consent is problematic when the subject is a child.

A. Human Autonomy and the Nature of Informed Consent

The Western liberal tradition in general and especially the Anglo-American system of common law have placed a great deal of emphasis on the concept of autonomy. The understanding of individual choice and freedom has developed in terms of this notion of autonomy.[33] U.S. courts, for example, have consistently ruled against anything that they have considered to be an infringement upon a person's autonomy by others, including even the person's family. Recently, in the famous Cruzan case, the U.S. Supreme Court cited favorably a 1891 judgment stating that "no right is held more sacred, or is more carefully guarded, by the common law, than the right of every individual to the possession and con-

29. Arthur Kleinman, *Patients and Healers in the Context of Culture: An Exploration of the Borderland between Anthropology, Medicine, and Psychiatry* (Berkeley: University of California Press, 1980), pp. 24-25.

30. See ibid., pp. 53-59.

31. Ibid., pp. 59-60. For a description of an African "folk" system, see John M. Janzen, "Health, Religion, and Medicine in Central and Southern African Traditions," in *Healing and Restoring: Health and Medicine in the World's Religious Traditions,* ed. Lawrence Sullivan (New York: Macmillan Publishing Company, 1989), pp. 225-54. See also John M. Janzen, *The Quest for Therapy in Lower Zaire* (Berkeley: University of California Press, 1978).

32. See, for example, one of the earliest books on experimental medicine: Claude Bernard, *An Introduction to the Study of Experimental Medicine* (1857): "It is our duty and our right to perform an experiment on man whenever it can save his life, cure him or gain him some personal benefit. The principle of medical and surgical morality, therefore, consists in never performing on man an experiment which might be harmful to him to any extent, even though the result might be highly advantageous to science, i.e., to the health of others." Trans. Henry Copley Greene (New York: The Macmillan Company, 1927), p. 101.

33. See, for example, Ruth R. Faden and Tom L. Beauchamp, *A History of Informed Consent* (Oxford: Oxford University Press, 1986), pp. 7-9.

trol of his own person, free from all restraint or interference of others, unless by clear and unquestionable authority of law."[34]

When the understanding of autonomy is used to refer to actions, certain generally accepted components of autonomous action emerge. Faden and Beauchamp, for example, describe such action as follows: "X acts autonomously only if X acts (1) intentionally, (2) with understanding, and (3) without controlling influences."[35] While each of these elements are themselves open to further interpretation, one can begin to see the relation between the notion of autonomy and that of informed consent. Such consent is seen as necessary both to protect the dignity of the subject and to help ensure that the person is treated as an end and not merely as a means to another person's end. Thus the Nuremberg Code demands that for one to consent to participate in any research, that person must "(1) be so situated as to be able to exercise free power of choice; (2) have the legal capacity to give consent; (3) have sufficient . . . comprehension to make an enlightened decision; and (4) have sufficient knowledge on which to decide."[36]

However, if the exercise of informed consent is situated in a context of competency and sufficient comprehension, a further question arises regarding the manner in which one may protect the rights of one judged not competent of exercising this autonomy. If the subject in question had at one time been deemed competent, one may have recourse to some form of transmitted judgment, by which that individual's previously expressed desires may be made known. A problem ensues, however, when the subject has never been in a position to exercise autonomous judgment.

B. Autonomy, Consent, and Experimentation with Children

Attempts to deal with this problem have focused around the understanding of what is in the "best interest" of the individual. Although concrete judgments of "best interest" differ, the notion itself, as that element that protects one's rights and dignity from unreasonable claims by others, is preserved both in law and in ethics. It is the same notion of dignity that imposes upon adults, and especially upon a child's parents, the duty to protect the child: "For their part, children have a right as persons to freedom from conditions that might impair the full development of their human capacities, especially their autonomy."[37]

As framed in U.S. law,[38] a child as a minor legally requires a parent's or guardian's permission to participate in research, even though he or she may be old enough to be of sufficient capacity to understand the nature of research and thereby able to consent to his or her own participation in the research project.[39] By demanding parental permission, the law does not thereby give parents absolute discretion regarding proxy consent. Traditionally there have been two limits on proxy consent for a minor, (1) the "best interest" judgment already discussed and (2) the understanding of a "reasonable person" or a "reasonable parent."[40] Thus, for example, there are certain medical procedures, such as a blood transfusion, that must be performed upon a child even if the procedure is against a parent's religious beliefs.

Even these concepts have been open to debate, however, and there is a spectrum of points of view regarding what constitutes the "best interest" of a child and consequently to what forms of experimentation a "reasonable parent" would give proxy consent. The classic expression of this debate has been that between Paul Ramsey and Richard McCormick.[41] Ramsey has argued that any experimentation on a child which does not directly benefit the child is not ethically permissible. Parents simply do not have the right to give such proxy consent:

> It is better to say of the consent-requirement or of the ethics of consent that this basically means that the *power* of proxy consent is not a *right;* that if men are in some sense capable of granting consent by proxy they should not for that reason do so; and that no one ought to consent for a child to be made the subject of medical investigations primarily for the accumulation of scientific knowledge, except in the face of epidemic conditions that bring upon the individual child proportionately the same or likely greater dangers. . . . A parent's decisive concern is for the care and protection of the

34. U. S. Supreme Court, "Cruzan v. Director, Missouri Department of Health," *Origins* 20 (5 July 1990): 128. The Court continues, "This notion of bodily integrity has been embodied in the requirement that informed consent is generally required for medical treatment."

35. Faden and Beauchamp, *A History of Informed Consent,* p. 238.

36. The Nuremberg Code, quoted in Karen Lebacqz and Robert J. Levine, "Informed Consent in Human Research: Ethical and Legal Aspects," in *Encyclopedia of Bioethics* (New York: The Free Press, 1978), p. 757.

37. Robert Proulx Heaney and Charles J. Dougherty, *Research for Health Professionals* (Ames: University of Iowa Press, 1988), p. 224.

38. Code of Federal Regulations, 45 CFR 46, revised March 8, 1983.

39. See Dennis M. Maloney, *Protection of Human Research Subjects: A Practical Guide to Federal Laws and Regulations* (New York: Plenum Press, 1984), p. 315.

40. See J. K. Mason, *Medico-Legal Aspects of Reproduction and Parenthood* (Brookfield, Vermont: Gower Publishing Company, 1990), pp. 283-90.

41. See Paul Ramsey, *The Patient as Person* (New Haven: Yale University Press, 1970), pp. 1-58; Richard A. McCormick, "Sharing in Sociality: Children and Experimentation," in *How Brave a New World?* (Garden City, New York: Doubleday and Co., 1981), pp. 87-98. It is interesting to note that the National Commission for the Protection of Human Subjects of Biomedical and Behavioral Research framed its own discussion of recommendations for the protection of children around this same debate. See *Research Involving Children: Report and Recommendations* (Washington, D.C.: U.S. Government Printing Office, 1977), pp. 95-104.

> child, to whom he owes the highest fiduciary loyalty, even when he also appreciates the benefits to come to others from the investigation and might submit his own person to experiment in order to obtain them.[42]

For Ramsey, any permission for nontherapeutic experimentation is necessarily treating the child not as an end but merely as a means to another's end and is thus a breach of the parent's fiduciary trust.

McCormick, on the other hand, uses the concept of sociality to argue that there are certain forms of experimentation in which a child ought to participate and for which a parent ought to give consent, even if there is no direct benefit to the child. If there is reason why adults are not able to participate in a particular experiment, if there is only "minimal risk" to the child, and if the experiment would contribute to benefits for others, then proxy consent is moral.[43] McCormick takes this position because there are things "that the child *ought,* simply as a human being, to choose."[44] It should be noted, however, that the language used in McCormick's argument contains terms such as "minimal risk," "no discernible risk," and "no notable inconvenience."[45] Thus McCormick's position by no means gives a parent carte blanche for proxy consent.

C. Zagury's Experiment

If one were to judge the ethics of Zagury's experimental protocol solely on the basis of the Western tradition of autonomy, informed consent, and proxy consent for minors, one would probably describe the research as unethical. One reaches this conclusion by recourse to both considerations discussed above. Regarding the issue of proxy consent, although the experimenter paid attention to the procedural details involved in obtaining signed "informed consent" forms, it is quite dubious whether he ever really obtained the mothers' informed consent. A signed consent form must not be equated with informed consent. Rather, the criteria for informed consent, which the tradition (especially as enshrined in the Nuremberg Code) demands, include sufficient knowledge, comprehension, capacity, and ability to exercise free choice. Zagury might have followed the protocol that demands that the proper forms be obtained, but it is by no means evident that the criteria for obtaining true informed consent were fulfilled.

An even more basic ethical question, however, is why a researcher would use children in a phase I study such as that described above. It does not seem that Zagury received special information by using children that he would not have received by using only adult subjects. Despite his protests to the contrary, children were put at risk without a concomitant benefit either to themselves or to other children. Given Zagury's seeming inability to explain the need for children in a phase I experimental protocol, one must have strong doubts regarding the morality of such experimentation.

V. Experimentation with Children Revisited: An African Perspective

These conclusions regarding the morality of Zagury's research solely from the point of view of the Western ethical tradition does not complete our task. A valid question remains regarding how Zagury's work might have been understood by those from whom he obtained consent. The discussion in this section will be more suggestive than definitive for two reasons. First, given the nature of the relation between anthropology and ethics, it seems more appropriate to conduct this investigation as a series of questions that can guide the ethicist rather than offer definite conclusions. Second, since Dr. Zagury has refused to release information about the children he used as subjects, it is difficult to reach particular conclusions, especially in the section on consent.

We have seen how anthropology can help to provide a context within which the ethicist may ask even more basic questions. From this discussion, one sees how the ethical norms that proscribe certain forms of experimentation on children arise from a particular Western point of view, which places a high value on autonomy. How does an experimenter translate this concern into a Zairian context with its own particular understanding of personhood and of childhood?

A helpful tool may be the distinction developed by anthropologist Richard Shweder between "egocentric-contractual" understandings of the person and "sociocentric-organic" understandings. While the former expresses

> features of the context-dependent, occasion-bound concept of the person: (1) no attempt to distinguish the individual from the station she or he occupies; (2) the view that obligations and rights are differentially apportioned by role, group, and so on; (3) a disinclination to ascribe intrinsic moral worth to people merely because they are people.[46]

Anthropologists who hold this distinction suggest, for example, that our notion of autonomy is not the result of a quasi-metaphysical discovery of the way things really are nor an inductive generalization. Rather it is a "creation of the collective imagination" of the West.[47] It "fits" into our way of seeing the world, but there is no reason why it must be accepted by a member of a sociocentric-organic culture. Shweder further explains:

> To members of sociocentric-organic cultures the concept of the autonomous individual, free to choose and

42. Ramsey, *The Patient as Person,* p. 25.
43. McCormick, "Sharing in Sociality," pp. 89-90.
44. Ibid., p. 89.
45. Ibid., p. 95.

46. Richard A. Shweder, *Thinking Through Cultures* (Cambridge, Mass.: Harvard University Press, 1991), p. 151.
47. Ibid., p. 153.

> mind his or her own business, must feel alien, a bizarre idea cutting the self off from the interdependent whole, dooming it to a life of isolation and loneliness.[48]

A. Personhood and Childhood in Zaire

The Zairian person is constituted by means of a web of relations, incorporating lineage, clan, and tribe. An ethicist may properly ask how the ethical principle of respect for persons, enshrined in Western tradition, might play itself out within a sociocentric-organic context. What would the very process of decision-making look like? For example, someone from a sociocentric-organic culture would very likely take exception to a Western framing of the notion of human rights in terms of noninterference. Such noninterference would itself be construed as immoral.

In Africa, the very reason given for having children differs from those usually given in the West. As Kilbride and Kilbride note, "the parent . . . literally has children for the group."[49] Considerable importance is attached to having children, not only for the parents but especially for the clan. At the same time, there is what a Westerner might see as ambivalence regarding the child. On the one hand, the child is not yet seen as a person. On the other hand, the young child is linked to the divine. Pierre Erny notes:

> To say that a small child is "water" is equivalent to saying that he is not yet a person, that he has no social meaning yet. "He is not solid yet," . . . and he is put in the category of things. Belonging still to the cosmos, he must grow tough before he asserts himself as a social being, and this process involves many dangers.[50]

Within this context, one understands the process of maturing in a different light. Willy De Craemer, for example, portrays a dynamic notion of person in which a child grows into personhood: "becoming a person is seen developmentally — as a state that is progressively achieved through stages, and by degrees, including ancestorhood."[51] Personhood, furthermore, becomes something that some individuals may never attain.

Certain situations that seem to go counter to our own Western sensibilities may seem quite normal to an African. In discussing the decisions of the Akamba tribe of Africa, for example, John Kilner relates:

> Whereas in the United States we tend to value the young more highly than the old because they are more productive economically, these Akamba espouse a more relational view of life. Life, they insist, is more than atomistic sums of individual economic contributions; it is the social fabric of interpersonal relations. The older a person becomes, the more intricately interwoven that person becomes in the lives of others, and the greater the damage done if that person is removed. At the same time, the older person has wisdom — a perspective on life that comes only with age — which is considered to be a particularly important social resource.[52]

I am not trying to suggest, however, that in certain African cultures children are expendable. Precisely because a child is not yet integrated into society, the child is seen as linked to the divine and to the other world.[53] The death of an infant is often interpreted as a curse to the family or clan from the spirits of the dead.[54]

This investigation seems to indicate that in whatever way a child is seen in Zaire, he or she is *not* viewed in the way typically understood in the West. The child is in a process of becoming related to its parents, clan, tribe, and society, in a process of becoming a person. At the same time, it is seen as already linked to God and to the cosmos. Prior to asking the relevance of this understanding for ethics, it may be helpful to also raise the question of what proxy consent might look like in Zaire.

B. The Question of Proxy Consent

The distinction between egocentric-contractual and sociocentric-organic cultures also affects the understanding of the nature of consent. To repeat a question raised earlier, what is the likelihood that what Zagury claims he understood as occurring between him and the mothers is similar to what the mothers of these children understood as occurring? Since traditional societies attach importance to one's answering questions in terms of the authority's expectations, there is a high probability that signing such a form was merely a form of deference, signing because an authority desired it rather than as an act of freedom and knowledge.

One may next ask whether the *mothers* of the children were even the proper people from whom to obtain proxy consent. This question is itself multifaceted, eventually raising a final question regarding the very nature and possibility of proxy consent in an African context. At one level, one must ask regarding the nature of kinship and responsibility in Zairian clans and tribes. In Zaire, tribes may be matrilinear or patrilinear. Information regarding the particular tribes and clans of the children who served as subjects is not available. Yet this knowledge is quite important in assessing the suitability of any consent

48. Ibid., p. 154.

49. Philip L. Kilbride and Janet C. Kilbride, *Changing Family Life in East Africa: Women and Children at Risk* (University Park: The Pennsylvania State University Press, 1990), p. 85.

50. Pierre Erny, *Childhood and Cosmos: The Social Psychology of the Black African Child* (Rockville, Maryland: Media Intellectics Corporation, 1973), pp. 166-67.

51. Willy De Craemer, "A Cross-cultural Perspective on Personhood," *Millbank Memorial Fund Quarterly/Health and Society* 61, 1 (1983): 24.

52. John F. Kilner, "Who Shall Be Saved? An African Answer," *Hastings Center Report* 14, 3 (June 1984): 19.

53. Erny, *Childhood and Cosmos*, pp. 82-85.

54. Kilbride and Kilbride, *Changing Family Life in East Africa*, p. 116.

given. For example, it is at least somewhat likely that members of one of the dominant tribes in Zaire, the Kasai, were among the experimental subjects. As a patrilinear tribe, a parental uncle of these children may have been much more significant than the mother in any decision to consent to experimentation.

This line of reasoning, however, leads to still another set of questions. We have already mentioned that in a sociocentric-organic culture, the relation between person and society must be seen differently from that understood in the West. John Janzen has described the social components in medical decision-making in Zaire as involving the sufferer, the specialist or professional, kinship factions, and nonkinship factions. This is further complicated by various supportive and antagonistic relationships between the sufferer and other members of the kinship and nonkinship factions and similar relationships between the other members of the kinship and nonkinship factions themselves.[55] It is this nexus of complicated relationships that forms the Zairian culture and from which the person cannot be extricated. Thus there are many legitimators of decisions, extending to kin, clan, tribe, and even to ancestors.

Janzen refers to these kinship groups that mediate between the sufferer and the specialist as "therapy management groups."[56] Our Western understanding of privacy and the authority of the specialist are antithetical to this kinship organization. Therapy is usually performed in the presence of the sufferer's kin. The relationship between the specialist and the therapy management group is an egalitarian one. In fact, the group often amends or even rejects the specialist's suggestion for therapy.[57] It is also common for the second and third parties in the management group to take the dominant role in decision-making, with the sufferer accepting a passive role.[58]

For therapy to be effective, there must be consensus among members of the therapy management group, though the scope of participation among kin is partly determined by the significance of the problem. Routine therapeutic questions focus the decision-making around few persons. Crisis situations, however, demand extensive consultation and participation. Disagreement within a management group can itself precipitate a crisis, until agreed-upon norms and relationships can be reestablished.

Thus, in a Zairian context, "consent" necessarily means more than that of an individual and definitely more than one other individual serving as "proxy." This seems prima facie to run counter to Western values regarding experimentation, enshrined, for example, in the Helsinki Declaration, which states: "Concern for the interests of the subject must always prevail over the interests of science and society."[59] Nevertheless, if what was said above is true, it is impossible to delineate how the interests of a Zairian individual conflict with those of his or her kin, clan, or tribe. As O. O. Ajayi states, it is difficult for an African "to see how the interests of the subject conflict with the interest of the society except, of course, if the society is not his own."[60] If the above is correct, the very notion of *proxy* consent is meaningless in a Zairian context. Important decisions simply cannot be made by an individual and must involve the family, clan, and possibly even the tribe.

VI. Conclusion: The Ethics of Dr. Zagury's Experiment

It may seem to some that this foray into anthropology has been irrelevant, complicating matters so much that no ethical decision can be made, or thrown ethics into a sea of cultural relativism. On the contrary, I believe that such a detour ultimately proves to be clarifying. I believe that one may come to four conclusions regarding the ethics of Zagury's research protocol.

1. Dr. Zagury's claim that the experiment was performed out of compassion seems to be contradicted by the fact that it was a phase I vaccine experiment. Phase I research, *ipso facto,* exposes experimental subjects to risk, with any direct benefit to a seronegative person being accidental. One does not yet know enough about the proposed vaccine to ascertain that it would be beneficial. Furthermore, the burden of proof rests upon Zagury to demonstrate the necessity of using seronegative children. To date he has never given any reason for this choice.

2. Ethicists representing a variety of points of view within the Western philosophical tradition would judge Zagury's research protocol unethical for two reasons. On the one hand, even though the experimenter obtained signed consent forms, it is not obvious that he received free and informed consent. Even more basically, however, given his seeming inability to explain the necessity of using children in a phase I study, great ethical difficulties arise from the very fact that he used children in a phase I study.

3. When these same facts are viewed from an African point of view, however, some ambiguity arises. Can one both respect the person of the child and also respect a culture which might have fewer difficulties in allowing a child to participate in an experiment that would in turn have benefit for the society as a whole? If one takes seriously the sociocentric-organic nature of Zairian culture, a negative answer to this question is not automatic.

55. Janzen speaks of this as the "triangle of truth." See Janzen, *The Quest for Therapy in Lower Zaire,* p. 145; for a discussion of these various components, see pp. 139-50.

56. Ibid., p. xviii.

57. Ibid., p. 142.

58. This is true even when the sufferer is an educated adult, whether male or female. See ibid., p. 90.

59. The Helsinki Declaration, in *Handbook of Declarations* (Paris: World Medical Association, 1992), 17C, p. 2, #5.

60. O. O. Ajayi, "Taboos and Clinical Research in West Africa," *Journal of Medical Ethics* 6 (1980): 61. See also Cristakis, "The Ethical Design of an AIDS Vaccine Trial in Africa," p. 35.

In fact, the question itself lays bare a difficulty inherent in some ways in which bioethics has been understood. Often this notion of ethics has become too closely equated with a rather literal adherence to published codes. Thus Zagury was concerned that the mothers of the children sign consent forms. Yet, at the same time he seems to have been oblivious to the values that provide the justification for the norms themselves.

Several contemporary, usually Catholic, ethicists, generally grouped together under the term of proportionalists, suggest that at times "it is necessary to contemplate true departures from norms as well as unusual applications of them."[61] It seems to me that nowhere is this more clearly the case than when one is working in a cross-cultural context. In such a situation, it is important to know what the rules are, but even more important to know the values that the rules are trying to protect. It becomes crucial to have an attitude both respectful and critical, acknowledging that some basic moral understandings that we use as guides may look quite different when applied in cross-cultural situations.

Yet, in trying to respect the values of another culture and the way those values are protected by norms and rules, it is equally important to understand the interrelation among the norms and values of a culture. Thus one must not stop by merely asking how the culture sees decision-making in general. Respect for the culture would seem to demand a general respect for decisions made by kinship groups and the acceptance not only of the presence but also the authority of such forms of decision-making.

4. This leads to my fourth conclusion. A researcher should not pick and choose which elements of a culture he or she accepts based upon the way in which it will help or hinder the research. "Cross-cultural sensitivity" does not give an experimenter license to bend and break norms of professional conduct merely for the sake of research. In fact, the opposite is probably more true. While an ethical researcher would avoid the extremes of playing loose with the rules and never going beyond the strict norm, she or he would at least be tentative and self-critical regarding the necessary superiority of his or her ethical stance. Such an experimenter would attempt to be true to his or her own conscience while being at the same time respectful of the culture of those who are the experimental subjects. Experimental protocols may need to pass two ethical tests, a general ethical test of respect for persons and a more specific test of how true respect may be obtained in a particular culture.

This specific ethical test would not abandon basic values but rather ask how such values are to be enfleshed in culturally different contexts. Often this may mean that protocols that appear to run counter to expressed norms may, upon closer analysis, reveal better ways of protecting the values in question. On occasion, however, a true impasse might arise because of a genuine clash of values themselves. At such times, the experimenter may very well find it ethically necessary to abandon a particular experiment in a particular culture. Such cross-cultural sensitivity may benefit not only the subjects of the experimentation but the ethical person who is the experimenter as well.

61. Lisa Cahill, *Between the Sexes: Foundations for a Christian Ethics of Sexuality* (Philadelphia: Fortress Press, 1985), p. 148. See also Richard Gula, *What Are They Saying About Moral Norms?* (New York: Paulist Press, 1982).

CHAPTER FOURTEEN

Embryonic Stem Cell Research and "Therapeutic" Cloning

The controversy surrounding embryonic stem cell research and cloning erupted into the public sphere in the late 1990s with twin technological developments. In 1997, Scottish scientist Ian Wilmut cloned Dolly the sheep, the first mammal to be cloned using a technique known as somatic cell nuclear transfer (SCNT). Immediately, commentators raised the specter of the cloning of human beings. Just over a year later, in November 1998, two researchers — John Gearhart at Johns Hopkins and James Thompson at the University of Wisconsin — announced that they had isolated human stem cells from embryonic and fetal tissue and cultivated them in their laboratory for up to nine months. Stem cells, it is argued, promise significant medical benefits owing to their ability to develop into any kind of human tissue or organ — bone, muscle, blood, brain. Medical research imagined possibilities of organ replacement or restoration therapies for destroyed tissue, such as could be used to treat Parkinson's disease, diabetes, or even Alzheimer's disease.

Unlike many issues in bioethics, however, the closely related issues of human cloning and human embryonic stem cell research instantly found themselves enmeshed in questions of public policy. For in 1995, Congress explicitly prohibited the use of federal funds for research involving human embryos. This deliberately extended a decades-long *de facto* ban on such funding. Stem cells, in Gearhart's and Thompson's procedure, were harvested primarily from embryos created through *in vitro* fertilization; human embryonic stem cell research would count as research involving human embryos. Wilmut's method of cloning involved the creation via modification of human embryos, a highly experimental procedure. While the public initially seemed more skeptical of cloning, embryonic stem cell research appeared to have broad support. But would funds from the National Institutes of Health (NIH) be available to support embryonic stem cell research? If not, it seemed certain that the goods promised by this research would remain out of reach.

To date, the questions of public policy have not been entirely resolved. In 1999, the Director of the NIH, Harold Varmus, announced that the NIH would indeed, in spite of the ban, fund research on stem cells, or more specifically on "cell lines" derived from embryonic stem cells. Varmus argued that there was a difference between conducting research on embryos themselves and conducting research on cells derived from embryos. In other words, while it would remain illegal for researchers to use federal funds to isolate and cultivate their own stem cells from embryonic or fetal tissue, researchers could receive federal money to conduct stem cell research as long as the cells themselves were derived using private funds. Many found this distinction to be not entirely credible.

In the meantime, the National Bioethics Advisory Commission — known as the NBAC — had been instructed by President Clinton to conduct a thorough review of human stem cell research. President Clinton's request was also spurred in November 1998 by the announcement of a company called Advanced Cell Technology (ACT), which claimed that by using SCNT — or cloning — they had created an embryo that was "part human, part cow," for the purposes of obtaining embryonic stem cells. As the then-President noted with uncharacteristic understatement, this research "raises the most serious of ethical, medical and legal concerns" (NBAC, 1999).

The NBAC report, *Ethical Issues in Human Stem Cell Research,* was issued in September 1999 and outlined a series of recommendations that were quickly translated into policy for the NIH, which was subsequently promulgated in August 2000. This policy followed Varmus's position: that the NIH would fund research using pluripotent stem cells obtained from embryos "left over" after infertility treatments or obtained from aborted fetuses, but would not fund research that would itself obtain those cells or fund research with cells obtained from embryos created specifically for research purposes.

Yet this was not the end of the story. In August 2001, shortly after election to his first term, President George W. Bush issued a decision that NIH funding would be made available for research with the sixty to seventy human embryonic stem cell lines in existence at that point, but not for research that derived the stem cells and not for research with cells or cell lines created from embryos after August 9, 2001. The revised NIH guidelines for human pluripotent stem cell research were subsequently promulgated on November 14, 2001, and remained in place during Bush's presidency. In 2009, at the beginning of his first term, President Barack Obama promised to overturn the Bush decision and allow federal funding for research with human embryonic stem cells and perhaps embryos.

Three additional developments are important to note. Earlier in 2001, the British government approved research on embryos created solely for research purposes — a policy that differed from the U.S. policy. It also approved what is called "therapeutic cloning" — using cloning techniques to create embryos for research. In response, on July 31, 2001, the U.S. House of Representatives passed by a margin of 265-162 a bill prohibiting human cloning for any purpose. The key difference between this and the items above pertaining to stem cells is as follows: at issue with stem cells was only the question of whether federal funding would be made available through the NIH for research; the cloning legislation seeks to make cloning illegal. Following the House's action in July 2001, a similar bill was introduced into the Senate. But before it came to the floor Congress unexpectedly had to deal with the aftermath of September 11th.

This legislative and policy struggle has been driven by deeply held moral commitments about human embryonic life, caring for the sick, and social justice. Yet while the policy struggles might be new, the conversation around human cloning is not. Cloning, in fact, was one of the issues engaged by the early shapers of the field of medical ethics. Important figures such as Paul Ramsey and Leon Kass were the first to raise concerns about proposals for human cloning (based on experiments with amphibian cloning) and to advance moral arguments.[1] Until the announcement by Wilmut, however, the question had only sporadically engaged public or professional attention.

Embryonic stem cell research, even more than other issues in medicine, has highlighted the question of the relationship between religious convictions and public discourse and policy-making. Two arguments have provided the contours of the embryo/stem cell research debate within the theological community: on the one hand, opponents cite inviolability of life; on the other, proponents cite the potential of such research and subsequent therapies to relieve human suffering. We open this chapter with the latter perspective. In "A Plea for Beneficence: Reframing the Embryo Debate" (selection 89), Ted Peters and Gaymon Bennett resurface one of the four principles of bioethics (autonomy, beneficence, nonmaleficence, and justice), one that largely receded to the background in the 1980s and 1990s as the principles of autonomy and utility gained hegemony. Peters and Bennett invoke the principle of beneficence — "doing the other's good" — as the central concept for reframing the public debate around embryo and stem cell research. They believe, moreover, that such a reframing has theological grounding, if Christians would rethink their anthropology as grounded in eschatology.

One of Peters and Bennett's main arguments is that Christians erroneously ground their arguments and anthropology "archonically," or by looking to the past. The authors of "A Theologian's Brief" provide a different perspective on this claim as well as offer an argument about the relationship between theological claims and public policy (selection 90). This ecumenical group of Christian theologians, responding to the policy developments in the U.K. mentioned above, ask: What is the role of arguments from the Christian tradition in a multicultural and multi-religious society? These authors contend that such arguments are important, not only because of the significant role Christianity has played in shaping our society's moral categories, but also because a large percentage of the public claims Christian identity. If discourse is to be truly public, encompassing the whole public, a place certainly must be made for the voices and perspectives of religious convictions.

These theologians offer a succinct yet nuanced and substantive overview of the Christian tradition on the question of the moral status of the embryo and human persons. They draw on the breadth of the scriptural and doctrinal witness, citing not just Genesis but broadly from the Hebrew and Christian Scriptures. They demonstrate that Christian convictions about the human person are grounded not only in the doctrine of creation but equally, and perhaps more centrally, in Christology — in our understanding of who Christ was and is, of the doctrines of incarnation, redemption, and resurrection. Beyond Scripture, they turn to the patristic writers and connect their witness to later Christian history. In short, these theologians create a substantive argument that weaves together Scripture, tradition, and doctrine, ultimately centering it all in the person of Christ.

The public debate into which the theologians entered has been complex both in the U.K. and in the U.S., with many competing voices. The remaining essays in this chapter serve two purposes. First, they seek to provide an overview of the debate itself. Here we turn to the essays by Gene Outka and Lisa Sowle Cahill. Outka in "The Ethics of Human Stem Cell Research" (selection 91) systematically lays out and analyzes three major positions on the issue, those that he identifies as the "right," "middle," and "left," pushing them to critically engage one another toward a new synthesis. Cahill in "Stem Cells and Social Ethics" (selection 92) analyzes the issue via five general values that structure the debate: the value of nascent life, the meaning of moral agency, the question of medical benefit (returning to Peters and Bennett's emphasis on beneficence), the challenge of distributive justice within our own context as well as internationally, and finally our

1. Paul Ramsey, *Fabricated Man* (New Haven: Yale University Press, 1972); Leon R. Kass, "Genetic Tampering" [Letter to the Editor in response to Joshua Lederberg], *Washington Post* (October 30, 1967).

broader social ethos. Cahill demonstrates the intellectual power provided by the Catholic moral tradition — with its principles of probabilism, cooperation, double effect, the common good, and preferential option for the poor — in making nuanced moral analyses.

With this overview of the issues in hand, the essays turn to a second task: to probe behind the standard arguments and public rhetoric. Amy Laura Hall in "Price to Pay" (selection 93) notes how behind the emotive appeals of personal stories lie a number of flawed assumptions and hidden factors that continue to shape the debate. She challenges the facile equation of embryonic stem cell research and abortion. She insists — as few are bold enough to do — that new technologies like embryonic stem cell research and "therapeutic" cloning must rightly be understood as for-profit industries rather than simply as individual moral decisions or choices, and that this economic reality must factor into our moral evaluation. Finally, she raises hard questions about the ways in which these technologies impact women, particularly women's bodies, making clear how easily, even in the twenty-first century, women can become objects of exploitation.

But which bodies are we talking about, speaking theologically? Stanley Hauerwas and Joel Shuman in "Cloning the Human Body" (selection 94) take up this question. Without fail, in questions of cloning the debate focuses on the propriety of cloning the human body and what this means for personhood, for identity, for relationality, and more. Hauerwas and Shuman step back from the standard debate on this question to ask, theologically: Which body? Drawing on St. Paul and Wendell Berry, they demonstrate that contemporary individualistic notions of the human body are, in many ways, foreign to the Christian tradition. Christian accounts of embodiment, as we saw in Chapter Eight above, are far more complex, stressing the tangible, material connection between our bodies and the bodies of others, the materiality of creation, and, most strikingly, the body of Christ. Christians, they claim, are called to clone the body — to nonsexually reproduce Christ's body. If this is the case, how might we think differently about technologically mediated somatic cell nuclear transfer?

The debates over embryonic stem cell research and "therapeutic" cloning have been driven not only by different perspectives but also by a rhetoric of desperation and, as Hall has noted, emotive appeals to human suffering. M. Therese Lysaught in "What Would You Do If . . . ? Human Embryonic Stem Cell Research and Defense of the Innocent" (selection 95) explores this aspect of the public rhetoric surrounding these technologies. She finds in the debate a familiar dynamic — an analogy to war that has become a standard component of public rhetoric surrounding medicine and technology, as well as an increasing number of political ventures for which factions in the U.S. seek public support. The end of the Cold War unleashed a series of wars on the U.S.: the War on Poverty, the War on Cancer, the War on Drugs, the War on Terror, and more. Lysaught explores how this rhetoric has functioned within the debate on embryonic stem cell research and then evaluates it in light of three positions from the Christian tradition on war and peace. In doing so, she demonstrates how questions of bioethics cannot be separated from questions of social ethics, be those questions about economics or about violence.

The discerning reader might ask: Why is this chapter on embryo and stem cell research located in the section entitled "vulnerable populations" rather than, say, "beginning of life"? To this we give two answers. Insofar as there is near unanimity within the theological community and U.S. public against the cloning of human beings for the purposes of reproduction, questions of embryo and stem cell research are not, at this time, primarily questions on the "beginning of life." They are more properly questions of research, and so it seemed best to locate this chapter next to the chapter on experimental subjects. For, as is clear from the readings in this chapter, at issue is the question: Does embryo and stem cell research constitute a subset of human subjects research or not? At the same time, questions of embryo and stem cell research concern another "vulnerable population" — the population of patients and those who might benefit from eventual cures. Thus, we locate this chapter at a tenuous interface — between medical ethics' concern for vulnerable populations (Part IV) and its engagement with questions at the beginning of life (Part V). We hope this chapter provokes lively and substantive discussion around both sets of questions.

SUGGESTIONS FOR FURTHER READING

Cahill, Lisa Sowle. "Realigning Catholic Priorities." *America* 191, no. 6 (September 13, 2004).

Campbell, Courtney. "Prophecy and Policy." *Hastings Center Report* 27, no. 5 (September/October 1997): 15-18.

Demopulos, Demetri. "A Parallel to the Care Given the Soul: An Orthodox View of Cloning and Related Technologies." In *Beyond Cloning: Religion and the Remaking of Humanity,* ed. Ronald Cole-Turner (Harrisburg, Pa.: Trinity Press International, 2001), pp. 124-36.

Kass, Leon R. *Human Cloning and Human Dignity: The Report of the President's Council on Bioethics* (New York: PublicAffairs, 2002).

Kass, Leon R. "The Wisdom of Repugnance: Why We Should Ban the Cloning of Human Beings." *The New Republic* (June 2, 1997).

Lustig, Andrew. "Human Cloning: Co-Creation or Hubris." In *Considering Religious Traditions in Bioethics: Christian and Jewish Voices,* ed. Mary Jo Iozzio (Scranton, Pa.: University of Scranton Press, 2005), pp. 31-51.

Meilaender, Gilbert. "Some Protestant Reflections." In *The Human Embryonic Stem Cell Debate: Science, Ethics, and Public Policy,* ed. Suzanne Holland, Karen Lebacqz, and Laurie Zoloth (Cambridge, Mass.: MIT Press, 2001), pp. 141-47.

Pontifical Academy for Life. *Declaration on the Production and the Scientific and Therapeutic Use of Human Embryonic Stem Cells,* 2000.

Snow, Nancy, ed. *Stem Cell Research: New Frontiers in Science and Ethics* (Notre Dame: University of Notre Dame Press, 2004).

Waters, Brent, and Ronald Cole-Turner, eds. *God and the Embryo: Religious Voices on Stem Cells and Cloning* (Washington, D.C.: Georgetown University Press, 2003), pp. 99-107.

89 A Plea for Beneficence: Reframing the Embryo Debate

Ted Peters and Gaymon Bennett

The birth of Dolly the sheep in 1997 inspired a rare phenomenon: near moral unanimity. Since that fateful February day, virtually everyone on the planet has been opposed to bringing children into the world through reproductive cloning. In June and July 2002, two high-level government reports, one in Singapore and the other in the United States, reiterated this shared opposition, recommending a total ban on the use of somatic cell nuclear transfer in human reproduction.[1] The bans have met almost no resistance. Whether the explanation is found in a shared worldwide ethical sensibility or in the lack of imagined ways to turn a profit from reproductive cloning, something close to unanimity reigns.[2] Despite the actions of renegade off-shore cloners, theological ethicists have found influencing public policy to be easy. In such a situation, ethical arguments tend not to be carefully examined, and rhetoric is rarely scrutinized. What may become public policy in many countries will be established on consensus, to be sure; yet, when in later years philosophers look back for fundamental premises, they may not find a solid foundation.

By contrast, the stem cell debate — entailing the question of whether cloning should be used for research — continues to be vigorous, spirited, and sometimes acrimonious. Venture capitalists with eyes fixed on potential big profits mix with laboratory scientists, theological

1. Bioethics Advisory Committee Singapore (hereinafter BAC), *Ethical, Legal and Social Issues in Human Stem Cell Research, Reproductive and Therapeutic Cloning.* Report submitted to the Ministerial Committee for Life Sciences, June 2002. And President's Council on Bioethics, *Human Cloning and Human Dignity: An Ethical Inquiry.* Report submitted to U.S. President George W. Bush, 10 July 2002.

2. Ian Wilmut, along with Donald Bruce, describe current nuclear transfer technology as a hit-and-miss affair; and the Roslin Institute has declared that cloning human beings is ethically unacceptable. See Wilmut and Bruce, "Dolly Mixture," in Donald Bruce and Ann Bruce, eds., *Engineering Genesis: The Ethics of Genetic Engineering in Non-Human Species* (London: Earthscan Publications, 1998), 71-76.

ethicists, secular ethicists, and public policy makers. The public square is riddled by crossfire from ethical guerrillas, each faction contending for the disputed laboratory territory. The stem cell itself is not the turf to be won; rather, it is the moral status of the embryo from which the stem cell is derived. The public battle requires that each faction return frequently to its philosophical armory to load up and strengthen its position in combat. In the case of theological ethics, theologians must return again and again to fundamental convictions about God's intention for human nature and destiny.

Though still exchanging shots, the factions have reached a stalemate, neither retreating nor advancing. This is due in large part to a combination of ideological entrenchment and the incommensurability of differing principles; however, it is also due to the caliber of ammunition being used in the exchange. In the rush to defend and advance, scientists, philosophers, and theologians alike have often not reached deep enough into the resources of their respective traditions. The result has been that the weighty ethical payload of moral arguments has been launched from less than stable foundations. Moral advances are weakened by incomplete ethical reflection.

In the present chapter, we will examine a crucial cause of this ethical incompleteness: the failure of beneficence to count substantively in ethical deliberation assessing the moral status of the embryo. We will outline this failure by examining the conclusions and supporting arguments of the two government reports from nearly opposite sides of the planet, the Singapore Bioethics Advisory Committee (the BAC) and the American President's Council on Bioethics (the Kass council). We will show how both reports found it easy to recommend government bans on reproductive cloning, and how that ease can belie a negative disposition toward moral responsibility. We will show further how much more difficult the respective investigations found the issue of cloning for research, with its implications for stem cell derivation and how this difficulty results in ambivalence. Although the Singapore report recommends support for stem cell research, ambivalence is reflected in its preference list for sources of research embryos. Although the American report includes a majority recommendation for a four-year moratorium on cloning for use in stem cell research, it includes a minority recommendation to support such research.

This nearly irresolvable situation in public policy compels church leaders to reexamine theological commitments, to reconsider what is foundational and what might be applicable or helpful. This reexamination begins with theological anthropology. It is our contention that Christian anthropology is characterized by (1) eschatological destiny, (2) the morally compelling value of the human person, or what is more commonly articulated as the affirmation of human dignity, and (3) the fundamental (meaning both primordial and universal) imperative of *agape* or neighbor love. This definition suggests to us that beneficence should play a basic role in bioethics.

Our support of beneficence will not resolve the stem cell debate to everyone's satisfaction. Our arguments are neither airtight nor, for that matter, complete. They are in process, our articulation inspired by a perceived lack in the current debate. Yet, we have something to offer to theologians and other church leaders involved in the public policy conversation. Our immediate contention is that the public policy debate would be healthier if all commentators would allow beneficence to count more significantly in their ethical calculus.[3] We would like to see the potential leap forward in human health and well-being promised by stem cell research play a role (at minimum) equal to that of nonmaleficence — that is, equal to a guarding against future harms and the protection of the embryo. Responsibility cast in positive terms inspires a move beyond the status quo of human suffering. Though the prevention of harm is crucial, proscriptions against crossing moral bright lines should be balanced by prescriptions for active stewarding of resources to improve human life.

Our more long-range contention is that theologians should be reminded that definitions of what makes us human rely less on our origin and more on our destiny, less on our creation and more on our new creation. In other words, what is significant about who we are now is not found in our genetic past, but in God's future — a resurrected future where suffering is transformed and life is had to the fullest.

Eschatology, Dignity, and Beneficence

The stem cell and cloning debates reveal inconsistencies in contemporary Christian anthropology and its application to bioethics. Beneficence often fails to function substantively in theological assessments of the moral status of the embryo and, hence, in the stem cell and cloning debates. We are persuaded that this has less to do with ignorance or ill will and more to do with poorly developed anthropology. Theological contributions to public debate are frustrated by dissonant interpretations of what constitutes ethical responsibility and morally protectable human life.

A curious phenomenon pervades virtually all human cultures and traditions. When seeking identity and meaningfulness, our minds tend to gravitate toward the past, toward origins. Whatever the reason for this phenomenon, we find a coincidence of the questions "Who am I?" and "Where did I come from?" In the stem cell debate, these anthropological questions become "When did life begin?" and "How is each person's unique human potential established?" and "What does that establish-

3. "The principle of beneficence in its simplest form is that we ought to do good or, if expressed as an obligation, that there is an obligation to help others." Marvin Kohl, "Beneficence," in Lawrence C. Becker and Charlotte B. Becker, *Encyclopedia of Ethics,* 2d ed., 3 vols. (New York: Routledge, 2001), 1:128.

ment tell me about how humans should be treated?" The unexamined assumption in this line of questioning is that, once we have located the ontogenesis or beginning, we will have located the defining source of our moral selfhood. In other words, if we discover just where it is that we come from, we will be compelled in the ethical direction we ought to be moving.

The Roman Catholic Church, with its modern history of commentary on the status of the embryo, was well positioned to be the first to define the theological agenda for the stem cell debate. Pope John Paul II and the Congregation for the Doctrine of the Faith had already, in 1987, provided answers to the question of moral ontogenesis.[4] In *Donum Vitae* the Vatican reiterates a previously articulated conclusion: that protectable human life begins at conception. *Donum Vitae*, however, takes what was formerly a philosophical/theological conclusion and spells it out in semiscientific terms. The recipe for personhood requires three ingredients: sperm, egg, and soul. At conception, when the sperm and egg join, God creates and imparts an immortal soul. The united gametes and soul constitute a new human individual endowed with dignity and worthy of the respect and protection due any adult or child. Of course, the conceptus is not at this early stage in itself a human person. It is, however, a human person in potential. Its genetic code is new, neither its mother's nor father's alone. It can become this person and no other.

This genomic novelty carries anthropological and ethical weight for the Vatican. It designates at what point we should apply the principle of inviolability, a universal marker of a morally protectable person. Evangelical Protestants, whose traditions may not have traveled the same arduous course of ethical deliberation, tend to respond intuitively to the Roman Catholic arguments. They affirm that the Vatican has it right.

The conclusions of other early commentators on embryo research have also helped set the moral agenda of the stem cell debate. Though with less appeal to metaphysics, these too answered the question of moral origins. Some have argued that morally protectable human dignity begins at fourteen days. This fourteen-day rule argues that, prior to the appearance of the primitive streak, a precursor to the central nervous system, and adherence to the uterine wall, the embryo is not truly individuated. Prior to fourteen days, the embryo can still become twins. Thus, it is not until fourteen days that we have the clear appearance of the individual human life.

Much like the Vatican, the fourteen-day rule looks for the origins of personhood in individuation. Though the appeal is not made to genetic uniqueness, the fourteen-day rule seems to concur that characteristics of respect and inviolability are meaningless until we have an individual person to whom we can apply those characteristics.

We find it significant that both an appeal to genetic uniqueness and the fourteen-day rule exemplify archonic reasoning. Archonic reasoning privileges the point of origin. It assumes that the essence of a thing is found in its beginnings. Archonism looks to the past for metaphysical or physical grounding of moral authority. The essence of the origin, it is presumed, will serve as ethical edict for the present situation.

The Greek word *arche* means both beginning and governance. The way in which a thing begins decrees or governs the direction in which it ought to continue. Contemporary genetic research seems to provide a new means of grounding archonic reasoning. By researching the biological "blueprint" for the beginnings of human life, we should be able to fashion moral prescriptions directing our human future. Both the appeal to genetic novelty and the fourteen-day rule appear to draw out of biology the moral authority of archonism.

We have suggested that theological anthropology needs to be reexamined. This reappraisal begins with the question, "Should archonic reasoning be privileged by Christian theologians?" Our answer is flatly, "No." What is distinctive about Christian anthropology is that it is oriented toward the future, a transformed and just future. The Christian understanding of the human person, counterintuitively, begins not in creation, with who we are, but in redemption, with who we are intended to be.

For the Christian, the identity, value, and meaningfulness of the human person are inextricably bound up in Jesus of Nazareth. Jesus announces and proleptically realizes God's eschatological destiny for creation. That announcement and realization reveals God's active, self-giving, and redemptive love and in doing so reveals the truth of human identity. The character of God's love for creation testifies to the true nature of who we are. The Kingdom of God, according to Jesus, is characterized by sight for the blind, functioning limbs for the lame, healing for those with leprosy, hearing for the deaf, new life for the dead, and good news for the poor (Luke 7:22-23). Jesus locates our fundamental identity not in the archonic roots of injustice, but in God's graceful future, a future which responds to human suffering, promising healing and offering the flourishing of life.

What anthropological generalizations can be drawn here? Jesus' vision of God's love suggests that who we are is inextricably tied up in who we are becoming, who we will be. Who we will be, in turn, is inextricably tied up in who the Easter Christ is — that is, we will realize who we truly are in the resurrection. In sum, what is most true about us is not revealed in our genetic origins but in the epigenetic history of God's relationship to each person in Christ. Eschatologically, we will become one with Christ and like Christ and live in Christ.

The vision of God's eschatological destiny for creation is morally compelling. It reveals not only the truth of human identity, but also the significance of human value and the imperative of neighbor love. God's love confers dignity on creatures. That conferring testifies to the way

4. Congregation for the Doctrine of the Faith, *Donum Vitae* (Vatican City, 1987), in Thomas A. Shannon, ed., *Bioethics* (New York: Paulist Press, 1987); also available at www.vatican.va.

in which the human person ought to be valued and related to.

Human dignity seems to imply individuality, even radical independence. After all, our concept of dignity as formulated by Immanuel Kant makes it clear that we treat a person — an individual person — as an end and not merely as a means.[5] Yet the individuality of dignity has a relational dimension to it. It is in the relationship that a person experiences being treated by someone else as an end and not a means; once dignity has been conferred by someone else, one's own internal sense of dignity arises. Dignity is first conferred, and then it is claimed. Dignity is conferred on individuals, but it is established in relationship.

For the Christian, God's relationship to creation, described and exemplified by Jesus, represents the conferring of dignity par excellence. In the Gospel of Luke (6:27-36), Jesus' understanding of God's relationship to human persons is described in this way: Jesus proclaims that we should love persons not as we think they deserve to be loved, but indiscriminately, as God loves them. God, Jesus reports, loves the good and wicked alike. Again, human value is revealed not in an archonic assessment of human worth — where people have come from — but according to the human person's future as beloved, completed and redeemed by God. Human dignity is measured by God's perfect and perfecting love.

A Christian anthropology that begins with Jesus is morally compelling in a second way. Danish philosopher Knud Løgstrup points out that Jesus' proclamation is concerned with the individual's relationship to the neighbor.[6] According to Løgstrup, this concern can be concisely described: the individual's relationship with God is determined at the point of the individual's relationship to the human neighbor. Moreover, it is precisely at the point where God determines his relationship to me that he cares for the other person. God's eschatological love for the other person is bound up in my relationship to that person. Face to face with the human other, I am confronted with a tremendous obligation — to participate in God's redemption of the world through what Martin Luther refers to as "neighbor-love."

Jesus articulates this primordial obligation in the parable of the Good Samaritan. When asked what it takes to participate in the Kingdom of God, Jesus answers, Love God and love your neighbor. Jesus' interrogator pushes the question: what does that love look like? Jesus replies with a story. The Samaritan (born of the wrong nation, subscribing to the wrong theology) single-mindedly purses one goal, to bring healing to someone suffering and in need. This is an active, aggressive form of love, one that takes initiative and acts creatively. In short, when asked what is most significant about human existence Jesus points to a commandment, an imperative to participate in God's healing of the world through the love of one's neighbor.

Christian anthropology does not begin with Adam (Genesis 1:26-29; 2:7), but with Jesus Christ (Romans 5). The problem with archonic anthropology when pursued by Christian theologians is that it looks to Adam rather than Christ, to creation without redemption. Proleptically, humans participate in the grace of God's eschatological destiny. Ethically speaking, grace appears to reorder reason. God's love identifies us with the future truth of who we are becoming, not with the merits of our genetic inheritance. Taking this vision of human dignity as our moral norm, we find ourselves responsible not only for what we did or willed, for our own faults and misfortunes. But, with Jesus, we find ourselves called to account for that which we may not have willed or done: the faults, misfortunes, and suffering of others.

In the end, it is not enough for Christian anthropology merely to inspire an ethic of proportionality, fairness, just deserts, or distributive equality, even if, relatively speaking, an ethic of equality lends itself well to public policy recommendations in a democratic context. Rather, Christian anthropology should inspire the pursuit of the other person's well-being toward the end of that person having what Jesus referred to as life, and having it to its fullest (John 10:10). Christian anthropology depicts the truth of human ethics as a going out of one's way for the healing and wholeness of one's most intimate friend, one's most feared enemy, and even for the faceless stranger.

The bioethical correlative of this active and determined neighbor-love is beneficence. The degree to which bioethical reflection fails to treat beneficence as a substantive factor in its moral calculus determines the degree to which it fails to draw on distinctively Christian resources.

The Singapore BAC

In June 2002, the BAC, chaired by Professor Lim Pin, submitted its report to Deputy Prime Minister Tony Tan. The report describes its central task in terms of ethical balancing. The gravity of questions concerning the moral status of the embryo is weighed against the need to harness potential medical benefits. This task is framed according to two guiding principles. When exploiting the benefits of science and technology, the pursued ends must be (1) just and (2) sustainable.[7]

The BAC clearly saw the potential benefits of embryonic stem cell research and promotes investment in this area. The promotion, however, is wed to substantial caveat. Note the language in Recommendation 3: "Research involving the derivation and use of ES [embryonic stem]

5. Immanuel Kant, *Groundwork for the Metaphysics of Morals,* ed. and trans. H. J. Patton (New York: Harper, 1948).

6. Knud Løgstrup, "The Radical Character of the Demand and the Social Norms," in Hans Fink and Alasdair MacIntyre, eds., *The Ethical Demand* (Notre Dame, Ind.: University of Notre Dame Press, 1997), 44-63.

7. BAC, iv.

cells is permissible only where there is strong scientific merit in, and potential medical benefit from, such research."[8] This would seem to go without saying. Without potential benefit, why pursue any course of medical research? The caveats become increasingly interesting as the BAC constructs a hierarchy of preferred sources for human embryonic stem (hES) cell derivation. According to Recommendation 4, "Where permitted, ES cells should be drawn from sources in the following order: (1) existing ES cell lines, originating from ES cells derived from embryos less than 14 days old; and (2) surplus human embryos created for fertility treatment less than 14 days old."[9] But could a scientist create a fresh embryo to obtain hES cells as will probably be needed if stem cell research goes to therapy? Only after these first two options would be exhausted.

Recommendation 5 expands the hierarchy, offering a third option, namely, the controversial creation of fresh embryos for research purposes: "The creation of human embryos specifically for research can be justified only where (1) there is strong merit in, and potential medical benefit from, such research; (2) no acceptable alternative exists, and (3) on a highly selective, case-by-case basis, with specific approval from the proposed statutory body."[10]

With consistent emphasis on both the potential benefits of stem cell research and the need for ethical caution concerning the status of the embryo, ambivalence seems to be at work. On the one hand, the Singapore BAC is convinced that research on stem cells, even if it involves therapeutic cloning, should go forward. Further, the assumption is made here that, prior to fourteen days, when the embryo adheres to the uterine wall and the primitive streak appears, we do not have a morally protectable human being — that is, no moral proscriptions deny the blastocyst to researchers. On the other hand, the Singapore BAC grants a degree of respect to the conceptus; it is reluctant to allow embryos at the blastocyst stage to be treated without any moral regard. The BAC introduces a calculus, namely, a preferential list of approvable derivations ranked according to levels of respect shown to the early embryo. The ambivalence at work here is one that we all feel, but it is difficult to move ethical deliberation forward when caught between competing moral obligations. The task of ethicists in this situation is to help us work through the ambivalence. Establishing weight-bearing foundations, ethicists need to construct arguments capable of informing firm decisions and setting public policies.

The U.S. President's Council on Bioethics

On 9 August 2001, U.S. President George Bush addressed his nation on the controversial matter of stem cell research and the public policy debate surrounding it. In the months that followed, he appointed members to serve on the President's Council on Bioethics, directed by Leon Kass, a professor at the University of Chicago. After six months' work, on 10 July 2002, Kass and appointees sent to the White House a report titled "Human Cloning and Human Dignity: An Ethical Inquiry."[11]

Concerning what it calls "cloning-to-produce-children," the U.S. report agrees with the Singapore document. The council unanimously recommends an indefinite federal ban. On what the report calls "cloning-for-biomedical-research" and its integral relationship to embryonic stem cell research, the council splits. The majority recommends a four-year moratorium, and the minority that cloning techniques be used to support stem cell research.

In the report's cover letter to President Bush, Kass cautions, "Cloning represents a turning point in human history . . . [carrying] with it a number of troubling consequences for children, family, and society."[12] It is noteworthy that this letter mentions only the troubling consequences of this historic turning point. Unacknowledged is the possibility of scientific breakthroughs; no suggestion is made that the advance of cloning technology could yield benefits to animal breeding or that cloning used for research might contribute to medicine's alleviation of human suffering.

The consideration of potential harms is crucial to responsible ethical reflection; both the majority and minority recommendations rightly grapple with the possible consequences of unexamined pursuit of science-based technology. But proscriptions against harm must be balanced by prescriptions for healing. One need not disagree with their conclusions to recognize that the majority's ethical reflection is guided almost exclusively by nonmalfeasance, a careful guarding against forecasted harm. By contrast, concern for stewarding resources to improve human well-being, or beneficence, is demoted to a secondary consideration. This demotion effectively disallows serious consideration of primary concerns related to theological anthropology as we understand it. It exemplifies the narrowing of ethics from active responsibility for healing to concern for not making matters worse.

Cloning and Babies

The council found unanimity on the one issue where everyone seems to agree: we should not use cloning to make human babies.[13] Six reasons were offered. The first is familiar cloning debate fare: safety. The council con-

8. BAC, vii.
9. Ibid.
10. Ibid.

11. See *Human Cloning and Human Dignity: The Report of the President's Council on Bioethics,* Foreword by Leon R. Kass (New York: PublicAffairs, 2002).
12. Leon R. Kass and James Q. Wilson, *The Ethics of Human Cloning* (Washington D.C.: AEI Press, 1998).
13. Kass report, iii.

tends that cloning to produce children is unethical and recommends that it be banned by law. The Kass council attends to two previous reports, President Clinton's National Bioethics Advisory Commission, 1997, and the National Academy of Sciences, 2002. These reports oppose reproductive cloning for safety reasons. The Kass report follows suit.[14]

The five additional reasons are less familiar: (1) identity — cloned children may be expected to copy in every respect the life of the "original"; (2) manufacture — cloned children may be considered products rather than "gifts" to be treasured; (3) new eugenics — cloned children might be designed to avoid genetic defects or enhance their genetically influenced life chances; (4) troubled family relations — cloning could "confound" and "transgress" "natural boundaries" between generations, allowing fathers to be genetic twins of sons, mothers of daughters; (5) society — cloning might affect the way we look at children, introducing novel forms of intergenerational control.[15]

A notable characteristic of these five reasons is that they all depend on possible future scenarios; they worry about what might happen should reproductive cloning be practiced. This argument against cloning is an argument based on imagined deleterious effects. These arguments do not appeal to any intrinsic violations of human dignity; nor do they appeal to any identifiable theological criteria. None is based on repugnance or natural law theory or God's will. In light of what we said earlier about the contrast between archonic and future oriented reasoning, we simply observe that on this issue the Kass council bypasses archonic assumptions. The domain of its concern is the future, in this case a speculative future.

Although we can concur with the Kass council that a ban on cloning to produce children is morally advisable at this time, we find the argumentation to be tendentious and at places superficial. Little or no medical benefits will come of reproductive uses of cloning. Moreover, those who do support reproductive cloning usually justify their views with some form of parental narcissism, that is, they seek a cloned child for selfish reasons, treating the cloned child instrumentally. The fact that the council's majority turns their moral attention almost exclusively toward potentially negative scenarios might seem unproblematic, yet it discloses a strictly negative disposition toward moral responsibility in general.

Cloning and Stem Cells

Unanimity against reproductive cloning was easy to achieve; the council, however, could not obtain unanimity on therapeutic cloning, on what it calls *cloning for biomedical research.* Like the rest of society, the council could not resolve the stem cell controversy.

Two positions within the council offer moral arguments in support of cloning for biomedical research.[16] Seven members (a minority) articulated what the report calls "position one," advocating that research proceed under strict federal regulation. Position one displays a mood of serious moral concern. The support offered does not advocate research at any cost, nor does it offer up the potential scientific gain as a moral trump card. Keeping with the tone of the entire report, they carefully acknowledge the ethical difficulties of this research while tentatively recommending that we go forward. Some of the poignant ambivalence seen with the Singapore BAC appears here as well.

Position one wrestles with four ethical difficulties: intermediate moral status, deliberate creation for use, going too far, and other moral hazards.

Intermediate Moral Status

The eye of the hurricane in public policy debate over research on hES cells has been the moral status of the early embryo. The position one minority speaks to this cautiously but clearly: "We believe there are sound moral reasons for not regarding the embryo in its earliest stages as the moral equivalent of a human person. We believe the embryo has a developing and intermediate moral worth that commands our special respect, but that it is morally permissible to use early-stage cloned human embryos in important research under strict regulation."[17]

Deliberate Creation for Use

Like the Singapore BAC, the U.S. council felt it needed to address the derivation question: should we limit research to discarded frozen embryos, or should we deliberately create fresh embryos that will be taken apart when retrieving hES cells? Most existing stem cell lines were derived from frozen excess embryos, although at least one was derived from a fresh embryo. It appears that fresh embryos have research advantages over frozen ones, meaning that we can expect future pressure to produce embryos for research purposes. The language used by the council minority instructs us here: "These embryos would not be 'created for destruction,' but for use in the service of life and medicine. They would be destroyed in the service of a great good, and this should not be obscured."[18]

Going Too For

Minority position one wants to prevent early embryos from developing so long that they approach the fetal stage. "We approve, therefore, only of research on cloned embryos that is strictly limited to the first fourteen days

14. Ibid., xvii.
15. Ibid., xvii-xviii.
16. Ibid., xviii.
17. Ibid., xix.
18. Ibid.

of development."[19] Minority position one within the Kass council supports the fourteen-day rule.

Other Moral Hazards

More and more voices in the public debate can be heard registering concern over the justice implications of gathering human eggs for scientific research, justice concerns that focus on the health and well-being of women who donate the eggs. In addition, a slippery slope fear has arisen. Some fear that, if we approve cloning in stem cell research, we could slide gradually toward approving reproductive cloning as well. Position one confronts these matters: "We believe that concerns about the exploitation of women and about the risk that cloning-for-biomedical-research could lead to cloning-to-produce-children can be adequately addressed by appropriate rules and regulations. These concerns need not frighten us into abandoning an important avenue of research."[20] Much like the Singapore BAC, position one recommends that the potential for future harms be guarded against by means of careful regulation. Thus qualified, position one recommends support of therapeutic cloning and related areas of research such as stem cells.

Minority "position two" within the Kass council offers similar support for cloning for biomedical research, but this position is much less timid about the moral reservations defined and dealt with above. Position two accords no special status to the early embryo. As such, it sees little reason to impede research that may revolutionize medicine. Position two argues that the cloned embryo "should be treated essentially like all other human cells."[21] In short, they do not accept the assumption that research involving cloning for biomedical research involves substantially novel moral issues, but rather that it involves concerns that accompany all human biomedical research. Position two offers categorical support for stem cell research.

Ten members of the Kass council, a majority, make the case against cloning for biomedical research. They do not recommend a total ban, but instead advocate a four-year moratorium applicable to all researchers regardless of whether federal funds are involved. The majority recommendation argues that it is morally wrong to "exploit and destroy developing human life, even for good reasons."[22] They see this research as opening doors to a morally unwise future. Moreover, they believe research on embryos is viscerally unsettling: "We find it disquieting, even somewhat ignoble, to treat what are in fact seeds of the next generation as mere raw material for satisfying the needs of our own."[23]

This argument against therapeutic cloning swings on a two-piece moral hinge. The weight-bearing piece of the hinge is the moral status of the cloned embryo. The majority rejects the claims of minority position two. They argue that the early-stage embryo is indeed quite unlike other human cells. Position two, according to the majority, "denies the continuous history of human individuals from the embryonic to fetal to infant stages of existence."[24] The majority position finds similar fault with the arguments invoked in position one, judging the concept of the intermediate status of the embryo to be unconvincing. They find invoking "special respect" for nascent human life "to have little or no operative meaning if cloned embryos may be created in bulk and used routinely with impunity."[25]

The cooperative piece on which the majority argument hinges concerns the deleterious affects resulting from a misunderstanding of the significance of potentiality. Failing to recognize the potential human life of the embryo as, de facto, a prohibition against embryonic research exhibits an ignorance of "the hazardous moral precedent that the routinized creation, use, and destruction of nascent human life would establish."[26]

What worries the Kass council majority is that we as a society will instrumentalize early human life and lose our sense of awe and respect, and that this instrumentalization could dull our social sensitivities. Cloning even for biomedical research risks crossing a "significant moral boundary. . . . Doing so would coarsen our moral sensibilities and make us a different society: one less humble toward that which we cannot fully understand, less willing to extend the boundaries of human respect outward, and more willing to transgress moral boundaries once it appears to be in our own interests to do so."[27]

While appreciating the majority's careful concern for the future well-being of society's moral sensitivity, we question the social naïveté that lends rhetorical strength to their position. Implied in their argument is that, generally speaking, society's corporate conscience is attuned to the noninstrumental value of human life. Unfortunately, this is often not the case. The ethical status quo worldwide is already quite unacceptable. We live in a society marred by a good deal of exploitation, instrumental abuse, and manipulation of human life. If cloning exacerbates these undesirable conditions, society will not be different, only sadly worse.

As thoughtfully articulated and reasonable as they may be, the possible troublesome consequences enumerated by the majority are nothing more than speculative possibilities. Can we, with any degree of certainty, know that through the use of cloning a society, which does not guarantee health insurance for many of the sick children already living among us, will have its moral sensitivity to the value of developing life coarsened beyond what it al-

19. Ibid.
20. Ibid.
21. Ibid.
22. Ibid., xx.
23. Ibid.
24. Ibid.
25. Ibid.
26. Ibid.
27. Ibid.

ready is? If not, should we invoke this troubling possibility as justification for shutting down potentially lifesaving research?

This existing state of suffering and injustice thrusts on us a profound moral obligation to make things better. Implied in making things better is not letting things get worse (i.e., concerning ourselves with the prevention of future harms). The opposite does not hold true: concern for not doing further harm does not carry with it a mandate to make existing ills better.

Back to Beneficence

The leadership Leon Kass has shown in producing such a thorough piece of scholarship over a relatively short period of time is admirable. So also is his willingness to report both the majority and minority positions so that the public can see the level of difficulty at producing consensus. It is also pleasurable to think that the White House will likely be reading an eloquent articulation of wholesome values protecting the dignity of children and warning society away from insensitivity toward the value of human life.

Yet, minority position one in this report has distinct merit. It stands in contrast to much of the report in the way it frames its basic argumentation, and its attentiveness to beneficence accords well with our view that beneficence should be central to a theologically based ethic. Whether articulated as the Jewish mandate to heal or the Christian commitment to love of neighbor, theologically informed beneficence reframes bioethics. Here beneficence begins with the constructive vision of God's desire to heal the world. The vision is basic, foundational. Hence, the first and framing question beneficence asks in the cloning debate is, Can biomedical technology be pressed into the service of healing and human well-being?

In light of injustices associated with for-profit medicine, where research dollars are usually poured into the development of treatments that offer the best return on investment, there are those that might answer "no" to the first beneficence question. These might argue that resources should be spent in meeting basic medical needs rather than pursuing therapies on the frontier of genetic science. While recognizing endemic problems with the current medical system, we choose to answer "yes." Stem cell research and cloning for research purposes can and should be pressed into the service of healing.

The model here is the Good Samaritan in Jesus' parable (Luke 10:29-37). The Samaritan pursues one goal: healing for the suffering stranger. This is an other-seeking form of love, one that takes the initiative and acts to bring about constructive change. This love defines its task according to the needs of the neighbor.

Medical science and its taxpayer support can be seen as a social form of neighbor loving, an investment on the part of the present generation for the health and welfare of the coming generation. What's more, medical research science, in its own way, contributes to God's healing work on earth. To ignore this divine mandate is itself an ethical concern. So many human diseases that shorten life and cause suffering could possibly find therapies through stem cell research: heart disease, cancers, organ deterioration, Alzheimer's and other brain malfunction.

Could we ask that beneficence count more in the public debate? If so, what would happen? Appeal to beneficence does not promote cloning to produce children; so living with the unanimous Kass council recommendation will be easy. In fact, theological beneficence does not necessarily require support of cloning for research, though it certainly encourages us in this direction; however, marginalizing beneficence when arguing against stem cell research, in this case against cloning for biomedical research, is lopsided. The Kass council report certainly acknowledges the potential medical benefits to which such research may lead, but this fails to function substantively in the majority argument.

Regardless of the role of the beneficence principle, there is no way to avoid facing a decisive question: when does morally protectable individual human life begin? The question invokes archonic reasoning. As such, it will significantly affect every other component to an ethical argument. Whether we date morally protectable dignity prior to the blastocyst stage or later than the blastocyst stage will determine whether we advocate hES cell research.

Keep in mind that our warrant for support of beneficence is an eschatologically informed theological anthropology. This understanding of the human person serves to answer the question behind the question of the status of the embryo, an alloyed question composed of equal parts ethics and anthropology: How ought we to understand moral responsibility for other people?

We argue that ethics should be future oriented, seeking to transform suffering into justice. A relational understanding of human dignity and the obligation to love actively and creatively underwrite this ethics. Our argument differs in form from the Vatican's appeal to genetic novelty and even to the fourteen-day rule, both of which are reasoned archonically. According to both positions, dignity is tied up in being an individual. Responsibility, here, risks being cast in strictly negative terms, as a prohibition against violating the intrinsic dignity correlative to the human individuation.

Better Safe than Sorry

We cannot, however, avoid the question, At what point during embryonic development does moral responsibility kick in? We recognize that human dignity is revealed in God's redemptive love, but when along the developmental pathway do we believe God's concern for a person's eschatological destiny begins? Is it at conception? Is it at four days, ten days, or fourteen days?

Though we do not appeal to it as a foundation for a theologically informed assessment of the cloning and stem cell debates, we find the fourteen-day rule to be more persuasive than arguments for conception. It is sufficiently convincing to warrant support as a subpremise within the larger beneficence framework. One can fully understand and appreciate Pope John Paul II and others who are convinced that dignity begins at conception; yet a closer look at what science tells us about embryo development makes the gastrulation threshold more defensible. (One can, by the way, hold to the fourteen-day rule and still hold to a prolife position on abortion.)

The belief that the embryo should be protected from the moment of conception is argued in various ways. Two arguments appear frequently. First is the argument from potential. This is the argument appealed to by the Kass council majority. The majority points to the seamless trajectory of development from conception to birth. In light of this continuum, the Kass council holds the conceptus to be nascent human life and deserving of a "shared obligation to protect it."[28]

As many supporters of embryonic stem cell research have rightly pointed out, the argument from potentiality assesses the status of the embryo in accordance with the presumption that the embryo can and will be placed in vivo. Stem cell research is conducted on embryos in vitro. The potential for an embryo in the lab to become a baby is nil. This is not a criticism, moral concession, or an argument from geography (as critics rhetorically put it). It is an ethically relevant fact. An embryo in vitro has many intrinsic qualities that are needed for baby making, but it does not have all of the necessary qualities. Although it has DNA, at minimum it still needs a womb to proceed down the developmental pathway.

The second argument is that articulated by the Vatican in *Donum Vitae*. This argument holds that with conception a genuinely new human individual comes into existence. When this argument appeals to genetic novelty for support, it fails to account for current embryology. It makes little sense to associate the appearance of the individual with novel DNA. If the existence of twins had not already made this clear, the birth of Dolly should certainly put the matter to rest.

It is difficult to hold to the fourteen-day rule with the same level of dogmatic fervor that the pope and, by implication, the Kass council hold to conception; it is subject to changes in perspective as embryology expands our knowledge. It is a finite human judgment call to combine beneficence with the fourteen-day rule when orienting public policy.

The recognition of the finitude of our ethical judgments could be incorporated into both sides in the stem cell or therapeutic cloning controversy. Science alone does not tell us when morally protectable personhood begins. We bring our ethical criteria for personhood to the science, to be molded, confirmed, or disconfirmed. Science itself plays the limited role of corroborator or critic.

In granting that the science of embryology in itself cannot supply the decisive biological fact that resolves the debate between the Vatican protection of the fertilized egg and the fourteen-day rule, the policy decision we would make here would have to take the form of an ethical leap of faith. In making this leap, we could imagine some sort of "better-safe-than-sorry" principle being invoked. The embryo protection position as defended by the Vatican and by the Kass council's majority might say, When in doubt about the moral status of the blastocyst, it is safer to assume it has protectable duty and avoid doing harm. In contrast, the Singapore BAC report and the minority within the U.S. report might say, When in doubt about the moral status of the blastocyst, it is safer to assume the appropriateness of the fourteen-day rule and proceed with this potentially life-saving and life-enhancing research. The former would appeal primarily to nonmaleficence, the latter to beneficence.

If the Vatican could convince us beyond a doubt to support its position regarding morally protectable dignity at conception, this would be sufficient to persuade us to join the antitherapeutic-cloning forces. The fourteen-day rule, to our reading, however, holds at least equal if not superior merit, even if it falls short of being absolutely decisive. Our fundamental commitment is to beneficence. So, in order to be safe rather than sorry (vis-à-vis the potential risk of failing to act decisively on behalf of those suffering from degenerative diseases), we join with those who wish to encourage stem cell and related research on the grounds that there exists here a potential for future healing that will relieve human suffering on a large scale. To elect an unsure commitment to nonmaleficence rather than an unsure commitment to beneficence would be, as in Jesus' parable of the Good Samaritan, passing by on the other side.

This amounts to a contingent ethical argument in support of laboratory research on therapies employing stem cells and cloning. While affirming this contingent ethical judgment, we remain somewhat unsatisfied about unfinished theological business. Despite all we said in our introduction regarding the important role that eschatology should play in defining human life, we find ourselves arguing along with everyone else in the archonic playground. For the sake of the public policy debate, we find ourselves conceding that biological origin — whether at conception or at adherence to the mother's uterus — determines moral status. Within the framework of the archonic assumptions, we believe the fourteen-day rule edges out the moment of conception position, and we still more earnestly believe that beneficence should be given larger place in ethical argumentation.

28. Ibid., xx.

90 A Theologian's Brief

Reverend David Jones et al.

Basis of This Submission

1. In a multi-cultural and multi-religious society, it is appropriate to take account not only of secular arguments concerning the place of the human embryo but also of arguments expressed in the religious language of some sections of the community. It is particularly important to understand the *Christian* tradition in this regard because of the place Christianity has had in shaping the moral understanding of many citizens in this country, and because this tradition has already been invoked in the context of public debate.[1]

2. The Human Fertilisation and Embryology (Research Purposes) Regulations 2001 greatly expand the purposes for which research using human embryos can take place, and thus, if implemented, will inevitably lead to a massive increase in the use and destruction of embryos. The Select Committee has expressed its wish not "to review the underlying basis of the 1990 Act";[2] however, the ethical and legal issues surrounding "the Regulations as they now stand" *cannot* adequately be addressed without considering the moral status of the human embryo. Similarly, the "regulatory framework established by the 1990 Act" *cannot* operate effectively if it is flawed in principle.

3. Adding more purposes for which human embryos can be created for destructive use builds upon a mistake that has already been made in the existing legislation. By far the most important ethical issue involved in the Regulations "as they now stand" relates to the ethical significance of embryonic human individuals whether produced by cloning or by the ordinary process of fertilization. The spectacle of thousands of stock-piled frozen human embryos being destroyed at the behest of this legislation bore witness that, even in the area of fertility treatment, too little consideration had been given to regulating the initial production of human embryos, as opposed to their subsequent disposal. The Regulations 2001 make the situation even worse in this regard.

1. Hansard (House of Lords Debates), Vol. 621, No. 16, column 35-37 (22 January 2001).

2. In its "Call for Evidence."

This statement on the place of the human embryo in the Christian tradition and the theological principles for evaluating its moral status was submitted to the House of Lords select Committee on Stem Cell Research on June 1, 2001, by an ad hoc group of Christian theologians from the Anglican, Catholic, Orthodox, and Reformed traditions. From Reverend David Jones et al., "A Theologian's Brief," in the issue on cloning, *Christian Reflection: A Series in Faith and Ethics* 16 (2005): 37-48. Used by permission of The Bioethics Press Ltd.

The Christian Tradition

4. Some scholars, considering the prospective benefits to be derived from experimenting on human embryos, have alleged that the Christian tradition had already set a precedent for treating the early human embryo with "graded status and protection."[3] In support of this it has been noted that there were seventh-century books of penance ("Penitentials") which graded the level of penance for abortion according to whether the foetus was "formed" or "unformed." The same distinction was invoked in Roman Catholic canon law, which, from 1591 to 1869, imposed excommunication only for the abortion of a "formed" foetus. Furthermore, St. Thomas Aquinas, one of the most authoritative theologians of the Middle Ages, explicitly held that the human embryo did not possess a spiritual soul and was not a human being *(homo)* until forty days in the case of males or ninety in the case of females.[4] Texts from the Fathers of the Church could easily be found to support a similar conclusion.

5. Nevertheless, the contention that for most of Christian history (until 1869) the human embryo has been considered to possess only a relative value — such as might be outweighed by considerations of the general good — relies on a misreading of the tradition. Even in the Middle Ages, when most Western Christians held that the early embryo was not yet fully human, it was held that the human embryo should never be attacked deliberately, however extreme the circumstances. To gain the proper historical perspective it is necessary to supply a wider context by incorporating other elements of that tradition.

6. The earliest Christian writings on the issue declared simply, "you shall not murder a child by abortion":[5] the embryo was held to be inviolable at every stage of its existence.[6] The first Christian writings to consider the question of when human life began asserted that the spiritual soul was present from conception.[7] As one account

3. Cf. G. R. Dunstan, "The Human Embryo in the Western Moral Tradition" in G. R. Dunstan and M. J. Sellers, *The Status of the Human Embryo* (London: King Edward's Hospital Fund, 1988), 55.

4. *Commentary on the Sentences,* book IV, d. 31 exp. text.

5. *Didache* 2.2; *Epistle of Barnabas* 19.5.

6. See also *Apocalypse of Peter* 2.26; St. Clement of Alexandria, *Teacher* 11.10.96; Athenagoras, *Legatio* 35; Municius Felix, *Octavius* 30.2; Tertullian, *Apology* 9.4-8; Hippolytus, *Refutation of All Heresies* 9.7.

7. St. Clement, *Prophetic Eclogues* 41, 48-49; cf. M. J. Gorman, *Abortion and the Early Church: Christian, Jewish & Pagan Attitudes in the Greco-Roman World* (Downers Grove, IL: InterVarsity Press, 1982), 52; and Tertullian, *On the Soul* 27. "Now we allow that life begins with conception, because we contend that the soul also be-

puts it: "The Early Church adopted a critical attitude to the widespread practice of abortion and infanticide. It did so on the basis of a belief in the sanctity of human life; a belief which was in turn an expression of its faith in the goodness of creation and of God's particular care for humankind."[8]

7. The earliest Church legislation also contains no reference to the distinction of formed and unformed,[9] and St. Basil the Great, who did consider it, saw it as a sophistical exercise in splitting hairs: "We do not consider the fine distinction between formed and unformed."[10]

8. In the fourth and fifth centuries some theologians argued that human life began at conception,[11] some held that the spiritual soul was "infused" at forty days or so[12] (following Aristotle)[13] and some held that the timing of the infusion of the soul was a mystery known to God alone.[14] However, whatever their views about the precise moment when human life began, all Christians held that abortion was gravely wrong,[15] an offense against God the Creator and either the killing of a child, or something very like the killing of a child. If it was not regarded as homicide in the strict sense, "it was looked upon as anticipated homicide, or interpretive homicide, or homicide in intent, because it involved the destruction of a future man. It was always closely related to homicide."[16]

9. In the Anglo Saxon and Celtic "Penitentials" (from the seventh century) and in the canon law of the Latin Church (from the eleventh century), abortion of a formed foetus sometimes carried heavier penalties than did abortion of an unformed foetus. Yet canon law has an eye not just on objective harm done but also on subjective culpability and on enforceability. The decision of Gregory XIV in 1591 to limit the penalty of excommunication to the abortion of a formed foetus was expressly due to problems enforcing earlier legislation.[17] Abortion of an unformed foetus was sometimes regarded as, technically, a different sin — and sometimes (though not universally) as a lesser sin — than abortion of a formed foetus, but it continued to be regarded as a grave sin closely akin to homicide.

10. From the twelfth century until the seventeenth century, convinced by the anatomy of Galen and the philosophy of Aristotle, most Christians in the West came to believe that the spiritual soul was infused forty days or so after conception. Nevertheless, during this whole period, there was no suggestion that the unformed foetus was expendable. The unformed foetus continued to be regarded as sacrosanct. It was *never* seen as legitimate to harm the embryo directly, only incidentally, and only then in the course of trying to save the mother's life.[18]

11. The first theologian to suggest explicitly that the embryo had a graded moral status, that is, a relative value that could be outweighed by other values, was Thomas Sanchez in the late sixteenth century.[19] He and other "laxists" proposed that a woman could legitimately abort an unformed foetus to avoid public shame of a kind which might endanger her life. This suggestion constituted a radical departure from the thinking of previous moralists such as St. Raymond of Penafort or St. Antoninus of Florence and provoked the criticism of Sanchez's contemporaries, the scandal of the faithful and, in 1679, the condemnation of Pope Innocent XI.[20]

12. Between this discredited school of the seventeenth century and the re-emergence of similar views in the late twentieth century, there is no significant or continuous strand of Christian tradition — either in the Catholic or the Reformed churches. The most balanced and representative Catholic moralist of the eighteenth century, St. Alphonsus Liguori, allowed no exception to the prohibition on "direct" (intentional) abortion and allowed "indirect" (unintentional) abortion only in the context of attempting to save the mother's life. In a statement reminiscent of St. Basil he declared that the distinction of formed and unformed made no practical difference.[21] He is the last great moralist to consider the inviolability of the "unformed" foetus as such, because, during his time, the prevailing medical opinion moved away from the distinction between formed and unformed. In his later writing (on baptism) St. Alphonsus also became sympa-

gins from conception; life taking its commencement at the same moment and place that the soul does."

8. "Some Current Ethical Issues Concerning the Treatment of the Pre-Implantation Human Embryo," a briefing paper prepared by the General Synod Board for Social Responsibility; cf. G. Bonner, "Abortion and Early Christian Thought" in J. H. Channer, ed., *Abortion and the Sanctity of Human Life* (Exeter: The Paternoster Press, 1985); M. J. Gorman; L. Crutchfield, "The Early Church Fathers and Abortion" at www.all.org/issues/ab99x.htm.

9. Elvira (305 CE) canons 53, 65; Ancyra (314 CE) 21; Lerida (524 CE) 2; Braga (527 CE) 77; Trullo (692 CE) 91; Mainz (847 CE) 21; cf. S. Troianos, "The Embryo in Byzantine Canon Law."

10. Basil, *Epistle* 118.2.

11. St. Gregory of Nyssa, *On the Making of Man* 29; cf. St. Maximus the Confessor, *II Ambigua* 42.

12. Lactantius, *De Opificio Dei* 12; Ambrosiaster, QQ *Veteris et Novi Testamenti* 23.

13. *On the History of Animals* VII.3, 4:583.

14. St. Jerome, *On Ecclesiastes* 2.5; *Apologia adversus Rufinum* 2.8; St. Augustine, *Enchiridion* 85, *On Exodus* 2.80; though each of these sometimes states that the foetus is not a man *(homo)* until he is fully formed.

15. St. Augustine, *On Marriage and Concupiscence* 1.15; St. Ambrose, *Hexameron* 5.18; St. Jerome, *Epistle* 22, 13; St. John Chrysostom, *Homily 24 on the Epistle to the Romans;* Caesarius of Arles, *Sermons* 9, 91.

16. J. Connery, *Abortion: The Development of the Roman Catholic Perspective* (Chicago, IL: Loyola University Press, 1977), 306; cf. G. Grisez, *Abortion: The Myths, the Realities, and the Arguments* (New York: Corpus Books, 1970); J. T. Noonan, "An Almost Absolute Value in History," in J. T. Noonan, ed., *The Morality of Abortion: Legal and Historical Perspectives* (Cambridge, MA: Harvard University Press, 1970).

17. Bull of 1591, *Sedes Apostolica;* cf. Connery, 148; Grisez, 167-168; Noonan, 33.

18. Connery, 114-134; Grisez, 166-168; Noonan, 26-27.

19. Connery, 134-141; Grisez, 168-169; Noonan, 27-31.

20. Denzinger-Schoenmetzer, *Enchiridion Symbolorum* (Rome: Herder, 1965), 2134-2135; cf. Connery, 189; Grisez, 174; Noonan, 34.

21. *Theologia Moralis* III, 4.1, n. 394.

thetic to the view that the spiritual soul was infused at conception.[22]

13. From the seventeenth century the classical biology of Galen and Aristotle had begun to be displaced by a variety of other theories. One, in particular, gave a more equal role to the female and male elements in generation, and therefore increased the significance of "fertilization," that is, the moment of the union of male and female gametes.[23] This theory was finally confirmed in 1827 with the first observation of a mammalian ovum under the microscope, a scientific development which informed the decision of Pius IX in 1869 to abolish the distinction in legal penalties between early and late abortions. By the mid-nineteenth century the prevailing opinion, among both Reformed and Roman Catholic Christians, was that, most probably, the spiritual soul was infused at conception.[24]

14. In asserting that "life must be protected with the utmost care from conception"[25] and rejecting "the killing of a life already conceived,"[26] twentieth-century Christians were in continuity with the belief of the Early Church that all human life is sacred from conception. This had remained a *constant* feature of Christian tradition despite a variety of beliefs about the origin of the soul and a similar variety in what legal penalties were thought appropriate for early or late abortion.[27]

15. In the tradition, the only precedents for attributing a "graded status and protection" to the embryo can be found in the speculations of some of the Roman Catholic laxists of the seventeenth century and the re-emergence of similar and even more radical views among some Protestant and Roman Catholic writers in the late twentieth century.[28] The great weight of the tradition, East and West, Orthodox, Catholic, and Reformed, from the apostolic age until the twentieth century, is firmly against any sacrifice or destructive use of the early human embryo save, perhaps, "at the dictate of strict and undeniable medical necessity";[29] that is, in the context of seeking to save the mother's life.

Some Theological Principles

16. For a Christian, the question of the status of the human embryo is directly related to the mystery of creation. In the context of the creation of things "seen and unseen"[30] the human being appears as the *microcosm,* reflecting in the unity of a single creature both spiritual and corporeal realities.[31] The beginning of each human being is therefore a reflection of the coming to be of the world as a whole. It reveals the creative act of God bringing about the reality of *this* person (of me), in an analogous way to the creation of the entire cosmos. There is a mystery involved in the existence of each person.

17. Often in the Scriptures the forming of the child in the womb is described in ways that echo the formation of Adam from the dust of the earth (Job 10:8-12; Ecclesiastes 11:5; Ezekiel 37:7-10; cf. Wisdom 7:1, 15:10-11). This is why Psalm 139 describes the child in the womb as being formed "in the depths of the earth" (139:15). The formation of the human embryo is archetypal of the mysterious works of God (Psalm 139:15; Ecclesiastes 11:5). A passage that is significant for uncovering the connections between Genesis and embryogenesis is found in the deutero-canonical book of Maccabees, in a mother's speech to her son:

> I do not know how you came into being in my womb. It was not I who gave you life and breath, nor I who set in order the elements within each of you. Therefore the Creator of the world, who shaped the beginning of man and devised the origin of all things, will in his mercy give life and breath back to you again (2 Maccabees 7:22-23).

18. The book of Genesis marks out human beings from other creatures. Only human beings — male and female — are described as being made in "the image and

22. *Theologia Moralis* VI, 1.1, dubia 4, n. 124; cf. Connery, 210; Grisez, 176; Noonan, 31.

23. The theory developed by Fienus (1567-1631), Zacchia (1584-1659), and Cangiamila (1701-1763); cf. Connery, ch. 10-11; Grisez, 170-172; Noonan, 34-40.

24. This has also become the prevailing opinion among followers of St. Thomas Aquinas; cf. B. Ashley, "A Critique of the Theory of Delayed Hominization" in D. McCarthy and A. Moraczewski, *Evaluation of Fetal Experimentation: An Interdisciplinary Study* (St. Louis, MO: Pope John Center, 1976); B. Ashley and A. Moraczewski, "Cloning, Aquinas, and the Embryonic Person," *The National Catholic Bioethics Quarterly* 1 (2000), 189-201; S. Heaney, "Aquinas and the Presence of the Human Rational Soul in the Early Embryo," *The Thomist* 56 (1992), 1; M. Johnston, "Delayed Hominization," *Theological Studies* 56 (1995); R. Joyce, "The Human Zygote Is a Person," *The New Scholasticism* 51 (1975).

25. Second Vatican Council, *Gaudium et Spes,* 51.

26. Lambeth Conference 1958 report, "The Family in Contemporary Society," in *What the Bishops Have Said about Marriage* (London: SPCK, 1968), 17.

27. "The Church has always held in regard to the morality of abortion that it is a serious sin to destroy a fetus at any stage of development. However, as *a juridical norm* in the determination of penalties against abortion, the Church at various times did accept the distinction between a *formed* and a *non-formed,* an *animated* and a *nonanimated* fetus." R. J. Huser, *The Crime of Abortion in Canon Law* (Washington DC: Catholic University Press, 1942), preliminary note.

28. An ill-tempered but perceptive critique of some recent attempts to reread the Christian tradition on abortion as "relatively tolerant" to abortion of an unformed foetus is D. DeMarco, "The Roman Catholic Church and Abortion: An Historical Perspective," in *Homiletic & Pastoral Review* (July 1984), 59-66 and (August-September), 68-76; cf. www.petersnet.net/research/retrieve.cfm?RecNum=3362.

29. Lambeth Conference 1958 report, 17.

30. Creed of Nicaea, in N. Tanner, *Decrees of the Ecumenical Councils* (London: Sheed & Ward, 1990) I, 5.

31. Gregory of Nyssa, *On the Making of Man;* John Damascene, *Exposition of the Orthodox Faith* 11.12; Creed of Lateran IV, Tanner, 230.

likeness of God"; only they are given dominion over creation; only Adam is portrayed as receiving life from God's breath and as naming the animals (Genesis 1:26-28; 2:7, 19-20). However, at the same time, it is clear that human beings are earthly creatures, made on the same day as other land animals, made from the dust of the earth, not descending out of heaven. Because they are earthly, human beings are mortal: "Dust you are, and to dust you will return" (Genesis 3:19). There is no sign in these stories of the dualism of body and soul that is found in Pythagoras or in the ancient mystery religions. The soul is not a splinter of God that is trapped in a body. The soul is the natural life of the body, given by the life-giving God.

19. It was because of the Jewish conviction of the unity of the human being that, when hope was kindled within Israel for a life beyond the grave, it was expressed as a hope for the resurrection of the body (Daniel 12:2-3; cf. Ezekiel 37:1-14; John 11:24). The disembodied life of the shades in the gloomy underworld of Sheol (Job 10:21-22; Psalms 6:5, 88:10, 115:17; Ecclesiastes 9:3-6; cf. Homer *Odyssey* XI.485-491) was not an image of hope but an image of death. The resurrection of the body was presented as the triumph of the Lord over death, the vindication of those who had been faithful to the Lord, even unto death (Isaiah 26:19; Hosea 13:14; cf. 2 Maccabees 7:9-14), and for Christians was given new meaning and foundation in the resurrection of Jesus (John 11:1-44). The story of the empty tomb and the description of the resurrection appearances emphasized the bodily reality of the life of the resurrection. Jesus walked with the disciples and ate with them and invited them to touch his hands and his feet. "Handle me and see that I am no bodiless phantom."[32]

20. The Fathers of the Church attempted to do justice to the scriptural truths of the bodily resurrection and of the mysterious parallel between the origin of each human individual and the origin of the entire cosmos. From different competing beliefs, the doctrine which prevailed was that the spiritual *soul* — what makes each individual human person unique, and gives each one the ability to know and to love — is neither generated by the parents nor does it pre-exist the body, but it is created directly by God with the coming to be of each human being.[33] Throughout the history of the Church, Christians have used the language of "body and soul" to understand the human being, but in such a way as not to deny the unity of God's creation. In the fourteenth century, in an attempt to defend this human unity, the Ecumenical Council of Vienne defined the doctrine that the soul was "the form of the body" *(forma corporis)*,[34] by which it meant: what gives life to the body. Christians held, and continue to hold, that the spiritual soul is present from the moment there is a living human body[35] until the time that body dies.

21. The Scriptures also emphasize how God's provident care for each person is present before he or she is ever aware of it. The Lord called his prophets by name before they were born: "The LORD called me from the womb, from the body of my mother he named my name" (Isaiah 49:1). "Before I formed you in the womb I knew you, and before you were born I consecrated you" (Jeremiah 1:5). It is possible to understand these passages as referring not only to the prophets, but to each one of God's children. The Lord calls each one from the womb, forms each one, gives each one into the care of his or her mother, and will not abandon his creature in times of trial (Psalms 22:10-11, 71:6; Job 10:8-12).

> For it was you who created my being,
> knit me together in my mother's womb.
> I thank you for the wonder of my being,
> for the wonders of all your creation.
>
> Already you knew my soul,
> my body held no secret from you
> when I was being fashioned in secret
> and moulded in the depths of the earth. Psalm 139

22. Such passages do not establish *when* human life begins, but they establish God's involvement and care from the very *beginning*, a concern that is not diminished by our lack of awareness of him.

23. "In reality it is only in the mystery of the Word made flesh that the mystery of the human being truly becomes clear."[36] To illuminate the mystery of the origin of human persons it seems reasonable to turn to the mystery of the Incarnation. In order to do justice to the infancy narratives, especially that of the Gospel of Luke, one must believe that, from the moment of the Annunciation to Mary of Jesus's birth, Mary conceived by the Holy Spirit and carried the Saviour in her womb. This is emphasized by the story of the Visitation — where one pregnant mother greets another, and the unborn John bears witness to the unborn Jesus.

24. The Incarnation was revealed to the world at the Nativity when Jesus was born, but the Incarnation *began* at the Annunciation, when the Word took flesh and came to dwell within the womb of the Virgin. This understanding of the text of Scripture is confirmed by the witness of the Fathers of the Church,[37] by the development of the feast of the Annunciation and, not least, by the solemn declaration of the Fourth Ecumenical Council, the Council of Chalcedon (451 CE):

> We profess the holy Virgin to be Mother of God, for God the Word became flesh and was made man and

32. Ignatius of Antioch, *Smyrneans* 3; cf. Luke 24:13-51; John 20:19-29.

33. John Damascene; Peter Lombard; St. Thomas Aquinas, *Summa Theologiae* Ia Q. 118 AA. 2-3; Pius XII, *Humani Generis*.

34. Council of Vienne, *On the Catholic Faith;* Tanner, 361.

35. The debate about the timing of the "infusion of the soul" was a debate about when the living human body came into existence.

36. Second Vatican Council, *Gaudium et Spes*, 22.

37. J. Saward, *The Redeemer in the Womb* (San Francisco: Ignatius, 1993), chapter 3.

> from the moment of conception *(ex auteis teis sulleipseoes / ex ipso conceptu)* united himself to the temple he had taken from her.[38]

25. In the Eastern Church, St. Maximus the Confessor turned to the Annunciation[39] to illuminate the intractable problem of when human life begins. Jesus is said to have been like to us in all things but sin (Hebrews 4:15), and Christians believe that Jesus was a human being from the moment of conception: therefore, it seems, every human being must come into existence at the moment of conception.

26. In the West, Christians were more strongly influenced by the biology of Galen and the philosophy of Aristotle and held that the spiritual soul was only infused at the moment when the body was perfectly formed, forty days after conception. The great medieval Christian thinkers all held that the conception of Jesus was an exception, and that he was unlike us in the womb.[40] This was an unhappy conclusion, forced upon theologians by an erroneous biology. Is it really sustainable to argue that Jesus was unlike us in his humanity? A more adequate vision was supplied by the seventeenth-century Anglican theologian Lancelot Andrewes, in a sermon on the Nativity:

> For our conception being the root as it were, the very groundsill of our nature; that he might go to the root and repair our nature from the very foundation, thither he went?[41]

27. The words of this sermon bring our attention, not only to the work of the Redeemer from the beginning of his life, but also to our need for redemption from the beginning of our lives. It was this need that David recognized in himself according to the psalm, "Behold, I was brought forth in iniquity, and in sin did my mother conceive me" (Psalm 51:5), where these words refer not to his mother's sinfulness, but to the complete extent of his own sinfulness. This psalm and the Eden story were given a deeper sense by Christians in light of the redemption accomplished by Jesus. As Jesus had achieved a total transformation, so all human beings were in need of a total transformation: total in the sense of including their very origins. In his letter to the Romans, St. Paul drew out the parallel between Adam and Christ and so asserted the involvement of all human beings in Adam's sin (Romans 5:12-21).

28. This association of sin and conception is also shown within the Roman Catholic tradition in the development of the doctrine of Mary's complete redemption from sin. The doctrine of the Immaculate Conception appears to imply that Mary was receptive to grace from the moment of her conception in her mother's womb. This Roman Catholic argument is simply an expression of a more widely accepted argument from the Christian doctrine of original sin. Both arguments express the general truth that each and every human being needs the help of God from the very first — which is constantly and, it seems, inevitably expressed as "from the first moment of his or her conception."

29. The Christian churches teach not that the early embryo is certainly a person, but that the embryo should always be treated as *if* it were a person.[42] This is not only a case of giving the embryo the benefit of the doubt — refraining from what might be the killing of an innocent person. It is also that the ambiguity in the appearance of the embryo has never been thought of as taking the embryo out of the realm of the human, the God-made and the holy. When Pope John Paul II asks, "how can a human individual not be a human person?"[43] he is not denying the mysteriousness of the implied answer. Christians recognize the embryo to be sacred precisely because it is inseparable from the mystery of the creation of the human person by God.[44] What is clear, at the very least, is that the embryo is "a living thing — under the care of God."[45]

30. The following, then, are five principal considerations which should inform any Christian evaluation of the moral status of the human embryo:

I. Though penalties have varied, the Christian tradition has always extended the principle of the sacredness of human life to the very beginning of each human being, and never allowed the deliberate destruction of the fruit of conception.
II. The origin of each human being is not only a work of nature but is a special work of God in which God is involved from the very beginning.
III. The Christian doctrine of the soul is not dualistic but requires one to believe that, where there is a living human individual, there is a spiritual soul.
IV. Each human being is called and consecrated by God in the womb from the first moment of his or her existence, before he or she becomes aware of it. Traditionally, Christians have expressed the human need for redemption as extending from the moment of conception.
V. Jesus, who reveals to Christians what it is to be human, was a human individual from the moment of his conception, celebrated on the feast of the Annunciation, nine months before the feast of Christmas.

31. Jesus reveals the humanity especially of the needy and those who have been overlooked. Concern over the fate of embryos destined for research is inspired, not only by the narratives of the Annunciation, the Visita-

38. Epistle of St. Cyril to John of Antioch; Tanner, 70.
39. *II Ambigua* 42.
40. Cf. Thomas Aquinas, *Summa Theologiae* IIIa Q.6 A.4.
41. Sermon IX on the Nativity in J. Saward, 100.
42. For example, "The human being is to be respected and *treated as* a person from the moment of conception." Pope John Paul II, *Evangelium Vitae* 60, emphasis added.
43. Ibid.
44. Cf. O. O'Donovan, *Begotten or Made?* (Oxford: Clarendon Press, 1984), ch. 4.
45. Athenagoras, *Legatio* 35.

tion and the Nativity, but also by the parable of the good Samaritan and the parable of the sheep and the goats: "Just as you did it to one of the least of these little ones, you did it to me" (Matthew 25:40). The aim of an ethically serious amendment to the 1990 Act should be to regulate the procedures in fertility treatment and nondestructive medical research on human embryos such that these human individuals are adequately protected.

91 The Ethics of Human Stem Cell Research

Gene Outka

Hype tempts us all. It would be naïve to exempt scientists from sometimes overstating the promise of their research. Early claims about what gene therapy would accomplish, for example, arguably were exaggerated and eroded public confidence. Yet claims about what stem cell research may accomplish belong in a class by themselves. The general public is now convinced that something momentous is occurring.[1] Both professional and popular publications register the excitement scientists evidence. This research, it is routinely said, not only will expand significantly what we know about cellular life, but also will bring dazzling clinical benefits. Those who suffer from Alzheimer's disease, Parkinson's disease, and the like are regularly identified as eventual beneficiaries. The cumulative effect is to raise expectations generally to a high pitch.

Whether these claims will prove exaggerated awaits research efforts that have only just begun.[2] As a society, we long for such benefits and sense a genuinely other-regarding motive among those who make these claims. That is, the prospect that such research will bring concrete benefits to numerous human sufferers motivates scientists to engage in it. At the same time, we recognize that less altruistic considerations — e.g., a search for windfall financial profits — sometimes operate as well.

1. For one early, engaging indication, see Gregg Easterbrook, "Medical Evolution: Will Homo Sapiens Become Obsolete?" *New Republic,* vol. 220, no. 9, 20-25.

2. Scientific uncertainties may go deeper than the public realizes. Maureen Condic (see "The Basics About Stem Cells," *First Things* 119 [January 2002]: 30-39) asks whether the merit of embryonic stem cell research is as widely accepted by researchers as it is routinely alleged to be. She emphasizes the scientific and medical disadvantages of using embryonic stem cells and their derivatives in treating disease and injury and on the advantages of using adult stem cells, even though the latter field is not as far advanced. For a report that testifies to the volatility of current scientific judgments about the respective merits of adult stem cell and embryonic stem cell research, see Alex Dominguez, "Studies Cast Doubt on Efficacy of Stem Cells," *Nando Times* (13 March 2002) [available at http://nandotimes.com/healthscience/v-text/story/302144p-2637767c.html].

From Gene Outka, "The Ethics of Human Stem Cell Research," *Kennedy Institute of Ethics Journal* 12:2 (2002), 175-213.

Yet, concern about profits figures only marginally in the ethical controversies that this research has generated so far. Rather, the controversies show how a single other-regarding motive that accents benefits to human sufferers cannot and should not go unexamined. Even as we praise the motive, we confront a host of complicating questions. May research that accents benefits to human sufferers trump all other considerations as it seeks to secure these benefits? What of embryos and aborted fetuses? Should their value reduce *totally* to their importance for relieving the suffering of *third* parties? Can a readiness to do anything with and to embryos and aborted fetuses be acceptably other-regarding after all? What other moral considerations count, and how much should they count?

I approach these questions by assuming a diagnosis of ourselves as human beings that sets the terms for appraising even novel developments. Two basic generalizations about us that derive from this diagnosis influence my reflections in what follows.

First, we are *morally capable* creatures, *accountable* beings. We should assume responsibility for what we are doing, and we go wrong when we seek to deny our agency. Not every outcome in stem cell research is foregone; we may shape, as well as be shaped by, developments, and much may depend on initiatives we take that accord with our own convictions. Second, we are creatures who can *exalt ourselves inordinately* — i.e., in ways that flout God and manipulate others. This condition is called sin and *moral evil* in many religious communities. Reinhold Niebuhr takes sin to extend in two directions:

> The Bible defines sin in both religious and moral terms. The religious dimension of sin is [our] rebellion against God, and [our] effort to usurp the place of God. The moral and social dimension of sin is injustice. The ego which falsely nukes itself the center of existence in its pride and will-to-power inevitably subordinates other life to its will and thus does injustice to other life.[3]

To be tempted to usurp and to do injustice is endemic to human life as we know it. In my own identity as an Augustinian Christian, I take it that we are continually in danger and that everything is corruptible.[4] If this is right, one should expect that stem cell research is itself not immune to pressures that may usurp and do injustice. In short, stem cell research presents novel opportunities and challenges and manifests permanent capabilities and dangers.

In examining the ethical controversies that surround stem cell research, I canvass a spectrum of value judgments on sources, complicity, adult stem cells, and public and private contexts and explore how debates about abortion and stem cell research converge and diverge. I propose extending the principle of "nothing is lost" to current debates, and I locate a definitive normative region to inhabit, within a larger range to rival value judgments. The creation of embryos for research purposes only should be resisted, yet research on "excess" embryos is permissible.

Recurring Ethical Controversies

Four points assume special salience in discussing the collision of value judgments pertaining to stem cell research. Three points concern the "sources" of stem cells. Particular evaluations of the three tend to cohere internally. That is, how disputants evaluate the "status" of the embryo and aborted fetus (point one) relates to how they evaluate "complicity" (point two) and "the alternative of research on adult stem cells" (point three). Comparison of a spectrum of particular evaluations increases understanding of where disagreements lie.

The fourth point concerns the political and legal contexts in which this research proceeds, and specifically proposals about how such research should be organized, financed, and overseen. They do not receive the rigorous examination that characterizes debates about "sources," but their importance is obvious. They impel us to mesh what is ethically desirable with what is politically viable. I can only touch on such an immense subject in this paper. But to ignore institutional realities altogether, including institutional lacunae, amounts to a certain kind of ethical failure, one that holds at bay questions about which institutional arrangements conduce to the "common good."

Moral Judgments Pertaining to the Sources of Stem Cells

In this section, I review a spectrum of moral positions that pertain to the *status* of the fetus and of the embryo; the question of *complicity,* where research depends on *someone* destroying a fetus or an embryo; and the *alternative* of concentrating on stem cells found in *adults.*

Views on the "Right" Here I refer mostly to Richard Doerflinger, who defends in lucid prose Vatican instruction on human procreation. Yet, other communities, including many evangelical Protestants and (Eastern) Orthodox Christians, hold these views as well.[5]

THE STATUS OF FETUSES AND EMBRYOS. Doerflinger considers the moral status of the human embryo in light

3. Reinhold Niebuhr, *The Nature and Destiny of Man,* I (New York: Charles Scribner's Sons, 1949), 179.

4. See Gene Outka, "Universal Love and Impartiality," in *The Love Commandments: Essays in Christian Ethics and Moral Philosophy,* edited by Edmund S. Santurri and William Werpehowski (Washington, D.C.: Georgetown University Press, 1992), 1-103.

5. See Gilbert Meilaender, "Remarks on Human Embryonic Stem-Cell Research," in *Ethical Issues in Human Stem Cell Research,* vol. 3, *Religious Perspectives* (Rockville, Md.: National Bioethics Advisory Committee, 1999), E1-E6, and Demetrios Dernopulos, "An Eastern Orthodox View of Embryonic Stem Cell Research," in *Ethical Issues in Human Stem Cell Research,* vol. 3, *Religious Perspectives,* BI-B4.

of the historic conviction that each human individual has basic and equal human worth. No differences in talents or other conditions should overturn this evaluation. If one takes this evaluation to heart, one infers that no one should be treated, exhaustively and without remainder, as a means or instrument. "The human individual, called into existence by God and made in the divine image and likeness, . . . must always be treated as an end in himself or herself, not merely as a means to other ends. . . ."[6] It is cogent to infer inviolability, too. To kill the innocent deliberately and directly is the prime instance of going against such inviolability. Fetuses and embryos are assuredly innocent. Doerflinger sees both abortion and the destruction of embryos merely as means to other ends and as going against inviolability.

By maintaining that the moral status of fetuses and embryos is decisively similar, he combats a view that certain liberal Catholics (among others) espouse, in which "conception" differs from "individuation." In this view, the early embryo is relevantly formless until the "primitive streak" appears at about 14 days of gestation. Proponents argue that one otherwise cannot account for the possibilities of "twinning" and "fusion" that occur after conception.[7] Consequently, this view allows moral room for maneuver up to 14 days. Doerflinger replies that the most recent studies show that the early embryo is not simply formless, that the capacity for twinning is established very early indeed, and, in any event, that the overwhelming majority of embryos lack the property of spontaneously producing twins. A more general concern surfaces as well. Some hold that, *even* if the argument from "twinning" allows for nontherapeutic experimentation, it remains the case that stem cell research regards early life only as "manipulable stuff" — not as a child, but as an entity that merely serves other, albeit perhaps laudable, ends. Such attention, it is argued, jeopardizes the ability to welcome children into the world and to care for them.[8]

Complicity. Doerflinger reviews and assesses various arguments about complicity in the act of harvesting stem cells. Here certain differences between abortion and the destruction of embryos *do* appear, but they give no comfort to the advocates of research on embryos.

Doerflinger considers efforts that Congress has made since 1993 to distinguish the actions and intentions of those who abort fetuses from the actions and intentions of federally funded researchers who use the resulting fetal tissue in human transplantation.[9] Although he does not altogether approve of these efforts, or of some of the arguments urged on their behalf, he grants that a researcher who uses fetal tissue does not necessarily support the decisions to request or to perform an abortion.

He refuses to say the same, however, about the derivation and use of stem cells from embryos.

> Here those who harvest and use the cells are necessarily complicit in the destruction of the embryo. This is illustrated by the fact that, if embryonic stem cell research were governed by the same legal conditions that now govern the use of fetal tissue from abortions in federally funded research — e.g., harvesting to be done only after death, researchers' needs may not determine the timing and manner of the destruction of the fetus — the research could not be done at all. These stem cells are taken from embryos while they are still living. In effect, the harvesting of cells is itself the abortion — i.e., it is the act that directly destroys a live embryo — and the method of destruction, using microsurgery to extract the embryo's inner cells from the outer trophoblast, is determined entirely by the needs of the stem cell researcher.[10]

Given this assessment, he rejects as incoherent any claim that government funding of research on embryonic stem cells does not involve complicity in the destruction of embryos as long as researchers did not participate directly in such destruction. This distinction strikes him as little more than a "bookkeeping exercise," since the act of destruction is not only *presumed* as with research on aborted fetuses, but is directly *undertaken* as part of the research protocol.

He also criticizes the argument that derivation of stem cells from "spare" embryos donated by fertility clinics differs morally from using embryos created *solely* for research purposes and that only the latter uses embryos as a mere *means* to other people's ends. Doerflinger maintains that destruction of an entity for body parts because that entity will die in any case is not the same as using cells from an entity that is already dead. In addition, "a policy that permits research only on 'spare' embryos is virtually impossible to maintain in practice. Fertility clinics easily can produce a few more embryos from each couple, ostensibly for reproductive purposes, to ensure that there will be 'spares' for research at the end of the process."[11]

The alternative of adult stem cells. Doerflinger accents the advances that researchers have made in the work on adult stem cells. One major advantage of using adult cells on which everyone agrees is the avoid-

6. Richard M. Doerflinger, "The Ethics of Funding Embryonic Stem Cell Research: A Catholic Viewpoint," *Kennedy Institute of Ethics Journal,* 9 (1999): 138.

7. This view holds that embryos up to 14 days are preindividual and prepersonal (see, e.g., Thomas A. Shannon, "Remaking Ourselves? The Ethics of Stem Cell Research," *Commonweal,* vol. 125, no. 21 [1998]: 2-3, and Richard A. McCormick, "Who or What is the Preembryo?" *Kennedy Institute of Ethics Journal,* 1 [1991]: 1-15). Shannon sees a distinction between cells drawn from a preimplantation embryo and cells drawn from an aborted fetus. I later compare stem cell research on embryos and fetal cadavers.

8. See William Werehowski, "Persons, Practices, and the Conception Argument," *Journal of Medicine and Philosophy* 22 (1997): 479-94.

9. See Doerflinger.

10. Ibid., 141.

11. Ibid., 143.

ance of possible tissue rejection by treating a patient with his or her own cells. That researchers cannot say with certainty that research on embryonic cells will yield clinical applications that would not be available otherwise strengthens the case on practical grounds for limiting research attention to adult stem cells. We as a society thereby avoid putting *firmly,* and probably *irrevocably,* into place morally contestable practices that may not be clinically necessary.

Views in the "Middle"

The status of fetuses and embryos. A more liberal case is made within the Catholic tradition that favors human embryo stem cell research. It requires one to distinguish, as I mentioned earlier, between conception and individuation. Margaret Farley[12] accepts this distinction. For her and a number of other Catholic moral theologians, the human embryo is not considered in its earliest stages (prior to the development of the primitive streak or to implantation) to constitute an individualized human entity with the settled inherent potential to become a human person. The moral status of the embryo is, therefore (in this view), not that of a person, and its use for certain kinds of research can be justified. (Because it is, however, a form of human life, it is due some respect; for example, it should not be bought or sold.)[13] While accepting some embryo research, she commends certain safeguards — e.g., donors may not specify who is to receive stem cells for therapeutic treatment, and an "absolute barrier" should be maintained between therapeutic and reproductive cloning.

Complicity. Those who occupy positions in the middle may disagree about the moral standing of fetuses, but they tend to agree on the moral relevance of one distinction respecting embryos. They refuse to equate the destruction of embryos who already exist, but who will either be frozen in perpetuity or discarded, with the creation of embryos solely for the purpose of destroying them in an effort to benefit third parties. Complicity in the former instance looks morally less ominous. For the decisive role here is played by those responsible for the existence of embryos and for the decision to freeze or discard them. Researchers react rather than initiate, after those responsible have reached their fateful determinations. Some estimate that at least 100,000 frozen spare embryos in the United States alone now languish in *in vitro* fertilization clinics. The majority are no longer wanted or claimed. They will never be implanted. Judging complicity should reckon with this datum.

12. See Margaret Farley, "Roman Catholic Views on Research Involving Human Embryonic Stem Cells," in *Ethical Issues in Human Stem Cell Research,* vol. 3, *Religious Perspectives,* D1-D5.

13. Ibid., D-4. Papers prepared for a meeting of the National Bioethics Advisory Commission (7 May 1999) display the diversity of views within religious traditions (National Bioethics Advisory Committee, 2000). (In addition to the papers already cited by Farley, Meilaender, and Demopulos, see Dorff, Pellegrino, Sachedina, Tendler, and Zoloth, in the same volume.)

The alternative of adult stem cells. Those who occupy middle places along the spectrum are disposed generally to accept — though sometimes reluctantly — a verdict that many scientists have reached. Stem cells derived from adults are necessary but not sufficient — if one wants to maximize the data available and hence the possibility of breakthroughs — to support all clinically important areas of research. Research using each of the "sources" should go forward, for each has its own advantages and disadvantages, and they complement one another. The settled verdict is that embryonic stem cell research holds promise for which at the present there is no adequate substitute.

Views on the "Left" Here I refer mostly to the work of John Robertson.

The status of fetuses and embryos. Those who stand on the left side of the spectrum characteristically deny that the value accorded to previable fetuses should *ever* override pregnant women's choices to terminate their pregnancies for whatever reason. To attribute basic and equal human worth to each human individual requires more than the presence of cells that have the potential to develop into a person. Robertson extends this value judgment to embryos in the following way:

> [Those] holding this view about pre-viable fetuses view preimplantation embryos, which are much less developed than fetuses, as too rudimentary in structure or development to have moral status or interests in their own right. . . No moral duties are owed to embryos by virtue of their present status and . . . they are not harmed by research or destruction when no transfer to the uterus is planned.[14]

Robertson refuses to say, however, that because embryos lack moral status in their own right one may do anything *at all* with them. They are not "means" in this sense or to this extent — e.g., one may not use them "for toxicology testing of cosmetics" or buy and sell them. One can deny intrinsic value to all embryos and still accord them "symbolic" value and "'special respect' because of their potential, when placed in a uterus, to become fetuses and eventually to be born."[15] Nevertheless, this symbolic value should be trumped when necessary to pursue a good scientific or medical end that cannot be pursued by other means.

Complicity. Robertson thinks that any distinction between the derivation and the use of embryonic stem cells does not survive critical scrutiny. Researchers who use stem cells derived from embryos are complicit in their destruction, regardless of whether they participate directly in the act of destruction. Moreover, those who support the use of cells from spare embryos from *in vitro*

14. See John A. Robertson, "Ethics and Policy in Embryonic Stem Cell Research," Kennedy *institute of Ethics Journal,* 9, no. 2 (1999): 117-18.

15. Ibid., 118.

fertilization clinics should *also* support the creation of embryos for the purpose of research. In both cases, embryos *do* become a means to address the needs of others, once one decides to use them in research. In this regard, Robertson displays an ironic affinity with Doerflinger. Both insist on an either/or scenario, though of course each draws the opposite normative conclusion. *Either* one should stop opposing the creation and destruction of embryos for research purposes only (in Robertson's view), *or* one should oppose not only the creation and destruction of embryos for research purposes, but also the research on spare embryos from *in vitro* fertilization clinics (in Doerflinger's view). Pressures are exerted on those in the "middle" from the "left" as well as from the "right."

THE ALTERNATIVE OF ADULT STEM CELLS. Those who take the position Robertson does can prefer limiting research to adult stem cells only *if* such a limit in fact will yield superior therapeutic benefits overall. The criteria for making this determination are, it seems, empirical and consequentialist: what research on which sources will produce the greatest benefit overall? Given this, Robertson insists that at present no definitive empirical-consequentialist case exists for limiting research to adult stem cells. The most promising course is to pursue research using cells from each of the three "sources" — fetuses, embryos, and adults.

Ethical Considerations in Political and Legal Contexts

I now turn to the fourth realm in which ethical controversies recur, the political and legal realm. Two areas of controversy figure most prominently here. The first concerns controversies about federal funding of stem cell research. These consume the bulk of disputants' energies to date. Passions rise highest where taxpayer dollars figure centrally. Disputants perceive federal expenditures to attest to society-wide convictions. Those who occupy particular positions along the spectrum characterized in the foregoing sections battle on behalf of criteria for federal funding that support their respective normative conclusions about "sources." A pastiche results.

The second area concerns controversies about the absence of coordination between research permitted in the public and private sectors. I find it worrisome that research possibilities lack any sort of society-wide oversight. Yet many either welcome the status quo or appear resigned to it. Some judge the current arrangements to be desirable on the whole, at least they prefer to leave well enough alone, so long as researchers are free *somewhere* to pursue various research possibilities. To enjoy liberty from scrutiny allows those in the private sector to conduct research that might achieve a major breakthrough, but which societal scrutiny might forestall. Others judge the present situation to be ad hoc to a fault. They accept that publicly and privately funded research should be coordinated somehow. Nevertheless, they view the practical chances of coordination to be distressingly slight.

Normative Assessments

In this section, I evaluate more fully the positions described so far, which requires that I also indicate positions I am myself disposed to take.

I commend as a normative point of departure the conviction that Doerflinger[16] cites: "the human individual, called into existence by God and made in the divine image and likeness, . . . must always be treated as an end in himself or herself, not merely as a means to other ends." Many hold this conviction, not only those on the "right." To regard each person for his or her own sake, as one who is irreducibly valuable, authorizes a sphere of inviolability, as previously noted. It also heightens sensitivity to multiple ways one may go wrong — e.g., when one dominates, manipulates, and self-aggrandizes. To affirm inviolability and to abjure domination captures deeply important commitments. They direct moral attention along lines I take to be permanently valid.

Many likewise draw on the language of ends and means to evaluate cases of "killing and saving."[17] To commit murder is arguably the quintessential instance of going wrong. Those who murder arrogate to themselves a position of false superiority. They usurp or perversely imitate God, who alone is the "Author of life and death." Yet they possess the power to accomplish this. That is, in the case of murder, they *can* do what they *ought not* to do. They also effectively claim that they are better than their victims, so much better that they are prepared to "instrumentalize" them through and through. Murderers do their victims *incommensurable* harm; in depriving them of life, they reduce them to "mere means" to their own aims and projects. Those who save life do the opposite. They pay homage to what they take the character of God's love to be, by attesting that the one saved is not a mere means, but someone for whom they should care, whose well-being they should protect and promote.

To mix theological and Kantian ingredients in this way deserves a degree of examination that I cannot pursue here.[18] I focus now on how far this evaluation extends. Is it cogent to claim that abortion and embryonic stem cell research are morally indistinguishable from murder?

16. Doerflinger, 138.

17. See John P. Reeder, Jr., *Killing and Saving: Abortion, Hunger, and War* (University Park: Pennsylvania State University Press, 1996).

18. I try to sort out these ingredients elsewhere. (See Gene Outka, "Respect for Persons," in *The Westminister Dictionary of Christian Ethics,* edited by James F. Childress and John Macquarrie [Philadelphia: Westminster Press, 1986], 541-45, and "Universal Love and Impartiality," in *The Love Commandments: Essays in Christian Ethics and Moral Philosophy,* edited by Edmund S. Santurri and William Werpehowski [Washington, D.C.: Georgetown University Press, 1992], 1-103.) To employ Kant's second formulation of the categorical imperative here does not imply acceptance of Kant's moral theory as a whole. The formulation, as I treat it, distills Christian depictions of neighbor-love.

Posing so blunt a question concentrates our thoughts, but it also encourages an unfortunate tendency to restrict evaluative possibilities to a single either/or. Either one judges abortion and the destruction of embryos to be *transparent* instances of treating fetuses and embryos as mere means to others' ends or one judges abortion and embryonic stem cell research to be, *in themselves,* morally *indifferent* actions that should be evaluated solely in terms of the benefits they bring to others. I reject such a simplifying restriction. The most fitting place to inhabit is, I think, a *particular* region in the "middle." Here one engages the formidable arguments from both the "right" and the "left" and appropriates as much as one consistently can, but still retains a distinctive vantage point. From this point, one finds a position *less* cogent than many conservatives do that extends *simpliciter* (morally, if not legally) the prohibition of murder to the prohibition of abortion and embryonic stem cell research. But one ascribes greater importance to fetuses and embryos than many liberals do, an importance not reduced to the benefits that research on them may bring to third parties. I shall say more about this region as the most fitting place to be, while acknowledging the dangers in locating oneself there.

From the "Right": Specificity and Stringency The tradition of moral reflection that shapes conclusions on the "right" emphasizes two considerations, specificity and stringency, that those in the "middle" should heed as well.

Specificity. I am drawn to the strand in the tradition that endeavors to identify certain actions — which persistently affect our weal and woe — in a definite and nontautological way. To consider the action that concerns us most: murder is prohibited, but not all killing is murder. How should one discriminate? One should not do so by writing morally evaluative references into the characterization of what murder is, for then one renders this characterization morally decisive by definition. So, for example, murder is defined as "wrongful" or "unjust" or "irresponsible" killing. But resorting to tautology forecloses debate. The tradition favors instead specification that leaves the wrongfulness of the action open, to be "settled only by a further nondefinitional judgment."[19] The prohibition of killing in the Decalogue is construed more precisely to mean that one should *not intentionally kill innocent human life.* This construal specifies what "murder" is. It is a delimited action-kind. The judgment that murder in *this* sense is wrong purports to be true, yet is not a tautology. (I accept that who is requisitely "innocent" is sometimes difficult to ascertain and deeply controversial, but not in the cases before us here.) It is the judgment under scrutiny, and it remains possible to dispute it.

To construe more precisely the prohibition of killing introduces, on the one hand, a certain flexibility. It helps to make sense of society's organized efforts to provide security for its citizens against arbitrary, unprovoked, or otherwise unjust assaults on life and limb and to accommodate policing, courts of law, and soldiering. We should by no means idealize here; activities that fall under these organized efforts are always corruptible, and, in some measure, distinctively so. Recognition of corruptibility, however, need not undermine the efforts. Yet, on the other hand, this construal limits flexibility. When one meets cases that fall within its range of applicability, one may not go roaming around redescribing at will. Instead, one acknowledges the moral feature of the case at hand and either condemns the action or seeks special justification or mitigation.

Stringency. To reiterate an ancient question: May we (ever) do evil to achieve good?[20] Cases that fall within the prohibitions range of applicability present one with two choices: the prohibition against killing as precisely construed possesses either *absolute* or *prima facie* authority in any circumstance to which it applies.

A familiar historical example brings out the difference between the two kinds of authority. President Truman reasoned that to drop atomic bombs on Hiroshima and Nagasaki would serve to hasten the end of the war and cost fewer lives than a full-scale invasion of Japan.[21] We cannot ascertain whether he was empirically correct, but we can ask whether he was morally right that the criterion of "fewer lives lost" should trump. Those who adhere to the prohibition against killing as precisely construed normally extend it in circumstances of war to forbid the direct and intentional killing of noncombatants (as "material innocents"). To accord *absolute* authority to the prohibition thus extended means that Truman erred morally when he calculated total outcomes in the fashion he did. No argument from outcomes — which includes Truman's readiness to pursue a "counter-city" rather than "counter-force" strategy to shorten the war and to kill fewer persons — can override what by prior determination is judged to be wrong in itself to do, whoever does it. In this sense, one may never do evil to achieve good. To accord prima facie authority to the prohibition thus extended means that noncombatant immunity has presumptive validity. This is strong enough to query Truman's decision. There is a presumption in the

19. See John Finnis, *Moral Absolutes: Tradition, Revision, and Truth* (Washington, D.C.: Catholic University Press of America, 1991), 37.

20. See Richard A. McCormick and Paul Ramsey, eds., *Doing Evil to Achieve Good* (Chicago: Loyola University Press, 1978).

21. Moral assessments of Truman's decision are legion (see, e.g., G. E. M. Anscombe, "Mr. Truman's Degree," in *Ethic, Religion and Politics: The Collected Philosophical Papers of G. E. M. Anscombe,* vol. 3, 62-71 [Minneapolis: University of Minnesota Press, 1981]; Michael Walzer, *Just and Unjust Wars* [New York: Basic Books, 1977], 263-68; Jonathan Glover, *Humanity: A Moral History of the Twentieth Century* [New Haven, Conn.: Yale University Press, 2000], 89-112; and, with reference to stem cell debates, Gilbert Meilaender, "The Point of a Ban; Or, How to Think about Stem Cell Research," *Hastings Center Report,* vol. 31, no. 1 [2001]: 9-16).

prohibition's favor, and any violation has the burden of proof. The prohibition retains authority in that it may never be disregarded in a circumstance to which it applies, but only overridden, and always with compunction. Still, one may consider in tragic cases whether one should do something morally repellent — something one would not do for its own sake — to prevent something far worse.

Unless one understands how the prohibition against killing is construed, and that it may be accorded absolute authority, one fails to grasp where and why many on the "right" judge abortion and embryonic stem cell research as they do, and where and why many on the "left" demur.

Those on the "right" judge that the prohibition extends to fetuses and embryos. Both are *innocent,* and aborting a fetus and disaggregating an embryo are *direct* actions that kill. Whether death is strictly *intended* is a more complicated question in the case of abortion. Certain defenders of abortion claim that a pregnant woman may justly withdraw her bodily life support from the fetus, but that she may not thereby have a "right" to the fetus' death, if the fetus can survive outside her womb.[22] Before 20 weeks of the pregnancy, however, this distinction has strictly theoretical interest. Death accompanies withdrawal of bodily life support, whatever hypothetical speculations one appends. Death also accompanies the disaggregation of embryos, which affords no room for distinguishing between intending withdrawal but not death. As for "human life," the last part of the specified prohibition, those on the "right" maintain that each human entity, from the time of conception, is irreducibly valuable. Indeed, each is judged to have an equally protectable status. If embryos are currently genderless and removed from the naked eye, they differ from the rest of us only in that they await implantation, growth, and subsequent entry into the world of social interaction.[23] They contain the requisite genetic information that renders each unique, and all of us began at this stage. Why then discriminate? Does self-absorption blind us to injustices we may commit because at present we enjoy superior power? Assuredly, fetuses and embryos cannot fight back on their own behalf, but *none* of us could at the point of our origins. We transcend self-absorption when we revere human entities by doing nothing that would jeopardize their inviolable status, just as our parents earlier revered ours and fought for our survival when necessary. To intervene and destroy fetuses and embryos palpably intrumentalizes them for the sake of those who are presently stronger. We would do well to remember what our parents did, and show that we are grateful for what they did, when we evaluate abortion and embryonic stem cell research.

Those on the "right" move from specificity to stringency. One should make others' ends one's own, *provided that these ends are morally permissible.* Violating the prohibition against killing as precisely construed is an impermissible end. One may not do or approve *this* evil, even when it achieves good. For one should always relate any benefits one aims to secure to what one is prepared to do to obtain them, One does best to consider *first* what *one does* and forbears, and not simply what will *happen,* and to live within the absolute limits that the prohibition against murder sets for us.

In the "Middle": Potentiality and When "Nothing Is Lost" I have identified arguments from the "right" that I find formidable, yet I also find certain extensions of them less cogent than their defenders assume. Two lines of argument prevent my concurring that abortion and embryonic stem cell research are morally indistinguishable from murder and permit my occupying a particular region in the "middle."

POTENTIALITY. The first line of argument concerns "potentiality," as applied to fetuses and embryos. This word recurs in the literature, yet is a red flag to many on the "right" and on the "left." Conservatives think it nullifies a serious commitment to fetuses and embryos; liberals deride it as "mere" potentiality, a referent too indeterminate ever to be permitted to trump decisions to abort and to conduct research on embryos. The truth, it seems to me, is complicated in ways these contrary evaluations neglect.

I claim that "potentiality" is double-sided in a way that leads me to draw back from unqualified extensions of moral status, but to draw back a lesser distance than do those on the "left." It yields appraisals that show how debates about abortion and about embryonic stem cell research are sometimes allied and sometimes not. How they diverge especially needs to be recognized. I consider these claims in turn, and attend first to fetuses.

One side of "potentiality" registers what fetuses *are not yet,* at least during the first 20 weeks of the fetus' existence (or until the lungs are sufficiently developed). The fetus *cannot* live absent total physical dependence on one and only one person in all the world. Assuming the medical technology available now and in the foreseeable future, pregnancy involves unique physical dependence. Every pregnant woman is noninterchangeable. *No one and nothing else can take her place.* This state of affairs is not at all odd (not numerically uncommon), yet it is distinctive (though numerically common). The distinctiveness means that in certain respects pregnancy is *sui generis.* Analogies that are entirely satisfactory do not exist.

Consider two sorts of cases in which this total dependence leads on to ascribe to the fetus a status less than that of equally protectable human life when weighed against the pregnant women, who also is *an end in herself.*

The first sort of case involves parity-conflicts in which one physical life collides with another, and it is impossible to save both. Such cases include conflicts between the

22. See Judith Jarvis Thomson, "A Defense of Abortion," *Philosophy and Public Affairs,* 1 (1971): 47-66.

23. See Andrew Sullivan, "Only Human," *New Republic,* 30 July 2001, 8.

pregnant woman and her fetus, where the pregnant woman will die unless the life of the fetus is terminated (though thankfully such cases are now rare). A random lottery solution lacks advocates in this set of circumstances. In brief, such a case differs from lifeboat scenarios, because, unlike the latter, one does not propose drawing straws. Rather, one unhesitatingly saves the pregnant woman. "Potentiality," here, captures the sense that commitment to fetal life is prima facie, not absolute. One may override the commitment when the fetus imperils the pregnant woman's physical life. Parity-conflicts of this sort are resolved in one way.

The second sort of case involves encounters with evil, where a woman is pregnant as a result of rape or incest. Here the absence of satisfactory analogies asserts itself most forcefully. No one except the pregnant woman can carry in her body someone conceived in rape, but nontransferable just the same, who combines her own genes with those of her violator. She is uniquely near the fetus, yet is alienated from it by virtue of the crime, which affects her intimately and in which she is not complicit. This evil case brings three factors together. The first concerns unique dependency. The woman can help in a way no one else can. The second concerns agency. She is not responsible for being pregnant. The third concerns cost. She carries the offspring of violence. The first holds for all pregnancies. The second and third do not, and they go together. How far these three factors are severally necessary as well as jointly sufficient to set this case apart points to the intricacies of debates about abortion as such that I cannot address here.[24] But at least in this case, to judge that a woman is obliged to bring the fetus to term exceeds what the conditions of her own inviolability accommodate. Potentiality again stops short of equal protectability that would prohibit termination in every such instance.

The second side of "potentiality" registers what fetuses *are*. Here I take potentiality to be something more than mere possibility. The "more" refers to an entity actually in motion, a force that is there, a *power underway* (after the primitive streak and implantation). This power includes *existent* capacities to *acquire* in the future various characteristics typically attributed to those who "bear the human countenance" — e.g., self-awareness, personal accountability, and conscious relations with other human beings. Since fetuses possess the capacities to acquire these characteristics, traditional appraisals are correct that fetuses have a value greater than zero, a value separate and independent from their parents.[25] In short, they *are* irreducibly valuable. I take this to mean that, from conception forward, a presumption holds that they should come to term. Overriding this presumption carries the burden of proof.

Such commitment to fetal life makes theological sense to many for whom biblical passages count in weighing matters of life and death. Believers adduce passages that trace the working of providence back to the womb (see, for example, Isa. 44:2; Ps. 138:13, for Jews and Christians; Luke 1:31-39, 42-44, for Christians). One should not dismiss citations like these as mere "proof-texting." For they cohere with a conviction that God's covenant love stands as our alpha and omega. In this case, human love should correspond to far-reaching providential action. To err on the side of inclusiveness looks fitting. That a biblical depiction of providence encompasses potentiality implies that human love should start before recipients become self-aware.

These evaluations of the status of the fetus locate me on the right side of the tortured "middle," within the vast territory of debates about abortion. It is essential to make these evaluations explicit, if one hopes to add anything useful to the widely-voiced opinion that debates about stem cell research chiefly reprise debates about abortion. This opinion is right in that both fetuses and embryos *are* irreducibly valuable — i.e., both have a value greater than zero, a value separate and independent from their parents; and still neither can live and develop without total physical dependence for a period of time on one and only one person in all the world.

Yet the opinion misses divergences that I find important in staking out a particular region in the "middle" of the smaller but rapidly expanding territory of debates about stem cell research. I allude to three such divergences here. The first concerns the kinds of *conflict* at issue. The second concerns the parameters of *cost*. The third concerns the range of *choices* that present themselves. I discuss each in turn.

First, debates about embryos *in vitro* miss the characteristic tensions resident in the two sorts of cases just reviewed, where total dependence allows one to ascribe to the fetus a status that is less than equally protectable human life when weighed directly *against* the pregnant woman. For these cases focus on conflicts between two parties where a one-to-one correspondence obtains. While the stakes differ — saving one physical life by ending another and deciding whether a fetus conceived in rape should be brought to term and parented with all of the deep and permanent commitments this carries — the correspondence does not. It is otherwise with *in vitro* embryos. In typical circumstances, no similar conflicts exist. Although one takes an active step by transferring the embryo, an act that the two conflict cases do not require and a stage that they have, in any event, passed be-

24. I gesture elsewhere to the intricacies of these debates (see Gene Outka, "The Ethics of Love and the Problem of Abortion." Second Annual James C. Spalding Memorial Lecture, printed in booklet form by the School of Religion, University of Iowa, Iowa City, 1999). Although I incorporate several sentences from this booklet in my present account of abortion, I simplify the issue by focusing on the case of rape; I do not consider here the moral responsibilities that arguably arise from requisitely voluntary sexual relations.

25. See John T. Noonan, Jr., "An Almost Absolute Value in History," in *The Morality of Abortion: Legal and Historical Perspectives,* edited by John T. Noonan, Jr. (Cambridge, Mass.: Harvard University Press, 1970), 1-59.

yond, the decision to transfer is not a conflicted one. The circumstances here center on infertile couples who want a child and who embrace emphatically the deep and permanent commitments parenting brings. If a conflict emerges, it is neither immediate nor one-to-one between the fetus and the woman. Rather, it is between those embryos who are not transferred and are to be frozen in perpetuity or discarded and the needs of *third* parties who suffer from various maladies that research on embryos *may* eventually alleviate.

Second, the costs (harms) are the same for fetuses and for embryos but diverge notably in the case of pregnant women and third parties suffering from maladies mentioned earlier. Fetuses aborted and embryos disaggregated both undergo *incommensurable* physical harm — i.e., lethal harm beyond human powers to reverse or compensate. I argue elsewhere that this incommensurable harm constitutes a decisive similarity between abortion and infanticide, and one may extend this argument to embryos.[26] As already discussed, conservatives judge this similarity to fall under the prohibition against murder and accord the prohibition absolute priority. I do not go so far. At the same time, one should not shrink from soberly acknowledging the similarity itself. By contrast, important divergences surface when considering costs to pregnant women and third parties suffering from maladies. Recall the instance of pregnancy following rape. The woman is not *obliged* to carry a fetus conceived in these circumstances to term. Yet she may choose to do so out of extreme generosity and despite excruciating personal cost. The sacrifices she makes are hers, though after the fact. That is, the rapist deprives her of the exercise of her agency, and yet she exercises it *post eventum;* she may choose voluntarily to bear the cost. This sort of personally incurred cost disappears in case of third parties suffering from maladies that stem cell research may alleviate. I do not deny that they suffer excruciatingly as well and that alleviating their suffering is something to be lauded. Still, their standing as possible beneficiaries of embryonic stem cell research is unrelated to the circumstances of conception. They are not actors within *these* circumstances. Unlike a pregnant woman, they cannot connect the plight they face with what they *do,* at voluntary cost to *themselves.* Moreover, no researcher on stem cells currently suffers, or faces permanent changes to his or her future life, that compare at all with the suffering a woman knows whose pregnancy is due to rape, and who elects to bear and parent a child.

Third, the choices a woman confronts whose pregnancy is the result of rape are stark. Either she elects to terminate the pregnancy or she does not, and, if she does not, she bears the child and may either place the child for adoption or parent. Her reasons for deciding as she does may vary, from honoring her own inviolability to honoring the well-being of the fetus who is another innocent. Yet some one reason must trump these others. And the time to decide is short: if she does not terminate, she will bear, by affirmation or default. Whatever she decides, she will live with a host of physical and emotional affects, from a single point of origin. Once more, the circumstances surrounding stem cell research diverge markedly from her case. The reasons to conduct such research include the alleviation of suffering and the advancement of scientific knowledge. Neither reason must trump; they may reinforce each other. And the choices of how to pursue such research are several, as the debates about stem cell "sources" make clear. No one source is the narrow gate through which all promising lines of research *must* pass. One can debate the relative advantages and disadvantages of each, as well as the place of moral constraints. Finally, the decision is not forced by a fixed timeline. And these are early days of such research.

The respects in which debates about abortion and about stem cell research converge and diverge push those in the "middle" in contrary directions, as already observed. Some are disposed to be more permissive about embryonic stem cell research than about abortion for these reasons: (1) Prior to implantation one may distinguish conception from individuation; and (2) after implantation the fetus is indeed a "power underway," who, left to self-elaborating processes, is likely to become "one of us." Abortion actively intervenes to terminate "a force that is there" and has the burden of proof, whereas an embryo *in vitro* must still be transferred, and, until it is, one cannot describe it *now* as a self-elaborating power underway.

Others are disposed to be *less* permissive about embryonic stem cell research than about abortion, for this reason: abortion may involve bona fide direct conflicts between two entities who *are* both ends in themselves, whereas embryonic stem cell research is *morally* simpler. It concerns only one entity about whom one can say with certainty, here and now, that the action one takes, disaggregation, causes incommensurable harm. That third parties may benefit from the research subsequently done is an outcome for which one fervently hopes, but such benefit lies in the future. And we cannot gainsay the possibility that it may be attained without taking any lethal step — e.g., through research on other, morally unambiguous, sources of stem cells (from adults, umbilical cord blood, and the like). The doubled-sidedness of potentiality supports the less permissive side, it seems, yet one should weigh a further argument that furnishes some room for maneuver and nuances the distinctiveness of debates about embryonic stem cell research.

"Nothing Is Lost" A second line of argument prevents my saying that abortion and embryonic stem cell research are morally indistinguishable from murder and permits me to occupy the particular region in the "middle" I do: "nothing is lost."

Here I invoke and extend the "nothing is lost" principle. I first learned of this principle from Paul Ramsey.

26. Outka, "The Ethics of Love and the Problem of Abortion."

While he was committed to an absolute prohibition against murder as the intentional killing of innocent life, he was prepared to attach two *exempting conditions* to it. One *may* directly kill when (1) the innocent will die in any case and (2) other innocent life will be saved.[27] These two conditions stipulate what "nothing is lost" means. They originally extend to parity-conflicts, where one physical life collides directly and immediately with another physical life, and one cannot save both. (Ramsey may not have continued to uphold the principle in later writings, and I doubt in any case that he would have accepted the further extension I now offer.) I will argue, however, that it is correct to view embryos in reproductive clinics who are bound either to be discarded or frozen in perpetuity as innocent lives who will die in any case and those third parties with maladies such as Alzheimer's and Parkinson's as other innocent life who may be saved by virtue of research on such embryos.

I grant this extension *at best* stretches the "nothing is lost" principle nearly to the breaking point. For I defend the extension (and perhaps the original principle) as a move to the effect that (1) nothing *more* is lost, and (2) *less* is lost, or, at least, *someone* is saved. This extension is worth considering because stem cell research represents a particular instance of a general phenomenon, namely, that novel developments arise for which no clear moral precedents suffice to guide us. In such cases, one should seek both to extend traditional moral commitments and to incorporate new developments as cogently as possible. To labor the obvious: some of the controversies have arisen only *after* the age of *in vitro* fertilization dawned. *It* stands behind them, amplifying questions about "ends" and "means" that our forebears could not foresee. Unless one is prepared now to repudiate *in vitro* fertilization as such, so that one sympathizes with infertile couples but refuses them a *right* to overcome their condition by any means that science and their financial resources make available, one must take the moral measure of these new possibilities.

In the instance before us, I sympathize with the plight of infertility, but I am disquieted by the way *in vitro* fertilization is practiced in our culture. I will return to this disquiet. But, rightly or wrongly, "excess" embryos are a tenacious datum, for they are a result of the practice as it currently exists in the United States. I welcome the day when such necessity vanishes and welcome in the meantime "adopting" mothers willing to implant embryos, when the genetic couple consents.[28] Not to welcome these events belies the claim that embryos as well as fetuses are irreducibly valuable. Nevertheless, it looks at present as if embryos in appreciable numbers will continue to be discarded or frozen in perpetuity. *They will die, unimplanted, in any case.* (Nothing *more* will be lost by their becoming subjects of research.) Again, it is the absence of prospects for *these* innocents that partly extends the first exempting condition. It is the enhancement of prospects for *other* innocent life that partly extends the second exempting condition. (*Less* will be lost, or, at least, *someone* may benefit.) These judgments taken together summarize the case I wish to make.

I say "partly" extends, not "wholly" and certainly not "transparently." The case for extension I put forward shows both continuities and discontinuities with prior judgments on the ethics of direct killing. I take the prior judgments seriously and extend them to novel situations as far as I can. But I also acknowledge that the present debates on embryonic stem cell research involve a moral space that is, to a degree, unprecedented. I shall give two examples of the continuities and discontinuities I have in mind.

First, a point of continuity: My extension goes so far, and no further. It includes embryos conceived to enhance fertility, but who will never be implanted. It excludes embryos created exclusively for research, where one intentionally creates them for the sake of benefits to third parties that one hopes to secure and where one *embraces* the disaggregation of embryos as necessarily part of what *one does.* This limited extension accords with the "timbre" of "nothing is lost" in that one encounters circumstances that one did not initiate and that one wishes were otherwise. That one contemplates doing repellent things, things that one would not do for their own sake, indicates how intentional killing was not "part of the plan" from the start. This timbre matters, yet a difference presents itself even here. The parity-conflict cases assume a contingent disaster that no one intends or foresees, nor that is part of any established procedure. The circumstance of *in vitro* fertilization includes a recognition that "excess" embryos are, to date, endemic to the

27. See Paul Ramsey, *War and the Christian Conscience: How Shall Modern War Be Conducted Justly?* (Durham, N.C.: Duke University Press, 1961), 171-91.

28. It is important to qualify any generalization that the creation of spare embryos is endemic to *in vitro* fertilization procedures as such. Consider the case of Germany since the passage of the 1990 Embryo Protection Act (Embroynenschutzgesetz [EschG]); the text is available online at www.bmgesundheit.de/rechts/genfpm/embryo/embryo.htm). Germany allows during an *in vitro* fertilization procedure only the number of embryos to be developed beyond the pronucleus stage that will later be transferred. And three is the maximum number of transfers permitted. The striking result is that Germany faces no "plight" of excess embryos. To be sure, there is a drawback. "Success rates" are lower than they are in the United States. Nevertheless, I conclude two things. First, the normative position I espouse in this chapter effectively pushes closer toward the policies that Germany follows. These would require, however, a degree of regulation that is needed but missing in the United States. Second, this same normative position requires that I attend to the large number of excess embryos that exist already in the United States and in certain other countries. Their "plight" is a fait accompli. The "nothing is lost" principle that I invoke here pertains chiefly to their plight. To ignore the existence of these excess embryos, to fail to reflect on their significance, would subtly belittle the moral quandaries they pose. I am indebted to Sabine Hermission for information about policies in Germany. More generally, see also my last remark in the final section of this chapter.

procedure in the United States. At a minimum, this is foreseen. Still, the intention of the procedure is to alleviate infertility, not to create embryos for research. Thus, a significant continuity holds, despite this difference.

Second, a point of discontinuity: The "nothing is lost" principle, as originally formulated, is narrower and more exact than an extension of it to the novel case of unimplanted embryos can be. In the sort of parity-conflict cases that goaded those in the past to articulate the "nothing is lost" principle in the first place, unless one directly kills one of the parties, one cannot save the other. This allows for the claim that one *would* save both if one *could*. No similar temporal and causal limits apply to the case of unimplanted embryos. No other party will directly and immediately die if one elects to save embryos by freezing them. Any "conflict," as previously stated, is much further removed and comparatively indeterminate, plainly from parity-conflict cases, and arguably from abortion decisions more generally.

From the "Left": Derivation and Use and Ends and Means Although the particular location in the "middle" that I seek to inhabit has led me so far to pursue boundary questions on the "right" side, what I have said anticipates how I shall pursue boundary questions on the "left" side as well. I noted previously that Doerflinger and Robertson, as representatives of each side, sometimes concur that the moral choices are less complicated than I take them to be. They hold respectively that *either* one should oppose not only the creation and destruction of embryos solely for research purposes, but also the employment of spare embryos in research, *or* one should stop opposing the creation and destruction of embryos for research purposes only. I have sought to show morally relevant differences between the creation and destruction of embryos for research purposes and the use of spare embryos in research. To the degree these differences make sense, they suggest how those in the "middle" differ from those on the "left" as well as from those on the "right." I now examine these boundary questions more closely.

Derivation and Use Robertson makes two claims, noted previously in the discussion of "complicity," that should not be conflated. He contends first that the distinction between derivation and use is chimerical. Researchers are complicit in destroying embryos when they use stem cells derived from them, regardless of whether they personally engage in the act of destruction. So far, I agree. The NIH guidelines promulgated during the Clinton administration split the difference, perhaps for legal reasons and to promote civil peace by not ignoring conservatives' concerns altogether, while funding research all the same.[29] Second, Robertson contends that, if one supports research on "spare" embryos, one should support the creation and destruction of embryos solely for the purpose of research. For embryos do become "mere means" once one decides to use them in research. I think one may compatibly accept Robertson's first contention and reject his second. And if I am right to extend, in a qualified way, the "nothing is lost" principle, one has important reasons to reject the second.

To recount the reasons clarifies where boundaries lie. Such reasons focus on what status one ascribes to embryos and on how one interprets the injunction to treat persons as ends in themselves.

Ends and Means Regarding status, recall that Robertson holds, along with many others, that embryos are too rudimentary to have moral status in their own right. He ascribes "symbolic" value to them, which means, for example, that they may not be bought and sold, but they lack "intrinsic" value. By contrast, the account of potentiality and irreducible value that I have offered does ascribe status to them in their own right. This account warrants resistance to such a thin view of their value that virtually any reason — except qualms about commercialization — trumps it. I intend potentiality to be robust enough, in the case of both fetuses and embryos, to resist the view that fetal life and embryonic life lack any weight that might ever be determinative *as soon as* their value conflicts with other values. Without such resistance, concern for such life is reduced to a platitude, a mere expression of goodwill, that never has efficacy, that can always be trumped.

Regarding the injunction to treat persons as ends in themselves, Robertson insists that, once we decide to use embryos in research, they do become a "mere means." This announces moral equivalence between two circumstances that I have argued differ relevantly. It is one thing to say that innocent life "will die" in any case, when one refers to a condition that one did not, by one's own hands, bring about and that in most instances one cannot alter. It is another thing to say that innocent life will die at one's own hands, a condition that one plans and brings about from the beginning and where one could have done otherwise. This latter procedure does reduce embryos to a menial status through and through. One would distort the "nothing is lost" principle beyond recognition if one proposed to "extend" it to say that nothing is lost when one creates an entity whose prospects are nil because of what one intends from the start.

29. These NIH guidelines have now been withdrawn. On 20 November 2001, the NIH posted the Human Embryonic Stem Cell Registry. It lists the human embryonic stem cell lines that satisfy the eligibility criteria specified by President Bush on 9 August 2001. These criteria are more restrictive than required by the position I defend here, for they "allow Federal funds to be used for research on existing human embryonic stem cell lines as long as prior to his announcement . . . the derivation process . . . had already been initiated" (see National Institutes of Health, NIH Human Embryonic Stem Cell Registry [Bethesda, Md.: NIH, 2001]. Available at http://grants.nih.gov/grants/guide/noticefiles/NOT-OD-02-005.html and at http://escr.nih.gov/.) This should be compared to the earlier comprehensive report and recommendations of the National Bioethics Advisory Committee.

The difference is there, yet Robertson's insistence valuably presses one to ask: How much remains of the injunction to treat persons as ends in themselves when one allows research on frozen and eventually-to-be-discarded embryos? I reply that the normative force of the injunction diminishes significantly when one takes to heart *their* prospects. It diminishes for every one, not only for those who allow research. Some seek to witness to the dignity of embryos by refusing to do anything to them other than to freeze them. They adhere to the norm I mentioned when canvassing conservative views, that one does best to consider *first* what one does and forbears, and not simply what will *happen.* Although this norm counts for me across a range of other circumstances, I find in the present circumstance that such a witness threatens to idle in relation to what the injunction paradigmatically summons us to undertake. It is difficult to specify what interest one *protects and promotes,* for example, when freezing and discarding are all that one can seriously envisage. To honor potentiality, where there is no hope of implantation, is to honor *perpetual potentiality.*[30] It diminishes *action-guiding content,* either present or future, in the injunction to treat as an end. It even affects what is said in the theological context to which I alluded earlier concerning providence and corresponding love. For one cannot precisely equate the affirmation that love should start before recipients become self-aware with an affirmation that one should love recipients who will *never* become self-aware. To deny the equation is emphatically not to disbelieve in providence in both cases, and it is not to withhold corresponding love in both cases. It aims only to acknowledge that the room for exercising fidelity in action over time may differ. What one can and cannot do in treating persons as ends will be affected by *their* prospects. Love for an embryo who will live at most in a perpetually frozen state without self-awareness has less prospective room than love for a fetus who is a power underway and who eventually *will* acquire self-awareness. What one can envisage and do, now and later, has a greater scope in the latter instance, which is why termination obliterates a future that the fetus now *has* in prospect, a future that an embryo frozen in perpetuity *lacks.*

This severely diminished force bears on the second exempting condition, that other innocent life will be saved. The case to extend this condition is imperfect as well, indeed more so, for reasons already given. I observe, however, that as one disallows the intentional creation of embryos for research purposes, one draws more closely together the moral considerations weighted in judging the permissibility of research on fetal cadavers and certain-to-be-discarded embryos. In both cases, the genetic parents decide whether to donate them for research. Researchers play a lesser role — they lack a voice in the decision to abort or to attempt *in vitro* fertilization — than when *they* guide the intentional creation and destruction of embryos.

Political and Legal Contexts I ask next how the normative orientation of locating oneself in the "middle" affects one's engagement in the political and legal contexts in which stem cell research proceeds. Four broad observations must do for the present.

Range of applicability. First, the range of applicability of such an orientation needs to be clarified. Do I take it to be relevant to the entire body politic, at least in the United States, or only to certain segments of it? I divide this question into two parts.

(1) Since I referred to Augustinian Christian convictions at the start, do I address persons in the church only, or persons in the wider society also? The answer is that, in this instance, I address neither audience exclusively. On the one side, particular convictions influence how I depict the orientation in various ways. For example, I have in view certain Christian accounts of agape-love as I interpret the notion of persons as ends in themselves;[31] I extend a principle from Ramsey, a Christian writer who claimed that his own formulation of "nothing is lost" came from a Christian understanding of charity; I dwell on the prohibition against murder as precisely construed; and my senses of "intentional" and "innocent" are influenced by my own tradition. On the other side, the subject of stem cell research demonstrably engages the wider society, and much of the literature on moral issues and scientific developments that I have read and incorporated focuses on no religious tradition. Moreover, to cite examples again, the prohibition against murder is one on which Jews, Muslims, and secularists likewise have innumerable things to say, from which I have learned; the protection of citizens from murder is a basic duty of *any* political government, which partly explains the urgency of debates about whether abortion and/or embryonic stem cell research are morally indistinguishable from murder; and the maladies that may be cured or ameliorated through stem cell research fall within the range of common human woes — e.g., Alzheimer's disease may strike anyone, regardless of whether one is a religious believer.

(2) Does the orientation apply with equivalent normative force in the public and the private sectors? It does, "in principle," but insofar as "ought implies can," the prospects in American society for de facto adherence differ greatly. I alluded to some of the reasons much earlier. Disputants from all parts of the spectrum have concentrated chiefly on what federally funded research should include. Comparatively little has been said about research conduct in the private sector. Some liberals especially look now to the private sector for much of the most promising and innovative research. As they see it, for the government to issue and enforce rules that would apply to *all* research would be a poison gift. To implement such

30. Brian Sorrells suggested this phrase while reading an earlier draft, and I thank him for this as well as other suggestions that improved the paper significantly.

31. See Gene Outka, *Agape: An Ethical Analysis* (New Haven, Conn.: Yale University Press, 1972).

a step would curtail substantially the kinds of research presently allowed in the private sector. They prefer to rely instead on ethical standards propounded by the professional bodies most directly involved and on the type of ethics advisory committees that Geron and the Advanced Cell Technology group, for instance, have established. These matters are beyond the scope of the present enquiry. I add only that one need not attack indiscriminately all free market undertakings in this area to entertain certain justified worries. The results of privately funded research may not be immediately or universally available to the general public in the fashion that federally funded research is. In addition, "commercial organizations" are, of course, designed to make money. Neither in their objectives nor in their management are they designed to balance conflicting interests or to pay homage to the distinctive noncommercial qualities of medical research and medical care. The government, at a minimum, should not ignore the paucity of coordination I mentioned previously or permit so many decisions to be made by default.

Ongoing moral debates. Second, the subject of stem cell research remains volatile. It so far resists any repetition of the pattern that one sometimes sees, where theorizing about moral matters yields divergent and rival points of departure and lines of argument, but weighing political possibilities and institutional policies yields more agreements and points of consensus (a modus vivendi of sorts). One should beware of assuming here that, once one turns to institutional policies, there is no longer a need to engage in "theoretical" debates. One's moral point of departure determines, in key part, what one takes desirable and undesirable institutional policies to be. One makes claims, as I have done here, weighing arguments about where to place oneself along a spectrum and exploring how far judgments about abortion and stem cell research diverge, and so on. If one gives these enduring moral concerns short shrift, one enters the political fray with undefended assumptions that one merely announces.

To avoid such an outcome, one must not grow weary of moral debates. They matter, and views taken exert vast influence. Between those who evaluate embryos as equally protectable human life and those who evaluate embryos as only "clumps of cells in petri dishes," there is no peace. I have tried to suggest why neither of these evaluations is adequate, and I must continue to attempt to address conservative and liberal objections to my position. For example, conservatives may discern a consequentialist flavor in the "nothing is lost" principle (the innocent *will* die in any event; other innocent life *will be* saved). I claim it is fitting to ask, in the case at hand, what *actual* benefits are or might be conferred and on whom. Yet I hardly comment on the intricacies of consequentialist theories. I only consider actual benefits in the case presented by the anomalous practice of *in vitro* fertilization, which results in entities whose destruction was not directly intended from the start. Liberals may protest my refusal to keep concern about the status of embryos in circuit with every other morally estimable consideration, without benefit of even prima facie ranking. While I extol possible benefits to third parties from embryonic stem cell research, I resist allowing concern about the status of embryos to recede again to a platitude, where it never has efficacy and can always be trumped.

Overall orientation. Third, I should specify further the overall orientation that emerges from the particular location in the "middle" that I inhabit. To extend the "nothing is lost" principle in the way I do sets a deontological constraint on "sources" that applies in principle to stem cell research in the public and private sectors. It draws a line between research on embryos created solely for this purpose and research on embryos from *in vitro* fertilization clinics that are to be discarded or frozen in perpetuity. It disallows the first sort of research and allows the second. This constraint makes concern about embryos more than an ineffectual afterthought. One should acknowledge any costs it may incur. Some liberals worry, for instance, that such a limit might affect adversely the "quality" of available embryos for research, a difficulty that intentional creation for research would surmount. Researchers debate whether this worry is well-founded empirically, but if one is unwilling to risk this much, one again transmutes concern about the status of embryos into a mere expression of goodwill. If one holds the constraint hostage to interminable bargaining, one deprives it of a normative force that makes a discernible difference. The line should remain intact, and one should be content to derive as many scientific and medical benefits as possible from research on "excess" embryos.

The constraint matters as it marks the drawing of a line. It matters also as it registers an attitude of ongoing mourning for a plight. One thus regards research, even on excess embryos, as something to which one only reluctantly acquiesces. This attitude begins in sympathy for those who view their own infertility as an affliction they seek to overcome. It continues in allowing unprecedented *in vitro* technology that sometimes triumphs over this affliction, but such technology brings with it one foreseeable and lamentable outcome, namely, the presence of embryos to be discarded or frozen in perpetuity. One welcomes neither infertility nor excess embryos. The attitude concludes in a desire that one day there will no longer be a need to destroy embryos. That is, one looks forward to a time when it is possible to reprogram adult stem cells so that embryos are no longer required as a source. One further hopes that this time comes quickly, that the establishment of cell lines will make the use of donated embryos a transitional matter. In short, to destroy embryos *never* should leave one at ease or become simply unproblematic, a permanently acceptable part of routine procedures. Our society's research priorities should attest to such an attitude.

A "performative" danger. Fourth, when I

claimed initially that the most fitting place to inhabit is a particular region in the "middle," I said there were dangers associated with that position. Let me give one example of such a danger.

This example falls within my third broad observation, that the constraint draws a line and registers an attitude. The danger derives from practical undermining more than from outright repudiation. Here the overused metaphor of "slippery slope" comes into play. One recalls Doerflinger's contention that researchers and those in charge of *in vitro* fertilization clinics might in effect collude to produce by the "back door" spare embryos in accordance with research needs rather than an intention to alleviate infertility. The "slope" at issue is not so much one of theoretical argument, where the "logic" of a position one takes moves inexorably to conclusions one deplores. It is more "performative." That is, the line — between research on embryos created solely for this purpose and research on embryos slated to be discarded or frozen in perpetuity — is accepted provisionally by some on the "left," perhaps because fewer public qualms presently accompany concentration on spare embryos, but their passion lies in the benefits to third parties this research promises. To participate in collusion, therefore, occasions no crisis of conscience on their part. Their governing aim is to secure embryos for research. If the line one day evaporates, they will have little to lament. In the meantime, their task is to exploit the distinction as far as possible, to make the most of all the opportunities for research it can possibly yield. The pressure to go down this slope shows how a line is harder to maintain when the attitude of permanent unease toward research on embryos is not shared.

Concluding Remarks on "Nothing Is Lost"

I said at the beginning that two basic generalizations about human beings inform my reflections in these pages. We are morally capable creatures, accountable beings, and we are creatures who can exalt ourselves inordinately, in ways that usurp and do injustice. The debates about stem cell research that I have canvassed and evaluated attest to the relevance of both generalizations in one particular space where, as I also said, one meets novel opportunities and challenges, as well as permanent capabilities and dangers.

Yet the results of canvassing and evaluation here display varying grades of moral clarity and accountability and different kinds of usurpation and injustice. I conclude by summarizing and elaborating such results in one concrete instance, my attempt to apply the "nothing is lost" principle to debates about stem cell research.

I proposed to apply the principle against a background of claims about *the status of human life from conception forward.* I take conception and all that it alone makes possible as the point at which one should ascribe a judgment of irreducible value. Once conceived, each entity is a form of primordial human life, a being in its own right, that should exert a claim upon others to be regarded as an end rather than merely means *only.* One should view its potentiality as constituting a presumption in favor of its coming to term. If this presumption is not robust enough to trump other claims on at least some occasions, the judgment of irreducible value becomes a platitude. "Symbolic respect" stands too near the chimerical because it trumps little or nothing *whenever* conflicts occur.[32]

After conception, I find no comparable bright line, but defend some proximate discriminations. Before individuation and implantation, the entity does not yet have the full-fledged moral standing of a fetus. Yet, for its part, a fetus' value is not equally protectible with the pregnant woman's, for she too is an end in herself and has devel-

32. Those who endorse "symbolic respect" for embryos rarely ask directly whether this respect should ever trump when it conflicts with the welfare of third parties, except for repeating qualms about commercialization. Michael Meyer and Lawrence Nelson (see "Respecting What We Destroy: Reflections on Human Embryo Research," *Hastings Center Report,* vol. 31, no. 1 [2001]: 16-23) offer a fuller discussion, however, as they defend the claim that one may respect embryos even as one intentionally destroys them. One may, because the moral status of embryos is "weak or modest." Although they are "alive" and "valued, in some cases very highly, by many people," they are not "agents," or "persons" — prior, at least, to "individuation" around 14 days — and they lack "ecological significance" (18). Destruction should occasion, nevertheless, a sense of "regret and loss" (20). My judgments differ from theirs at two points. First, I claim that the irreducible value embryos have trumps the possible welfare of third parties in that one may not create embryos where one embraces their disaggregation from the start as necessarily part of what one does, for this instrumentalizes them through and through. Meyer and Nelson (21) stress that as necessarily part of what one does the "gamete sources" must give voluntary and informed consent "for any disposition of their embryos," but they neglect the distinction between creation that embraces destruction and employment where creation has another rationale. Nothing they say about "respect" strictly forbids taking the former step, as far as I can tell. If this is right, their case permits more than I do, at the end of the day. Second, my appeal to the double-sided nature of potentiality yields an account of how embryos and fetuses are similar and dissimilar that retains the following link. Like fetuses, they are not yet a self-elaborating power underway. Meyer and Nelson approach this account but then draw back from it. They hold that embryos are not yet "effectively a stage in the early development of a person." I accept their "effectively," if it means "not now a self-elaborating power underway." But then they add: "Put differently, an extracorporeal embryo — whether used in research, discarded, or kept frozen — is simply not a precursor to any ongoing personal narrative. An embryo properly starts on that trajectory only when the gamete sources intentionally have it placed in a womb" (18). This is a distinct appraisal; it is not the same point "put differently." I take embryos to be the precursors to any ongoing personal narrative by virtue of the genetic properties they already have. Implantation does not create these properties or start the "trajectory" that only these properties make possible. It allows them to develop "properly." Thus, it seems more cogent to take conception and all that it alone makes possible as the point at which one should ascribe a judgment of irreducible value, for once conceived, each entity is a form of primordial human life.

oped beyond the potentiality that still characterizes the fetus. Equal protectability holds after the fetus becomes capable of in dependent existence outside the womb.

These claims about status indicate why I deny that abortion and embryonic stem cell research are morally indistinguishable from murder and why I deny that abortion and embryonic stem cell research are morally indifferent actions in themselves, to be evaluated wholly by the benefits they bring to others.

The claims indicated as well why I object to the sort of embryonic stem cell research that creates embryos for the sake of benefits to third parties, where one *embraces* the disaggregation of embryos as *necessarily* part of what *one does*. To conduct such research clashes directly with the judgment that entities conceived have irreducible value. It is one thing to accept that one need not ascribe full moral standing or equal protectability to embryos. It is another thing to "instrumentalize" them completely through actions that are performed solely for the potential benefit of *third* parties. But the claims also indicate why I object to the ironic alliance that those on the "right" and "left" sometimes form, to the effect that one either should forbid all embryonic stem cell research or permit it all. There is, I believe, a more nuanced possibility, where one may distinguish *creating* for research from *employing* for research. The latter allows consideration of the tangled aftermath of *in vitro* fertilization as a practice in our culture. Employment for research connects with the datum of discarded embryos, where the original creation of those embryos possesses a noninstrumental rationale, namely, the promotion of fertility. In this case, what one intends does not exhaustively concern benefits to third parties, yet the aftermath allows one to pursue benefits to third parties without embracing the disaggregation of embryos *from the start* as necessarily part of what one does. These differences lead me to argue that the "nothing is lost" principle illumines a morally significant distinction between creation for research and employment for research.

I offer four concluding observations that illustrate varying grades of moral clarity and accountability and different kinds of usurpation and injustice.

First, an appeal to "nothing is lost" remains distinct from the kind of calculus President Truman favored. He elected to take certain innocent lives intentionally for the sake of saving many more. If this kind of calculus operates in stem cell debates, as it surely does in certain circles, it should not be run together with "nothing is lost." The latter principle limits itself to two sorts of cases, neither of which possesses the type of balancing of lives lost and saved that Truman's calculus encompassed. In the first sort of case, one *can* choose whom to save, but one *cannot* save all. This sort of "lifeboat" scenario requires the invocation of some distributive criterion — e.g., a lottery. In the second sort of case, one *cannot* choose whom to save. The embryos in question fall under the second case. They will be *lost* no matter what one does. They will die if one does nothing — one may assume that the embryos will be frozen and eventually destroyed, or at least that they cannot be kept in limbo forever — and one cannot save them by killing others or letting others die.[33]

Second, consider another reasonably clear but less widely recognized distinction regarding the status of moral claims. I believe my appeal to "nothing is lost" reaches a moral judgment that should endure rather than one that holds only "for the time being." It is one thing to seek both to extend traditional moral commitments and to incorporate new insights as cogently as possible in the development of enduring moral judgments regarding novel moral issues. It is another thing to seek the most judicious judgment deemed acceptable at the present time, where the judgment remains provisional and revisable in response to shifting social consensus. In the latter case, disputants sometimes tacitly assume and hope that what is beyond the pale now may not be later. I follow the former route. Once one takes the step of combining traditional commitments and incorporating new developments, one should reach definite moral judgments. If the principle that "nothing is lost" rules out the creation of embryos for research, but permits research on spare embryos, shifts in public opinion should not cause a change in course.

Third, consider a possible difficulty internal to the "nothing is lost" principle itself. Here clarity is harder to attain. The difficulty is that "nothing is lost" may permit more extensions than I seek. Recall the difference Doerflinger cites, which I noted much earlier: destruction of an entity for body parts because that entity will die in any case is not the same as using cells from an entity already dead. Some may worry that the principle may allow the general "harvesting" of organs or tissues from the living who are, for example, terminally ill, permanently comatose, or condemned to die by authorities of the state as criminals. The specter of Nazi doctors may well appear: If certain people are slated for death anyway, why not experiment on them to the point of ending their lives to acquire knowledge?[34] These possible extensions differ from the one I propose because the embryos in question are in physical limbo without history or prospects. I judge that the general difference Doerflinger cites should *otherwise* continue to claim allegiance. It *is impermissible* to destroy *any* entity for body parts who has an agential history even if he or she does not now have any considerable future — e.g., entities whose maturity — their "potentiality" has *long since* been realized — deprives their genetic parents of authority to end their existence or to elect to donate them for research. But the "perpetual potentiality" of the embryos in question dis-

33. For my subsequent account of the "nothing is lost" principle, I owe a great debt to John Reeder's volume *Killing and Saving: Abortion, Hunger, and War* and to his detailed comments on an earlier draft of this chapter.

34. This question was helpfully posed to me by Gilbert Meilaender in correspondence.

tinguishes them markedly enough from these other entities. "Perpetual potentiality," assuming the claims I made about the double-sidedness of potentiality, permits one intelligibly to find more affinities than differences between fetal cadavers and the embryos in question. Whatever other extensions "nothing is lost" may warrant — e.g., in cases of tragic forced choices, which I have not considered at any length — the extension I offer here pertains to a peculiar case by virtue of what the embryos in question currently are and are not. John Reeder[35] observes in quoting Baruch Brody that "the basic point of nothing is lost is that, as Brody puts it, the one to be killed does not 'suffer any significant losses . . . in unrealized potential.'"[36] I claim that "unrealized potential" carries for the embryos in question *distinctive* finality that resists generalization.[37]

Fourth, another difficulty for "nothing is lost" derives from the very features that render this case peculiar. I ask now whether these features may complicate my proposed extension beyond what I have so far allowed. I only touched on what complicates when I registered "disquiet" over the way in which *in vitro* fertilization is practiced in our culture. It is the practice itself that gives possible trouble for my proposed extension.

The original conflict, as I noted earlier, is that one welcomes neither infertility nor excess embryos. Those who are spared infertility should show "epistemic humility" toward those not spared and should try to understand from a respectful distance their sense of deprivation. One thus rejoices in what is hardly a trivial gain: *in vitro* fertilization has overcome a condition that would have otherwise consigned many to having no genetic children of their own. One should remember this and feel the force of the conflict that has ensued.

Yet excess embryos remain a tenacious datum, too, and it is here that the disquiet centers. It persists on three levels. The first I noted when I contended that one should never regard as simply unproblematic the destruction of embryos or the consignment of them to perpetual storage. Furthermore, one should extend this attitude of permanent unease to research on them as well. Something inestimably valuable is at stake and at risk. A second level pertains to current practices in American society. Approximately 10,000 embryos are added each year in procedures and processes that are substantially free of society-wide oversight — a general circumstance I lamented previously — and in which the profit motive plays a large but ill-considered role. Although many embryos will be transferred, it is certain that many more embryos are generated than will be transferred. A third level concerns the moral diagnosis that accompanies these practices. Such practices are a human achievement, not a contingent natural disaster. Matters could have been otherwise.[38]

It would be idle to deny that such disquiet complicates my proposed extension. At a minimum, the permanent unease that I defend should not end in passive resignation to these status quo practices. Such unease should prompt instead far more critical and skeptical appraisals of the practices presently in place. Again, in this area the government is permitting too many decisions to be made by default.

Yet I continue to uphold my extension of "nothing is lost," albeit in a chastened mood, rather than jettison any distinction between the creation and the employment of embryos, as those on the "right" and "left" propose. My reasons are also three.

Above all, one should not avoid the brute fact of the 100,000 embryos or more who are languishing in vats and whose prospects for implantation are nil (and many are unviable). Even if *in vitro* fertilization stopped the creation of excess embryos immediately, this phenomenon confronts us. Accounts of "nothing is lost" allow for circumstances in which the fact that innocents will die is seen as a moral evil and not a natural accident — e.g., situations a tyrant creates. The reasoning is this. One need not approve of how the situation was created in order to judge that it is better to save some than none when those who die would die anyway. I regard employment of discarded embryos for research as morally tolerable, and no more. It remains difficult for me to see what treating them as ends summons us to do, how flushing them respects them more, or is less evil, than employing them for research.

Second, I grant that recognition of human construction of the *in vitro* fertilization industry puts pressure on my earlier distinction between a condition we did not, by our own hands, bring about, and in most instances can not alter, and a condition where we plan and bring about the death of an innocent life at our hands when we could have done otherwise. Yet I draw back from any grand use of the societal "we" in this prior account of human construction. We, as individuals, may now become complicit if we do not criticize, yet the circumstances of the original construction attest to the realities of our social pluralism. Those most deeply affected — the infertile — and those prepared to respond — the organizers of the industry — were the driving forces behind such construction. So it continues to matter whether one creates these particular embryos and embraces their disaggregation from the start as necessarily part of what is done, or whether one only knowingly foresees that excess embryos form part of the practice.

Third, the particular region of the "middle" that I extol averts the excesses of a debate that engages those on

35. Reeder, *Killing and Saving*, 62-63.

36. See Baruch Brody, *Abortion and the Sanctity of Human Life: A Philosophical View* (Cambridge, Mass.: MIT Press, 1976), 151.

37. Conversations with Richard Fern shed light on the matter I raise in this paragraph, and on much else besides.

38. Sondra Wheeler led me to see that the normative position I defend requires a critical assessment of *in vitro* fertilization as currently practiced in the United States, and I thank her for perceptive counsel.

the "right" and the "left" concerning the *necessity* of embryonic stem cell research. The former denies such necessity — there are alternative ways, even if slower ones — e.g., research on adult stem cells — that will bring the desired benefits — and the latter insists on it in order to alleviate immediate mass suffering as quickly as possible. I opt for something less sweeping. I bracket the debate about necessity. Instead, let us not elide the difference between creation and employment, but rather draw this line for good and permit research in accordance with it.[39]

The performative danger to which I have alluded will endure. Yet one may nevertheless defend certain commitments as always in force, such as the injunction to treat persons as ends in themselves. I think that the constraint I identified that follows from this injunction continues to do important normative work in calling attention to a limit and in lauding research within it. There is still lasting value in seeking moral integrity, after one engages — with critical respect — points on the spectrum.

39. This position stands closer to the guidelines that the Canadian Institutes of Health Research released in March 2002 than to the more restrictive policies of the United States and the more permissive policies of the United Kingdom. "In Canada, publicly funded researchers can derive and study pluripotent human stem cell lines from embryos, fetal tissue, amniotic fluid, the umbilical cord, placenta, and somatic tissues (either from persons or cadavers). . . . Research not eligible for public funding will include studies involving the creation of clones for further research or for reproductive purposes, research involving the creation of embryos strictly for research purposes, and research in which non-human stem cells are combined with a human embryo or fetus" (see Françoise Baylis, "Canada Announces Restrictions on Publicly Funded Stem Cell Research," *Hastings Center Report,* vol. 32, no 2 [2002]: 6).

92 Stem Cells and Social Ethics: Some Catholic Contributions

Lisa Sowle Cahill

Many theologians and philosophers, politicians and members of the public find stem cell research to be full of ethical perplexities and imponderables. In the 1960s, John Noonan, the Catholic historian and legal scholar, confronted a similar situation as the birth control debate was heading toward the crisis of *Humanae Vitae.* Placing the evolution of Catholic teaching on contraception in a social context extending over time, Noonan defines "the moralist's business" as "the drawing of lines"[1] — not necessarily indelible lines, but prudential determinations of how to protect values while negotiating ambiguity, uncertainty, and conflict.

In the instance of sex, Noonan identifies the enduring values as procreation, education, life, personality, and love. In stem cell research, the two most obvious values at stake are nascent life and medical benefits. But constellations of values, the dangers to which they are subject, and specific opportunities for their defense and enhancement change over time and in relation to historical factors.[2] In assessing the ethics of embryonic stem cell research, advocates and opponents both tend to assert more clarity than the situation warrants. Drawing lines about specific ethical stances and policies will not be easy.

I will propose that embryonic stem cell research ought to be approached very cautiously and in a spirit of great moral reservation; the lines we draw are prudential and call for practical wisdom. Ultimately, I think our key concerns should be advocating for basic health care and drawing the firmest line possible on the creation or cloning of embryos for research purposes. The research use

1. John T. Noonan, Jr., *Contraception: A History of Its Treatment by the Catholic Theologians and Canonists,* enlarged ed. (Cambridge, Mass., and London: Harvard University Press, 1986), 459.

2. Of Paul VI's reconsideration of acceptable means of controlling fertility, Noonan remarks, "The campaign of the Church to outlaw some forms of contraception must be read in conjunction with [a] doctrinal development that came eventually to allow, for example, the deliberate use of the sterile period to avoid pregnancy." Ibid., 473.

From Lisa Sowle Cahill, "Stem Cells and Social Ethics: Some Catholic Contributions," in *Stem Cell Research: New Frontiers in Science and Ethics.* Ed. Nancy E. Snow (Notre Dame, Ind.: University of Notre Dame Press, 2003), 121-42. Used by permission of University of Notre Dame Press.

of embryos that are to be discarded in any event may be justifiable, but it is not unproblematic.

Values in the Stem Cell Debate

I will begin by identifying, like Noonan, five general values that we should be committed to protect in the moral debate about embryonic stem cell research. These are: the value of nascent life, the value of moral virtue or moral integrity, the value of medical benefits, the value of distributive justice or just institutions, and the value of a social ethos of generosity and solidarity. To illuminate the ways in which these values and general moral principles advancing them might be represented in detailed judgments and practices, I will draw on five principles of traditional Catholic theology (one in the case of each value). These are probabilism, cooperation, double effect, common good, and preferential option for the poor (a more recent emphasis in Catholic thought).

1. The Value of Nascent Life

This value yields a principle of respect for and protection of early human life, furthered under the traditional prohibition of directly taking innocent human life. Does the life of the embryo fall directly under this prohibition? Is the prohibition absolute in this case?

One of the crucial moral conflicts posed by the use of an embryo's stem cells for research is that the benefits it offers must be obtained at the price of its life. But the precise moral status of the embryo is a highly contentious matter. Although it is hard to deny that even a recently fertilized human egg is a living organism and a member of the human species, it is not so clear that very early human life has the full moral status of a person. Nonetheless, official Catholic teaching asserts that the earliest embryo, the blastomere, is morally the same as a person for all practical purposes. For example, referring specifically to the use of embryonic stem cells, John Paul II has ruled out "the manipulation and destruction of human embryos," on the grounds that "methods that fail to respect the dignity and value of the person must always be avoided."[3] On the other end of the spectrum are *New York Times* editorials that have referred repeatedly to the stem cell source as just "a microscopic clump of cells."[4]

Somewhere in the middle are a variety of other positions that see embryonic value as developing over time. The late Richard A. McCormick popularized the phrase "nascent human life" to refer to developing life whose value is not merely potential but that also is not fully realized individual human life until later.[5] Since at least the late 1960s, Catholic authors have proposed that the time of "individuation" and "implantation," in the second week after fertilization, offers a reasonable line defining the emergence of decisive value in embryonic life.[6] At this point, the time of possible twinning is past, the embryo implants in the uterine wall, and its chances of survival to birth increase enormously. In Great Britain and Australia, research on embryos younger than fourteen days is permitted for these reasons.

Restating this position in light of the stem cell debate, Kevin Wildes defends a "developmental school," holding that "while the early human embryo is worthy of respect, it ought not to be given personal moral status until there has been sufficient development of the embryo."[7] This development has not yet occurred, in his view, during the time at which totipotent stem cells can be extracted from the blastocyst and still develop into different human organisms. Thomas Shannon has defended a similar view.[8] The National Bioethics Advisory Commission adopted a loose version of the developmental position in its 1999 report on the federal funding of stem cell research: "We believe that most Americans agree that human embryos should be respected as a form of human life, but that disagreement exists both about the form that such respect should take and about what level of protection is owed at different stages of embryonic development."[9] Among the "shared values" that became part of the framework of their report, the commissioners included "respecting human life at all stages of development."[10] The report, however, went on to approve the destruction of embryos for research purposes, though not their creation for research. This limit was phrased in nonabsolute terms, however, depending on the fact that "at this time" there is no "public support for creation of research embryos."[11]

In a well-nuanced discussion in the *Hastings Center Report,* Michael Meyer and Lawrence Nelson show how respect and regret can and do surround the destruction of some types of valuable entities, including cadavers, animals, and even fetuses. However, the authors ultimately must ground their view that embryos can be destroyed respectfully on the premise that their status is "weak or

3. John Paul II, "Address to the 18th International Congress of the Transplantation Society," 29 August 2000, available at the Vatican website, www.vatican.va.

4. For example, editorial, "Sensible Rules for Stem Cell Research," *New York Times,* 25 August 2000, A2.

5. Richard A. McCormick, S.J., "Notes on Moral Theology: 1978," *Theological Studies* 40 (1979): 108-9.

6. See Joseph Donceel, S.J., "Immediate Animation and Delayed Hominization," *Theological Studies* 31 (1970): 79-80; and Thomas A. Shannon, "Human Embryonic Stem Cell Therapy," *Theological Studies* 62 (2001): 811-24. For an overview of some other literature on the topic, see Lisa Sowle Cahill, "The Embryo and the Fetus: New Moral Contexts," *Theological Studies* 54 (1993): 124-42.

7. Kevin Wm. Wildes, S.J., "The Stem Cell Report," *America,* 16 October 1999, 14.

8. See Shannon, "Human Embryonic Stem Cell Therapy," 816-19.

9. National Bioethics Advisory Commission, *Ethical Issues in Human Stem Cell Research,* vol. 1, *Report and Recommendations* (Rockville, Md.: National Bioethics Advisory Commission, 1999).

10. Ibid., 4.

11. Ibid., 55.

modest."[12] They recommend that only embryos less than fourteen days old be used, that they be used only as a last resort for important research (which might rule out embryonic stem cell research, since its advantages over adult stem cell research have not been well demonstrated), that they not be sold, and that the actions of researchers should demonstrate loss, regret, and seriousness.

A subsequent issue of the *Report* featured two letters of objection, testifying to the paradoxical, even if not incoherent, nature of a policy of "respect and destroy." Daniel Callahan calls this a mere "cosmetic ethics . . . of no value whatever to the embryos," serving "only to make the embryo donors and the researchers feel better." Cynthia Cohen suggests that "it is difficult, even across cultures, to escape the nagging realization that a human embryo is a human being in process" and that as "a potential human being, it has more than weak moral status."[13]

Although drawing lines at fertilization, fourteen days, or even birth can provide clear moral and policy guidance, this guidance might come at the price of consistency with objective reality: for instance, the contradiction in seeing the embryo as a human but "nascent" or developing entity that has significant value from fertilization but does not fall within the category "person." It is very difficult to recognize the moral relevance of embryonic development in a clear and coherent formula that can connect with meaningful moral and policy requirements prescribing and limiting the ways in which embryos can actually be treated, beyond just the attitudes accompanying destructive research.

The clarification of the value of embryonic life in the 1987 Vatican *Instruction on Respect for Human Life in Its Origin and on the Dignity of Procreation* is interesting in light of the above uncertainties. Its position on the personal status of the embryo is more nuanced than some might think. First, the opening sections of the document refer to the specific problem of infertility therapies, biomedical research, and science and technology. The concluding paragraphs refer to civil society, political authority, legislation, and the courts. The specific guidelines on treatment of the embryo are thus set in a context that envisions and takes into account the larger implications for science, society, and policy of rulings that are made. The document asserts in seemingly unqualified terms that "from the moment of conception, the life of every human being is to be respected in an absolute way."[14]

Shortly thereafter, however, the document observes that, although "the human being is to be treated as a person from the moment of conception," the presence of a human soul cannot be proven by any "experimental datum," nor has the magisterium "expressly committed itself to an affirmation of a philosophical nature."[15] I infer from this that the embryo, while not proved scientifically or philosophically to be a person, is still to be given the benefit of the doubt and treated as a person, not for special religious reasons, but because the preponderance of scientific and reasonable evidence is judged to fall on the side of personhood. (". . . The conclusions of science regarding the human embryo provide a valuable indication for discerning by the use of reason a personal presence at the moment of the first appearance of a human life: how could a human individual not be a human person?"[16])

But what if doubt in the matter is more significant than this document concedes? What if doubt as to the early embryo's full personal status is substantial? How does the ambiguity of the status of the embryo interact with other conditions and social factors that come into play in practical decision making? Probabilism, cooperation, double effect, and common good are all traditional ways of acknowledging the social and practical character of moral discernment. First, probabilism. Catholic moral tradition has not treated degrees of doubt as all having the same moral bearing on the permissibility of a given action. The larger the doubt as to the rectitude of a certain moral teaching or the facts upon which it relies, the greater the room there is for flexibility in the application of the teaching. The pertinent traditional debate was over when freedom from obedience to a doubtful law could be justified. How is it possible to move from a state of uncertainty about the application of a law to a choice about a right course of action?[17] The name most often attached to this debate is that of Alphonsus Liguori, an eighteenth-century defender of the moderate position that a solid opinion against the law is sufficient to justify freedom, even if other opinions are also probable. But the roots of this solution go back to the sixteenth-century Dominican, Bartolomeo de Medina, who wrote in his commentary on Aquinas that "'if an opinion is probable . . . it is permissible to adopt it, even if the opposite be more probable.' And if one wishes to know what constitutes a probable opinion, it is one 'stated by wise men and confirmed by good arguments.'"[18] In the view of a pre–Vatican II commentator, "Probabilism is common sense; it is a system used in practical doubt by the majority of mankind."[19]

12. Michael J. Meyer and Lawrence J. Nelson, "Respecting What We Destroy: Reflections on Human Embryo Research," *Hastings Center Report* 31, no. 1 (2001): 18.

13. Daniel Callahan and Cynthia B. Cohen, "Letters: Human Embryo Research: Respecting What We Destroy?" *Hastings Center Report* 31, no. 4 (2001): 4 and 5, respectively.

14. Congregation for the Doctrine of the Faith, *Respect for Human Life in Its Origin and on the Dignity of Procreation: Replies to Certain Questions of the Day* (1997), "Introduction," 5; see *New York Times,* 11 March 1987.

15. Congregation for the Doctrine of the Faith, *Respect for Human Life in Its Origin . . . ,* part I.1.

16. Ibid.

17. Charles E. Curran, *The Catholic Moral Tradition Today: A Synthesis* (Washington, D.C.: Georgetown University Press, 1999), 63.

18. Quoted by John Mahoney, *The Making of Moral Theology: A Study of the Roman Catholic Tradition* (Oxford: Clarendon Press, 1987), 136.

19. Henry Davis, S.J., *Moral and Pastoral Theology,* vol. 1, *Human Acts, Law, Sin, Virtue* (New York: Sheed and Ward, 1946), 93.

In the case of stem cell research, it is not necessary to reject the general principle that it is wrong directly to kill an innocent human person in order to call into question the application of the law in the case of the early embryo. Yet, according to at least some interpretations of probabilism, the maxim that "a doubtful law does not oblige" is meant to cover only some types of doubt. It does not apply in cases in which, rather than there being a doubt about whether the law is meant to cover a given sort of case (a doubt of law), there is a doubt of fact about the real circumstances to which the law is to be applied, a doubt which would put natural rights in question, particularly the right to life. For example, one may not shoot at movement in the brush that might probably be a man, even if it is more probable that it is not.[20] In a lengthy article on probabilism and the early embryo, Carol Tauer has argued that probabilism does apply to doubt whether the early embryo must be treated as a person, since its status is not a matter of "fact" in the sense used by the theorists of probabilism. The status of the embryo cannot be settled as matter of empirical fact, but requires a philosophical judgment; yet all the examples of doubts of fact given by traditional moralists refer to empirically verifiable states of affairs. It would be "ludicrous," Tauer concludes, to apply the law against taking human life in such a way that "if there is the slightest chance that some type of being falls under the law, then we may not kill it."[21]

An issue that deserves perhaps further attention is the problem of weighing the probability that the principle of the inviolability of innocent human life *does* apply in the case of the early embryo, both against the certitude or risk of harm that will follow from insisting on a strict application and against indirect deleterious effects on the social ethos that could result from a lenient interpretation. In the case of stem cell research, to treat the embryo as a person is possibly to forego lifesaving benefits to undoubted persons; but to not treat it as a person may lead to the instrumentalization and commodification of life, if firm standards for the treatment of nonpersonal "nascent" life cannot be established. We shall return to these matters below, in considering the values of medical benefits, distributive justice, and solidarity.

2. *The Value of Moral Virtue*

This value may be translated into the principle that one ought always to act with moral integrity and never to act against one's conscience. Conscience, in turn, should be informed with reference to a reasonable interpretation of one's objective moral circumstances and the effects of one's actions on others and on society.

The value of moral integrity impinges on the stem cell debate by way of the prospect of cooperation with or complicity in the evil of destroying embryos. Whether this is a moral evil remains to be decided on the basis of a more complete discussion, but few would deny that ending the lives of embryos is at least a prima facie strike against the justifiability of stem cell research. To be involved in or to support the destruction of embryos thus poses a danger to the virtue and integrity of moral agents who otherwise would support this research. The object of moral concern here has recently been identified in the press and in policy debates as "complicity" in evil. The reason President Bush limited the cell lines to be studied with federal funding to the sixty or so existing as of August 9, 2001, was to avoid encouraging the derivation of more cell lines through the destruction of additional embryos in the future. While many have objected that this degree of availability is far too inadequate, others have criticized Bush's decision as permitting undue "complicity" in the evil of the original derivation.

What sorts of moral concerns are denoted by the term "complicity"? They fall into two essential categories: (1) the moral standing of the agent who proposes to be in some way associated with evil actions undertaken by another and (2) the effects of complicity on the social context or community in which the actions take place. In Catholic moral theology, a principle that addresses similar but not exactly identical concerns is that of cooperation.[22] Like the principle against complicity, the principle of cooperation addresses both the intention and hence moral posture of the agent as well as his or her role as a possible facilitator of evil whose actions have an unjust impact on others. One difference between cooperation and complicity is that the former judges action prospectively, while the latter also looks back to past immoral actions whose consequences one now appropriates as part of one's own action. While it is clear that participating in a proposed immoral act in order to achieve some good is likely to have the objectionable effect of facilitating or encouraging the evil, it is less clear that using the results of a past bad act to achieve some subsequent good entangles the second agent in the original evil in the same way. The past evil is over and done, and later choices cannot prevent it. Nonetheless, as debates about the moral justifiability of using the results of Nazi medical experiments have shown, complicity in past evildoing, even by those who do not approve of it, is a serious moral possibility.[23] Important to consider is the

20. Ibid., 99.

21. Carol A. Tauer, "Probabilism and the Moral Status of the Early Embryo," in *Abortion and Catholicism: The American Debate*, ed. Patricia Beattie Jung and Thomas A. Shannon (New York: Crossroad, 1988), 78.

22. See Shannon, "Human Embryonic Stem Cell Therapy," 814-21; James F. Keenan, S.J., "Prophylactics, Toleration and Cooperation: Contemporary Problems and Traditional Principles," *International Philosophical Quarterly* 29 (1989): 205-20; James F. Keenan, S.J., "Institutional Cooperation and the Ethical and Religious Directives," *Linacre Quarterly* 63, no. 3 (1997): 44-67; and James F. Keenan, S.J., and Thomas R. Kopfensteiner, "The Principle of Cooperation: Theologians Explain Material and Formal Cooperation," *Health Progress* (April 1995): 23-27.

23. See Robert L. Berger, "Nazi Science — The Dachau Hypothermia Experiments," in *Medicine, Ethics, and the Third Reich:*

likelihood that present use of past immorality will encourage similar wrongdoing now or in the future, by seeming to give it moral, practical, and social acceptability. While one would hope that there exists a strong social consensus about the immorality and intolerability of Nazi-like experiments, the same cannot be said for the destruction of embryos in pursuit of stem cells, which is already occurring at a considerable rate in privately funded laboratories.

What light can the principle of cooperation shed on the stem cell dilemma? According to a moral theology text widely in use before Vatican II, cooperation is "concurrence with another in a sinful act," which is always wrong if it is "formal," i.e., if both agents fully intend and desire that the act occur. In cases of "material" cooperation, the cooperating agent shares in or facilitates a wrong deed, without necessarily wanting it to occur. Not only may the cooperating agent be acting under pressure, but his or her cooperation can be tied to the wrongful act by degrees: direct participation (immediate material cooperation), "secondary and subservient" participation (mediate material cooperation), and secondary participation that is also removed in time and place from the wrong act itself (remote mediate material cooperation).[24] Fairly clearly, the use of embryonic stem cells derived by others falls into the latter category, with the additional distancing factor that the objectionable act with which one "cooperates" (or better, is complicit) has already occurred.

According to Henry Davis, the author of the widely used text, cooperation of this sort can be justified if the cooperating act (here, research on the stem cells) is not in its own right sinful, and if there is a sufficient cause (here, development of therapies for disease, the prestige of cutting-edge research, and the financial gain to ensue). Of course, the "sufficiency" of the cause must be determined in relation to the weightiness of the wrongful act, which, in the case at hand, returns us to the debated question of the precise status of the embryo.

Leaving the complicity question to one side for the present, as not in itself definitive of the ethics of stem cell research, we shall move on to the next point.

3. *The Value of Medical Benefits*

The rationale for destroying an entity that deserves, at the least, "special respect" turns on the immensity of the health benefits that supporters of the research envision for the future. The basic ethical principle of beneficence implies that we should serve the health of human beings by developing medical science and technology.

The report on the current state of the science of stem cells prepared by the National Institutes of Health (NIH) for President Bush in June 2001 describes research on stem cells as having "extraordinary promise."[25] More specifically, the report mentions the hope that cells may be replaced in "many devastating diseases," such as Parkinson's disease, diabetes, chronic heart disease, end-stage kidney disease, liver failure, and cancer. Replacement tissue may be generated to treat neurological diseases, including spinal cord injury, multiple sclerosis, Parkinson's disease, and Alzheimer's disease.[26] Yet the magnitude of these projections is mitigated by their degree of uncertainty. To date, there are no diseases for which stem cell therapy has been proven effective in humans. *Commonweal* magazine entitled an editorial "The Stem-cell Sell" and, perhaps hyperbolically, compared "scientists clamoring for federal funds" to "that quintessential American huckster, the snake oil salesman."[27] The fact is that profits as well as humanitarianism motivate stem cell science advocates, as will be discussed in the next section. Promises should be received with a healthy dose of skepticism. At the same time, it is hard to doubt that the medical advances to be achieved through such research could be significant.

Catholic moral tradition has developed tools for judging when it is justified to cause some evil in the pursuit of a good. For a utilitarian ethic, the sole moral criterion is a balance of good over evil effects, the greatest good for the greatest number. In its more subtle invocation of multiple criteria, Catholic tradition concurs in the moral value of seeking to bring about good as widely as possible, but sets limits on the means that may be used in so doing. The traditional principle through which this is accomplished is called double effect. The principle of double effect has been the subject of a huge amount of intra-Catholic debate since the 1960s because, taken together, its criteria seem to rule out good-producing actions that common sense would condone, and because the principle's constituent criteria do not, in fact, hang together all that coherently. The principle may perhaps best be understood as a practical summary of the common features of situations in which promoting good at the cost of some evil should be permitted. It is not a mathematical formula for guaranteeing moral rectitude, nor even for ruling out classes of actions beyond a shadow of a doubt. But as a practical, prudential guide to moral discernment, it is still useful.

The conditions of double effect can here be set out only briefly and with admittedly inadequate exposition

Historical and Contemporary Issues, ed. John Michalczyk (Kansas City, Mo.: Sheed and Ward, 1994), 87-105.

24. Davis, *Moral and Pastoral Theology,* 1:341-42. See also Thomas J. O'Donnell, *Medicine and Christian Morality* (New York: Alba House, 1976), 31-40; Benedict M. Ashley, O.P., and Kevin D. O'Rourke, O.P, *Health Care Ethics: A Theological Analysis* (St. Louis, Mo.: The Catholic Health Association, 1978), 197-99; and Russell E. Smith, "Formal and Material Cooperation," *Ethics and Medics* 20, no. 6 (1995): 1-2.

25. National Institutes of Health, *Stem Cells: Scientific Progress and Future Research Directions* (Bethesda, Md.: National Institutes of Health, 2001), i. Available on the NIH website, www.nih.gov/news/stemcell/sireport.htm.

26. Ibid., "Executive Summary," 4.

27. Editorial, "The Stem-Cell Sell," *Commonweal,* 17 August 2001, 5.

and critique. According to the Jesuit medical moralist Gerald Kelly, who published a widely used commentary on the *Ethical and Religious Directives for Catholic Hospitals* in 1957, double effect is a basic tool of moral reasoning. An action that brings about good while producing an evil effect is permitted if the following conditions are met: (1) the action, considered by itself and independently of its effects, must not be morally evil; (2) the evil effect must not be the means of producing the good effect; (3) the evil effect is sincerely not intended but merely tolerated; (4) there must be a proportionate reason for performing the action, in spite of its evil consequences.[28] The debates about this principle have centered primarily on an implied category of absolutely forbidden "intrinsically evil" acts, under the first criterion; and on the necessity of ensuring that the evil effect not be the means to the good, as required by the second criterion. Some revisers of the principle have offered the opinion that double effect's core lies in the third and fourth criteria, so that if the main object of one's intention is the accomplishment of the good effect, and if that effect is greater than the harm caused, then the act is permitted.[29]

Assuming that the "evil effect" under consideration is the death of embryos, the results of applying double effect will differ, depending on the status or approximate status assigned the embryo. Those who view it as a person would rule out research even to bring great benefits, since killing an innocent person is regarded as an "intrinsically evil act" and in violation of the first criterion of double effect. However, moving to criteria (2), (3), and (4), the research on the stem cells is not in itself the means of killing the embryo; the death of the embryo is in fact not wanted in its own right, but only as a means to a good end; and the saving of many lives could be seen as proportionate to the deaths of a more limited number of embryos. Thus, if the status of the embryo is less than clear, the force of the first criterion prohibiting intrinsically evil acts is equally in doubt, and the application of the principle follows suit. Killing a living being, perhaps even a nascent human being, is not necessarily intrinsically evil, if that being is not a person. The other criteria can be met. Thus, perhaps destroying embryos could be justified by anticipated benefits. But ambiguity about this result is commensurate with the remaining levels of uncertainty about the status of the embryo itself and the real potential of stem cell research to result in major advances. Still, the principle of double effect serves as a reminder that "the greatest good for the greatest number" is a valid but not self-sufficient moral principle. There must be limits on the means used to bring about even the best of consequences, however difficult these limits may be to set and maintain.

4. The Value of Distributive Justice

Equitable sharing in social goods, including the goods of health and health care, is a value protected under the larger value and virtue of justice. The Catholic common good tradition upholds distributive justice as a requirement of social ethics.

While commutative justice calls for fairness in the relations between individuals, for example, in undertaking and fulfilling contracts, distributive justice focuses on the community as a whole and its distributions of benefits and burdens to all through its government and institutions. Distributive justice is implied by and furthered through the principle of the common good. The common good has a long history in Catholic social ethics, from Thomas Aquinas to the modern papal social encyclicals. The common good is a concept of justice that begins from the sociality of the person and includes mutual rights and duties of all members of society; the cooperation and participation of all in the common good of society, so that all contribute to and share in society's material and social benefits; and the moral and legal responsibilities of the state, which extend beyond guaranteeing civil liberties and freedom to ensuring that the basic needs of all are met. Substantive goods in which all are entitled to share include food, shelter, education, employment, private property, and political participation. The right to own private property is limited by the rights of all to basic goods and the duties of all to contribute to the common welfare. Since the 1960s the concept of the common good has been expanded to include a global dimension. John XXIII called for international cooperation to end the threats posed by nuclear deterrence and the cold war; Paul VI called for more responsibility on the part of the industrialized nations to aid in development through trade, aid, debt relief, and investment; John Paul II has noted repeatedly how the consumerism and materialism of some countries results in economic and cultural deprivation for others, and he has called for a new spirit of solidarity to inform renewed commitment to the common good. Bioethicist Andrew Lustig applies this ethic of the common good to health care, stressing that social justice has an institutional and structural meaning. Societies and governments are under a moral requirement to mediate the claims of individuals, to advance the right to medical care, to address social inequities through institutional change, and to prioritize the dignity of the most disadvantaged in society.[30]

Although John Paul II's remarks to President Bush on the inviolability of the embryo have been quoted fre-

28. Gerald Kelly, S.J., *Medico-Moral Problems* (St. Louis, Mo.: Catholic Hospital Association, 1957), 13-14. See also Ashley and O'Rourke, *Health Care Ethics,* 194-97.

29. For some of the debates, see Charles A. Curran and Richard A. McCormick, S.J., eds., *Moral Norms and Catholic Tradition,* Readings in Moral Theology, no. 1 (New York: Paulist Press, 1979).

30. B. Andrew Lustig, "The Common Good in a Secular Society: The Relevance of a Roman Catholic Notion to the Healthcare Allocation Debate," *Journal of Medicine and Philosophy* 18 (1993): 569-87.

quently, less attention has been given to his accompanying words on justice and the common good. Yet these have an equally important bearing on the social ethics of stem cell research. Meeting with Bush, the pope called for

> a revolution of opportunity, in which all the world's peoples actively contribute to economic prosperity and share in its fruits. This requires leadership by those nations whose religious and cultural traditions should make them most attentive to the moral dimension of the issues involved. Respect for human dignity and belief in the equal dignity of all the members of the human family demand policies aimed at enabling all peoples to have access to the means required to improve their lives. . . .[31]

Meanwhile, national and international patent law are expanding to permit highly remunerative development and marketing of discoveries in genetic science and biotechnology, including stem cell science. Investment in new scientific research in the biomedical sciences will guide such research toward the most profitable potential consumers. Those with the best ability to pay will have the most, or even exclusive, access to the benefits promised. Corporations are increasingly gaining control over research, new technologies and treatments, targeted audiences, and profits. A recent cover story in the *New York Times* "Money and Business" section featured the legal toehold of Geron Corporation in the stem cell market, while it also emphasized that Geron has as yet no real stem cell products to sell.[32] Geron controls the commercial rights to most of the stem cell lines that now exist in the United States, and it has already been involved in disputes over how widely they will be available and at what price. Dr. Thomas Okarma, Geron's president, asserts that his company "is going to dominate regenerative medicine." Although he claims not to want to impede others from doing research, he also intends to charge royalties for the development of stem cell–based therapies for diseases like diabetes. "I'm not apologetic for our intellectual property. We paid for it, we earned it and we deserve it." Vouching that he was raised a Catholic, Okarma questions why his work is being challenged by the pope. "'What is the objective of religion?' he asks. 'To make society better. Isn't that what we're trying to do here?'"[33] The distributive justice question is who belongs to the society of recipients of the improvements at which stem cell researchers aim. In a nation with forty-four million medically uninsured persons, the society of beneficiaries is not going to be inclusive. In a world in which millions of people live on less than a dollar a day and die from lack of clean drinking water, nutrition, basic health care, and diseases like malaria, tuberculosis, and AIDS, the regeneration of tissue by stem cell techniques is as exotic as it is expensive.

Before returning to that issue in the next section on social ethos, let me make a final observation on distributive justice in access to stem cell therapies. Finally, to the extent that stem cell lines are taken from embryos left over from in vitro fertilization (IVF), they are unlikely to provide the best tissue matches for a diversity of populations, even if wide access were financially available. Patients seeking treatment at infertility clinics are overwhelmingly white. Most of the cell lines were cultivated from embryos in the United States, Sweden, Israel, Singapore, and India. This provides for very limited genetic diversity in any therapies eventually developed from the cells.[34] While humans are 99 percent the same genetically, and while race is an unreliable, loose, and overlapping category on which to make human distinctions, it is still true that propensity to disease varies significantly according to ethnic and racial backgrounds. For example, those of white European ancestry are more susceptible to cystic fibrosis, light-skinned women to osteoporosis, whites more than blacks to Alzheimer's, blacks to sickle-cell anemia, and Ashkenazi Jews to Tay-Sachs disease.

5. The Value of a Social Ethos of Generosity and Solidarity

Speaking from a religiously informed standpoint and drawing on liberation theology and the Polish solidarity movement, John Paul II and others adopt the principle of a "preferential option for the poor" and see solidarity as the social virtue most important to the common good. Generosity and solidarity can help create a social ethos endorsed and shared by persons from many moral and religious traditions, for they reflect the highest ideals of humanity and social justice.

In the 1980s and 1990s, during the current pontificate, the "preferential option for the poor" became an increasingly visible part of the common good tradition, often imaged in gospel terms and associated with the virtue of "solidarity." John Paul II has been a strong critic of consumerism, materialism, and the excesses of market capitalism. In *Evangelium Vitae* (Gospel of life), he rejects "a completely individualistic concept of freedom, which ends up by becoming the freedom of 'the strong'" (no. 19), commends greater international availability of medical resources as "the sign of a growing solidarity among peoples" (no. 260), and reminds us that "it is above all 'the poor' to whom Jesus speaks in his preaching and actions" (no. 32).[35] A couple of weeks prior to his meeting with George Bush to discuss stem cell research, he had addressed a congress of Catholic doctors, urging "researchers in the biomedical sciences" to "make a gener-

31. John Paul II, "Remarks to President Bush on Stem Cell Research," *National Catholic Bioethics Quarterly* 1 (2001): 617-18; summarized and cited in "Remarks by John Paul, Rome, July 23, 2001," *New York Times*, 24 July 2001, A8.

32. Andrew Pollack, "The Promise in Selling Stem Cells," *New York Times*, 26 August 2001, sec. 3, p. 1.

33. Ibid., 11.

34. John Entine and Sally Satel, "Race Belongs in the Stem Cell Debate," *Washington Post*, 9 September 2001, B1, B6.

35. John Paul II, *The Gospel of Life* (Boston: Pauline Books, 1995).

ous contribution to providing humanity with better health conditions" and to cultivate "a deeper concern for your neighbor, a generous sharing of knowledge and experience and an authentic spirit of solidarity. . . ."[36]

The development of profitable medical miracles for the elite extends as an ethical problem across the spectrum of biotechnology and genetics research. The legal scholar and philosopher Margaret Jane Radin notes the growing prevalence of market rhetoric in many spheres of cultural and political life. While granting that commodification is not always inappropriate, and that commodification admits of degrees, sometimes acceptable ones, she warns that "commodification of significant aspects of personhood cannot be easily uncoupled from wrongful subordination," and that the commodification of persons and of significant personal relationships can result in "dehumanization and powerlessness."[37] A Canadian legal scholar, commenting on genetics research, notes similarly a "commercialization environment" that can be seen worldwide, but which he finds most clearly present in the United States, where individual choice and the right to buy and consume products is so key to the national culture.[38]

Instances of excessive commodification and subordination can be hard to identify with precision, and there may be legitimate disagreement in this regard.[39] Yet, to the extent that basic human goods are commodified, and that their availability depends on their purchase as commodities, some persons who need them are certain to be excluded. When embryos are destroyed and their cells sold to provide saleable research material and to promote biomedical business, commodification increases in the sphere of procreation, which should generally be an expression of sexual, parental, and familial commitments.

A social ethos of generosity and solidarity does not require that the market in biotechnology and medicine be eliminated, but that it be limited by a sense of the common good, mutual rights and duties, and the participation of all in goods to be shared. Solidarity and generosity, rather than commodification and the profit motive, seem particularly important as virtues to guide the treatment of early human life as well as of lifesaving medical measures.

Concluding Reflections

A German colleague with whom I have participated in an international bioethics seminar, Dietmar Mieth, is a bioethicist at the University of Tübingen. He serves on ethics committees for UNESCO (United Nations Educational, Scientific, and Cultural Organization) and the European Parliament, and has labored for years in a religiously, ethically, culturally, and politically pluralistic environment to create an international ethos that is more protective of embryos, less willing to accept genetic interventions whose results for future generations are unknown, and less willing to sacrifice moral values for the sake of scientific advances and investments. Working in the midst of differing ethical perspectives, factual uncertainties, moral ambiguities, and policy limitations, he has come to rely on what he calls a "convergence argument": an ethical position based on several arguments, none of which is conclusive in itself, but which together "form a sort of cable made of different cords."[40]

On the ethics of stem cell research, I have woven together five cords: the special status of the embryo, moral integrity, medical benefits, distributive justice, and an ethos of generosity and solidarity, to form what is a suggestive rather than a conclusive argument. In the case of leftover IVF embryos, the fully personal status of the embryo is in question, as was demonstrated above in the discussion of the value of nascent life. I see the fact that frozen embryos have virtually no prospects for gestation and birth as a relevant consideration, since it means that their destruction deprives them, at most, of indefinite existence in an arrested state of development, and not of the development of personhood. Perhaps an analogy to brain-dead patients who become organ donors could be made. It is important to draw our firmest lines against the creation of embryos for research, since it is a proximate social danger and since it constitutes a major step toward the commodification of developing human life and of the procreative process.

The thrust of this paper has been to show that the ethics of stem cell research is a complicated and ambiguous territory that cannot be negotiated by any simply scientific or philosophical argument. The Catholic tradition does provide tools — like the principles of double effect and cooperation — to guide moral decision making in gray areas. However, in the case of stem cell research, not even traditional principles and values are able to provide incontrovertible answers. The most important role of thoughtful ethicists, Catholic and otherwise, may be to support the emergence of a different ethos, one more attuned to social interdependence and reciprocity regarding basic needs and less trusting of technological and scientific predictions and marketing propaganda. Certainly, this would mean more attention to distributive justice, and more caution in using embryos for what is claimed to be scientific necessity, at least until other avenues,

36. "Holy Father to Catholic Doctors Congress," 7 July 2000, at the Vatican website, www.vatican.va.

37. Margaret Jane Radin, *Contested Commodities* (Cambridge, Mass.: Harvard University Press, 1996), 163, 82.

38. Timothy Caulfield, "Regulating the Commercialization of Human Genetics: Can We Address the Big Concerns?" in *Genetic Information,* ed. Ruth F. Chadwick and Alison K. Thompson (New York: Kluwer Academic / Plenum Publishing, 1999), 153.

39. Margaret Jane Radin, "Response: Persistent Perplexities," *Kennedy Institute of Ethics Journal* 11 (2001): 305-15.

40. Dietmar Mieth, "The Ethics of Gene Therapy: The German Debate," paper prepared for a meeting of the Genetics, Theology, and Ethics Group, Boston College, October 1999. This was a five-year international study group sponsored by the Porticus Foundation.

such as adult stem cell research, have been explored. The centerpiece of the Catholic agenda for medical research should be basic health care and solidarity. Concerns about the embryo should be framed, as the words of John Paul II suggest, within a larger call for "respect for human dignity and belief in the equal dignity of all the members of the human family," achieved through "policies aimed at enabling all peoples to have access to the means required to improve their lives. . . ."[41]

41. John Paul II, "Remarks to President Bush," 618.

93 Price to Pay

Amy Laura Hall

A 43-year-old woman rolls slowly out of bed, having dreamt the night before of her fifth-grade classroom — a room she knew well before taking disability leave. She makes her daily plea for a treatment that will allow her to get to the grocery store without tripping over her own feet. Meanwhile, a seven-year-old girl wakes up to check her insulin level. She adjusts the pump attached to her abdomen and wonders whether she will be able to eat the school lunch today, and whether she will eventually lose her sight.

These stories of people suffering from Parkinson's disease and juvenile diabetes represent the plight of real people. Stem cell research using human embryos might mean new mornings for people like these — people you and I know by name. If embryonic stem cell research (ESCR) can alleviate such suffering, then is it not consonant with the Good News?

I have come to believe, on the contrary, that ESCR is not consonant with Christian faith because of the moral costs involved. To count these moral costs requires us to take several heart-wrenching steps away from the names, faces and complicated narratives of those who might benefit from ESCR.

The default mode of bioethical reasoning in popular Christian culture — a sentimental version of utilitarianism — deems such reflective distance unfeeling and cruel. It was at the risk of such apparently cruel abstraction that a small group of pastors and scholars worked on a United Methodist Bioethics Task Force convened by the church's General Board of Church and Society to consider ESCR.

After months of discussion, the group drafted a call to ban all human cloning and to limit ESCR to the use of the "excess" embryos created in the process of in vitro fertilization (IVF). Most controversially, the group took on the question of IVF and the production of "excess" embryos and counseled United Methodists to pursue adoption and foster care rather than IVF.

When the United Methodist General Conference discussed the proposal at its Pittsburgh convention in May, it vitiated the original document. The revision committee rewrote the report by striking in particular the contributions of the moral theologians.

As a member of the initial task force, I submit that we posed several distinctions, questions and answers that are crucial for evaluating ESCR. What follows is my own interpretation of the issues involved. It does not necessarily represent the reflections of the other members.

The left and right wings of the UMC tried originally to ferret out whether the composition of the original task force was "pro-life" or "pro-choice." That approach reflected a misunderstanding of the question at hand. The debate about ESCR must be distinguished from prior debates on abortion. Naming abortion a sui generis conflict of life with life, most mainline Protestant denominations have affirmed that abortion should be rare but also legal.

Unlike abortion, ESCR involves neither a conflict between two physically interconnected lives nor the rare, unplanned and deeply regrettable destruction of incipient human life. When advocates of ESCR rhetorically evoke prior debates on abortion by presenting ESCR as a choice between a living person and an early human embryo, we are distracted from the broader context of ESCR.

A multimillion-dollar medical industry surrounds the supposedly simple "which of these two entities matters more?" approach. Endorsing ESCR means endorsing an elaborate, systematic, routine industry of embryo production and destruction, an industry not likely to limit itself to therapies for chronic disease. To suggest that we will not also see the emergence of more generally applicable, and more widely lucrative, products defies common sense.

THE ORIGINAL United Methodist proposal recognized that the fertility industry already engages in the routine production, cryopreservation (freezing) and disposal of human embryos in the process of IVF. Mainline Protestants have largely avoided this set of questions attached to IVF, perhaps because we are justifiably reluctant to question the process by which many (rightly) beloved and (rightly) baptized children have been conceived.

But there are two related problems with this avoidance. Not only is IVF the most obvious source of "fresh" and cryopreserved embryos, but the growing acceptance of embryo creation and disposal through IVF has shaped our moral imagination, rendering us less and less capable of seeing any relevant moral claims attending the early embryo as incipient human life.

Once early embryos become something less than incipient human life, once they are treated in vitro as a means toward the end of pregnancy, once they are cryopreserved in thousands of vats across the country, ESCR with "excess" embryos may be predictably the next step. Given that so many good Protestant couples have accepted the creation, cryopreservation and disposal of early embryos, it may be almost impossible for an argument against ESCR to gain traction.

It may also become increasingly difficult for any argument against any research on early embryos to command a hearing (including arguments against "therapeutic" cloning) as other procedures that involve embryo selection and disposal become more common. As use of preimplantation embryo selection grows, for example, there is a diminishing chance that anyone in the mainline will remain willing to throw the first stone at the Goliath of embryonic biotechnology.

Meanwhile, the next stage of the debate on ESCR is upon us. While the initial UM proposal tried to catch up with issues surrounding "excess" embryos, a team in South Korea brought into being the first cloned human embryo to be used for ESCR. If ESCR using "excess" embryos from IVF continues, the next step will likely be the pursuit of such "therapeutic" cloning — the creation of embryos through somatic cell nuclear transfer (SCNT) to provide individually tailored stem cell therapies.

The original and adopted United Methodist documents both oppose such so-called "therapeutic" cloning, but the adopted UM document strikes all moral and theological reasoning for such opposition. I suspect that the revision committee hoped thereby not to preclude future acceptance of SCNT.

The original document explained that to craft incipient human life precisely in order then to disaggregate it for materials crosses a moral boundary set when the first in vitro experiments took place. Why did Western bioethicists of almost every ilk develop this boundary? They recognized, as United Methodists on either side of the abortion debate have recognized until recently, that the in vitro human embryo makes, at the very least, an iconic moral claim. Put more theologically, both pro-life and pro-choice Protestants have agreed that Christians should assume and hope that even incipient life is indeed life bound for blessing. To bring into being a human embryo solely in order to divide up its constitutive parts for research threatens fully to erode the sense that incipient human life is never simply, or primarily, a tool.

The specter of treating human life simply as fodder for research is relevant for the discussion of "therapeutic" cloning for another reason not discussed in either UM document. Some feminists who have no problem with the creation or research use of "excess" IVF embryos adamantly oppose "therapeutic" cloning for ESCR. Why? Ova. The intricate work of "therapeutic" cloning will require not only millions of dollars but thousands of eggs.

WHICH RAISES another set of disquieting questions: Why was the research team (led by a Methodist) in South Korea able to cross the scientific barrier while researchers in the U.S. were not? They were able to harvest a large supply of "fresh" eggs — 247 of them, apparently from 16 women who volunteered for the process. How were these 16 women in South Korea recruited for this research? To what procedures did they consent in order to produce this unusually high number of ova?

To date, no one outside of the research team itself seems clear whether basic guidelines for gamete donation were breached. At this point, some in the pro-research camp are suspiciously eager to propose that the U.S. should not force its more stringent research guidelines on a developing country.

This brings me to what I consider to be the most compelling reason to oppose ESCR. With other feminists, I believe that we must consider the likelihood a) that countries with less stringent guidelines for ova donation will proceed more efficiently with research; b) that countries in the one-third world will likely benefit from research using ill-gotten gametes; and c) that advocates for ESCR will argue that, for the sake of justice, the U.S. needs to implement more liberal guidelines for gamete procurement so as to avoid the injustice inherent in situation b).

The guidelines by which research groups in the U.S. have had to proceed were developed to protect vulnerable populations in the U.S. from one of the most intimate forms of exploitation. Relatively privileged Christians in the U.S. must consider the likelihood that the procurement of requisite ova will follow the predictable patterns of women's labor in an exploitative global market. A moral analysis of ESCR, as it is likely to proceed, therefore requires reckoning not only with the lives of those who suffer from juvenile diabetes or Parkinson's, but also with the specter of women sacrificing their bodily integrity for our sakes.

In debating ESCR, we have the opportunity to ask anew whether we will encourage the routine, systematic creation and destruction of embryonic life. Will we continue to pursue a form of fertility treatment that has led to vat after vat of incipient human life? Will we allow for the creation of incipient human life merely for the sake of its destruction? Will we countenance the systematic and industrialized harvesting of human ova?

The entire conversation around ESCR is ineluctably complicated by our love for friends and family with chronic illnesses and by our love for family and friends who have been blessed through the process of IVF. The original UM document nonetheless called for self-interrogation, repentance and even sacrifice. To ask probing questions about the current trajectory of reproductive biotechnology would have given us a chance to reflect with humility on the ways that our moral imaginations have been shaped by new "givens."

The original UM document called one body of mainline Protestants to affirm at the most basic level that all forms of human life are worth incalculably more than their industrial, market, scientific or even therapeutic use value. This reasoning may initially seem cold and overly distanced, but the underlying issues touch on the most fundamental questions of what it means to be human, of what it means to love.

94 Cloning the Human Body

Stanley Hauerwas and Joel Shuman

. . . now we are children of God, and what we will be has not yet been made known. But we know that when he appears, we shall be like him, for we shall see him as he is.

1 John 3:2 (NIV)

We know that the whole creation has been groaning as in the pains of childbirth right up to the present time. Not only so, but we ourselves, who have the first fruits of the Spirit, groan inwardly as we wait for our adoption as sons, the redemption of our bodies. For in this hope we were saved. But hope that is seen is no hope at all. Who hopes for what he already has? But if we hope for what we do not yet have, we wait for it patiently.

Romans 8:22-25 (NIV)

In the circle of the human we are weary with striving, and are without rest. Order is the only possibility of rest.

Wendell Berry

Cloning — the nonsexual reproduction of an organism using the genetic material of another organism — has been a theoretical possibility for some time. As such, it seems to have elicited very little in the way of moral argument. Recent laboratory developments in mammalian cloning indicate, however, that we soon may have the capacity for human cloning, the nonsexual reproduction of the human body, using the genetic material of another human being. This prospect has evoked a loud and somewhat alarmed call for public moral debate, ostensibly to be led by "experts" in the field of bioethics. Our imaginations, however, do not seem ready for such challenges. As a result, the first question we ask of them always seems be, "Should we do what we now can do?"

We do not think we should do what we now can do. Christians, we believe, should resist the technological imperative that gives rise to such questions. However, we also think it a mistake to begin arguments about cloning with questions about whether we should do what we now can do. To begin in this way presupposes that we know who is asking such questions and why they are being asked. As a result, the politics producing the technologies that give rise to the questions are hidden from view.

For example, consider this sentence: "Our imaginations do not seem ready for such challenges." Who is indicated by the "our" in that sentence? Confronted by such an "our," Christians assume that we are included in the "our." As a result we — that is, we Christians — think we must then say what, if any, particular insights we have about these matters correlative to our convictions about God's created order or some other relatively benign set of beliefs. This is particularly challenging to Christians living in modernity, who are afraid of appearing to be against human progress. After all, does not cloning promise to cure genetically carried diseases or even to eliminate human hunger? Surely Christians cannot be against a technology that promises such results simply in the name of not messing around in God's creation. Christians, especially given our relatively insignificant status in modernity, simply cannot afford another Galileo affair.

Such challenges certainly may need to be addressed, but we think to begin with such statements of the "problem" is to rob ourselves of the resources of the Christian imagination. In short, the question for us is not whether cloning is a good or a bad thing, but rather how Christians, given the character of the Christian community and in particular the way that community understands the human body, are to understand cloning. "Cloning" is not a new thing for Christians, since we believe we have been made part of Christ's body. But because the promised redemption of our bodies seems so slow in coming, we may be tempted to compromise the body we have in Christ by subjecting that body to biomedical technologies promising immediate relief from all forms of human suffering. Ironically, from the standpoint of the Christian body, biological cloning then becomes but another gnostic technique designed to avoid or to overcome our bodies as Christians.

This very way of putting the matter in fact challenges the presumption that what makes Christians Christians is the beliefs they hold. The same practices that have reduced Christianity to a set of beliefs freely chosen by the individual make cloning seem like such a humane technology. The modern presumption, formed by the practices of capitalism, that the "I" names a self apart from and reigning over my body also produces a Christianity that is mainly about satisfying my "I." In contrast to this view, we assume that what makes Christians Christians is that through baptism they are made part of Christ's body.

We believe, accordingly, that the question Christians must ask about nonsexual reproduction of the body is not whether it should be done, but whose body, exactly, should we be nonsexually reproducing? For Christians have for nearly two thousand years been about the business of nonsexually reproducing the one body that matters most, and indeed the only one that must be reproduced in pursuit of the human good, and that is Christ's body. We are part of a community of people comprised of many very diverse members that is itself that body, and we understand that it is our baptism and our discipleship as members of that body, and not the information encoded in our genes, that finally determines our lives.

The apostle Paul, though he was never tempted by the possibility of cloning, nonetheless saw the reproduction of his body as being essential to his life as a minister of the gospel. The body matters to Paul; he knew no spirit, no soul, and no self that existed apart from the body. It is in and through the bodies of Christians, he claimed, "whether, by life or by death" (Phil. 1:20, NIV), that Christ would be made redemptively present to the world. This presence, moreover, was to be transmitted — or reproduced — in a very particular way, through a particular kind of pedagogy that is perhaps best understood as a profound friendship. "Whatever you have learned or received or heard from me, or seen in me," Paul wrote, "put into practice. And the God of peace will be with you" (Phil. 4:9, NIV). Therefore Paul did not hesitate to exhort those in the young churches under his guidance to imitate him. For in that imitation he understood that the disciples were being formed into a body determined by something far more substantial than a DNA sequence. This is evidenced by the language he uses in corresponding with those troublesome Christians in Corinth, to whom he wrote:

> Even though you have ten thousand guardians in Christ, you do not have many fathers, for in Christ Jesus I became your father through the gospel. Therefore I urge you to imitate me. For this reason I am sending you Timothy, my son whom I love, who is faithful in the Lord. He will remind you of the way of life in Christ Jesus, which agrees with what I teach everywhere in the Church (I Cor. 4:15-17, NIV).

This passage suggests that Paul not only expected his life to be imitated by those converted in response to his witness, but that he understood that this imitation would constitute their lives in a way so substantial that he freely used frankly "biological" language — the language of father and child — to express the relationship between himself and Timothy and himself and the Corinthian Christians. Our tendency as moderns is to make light of such language, to say that it is a "mere" metaphor for what Paul understood to be occurring in the "spiritual" realm — the realm of "belief." But to understand Paul's writing in this way is to weaken his understanding of the church by imposing upon him an incorporeal dualism he probably would have rejected.

Dale Martin argues that when we read Paul we need to leave behind distinctions between the physiological and psychological that we in modernity have come to accept as obvious.[1] Paul assumes the church is Christ's body in

1. Dale Martin, *The Corinthian Body* (New Haven, Conn.: Yale University Press, 1995).

such a way that immorality is not *like* the body becoming ill or polluted; it *is* the body becoming ill or polluted. So questions of a man having sexual relations with his stepmother (1 Cor. 5:1), of Christian men visiting prostitutes (6:12-20), of eating meat sacrificed to idols (chapters 8–10), and of the proper eating of the Lord's Supper (11:17-34) are all connected. For Paul, each of these are questions of the purity of the body and consequently of the avoidance of pollution. A Christian man visiting a prostitute is the exact equivalent of the body being invaded by a disease that threatens all its members, since in fact every member is the body.

Paul understood that in this life there is no genuine spirituality that does not take the body seriously. Speaking as if things were otherwise, suggests Wendell Berry, tends to "imply that the Creation is divided into 'levels' that can readily be peeled apart and judged by human beings." Some version or another of this very compartmentalized view seems to prevail in modernity, and we typically understand the spiritual as another means of escape from the banality of the everyday. Against this perspective, Berry posits an alternative that clearly derives from his Christianity: "I believe that the Creation is one continuous fabric comprehending simultaneously what we mean by 'spirit' and what we mean by 'matter.'"[2]

Only when Paul is read in this manner do we understand the radical challenge he presents to the assumption that what makes us Christian and/or human is our "self-understanding." Paul really expected those converted by his preaching to display in their bodies the same way of life he displayed in his own. This expectation was rooted not in any sort of megalomania, but in Paul's faith that his body had been transformed by his baptism in so profound and so mysterious a way that he could not speak of that transformation except paradoxically: ". . . I no longer live, but Christ lives in me. The life I live in the body, I live by faith in the Son of God, who loved me and gave himself for me" (Gal. 2:20, NIV).

Paul's expectation that his body would be reproduced in the bodies of others was based on his understanding that "all of us who were baptized into Christ Jesus were baptized into his death. We were therefore buried with him through baptism into death in order that, just as Christ was raised from the dead through the glory of the Father, we too may live a new life" (Rom. 6:3-4, NIV). This is to say that Paul understood baptism into the church as the beginning of a process of transformative reproduction through which the Christian body would be "conformed to the likeness of his Son, that he would be the firstborn among many brothers" (Rom. 8:29, NIV). Paul knew that the body being reproduced in those he baptized and taught was not his own, but Christ's. In this sense Paul understood the body more thoroughly than those who see genetic cloning as being a sufficient means of reproducing the body. Really being a body, he understood, requires certain kinds of relationships with others. Berry makes a similar point in arguing:

> . . . the body is not so formally self-contained; its boundaries and outlines are not so exactly fixed. The body alone is not, properly speaking, a body. Divided from its sources of air, food, drink, clothing, shelter, and companionship, a body is, properly speaking, a cadaver. . . . Merely as an organism (leaving aside issues of mind and spirit) the body lives and moves and has its being, minute by minute, by an interinvolvement with other bodies and other creatures, living and unliving, that is too complex to diagram or describe.[3]

We believe that we are speaking here, lest anyone think otherwise, of the very moral issues that surround technologies of cloning. Berry's broad point is that our bodies are constituted by an extraordinary web of contingencies on a multitude of levels. What Christians should believe about the way these contingencies, especially baptism and discipleship, constitute the body seems not only consistent with what Wendell Berry is saying, but also analogous with the point the philosopher of science Michael Polanyi was trying to make in his critique of modern science's strong tendency toward mechanistic reductionism. Polanyi opposed the insistence of certain scientists that a thing's ontology lay not in its being a comprehensive structure functioning in a given environment towards a particular end, but in an analysis of its constituent parts. This view, he argued, although valuable in its place, is finally inadequate:

> Indeed, nothing is relevant to biology, even at the lowest level of life, unless it bears on the achievements of living beings — achievements such as their perfection of form, their morphogenesis, or the proper functioning of their organs — and the very conception of such achievements implies a distinction between success or failure — a distinction unknown to physics and chemistry.[4]

How this point is analogous to Berry's becomes clear when restated in explicitly theological terms: Any theological discussion of the human body, at any level, must include a consideration of the body's goods and the relationship of those goods to the highest Good — its ultimate purpose — which is eternal friendship with God in the new creation. Such friendship is attained through the process of baptism into the life, death, and resurrection of Jesus of Nazareth, through which the body is transformed and made part of Christ's body, which is itself at once both an organism and a network of friendships which make Christ redemptively present to the world.

We cannot then speak of the body's goods — including the physical health of any one individual body — apart from its Good; for to do so is to attenuate the body's health, which cannot be properly considered apart

2. Wendell Berry, *Another Turn of the Crank* (Washington, D.C.: Counterpoint, 1995), 91-92.

3. Ibid., 94-95.

4. Michael Polanyi, "Scientific Outlook: Its Sickness and Cure," *Science* 125 (1957): 480-84, at 482.

from its relationship with other bodies. As Christians, we find our bodies taken up — "cloned," if you will — through baptism and discipleship into the one body whose presence the world cannot do without, a presence that affords the possibility of finally bringing order to chaos and giving rest from our striving in God's new creation. It is thus imperative that we continue first of all to reproduce that body — a reproduction that cannot be effected genetically — and to wait patiently for the final redemption of our individual bodies.

From this perspective biological cloning represents but another attempt at perfection in a world that no longer acknowledges God. No longer trusting in our ability to make sense of our sufferings through the sharing of our bodies with one another, we now seek to perfect our isolated bodies as if such bodies were intelligible in themselves. In the name of eradicating suffering, we use technological power to avoid being with one another in illness and death. Cloning thus becomes simply another means to escape the knowledge that, when all is said and done, we will each have to die alone.

Ironically, the high humanism used to justify cloning as a means to overcome the limits of our condition as creatures reproduces the very presumptions that are at the heart of the environmental crisis. When all life is seen to exist for the sole purpose of serving *human* life, then humans presume that we can instrumentally subject all life to our purposes. The widespread assumption is thus that human cloning is wrong because it violates the uniqueness and the autonomy of the individual, but that cloning animals is a fundamentally good thing insofar as it contributes to the elimination of human suffering. But this assumption is highly questionable from the perspective we have developed in this chapter.

The redemption Paul says has begun in our bodies is cosmic. Animals and humans are equally creatures of a good Creator, and the ultimate purpose of both is nothing less than to praise God. The idea that animals exist for no other purpose than to supply human needs and desires cannot be justified theologically. Given the practices of the Christian community with regard to the body, we can see no reason why Christians might think animals — much less humans — can be cloned in the name of human progress. Any "progress" that is not found in the joining of our bodies into the one body of Christ, we suspect to be an idolatrous attempt to perfect the created order in a manner that denies our lives have already been perfected in Christ.

95 What Would You Do If . . . ? Human Embryonic Stem Cell Research and the Defense of the Innocent

M. Therese Lysaught

Into whatever city you go, after they welcome you, eat what they set before you, and cure the sick there. Say to them, The reign of God is at hand.

(Luke 10:9)[1]

This passage, and St. Luke's continuing presence to us in the communion of saints, issues an important reminder that should shape our inquiry into the ethics of human embryonic stem cell research. That reminder is this: healing is a sign of the Kingdom of God. Healing was a fundamental component of Jesus' ministry, as witnessed in the gospels. Healing is central to God's identity as disclosed through revelation. As this particular passage from Luke notes, healing is part of the commission Jesus gives to those he sends out into the world to preach the good news of the kingdom. Healing, therefore, ought to be central to the ways of discipleship and Christian reflection today.

The centrality of healing to the mission of Christian discipleship is witnessed not only in Scripture but in the historic commitment of the Roman Catholic tradition to the practice of healing and support of health. Nowhere is this commitment more evident than in the marked presence of Catholic hospitals and allied health care organizations. The origin of hospitals can be traced to Christian practices of caring for the sick, and for centuries communities of religious women and men in the church have

1. As a theologian and the first speaker in a three-day conference on new frontiers opened in science and ethics by human embryonic stem cell research (and sponsored by Marquette University, the Archdiocese of Milwaukee, and the Wisconsin Catholic Conference), I thought it seemed particularly fitting to begin this paper with a passage from the day's lectionary readings. Little did I anticipate that October 18, 2001 — the day the conference opened — would turn out to be the Feast of St. Luke, Evangelist, who was reputed to be (among other things) a physician. Physicians, accordingly, claim him as one of their patron saints.

From M. Therese Lysaught, "What Would You Do If . . . ? Human Embryonic Stem Cell Research and the Defense of the Innocent," in *Stem Cell Research: New Frontiers in Science and Ethics.* Ed. Nancy E. Snow (Notre Dame, Ind.: University of Notre Dame Press, 2003), 167-93. Used by permission of the publisher.

dedicated themselves to the apostolate of caring for the sick and the dying.[2] Currently, Catholic hospitals constitute over 16 percent of all community hospital beds and admissions in the United States. Not simply an ideal, the Catholic commitment to healing is concretely embodied and enacted in our contemporary context.[3]

I begin with this reminder because the Christian commitment to healing is often obscured or ignored by those who caricature and dismiss Catholic arguments against human embryonic stem cell research. The arguments of Catholics or other groups who inveigh against human embryonic stem cell research, in the words of Glenn McGee and Arthur Caplan, are illogical and bizarre. McGee and Caplan accuse opponents of holding that embryos are special people who can never be allowed to die and of ascribing to embryos a sort of super status that outweighs the needs of others in the community.[4] Not only do such claims distort the arguments in question, but they abstract Catholic claims and arguments against human embryonic stem cell research from the broader narratives and practices out of which they emerge. This cannot but render them unintelligible. In order to avoid such misrepresentation, we need to be mindful of the centrality of healing to the practice of the Christian life and the historic embodiment of this commitment in the Catholic tradition in the broader context of the debate about the moral propriety of human embryonic stem cell research.

This said, in this paper I will examine what has emerged as the central moral question surrounding human embryonic stem cell research, at least within the public debate.[5] The question has been phrased in different ways, so I will offer three versions. First, Kenneth Woodward summarizes the issue in *Newsweek:* What value should we place on human embryos, he asks, and how should their well-being be balanced with that of the millions whose acute suffering might be alleviated through stem cell research and development?[6] The logic of this appeal is undilutedly utilitarian. But, as savvy proponents of human embryonic stem cell research know, utilitarian calculus, while inescapably operative for most moral agents, is generally deemed insufficient, especially when human lives occupy both sides of the equation. Consequently, a second appeal is often launched, one that more subtly individualizes the question. It is usually presented as an image or a narrative rather than as a direct question. Those who followed the controversy as it evolved may remember Mollie and Jackie Singer, 12-year-old twins who spoke at a congressional hearing in July 2001, urging President Bush to permit federal funding for human embryonic stem cell research. Mollie is afflicted with diabetes, and Jackie appealed for stem cell research to advance in order that her sister might be spared the debilitating effects of the disease.[7] Or one may remember the photo dominating the extended coverage by *The New York Times* of President Bush's decision the Sunday after his announcement. In the photo, Charles and Jeri Queenan and their four children soberly watch Bush's August 9th address. The Queenans' daughter Jenna, also twelve years old, struggles with juvenile diabetes, too, and they hope human embryonic stem cell research might cure her.[8]

Mollie, Jackie, Jenna — this second appeal comes in the images and stories of children whose acute suffering might be alleviated through stem cell research. The crux of this appeal is simple. The images whisper: What if this were your child? Indeed, this question is not only whispered. Sooner or later, in any effort to question the moral propriety of human embryonic stem cell research, one can expect a challenge that seems, for the challenger, to be the moral trump card: What would you do if one of your children needed therapy generated by human embryonic stem cell research? What if your child had a terrible disease, and stem cell research provided the only or best possible hope for the alleviation or eradication of the disease? Could you stand against it then?[9] The challenge brings argument to an end. Only a moral barbarian could argue against pursuing a therapy that could possibly relieve the suffering or forestall the early death of a child, particularly one's own child.

2. Charles Curran, "Roman Catholic Medical Ethics," in *Transition and Tradition in Moral Theology* (Notre Dame, Ind.: University of Notre Dame Press, 1979), 175.

3. For these and other statistics on the Catholic presence in U.S. health care, see the website of the Catholic Health Association of the U.S. at: www.chausa.org/aboutcha/chafacts.asp.

4. Glenn McGee and Arthur Caplan, "The Ethics and Politics of Small Sacrifices in Stem Cell Research," *Kennedy Institute of Ethics Journal* 9, no. 2 (1999): 157, 151.

5. This essay takes the ordinary moral language of the public debate as its starting point. In preparing for the conference, I informally "surveyed" friends, colleagues, and students, asking them, "What do you think about research with human embryonic stem cells?" I was surprised by how often we ended up at the "what would you do if?" question discussed below. As John Howard Yoder notes in his analogous context, "The way the question is put arises very naively and authentically from ordinary language of lay ethical debate" ("What Would You Do If?" *Journal of Religious Ethics* 2, no. 2 [1974]: 82). The anomaly revealed simply in this anecdotal experience led me to the questions posed below, since, as Yoder further notes, "Ethical discourse properly arises out of the deepening self-critique of ordinary argumentation." The ordinary language of public discourse as presented in the media powerfully shapes the opinions of so many, especially on issues of bioethics. Insofar as public debate itself is informed and shaped by "bioethics communicators" like Glenn McGee (self-description at the conference "Stem Cell Research: New Frontiers in Science and Research," Milwaukee, 19 October 2001), it provides an important point of entry for engaging both the rhetorical and philosophical components of the discussion.

6. Kenneth L. Woodward, "A Question of Life or Death," *Newsweek* (9 July 2001): 31.

7. Sheryl Gay Stolberg, "Stem Cell Debate in House Has Two Faces, Both Young," *New York Times,* 18 July 2001, A1.

8. John W. Fountain, "Stem Cell Decision Does Not End the Debate," *New York Times,* 12 August 2001, 1, 26. Interestingly, the Queenans and the Singers are listed as Roman Catholics and "devout Catholics," respectively.

9. Sometimes, of course, the question concerns another member of one's family: spouse, parent, sibling. The appeal to one's children is, of course, the most powerful.

Prescinding for a moment from the obvious emotive appeal to feelings of parental succor and obligation, one could argue that this challenge, as well as the utilitarian version of the question stated earlier, paints the situation as one of defense of the innocent. Here we have an innocent: a family member, a child, a multitude that is threatened by an aggressor (in this case, a disease).[10] The individual is appealed to as the one who has the power or ability to come to the defense of the innocent victim.[11] The defense of the innocent victim against the aggressor requires, unfortunately, the sacrifice of a human life.[12]

Is this a situation where the sacrifice of human life might be justified? McGee and Caplan, offering a third version of our question, claim that the central moral issues in stem cell research have to do with the criteria for moral sacrifices of human life.[13] What might such criteria look like? Where might we find moral criteria for justifying the sacrifice of one human life in order to save another or to protect the common good?

Three classic examples, centrally located within the Christian tradition, provide a starting point from which to begin to address this question. These are, (1) the justification of self-defense, offered in one instance by Thomas Aquinas; (2) the classic situation of defense of one's family member or neighbor against a malicious attacker, helpfully analyzed by the late Mennonite theologian John Howard Yoder; and (3) the just war tradition.[14]

These three situations share certain structural features with the current debate. First, in each situation, an "innocent" (i.e., the self, the family member, one's nation) has been or is being attacked. Second, in each situation, the taking of human life is presented as the only, primary, or last option, and it is required to defend the life of an "innocent" third party. Thus, each scenario can be described as one in which the taking of human life might be justified in defense of the innocent, and each provides a classic site within the Christian tradition where moral theologians have struggled with the question of the justified taking of human life.

One might object that these analogies will be of limited relevance to human embryonic stem cell research insofar as they concern, not health care, but violence or war. I would suggest, however, that they are fitting for precisely this reason. For the rhetoric surrounding the human embryonic stem cell debate is rife with images of war. This is not, of course, necessarily specific to the human embryonic stem cell debate: much of this sort of rhetoric arises whenever a new biotechnology is developed and needs to be sold to political and public audiences in the U.S. While I will not create an exhaustive account of this here, a few examples will illustrate.

Consider, for example, McGee and Caplan's article, "The Ethics and Politics of Small Sacrifices in Stem Cell Research." One finds at least seven war-related images in as many pages. Those who seek to develop therapies from human embryonic stem cells are characterized as fighting a just war, a war against suffering caused by the whole gamut of diseases from Parkinson's to cancer to heart disease and more.[15] The annual mortality of cancer, which might potentially be alleviated through human embryonic stem cell research, is compared to the number of people killed in both the Kosovo and Vietnam conflicts.[16] Human embryonic stem cell research advocates plan to sacrifice embryos for a revolutionary new kind of research.[17] Parkinson's disease is likened to a dictator dreaming up the most nefarious chemical war campaign.[18] Resonating with our current political situation, they note that adults and even children are sometimes forced to give life, but only in the defense, or at least interest, of the community's highest ideals and most pressing interests.[19]

McGee and Caplan are far from alone in employing

10. For an account of disease as an aggressor in the context of a theological response, see Arthur C. McGill, *Suffering: A Test of Theological Method* (Philadelphia: Westminster Press, 1982).

11. Terrence W. Tilley helpfully argues that much confusion in the Catholic attempt to forge a "consistent ethic of life" stems from equivocation on the term "innocent," especially between and within discussions of abortion and just war. He notes that there is a difference between the innocence of moral agents — those who act — and the innocence of moral *patients* — those upon whom an act is performed. See his "The Principle of Innocents' Immunity," *Horizons* 15, no. 1 (1988): 43-63. For the purposes of this essay, I will use it in its traditional undifferentiated sense.

12. Throughout this essay, of course, I will presume that human embryos are one of a class of creatures that come under the heading "human life." That this is now questioned is evidenced by the opening of Ken Woodward's question ("what value do we place on human embryos . . . ?"). Others more explicitly raise the question of whether we should consider thawed embryos "alive" or whether embryos prior to twenty-one days even ought to be identified as "organisms." See David Hersenov, "The Problem of Potentiality," *Public Affairs Quarterly* 13, no. 3 (July 1999): 255-71, or his subsequent piece, "An Argument for Limited Human Cloning," *Public Affairs Quarterly* 14, no. 3 (July 2000): 245-58. However, if one presumes that human embryos do not qualify as "human life," the main moral question with regard to human embryonic stem cell research essentially evaporates. One might still explore questions of cow-human chimeras or similar entities created through in vitro techniques, but it would render the moral question of human embryonic stem cell research moot. This is one strategy pursued by advocates of the research.

13. McGee and Caplan, "The Ethics and Politics of Small Sacrifices . . . ," 151.

14. One might also look to three analogous situations within the broad umbrella of health care: triage, human experimentation, and maternal-fetal conflict. Each of these situations wrestles with the possibility that one life might be lost or sacrificed in order to benefit others. How is this situation like or unlike these three other situations? Might they provide insight for understanding when the claims of particular human lives might override the concern for the protection of embryonic life? Answers to these questions await a subsequent essay.

15. McGee and Caplan, "The Ethics and Politics of Small Sacrifices . . . ," 156.

16. Ibid., 154.

17. Ibid., 152.

18. Ibid., 156, 154.

19. Ibid., 153.

this sort of rhetoric to frame the discussion about human embryonic stem cell research. For many, and certainly for the media, clinical medicine through the auspices of biotechnology is engaged in a war against disease, disability, suffering, and death. Regenerative technologies are referred to as revolutionary. The tools of research and the clinic are the medical armamentarium. Those who suffer from particular illnesses are survivors. Moreover, the hyperdrive politicization of this current issue points to the familiar adage that politics is but war waged by other means. As Katharine Seelye notes, on August 9, 2001, when George W. Bush finally revealed his decision about federal funding of human embryonic stem cell research, they chose to have Mr. Bush announce his decision in prime time on national television, a format that presidents traditionally reserve for explaining military actions or trying to extract themselves from difficult political binds.[20]

This rhetoric of war is, I think, not accidental. In a time of war, different rules apply. Rights and lives can be abrogated in ways that would be considered an outrage in peacetime. For reasons that will become clear, I would challenge the metaphor of war as the proper way of framing our understanding of clinical research. Yet that argument must wait. Instead, for the moment I will accept the terms of the debate offered by advocates of human embryonic stem cell research: that we are at war and that this creates a situation in which the sacrifice of human life may, nay must, be justified.

If so, those who earnestly seek to justify the sacrifice of human life on moral grounds and who wish to do so in terms that transcend bald utilitarianism would do well to begin with traditional arguments that justify such sacrifice in analogous contexts. Traditional arguments have stood the test of time, have proved their power by admitting analogous transfer in other contexts, and have done so in a way premised on substantive moral claims. Should human embryonic stem cell research fit with the structure of these arguments, a compelling case could be made to advance its cause. With this in mind, I turn now to consider the three analogies outlined above: (1) Aquinas' justification of self-defense; (2) the defense of one's family member or neighbor against a malicious attacker; and (3) just war. Each of these cases could be the subject of this paper in its own right, and my remarks will therefore be far from exhaustive. Instead, I will highlight the morally relevant features of each case and show how they illuminate the rhetoric that attends human embryonic stem cell research.

Thomas Aquinas and the Justification of Self-defense

A first case where the Christian tradition has permitted the sacrifice of one human life to save another is self-defense. The question of self-defense is worth examining not only as an instance where killing might be justified in defense of the innocent (i.e., the self), but insofar as arguments for the natural right to self-defense and protection of the common good form the basis of the just war tradition that will be examined below.

The classic treatment of self-defense is found in Thomas Aquinas's *Summa Theologica* (II-II, q. 64, a. 7). Here Aquinas considers the question: Is it lawful to kill a man in self-defense? After noting that the tradition does not speak with one voice to this question, he concludes that it can be not unlawful. He notes:

> Nothing hinders one act from having two effects, only one of which is intended, while the other is beside the intention. Now moral acts take their species according to what is intended, and not according to what is beside intention, since this is accidental as explained above (43, 3; I-II, 12.1). Accordingly, the act of self-defense may have two effects; one is the saving of one's life, the other is the slaying of the aggressor. Therefore, this act, since one's intention is to save one's own life, is not unlawful, seeing that it is natural to everything to keep itself in being, as far as possible. And yet, though proceeding from a good intention, an act may be rendered unlawful, if it be out of proportion to the end. Wherefore, if a man, in self-defense, uses more than necessary violence, it will be unlawful: whereas if he repel force with moderation, his defense will be lawful. . . . Nor is it necessary for salvation that a man omit the act of moderate self-defense in order to avoid killing the other man, since one is bound to take more care of one's own life than of another's. But as it is unlawful to take a man's life, except for the public authority acting for the common good as stated above (3), it is not lawful for a man to intend killing a man in self-defense, except for such as have public authority, who while intending to kill a man in self-defense, refer this to the public good, as in the case of a soldier fighting against the foe, and in the minister of the judge struggling with robbers, although even these sin if they be moved by private animosity.[21]

Aquinas's analysis provides two possible starting points for those interested in developing criteria for sacrificing one human life for the sake of another, specifically, intention and public authority.

Intention, for Aquinas, does not in itself justify an act, in this case, the act of self-defense. Rather, intention is that aspect of an action by which we can determine how it ought to be described or categorized. As any good ethicist knows, 90 percent of the solution to a question lies in how it is described or (we could say) narrated. Our descriptions locate questions within a larger narrative,

20. Katharine Q. Seelye, "Bush Gives His Backing for Limited Research on Existing Stem Cells," *New York Times*, 10 August 2001.

21. Thomas Aquinas, *Summa Theologica*, trans. Fathers of the English Dominican Province, 2d rev. ed. (London: Burns, Oates, and Washburn, 1920-1942). Available at www.newadvent.org/summa/.

placing the question in proper relationship to relevant substantive claims that, taken together, point to the morally pertinent dimensions of the issue.

In this case, then, an action whose direct intention is to save one's own life is (somewhat tautologically) properly categorized as an act of self-defense. Self-defense is justified by a broader web of concepts within Aquinas's system: the natural propensity toward self-preservation, our duty to care for one's own life more than for another's, the virtue of justice (under which this discussion is located), and so on. Might advocates of human embryonic stem cell research be able to define the intention of the practice such that it naturally falls under a category that finds itself justified in relationship to substantive moral claims present in contemporary culture? Clearly, advocates argue that, while human embryonic stem cell research requires the destruction of embryos, the intention of ameliorating suffering and preserving the lives of those with serious illness ought to locate it under a different heading — for example, promotion of the common good.

Equally interesting, Aquinas allows public authorities to do what an individual cannot do, namely, to intend to kill a man in self-defense. In order for them to do so lawfully, they must refer the action to the public good. Given the recent controversy over the role the federal government ought to play in funding and oversight of human embryonic stem cell research, advocates might make a case that a Thomistic framework could support the claim that human embryonic stem cell research would be more properly administered by public authorities aiming at the common good — i.e., the NIH and federal funding — than by the private sector. However, while the traditional case for self-defense seems to hold promise for constructing a justification for human embryonic stem cell research, the analogy between such research and self-defense breaks down at a significant number of points, rendering the self-defense argument of doubtful utility.

First, the act or practice of human embryonic stem cell research and an act of self-defense are structurally quite dissimilar. Most obviously, human embryonic stem cell research lacks the binary nature of the act of self-defense: it is necessarily mediated by third parties (researchers, lab technicians, physicians). Moreover, for Aquinas, in an act of self-defense the one justifiably killed is an aggressor. Human embryos clearly are not. For Thomas, even public authorities are limited in their ability to sacrifice life for the common good, being granted permission by Aquinas only to take the lives of aggressors and sinners (II-II, q. 64, a. 3).

Second, it is clear that in Aquinas's analogy, the effects of the one act are immediately related, if not simultaneous: in the same action by which I defend myself I simultaneously kill you. It is this simultaneity that allows Thomas to create what would otherwise rightly be called a fiction — the claim that there is only one direct intention, in spite of the two inseparable effects. As the two effects of an act become separated from each other in time, with subsequent actions required to effect the second outcome, our ability to ascribe a single intention disappears. Some might wish to construe human embryonic stem cell research as one act or practice that has two inseparable effects: one desired and intended, the relief of suffering and the avoidance of death, and one not desired and therefore not directly intended — the destruction of embryos. However, given that these two effects are far removed from each other in time, the legitimacy of this move becomes doubtful.

Third, the intention to save one's own life — while helping one place the action in the proper moral category — is not itself sufficient to render the act lawful. As he notes, "and yet, though proceeding from a good intention, an act may be rendered unlawful, if it be out of proportion to the end. Wherefore if a man, in self-defense, uses more than necessary violence, it will be unlawful: whereas if he repel force with moderation his defense will be lawful." Rather than being a loophole through which one might justify violence, Aquinas is clearly concerned not to give license even toward the pursuit of a good end. The violence that is justified must be *necessary* to save one's own life. If, by any means, violence or the death of the aggressor may be avoided, the act becomes unlawful. With regard to human embryonic stem cell research, the *necessity* of using embryonic stem cells and the ready availability of promising alternatives are precisely what is at issue. I will discuss both of these in more detail below.

In the interest of space, I will simply mention, rather than elaborate on, three additional points of difference. For Aquinas, a justified act of self-defense is an exception for both individuals and for public authorities. As Paul Ramsey notes: he does not say that it is intrinsically right to intend to kill an onrushing, unjust assailant, and then apply this general rule to the case of action in defense of the common good. Intending to kill a man as a means to the public good is clearly an exception to the basic rule (which still remains in force) that no Christian shall intend to kill any man.[22] Relatedly, Aquinas is here attempting to justify actions, not practices. As exceptions, these are seen as ad hoc, one time, unavoidable acts — not as a systematically developed program of activity. Likewise, the actions are considered retrospectively rather than prospectively. The question is: Is this action that has already occurred, unfortunate though it may be, justifiable? The requirements of intention, simultaneity, and proportion render it difficult to imagine how one might prospectively structure an act or practice that would not fall short on any of these measures.[23]

22. Paul Ramsey, *War and the Christian Conscience* (Durham, N.C.: Duke University Press, 1961), 40-41.

23. Those familiar with the Catholic tradition will have undoubtedly noticed that I have studiously avoided using the phrase "double effect." Though the classic principle of double effect takes its origins from Aquinas's account of self-defense, the principle as now articulated radically departs from his limited account. Since the sixteenth century, the principle has been articulated as an at-

Even the promise of intention dissolves upon closer analysis. For Aquinas, once intention shifts from self-defense to any other intention, it becomes immediately unjustified. In the case of human embryonic stem cell research, advocates identify a range of possible uses for stem cell lines (e.g., basic research into the processes of human development, the testing of cosmetics and household products, and so on) in addition to curing diseases and saving lives. Most if not all of these additional outcomes will likely be more immediate. Moreover, as has been the case with so many other recent developments in biotechnology over the past fifteen years, it is more likely than not that we will find ourselves faced with yet another instance of what one might call the therapeutic shift, wherein the initial rhetoric presented in order to marshal public opinion and funding focuses almost exclusively on the therapeutic potential of the new technology in question. After securing public support and becoming feasible, however, the technology takes on a life of its own and becomes made available for any purpose for which those with money can pay.[24]

In the end, the classical justification of self-defense, as found in Aquinas, fails to provide a moral framework for the sacrificing of one human life for the sake of another in the practice of human embryonic stem cell research. Instead, it offers a framework that seeks to minimize the violence we might naturally inflict on one another in the name of our own needs, desires, or even justice.

What Would You Do If . . . ?

A second case where some within the Christian tradition have attempted to justify sacrificing one life to save another would be that of killing an assailant in order to defend not the self but an innocent third party. This question is often raised, as John Howard Yoder notes, as a rejoinder to pacifist objections to war. As he observes at the beginning of his short book What *Would You Do?*:[25]

> Sooner or later, in almost any serious discussion about peace and war, someone is sure to ask the standard question: "What would you do if a criminal, say, pulled a gun and threatened to kill your wife?" (or daughter or sister or mother, whichever one the challenger decides to use). It's uncanny how many persons see this question as a way to test the consistency of the pacifist's convictions that war is wrong.[26]

Yoder tackles this question from two directions. He first unpacks the assumptions implicit in the question, and then goes on to show how the situation of defense of a loved one differs significantly from the situation of war. The analogy, in other words, breaks down.

The parallel in the questions raised between the situations of war and human embryonic stem cell research is uncanny. And like the attempt to analogize the defense of the innocent third party to the question of war, the attempt to draw this analogy to human embryonic stem cell research likewise breaks down.[27] Therefore, rather than proceeding as I did with the question of self-defense (i.e., outlining the analogy, identifying points of contact, and showing how it breaks down), I will instead follow Yoder's lead and analyze the assumptions and dynamics at work in the rhetorical apparatus employed by advocates of human embryonic stem cell research. Yoder identifies six assumptions that underlie the "what would you do if" question. Four will be explored here: determinism, control, knowledge, and alternatives.

Determinism is a problem that afflicts the rhetoric surrounding almost every new development in biotechnology.[28] Not surprisingly, then, we find it in the human

---

tempt to provide justifications for killing innocent persons. (See Ramsey, ibid., p. 47. Ramsey cites Joseph T. Mangan, "An Historical Analysis of the Principle of Double Effect," *Theological Studies* 10, no. 1 [1949]: 41-61.) Such a shift demonstrates the sorts of problems that can occur when one attempts to lift a "principle" out of its narrative context. As mentioned earlier, the narrative context anchors a question within a web of substantive moral concepts that are necessary for making the argument. If, for Aquinas, it is not just to intend to kill an *unjust* aggressor in order to save one's own life, how much less so would it be to kill innocent life in order to save one's own? Thomas's discussion of self-defense not only does not help us in creating criteria for justifying the sacrifice of innocent human life; it provides a compelling argument against it.

24. One might less charitably refer to this as "the therapeutic bait-and-switch." Examples of technologies that argue from the therapeutic premise would be gene "therapy" (the promise embedded in the very term), the cloning rhetoric that followed upon Dolly and other ventures in the 1990s, the development of sperm-sorting techniques for sex selection, and so on. Sperm sorting, or "Microsort" as it is marketed, is an example of how quickly a developed technique can leave its "therapeutic" context and be made available for other purposes.

25. John Howard Yoder, *What Would You Do?* (Scottsdale, Pa.: Herald Press, 1983). See also Yoder, "'What Would You Do If . . . ?' An Exercise in Situation Ethics," *Journal of Religious Ethics* 2, no. 2 (1974): 81-105. Gilbert C. Meilaender also draws on Yoder's essay in his testimony before the National Bioethics Advisory Commission (NBAC). See *Ethical Issues in Human Stem Cell Research,* 3 vols. (Rockville, Md.: June 2000), 3:E1-E6.

26. Yoder, *What Would You Do?,* 13.

27. For example, as with the analogy to self-defense, embryos cannot be properly described as "aggressors," which is morally relevant for this second situation. Likewise, the situation of defense of the innocent compels agreement because of the immediacy and magnitude of the harm that will befall the victim. The killing of the aggressor is allowed in order to prevent a harm from occurring, not to redress a harm that has already taken place. And so on.

28. Yoder identifies three deterministic elements of the standard question. First, "the way the question is usually asked assumes that I alone have a decision to make." Second, the scenario "unfolds mechanically"; once the situation is engaged, the actions of the actors are predetermined. Neither the potential attacker nor the potential victim can exercise any other role than the one predetermined. Third, "the assumption is that how I respond solely determines the outcome of the situation." In the end he notes, "This deterministic assumption is in some sense self-fulfilling. If I tell

embryonic stem cell debate in spades. On a first level, advocates of human embryonic stem cell research paint a scenario that unfolds mechanically. Something like the claim that "millions of people will suffer and die unless human embryonic stem cell research is pursued" is often made explicitly or by implication. For example, Stanford biologist Irv Weissman has been quoted as saying: "Anyone who would ban research on embryonic stem cells will be responsible for the harm done to real, alive, postnatal, sentient human beings who might be helped by this research. Opponents are sacrificing these people to keep from destroying embryos in fertility-clinic freezers that will be thrown out anyway."[29] Or John Gearhart, one of the two researchers whose work initiated the public debate, notes that banning research on embryonic stem cells could make "a lot of people in the future suffer needlessly and maybe even die."[30] The converse, "if we agree to allow the research, these people will be spared," is implied as well.

The argument is not only deterministic in structure, it is also deterministic in time. In making their pitch, biotech advocates often like to work in factors of five, positing clinical therapies "within five years," or "in a decade." Ron McKay, a stem cell expert at the NIH, was, in November 2000, even more optimistic, promising that "in a few months it will be clear that stem cells will regenerate tissues. In two years, people will routinely be reconstituting liver, regenerating heart, routinely building pancreatic islets, routinely putting cells into the brain that get incorporated into normal circuitry. They will routinely be rebuilding all tissues."[31]

Such deterministic claims, of course, ignore important components of the situation. Essentially dismissing the wide range of other research endeavors that have been in process for decades, they ignore the possibility that other interventions might be developed to ameliorate the suffering of those afflicted by particular diseases. In creating the fiction of imminent clinical application, they pretend that the untold millions cited will not, most likely, suffer and die an early death from their conditions, since so much of research bears so little clinical fruit. Witness, for example, the unfulfilled promise of gene "therapy." Moreover, these deterministic claims obscure the troubling practical reality that, should therapeutic applications be developed from human embryonic stem cell research, they will probably not be made available to most of the people who could benefit. The intractable issues of access to health care, social justice, and global inequities will not simply evaporate should human embryonic stem cell research bear fruit.

Yoder's second charge is that the challenge "what would you do if" assumes "if not my omnipotence, at least my substantial control of the situation. It assumes that if I seek to stop the attacker, I can. Now in some cases," he admits, "this may be true, but in many it is by no means certain."[32] This assumption likewise animates biotech rhetoric, of which advocacy of human embryonic stem cell research is but one example. The rhetoric assumes that if we seek to remedy a particular disease, we can. It is only a matter of enough money, time, freedom, collaboration, and scientific ingenuity.

Moreover, in the case of human embryonic stem cell research, this unwarranted optimism posits control not only over one particular disease or condition, which might be more realistic and achievable, but over the entire gamut of morbidity and mortality. It is the ultimate panacea, the cure for everything. An historian of biotechnology might caution that human embryonic stem cell research falls in line as only the most recent Holy Grail, a cousin of practices spanning organ transplantation to gene therapy that have met with limited or minimal success.

This is not to suggest that human embryonic stem cell research might not lead to the development of therapeutic options for specific diseases. It very well may. But, as Yoder reminds us, the classic theory of just war (to skip ahead for a moment) requires that the criterion of "probable success" be met before innocent lives can be taken. In light of the difficulties that well-funded, novel therapeutic paradigms have historically encountered, coupled with the primitive state of embryonic stem cell research, the probability of moving from theory to therapy, at least at this time, cannot be predicted.

In making this point, however, I am getting ahead. Before elaborating on the difficulty of characterizing the therapeutic success of human embryonic stem cell research as probable, we need to consider a third assumption, namely, that of knowledge. As Yoder notes, "The 'what if?' question presupposes, if not omniscience, at least full and reliable information."[33] Likewise, the kinds of claims made in support of human embryonic stem cell

myself there are no choices, there are less likely to be other choices. Still less will I feel a creative capacity (or duty) to make them possible if I don't expect them. But then the limit is in my mind, not in the situation." Yoder, *What Would You Do?,* 14-15.

29. *Newsweek* (9 July 2001): 24. See also McGee and Caplan, "The Ethics and Politics of Small Sacrifices. . . ," 153-54: "Stem cell research consortium Patient's CURe estimates that as many as 128 million Americans suffer from diseases that might respond to pluripotent stem cell therapies. Even if that is an optimistic number, many clinical researchers and cell biologists hold that stem cell therapies will be critical in treating cancer, heart disease, and degenerative diseases of aging such as Parkinson's disease. More than half of the world's population will suffer at some point in life with one of these three conditions, and more humans die every year from cancer than were killed in both the Kosovo and Vietnam conflicts."

30. *Newsweek* (9 July 2001): 27.

31. Nicholas Wade, *Life Script* (New York: Simon and Schuster, 2001), 121.

32. Yoder, *What Would You Do?,* 15.

33. He continues: "Not only does it assume on my part that events will unfold in an inevitable way, but it also presumes that I am reliably informed about what that unfolding will be like. I know that if I do not kill the aggressor, he will rape my wife, kill my daughter, attack me, or whatever. And I know I will be successful if I try to take his life." Ibid., 16-17.

research require a level of knowledge that is certainly not at hand and may well never be, even should such research be funded. For example, as those pursuing the promise of gene therapy have discovered, what one can coax human cells to do in the laboratory often proves impossible to convince them to do in the human body. After much effort, researchers have succeeded in preventing human embryonic stem cells from differentiating in culture long enough to establish cell lines. This outcome has been achieved. What is still lacking is knowledge of precisely what mechanism is at work in preventing differentiation; how to direct cells to differentiate into specific tissue types; how to control cell growth (suppress tumorogenesis) once differentiation has been achieved; how to get cultured tissues to properly engraft; and then, the most difficult piece, how to get them to achieve function in vivo.

As with the field of gene therapy, the rhetoric advocating human embryonic stem cell research steamrolls ahead, hyping the promise of application, while the state of the science and the fundamental understandings of how relevant processes work is itself embryonic. Without first conducting more basic research, the promise has a higher probability of being broken than fulfilled. Of course, perhaps such knowledge is not necessary. As Nicholas Wade exults: "The magic of regenerative medicine is that the physician does not have to know everything, only how to create the right conditions for the body's cells to respond to the appropriate signals."[34] In addition, one might counter that, without the sacrifice of a few frozen embryos, we will not be able to conduct basic research and gain the knowledge necessary to better envision and enact the end. The response to this claim leads us to the last of Yoder's assumptions, namely, that of alternatives.[35] As Yoder notes, the question of "what if" is designed to limit the respondents' options to two: yes or no, for or against, all or nothing. To set up the discussion as if there were only two possible kinds of outcomes (millions suffer and die vs. all are saved) or only one route (human embryonic stem cell research) to the desired outcome is to prejudice the argument. The situation has been descriptively constructed so as to predispose to a particular outcome.

The posing of alternatives, of course, has been one strategy of those who oppose human embryonic stem cell research. To advance basic science, many call for further animal research, noting that the trajectory in animal studies from in vitro to in vivo to therapy is far from complete. Others call for work to first be completed, or at least further advanced, with adult stem cells before moving to human embryonic stem cells. But the rhetoric of the debate will not brook alternatives. Adult stem cells are dismissed by researchers as not totipotent and therefore deficient; they are dismissed because (ironically enough) not enough research has been done to assess their promise. In the media, adult stem cell research becomes "a canard,"[36] "crap science," or "baloney."[37] Alternative means to a shared goal will not be taken seriously. As in most wars, there will be no negotiations; there is no middle ground. Thus, ironically, advocates of human embryonic stem cell research become absolutist, while their opponents emerge as those searching for a compromise that will seek to achieve the ends of protecting innocent life and of working to ameliorate the suffering and mortality associated with the human condition.

In the end, the crux of the "what if" question, as well as the case made in favor of human embryonic stem cell research, lies largely not in rational argument but in emotional appeal. As Yoder notes, the question

> appeals to family connections and bonds of love so that it becomes a problem of emotions as well as thought. Instead of discussing what is generally right or wrong, it personalizes the situation by making it an extension of my own self-defense. Especially is this emotional dimension of the question more visible when the discussion centers on one's duty to protect someone else. Often the questioner will heighten this aspect of the argument by saying, "Perhaps as a Christian you do have the right to sacrifice your own welfare to be loving toward an attacker. But do you have the right to sacrifice the welfare of others for whom you are responsible?"[38]

Classically, these questions are taken up in the just war tradition, and so to our third analogy I now turn.

Jus in Bello: Human Embryonic Stem Cell Research and the Just War Against Disease

A third case where the Christian tradition has justified the sacrifice of human life would be the just war tradition.[39] As noted at the outset, the language of the just war is invoked by McGee and Caplan. They attempt to argue that, in human embryonic stem cell research, the essence of the embryo — that is, its DNA — is not destroyed but actually lives on in the cell lines and potential tissues developed therefrom. What is destroyed, they claim, are simply the "inessential components" of the embryo — its cytoplasm, external wall, and mitochondria. The reduc-

34. Wade, *Life Script*, 168.

35. I am here collapsing his discussion of "other options" under the heading of "alternatives."

36. Sheryl Gay Stolberg, "A Science in Its Infancy, but with Great Expectations for Its Adolescence," *New York Times*, 20 August 2001, A17.

37. *Newsweek* (9 July 2001): 27.

38. Yoder, *What Would You Do?*, 19-20.

39. Gilbert C. Meilaender examines a different set of "war"-related arguments in relation to human embryonic stem cell research, taking as his interlocutors both the NBAC report and McGee and Caplan. See his "The Point of a Ban: Or, How to Think about Stem Cell Research," *Hastings Center Report* 31, no. 1 (2001): 9-16.

tionistic and gnostic character of these claims aside, they conclude: "It is difficult to imagine those who favor just war opposing a war against such suffering given the meager loss of a few cellular components."[40]

How might the just war tradition illuminate our question? In the interests of space, I will limit my observations to three. First, of our three analogies, the just war tradition provides the closest fit with the situation of human embryonic stem cell research. In the model for a just war, a nation — a multitude — has been attacked or has had its interests threatened. The war may entail the loss of innocent life in the defense of the innocent and the common good. Those who answer the call to fight do so from a position of innocence, and it is recognized that in pursuing the aggressor, innocent civilians on both sides might be killed as well as combatants. But, at the same time, an obligation to protect those unjustly attacked and to work for justice on their behalf is invoked.[41]

Furthermore, the context of human embryonic stem cell research mirrors a number of *jus ad bellum* criteria, the conditions that must be met for a war to be legitimately declared. One could make a case that the cause is just — humanity has a right to defend itself against the onslaught of disease. The war must be declared by a competent, public authority — in this case, perhaps the NIH. The intention must be right, namely, the restoration of peace — which a world free of the ravages of disease approximates. Success must be probable. Apart from my earlier skepticism about the probability of moving from the laboratory to clinical applications, one could grant, for the sake of argument, that human embryonic stem cell research has a sufficient prospect of probable success. In light of this, one could argue that the principle of proportionality is likewise met — the good expected by pursuing the research outweighs the damages to be inflicted in the loss of embryonic life.[42]

However, two important criteria remain, both of which are essential for validating a particular war as just. The first is a final *jus ad bellum* condition: that all peaceful alternatives must first be exhausted. This is also known as the condition of last resort. The debate over alternatives — further animal studies, the use of adult stem cells or placental stem cells — has been discussed above. Until it can be definitively established that all nonviolent alternatives have been exhausted, that human embryonic stem cell research truly is a last resort, the analogy to a "just war" will fail. This is a process that will take time.

In addition to the exhaustion of all peaceful alternatives as a crucial condition for going to war, the just war tradition also provides conditions that must be met during combat, the *jus in bello* criteria. For our purposes, the key condition is that of discrimination or noncombatant immunity. The principle of discrimination protects the immunity of noncombatants by restricting direct targeting to combatants, military installations, and factories whose products are directly related to the war effort. As Aquinas notes in his discussion of war: "those who are attacked should be attacked because they deserve it on account of some fault."[43] Noncombatants are not to be targeted. Just warriors realize that, in the course of attacking legitimate targets, innocent noncombatants may be killed. But within the tradition, a most important moral distinction obtains between recognizing that noncombatants may accidentally and tragically be killed and directly targeting those noncombatants.

In the case of human embryonic stem cell research, frozen embryos occupy the place in the analogy of noncombatants. It cannot be argued that the loss of embryonic life is an unintended, indirect, and accidental byproduct of the activities of the research. For this is what is at stake, the ending of embryonic life — not, contra McGee and Caplan, simply the loss of embryonic identity. Human embryonic stem cell research directly targets the lives of human embryos — frozen though they may be, slated for disposal though they may be — in order to achieve the ends of the war. Within the just war tradition, this means to a good end would not be licit. It would be total war.

Finally, the just war tradition reflects the commitments of the Christian tradition from which it emerged. As Aquinas notes, "Those who wage war justly aim at peace."[44] The imperfect peace obtainable in this world is considered to be the normative human condition, and war is reluctantly admitted into the realm of possibility in order to restore natural order and harmony. Aquinas's discussion of war is located, in the *Summa,* not under the heading of justice, where one might expect to find it, but rather under the heading of charity. War is properly categorized as sin, a vice, a violation of the virtue of charity, of the friendship between humans and God that is, within the human community, made possible by the incarnation. Cognizant of this, the just war tradition seeks not as much to carve out a space for the legitimacy of war but rather to create parameters that will severely limit it.

War and Peace

In so limiting the legitimate taking of human life in war or self-defense, the Christian tradition fails to provide moral criteria that would justify directly and intentionally taking innocent human life. By illuminating the operative assumptions of the human embryonic stem cell

40. McGee and Caplan, "The Ethics and Politics of Small Sacrifices . . . ," 156. The claims made here are not only reductionistic — reducing human identity to DNA — but also gnostic and dualistic insofar as our actual concrete embodiment is deemed not an essential part of who we are.

41. In other words, the human embryonic stem cell debate may approximate the question: "Can an otherwise neutral nation intervene in defense of an innocent party that is attacked by some other nation?"

42. Again, I am making this latter claim for the sake of argument.

43. ST II-II, q. 40, a. 1.

44. Ibid., reply to obj. 3.

debate, analysis of the classic situation of defense of the neighbor renders that particular analogy similarly unhelpful. In each of the three analogies, a case might be made for taking the life of the aggressor. But no moral criteria emerge that would justify sacrificing the life of one not party to the conflict, even in order to save the life of another. One is free to sacrifice one's own life — one may find oneself called to be a martyr — but neither an individual nor public authorities may justifiably sacrifice the life of even one innocent person, even for the sake of the common good. Therefore, as long as we hold that human embryos qualify as human life, "sacrificing" them is not an available moral option.

Ken Woodward reminds us that "the words we choose to frame our arguments reveal the moral universe we inhabit," and it is with this thought that I would like to close.[45] McGee and Caplan end their article echoing Woodward's claim. They state:

> The issues here are novel and they are hard, but mostly they require philosophical innovation about what an embryo is and how we are to treat embryonic material in a time of stem cell research [one hears the resonance: "in a time of war"]. Our argument here is that no embryo need be sacrificed, but we must alter the terms and goals of our debate to frame an appropriate moral framework for dealing with embryos.[46]

In other words, McGee and Caplan propose to resolve this particular moral controversy by redefining the terms — what an embryo is, what it means to kill. They propose to create a different story to describe what we are doing. This is a classic tactic in wartime: to dehumanize the other, to craft a narrative that justifies the necessary use of lethal force, and to tell ourselves that we do it in order to protect the community's highest ideals and most pressing interests. They suggest that the way out of the dilemma is to descriptively construct the practice of human embryonic stem cell research so as to predispose to a particular outcome.

I cannot but agree that a necessary step forward toward resolving the debate over human embryonic stem cell research is the narrative task of redescription. I opened this paper with a passage from St. Luke, and that passage points to a fundamentally different narrative frame for the debate about human embryonic stem cells, in particular, and biotech and clinical research more generally. St. Luke reminds us that, for Christians, healing is understood not in relation to war but in relation to peace.[47] Healing, that practice rightly privileged as a central and enduring commitment for Christian identity and communities, is not, within a Christian narrative, an end in itself. Rather, healing is a sign of the "reign of God," a practice rooted in the identity and actions of the God of peace. For Christians, the healing that we pursue must be anchored in the broader context of God's work in the world and our participation therein. If we abstract the commitment to healing from its narrative context, we are left with a formal claim that becomes an end in itself, to which any and all means might be fitted, even the means of killing embryos. In the end, to paraphrase Yoder, I do not know what I would do if one of my children needed the products of human embryonic stem cell research. But I know that what I ought to do should be illuminated by the story of the Trinitarian God, whose story is one of peace, healing, and compassion — the difficult activity of suffering with those who suffer precisely because, want as we might, we cannot eliminate that suffering.[48]

45. Woodward, "A Question of Life or Death," 31.

46. McGee and Caplan, "The Ethics and Politics of Small Sacrifices . . . ," 157.

47. On a similar note, Mark Kuczewski suggested a similar critique of the tendency to construe science and clinical research as a "war against nature," rather than situating it in the context of the "story of creation" (comment at the conference "Stem Cell Research," Milwaukee, 18 October 2001).

48. I would very much like to thank Nancy Snow for inviting me to participate in what was such a vital and thorough conference. It was an honor to be part of such an esteemed slate of presenters and a privilege to be able to offer my thoughts to the Wisconsin Catholic Bishops Conference and the Archdiocese of Milwaukee. I must also thank my colleagues who read and so helpfully commented on previous drafts of this paper: Michael Barnes, Una Cadegan, Dennis Doyle, James Heft, Brad Kallenberg, Jack McGrath, Sandra Yocum Mize, Maureen A. Tilley, and Terence W. Tilley. In them, I am richly blessed.

V. The Beginning of Life

CHAPTER FIFTEEN

Life and Its Sanctity

Shall we abort a fetus diagnosed as suffering from a fatal genetic defect? Shall we strive to keep a terminally ill patient alive? Is research using embryonic stem cells morally appropriate, given that it requires the destruction of embryos? What should we make of the health discrepancies between racial/ethnic groups? Is there a moral claim to universal health care?

Such difficult questions run throughout this volume. While these questions are disparate and wide-ranging, our basic disposition toward life underlies them all. Notions about the "sanctity of life" are being addressed implicitly, and sometimes explicitly, as we wrestle with these tough questions. For example, what does it mean to affirm the "sanctity of life" as we struggle with the potential benefits of embryonic stem cell research? Is there something sacred or holy or awe-inspiring about a human embryo? If so, what protection should that afford? And what of the sacredness or sanctity of the lives that would benefit from the research? Or, for example, what does it mean to affirm the sanctity of life as we contemplate the removal of nutrition and hydration from a patient in a persistent vegetative state? Is the removal of nutrition and hydration a denial of that sanctity? Or might removal actually be an affirmation of the life that had been led? Given the remarkable powers of modern medicine, we often wrestle with what it means to affirm the sanctity of life.

The Hebrew and Christian Scriptures reveal a God who creates and values life. This divine viewpoint is witnessed in the creation stories where God creates humanity in God's own image (Genesis 1:26-27) and breathes life into us (Genesis 2:7). It is likewise discernible in a covenant signified by a rainbow (Genesis 9:1-17), in a commandment (Exodus 20:13), in an empty tomb (John 11:20-26; 1 Corinthians 15), and in a vision of a new heaven and a new earth (Revelation 20:1-8). So, too, God's stance toward life is glimpsed when the Psalmist exclaims that God has crowned humanity with glory and honor (Psalm 8:5) and when Jesus proclaims that God's concern for us exceeds God's obvious care for the birds of the air and lilies of the field (Matthew 6:25-32).

Earlier editions of this volume observed that affirming the sanctity of life is not unambiguous. Are we affirming all of life or only human life as sacred? With sanctity of life, do we mean to afford respect to *bios* or *zōē*, biological or spiritual life? Are we affirming something inherent within the human individual or something that is bestowed from outside the self? And what is the relationship between the good of life and other goods, such as freedom or creativity or community? In short, affirming the "sanctity of life" raises as many questions as it answers and seems but a shorthand way of asking about our most basic predispositions toward life.

Christian theologians give different accounts of the "sanctity of life," accounts that may bear in different ways on the questions posed by the power of modern medicine. While many essays within this volume touch on the theme of the "sanctity of life," the selections gathered in the current chapter help us to think more directly about this notion. For example, one set of themes concerns how we know the sanctity or sacredness of life and from whence it is derived. In "Respect for Life" (selection 97), Karl Barth locates the "respect" due to life in the command of God. The election and love of humanity by God, seen most decisively in Christ's incarnation, confronts us with the respect that is owed to life. Barth also claims that appeals to nature or reason are ultimately unable to respect life in its full psycho-physical existence but will instead value one aspect over the other. Likewise, Barth wonders whether any natural account of the respect due to human life can fully appreciate what is owed to each individual, including to one's self, in his or her full solidarity and coexistence with others.

A related argument is seen in Karen Lebacqz's retrieval of Helmut Thielicke's notion of "alien dignity" (selection 98). For Thielicke, every human life is of "incommensurable, incalculable worth." This worth is not derived from specific human characteristics such as rationality or freedom, which are limited and sometimes fleeting. Rather, each human life is of inestimable worth because each has that standing before God. God creates us in love, redeems us in love, holds us in love. The infinite God loves us and calls us into relationship with God and with all of God's other children. It is from this divine relationship and evaluation that "even the most pitiful life" is rightly seen as in the *imago Dei* and thus of incalculable worth.

Lebacqz contends that such God-given "alien dignity" provides more protection and higher worth for human life than notions of intrinsic value. In medicine, this value can help protect us from being reduced to our utility for others or "being swept up in the instrumentalization of human life." Such dignity, says Lebacqz, also equalizes people, calls for both personal responsibility and structures that support human flourishing, and "requires a relational view of human beings" that is both "consonant with many feminist approaches to ethics, and provides an important corrective to the contemporary stress in bioethics on autonomy."

By contrast, Richard Stith's essay, "Toward Freedom from Value" (selection 99), explicates the "sanctity" of life by drawing on moral intuitions and the way we use other terms, such as "value," "love," "respect," and "reverence." Stith argues that the reverence that is due to the sanctity of life is a bedrock or foundation for other moral commitments, including justice. It especially grounds claims that we cannot aim to kill (individually or as public policy). Interestingly, Stith makes this case without Barth's appeal to God's command or Thielicke's notion of alien dignity.

In his essay, "Suffering, the Body, and Christianity: The Early Christians Lived the Theological Basis of Catholic Health Care" (selection 100), James F. Keenan enters this debate at a different point. Keenan worries that older Catholic accounts of life's sanctity depended too heavily on notions of God's dominion and God's ownership of life. In those accounts, we are not to trespass on life because it belongs to God. But, says Keenan, Pope John Paul II developed a richer and more adequate account of life's sanctity by appealing to humanity as made in God's image, made for relationship with God. The inviolable character of human life is now seen not merely as external but also as lying within the human. In this account, sanctity of life means that human life is not only an object that belongs to God but also a subject, meant for relationship, whose value is intrinsic to the subject as one having been made in God's image. Part of Keenan's concern is that, while seeing life as God's dominion might provide a type of protection from intrusion, it provides an inadequate foundation for the compassion toward, and listening to, others that is part of life's true sanctity.

Interestingly, Keenan's resistance to dominion language sparks some tension with the "command" and "alien dignity" language of Barth and Thielicke/Lebacqz, but Keenan depends more on overt theological language than does Stith, including the same "image of God" language that is so important to Thielicke/Lebacqz. Keenan also develops a notion of sanctity that is self-consciously focused on embodiment and relationality. These elements are not absent from Stith, but they are more evident in the accounts offered by Barth and Thielicke/Lebacqz.

A related set of issues concerns how we talk about and defend the "sanctity" of life. Stith shows us that the language of "valuing" life ends up commodifying it and provides little actual protection. He also suggests that alternative notions, such as "love," do not get at the reverence due to all life, which is better captured as life's sanctity. Barth claims that only God's command can grant life its due and protect it from an overemphasis on the spiritual or on the physical, the individual or the social. Thielicke/Lebacqz assert that it is precisely the "alien dignity" of God's love for us from our very creation that provides the protection, equality, relationality, and structural support due to all those made in the image of God. Keenan emphasizes that the one made in God's image is an embodied human subject, not just an object, who has a voice that deserves to be heard, especially in voicing suffering or marginalization. Thus, even if we agree to life's sanctity, we are left with the question of how to best frame it: primarily in terms of reverence and sanctity, or command and respect, or alien dignity and God's image, or the embodied human subject?

The last essay in this chapter, Chris Huebner's "Bioethics and the Church: Technology, Martyrdom, and the Moral Significance of the Ordinary" (selection 101), could have appeared in this volume in the chapters on method or beginning of life. We include it here for several reasons. First, Huebner warns that technology, including medical technology, is far from morally neutral. Instead, such technology goes hand in hand with a view of the good life that is focused on gaining control of contingency and on providing individuals with the means for seeking their desires. This concern about technology's moral direction dovetails well with Lebacqz's conviction that "alien dignity" can provide a counterweight to "increasing technological imperatives." Second, Huebner's appeal to martyrdom reflects the view that we are not our own possession. Life comes to us as a gift, and we are invited to return that gift to God and to others. This sense that we are not our own fits well within the debate regarding the "whence" of life's sanctity. Finally, the appeal to martyrdom reminds us that life's value does not proscribe that there are values and relationships worth dying for. Sometimes those who most value life as a gift are also those most willing to give it up.

Our basic posture toward life underlies many of the challenges that confront us in the power of modern medicine. The essays gathered here help us to think more carefully about life's sanctity. Of course, learning how to think and talk about life's sanctity does not always answer the question of how to apply those convictions. For this reason we need the many additional discussions suggested by the other chapters in this volume.

SUGGESTIONS FOR FURTHER READING

Amundsen, Darrel W. *Medicine, Society, and Faith in the Ancient and Medieval Worlds* (Baltimore: Johns Hopkins University Press, 1996).

Bayertz, Kurt, ed. *Sanctity of Life and Human Dignity* (Dordrecht: Kluwer Academic Publishers, 1996).

Callahan, Daniel. "The Sanctity of Life." In *Updating Life and Death,* ed. Donald R. Cutler, with commentaries by Julian Pleasants, James M. Gustafson, and Henry K. Beecher (Boston: Beacon Press, 1969), pp. 181-250.

Callahan, Daniel, et al. "The Sanctity of Life Seduced: A Symposium on Medical Ethics." *First Things* 32 (April 1994): 13-28.

Clouser, Danner K. "The Sanctity of Life: An Analysis of a Concept." *Annals of Internal Medicine* 78 (1973): 119-25.

Crane, Diana. *The Sanctity of Social Life: Physician's Treatment of Critically Ill Patients* (New York: Russell Sage Foundation, 1975).

Hartt, Julian. "Creation, Creativity, and the Sanctity of Life." *The Journal of Medicine and Philosophy* 4 (December 1979): 418-34.

Kilner, John F. *Life on the Line: Ethics, Aging, Ending Patients' Lives, and Allocating Vital Resources* (Grand Rapids: Eerdmans, 1992).

Meilaender, Gilbert. *Neither Beast nor God: The Dignity of the Human Person* (New York: Encounter Books, 2009).

Mitchell, C. Ben, et al. *Biotechnology and the Human Good* (Washington, D.C: Georgetown University Press, 2007), pp. 58-86.

Nelson, Robert J. *Human Life: A Biblical Perspective for Bioethics* (Philadelphia: Fortress Press, 1984).

Ramsey, Paul. "The Sanctity of Life." *Dublin Review* 241 (Spring 1967): 3-21.

Shils, Edward, et al. *Life or Death: Ethics and Options* (Seattle: University of Washington Press, 1968).

Song, Robert. "Whose Sanctity of Life? Ricoeur, Dworkin and the Human Embryo." *Holiness Past and Present* (2003): 460-76.

Thomasma, David C. *An Apology for the Value of Human Life* (St. Louis: Catholic Health Association of the United States, 1983).

Weber, Leonard J. *Who Shall Live?* (New York: Paulist Press, 1976).

96 Genesis 1:26-27; Psalm 8; Matthew 6:25-32

Genesis 1:26-27

Then God said, "Let us make humankind in our image, according to our likeness; and let them have dominion over the fish of the sea, and over the birds of the air, and over the cattle, and over all the wild animals of the earth, and over every creeping thing that creeps upon the earth."

So God created humankind in his image,
in the image of God he created them;
male and female he created them.

Psalm 8

O Lord, our Sovereign,
how majestic is your name in all the earth!

You have set your glory above the heavens.
Out of the mouths of babes and infants
you have founded a bulwark because of your foes,
to silence the enemy and the avenger.

When I look at your heavens, the work of your fingers,
the moon and the stars that you have established;
what are human beings that you are mindful of them,
mortals that you care for them?

Yet you have made them a little lower than God,
and crowned them with glory and honor.
You have given them dominion over the works of your hands;
you have put all things under their feet,
all sheep and oxen,
and also the beasts of the field,
the birds of the air, and the fish of the sea,
whatever passes along the paths of the seas.

O Lord, our Sovereign,
how majestic is your name in all the earth!

Matthew 6:25-32

"Therefore I tell you, do not worry about your life, what you will eat or what you will drink, or about your body, what you will wear. Is not life more than food, and the body more than clothing? Look at the birds of the air; they neither sow nor reap nor gather into barns, and yet your heavenly Father feeds them. Are you not of more value than they? And can any of you by worrying add a single hour to your span of life? And why do you worry about clothing? Consider the lilies of the field, how they grow; they neither toil nor spin, yet I tell you, even Solomon in all his glory was not clothed like one of these. But if God so clothes the grass of the field, which is alive today and tomorrow is thrown into the oven, will he not much more clothe you — you of little faith? Therefore do not worry, saying, 'What will we eat?' or 'What will we drink?' or 'What will we wear?' For it is the Gentiles who strive for all these things; and indeed your heavenly Father knows that you need all these things."

97 Respect for Life

Karl Barth

Those who handle life as a divine loan will above all treat it with respect. Respect is man's astonishment, humility and awe at a fact in which he meets something superior — majesty, dignity, holiness, a mystery which compels him to withdraw and keep his distance, to handle it modestly, circumspectly and carefully. It is the *respicere* of an object in face of which his attitude cannot be left to chance or preference or even clever assessment, but which requires an attitude that is particularly appropriate and authoritatively demanded. This compulsion does not derive from life itself and as such. Life does not itself create this respect. The command of God creates respect for it. When man in faith in God's Word and promise realises how God from eternity has maintained and loved him in his little life, and what He has done for him in time, in this knowledge of human life he is faced by a majestic, dignified and holy fact. In human life itself he meets something superior. He is thus summoned to respect because the living God has distinguished it in this way and taken it to Himself. We may confidently say that the birth of Jesus Christ as such is the revelation of the command as that of respect for life. This reveals the eternal election and love of God. This unmistakably differentiates human life from everything that is and is done in heaven and earth. This gives it even in the most doubtful form the character of something singular, unique, unrepeatable and irreplaceable. This decides that it is an advantage and something good and worthwhile to be as man. This characterises life as the incomparable and non-recurrent opportunity to praise God. And therefore this makes it an object of respect.

It is really surprising that the Christian Church and Christian theology have not long ago urged more energetically the importance for ethics of so constituent a part of the New Testament message as the fact of the incarnation, instead of resorting, in the vital question why man and human life are to be respected, to all kinds of general religious expressions and to the assertions of non-Christian humanism. The assurances of the latter that the value of human life rests on a law of nature and reason sound quite well. But on this basis they are extremely insubstantial, and it is clear that nature and reason can always be used to prove something very different from respect for man. They also have the disadvantage

From Karl Barth, *Church Dogmatics,* III/4, trans. A. T. Mackay et al. (Edinburgh: T&T Clark, 1961), pp. 336-43. Used by permission.

that by "human life" they understand either his very one-sided intellectual existence, "the infinite value of the human soul," on the one side, or his equally one-sided material existence and prosperity on the other. They have the further drawback of always being bound up with illusory overestimations of his goods, abilities and achievements which can only prove detrimental to the respect which ought really to be paid. And somewhere there obviously lurks the ambiguity that, although reference is made to man, humanity, the dignity of man, etc., it is not really man himself who is intended but all sorts of things, ideas, advances and aims which in effect man has only to serve, for which he has only to let himself be used, and for the sake of which he can at any moment be dropped and sacrificed.

In contrast to every other, the respect of life which becomes a command in the recognition of the union of God with humanity in Jesus Christ has an incomparable power and width. For in this recognition it is really commanded with the authority of God Himself and therefore in such a way that there can be no question whatever of disregard as an alternative. Intellectualistic and materialistic one-sidedness in answer to the question of what human existence is all about is thus excluded by the grounding of the command in this recognition because the human life in question, the life of the man Jesus, cannot be divided into psychical or physical but compels us to offer the respect demanded by God to the whole man in his ordered unity of soul and body. The usual overestimations of man and human nature are also excluded, because the distinction of human existence brought about in Jesus Christ is to be seen wholly as grace and therefore only in humility. And finally on the basis of this recognition there can be no question of man's life being secretly honoured again as only the vehicle and exponent of an idea or cause superimposed upon him. For human life itself and as such is seen in the person of the man Jesus to be the matter about which God is concerned, and therefore man must also be concerned in His service. In respect of the recognition of the command in the sense which now occupies us the Christian Church and Christian theology have an incomparable weight to throw into the scales. They and they alone know exactly why and in what sense respect for life is demanded from us, and demanded in such a way that there can be no evasions or misunderstandings.

But what does respect for life mean? We have spoken of astonishment, humility, awe, modesty, circumspection and carefulness. Application must now be made to our particular theme. What matters is not something but someone, the real man before God and among his fellows, his individual psycho-physical existence, his movement in time, his freedom, his orientation to God and solidarity with others. What matters is that everyone should treat his existence and that of every other human being with respect. For it belongs to God. It is His loan and blessing. And it may be seen to be this in the fact that God himself has so unequivocally and completely acknowledged it in Jesus Christ. What, then, can be the meaning of respect in relation to this object?

First, it obviously means an adoption of the distance proper in face of a mystery. It is a mystery that I am, and others too, in this human structure and individuality in which we recognise one another as of the same kind, each in his time and freedom, each in his vertical and horizontal orientation. This is indeed an incomprehensible and in relation to ourselves intangible fact, inexhaustible in its factuality and depth and constantly adapted to give us pause. Those who do not know *respicere* in face of it, those who are not startled and do not feel insignificant and incompetent in its presence, those who think they can understand and master and control it, do not know what obedience is. All human life as such is surrounded by a particular solemnity. This is not the solemnity of the divine, nor of the ultimate end of man. Life is only human and therefore created, and eternity as the divinely decreed destiny of man is only an allotted future. But within these limits it is a mystery emphasised and absolutely distinguished by God Himself. As such it must always be honoured with new wonder. Every single point to be observed and pondered is in its own way equally marvelous — and everything is equally marvelous in every human existence. First, then, we have simply to perceive this, and once we have done so we have not at any price to relinquish or even to lose sight of this perception. We must be awake to this need to keep our distance, and always be wakeful as we do so.

But a mere theoretical and aesthetic wonder is not enough. On the contrary, the theoretical and aesthetic wonder which rightly understood forms the presupposition for everything else, must itself have a practical character if it is to be the required respect. And this means that human life must be affirmed and willed by man. We hasten to add that it must be affirmed and willed as his own with that of others and that of others with his own. Egoism and altruism are false antitheses when the question is that of the required will to live. My own life can no more claim my respect than that of others, but neither can that of others. Although they are not the same, but each distinct, the homogeneity and solidarity of all human life is indissoluble. But what is the will to live understood in this sense? Obviously, because to life there also belongs the freedom of this will, it is determination and readiness for action in the direction of its confirmation. That we should spontaneously perceive and affirm the reception of life as a divine loan in its character as a favour shown, a possession entrusted and an opportunity offered to us, is obviously what is expected of us as those who possess it, who are alive. But if this perception and confirmation is our act, it must consist in our making of our life the use prescribed by its nature as seen in these points. What is important is that according to the measure and within the limits of his individuality, and in the time granted to him, each should exist — always in orientation to God and solidarity with others — as this rational creature, attentively, unreservedly and loyally confessing his human existence in willing responsibility to the One to whom he owes it. We cannot live in obedience accidentally, irresolutely, without plan or responsibility. We cannot in obedience let ourselves go or be driven. We cannot and must not seriously tire of life. For it is always an offer waiting for man's will, determination and readiness for action. And it is to be noted that this is real respect for life. In this form as the will to live it is more than passive speculation in face of its mystery. It is the respect which its mystery demands. We really see it as the mystery it is in the fact that we will to live it and accept it responsibly. A life which is not affirmed and willed, which is irresolute, irresponsible and inactive, is necessarily a life without mystery. And against the constant threat of egoism, there is always the safeguard and corrective of recollection that the real human life is the one which is lived in orientation to God and co-ordination with others. The last is particularly important from the practical standpoint. The will to live which is the form of respect for life will always be distinguishable from an inhuman and irreverent will to live contrary to the command, by the fact that it considers the existence and life of others together with its own, and its own together with that of others.

But having considered and said this, we must also show that the commanded respect for life includes an awareness of its limitations. We have already mentioned these. We refer to the creaturely and the eschatological limitations. These cannot diminish respect for life, much less abrogate it. But it is necessarily modified and characterised by the fact that the life to which it is paid has these limitations. As the reverence commanded of man it is not limitless. As such it has within itself its own limitation. Its limitation is the will of God the Creator Himself who commands it, and the horizon which is set for man by the same God with his determination for eternal life. Life is no second God, and therefore the respect due to it cannot rival the reverence owed to God. On the contrary, it is limited by that which God will have from the man who is elected and called by Him. For the life of man belongs to Him. He has granted it to him as a loan. And He decides in what its right use should consist. He also decrees and decides in His command in what man's will to live should at any moment consist or not, and how far it should go or not go as such. And what God will have of man is not simply that he should will to live for himself and in co-existence with others. God can also will to restrict man's will to live for himself and in co-existence with others. He can weaken, break and finally destroy it. He actually does this. And when He does, obedience may not be withheld from Him. As Creator and Lord of life, He has also the right to will and do this, and if He does, then He knows well why it must be so, and in this too He is man's gracious Father. In relation to man, He has much more in mind than what man can see here and now in the fulfilment of his life-act. He has determined him for eternal life, for the life which one day will finally be given him. He is leading him through this life to the other. The respect for life commanded by Him cannot then be made by man a rigid principle, an absolute rule to be fulfilled according to rote. It can only try to assert and maintain itself as the will to live in the one sense understood by man, whether in relation to his own life or that of others. Respect for life, if it is obedience to God's command, will have regard for the free will of the One who has given life as a loan. It will not consist in an absolute will to live, but in a will to live which by God's decree and command, and by *meditatio futurae vitae,* may perhaps in many ways be weakened, broken, relativised and finally destroyed. Being prepared for this, it will move within its appointed limits. It can always be modest. And it will not on this account be any the less respect for life. It will be so in this modesty and in readiness for it. When we come to questions of detail, we shall see how important it is to remember this reservation, or rather this closer definition. Respect for life without this closer identification could be the principle of an idolatry which has nothing whatever to do with Christian obedience.

But this reservation must now be strictly and sharply qualified. This inwardly necessary relativisation of what is required of us as respect for life, this recollection of the freedom of the controlling and commanding God and of eternal life as the limitation of this present life, must not be forgotten for a single moment. But the application of this reservation, the reference to it and the corresponding modesty, cannot have more than the character of an *ultima ratio,* an exceptional case. They arise only on the frontiers of life and therefore of the respect due it. Hence it is not true that respect for life is alternately commanded and then not commanded us. Neither is it true that alongside the sphere of this respect there is a sphere in which it is not normative, or only partially so. However much we understand by this respect and therefore by the commanded will to live is limited and relativised by God's free will and man's determination for a future life, this relativisation never means that man is released from this respect. The one God, who is of course the Lord of life and death, the Giver of this life and that which is to come, will in all circumstances and in every conceivable modification demand respect for life. He will never give man liberty to take another view of life, whether his own or that of others. Indifference, wantonness, arbitrariness or anything else opposed to respect cannot even be considered as a commanded or even a permitted attitude. Even the way to these frontiers — the frontiers where respect for life and the will to live can assume in practice very strange and paradoxical forms, where in relation to one's own life and that of others it can only be a matter of that relativised, weakened, broken and even destroyed will to live — will always be a long one which we must take thoughtfully and conscientiously, continually asking and testing whether that *ultima ratio* really applies. The frontiers must not be arbitrarily advanced in any spirit of frivolity or pedantry; they can be only reached in obedience and then respected as such. Recollection of the freedom and superior wisdom, goodness and controlling power of God, and recollection of the future life, cannot then form a pretext or excuse for attitudes and modes of action in which many may actually evade what is commanded within these limits. They are frontiers which are necessarily set by God, and cannot be claimed as emancipations of man. This will be best understood by those who do not treat respect for life as a principle set up by man. Even on these frontiers they will not see a relaxation of the command or exception to the rule, but only a relaxation of that which they think they should understand and offer as obedience when they accept it as a summons to the will to live. Even here there will be required of them a new and deeper understanding of the will to live, which *ultima ratione* can now take the form of a broken and even destroyed will to live, and, if it be the will of God, must necessarily do so. Yet if it is an obedient and not frivolous will, if it is not wantonness and self-will, it must always be the will to live, and therefore the practical form of respect for life.

98 Alien Dignity: The Legacy of Helmut Thielicke for Bioethics

Karen Lebacqz

This experience of rejection made me think that there was no God, because in moments of rejection like that one I feel I am no good. And if I am no good, how can there be any God? Am I not made in the image and likeness of God?[1]

With these haunting words, Ada Maria Isasi-Diaz points not only to the painful realities of racism and sexism in our midst but also to the centrality of the image of God for theological ethics and to the intimate link between that image and the valuation of human beings. "If I am no good, how can there by any God? Am I not made in the image and likeness of God?" What does it mean to be made in the image and likeness of God and how does it relate to our valuation as persons?

No modern ethicist has elaborated the link between the image of God and the valuing of persons with more care than the great German theologian Helmut Thielicke. Twenty-five years ago Thielicke provided the reflections on theological foundations for Houston's first international conference on ethics in medicine and technology. In "The Doctor as Judge of Who Shall Live and Who Shall Die,"[2] Thielicke suggested that there are two ways to view people: in terms of their utility, or in terms of their "infinite worth." Thielicke opted for their infinite worth, and based that option on his understanding of the "alien dignity" of persons.

In this essay, I will explore briefly the theological roots and meaning of "alien dignity" in Thielicke's thought, and then develop the legacy of this term for the task of health care ethics today by illustrating its implications in several arenas of medicine and health care. Although there are problems with the concept of alien dignity, I will argue that it provides a rich legacy for protecting and equalizing human beings, for requiring personal responsibility, for attending to structural prob-

1. Ada Maria Isasi-Diaz, "Las Palmas Reales de Ada," in Katie G. Cannon et al. (The Mudflower Collective), *God's Fierce Whimsy* (New York: Pilgrim Press, 1985), 106.

2. Helmut Thielicke, "The Doctor as Judge of Who Shall Live and Who Shall Die," in Kenneth Vaux, ed., *Who Shall Live? Medicine, Technology, Ethics* (Philadelphia: Fortress Press, 1970).

From Allen Verhey, ed., *Religion and Medical Ethics: Looking Back, Looking Forward* (Grand Rapids: Eerdmans, 1996), pp. 44-60.

lems in health care, and for seeing humans as fundamentally relational.

Alien Dignity and the Image of God

The "incommensurable, incalculable worth of human life,"[3] argued Thielicke, does not reside in any immanent quality of human beings, but in the fact that we are created and redeemed by God. Our worth is imparted by the love bestowed on us by God. Human worth is thus an "alien dignity," given in the relationship between humans and God. It is the image of God in us that gives us our alien dignity.

The image of God in humans was not, for Thielicke, a given attribute or property, such as rationality or even freedom.[4] Rather, "the divine likeness rests on the fact that God remembers [us]. . . ."[5] The image of God is not our own immanent or ontic dignity, not some quality such as rationality that "imitates" the character of the divine, but rather a statement of our relationship to God. To speak of the *imago Dei* is to speak of God's love for us. God creates us in love, calls us in love, and redeems us in love; and it is this love that creates the image of God in us and gives us our worth. The image of God is not substantive, but relational.

Human worth is therefore "alien" in the sense that it comes to us from God. It is "that alien dignity which is grounded in and by [the one] who does the giving."[6] As a *proprium,* a true ontic possession or attribute in the strict sense, it belongs only to Christ.[7] The divine likeness of human beings is fulfilled only in Christ. Only in Christ is there the immediacy of relation to God that constitutes the *imago Dei,* and that was destroyed in the "Fall." The immediacy thus lost is restored in Christ, and so we participate in this divine likeness through Christ. God "remembers" us and draws us back into proper relationship, and herein lies the image of God.

The image of God is therefore ineffable and difficult to describe concretely, since it does not consist in specific characteristics or attributes that can easily be named.[8] For Thielicke, the divine image in humans was like a mirror reflecting the glory of God. Like a mirror, the image goes dark when the source of light is withdrawn: "it possesses only borrowed light."[9]

The *imago Dei* is thus, substantively, a representation of agape — of God's love for humans. It is therefore also agape that recognizes and realizes the *imago Dei,* seeing the other person in her standing before God rather than in her "utility" value for me. It is agape that allows us to love our enemies, not identifying them with their opposition to us, but seeing in them the children of God.[10]

For Thielicke, then, to speak of the alien dignity of human beings is to speak of their infinite worth. It is to speak of their relationship to God, and of the love with which they are held by God. It is to speak of what God has "spent" on human beings, the love poured out that creates an unimpeachable worth possessed by "even the most pitiful life."[11] To speak of alien dignity is to speak of the individual destiny received from God, of the indivisible totality of the person, of the person's standing in the eyes of God.

Problems with Alien Dignity

"Alien dignity" may not be a comfortable term today, especially for feminists and others from oppressed groups. Two problems are immediately evident. First, to speak of dignity as "alien" is to imply that it is not truly "ours." If the source is outside humans, then it seems something that is "not us." If it is only reflective of a light that originates elsewhere, then it seems that it could too easily be removed. To see dignity as "alien" thus seems to remove it too much from the *humanum* and to make it precarious.

In our post-Enlightenment world, and particularly since the human potential movement, the Western world has tended to stress the dignity and potential that are inherent to humans. We want a dignity that is *precisely* ours, that is so much a part of us that there can never be any recognition of us without an acknowledgment of that dignity. To suggest that one's dignity is "alien" and comes from outside may perhaps make us think that it is therefore more vulnerable to attack or erosion. We are probably more comfortable today with a notion of *intrinsic* dignity, as this notion would imply something so inbuilt that it can never be taken away.

Second, Thielicke's notion that alien dignity is like the reflection of a mirror in which all light comes from outside may appear to posit human beings as empty vessels. All value, all light, all dignity appear to come from God and from God alone. Thielicke's God seems distant and omnipotent. The gulf between the divine and the human seems virtually unbridgeable. Thielicke's alien dignity, the mirror reflecting God's light, seems to pose an all-powerful God and an all-empty human being: "the *imago Dei* depends on the reflecting of alien light, a process which is always under the control of the glory of God which casts the reflection."[12] Any sense of divine-human partnership seems fragile at best. We appear to have a process in which humans are at most pawns in a game controlled by God.

Such a transcendent, omnipotent God has been aban-

3. Thielicke, "Doctor as Judge," 170.

4. Helmut Thielicke, *Theological Ethics, Volume 1: Foundations,* ed. William H. Lazareth (Philadelphia: Fortress Press, 1966), 151.

5. Helmut Thielicke, *Theological Ethics,* vol. 1, 165.

6. Helmut Thielicke, *Theological Ethics,* vol. 1, 170.

7. Helmut Thielicke, *Theological Ethics,* vol. 1, 171.

8. Helmut Thielicke, *Theological Ethics,* vol. 1, 159.

9. Helmut Thielicke, *Theological Ethics,* vol. 1, 177.

10. Thielicke, *The Ethics of Sex,* trans. John W. Doberstein (New York: Harper & Row, 1964), 32.

11. Thielicke, "Doctor as Judge," 172.

12. Helmut Thielicke, *Theological Ethics,* vol. 1, 180.

doned in many contemporary theologies. Liberation and feminist theologians tend instead to speak of a vulnerable God who suffers with us or of a partnership between humans and God. How else are we to explain the suffering of children who are abused by their parents or of oppressed peoples everywhere? An omnipotent God who fails to intervene in human suffering seems a cruel hoax.[13]

We might wonder, then, whether Thielicke's notion of alien dignity is theologically and ethically adequate. Does it create too fragile a dignity, not sufficiently rooted in human nature itself? Does it pose a God too remote and removed for an age of liberation that needs a God who suffers with us?

Within the scope of this essay, I cannot fully address these questions. Nonetheless, I believe that such doubts may arise from a misreading of the implications of Thielicke's work, and that Thielicke's core notion of alien dignity offers protections and insights badly needed today. I will illustrate this claim by pointing to five implications of alien dignity and their application in bioethics.

Implications of Alien Dignity for Ethics

1. Alien Dignity Protects People

That human dignity is "alien" does mean that it comes from outside me; it does not arise from within me. But for Thielicke, it is also integral to me. Since it is given to me in my very creation by God, since it is bestowed from the beginning with God's love, it is always present with me. It is therefore intimately mine, as truly mine as any of my characteristics and far more enduring. My youth will surely pass, my beauty will fade, but my alien dignity does *not* dim, in Thielicke's view.

Precisely because human dignity is "alien," it does not have to be *earned,* and it cannot be *lost.* It does not depend on my skin color, my sex, my sexual orientation, my intelligence, or any other particular characteristic or achievement. It does not depend on "works."[14] Precisely because it is "alien" to me, it cannot be given away by me or taken away by others. It is both alien and inalienable. It is indelible, a mark put on us by God's love that permeates our being to the core. Since the alien dignity of humans depends only on God's love, and since God's love is constant and enduring, so is the dignity of each person.

To speak of alien dignity is therefore precisely a way of securing the basic inalienable worth of every person. Alien dignity *protects* people. They are inviolable. "Even the most pitiful life" retains its dignity, and its incommensurable, incalculable worth. Because of this worth, humans may not be subjected to the dictatorial rule of technical capacities.[15]

The concept of alien dignity thus provides a strong base for responding to difficult bioethical questions such as when to cease treatment. In "House Calls to Cardinal Jackson," David Schiedermayer struggles to explain why he continues to treat a 79-year-old woman who has been "mindless, lights-on-but-nobody's-home" for over ten years.[16] In trying to explain why he does not withdraw her feeding tube, Schiedermayer speaks of the daughter's love for the old woman and also of the fire that still burns in her green eyes. Then he asks:

> What is it that gives a person dignity? What is that inner grace that projects out toward the doctor, so that he, despite his intellect and education and training and skills, is taken aback? . . . The dignified are above reproach. You can't take dignity away from the dignified.[17]

Schiedermayer speaks here of the dignity of a woman who no longer functions as she once did. There is something about Cardinal Jackson that makes her inviolable to him, in spite of her advanced age and her mental incompetence. This something, which Schiedermayer calls her dignity, is what Thielicke would have called her alien dignity. For Thielicke, it is the worth that does not fade with age nor dim with incompetence because it comes from God.[18] Schiedermayer finds it harder to name the source of the dignity. He mentions not the love of God but the love of Cardinal Jackson's daughter, the hardship of Cardinal Jackson's life, the sense that we cannot abandon her after her history of discrimination and mistreatment.

While Schiedermayer does not name the same source of dignity that Thielicke would name, his understanding of the inviolability conferred by that dignity comes very close to Thielicke's. For Thielicke, alien dignity of humans means that others can never be treated simply for their instrumental value. They cannot be a means to an end for me. Their technical or utilitarian capacities do not define their worth. Hence, they do not lose their worth when they cease to function or when their capacities diminish.

In *The Ethics of Sex,*[19] for example, Thielicke argues against prostitution because it entails the instrumentalization of a human being. Such instrumentalization — turning the other into an instrument for my pleasure or satisfaction — is contrary to the alien dignity that prevents another from being simply a means to my ends.

Elsewhere, Thielicke argues that one can never fully possess another human being. To try to do so would be to destroy him at the center of his being.[20] One cannot

13. See, e.g., Wendy Farley, *Tragic Vision and Divine Compassion: A Contemporary Theodicy* (Louisville, Ky.: Westminster/John Knox Press, 1990); Joanne Carlson Brown and Carole R. Bohn, eds., *Christianity, Patriarchy, and Abuse: A Feminist Critique* (New York: Pilgrim Press, 1989).

14. It also does not depend on faith, but only on the image of God. Thus, even the nonbeliever would have dignity.

15. Thielicke, "Doctor as Judge," 186.

16. David Schiedermayer, "The Case: House Calls to Cardinal Jackson," *Second Opinion* 17, no. 4 (April, 1992): 35-40.

17. Schiedermayer, "The Case," 39.

18. Indeed, for Thielicke, her dignity would remain even if there was no fire in her eyes and no love proffered by her daughter.

19. Thielicke, *Ethics of Sex,* 33.

20. Thielicke, *Ethics of Sex,* 61.

split off parts of a person or objectify that person, but must deal with the whole person, with the "indivisible totality of a human being."[21] Only this is recognition of the alien dignity of the other.

Nor are others subject to the fickle nature of our emotions. To see another as the bearer of an alien dignity means that our regard for that other will remain even when her or his importance for us diminishes.[22]

Thus, in none of these ways can we take away the dignity of the other. Alien dignity protects the other from our vagaries, from objectification or instrumentalization, from our lust for possession or for power, from our imposition of our goals and purposes. If Cardinal Jackson's daughter tired of caring for her mother and ceased to love her, the old woman would not lose her dignity, in Thielicke's view.

In the medical arena, the inviolable worth of the other means that no one could simply be used, for example, as an organ bank. It means that research on human beings must respect those persons as whole beings, even if they are convicted criminals or the "most pitiful" of mental patients.[23] The notion of alien dignity provides fundamental protections against using persons as means to the ends of others, against objectifying people, against the intrusions of power to oppress the powerless.

2. *Alien Dignity Equalizes People*

If the first implication of alien dignity is the protection of persons, the second is the equalization of persons. Since human worth is not earned or achieved, but given by God, no one is "worth" more than others. All were bought for a price, and therefore all carry an incalculable value. The worth of human life for Thielicke was "incommensurable" — it is not possible to measure one person's worth against another. Genuine agape, which recognizes the alien dignity in the other, "does not degrade the other person." Rather, it honors the other, and puts the other "on the same level" as the one doing the loving.[24] Alien dignity has an equalizing effect.

This is reinforced by understanding that alien dignity would never allow the other to be dealt with simply in utilitarian terms. The "use value" or "social contribution value" of the person is not the person's true value. Only the alien dignity, the love poured out by God, represents the true value of the person. This value is unique, individual, incommensurable.

Operating out of this understanding of alien dignity would therefore prevent some approaches to the allocation of health care resources. In his study of medical directors of kidney dialysis and transplant facilities, John Kilner found that "more than half of the directors would assess the different social value of various candidates" for dialysis or transplant, and "less than a third would institute a more egalitarian random selection."[25] Thielicke's understanding of alien dignity would suggest that such attempts to measure the social worth of candidates for dialysis violates the incommensurable dignity of each.

In "The Doctor as Judge of Who Shall Live and Who Shall Die," Thielicke tackled directly the problem of insufficient resources to help those who might live with medical intervention. He recognized explicitly that at times, difficult choices must be made and some must be chosen to live while others die. Under these circumstances, humans will make the best choices they can. Considerations of social worth may in fact enter those choices. But there can never be, for Thielicke, an easy conscience about this choice. "One must simply run the risk of making the decision — and be prepared in so doing to err, and thereby to incur guilt."[26] When we must choose some to live at the price of death for others, we should experience that choice as wounding. These are the wounds that "must not be allowed to heal."[27] They touch on a deep "metaphysical" guilt that is built into the very structure of human existence[28] and that, ironically, makes us sound and healthy. Not to experience such guilt would be a sign that we forget the alien dignity and hence equality of all; to experience it is a sign that we recognize the alien dignity and equal worth of each. To do so is to be in partnership; thus, experiencing metaphysical guilt means that we remain fundamentally in relationship and hence healthy.

To say that alien dignity equalizes people is not to say that it makes everyone the same. The great diversity of human life is never denied by Thielicke. Indeed, he held to some traditional notions, for example, of the differences between men and women and of the roles appropriate to them. But even in the midst of recognizing these differences, Thielicke held that women were right to demand respect because their alien dignity makes them "equal before God."[29] Women's different *roles* did not affect women's basic *worth* or *equality* with men, which is secured by their alien dignity. Similarly, people's different roles or status in life do not affect their basic value, which is secured by their alien dignity. Precisely because we are made in the image and likeness of God, we cannot be rejected as being "no good." Whatever our race, color, sex, class, or social status, we are all equal in the eyes of God.

From the notion of alien dignity, then, might come

21. Thielicke, *Ethics of Sex*, 63.

22. Thielicke, *Ethics of Sex*, 27.

23. See The National Commission for the Protection of Human Subjects, *Research Involving Those Institutionalized as Mentally Infirm*, DHEW #OS-78-0006, and *Research Involving Prisoners*, DHEW #OS-76-131.

24. Thielicke, *Theological Ethics, Volume 2: Politics*, ed. William H. Lazareth (Philadelphia: Fortress Press, 1969), 305.

25. John K. Kilner, "Selecting Patients When Resources Are Limited: A Study of U.S. Medical Directors of Kidney Dialysis and Transplantation Facilities," *American Journal of Public Health* 78, no. 2 (1988): 146.

26. Thielicke, "Doctor as Judge," 166.

27. Thielicke, "Doctor as Judge," 173.

28. Thielicke, "Doctor as Judge," 164.

29. Thielicke, *Ethics of Sex*, 12.

an appreciation not only of the protectability of humans, but of their equality without diversity. As the Human Genome Project continues to locate and define the many genes that make up human beings, it will be increasingly important to find a grounding for understanding equality in the midst of diversity. Our history of genetic discrimination indicates all too graphically how easy it is for human communities to establish genetic norms and discriminate against those who do not fit the norm.[30] As the Human Genome Project progresses, there is the danger that we will make judgments of social worth based on individual genomes. Troy Duster charges that we are opening a "backdoor" to eugenics, legitimizing social discrimination under the name of genetic science as we seek to correct "defective" genes.[31] Some will be judged not to have "normal" genes, others to have "superior" genes. Such judgments are exactly what the concept of "alien dignity" prevents. To accept diversity and yet affirm equality may be the most important challenge that lies before us in the realm of genetics. Thielicke's notion of alien dignity captures the underlying premise of equal worth amidst differing manifestations of human life.

3. *Alien Dignity Requires Personal Response*

For Thielicke, the alien dignity of the other required an "I-Thou" relationship. Agape must be immediate, improvisational, non-routinized.[32] For Thielicke, there is no escaping personal responsibility by assuming that institutions or others will take over. The institutionalization of agape was therefore problematic: "Does not the Samaritan's ministry of mercy become inconceivable, is it not altered in its very substance, the moment it is institutionalized? . . ."[33] Thielicke cautioned against the "welfare state," because "no one is ever summoned personally" or need take personal responsibility in it.[34] In the welfare state, care would be "rationalized," and this very rationalization would kill the agape element in it.[35] Thus, the agape that responds to the alien dignity of the other, and in so responding realizes that dignity, must always be a personal response.

In the arena of health care, such a view may be an important corrective to the assumption that "others" or "the system" will provide. In the United States, for example, 95 percent of elderly people live not in nursing homes but in the community, dependent on care by family, friends, or hired workers. More than 80 percent are cared for by families, and in 75 percent of these cases, the caregiver is a woman. Most of these women are over the age of fifty and not always in the best of health themselves.[36]

On the one hand, Thielicke would probably applaud these women. They have chosen positively, lovingly, and willingly to care for elderly spouses or parents. They exhibit agape. They assume personal responsibility.

On the other hand, the fact that 75 percent of the care is being done by women should make us ask, Where are the men? In Thielicke's view, no one should escape from personal response to and responsibility for the needs of others. A society that allows some to escape responsibility while others carry the burden would not meet with Thielicke's approval. Since Thielicke did not believe that a ministry of mercy could be institutionalized without losing something of its basic character, the institutionalization of caring as "women's work" or a "female function" might also violate his understanding of the need for personal responsibility. Thus, alien dignity could provide correctives to some societal arrangements.

4. *Alien Dignity Requires Structural Response*

Thielicke's resistance to the institutionalization of care might be particularly problematic today for liberation theologians who stress the structural nature of injustice. It might seem at first glance that Thielicke's understanding of alien dignity would militate against nationalized health care or against a universal program such as that currently proposed by the Clinton administration. True, Clinton stressed personal responsibility in presenting his proposal to the nation. Responsibility is one of the principles presumably embedded in the design of the program.[37] Nonetheless, Clinton's program would require massive intervention on state and national levels to ensure access to health care for all American citizens and legal residents. Since Thielicke argued against routinization of care, one might wonder whether this I-Thou approach to alien dignity would undercut the Clinton plan.

Yet before we draw this conclusion, some nuancing is in order. It is true that Thielicke argued against the welfare state. The rationalization or routinizing of care, he asserted, ran counter to what is characteristic of Christian love of the neighbor.[38] He was particularly troubled by the argument that the welfare recipient could "claim" welfare as a right, and that claiming such a right would be seen to honor the dignity of the person in ways that offering charity or agape does not.[39] But one must understand why Thielicke was troubled in order to understand the structural implications of his reflections on the welfare state. In spite of his reservations, his under-

30. Troy Duster, *Backdoor to Eugenics* (New York: Routledge, 1990). See also John Horgan, "Eugenics Revisited," *Scientific American* 268, no. 6 (June 1993): 122-31.

31. Duster, *Backdoor to Eugenics,* 122-31.

32. Helmut Thielicke, *Theological Ethics,* vol. 2, 291.

33. Helmut Thielicke, *Theological Ethics,* vol. 2, 291.

34. Helmut Thielicke, *Theological Ethics,* vol. 2, 292.

35. Helmut Thielicke, *Theological Ethics,* vol. 2, 294.

36. See Tish Sommers and Laurie Shields, *Women Take Care: The Consequences of Caregiving in Today's Society* (Gainesville, Fla.: Triad Publishing, 1987), 21.

37. *American Health Security Act of 1993,* Sept. 7, 1993, section 10 (Washington, D.C.: Bureau of National Affairs, 1993).

38. Helmut Thielicke, *Theological Ethics,* vol. 2, 300.

39. Helmut Thielicke, *Theological Ethics,* vol. 2, 304.

standing of the implications of alien dignity pushes in the direction of a structural response to social and personal ills.

Thielicke's resistance to "rights" and preference for agape or charity was based on the understanding that love never degrades the other, but must treat the other as a true partner. "Rights" or claims separate people and force them into antagonistic relationships. Not antagonism, but a partnership "in the ultimate dimension" was, for Thielicke, the goal of all Christian action.[40] Precisely because of the alien dignity of the other, that other is meant to be seen as a person in the sight of God, never merely as an object. But if the other is a subject, contended Thielicke, then the other can never be left as the mere passive recipient of our actions. To do so is to degrade the other.

By the same token, poverty can never be accepted as the other person's fate.[41] The other must not simply be helped or sustained in poverty, but must "be restored to economic independence."[42] I have argued elsewhere that such restoration is implied by the Jubilee image of justice.[43] Such restoration requires structural undergirding. Rehabilitation was, for Thielicke, a proper undertaking of the state.[44]

In fact, for Thielicke the other must not simply be restored and helped to move out of poverty, but must be prevented from moving into poverty in the first place. "What is more urgently needed is preventive action."[45] Prevention, however, requires structural response: "a social order in which the right to gainful employment is assured and in which possibilities are created for the attainment of economic independence by way of education, financial credits, and the like."[46] Only such a structural, preventive response would constitute in Thielicke's view a genuine partnership or expression of agape.

Thus it is true that Thielicke argued for a limited role for the state and would not have condoned either the Marxist analysis or the more extensive welfare state supported in some liberation treatises today. At root, he understood agape to be a deeply personal response, and he shied away from any institutional response that would relieve personal responsibility. He feared the "impersonal machine" that would take away direct person-to-person care.[47] Nonetheless, his understanding of alien dignity also required preventive and structured response, in order to support the dignity of the other and the true partnership between people and between people and the state. Most significantly, it required not simply "charity" but moving people to a place of restored autonomy and self-support. Thielicke recognized the structural components of poverty and other human ills, and his understanding of alien dignity required attention to these components. To argue that the social order must guarantee a "right to gainful employment" is to take a large step toward structural justice.

By extension from this reasoning, I believe that we could also see in Thielicke's work the structural demands for a system of universal health care. If, as President Clinton said in his address to the nation, health care is crucial to the security necessary in order for people to make free choices and take risks for the future, then health care would be one of the structural demands of agape. Universal access to basic health care would recognize the alien dignity of all.

5. *Alien Dignity Is Relational*

It is clear by now that Thielicke's concept of alien dignity is relational through and through. To have dignity is to be in relation.

First, it is to be in relation to God, who gives the dignity by investing love in people. Thus, one cannot speak of alien dignity without speaking of God's relationship to humankind. The very concept depends on relationality. Indeed, it connotes relationality, since for Thielicke alien dignity is not an "ontic" possession but precisely a statement of our relationship to God.

Second, to have alien dignity is to be in relation to people. It is others who realize our dignity by acting out of agape, out of a perspective of who we are before God. The term thus implies not only our "vertical" relation to God but also our "horizontal" relation to others.

Alien dignity is therefore very *personal,* but it is not *private* or atomistic. Dignity derives *between* beings — between humans and God, between humans and other humans. Thielicke called alien dignity "teleological, not ontological."[48] By this he meant that it does not refer to human characteristics or status, but to the purposes for which we are created by God. The term implies connections between beings and a fundamental covenant of life with life. To speak of alien dignity is therefore always to point us to relationship, interdependence, and covenant.

In this relationality, love is central. It is God's love that establishes the alien dignity of humans. It is human love that recognizes and realizes it. Once we know that God, like every mother, loves precisely the vulnerable and weak ones, then we know how irrevocable is the dignity of the poor and outcast. "If I am no good, how can there be any God? Am I not made in the image and likeness of God?" Our fate is not sealed by our actions or by the judgments of others about us, but by the love of God for us. Alien dignity is a Christological concept for Thielicke.

This notion of relationality also has important implications for contemporary bioethics. Criticisms of the

40. Helmut Thielicke, *Theological Ethics,* vol. 2, 305.
41. Helmut Thielicke, *Theological Ethics,* vol. 2, 306.
42. Helmut Thielicke, *Theological Ethics,* vol. 2, 306.
43. See Karen Lebacqz, *Justice in an Unjust World* (Minneapolis: Augsburg Publishing House, 1987), ch. 7.
44. Helmut Thielicke, *Theological Ethics,* vol. 2, 307.
45. Helmut Thielicke, *Theological Ethics,* vol. 2, 306.
46. Helmut Thielicke, *Theological Ethics,* vol. 2, 306.
47. Helmut Thielicke, *Theological Ethics,* vol. 2, 313.
48. Helmut Thielicke, *Theological Ethics,* vol. 1, 154.

current stress on "autonomy" are now legion.[49] Increasingly, bioethicists are searching for an approach to ethics that neither isolates the individual nor manufactures a false autonomy, but places the individual in social context, recognizing the role of family, of fiduciary relationships, of diminished autonomy. Feminists have been particularly keen on stressing caring and relationship as central to the tasks of ethics.

Thielicke's notion of alien dignity fits well with these concerns. Cardinal Jackson's dignity was not dependent on her mental capacity, but rather on her relationships. Significantly, as Schiedermayer struggled with what gave Jackson her dignity, he pointed both to past relationships and to present ones, both to relationships of harm and to relationships of love. Cardinal Jackson's unassailable dignity came for him in part because of the love that her daughter still held for her. But it also came because a history of discrimination and mistreatment required a form of reparations — of refusing to abandon now one who had been abandoned in the past. In his own way, Schiedermayer attempts to establish a covenant that would assure Cardinal Jackson and her family that her dignity remained evident and appreciated. Cardinal Jackson does not have to have autonomy in order to be in relationship, to be the recipient of duties such as reparations on the part of others, to be loved and recognized. Her dignity — what Thielicke would call her alien dignity — is relational and implies covenant.

In response to Isasi-Diaz, Schiedermayer might say that the fact that she has experienced racist rejection in the past is precisely what gives her an inviolable dignity, just as it has contributed to that dignity for Cardinal Jackson. A relationship need not be one of love in order to remind us of the inviolable dignity of the other. Alien dignity requires a relational understanding of human life.

Conclusions

When Helmet Thielicke spoke to the first international conference on ethics in medicine and technology twenty-five years ago, health care ethics was in its infancy. The Human Genome Project, Kevorkian's "suicide machine" — these were unknowns. Abortion was not legal in the United States, in vitro fertilization clinics were not dotting the landscape as they now do. Much has changed in the intervening years.

Yet much has also remained the same. The genome project, assisted suicide, legalized abortion, in vitro fertilization — these modern developments raise ancient questions: should there be limits to human intervention in nature; when if at all is it permissible to take human life; should human bodies be bought and sold? At the root of these questions lies the ever present dilemma of the valuing of human life. What does it mean to be human, and what gives human life its worth?

It is to these foundational questions that Thielicke addressed his understanding of alien dignity. "If I am no good, how can there be any God? Am I not made in the image and likeness of God?" queries Isasi-Diaz. For Thielicke, being made in the image and likeness of God meant that each person gained an alien dignity that stamped a fundamental worth on that person — a worth so central and ineradicable that nothing done by oneself or by others could ever remove it. If there is a God, and if God is good, then so are we, for we are made in the image of God.

To be sure, Thielicke's precise formulation of alien dignity raises some problems. Although he speaks of partnership "in the ultimate dimension," it is not clear whether his understanding of alien dignity implies a true partnership between humans and God. His God seems distant and wholly "other," his human beings perhaps a bit too empty. Human dignity seems removed, perhaps a bit too alien.

Yet in spite of these problems, there is an enduring legacy here to which we would do well to attend. The notion of alien dignity provides considerable protection to human beings. It keeps us from being used as objects of others' desires or schemes and from being swept up in the instrumentalization of human life. This may be important for our consideration as we move toward increasing technological imperatives. Alien dignity also has a powerful equalizing vector, which may be important as we struggle to understand how to do ethics in the midst of diversity. Alien dignity requires both the immediacy of love and personal responsibility on the one hand, and on the other hand structures that undergird true partnership. It neither lets us off the hook nor reduces ethical action to mere sentimentality.[50] Finally, alien dignity requires a relational view of human beings. Such a focus on relationality is consonant with many feminist approaches to ethics, and provides an important corrective to the contemporary stress in bioethics on autonomy.

49. See, e.g., Marshall B. Kapp, "Medical Empowerment of the Elderly," *Hastings Center Report* (July-August, 1989): 5-7, George J. Agich, "Reassessing Autonomy in Long Term Care," *Hastings Center Report* (November-December 1990): 12-17.

50. Some feminist texts that take "caring" or love as central to ethics do run the risk of dealing only with immediate relationships and failing to provide structural supports. See, for example, Nel Noddings, *Caring: A Feminist Approach to Ethics and Moral Education* (Berkeley: University of California Press, 1984).

99 Toward Freedom from Value

Richard Stith

Introduction

Few would wish for a world where life would always be preserved indefinitely and at all costs, for we feel that life ought sometimes to give way to other human aspirations. At the same time, most of us hold inviolable the life of every individual, regardless of its usefulness for the achievement of our heart's desires.

We have, then, two intuitions: that life must not be destroyed, but that it need not be always preserved; that every person's life is infinitely valuable, but that other things may sometimes be more valuable; that human life has sanctity, but that death may occasionally be welcomed. As we seek to map out even a crooked frontier separating these two sovereign intuitions, we soon learn that each lays claim to perhaps the entire territory of the other, and that neither will remain satisfied for long with those apparently "convenient" compromises represented by distinctions between "active and passive" or "ordinary and extraordinary." If life has infinite value, how can we passively abandon it when its preservation becomes burdensome? Or, if we can indeed abandon it, perhaps it has little value after all, and therefore may be violated. So we discover not only that we cannot easily draw a clear line of separation between our two intuitions, but also that each seeks to annihilate the other.

If we wish to intervene to prevent either side from suffering a total rout, we must begin by finding high ground from which we can describe the proper limits of each. That is, we must develop an appealing and understandable theory of the nature and limits of the prohibition on taking human life.[1]

Here again is our dilemma: if we set the value of life low enough to account for the moral[2] intuition that we need not preserve life at all costs, we have set it too low to account for our other intuition that we ought not to kill no matter what benefits we might gain. On the other hand, if we raise the value of life to the point where no benefits are weighty enough to justify killing, we soon discover that we have committed ourselves to a surely excessive effort to eliminate death. It is my belief that our error here does not lie in valuing "mere" life or "quality" life too highly or too lowly, but rather springs from the ordinary use of the word "value." Is there no other word available? Is there no attitude, besides that of "valuing," which we take to life? I suggest that we already know and name the attitude for which we are searching: "reverence." And we also speak often about the aspect of life which accounts for our attitude of reverence: "sanctity." Unfortunately, life's *sanctity* is ordinarily confounded, or even identified, with its *value* — so that to say that life has sanctity is popularly taken to mean that it has great (or even absolute or infinite) value. Yet it is my contention that sanctity and value are radically different, and that it is precisely thinking in terms of value which obscures and may destroy our sense of the demands of human life. Only by first overthrowing the rulership of value-thought can contemporary man hope to *think* clearly about what he still already knows.

Why not kill? This essay seeks to say what there is about human life[3] as we perceive it which could account for our moral intuition that killing is wrong. In the first part of the essay, it will be argued that the value of life cannot account for the prohibition on killing for two reasons: (1) we often give life such a low "value" that this value alone would be insufficient to preclude permission to kill, and (2) we would not feel killing to be forbidden even if we were to value life infinitely. The value of life, even when made absolute, cannot preclude the taking of life. This is so not because of any defect in life, but because of the impotence of the concept and attitude called

1. By "life" or "human life" I mean "living humans." This meaning, I take it, is that most commonly understood in speaking of the value or sanctity of human life. To "value human life" thus means to "value people" — except that the first phrase focuses upon those valued as simply alive, while the second pulls us away from the question of life or death and toward the complexities of social existence. Put another way, human life is the foundation which all people have in common; to value life is thus to value people simply because of this foundation rather than because of their maturity, personality, or whatever. A newborn baby is perhaps the clearest example of naked human life.

By contrast, I do not in this essay take seriously the frequent way of speaking which treats life as a thing which may be "given to" or "taken from" someone. For an organism, to live is to *exist*. The idea that existence (life) is a separate entity which can be added to or subtracted from a person seems to me a worthy subject for reflection, but only indirectly and confusedly applicable to the question of whether or not we may destroy people. When I say "taking human life," I mean eliminating it, not removing it.

2. Except where otherwise stated, this essay deals entirely with morality, and with the moral underpinning of law, rather than with law itself.

3. Implicit here is that there is phenomenologically something *about life* which makes us reluctant to kill. We do not refrain from killing *only* out of obedience to a disincarnate moral rule not to kill, whether that rule derived from God or from ourselves. We genuinely care about not harming people, and therefore are already reluctant to destroy them prior to explicit reflection upon God's commands or upon the moral rules which we personally would like everyone to follow.

Furthermore, we do not feel such rules themselves to be arbitrary or to have a status no higher than our desires. Rightly or wrongly, we feel that they are an expression of human dignity rather than *only* of formalized self-interest or will. In this essay, I argue that this dignity cannot be called "value."

From *The Jurist* 38 (Winter 1978). Used by permission.

valuing. Because all valuing is for a type (or essence), I will argue, it can demand only that a quantity or quality of life exist, but never that a particular person live or be allowed to live. (To debate quantity vs. quality of life is thus *already* depersonalizing, no matter which side one takes.)

Having attacked the notion of valuing and having demonstrated the inadequacy of the attitude we take to life when we value it, in the second part of this essay I shall describe and distinguish the attitude of reverence, the object of which has sanctity rather than value. Here it will be argued that the sanctity of life primarily demands nonviolation — rather than preservation — of life, and therefore can both forbid the taking of life and coexist with the nonpreservation of life. Thus, both of our original intuitions can be affirmed: sanctity makes the individual *matter,* in a way which value does not, and yet does not demand his preservation at all costs.

Dependency, however, raises difficult problems for the meaning of sanctity. If someone's life is dependent upon our actions, is there a difference between causing death and not preserving life? This dilemma is most often currently discussed in the medical context, but it is surely as ancient as the helplessness of every newborn. Its solution, I shall argue, lies not in behavioral but in intentional criteria for actions violative of the sanctity of life.

Finally, some practical consequences of the theory of sanctity will be developed. The demands of sanctity will be described first vis-à-vis medical patients and then as a guide to social and economic planning.

I. The Insufficiency of Value

Not all of us regard killing as always wrong. Most make an exception for self-defense; many do so in cases ranging from war and capital punishment to selective euthanasia. But all of us are *reluctant* to kill. Why?

Perhaps the most frequent answer to this question is "because of the value of life." Indeed, advocates of an absolute prohibition on, say, capital punishment or euthanasia are wont to cite "the *infinite* value of life." And for people used to translating all ethical and policy issues into "value" terminology, these answers are quite understandable. After all, why *would* we protect life unless it had value? And how could the value of life *never* be outweighted unless it were infinite?

Nevertheless, it is my contention here that the value of life cannot adequately explain our reluctance to kill, that some other factor is at work. I shall try to demonstrate this thesis by first showing that even where life's value is clearly insufficient to outweigh other relevant values, we do not kill. Therefore, more than the *value* of life must matter to us. Further, I shall show that even if life had infinite value, this alone could not make killing wrong in many situations where we refrain from killing. And so, again, I conclude that we regard life as having more than value and in subsequent sections will move beyond value in search of the missing element that explains our intuitions.

Sometimes life is not valued highly. For example, many doctors would be willing not to use "extraordinary" measures in order to preserve the lives of persons able to live only a very short time in any event.[4] Such minimal amounts of life are seemingly considered not valuable enough in themselves to require the costs of heroic treatment. Yet at the same time, these physicians are apparently reluctant to kill actively and deliberately in order to avoid equivalent future costs. Why? Do these doctors see something else in life besides its value?

Even a healthy normal life may have insufficient "value" to outweigh other considerations. I am not referring here to the oft-cited case of martyrdom where someone sacrifices his own life for the sake of some noble ideal,[5] but rather, I am speaking of those instances where we value our own *and others'* lives less than comfort and convenience — as is the case with all limitations on "safety." Without a doubt we could individually and collectively live far more safely and so protect life better if we were willing to put up with the accompanying decline in life's "quality."

Nowhere is this fact more obvious than in the question of speed limits. By not drastically lowering the speed limit, our various governments and their constituencies are with statistical *certainty* allowing tens of thousands of violent deaths to occur. Nor do these deaths occur only to those who have chosen to "assume the risk" of driving. Pedestrians and dependents (e.g., children) are also killed; and given our society and economy, even those who "choose" to drive can hardly be said to have much choice in the matter. The simple fact is that thousands upon thousands of innocent and unwilling victims of traffic accidents die each year because our society and government do not want the decline in mobility and in GNP which would be caused by a speed-limit reduction.

And yet my torts teacher, Guido Calabresi, found no takers when he presented to our law school class the hypothetical case of a god who offered us an equivalent increase in societal well-being if we would agree to kill one

4. See the 1973 A.M.A. statement condemning intentional mercy killing but allowing cessation of extraordinary life support, reprinted and criticized for inconsistency in the important article by J. Rachels, "Active and Passive Euthanasia," *New England Journal of Medicine* 292:2 (January 9, 1975): 78-80. Rachels in turn has been criticized (rightly, in my opinion) by T. Sullivan for misunderstanding the A.M.A. position. See "Active and Passive Euthanasia: An Impertinent Distinction?" in *The Human Life Review* 3:3 (Summer, 1977): 40-46. Sullivan's distinctions are similar, but not identical, to those developed below.

5. Nor am I here or elsewhere in this essay thinking of intentional suicide. The primary method of this essay (placing human life before us, and asking our attitude toward it) is simply not easily adaptable to an examination of self-killing. Perhaps our conclusions are nevertheless applicable to suicide: See the powerful attempt by Germain Grisez to grapple with suicide within a project in many ways similar to that of this essay in "Suicide and Euthanasia," *Death, Dying and Euthanasia,* edited by D. Horan and D. Mall (Washington: University Publications of America, 1977), pp. 742-817.

thousand persons on an altar each year. Why this difference? Why was the class simultaneously willing (albeit with qualms) to let many die in traffic deaths and unwilling to produce the same benefits by the "sacrifice" of a lesser number?[6]

No adequate answer to these questions is possible, I submit, as long as we persist in treating human lives merely as valued objects. The way we regard people, which includes a reluctance to destroy them, has very little analogy to the way we treat that which we value, as we can see again by turning to the "potentiality-actuality" continuum — first in regard to things we value (money and justice, for example) and second in regard to human life.

Now, an object which is valued when we have it (in "actuality"), is also valued when we *could* have it (in "potentiality"). True, we discount the value of the latter by the time, trouble, and uncertainty involved. But we would surely think someone at least confused who were stingy with money that he did not wish to have it in the first place. Or again, we would doubt the sincerity of someone who strongly resisted increased injustice and yet also opposed increased justice.

But in an age of individualism and of possible overpopulation, this strange stance seems to be exactly what many people take toward other human beings. As individuals and as a society, many of us do not wish more children, do not consider them a net value when considering their possible existence. Yet once a child is born (or once it is conceived), killing is for most of us out of the question — even if the child is still "unwanted." This reluctance to destroy that which we never wanted to begin with would border on insanity if we were speaking of something we merely valued. We cannot explain our disinclination to kill by saying simply that we value human life, because sometimes we do not value it and yet are still reluctant to kill.

I have so far argued that life's value is sometimes relatively too low to be sufficient to prevent killing and that we should look elsewhere for reasons not to kill. However, I suspect that at least some of us will not be ready to give up on value this easily. Not knowing what else we may find, some may be appropriately cautious about casting loose from what may seem the only firm mooring for the protection of life. "Should we not," some of us might ask, "find ways instead to increase the value we give to life, even at the cost of a larger population, more respirators, and even more bicycles?"

I want to cut off this last hope in the value of life by arguing that even if we somehow could agree that human life had *infinite* value, we would not necessarily prohibit killing. Only when this has been shown will the inadequacy of value be sufficiently clear to send us in search of a new base on which to anchor the protection of life.

Let us assume, then, for the sake of argument, that human life has infinite value, meaning that a human being is so valuable, of such great worth, that no other kind of entity (thing, relationship, or whatever) or combination of entities can ever be preferable to such a being. In other words, insofar as we choose rationally that which is most valuable, we would *never* choose something else instead of a living human being. Consequently, we would never destroy such a being, no matter what other kinds of benefits we might realize.

But, I submit, we might well destroy such a being for the sake of the *same* kinds of benefits (i.e., human life). Indeed, if we felt that human life were of infinite value, we might well feel morally compelled to kill, whenever such killing would save more lives than those lost.[7] We would promote capital punishment, for example, if it were the only effective means of deterring a greater number of killings. We also would kill a healthy person if his vital organs were needed to save his two ailing siblings.

We might also kill for reasons other than saving life. If life were really of infinite value but our resources were limited, would we not favor those who were more fertile and/or lived longest at least cost? Would we not like some kind of "breeder," to put to sleep the fat and the sick to make room for more people to replace them? If every single life had tremendous value, we would want as many as we could afford, for as long as possible, even if this meant destroying those requiring greater care, resources, or space.

Nor would we avoid comparing the lives we valued, and perhaps killing would result. Even if all lives had infinite value, we would have no rational objection to killing whenever an equal *substitute* were available. Even if I valued Austro-Hungarian gold coins infinitely, I would not have any objection to exchanging equivalent coins. So, too, I would not object, say, to killing the newborn if they could be quickly replaced and extra inconvenience compensated for. Moreover, I would actually *prefer* to destroy and replace if the quality of what I have could be in any way improved. Even if I valued those coins infinitely (in that I would give *anything* else to have even one), I no doubt would rather have one without a scratch. Similarly, even though I value every baby infinitely, I would prefer to have one of maximum quality, as long as it is easy to have "defective" ones sent back to their maker and new ones substituted. No value of human life can preclude killing simply to improve life's quality.

These last examples begin to reveal the reason why no amount of *valuing* of human life, not even infinite valuing, can be in harmony with our intuitive regard for life:

6. For Calabresi's own explanation of this kind of discrepancy, which differs from my own, see "Reflections on Medical Experimentation in Humans," *Daedalus* 98:2 (Spring, 1969): 387-405.

7. Note that I am here assuming only that life has an infinite *exchange* value, i.e., that we would exchange an infinite amount of anything else for one life. If one life were taken to provide infinite *satisfaction,* then we might be indifferent between preserving one life or many. Such infinite satisfaction-value would be even less able to prevent killing than would infinite exchange value, for although it would refute the claim that we ought to kill one person to save 2 or 50 (by affirming that one person has as much value as 50), it would also be indifferent to killing 50 to save one — i.e., it would affirm that no value would thus be lost.

we think that the *individual* matters, whereas anything which we merely value can be *substituted* for something relevantly identical. In other words, all valuing (in common with many other attitudes) is and must be for *types* (or essences), and not for mere particular examples of such types. No matter how highly I value gold coins, there is no possible reason I would prefer one to another if both partook equally of value-conferring characteristics. If we only *valued* human life, we would otherwise treat people as substitutable; since we do not so treat them, we must do more than value them.

Nor can we make do with value by saying that we value the individual examples of the type, rather than the type itself. Such a clarification is no doubt true, in that we do not value some kind of disincarnate type called "human life" any more than I value the abstract type of gold coins. But my point is that as long as the individuals are described as valuable only because they are human beings (i.e., examples of this type), they become substitutable. That is, if I value the set called "individual human beings," I cannot object to the substitution or maximization of the members of this set, even where this involves killing.

Someone might object here that I have misunderstood the way we value human beings; we do not value them merely as examples of the human species, but for their qualities as "unique" persons. Now, although it is certainly commonplace to hear that everyone is unique and therefore valuable, I regard such talk as a meaningful intuition seeking to express itself in meaningless value terminology. For even if people are all unique (which is quite uncertain except in the sense that they are not identical), it seems impossible that we could value them infinitely for their unique characteristics, primarily because the differences are just not so important. I do not care about a stranger in his uniqueness (his never-to-be repeated fingerprints, or his special facial appearance), but in his humanity. It is only his humanity, in fact, which I know with any degree of certainty, but this knowledge suffices to make me reluctant to kill him. Again, even if all people are unique, we can hypothetically imagine the existence of absolutely identical siblings. Would our reluctance to kill one to save the others be in any degree lessened by their lack of uniqueness? I think not, but obviously something other than valuing their individual or collective uniqueness must be at the root of our reticence. We must somehow explain how the *individual* thus matters to us, in the sense that we are reluctant to kill him even when he is exactly identical to his fellows.

II. The Alternative of Sanctity

What is the moral status of human life? What is there about human life, as we perceive it, which makes us reluctant to destroy it even where we are not interested in producing or preserving it? We have seen that "the value of life" cannot adequately explain our deference to life: Even if human life had an infinite value, *individual* human beings would not necessarily be morally protected. But in fact the value of life is often treated as far less than infinite. *A fortiori* valuing of life cannot give it the protection we think it deserves.

We need, therefore, an alternative way to conceptualize our moral recognition of life, a way different from saying "we value life" or "life has value." Before we can even begin to argue about whether or not we *ought* to have the attitudes we have to human life, we must adequately describe the attitudes we *do* have, and "valuing" is not an adequate description.

In particular, we need to explain how we can at once not wish to maximize the quantity (in numbers of years) of life, and yet seek to prevent the killing of every individual simply because he belongs to the type we call "people." We need to find an attitude which is both universally applicable to all human beings and particularly applicable to every individual, making us reluctant to kill even those we do not highly value. We already experience this attitude: I submit that when we contemplate killing someone, our mind does in fact recoil in a way unrelated to any worry about the destruction of something valuable. We feel that we simply ought not to kill, that life is not to be *violated* by us, that life is not entirely subject to our value-judgment and disposal. What name can we give to our regard for life?

Perhaps the first hurdle we must overcome is the modern tendency to identify all affirmative attitudes with some sort of valuing. The world and thought are today assumed to consist entirely of "facts" and "values." Is our reticence about killing due to some empirical fact of life? If not, conventional thought takes it to be a "value-judgment" about life. For such a mind-set, our proof that life cannot be consistently valued sufficiently to prevent killing could be evidence only that our reluctance is irrational and arbitrary.

Against such narrowness, we must show that value-language is a trap and prison of the mind, and that the moral world has a multitude of curious creatures in it — many of whom are at least as fascinating as those two beasts of burden called "fact" and "value."[8]

8. Further political and historical studies would be of immense help in a struggle for liberation from value, perhaps along the lines suggested by Karl Mannheim in *Ideology and Utopia* (New York: Harcourt, Brace and World, 1936), p. 82:

> . . . [T]he fact that we speak about social and cultural life in terms of values is itself an attitude peculiar to our time. The notion arose and was diffused from economics, where the conscious choice between values was the starting point of theory. This idea of value was later transferred to the ethical, aesthetic, and religious spheres, which brought about a distortion in the description of the real behavior of the human being in these spheres. Nothing could be more wrong than to describe the real attitude of the individual when enjoying a work of art quite unreflectively, or when acting according to ethical patterns inculcated in him since childhood, in terms of conscious choice between values.

Our method, then, in the following few pages will be to look at three further attitudes which it is often claimed we take or should take to life: love, respect, and reverence. In each case, we shall first seek phenomenologically to distinguish the given attitude from valuing, in order both to prove that there do exist moral stances other than valuing and to get a better hold on the particular proposed alternative. Then, second, we shall ask whether the suggested attitude is one which would describe adequately our feelings and behavior toward human life.

Love

There is, of course, a loose sense of the word "love" which would seem to apply to many valued objects. I might say that I love steak or horses or diamonds — and mean little more than that I value them.

But love in the full sense in which we say we love God, or a spouse, or a friend, is not normally used for *things,* no matter how highly we value them. We cannot translate all value into love. More surprisingly, the converse is also true: we cannot translate our feelings for those we love into value terminology. "I love my wife" has a very different feel to it than "I value my wife." The latter, of course, seems at first objectionable because of its instrumentalist connotation; one suspects that I care about my wife only because I have some *use* for her. But the antagonism between love and value is even deeper. If anything, it sounds more inappropriate to eschew instrumentalism and to say "I consider my wife to have intrinsic value."

No doubt I can speak of valuing our marriage, but to speak of my wife herself having value seems to demean her — not because of a connotation of instrumental value, but because the very idea of valuing her seems to reduce her to a good or commodity to be prized and even priced. Such an attitude is at least different from, if not incompatible with, love. I appear in some way to have set myself above her and to be evaluating and preferring her, rather than unselfconsciously delighting in her in the way of *eros* and giving myself to her in the way of *agape.* Indeed, to speak solely in value terms of a beloved seems so misguided as to be nearly absurd.

Love is radically different from valuing. Moreover, at least some loves care about the beloved as an *individual,* while valuing regards only types. As we saw earlier, valuing is willing to *exchange,* to accept substitutes of at least equal value. Such willingness is quite appropriate for value since, as we have noted, valuing proceeds from a value-judgment, an evaluation, and it would be silly not to value two entities equally if both were judged to have the same valued characteristics — i.e., to be the same value type. Love, by contrast, is often not willing to accept substitutes, even identical ones. Even if God were to promise me that He would immediately substitute an identical person (or more than one) for my wife if I would let Him take her away, I would refuse. I do not want someone *like* her; I want *her.*

The fact that one cannot give sufficient reasons for one's love is directly related to the fact that one cares about the beloved as an individual and not as a type. If one were to claim that any characteristics of the beloved could fully account for one's love, then one would be saying that anyone else of the same type would be equally loved. But many lovers would not say this. Love can be for particular individuals instead of for types.[9]

Could this love be the alternative to valuing for which we are searching? Could it be that we are reluctant to kill because we love other people, even strangers? Without even beginning to discuss the complex question of whether love precludes killing but allows not preserving life, which the attitude for which we are looking must do, we must reject love. For although love may indeed care for individuals, in a way which valuing does not, this love cannot be extended to all human beings. This is so, not only because such love is too intimate and too scarce a commodity, but also because to universalize it is to destroy its particularity. That is, if we were to love all people simply as people rather than as "John" and "Mary," we would be treating the object of love as a type — i.e., "people." But it is the very non-type caring of love which makes the individual matter. Therefore, we can never fully love individuals simply because they are people. Someone who says he loves people cannot mean love in our sense here and may mean rather in the sense of liking a type.[10] Such "people-liking" may well be no more incompatible with killing individuals than is the people-valuing which we have discussed at length above.

The love alternative, then, will not work, but it has shown at least this much: We are looking for an attitude which finds significance in individuals, but not *only* in individuals — because it must be an attitude which can be for all human beings simply because they are such. We must somehow find a way to respond to this *type* called "people" in a way which nevertheless cares about individual examples of this type.

9. A particular entity is distinguished not by *what* it is but by *where* it is in space-time. I can think abstractly of a table, but I cannot think of, say, the third identical table I am about to build unless I mentally insert it into space-time and imagine it existing sequentially with the first two. Only if they have differing space-time coordinates can two entities of the same type be distinguished. Only if they so exist, consequently, can they be *thought* of as particular individuals; the mind otherwise knows only quantity and quality, not particulars.

Put another way, one might say that "location" is part of the essence of an individual. In searching for a way of thinking which can respect the individuality of people, we are thus looking for a mode of thought which can take such location seriously.

10. The religious person, however, may mean that he loves God, that God loves all persons individually, and that he thus indirectly loves all those loved by his Beloved as individuals. This alternative to valuing is not insignificant, but its exploration here would take us too far from the common realm of philosophy and phenomenology.

Respect

Let us look at the *feeling,* similar to admiration and esteem, which we call "respect."[11] In many circumstances, this feeling cannot easily be translated into value-talk.[12] I might tell a judge of my respect for his court, but I would be unlikely to tell him how I valued it. Valuing again seems connected to using, or at least implies congruence with one's desires; the judge is normally not interested in how desirable I find his court's judgments. Just as valuing seemed unloving in regard to a spouse, so here it seems disrespectful in regard to a court. Its evaluative boldness seems necessarily to obscure a court's particular kind of dignity, no matter how highly I finally rank the court in my scale of values.

Nor can we respect just anything we value. I can value diamonds, but do I make sense if I say "I respect diamonds"? The answer is obvious. The important point is not that I am silly or overly materialistic, but that the sentence does not make sense. It would perhaps be wrong of me, but certainly not senseless, to say, "I value diamonds more than anything else in the world." Nor is the problem that diamonds cannot be valued as ends in themselves, or that they are merely desired but not obligatory ends. I can say, "I think diamonds ought to exist for their own sake," or "Everyone has an obligation to produce a maximum number of diamonds." Yet it sounds like gibberish to say, "I respect diamonds." We would be dumb-founded by such a statement during a conversation.

Similarly, we cannot sensibly say, "I respect honor," though certainly many value it. Honor and diamonds just do not seem to be the proper *kind* of object for respect. The same holds for happiness, which has been proposed again and again as the final end of all action. We cannot say, "I respect happiness." Whether or not eudaemonism or hedonism has been refuted is irrelevant here. It certainly is possible to think of happiness as having great value, yet it is not possible even to imagine it as an object of respect.

If someone were to ask why we could not feel respect for goods of such obviously high value, we might well respond, "But they don't *do* anything! How can I say I respect them?" Agency, the ability to act or to participate in action, seems necessary (though not sufficient) for respect. So we can respect intelligence but not good looks, and courage but not honor. We respect not goods or goals, but virtues — not only moral virtues but also what might be called "directed powers."

Moreover, even where the object of valuing appears to be the same as the object of respecting, our stance toward it is quite different. "I value intelligence" has a different feel from "I respect intelligence." The former puts intelligence into my sphere of action and speaks of the preference it has; the latter steps back and accords the virtue of intelligence its own proper sphere of action. The first is a holding and the second a releasing.

Undoubtedly, to respect people means something important other than to value them. In a sense, respect discerns the personhood of human beings as creatures able to persevere powerfully and creatively in their aims. And although this agency is usually discovered in people one-at-a-time, it might be that all human beings are at least potentially capable of some kinds of "virtue" (e.g., moral virtue).[13] If potential virtue is sufficient for respect-worthiness, then perhaps respect is the individual and universal attitude to human life which we are seeking. Or, again, if the human *species* generates respect in us, perhaps this feeling can be appropriate even for individuals in themselves unworthy of respect. In this way, too, respect might be the feeling we seek toward human life.

Without denying the tremendous human importance of respect felt for others (and the even greater importance to human dignity of respect *shown* — i.e., treating people as though they had various virtues even when they may not), we cannot accept respect as an adequate description of our attitude to human life primarily because respect not only does not prevent killing, but it also may even cause it. Someone we respect, after all, may be a friend or an enemy. If he is the latter, then our feeling of respect for his prowess can only increase our determination to act well against him. True, we would do so with appropriate acknowledgment and consideration for his ability, and thus our opposition would not demean him, but it might lead to his destruction. Surely among the greatest epic stories are those in which two heroes seek with all due respect to kill each other.

11. The word "respect" is also used for actions which may be quite unconnected to *feeling* respect. So, for example, one might "act respectfully" in church, even though one felt reverence rather than respect. Or one might treat an authority with respect, even though one felt only fear. Or one might respect someone's rights, in the sense simply of not violating them, while feeling nothing at all or even contempt for them. Our concern here is to describe only the feeling we call respect, not the many actions we call by the same name.

12. Certainly value requires more to be treated as a component of respect and a measure of human dignity, as happens in Marvin Kohl's "Voluntary Beneficent Euthanasia," in *Beneficient Euthanasia* (Buffalo: Prometheus Books, 1975), p. 133.

13. So Michael Polanyi, in *The Tacit Dimension* (Garden City: Doubleday, 1966), pp. 51-52, writes:

> ". . . [H]owever greatly we may love an animal, there is an emotion which no animal can evoke and which is commonly directed toward our fellow men. I have said that at the highest level of personhood we meet man's moral sense, guided by the firmament of his standards. Even when this appears absent, its mere possibility is sufficient to demand our respect.
>
> "[B]oth this moral sense and our respect for it presuppose an obedience to commands accepted in defiance of the immemorial scheme of self-preservation which had dominated the evolutionary process up to this point."

Kant, too, makes the capacity for moral action a basis for respect for humanity, although he sometimes appears to be thinking of a feeling more akin to what is below called "reverence," rather than to what is here called respect. See, e.g., *Critique of Practical Reason* (Indianapolis: Liberal Arts Press, 1956), pp. 99ff.

Reverence

Valuing feels demeaning in contrast to revering, just as it did in contrast to loving and to respecting. The sentence "I value God" seems rather presumptuous and can hardly mean that I revere Him. To talk of valuing art or law, again, is to give them less importance than to speak of reverence for them. Reverence acknowledges a nobility in its object which valuing does not, a quality we may call "sanctity."[14]

The inequality of value and sanctity can be shown in still another way: As with respect, reverence for many objects of value would be nonsensical. Happiness and honor can no more be revered than they can be respected. They are just not the proper *kind* of object for reverence. We do not and cannot revere goods or goals *as such*.[15] Therefore, we cannot revere those entities which can never present themselves to us except as desired goods or goals, and we can revere other entities which we value, such as people, only by seeing them differently than we do when valuing them.

Value is not necessary for sanctity, any more than it is sufficient. One may well not like going to church, yet behave reverentially each Sunday. One might even resent an ugly church while feeling reverence once inside. Reverence, after all, harkens back a bit to its linguistic root of *vereri* — "to fear." There is no necessary correlation between that which we revere and that which we like or value. Consequently, we may well not seek to produce or preserve many objects which partake of sanctity for us — e.g., ugly churches.[16]

Nor does the revered have to have the "virtues" of the respected. I can feel reverence for churches, even if at the same time I do not have a feeling of respect for them (because I regard them as inert objects). Only if I attribute some dynamic qualities to churches in addition to their sanctity can I also feel respect for them. That which we revere does not have to have actional virtues, as did that which we respect.

And unlike love, reverence does not need to fasten *only* upon the individual in order to make him matter. Reverence can be for types, e.g., "churches" or "people." But instead of making and having its types, as does valuing, reverence lets them be. Reverence is reticent and hesitant before that which has sanctity. It seeks to leave room for its object. Above all, it seeks not to violate the object of its concern. But not to violate that which we revere means necessarily not to violate any individual examples of the revered. Because valuing seeks actively to promote its type, it cannot be bothered with individuals, but seeks to use them in furtherance of its goal. Because reverence is a largely passive withdrawing, a "letting be" of its type, it must move back from every individual instance of that type. The only way not to destroy human life is not to destroy *any* human lives.

All valuing seeks to dominate the world. Individual entities as they exist have no significance; what matters is the production and preservation of various valued types. People, facts, matter, the stuff of being become mere resources to be used in the maximization of values. All that exists is expendable, because only the abstractions we have here called "types" count. Even if these types are considered to have intrinsic or infinite value, rather than only an instrumental value, the individual examples of these types (including human beings) are reduced to the status of desired goods and can be destroyed and exchanged at will. No wonder, then, that valuing feels bold and arrogant in contrast to the other attitudes we have examined; a world we only value is a world entirely subject to our evaluation and control.

Reverence, by contrast, eschews domination. It steps back before the "sanctity" of that which is revered, and thus necessarily before every particular which has sanctity. A limit is given to us and to our schemes of domination. We can no longer destroy and rebuild as we wish, but must accept and accommodate being, even the being of individuals. If I revere human life, if I say it has sanctity, then rather than making and controlling it, I acknowledge and defer to it; I let it be. That which has sanctity is beyond the scope of our rightful judgment; even to evaluate it seems presumptuous and wrong. True, I may sometimes (but not necessarily or always) have a kind of attraction to what I revere. But even here my feeling is not the achieving and holding stance which accompanies valuing, but is rather an appreciative awe or delight.

14. D. Callahan, in *Abortion: Law, Choice, and Morality* (New York: Macmillan, 1970), may be correct about some of the behavioral consequences of the sanctity of life, but he and others he cites (e.g., Gustafson at p. 325) too quickly assume that sanctity can be only a kind of value. He simply asserts that "when we speak of 'the sanctity of life,' we are . . . speaking of . . . the value we attach to human life" (p. 326). Daniel Maguire, too, despite his seeming awareness of the nature of sanctity, seems to equate it with value. *Death by Choice* (New York: Schocken Books, 1974), pp. 92-93, 156-57.

15. The sanctity of life may, however, be to some degree analogous to the "sanctity" of goods which are owned by another. We leave such goods alone, or feel numinously uneasy with them if we steal them, not because we value them *or* disvalue them, but simply because they are not properly within our control. Note that such "sanctity" necessarily has a transcendent origin: a book is more than a mere book if it is someone else's book. God's ownership of life could be the explanation of *this* kind of sanctity, or there might be a better explanation. In any event, our experience of human life seems not identical to our rather more cool and uncaring deference to the property of others. The sanctity of life may be thus not reducible to the sanctity of property, even of divine property.

16. Churches are used here as a familiar example of that which appears to have sanctity. However, sanctity need not be found only in religious contexts. A history of art teacher has told me of a recent sale of a large piece of land in which buyer and seller quarreled over who should pay the enormous costs of removing certain unsaleable monumental sculptures which neither party wanted or valued. Clearly the simplest and cheapest solution would have been to destroy the sculptures and cart away the pieces. But "the sanctity of art" made this impossible. At the same time, the low value of the works of art justified doing little or nothing to preserve them from gradual destruction by the weather.

Both universal and individual, both not violative and not necessarily preservative, reverence remedies the deficiencies of valuing, loving, and respecting and provides an adequate concept descriptive of our feelings and behavior toward human life and, in particular, of our reluctance to kill.

Are there no exceptions to the demand that human life not be violated? At first sight it may seem that there is no kind of human killing with which we feel totally at ease, that reverence always shrinks before violence toward human life.

Still, the existence of many traditional permissions to kill must give us pause. The sanctity of life in itself would seem to prohibit capital punishment, for example: Although one can argue that such punishment does not reduce the "value" of life (because by treating the destruction of life as the greatest deterrence and retribution, capital punishment obviously treats life as the greatest good), it clearly does not treat life as something inviolable. So there must be in the minds of ardent supporters of capital punishment some exceptions to the sanctity of human life — perhaps the notion that one voluntarily forfeits one's sanctity by committing a capital crime. Proponents of voluntary euthanasia or assisted suicide would likewise seem to be arguing that one can by choice give up the sanctity of one's own life. Perhaps they are right, although sanctity seems to me something one cannot easily turn off.

But it is at least clear that a low value alone cannot destroy sanctity, cannot create exceptions to reverence for life. Valuing and revering are two separate stances toward the world. One cannot argue from the judgment that a handicapped newborn has a low value life to the conclusion that his life has no sanctity and may be taken. (Nor, of course, can one make the opposite argument that because his life has sanctity it has a high or infinite value, and so an indefinite amount of resources must be expended in keeping him alive.) Moreover, there seems no obvious way to "balance" a life's low value against its sanctity; being entirely different creatures, value and sanctity have no common scale (such as "usefulness" or "satisfaction") by which they could be weighted against each other. We return to a much more specific discussion of practical policy toward life below. Here our only point is to say that the sanctity of life creates at least a prima facie demand not to kill anyone, and that the mere fact that life sometimes lacks highly valued qualities cannot create an exception to this demand.

The same point should be noted with regard to respect and virtue: Because we can revere that which we do not respect, the fact alone that a coward does not call forth respect in everyone cannot prove that everyone does not or should not feel reverence for his life. Human life may have sanctity even when it is neither valued nor respected.

Is the moral significance of the sanctity of life exhausted by a rule forbidding killing? Does reverence for life demand only that we not kill? It would seem not. Rather, the sanctity of life is a foundation, perhaps the only foundation, for all ethical principles which make individual people a matter of moral significance.

All moral attitudes which, like valuing, *demand* something must be indifferent as between individual examples of that which they seek. Only an attitude, such as reverence, which seeks to *respond* to something necessarily has regard for every individual example of the object of its concern. Only a responding can make individuals even have "reality," in the full sense of that which must necessarily be accepted and taken into account in planning how to use the things of the world. Now the word given to individuals who have this reality, who have a final and fundamental moral significance, is "persons." Reverence, by requiring the nonviolation of human life, raises in the soft clay of value the hard rocks of persons. We can *recognize* persons, we can distinguish and make each one matter, not only in spite of the fact that they are all identical *qua* human but because of this fact. Because we revere people's lives, we cannot care only about their quantity or quality; we are suddenly aware of them as individuals who cannot be sacrificed to the whole.

What does the sanctity of human life then entail, besides not killing? The answer to this question may be: everything. All interpersonal morality and all human rights may be derivable from the sanctity of life. For that which has sanctity must be seen as always also an end in itself. Our deference to it prevents us from using it in any destructive way. Metaphorically, we are forced to leave a "space" around persons, not unlike the empty and unused space in churches, within which they can manifest themselves. "Rights" demarcate this space: The necessary supports for personal integrity, such as health, acquire a derivative sanctity which demands their nonviolation. And reverence is not indifferent to personal flourishing in this space, but in service and in delight waits for human fulfillment.

Unfortunately, the attempt to construct an entire moral system founded solely on sanctity is beyond the hope of this article. And it may well be that there are other appropriate objects of reverence (such as nature, truth, or beauty) whose sanctity is not derived from that of human life. Yet even if the sanctity of life could not stand alone, it could provide an invaluable basis for other moral principles. Justice, in particular, requires as its necessary starting point the identification of those *to whom* one must be just. It needs both to know the type on which it is to operate, i.e., human life, and to separate this type into persons. It needs to operate on individuals, but in a world of pure value, individuals cannot easily matter. Reverence for human life lets justice know where to start, lets it know for whom to ready its tools of equal regard.

Perhaps such explanation of the significance of life's sanctity seems overly abstract. Let us then speak frankly of some of the direct effects which a rule against killing may have on our moral life.

Without the sanctity of life, justice is a sham. If we must be fair to the interests of everyone existing, but need not let them remain existing, we effectively undercut all demands of justice. If we must relieve the oppressed unless we kill them, then we will probably choose the latter and easier way. The idea of justice to the weak might never even occur to us if we could get rid of others, instead of having to deal with them, when they get in our way. That justice must be founded on the inviolability of the individual is so obvious it would not be worth stating were it not sometimes overlooked in the way we treat the handicapped. On the one hand, we have today a great awareness of our responsibility for just treatment of those dependent on us as evidenced, for example, by frequent declarations of child and handicapped rights. But on the other hand, we have the "common practice" of infanticide of handicapped newborns.[17] We seem to take a schizophrenic attitude toward these dependent people: we insist that we must treat them justly if they are around, but that we may make sure they die when they first arrive. I submit that the latter allowance must in the long run either destroy the rights even of the older handicapped or else convert these very rights to a pressure to kill them while they are young.

Similarly, the demand for a universal high "quality of life" masks a monstrous choice unless it is accompanied by the recognition of life's sanctity. For there are two ways to ensure that everyone living has a high quality of life: raise the quality of all lives, or eliminate those of low quality. Without the sanctity of life to exclude the less arduous second alternative, any increase in the urgency or degree of the quality of life demanded may lead to mass killing. Achieving top quality life may be felt too expensive, drawn-out, and problematic a process, and death may be found preferable. Already this seems the plight of the "defective" newborn, but unless at some point the quality-of-life ethic is supplemented by the sanctity of life, no one with any quality deficiency can be secure. Without sanctity, we are all likely to be aided only when and to the extent that aid is cheaper than poison. Whether our "defects" are physical or mental, economic or educational, only sanctity can ensure that others see these lacks as reasons to help us rather than to destroy us.

Lastly, the sanctity of life grants us an appreciation of the dignity and meaning of the human condition which we could not otherwise have. This fact was brought home to me last year when I spoke to a meeting of an association of parents of retarded children. During my speech, I had gingerly expressed sympathy for the "burdens" of such children. Afterwards a number of parents came up to me to say that they did not think of their children as "burdens"; they were just "their children," although they did have needs others did not.

Yet surely, I thought, any parent deciding whether or not to let such a newborn child die would perceive these burdens. And then I realized that these people were *not* making such choices. For them, their children were a *given,* something they simply accepted and, indeed (as I later saw), came to delight in.

Now this prochild attitude is possible, I submit, because the sanctity of life not only does not correspond to life's value but also tends to exclude a consideration of its value. Valuing is preferring; preferring is choosing. All valuation implies the possibility of an alternative to the thing valued. But here there is no occasion to compare the child's existence with its nonexistence, and to come up with the feeling that it is a burden, because the sanctity of life excludes the possibility of killing the child.

Would we be likely to call these children "vegetables," or otherwise to denigrate them, if we accepted them and sought to help them? I think not. Yet if we saw killing as an option, could we avoid comparison and evaluation?[18] To allow killing leads us to evaluate and so to "devaluate" those whom we might kill, even if we do not do so. To eliminate the option of killing does not so much cause handicapped life to be given an erroneously high "value" as place it beyond all valuation and valuing. Handicapped lives become not merely valued, highly or lowly, but appear as the given objects of appreciation and delight.

Sanctity, in sum, by asserting the reality and importance of the individual, makes possible or at least facilitates all attitudes which focus on particular persons.[19] It overthrows the depersonalizing tyranny of value, and presents others insistently to us. We must then take them into account and perhaps respond with delight, compassion, justice, or respect. Without the sanctity of human life, could even love long survive? Would it make any sense at all, say, to love a handicapped newborn if he were thought of only as a defective human-type specimen? But if we revere him first, perhaps we will come also to love him.

III. "Do Not Act or Fail to Act in Order to Have Someone Die"

Taking as data our usual feelings and behavior toward human life, we have sought to give them a name. We have

17. Robertson, "Involuntary Euthanasia for Defective Newborns: A Legal Analysis," *Stanford L. Rev.* 27 (1975): 213, 214. Robertson is speaking primarily of passive (or "negative") euthanasia; but see *Pediatric News,* February, 1977, for a report of the 1974 Sonoma Conference on neonatal ethics where seventeen out of twenty panelists approved the possible use of active (or "positive") intervention to end the life of a presumably handicapped infant. Most graphic is the documentary film "Who Should Survive?" produced by the Kennedy Foundation in 1971, in which a mongoloid newborn is intentionally let die by his parents and the hospital staff.

18. See David Mall's analysis of human objectification in his essay "Death and the Rhetoric of Unknowing," in *Death, Dying, and Euthanasia, op. cit.,* pp. 659-61.

19. Such tremendous functional significance cannot, of course, justify a personal or societal belief in the sanctity of life. If one "believes" in life's sanctity only because such a belief is useful, then one in fact is only *pretending* to believe — and this pretense will be dropped in private at any time, and in public whenever it becomes too costly. Only if we believe that life *really* has sanctity can we reap the full benefits of this belief.

focused on the curious fact that we often do not desire human life as a good or goal, and yet are deferentially reluctant to violate it in general or in its individual examples. "Valuing" was rejected as a name for this stance, primarily because such a bifurcated regard for valued objects would be irrational. Exploring more deeply, we also discovered that valuing seems improperly demeaning to human life and this fact likewise demanded an alternative to value. At the same time, love, respect, and reverence were examined; of these, reverence matched up best with the way we treat human life. Reverence does not treat life as a desired good to be achieved (as valuing would), but rather bows before the sanctity of human life, refusing to destroy any individual people (as valuing would not).

What behavior results from reverence for life? What pattern of actions is compatible both with the demand to accept life and with the permission not to achieve or maintain it? How can we both not act destructively against life and also not prolong it indefinitely?

The simplest answer to these questions is no doubt that we must not ourselves cause death, but also need not preserve life. The inviolability of life gets interpreted in a kind of spatial metaphor, so that as long as we do not "trespass" upon life we have not violated it, even though at the same time we do not come to its rescue when we see it threatened. In other words, we may not "kill," but may "allow to die"; we may not "actively" terminate life, but may "passively" stand back and let it end. Life, in this view, sets limits to our action, but not to our inaction.

Now we shall see shortly that this concept of the demands of life is quite inadequate, but we should first recognize that it is clearly founded upon more than life's value. It seeks reverently to step back before life, not to violate it. No moral theory based solely upon the *value* of life could explain such behavior; to distinguish a causing and an allowing which have the same valued (or disvalued) consequences for life would be highly irrational.

Therefore, we can already conclude that all valid criticism even of these crude distinctions must take into account the attitude of reverence out of which they may arise. That is, no one can validly be driven to support active killing simply because he believes that passive letting die is permissible. To make such a distinction, he may be operating out of a sense of life's sanctity. He is against active killing because it clearly violates life; he approves of passive letting die because he *thinks* it does not. If one argues that he is inconsistent in the way he *values* life, one has missed his point. If one argues that the active-passive distinctions themselves are meaningless, then one forces him to reevaluate his approval of letting die, rather than his disapproval of killing.

Put generally, the common moral allowance of lethal inaction, omission, passivity and the like cannot be used as a persuasive moral precedent for active killing. No refutation of the distinction between these two types of behavior can justify the latter, because the very reason the former is allowed is that it is thought to be distinguishable from the latter.

With all this said, we must nevertheless insist upon the inadequacy of all interpretations of reverence for life solely as "not causing death." Such an approach would work only if the meaning of "cause" were clear and if the intention of the moral agent were irrelevant to reverence. However, neither of these propositions is true: Causal terminology is highly elastic, and reverence involves an *attitude* of deference as well as nonviolative *behavior* toward life.

All conditions "but for" which a given death would not have occurred are necessary causes of death. Yet few are sufficient causes of death. My driving a car today may well be the *sine qua non* precondition of someone else's death. At the same time, my firing a bullet at someone would not cause his death if he were wearing a bulletproof vest. If the sanctity of life precluded all necessary causes of death, it would prohibit the automobile; if it demanded only that no person act in a way sufficient to cause death, shooting people in the chest would not violate that sanctity.

Of course, death is far more *likely* in the latter than in the former case. Could we simply say that we must not act in such a way that we make death highly probable for others? Unfortunately, no. If I carefully hide a vial of poison in a tree, hoping that some child will find it and drink it, I have surely violated the sanctity of life even if it is extraordinarily unlikely that my wish will be fulfilled. But at the same time, few would condemn me equally for voting no to lower the speed limit to 20 m.p.h., or for giving my dying aunt requested pain-killing medication, even where these actions probably or even certainly will cause death.

The difficulty in causal terminology is even clearer if we move to the situation of *dependency,* whether another person needs my help to survive. If I fail to feed my child, I can be simultaneously and correctly said to have "caused her death" and to have "let her die." The "no trespassing" metaphor for the sanctity of life does not work here. We live in constant interaction with others; human life is not like some holy altar which we could refrain from touching at all. Indeed, "not touching" may itself violate life. That is, as long as anyone in any way depends upon my actions (a most frequent occurrence), then any omission by me may be as much a necessary or sufficient cause of death as an action could be. To say that dependent persons need not be helped is to say that we may cause their death by omission just as surely as we cause the death of independent persons by action. Yet requiring of us that we never omit any treatment where this omission tends to result in death is equivalent to requiring that we never cease any treatment which preserves life — something which our reverent intuition tells us is not demanded by life's sanctity. Causal terminology either permits killing or demands preserving life. But both are intuitively wrong. Therefore, such terminology is inadequate.[20]

20. That is, it is inadequate unless one adopts and uses highly conventional definitions of "cause." So, for example, one could say that only the omission of a pre-existing duty can "cause" death. But

Moreover, regardless of whether or not a particular action is labeled a "cause," I seem a trickster if I aim effectively to bring about someone's death, but claim not to have violated the sanctity of life. If I let my child run in the street hoping that she will be run over, I have killed her even if I could be said not to have "caused" her death. If I fail to give my wife the medicine she needs to survive, in order to collect her insurance, again I cannot honestly claim to abide by the sanctity of life, even if her disease is officially listed as "cause" of death. Both our idea of morality, which focuses on the intention of the moral agent, and reverence for life itself, which is an inner deference to the sanctity of life before it is an outer step back, seem to preclude my intent to bring about another's death by the clever use of inaction to produce a lethal situation under my control.

Should we then throw out the use of the word "cause" in explaining the demands of sanctity, and substitute the word "intent"? I do not think so. "Not causing death" is too fundamental a human response to ignore. But the word "intent" itself has a causal content: I cannot be said to place my pen in my pocket with the intent that it reach the moon unless I have posited some causal connection between my pocket and the moon. And at the same time, our analysis has been frustrated by our inability to label the morally significant causes of death. Could we not use *intent* to identify *cause?* Could we not say that an action or omission causes death if it is intended to result in death or does so? The vial of poison may be far less dangerous than my car, but I *intend* it, *wish* to kill children. Therefore, placing it in the tree is contrary to the sanctity of life even if driving is not.

In other words: if I see myself wishing for someone's death and choosing means which I hope will bring about his death, then I have acted against the sanctity of life even if the means chosen consist only in a passive withholding of life supports. More concisely, the practical rule resulting from life's sanctity is the following: "*Do not act or fail to act in order to have someone die.*"

Again, let me emphasize that we have not claimed that the sanctity of life is absolute; if it is not, then clearly no rules derived from it can be absolute. This rule would then be only a *prima facie* one, with some exceptions. However, we have not here discovered any exceptions. No one I know of has explained convincingly how life can lose sanctity or how sanctity can be weighed, say, against value. And in any event, description of the operation and limits of this rule is simpler if we state it without exceptions, and we shall adopt this simpler treatment in the rest of this essay.

Perhaps the most troublesome aspect of this rule is not what it prohibits, but what it permits. Purposely bringing about someone's death surely seems to violate the sanctity of life however it is accomplished. But we may well feel that knowingly causing someone's death, even if his death is not desired, also shows a lack of reverence for life. If I fail to give my wife her medicine simply out of laziness rather than out of malice, knowing, however, that she will die as a result, have I not killed her? If I shoot a burglar in the head, is my action in accord with reverence for his life, even if I only wish to stop him from stealing my watch and hope by some miracle that he survives? In other words, is intent here only a matter of purpose (the "in order to" is the rule formulated above), or is it also a matter of "forseeable consequences"?

It seems to me that there may be at least some sets of foreseeable consequences which are so bound up with our desired goals that they cannot be morally separated. Can I blow up a fat man stuck in the entrance to a cave, wishing only that the cave be opened and not that he be killed? I think not. But still our rule may stand, because if I do intend consequences bound up tightly with my immediate desires, I am held back by the rule. Perhaps the scope of protection afforded by the sanctity of life varies from person to person; some people may sincerely feel themselves wishing for certain foreseeable consequences of their actions while others sincerely do not. Reverence for life could still be said to require that we not act or fail to act with lethal intent. Besides, we are not here claiming that reverence for life means *only* not acting in order to bring about death, but rather that it means *at least* not so intending death. It may mean more, or it may not.

Moreover, I think that the force of this objection to the permissiveness of our rule is greatly diminished by pointing out that a given consequence of an action or omission does not automatically become moral merely because it is not prohibited by this particular rule. We are clearly responsible for all the foreseen and foreseeable results of our moral decisions. But our responsibility may be formulated in terms other than those involving reverence for life alone. Do love and familial obligation allow me to put my laziness ahead of my wife's life? I should think not, even if I in no way can be said to wish her to die. May I shoot a burglar in a fashion obviously likely to result in his death? Justice and prudence might condemn me, even if reverence did not. May we leave a worker trapped in a coal mine as long as we do not *wish* for his death? Surely human sympathy, as well as economic justice, demand that we save him, even if neglecting him is not intentional murder. In other words, our rule is intended to be supplemented by other moral norms, based perhaps on justice, sympathy, and charity. It says only, for example, that I may not fail to give alms to a beggar hoping that he will die.[21] It does not

then one must develop a full description of all prior duties to others before one can make sense of a requirement not to cause death. Such a prerequisite does not seem in keeping with the immediacy of the demand for reverence for life and seems difficult or impossible to fulfill in the area of morality. But cf. the excellent application of this data to the conventions of legal causation in G. Fletcher, "Prolonging Life," *Wash. L. Rev.* 42 (1967): 999-1016.

21. Note that such a hope would be joined here with an attempt to effectuate it. A *mere* hope for someone's death, which is not the motive for an action or an omission, might not be precluded by reverence for life.

say that I may withhold alms hoping to buy a chocolate sundae. Surely I ought to help him, or at least do my fair share to meet a societal obligation to help him, if his death is otherwise imminent. But unless I ignore him out of a death wish, out of malice against his life, I have not clearly shown a lack of reverence for life.

Perhaps the prime contrast between valuing and revering is that the first seeks to preserve its object while the second does not. The first controls, the second does not. Our maxim prohibiting an antilife intention, but permitting unintended effects harmful to life, is an application of reverence to the complexity of causation and of human dependency which is quite in keeping with the noncontrolling ethos of the principle applied.

"Do not act or fail to act in order to have someone die" both liberates and disciplines us. It frees us from the idea that life is so precious that it must receive priority in all our hopes and plans. It tells us that as long as we never wish for someone's death or act on this wish, we may strive for things other than life. Life is revered while the good life is pursued. Yet the maxim also keeps us away from the countermistake of thinking that because death is sometimes acceptable, human lives may be taken for the sake of noble aims. By making sense of our intuition that life must not be destroyed but need not be preserved, it keeps us off the slippery slope to the dangerous moral abyss where human life is as expendable as the individual things we value.

IV. Applications of the Maxim

Much more investigation needs to be done into the implications of the sanctity of human life. We have in this article described at length only a "nonviolation" requirement of reverence for life, and have specified only the minimal maxim "Do not act or fail to act in order to have someone die." The sanctity of human life surely grounds behavior other than this alone, just as the sanctity of churches demands more than not intentionally vandalizing them. Nevertheless, in an effort to provide as much help as possible in matters of life and death, we shall now seek to understand some ethical consequences of the sanctity of life, as we have so far discerned it, in two areas: medical care and public policy.

The Ethics of Medical Care

A tripartite decision procedure (in all cases where death of the patient is a possibility) would seem adequately to adhere to the maxim developed above.

First of all, medical choices must be for the sake of something other than death. According to our maxim, we may never choose to act or not to act in order to bring about death. Therefore, if we assume that all choices are motivated, there must be some end other than death motivating our choice of treatment. Now, this requirement is not particularly onerous. Other ends are almost always present as possible motivating factors. But it does mean that the hypothetical "costless" patient, whose continued existence was no burden at all to himself or to anyone else, could not be gratuitously dispatched because of, say, the low value or quality of his life. We must always be acting *for* something else, not simply *against* life. And this means also, for example, that a parent or doctor caring for a handicapped newborn could not act or fail to act in any degree out of an elitist desire to put an end to such a life because it is undignified or embarrassing. Wherever a death wish is operative in a decision not to care for a newborn, the decision violates the sanctity of life.

Second, that for the sake of which the decision is made may never be something which can be obtained only by means of the patient's death. I cannot say, for example, "I didn't pull the plug to kill him, but only to collect his insurance" (or ". . . to collect his heart"). Since there is no way I can collect the insurance unless he dies, and since I know death is a necessary means to my end, I do intend death in pulling the plug. The point seems obvious in this case, but it can be more subtle. For example, it might well be in keeping with our maxim for the parents of a handicapped child to refuse a life-saving operation which is so expensive that it would economically ruin the family; there it is quite possible that the parents are still hoping and praying that their child will live. But it would not be permissible to refuse a life-saving operations because the expenses of bringing up the surviving child would be too great; here the parents are in fact wishing the death of the child. Note that in both cases, the motivation for refusal of the operation is to save money, and the almost certain consequence is death. Nevertheless, there is an important moral difference between them. Only in the second case are the costs the parents seek to avoid the "costs of continued life" (rather than only "costs of the operation"); only in the second case are the money benefits the "benefits of death" (rather than only the "benefits of not operating"). Only in the second case do the parents omit the operation *in order* to have death occur.

Third, our maxim must never be applied alone, must always be used together with other moral norms. We must never assume that a particular action or omission is permissible simply because it is not done in order to have someone die. Social justice, contract, sympathy, charity, and all the relevant norms of a complex moral universe must be at least tacitly considered before fatal damage is done. So, for example, besides not seeking to get rid of burdensome newborns, one should also not unjustly neglect them, especially where such neglect is likely lethal.

Pope Pius XII, in his oft-quoted medical address of November 24, 1957, seems to address himself to this third point. He there declares that only failure to provide the "ordinary" means of support would constitute what we have here called "neglect." "Extraordinary" supports would go beyond what justice and charity demand, and so they need not be provided:

"Natural reason and Christian morals say that man (and whoever is entrusted with the task of taking care of his fellowman) has the right and the duty in case of serious illness to take the necessary treatment for the preservation of life and health. This duty that one has toward himself, toward God, toward the human community, and in most cases toward certain determined persons, derives from well ordered charity, from submission to the Creator, from social justice and even from strict justice, as well as from devotion toward one's family.

"But normally one is held to use only ordinary means — according to circumstances of persons, places, times, and culture — that is to say, means that do not involve any grave burden for oneself or another."[22]

The Pope's permission here to withhold extraordinary life supports is, I suggest, misinterpreted if it is taken to mean that supports may be withheld *in order* to have someone die. Note that he does not even directly mention the sanctity of life in his above enumeration of the norms governing withholding of care. Apparently, he is taking for granted that no actual attack on life is involved, and therefore he considers only the moral principles governing the extent of affirmative duties of care. Indeed, he later adds that even the withholding of extraordinary means (specifically, resuscitation attempts) is subject to two additional norms, both directly relevant to our concept of the sanctity of life:

> Even when it causes the arrest of circulation, the interruption of attempts at resuscitation is never more than an indirect cause of the cessation of life, and one must apply in this case the principle of double effect and of '*voluntarium in causa.*'[23]

Double effect and *voluntarium in causa* are roughly equivalent to the maxim of intention developed in this essay.[24] What the Pope seems to be saying is that if life supports involve extraordinary hardship, then justice *et al.* do not require that they be given — provided, of course, that the intention of the omission is to avoid the hardship rather than to achieve death.

The simple "ordinary-extraordinary" distinction is no doubt a useful rule of thumb, which normally would sufficiently protect life. It is quite unlikely that one would omit the ordinary means of life (e.g., food) unless one's purpose were to kill; and it is quite likely that extraordinary means would be omitted to avoid hardship to the patient or to others. Nevertheless, ordinary means *might* be withheld from a patient without an operative death wish by the physician (e.g., out of deference to the patient's wishes). Similarly, extraordinary means *might* be withheld in order to have a dependent patient die. So, if one treats the papal distinction as authority, one should always point out that even extraordinary care must not be withheld in order to have death occur.

Are these guidelines unduly restrictive? On the contrary, they are at once a protection for the patient and a freedom for those caring for him. The patient knows that he will not be purposely violated in his weakness, though he must also modestly acknowledge that his welfare is not the center of the moral universe. The physician knows that he is free to seek the good of the patient, of his family, and of all others affected, without the fear of death as the ultimate evil — as long as he never wishes for death and acts on this wish. He might, in my opinion, accede to the family's wish to care for a handicapped child at home rather than at the hospital, even if he thought this meant certain death for the child. His goal here might well be to provide a more loving environment for the child, and a wish for death might be far from his mind. Or, as already suggested, he could discontinue a necessary life-saving treatment at the request of a competent patient, having in mind only respect for the patient's autonomy and not a desire for the patient's death. He could, perhaps, inject a dose of morphine into a dying patient, where no other pain-killer were available, even though he knew that the dose were sufficiently high eventually to cause death. He would be acting to relieve suffering, not to achieve death, and would not be disappointed if the patient survived. Or he could disconnect "unnatural" or "undignified" life supports from a comatose patient, out of deference to aesthetic sensibilities, as long as no intent to achieve death were present and no injustice or other wrong were being done.

"Quality of life" criteria might be relevant to such decisions. The fact that a dying patient has at best only a short and/or comatose existence left could be taken into account in deciding whether further burdens on patient, family, medical personnel, and society are worthwhile. Additional resuscitations might seem to do little good where the patient could at best gain only a few hours more of possible unconscious life; and avoiding pointless draining of the hospital staff and perhaps physical abuse of the patient (e.g., broken ribs) might seem a sufficient reason not to resuscitate. In other words, the low benefits to be gained by treatment could be considered as well as the costs to be avoided. Where the sum were negative, the treatment might be discontinued in order to save these costs rather than in order to achieve death.

However, we must again emphasize that this calculus is subject to two very important strictures. First of all, in this cost-benefit weighing neither the "costs of life" nor the "benefits of death" can have any place whatsoever. It is one thing to discontinue a procedure which is a burden and is doing little good; it is quite another to terminate a life which is itself thought burdensome. Second, justice and other moral norms must be brought into play. If parents refuse an expensive operation on their handicapped newborn because they do not want to waste

22. "The Prolongation of Life," reprinted in *Death, Dying and Euthanasia, op. cit.*, pp. 283-84.

23. Ibid., p. 286.

24. For a summary of the meaning of these terms in traditional Catholic moral theology, see T. O'Donnell, *Morals in Medicine* (Westminster: Newman Press, 1960), pp. 39-44.

their resources on what their doctor calls a "defective," they are not clearly failing to revere life. They are not trying to kill him, just to save money. Nevertheless, although such a parental decision is not the moral equivalent of murder, it does seem to me quite probably a violation of familial obligation, and a gross injustice if not by the parents then by the society which does not fairly share this financial burden. In not falsely calling such calculated neglect murder, we do not and must not forget the callous selfishness which may motivate our abandonment of those who depend on us for their lives. Here again the sanctity of life must be considered not alone, but as the undergirding of justice. Without the sanctity of life, talk of justice is a sham because we can eliminate those with a claim on us. But without justice, lethal discrimination is easy. Both are necessary. Sanctity must guarantee that individual persons are recognized and not destroyed, and then justice must ensure all persons are treated fairly.[25]

25. Adequately to develop the proper medical-legal applications of this moral rule would require an additional article. Nevertheless, a few remarks can be made on its legal usefulness and limits.

Because of the extremely subjective nature of the "in order to," it may well be that our legal institutions are unsuited to the full enforcement of the maxim. Even so, the maxim could be a legislative guide in that lawmakers could ask themselves whether or not a proposed legal rule would make it *easy* for those with lethal intent to be successful. "Death with dignity" legislation could be carefully limited to ensure that it is at least *likely* that treatment withdrawals occur to achieve dignity rather than to achieve death. "Proxy" or "substitute" decisions (especially by interested parties) for an incompetent patient could, for example, be strictly limited, in keeping with fiduciary principles. The "trustee" for the patient's life should have far less freedom to refuse life-saving treatment than the patient himself would have, in order to avoid the possibility of the patient being taken advantage of.

But the idea of "specific intent" is not entirely unheard of in our law. It has had a place in the criminal law (see, e.g., Rollin M. Perkins, *Criminal Law,* Second Edition [Mineola, New York: Foundation Press, 1969], pp. 762-64) and in recent constitutional law dealing with the intent to segregate (see *Village of Arlington Heights v. Metropolitan Housing Development Corporation,* 97 S.Ct. 555, 563-66 [1977]). Enacting into law a prohibition on the withdrawal of even "extraordinary" or "undignified" life-supports with the specific intent to end life could serve the salutary function of clarifying and guiding medical decisions, even if because of evidentiary obstacles the laws were seldom if ever enforced. To omit such a prohibition could promote the misunderstanding that the more dependent a person becomes, the less sanctity his life has.

Yet there can never be full legal-moral congruence. The law can never forbid all omissions designed to cause death, but only lethal omissions of a prior legal duty. Law would over-extend itself if it were to prohibit, say, failure to give money to beggars with the secret intent that they die. And, too, it might be appropriate legally, by way of excuse rather than of justification, to allow intentional killing *in extremis* (e.g., lifeboat cannibalism) and/or to show mercy for merciful motives. For all these reasons, our maxim seems most appropriately considered only a guide for law making, rather than an absolute legal rule.

The Ethics of Public Policy

A similar procedure would be applicable to political decision-making.

First, the sanctity of life would preclude any policy choices, whether by action or omission, done in order to bring about death. Most obviously, capital punishment would not be permissible, unless some relevant exception to life's sanctity exists. Its immediate purpose is without a doubt the taking of human life. But more subtle uses of death would likewise be disallowed. We could not individually or collectively withhold food from drought-stricken foreigners, even if they are our enemies, if our purpose is to have them decimated. We also could not allow famine in order to "teach a lesson" to other countries about the benefits of birth control. One cannot judge the morality of private or governmental actions only by their efforts; it is not that we must never allow anyone to die around the world, but rather that we cannot make death a goal of our programs or nonprograms.

And even where death is not obviously a goal, we must be very careful not to include in our cost-benefit calculations any of the "costs of life" or the "benefits of death," because if we do we are unavoidably intending the deaths necessary to eliminate such costs or to achieve such benefits. So, for example, as far as our maxim is concerned, it would seem permissible to leave the speed limit at 55 m.p.h. in order to maintain economic efficiency, even knowing that thousands of persons will thus be killed. We do not here desire their deaths, and may even impose safety requirements to minimize the number of fatal accidents. Death is acquiesced in rather than hoped for. However, it would be impermissible to include in a cost-benefit analysis of various suggested speed limits items such as savings on Social Security benefits as the old are killed or the net economic gain by the elimination of other "marginal" members of society, i.e., members whose consumption is expected to be greater than their production (such as the chronically unemployed). This point cannot be overemphasized, because an advancing medical technology and an increasing marginal population may soon force difficult decisions upon us. Even though these "benefits of death" are real, they must be ignored in policy-making. We must simply shut our eyes to such benefits, and of regard for the sanctity of life, in policy-making for highways, hospitals, and the care of the dependent — at home and abroad. Analysts must, when necessary, submit "inaccurate" figures on the total costs and benefits of various proposed policy options, in order not to allow the benefits of death to have any weight in public planning.[26]

26. Cost-benefit analysts, in other words, must go beyond a pluralistic willingness to have their findings considered only one factor, along with morality and other influences, in policy decisions. If the "benefits of death" are to have zero weight in such decisions, but if other costs and benefits are to be taken into account, then the proposed "inaccurate" figures must at some point be made available. See M. W. Jones-Lee, *The Value of Life: An Economic Analysis*

Lastly, and as always, we must never think only of life's sanctity. A high speed limit may be imprudent or unjust even if not irreverent to life. Do pleasure and profit outweigh the enormous violence of traffic deaths? We cannot honestly avoid this question simply by pointing out that we are sorry about these deaths, are looking for means to prevent them, and are compensating those who survive.

We can speak clearly about the ways we act toward other people only if we do not force all morality into value-talk, but allow words such as "sanctity" to develop an independent resonance. The ethical norms developed in this essay are the echoes of sanctity, and, as such, are meant to be taken seriously. Yet words are prior to echoes, and first of all is freedom of value-free speech.

(Chicago: The University of Chicago Press, 1976), pp. 3ff for a discussion of the pluralistic or "restricted" theory of policy decision. Mr. Jones also provides an excellent review of the literature on value of life vs. value of safety which is sensitive at various points to the possibility that some people's lives might be found to have a net negative economic value under those modes of analysis which do not rely entirely on gross output measurement, e.g., pp. 33, 43-46.

100 Suffering, the Body, and Christianity: The Early Christians Lived the Theological Basis of Catholic Health Care

James F. Keenan

No term in current Catholic thought is more frequently invoked as the theological foundation for health care than "sanctity of life." Surprisingly, the term itself is rather new: No Catholic dictionary or encyclopedia before 1978 had an entry on it. For instance, in the 15-volume *New Catholic Encyclopedia* of 1967, the term has no entry.[1] (It appeared as a modest afterthought in the later supplement.[2]) Nor is it found in new theological dictionaries from the United States, England, or Germany.[3] It did not appear in the *German Concise Dictionary of Christian Ethics,* although there was a passing reference in the Italian counterpart.[4]

"Sanctity of life" certainly has its roots in modern Christian writings, however. In 1908, the Jesuit moralist Thomas Slater discussed suicide and declared, "The reason why suicide is unlawful is because we have not the free disposal of our own lives. God is the author of life and death, and He has reserved the ownership of human life to Himself."[5] At its roots, sanctity of life is about God's ownership: We do not own our lives; God does. Therefore, we are not free to dispose of them.

Later, Pope Pius XI declared in *Casti Connubii,* "The life of each is equally sacred and no one has the power,

1. *New Catholic Encyclopedia,* McGraw-Hill, New York City, 1967.
2. *New Catholic Encyclopedia: Supplement, 1967-1978,* McGraw-Hill, New York City, 1978, vol. 16, pp. 400-401.
3. Joseph Komonchak, ed., *New Dictionary of Theology,* Michael Glazier, Wilmington, DE, 1987; F. Cross, ed., *The Oxford Dictionary of the Christian Church,* Oxford University Press, Oxford, England, 1974; and K. Rahner and H. Vorgrimler, *Theological Dictionary,* Herder and Herder, New York City, 1965.
4. Bernhard Stoeckle, ed., *The Concise Dictionary of Christian Ethics,* Seabury, New York City, 1979; P. Palazzini, ed., *Dictionary of Moral Theology,* Newman Press, Westminster, MD, 1962.
5. Thomas Slater, *A Manual of Moral Theology, I,* Benziger Brothers, New York City, 1908, p. 302.

From James F. Keenan, "Suffering, the Body, and Christianity: The Early Christians Lived the Theological Basis of Catholic Health Care." *Health Progress* (St. Louis) 86.3 (May-June 2005): 53-59.

not even public authority, to destroy it."[6] In a manner of speaking, our life is an object: Human life is something that, because God owns it, only God can dispose of. We, on the other hand, have only the use of life, not dominion over it.[7]

The phrase "sanctity of life" first explicitly appeared in papal writings in the encyclical *Mater et Magistra.*[8] In its original form, "sanctity of life" functioned as a euphemism for God's dominion.[9] Thus, in *Humanae Vitae,* life is sacred because its owner, God, willed it so; like other objects that God owned and sanctified — the marriage bond and the temple, for example — life cannot be violated.[10] The sacredness rests not in anything intrinsic to the marriage bond, the temple, or human life; it rests on the claim of God, who made and owns the sacral quality of the marital bonds, temples, and human lives.[11]

Pope John Paul II has significantly developed the term. In 1987, in his apostolic exhortation, *Christifideles Laici,* he speaks at length about the inviolable right to life, saying, "The inviolability of the person, which is a reflection of the absolute inviolability of God, finds its primary and fundamental expression in the inviolability of human life."[12] Nowhere does he refer to God's dominion or prerogatives. Rather, the argument is simply that we are in God's image; as God's person is inviolable, so is God's image.

In the same year, in *Donum Vitae,* the pope wrote: "From the moment of conception, the life of every human being is to be respected in an absolute way because man is the only creature on earth that God has 'wished for himself' and the spiritual soul of each man is 'immediately created by God'; his whole image bears the image of the Creator."[13] The document continues: "Human life is sacred because from its beginning it involves the 'creative action of God' and it remains forever in a special relationship with the Creator, who is its sole end. God alone is Lord of life from its beginning until its end: no one can, under any circumstance, claim for himself the right directly to destroy an innocent human being."

This latter section is repeated later in paragraph 53 of *Evangelium Vitae* and becomes the single text in the *Catechism of the Catholic Church* (paragraph 2,258) to interpret the Fifth Commandment. The entire paragraph was John Paul II's most extensive statement, before *Evangelium Vitae* itself, on both the sanctity of life and God as Lord of life.[14] In it we see some of the key elements that later appear in the encyclical: that human life is singular; that it is created in God's image; that it is uniquely created by God for a special relationship with God, which is, in turn, the human's destiny; and that, finally as source and end of human life, God is Lord of life. While not at all abandoning the "God's ownership or dominion" argument, the pope gives it newer meaning by highlighting the uniqueness of the human subject.[15]

The act of creation is where God invests each human life with its inviolable character that now lies *within* the human, the image of God.[16] The human is not to be killed, therefore, because of who the human is. Human life is not an object that God owns: Human life is a sub-

6. Pope Pius XI, *Encyclical Letter on Christian Marriage,* St. Paul Editions, Boston, 1930, p. 32.

7. The same position is found in more recent teaching. Suicide, like murder, "is to be considered a rejection of God's sovereignty and loving plan," said the Second Vatican Council ("Declaration on Euthanasia," in Austin Flannery, ed., *Vatican Council II: More Post Conciliar Documents,* Costello Publishing Co., Northport, NY, 1982, p. 512). Gerald Coleman sums up the tradition well: "Human persons, then, have only a right to the use of human life, not to dominion over human life. What makes killing forbidden is that it usurps a divine prerogative and violates divine rights" (Gerald Coleman, "Assisted Suicide: An Ethical Perspective," in Robert Baird and Stuart Rosenbaum, eds., *Euthanasia,* Prometheus Books, Buffalo, NY, 1989, p. 108).

8. "All must regard the life of man as sacred, since from its inception, it requires the action of God the Creator. Those who depart from this plan of God not only offend His divine majesty and dishonor themselves and the human race, but they also weaken the inner fibre of the commonwealth" (Pope John XXIII, *Mater et Magistra,* 1961, para. 194). The "sanctity of life" phrase became key in *Humanae Vitae* (1968, para. 13). There Pope Paul VI used it to affirm the limited dominion that the human has over human life and human generativity.

9. Richard M. Gula writes: "Closely related to the principles of sanctity and sovereignty is the divine law prohibiting killing as found in the fifth commandment" (*Euthanasia,* Paulist Press, New York City, 1994, p. 26).

10. See James Keenan, "Sanctity of Life and Its Role in Contemporary Biomedical Discussion," in Ken Bayertz, ed., *Sanctity of Life and Menschenwurde: Ethical Conflicts in Modern Medicine,* Kluwer Academics, Boston, 1996; and Joseph Boyle, "Sanctity of Life and Suicide: Tensions and Developments within Common Morality," in Baruch Brody, ed., *Suicide and Euthanasia,* Kluwer Academics, Boston, 1989, pp. 221-250.

11. St. Thomas Aquinas underlined this positivistic nature of "sanctity." In distinguishing one meaning of sanctity as purity, he wrote of the other, "it denotes firmness, wherefore in older times the term *sancta* was applied to such things as were upheld by law and were not to be violated. Hence a thing is said to be sacred when it is ratified by law" (*Summa Theologica,* II-II, 81, 8c).

12. John Paul II, "Christifideles Laici," *Origins,* February 9, 1989, p. 579.

13. Congregation for the Doctrine of the Faith, *Donum Vitae,* 1987, Introduction, para. 5, available at www.nccbuscc.org/prolife/tdocs/donumvitae.htm.

14. See James Keenan, "The Moral Argumentation of Evangelium Vitae," in Kevin Wildes, ed., *Choosing Life: A Dialogue on Evangelium Vitae,* Georgetown University Press, Washington, DC, 1997, pp. 46-62; and "History, Roots and Innovations: A Response to the Engaging Protestants," in Reinhard Hütter and Theodore Dieter, eds., *Ecumenical Ventures in Ethics: Protestants Engage Pope John Paul II's Moral Encyclicals,* Eerdmans, Grand Rapids, MI, 1997, pp. 262-288.

15. Pope John Paul II, "Evangelium Vitae," *Origins,* April 6, 1995, pp. 689, 691-727.

16. Early, in "Celebrate Life," John Paul II quoted from his address in Poland: "The Church defends the right to life, not only in regard to the majesty of the Creator, but also in respect of the essential good of the human person" (*The Pope Speaks,* vol. 24, no. 4, 1979, p. 372). In the pope's thinking, the essential good of the person emerges more clearly as the years of his pontificate advance. Often it appears in language regarding the sanctity of life.

ject that bears the inviolable image of God. This image of God is hardly extrinsic. Speaking of the Yahwist account of creation, the pope writes in *Evangelium Vitae* that we have within us that divine breath that draws us naturally to God.[17]

Elsewhere in the encyclical we read: "At this point we come to the decisive question, Why is life a good? Why is it always a good? The answer is simple and clear: because it is a gift from the Creator, who breathed into man the divine breath, thus making the human person the image of God."[18] In John Paul II's personalist writings, all people are invited to see within human life an indelible mark of its sacredness. The pope breathes life into the concept of "sanctity of life."

Sanctity of life now means that the human life as created in the image of God is no longer primarily an object that belongs to God, but, rather, a subject whose inviolability is indisputable. With this understood, I now turn to the notion of body.

The Human Body

Ask ordinary Catholics whether the church has a positive or negative stance on the human body, and invariably we answer, "Negative."[19] We shouldn't. The church's tradition has been intractably invested in the human body since the church was first established. First consider, for instance, that the central mystery concerning Jesus Christ is the incarnation! Our religion boasts that God became incarnate, that is, that God became human flesh.

Second, consider that our central sacramental celebration is the Eucharist, a thanksgiving meal in which we eat (!) the body of Christ and drink (!) his blood. We partake in his life through this sacrament, which concretely underlines the incarnateness of God.

Third, consider that the overriding promise for all Christians is the resurrection of the body. Through that promise we understand that who we are now is who we will be in glory: We will be *glorified in our bodies.* The Scripture scholar Wayne Meeks makes a similar point in quoting St. Paul: "Christ will be magnified *in my body,* either by life or by death" (Phil 1:20).[20] The resurrection of the body makes sense when we understand that God continues to love us precisely the way God made us — in our bodies.[21]

Fourth, consider how we call the church the Body of Christ. Inasmuch as we are in the church through Christ's incarnation, passion, death, and resurrection; inasmuch as, by eating his body, we are made one in Christ; and inasmuch as we share the same promise of participating in his resurrection; then what we are — church — ought to be identified with the Body of Christ.

The body is central for understanding Christianity. Through the body we understand God, our worship, our destiny, and our communal identity. Moreover, as the Jews, who preceded us, taught us, we should, as believers, take human bodies seriously.[22]

Catholics take the appreciation of the body even further, in part, because we have our emphasis on the sacramental, which accentuates our regard for the physical — particularly, the human body. Our language, art, and culture are, therefore, extraordinarily corporeal. Think for a minute of the Sistine Chapel, a very Catholic place. Here is the most important political room in Roman Catholicism: It is where our cardinals, surrounded by the images of nude bodies, meet to elect the Vicar of Christ, the pope.

Consider, also, our respect for relics, in which we locate our attachment to another's holiness precisely through the person's flesh. In her brilliant book, *The Resurrection of the Body,* Caroline Walker Bynum traces how early and pervasive our concern for relics has been.[23] Through relics, we become close to the saints, whose hair, skin, or clothing we can still touch. Through them, we "preserve" the presence of their holiness.

Clearly, then, we Christians take the body seriously. We always have. Paul, for instance, held that the body *(soma)* was so constitutive of being human that the only way we could conceive of the human was as bodily. The body was not something the human being *had;* it was,

17. Pope John Paul II, *Evangelium Vitae,* para. 35. Of course, for the pope all this must be understood by locating in God not only the source of this initiative but the end as well. "The plan of life given to the first Adam finds at last its fulfillment in Christ" (para. 35). By Christ's blood we are both strengthened and given the ground of hope that God's plan will be victorious. In fact, in that piercing by which Christ gives up his spirit, he gives *us* his spirit; through his death, he gives us life. "It is the very life of God which is now shared with man" (para. 51). Because of its origin and destiny, human life remains from its very beginning until its end sacred.

18. "The Vatican's Summary of *Evangelium Vitae,*" *Origins,* April 25, 1995, p. 729.

19. See, for example, James Nelson, who writes, "For most of the Christian era we have mistrusted, feared, and discounted our bodies" (*Body Theology,* Westminster/John Knox Press, Louisville, KY, 1992, p. 9).

20. Wayne Meeks, *The Origins of Christian Morality: The First Two Centuries,* Yale University Press, New Haven, CT, 1993, p. 134.

21. But this resurrection is established by the resurrection of Jesus: In the Risen Jesus, made in the image of God, we see our beginning and our end. Michelangelo caught this brilliantly when, in painting the famous ceiling of the Sistine Chapel, he depicted the newly created Adam with the same face as the Risen Jesus in the adjoining Last Judgment.

22. For recent Jewish literature, see Howard Eilberg-Schwartz, ed., *People of the Body: Jews and Judaism from an Embodied Perspective,* State University of New York, Albany, NY, 1992; and Paul Morris, "The Embodied Text: Covenant and Torah," *Religion,* vol. 20, no. 1, 1990, pp. 77-87.

23. Caroline Walker Bynum, *The Resurrection of the Body in Western Christianity, 200-1336,* Columbia University Press, New York City, 1995; see also "Material Continuity, Personal Survival and the Resurrection of the Body," in Caroline Walker Bynum, *Fragmentation and Redemption: Essays on Gender and the Human Body in Medieval Religion,* Zone Books, New York City, 1991, pp. 239-297.

rather, the only way humans could understand themselves. From Paul to contemporary theologians, an attentiveness to the human body can be seen in Christian thought. Robert Brungs, for instance, remarks that "all the major issues agitating the Church today . . . revolve about the meaning of our bodiedness."[24] Not surprisingly, the body is centrally important for Christians. Walter Kasper provides us an important summary:

> According to Scripture the body is so vital to humanity, that a being without a body after death is unthinkable (1 Cor 15.35ff; 2 Cor 5.1ff). For the Hebrew the body is not the tomb of the soul as it is for the Greek *(soma-sema)* and certainly not the principle of evil from which humanity's true self has to set itself free, as it was for the Gnostics. The body is God's creation and it always describes the whole of the human and not just a part. . . . The body is the whole human in relationship to God and humanity. It is human's place of meeting with God and humanity. The body is the possibility and the reality of communication.[25]

Christianity has traditionally held that the human body constitutes human identity and has combated vigorously any attempts to make the human body an object.[26]

The issue of the body as object, as some *thing* we can treat as opposed to some *one* we meet, is a real problem, however, in contemporary medicine. The notion of treating the patient as person — but the body as object — is rooted in the Enlightenment. Barbara Stafford, for instance, argues that considering the body as an object resulted from the Enlightenment's championing of reason and its devaluation of human feeling or sentiment.[27] Eighteenth-century thinkers sought to subdue the visible (the body) for the sake of the invisible (the mind). As a result, an anthropology developed in which mind dominated body, and the dualistic insights of Plato returned.[28]

The Enlightenment inclination for dualism helped cause modern medicine's tendency to objectify the human body.[29] As S. Kay Toombs puts it, "Medicine has, for the most part, adopted a 'Cartesian' paradigm of embodiment (i.e. a dualistic notion that separates mind and body and which conceptualizes the physical body in purely mechanistic terms). . . . This paradigm has been successful in many ways. The body-as-machine is susceptible to mechanical interventions."[30] Emily Martin writes, "Many elements of modern medical science have been held to contribute to a fragmentation of the unity of the person. When science treats the person as a machine and assumes the body can be fixed by mechanical manipulations, it ignores, and it encourages us to ignore, other aspects of our selves, such as our emotions and our relations with other people."[31]

In this light, we can say that Christianity and Judaism offer medicine a healthy reminder that when we recognize human life as sacred, we also understand that the sacrality is in our being embodied.[32] We must aim to respond to our neighbors as integrated whole persons, as subjects in their bodies, especially in their suffering.

Suffering

One way to recognize the importance of an integrated person is to appreciate the important role that a patient's voice plays in our response to her or his suffering. I came to appreciate that role by reading an essay about torture by Elaine Scarry. She argues that torturers derive their power from the voices of the tortured. The real object of torture is neither to exact a confession nor to learn information, but rather to make the tortured person blame his or her very self; the voice betrays the body when, so broken with pain, the body is unable to keep the voice from submitting to the power of the torturer. The aim of torture, then, is dualism: to tear the voice from its body. As Scarry puts it, "The goal of the torturer is to make the one, the body, emphatically and crushingly *present* by destroying it, and to make the other, the voice, *absent* by destroying it."[33] The tortured body is left voiceless, once it acknowledges the torturer's "authority."

Scarry notes that, of the tortured person's wounds, the most difficult to heal is his or her voice. To this end, Amnesty International helps tortured people, unable because of shame to tell their own stories, to read and understand the record of what was done to them, so that

24. Robert Brungs, "Biology and the Future: A Doctrinal Agenda," *Theological Studies,* vol. 50, no. 4, 1989, p. 700.

25. Walter Kasper, *Jesus the Christ,* Paulist Press, New York City, 1976, p. 150.

26. See Gedaliahu Stroumsa, "*Caro salutis cardo:* Shaping the Person in Early Christian Thought," *History of Religions,* vol. 30, no. 1, 1990, p. 25. See also my bibliographical survey: James Keenan, "Christian Perspectives on the Human Body," *Theological Studies,* vol. 55, 1994, pp. 330-346.

27. Barbara Stafford, *Body Criticism: Imaging the Unseen in Enlightenment Art and Medicine,* MIT Press, Cambridge, MA, 1991; see also Raymond J. Deveterre, "The Human Body as Philosophical Paradigm in Whitehead and Merleau-Ponty," *Philosophy Today,* vol. 10, no. 4, 1976, pp. 317-326.

28. Mark Johnson argues, against the claims of the Enlightenment, that "any adequate account of meaning and rationality must give a central place to embodied and imaginative structures of understanding by which we grasp our world" (*The Body in the Mind: The Bodily Basis of Meaning, Imagination, and Reason,* University of Chicago Press, Chicago, 1988, p. xiii). Johnson's aim is simple: to "put the body back into the mind" (p. xiv).

29. Richard Zaner, *The Context of Self: A Phenomenological Inquiry Using Medicine as a Clue,* Ohio University Press, Athens, OH, 1981.

30. S. Kay Toombs, "Illness and the Paradigm of Lived Body," *Theoretical Medicine,* vol. 9, no. 2, 1988, p. 201.

31. Emily Martin, *The Woman in the Body: A Cultural Analysis of Reproduction,* Beacon Press, Boston, 1987, pp. 19-20.

32. See, for instance, Joel Shuman, *The Body of Compassion: Ethics, Medicine and the Church,* Westview Press, Boulder, CO, 1999.

33. Elaine Scarry, *The Body in Pain: The Making and Unmaking of the World,* Oxford University Press, New York City, 1985, p. 49.

they may one day articulate the truth of the atrocities. Scarry's work convincingly demonstrates the centrality of the human voice in attaining the integration of body and soul. Her book demonstrates that silencing and other forms of exclusion are physically and personally destructive acts, but that the body as subject can still express selfhood through a verbalized narrative.

Listening thus has an enormous role to play in the ethics of healing, because the healer, in the act of listening, encourages the sufferer to speak.[34] Encouraging the sufferer to speak is a very biblical stance. One such instance is found in *The Book of Job*. J. David Pleins notes that God, unlike those so-called friends of Job who do not allow him to speak and who try to redirect the purpose of his discourse, allows Job to speak. Not God's absence but "God's silence dominates the discussions of Job with his friends."[35] The same listening stance is also apparent in those who, standing helpless at the cross of Jesus, heard his words, even his cry to God: "My God, my God, why have you forsaken me?" They, like God, listen to the cry of the sufferer. Of course, in the face of God's silence, we, like the Psalmist, might ask God, "Are you asleep?" But God's silence, both in Job and at the crucifixion, seems to convey a God both attentive and listening.

This listening stands as an alternative to the all-too-frequent Christian urge to interpret in the face of suffering, which has led, in this decade, to some really terrible remarks.[36] I am thinking specifically here of unfortunate moments in which certain Catholic leaders, known for wanting to better Christian-Jewish relations, let their own theology of suffering interpret the Jewish suffering in the Holocaust.[37] Worse still is the insistence, on the part of some Christians, on speaking of another's suffering — especially when Christians were the *cause* of that suffering. Marcel Sarot brings this point out poignantly in his essay "Auschwitz, Morality and the Suffering of God."[38] There Sarot calls on his fellow Christian theologians to call a moratorium on invoking Auschwitz as providing testimony necessary for the understanding of faith and suffering. Sarot especially addresses the Christian insistence on answering the Jewish sufferer who asks, "Where is God in all this?" Sarot contends that the primary question Christians should ask in the face of Auschwitz is not, "What concept of God gives most comfort to those who suffer?" Instead, Auschwitz should prompt Christians to ask, "How can we prevent Christianity from ever again providing fertile soil for antisemitism and kindred movements?"[39]

The Christian insistence on interpreting in the face of suffering must be challenged by the Jewish insistence on listening. The Scriptures urge us in this direction. As Paul Nelson notes, "The psalms of lament . . . make no attempt to explain or palliate. Instead they give voice to human anguish, rage and despair on the apparent assumption that the God of Israel is strong enough to take it."[40]

The sufferer's need to express his or her suffering is manifold, apart from obeying the religious prescription to encourage lament. As Eric J. Cassell, author of *The Nature of Suffering and the Goals of Medicine,* puts it, "Suffering is necessarily private because it is ultimately individual."[41] Cassell describes suffering as "the distress brought about by the actual or perceived impending threat to the integrity or continued existence of the whole person."[42] Suffering begins, not so much when we become aware of the fact that we cannot do something, as when we become aware of what our future holds. Suffering arises with "the loss of the ability to pursue purpose."[43] In the face of such vulnerability, we face the loss of the self that organizes purposeful action. The loss of our ability to continually move forward in an integrated manner is the ground of our suffering.

The call to listen to a suffering person is not necessarily easy to respond to, especially when the sufferer cannot or will not speak. Meredith McGuire reminds us, for instance, that suffering results precisely because the body in pain is often unable to express itself.[44] Paul Brand captures this phenomenon by considering the way chronic pain constrains the sufferer from doing the only thing that he or she wants to do — communicate the pain.[45] Brand highlights the empathetic quality of pain, arguing that a witness to someone in pain can sometimes communicate and articulate the depth of the suffering. In the same spirit, Cassell invites medical practitioners to de-

34. This idea is developed further in James Keenan, "The Meaning of Suffering," in Edmund Pellegrino, ed., *Issues in Biomedical Ethics: Comparison of Jewish and Christian Perspectives,* Georgetown University Press, Washington, DC, 1999, pp. 83-96; and in James Keenan, "Listening to the Voice of Suffering," *Church,* vol. 12, no. 3, 1996, pp. 41-43.

35. J. David Pleins, "'Why Do You Hide Your Face?' Divine Silence and Speech in the Book of Job," *Interpretation,* vol. 48, July 1994, p. 230.

36. Some Christians differentiate *suffering* from *pain* by noting that, as Joseph Selling argues, "pain demands a response, while suffering demands an interpretation" (Joseph Selling, "A Credible Response to the Meaning of Suffering," in Jan Lambrecht and Raymond Collins, eds., *God and Human Suffering,* Peeters, Louvain, Belgium, 1990, p. 181).

37. See, for example, Robert Hirschfield, "Rabbi Marshall Meyer: A Prophet's Agenda," *The Christian Century,* April 26, 1989, pp. 438-439.

38. Marcel Sarot, "Auschwitz, Morality and the Suffering of God," *Modern Theology,* vol. 7, no. 2, 1991, pp. 135-152.

39. Sarot.

40. Paul Nelson, "The Problem of Suffering," *The Christian Century,* May 1, 1991, p. 491. See also Daniel Simundson, *Faith under Fire: Biblical Interpretations of Suffering,* Augsburg Publishing House, Minneapolis, 1980, p. 144.

41. Eric J. Cassell, *The Nature of Suffering and the Goals of Medicine,* Oxford University Press, New York City, 1991, p. 31.

42. Cassell, p. 24.

43. Cassell, p. 25.

44. See Meredith McGuire, "Religion and the Body: Rematerializing the Human Body in the Social Sciences of Religion," *The Journal for the Scientific Study of Religion,* vol. 29, no. 3, 1990, pp. 283-296, especially pp. 287-289.

45. Paul Brand, *In His Image,* Zondervan, Grand Rapids, MI, 1987, pp. 226-291.

velop an aesthetic sense through which they can try to apprize the suffering of a patient who cannot speak but who can communicate his or her suffering through a variety of movements.[46]

That the body becomes the expresser of suffering is very important. We should, rejecting any soul and body dualism,[47] recognize that even when there is no voice to express the suffering, the body, as Eli Yasif puts it, "never lies."[48]

Why Christians Are Involved in Healing

Listening and responding to the sufferer as an embodied subject has always been the vocation of the Christian disciple, as Rodney Stark argues in a brilliant work on the rise of Christianity. "Christianity," Stark writes, "was an urban movement, and the New Testament was set down by urbanites."[49] Biblical cities were dreadful — "social chaos and chronic urban misery," in Stark's words. The dreadfulness was in part due to population density. At the end of the first century, Antioch's population was 150,000, or 117 persons per acre. Today's New York City has a density of 37 overall; Manhattan, with its high-rise apartments, has 100 persons per acre.[50]

Moreover, contrary to early assumptions, Greco-Roman cities were not settled places whose inhabitants descended from previous generations. Because of high infant mortality and brief life expectancy, these cities required "a constant and substantial stream of newcomers" in order to maintain their population levels. As a result, the cities were composed of strangers.[51] These strangers were well-treated by Christians who, again contrary to assumptions, were anything but poor.[52]

Moreover, the Christians' religion was new. Although the gods of the pagan religions had imposed ethical demands on their worshipers, these demands were substantively ritual; they were not neighbor-directed. And, although pagan Romans could be generous, that generosity did not stem from any divine command. Consider, for example, a nurse who cared for the victim of an epidemic, knowing that doing so might result in her own death. A pagan nurse could expect no divine reward for her generosity. A Christian nurse, however, knew that this life was but a prelude to the next, in which the generous were united with God.[53]

And, although Romans practiced generosity, they did not promote mercy or pity. Since mercy implied "unearned help or relief," it was considered a contradiction of justice. Roman philosophers opposed mercy. "Pity was a defect of character unworthy of the wise and excusable only in those who ha[d] not yet grown up. It was an impulsive response based on ignorance."[54] Concurring, Stark writes:

> This was the moral climate in which Christianity taught that mercy is one of the primary virtues — that a merciful God requires humans to be merciful. Moreover, the corollary that *because* God loves humanity, Christians may not please God unless they *love one another* was entirely new. Perhaps even more revolutionary was the principle that Christian love and charity must extend beyond the boundaries of family and tribe, that it must extend to "all those who in every place call on the name of our Lord Jesus Christ" (1 Cor 1:2). . . . This was revolutionary stuff. Indeed, it was the cultural basis for the revitalization of a Roman world groaning under a host of miseries.[55]

Elsewhere, Stark summarizes his argument: "Christianity revitalized life in Greco-Roman cities by providing new norms and new kinds of social relationships able to cope with many urgent urban problems. To cities filled with the homeless and impoverished, Christianity offered charity as well as hope. To cities filled with newcomers and strangers, Christianity offered an immediate basis for attachments. To cities filled with orphans and widows, Christianity provided a new and expanded sense of family."[56]

Stark, with writers such as Meeks and Abraham Malherbe, identifies hospitality and mercy as among the key traits of early Christians.[57] More recently, the Christian ethicist Christine Pohl has taken a critical look at these virtues and has analyzed the power inequities that

46. Eric Cassell, "Recognizing Suffering," *Hastings Center Report,* vol. 21, no. 3, 1991, pp. 24-31, especially pp. 29-31.

47. See Keenan, "Christian Perspectives on the Human Body," as well as James Keenan, "Dualism in Medicine, Christian Theology and the Aging," *Journal of Religion and Health,* vol. 35, no. 1, 1996, pp. 3-46.

48. Eli Yasif, "The Body Never Lies: The Body in Medieval Jewish Folk Narratives," in Eilberg-Schwartz, *People of the Body: Jews and Judaism from an Embodied Perspective,* pp. 203-222.

49. Rodney Stark, *The Rise of Christianity: A Sociologist Reconsiders History,* Princeton University Press, Princeton, NJ, 1996, p. 147.

50. Stark, pp. 149-150.

51. Stark, p. 156.

52. Stark, pp. 28-47. See also Robin Scroggs, "The Social Interpretation of the New Testament," *New Testament Studies,* vol. 26, no. 2, 1980, pp. 164-179; and Marta Sordi, *The Christians and the Roman Empire,* University of Oklahoma Press, Norman, OK, 1986. Stark, pp. 73-94, describes the effect of Christian nursing during two epidemics in the first three centuries of the Christian era.

53. Stark, p. 88.

54. E. A. Judge, "The Quest for Mercy in Late Antiquity," in P. T. O'Brien, ed., *God Who Is Rich in Mercy,* Macquarie University Press, 1986, Sydney, Australia, p. 107. Quoted in Stark, p. 212.

55. Stark, p. 212.

56. Stark, p. 161.

57. Meeks, *Origins of Christian Morality* and *The First Urban Christians: The Social World of the Apostle Paul,* Yale University Press, New Haven, CT, 1983; and Abraham Malherbe, *Social Aspects of Early Christianity,* Louisiana State University Press, Baton Rouge, LA, 1977. See also James Keenan, "Jesuit Hospitality," in Martin Tripole, ed., *Promise Renewed: Jesuit Education for a New Millennium,* Loyola University Press, Chicago, 1999, pp. 230-244.

occur in any guest/host relationship.[58] But Pohl turns to the Scriptures, discovering in both the Hebrew and Christian Bibles that the hosts were often themselves once aliens — and thus understood the normative significance of being marginal. In noting this, Pohl captures what so many who write about hospitality and mercy miss — that the host must understand the perspective of the alien, by allowing the newcomer to *voice* his or her concerns. This was precisely the richness of hospitality in both Bibles.

Quintessential Mercy

I want to close with Pohl's insight, which cannot help but remind us of the Good Samaritan parable, the quintessential story of mercy (Lk 10:29-37). Major theologians from Augustine to Venerable Bede have commented on this parable's evident Christological structure, in which the Samaritan is Christ himself. Christ encounters the wounded stranger (the exiled Adam) lying on the road outside the city (Paradise) and bears him to the inn (the church) where he pays (that is, redeems) the stranger and promises to return. The Good Samaritan parable is a story of Christ as the merciful one who enters into humanity's chaos and brings us into the church, where we await his return.[59]

I began this essay by looking at ourselves in God's image: Therein we derive the notion of sanctity of life. I close looking at ourselves as called to imitate Christ: Therein we derive the practice of mercy. The ethics of healing fits between these two assertions: Recognizing the dignity of the embodied human, we are called to respond to those who suffer and fear the loss of their integrated selves by assuring them that we shall always treat them as they are, subjects and fellow citizens of the kingdom of God.

58. Christine Pohl, "Hospitality from the Edge: The Significance of Marginality in the Practice of Welcome," *The Annual of the Society of Christian Ethics,* Society of Christian Ethics, Boston, 1995, pp. 121-136.

59. In James Keenan, "What's New in the Ethical and Religious Directives?" *Linacre Quarterly,* vol. 65, no. 1, 1998, pp. 33-40, I argue that the Good Samaritan parable is the scriptural foundation of the *Ethical and Religious Directives for Catholic Health Care Services.*

101 Bioethics and the Church: Technology, Martyrdom, and the Moral Significance of the Ordinary

Chris K. Huebner

This essay examines the question of ethics at the beginning of life by bringing together three areas of consideration not normally associated with each other. The approach I will be defending turns on an appreciation of the close connection between the three references that converge in the subtitle: technology, martyrdom, and the moral significance of the ordinary. I will draw attention to the fact that technology is central to contemporary bioethics and will suggest that we need a better appreciation of the way our many technological investments in medicine imply deeply held moral convictions that often go unrecognized. The reference to martyrdom is meant to suggest that we will make little progress in thinking about ethics at the beginning of life unless our thinking on this matter is informed by reflection on the end of life. Martyrdom is significant in this regard, as it captures a particular understanding of what it means to die well that has been central to Christian tradition. And finally, I am suggesting that in order to better appreciate how these first two themes are in fact connected, we require a greater appreciation of the moral significance of the ordinary.

Many beginning-of-life issues — abortion, in vitro fertilization, stem cell research, to name a few — fall within the domain of the relatively new discipline of bioethics. The beginning of this discipline's life is sometimes traced to 1962, when a special committee of experts in Seattle was formed to determine which patients would be eligible to receive newly available chronic kidney dialysis treatments.[1] The problem these ethicists wrestled with was a situation in which the demand for dialysis technology exceeded the available supply. The committee deliberated about how to allocate these limited resources to people whose lives depended on them. From its origins, then, contemporary bioethics has been concerned with technology. The discipline was invented to

1. For a helpful account and interpretation of this story of the birth of bioethics, see Joel James Shuman, *The Body of Compassion: Ethics, Medicine, and the Church* (Boulder: Westview Press, 1999), 52-6. See also Carl Elliott, *A Philosophical Disease: Bioethics, Culture and Identity* (New York: Routledge, 1999), 6-7.

From Chris K. Huebner, "Bioethics and the Church: Technology, Martyrdom, and the Moral Significance of the Ordinary." Reprinted, by permission of the publisher and the author, from *Vision: A Journal for Church and Theology* 4.1 (Spring 2003).

deal with new medical technology, which creates new therapies but simultaneously introduces a new and troubling set of problems.

Notice that this narration of the birth story of bioethics is built on certain assumptions about both ethics and technology. One of the defining characteristics of life in contemporary liberal democracies is that we have learned to associate ethics with a breakdown in the fabric of everyday life. Ethics is thus understood as taking the form of an emergency response, usually to something we attribute to the complex character of contemporary existence. Put differently, the very idea of the ethical has become "exoticized" to the extent that we assume it deals with what is out of the ordinary.

Furthermore, we assume that ethics is primarily concerned with telling us what to do in these extraordinary situations. The debate about what to do with respect to our paradigmatic moral dilemmas — abortion and stem cell research, for example — appears interminable, admitting of no clear and easy answers. Still, we tend to assume that with more impartial, rational reflection, and better, more historically informed biblical interpretation, we could identify ethical principles that would enable us to resolve these dilemmas.

The discipline of bioethics reflects these pervasive assumptions about ethics in general. We expect it to help us respond to — make decisions about — certain problems generated by medical technology. The need for bioethics grows out of the perception that a new space is opened up because technological possibilities outrun the capacity for ethical judgments. Bioethics comes to name a process whereby that space might be filled in. As Donald Kraybill has written,

> We are caught in the lurch — in an ethical gap — as technology races far ahead of our ethical formulas of bygone years. Ironically, as the technological precision increases, the moral precision wanes. The old answers that prescribed the boundaries between right and wrong, good and evil, are suddenly blurred by the provocative questions stirred by the spiraling genetic technology. After four decades of playing theological catch-up with the nuclear age, we finally have realized that the old "just war" formula is archaic for fighting nuclear wars. Now we face a new game of ethical catch-up as we try to maintain stride with the technological leaps in genetic engineering.[2]

Kraybill's words about genetic engineering also typify how bioethics often responds to beginning-of-life issues, when our standard ethical and theological responses do not seem to apply directly to technological innovations such as in vitro fertilization and stem cell research. Ethics is seen as a distinct realm into which we step when the rest of life somehow cracks under the pressure of certain "non-moral" facts, such as our inability to have biological children, or the realization that we are about to have a child who is not wanted. We name in vitro fertilization and abortion as ethical issues because they represent difficult decisions that must be made when the ordinary way of having children does not work.

Just as the story of the birth of bioethics makes certain assumptions about the nature of ethics, it also makes assumptions about the nature of technology. Donald Kraybill's words, quoted above, suggest that ethical questions do not apply to technology itself, but only to the new situations made possible by technological developments. When ethics is defined in terms of extraordinary problems, such as those generated by new technologies, the implication is that the technology itself remains morally neutral.

This assumption misses the sense in which technology in general and medical technology in particular presuppose a set of specific moral convictions. Technology, in other words, gives expression to a conception of the good life: the goal of technology is to master contingency. It promises the capacity to escape from luck, finitude, and vulnerability. Medicine harnesses technology to provide us with a means to exercise ever greater and more efficient control over our lives. As Gerald McKenny puts it, the technological imperative of contemporary medicine is "to eliminate suffering and to expand the realm of human choice — in short, to relieve the human condition of subjection to the whims of fortune or the bonds of natural necessity."[3]

Such a conception of medicine is grounded in assumptions about autonomy and radical individualism. Our lives are understood as possessions over which we alone are finally in control. And technology is seen as a tool that enables us to better satisfy whatever desires we may happen to have. Among other things, these assumptions are reflected in the way we view both doctors and bioethicists as agents of technical expertise. They coexist in a delicate balance of power designed to ensure that our ability to choose and to exercise control over our lives is never seriously compromised.

When we see technology as a morally neutral tool that is merely at the service of individuals, we have bought the self-legitimating story that those captured by the technological imagination have learned to tell themselves. This view of technology is tied up with the creation of a particular kind of people. It produces a people who have come to understand themselves as autonomous individuals who are in need of protection against whatever they see themselves as vulnerable to. Technology is thus not simply a tool for the more efficient satisfaction of desires; it involves a specific ordering of de-

2. Donald B. Kraybill, "Communal Responsibilities," in *Bioethics and the Beginning of Life,* ed. Roman J. Miller and Beryl H. Brubaker (Scottdale: Herald Pr., 1990), 194; quoted in Keith Graber Miller, "Bringing infertility out of the shadows," in this issue [of *Vision: A Journal for Church and Theology*], pp. 20-21.

3. Gerald P. McKenny, *To Relieve the Human Condition: Bioethics, Technology, and the Body* (Albany: State Univ. of New York Pr., 1997), 2.

sires. In short, technology names an account of identity that orders human desires toward the ends of mastery, possession, and control.

Technology fosters an account of identity which exists in tension with Christian identity. Understanding how that is so and why it is important is related to exploring the limitations of our society's understanding of the task of ethics in general and bioethics in particular. We misunderstand what ethics is about when we assume that it is primarily concerned with telling us what to do when we face moral dilemmas. Such an approach to ethics presupposes a faulty moral psychology that understands the self as nothing but a collection of discrete decisions. It disconnects what we do from who we are.

A more adequate moral psychology would appreciate the sense in which the self is constituted by histories, stories, and social practices. Such an understanding of selfhood presumes that the stuff of ordinary experience — what happens between, beyond, and under our dilemmas and decisions — is as important, morally speaking, as facing decisions and making difficult choices. Put simply, our decisions and choices flow from somewhere. Ethical issues and moral dilemmas, not to mention decisions and choices, do not exist in and of themselves, but only as interpreted. And we interpret them by locating them in the context of the larger story of our lives.

It follows that ethical issues are best approached not so much as problems to be solved by the application of principles, but as exercises in self-understanding. Of course, our lives do involve decisions, many of them difficult. My claim, though, is that ethics is primarily about the formation of a character and an identity out of which our decisions flow. Our paradigmatic ethical issues are at least in part the reflection of our identities. They are at least in part the product of moral convictions we all too often fail to acknowledge about ourselves. The issues and dilemmas that preoccupy contemporary bioethics can be read as reflecting a profound confusion about who we are: Are we a people whose identity is shaped by the good life as defined by technology, or by the good life as defined by Christian faith?

Our technological world forms us, often without our awareness, as people with a certain set of desires. The church, too, is involved in the creation of a people with a particular identity, whose character is shaped by a different ordering of desires. To be a Christian is to have one's desires ordered not toward mastery and possession but toward participation in the life of Christ. Among other things, this involves a call to live "out of control." The Christian life is not a possession over which we are masters, but a gift we receive in spite of ourselves, which we are in turn invited to give back. Nor is the Christian life finally that of autonomous individualism. Christian life is shared. It is an exchange of gifts with many others, including God and friends, but also strangers and enemies.

It is at this point that the practice of martyrdom is significant. For martyrdom is a way of dying that only makes sense in the context of a larger way of life that characterizes a people who have come to understand that their lives are not finally their own. Too often, appeals to martyrdom have functioned as yet another attempt to secure power and control. This dynamic is at work, for example, when martyrs are turned into heroes who are seen as having effectively seized power from the hands of their enemies. But the meaning of martyrdom is misunderstood when it is read in this way. Rather, what the practice of martyrdom names is the recognition that life is not a possession to be protected at all costs.

One of the most striking features of contemporary life is that our deaths so often happen in a way that marks a stark contradiction to the way our lives have been lived.[4] By contrast, the martyr is one — though not the only one — whose death is meaningful precisely because it is consistent with the Christian life, marked as it is by the virtues of charity and humility, both of which name a stance of vulnerability to the world of the other.

Martyrdom as an intelligible Christian practice is thus correlative to the Christian confession that life is a gift received and given. To say that life is a gift is to say that it is not ours to control. But this conviction places the Christian life in direct conflict with the conception of the good life assumed by the technologically-driven medical establishment. Martyrdom is thus significant in that it names a counter-practice to medicine and other practices informed by the technological imperative. It is not accidental, I think, that as the church becomes more and more familiar with technology, it has largely lost the ability to think intelligibly about martyrdom.

Martyrdom is, of course, a way of dying. As such, it may seem irrelevant to a discussion of the beginning of life. But part of the problem underlying our difficulty concerning ethics at the beginning of life is that it has been divorced from an understanding of the end of life. What martyrdom names about the end of life is especially relevant for how it might help us think about ethics at the beginning of life.

We want biological children rather than adopted ones because we feel that they are somehow more significantly ours. We thus invest in in vitro fertilization and other reproductive technologies in order to facilitate the desire to have children of our own. We want prenatal diagnostic testing to ensure that the children we have will not suffer. We support stem cell research because it promises to give us better control in managing other illnesses. I highlight the significance of martyrdom in an attempt to help us recognize that each of these desires is but the manifestation of an underlying desire to master and control the lives we have been given.

I do not mean to trivialize the profound struggles and painful emotions many of us have surrounding these matters. Rather, I am attempting to recognize that those feelings are to an extent the product of the way our lives exist in the midst of deep tensions concerning rival vi-

4. This is the central claim of Joel Shuman's remarkable book, *The Body of Compassion*.

sions of the good life. In many ways, the confusions we experience can be read as evidence of the church's failure to be the church. In particular, they are the result of a failure of the church to understand that it names a specific way of life, and thus that it is engaged in creating a particular people.

At the same time, the church has failed to be the church to the extent that it relegates these concerns to the private realm, leaving individuals or couples to negotiate these difficult matters on their own. So long as the church sees itself as dedicated to the work of the soul to the neglect of the body, we will make no meaningful progress on thinking ethically about the beginning of life.

I do not propose that we should do away with technology. Nor am I calling for a church-wide boycott of doctors and other medical professionals. Rather, I am suggesting that we need to be more aware of the fact that medicine and technology are not neutral things that people may use to satisfy whatever desires we happen to have. Technology uses us as much as we use it. It uses us precisely to the extent that it gets us to see ourselves in particular ways. This shaping of identity happens especially with respect to the kinds of questions that preoccupy contemporary bioethics, such as those related to the beginning of life.

Much of our ethical inquiry into the beginning of life misleads us because it fails to understand that the problems with which it deals are the products of cultures and identities. To approach these matters in yet another ethics-as-emergency-measure way is to miss the point. Difficult as these problems may be, their difficulty does not arise from the fact that the rest of life has broken down. Rather, they are questions of everyday life, of identities and cultures we already live in the midst of. And they are difficult because they represent versions of everyday life that we live even as we fail to recognize the extent to which we do so.

The primary task for the church with respect to the beginning of life is not to develop new ethical principles that might enable ethics to keep pace with new technological innovations and the procedures they enable. Rather, the task facing the church is to understand why we ever assumed that technology might save us in the first place.

CHAPTER SIXTEEN

Children

Children do not always make the pages of medical ethics texts. When they do, the concern is usually of two related types: Who decides for children, and by what criteria? Should the decision making focus be on parents or physicians or review boards? Should the decision making depend on "substitute judgment" or "best interest" or some other criteria?

These are important concerns that play out in sometimes dramatic ways: When an infant is born severely premature, who decides between life support and comfort care? And by what criteria? Who decides, and how, when to discontinue treatment for a child losing the battle against leukemia? And what of medical research involving children? Who decides and what standards determine that exposing a child to the risks of research is justified?

These are weighty matters, but with this section we suggest that theological medical ethics must also consider "broader" or "background" concerns that are of even greater significance. For example, what is the role or place of children in the family or in the church? Or, are current cultural assumptions about children at odds with how Christians should view them? Or, where do we place the good of having children among other goods, especially the good of Christian fidelity?

Frankly, to address as Christians topics such as abortion or assisted reproductive technologies or neonatal care or medical research, we need a deep sense of how Christians are to think about the role, place, or significance of children. We cannot confidently think about such matters if we do not know what to make of children in the first place. Indeed, even the dual issues of who decides and by what criteria cannot be answered if we have not addressed the even more basic and contentious question asked by theologian, parent, and foster father Joel Shuman and pediatrician, parent, and adoptive father Brian Volck: "What Are Children For?" (selection 103).

Shuman and Volck suggest that we have children for reasons other than are often presumed. Evidence — ranging from abortion rates to medical terminology to contemporary artwork — suggests that our society views children as commodities whose value is dependent upon adult intentions and desires, giving the lie to the idea that children are ends in themselves. This trend toward the commodification of children is driven in part by technological medicine itself, which promises to give us what we want. Christians, say Shuman and Volck, cannot accept this implicit notion of children as commodities. But Christians ought not to buy into the alternative suggestion that children are a hedge against the future. We do not control the future, ours or our children's; instead, our future is secured by Christ.

Rather than our possession or our future salvation, children are the often-demanding gifts temporarily entrusted to our care by God. As such, children are a type of stranger, and the appropriate response to strangers is the practice of hospitality. As we offer hospitality to children, we become the recipients of gifts, including opportunities to grow in characteristics such as love, gentleness, patience, and dependence on God.

Shuman and Volck further frame discussion of children by attending to images of the church as body and family. These images suggest that raising children is never a solitary activity; it should be one shared by the entire church community. Thus, childless couples are never really childless, and single parents should never really be alone in their efforts to raise their children. Moreover, the practice of hospitality and the images of body and family challenge us to see "our children" in atypical places — for instance, funneling through the foster care system or suffering in the "developing world" from treatable maladies such as diarrhea and malaria.

In Flannery O'Connor's introduction to *A Memoir of Mary Ann* (selection 104), we meet the Dominican nuns who took in the then three-year-old disfigured girl. Here we see an example of the practice of hospitality described by Shuman and Volck. We likewise see in that practice the way lives are changed unexpectedly, including wonderful surprises and growth in character and virtue. O'Connor also entwines the story of Mary Ann with that of author Nathaniel Hawthorne and his daughter Rose Hawthorne, the latter eventually becoming Mother Mary Alphonsa, the founder of the community of Dominican religious that years later will welcome Mary Ann into their midst. O'Connor uses the story of Nathaniel Hawthorne to suggest that our response to the needs of a single child may well be our response to God's offer of salvation. The interlaced stories of Nathaniel Hawthorne, Mother Mary Alphonsa, the Dominican nuns, and Mary Ann remind us that within the communion of saints our lives are connected in unpredictable, grace-filled ways.

"Being Mickey's Doctor" (selection 105) is a moving narrative of Dr. Margaret Mohrmann's engagement with twelve-year-old Mickey and her family. Shuman and Volck suggest hospitality to strangers as an applicable practice to the task of child-raising. One aspect of hospitality to strangers is that we grow by having our view of the world challenged and extended by the stranger. One way to read the story of Mickey is to notice some of the things Dr. Mohrmann learned from this particular child: the deep interconnectedness of families means you are never treating only the child but also the family members; suffering is multifaceted, including being cut off from loved ones and being talked about instead of to; the importance of treating the particular child in his or her irreplaceable uniqueness and not simply as an "Everypatient"; and the moral importance of remembering.

Shuman and Volck see our society as commodifying children. In "Pastoral Concerns: Parental Anxiety and Other Issues of Character" (selection 106), Joseph Kotva worries about a potentially related social phenomenon: Christian parents who unconsciously sacrifice their Christian commitments because they are anxious to maximize their children's opportunities and chances to get ahead. Kotva suggests that such parents are ill-equipped to confront the current and future powers of biotechnology, such as genetic screening and enhancement. Parents driven by fear that their children will miss out or fail to get ahead will too quickly and uncritically adopt such technology. Kotva argues that the biblical call to love and provide for our children is not to be at the expense of Christian faithfulness. He also suggests that resources for challenging such parental anxiety can be found in communal discernment and in the stories of Christian missionaries and relief workers who spent significant time outside the anxious and competitive environment of North America.

The essays by Shuman and Volck and by Kotva contrast contemporary social norms with Christian convictions and practices. Darrel Amundsen's "Medicine and the Birth of Defective Children: Approaches of the Ancient World" (selection 107) contrasts early Christianity with classical Greek and Roman society. In classical antiquity, the killing of defective newborns was a common, unquestioned practice, and even healthy children were valued merely as potential adults, for what they would become. By contrast, early Christianity was oriented to helping the weak and the marginalized and was shaped by Jesus' revolutionary teaching that it is necessary to become like children to enter the kingdom of God. The resulting universal Christian condemnation of abortion and infanticide, regardless of the infant's health, is a striking contrast to classical society. Moreover, by the time of Clement of Alexandria and then Augustine, all children, regardless of health or physical defect, were viewed as born in the image of God. This notion of being in the divine image provides a foundation for a child's value and rights unthinkable in pagan antiquity.

Allen Verhey's "The Death of Infant Doe" (selection 108) offers yet another contrast between developing social norms and Christian convictions and practices. Verhey reviews the 1982 case where parents refused corrective surgery for an infant with Down's syndrome who had a malformation of the esophagus; the infant was allowed to die. In striking contrast, Verhey calls our attention to the story of Jesus welcoming children in Mark 10. Jesus welcomes real children, sweaty, silly, obnoxious kids, and puts the pretentious disciples in their place. Jesus welcomes those who do not count (women and children), even making children the kingdom model of discipleship. In light of Mark 10, the role of parents and physicians in the case of Infant Doe is called into question. Physicians too readily deferred to the parents instead of protecting the child. Instead of uncalculating nurture and trust, the parents' actions reflect a culture that does not know what to do with parenting and increasingly focuses on having perfect children. As with Shuman, Volck, and Kotva, Verhey worries about a culture that misconceives the roles of children and parents.

The last essay, Bruce Birch's "Biblical Faith and the Loss of Children" (selection 109), is different from the rest. As in the cases of Mary Ann and Mickey, we are dealing here with the death of a loved child. Unlike those cases, the focus here is on biblical images of God and community that sustain us in the face of such loss. Drawing on his own experience, Birch offers the images of God as hearer of our cries and laments; God as life-giver, seen preeminently in the exodus and resurrection; God as one who enters our suffering, especially in the crucifixion; and church community as the body that is present, holding up the symbols of faith, and mediating the word. Birch's reflection on the death of his daughter is a fitting reminder that we do not own our children or control their future. The focus on God and church is a fitting context for asking, What are children for?

SUGGESTIONS FOR FURTHER READING

Breck, John. "The Sacredness of Newborn Life." *St. Vladimir's Theological Quarterly* 47, no. 2 (2003): 211-27.

Bunge, Marcia J. "A More Vibrant Theology of Children." *Christian Reflection: A Series in Faith and Ethics* 8 (2003): 11-19.

Bunge, Marcia J., ed. *The Child in Christian Thought* (Grand Rapids: Eerdmans, 2001).

Bunge, Marcia J., Terence E. Fretheim, and Beverly Roberts Gaventa, eds. *The Child in the Bible* (Grand Rapids: Eerdmans, 2008).

Guillemin, Jeanne, and Lynda Lytle Holmstrom. *Mixed Blessings: Intensive Care for Newborns* (New York: Oxford University Press, 1986).

Gustafson, James M. "Mongolism, Prenatal Desires, and the

Right to Life." In *On Moral Medicine: Theological Perspectives in Medical Ethics,* 2nd ed., ed. Stephen E. Lammers and Allen Verhey (Grand Rapids: Eerdmans, 1998), pp. 693-708.

Gustaitis, Rasa. *A Time to Be Born, a Time to Die: Conflicts and Ethics in an Intensive Care Nursery* (Reading, Mass.: Addison Wesley, 1986).

Hall, Amy Laura. *Conceiving Parenthood: American Protestantism and the Spirit of Reproduction* (Grand Rapids: Eerdmans, 2007).

Hauerwas, Stanley. "The Demands and the Limits of Care: On the Moral Dilemma of Neonatal Intensive Care." In *Truthfulness and Tragedy* by Stanley Hauerwas and Richard Bondi (Notre Dame: University of Notre Dame Press, 1977), pp. 169-83.

Hauerwas, Stanley. *Naming the Silences: God, Medicine, and the Problem of Suffering* (Grand Rapids: Eerdmans, 1990), pp. 1-38.

Hauerwas, Stanley. "Rights, Duties, and Experimentation on Children." In *Suffering Presence: Theological Reflections on Medicine, the Mentally Handicapped, and the Church* (Notre Dame: University of Notre Dame Press, 1986), pp. 125-41.

Johns, David L. "Parenting Virtues for Today." *Christian Reflection: A Series in Faith and Ethics* 8 (2003): 53-60.

Lammers, Stephen E. "Tragedies and Medical Choices." In *On Moral Medicine: Theological Perspectives in Medical Ethics,* 2nd ed., ed. Stephen E. Lammers and Allen Verhey (Grand Rapids: Eerdmans, 1998), pp. 723-24.

Lysaught, M. Therese. "Becoming One Body: Health Care and Cloning." In *The Blackwell Companion to Christian Ethics,* ed. Stanley Hauerwas and Samuel Wells (Malden, Mass.: Wiley-Blackwell, 2004), pp. 263-75.

Maher, Daniel P. "Parental Love and Prenatal Diagnosis." *National Catholic Bioethics Quarterly* 1, no. 4 (Winter 2001): 519-26.

McCormick, Richard A. "To Save or Let Die: The Dilemma of Modern Medicine." *Journal of the American Medical Association* 229 (1974): 172-76.

McMillan, Richard C., H. Tristram Engelhardt Jr., and Stuart F. Spicker, eds. *Euthanasia and the Newborn: Conflicts Regarding Saving Lives* (Dordrecht: Kluwer, 1987).

Miller, Richard B. "Love and Death in a Pediatric Intensive Care Unit." *The Annual of the Society of Christian Ethics, with Cumulative Index, 1996,* ed. Harlan Beckley (Washington, D.C.: Georgetown University Press, 1996).

Mohrmann, Margaret E. "It's What Pediatricians Are Supposed to Do." In *Caring Well: Religion, Narrative, and Health Care Ethics,* ed. David H. Smith (Louisville: Westminster John Knox, 2000), pp. 89-116.

Murray, Thomas H. "What Are Families For? Getting to an Ethics of Reproductive Technology." *Hastings Center Report* 32, no. 3 (May-June 2002): 41-45.

Murray, Thomas H. *The Worth of a Child* (Berkeley: University of California Press, 1996).

Murray, Thomas H., and Arthur L. Caplan, eds. *Which Babies Shall Live? Humanistic Dimensions of the Care of Imperiled Newborns* (Clifton, N.J.: Humana Press, 1985).

Nolan, Kathleen. "Imperiled Newborns." *Hastings Center Report* 17 (December 1987): 5-32.

Ramsey, Paul. "Justice and Equal Treatment." In *On Moral Medicine: Theological Perspectives in Medical Ethics,* 2nd ed., ed. Stephen E. Lammers and Allen Verhey (Grand Rapids: Eerdmans, 1998), pp. 725-28.

Shelp, Earl E. *Born to Die? Deciding the Fate of Critically Ill Newborns* (New York: Free Press, 1986).

Smith, David H. "Our Religious Traditions and the Treatment of Infants." In *Which Babies Shall Live? Humanistic Dimensions of the Care of Imperiled Newborns,* ed. Thomas H. Murray and Arthur L. Caplan (Clifton, N.J.: Humana Press, 1985).

Weir, Robert F. *Selective Nontreatment of Handicapped Newborns: Moral Dilemmas in Neonatal Medicine* (New York: Oxford University Press, 1984).

Wyatt, John S. "Ethical Issues in the Application of Medical Technology to Pediatric Intensive Care: Two Views of the Newborn." *Science & Christian Belief* 8, no. 1 (April 1996): 3-20.

102 Mark 10:13-16

People were bringing little children to him in order that he might touch them; and the disciples spoke sternly to them. But when Jesus saw this, he was indignant and said to them, "Let the little children come to me; do not stop them; for it is to such as these that the kingdom of God belongs. Truly I tell you, whoever does not receive the kingdom of God as a little child will never enter it." And he took them up in his arms, laid his hands on them, and blessed them.

Mark 10:13-16 from the New Revised Standard Version of the Bible,

103 What Are Children For?

Joel James Shuman and Brian Volck

Were this a conventional book on medical ethics, we might spend a few paragraphs on the matter of "normal" childbearing before moving on to "real issues" like abortion, assisted reproduction, or cloning. Medical ethicists are no different from the rest of us in assuming that, after a million years of practice, humans know all about making babies, why we do it, and what it's for. Having never planned to write a conventional book, we want to pause a moment to consider these apparently settled questions.

One way the powers and principalities maintain control is to limit our imagination, to stifle impertinent questions like, "Why do things this way?" If we already know why children are desired, our imaginations and energies can remain fixed on obtaining them. Yet the technological power of medicine also changes the ways in which we think about things, gradually altering our expectations by promising to provide "what we want."[1] Technological medicine, always good at providing what we want, is increasingly able to deliver not just any children, but made-to-order ones. This is something quite new. Can the advent of in vitro fertilization (IVF), surrogate pregnancy, and pre-implantation genetic diagnosis (PGD) to screen for and eliminate embryos with unwanted traits possibly leave our understanding of "normal childbearing" unaffected?

New technologies bring more and more of the particulars of our children within the control of those who can afford such "treatments," which, in turn, alters the way we see our children. Jackson Lears, reflecting on the nineteenth century's nearly idolatrous image of childhood, remarked that Victorians transformed children from miniature adults to superior pets.[2] The subsequent hundred years has further transformed children into something more like a consumer item. Ethicist Amy

1. George Orwell, in *1984,* understood that a limited language (i.e., "Newspeak") limits the imagination. If there is no word to express "resistance," resistance itself is unsustainable, and if each word has only one approved meaning, there will be no variability of opinion or belief. Aldous Huxley, in *Brave New World,* understood that a people given everything they want will come to love their servitude.

2. Jackson Lears, *No Place of Grace: Antimodernism and the Transformation of American Culture, 1880-1920* (Chicago: University of Chicago Press, 1981), 144.

From Joel Shuman and Brian Volck, "What Are Children For?" in *Reclaiming the Body: Christians and the Faithful Use of Modern Medicine* (Grand Rapids: Brazos Press, 2006).

Laura Hall notes how contemporary sentimental images of children differ from those only a few decades earlier:

> Look at the Ann Geddes pictures, an image of a child as pumpkin, or a child as flower: the baby as the commodity you get to consume or pluck and put in your vase, versus the kind of images you have with Norman Rockwell. Almost all of his images of children are children with skinned knees, are of the chaos of kids — I think about the one with the boys running and trying to pull up their pants, they've been swimming in the water hole with their dog. The images of children that he depicts are children with other children, who are showing signs of mess, which children inevitably are. . . . [Anne Geddes's images are] . . . a kind of really dangerous idolatry . . . a kind of purely platonic form of "baby," the "baby" one can fashion according to one's own desires, the "baby" as consumable. And notice that those babies never have a sign of food on themselves; if you know anything about toddlers they are constantly covered in food. These pictures are children that do not consume; *these are babies that we consume.* And those icons of childhood are indicative of a dominant culture in America that sees children as a way to accessorize and fulfill one's own life, rather than as interruptions into our own hopes, dreams and goals.[3]

The power of our technologies and the images they generate turn children from people to pets to consumable accessories, and each step is taken with our consent and approval. Christians ought not fall for this. Our lives are reshaped in Christ through baptism and Eucharist, making us misfits in a world still under the yoke of powers and principalities. If Christ transforms all creation, surely among the transformed is our answer to the question, "What are children for?"[4]

That's a rude question to ask in public. If we ask anyway, after the sputtering and uneasy laughter quiet down we may be told something like, "Children aren't *for* anything; they're ends in themselves." This may be true, but there's scant evidence we believe it. In oral presentations on pediatric hospital rounds, for instance, a child is often described as a "product of a planned pregnancy," with the implicit understanding that "unplanned" pregnancies are problematic. What matters in this view are the adult intentions behind the child's existence. In this and other ways, children are subjected to unspoken tests of value, both to the parents and to "society." In contemporary North American society, children — at least the children of the materially comfortable — are technologically spaced and provisionally accepted pending the results of prenatal diagnostic tests.

Such calculations of value are shot through with tacit assumptions and myths. To begin with, it's unclear what "society" might be under consideration here — the world, North America and its economy, the "consuming public," or the medical-industrial complex. There is also broad room for interpretation in calculating "cost" and "value" in human life. One medical article proposing the "triple screen" as standard of care in pregnancy (the triple screen is a group of prenatal tests used to diagnose Down syndrome and other conditions, providing prospective parents with information with which they can decide whether or not to abort a fetus) included in its analysis a dollar amount as the "cost to society for raising a child with Down Syndrome."[5] Two obstetrician/gynecologists, both parents of children with Down syndrome, offered a rebuttal that cleverly included a proposed "cost to . . . society of a 'normal' person who becomes a physician."[6] While there is yet no reliable prenatal diagnostic test to determine whether a fetus will become a physician, the "triple screen" and other such prenatal quality assurance tests are used widely and often. In the United States, it is estimated that 90 percent of all Down syndrome fetuses diagnosed in utero are aborted.[7] So much for children as "ends in themselves."

Planned Parenthood claims its goal is to ensure every

3. From "An Interview with Amy Laura Hall," in *The Other Journal,* no. 4; italics ours.

4. We hope our debt to Wendell Berry is obvious here. His essay collection, *What Are People For?* (New York: Farrar, Straus, and Giroux, 1990), is one among many places in which he steps back from the modern enthrallment to technology and asks, "To what end are we doing this? Whom does this serve?"

5. Owen P. Phillips, Sherman Elias, Lee P. Shulman, et al., "Maternal Serum Screening for Fetal Down Syndrome in Women Less than 35 years of Age Using Alpha-fetoprotein, HCG, and Unconjugated Estriol: A Prospective Two-Year Study," *Obstetrics and Gynecology* 80 (1992): 353-58.

6. Thomas Elkins and Douglas Brown, "The Cost of Choice: A Price Too High in the Triple Screen for Down Syndrome," *Clinical Obstetrics and Gynecology* 36, no. 3 (1993): 532-40. In their discussion, Elkins and Brown cite Barbara Katz Rothman's largely ignored warning: "The technologies of prenatal diagnosis are offered to people in terms of expanding choices. However, it is always true that although new technology opens up some choices, it closes down others. . . . Prenatal diagnosis serves as a technology of quality control, based on a given society's ideas about what constitutes 'quality' in children. The ability to control the 'quality' of our children may ultimately cost the choice of not controlling that quality. . . . Issues of basic values, beliefs, and the larger moral questions will be lost in this narrowing of choices as decisions become more pragmatic, often clinical, and always individual" (From Barbara Katz Rothman, "Prenatal Diagnosis," in J. M. Humber and R. F. Almoder, eds., *Bioethics and the Fetus: Medical, Moral and Legal Issues* [Totowa, NJ: Humana Press, 1991], 173-75).

7. Hard statistics are difficult to come by, but almost every review acknowledges that the vast majority of prenatal diagnoses of Down syndrome result in abortion. The U.K., which documents this far better than the U.S., had a 92 percent abortion rate between 1989 and 1997 (David Mutton, Roy Ide, Eva Alberman, "Trends in Prenatal Screening for and Diagnosis of Down Syndrome: England and Wales 1989-1997," *British Medical Journal* 317 [1998]: 922-23). A 91 percent rate was observed at Boston's Brigham and Women's Hospital between 1988 and 1990 (T. M. Caruso and L. B. Holmes, "Down Syndrome: Increased Prenatal Detection and Dramatic Decrease in Live Births: 1972-1990," *Teratology* 49 [1994]: 376). Prenatal diagnosis is more frequently offered to "older" women, who have a statistically higher risk of bearing a child with Down syndrome (see *Morbidity and Mortality Weekly Report* 43 [33]: 617-23).

child born is a wanted child,[8] which still begs the question of why we might want children in the first place. Stanley Hauerwas asked his students in a Notre Dame course on marriage, "What reason would you give for you or someone else wanting a child?":

> I would get answers like, "Well, children are fun." In that case, I ask them to think about their brothers and sisters. Another answer was, "Children are a hedge against loneliness." Then I recommended getting a dog. Also I would note that if they really wanted to feel lonely, they should think about someone they had raised turning out to be a stranger. Another student reply was, "Kids are a manifestation of our love." "Well," I responded, "what happens when your love changes and you are still stuck with them?" . . . It happened three or four times that someone in class, usually a young woman, would raise her hand and say, "I don't want to talk about this anymore," . . . they know that they are going to have children, and yet they do not have the slightest idea why. And they do not want it examined. You can talk in your classes about whether God exists all semester and no one cares, because it does not seem to make any difference. But having children makes a difference and the students are frightened that they do not know about these matters.[9]

As Christians, then, we must push into frightening territory, trusting that even here, when we seem most confused, we will discover the God who calls us together into the body of Christ. For Christians, life must first and always be seen as God's gift, incomprehensible outside of relationship with God. Life itself, though deserving the utmost respect, is not "sacred." Only God, who gives each one of us life, is sacred. Christians must, therefore, respect life but not worship it. "Life" is never encountered in disembodied abstraction, but always and everywhere in particular bodies.[10] If a particular life can be called "sacred," it is only in the awareness that this particular body is God's unique, irreplaceable gift.

Likewise, if we asked God what children are for, the answer may well be, "Which child do you have in mind?" Fashionable idolatries of children and childhood have no place in Christian life. Children — who will, in time, die just like us — are not "our hope for the future," since our hope is in the Lord (1 Tim. 1:1; Ps. 39:7, 146:5). Thus, even biological imperatives to reproduce and "perpetuate the species" wither under theological inspection. Karl Barth spells this out:

> It is one of the consolations of the coming kingdom and expiring time that this anxiety about posterity, . . . that we should and must bear children, heirs of our blood and name and honor and wealth . . . is removed from us by the fact that the Son on whose birth alone everything seriously and ultimately depended has now become our Brother. *No one now has to be conceived and born.* We need not expect any other than the One of whose coming we are certain because He is already come. *Parenthood is now only to be understood as a free and in some sense optional gift of the goodness of God.*[11]

Here, after clearing away thickets of sentimentality and cliché, we are at last able to see children properly: extravagant gifts, yet subordinate to the greatest gift of salvation through Christ: "No one has to be conceived or born . . . because He has already come." With Jesus as Brother, we have all the kinship we shall ever need. The early Christians, who sustained hope in Christ while living in a hostile empire, understood this far better than we. In a society where women produced children useful to the emperor, the refusal to bear children was a threat to imperial "family values." Incorporated into the body of Christ, early Christians saw the church as their family and rejected the traditional, imperial model. Rowan Greer observes:

> The rejection of the family that often characterized Christianity in the age of martyrs often carried with it the notion of the Church as a new and true family. In one respect the Church was a family not only in theory but in practice. . . . The New Testament shows us that from the earliest times the Church took under its protection widows and orphans, and there seems also to have developed an institutionalization of virgins, single women who found their family in the Church.[12]

It is in this confidence that Christ, our Brother, has made the bearing of children unnecessary for the survival of our new family, that we may best understand the earliest practice of Christian vowed virginity.[13] Yet early

8. Margaret Sanger, the founder of Planned Parenthood, spoke in a less politically correct era when she advocated the segregation and sterilization of "human weeds," while encouraging the planned breeding of "human thoroughbreds," as in *The Pivot of Civilization* (New York: Brentano's, 1922). Sanger's embrace of and complicity in the American eugenics movement is briefly reviewed in chapter 7 of Edwin Black's *War against the Weak: Eugenics and America's Campaign to Create a Master Race* (New York: Four Walls Eight Windows, 2003). Black's book catalogs in painstaking detail the "scientific" origins of eugenics, its champions throughout American secular progressive movements, and its deliberate exportation to other countries, particularly Germany. How "liberal" and "progressive" American Protestants enthusiastically embraced this movement — which involuntarily sterilized more than 60,000 of the "unfit" in the United States — is documented in Christine Rosen's *Preaching Eugenics: Religious Leaders and the American Eugenics Movement* (Oxford: Oxford University Press, 2004).

9. From "Abortion, Theologically Understood," in Hauerwas and Pinches, *Hauerwas Reader,* 618.

10. Such bodies include our own, those of our loved ones, our enemies, and the animals, plants, fungi, and unicellular organisms with which we share this planet.

11. Karl Barth, *Church Dogmatics,* III/4: The Doctrine of Creation, G. W. Bromiley and T. F. Torrance, eds. (Edinburgh: T & T Clark, 1961), 266. Italics ours.

12. Greer, *Broken Lights and Mended Lives,* 104.

13. Compare this to the Stoic extinction of the passions. Stoics typically understood producing heirs as a duty proper to the virtu-

Christians, in contrast to some Gnostics, did not insist upon virginity or view the birth of children as the tragic imprisonment of spirit within gross matter. Rather, they saw the gift of children in the light of the God who is their source. Again, Rowan Greer:

> Only God is the proper object of love; all other loves are of value only to the degree that they are ordered under the love of him. This means that the family, and indeed any human relationship, can never be regarded as an end in itself. At the same time, human loves receive their meaning and value when ordered by the love of God. They are transfigured by him and are vehicles through which we may find him. And so we find a warrant in Augustine for the notion that the Christian ideal can transform the meaning of the family.[14]

As we have learned, all gifts — including the gift of children — are to be received in confidence and gratitude. That's easy enough to say, much harder to embody. How, though, can we foster this response? Through what communal practices can we school one another in gratitude?

Children as Strangers

The Christian practice most applicable to the daunting tasks of child raising is, once again, hospitality toward strangers. If children are God's unnecessary gift, then they are never "ours" in any real sense.[15] Our care of and responsibility for them does not translate into ownership, and any parent of teenagers can confirm that children — even "biological" children[16] — are strange creatures. Given the North American fetish for independence and "autonomy," these strangers occupy space in a family's life very briefly, temporary boarders on the road to another country. But children are always already strangers to us, springing from the womb with characters and callings beyond our control. The first lesson of parenthood, we've noted before, is: "You are not in control." Sitting with parents whose children are dying, knowing there are no words to "make it better," will convince even the most skeptical person this is true. To welcome a child into one's home makes one vulnerable.

It's a lonely practice, even for those who aren't single parents, and such loneliness can grow unbearable. Yet, if the church acts as it is called to, there should be no "single parents," since raising children is thoroughly communal. That is, it takes a church to raise a (Christian) child. The *Catechism of the Catholic Church* states that the godparents' task is "a truly ecclesial function. . . . The whole ecclesial community bears . . . responsibility for the development and safeguarding of the grace given at Baptism."[17]

This statement contains the kernel of an important Christian truth: the body of Christ does not grow through sexual reproduction, but through lifelong practices of conversion. Conversion is itself a gift, one which demands much hard work from the recipient. Seen this way, childraising becomes an opportunity for conversion, presenting opportunities to love when one prefers independence, to practice gentleness before efficiency, mercy rather than control. In time, we may learn to be grateful for these interruptions. Such work must be shared by the entire body. Part of what the gathered body remembers is the body itself, in precisely the ways we discussed in chapter 3 [of *Reclaiming the Body*]. Children, remember, come to us not as ideas or emotions, but as bodies, and it may be hard to see them as a gift from God when they disrupt our ideas of what "the good life" might look like. Furthermore, they enter with us into the Body of Christ, becoming part of a story reaching back past David, Moses, and Abraham to the very creation of the universe and forward to the gathering of all things in Christ.

Discerning the Body: Two Very Different Stories

If the destiny of Christ's body is to gather all things within it, then Christians must discern the body past boundaries of genetic kinship. That reminds us of a story, namely Flannery O'Connor's "A Good Man Is Hard to Find." A tale in which an entire family is brutally murdered by a psychopathic killer named The Misfit seems an unlikely place to learn about recognizing children in the stranger, but O'Connor was never one to pretty up the facts of Christian life with sentimentalities. Near the end of the story, the grandmother — an entirely unsympathetic character — and The Misfit engage in an unlikely theological discussion, engendered by her plea: "I know you

---

ous man — a virtue that, of course, required the participation, if not necessarily the cooperation, of women. It's interesting here to recall that the Stoic philosopher-emperor Marcus Aurelius rejected the practice of adopting a suitable heir to the imperial throne — a practice that fostered the political stability necessary to create the admittedly mixed blessings of "Pax Romanum" — in favor of his biological son, the megalomaniacal Commodus, whose reign was anything but virtuous. In a modern Christian context, Hauerwas notes, "the 'sacrifice' made by the single is not that of 'giving up sex,' but the much more significant sacrifice of giving up heirs. There can be no more radical act than this, as it is the clearest institutional expression that one's future is not guaranteed by the family, but by the church" (from "Sex in Public: How Adventurous Christians Are Doing It," in Hauerwas and Pinches, *Hauerwas Reader,* 498).

14. Greer, *Broken Lights and Mended Lives,* 116.

15. Nor can the Christian be satisfied with Kahlil Gibran's vague and airy references to children as "Life's longing for itself."

16. Those familiar with contemporary adoption practices and parlance know how quickly "correct" terminology comes and goes, yet people have adopted children for millennia. Apparently the practice still mystifies us enough to fall back on scientific-sounding euphemisms.

17. *Catechism of the Catholic Church,* no. 1255. English trans. (Vatican City: Libreria Editrice Vaticana; Chicago: [distributed by] Loyola University Press, 1994).

come from nice people! Pray! Jesus, you ought not to shoot a lady."[18] The Misfit blames his sorry life on punishment for things he can't remember doing. When told to pray, he says, "I don't want no hep. . . . I'm doing all right by myself."[19] He particularly blames Jesus for raising the dead, which "thown everything off balance." He continues, "If He did what He said, then it's nothing for you to do but thow away everything and follow Him, and if He didn't, then it's nothing for you to do but enjoy the few minutes you got left the best way you can. . . ."[20]

In the end, just as The Misfit's buddies return from killing the last of the grandmother's family, her head "cleared for an instant":

> She saw the man's twisted face close to her own as if he were going to cry and she murmured, "Why you're one of my babies. You're one of my own children!" She reached out and touched him on the shoulder.[21]

In the unlikeliest of circumstances, the grandmother, perhaps for the first time in her life, sees the stranger — The Misfit — as her own child. In some parts of the Old South, shoulder blades were referred to as "wing buds," the spot where one's heavenly wings might eventually sprout.[22] The Misfit will have none of it. He shoots the woman three times through the chest.

When his small gang returns, the eerily calm Misfit tells them, "She would of been a good woman . . . if it had been somebody there to shoot her every minute of her life."[23] Most of us would prefer a subtler reminder of our kinship with the stranger, but can something other than a loaded gun to the head call us to our senses? For Christians who have forgotten the terrifying scandal of the cross, maybe not. Still, there are signs of hope.

Friends of ours shared with us the story of their own struggle to recognize who their children were. They recall their frustrated desire to have children while in graduate school, and their initial, awkward encounters with "infertility specialists." When the couple

> visited a local hospital twice to see an older guy at an infertility practice, we were intrigued with the range of possible strategies and open to learning more about them. . . . [T]his fellow seemed to have acquired some wisdom over the years and noticed our hesitancy. The high tech methods at which we balked seemed to begin at pouring a semen sample onto a single ovum on a Petri dish and stirring it up, or something like that, which must have been no more complex to him than putting Miracle-Gro on his tomatoes. He calmly asked, "Are you Catholic?" in a tone of voice that indicated he doubted our willingness to do whatever needed to be done to solve this problem. He assured us that he had participated in IRBs [institutional review boards] with priests who approved of these methods.[24] We so wanted a happy ending and found ourselves already on the border of this brave new world, thinking about it and looking across but not actually . . . plung[ing] in. The next likely steps seemed morally manageable and were tempting indeed.[25]

Unable to afford expensive technological solutions, they held off awhile, consulting a priest, who referred them to a number of articles by contemporary theologians, which suggested that

> anything short of (technologies involving) abortion seemed to be in play and to some degree even morally good. If you wanted kids, technology, or at least some approvable technologies, could provide them, and that was that. Why not put some Miracle-Gro on those tomatoes? . . . The flip-side of this freedom . . . was that we were on our own. It was a lonely place to be. There wasn't much in the way of tradition here — after all, who needed Aquinas or Augustine on GIFT when we have those clerically approved IRB decisions?[26] No scripture either, except perhaps the thought that at least we wouldn't be roping any Hagar . . . into the process?[27]

Then the couple did some very strange things. They read, among other things, the *Catechism of the Catholic Church,* surprised and "grateful for its severely skeptical stance on these applications of biotechnology." They also prayed. They talked. They went to church and joined in the liturgy. They began to ask where God fit into this world technological medicine was inviting them to enter:

> At our last appointment the older physician used the term "selective reduction" to describe the abortion of

18. "A Good Man Is Hard to Find," in Flannery O'Connor, *The Collected Stories* (New York: Farrar, Straus, and Giroux, 1971), 132.

19. Ibid., 130.

20. Ibid., 132.

21. Ibid., 132.

22. We owe this insight to Gil Bailie.

23. O'Connor, "A Good Man," 133.

24. "Institutional review boards" are the committees that review human research proposals for practical and ethical concerns within a hospital, university, or corporation.

25. The following quotations are taken from a private communication and used with permission from the original author. Names are withheld for reasons of privacy.

26. GIFT is an acronym for gamete intra-fallopian transfer, a technological procedure requiring ovarian stimulation and egg retrieval — rather like in vitro fertilization (IVF), but without fertilization outside the body. Instead, the collected ova are placed directly into the woman's fallopian tubes along with the man's sperm.

27. Ibid. The reference to Hagar, of course, recalls Abram's "technological fix" to the problem of Sarai's infertility, an approach that Sarai herself suggested, then regretted (Genesis 16). Margaret Atwood's *The Handmaid's Tale* (New York: Anchor, 1998) skillfully imagines an American theocracy where fertile "handmaids" are forced to bear children for infertile "mistresses." In this case, the biblical reference is to Rachel's infertility, and her suggestion that Jacob bear children through her maid, Bilhah. We await a similarly well-told novel of the dystopia we have already entered, in which the wealthy buy the means to desirable offspring while selectively exterminating the undesirable, even as the poor are vilified for having "unwanted children" and left to fend for themselves. We hope it is clear by now that this is a problem the church must decisively respond to.

technologically-induced multiple conceptions. We both knew then that we were well into the dystopia that right wing Catholic moral theologians had warned everyone about all along. We did not want to take part in any further dehumanization of family life, and mutually agreed to end our consideration of technological solutions to our infertility.

As strong as our desire to beget a child had been, that was how firmly sealed this issue was. I was really kind of surprised that my wife and I came to the same conclusion at the same time with the same strength of conviction. And for the same reasons. I began to see what faith in God was — not just a belief that, "Sure, He's out there somewhere," but a characteristic of a continuing relationship. . . . That took me a long time to understand. Eventually, when we adopted our twin girls I could see at least a little of what I had been blind to during our fertility misadventures: God's love for us, our helplessness to force His grace to come our way the way we want it when we want it, and His inescapable presence among us all the same.[28]

There is much here worth exploring, but we will limit ourselves to these brief comments. First, this couple didn't peer into the display case of assisted reproduction because they were self-absorbed or greedy. They wanted the good that childbearing is. What they learned along the way, though, was how to properly order such gifts in the light of God. They came to this understanding in large part through the practices of the church; prayer, shared and private reflection, reading, and the sacraments.

Second, the older doctor who wanted to "solve this problem" sniffed them out as odd. The couple is, in fact, Catholic, and their allegiance to a people gathered by God qualified any allegiance to technological medicine. Would that more Catholics were sufficiently odd to be found out, not to mention more Episcopalians, Lutherans, Methodists, Baptists, and Presbyterians.

Third, when they acknowledged their inability to fit into a world determined by medicine (having been shaped by the practices of the church into misfits), they recognized their children in the stranger: they adopted twin girls. Their children were waiting for them in a place they hadn't been looking. For those who know the proper stories, this should not be at all surprising: God's people have always been built up through extraordinary and surprising means.

Reclaiming the Body in Unexpected Ways

The "genealogy of Jesus Christ," with which Matthew begins his Gospel (Matt. 1:1-17), includes four unusual women: Tamar, Rahab, Ruth, and "the wife of Uriah" (i.e., Bathsheba). As scripture scholar Raymond Brown notes,

> there is something extraordinary or irregular in their union with their partners — a union which, though it may have been scandalous to outsiders, continued the blessed lineage of the Messiah, . . . (and) the women showed initiative or played an important role in God's plan and so came to be considered the instrument of God's providence or of His Holy Spirit.[29]

Joseph, Mary's husband, understands the "extraordinary and irregular" nature of Jesus's begetting and chooses to stand with his betrothed, welcome the child, and protect him from Herod's murderous power. The salvation of the world is effected outside of what we've come to consider "normal circumstances."

One of the most powerful temptations offered by the power that is medicine is the illusion that, through medical technology, we can restore unpleasant situations to "normal circumstances."[30] The couple who in other times might have been considered "barren" can now have the baby they've always dreamed of, free of genetic diseases and even undesirable "normal variants," while still looking like Mama or Papa. "Problematic" and "unwanted pregnancies" — some from situations so horrific any reasonable individual would understandably seek an escape — can be "terminated." Fetuses and now embryos can be examined for defects that might require more attention and resources than the parents believe they are able to give, the undesirables being aborted or discarded.

By appealing to our desires for certain qualities in children — we want our children to be happy, successful, attractive, independent, and smart — technology has redefined the sad, the unpromising, the imperfect, the dependent, and the slow as abnormal. While the rhetoric of choice suggests an explosion of options, increased control often brings a narrower range of publicly acceptable outcomes, and our understanding of what constitutes normal is diminished. A line is drawn, the human circle is shrunken, and technology offers to dispose of those who don't make the cut. By framing the use of technology in individual terms, the powers distract us from communal resources that might help us welcome the less than optimal child. Arguments for enhancing "human flourishing" over "needless suffering" often rely on this seductive narrowing of imagination.[31] Even some Christians have argued that all means available should be used to eliminate suffering, including the unasked-for elimination of the sufferer. The powers encourage us to reframe this destruction as "collateral damage" or a "tragic choice," keeping us focused on the desired ends

28. Ibid.

29. Raymond Brown, *The Birth of the Messiah* (New York: Doubleday, 1993), 73.

30. Is it still possible to write satire in an age where none blink at restoring the "normal" through expensive, intricate, and artificial means? As one of us is fond of saying, "No wonder Kurt Vonnegut doesn't write much anymore."

31. While a bit grim, it's worth remembering how the still-disguised Wesley rebukes Buttercup in *The Princess Bride*, "Life is pain, Highness. Anyone who says differently is selling something."

of individuals. The Christian story does not claim that all temporal suffering should end with the Christ's victory but rather that, as we wait in hope for the eschatological fullness of that victory, all suffering is shared in Christ's body.[32]

Naming abortion as an "individual choice" or even an "individual sin" fails to discern the body. Each abortion is a negation of community, a failure of the gathered body to find room for even the most unpromising of children. It is a communal failure to say clearly to the pregnant mother and her growing child, "You are welcome here." The principal way in which the church can reduce abortions — a goal even "pro-choice" organizations claim to favor — is less by becoming an organized voting bloc championing certain individual rights than by reclaiming the body in all its forms. The pregnant woman, frightened and battered by the powers, is not an individual who simply needs to behave in a morally upright fashion. She is part of *our* body. The child she carries is not any child — he or she is *our* child.

William Willimon describes hearing an African-American pastor's response to the grim realities of teen pregnancy:

> "We have young girls who have this happen to them. I have a fourteen-year-old in my congregation who had a baby last month. We're going to baptize the child next Sunday," he added.
>
> "Do you really think that she is capable of raising a little baby?" another minister asked.
>
> "Of course not," he replied. "No fourteen-year-old is capable of raising a baby. For that matter, not many thirty-year-olds are qualified. A baby's too difficult for any one person to raise by herself."
>
> "So what do you do with babies?" they asked.
>
> "Well, we baptize them so that we all raise them together. In the case of that fourteen-year-old, we have given her baby to a retired couple who have enough time and enough wisdom to raise children. They can raise the mama along with her baby. That's the way we do it."[33]

What this church has done is not merely discerned the body, but reclaimed it from the individualistic, technological solutions medicine as power offers. Heeding the warning of James, they have become doers of the word rather than merely hearers.[34] This may not be the ideal American nuclear family, but, as Matthew's genealogy recalls, salvation often is carried out in irregular circumstances.

Baptizing one fourteen-year-old's child doesn't eliminate the perceived need for more than a million abortions in the United States every year. Nor does it respond to the heartbreaking circumstance of a child born with severe, even lethal, abnormalities. Welcoming such children, and in such numbers, would require an even stronger sense of gathering in Christ, a much deeper network of support empowered by the Holy Spirit. Welcoming the fourteen-year-old's child is, however, a start — one which the church might grow accustomed to. Such a practice of hospitality to the stranger may well lead to the situation Bill Tilbert imagines: "What if there were abortion clinics but nobody went in? What if abortion was a legal choice, but it was a choice nobody took?"[35]

Christians should not fool themselves into believing that reclaiming the body will drive abortion clinics out of business. Abortion, like war, is a human invention of great antiquity, arising from the deepest brokenness within humanity. Like any other violent rupture of community, abortion requires sustained, patient, and nonviolent communal witness to women and men across generations.[36] While less gratifying than angry condemnation and less flashy than political power plays, such quiet resistance to the powers shows — instead of merely telling — those contemplating abortion, "There are other ways."

32. In this respect, the King James translation of Mark 10:14, "Suffer the little children to come unto me," takes on special resonance.

33. William H. Willimon, *What's Right with the Church?* (New York: Harper and Row, 1985), 65.

34. Cf. James 1:22. Read as an entirety, the Letter of James is a powerful rebuttal to the Gnostic claims of the powers, particularly those of medicine. As we noted in the previous chapter, even the sick person's body is reclaimed from alienation through anointing and prayer.

35. Bill Tilbert, from an unpublished sermon cited by Richard B. Hays in *The Moral Vision of the New Testament* (San Francisco: HarperCollins, 1996), 458.

36. Like pacifism, embodied witness to real abortion alternatives is largely dismissed in North American society as "unrealistic," often painted as "doing nothing" in the face of horrible circumstances. Unlike pacifists, though, many so-called conservatives fit the bill of their detractors, frequently ignoring women's lived experiences and imagining that answers to such conditions are simple or available with the stroke of a presidential pen. Liberals have a better record of listening to women in crisis, but are — in our view — overly fond of technological solutions. If the gathered body is to respond to the realities of North America culture, it will need to begin its lived witness long before crises occur, showing children there is more to intimacy than genitals, that "what people do in their bedrooms" is deeply connected to the health of the community, and discussing openly, honestly, and with respect for both communal tradition and real circumstances, roles for contraception and abstinence. The rest of this chapter will gesture at the community's responsibility once children are begotten. To do justice to this communal witness across generations would take an entire book, but we can suggest some places for the interested to start their reading. Years before Hillary Clinton stumbled upon the idea that pro-choicers and pro-lifers might work together to reduce the number of abortions, Frederica Mathewes-Green and others were already engaging in that conversation. The news industry predictably ignored such endeavors in favor of juicier stories, but Mathewes-Green's book *Real Choices: Listening to Women; Looking for Alternatives to Abortion* (Ben Lomond, CA: Conciliar Press, 1997) is well worth reading. Wendell Berry's conviction that nothing, not even food or sex, falls outside community concern, runs throughout his work. We particularly recommend the title essay in his collection, *Sex, Economy, Freedom & Community.* Anne Tyler's wonderful novel *Saint Maybe* (New York: Fawcett Columbine, 1991) describes how costly responsibility for another's children might be embodied.

Which Children Are Ours?

Welcoming children is a good thing. Wanting one's own children is part of the human experience. What if having "one's own" children is difficult, not because of financial or social reasons, but — as in the case of the couple who eventually adopted — for medical reasons?

Medicine answers this challenge through the new technologies of assisted reproduction: IVF, PGD, GIFT, ZIFT: an entire alphabet soup of techniques. The United States Centers for Disease Control and Prevention documented in one recent year 107,587 "procedures," resulting in 29,344 deliveries and 40,687 live births.[37] No calculations of monetary cost were included in the report. We realize many Christians welcome and baptize children born following assisted reproduction technologies each year. We agree such children should be baptized, but how is the body being discerned in their begetting? Are Christians properly ordering goods in this respect?

Perhaps a place to begin is to place the number of assisted reproduction procedures side by side with three other statistics. First, in the year 2000, there were 1.31 million abortions in the United States, making induced abortion one of the most commonly performed surgical procedures in the United States.[38] Second, as of September 30, 2001, there were 542,000 children in foster care in the United States, with 290,000 entering the system and 263,000 leaving in the previous twelve months.[39] Third, the estimated number of children less than five years of age who died in the year 2000 worldwide was 10.8 million.[40] The British journal *Lancet* asked, "Where and why are 10 million children dying every year?"[41] The short answer is in mostly poor, so-called developing countries, and for entirely preventable reasons, such as diarrhea, malnutrition, and measles.

In this context, the welcoming of children through assisted reproduction techniques becomes much more problematic. Without even considering the ethical concerns raised by the techniques themselves, can Christian communities justify the pursuit of children through such costly means when millions conceived naturally die by "choice" or from causes most North Americans consider ancient history? And what of the thousands in foster care, waiting for a home?

We will consider the church's response to medical disparities between rich and poor nations in the following chapter, but it is worth noting here that if, in Christ, there is neither male nor female, Jew nor Greek, slave nor free, then surely there is also neither white nor black, American nor Sudanese, able-bodied nor handicapped. Furthermore, if all children are gifts from God, and never truly our possessions, then pondering the ethical complexities of embryo disposal and selective reduction while ignoring the gift of children already present but strangely invisible to us seems a luxury we can neither afford nor justify.

Given this incredible worldwide death toll, how might Christians properly welcome children? The struggling graduate-school couple whose story we shared above found one: adoption. Full of moral complexity and potential for abuse itself, adoption nonetheless provides a home for tens of thousands of children each year. Many of these children do not meet North America's changing standards for ability or promise, but some brave women and men adopt them anyway. Most arrive at a decision to adopt as isolated couples, often after meeting another adoptive family. Churches generally endorse the practice, but it is harder to find a church that actively encourages and supports these families. How many churches consider adoption integral to its communal witness to the world? How many churches support birth mothers in their heartbreaking courage, as they witness to the life we share? Or, as happens all too often in the churches of the rich and materially comfortable, is the subject mentioned only when convenient, as part of the parish "outreach report," or on "Respect Life Sunday"? The church's failure to witness communally this response surely implicates Christians in the ten million child deaths around the world and more than a million abortions in the United States each year.

One small church that has taken up this calling is Bennett Chapel Missionary Baptist Church in the wonderfully named town of Possum Trot, Texas. Pastor William C. Martin and his wife, Donna, led the congregation by example, adopting several children themselves.[42] Susan Ramsey, a caseworker for the Texas Department of Protective Services, was then contacted by Pastor Martin:

> "I told him I would come to teach the training classes for prospective adoptive and foster parents if he could get 10 potential families to attend," Ramsey explained. "When I arrived there were 24 families at the first meeting. It was incredible. And Reverend Martin let us hold the meetings in the church, which is the center of the community."

The small church has since surpassed one hundred total adoptions and foster care placements, including

37. "Assisted Reproduction Technique Surveillance — United States, 2001," *Morbidity and Mortality Weekly Report,* April 30, 2004/53 (SSOI), 1-20.

38. Alan Guttmacher Institute, www.agi-usa.org/presentations/abort_slides.pdf.

39. From *Foster Care National Statistics,* National Clearinghouse on Child Abuse and Neglect Information (HHS), 2003, www.nccanch.acf.hhs.gov/pubs/factsheets/foster.cfm.

40. UNICEF Child Mortality Statistics, www.childinfo.org/cmr/revis/db2.htm.

41. Robert E. Black, Saul S. Morris, and Jennifer Bryce, "Where and Why Are 10 Million Children Dying Every Year?" *Lancet* 361 (2003): 2226-34.

42. Brendan Kramp, "Rural Texas Church Makes Adoption a Community Affair," available through the North American Council on Adoptable Children, www.nacac.org/newsletters/faith/texaschapel.html. All subsequent references to Bennett Chapel are from this article.

abused, special needs, and other "hard-to-place" children. In reflecting on the Bennett Chapel witness, Ramsey noted:

> The people in the Bennett community are comfortable with who they are. . . . They are good, honest, hardworking people who aren't threatened by the idea of bringing children into their homes. They don't view themselves as a blessing for the child. They view the child as their blessing.

Adopting a child will not solve the world's problems, and the world might well do without more North Americans, whose aggressive consumption of God's gifts severely taxes the earth's material bounty. Yet adoption can be a first step beyond the comfortable boundaries of biological and even national kinship, toward a fuller understanding of our kinship in Christ. For example, one of us is the adoptive father of a girl from Guatemala. Part of our family for over eight years now, she still calls us to deeper conversion and reminds us of undeserved privileges in an unfair world. One of those privileges, the freedom to choose when and if to challenge racism and poverty, was lost the moment we stepped into the Houston airport with her. There, everyone who looked like her new parents was hurrying to catch a flight, while everyone who looked like her was pushing a broom. Whenever we encounter racism — in institutions, in others, in ourselves — we know silence hurts her, and that hurts us as well.

But what about the many millions more who are not being adopted, and whose parents might well wish for some less drastic solution? The adoption experience connects us, in a surprisingly visceral, embodied way, to the needs of our daughter's people. We sponsor another Guatemalan child, so her family can feed her and send her to school without leaving her parents or her village. For several years now, one of us has worked with a medical team in rural Honduras, in what has become a permanent, Honduran-staffed and -run medical-dental clinic with locally designed nutrition and education projects. We also work to educate medical students and residents how to bridge the cultural, linguistic, and economic divides immigrants encounter upon entering the American medical-industrial system. We have not done enough. We can't do it alone.

Parenting When One Has No Children

The enormity of this cosmic woundedness overwhelms us. How do we answer the world's need if every child is our responsibility? If we are dazzled by "global problems" and only ponder individual responses, there is no hope. Yet the world's woundedness, like life, is never encountered in the abstract, but in particular, embodied manifestations — some of them very close to home. We best not engage in "telescopic philanthropy," as did Mrs. Jellyby, in Charles Dickens's *Bleak House*, who devoted her energies to assisting natives of "Borrioboola-Gha, on the left bank of the Niger," while her own neglected children picked their way through her crumbling house. Knowing where and with whom to begin requires wisdom, discernment, and ultimately a choice, recognizing that faithful Christians may be called to different, particular needs. What is important is to ground each response in the community while acknowledging the diversity of the body.

The parish with whom one of us worships sponsored an Afghan family that arrived in our town after the American invasion of their country. In getting to know them, we learned the children were forced to watch as the Taliban assassinated their father outside their home in Afghanistan. We assisted them in finding an apartment, schools for the children, and a job for the mother. We helped them move twice, once to a larger house and again when they experienced repeated acts of prejudice and intolerance in that neighborhood, which sadly did not welcome "foreigners." We took the family to local parks, giving the children a change of scenery and their mother a break. Our kids and theirs played soccer and flew kites together, overcoming barriers of language, nation-state, and religion. After a few years, they no longer needed help from us, having established their own networks of support and care — and that was as it should be. The kids were doing reasonably well in school, made friends, and embraced — for good or ill — American tastes. Once again, we wonder how many North American consumers the world can survive, yet a mother and her children were materially and spiritually supported in time of great need.

During this time, the parish sustained its other witnesses — some local, some distant — each connected to the church by one or more bodies seeing a need and responding to it. In reclaiming the body wherever and however it manifests itself, we reclaim the essential practice of hospitality and recover the meaning of sanctuary so all can find safety and support in the house of the church. The possibilities are limited only by the boundaries of Christian imagination.

Some may insist that hospitality as "mere charity" prolongs suffering without eliminating its cause. Indeed, a crude form of this argument was used by American progressives to justify the eugenics campaigns of the twentieth century. Christians, we contend, should embrace efforts to reform structural evils to the extent that such actions are nonviolent and respect each life as God's gracious gift. But the Christian practice of hospitality can never be "mere charity," a bureaucratic warehouse of undesirables into which the affluent toss occasional offerings to salve their conscience. Hospitality, like the medical buildings named for the practice, involves bodies. Real bodies are harder to face than the idea of the poor. Real encounters leave people changed — unpredictably so — but rarely in ways the powers encourage. The messy reality of bodies is a powerful antidote to the dehumanizing dreaminess that makes it easier to love the poor in the abstract than to be present to the poor person in the flesh. As Dostoyevsky warns, "Love in action is a harsh and dreadful thing compared to love in dreams."[43] Without direct encounter, hospitality grows Gnostic, as indeed much of the contemporary church's "social action" has already done.

What the church proclaims is Christ crucified for the salvation of the entire world. What it exemplifies is often quite different. Though we are gathered into one body in Christ, our history as sinners does not permit dividing humanity into "us" and "them." If we do, then only too late and to our infinite regret will we realize, like Joe Keller in Arthur Miller's *All My Sons,* that they — all sons and daughters — really are ours. Most parents learn — and often to their embarrassment or regret — that their children are forever watching them. Adolescents, in particular, are vigilant for signs of hypocrisy and, like *The Catcher in the Rye's* Holden Caulfield, they quickly sniff out phonies. Rather than take this as a threat, Christians might welcome another call to conversion. In welcoming children into our families, into our churches, and into the families we support and nourish, we become more than vulnerable, we become *accountable to them.* Children's powers of observation are incentives to live up to our call, to embody the life we say we live. In turn, we witness back to those who watch us.

Becoming doers of the word and embodying the way of life we call Christian have never been easy. Where once there were violent threats from a hostile empire, now Christians are surrounded by the temptations of a culture and economy in bondage to the powers. We, too, are at least partially enthralled by these same powers, and only by living as the body can we begin to resist them. We will, at times, fail — that much is certain this side of the grave — but God forever calls us back to the gathered body, where we hope to be supported, hope to gather strength, hope to be witnessed to and to witness. For our innumerable children, even our repentance, our returning to reclaim the body we lost and denied, can be a witness, an invitation to their conversion as well as our own.

43. Fyodor Dostoyevsky, *The Brothers Karamazov,* trans. Constance Garnett, rev. Ralph E. Matlaw (New York: Norton, 1976), 49. Even more troubling is the warning a few paragraphs earlier:

> The more I love humanity in general, the less I love man in particular, that is separately, as single individuals. In my dreams . . . I have often come to making enthusiastic schemes for the service of humanity, and perhaps I might actually have faced crucifixion if it had been suddenly necessary; and yet I am incapable of living in the same room with anyone for two days together, as I know by experience. As soon as someone is near me, his personality disturbs my self-esteem and restricts my freedom. In twenty-four hours I begin to hate even the best of men: one because he's too long over his dinner, another because he has a cold and keeps blowing his nose. I become hostile to people the moment they come close to me. But it has always happened that the more I detest men individually the more ardent becomes my love for humanity. (Ibid., 48-49)

104 Introduction to *A Memoir of Mary Ann: By the Dominican Nuns Who Took Care of Her*

Flannery O'Connor

Stories of pious children tend to be false. This may be because they are told by adults, who see virtue where their subjects would see only a practical course of action; or it may be because such stories are written to edify and what is written to edify usually ends by amusing. For my part, I have never cared to read about little boys who build altars and play they are priests, or about little girls who dress up as nuns, or about those pious Protestant children who lack this equipment but brighten the corners where they are.

Last spring I received a letter from Sister Evangelist, the Sister Superior of Our Lady of Perpetual Help Free Cancer Home in Atlanta. 'This is a strange request,' the letter read, 'but we will try to tell our story as briefly as possible. In 1949, a little three-year-old girl, Mary Ann, was admitted to our Home as a patient. She proved to be a remarkable child and lived until she was twelve. Of those nine years, much is to be told. Patients, visitors, Sisters, all were influenced in some way by this afflicted child. Yet one never thought of her as afflicted. True she had been born with a tumour on the side of her face; one eye had been removed, but the other eye sparkled, twinkled, danced mischievously, and after one meeting one never was conscious of her physical defect but recognized only the beautiful brave spirit and felt the joy of such contact. Now Mary Ann's story should be written but who to write it?'

Not me, I said to myself.

'We have had offers from nuns and others but we don't want a pious little recital. We want a story with a real impact on other lives just as Mary Ann herself had that impact on each life she touched. . . . This wouldn't have to be a factual story. It could be a novel with many other characters but the outstanding character, Mary Ann.'

A novel, I thought. Horrors.

Sister Evangelist ended by inviting me to write Mary Ann's story and to come up and spend a few days at the Home in Atlanta and 'imbibe the atmosphere' where the little girl had lived for nine years.

It is always difficult to get across to people who are

From Flannery O'Connor, "Introduction," in *A Memoir of Mary Ann: By the Dominican Nuns Who Took Care of Her* (Savanna: Frederic C. Beil, 1991), 3-20. Used by permission.

not professional writers that a talent to write does not mean a talent to write anything at all. I did not wish to imbibe Mary Ann's atmosphere. I was not capable of writing her story. Sister Evangelist had enclosed a picture of the child. I had glanced at it when I first opened the letter, and had put it quickly aside. Now I picked it up to give it a last cursory look before returning it to the Sisters. It showed a little girl in her first Communion dress and veil. She was sitting on a bench, holding something I could not make out. Her small face was straight and bright on one side. The other side was protuberant, the eye was bandaged, the nose and mouth crowded slightly out of place. The child looked out at her observer with an obvious happiness and composure. I continued to gaze at the picture long after I had thought to be finished with it.

After a while I got up and went to the bookcase and took out a volume of Nathaniel Hawthorne's stories. The Dominican Congregation to which the nuns belong who had taken care of Mary Ann had been founded by Hawthorne's daughter, Rose. The child's picture had brought to mind his story *The Birthmark*. I found the story and opened it at that wonderful section of dialogue where Aylmer first mentions his wife's defect to her.

> One day Aylmer sat gazing at his wife with a trouble in his countenance that grew stronger until he spoke.
>
> 'Georgiana,' said he, 'has it never occurred to you that the mark upon your cheek might be removed?'
>
> 'No, indeed,' said she, smiling; but perceiving the seriousness of his manner, she blushed deeply. 'To tell you the truth it has been so often called a charm that I was simple enough to imagine it might be so.'
>
> 'Ah, upon another face perhaps it might,' replied her husband, 'but never on yours. No, dearest Georgiana, you came so nearly perfect from the hand of Nature that this slightest defect, which we hesitate whether to term a defect or a beauty, shocks me, as being the visible mark of earthly imperfection.'
>
> 'Shocks you, my husband!' cried Georgiana, deeply hurt, at first reddening with momentary anger, but then bursting into tears. 'Then why did you take me from my mother's side? You cannot love what shocks you!'

The defect on Mary Ann's cheek could not have been mistaken for a charm. It was plainly grotesque. She belonged to fact and not to fancy. I conceived it my duty to write Sister Evangelist that if anything were written about this child, it should indeed be a 'factual story,' and I went on to say that if anyone should write these facts, it should be the Sisters themselves, who had known and nursed her. I felt this strongly. At the same time I wanted to make it plain that I was not the one to write the factual story, and there is no quicker way to get out of a job than to prescribe it for those who have prescribed it for you. I added that should they decide to take my advice, I would be glad to help them with the preparation of their manuscript and do any small editing that proved necessary. I had no doubt that this was safe generosity. I did not expect to hear from them again.

In *Our Old Home,* Hawthorne tells about a fastidious gentleman who, while going through a Liverpool workhouse, was followed by a wretched and rheumy child, so awful looking that he could not decide what sex it was. The child followed him about until it decided to put itself in front of him in a mute appeal to be held. The fastidious gentleman, after a pause that was significant for himself, picked it up and held it. Hawthorne comments upon this:

> Nevertheless, it could be no easy thing for him to do, he being a person burdened with more than an Englishman's customary reserve, shy of actual contact with human beings, afflicted with a peculiar distaste for whatever was ugly, and furthermore, accustomed to that habit of observation from all insulated standpoint which is said (but I hope erroneously) to have the tendency of putting ice into the blood.
>
> So I watched the struggle in his mind with a good deal of interest, and am seriously of the opinion that he did a heroic act and effected more than he dreamed of toward his final salvation when he took up the loathsome child and caressed it as tenderly as if he had been its father.

What Hawthorne neglected to add is that he was the gentleman who did this. His wife, after his death, published his notebooks in which there was this account of the incident:

> After this, we went to the ward where the children were kept, and, on entering this, we saw, in the first place, two or three unlovely and unwholesome little imps, who were lazily playing together. One of them (a child about six years old, but I know not whether girl or boy) immediately took the strangest fancy for me. It was a wretched, pale, half torpid little thing, with a humour in its eye which the Governor said was the scurvy. I never saw, till a few moments afterward, a child that I should feel less inclined to fondle. But this little sickly, humour-eaten fright prowled around me, taking hold of my skirts, following at my heels, and at last held up its hands, smiled in my face, and standing directly before me, insisted on my taking it up! Not that it said a word, for I rather think it was underwitted, and could not talk; but its face expressed such perfect confidence that it was going to be taken up and made much of, that it was impossible not to do it. It was as if God had promised the child this favour on my behalf, and that I must needs fulfil the contract. I held my undesirable burden a little while, and after setting the child down, it still followed me, holding two of my fingers and playing with them, just as if it were a child of my own. It was a foundling, and out of all human kind it chose me to be its father! We went upstairs into another ward; and on coming down again there was this same child waiting for me, with a sickly smile around its defaced mouth, and in its dim-red eyes. . . . I should never have forgiven myself if I had repelled its advances.

Rose Hawthorne, Mother Alphonsa in religious life, later wrote that the account of this incident in the Liverpool workhouse seemed to her to contain the greatest words her father ever wrote.

The work of Hawthorne's daughter is perhaps known by few in the United States where it should be known by all. She discovered much that he sought, and fulfilled in a practical way the hidden desires of his life. The ice in the blood which he feared, and which this very fear preserved him from, was turned by her into a warmth which initiated action. If he observed, fearfully but truthfully; if he acted, reluctantly but firmly, she charged ahead, secure in the path his truthfulness had outlined for her.

Towards the end of the nineteenth century, she became aware of the plight of the cancerous poor in New York and was stricken by it. Charity patients with incurable cancer were not kept in the city hospitals but were sent to Blackwell's Island or left to find their own place to die. In either case, it was a matter of being left to rot. Rose Hawthorne Lathrop was a woman of great force and energy. A few years earlier she had become a Catholic and had since been seeking the kind of occupation that would be a practical fulfilment of her conversion. With almost no money of her own, she moved into a tenement in the worst section of New York and began to take in incurable cancer patients. She was joined later by a young portrait painter, Alice Huber, whose steady and patient qualities complemented her own forceful and exuberant ones. With their concerted effort, the gruelling work prospered. Eventually other women came to help them and they became a congregation of nuns in the Dominican Order — the Servants of Relief for Incurable Cancer. There are now seven of their free cancer homes in the United States.

Mother Alphonsa inherited a fair share of her father's literary gift. Her account of the grandson of her first patient makes fine reading. He was a lad who, for reasons unpreventable, had been brought to live for a while in the tenement apartment with his ailing grandmother and the few other patients there at the time.

> The boy was brought by an officer of the institution, to remain for a visit. My first glance at his rosy, healthy, clever face struck a warning shiver through my soul. He was a flourishing slip from criminal roots. His eyes had the sturdy gaze of satanic vigour. . . . I began to teach him the catechism. With the utmost good nature he sat in front of me as long as I would sit, giving correct answers. 'He likes to study it better than to be idle,' said his grandmother; 'and I taught it to him myself, long ago.' His eyes took on a mystic vagueness during these lessons, and I felt certain he would tell the truth in future and be gentle instead of barbaric.
>
> Food was hidden away in dark corners for the cherubic, overfed pet, and his pranks and thefts were shielded and denied, and the nice clothing which I provided him with, out of our stores, with a new suit for Sundays, strangely disappeared when Willie went to call upon his mother. . . . In a few weeks Willie had become famous in the neighbourhood as the worst boy it had ever experienced, although it was lined with little scoundrels. The inmates of the house and adjacent shanties feared him, the scoundrels made circles around him as he flew from one escapade to another on the diabolical street which was never free from some sort of outrages perpetrated by young or old. Willie built fires upon the shed roofs, threw bricks that guardian angels alone averted from our heads, and actually hit several little boys at sundry times, whom we mended in the Relief Room. He uttered exclamations that hideously rang in the ears of the profane themselves. . . . He delighted in the pictures of the saints which I gave him, stole those I did not give, and sold them all. I preached affectionately, and he listened tenderly, and promised to 'remember,' and was very sorry for his sins when he had been forced by an iron grasp to accept their revelation. He made a very favourable impression upon an experienced priest who was summoned to rescue his soul; and he built a particularly large bonfire on our woodshed when let go. The poor grandmother began to have severe haemorrhages, because of the shocks she received and the scoldings she gave. Before he came she used to call him 'that little angel.' Now she wisely declared that he was goodhearted.

Bad children are harder to endure than good ones, but they are easier to read about, and I congratulated myself on having minimized the possibility of a book about Mary Ann by suggesting that the Sisters do it themselves. Although I heard from Sister Evangelist that they were about it, I felt that a few attempts to capture Mary Ann in writing would lead them to think better of the project. It was doubtful that any of them had the literary gifts of their foundress. Moreover, they were busy nurses and had their hands full following a strenuous vocation.

THEIR MANUSCRIPT arrived the first of August. After I had gathered myself together, I sat down and began to read it. There was everything about the writing to make the professional writer groan. Most of it was reported, very little was rendered; at the dramatic moment — where there was one — the observer seemed to fade away, and where an exact word or phrase was needed, a vague one was usually supplied. Yet when I had finished reading, I remained for some time, the imperfections of the writing forgotten, thinking about the mystery of Mary Ann. They had managed to convey it.

The story was as unfinished as the child's face. Both seemed to have been left, like creation on the seventh day, to be finished by others. The reader would have to make something of the story as Mary Ann had made something of her face.

She and the Sisters who had taught her had fashioned from her unfinished face the material of her death. The creative action of the Christian's life is to prepare his death in Christ. It is a continuous action in which this world's goods are utilized to the fullest, both positive gifts and what Père Teilhard de Chardin calls 'passive diminishments.' Mary Ann's diminishment was extreme, but she was equipped by natural intelligence and by a suitable education, not simply to endure it, but to build upon it. She was an extraordinarily rich little girl.

Death is the theme of much modern literature. There is *Death in Venice, Death of a Salesman, Death in the Afternoon, Death of a Man.* Mary Ann's was the death of a child. It was simpler than any of these, yet infinitely more knowing. When she entered the door of Our Lady of Perpetual Help Home in Atlanta, she fell into the hands of women who are shocked at nothing and who love life so much that they spend their own lives making comfortable those who have been pronounced incurable of cancer. Her own prognosis was six months, but she lived nine years, long enough for the Sisters to teach her what alone could have been of importance to her. Hers was an education for death, but not one carried on obtrusively. Her days were full of dogs and party dresses, of Sisters and sisters, of Coca Colas and Dagwood sandwiches, and of her many and varied friends — from Mr. Slack and Mr. Connolly to Lucius, the yard man; from patients afflicted the way she was to children who were brought to the Home to visit her and were perhaps told when they left to think how thankful they should be that God had made their faces straight. It is doubtful if any of them were as fortunate as Mary Ann.

The Sisters had set all this down artlessly and had devoted a good deal of their space to detailing Mary Ann's many pious deeds. I was tempted to edit away a good many of these. They had willingly given me the right to cut, and I could have laid about me with satisfaction but for the fact that there was nothing with which to fill in any gaps I created. I felt too that while their style had been affected by traditional hagiography and even a little by Parson Weems, what they had set down was what had happened and there was no way to get around it. This was a child brought up by seventeen nuns; she was what she was, and the itchy hand of the fiction writer would have to be stayed. I was only capable of dealing with another Willie.

I later suggested to Sister Evangelist, on an occasion when some of the Sisters came down to spend the afternoon with me to discuss the manuscript, that Mary Ann could not have been much *but* good, considering her environment. Sister Evangelist leaned over the arm of her chair and gave me a look. Her eyes were blue and unpredictable behind spectacles that unmoored them slightly. 'We've had some demons!' she said, and a gesture of her hand dismissed my ignorance.

After an afternoon with them, I decided that they had had about everything and flinched before nothing, even though one of them asked me during the course of the visit why I wrote about such grotesque characters, why the grotesque (of all things) was my vocation. They had in the meantime inspected some of my writings. I was struggling to get off the hook she had me on when another of our guests supplied the one answer that would make it immediately plain to all of them. 'It's your vocation too,' he said, to her.

This opened up for me also a new perspective on the grotesque. Most of us have learned to be dispassionate about evil, to look it in the face and find, as often as not, our own grinning reflections with which we do not argue, but good is another matter. Few have stared at that long enough to accept the fact that its face too is grotesque, that in us the good is something under construction. The modes of evil usually receive worthy expression. The modes of good have to be satisfied with a cliché or a smoothing down that will soften their real look. When we look into the face of good, we are liable to see a face like Mary Ann's, full of promise.

Bishop Hyland preached Mary Ann's funeral sermon. He said that the world would ask why Mary Ann should die. He was thinking undoubtedly of those who had known her and knew that she loved life, knew that her grip on a hamburger had once been so strong that she had fallen through the back of a chair without dropping it, or that some months before her death she and Sister Loretta had got a real baby to nurse. The Bishop was speaking to her family and friends. He could not have been thinking of that world, much farther removed yet everywhere, which would not ask why Mary Ann should die, but why she should be born in the first place.

One of the tendencies of our age is to use the suffering of children to discredit the goodness of God, and once you have discredited His goodness, you are done with Him. The Aylmers whom Hawthorne saw as a menace have multiplied. Busy cutting down human imperfection, they are making headway also on the raw material of good. Ivan Karamazov cannot believe, as long as one child is in torment; Camus' hero cannot accept the divinity of Christ, because of the massacre of the innocents. In this popular pity, we mark our gain in sensibility and our loss in vision. If other ages felt less, they saw more, even though they saw with the blind, prophetical, unsentimental eye of acceptance, which is to say, of faith. In the absence of this faith now, we govern by tenderness. It is a tenderness which, long since cut off from the person of Christ, is wrapped in theory. When tenderness is detached from the source of tenderness, its logical outcome is terror. It ends in forced labour camps and in the fumes of the gas chamber.

These reflections seem a long way from the simplicity and innocence of Mary Ann; but they are not so far removed. Hawthorne could have put them in a fable and shown us what to fear. In the end, I cannot think of Mary Ann without thinking also of that fastidious, sceptical New Englander who feared the ice in his blood. There is a direct line between the incident in the Liverpool workhouse, the work of Hawthorne's daughter, and Mary Ann — who stands not only for herself but for all the other examples of human imperfection and grotesquerie which the Sisters of Rose Hawthorne's order spend their lives caring for. Their work is the tree sprung from Hawthorne's small act of Christlikeness, and Mary Ann is its flower. By reason of the fear, the search, and the charity that marked his life and influenced his daughter's, Mary Ann inherited, a century later, the wealth of Catholic wisdom that taught her what to make of her death. Hawthorne gave what he did not have himself.

This action by which charity grows invisibly among us, entwining the living and the dead, is called by the Church the Communion of Saints. It is a communion created upon human imperfection, created from what we make of our grotesque state. Of hers Mary Ann made what, like all good things, would have escaped notice had not the Sisters and many others been affected by it and wished it written down. The Sisters who composed the memoir have told me that they feel they have failed to create her as she was, that she was more lively than they managed to make her, more gay, more gracious, but I think that they have done enough and done it well. I think that for the reader this story will illuminate the lines that join the most diverse lives and that hold us fast in Christ.

105 Being Mickey's Doctor

Margaret E. Mohrmann

None of the stories in this book is more wrenching than Mickey's. It was through my encounter with Mickey and her family that I most clearly and most unforgettably discovered the nature of doctoring. It is the grounding story of my career — perhaps of my adult life — and the one that encapsulates everything else I have to say. I remember Mickey more clearly than any other patient I have ever cared for, even now, some thirty years later. I owe more to her and her parents than I can tally. I have thought and rethought these scenes since they happened, but it took many years for me to grasp their fundamental significance in the understandings of doctoring that I bring to my work as a teacher of medicine, in the perspectives on suffering and human relationships that I bring to my teaching and scholarship in Christian ethics, and in my sense of myself as doctor, teacher, believer, friend, and family member.

I first met Mickey in May of my internship year. I had survived ten months: only two months left before reaching the relative calm of the second year, with its emphasis on general and specialty outpatient clinics, which I looked forward to as a virtual vacation. Coming back to the service with the two- to twelve-year-olds that month was something I welcomed. They were the age group I felt most comfortable working with. Procedures (placing intravenous lines, drawing blood, doing lumbar punctures) on babies and toddlers were more technically difficult, and the adolescents — well, they just asked too much and gave too little by my naïve calculation, plus that service had included a couple of patients who had left me exhausted and chastened. The fact that I had recently finished two consecutive months in the N.I.C.U. and nursery made this rotation look even better. I was ready for anything, fortunately.

Mickey had been admitted a week before, referred in by her pediatrician. She had had a particularly painful, refractory ear infection — unusual in a twelve-year-old — that led her doctor to check her blood counts and thereby discover the reason for her inability to rid herself of the infection: Mickey had leukemia. In the week during which she had been in the hospital, she had had all the necessary evaluations, had the ear infection successfully treated, and had been started on the standard chemotherapy for her type of cancer, acute myelogenous leukemia, or A.M.L. Of the two most common types of childhood leukemia, the other being acute lymphocytic leukemia (A.L.L.), A.M.L. was definitely the worse, less likely to respond to treatment, and, in 1974, offering a dismal chance of long-term survival. In the early 1970s we were just beginning to see that A.L.L. might in fact be a curable cancer, as it has proven to be. A.M.L. was notorious not only for the short life span of its victims but also for its association with dreadful complications before death, such as widespread and uncontrollable bleeding, and its requirement for particularly nasty chemotherapeutic agents — a terrible diagnosis, a grim outlook.

I do not remember our first meeting specifically, except that I was struck from the outset by Mickey's intelligence, wit, spark, and willingness to engage with me well beyond what I then expected of twelve-year-old girls. She was a tall, well-built child, with lots of curly auburn hair and a scattering of freckles over her nose and cheeks. Developmentally mature and athletic (she ran track at school), Mickey used to really enjoy food. Now, however, she was wracked by the side effects of the chemical bludgeons being used against her disease: nausea and vomiting, mouth sores, and a not surprising loss of appetite. She was not an uncomplaining child — no saint, but a real twelve-year-old — and made no bones about the fact that she hated this, all of it. She hated being in the hospital, missing school (as she was missed: her room was lined with get-well cards crafted by her classmates and teachers), and feeling sick all the time. More than anything, she often half-cried at me, she hated being talked about so much. Mickey had the shyness of a "big-boned" adolescent girl — I recognized that kind of deep-down introversion, having been one of those myself — and anything was better than being in the spotlight, especially because the spotlight in this case was more like a searchlight scouring the grounds of a prison compound.

The medical team made rounds first thing each morning and last thing each afternoon. The group included six residents and interns, plus a nurse (if one could get free from other duties to accompany us), and a student or two; in the afternoon we were joined, and led, by the chief resident. Twice a day a sizeable knot of people would stand beside Mickey's closed half-glass door, just outside the mostly glass walls of her room, where she could see us talking, watch me telling them about her, and register our unguarded (because generally oblivious) expressions of who knows what? Frustration and fear, indifference and weariness, love and concern? Who knows if I shook my head in despair of her future, there where she could watch me do it, or if she might have read my gestures that way at a time when I was actually despairing of my own future, having given a poor impression of my competence as the chief resident grilled me on the pathophysiological details of her disease and the pharmacological intricacies of its treatment.

It was only after a couple of weeks of this routine that Mickey mustered the courage, one day when she was perhaps feeling particularly body-sick and homesick, to blurt out, "I *hate* it when you all stand outside there and talk about me! What are you saying? Why can't you say it in here to me? I *hate* it!"

In my groping attempts to take care of her and of myself, and having yet formed no inner mechanism — of integrity? of confidence? — that would allow me to question or try to change the way things were done in this august place I had come to for training, I reached for some accommodation. I asked, "What if we did our talking down the hall where you can't see us? Would that be better?"

She muttered a grudging "Yeah, I guess."

From then on, when I remembered to do so, I had the team talk about Mickey while we were still standing in front of the room before hers. I have no idea, nor did I ask myself then, what the children and parents in *that* room thought when we began standing there so much longer than we had before, deep in earnest conversation — about them? Mickey could then watch us sail by, clipboards in hand, faces intent on the next task, no one acknowledging her with a glance or a wave. So determined were we to leave her in peace that we simply left her. She did not mention the issue again, at least not during that hospitalization. But I had reason, more than once, to recall the intensity of her anguished cry.

Two years later, I was once again on this service, this time as the senior resident, running those rounds that still went door-to-door, stopping outside each glass-walled room as though we were sightseers at the zoo. One day a woman accosted my fellow senior resident during rounds as we left our post outside the room she was in to move on to the next. I expect she picked him as the focus of her anger because he was male and probably looked as though he were in charge. She was a friend of the parents of the child in that room — perhaps a frequent visitor, perhaps on her only visit; I had not noticed her before and did not see her again. She was very angry, almost spitting, as she railed at my colleague for this rounding practice of ours. I do not remember her argument particularly, only the word she kept using over and over: *dehumanizing.*

After saying her piece, while my colleague looked at her sternly and repeated something about doing our job, she stalked off in tears. We glanced at each other, in her wake, employing that patronizing shrug and wry smile we had so easily assumed years before as the stance of the professional against the unenlightened. "Dehumanizing? What is she talking about? She doesn't have a clue what we're doing out here, does she? What's her problem?" My colleague looked as uncomfortable as I felt, but we never discussed it, then or later. In the back of my mind, though, I remembered Mickey and how she had felt about these rounds. There was something here to think about someday, when I had time and might not be called on to act in ways for which I lacked courage, wit, and energy.

During Mickey's hospitalization, I also came to know her family well. Her mother, Mary, was there most of the time. She was a native of the city, her speech redolent of the characteristic intonations and phrasings of her hometown (she usually called me "hon"), and a full-time stay-at-home mother. Her exuberant, enfolding personality was floored by this disastrous turn, but was no less embracing for all that. We hit it off; she took me in as friend and ally in this crisis situation, even to the point of letting me in on family jokes — both old ones and the new ones that present events gave rise to — and family idiosyncrasies. Through her eyes first, and then through my own, I got to know Mickey's father, Marshall. (Marshall was also called by his first name, Fred, at times, but the joke that seemed clearly to be associated with calling him "Fred" was never revealed to me. It appeared to be what Mary called him when she had a minor beef with him, and Mickey had adopted that usage, along with many other of her mother's mannerisms. "Fred" was always said with a sarcastic lilt and accompanied by a teasing needle.) Marshall was not around quite as much as Mary, given his full-time day job as a butcher at the A&P, but he came every evening, and, given my every-other-night call schedule, I got to see a lot of him. He was a gentle and affable man, in love with his family and the Baltimore Orioles, in that order, and overwhelmed by what was happening to his beloved Mick.

Then there were Flo and Joe, Mary's parents. Flo was a smaller, grayer Mary, equally intense and embracing. Joe, like Marshall, was quiet — and seemed older than his wife, not in such good health — with a down-to-earth manner and a sweet and warming smile. I saw Mickey's siblings only infrequently during this hospitalization, when they visited on occasional evenings and weekend days. Her brother Chris was fourteen or fifteen then, Joey ten, Jenny eight.

Mickey's leukemia went into remission just as it was intended to, a victory for the chemo, a great relief for all of us. She went home early in June, soon after I had left the service and turned her over to another intern for the rest of her stay. Before I signed off, however, I made it clear to the new intern that Mickey was mine and that I would be following her through her outpatient visits, monitoring her disease. That is, as was the practice in this residency program, whatever rotation I was on, I would come to the cancer clinic to see her on her appointed day, and I would be the one to draw the blood, perform the lumbar puncture or bone marrow aspiration. I would also be the one to discuss with Mickey and her parents the results of those studies, plans for treatment, effects of medications, everything — the one they would call, at any time, if they had questions or concerns.

Moreover, neither Mickey nor her parents wished to have our oncologist be their primary caregiver. Mary's initial encounter with the oncologist had become the stuff of family legend, another family "joke," this one grounded in intense pain. On the day Mickey was first admitted to the hospital, Mary accompanied her. Marshall was at work and could not join them until he got off at the end of the day. That day was a nightmare for Mary. From the pediatrician's initial concern about the ear infection to the whirl of activity that followed Mickey's entrance into the hospital — lengthy history taking, meticulous physical examinations, blood drawing, lumbar puncture, bone marrow aspiration, even a tap of her infected middle ear — the significance of the day could scarcely be fathomed in the midst of it all, only experienced. The word *leukemia* had been uttered as justification for all the testing, accompanied by modifiers denoting uncertainty and the existence of other, less devastating, possible diagnoses. Mary had longed for Marshall's presence through this but knew he could not leave his job until later. By late afternoon she knew he would arrive soon, when they could face together whatever it was they had to face.

The oncologist — forever after in this family referred to only as "Les," a diminutive of his first name, which no one else ever used — appeared at Mickey's door, Mickey now asleep, exhausted by the unimaginable assaults on her body, the utter confusion of it all, the fever and the pain in her ear. Les asked Mary to come with him to the conference room to talk. She asked him to wait until Marshall arrived. Les looked at his watch and said he really needed to talk with her now. Reluctantly, she went with him to the conference room. Before he could begin, she said, "If you've got something to tell me, please wait until my husband gets here. Please don't tell me without him here."

Les started talking, reviewing the day's course, the tests that had been done. Mary interrupted him to plead, once again, "Please don't tell me anything before Marshall gets here. Please don't tell me this while I'm alone."

Les continued as though she had not spoken. He told her Mickey had leukemia. He explained the type of leukemia, the prognosis, and the treatment plans. And then he left Mary in the conference room, alone.

Mary told me this story late in May, when we were making plans for Mickey's discharge and I was explaining to her the follow-up routine. She was so relieved to hear that they would be seeing me on their return visits and not Les, who would be calling the shots from some distant control booth, so adamant that she did not want to see Les any more than necessary, that I had to ask why. She wept as she told me, reliving the awful pain of hearing that Mickey had leukemia and of being so terribly alone, treated so callously. "Why couldn't he just wait like I asked him to? I told him not to tell me, but he did anyway. Why?" I could only shake my head. What possible answer would suffice? I knew that, had I had the opportunity, I could have been guilty of a similar crime.

A day or so before Mickey was discharged, I came by to visit. Marshall walked out with me as I left and asked if I would tell Mickey her diagnosis — the name of her disease, as he put it — before she went home. Weeks before, I had talked with her parents about how they wanted to handle information, how much to say to Mickey, how much to dance around real issues. I had given them my naïve canned spiel about the problems of lying to children, who almost always know some version of the truth anyway and are deprived of the chance to talk about it if the adults around them will not acknowledge the truth. So now they were certain that they wanted Mickey to have the truth — how could they justify all the follow-up visits if all she had was the "anemia" they had been using as the code word for her illness? — and they wanted me to be the one to tell her. They would be there, of course, but they did not know how to say the words, so would I please do it?

"Of course," I said quickly. "I'll come visit this same time tomorrow, if you can be here then, and that's when I'll tell her." I walked off, quietly moved that they had asked me to do this, that they really regarded me as Mickey's doctor. Then I began thinking of what I might say, what it might be like to do it, and my heart sank. This would be a new experience for me.

Although during that year of internship I had had to tell parents that their child had died, those experiences could in no way assure me of my competence in giving bad news — quite the opposite. And I had never had to give parents a bad diagnosis, much less to tell a child of any age the news of his or her grim disease, to pronounce the doom that words like *cancer* and *leukemia* portended. How to do this? I spent that evening thinking about it, planning how to explain; at the level of an intelligent twelve-year-old, the nature of her disease, I worked it out in great detail. I went to Mickey's room the next day with a well-rehearsed account in mind, in which I would show her — even draw pictures (my pad was ready in my pocket) — how the renegade white blood cells pushed out the red cells and the tiny platelets and thus created problems of infection, anemia, and bleeding. I would explain something of how all the nasty medicines she had endured had done their work against her particular traitorous cells and why they had also made her so sick and made her hair fall out. I was rather proud of what I had put together, but that did not stop me from feeling apprehensive as I entered her room.

I had established a good relationship with Mickey, mostly by being around a lot, available and willing to talk with her about schoolwork or to compare the merits of her favorite nurses or to puzzle over the style of wig that would be both flattering and unremarkable. I had listened when she had something to complain about (which was, of course, often — we gave her plenty to complain about), and I had entered into her family's mode of humor and coping. Perhaps most important, I had been as honest as I could about what she could expect from a new medicine or test — or me. I wanted very much to keep her trust and respect, to continue to be honest with her but not to overwhelm her with information beyond her capacity to handle.

When I came into the room, I saw she was in good spirits. Now that she was done with the chemotherapy, she was feeling so much better. Plus, she knew she was going home the next day, and she was happy. The get-well cards had been taken down from the walls and packed away to take home. She was in her own pajamas instead of a hospital gown and wearing her new wig, the one her mother and grandmother had found for her that matched her own hair amazingly well, although it was styled in a way that was jarringly adult and formal next to her young adolescent face. She was sitting up in bed, talking with her parents. They all turned to me as I entered, and her parents' anxiety was almost palpable. It was clear there would be no small talk. I needed to get right to the point before Mickey started sensing the fear in the room.

I sat on the edge of her bed; she scooted over to make room for me. "Before you head home, Mick, we need to talk about when I'll be seeing you back for checkups. And we need to talk about why I need to see you back in the clinic. What have you been told you've been in the hospital for?"

She looked at me warily. "Some kind of anemia?"

"Well," I said, "you do have anemia, but the reason you're anemic is that you have leukemia." I was prepared to keep talking, but I saw her eyes widen in surprise, so instead I waited to hear her reaction.

She stared at me for a long moment, shifted her gaze to her parents then back to me. "But that means it can come back!" she wailed and settled into her now-familiar pout, the firm set of her jaw and protrusion of her full lower lip that signaled both her displeasure and the effort it took to be brave.

I regrouped, discarding my script. "Yes, it can. We don't know if it will; it may not. That's what we're hoping for, and that's why we'll keep checking you and giving you medicine at home — to keep that from happening, if we can."

Her lower lip trembled, then stiffened again. "I thought I was through with all this. I don't ever want to come back here again."

I felt that frisson of rejection that I was only beginning to get used to: the repeated, but still jarring recognition that, no matter how close I became to my patients and their families, no matter how intensely good the interaction, I nevertheless worked in a place that they wanted to put behind them forever — and thus leave me behind too. Now this child I loved, part of this family I loved, was saying the same thing: Let me out of here! How hard it is to keep their perspective separate from mine. My job is their torture. The place where I find such fulfillment and satisfying relationships is a place that they, no matter how sincerely they treasure the relationship, would much rather never have entered. The good of the encounter cannot outweigh, even though it may ameliorate, the evil of the situation. I keep forgetting that because, for me, it can and does. But that can be true only because the evil of the situation is not mine to bear.

I swallowed hard against my own feelings so I could agree with her entirely appropriate reaction and assure her again that her goal was, indeed, our common goal: to keep her healthy, out of the hospital, back in school, even able to run track again. I never got the chance to do my junior high pathophysiology lecture. The conversation was clearly over. I stayed around a bit longer to see if she had questions, but Mickey had nothing else to say or to ask. Her parents glanced my way, with shrugs and tentative smiles, as if to reassure me that I had done my best, and returned their focus to their daughter, as they prepared themselves to take care of her. I left, feeling both relieved that the deed had been done and troubled by how much I did not know about Mickey in particular and doctoring in general. Good grades in medical school do nothing to make one worthy to serve the suffering.

I saw Mickey, usually accompanied by her mother, off and on for checkups over the next few months. She gradually regained strength and started doing whatever twelve-year-old girls did during hot city summers in the 1970s. She continued to wear her wig, despite discomfort from the heat, as her hair slowly grew in. A few times that summer I was a guest in their house — lovely, embracing times of family meals, with lots of laughter. On one such occasion, Marshall brought home a batch of seasoned steamed crabs and spread them out on a table in the basement. Mickey's parents, siblings, and I tore into them, wielding mallets and picks with abandon, rapidly diminishing the pile of crabs. Then I noticed that Mickey was still picking at her first crab very slowly. I was concerned. I had thought her appetite had returned; she certainly seemed full of energy and did not appear to be losing weight. What was the problem?

Just then everyone else seemed to notice my noticing, and the teasing began. Apparently this was Mickey's traditional way of eating steamed crabs — excruciatingly slowly, carefully picking out every shred of crab meat while avoiding every shard of shell and any taint of "mustard" (the oddly tasty name given to what amounts to the crab's steamed viscera, prized by some as a piquant bonus, like the condiment its name suggests, and disdained by others who cannot forget its previous role in the crab's life). They were quite used to Mickey's eating a single crab in the time it took the rest of us to down four or five. She smiled slightly at their scoffing, holding herself above it, focused on the fine art of crustacean demolition. It was good to see her being recognizably, irreducibly Mickey among those who knew and loved her, idiosyncrasies and all. It was a very happy evening.

Late in October came the clinic visit I had dreaded. Mickey felt fine and was well into the school year, rejoicing in normalcy regained. It was a routine checkup, but this time the lab results showed that the leukemia had returned: the remission was over. Les was there, and we told Mickey and Mary together that she would have to come back into the hospital for another round of intensive chemotherapy. Mickey was stunned. She and her mother shed a few tears but then went about the business of facing the next step, starting the climb all over again. In retrospect, I suspect they were resigned to having to go through it all again, but expected the same outcome as before. Neither of them could have known what I knew: the first remission was the only remission. In 1974, for a patient's A.M.L. to relapse was to lose virtually all hope of cure or even long-term remission. Mickey's first remission — the first was almost always the longest — had lasted fewer than five months. The most we could hope for now was a few more good months at home, nothing more. I did not say that to them, and I believe they were not thinking it. I began then to comprehend that knowledge itself is one of the burdens a doctor is obligated to bear.

As it happened, that month I was once again working on the floor to which Mickey would be readmitted. She would be my inpatient again. When she arrived in the ward a few hours later, after she and Mary went home long enough to pack a bag and notify the rest of the family, I took her into the treatment room to do her admission physical examination and get started on the tests and treatments that were dictated by the study protocols for her disease. This time the chemotherapy would be more brutal than before, but I did not intend to warn her of that. She would find out for herself in time; no need to have to suffer through the anticipation of it too.

While I did the exam in the treatment room, Mary sat in the hospital room that would be Mickey's, talking to the senior resident, giving Mickey's history yet again. Mickey and I chatted some as I worked, but it was awkward — I resolutely cheery, Mickey uncertain, quiet, a bit disoriented. In a weak attempt to take some of the bite out of this hospitalization, I talked of nurses and Child Life workers she would enjoy seeing again. I suspect that ploy triggered her question: "What about LaTanya? How's she doing?"

Eight-year-old LaTanya, who had also had leukemia, had been Mickey's roommate for a few weeks in May, until each girl had required a room of her own to protect her from infection. Mickey and her mother had "adopted" LaTanya, whose own mother could not be with her during weekdays, and the two girls chatted, played board games, watched TV, complained about the food, and cried over needle sticks together. LaTanya's disease had not gone into remission. She had never left the hospital, but had died during the summer.

"She died, Mickey. I'm sorry. It happened a couple of months ago."

"She died!" Mickey's eyes practically jumped out of her head as she stared at me in stricken disbelief. "Am I going to die?"

Oh, no. Not that question. I'm not ready for this. She's boring holes through me with her eyes. There is no evasion possible. I cannot deflect this. Oh God, I want to. I'm the one she's asking. I'm the one who has to answer. Any number of possible replies zipped through my head, each discarded as soon as it appeared: too dishonest, too hokey, too obviously an escape. This girl deserves better from me. Do I have better to give her?

"You have a disease people can die from, Mick, but that's not what's happening right now. And we're doing everything we can to be sure that doesn't happen. LaTanya did have leukemia, but it was a different kind from yours, and she didn't respond to the treatment. The medicines didn't work for her. They've been working for you, and we think they'll work again."

"Okay. They'd better work," she said with all the defiance of a child who knows she is trapped in an unfair world.

She never asked me The Question again. Over the next few weeks, she talked around the subject with an art therapist who helped her draw and paint her way out of the isolation that had to be imposed to protect her from infection as her immune defenses succumbed to the chemotherapy. She even, so the therapist reported, got to the point of calling it "The Big Question," acknowledging its existence in the room and in her mind, but she did not ask directly again about the possibility of her dying — not until a week or so before death came, and then it was to her parents that she posed it.

Mickey was readmitted to the hospital, and the routine began again. Toxic medicines, intravenous lines that were increasingly difficult to place and maintain, nausea and vomiting, days of feeling rotten — better just slept away — alternating with days of feeling feisty and homesick at the same time. The room filled quickly with cards from classmates again, taped to every available space on walls and curtains alike. Within a week of her admittance, her white blood cell counts were too low to risk exposing her to all the germs abroad on our lips and our hands, which meant protective isolation. Everyone who entered her room, family and staff alike, donned yellow gowns and surgical face masks covering nose and mouth. She did not like it a bit, but soon gave up complaining; it took too much energy, and she never won.

On Halloween night I was on call, my last night on before leaving the service for an elective month without call, a precious rarity in this residency. Flo, Mickey's grandmother, came to be with her while Mary and Marshall stayed home so the younger children could go trick-or-treating. Flo had decided that Halloween needed to come to Mickey too — so she brought *me* a costume. Black curly wig, black lacy shawl, elbow-length black gloves: I was to be a "lady of the evening" that night, she informed me. Mickey was delighted; she seemed to think it the perfect role for me. I looked askance at Flo's bagful of black clothing, especially at the rather dreadful wig, but neither Flo nor Mickey would let me back out. I still have the photo Flo took of me in Mickey's room, in yellow gown and surgical mask, long black gloves, absurd black wig, the black shawl draped suggestively over my shoulders. I am standing against a backdrop of some of the numerous get-well cards plastering the room. My left hand is resting coyly on a carved pumpkin. Perched on top of the black wig is my addition to the costume, one of my prized possessions: a dimestore nurse's cap emblazoned with "Dr. Mohrmann, R.N." — a gift the N.I.C.U. nurses had given me that spring at the end of my two-month stint there.

The three of us laughed — or, more accurately, I pranced and postured, Flo made bawdy remarks, and Mickey guffawed — until I was called away to the telephone. When I left the room still in full regalia, we laughed even harder. I came back later to tell them about the odd looks I had received from the other patients and their parents as I traipsed through the halls. No one could figure out who that odd woman was.

With Mickey's reentry into the hospital, her siblings began to fall apart in their own ways. Chris, her older brother, had been given the opportunity to attend an excellent prep school just outside the city. He boarded there during the week and came home on weekends. But, as he later said quite clearly, he could not tolerate being away from home while Mickey was so sick, so he ran away from school one night and turned up at home, refusing to go back. Joey began doing poorly, academically and behaviorally, in his school, a real change for him. Jenny went skating and broke her leg.

I asked Mary, after she recited this litany of mishaps to me, what the children knew about Mickey's illness. She said that she and Marshall had told Chris Mickey's diagnosis and thought he probably understood what was going on, although he did not talk about it. They had not told the younger ones anything except that Mickey was sick; they were not sure what they knew or guessed. Later I talked with Kathryn, the social worker on the oncology service, who made the wise suggestion that she and I offer a home visit to talk with the children. Mary and Marshall jumped at the suggestion, pleased and relieved that we would take on the task they had been avoiding, while knowing it had to be done. We set a date for one evening early the following week.

When we arrived at their house, Mary ushered us into the dining room, and we all sat around the table, with coffee and sodas and cake before us, to have our conversation. Kathryn and I had done some earlier planning, so, on cue, I launched into an explanation of Mickey's illness, including an abbreviated version of the pathophysiology lecture I had prepared for her in June but had never delivered. I explained the treatment, why she had to be in the hospital so long, and what the isolation was intended to accomplish. And then I told them the possible outcomes, including death, while trying to be as optimistic as I could. They listened attentively; no one fidgeted or giggled. Kathryn spoke directly to Chris about how difficult it must have been for him to be away from home when so much was going on. She acknowledged the significant additional pain for the children caused by their parents' being so preoccupied with Mickey's illness and by the loss of the usual routines and expectations of life at home.

Joey, who was sitting next to me, had kept his head down throughout the discussion; he had not touched the cake on his plate. I looked at him and, all at once, knew what else needed saying. To the table in general I said, "You know, a lot of times kids say mean things to each other. Things like, 'I wish you were dead.' Or sometimes you just think it and don't say it. I want you guys to know that saying or thinking that kind of stuff doesn't make people sick. Mickey did not get sick because you wished something bad on her. This isn't your fault."

Joey expelled a great rush of air and slid halfway down in his chair like a man who had just been acquitted by the jury. I cannot pretend that everything was rosy for the children from that night on — of course it was not — but Joey's school performance improved noticeably, and there was no further trouble among Mickey's siblings.

Mickey was another matter. I had told her ahead of time about the planned meeting at her house, why we thought it was a good idea, and what I was going to tell her brothers and sister about her illness. She had little to say, just nodded solemnly as she received the information. The day after the meeting she was tearful and angry. "I don't see why you had to go talk to them. What did you tell them about me? Why aren't you telling me those things?"

"I didn't tell them anything I haven't told you, Mick." (That was not quite true; I had not been nearly as forthright with her about the possibility of death.) I went over most of what I had talked about the night before, but she was not mollified.

"But why did you do it? I hate being talked about." And so it dawned on me. This was like the problem with making rounds outside her room, talking about her instead of to or with her, treating her as patient-on-display and not as Mickey, the human being most intimately involved in the subject matter of the discussion. But there was more. Her separation from her family (she saw her siblings no more than twice a week during this time) was a significant part of her suffering, and I had intensified it by going to her house — something she could not do — and talking with them *about* her, as though she were no longer part of the family. Worse, I had talked mostly about her *disease,* as though it had now taken the place of their sister Mickey. I could only apologize and assure her, although I doubt she was reassured, that I was not hiding anything from her, not sharing information with Chris and Joey and Jenny that I was not also giving her.

Soon after that the treatment and the disease together began to take their toll. I left the service at the beginning of November to begin a "reading" elective I had arranged months before with our neonatologist. It was to be an opportunity to immerse myself in what was known about the health problems and medical care of premature infants. I did end up reading a couple of books and many journal articles about premies that month, but my more enduring educational experience took place in the P.I.C.U., where Mickey took up residence early in November.

Mickey's move to the P.I.C.U. was deemed necessary because of the many devastating consequences of leukemia and its fearful treatment, which could include infection, bleeding, neurologic abnormalities . . . the list goes on. At some point she became much less alert than she had been, and it was concluded that she had bled someplace, probably several places, in her brain. The severity of her illness and the combination of fears and distresses, ours and hers, resulted in her transfer from the room with all the bits of home in it to the room with nothing but cold tiled walls and a television — card art, stuffed animals, and flowers not allowed.

One night soon after her transfer I was in the P.I.C.U. with her. I cannot now recall if I was taking call for someone else, or just there because I wanted to be. It was late, 1 or 2 A.M.; her parents had gone home hours before. Something about Mickey that night made me think her death was imminent. In retrospect, I wonder if what I realized that night was that her death was inevitable. Perhaps I had not let myself think that far before. Whatever the illumination was, I remembered the importance to Mickey and her family of their Roman Catholic faith — the children enrolled in parochial school, the family an integral part of the parish, the priests spoken of familiarly as vital parts of their lives. (Among those priests was the one whom Mickey insisted looked like Ted Baxter, a character on the then-popular *Mary Tyler Moore Show.* If I was around when he came to visit, I inevitably got an elbow nudge and wink from whichever family member was standing closest to me and was invited to participate in the general, gentle laughter after he left. He did look like Ted Baxter, complete with the air of unwarranted self-confidence that characterized that bumbling, pompous TV newscaster. Mick was right on target.)

That night, watching a stuporous Mickey take big, halting breaths, I feared she was dying and, all of a sudden, I was certain that it was necessary to call a priest now. My reasoning, such as it was, was that it would be important to Mary and Marshall to know that she had had last rites: thus my knowledge of Catholicism. But I did not know the names of the priests ("Ted Baxter" would surely not do) nor even the name of the parish. So, mea maxima culpa, I called Mickey's parents, in the dead of night, to ask the name of their priest.

"No, she hasn't changed any. No, nothing's happened. No, you don't need to come. I just thought that, as sick as she is, anything could happen any time, and I thought it would be important for her and for you to have had the priest here."

"Are you talking about last rites?!"

"I guess so, although I don't really think you need to worry." They gave me the priest's name. I called him and he came right over. What could I have been thinking? Who knows? How does one learn, in this business, not to mistake one's own epiphanies for meaningful changes in the lives of patients? I expect this was some mix of wanting to do it all correctly, to be the complete doctor, sensitive to this family's particular needs, not missing an opportunity to care for them, coupled with my unacknowledged, indeed unrecognized, difficulty dealing with the midnight realization that Mickey was going to die sooner rather than later.

I told the priest my concerns, as far as I understood them at that moment, and he explained to me, quite patiently given the hour, that the issue was not "last rites," as popularly understood by non-Catholics such as I, but prayers for the sick — which were always appropriate and carried no necessary association, subtle or otherwise, with imminent death. That sounded just right to me, as I had now begun to think I might have erred in calling him out in the middle of the night. He went into her room to pray.

Just then Mickey's parents came rushing in from the elevators. "What's going on? Is the priest here? What's happening with Mickey?"

"He's in there now. She's the same as when you left this evening. You can go in with him if you want."

Marshall went in to join the priest in his prayers. Mary just shook her head silently and retreated to the waiting room — to wait. I sat there with her, but there was little to say. I had no way to explain, much less justify, what I had done to them that night. I was still not sure that it had been an entirely wrong thing to do, but it had certainly mushroomed out of my control, gone well beyond what I had imagined when I embarked upon this putatively sensitive acknowledgment of what I presumed to be their religious concerns. What an ass! In that episode I recognize the seeds of my later insistence upon clarity on such matters long before they were called for. It would take more clumsy errors — perhaps none of this magnitude, but errors nonetheless — before that lesson would alter my behavior and my understanding, but I have never forgotten this scene or the feeling of having intensified their suffering because of my needs, my ignorance, and my ineptness.

The priest — he was not Ted Baxter but one of the younger clergy, the one Mickey thought was drop-dead gorgeous — came to find Mary after he had finished the prayers. He squatted in front of Mary and put his hand on hers. She had been crying, not something she did much of when others were around, and she looked up at him with as bleak a face as I had seen on a human being. With great conviction, she said softly, "I hate this place."

Immediately, the young priest said, "No, you don't, Mary. This is a good place."

"I do. I do. I hate it."

To my surprise, I found myself saying, "Of course she does. Of course you do, Mary. How could you not?"

The priest flicked a glance at me, rose to his feet, patted Mary's hand one last time, and left. And at that moment I hated the place too, and me in it.

Mickey lived another two weeks or so after that night. The days that remained were a gray, unchanging scene. We had stopped Mickey's chemotherapy because her counts were so low — and because we were, in essence, waiting for her to die from the neurologic damage wrought by the bleeding, if not from some new assault. There was no longer any reasonable hope that she would survive for long, much less that she would be able to return to anything like her old self. Not that we ever said as much, to each other or to her parents. We just settled into the grim routine of daily neurologic exams and blood counts (why? because that was the routine), donning our yellow gowns and surgical masks each time we entered her P.I.C.U. room.

Mickey slept a lot or, perhaps more accurately, slipped in and out of consciousness. When she was awake, she was coherent, mostly; she knew people and could still muster a smile at a Ted Baxter joke. At some point she let us know that she could no longer see anything except some contrast of light and darkness. She did not announce this as a sudden or frightening revelation, just a point made in passing, thinking we might be interested. Again, bleeding was the culprit; her retinas could not be seen for the blood that filled her eyeballs. As the consulting ophthalmologist said rather bluntly, it did not really matter whether the bleeding was only in her eyes or also in the part of her brain that received nerve impulses from the eyes and presented them to the rest of the brain as visual images. She was dying; nothing was going to be done, or could be done, about her vision. She was in no apparent pain, for which I remain deeply grateful, especially given how little we understood about pain control in 1974. Mickey spent the last two weeks of her life quite blind and mostly asleep.

Each day I joined Mary for a while as she kept vigil by Mickey's bedside, each of us wearing the regulation isolation gown and face mask, talking little. On one of those days, Mickey woke up while I was there, and we talked a bit, mostly my checking to see if she was comfortable, if she needed anything. I stood by the bed, my hand resting lightly on her pale, bald scalp. She mumbled, "I want to kiss someone."

I thought I had not heard her correctly. "What did you say, Mick?" Clearly and forcefully this time, with a tinge of desperate tears in it: "I want to kiss someone." I felt my heart break. So this is what it feels like, I thought.

I called Mary over and told her to take her mask off, that her daughter wanted a kiss.

"Is it all right?"

"You bet it is. Go right ahead."

Mary untied the mask and let it drop. She bent down and kissed her daughter's swollen, crusted lips and then put her cheek on Mickey's for a long moment. Mickey smiled and slipped back into sleep. Mary turned away from me as she redid her mask. Watching her, I received another revelation of the obvious.

"Mary," I said, "you don't need to put it back on. You've kissed her. What's the point?"

Indeed, what was the point? We knew she was dying. We knew that infection could be the final blow, as much as bleeding could be, but that the name of the final blow did not much matter. Why maintain this isolation, keeping her from the human contact she needed? Why had her last sight of her parents been of their eyes only, the rest of their faces hidden, their old familiar clothes covered, their hands hesitant to hold hers lest they harm her somehow? Why indeed? I began, tentatively at first, then with increasing conviction, to lobby with the residents on the service to end the isolation. Yes, it was what one did for someone with counts as low as hers, but to what end in this case? How could it be justified? They were skeptical, and I too was a bit afraid of this novel idea. Although her doctors resisted overturning established protocol, I encouraged Mary and Marshall not exactly to flout the rules, but not to hold back from holding, touching, and kissing their child.

Kathryn, the social worker with whom I had made the visit to Mickey's home, also kept vigil with Mary during those days. As her schedule allowed, she would join Mary at Mickey's bedside for an hour or so. Sometimes I was there too and observed the behavior that Mary talked about later. Kathryn and Mary would sit quietly, saying little. This was not a venue for chatting; it was a sacred space of watching and waiting. Periodically, Kathryn would sigh, shake her head back and forth a few times, and murmur into the full silence, "I don't know." She would then be quiet again, only to repeat her puzzled lament after several more minutes of contemplative silence. After Mickey's death, Mary recalled this behavior with a laugh, a sort of fond perplexity about what was going on there. Despite the humorous turn she gave it, the tale of Kathryn's repeated hushed elegies was the only story Mary told from those dark days. Something in Kathryn's action was a touchstone for her, encapsulating the nature of the vigil and its grief. "I don't know." No questions or answers, no explanations and no demands. Only presence, faithfulness, and honesty.

During this period of watchful waiting, I left town for a long-planned weekend in New York City. I was anxious about leaving Mickey but decided to handle my concern by calling the P.I.C.U. each morning to talk with her parents. Saturday morning it was Mary who came to the phone. She told me that the evening before, when it was just Mary and Mickey in the room, Mickey had asked, "Am I going to die?"

"What did you say, Mary?"

"Well, jeez, I mean, what do you say? I said I hoped not, that we were trying to keep that from happening. But that, whatever was happening, we were going to be right there with her. No matter what, we're in this together."

"Good, good. So, what did she say then?"

"Nothing really. Just like 'okay,' and then she went back to sleep." We talked a bit more, then I hung up and went on with a day of museums and theater, pleased that Mickey had been able to ask the question and that Mary had been able to allow it, without veering away, and to tell her what I thought was most important: that she would not be alone. I wondered whether, had Mickey asked me, I could have been honest (and brave) enough to say simply "Yes," and whether or not that reply would have been a better way to respond to this particular twelve-year-old. I was glad Mary had been the one she asked.

I called again Sunday morning, and this time it was Marshall who came to the phone. "Dr. Mohrmann, Mickey asked me something just now, and I don't know if I said the right thing."

"What was it?"

"She asked me if she was gonna die. And I just said, 'No way, Mick. Don't think about stuff like that. You just think about getting better.' I couldn't tell her the truth, Dr. Mohrmann. Did I do the right thing?"

"Sure," I said, "if that's what you were comfortable telling her." How could I chastise this heartbroken man? How could I ask him to say to his daughter what he could scarcely admit to himself? Besides, how do I know his answer was not just right, exactly what Mickey expected and wanted from her dad?

When I returned from that weekend I started agitating in earnest not only to end the isolation but to transfer Mickey out of the P.I.C.U. and back to her old room, which had been kept for her, cards still on the walls (fortunately, her bed had not been needed). Mickey's constant theme since entering the P.I.C.U. had been her desire to return to that room. Each time she roused from sleep, she asked the same question: "Why can't I go back to my room? I don't like this room. All my stuff is up there. I want to go back."

I could speculate about what a move back to her old room might mean to her. It contained as much of home as she could take with her, so it was as close to home as she could get. Plus, she had been in the hospital long enough to have learned the pediatric patients' conventional wisdom: a kid who gets "transferred to the P.I.C.U." never comes back — it's just the way adults get around telling us that that kid died. So if going to the P.I.C.U. is the euphemism for death, perhaps being transferred back to one's old room means survival. Or maybe Mickey just needed to yearn for something potentially attainable, knowing that her deepest wishes would not be granted.

The P.I.C.U. nurses said they would be willing to check in on her and supplement the floor nursing staff if her care became too much for them; the floor nurses wanted her back. Even with that, it took days of diplomacy and pleading, but finally all agreed that Mickey could be moved back to her old room, without isolation precautions. We all acknowledged that she was dying, that her death would come soon, that there was nothing more to be done by way of treatment and nothing to be gained by continuing intensive care.

She greeted the news of her impending move with as much enthusiasm as she could manage: "Good." That single syllable, spoken with the old asperity directed at those whose mental processors did not work as rapidly or precisely as hers, reminded us of who this child was, of the Mickey who was still there, still inhabiting the wracked body rapidly moving toward its end. She was awake for the move and, like a queen on her throne, received graciously the warm farewells of the P.I.C.U. staff and the welcoming embrace of the floor nurses. Once she was installed in her room, her parents pointed out to her that all the old decorations were still in place, envisioning them for her, assuring her that this was indeed the same old, familiar place. Mickey was home, such as it was. She broke into a broad grin, turned on her side, and fell deeply asleep.

Her parents and I watched her sleeping and spoke briefly, hesitantly of what we believed to be true, that Mickey would surely die soon, perhaps even that night or tomorrow — perhaps assisted on her way by her victory over pediatric protocol, by being the one kid who actually came back from the P.I.C.U. Her parents agreed: "This is where she should be. We won't be going back to the P.I.C.U., will we?"

"No," I said, "we won't. This is it."

It was now early evening, and I was not on call. I left and went home. I felt certain Mickey would die that night, but I had no official role on the team, and, for all my feelings of closeness to her parents, I was not so much part of her family that I should stay the night there. I was at a loss about where I should be, what I should do, even who I was now. I had done my final doctor act for Mickey by getting her transferred. What could my role be now? I knew nothing else to do but go home. Driving the thirty minutes to my apartment with a painful weight in my chest, I felt I was running away from something, something unfinished, undone, but I could not grasp what it might be. I was somehow failing to measure up but could not fathom what the missed standard might be. I knew only that I felt bad, really bad. The idea that this might be what grief is like did not occur to me.

At home I changed into more relaxed clothes, fixed and ate dinner; and watched television. Then the phone rang. It was the resident on call. Mickey had arrested. The team had resuscitated her, moved her back to the P.I.C.U., and hooked her up to a ventilator. "You *what?*" I screamed — but I think that was in my head only. I think I actually said something more like, "Oh, gosh. I'm on my way."

A thirty-minute drive back to the hospital — thirty minutes in which to deal with the turmoil of questions in my head. Why had I not stayed? Why had they resuscitated her? Why had I not foreseen this? I knew my colleagues, I knew that was what they would do. I just had not put it all together, had not imagined what the night would be like, what would actually happen when Mickey stopped breathing. And, I realized with sickening suddenness, I had never talked explicitly with the residents on call about how Mickey's parents and I understood the significance of her move out of the P.I.C.U. I had not said to them, "We think she'll die tonight, and if not tonight, very soon. She's ready; they're ready. When she dies, let her go. It's time. Let it happen here, in this room, with her parents here with her." I did not say it. Truth to tell, I did not think it, not that clearly. I had indeed left something undone.

Matt, the senior resident on call that night, met me at the entrance to the P. I.C.U. "She's gone," he said. "She arrested again, and we couldn't get her back."

"Yes," I thought, "good. It's over, Finally. Good, Mick, good." What I said was, "Where is she?"

"There." Matt gestured toward the door of her old P.I.C.U. room, the one she had triumphantly sailed out of just a few hours before. "Her parents are back in the conference room. Curtis was on tonight too and happened to be up here seeing another patient when we were working on her. He knows them. He's in there with them." Curtis was the resident who had admitted Mickey the first time, back in April, and cared for her until I took over in May. He had never failed to ask about her when he saw me. I was glad he was there, someone they knew and knew cared about Mickey.

As I turned to go into the room to see her, Matt put his hand on my arm. "Wait a minute. Why don't you just take a minute to deal with this before you go in there." He said it with real concern, but I bristled at what I read as a patronizing tone, with the implication that I was less than professional, that I had crossed that bright line, dear to those who think they can see where it is, between caring about my patients and being overly involved with them.

"I'm fine," I said abruptly. "I want to see her, and then I'll go talk with her parents." He shrugged and turned away.

"Why did you do it, Matt?" I asked of his departing back. "You knew she was going to die. Why the code?"

"Every patient deserves our best efforts, Margaret," he said over his shoulder. "Of course we had to do it. We didn't even consider not doing it." He walked away.

I closed my eyes a moment, feeling the grief wash over me — grief at Mickey's death, certainly, but also grief that I had failed her and her parents at this most critical moment and left her in the hands of those who saw her only as Everypatient, not as beautiful, irreplaceable, dying Mick who needed to leave.

I entered her room — the room she had so wanted to be shut of — and saw her body lying on the bed, surrounded by the familiar detritus of a failed code. The board still under her torso; ripped-open packages of gauze, syringes, tubing scattered on the floor; the "crash cart" gaping open, standing at an angle to her bed. It was the kind of scene I had walked away from many times before. I knew what the room had been like a half-hour before when it was a live-action drama. I could imagine the clipped orders, the barked questions — "Can you get a pulse? Stop a minute and let me listen! How long has it been? Haven't you got that line in yet? Give me another epi!" — bouncing off the ugly tile walls that had been the last thing Mickey's eyes ever gazed upon.

The silence now was ripe and heavy. I walked over to the bed and gazed down at her. The endotracheal tube that had connected her to the ventilator was still in place, its anchoring tape obscuring much of her lower face. Her naked body was arrayed as it had been left, arms out to receive intravenous lines, disregarding her twelve-year-old girl's modesty, which she had emphatically taught me to honor months before when I had performed her first (and last) rectal exam. I arranged the tangled sheet as well as I could without removing the equipment from the bed, but I could only get it up to her waist. I caressed her bald head, told her goodbye, and left the room.

I walked slowly down to the conference room to see Mickey's parents. They were seated facing each other, with Curtis squatting in the space between, a hand reached out to each of them. I eased in quietly. Mary, facing the doorway by which I stood, kept her head down, weeping. Marshall's back was to me, his head bowed. As I walked around him, I put my hand on his shoulder. He jumped up and hugged me, crying, "She did it, Dr. Mohrmann. She beat 'em." He crumpled back into his chair, face in his hands. I reached over to Mary, who just nodded and grasped my hand. Then I sat in the chair between them.

"Dr. Evans here has been wonderful," Mary said, as she got control of her voice. "He knew Mickey from the beginning, you know, and he's here tonight."

I nodded my appreciation to Curtis, whose brimming eyes mirrored my own.

Then Marshall grabbed my hand, needing to explain. "We tried to tell 'em, Dr. Mohrmann. We knew she was going to die. She didn't want to leave her room. We tried to tell 'em it was all right, but they did it anyway. They brought her back down here and did all that stuff to her. And the whole time they were working on her, I sat there in that waiting room, saying 'Beat 'em, Mick! Beat 'em!' And she did!"

Thus the grieving father, forced to cheer on his daughter's death, pleading for absolution — "We tried to tell 'em! We tried!" — for having failed to protect her from this last insult, and asking it of me, who felt the same sense of failure and did not know how to separate it from grief for the loss of Mickey. Mary, the one who had always had so much more to say, was now the silent one, locked in a world of loss, ready to leave this place she hated.

At their request, I followed Mary and Marshall to their house, where Chris was waiting, keeping solitary vigil. Joey and Jenny were spending the night with Flo and Joe, but Chris had refused to leave the house, insisting on being dealt with as an adult in this crisis. They told him the news; he ducked his head and nodded, let himself be hugged, then got in the car with all of us to drive over to his grandparents. They knew when they saw us at the door. We tiptoed through the dining room where the children lay on cots — supposedly asleep, but I was unconvinced — to the kitchen, where we sat around the table and talked aimlessly. I do not remember whether we talked about the events of that evening or about Mickey herself or about necessary plans. I recall periods of silence and staring; attempts to take care of Chris, whose red-rimmed eyes belied his stoic demeanor; and studious ignoring of Joey and Jenny, lying prone on their cots on either side of the kitchen door, just outside the ring of light over the table, their heads propped up on their hands, eyes wide, staring solemnly back at me each time I glanced their way.

When we left after an hour or so, the children slept, or feigned sleep, once more, so we again tiptoed our way across the floor. They offered me a room for the night, but I insisted on returning to the hospital. I felt some need to be there; it was more my home than my apartment was. Back at the hospital, I determinedly set about taking down the cards from the walls of Mickey's room, packing them away with the stuffed animals and other souvenirs of home to return to her parents.

A few days later I went to the wake at the funeral home and the following day, along with some of the nurses who knew Mickey well, to the funeral at the family's parish church. At the wake, there were little cards of remembrance in the room, each with a poem about God's tendency to pluck the fairest flowers from Earth to beautify a heavenly garden. When I walked over to speak to the family, I could see that the casket was open. Flo immediately began urging me to go over and see how good Mickey looked. I resisted. Although open caskets are the practice in my own family, and I had not shied away from them before, this time I did not think I wanted to see her rehabilitated but dead face. However, by the time I was ready to leave, I realized how important it was to Flo, and possibly to Mary, that I pay my respects, so I went over to the casket and knelt on the prie-dieu set up in front of it. Out of the corner of my eye, I could see Flo nudge Mary and point to me, a smile of pleased satisfaction on her face. Mickey looked remarkably well, remarkably like the child I had first met in May, before the real tortures had begun. She was wearing the wig she had sported all summer. I remember, Mickey.

106 Pastoral Concerns: Parental Anxiety and Other Issues of Character

Joseph J. Kotva Jr.

The Case

Lyle and Judy Smith are Mennonites by conviction. Neither grew up in an Anabaptist-related church setting, but both are drawn to Mennonite convictions about following Jesus, discipleship, community, and so on. Judy is a schoolteacher. Lyle is primary caregiver for their seven-year-old daughter, Tiffany.

The Smiths live in a small, two-bedroom home in a quiet suburban neighborhood. They have a large yard and a park nearby. Their neighborhood includes two other families from their church and several children that are Tiffany's age.

Lyle and Judy recently decided to buy a new, much larger home in an exclusive development in a neighboring suburb. They are moving to get Tiffany into a better school system. Their current school system scores slightly below average in state tests and has above average class size. Although Tiffany is doing well in school, Lyle and Judy believe she could be doing better.

This move will put them geographically farther from both Judy's job and their church. The new house is expensive; to swing the payments, Lyle is getting a half-time job and they are significantly reducing their charitable giving. The Smiths also feel a bit guilty that the new house does not fit their ideals of simple living, but they are anxious to get Tiffany the best education possible. Lyle and Judy did not deliberate about this move with their small group or pastor. Instead, they announced the move during the Sunday service sharing time. This announcement was greeted after the service with many congratulations and several offers to help with the move.

This brief description of Lyle and Judy's decision will strike many as an odd place to start discussing pastoral concerns about biotechnology. I begin here to move our attention to the larger contexts in which our appropriation of this technology will take place. One such context is the anxiety exhibited by many Christian parents to do everything possible for their children to get ahead. Such parents are driven by the commendable desire to do right, but this desire (fueled by assorted social pressures) too often leads parents to make decisions at odds with the rest of their Christian commitment. Thus, although minimally aware of it, Lyle and Judy's move requires that they modify, if not outright reject, many of the Anabaptist-Christian convictions that brought them to the Mennonite church — including stewardship, simple living, and communal discernment.

Of course, the Smiths are not alone in loosening other commitments to fulfill their desire to do everything for their children. Most pastors know families where each child is involved in multiple extracurricular activities. These good parents worry that their children will miss out. Although often unnoticed by these parents, such programming means their children have little time for unstructured, imaginative play, and the family has little money and less time for the church and its ministries.

My recognition of such parental anxiety and its resulting life choices leaves me doubly troubled when I consider the new powers coming with biotechnology. As parents within Christian communities, do we exhibit the habits, skills, convictions, qualities of character, and choices that will allow us to judge these new powers rightly? Or is it more likely that these new powers will further fuel our parental anxiety so we will genetically screen, select, and enhance our children with little regard for the effects on our lives together as a Christian community?

Questions of Character

As a pastor, I frequently consider a series of interrelated questions to evaluate our moral lives together: (1) Who does Christ call us to be? What qualities of character, types of relationships, patterns of behavior, and choices are expected from faithful followers of Christ? (2) Based on our habits, choices, and actions, who are we now with respect to that calling? (3) Are our current practices, patterns of behavior, relationships, and choices likely moving us toward or away from Christ's calling? (4) If we are contemplating some particular course of action, pattern of behavior, or choice, will it likely move us toward or away from Christ's calling? (5) In our life together, both within and outside the worship service, what practices, activities, social settings, discussions, and relationships can the congregation promote to encourage our growth toward Christ's calling?[1]

Directing these questions to the issue at hand is instructive. I believe shorthand answers would be something like the following:

(1) As a church community and Christian parents, we

Reprinted from Joseph Kotva, Jr., "Pastoral Concerns: Parental Anxiety and Other Issues of Character," in *Viewing New Creations with Anabaptist Eyes: Ethics of Biotechnology* (Telford, PA: Cascadia Publishing House, 2005), pp. 224-29.

1. Cf. MacIntyre's account of the tripartite structure of an Aristotelian ethic: Alasdair MacIntyre, *After Virtue,* 2nd ed. (Notre Dame: University of Notre Dame Press, 1984), pp. 52-55.

are called to welcome all children with unconditional love as gifts from God. Jesus blesses children[2] and elevates children as models to be emulated.[3] Our own raised status is that of children of God.[4] Parents are instructed to care for their children,[5] and raising children is listed first among the good deeds of widows.[6] Born in the image of God, all children, healthy or sick, deserve our care.[7]

Yet our care for our children is to be limited by our faithfulness to God. God tests Abraham's faithfulness by calling for the surrender of Isaac.[8] Jesus tells us fidelity to him will bring conflict into the family, including between parents and their children.[9] We are told that the reward in heaven will justify the possible need to leave our children for Christ's sake.[10] In a typical hyperbole, Jesus says discipleship may even require us to hate our children.[11] In short, we are to love and provide for our children, but not at the expense of faithfulness.

(2) We are loving, anxious parents who frequently (though unconsciously) qualify our fidelity to Christ in the name of our children's enrichment and well-being.

(3) Many of our current patterns of behavior, such as moving to better school districts and over-scheduling our children, likely reinforce our parental anxieties and willingness to sacrifice faithfulness. Each time we make such choices, we reinforce in ourselves and model for others the notion that our children's advancement is a preeminent concern. These distortions are further encouraged in all of us when such choices are met with congratulations and offers of help.

(4) We must recognize that parents already anxious for their children to get ahead have a built-in predisposition to avail themselves of various biotechnologies when they become available. Parents who see their children's advancement as such a preeminent concern are ill prepared to judge the Christian fidelity of such developments as genetic screening, selection, and enhancement. Parents face enormous social pressure to ensure that their children get ahead. In this climate, instead of careful Christian discernment, it seems likely that parental anxiety "will be readily exploited when they hear what other parents, more committed to their children, are doing to improve their offspring's [genetic] inheritance."[12] Moreover, it seems likely that our use of such technologies will further reinforce our anxious pursuit of our children's advancement. Even if the technologies themselves are morally acceptable from some supposedly "neutral" or "objective" perspective, when chosen by parents anxious for their children to get ahead, that choice will reinforce the tendency to make future choices out of the same anxious posture. In short, I believe that in the current context the arrival of these technologies will likely further corrupt our understanding of parenting and its relationship to Christian fidelity.

(5) The many parents who are/were missionaries and relief workers constitute one resource that might help move us toward a more balanced, Christian practice of parenting. Missionaries and relief workers spend significant time outside the anxious, competitive climate of North America. In addition, many have engaged in specific practices and made specific choices that reflect the priority of Christian fidelity over offspring advancement. Encouraging these folks to tell their stories in our midst is one Christian way to challenge our parental anxiety.

While many other things should be said about moving us toward Christ's calling regarding Christian parenting, I here note only one: The new powers of biotechnology again confront us with the need for communal discernment. We should be talking together about these issues before we ever confront them as choices, and we should repeatedly encourage parents in advance to bring such decisions to a communal forum that includes brothers and sisters free of parental anxieties. After all, Christ promised to join such gathered discernment.[13]

Conclusion

I was asked to address "pastoral concerns" about biotechnology. One tack on such concerns is to attend to the larger contexts in which we will appropriate that technology, an approach illustrated by focusing on parental anxiety. If space allowed, I would raise similar concerns about another dimension of parenting: our culture's tendency to view children as our right and our possession (a tendency seen in both the frequency of abortion and in many forms of reproductive technology). I fear that in the current context, the emerging biotechnologies will feed our tendency to view children as possessions rather than gifts.

I would raise similar concerns about our capacity for suffering and for justice. That is, I would argue that the rhetoric and expectations surrounding the emerging technologies will likely further degrade our already diminished capacity to recognize struggle and suffering as an inevitable part of finitude and of fidelity to Christ.

2. Matt. 19:14.
3. Matt. 18:13.
4. Rom. 8:16; 1 John 3:1.
5. Col. 3:21; Eph. 6:4; cf. 2 Cor. 12:14.
6. 1 Tim. 5:10.
7. Darrel Amundsen reminds us that early Christian attitudes toward children and newborns were strikingly different from much of Greco-Roman culture: Darrel W. Amundsen, "Medicine and the Birth of Defective Children: Approaches of the Ancient World," in *On Moral Medicine: Theological Perspectives in Medical Ethics,* ed. Stephen E. Lammers, Allen Verhey (Grand Rapids: William B. Eerdmans Publishing Company, 1998), 681-92 [included as article 107 in the present volume].
8. Gen. 22.
9. Mark 13:12.
10. Matt. 19:29.
11. Luke 14:26.
12. Ronald Cole-Turner, "The Era of Biological Control," in *Beyond Cloning: Religion and the Remaking of Humanity,* ed. Ronald Cole-Turner (Harrisburg: Trinity Press International, 2001), 11.
13. Matt. 18:20.

I would similarly argue that our capacity for justice is at stake. The technologies are largely emerging in an individualistic, consumer-oriented, capitalistic system that accepts high rates of child poverty and infant mortality, let alone the 43 million Americans who lack health insurance. Despite the best intentions of scientists and researchers, there are good reasons to believe that the inevitable limited access to these technologies will further the gross disparities in our system and further diminish our capacity to struggle for justice. In short, I am less pastorally concerned about the technologies themselves than I am about the contexts in which they are emerging and their likely negative effects on our Christian capacities to parent, to suffer, and to strive for justice.

Still, I remain hopeful, not because I believe in the inevitable progress of science or in the fundamental goodwill of our culture, but because I believe in God and God's church. If we are willing, the church can be the context in which we learn the skills and virtues (such as humility, wisdom, patience, integrity, and courage) necessary to chart these waters well. We can learn something about parenting from missionary and relief workers, and the church is full of similar resources through which God may yet teach us how to faithfully engage these new technologies.

107 Medicine and the Birth of Defective Children: Approaches of the Ancient World

Darrel W. Amundsen

So diverse are the varied strands of ancient Greek and Roman cultures that it is dangerous — indeed, probably irresponsible — to speak of any universal ancient attitudes and practices, unless significant qualifications are placed upon any assertions other than the most specific and limited. In attempting accurately to describe — or more correctly, to reconstruct — the response of people in antiquity to the defective newborn, it is necessary first to provide the broader context of values that informed, or actually formed, that response. And that broader context of values involves such issues as human worth, human dignity, the value of life, and human rights, inalienable and otherwise.

In the introduction to his very perspicacious monograph *Human Value: A Study in Ancient Philosophical Ethics,* John M. Rist maintains that the view that such rights as "the right to life, to have enough to eat, to live without fear of torture or degrading punishments, the right to work or to withhold one's labour," or any other rights, "are the universal property of men as such was virtually unknown in classical antiquity." He further asserts that classical antiquity had no theory "that all men are endowed at birth (or before) with a certain value . . . though some of its philosophers took certain steps toward such a theory."[1]

It is especially in the literature of political philosophy that theories of human value are developed. The most famous representative of this genre is Plato's *Republic,* which must be supplemented by the *Statesman* and the *Laws* to provide a thorough picture of Plato's conception of human value within the ideal state. Does the ideal state exist for its inhabitants, or do the latter exist for the sake of the state? It seems as though both are true in Plato's view. Private worth, which is possession of the virtues, will inevitably lead to the seeking of the public good. While personal worth or value is always manifest in one's social utility, and is thus contributory to the common good, Plato seems to hold that personal worth

1. John M. Rist, *Human Value: A Study in Ancient Philosophical Ethics* (Leiden: E. J. Brill, 1982), p. 9.

From Darrel W. Amundsen, *Medicine, Society, and Faith in the Ancient and Medieval Worlds.* © 1996 The Johns Hopkins University Press. Used by permission.

is the *telos* of the ideal state (as the best environment for growth in personal virtue), rather than that the state is the telos of personal value. But the relationship is transparently circular, cause and effect, means and end being inextricably interwoven.

Within Plato's ideal state, failure to contribute renders one worthless. And there are levels of worth; some people are superior to others. The Guardian class, of course, has an intrinsic value that exceeds that of slaves, whose only value is in their material contributions to the state. But slaves aside, even among the Guardian class there are grades of worth. Although Plato views men and women of the Guardian class as fully equal, the qualities of this class are starkly masculine, suggesting that the most virtuous (i.e., valuable) women are those who are most like men in their developed character. The children of superior adults clearly possess a potential worth that increases as they come closer to maturity. However, children's worth is not intrinsic but only potential, and children are valued in proportion to their approximation to the ideal adult. They must be malleable, disposed to virtue, and physically fit.

Plato's concern for healthy children is clearly seen in his marriage regulations. The maximum number of superior adults should couple with others of equal worth. The number of inferior types coupling with others of similar value should be kept at a minimum. Since adults who are too young or too old produce less vigorous children than do those who are of ideal age for procreation, people should be prevented from having children except during their ideal years for producing robust offspring.[2] Indeed, the purpose of marriage is first to produce children to ensure the continuity of the state, and second to improve human stock.[3]

In a society in which absolute value is always seen through the grid of social value, those who are physically defective, or at least those who are chronically ill, should not be kept alive by diet, drugs, and regimen, since such people will likely reproduce similarly wretched offspring and be of use neither to themselves nor to society.[4] Indeed, the only legitimate claim to medical care is the continued social usefulness of the one desiring care.

Aristotle's view of human value is expressed in a variety of his works, ranging from the biological to the political and ethical. He clearly postulates a hierarchy of worth within the species. Men with fully developed virtue(s) are most fully human, and thus of the greatest value both to themselves and to society. There are, of course, gradations within this group. All other humans are, by comparison, defective by nature or in their present state. Those who are defective by nature include especially those whom Aristotle calls "natural slaves," that is, individuals who have a capacity to acknowledge reason but not to conceptualize or to engage in rational activity. They are somewhat like domesticated animals: defective by nature. Also defective by nature, but having considerably greater range of capacity for virtue than natural slaves, are those women who themselves are not natural slaves. They are naturally defective by virtue of being women but yet, in unnatural or unusual circumstances, may demonstrate a kind of female excellence. But at the best they are defective males.

Quite distinct from natural slaves and women are children. Children may be natural slaves — a condition not immediately discernible — or female, and thus limited in potential. But all male children, except for those who prove to be natural slaves, are potentially virtuous men, therefore potentially fully human. Children, however, resemble natural slaves and animals more than they do virtuous men, because they lack the developed capacity for rational thought and behavior.

For both Plato and Aristotle, then, human value is primarily social value and is determined by potentiality.[5]

Do the positions taken by Plato and Aristotle reflect the values of classical society? The answer to that question must be a highly qualified, yet hearty, affirmative; qualified, because there was a tremendous diversity of values in classical antiquity; a hearty affirmative for two reasons: (1) No pagan, whether philosopher or jurist, appears to have asked whether human beings have inherent value, or possess intrinsic rights, ontologically, irrespective of social value, legal status, age, sex, and so forth. (2) Connected with the first reason is a fundamental, though primitive and residual, principle that, as Thrasymachus expresses it, "justice is the will of the stronger." Rights are recognized only by their enforceability. It was against the idea that might makes right that various philosophers, including Plato and Aristotle, reacted. Power must be checked by justice, justice being essentially the definition and enforcement of rights. Rist observes that, "instead of starting with a consideration of human rights, or of basic rights, [the ancients] start with theories of power and of how power shall be tempered by justice. As their thought proceeds, they come to recognize that certain types of people, for various reasons, are in fact possessed of rights. . . . The moral problem is not viewed in terms of enlarging or protecting the rights of the weak, but of controlling and rationalizing the power of the strong."[6]

Rist's comments certainly appear valid when one considers the various legal systems of classical antiquity. Among the Greeks the exclusivistic atmosphere of the polis fostered a definition of rights focusing on citizens — more on males, who possessed the franchise, than on

2. Plato, in the *Republic,* recommends that women not bear children before age twenty (460E), but in *Laws* he sets the age at sixteen (785B). Aristotle recommends eighteen as the minimum age (*Politics* 1335a). Their concern is with eugenics.

3. Plato, *Laws* 773D, 783D-E.

4. Plato, *Republic* 407D-E, 410A.

5. For a discussion of Plato's and Aristotle's views on human value, see M. P. Golding and N. H. Golding, "Population Policy in Plato and Aristotle: Some Value Issues," *Arethusa* 8 (1968): 345-58; and Rist, *Human Value* (n. 1).

6. Rist, *Human Value* (n. 1), p. 131.

females, who did not. The rights of adult male citizens' dependents (wives, to a certain degree, and children) and human possessions (slaves) were essentially developed with a view to protecting the rights of the adult males on whom those persons depended or to whom they belonged. This prevailed even in the highly developed law of the Roman Empire, though its more cosmopolitan character is reflected in its extension of various, if limited, rights to a broader spectrum of society than had typically been the center of Greek attention. Yet the emphasis remains on the rights of the adult male citizen primarily, with a variety of rights defined for women (these rights essentially comprising limitations of their fathers' or husbands' power and authority), and even for slaves (slight limitations being placed on the absolute power of owners).

Human Value and Newborns

In part, some of the changes that we see during the early centuries of the empire were the result of what some have hailed as a growing humanitarianism, a by-product of a sentiment not of egalitarianism, but at least of the brotherhood of man, proclaimed by the Stoicism of this period. This found its way into the medical ethics of probably a minority of physicians in an ethic of respect for life that condemned both abortion and active (although not passive) euthanasia, and a broader sentiment of generosity and altruism, a philanthropy predicated upon the unexpressed and ill-defined feeling that somehow people have a value to which our compassion is owed.

Even this pagan humanitarianism, however, was not grounded on a principle of inherent value of life. A stand against abortion and active euthanasia by the probably Pythagorean author of the so-called Hippocratic Oath, and by such physicians as Scribonius Largus and Soranus, both of whom lived in the early empire, was based less upon an idea of inherent value or sanctity of life than on an abhorrence of a physician's using his art in actively terminating life (fetal or otherwise); and especially in the case of abortion, an enduring, if not always articulated principle that value is more potential than ontological.

The strongly held idea that human value is acquired rather than inherent was nearly pervasive in classical antiquity, even among those pagans who condemned abortion. It was so central to ancient conceptions of value that a fully developed principle of sanctity of human life was never achieved in pagan society. This is particularly easily demonstrated by considering the status of newborns and their treatment. Once more I quote John Rist:

> It was almost universally held in antiquity that a child has no intrinsic right to life in virtue of being born. What mattered was being adopted into a family or some other institution of society. Both Plato and Aristotle, as well as the Stoics, Epicurus, and presumably Plotinus, accept the morality of the exposure of infants . . . on eugenic or sometimes on purely economic grounds. . . . We see here further clear evidence of the ancient view that somehow value is acquired, either by the development of intelligence or by the acceptance into society. There is no reason to think that the philosophers made substantial advances on the assumptions of the general public in this regard.[7]

Rist is absolutely correct in this assertion. Some clarification, however, is necessary. It is misleading to say that in antiquity the attitude that "a child has no intrinsic right to life in virtue of being born" was "almost universal." There were indeed some pagans who did condemn exposure[8] of healthy children for any reason: is Rist referring to these by his qualifying "almost"? That would imply that such individuals condemned exposure of healthy infants on the grounds that there is an "intrinsic" right to life in virtue of being born. Or is Rist suggesting that there were some — that few permitted by his "almost" — who unequivocally condemned all infanticide, including exposure of healthy infants and the disposal of the defective? If there actually were any pagans in the second of these categories, they most certainly had not formulated an ethic of intrinsic human value, any more than had those who were in the first category. His "almost" cannot include any — even the most humanitarian — pagans, not even those were were adamant in condemning abortion.

Although Rist's first qualifier, the adverb *almost* can

7. Ibid., pp. 141-42.

8. The prevalence of exposure in classical antiquity has been debated by modern scholars. For some specialized studies see H. Bennett, "The Exposure of Infants in Ancient Rome," *Classical J.* 18 (1923): 341-51; H. Bolkestein, "The Exposure of Children at Athens and the ἐγχυτρίστριαι," *Classical Philol.* 17 (1922): 222-29; A. Cameron, "The Exposure of Children and Greek Ethics," *Classical Rev.* 46 (1932): 105-14; D. Engels, "The Problem of Female Infanticide in the Greco-Roman World," *Classical Philol.* 75 (1980): 112-20; R. H. Feen, "Abortion and Exposure in Ancient Greece: Assessing the Status of the Fetus and 'Newborn' from Classical Sources," in *Abortion and the Status of the Fetus,* ed. W. B. Bondeson and H. T. Engelhardt, Jr. (Dordrecht: D. Reidel, 1983), pp. 283-99; M. Radin, "Exposure of Infants in Roman Law and Practice," *Classical J.* 20 (1925): 337-42; and L. Van Hook, "The Exposure of Infants at Athens," *Trans. Amer. Philol. Soc.* 51 (1920): 134-45. Engels' assessment appears correct: "After careful analysis of the literacy evidence, earlier studies concerning the exposure of children (and any resultant infanticide) have established that the practice was of negligible importance in Greek and Roman society" (Engels, "Female Infanticide" [n. 8], 112). It has been popularly assumed that the exposure of female newborns was extremely common. Engels convincingly argues that the high level of female infanticide assumed for classical antiquity by some scholars would have produced demographic consequences of a catastrophic nature. It is, of course, important to bear in mind that exposure is an ambiguous word, and that very likely exposure, unless excessive, may well have affected the population relatively little since probably the majority of exposed infants were reared. Sometimes exposure is infanticide; sometimes it is simply abandonment.

be misleading, his second qualifying phrase is more helpful, namely, that various philosophers accepted the morality of exposure of infants "on eugenic or sometimes on purely economic grounds." If we take the term *eugenic* in a broad sense, we can apply it to the disposal of defective infants, as distinct from the exposure of healthy infants for economic (or other non-eugenic) reasons. These two categories must be kept distinct if we are to understand the response of pagans in classical antiquity to defective infants.

First of all, it can be categorically asserted that there were no laws in classical antiquity, Greek or Roman, that prohibited the killing, by exposure or otherwise, of the defective newborn. Further, it is unlikely that there actually were any laws that classified exposure (as distinct from other forms of killing) of the healthy newborn as parricide or homicide, or prohibited the practice on other grounds, except, perhaps, in some limited regions or under unusual circumstances before the Christianization of the Roman Empire. If any such law or laws existed, there appears to have been little or no effort to enforce them.[9]

As already mentioned, there were some pagans who opposed the exposure of healthy infants. Aristotle implies in the *Politics* that there was in Greece some sentiment against exposure of healthy infants or traditions hostile to the practice, when he recommends that, if there are already too many children, abortion — before sensation *(prin aisthēsin)*[10] — be practiced in those regions where "the regular customs hinder any of those born being exposed" *(ean hē takis tōn ethōn kōlyę mēden apotithesthai tōn gignomenōn).*[11] The second-century B.C. historian Polybius criticizes the practice of child exposure, which he saw as one of the causes of the serious depopulation of Greece that occurred in the second century B.C., attributing the act to people's "pretentious extravagance, avarice and sloth."[12] The stoic philosopher Epictetus, who lived in the late first and early second centuries A.D., criticizes Epicurus for approving the exposure of children, saying that even a sheep or a wolf does not abandon its own offspring. His argument is that we ought not to be more foolish than sheep or more fierce than wolves, but rather should yield to our natural impulse to love our own offspring.[13] It is significant that he uses *stergein* here, the obvious word for having "natural affection," as distinct from other Greek words that are translated by the English word *love.*

Many of the examples of condemnation of child exposure found in classical authors are in descriptions of the practices of other cultures. The novelist Heliodorus (third century A.D.), in *An Ethiopian Romance,* has an

9. J. W. Jones writes of ancient Greece generally that "neither Greek public opinion nor Greek law frowned on the practice [of exposure], if the exposure was not delayed beyond a few days after birth" (*The Law and Legal Theory of the Greeks* [Oxford: Clarendon, 1956], p. 288). Thebes, during the early centuries of the Christian era, may possibly be an exception, if Aelian (*Varia historia* 2.7) can be trusted (for which see Feen, "Abortion and Exposure" [n. 8], 289). Speaking only of Athens, A. R. W. Harrison says that while "there seems general agreement that there was probably no explicit enactment conferring the right to expose," nevertheless there is "no reason to doubt that the father had this absolute discretion and that the right of exposure was more than a purely formal one" (*The Law of Athens: The Family and Property* [Oxford: Clarendon, 1968], p. 71, and n. 1). Putting this in other terms, he says that an Athenian father's right to expose his child is "perhaps better expressed as the absence of a duty to introduce it into the family" (73), or "the right to expose should perhaps be thought of as the absence of a duty to rear" (74, and n. 2). The assertion made by the late-second-century or early-third-century A.D. physician-philosopher Sextus Empiricus, in his *Outlines of Pyrrhonism* 3.211, that "Solon gave the Athenians the law . . . by which he allowed each man to slay his own child" can be confidently rejected (Harrison, *The Law of Athens* [n. 9], p. 71 and n. 2). It can be categorically asserted that the Athenian father never "enjoyed a power remotely resembling the Roman father's *ius vitae ac necis*" (74), that is, "power of life and death" over his children. That power is, of course, the well-known Roman father's *patria potestas.* The question of the legality of exposure in Roman law is entangled in the complexity of the changing patria potestas during the imperial period as well as the development of laws governing the parental reclaiming of exposed children reared by others, either as free children or as slaves, and the sale of free newborns as slaves. The Roman father's authority to put his children to death appears not to have been rescinded until the reign of the first Christian emperor, Constantine, who in 318 promulgated a law concerning parricide, that is, the killing of parents and children (*Codex Justinianus* 9.17.1). In 374, Valentinian enacted a statute concerning homicide which made the killing of an infant a capital offense (*Codex Justinianus* 9.16.7). In the same year he issued another statute that seems unambiguously to forbid exposure of infants. It begins, "Unusquisque subolem suam nutriat. Quod is exponendam putaverit, animadversioni quae constituta est subiacebit" (Everyone should support his own offspring, and anyone who thinks that he can expose his child shall be subject to the penalty prescribed by law [*Codex Justinianus* 8.51.2]). While this seems clear enough, is the penalty referred to here that of Constantine's law of 318 concerning parricide, or is there an even earlier law to which this legislation of 374 has reference? This question is raised in great part by a statement made by the great Roman jurist Paul in his *Sententiae* (third century): "Necare videtur non tantum is qui partum praefocat, sed et is qui abicit et qui alimonia denegat et is qui publicis locis misericordiae causa exponit, quam ipse non habet" (Not only he who strangles a child is held to kill it, but also he who abandons it, or denies it food, as well as he who exposes it in a public place for the purpose of arousing the pity which he himself does not feel. [The better manuscripts read *praefocat* = strangle; some read *perfocat* = smother. *Digest* 25.3.4.]) Paul is here obviously defining *necare.* The exact significance of the passage for the right of the Roman father to kill his children — or to expose them — cannot be dogmatically asserted. For a discussion, see Radin, "Exposure of Infants" (n. 8). On *patria potestas,* see W. W. Buckland, *A Text-Book of Roman Law from Augustus to Justinian,* 2d ed. (Cambridge: Cambridge University Press, 1952), sec. 38.

10. On which see J. M. Oppenheimer, "When Sense and Life Begin: Background for a Remark in Aristotle's *Politics* (1335b24)," *Arethusa* 8 (1975): 331-43.

11. Aristotle, *Politics* 1335b, trans. H. Rackham (Cambridge, Mass.: Harvard University Press, 1932).

12. Polybius, *The Histories* 36.17, trans. W. Paton (Cambridge, Mass.: Harvard University Press, 1922-27).

13. Epictetus, *Discourses* 1.23.

Ethiopian gymnosophist say that he found and reared an exposed girl "because for me it is not permissible to disregard an imperiled soul once it has taken on human form. This is a precept of our gymnosophists."[14] These attitudes were divergent enough from typical classical values that some authors were sufficiently intrigued to tickle their readers by relating such strange customs of exotic peoples. Others who decried various practices of their own societies describe the contrasting purity of other cultures. Tacitus, a contemporary of Epictetus, does both. He finds it remarkable that among the Germans it was regarded as shameful to kill any "late-born" child, that is, an unwanted child.[15] He uses nearly an identical sentence when he attributes the same peculiarity to the Jews, a people whose customs he usually finds strange and obnoxious.[16]

That Jews of Tacitus' time regarded the killing of infants as a reprehensible act, violating sacred law, is evident from the writings of Philo Judaeus[17] and Josephus.[18] Relying on the writings of Hecataeus of Abdera (sixth/fifth centuries B.C.), Diodorus Siculus remarks that Moses required the Jews "to rear their children" *(teknotrophein),*[19] and says virtually the same thing about the Egyptians, that is, that they are required "to raise all their children" *(ta gennōmena panta trephousin).*[20] Oribasius (personal physician to Julian "the Apostate") maintains that Aristotle also attributed this same practice to the Egyptians *(to trephein panta ta ginomena).*[21] And the geographer Strabo (first centuries B.C./A.D.) asserts that the Egyptians most zealously observe the custom of raising every child who is born *(to panta trephein ta gennōmena paidia).*[22]

The expressed or implied motivations behind these condemnations of exposure differ. Epictetus obviously regards exposure as a violation of natural law. Polybius regards those who engaged in it as selfish and immoral. Tacitus says that the Germans held this practice (as well as any limitation of the number of their children) as *flagitium* (a disgraceful or shameful deed) and says of the Jews that they saw it as *nefas* (contrary to divine law, impious), a word much more charged with moral principle than that descriptive of German sentiment. Josephus maintains that it was forbidden by the Law, and Philo condemns it as murder, a perversion of natural law. Diodorus Siculus implies that the Jews were motivated to condemn the practice by a desire to increase their population, the motive specified by the same author for the Egyptians' forbidding the act. And Heliodorus' imaginary Ethiopian gymnosophist regarded it as morally wrong, at least for his exclusive group of gymnosophists.

The Killing of Defective Newborns

These instances of condemnation of child exposure, or of infanticide in the broader sense of the word, whether by some few Greeks or Romans or by exotic peoples, both Jews and pagans, can be taken to include the condemnation of the killing of the defective newborn, and not only the exposure of healthy infants. There is no qualifying phrase introduced by "except." The statements are generally quite specific and seem to imply that all that are born are raised, the word translated "raised" meaning "nourished," and the word translated "born" either the word commonly used for giving birth, or else the word for becoming or coming into existence. These phrases certainly would, on the surface, seem all-inclusive. Aristotle, you recall, recommends early abortion as a means of population control in the event that "regular customs hinder any of those born being exposed."[23] Such a statement seems inclusive, even in the English translation. But it most certainly is not, for it follows directly on this: "As to exposing or rearing the children born, let there be a law that no deformed child shall be reared" *(peri de apotheseōs kai trophēs ton gignomenōn estō nomos mēden pepērōmenon trephein).*

Aristotle, writing in *Politics,* is describing "the best state." As we have just seen, in such a state he thinks there should be a law that no deformed child should be reared. While the practice of exposing or killing deformed infants was, as we shall see, common enough in classical antiquity, suggesting a law that would make it mandatory was not by any means typical. Quintus Curtius, writing in the first century A.D., thought it was worthy of note to inform his readers that at the time of Alexander the Great it was supposedly the custom in part of India not to permit parents to determine whether their children should be reared; the decision was in the hands of "those to whom the charge of the physical examination of children had been committed. If these have noted any who are conspicuous for defects or are crippled in some part of their limbs, they give orders to put them to death."[24] This sounds very similar to the well-known custom ascribed to the Spartans in Plutarch's *Life of Lycurgus:* "Offspring was not reared at the will of the father, but was taken and carried by him to a place . . . where the elders . . . officially examined the infant, and if it was well-built and sturdy, they ordered the father to rear it . . . but if it was ill-born and deformed, they sent it

14. Heliodorus, *An Ethiopian Romance,* trans. H. Thackeray (Ann Arbor: University of Michigan Press, 1957), p. 61.

15. Tacitus, *Germania* 19.

16. Tacitus, *The Histories* 5.5.

17. E. R. Goodenough, *The Jurisprudence of the Jewish Courts in Egypt: Legal Administration by the Jews under the Early Roman Empire as Described by Philo Judaeus* (Amsterdam: Philo, 1968), pp. 115-16.

18. Josephus, *Against Apion* 2.24.

19. Diodorus Siculus, *Library of History* 40.3, trans. C. H. Oldfather (Cambridge, Mass.: Harvard University Press, 1933-57).

20. Ibid., 1.80.

21. Oribasius, *Collectiones medicae,* ed. I. Reader (Amsterdam: Hakkert, 1928-33), 4: 99-100.

22. Strabo, *Georgraphy,* 172.5.

23. Aristotle, *Politics* (n. 11), 1335b.

24. Quintus Curtius, *History of Alexander* 9.1.25.

to . . . a chasm-like place at the foot of Mount Taÿgetus, in the conviction that the life of that which nature had not well-equipped at the very beginning for health and strength, was of no advantage, either to itself or to the state."[25]

The explanation given for this practice is a concern for eugenics. We can assume the same in the case of Aristotle's ideal state and the supposed custom in India. Another feature that they have in common is that the parents have no say in the matter. Both of these aspects are present in a passage from Plato's *Republic:* "The offspring of the inferior, and any of those of the other sort who are born defective, they will properly dispose of in secret, so that no one will know what has become of them."[26] This passage has been the focus of much controversy, with some scholars maintaining that it has nothing to do with exposure.[27] Irrespective of that debate, we need to step back for a moment and look at the vocabulary in these four passages used to describe the infants in question.

The child is described as *anapēron* (maimed, crippled) by Plato. Aristotle uses a related word, *pepērōmenon,* meaning essentially the same thing. The text of Quintus Curtius is somewhat corrupt, but the basic meaning is "defective" or "crippled." Plutarch uses two terms, the first of which, *agennes,* is quite unusual, having the meaning "unborn" or "uncreated," *perhaps* "grossly deformed"; the second, *amorphon,* means "misshapen" or "disfigured." Aside from the fact that the vocabulary is frustratingly imprecise, we should note that there appears to be nothing superstitious in the procedures or decision making described. The conditions are assumed to be natural defects, of no numinous or ominous character. The situation changes when we look at the Roman scene.

The first-century B.C. historian Dionysius of Halicarnassus attributes to Romulus, the legendary founder of Rome, the following law. Explaining how Romulus had made the city large and populous, Dionysius maintains that "he obliged the inhabitants to bring up all their male children and the first born of the females, and forbade them to destroy any children under three years of age unless they were maimed or monstrous from their very birth. These he did not forbid their parents to expose, provided they first showed them to their five nearest neighbors and these also approved."[28] Irrespective of the very questionable historicity of this "law," an important element is introduced. There are two different categories of defective infants here: *anapēron,* the same word Plato used, translated as "maimed," and *teras,* a noun denoting a sign or wonder, a marvel, a portent, or anything that serves as an omen, as, for instance, here a strange creature or monster. What is probably meant is a grossly deformed infant, perhaps the type implied by Plutarch's word *agennes.* The significant difference is that Plutarch's adjective is devoid of superstitious meaning, while the word *teras* is supernatural to the core. While the infant in Plutarch's account is probably no more or less grotesque than that in Dionysius', the response that each elicits is different, the response at least of the two authors as revealed in their choice of vocabulary.

Much more common in Roman than in Greek society was the occurrence of *prodigia* (in Greek, *terata,* plural of *teras*), unnatural and inexplicable events, such as the birth of a lamb with five legs, a human hermaphrodite, and the like. While some prodigia on record are so bizarre that their historicity must be discounted, many, perhaps most, are well within the realm of possibility, especially after exaggeration is subtracted from the account. A prodigium had enormous significance; it was itself a message from the supernatural powers, more often than not a warning, eliciting a communal fear and guilt in Roman society, particularly during the Republican period. The message had to be discerned by *haruspices* (soothsayers), the unnatural thing destroyed, and a *piaculum,* that is, an expiatory rite performed. Consider the following event, which occurred in 207 B.C., as recorded by the first-century B.C. historian Livy:

> Relieved of their religious scruples, men were troubled again by the report that at Frusino there had been born a child as large as a four-year-old, and not so much a wonder for size as because . . . it was uncertain whether male or female. In fact the soothsayers summoned from Etruria said it was a terrible and loathsome portent; it must be removed from Roman territory, far from contact with earth, and drowned in the sea. They put it alive into a chest, carried it out to sea and threw it overboard. The pontiffs likewise decreed that thrice nine maidens should sing a hymm as they marched through the city.[29]

Such events abound in the extant literature.[30] The motivations for the killing of such newborns are different from the primarily eugenic concerns of the other authors whom we have considered thus far. The response to prodigia is rooted in some very deep-seated fear, guilt, and shame that are only slightly evident in the response to the birth of sickly, maimed, or moderately deformed infants. The maimed, the deformed, and the monstrous constitute a continuum that can accommodate both superstitious and eugenic concerns. A law requiring the

25. Plutarch, *The Parallel Lives: Life of Lycurgus* 16, trans. B. Perrin (Cambridge, Mass.: Harvard University Press, 1914-26).

26. Plato, *Republic,* 460C, trans. P. Shorey (Cambridge, Mass.: Harvard University Press, 1930-35).

27. See, for example, J. J. Mulhern, "Population and Plato's *Republic,*" *Arethusa* 8 (1975): 265-81.

28. Dionysius of Halicarnassus, *Roman Antiquities* 2.15, trans. E. Cary (Cambridge, Mass.: Harvard University Press, 1937-50).

29. Livy, *Histories* 37.27, trans. B. O. Foster, E. T. Sage, A. C. Schlesinger, and R. M. Geer (Cambridge, Mass.: Harvard University Press, 1919-59).

30. For an interesting discussion, see W. den Boer, "Prodigium and Morality," in his *Private Morality in Greece and Rome: Some Historical Aspects* (Leiden: E. J. Brill, 1979), pp. 93ff.

killing of deformed infants would include so-called monstrous births as well, motivated perhaps by both eugenic and superstitious responses. Such seem to underlie a law in the ancient Twelve Tables, a code thought to have been compiled in Rome in the fifth century B.C., to which Cicero alludes. This law required that a *puer ad deformitatem* be killed quickly.[31] While modern translators render this as "terribly deformed," that seems stronger than the Latin, which appears to accommodate the entire continuum described above.

The continuum broadens when we consider a passage in a treatise written by the first-century A.D. Stoic philosopher Seneca: "Mad dogs we knock on the head; the fierce and savage ox we slay; sickly sheep we put to the knife to keep them from infecting the flock; unnatural progeny we destroy; we drown even children who at birth are weakly and abnormal. Yet it is not anger, but reason that separates the harmful from the sound."[32] Here we see *portentosi,* that is, unnatural or monstrous births; *debiles,* that is, sickly or weak infants; and *monstrosi,* that is, deformed or abnormal newborns. We should note that Seneca is neither recommending nor condemning this practice. He simply gives it as an example, along with several others, of violence or ostensibly destructive activity, in which his society engaged as a matter of course, that did not involve anger or hatred but was motivated by a concern for individual or social good. The two sentences immediately preceding the section quoted say, "Does a man hate the members of his own body when he uses a knife upon them? There is no anger there, but the pitying desire to heal."

It should be clear that in Roman culture the killing of defective newborns was common, and was even apparently required in the case of those infants so grossly deformed or unusual as to appear to be *portentosi* or monstrous births. For Greece, however, we have seen only the anomalous conditions in Sparta and the "ideal" practices suggested by Aristotle and Plato. These really tell us little about conditions in Greek society during the classical period. There is, however, a passage in Plato's *Theaetetus* that is very revealing. The man whose name supplies the title for this dialogue has suggested that knowledge is nothing more than perception. Socrates wishes to subject this "brain-child" to examination to see whether it is worth rearing. Socrates had earlier warned him that that was precisely what he was going to do once Theaetetus gives birth to his idea:

> I suspect that you, as you yourself believe, are in pain because you are pregnant with something within you. Apply, then, to me, remembering that I am the son of a midwife and have myself a midwife's gifts, and do your best to answer the questions I ask as I ask them. And if, when I have examined any of the things you say, it should prove that I think it is a mere image and not real, and therefore quietly take it from you and throw it away, do not be angry as women are when they are deprived of their first offspring. For many, my dear friend, before this have got into such a state of mind towards me that they are actually ready to bite me, if I take some foolish notion away from them, and they do not believe that I do this in kindness.[33]

After Theaetetus elaborates his theory, Socrates says, "Shall we say that this is, so to speak, your newborn child and the result of midwifery? Or what shall we say?" Theaetetus replies, "We must say that, Socrates." Socrates then continues: "Well, we have at least managed to bring this forth, whatever it turns out to be; and not that it is born, we must in very truth perform the rite of running around with it in a circle — the circle of our argument — and see whether it may not turn out to be after all not worth rearing, but only a wind-egg, an imposture. But, perhaps, you think that any offspring of yours ought to be cared for and not put away; or will you bear to see it examined and not get angry if it is taken away from you, though it is your firstborn?"[34] First of all, it is self-evident that the whole comparison would be sheer nonsense unless a custom prevailed of disposing of defective newborns, even defective firstborns, at least at Athens at that time. Second, we may note that mothers typically were angry when their firstborn was taken from them. Apparently they were better able to cope with losing a defective infant if they already had at least one healthy child. Third, it is evident that the examination of a newborn infant was part of a midwife's responsibilities. There is relatively little attention given in ancient medical literature to the duties of midwives. However, Soranus, a physician who lived in Rome in the first and second centuries A.D., wrote a gynecological treatise — the best that has survived from antiquity — that was designed for midwives. A passage in this treatise is entitled "How to Recognize the Newborn That Is Worth Rearing." It reads:

> Now the midwife, having received the newborn, should first put it upon the earth, having examined beforehand whether the infant is male or female, and should make an announcement by signs as is the custom of women. She should also consider whether it is worth rearing or not. And the infant which is suited by nature for rearing will be distinguished by the fact that its mother has spent the period of pregnancy in good health, for conditions which require medical care, especially those of the body, also harm the fetus and enfeeble the foundations of its life. Second, by the fact that it has been born at the due time, best at the end of nine months, and if it so happens, later; but also after only seven months. Furthermore by the fact that when a woman puts it on the earth it immediately cries with proper vigor; for one that lives for some length of time without crying, or

31. Cicero, *Laws* 3.8.

32. Seneca, *On Anger* 1.15, in *Moral Essays,* trans. J. W. Basore (Cambridge, Mass.: Harvard University Press, 1928-35).

33. Plato, *Theaetetus* 151B-C, trans. H. N. Fowler (Cambridge, Mass.: Harvard University Press, 1921).

34. Ibid., 160E, 161A.

> cries but weakly, is suspected of behaving so on account of some unfavorable condition. Also by the fact that it is perfect in all its parts, members and senses; that its ducts, namely of the ears, nose, pharynx, urethra, anus are free from obstruction; that the natural functions of every [member] are neither sluggish nor weak; that the joints bend and stretch; that it has due size and shape and is properly sensitive in every respect. This we may recognize from pressing the fingers against the surface of the body, for it is natural to suffer pain from everything that pricks or squeezes. And by conditions contrary to those mentioned, the infant not worth rearing is recognized.[35]

While this passage from Soranus gives concrete evidence for what was undoubtedly a common practice both in Greek and Roman cultures, it is not, strictly speaking, a medical pronouncement upon the decision-making processes involving the care of the defective newborn. It is written on the assumption that a defective infant is *eo ipso* not worth rearing. The question is simply how to determine most easily and efficiently which infants are worth rearing. Even this was a question seldom addressed by ancient medical authors. It was a midwife's concern — which is why we encounter this guidance in a gynecological treatise written for midwives. Not that medical authors, as well as natural philosophers, were uninterested in why some infants were born defective, and how to try to prevent this. Various intriguing suggestions were advanced and theories developed that are not germane to this study.

Two conclusions can now be drawn. One is that the *care* of defective newborns simply was not a medical concern in classical antiquity.[36] The second is that the morality of the killing of sickly or deformed newborns appears not to have been questioned, at least not in extant sources, either by nonmedical or by medical authors. Interestingly enough, Soranus, who was atypical of the ancient medical authors in condemning abortion, not only raises no objection to the rejection of defective newborns but also, as we have seen, quite dispassionately provides the criteria to be used by midwives in determining which newborns are worth rearing.

The Christian Principle of the Sanctity of Life

I have earlier asserted that the idea that human value is acquired rather than inherent was so central to ancient conceptions of value that a fully developed principle of the sanctity of human life, one that includes even the defective newborn, was never achieved in pagan antiquity. For apparently no pagan raised the question of whether human beings have inherent value, or possess intrinsic rights, ontologically, irrespective of social value, legal status, age, sex, and so forth. The first espousal of an idea of inherent human value in Western civilization depended on a belief that every human being was formed in the image of God. We shall return shortly to this principle of *imago Dei* as a basis for inherent human value.

It is unlikely, however, that the earliest Christians formulated a concise definition of human value based upon the concept of imago Dei. The condemnation of acts that would later be viewed as violations of the rights that accrue to a person as one formed in God's image were, in the earliest Christian literature, part of a broad moral indignation against those aspects of Greco-Roman culture which stand in the starkest contrast to the most basic principles of the gospel of love, mercy, compassion, and salvation from sin to holiness and purity. All aspects of pagan brutality and immorality were condemned; they seemed to early Christian apologists to be common and related features of a society that was viewed as corrupted to its very core by the disease of sin. Apologists condemned in the same breath gladiatorial shows, grossly cruel executions conducted as spectator sports, abortion, infanticide, and a broad and imaginative variety of sexual deviations. Some apologists saw abortion as a sexual crime, in that it was done to destroy the results of a sexual act that was lust when engaged in for a purpose other than procreation. Infanticide had the same motive as did exposure, except that the latter created a potential for another sexual sin, incest, since exposed children often ended up in brothels.[37]

So common, indeed universal, among Christians in the early centuries of Christianity was the condemnation of abortion and infanticide, including exposure,[38] that I shall only mention a few features. Some apologists point out that the practice of infanticide among the pagans is not surprising, in light of a tradition of the sacrifice of infants in various cults — a practice in which some cults still engaged, although it was strictly forbidden by law; and a practice, incidentally, of which early Christians were themselves slanderously accused. Further, these apologists claim, the pagan myths are full of tales of infanticide, which set a precedent of approbation. Further, some early church fathers contrast active infanticide with exposure, asserting that exposing a baby to cold, hunger, and carnivorous animals is more cruel than simply strangling it. But, they tell us, many pagans, thinking that it is impious to kill the infant with one's own hands, kill it by the less messy means of a slow death out of their sight.

35. Soranus, *Gynecology*, trans. Owsei Temkin (Baltimore: Johns Hopkins Press, 1956), pp. 79-80.

36. For an interesting discussion of the minor role of pediatrics in ancient medicine, see R. Etienne, "Ancient Medical Conscience and the Life of Children," *J. Psychohist*, 4 (1976-77): 127-61.

37. See, e.g., Justin Martyr, *The First Apology* 27; Tertullian, *Apology* 9; Clement of Alexandria, *Christ the Educator* 21; and Lactantius, *The Divine Institutes* 6.20.

38. See, e.g., Minucius Felix, *Octavius* 30; Justin Martyr, *The First Apology* 27; Lactantius, *The Divine Institutes* 5.9; Tertullian, *Ad nationes* 1.15; idem, *Apology* 9; idem, *The Didache* 2; *The Epistle of Barnabas* 19.5; and *The Epistle to Diognetus* 5–6. For a discussion, see I. Giordani, *The Social Message of the Early Fathers*, trans. A. Zizzamia (Boston: St. Paul Editions, 1977), pp. 243-52.

None of the early Christian condemnations of infanticide make any reference to the condition of the baby, whether it is healthy or defective, or consider a possible eugenic motivation for the active or passive killing of a newborn. But while I asserted that the relatively rare instances of pagan condemnations of exposure would not have included the killing of the defective, I shall maintain even more categorically that early Christian condemnation of exposure and other forms of infanticide would have included any and every form of infanticide, active or passive, of newborns, whether they be healthy, sickly, or deformed.

There are three reasons that immediately come to mind for this attitude. The first, which I shall mention only in passing, is the significantly different attitude of Christianity to children generally. In classical society, even in its more humanitarian movements, children were essentially viewed as potential adults, their value residing in what they would become. We moderns, in a child-oriented society, generally do not appreciate just how revolutionary was Jesus' teaching that unless you become as little children you cannot enter the kingdom of God. Second, the social thrust of early Christianity was demonstrably and spectacularly oriented to helping the helpless, caring for the destitute, and succoring the deprived.

The third reason requires a little more space than the first two. I made reference earlier to the concept of people being created in God's image as ultimately providing the basis for a Christian theology of human value. I shall leave aside such questions as the relationship of image and likeness of God and the extent to which these concepts are entangled by patristic authors with the Platonic conception that likeness to God is the telos of human endeavor. The earliest Christian apologist who seems to imply the concept of imago Dei as a basis for the condemnation of abortion and infanticide is Clement of Alexandria (second century).[29] Even if the imago Dei may be defaced by human will, obstinacy, and sin, such could not be the case with the fetus and the newborn infant. Such an assertion obviously would include the sickly and deformed newborn. But what of the extreme end of the continuum of which I spoke earlier, the monstrous or grossly deformed?

Augustine, in the *City of God*,[40] comments on the tremendous diversity among people, enormous racial differences, and whole tribes of people who seem to us to be monstrous. He then says,

> If whole peoples have been monsters, we must explain the phenomenon as we explain the individual monsters who are born among us. God is the Creator of all; He knows best where and when and what is, or was, best for Him to create, since He deliberately fashioned the beauty of the whole out of both the similarity and dissimilarity of its parts. . . . I know men who were born with more than five fingers or toes, which is one of the slightest variations from the normal, but it would be a shame for anyone to be so silly as to suppose that, because he did not know why God did this, the Creator could make a mistake in regard to the number of fingers on a man's hand. Even in cases of greater variations, God knows what He is doing, and no one may rightly blame His work. . . . it would be impossible to list all the human offspring who have been very different from the parents from whom they were certainly born. Still, all these monsters undeniably owe their origin to Adam.[41]

Later in the same work, Augustine says that pagans mock the idea of the resurrection of the dead, referring to various physical defects as well as "all the human monstrosities that are born" and then asking, "What kind of resurrection will there be in cases like these?"[42] Augustine, in his *Enchiridion,* specifically addresses the question of the resurrection of the grossly deformed, or human "monstrosities":

> Concerning monsters which are born and live, however quickly they die, neither is resurrection to be denied them, nor is it to be believed that they will rise again as they are, but rather with an amended and perfected body. God forbid that the double-membered man recently born in the East — about whom most trustworthy brethren, who saw him, have reported, and Jerome the priest, of holy memory, left written mention — God forbid, I say, that we should think that at the resurrection there will be one such double man, and not rather two men, as would have been the case had twins been born. And so all other births which, as having some excess or some defect or because of some conspicuous deformity, are called monsters, will be brought again at the resurrection to the true form of human nature, so that one soul will have one body, and no bodies will cohere together, even those that were born in this condition, but each, apart, for himself, will have as his own those members whose sum makes the complete human body.[43]

The imago Dei, with its attendant value, rights, and responsibilities, attached in early Christian thought to the newborn, whether healthy or sickly, maimed, deformed, or monstrous, indeed to the whole continuum of the defective, in vivid contrast to the attitudes and practices of pagan antiquity. The Christian concept of imago Dei provided both the basis and the structure for the idea of inalienable rights and of intrinsic human value that has prevailed in Western society nearly until the present.

39. Rist, *Human Value* (n. 1), pp. 162-63.

40. Augustine, *City of God* 16.8.

41. Augustine, *City of God,* in *Writings of Saint Augustine,* various translators (Washington, D.C.: Catholic University of America Press, various dates), 7: 502-3.

42. Augustine, *City of God* 22.12, vol. 8, p. 459, in the edition cited in n. 41.

43. Augustine, *Enchiridion* 87, in *Writings of Saint Augustine* (n. 41), 4: 442-43.

108 The Death of Infant Doe: Jesus and the Neonates

Allen Verhey

I imagine it was a hot and sunny day, the kind of day when kids seem to have such boundless energy and grown-ups seem to wilt. The disciples, I suppose, were quite glad for the rest; at least they were a little peevish when women and children threatened to interrupt it. They rebuked them, the story in Mark 10 says. "Can't you see Jesus is an important person? What business do you have bothering him? Get back to your ovens, women! Return to your toys, children! Stay out of our way."

The disciples' response was conventional enough; surely understandable. Women and children were just not that important. They were numbered among the heathen and illiterate, with sinners and those who do not know the law, with slaves and property. They were not numbered at all when the members of the synagogue were counted. You needed ten *adult males* for a synagogue. Nine plus all the women and children of Galilee would not make a synagogue. Women and children just did not count for much. The disciples knew that and told them to go away.

Jesus gets angry too, but not with the women, not with the children. He gets angry with the disciples. He turns the conventional rules of pomp and protocol upside down. Those who don't count do count with him; he makes the last first! When will his disciples ever learn that? He says to them, "Let the children come to me. Do not hinder them. To them belongs the kingdom of God." The disciples must have been more than a little dumbfounded. Other strange behavior of this Galilean teacher had hardly prepared them for this.

There must have been babies there, and more than one dirty diaper, and Jesus takes them in his arms. There must have been toddlers and youngsters, curious and energetic, crying occasionally and interrupting often. "Women are meant to deal with them," the disciples thought, but Jesus blesses them. There must have been boys and girls, taking a break from playing tag and catch, and some who stood on the sidelines because of a limp or a disease or something else that made them unwelcome in the game, and Jesus lays his hands on them.

And as though all this is not enough, Jesus says, "If you want to enter the kingdom, become like one of these children." People have speculated endlessly about how we are supposed to be like children. It is their *trust,* some say; their *dependence,* others say; their *joy,* still others say; or their *simplicity.* There is perhaps some truth in each of those comparisons, but I really think they are beside the point. Jesus says in other places, "If any would be first of all, let him be last of all and the servant of all." And that's what he says here too. "Become like one of these children" means simply "become last — for such are first with me." That's the shocking thing. Jesus exalts the humble and humbles the exalted. He makes the last first. Those who don't count count with him. He blesses kids; dirty-diapered, sweaty, silly, obnoxious kids. He rebukes the disciples, impressed with their own importance and conventional prestige. And he makes it clear that to be his disciple, to welcome the kingdom, will mean to welcome, to serve and to help, these little children. Who is greatest in the kingdom? These little children and those who bless and serve them.

Soon after the death and resurrection of Jesus, that story was being told again and again in the young church. Pentecost had convinced the people of the church that Jesus continued to abide with them and that he continued to address them in their memory of what he had once said or done. Even as the church awaited the new creation, the redemption of their bodies and their adoption as sons, as Paul says, it was constantly informed and reformed by the stories about Jesus. Imagine, for example, Peter telling the story to settle the question of whether the children of believing parents should be baptized. Or Andrew telling the story in a slightly different way to exhort his hearers to a childlike faith. Or again, imagine some unknown preacher telling the story to protest the neglect and abandonment of children that was practiced in the Roman empire. The story found its way finally into Mark's gospel alongside sayings about marriage and riches to provide guidance for a Christian household.

The story continues to be told in the churches, of course. It is told in countless stained glass windows. We have all seen them. The only thing wrong with these windows is that the kids are too angelic. There are no runny noses or bruised knees or imperfections to be found in the stained glass representations of the story. The story has indeed become so familiar that we have to make an effort to stop and think about it, to contemplate what it would mean to make this story our story, to be informed and reformed by this story. I invite you to make that effort, specifically to think about what this story might mean for our care of neonates.

To do this there is another story that I want you to think about. It is a familiar story, too, the story of Infant Doe. It happened in Bloomington in 1982. Now Bloomington is a pleasant little city set in the lovely hills of southern Indiana. Bloomington Hospital is typical of hospitals in pleasant little cities; the daily human events of giving birth, suffering, and dying are attended to with

From *The Reformed Journal* 32 (June 1982): 10-15. Used by permission. Revised by the author for this volume.

the ordinary measure of professional competence and compassion. It seems unlikely that the story of birth, suffering, and death of a baby in Bloomington would capture national attention.

On April 9, 1982, a boy was born in Bloomington Hospital with Down's syndrome and esophageal atresia. Down's syndrome is a fairly common genetic defect which causes varying degrees of mental retardation and physical deformity. Esophageal atresia is a malformation of the esophagus, so that food taken orally cannot enter the stomach and instead causes choking.

The parents of this baby refused to consent to the surgical procedure necessary to correct the esophageal atresia. The obstetrician who had initially presented such "benign neglect" as one of the medical options supported the parents in that decision. A pediatrician who had been consulted to confirm the diagnosis dissented from such a course of "treatment." The Circuit Court in Bloomington and subsequently the Indiana Supreme Court in Indianapolis refused to override the parents' decision and to order the surgery to correct the esophagus of "Infant Doe." The baby lay in Bloomington Hospital for six days until his starving yielded to his death on April 15.

The obstetrician and the pediatrician disagreed not only about the recommended treatment but also about the chances for successful esophageal surgery, about the likelihood of other serious physical problems, and about the prognosis of retardation. The obstetrician, in presenting the options to the parents, said that the chances for successful surgery were about fifty-fifty, that other physical defects, including congenital heart disease, would subsequently have to be surgically corrected, and that the child would certainly be severely retarded. The pediatrician insisted that the likelihood of successful surgery was more like ninety percent, that there was no evidence of congenital heart disease, and that it was impossible to determine the severity of the retardation Infant Doe would have. The conflicting medical opinions and recommendations weighed heavily in the courts' decisions not to intervene, not to play either doctor or parent to the child.

The courts' hesitancy to pretend to either medical competence or parental compassion can be appreciated (especially by those schooled in something called "sphere sovereignty"). Moreover, the competence of the doctors and the compassion of the parents were widely attested. Still, the medical recommendation of the obstetrician and the decisions by the parents and by the justices were morally wrong — not just tragic, but wrong.

Decisions are tragic when goods come into conflict, when any decision brings in its train some wrong. This was not such a decision. The right decision would have been to do the surgery. I will undertake to defend that judgment in ways that are standard in medical ethics, in ways that rely on "impartial rationality" to formulate judgments and to solve dilemmas. One need not be a Christian to see that the decision not to treat Infant Doe was wrong. But I will also undertake to show that impartial rationality is inadequate, that it can provide only a minimal account of morality, and that when its minimalism is not acknowledged it can distort the moral life. Finally, because the conventional approach is inadequate, I will undertake another approach, a candidly Christian approach, an approach which owns the Christian story, including the story of Jesus and the children, as *our* story also in cases like Infant Doe's.

First, then, one need not be a Christian to see that the right decision would have been to perform the surgery to correct the esophagus so that Infant Doe could be fed. The impartial rational justification for saying this might be provided in a number of different ways. The most telling in my view is that if a "normal" child had been born with esophageal atresia, the surgery would have been performed — even if the obstetrician were right about the risks and the additional physical problems. The reason for "treating" Infant Doe differently was an irrelevant one, Infant Doe's Down's syndrome. (Furthermore, the obstetrician was simply wrong about the ability to predict so early the extent of retardation caused by Down's syndrome.)

Suppose that on April 9 two other babies were born in Bloomington. Suppose "Infant Smith" was born without Down's syndrome but with esophageal atresia. The consent to operate would surely have been given or ordered, and Infant Smith would probably be alive today. Suppose "Infant Jones" was born with Down's syndrome but without any life-threatening malformations of the esophagus. No consent to operate would have been necessary, and Infant Jones would probably be alive today. The difference between Infant Doe and Infant Smith, the difference between life and death, is that Infant Doe had Down's syndrome, nothing else. The difference between Infant Doe and Infant Jones, also the difference between life and death, is that Infant Doe had esophageal atresia in addition to Down's syndrome. If we ought to preserve and cherish the life of Infants Smith and Jones, then we ought also to have preserved and cherished the life of Infant Doe. The differences among these infants are irrelevant to the obligation to sustain their lives and to nurture their bodies and spirits.

This is not to deny that different conditions among infants may indicate different treatments or even in some cases the cessation of treatment. If a condition is terminal and if treatment would only prolong the child's dying and exacerbate his or her suffering, then treatment is not indicated. Anencephalic newborns are a clear case of legitimate neglect. There are tragic cases where a child's suffering from a disease and from the treatment of the disease is so profound as to put it outside the reach of human caring, let alone human curing. Such, however, was not the case with Infant Doe or other Down's syndrome youngsters. Down's syndrome is not a terminal condition; and if people who have it suffer more, it is not because surgery pains them more but because "normal" people can be cruel and spiteful. A Down's child can experience and delight in the reach and touch of human caring.

The neglect of Infant Doe was morally wrong. His death was caused by "natural causes," to be sure, but it was both possible and obligatory to interfere with those "natural causes." If a lifeguard neglected a drowning swimmer whom he recognized as his competition for his lover's affection, we would say he did wrong. That the drowned man died of "natural causes" would not prevent us from seeing the wrong done to him — or from invoking the category "murder." If the same lifeguard neglected a drowning wader whom he recognized as an infant with Down's syndrome, we should also say he did wrong. That the infant died of "natural causes" should not prevent us from seeing the wrong done to him — or from invoking the category "murder."

Someone may argue that "lifeguard" is a well-defined role with specific responsibilities and a tradition involving certain technical skills and moral virtues, and that the obligation to rescue the swimmer and the wader is really a role-obligation. Two replies might be made to this objection to our analogy. First, we might say that any person — lifeguard or not — who sees an infant stumble and fall face down in the water is obliged to attempt to rescue the child, Down's syndrome or not. The decision to neglect Infant Doe, by analogy, is simply morally wrong. The second reply is to acknowledge that "lifeguard" is a special role with special responsibilities and a tradition, and to insist that "physician" and "parent" are also such roles.

But here impartial rationality begins to fail us, for it tends to reduce role relations — for example, the relation of the doctors to Infant Doe or his parents or the relation of the parents to Infant Doe — to *contractual* arrangements between independent individuals. That is a minimal account of such roles at best, and when its minimalism is not acknowledged, it is an account which distorts the moral life and the covenants of which it is woven. The stance of impartial rationality cannot nurture any moral wisdom about these roles or sustain any moral traditions concerning them. And it is our confusion about these roles, our diminishing sense of a tradition concerning them, that accounts for the failure of a competent physician, compassionate parents, and duly humble justices to make the morally right decision with respect to the care of Infant Doe.

There are other inadequacies in the stance of impartial rationality which bore on the story of Infant Doe. The stance of impartial rationality tends to emphasize the procedural question, the question of who decides, rather than the substantive question of what should be decided. The first and final question in the care of Infant Doe was who should decide, and the answer was consistently that the parents should decide. I am not saying that that question or that answer is wrong, but I am saying that it provides only a minimal account of the moral issues, and that if its minimalism is forgotten or ignored, the moral life and particular moral issues can be distorted. I am saying that a fuller account of morality would focus as well on substantive questions — on the question of *what* should be decided — and on questions of character and virtue — on the question of *what* the person who decides should *be*.

Let me call attention to one other weakness (or inadequacy) of the approach of impartial rationality. This approach requires alienation from ourselves, from our own moral interests and loyalties, from our own histories and communities in order to adopt the impartial point of view. We are asked, nay, obliged, by this approach to view our own projects and passions as though we were objective outside observers. The stories which we own as our own, which provide our lives a narrative and which develop our own character, we are asked by this approach to disown — and for the sake of morality. Now, to be asked to pause occasionally and for the sake of analysis and judgment to view things as impartially as we can is in certain contexts not only legitimate but salutary, but neither physicians nor parents nor any Christian can finally live their moral lives like that with any integrity.

These remarks about the inadequacies of impartial rationality allow us to turn an important corner in this paper. My concern is not merely to make a moral judgment about the care of Infant Doe. The decision not to treat him was wrong, but the more interesting questions — and finally the more important questions, from my point of view — are, How could a competent physician, compassionate parents, and duly humble justices make such a decision? What stories and traditions make sense of such a decision? And how can the Christian story, explicitly the story of Jesus and the children, be brought to bear on such decisions? Can we begin to write a story of Jesus and the neonates? Let us examine briefly the stories and traditions of medicine, of parenting, and of society's attitude toward the handicapped.

The obstetrician, however competent and skillful he may have been, had apparently not been initiated into the tradition of medical care which insists that the practice of medicine involves more than techniques and skills, that it serves and embodies certain intrinsic goods. According to one witness to that tradition, the Hippocratic Oath, the end of medicine is "the benefit of the sick," not some extrinsic good like money or fame or the wishes of the medical "consumer."

The benefit of the sick does not stand as a motive for taking up certain ethically neutral skills. It does not identify an extrinsic good to be accomplished by means of ethically neutral technical means. Rather, the benefit of the sick is the *intrinsic* good of medicine. It governs the practice of medicine and entails certain standards which define medicine as a moral art. Medicine in this tradition intends to heal the sick, to protect and nurture health, to maintain and restore a measure of physical well-being. All the powers of medicine are guided and limited by those ends, and they may not be used to serve alien ends — and death is an alien end. In this sad world death will win its victories finally, but medicine which has identified with the tradition to which the Hippocratic Oath witnesses will not serve death or practice hospitality toward it. This tradition has its own stories, of course, stories about the great Hippocrates initiating his students into the art with an oath that they will indeed practice medicine for "the benefit of the sick," stories about dedicated physicians braving the elements or the opposition to help some sick scoundrel without worrying about the social utility of his patient or of his profession.

Medicine truly in the tradition formed and informed by such stories would and should have stood in the service of Infant Doe, the sick one, the patient, and braved the claims of any and all who wanted him dead. A physician initiated into such a tradition would not present the choice between possible life with Down's syndrome or certain death without esophageal surgery as an option to be contemplated, nor would he or she support the choice of death.

The obstetrician's failure to embody this tradition is symptomatic of our entire society's diminishing appreciation of this view of medicine and a growing confusion about the physician's role. These stories of medicine are today considered naive, sometimes foolish, both by physicians and by society. Properly impressed by modern medicine's technological accomplishments, we are tempted to view medicine as a collection of skills to get what we want, as a value-free enterprise which may be bought and sold to satisfy consumer desires, hired to do the autonomous bidding of the one who pays. Thus, a new model has taken over the understanding of medicine — that omnipresent model of the marketplace, where you get rich by supplying what the buyer wants.

The decision about Infant Doe is understandable, I think, within the marketplace model, but we are justifiably uncomfortable with this way of understanding medicine, for medical skills alone, removed from their original tradition, can make one either a good healer or a crafty murderer. The skills alone cannot provide the wisdom to make a morally right decision. Medicine formed by the model of the marketplace cannot and will not sustain the disposition of care and trust which have defined the characters of doctor and patient in the Hippocratic tradition. On the contrary, the marketplace model will end with medicine in the service of the rich and powerful, while the poor and weak watch and pray.

Infant Doe was too young to pray but not too young to groan with the rest of us "as we wait for . . . the redemption of our bodies" (Rom. 8:23). That eschatological vision of Christianity — and the entire Christian story, including the story of Jesus and the children — provides a resource to support the fragile Hippocratic tradition of medicine, for it enlists us on the side of life and health in a world where death and evil still apparently reign. It makes us suspicious of and repentant for human capacities for pride and sloth with respect to medical technology. And it calls us to identify with and to serve especially the sick and the poor, the powerless and the despised, and all those who do not measure up to conventional standards.

A note must be added with respect to another community that evidently has the resources to support the fragile tradition of medicine — nurses. The nurses at Bloomington Hospital who were first charged with the "care" of Infant Doe refused to participate in his nontreatment masquerading as care. It violated the ends of nursing as they understood them; it compromised their integrity as members of a nursing community and as heirs of a medical tradition. The immediate consequence of their protest was not great: Infant Doe was simply moved from the nursery to a private room on a surgical floor. But a worthy tradition of medicine was represented and protected by their action. These nurses and others like them are a precious resource if the medical professions and society are to remember and relearn the medical moral tradition.

Our society is also confused about the role of parent. The parents of Infant Doe, however compassionate they may have been, had apparently not been initiated into a tradition of parental care which insists that parents have a duty not only to care *about* their children but to care *for* them, to tend to their physical, emotional, moral, and spiritual needs, not because they "measure up," but because they are their children.

The parents' failure to represent this tradition is symptomatic of our society's growing confusion about parenting. The tradition has always been challenged by the contrary opinion (now usually unstated) that children are the property of parents to be disposed of as they wish, that children exist for the happiness of parents. Today, however, especially among the compassionate, the tradition is being challenged by a contrary opinion: the view that parents have the awesome responsibility to produce "perfect" children and to assure them a happy and successful life or at least the capacity to attain to and conform to the American ideal of "the good life."

All of us who are parents know we desire our children to be perfect. And all of us who are children know the pain that can be caused by that desire. The responsibility of making perfect children and making children perfect, which is now entering and forming a new model of medicine, will allow — or finally require — the abortion of the unborn who do not meet our standards and the neglect of newborns with diminished capacities to achieve *our* ideal of "the good life." Such a view of parenting will finally reduce our options to a perfect child or a dead child. The Infant Doe decision is understandable, I think, within a model of medicine that requires making perfect children and making children perfect, but that model will not and cannot coexist with the disposition of uncalculating nurturance and basic trust which have defined the relation of parent and child within the Christian story.

It is a commonplace to assert that the institution of the family is in crisis, but it can receive little support from conventional modern moral theory, whether utilitarian or formalist. Both have some power in dealing with our relation with strangers, but neither can deal adequately with the family or sustain it in a time of crisis.

Family loyalties are an embarrassment to our calculations of "the greatest happiness for the greatest number" and to our assertions of autonomy. The tradition of the family — and experience in a family — reminds us both that "happiness" is not what it's all about and that we are not as independent, self-sufficient, and autonomous as we sometimes claim.

The fragile tradition of the family, too, may be and should be supported by the Christian story, for the Father's uncalculating nurturance is still the model from which to learn parenting. In the Christian vision the family is seen as a gift and a vocation, providing opportunities to learn to love the *im*perfect, the runny-nosed, and the just plain obnoxious. The story of a Lord who welcomed little children (along with the sick and women and sinners and all others who did not measure up) is a resource for that sort of uncalculating nurturance that can love the child who is there, that would and should insist on the support of others to enable that child to live and — within the limits of his condition and the world's fallenness — to flourish. Infant Doe's groans awaited not only "the redemption of our bodies" but "our adoption as sons." Parental nurturance formed and informed by the story of Jesus and the children would think it curious — at best — to be told that it was *optional* to do the surgery necessary for the child's life and flourishing, as though one has a choice whether to attend to those things necessary for one's child's life and flourishing or to neglect and starve one's child.

The fundamental point is this: although the parents were, by all accounts, compassionate individuals, love is *not* all you need — no matter what popular songs and popular preaching may tell us. Compassion exercised outside the moral tradition of parenting is quite capable of pitying and killing ("mercy-killing," some would call it) those who do not measure up to the perfection we want for and from our children. Joseph Fletcher — whom no one may accuse of not emphasizing love enough — has (in spite of himself) at least one moral rule: "No unwanted child should ever be born." Compassion by itself may be quite capable of formulating another rule: "No unwanted child need be fed."

The Indiana judges were properly hesitant to intervene in the private arena of medical and parental decisions about the appropriate care of "defective neonates" (a neologism to help us forget that it is our children we are talking about). As we have observed, the decision not to treat is sometimes perfectly legitimate and sometimes legitimately controverted. In such cases that decision is best left to the parents and to the advice of physicians. The decision not to treat Infant Doe, however, was immoral; yet the court did not have the resources to call it illegal.

In part the court could not judge the decision illegal because of the simple lack of law governing such cases. But it is also true that the predominant legal theory today, quite self-consciously impartial and rational, emphasizes autonomy and privacy and contract in ways which make it difficult to give legal support to the interdependencies of a family or to the moral traditions of certain roles in which there is no formal contract. I do not deny the moral importance of this legal theory or the pluralism it sponsors and sustains, but I do claim that it can give only a minimal account of the moral life, and also that society and the courts dangerously distort the moral life and endanger our life together when they reduce morality to such legality.

The courts might still have intervened in the case of Infant Doe if not for our confusion about the rights of the retarded and the otherwise handicapped and the rights of others to be free from contact with them. On the one hand, there is physical evidence everywhere — ramps, special bathrooms, barrier-free doorways — of legislation to integrate the handicapped into our social life. On the other hand, many such people remain segregated in institutions acknowledged to be inhumane; and in fact a 1981 Supreme Court decision, *Pennhurst v. Haldemann,* overturned a state court's order to close one such institution and to establish smaller facilities integrated into the state's residential communities.

Integration verses segregation, the rights of a minority versus the rights of a majority not to be confronted with them — it all has a dismally familiar ring. In the case of Infant Doe and others like him, integration would entail welcoming their life without celebrating or romanticizing their condition. It would mean recognizing their right to equal treatment by the law and by medicine. It would mean acknowledging that even if we call them "defective neonates," they remain our children, and that attempts to cut off emotional and role relations with them are self-deceptive. And it would mean a willingness to pay the additional taxes necessary to support the care and nurturance of such children. Segregation, on the other hand, would mean a refusal to practice hospitality toward them or toward their lives, seceding from the obligations of community with them, and asserting our independence from them. The duly humble decision of the justices not to rule in the case is understandable in terms of the segregationist positions, and — however unwittingly — it strengthened that tradition for the future.

The Christian story — including the story of Jesus and the children — would support and sustain a tradition of including and welcoming society's outcasts, of serving and helping those who are last. If we keep telling the story of Jesus we may yet learn and live a life of joyful acceptance of people, including little people, who in other stories and other views don't count for much.

A competent physician, compassionate parents, and humble justices failed to make the right decision. The problem was not that the decision was extraordinarily difficult, a real moral dilemma. The problem was not that these people were mean-spirited or evil. The problem was rather that they had — however unwittingly or unconsciously — accepted the wrong models of medicine and parenting and relations with the handicapped. This is not altogether their fault: the traditions of caring and nurture and respect are fragile in contemporary culture. But those traditions have not completely broken down. Witness the statement of the pediatrician, "As a father and physician I can't make the decision to let the baby die." Witness the response of the nurses. Witness the offers to adopt Infant Doe.

Yet the traditions are weak. Babies are not even as fragile as the moral traditions that protect them. And the courts are apparently powerless to preserve those traditions. Infant Doe and all of us are dependent on moral traditions and communities, on covenants which can neither be reduced to contracts nor rendered legally enforceable means to legally enforceable ends.

Infant Doe now rests in peace. The sleep of many others is still disturbed by thoughts of his brief but real suffering and his calculated death. To judge these parents or these physicians will not ease our restlessness. But to resist the erosion of some ancient traditions about medicine and parenting and to establish a tradition of including the handicapped in our community is today part of our Christian vocation and our cultural mandate. Christians can, sometimes do, and should preserve and cherish a tradition about medicine that gives to doctors the worthy calling of healer, not the demeaning role of hired hand to do a consumer's bidding. Christians can, sometimes do, and should preserve and cherish a tradition about the family that gives parents the vocation of uncalculating nurturance and rescues them from the impossible obligation of making their children either perfect or "happy." Christians can, sometimes do, and should welcome and include those whom it is too much our impulse to shun and neglect.

Such medicine and such families and such a community may not always be "happy," but they will always be capable of being surprised by joy in caring for one they cannot cure. They will learn to tell and live a story of Jesus and the neonate. And when the groanings of all creation cease, they may hear, "As you did it to one of the least of these my brethren, you did it unto me."

109 Biblical Faith and the Loss of Children

Bruce C. Birch

Death always comes as an offense. Death is the end of life. For most of us life is good; death is the ultimate end of the touching, the sharing and the struggling together that make for wholeness. There has been much recent effort in the church to understand and deal with death, and we have been blessed by a great deal of helpful literature and attention in the communities of faith to the issues of death and dying.

There is something about the death of a child, however, which heightens the offense; we have not often faced that matter very directly in our churches. The death of a child is felt to be unacceptable. It seems unnatural. We can't use some of those bromides that we sometimes use to reassure ourselves; for example, "She lived a full life." Often a child's death becomes the occasion for a crisis of faith. Not only a matter of psychology of grief, a child's death is a challenge to our own deepest faith understandings. What kind of God would allow this to happen? What could faith possibly have to say to this experience?

These questions have been my own. In the fall of 1970 we were told that our daughter Christine had acute lymphocytic leukemia. This diagnosis came at the end of a difficult year for us. I had been fired from my first college teaching job because of antiwar activities. We had been unable to find a job and were forced to move out of our house. There was no place to go. We stored our furniture in a friend's basement and headed for parts unknown. I finally found a teaching job in August, one month before the beginning of school, and moved from Iowa, out on the plains where we had family close by, to South Carolina, a region of the country where we knew no one.

Six weeks after we arrived in South Carolina, we learned that our daughter had a potentially fatal illness. The nearest treatment center was in Atlanta, the Henrietta Eggleston Children's Hospital at Emory University. We traveled there to begin the arduous course of treatments which we hoped would put our daughter's disease into remission. A remission might have allowed her to receive the benefits of advancing medical knowledge in dealing with leukemia. But before Christine could be put into remission, she broke out in chicken pox, to which she had been exposed in the church nursery before we knew she had leukemia. Her diseased blood cells could not fight the infection, and she went into shock. One month after the diagnosis, she died, on her third birthday. The precipitating cause of her death and its timing seemed cruel ironies.

We were filled with anger and grief. Where was God? Where was justice? Where was meaning? I can only share with you out of my own knowledge of the power of those questions — and my conviction that in the biblical tradition of the Christian faith, we do have some resources which help us, even in times of such loss.

We can begin by talking about the problem of God. God is the easiest hook on which to hang blame. Many instinctively feel that God must somehow be punishing them. "Why did God do this to me? I must have done something to deserve this." Unfortunately, that notion is reinforced by a good deal of popular religion; but the punisher God is not a helpful concept. It either produces guilt that is undeserved and unrelated to the situation, or it leads to angry rejection of God altogether.

This concept of a punisher God does sometimes appear in the Bible, however. In the Old Testament, particularly in Deuteronomy and in the Wisdom literature, we find a God who dispenses rewards and punishments for every human action, as if life could be reduced to such mechanical blessings and curses. But a corrective to this view also appears in the Bible; the entire Book of Job is a protest against it, sweeping away its irrelevant and monstrous blasphemy. Job is a righteous man who has suffered great and grievous loss. In the traditional story (chapters 1-2; 42:7 ff.) He is patient and long-suffering, and God finally restores everything to him. This traditional tale of the patient sufferer was surely known widely in the ancient world of Israel. That is not the total picture in the Book of Job, however. The author has split the old story in half, inserting into the middle of it, alongside the traditional picture of the patient Job, the hurt, angry and rebellious Job. This Job argues with the friends and challenges God. The friends say all the pious things: "God's purposes are too great for us. You must have deserved this, so accept it." But Job argues that all people, whether righteous or not, are vulnerable to suffering, and that a hidden, uncaring God is no help at all.

The Book of Job helps us to reject the notion of the punisher God as inadequate. It calls us to look further for a God who does care and who identifies with our pain. Perhaps the God who finally appears to Job in a whirlwind at the end of the book is a pointer toward a deity who at least engages and is present with those who suffer — but the Book of Job is not intended to give us easy answers to that struggle. By sweeping away glib responses to the problem of God in times of deep pain and suffering, the book points to our own struggles and our own engagement with an even wider biblical tradition in which there does appear a caring God who is central to our faith tradition. I want to describe three aspects of this divine image over against that of the punisher God.

The first is *God as hearer.* Over and over again in Scripture, we find lines like these: "I have heard their cries. Their cries have come to me. Their cries have fallen on my ears." Dorothee Sölle, in her important book *Suffering* (Fortress, 1975), suggests that the outcry is the beginning of healing. Israel knew the importance of expressing pain and despair to God, and in the midst of the community. Nowhere is this seen more eloquently than in the laments of the Psalter. We think of the Psalter as a book of praises, but the largest number of Psalms are songs of lamentation. One cannot read these laments without being impressed that Israel had a rather different concept of worship than we commonly do. The psalms are gutsy and honest; they don't pull any punches. They express despair: "Out of the depths have I cried to thee, O Lord" (Ps. 130). They express doubts: "My God, my God, why hast thou forsaken me?" (Ps. 22). They express anger and bitterness. The 137th Psalm, which begins, "By the waters of Babylon we sat down and wept," ends with lines so terrible in their expression of anger and bitterness that we almost never read them in public worship: "O daughter of Babylon, you devastator! . . . Happy shall he be who takes your little ones and dashes them against the rock!" Anger, bitterness, despair, doubt — it is all there, not because the tradition desires to affirm those expressions as ends in themselves but because if the pain is not exposed the healing cannot begin. These Psalms are often shocking to us because so much of our own worship tries to conceal our deepest wounds. Our own worship so often takes place at the level of the lowest common denominator of our corporate experience.

The role of the pastor as counselor can also serve to hide our deepest wounds from the wider community. I once was in a church in which someone expressed very deep hurt and anger during the time set aside for the sharing of concerns in the worship service — only to have the pastor remark at the end of the service, "Well, Fred, if you had brought that to me we could have talked about it without imposing on everyone else's worship experience." If the hurt is not exposed, the healing word cannot be spoken.

My wife and I found many in the church especially reluctant to deal with the death of a child. One can speak of one's recently deceased parent for years; it is not unusual and is widely acknowledged as healthy. But to speak of one's lost child is often to evoke responses like "Hasn't he gotten over that yet?" One of the most frequent pieces of advice given to people who lose small children is to have another child as soon as possible — as though that could mask the hurt or take away the loss. Out of our own experience we came to understand that the death of a child is threatening to all in a way that our own death as adults is not. Thus many prefer to hide their pain.

The Hebrews understood instinctively that such pain had to be shared. They believed God heard; if our cries were not expressed, then they could not come to God. Their response to pain and loss was dialogic. It was offered up to God in the belief that God cared and would respond. The interesting thing about the laments of the Psalter is that, with one exception (Ps. 88), all the laments move toward praise. They begin with lines of despair and anguish such as "My God, my God, why hast thou forsaken me?" and move to expressions of confidence and trust. This was not because Israel thought God heard simply in order to grant our wishes. Israel knew that what we sometimes wish for in painful situations does not always take place — but it believed that God *would* respond. The Israelites ended their laments in praise, anticipating that out of God's response, new life could come from any crisis as God's gift, sometimes in unexpected ways.

This brings us to a second image of God which can aid us in times of loss: *God as life-giver.* Both the Hebrew Scripture and the New Testament know that God is the one who makes new life possible where only death seems to reign. It is important not to misunderstand this assertion. It does not remove the reality and the pain of death. That pain remains an offense. There are two great biblical symbols of God as life-giver out of the experience of death, which are also the great central symbols of salvation: the Exodus event in the Old Testament and the resurrection of Christ in the New Testament. Each of these central events witnesses to the faith conviction that life wins out over death, not because death is unreal or to be ignored or submerged but because God acts as the life-giver beyond death.

The deliverance from bondage in Egypt was a moment of birth for Israel as a people. They had come into being not out of their own efforts but as a result of God's gracious activity of deliverance. In bondage in Egypt and in the dramatic moment at the sea, death seemed to be the only possibility. Life came unexpectedly as God's gift, enabling a new future where none had seemed possible. To Israel this moment became a symbol of possibilities for new life beyond any experience of death. To be an Exodus people was not to live in a world without death; only God was without death. Exodus was a sign of God's gift of life despite death, beyond death, in the midst of death. One can give praise for life as God's gift even when the life of a child is ended prematurely, as was our daughter's. The three years of her life were a gift which her death cannot erase.

The resurrection symbol which is central to the Christian faith in the New Testament witness points to a message similar to that of Exodus. For the church, the resurrection has often lost its power because it is used to obscure the reality of death shown forth in the crucifixion. Our daughter's death came to us as a terrible offense and brought to us an immense sense of aloneness. No meaningful word could ever obscure that reality. It is present within me at this very moment. The disciples also knew the experience of pain and loss in Christ's crucifixion. The power of the resurrection is not in removing the offense of death but in saying, "This is not the final word." This is the good news which the community of faith is charged to carry to each new age.

The community of faith we knew in a house church in Iowa gathered around us again in Wichita, Kansas, to support us at the time of our daughter's death. Its members shared and received our sense of loss. With their support we chose to write a service of thanksgiving for Christine's life because we believed that her death could not be the final word, obscuring all that she had been in life. Her death could not be the final word for our lives either, and in the days after her death, church people helped us see the life that God makes possible beyond such painful moments.

Finally, I want to speak about *God as sufferer.* The biblical picture of God is of a God who suffers with us. This God not only hears and offers us the possibility of life-giving ways into the future; this God has shared our sufferings.

In the account of Moses' encounter with God in the burning bush, God says to Moses, "I have seen the affliction of my people, I have heard their cries. I know their sufferings" (Ex. 3:7). The Hebrew verb we translate as "know" is much broader than can be captured by any English word. It does not indicate "cognitive knowledge, knowledge in the head." Its meaning is closer to our verb "experience." It indicates interaction with and participation in the reality of that which is known. God's statement to Moses is one of the earliest points at which we can see the beginning of the tradition of a God who not only sees and hears from on high but who also chooses to enter into and experience our suffering with us.

The concept of the suffering God reaches a culmination in the crucifixion. There the divine Self shares our ultimate aloneness in pain and death in the form of the cross. Then God can say in the resurrection that death is not the final word, and say that not as a word from on high but as a word from our very midst. And we can better hear that word as meaningful.

We have been speaking of the problem of God. The Scriptures also address us at the point of affirming the life of a child. Our response to the death of a child often suggests that his or her death was more important than his or her life, however short. But Scripture is absolutely clear that all life is of God; all life should be valued as fully participating in God's creation.

One way the faith community can assist grieving parents is by honoring children in the first place. We need to examine our communities of faith in this regard. If we are attentive to the full personhood of our children, then when death tragically takes a child from our midst, we can celebrate the gift which has been among us and not just the life that might have been.

Finally, we must say a word about the role of the covenant community. It seems to me that the Scriptures uniformly witness to the importance of the corporate body of faith as the context of support in times of crisis. This was certainly our experience. In South Carolina, where we knew not a soul, people rose up to claim the privilege of ministering to our hurt. Even though we had no history with that community, we were part of the wider community of faith, and we received unqualified support. People also gathered to be with us in Kansas, where we went for our daughter's burial. If we had been alone, we might not have seen how important it was to affirm our daughter's life and not simply her death.

There seem to be three roles that the community of faith plays in such crises. First, the community helps to relieve the isolation suffered along with the anger and pain. A terrible sense of aloneness comes in the midst of such hardships; the community should surround us in those moments with a presence that it is a witness to the presence of God.

Second, the church should pass on and hold up symbols of our faith so that they are available to us in time of trauma as ways of seeing God's gift of life even beyond the offense of the moment. This function cannot be left until a crisis occurs. We have to labor constantly at the task of preparing people with the great symbol resources of our faith, in anticipation of the crises that come to us all.

We must know of Exodus and resurrection. We must learn of the God who hears, gives life to and suffers with us. In stories, hymns, liturgies and studies we equip ourselves with the resources of our faith. These resources will also help us bring the grief and pain out of the counselor's study and into the wider community, so that we all begin to draw on the faith symbols and words that speak to these experiences. We can then have recourse to those traditions when pain descends on us.

Finally, the community of faith mediates the healing word. The community helps to show us pathways into the future when we do not see them ourselves. It does this by receiving our pain and our loss, but also by refusing to believe that such pain and loss constitute the final word.

Out of these perspectives from Scripture and experience, has my daughter's death been made more acceptable? No! But is there a further word of meaning about her life and the life which goes forward for us? Through the grace of God and the support of the people of God, Yes!

CHAPTER SEVENTEEN

Contraception

Theological perspectives on life and children form the necessary background for the next four chapters in this book, each of which, in its own way, considers technological interventions in the processes of procreation. An overarching question for these chapters is: To what extent ought persons or couples be free to control their own reproduction? Or perhaps that very question is already shaped by particular assumptions about freedom, reproduction, individuality, and choice. An alternative way of framing the question would be: How do our theological and moral understandings of marriage and procreation shape our role or intervention in the reproductive process? How one asks the question will determine in large part the shape of one's answer.

In this chapter we look at the question of contraception. Many readers of this book might consider contraception to be something of a non-issue or at least not ethically significant. Admittedly, the Roman Catholic magisterium deems artificial methods of contraception intrinsically evil and therefore absolutely morally illicit. But so widespread is the use of contraceptives, even among Catholics, that the moral questions seem to be settled. We hope in this chapter to complicate this conventional wisdom. For as the structure of Part V of *On Moral Medicine* indicates, we believe that questions of technologically assisted reproduction or genetic intervention are of a piece with questions involved in contraception.

As is the case with most issues in bioethics, the public discussion around the question of contraception has largely been shaped by the principles of autonomy and utility. Sex, it is assumed, is an individual, personal, private matter, protected by the right to privacy. The right to reproduce — or not — is essential to one's personal identity or the private space of the family. Put more strongly, the right to reproduce constitutes one of the most fundamental components of the very self; the freedom to exercise this right must be untrammeled, as long as it does not impinge on the freedom or well-being of another.

Central to the exercise of this autonomy — or to societal restrictions on this autonomy — is the principle of utility and the weighing of costs/risks and benefits. In deciding whether or not to use contraceptives, individuals are urged to weigh the number and quality of life of children against a variety of other factors: the physical and emotional resources of the parents, the health of the mother, the burden on the ecosystem, and almost invariably money and professional progress. Freedom entails not only the decision of whether or not one wishes to be a parent, but also the freedom to advance one's education, to advance in one's career, and to achieve a certain socioeconomic status. Oftentimes, children are portrayed as an obstacle to these achievements.

But not all autonomy is equal, especially the autonomy of those lower on the socioeconomic scale. Where conventional wisdom holds that people of means ought to be free to contracept, it equally holds that people of straightened means ought to be obliged to contracept. Where people of means are free to weigh the burdens children may impose on themselves, people of straightened means (as well as people of color) are often asked to weigh the burdens such children will impose on society. The controversy surrounding the use of Norplant or other long-acting contraceptives within minority communities in the U.S. in the early- to mid-1990s stands as a case in point. Those who know the history of eugenics in the U.S., however, know that this controversy is only the most recent in a lengthy history of problematic uses of contraceptive technologies with regard to poor women and women of color.[1]

This, then, is the conventional framework for thinking about issues of contraception in the U.S. The theological framework for thinking about issues of contraception differs significantly. For example, in both its historic and contemporary phases, the theological conversation about contraception (Protestant and Catholic) starts not with the individual and his or her rights *vis-à-vis* reproduction but with a couple situated within the broader practice of marriage. In a way that might surprise contemporary sensibilities, the authors here (who represent a spectrum of

1. The literature on this topic is substantial. See, for one example, Kathleen E. Powderly, "Contraceptive Policy and Ethics: Illustrations from American History," *Hastings Center Report* 25, no. 1, Suppl. (1995): S9-11.

views) take as their focus not the question of whether contraception ought to be used outside of marriage but rather whether it ought to be used *by married couples.*

The first three essays provide some historical context for the contemporary conversation. Karl Barth, writing in the late 1950s, opens with "Parents and Children" (selection 110). Like his interlocutors, Barth situates the question of contraception within marriage, but he complicates it. He notes that while human beings are naturally drawn toward the bearing of children, *post Christum natum* (after the birth of Christ) Christians are freed from the natural or social necessity of bearing children. Marriage, therefore, does not necessarily entail the procreating of children, and those who remain childless, whether by nature or by decision, ought not to feel at fault. For Christians, having children is not an end in itself, beautiful and promising though it may be: "From a Christian point of view, the true meaning and the primary aim of marriage is not to be an institution for the bringing up of children. On the contrary, children may be at least a serious threat to what man and wife should together mean in marriage for the surrounding world." But neither is it simply a matter of personal autonomy based on the balancing of burdens and benefits. Rather, the bearing of children is a response to God's command to particular married couples at particular times and places for God's particular work in the world. And procreative or not, all Christians (single, married, widowed, or otherwise) are called to a parenting role within their localities. Notably, for Barth, whichever course is followed, the greater burden must fall upon the husband, since biologically and socially, the greater share of the costs and risks will be borne by the woman.

Barth, then, provides one classic and influential perspective on the contemporary conversation. The later articles by Elizabeth Bahnson and Julie Hanlon Rubio (selections 114 and 112, respectively) narrate two additional and important pieces of the debate about contraception in the twentieth century: the decision by the Anglican Church at the 1930 Lambeth Conference to permit the use of contraception by married couples under certain conditions; and the 1968 encyclical by Pope Paul VI, *Humanae Vitae,* which reiterated the Roman Catholic Church's prohibition on artificial means of contraception. Given the historic nature of this document, its continued authority within the Catholic Church, and its growing appreciation among many evangelicals, we recommend that readers of *On Moral Medicine* access the full text of *Humanae Vitae,* which can be found online at the Vatican website.[2]

The position taken by Paul VI in *Humanae Vitae* surprised many within the Catholic Church and has in many ways been a flashpoint for a growing rift within the Catholic Church between "liberals" and "conservatives." James Burtchaell's essay, "'Human Life' and Human Love" (selection 111), captures the anger and critique that animated much of the Catholic community in the U.S. immediately after the promulgation of the encyclical. Burtchaell's essay voices the major concerns of critics of *Humanae Vitae* — that the position was "physicalist," that Paul VI was working with a static and inadequate notion of nature, that to limit marital sexual expression endangers marriage. More importantly, however, Burtchaell argues that part of what is at stake in thinking about contraception is competing conceptions of marriage. In other words, how one thinks about marriage (theologically) is critical for how one evaluates the questions of children and of contraception. He invites us to consider Christian marriage as an exercise in adult education, as a school for virtue, and to think about our new powers over the beginnings of human life in that context.

Burtchaell's essay was penned in 1968. Thirty years later, younger, lay, married Catholics (and Protestants) began to take up the question of contraception in a much more nuanced manner. Julie Hanlon Rubio represents one such voice, continuing Burtchaell's focus on marriage as the context for considering contraception. Her "Beyond the Liberal/Conservative Divide on Contraception: The Wisdom of Practitioners of Natural Family Planning and Artificial Birth Control" (selection 112) describes well the continuing divide between "liberals" and "conservatives" on this issue but seeks to move beyond it. Her essay takes seriously the growing practice of natural family planning (NFP), a practice quite different from the "rhythm method" of the 1960s, and posits a novel idea, that of "sexuality as a dimension of discipleship." She attempts to take seriously the experiences both of those married couples who have used artificial contraception as well as of those who use natural family planning. Rubio focuses particularly on the claims of both camps with regard to the unitive end of marriage, highlighting questions of the total and mutual self-giving in Christian marriage, of the virtues of chastity and justice, on the ways in which the methods enhance communication and intimacy, and more.

While Rubio offers a more positive assessment of natural family planning, fellow Catholic David M. McCarthy, in his essay "Procreation, the Development of Peoples, and the Final Destiny of Humanity" (selection 113), argues for a more accurate understanding of *Humanae Vitae.* He insists that, for the most part, both opponents and defenders of the encyclical misread it theologically and contextually. McCarthy argues that *Humanae Vitae* and Paul VI's arguments on contraception must be read in the context of the rest of the pontiff's writings, particularly in the context of his encyclicals on "persistent social, political and economic themes." In other words, McCarthy is arguing that *Humanae Vitae* must be read as a document within the tradition of Catholic social teaching. Contraception, in other words, is a social question. What would *Humanae Vitae* look like if read in the context of *Populorum Progressio* (1967), for example?

McCarthy picks up on a point central to Burtchaell's critique — namely, how the rise in contraceptive practices is

2. http://www.vatican.va/holy_father/paul_vi/encyclicals/documents/hf_p-vi_enc_25071968_humanae-vitae_en.html (accessed February 25, 2012).

related to economic ambition and a certain story of economic progress that pits making money against making children. This story not only captures the imagination within America but also becomes the way in which we learn to read the world economically — "if only," we lament, "those poor benighted, backward people in developing countries could get a handle on their profligate procreativity, then they would be able to make some economic progress." Or, more negatively put, we believe that it is because of the "population explosion" that most of the world cannot eat, not because the world's resources are distributed so inequitably that we in the first world, with our profligate habits of overconsumption, consume far more than our fair share.

A final point of contest with *Humanae Vitae* is Paul VI's use of the notion of "nature" — both in describing the "natural" ends of marriage as unity and procreation and in terms of permitting natural methods of family planning while rejecting "artificial" methods. Many arguments have been lodged against this claim, with many arguing that all methods — natural or artificial — are morally equivalent insofar as all "intend" the same outcome, namely control of reproduction. Shared "motive" renders means equivalent.

But is "intention" or "motive" alone sufficient for moral evaluation? Might "method" make a difference? It is interesting that the two essays that address this question were authored by women. Rubio makes clear that practitioners of NFP do not see NFP primarily as a method — rather, they understand it to be a lifestyle, a radical form of Christian discipleship. And in our final selection, Elizabeth Bahnson, a Methodist, suggests that some methods — particularly the chemical approach to suppressing fertility, tricking a woman's body into thinking it is pregnant — might well be far more problematic than other (e.g., barrier) methods.

Bahnson's argument is rooted in a theologically thick notion of nature that derives in large part from her practical engagement with the natural world. In "The Pill Is Like . . . DDT? An Agrarian Perspective on Pharmaceutical Birth Control" (selection 114), Bahnson — a theologian, a mother, and an organic farmer — sees disturbing parallels between the industrial-chemical approach to agriculture, which many within and beyond Christianity are beginning to understand as deeply problematic for the well-being of the environment, for the food chain, and for human well-being, and the similar approach to women's bodies. Drawing on the work of Southern agrarian thinker Wendell Berry, Bahnson shows how oral contraceptives presume a particular attitude toward our bodies, and especially toward women's bodies. What is the connection between our bodies and nature? Does it have to be an either/or — all nature or all reason and control? Does contraception allow us to "think ourselves gods," to "live under the illusion that we are independent, disconnected beings that can and should pursue our individual self-interests at all cost," locked in a narrative of scarcity and competition? Does contraception pit us against our bodies, dividing our very selves?

Bahnson argues that from an ecological, social, and biblical perspective, these realities that contraception separates are actually deeply interconnected, all pieces of a "complex system of dependency that comprises the whole." Perhaps it is not insignificant that the question of technological, artificial, pharmaceutical contraception became a serious public question only in the twentieth century, a century in which humanity began to move away from the land in a way unknown in human history. Much of bioethics presumes a fundamental conflict between "nature" and "the human," that the normatively human is to be found in mastery over nature, when it is controlled and planned and directed to human ends. Bahnson and Berry challenge this facile anthropology, an anthropology that divorces the human from its context in creation, its fundamental relationship to the land and to the rhythms of the natural world, and its theological context of being a creature in relation to God.

Like the editors of *On Moral Medicine,* the authors in this chapter do not speak with one voice on whether contraception is morally licit. Rather, each raises important challenges to the assumptions that shape the conventional position that contraception is a non-issue, that the moral questions are settled, that it is simply an individual decision. The authors provide a more complex and theologically robust framework for thinking about these questions than simply autonomy and utility. And we hope they invite the reader into a further exploration of the complex social, political, and economic history of the question of contraception, one that will illuminate as well the subsequent issues of technological reproduction, abortion, and genetics.

SUGGESTIONS FOR FURTHER READING

Black, Edwin. *War Against the Weak: Eugenics and America's Campaign to Create a Master Race* (New York: Basic Books, 2008).

Cahill, Lisa. "Catholic Sexual Ethics and the Dignity of Persons: A Double Message?" *Theological Studies* 60, no. 1 (1989): 120-50.

Franks, Angela. *Margaret Sanger's Eugenic Legacy: The Control of Female Fertility* (Jefferson, N.C.: McFarland, 2005).

Gordon, Linda. *The Moral Property of Women: A History of Birth Control Politics in America* (Urbana and Chicago: University of Illinois Press, 2007).

Noonan, John T. *Contraception: A History of Its Treatment by Catholic Theologians and Canonists* (Cambridge, Mass.: Harvard University Press, 1986; originally published 1965).

110 Parents and Children

Karl Barth

Man can be father or mother. A husband and a wife can together become parents. Their relationship to their children in the light of the divine command must now occupy our attention. But first we must answer two unavoidable preliminary questions.

The first is posed by the fact that there are men who do not become parents. We are thinking of all those who broadly speaking might do so, and perhaps would like to do so, but either as bachelors or in childless marriage do not actually fulfil this possibility. What attitude are they to adopt to this lack? What has the divine command to say to them concerning it? In some degree they will all feel their childlessness to be a lack, a gap in the circle of what nature obviously intends for man, the absence of an important, desirable and hoped-for good. And those who have children and know what they owe to them will not try to dissuade them. The more grateful they are for the gift of children, so much the more intimately they will feel this lack with them. Parenthood is one of the most palpable illuminations and joys of life, and those to whom it is denied for different reasons have undoubtedly to bear the pain of loss. But we must not say more. If we can use the rather doubtful expression "happy parents," we must not infer that childlessness is a misfortune. And we must certainly not speak of an unfruitful marriage, for the fruitfulness of a marriage does not depend on whether it is fruitful in the physical sense. In the sphere of the New Testament message there is no necessity, no general command to continue the human race as such and therefore to procreate children. That this may happen, that the joy of parenthood should still have a place, that new generations may constantly follow those which precede, is all that can be said in the light of the fact which we must always take into fresh consideration, namely, that the kingdom of God comes and this world is passing away. *Post Christum natum* there can be no question of a divine law in virtue of which all these things must necessarily take place. On the contrary, it is one of the consolations of the coming kingdom and expiring time that this anxiety about posterity, that the burden of the postulate that we should and must bear children, heirs of our blood and name and honour and wealth, that the pressure and bitterness and tension of this question, if not the question itself, is removed from us all by the fact that the Son on whose birth alone everything seriously and ultimately depended has now been born and has now become our Brother. No one now has to be conceived and born. We need not expect any other than the One of whose coming we are certain because He is already come. Parenthood is now only to be understood as a free and in some sense optional gift of the goodness of God. It certainly cannot be a fault to be without children. . . .

The first point to be inferred as God's command to the childless is thus that they do not let themselves be misled about the matter. They must set their hope on God and therefore be comforted and cheerful. Their lack cannot be a true or final lack, for the Child who alone matters has been born for them too. And we must then continue that they may and must interpret their childlessness as something which specifically frees them for other tasks and cares and joys. To bring up children is a beautiful and promising thing, but the end and purpose of human life cannot and must not be sought in this, as all too happy parents would often have it, since the meaning of this activity is only earthly and temporary. One may and can and must live for God and one's fellows in a very different way. May not childlessness be an indication to those who are troubled by it that they should look all the more seriously to other and perhaps very obvious fields which might have lain fallow had there not been men and women without the desire or worry of bringing up children? And childless married couples in particular should feel the persuasion that as such they are all the more called and empowered to build up their life-companionship with particular care both outwardly and inwardly. Parenthood may be a consequence of marriage which is both joyful and rich in duties, but from a Christian point of view the true meaning and the primary aim of marriage is not to be an institution for the upbringing of children. On the contrary, children may be at least a serious threat to what man and wife should together mean in marriage for the surrounding world. From this point of view, childlessness can be a release and therefore a chance which those concerned ought to seize and exploit instead of merely grieving about it. And finally, should we not ask whether a man and his wife, and even those who are single, are any the less called to be elders, to fatherliness and motherliness, because they are not parents in the physical sense — elders who in regard to all young people have the same task as physical parents have toward their physical offspring? May there not be young persons in their locality whose physical parents may be dead, or for some reason do not fulfil their duty, so that they can help both them (and themselves) if they are willing directly or indirectly to fill the gap? Where the great message of divine comfort is not known and believed, such suggestions will be scorned as an offering of stones for bread. But where it is perceived and accepted, it is hard to see why the childless should not act upon one or other of these suggestions. The divine command, which is only the practical form of this comfort, will cer-

From Karl Barth, *Church Dogmatics,* III/4, trans. A. T. Mackay et al. (Edinburgh: T&T Clark, 1961), pp. 265-76. Used by permission.

tainly draw them out of their grief and warn them to take some such action.

The second preliminary question to be considered is posed by the fact that, while it does not depend on the wishes of a man and woman if their sexual intercourse leads to the birth of a child and therefore to parenthood, they do have the technical possibility of so guiding their sexual activity that it does not have this consequence. Hence in regard to the prolongation of their existence in that of children they have at least this negative power of control. We allude to the problem of what is called birth control. From a Christian point of view, is the exercise of this control permissible, and if so may it sometimes be obligatory? . . .

Our starting point is again the fact that *post Christum natum* the propagation of the race ("Be fruitful, and multiply," Gen. 1:28) has ceased to be an unconditional command. It happens under God's long-suffering and patience, and is due to His mercy, that in these last days it may still take place. And it does actually do so with or without gratitude to the One who permits it. There may even be times and situations in which it will be the duty of the Christian community to awaken either a people or section of people which has grown tired of life, and despairs of the future, to the conscientious realisation that to avoid arbitrary decay they should make use of this merciful divine permission and seriously try to maintain the race. But a general necessity in this regard cannot be maintained on a Christian basis. . . .

From this standpoint, then, there can be no valid objection to birth control.

The matter is rather different, however, when we consider the problem of marital fellowship.

We must first insist that this life-fellowship as such, whether or not it includes parenthood, is a relationship which is sanctified by the command of God. We do not refer to sexual intercourse in itself and as such. Sexual intercourse performed for its own sake, whether within marriage or without, whether with or without birth control, is a nonhuman practice forbidden by the divine command. We say deliberately, however, that according to the command this life-fellowship as such, including its physical basis in sexual intercourse, has its own dignity and right irrespective of whether or not it includes parenthood. It was always crude to define marriage as an institution for the production of legitimate posterity. Even sexual intercourse may have a first essential meaning simply in the fact that it is integral to the completion of marital fellowship. From the standpoint of this fellowship, then, it may not be generally and necessarily required that it should be linked with the desire for or readiness for children. It may rather be that from the standpoint of this fellowship sexual intercourse should be performed in a way which implies that its meaning is simply the love relationship of the two partners and excludes the conception and birth of children.

At this point there does, of course, arise a question which in my judgment is the only one which weighs against the acceptability of birth control. Sexual intercourse as the physical completion of life-partnership in marriage can always be, not merely human action, but an offer of divine goodness made by the One who even in this last time does not will that it should be all up with us. Hence every act of intercourse which is technically obstructed or interrupted, or undertaken with no desire for children, or even refrained from on this ground, is a refusal of this divine offer, a renunciation of the widening and enriching of married fellowship which is divinely made possible by the fact that under the command of God this fellowship includes sexual intercourse. Can we really do this? Should we do so? Do we realise what it means? Does not a real unwillingness at this point involve an imperiling of marital fellowship, slight perhaps but possibly more serious, to the extent that the latter includes the possibility of this broadening? Can even sexual intercourse as the physical complement of marriage be perfect within its limits if it is thus burdened by reluctance in the face of this possibility, or even its deliberate refusal? Or can it be neglected through such reluctance without intimately threatening the whole structure of marriage? Those who basically affirm freedom for birth control cannot too severely put to themselves this practical question. The exercise of this freedom must have valid reasons if the gravity of this renunciation and the seriousness of this threat are to be dispelled, and what one does is therefore to be done with a clear conscience. By this question all frivolity and expediency are excluded. If married life includes sexual intercourse, it means that the possibility of parenthood is a natural consequence. To be sure, the attempt to evade this consequence is not always the result of arbitrariness or sloth. Yet those who exclude this possibility and deliberately avoid this consequence must be asked whether they do so under the divine command and with a sense of responsibility to God, and not out of caprice. From this standpoint, therefore, a strong warning must be inserted which we must always consider. In the light of what marital fellowship demands, the use of this freedom may be something which the divine law strictly forbids. The fact remains, however, that even from this standpoint there can be no absolute denial of this freedom.

In favour of this essential freedom, we have to consider that not only the physical consummation of marriage in sexual intercourse as such, but within this the phenomena of procreation and conception, if they are not to elude the imperative of God's command, must be understood as a responsible action on the part of both those concerned. If marital fellowship, including sexual intercourse, has its own right and dignity, the same is true for the act of generation and conception. Just as the former is not merely an arrangement for the continuance of the species, so the latter are not to be regarded as merely the inevitable consequence of the physical intercourse which forms the climax of the fellowship. This means, however, that generation and conception are the effects of an action which is in its own particular way responsible. And as a responsible action it must and will be a choice and decision between Yes and No. Why should we not ask at this point concerning the divine command as though it were already known in this respect? Why should there not have to be a choice and decision at this point? With what right may it be said that these are not necessary here, but it is better to leave things to potluck, i.e., to chance? It might be objected that they should be left to the rule of divine providence. Man should not interfere with this and therefore with the course of nature. With this, and therefore with "the course of nature" — this is the flaw in the reasoning. For surely the providence of God and the course of nature are not identical or even on the same level. Surely the former cannot be inferred from the latter! Surely the providence and will of God in the course of nature has in each case to be freshly discovered by the believer who hears and obeys His word, and apprehended and put into operation by him in personal responsibility, in the freedom of choice and decision. Surely the specific question: May I try to have a child? has in each case to be given a specific answer as he sets himself in the hands of the living God. Surely he is not allowed to dispense with rational reflection or to renounce an intelligent attitude at this point. The very opposite is the case. At this point especially intelligent reflection may and must constantly and particularly prevail, and nothing must be done except in responsible decision.

I gladly quote what Ernest Michel (*Ehe*, pp. 189f.) says on this point: "Believing trust (in the government of providence) vouches also for the potential blessing given in the gift of children and adopts a responsible attitude with regard to the question of generation and conception, not a religiously masked naturalism. . . . To reveal its full potentiality as blessing, the blessing of children demands the responsible Yes of parents, just as every good gift of God is meant for the acceptance of the human being for whom it is intended, and only then is able to unfold its character as a gift and blessing. . . . We thus affirm birth control as a matter for responsible consideration. For it is part of the dignity of man that in responsibility he moulds nature intelligently to his purposes. It is hard to see why in the domain of sex he should simply accept the course of nature or even make it an ethical norm for himself."

The danger of such reflection and decision is obvious. We have already mentioned one of its forms. Broadly speaking, it may happen that in consequence of mistaken reflection an actual divine gift may be refused and a child who might have been the light and joy of its parents is not generated and conceived and does not come into existence. On the other hand, something may be affirmed which was not offered by God. Again in consequence of mistaken reflection, a child may be generated of whom it might well be said from the parents' standpoint that they would have been better without it. Thus the possibility of error exists on both sides. And both errors may mean an imperiling of marital and even sexual fellowship. Both may entail a divine judgment in some form. The danger of thus failing to do the will and command of God is no smaller, but also no greater, at this point than everywhere where responsible action and the venture of faith and obedience are required. The venture, however, is required at this point too. Hence it would be false to say that in view of the risk an unthinking *laissez faire* is better in this matter than action in free responsibility and decision.

It may be that in a given case the faith of a man and a woman will assume the form and character of a homely and courageous confidence in life. Thus the husband thinks that he is entitled to expect of his wife the ordeal of giving birth to children, and the wife believes that she may understand and accept this prospect not merely as a threat but also as a promise. Both of them believe that they are equal to the task imposed upon them with the possibility of generation and conception and therefore with that of the birth and existence of a child. When both together and each individually can believe this, then they ought to believe it, and therefore in all seriousness they should seek to have a child in the name of God, and what happens, even if they are mistaken, will at least happen in responsibility and therefore in a right relation to the divine command.

The idea of birth control can and should also and especially have this positive connotation. Birth control can also be the conscious and resolute refusal in faith of the possibility of refusing, i.e., the joyful willingness to have children and therefore to become parents. Undoubtedly it rests upon false ideas of the good old days to try to maintain that people were then so much more reckless with regard to procreation because they all had this confidence in life rooted in faith. Prudence, and a practice determined by it, were no less characteristic then than they are now. Yet in relation to the modern increase of carefulness in this direction, and the corresponding prevalence of birth control in the negative sense, the question arises why it is that to-day so many people obviously do not seem able to command this confidence in life. Changed social conditions are partly but not wholly responsible, for it was not among small farmers and workers that the modern habit arose and spread, but among the propertied middle and upper classes. It was, for example, an accompaniment of the high standard of living in modern America. A certain degeneration and impoverishment of faith rather than outward circumstances undoubtedly plays some part. And there can be no doubt that a positive choice and decision ought to be made far more often than they are today on the basis of this confidence in life grounded in faith.

Yet it is certainly not a Christian but a very heathen or even Jewish type of thought to try to make it an invariable rule that faith should self-evidently produce and exercise in all cases and circumstances this cheerful confidence in life. The fact may be that in certain circumstances a man cannot believe himself justified in expecting this of his wife. Indeed, various considerations regarding her physical and psychological health may forbid him to do so. There must be room for such considerations. Failure to take them into account was and is always to be described as male brutality. But the wife may also be forbidden to understand conception as a promise and therefore to desire it. And both may be prevented from believing that they can rightly assume responsibility for the birth and existence of a child. For both of them it may be impossible for one reason or another really to desire a child in the name of God and therefore in faith. It might also involve an imperiling of their marital fellowship if either or both were to do so in spite of these serious considerations. They must examine their consciences to be sure that these reasons are not merely pretexts of expediency and frivolity. But if their reasons stand this test, they ought not to desire a child (again at the risk of being mistaken), and what happens will happen in responsibility and therefore in a true relation to God's law.

Up to this point there is agreement today among all serious Christian moralists, whether doctors, theologians or ecclesiastics. It is accepted that, although the choice for or against generation and conception is not a matter for human caprice, it should not be left to chance and therefore lack the character of true decision, but must always be a matter of free obedience and therefore free consideration and decision. The disagreement that remains and cannot easily be overcome, especially between the Evangelical and Roman Catholic view, concerns the question how the negative decision, when taken in obedience to the divine command, is to be put into effect in harmony with this command and therefore in responsibility.

What is to happen when a man and woman actually believe they cannot accept the responsibility of generation and conception? Four possibilities arise: 1. the practice of complete sexual restraint; 2. sexual intercourse at periods when the woman cannot conceive; 3. *coitus interruptus;* and 4. the use of contraceptives. It must be said of all four, even of the first, let alone the second, (1) that in relation to the course of nature as such they have the character of human arrangement and control. To be consistent, those who on principle decline such a possibility must refuse all these possible courses of action. But if we cannot on principle refuse this possibility, we cannot basically and absolutely give one of these alternatives preference over another. Again, it must be said of all of them (2) that in each there is something painful, troublesome and we may say unnatural or artificial. Since it is a question of controlling the course of nature, and in this case its biological rhythm, this is not surprising. It is obvious that the negative decision in this matter must be paid for no less than the positive, and that the cost cannot be small either way, whichever possibility we choose on the negative side. The costliness is not in itself an argument against any of these four possibilities. If something preventive has to be done, then one of these four possibilities will be chosen in spite of their technical and therefore unnatural or artificial character and the painfulness inherent in each of them.

Sexual restraint or connubial asceticism, which was once the only possible course for Christians in the case of a negative decision, has been described in our times as at least the higher path and therefore to be recommended. The fact that it seems to be the most difficult and sometimes heroic makes it most impressive. It would be wrong to say that its practice is always impossible, and that it may not be obligatory for certain men in certain situations. Hence I do not think that it should be generally described as a terrible *tour de force* (so E. Brunner, *The Divine Imperative,* p. 369). But we must be clear that even this method is a matter of technique and therefore unnatural, artificial and painful. Where it is adopted we do not usually have to reckon seriously with injuries to the health of the two partners, but rather with undesirable psychological repressions which might have fatal consequences for the marital fellowship, which as such includes sexual intercourse. And what Paul says to married people in 1 Cor. 7:3f, and especially v. 5: "Defraud ye not one the other, except it be with consent for a time, that ye may give yourself to fasting and prayer; and come together again, that Satan tempt you not for your incontinency," hardly seems to point in this direction, although the reference is not, of course, to the problem of birth control. To strict but careful thinking this course cannot therefore claim to be the only possible solution to the problem.

In the second possibility, i.e., sexual intercourse at periods when there is no danger of conception, we have the great and so far the only concession which the Papacy can allow apart from complete continency. The relevant clause in the encyclical *Casti connubii* is put very guardedly and cautiously, but it is quite unmistakeable: *Neque contra naturae ordinem agere ii discendi sunt coniuges, qui iure suo recta et naturali ratione utuntur, etsi ob naturales sive temporis sive quorundam defectuum causas nova inde vita oriri non possit.* Apart from the main purpose of marriage (the procreation of children, as the encyclical firmly maintains), there are also certain *secundarii fines* such as the *mutuum adiutorium* and *mutuus amor* of the married partners, which they may freely cultivate, so long as the *intrinseca natura* of the sexual act remains intact, its centrality is preserved and it takes place normally. T. Bovet (*Die Ehe,* p. 162) recommends his Roman Catholic readers to keep strictly to this injunction, "for it is especially important that they should be in harmony with their Church." They may thus adopt this course, and others with them who see in it a right and happy *via media:* It is certainly feasible. Indeed, since it is distinct from the way of absolute asceticism on the one side, and obviously does less violence to the *intrinseca natura* of the sexual act on the other, it might well seem to be relatively the most feasible course of all. But we cannot take it too blithely. Why did not the papal pastor say expressly that the whole burden of the question whether we may exclude the possibility of procreation on our own judgment cannot be evaded even if we take this course, and that this question is really more serious than that with which he is clearly preoccupied, namely the normality or abnormality of the sexual act as such? And is not this, too, a painful course with its complicated technique and all the statistics and calculations which it involves? Indeed, does the *natura intrinseca* of the sexual act really remain unaffected when its performance, although quite normal, is cramped by so much calculation which seems open to objection even from the medical standpoint, and by all the anxious considerations and obvious fears of the participants? What becomes of its spontaneity if it necessarily involves a constant glancing at the calendar of conception? And what becomes of its character as the joyful consummation of marital fellowship if its spontaneity is threatened in this way?

The simplest and perhaps the oldest and most popular method of preventing conception is that of *coitus interruptus* (*copula diminuata*). In a decree of the Holy Office (22 Nov. 1922, Denz. 2240 note) the Roman Catholic Church forbids confessors spontaneously (*sponte sua*) and indiscriminately *(promiscue omnibus)* to advise this course, but according to the same text it does not seem to exclude it absolutely in individual cases, provided certain reservations are made by confessors. One cannot allege in objection to it the story of Onan the son of Judah (Gen. 38:7-10), because what is described as a sin worthy of death in that story does not consist in the substance of the act and therefore in what normally goes under this name today, but in his refusal to give adequate satisfaction to the Levirate law of marriage. We need not waste words, however, on the particularly unsatisfactory nature of this course. And there also seem to be medical objections to it on account of its psychological dangers. T. Bovet (*op. cit.*, p. 167) declares that for these reasons he must issue an emphatic warning against it, and that it can be harmlessly practised only for a time and by less sensitive married couples. In any event, we have always to reckon with the fact that it constitutes a special threat to marital fellowship.

It is obvious that with the fourth possibility, the use by man or woman of mechanical or chemical means of contraception, the technical and therefore unnatural or artificial character of the whole business is more immediately apparent than in the case of the previous alternatives. At this point, then, Roman Catholic moral and pastoral theology issues what is for the moment, at any rate in theory, an inflexible veto. The difficulty of the whole problem is again revealed in miniature by the fact that none of these means — assuming this fourth possibility is chosen — seems to be free from objection or even reliable, and that each of them is in some way suspect or even repellent. Some of them are even dangerous, so that they should not be used except on medical advice. And it is perfectly natural that even some who do not disallow birth control as such should feel a kind of instinctive or aesthetic repugnance to all the means suggested. The only thing is that they must not make their repugnance a law for others. Nor must it be supposed and asserted that at this point, where the artificiality is so apparent, we enter the sphere of what is evil and illegitimate. The use of these means is not evil just because they are so manifestly artificial. It is evil when it takes place for reasons of self-seeking, pleasure-seeking or expediency (cf. The Statement of the Lambeth Conference 1930). The earlier courses are no less evil when they are adopted for these reasons. And the same holds good not only of these courses, or of birth control as a whole in its negative sense, but of the failure to exercise it if this is grounded in self-seeking, pleasure-seeking or expediency.

Among the various possibilities of negative birth control there is thus none to which, all things considered, an absolute and exclusive preference can be given, but there is also none which can be flatly rejected. Hence it is impossible to formulate any general rule facilitating choice among the four possibilities indicated. Does this mean that we can only conclude that in this matter each individual must choose and decide for himself in the freedom which faith confers? This is true enough. Yet we may still mention and seriously insist upon certain universal principles which must govern the choice made.

1. The choice will be correctly made if it is made, not without difficulty of course, yet with a clear and not an uneasy conscience, with the realisation that in the special responsibility in which one finds oneself it must take the form it does and may therefore do so. Whatever the outcome of the choice may be, if it is to be right it must be made in this freedom of obedience, i.e., it must be made and executed in faith, not in fear, doubt or dismay. As a human act it may, of course, be mistaken. And in any case it will be made only in transition through a more or less difficult set of problems. Hence it can be made — otherwise how could it be related to the freedom of faith? — in reliance upon God's forgiving grace and therefore upon the fifth petition of the Lord's Prayer. But this does not mean that here any more than elsewhere we may desire to sin with a view to forgiveness, and therefore act with a bad conscience. What we can desire only as conscious sin, and can therefore do only with a bad conscience, we ought not to desire and do at all either here or elsewhere.

2. If it is to be correct, the choice must in any case be made only in joint consideration and decision by the two partners. There must be no dictation, overreaching or deceit on either side, but they must both act in full freedom, i.e., they must both take the decision in the free responsibility of their faith and in such a way that they can be open with each other both before and after. Their resolve and its execution must be a communal task, a product of their whole life of fellowship in marriage, so that they can rejoice together in spite of all difficulties, and their solidarity can remain unbroken even though later they may have cause to regard the step as an error and therefore have to repent of it together. What the two partners will and do together will be well willed and done for all the unavoidable problems and the possibility of better information later.

3. The choice must be made with due regard to the fact that so far as possible the inevitable painfulness of each available course must be the burden of the husband and not of the wife. In this whole question of positive and negative birth control, and in all the various possibilities mentioned, it is the wife who is directly and primarily affected and concerned. Here if anywhere there is an opportunity intelligently to respect the order of the relationship of man and woman, and therefore to express the priority and demonstrate the masculinity of the man in such a matter that in every possible choice he takes into decisive account, first individually and then in common discussion and decision with his wife, the fact that biologically she is always in greater danger than he is, and that she must therefore bear the lighter burden, he himself the heavier. It is on this assumption that the decision must then be made which of the alternatives is to be adopted and which rejected. This does not mean that the wife may not be ready for sacrifice as her love requires. But if the husband does not take the initiative in surrendering his own wishes and shouldering the dangerous burden, there can be no genuine achievement in concert, the conscience of the two parties cannot be free, and the decision to adopt a particular course cannot be a good one. No doubt the problem of birth control is not immediately envisaged in 1 Pet. 3:7, but this text is a valid criterion for genuine answers to the problem: "Ye husbands, dwell with them according to knowledge, giving honour unto the wife, as unto the weaker vessel, and as being heirs together of the grace of life; that your prayers be not hindered."

111 "Human Life" and Human Love

James T. Burtchaell

The Pope's veto upon artificial contraception, some fear, may provoke schism within the Roman Catholic Church. Others disagree: the issue is not a crucial dogma, it is not at the epicenter of the Christian faith. But these more sanguine observers forget that schism never was the outcome of dogmatic disagreement. It grows out of anger. . . .

The public debate has already known bitter moments and acid words. Many Catholics, according to the polls, could not believe their ears, and are outraged. The Shepherd, who for his part surely anticipated some unhappy bleating from his flock, must have been startled at the barking, howling, and baying, and must wonder what sort of flock grazes in his pasture. Numerous and loud have been the bishops who have instantly demanded unqualified acceptance of *Humanae Vitae;* one is puzzled why similar loyalty oaths were not required after the same pope published *Populorum Progressio.* Many theologians — impressively many — reacted swiftly and dissented from the encyclical. I have felt it necessary to hesitate a while longer, for fear of speaking too rudely. Whenever a responsible and venerable world leader ignores the wisest and most professional advice he can obtain, and throws his full reputation and public respect into jeopardy for a policy he knows will fly in the face of popular sentiment and comfort, one takes pause before criticizing him. But in the end one cannot be abject for the sake of courtesy. And so — surely without rancor, and hopefully with some small measure of the great courage that Paul VI has himself displayed — I must now take public issue with an encyclical that I consider to be disappointingly inadequate and largely fallacious. . . .

Roman documents, it should be remembered, have taken different stands on contraception and on birth control. They are, after all, not exactly the same. Birth control is the more general term, since it includes both contraception and also infanticide before birth. Since abortion has traditionally been viewed by most Catholic divines as occult murder, it is regarded with no tolerance by Rome as a method of birth control. Contraception, an alternative mode of birth control, has been differently considered by Rome, and in 1951 Pius XII executed a remarkable swerve in the course of recent tradition when

---

From *Commonweal* 89, no. 7 (15 November 1968): 245-52. Slightly abridged and edited from the original.

he accepted contraception on principle, in his famous allocution to the Italian Midwives' Society: "There are serious motives, such as those often mentioned in the so-called medical, eugenic, economic and social 'indications,' that can exempt for a long time, perhaps even for the whole duration of the marriage, from the positive and obligatory carrying out of the act. From this it follows that observing the non-fertile periods alone can be lawful only under a moral aspect. Under the conditions mentioned it really is so."

Once the Pope admitted in principle that married couples might have good and wholesome reasons for controlling their own fertility, discussion narrowed to the single question of method. Pius approved only two methods of contraception: total abstinence and periodic abstinence (unfortunately called "rhythm"). All other methods he unflinchingly proscribed.

My own opinion on total abstinence between husband and wife is that it would generally be repugnant and offensive. There would, I reckon, be a few instances when this denial — even by mutual consent — of one of the most appropriate embodiments of marital commitment and affection would not be judged immoral. As for all other means of contraception — withdrawal, rhythm, artificial devices, anovulant pills, temporary or permanent sterilization — I can see no imposing intrinsic ethical difference between them. All are obviously artificial. Some require cultural sophistication (rhythm, pills), others involve a modicum of risk (sterilization), still others are unpleasant (withdrawal, spermicides, devices). Catholic moralists have conventionally condemned all of them, and one ventures to suggest that much of their writing on the subject reads like treatises on sexual plumbing, with a devastatingly equivocal use of the term "unnatural."

Of all these methods I should be tempted to think of rhythm as the most unnatural of all, since it inhibits not only conception, but the expression of affection. It is, in my opinion, a base theology that would want intercourse to harmonize with the involuntary endocrine rhythm of ovulation and menstruation, while forsaking the greater spiritual and emotional ebbs and flows which should also govern sexual union. In the human species, especially, where coitus is freed from the estrous cycle, it is obviously open to personal meaning and depth quite independent of fertility. Different methods of contraception will be employed by couples in different circumstances. Medical advice and convenience will lead them to favor the surest and easiest means, although in certain instances they may have recourse to otherwise less preferable methods. All are artificial, of course, and artificiality in the biology of sexual intercourse need be no more loathsome than it is in synthetic fibers, vascular surgery, or musical composition.

According to the ethical model followed by *Humanae Vitae,* one must assign moral value to methods of contraception within the isolated context of a single event of coitus, rather than the full sequence and story of love and childbearing throughout the course of a marriage. The Pope parts company with his advisory commission, which reported: "The morality of sexual acts between married people takes its meaning first of all and specifically from the ordering of their actions in a fruitful married life, that is, one which is practiced with responsible, generous and prudent parenthood. It does not then depend upon the direct fecundity of each and every particular act."

The Pope rejects this view by stating simply that a single intercourse made intentionally infecund is intrinsically dishonest. But this begs the question. It is being argued precisely that the honesty of intercourse derives, not just from the individual act, but from the whole orientation of the marriage. There are certain features of intercourse which would always have to be present, like gentleness. Other features need to derive from the total sequence of sexual union, but are in no way attached to each event — conception would seem to be one such feature.

Consequently, it is difficult to follow the papal argument. I am unpersuaded that contraception is intrinsically immoral, and, what is more, I doubt that the question can be answered on the narrow, single-intercourse basis which the encyclical has taken to be normative.

Primary End

Customary Catholic theology has claimed that the primary end of marriage and of sex is the begetting and rearing of children. Listed as secondary ends: the satisfaction of desire and mutual support. Contraception — so the argument runs — violates this primary purpose by frustrating procreation.

Few non-Catholics accept this outline. Fewer Catholics are anxious to defend it publicly. . . . The argument's greatest weakness, it seems to me, is that it bespeaks of a stud-farm theology. What does "primary end" mean? If it is supposed to mean that the act of intercourse is basically a biological act whose immediate orientation is aimed at procreation, all would agree. But the preponderance of Catholic writers seem to take "primary end" to mean "principal purpose," "most important goal," "chief finality." This is quite absurd. We could as well say that the "primary end" of the Nobel Prize Award Banquet is nutrition, that the "primary end" of the Mexico City Olympic Games is exercise, and that the "primary end" of Baptism is hygiene.

There are plenty of indications that a broader view exists among Catholics. Pius XI, in his encyclical letter on marriage in 1930, cites the traditional Augustinian "reproductive" formula, but later goes beyond it: "This inward molding of spouse to spouse, this eager striving to draw each other to fulfillment, can in the truest sense be called the primary purpose and explanation of marriage, as the *Roman Catechism* teaches. Marriage would thus be considered, not in the narrow sense as created for the procreation and education of offspring, but in the broad sense as the sharing, the familiarity, and the companionship of life in its fullness."

Pius XII laid similarly heavy emphasis on the personal dimension of sex when he spoke out sharply in 1951 against artificial insemination: "To reduce the cohabitation of married persons and the conjugal act to a mere organic function for the transmission of the germ of life would be to convert the domestic hearth, sanctuary of the family, into nothing more than a biological laboratory. . . . The conjugal act in its natural structure is a personal act, a simultaneous and immediate cooperation of the spouses which, by the very nature of the participants and the special character of the act, is the expression of that mutual self-giving which, in the words of Holy Scripture, effects the union 'in one flesh.' "

And just a few years back, the late Msgr. J. D. Conway, former president of the Canon Law Society of America, called for the old Augustinian formula to be dropped: "Canon 1013, which defines the purposes — the philosophical ends — of marriage, should be worded with greater delicacy. The primary purpose, procreation and education of children, clearly relegates to second rank the mutual love, happiness and welfare of the spouses. And these secondary purposes are further slighted by defining them as 'mutual aid and the remedy of concupiscence.' Even though law is not romantic it should be able to recognize in marriage something more human, positive, spiritual and amorous."

There is no reason why the Church should not produce a restatement which gives personal values their proper due. *Humanae Vitae* might have been that restatement. Conjugal love is a many-splendored thing. Christian theology has no choice but to confront it in all its fullness: what Daniel Sullivan has called "psychospiritual union and abandon, the total orgasm of the natural body and spirit."

Natural?

Another weak point in the standard Catholic formula is the undefined and ambiguous way it uses the notion "natural." Everyone agrees that it is good to be natural; what that might mean is more difficult to agree upon. The average European will think it natural to smoke, live gregariously in cities, and discuss politics and religion in the pub; the Peruvian Indian may do none of these, yet not think himself unnatural. A child of three may feel it natural to suck his thumb, as he may feel it natural at fifteen to masturbate; his parents will think both activities are unnatural and immature. Anthropologists tell us it is natural for all peoples to worship a deity; theologians find this suggestive of the supernatural. Manuals of medical ethics teach that progestational steroids (the Pill) are unnatural because they inhibit ovulation; Dr. Rock replies that they are as natural as vitamins. Catholic moralists have claimed it unnatural to misplace, trap, kill, or block the seed in intercourse, but have labeled the rhythm method natural. Not all Catholic parents would agree, as witness this letter to the editors in *Commonweal* in 1964:

"Our second child had shown us that the calendar approach to rhythm was ineffective in our case, and so my wife moved on to the more sophisticated paraphernalia of the rhythm system — thermometers, tapes, tubes and the like. . . . We read and re-read the Catholic teaching on the natural law as it applied to marriage in general and to the Church's position on birth control in particular. Again and again the emphasis was found to be placed on what is 'natural'. And then we thought of the tapes and tubes and thermometers. This was natural?"

It seems hopeless to disentangle from this thicket of cross-purposes a working notion of "natural" that could serve the discussion of conjugal morality. For what it is worth, I should like to propose one from scratch.

Moral decisions in statecraft, economics, and jurisprudence are in constant flux, since the state, the economy, and the law are artificial institutions always on the move. There is something more perennial about the family. Marriage, it seems, has certain inbuilt requirements for success — requirements as complex as the intricate, constant makeup of man and woman. Though they have often failed to take the total view of marriage, Catholics have rightly insisted that it has its own ineluctable rules.

On the other hand, marital life is not automatically controlled as is digestion; a life of love must be a life of free choice. Any appropriate notion of "natural" will have to be correspondingly supple. There is perhaps no other human activity which so completely draws on the full range of forces in our nature: the will, the passions and affections, and the body. A restored vision of the "natural" would view the way in which these components of human nature are meant to respond to the conjugal situation: *What brings the personality of the spouses to full bloom, what promotes their growth to maturity, what brings husband, wife, and children to the highest pitch of happiness.*

Learning Generosity

It is unfortunate, not so much that the Pope has chosen to repeat such negative and unconvincing judgments on contraception, but that he continued to dwell almost exclusively upon the problem of method, without adequate attention to the far more crucial issue of motivation. Catholics have offered little insight into this more sensitive moral problem. Except for Pius XII's rather terse outline of reasonable causes, the conventional breeding theology has been about all we have had to give. On the other hand, I find the equally shrill and superficial sort of propaganda devised by those who promote contraception to be frighteningly deprived of any rich vision of marital growth in love. In any Dantesque view of the future, surely the canonist-moralists of the narrow tradition and the evangelists of the Planned Parenthood Federation will be consigned to each other's company.

My distress is that our quibbling over method fails to challenge the illusory motives which lead so many families to adopt contraception. This appears to be the case with individual couples, as also with entire peoples. In this country, for example, millions of families are pressed by medical urgency or financial crisis or similarly serious burdens that contraception can rightly relieve. And in numerous homes, births are timed to allow either for further self-growth in education, or for alternative forms of neighbor-service. But I would estimate that far more couples avoid or curtail children because they share the grudging national attitude that resents children as so many more drains on their generosity and budget. Bluntly: selfishness is perhaps the most frequent excuse for contraception in this rich county.

In this regard, one would fault the Pope for having said too little rather than too much. If a critic may be permitted to point out a passage in the encyclical which seems particularly well put, I would draw particular attention to the disappointingly brief remarks made in par. 9 about the characteristics of conjugal love: "This love is first of all fully human, that is to say, of the senses and of the spirit at the same time. . . . This love is total, that is to say, it is a very special form of personal friendship, in which husband and wife generously share everything, without undue reservations or selfish calculations. . . . Again, this love is faithful and exclusive until death."

Here was the vein of thought that could have been worked so much more. It is here, in throwing up to his readers the awesome challenges of marriage, that the pontiff could have confronted the world with its increasingly contraceptive mentality. This is a point which needs making, needs shouting from the rooftops.

Someone is responsible for foisting on our world the fantastic idea that marriage is easy. The Catholic Church has, I think, tended to think it frighteningly difficult. It is always moving for a priest to face a young couple before the altar and guide them through the awesome oaths of total abandonment. Like six-year-olds promising in their prayers to "love God with my whole heart," the bride and groom speak in hyperbole. They could hardly be expected to imagine what are the deeps of "for better, for worse, for richer, for poorer, in sickness and in health, until death do us part." Their parents in the front pews have a good idea; the Church knows, and prays that the young man and woman will find the generosity to learn, and will learn the generosity.

Real love, to men and women born as we all are with a selfish streak, doesn't come easily at all. When Paul tells husbands to love their wives as Christ loved the Church and gave himself up for her, he is haunted by the symbol and measure of that cherishing: the crucifixion. Love, says the Song of Songs, is as mighty as death. It is a struggle to the death to give self away. It has to be learned so very slowly. Marriage is that great adventure in adult education wherein parents have far more to learn and longer strides to make toward maturity than the children.

Growth in love — as all growth — means stress and sacrifice. The Church has never tried to conceal this. She simply says that marriage is glorious if you accept the stress and sacrifice. It is hell if you try short-cuts. And there are all sorts of short-cuts offered these days.

Barbara Cadbury, for instance, returned from a good-cheer tour in Asia for the Planned Parenthood Federation, wrote enthusiastically in *Family Planning in East Asia* (Penguin, 1963) of the "courageous sense of realism" with which Japanese kill their children. But the government, she says, now feels "that abortion is, as a regular method of birth control, harmful to the individual despite its benefit to the nation." The individual harmed is presumably the individual killing, not the individual killed. (I am reminded of the complaint made by the Commandant of Auschwitz, that the excessive shipments of Jews to be gassed and cremated worked unreasonable hardship on the prison guards.) But Mrs. Cadbury's most telling remark is this: "No other country in the world has so rapidly passed from fertility-motivated habits to producing only desired and cherished children." The two million or so children each year who are not "desired and cherished" are cut out of the womb and thrown away.

The Catholic Church should see it just the other way around from Mrs. Cadbury. If a man and woman have brought to life in the womb a child who is not desired or cherished, their problem is not how to murder the child but how to learn to desire and cherish him. The Church would concede that it is often easier to kill your child than to love him. But to the Japanese parents and to Mrs. Cadbury she recommends the latter.

A young woman at whose marriage I had officiated came to me several months later to tell me that every night during intercourse she was seized with fear that she might conceive. They couldn't possibly, she cried, afford a baby yet. Knowing that her parents had given them a house and land, and that both husband and wife were working for good wages, I was rather surprised. As it turned out, they had gone heavily into debt to buy an oak living-room suite, a maple bedroom set, a dining room ensemble, kitchen appliances, and laundry equipment. The unfortunate couple had been sold a bill of goods — not by the furniture salesman, but by the rotten and damned culture that had so persuaded a man and his wife that a child came just below laundry equipment on their list of needs. Before the year was out they would come to loathe the oaken and maple boredom.

There are plenty of other examples which betray the radical disagreement between the Church and our culture regarding marriage. We are chided by the realists of the day for our intransigent stand against divorce. Once the marriage relationship is dead — especially when it is violently killed by adultery — it is false to pretend otherwise. The Church replies that the marriage bond is grounded, not on the love of the moment, but on oaths made in view of love. Obviously the oath without the love is misery. But it is the very function of forgiveness to restore that love and breathe into it an even steadier life than before. The Church never ignored the cold fact that adultery kills love; but she recommends resurrection instead of cremation. The Church should know something of forgiveness and its power. The only love-bond she has as Christ's bridge is one of her repentance and his forgiveness. Says Jean Guitton: "The remedy for the ills caused by love is a summons to progress in love. In other terms, love can cure the wounds it inflicts, on condition that it rises to greater heights."

The source which has taught me the most about marriage is the 19th chapter of the Gospel according to Matthew. The chapter records two interviews with Jesus. In the second, he is asked by a young man what he must do to possess eternal life. This was a standard question that any Jew would ask a rabbi, and Jesus' answer at first is a very standard answer: "You must keep the Commandments." And he lists several of the very familiar commandments. The young man is pleased and replies that he has been observant since boyhood. Jesus then says that this is not enough. If he wants to go all the way, then he must sell everything, give it away, and follow after him. At this the young man is not so pleased because, as the evangelist points out, he has a great deal to sell. Somewhat disillusioned, he turns around and goes away. The point of the story is that he does not have eternal life even though he has kept the commandments from his youth.

Here Jesus is opposing to the religion of his day another type of faith which has no concrete terms or prior conditions. When a Jew purposely undertook the life of a Jew, he knew what he was undertaking. He was told in advance what were the terms of faith, and he accepted them with eyes open. When a man accepted to follow Jesus, he had no idea what the terms were. Nothing specific was told him in advance except that he must surrender to whatever claims Jesus, through all of his neighbors, would put on him. The young man rightly recognized that this was far more frightening since there was no way of calculating how much he was giving away. And so . . . he relinquished eternal life. After he leaves the scene, the disciples are somewhat nervous and ask, "Well, if this is the way it is, who on earth could get into the Kingdom of Heaven?" and Jesus says it is not for everyone, it is a gift.

In the earlier part of the chapter, a very similar interview takes place. Jesus is asked what are the terms for divorce. In the religion of his day, people entered marriage knowing in advance what were the limits of endurance: what things a man could be expected to tolerate and what things he need not accept. Jesus insists that in marriage, as he conceives it, there are no terms; there is no divorce. The people go away shaking their heads. Once again the disciples are a little bit upset, and they ask Jesus, "But if this is the way it is, who on earth could get married?" and he says, "It is not for everyone; it is a gift."

What I perceive from this chapter is that the unlimited surrender which a man very frighteningly makes to Jesus Christ in Baptism has as perhaps its closest imitation among men Christian marriage, wherein a man and a woman surrender to one another without terms. Jesus can say to a man in the crowd, "You! Follow me," and the man has no idea where that will lead. Just so, a man can say to a woman, "Follow me, with no idea where that will lead or what I will become." And the woman in her turn says to him, "And you follow me, not knowing where I will lead you." Marriage, like Baptism, begins in faith. It is a move based simply upon trust in a person — not a policy, a religion, a moral code, a set of requirements. It is an open-ended abandonment to an unpredictable person, who is known and cherished enough that one can make the surrender.

If this be so, then Christian marriage is not like all other marriages. Marriage is what you make of it, and Christian marriage is a particular, voluntary form which Christians have fashioned for themselves. There are many other forms of marriage, and we should not imagine that they are not legitimate. If in a certain culture it is accepted that a man has six wives, it is none of our business to constrain the man to discard five of them. If a man says to six women, "You are my wife," then they are indeed his wives. If in another culture it is understood that a man may exchange wives at whim, then it is none of our business to tell him he must marry for life. It is our calling to live our baptismal faith and our marriage faith before the eyes of all men and women so honestly and generously that the entire Christian commitment would in turn become their voluntary undertaking, also.

In fact, it is unfortunate that in our civil marriage ceremony, words are put into the mouths of men and women whereby they promise to one another things that they in no way intend to promise. In our society it is not understood that a man and a woman give themselves away for better, for worse, until death. They do not give themselves away unconditionally; they give themselves away indefinitely. Yet because our civil marriage form is descended from the Christian sacramental forms, couples are forced to say more than they mean.

Now if Christian marriage is a particular, extraordinary, peculiar way for a man and a woman to join together, then we must realize that it has particular obligations. The most important one is similar to the obligation to follow Jesus. When you tied yourself to a person, you cannot control your future. Every one of us has within himself an unbelievable potential for love and for generosity, but we do not bring it out very willingly. It has to be torn out of us. And the thing about Christian marriage is that the surprises encountered demand a love and generosity from us that we can in no way calculate or control. If that be so, then the incalculability of the demands of children fits very closely into the generosity that a man and a woman share in marriage. If a man and a woman can and do calculate and hedge the major claims made upon their generosity in the course of their marriage, then I fear that it is less a marriage of faith, and it will not blossom into a marriage of love such as Christians can enjoy.

The Church should not be interested in breeding. A

thoughtless priest said in the United States a few years ago that Catholics would put an end to religious discrimination in a generation or two by outproducing their contracepting opponents. Preachers have also suggested that the obligation to crowd heaven should stimulate Catholic parents to optimum production. Both statements breathe nonsense. Yet the Church has always had a smile for children, not because she is interested in population but because she is interested in love. And besides, she was once told that of such is the kingdom of heaven.

A first child, especially a boy-child, can easily be a threat to his father, for he seems to be a competitor for the wife's love that had been all his before. Similarly, each new child that swells the brood can seem a burden: the loaf must now be sliced just that much thinner. Faith sees another side to it. Bread may be sliced thinner, but love is sliced larger, and greater love sets about winning more bread. Every person, every parent is a fathomless well of love-potential. Children are not threats to love or competitors for it — they are new claims upon it, new tugs on the ungenerous heart to force it open further than it felt it could go. Children don't divide parents' love; they should invite it to multiply. Enormous resources of parent-love are let go stagnant in the heart's reservoirs for lack of children to make it gush and flow. Now obviously physical resources are not fathomless, and children must have bread. But in our age and culture, when parents feed their children cake and live in fear of a bread shortage, the Church weeps — and rightly so — that the children are starving in a famine of love.

One is so disappointed in the encyclical. One wishes the Pope had called parents to abandon themselves — in a way that would seem reckless to those without Christian faith — to their children as well as to one another. One wishes he had found a way to restore in husbands and wives so zestful an appetite for sons and daughters that when constrained to choose contraception for one strong motive or another, they would do so with reluctance and a sense of loss. Instead of grumbling that he has wrong-headedly forbidden artificial contraception, one regrets rather that he has not really preached to us the sort of good news that Matthew heard from Jesus.

If we have faith, we have hope. In this time of turmoil and contradiction, the Church will see its way through to a new and yet so very ancient understanding of what children do for their parents — of how they force them, in ways that surprise even themselves, to be greater men and women than they had planned. Jesus Christ has come to destroy all our plans — even those of parenthood.

112 Beyond the Liberal/Conservative Divide on Contraception: The Wisdom of Practitioners of Natural Family Planning and Artificial Birth Control

Julie Hanlon Rubio

I. Introduction

Because academic arguments about *Humanae Vitae*[1] are typically characterized by tension and intractability, conversation among those who disagree on sexual ethics has all but ceased. Discussions continue among conservatives, in forums removed from mainstream academic conferences,[2] while liberals sometimes use teaching on contraception as an example of various problematic tendencies in the church, but otherwise indicate by their silence that the issue has been settled. The language used to talk about the other side is almost always reductive and dismissive. Even the Common Ground Initiative, founded by Cardinal Bernadin in 1996 to encourage dialogue between liberals and conservatives in the church, only took up the issue of sexual ethics in 2004. Because of the delicate nature of the discussion, for the first time proceedings were not made public and participants were asked not to take the content of conversations outside the confines of the conference. Dialogue itself was a scandal!

Yet dialogue has never seemed more important. There is a groundswell of popular literature on natural family planning written by couples and those who work with them, and a small, but growing response from couples who use contraception.[3] Theologians in the post–Vatican II generation also seem somewhat more willing to give serious consideration to sexual ethics, as they move beyond narrowly focused discussions regarding the mo-

1. Pope Paul VI, *Humanae Vitae* (Washington, DC: United States Catholic Conference, 1968).

2. See, for instance, Kenneth D. Whitehead, ed., *Marriage and the Common Good* (South Bend, IN: St. Augustine's Press, 2001), proceedings from the Twenty-Second Annual Convention of Catholic Scholars.

3. See articles by Pamela Pilch and Leslie Tentler in *Commonweal*, 23 April 2004, and multiple responses in Correspondence sections in subsequent issues.

From Julie Hanlon Rubio, "Beyond the Liberal/Conservative Divide on Contraception: The Wisdom of Practitioners of Natural Family Planning and Artificial Birth Control," *Horizons* 32.2 (Fall 2005): 270-94. Used by permission.

rality of particular contraceptive acts and the question of dissent.[4] Their work suggests that the unnecessary and unhelpful divide between "liberals" and "conservatives" can be transcended. This new generation is much less invested in defending or criticizing *Humanae Vitae*; they are more interested in contributing to the development of sexual relationships that are as central a part of the life Christian discipleship as prayer, parenting, and social justice. A new sort of sexual ethics that fails to fit into the usual categories is beginning to emerge.

For participants, proving the other side wrong on contraception is not the point. Rather, dialogue is valued if it leads to recognition of areas of shared concern and contributes to more authentic Christian living. This paper, which examines the new theological conversation, is envisioned as a contribution to a new way of doing sexual ethics that focuses less on argument about norms and more on dialogue within a diverse Christian community about practices. While I will not claim to resolve the debate over contraception, I will suggest that reframing the dialogue around a new focus on sexuality as a dimension of discipleship is valuable in itself.

The method I will utilize is designed to encourage this new dialogue. After a brief review of the document at the heart of the modern debate, I will turn to experience,[5] analyzing the arguments of advocates of artificial contraception and natural family planning, pointing out key claims made by each group, identifying distinctive contributions, and searching for common ground. Listening to practitioners from both sides will allow for a new way of seeing the contemporary social map of sexual ethics. Contemporary Catholic writing on family planning differs from Vatican II–era discussions marked by competing concerns with resisting or adapting to the modern world by upholding or questioning moral norms. Younger writers both embrace the relational focus of contemporary culture and maintain a counter-cultural understanding of sexuality as a dimension of Christian discipleship. This is a good place for a new conversation to begin.

II. Humanae Vitae and Its Aftermath

Humanae Vitae is significant for the purposes of this article not only because it ignited the contemporary debate on contraception, but also because the commission appointed to decide if church teaching on contraception should change incorporated the experiences of married couples. Prior to the Second Vatican Council, some prominent Catholic theologians, including Bernard Häring, Edward Schillebeeckx, and Louis Janssens, raised questions about the official teaching against contraception, while others, notably Cardinal Suenens, Josef Fuchs, and John Ford, upheld the traditional view.[6] In order to deal with growing controversy, Pope John XXIII appointed a commission to study the subject. It started as a group of six men, most of them scientists, and eventually expanded to include over sixty members, including four women.

In *Turning Point: The Inside Story of the Papal Birth Control Commission,* Robert McClory details the crucial roles played by Pat and Patty Crowley, leaders of the Christian Family Movement (CFM), whose testimony was influential in pushing the majority of the commission toward acceptance of artificial birth control. Initially, the Crowleys did an informal survey of the membership of the CFM, a network of groups of lay Catholic couples who met weekly to discuss the role of faith in their daily lives. They were staggered to find that "even the most dedicated, committed Catholics are deeply troubled by this problem."[7] Frustrated users of the rhythm method testified in their letters that the method "seriously endangered [their] chastity," "[made them] obsessed with sex throughout the month," allowed them to show only "guarded affection" in fertile times (during which many women experienced their highest levels of sexual desire).[8] They urged the Commission to allow married couples to decide for themselves when sex was appropriate, taking account of all relevant dimensions of their sexual relationship and their married life.[9] According to Patty Crowley, at the end of the Commission's third meeting in 1964, Pope Paul VI urged the group to "continue its deliberations, listen to the anxiety of so many souls, and work diligently without worrying about criticism or difficulties."[10] Commission members dared to hope that change was imminent.

The Crowleys returned to the next meeting of the Commission with a more systematic survey of over 3000 couples in 18 countries that was to have an even greater effect. Though most couples said the method worked well enough, and 64% said it helped them grow in self-sacrificial love, 78% believed that it was harmful to their

4. See, for instance, Richard Gaillardetz, *A Daring Promise: A Spirituality of Christian Marriage* (New York: Crossroad, 2001), 101-11, and David McCarthy, "Procreation, the Development of Peoples, and the Final Destination of Humanity," *Communio* 26 (Winter 1999): 698-721.

5. Experience is a significant source for contemporary Christian Ethics for both liberals and conservatives, though its precise value is disputed. See Margaret Farley, "The Role of Experience in Moral Discernment," in Lisa Sowle Cahill and James F. Childress, eds., *Christian Ethics: Problems and Prospects* (Cleveland: Pilgrim, 1996), 134-51, and Karol Wojtyla, "The Problem of Experience in Ethics," in his *Person and Community: Selected Essays,* trans. Theresa Sandok (New York: Peter Lang, 1993): 107-28.

6. William Shannon, ed., *The Lively Debate: Responses to Humanae Vitae* (New York: Sheed & Ward, 1970).

7. Robert McClory, *Turning Point: The Inside Story of the Papal Birth Control Commission* (New York: Crossroad, 1995), 72. See also Robert Blair Kaiser, *The Politics of Sex and Religion* (Kansas City, KS: Leaven Press, 1985)

8. Ibid., 73. McClory notes that the studies of psychiatrist John Cavanaugh were also used to support the idea that rhythm was psychologically harmful, especially for women.

9. Ibid. This is a popular version of the principle of totality, proposed as an alternative to act-centered moral analysis.

10. Ibid., 78-79.

marriage, in that it increased tension and reduced spontaneity. As the Crowleys saw it, couples "were struggling to find something positive in what struck them as basically negative."[11] One woman questioned whether the sacrifice was worth it. "Rhythm leads to self-seeking, promotes excess in infertile times and strain in fertile times. Is contraceptive sex irresponsible when I have already borne 10 little responsibilities?"[12] The Crowleys' surveys, which were complemented by similar, smaller studies done by Commission members from Europe and Australia, significantly influenced members of the commission.[13] When a straw vote was taken among the nineteen theologians of the group at the Commission's final meeting, fifteen agreed that contraception was not intrinsically evil.[14] Commission members then asked the women to speak of their experience, and they did. Patty Crowley in particular testified to the negative psychological effects of rhythm, to the testimony of married couples that it did not foster married love or unity, to their belief that it felt unnatural.[15] In sum, said Crowley, "the sense of the faithful is for change."[16]

However, despite the Commission's official report, which reflected the views of the majority[17] of Catholics that the totality of the married relationship should be considered when analyzing the morality of contraception, a minority report (authored by Germain Grisez and signed by four Commission members) convinced the pope that the church could not have erred for centuries and that when the good of procreation is blocked by contraception, the integrity of the sexual act is violated.[18] In 1968, he issued *Humanae Vitae,* affirming that every sexual act must remain open to procreation.

Some liberal theologians argue that the document has never been received by lay Catholics. McClory notes that of all episcopal conferences in the world, 17% fully accepted the teaching, 56% were opposed, and 28% uncertain.[19] The Crowleys, who had been convinced the teaching against contraception would change, felt betrayed and, along with the other U.S. lay members of the Commission, urged couples to follow their consciences.[20] At Catholic University, Charles Curran authored a dissenting letter that was signed by over six hundred Catholic scholars within a few weeks.[21] This organized public theology was greeted with suspicion by the Vatican. Yet, the majority of American Catholics stopped using the rhythm method, and polls show that most believe they should be permitted to make their own decisions about family planning.[22]

As disagreement spread, many moral theologians wrote articles developing the idea of totality[23] or showing the legitimacy of dissent from non-authoritative specific magisterial moral teachings.[24] The controversial *Human Sexuality,* which resulted from a study commissioned by the Catholic Theological Society of America and is representative of liberal scholarly arguments of the time, promoted sex as a sign and means of growth in mutual perfection and characterized contraception as a dimension of responsible parenthood.[25] The faithful grew increasingly suspicious of official Catholic sexual teaching, and all but a small minority stopped listening altogether. According to Andrew Greeley, *HV* has been an important cause of decreasing mass attendance and commitment since Vatican II.[26] At every level, liberals argue, the teaching has been rejected.

Yet, the late John Paul II was a great defender of *HV,* and his new way of teaching about sexuality was an inspiration to many during his pontificate. Especially in his lectures on theology of the body and his writings on the family, he tries to provide a personalist understanding of sexuality.[27] Eschewing traditional natural law arguments, he promotes NFP as a method that is fully giving

11. Ibid., 91.

12. Ibid., 92. For an alternative view of the Commission, see George A. Kelly, *The Battle for the American Church* (Garden City, NY: Doubleday, 1979), 153-98, and James Hitchcock, "The Significance of the Papal Birth Control Commission," in Patrick G. D. Riley, ed., *Keeping the Faith: Msgr. George A. Kelly's Battle for the Church* (Front Royal, VA: Christendom, 2000). Both question the relevance and accuracy of the CFM surveys.

13. After listening to the lay women of the Commission, one bishop commented, "This is why we wanted to have couples on our Commission" (McClory, 106).

14. Ibid., 90. The final vote of the entire commission was fifty-eight to four.

15. Ibid., 103-4.

16. Ibid., 107.

17. Of course, a worldwide survey of Catholics has not yet been done. It is possible that such a survey would reveal a greater diversity than the current data suggests.

18. Ibid., 110-11.

19. Ibid., 145.

20. Ibid., 141.

21. Ibid., 140.

22. Eighty seven percent of Catholics agreed with this statement in a 1993 Gallup poll (*Los Angeles Times,* 7 January 1993, p. E6). Vincent Genovesi reports that only about 4% of couples use NFP, *In Pursuit of Love: Catholic Morality and Human Sexuality,* 2d ed., (Collegeville, MN: Liturgical Press, 1996), 206. The pro-NFP Couple to Couple League believes the figure may be even lower, perhaps three percent. See John Kipley, "How Many?" available at ccli.org/articles/howmany. See also Richard Fehring and Andrea Matovina Schlidt, "Trends in Contraceptive Use Among Catholics in the U.S.: 1985-1995," *Linacre Quarterly* 68/2 (May 2001): 170-85. Seventy percent of Catholic couples did not use contraception in 1955; see Kelly, 188, relying on demographic research from 1973.

23. See, for instance, Bernard Häring, "The Inseparability of the Unitive-Procreative Functions of the Marital Act," in Charles E. Curran, ed., *Contraception, Authority and Dissent* (New York: Herder and Herder, 1969), 176-92.

24. See Charles E. Curran and Robert E. Hunt, *Dissent In and For the Church: Theologians and Humanae Vitae* (New York: Sheed and Ward, 1969).

25. Anthony Kosnik et al., *Human Sexuality* (Garden City, NY: Doubleday, 1979), 131-37.

26. Andrew Greeley, *The American Catholic: A Social Portrait* (New York: Basic Books, 1977), 141.

27. See *Familiaris Consortio* (Washington, DC: National Conference of Catholic Bishops, 1981), #28-36, and Reflections on *Humanae Vitae: Conjugal Morality and Spirituality* (Boston: Daughters of St. Paul, 1984).

because fertility is offered to one's partner and lovingly received, fully human because it allows for transcendence of desire through self-control in the service of a higher good, and fully open to life in that children are graciously accepted rather than ruled out.

Catholic conservatives appreciate John Paul II's theology of the body and offer a different perspective on *HV*. As they see it, the document was a prophetic denunciation of a deeply problematic cultural move to de-emphasize the procreative end of sex and marriage.[28] The CTSA's *Human Sexuality* was a misguided attempt to remove procreation from its central place in sex and marriage.[29] Pope Paul VI, who saw clearly that contraception would lead to growing promiscuity, sexual diseases, abortion, divorce, and an increasing anti-life mentality, is to be celebrated for his prophetic wisdom.[30] If the pronouncements of *HV* were not fully supported by theological reasoning at the time, the theology of the body developed by John Paul II now more than suffices. While *HV*'s defenders acknowledge that the majority of the faithful disagree, they mourn this fact and celebrate the strong witness of couples who testify to the ways in which the practice of NFP enriches their marriage.[31] In their view, Pope Paul VI was right to defend the truth and reject the opinions of married couples, since the Magisterium is obligated to lead the faithful, not yield to the culture. If *HV* is not received by all Catholics, it is nonetheless true, fully accepted by some, and wholly supported by the Holy Father's theology of marriage and family. According to conservatives, the battles leading up to the issuing of *HV* are beside the point; what matters is the document that was promulgated and the prophetic witness of the faithful who live it out.

In sum, the Papal birth control commission was unique in that the experience of married couples was solicited and seriously considered over a three-year period of deliberation that culminated in a negative judgement on natural methods of family planning. Pope Paul VI's decision to affirm the traditional teaching is read by liberals as a rejection of the modern experience of the faithful and by conservatives as evidence of the enduring truth of Catholic tradition. However, if the conversation seems to stall here, it need not do so. Contemporary advocates of both natural family planning and contraception share a new approach and more common ground than is usually acknowledged. An analysis of their reflection on experience will bear this out and point toward a new kind of dialogue on sexual ethics.

III. Lessons from Experience: Natural Family Planning and Artificial Birth Control

The contemporary popular literature on natural family planning is vast, and one who studies it can only conclude that, for the majority of practitioners, the experience is extremely positive. The problems of couples in the Crowley's study seem largely absent. In order to understand why, it is important to note what has changed since 1968. NFP is more scientific than the traditional rhythm method, and, if strictly adhered to, much more effective (95-99% for dedicated users, though actual use rates are somewhat lower).[32] However, while increased effectiveness may account for some of the differences between the new literature and older accounts of rhythm users, theological developments are at least as significant. Indeed, the theology shapes the experience in profound ways.

New understandings of church authority and the role of conscience allow couples today to choose NFP as lifestyle rather than accept it as an externally imposed law. As John Grabowski points out, *HV* asserts the inseparable connection between the unitive and procreative ends of sex without explaining it, leaving couples to obey or dissent.[33] While few Catholic couples today believe that use of contraception would render moot their claim to Catholic identity, John Paul II's theology of the body invites the radical choice of NFP as a practice that fits in with a larger commitment to maintain a distinctively Christian marriage. As the pope sees it, sex is the sign of the total self-giving of the married couple, the language to communicate fidelity. The suppression of fertility (viewed as an essential dimension of the person) is a falsification of the inner truth of sexual love. It causes the body to say with its actions, "I give myself to you," but with fertility withheld, the fullness of self-gift is denied.[34] This understanding both rules out contraception and provides a theological framework for viewing sexuality as a crucial dimension of a radically self-giving marriage.

Theologians supportive of this view write about how the practice of NFP helps marriages of Catholic couples grow and deepen. John Grabowski, whose work is representative of this new trend, sketches a positive picture of

28. See Germain Grisez, Joseph Boyle, John Finnis, and William E. May, "Every Marital Act Ought to Be Open to New Life," in *The Teaching of Humanae Vitae: A Defense* (San Francisco: Ignatius Press, 1988), 33-116.

29. See "Morality in Sexual Matters: Observations of the Sacred Congregation for the Doctrine of the Faith on the Book *Human Sexuality*," *The Pope Speaks*, 13 July 1979, pp. 97-102.

30. Janet E. Smith, "Paul VI as Prophet," in Janet E. Smith, ed., *Why Humanae Vitae Was Right: A Reader* (San Francisco: Ignatius Press, 1993), 519-31.

31. See John Grabowski, *Sex and Virtue: An Introduction to Sexual Ethics* (Washington, DC: Catholic University of America Press, 2003), 10-14, 142-54.

32. Mercedes Arzu Wilson, *Love & Family: Raising a Traditional Family in a Secular World* (San Francisco: Ignatius Press, 1996), 250-55. How much lower is a matter of much dispute. NFP advocates like Wilson and the Couple to Couple League cite use rates of seventy to ninety percent, while others present evidence that failure is much more common. See Christina Traina, "Papal Ideals, Marital Realities: One View from the Ground," in Patricia Beattie Jung with Joseph Andrew Coray, eds., *Sexual Diversity and Catholicism: Toward the Development of Moral Theology* (Collegeville, MN: Liturgical Press, 2001), 277.

33. Grabowski, 130.

34. Ibid., 130-31. See John Paul II, *Familiaris Consortio* §32.

NFP as a practice that is confirmed by the majority of studies and testimonies today.[35] As Grabowski indicates, many NFP couples experience an increased capacity for total self-giving, growth in mutuality, better communication, higher levels of intimacy, increased sexual pleasure, and spiritual growth.

There is significantly less contemporary Catholic writing on the experience of using contraception, perhaps because while contraception makes possible certain sexual practices and life choices, it is not a radical lifestyle choice in itself. A method of family planning rather than a practice, contraception does not call forth the same level or type of reflection as does NFP. Still, Rosemary Radford Ruether's groundbreaking 1971 article, "Birth Control and Ideals of Marital Sexuality" (an older piece that nonetheless fits more with the newer conversation), and more recent work by Christina Traina, David McCarthy, Richard Gaillardetz, and others point in new directions.[36] Most agree with the traditional teaching that sex is for union and procreation. However, as Ruether suggests, "the procreational and the relational aspects of the sexual act are two semi-independent and interrelated purposes which both are brought together in their meaning and value within the total marriage project, although it is not only unnecessary but even biologically impossible that both purposes be present in every act."[37] While the marital relationship ought to be marked by mutual love and openness to children, a couple's sexual relationship is primarily oriented toward the former. These theologians assert that contraception is beneficial because it allows couples to grow in mutual love without worrying about conceiving more children than they can responsibly welcome. Though their arguments may fit with more theoretical claims about totality, they are deeply rooted in experiences of Christian spouses who want their sexual lives and their faith to be of one piece, and find contraception to be helpful rather than harmful.

Because popular accounts of the benefits of contraception for the relationship of Catholic married couples are rare, it will be difficult to evaluate these claims. Clearly, a precise comparative study of couples using NFP and artificial birth is yet out of reach. Still, it will be possible to glean insights into the goods of the practice of contraception by looking at contemporary Catholic and Protestant writing on sexuality, as most of this writing assumes (even if it does not explicitly acknowledge) the use of birth control. While these sources cannot provide evidence that the practice of birth control results in various goods, they can at least suggest that the practice does not impede their realization. Along with more direct writing on the difficulties of natural methods, these sources make possible an analysis that finds in the lives of couples who use contraception desire for and experience of many of the very same goods NFP advocates value. When this common ground is discerned, the future of sexual ethics (taken up in the conclusion of this article) will be easier to envision.

Total Self-Giving

Among the goods that couples on both sides of the divide claim to find, self-giving is possibly the most prominent. On one hand, NFP is reputed to both make possible self-giving in sexual relations and predispose couples to the sacrifice required for total self-giving in their marriage. Christopher West, perhaps the primary popular communicator of John Paul II's theology of the body, does not attempt to prove that contraception is intrinsically evil or sinful. Instead, he tells his audiences that since sex requires total self-giving, giving one's fertility is a reenactment of a couple's wedding vow.[38] Protestants Sam and Bethany Torode adopt a similar approach using their own experience. "Rather than pointing fingers," they say, "we want to point to a better way."[39] For them, birth control is wrong because, "[w]hen we should be saying 'I do,' contraception says, 'I do not.'"[40] Furthermore, they suggest that if fertility is reserved, couples are more likely to reserve themselves in other regards, while giving freely will lead to increased respect, truth, love and surrender.[41] Centering their argument on discipleship to Christ, the Torrodes ask, "[W]ould Christ ever withhold any part of himself from the Church, or sterilize his love?" Seeking to follow Christ's example, they advocate coming together in "an open embrace, withholding nothing from each other."[42] Many studies of NFP couples provide evidence of the opening effect of NFP.[43]

35. Grabowski, 152-54. Thomasina Borkman points out the limits of existing studies that focus, for the most part, on satisfied users. Comparison with artificial methods of contraception is also difficult because NFP is more of a way of life with training methods similar to those of self-help movements than a birth control method. See Borkman, "A Social Science Perspective of Research Issues for Natural Family Planning," *IRNFP* 3/4 (1979): 331-55.

36. Ruether's article appears in Charles E. Curran and Richard P. McCormick, eds., *Moral Theology No. 8: Dialogue about Catholic Sexual Teaching* (New York: Paulist, 1993), 138-52. See also Traina.

37. Ruether, 141.

38. Christopher West, *Good News about Sex and Marriage: Answers to Your Honest Questions about Catholic Teaching* (Ann Arbor, MI: Servant Press, 2000), 108.

39. Sam and Bethany Torode, *Open Embrace: A Protestant Couple Rethinks Contraception* (Grand Rapids, MI: Eerdmans, 2002), 8.

40. Ibid., 30. [Editors' note: We are aware that Mr. Torode and Ms. Patchin, formerly Mr. and Mrs. Torode, are now divorced and have reversed their positions on NFP. One account of that reversal is found at: http://www.nytimes.com/2011/07/09/us/09beliefs.html (accessed March 4, 2012). While Ms. Patchin's and Mr. Torode's past and present arguments regarding NFP are worth considering, their reversal does not substantially diminish Julie Hanlon Rubio's fine essay reprinted here.]

41. Ibid., 127.

42. Ibid., 25.

43. See Joseph Stanford, M.D., "My Personal and Professional journey with Regard to Moral Issues in Human Procreation," in Cleta Hartman, *Physicians Healed* (Dayton, OH: One More Soul, 1998), who says he learned from patients that abstinence strengthened couples' ability to sacrifice for each other, 115; Kimberly Kirk

Some advocates go even further, arguing that development of the virtue of chastity, which requires sacrifice in periodic abstinence, also predisposes couples to grow in the virtue of justice. Catholic philosopher Gregory Beabout states that "chastity forms sexual desires so that they are desires for sexual activity as a sign of the mutual and complete self-donation of persons and for reasons commensurate with its being that kind of sign." Practice in discerning what sorts of bodily actions are signs of self-giving helps couples become more open to self-donation in other areas of their lives. Chastity, according to Beabout, also opens families to more children, makes materialist living less thinkable, and leads to a prioritization of people over things. So while he agrees with Pope Paul VI that those who want peace should work for justice, he proposes, "If you want justice, work for chastity."[44] In this view, a sexual relationship shaped by natural family planning celebrates and encourages self-donation in the relationship of the couple, which spills over to the children, and, ultimately, to the world.

In the contrasting experience of couples who use contraception, self-giving is central to sexual relationships even when sex is not completely open. Ruether grants that in an ideal world, every sexual act would be totally open to procreation and totally loving, but claims that in reality, people are not free to have unlimited numbers of children, nor are they always capable of giving themselves fully to a spouse. Concerns about population and the limits of parental energies contribute to her sense that families ought to be limited.[45] Love is limited, in her view, by human capacity as well, for "[m]ost couples do not express the full mutuality of their persons in the sexual act for the simple reason that they have not achieved such mutuality, because their understanding of each other is distorted and fraught with petty tensions and dislikes."[46] Human beings do not always have a "total" self to give. Their self-understanding evolves over time and is incomplete. Thus, their ability to love with everything that they are in order to achieve oneness is limited by their humanity. Sex is ordinary much of the time, but over a lifetime the sexual relationship of a couple contributes to the total self-gift of their marriage.[47]

Self-giving in the marriages of couples who use contraception is also parental, according to advocates, even though spouses are not always open to procreation. Traina contends that intentionally procreative sex is not ideal, but extraordinary, in that "[t]here is a new focus, a shared delight in a common project that really is a 'total self-gift' to each other and our hoped-for future child."[48] Still, it is relatively rare for most couples and thus not normative in any way, since intentionally non-procreative sex is good in itself. Ordinary non-procreative sex centers on self-giving, and this is encouraged, rather than compromised, by the practice of contraception. For, argues Traina, "contraception does not impede self-gift but, like pregnancy, allows it the freedom to proceed unworried by consequences."[49] Just as the unitive and procreative goods of marriage are separable, so, too, the self to be given is distinct from fertility. One does not have to give oneself as a potential parent in order to give fully. Even with contraception, partners may still give themselves as parents to the ongoing sexual relationship. As Traina puts it, "[o]ur children have in a certain respect made us, have shaped our minds, spirits, and even bodies. This awareness is always implicit and sometimes explicit in our lovemaking."[50] Believing that many potential goods must be balanced when they choose to have sex, practitioners of contraception argue that birth control allows them to give themselves as fully as possible to each other and their existing children.[51]

Yet theologians who promote contraception do not stop here. They contend that sex "communicates to us our own goodness. That sense of goodness is essential if we are to understand ourselves as beloved by God, and thus able to communicate God's love to others."[52] According to Catholic theologian Christine Gudorf, experiencing sexual pleasure

> reinforces the lesson that it is OK, even good, to let go of control, to open oneself up to other people and experiences, to let down our protective barriers, our self-consciousness. When sex is not segregated from the rest of our lives, the pleasure of orgasm can reach far beyond the moment of intense pleasure itself, and change, a little at a time, the way we relate to our partner, and even to the larger society and world. It can encourage us to trust more, to be willing to risk more, to reach out to others more.[53]

Gudorf points out that sex makes people feel loved and loving, to their partners, their children, their community, and this is why many strongly advocate contraception, which may allow for more spontaneous, unworried sex among married couples.

In sum, contemporary NFP defenders and birth con-

Hahn, *Life-Giving Love: Embracing God's Beautiful Design for Marriage* (Ann Arbor, MI: Servant Press, 2001); Mary Shivanadan, *Crossing the Threshold of Love: A New Vision of Marriage* (Washington, DC: Catholic University of America Press, 1999), 262-70.

44. Gregory R. Beabout and Randall Colton, "If You Want Justice, Work for Chastity," unpublished paper, 2003. See also McCarthy, who highlights the connection between openness to procreation and solidarity, "Sexual Utterances and the Common Life," *Modern Theology* 16/4 (October 2000): 443-59.

45. Ruether, 141. Traina (275) also notes that other goods must be weighed when considering whether or not to be open to the good of procreation.

46. Ruether, 141.

47. On this theme, see also David McCarthy, *Sex and Love in the Home: A Theology of the Household,* 2d ed. (London: SCM Press, 2004), 46-48.

48. Traina, 274.

49. Ibid., 279.

50. Ibid.

51. Joseph A. Selling, "The 'Meanings' of Human Sexuality," *Louvain Studies* 23 (1998): 35.

52. Christine Gudorf, *Body, Sex, & Pleasure: Reconstructing Christian Sexual Ethics* (Cleveland: Pilgrim Press, 1994), 98.

53. Ibid., 109.

trol advocates both see self-giving (between spouses, to children, and to others) as a goal, even though they conceive of self-gift differently. Despite the disagreement about how best to achieve self-gift, there is a shared vision of marriage, and in particular the sexual relationship of a married couple, as an ongoing project of total self-giving. Sexual practices that contribute to this project are judged to be helpful, while those that hinder it are seen as harmful.

Communication and Intimacy

The framework for growth in self-giving is the marital relationship; thus it should come as no surprise that advocates of both NFP and contraception seek high quality marital relationships and embrace practices that enhance intimacy. Theologians who favor NFP are likely to cite sociological studies showing that NFP improves communication between husbands and wives. Many couples report that their need to communicate about their fertility translates into better communication about other matters. One physician notes that "As one of my male clients says, 'If you can talk about cervical fluid, you can talk about anything.'"[54] In addition, during fertile times when children are not desired, couples learn to communicate their love in other ways. Family therapist Gregory Popcak finds that couples "are forced to nurture their friendship more because they can't just 'throw sex' at their problems."[55] Popular NFP guides help spouses plan other ways of showing affection, such as sharing a candlelight dinner, meditating or praying together, and talking about feelings of love or desire.[56] Alternatives to sex (which may become less common as a marriage progresses) seem to increase intimacy in the lives of couples committed to NFP,[57] and better quality relationships may even contribute to more lasting marriages.[58] For contemporary NFP supporters, stronger, more intimate relationships are a key reason to adopt what may at first appear to be a difficult practice.

Advocates of contraception share this concern with communication and intimacy. However, they are more likely to emphasize that sex is a necessary part of maintaining intimacy in marriage. Ruether argues that "[m]an needs to express his mutuality with his partner, and in the sexual act this mutuality is both expressed and recreated"; thus abstinence can cause "extensive emotional damage to the basic stability of the marriage."[59] The cementing of love between the couple is necessary for the good of their relationship and the good of their already born children. Traina concurs, noting the importance of sex as a glue, especially in times of difficulty, "when words fail (or worse, harm)."[60] Ruether proposes that if couples really wanted to use times of abstinence for spiritual growth, they would abstain during Lent or at other religiously significant times.[61] Traina points out that the busy lives of modern married couples provide many opportunities for not having sex, making planned abstinence unnecessary.[62] Whatever the role of abstinence, when sex is possible, advocates of contraception claim that intimacy would be impeded by undesired abstinence. Early testimonies of those who switched from rhythm to the pill provide good illustrations of the experiential argument for the connection between intimacy and contraception. One woman relates:

> I can't begin to tell you the difference the pill made in our relationship within a week. Never before in our married life had either of us felt so free about our sexual love. We became immediately more physically affectionate outside of the marital act. We became more communicative, there was a greater feeling of family, we became less critical and less nagging about smaller everyday things, happier with our particular places in the world.[63]

Most contemporary Catholic couples who assume they will use contraception and use it consistently are not quite as ecstatic about its life-giving powers. However, one does find in the literature a recognition that NFP can impede intimacy in the lives of modern couples who "if they have children, are often struggling to keep sexual intimacy alive in their marriage."[64] Given the realities of modern family life, "the demands of periodic abstinence can be transformed from 'an opportunity to find other ways to express their love' into a major obstacle in the marriage relationship." If married sexuality is to "[make

54. Torodes, 50.

55. Ibid.

56. Merryl Winstein, *Your Fertility Signals: Using Them to Achieve or Avoid Pregnancy, Naturally* (St. Louis: Smooth Stone Press, 1989).

57. See Beverly McMillan, "Confessions of an Ob-Gyn," *New Oxford Review* 68/8 (September 2001): 17; K. J. Tompkins and Barbara Dwyer, "Experience with a Hospital-Based Natural Family Planning Service," *IRNFP* 10/4 (Winter 1986): 347; Thomasina Borkman and Mary Shivanadan, "The Impact of Natural Family Planning on Selected Aspects of the Couple Relationship," *IRNFP* 8/1(1984):63; M. Peter McCusker, "NFP and the Marital Relationship: The Catholic University of America Study," *IRNFP* 1/4 (1977): 333.

58. There is some evidence that NFP couples have lower divorce rates. See Nona Aguilar, *The New No-Pill, No-Risk Birth Control* (New York: Rawson Associates, 1986), and Jeff Brand, *Marital Duration and Natural Family Planning* (Cincinnati: Couple to Couple League, 1995), though systematic comparative studies have yet to be attempted.

59. Ruether, 143. See also Michael Novak, *The Experience of Marriage* (New York: Macmillan, 1964), quoting married couples, "We know that it [sex] is of fundamental importance to developing our personal relationship, to increasing that mutuality that we find is a very real analogy of Divine Love" (42).

60. Traina, 273.

61. Ruether, 150.

62. Traina, 280.

63. A letter from the Crowley surveys, quoted in John Kotre, *Simple Gifts: The Lives of Pat and Patty Crowley* (New York: Andrews and McMeel, 1979), 97. Testimony that abstinence distorts intimacy can also be found in Novak, *The Experience of Marriage*, and Mitch Finley, "The Dark Side of Natural Family Planning," *America*, 23 February 1991, pp. 206-07.

64. Gaillardetz, 110.

spouses] capable of play, delight, and the risk of vulnerability together," if it is to "ratify their covenantal love for one another," it seems to those who approve of contraception that it can assist couples seeking to strengthen their marital relationship through sexual intimacy.[65]

While the different conceptions of the value of abstinence are clear, it is perhaps more significant that advocates from both groups are deeply concerned with communication and intimacy. No one is claiming, as many earlier opponents of contraception did, that intimacy must be sacrificed for the sake of some other good, even procreation. Rather, both are convinced that their chosen method of family planning helps couples grow closer together and thus contributes to the good of marriage.

Enhanced Sexual Relationship

Advocates of both NFP and contraception agree that their practice benefits their marriages in part because it enhances their sexual relationships. NFP practitioners often speak of the courtship and honeymoon phases in each cycle as helpful for keeping sex interesting. Some couples who move from artificial means of contraception to NFP report that their sex life improves. In a typical statement, one couple testifies that, "[With the pill], we started to get bored. A thing of beauty loses its attractiveness when it is available at any time without any effort," while another claims that "[d]uring the waiting period, we find ourselves talking things over more, and when the infertile days come again, we experience supreme joy in our sexual union with each other. There is a natural creative tension present that is missing when you take the pill."[66] Paul Murray, a Catholic teacher and NFP user, concurs, noting that, "If intercourse is intimate sharing, then a conscious decision to abstain under such circumstances is intercourse in all but the physical sense of the word, and is utterly sexual in its nature."[67] Here, sacrifice is linked to pleasure, because rather than burdening a couple, it frees them to be creative in their expression of sexual desire for each other. Unlike most couples in the Crowley's study, today's NFP users overwhelmingly report that though abstinence can be difficult at times, it ultimately contributes to the good of their sexual relationship rather than diminishing it.

Similarly, practitioners of contraception believe that contraception enhances their sexual relationships. Methods such as the birth control pill and male or female sterilization allow for spontaneity and response to the sexual cycles of both males and females.[68] Neither partner is held back by fear of pregnancy or discomfort with disruptive barrier methods of contraception, thus both are better able to express themselves sexually and give and receive sexual pleasure. This is significant because both the desire for and experience of pleasure are viewed by most practitioners of artificial contraception as central to the goodness and holiness of sexual relationships. Mary Pellaur's now classic description of female orgasm, which acknowledges the role of an almost greedy desire for pleasure, reads differently from the theology of the body's definition of sex as total self-giving. Instead, Pellaur sees several important elements of sexual experience, including being here and now, ecstasy, and vulnerability. She writes of the difficulty of allowing herself to be vulnerable to her husband, "I experience an orgasm and all the impelling feelings before it as his power over me in order to receive this ecstasy, and this is not easy. It depends upon trust that is built up in many elements of our relationship — the mutuality growing, the confidence in reliability, the sense that this person will not hurt me on purpose, our abilities to forgive each other."[69] This is testimony that while human beings may sometimes find it hard to receive sexual pleasure because it requires vulnerability and trust, it is nevertheless fundamentally important. Contraception advocates emphasize the good of sexual pleasure and believe that birth control enhances their ability to become vulnerable enough to give and receive it.

Both NFP and contraception users are concerned with enhancing sexual pleasure, and many testify that their sexual relationships improved due to their chosen method of family planning. NFP promoters note that the sexual tension and creativity accompanying periods of abstinence enhance sexual relationships, while contraception advocates are more likely to recognize and name the centrality and complexity of desiring and receiving pleasure. However, neither group prioritizes pleasure in such a way that relationships outside of a mutually giving covenantal relationship would be legitimized, and both recognize its power and significance in the lives of married couples, not just because pleasure feels good, but because experiencing pleasure affirms the self-worth of individual spouses and calls them into deeper relation with each other.

Increased Mutuality

Within the marital relationship, both NFP and contraception practitioners seek mutuality. Though in earlier writing, NFP advocates may have appeared insensitive to potentially sexist implications of using this method, the

65. Ibid., 111. Note that Gaillardetz sees much wisdom in *HV* and believes that many couples can successfully adopt NFP.

66. Ingrid Trobisch and Elisabeth Roetzer, *An Experience of Love: Understanding NFP* (Old Tappan, NJ: Fleming H. Revell, 1981), 83. See also Torodes, 52.

67. Paul Murray, "The Power of 'Humanae Vitae': Take Another Look," *Commonweal,* 15 July 1994, p. 15.

68. Bjorn J. Oddens, "Women's Satisfaction with Birth Control," *Contraception* 59 (1999): 281-82. According to a large German study, compared to NFP users, women who used contraception reported higher satisfaction generally, higher sexual frequency, more spontaneity. Still, NFP users, though generally somewhat less satisfied (72% versus 83% of pill users, 90% of IUD users, and 92% of those who relied on sterilization), reported more pleasure and increased sex drive, along with decreased frequency and spontaneity.

69. Mary Pellaur, "The Moral Significance of Female Orgasm: Toward Sexual Ethics That Celebrate Women's Sexuality," *Journal of Feminist Studies in Religion* 9/1-2 (Spring/ Fall 1993): 174.

newer generation is convinced that they have a strong answer to modern concerns about gender equity in marriage. NFP advocates contend that use of the method increases mutuality, as both husband and wife are involved in making the decision to abstain or have sex and remain open to life. Whereas most contraceptive methods are the responsibility of women alone, NFP requires the participation of men and women, because it takes two to abstain. Shared responsibility for sexual decision making is related, in advocates' eyes, to mutuality in other dimensions of the relationship. Moreover, many studies report that NFP users, particularly women, have higher levels of self-esteem that they attribute to increased awareness of and control over their bodies.[70] The testimony of a woman in a recent study is typical, "I've learned more about myself as a woman since I've started. . . . I just feel better about it on the whole, my self-esteem. It caused me to have more control."[71] Men's growing knowledge of and respect for their wives also contributes to enhanced mutuality.[72]

Even still, contraception advocates argue that mutuality is more easily attained with contraception because as "accidental" pregnancies are less likely to occur, women are not necessarily limited in their career potential. In a time in which women as well as men feel the pull of multiple vocations, this freedom is seen as necessary to women's equality.[73] While some natural family planning advocates believe that contraception is disrespectful of a woman's sexuality,[74] accounts of the sexual relationships of couples using contraception attest to feelings of sexual empowerment and mutual respect.[75] There is no sense that using contraception is experienced as the opposite.

Moreover, mutuality is enhanced, according to contemporary writers who favor contraception, when growth through intimacy results in greater wholeness (understood as balance between the masculine and feminine sides of oneself) for both partners. To be fully human is to be in mature relationship and transcend the limits of gender roles,[76] and this is more possible in a sexual relationship unhampered by the female fertility cycle.[77] This cycle is relevant when conceiving children, and should be known in order to better understand emotional and sexual variances, but it fades into the background with contraception, and the significance of gender fades as well.[78] Practitioners of artificial birth control value mutuality unbounded by complementarity, and feel they draw closer to it with contraception.

While differing understandings of mutuality are apparent in the writings of the two groups, it is also clear that some sort of mutuality in relationships is valued by both. Most formal studies of NFP users show that women are even more satisfied with NFP than men, because of their enhanced self-knowledge, self-esteem, and sexual desire. Yet, practitioners of contraception see their method as the guarantor of enhanced sexual freedom and pleasure for women. Both seek to establish that women are valued and even liberated by their family planning practice for equality in relationships.

Sexuality Linked to Spirituality

Perhaps most importantly, both NFP and contraception advocates make the case that their practice predisposes couples to see the spiritual in the sexual. Nowhere do we see a hesitance to affirm the goodness of sex or a blindness to the potential of sex to serve as a conduit of God's grace. For NFP users, self-control is viewed as necessary to making sexual behavior fully human. In order to be truly free, human beings must act according to the will rather than blind or animal impulse. Knowing the truth and acting on it, they are better able to engage in sex in a fully human way. In the view of some advocates, NFP calls for virtue (chastity); thus it fits more easily into religious life. Influenced by the pre-papal writings of John Paul II, in their experience, the association of sex with virtue is freeing rather than stifling:

> The liberation of the person through chastity takes place not just exteriorly but in the depth of the will. It ensures that loving kindness takes precedence over the desire for enjoyment. Wojtyla states that 'only the chaste man and woman are capable of true love.' NFP couples experience this liberation.[79]

Theological ideals extolling self-control are complemented by thick descriptions of the open marital em-

70. Joseph Tortorici, "Conception Regulation, Self-Esteem, and Marital Satisfaction among Catholic Couples: Michigan State University Study," *IRNFP* 3/3 (1979): 197-98.

71. Richard J. Fehring and Donna M. Lawrence, "Spiritual Well-Being, Self-Esteem and Intimacy among Couples Using Natural Family Planning," *Linacre Quarterly* 61:3 (August 1994): 25.

72. Ibid.

73. On competing goods, see Traina, 275 and Lisa Sowle Cahill, *Sex, Gender, and Christian Ethics* (Cambridge: Cambridge University Press, 1996), 204-05.

74. Jim Ternier and Marie-Louise Ternier-Gommers, "Speaking Up for Natural Family Planning," *National Catholic Reporter* (13 February 2004), p. 19.

75. *HV*'s insistence that contraception will decrease men's respect for women denies the possibility that a woman could desire sexual gratification for herself and/or degrade a man, with or without contraception. Moreover, Barbara Andolsen makes the point that women "are asserting ever more strongly that an ability to direct their own reproductive power is essential for their well-being and that of their families" ("Woman and Roman Catholic Sexual Ethics," in Charles E. Curran, Margaret A. Farley, and Richard A. McCormick, eds., *Feminist Ethics and the Catholic Moral Tradition* [New York: Paulist, 1996], 226).

76. See Ruether, "Homophobia, Heterosexism, and Pastoral Practice," in James B. Nelson and Sandra P. Longfellow, eds., *Sexuality and the Sacred: Sources for Theological Reflection* (Louisville, KY: Westminster John Knox Press, 1994), 389.

77. Sylvia Chavez-Garcia and Daniel A. Helminiak, "Sexuality and Spirituality: Friends, not Foes," *Journal of Pastoral Care* 34/6 (June 1985): 160.

78. Traina, 280-82.

79. Shivanadan, "Natural Family Planning and the Theology of the Body," *National Catholic Bioethics Quarterly* 3/1 (Spring 2003): 25.

brace. Both inspire the religious imagination of adherents, making the practice of virtue both easier and more meaningful. One theologian argues that "[t]o reject the fertility of one's spouse as 'unwanted,' or unwanted right now is to reject his or her capacity, together with oneself, to image the Trinity.[80] Conversely, to accept the whole person including fertility is to allow for total oneness, and this one flesh union is the triune God embodied. It is not surprising this view of sex is associated with a positive response to NFP.[81] Mary Shivanadan calls the theology of the body a new discourse for married couples. It has a profound effect on them because it is "much more than a method of family planning. It is a way of discerning God's plan for the family. Many couples view it as a 'way of life.'"[82] Testimonies from NFP couples collected by Kimberly Hahn confirm this insight. "We don't 'have sex'; we give ourselves to each other," says one woman. NFP "added a sacredness to our marital relations that wasn't there when we were contracepting," claims another. As one woman sums up her relationship with her husband since they started using NFP, "I never felt so deeply loved and accepted by him nor so loving and accepting of him. We became keenly aware of the power of each act in a whole new way — a new life could result from *that* act of marriage."[83] NFP brings sex into the realm of the sacred because it links it to virtue, procreative power, and symbolic representation of God.

Writers who defend contraception also believe that practicing sexual virtue leads to spiritual growth. However, according to Ruether, most mature married couples do not struggle to contain desire. She asserts that though celibates might ask, "I have sublimated my sexual drive entirely. Why can't they do it for a little while each month?" married persons "have sublimated the sexual drive into a relationship with another person." It is no longer an abstract drive, but "the intimate expression of one's relationship with this particular other person."[84] It is not that couples cannot control their lust, but that at some moments, "they need to turn to each other for solace, reassurance, renewal of their bonds with each other, [and] it is precisely at this moment and not ten days later that they need to be able to use the sexual act."[85] They need to turn to sex when they feel called to.

Doing otherwise could be seen as ignoring the nature of chastity as a virtue, which calls for the right amount of sex at the right times for the right reasons.[86] Yet most writers who assume contraception do not explicitly invoke the virtue of chastity to inform their discussions of sexuality and spirituality; instead, they focus on the goodness of the body. Many believe that Christian spouses are held back from realizing their full sexual potential, not because they fail to control their desire, but because they are disconnected from their bodies and fail to recognize or respond to their desires.[87] Rejecting the traditional call to exercise self-mastery as unnecessary, James and Evelyn Whitehead ask couples to affirm their belief in the Incarnation ("in the flesh, we meet God")[88] by listening to the stirrings — emotional, intellectual, and sexual — of their own bodies and responding. For too long, the Whiteheads claim, the tradition denigrated non-procreative sex by describing it as "using another person for pleasure," rather than understanding, as married couples always have, that "sexual arousal is about more than lust, that sexual delight is not always selfish. . . . The sexual relationship . . . made life richer and more religious."[89] Desire is recognized as good and even godly, for human passion is connected to God's passion. The goal is to embrace this passion, exploring its depths and riches.[90]

Despite the fact that theologians with differing views on contraception find God in different aspects of the sexual experience, both seek to link sexuality to the divine. Sex between spouses is not just sex, as the culture would have it, nor is it something best avoided by those seeking holiness (unless one desires procreation), as earlier Catholic accounts may have implied. It is, rather, a part of one's Christian commitment, a practice through which married Christians live out their call to discipleship.

In sum, this analysis of experience and family planning shows that those who practice different methods nonetheless share a desire for, and claim the realization of, many of the same goods. True, differences persist. Those who support birth control advocate sex as a way

80. Paula Jean Miller, "The Theology of the Body: A New Look at *Humanae Vitae*," *Theology Today* 57/4 (January 2001): 507.

81. See Borkman and Shivanadan, "The Impact of NFP." Sixty percent of the couples studied found that NFP enhanced the religious or spiritual dimension of their relationship, (64). Sam and Bethany Torode claim that the abstinence required by NFP reminds them of the goodness of sex, making sex as prayer more of a possibility (54). A comparative study of twenty couples using NFP and twenty using contraception found higher spiritual and religious well-being in the NFP couples. See Fehring and Lawrence, 27.

82. Shivandan, "Natural Family Planning and the Theology of the Body," 24.

83. Kimberly Kirk Hahn, *Life-Giving Love: Embracing God's Beautiful Design for Marriage* (Ann Arbor, MI: Servant Press, 2001), 89, 26, 73. Hahn includes a moving meditation on the sacrifice of her own body scarred by numerous difficult pregnancies. She maintains, "through the marital act, we choose to be a living sacrifice," 122.

84. Ruether, 149.

85. Ibid., 150.

86. Christina Traina, "Roman Catholic Resources for an Ethic of Sexuality," unpublished paper, 2004.

87. See Chavez-Garcia and Helminiak, 161. The writers claim that orgasm breaks through human preoccupation with ideas and puts people back in touch with their bodies, opening them to the spiritual dimensions of reality. Many writers speak critically of the Christian tradition's negative view of the body as something to be overcome. See, e.g., Donal Dorr, "Rethinking Sexual Morality," *The Furrow* 53/12 (December 2002): 655. No NFP proponents I read had similar concerns.

88. Whiteheads, 12.

89. Ibid., 17.

90. On this theme, see also James Nelson, *Between Two Gardens: Reflections on Sexuality and Religious Experience* (New York: Pilgrim, 1983), and Fran Ferder and John Heagle, *Your Sexual Self: Pathway to Authentic Intimacy* (Notre Dame, IN: Ave Maria, 1992).

for married couples to grow as partners united in flesh and spirit. With the freedom to have sex when they desire it, practitioners of contraception find themselves more open to each other, their children, and their world. For NFP couples, openness to procreation is a fundamental part of openness to God. Advocates find in their practice a deeper willingness to sacrifice for the other leading to increased intimacy, sexual satisfaction, mutuality, and spiritual growth, all of which are tied to the fundamental willingness to give one's fertility to one's spouse throughout a marriage.

Still, the overlapping desires of contemporary writers seeking the goods of total self-giving, sexual pleasure, mutuality, and a sexual relationship that is deeply spiritual, are profound, and, in my view, ultimately more significant. There is a freshness in this conversation that allows for further growth in sexual ethics and practice, because instead of trying to prove each other's positions illegitimate, this new generation is simply attempting to situate their sexual practice in the context of Christian living.

IV. Conclusion: Sexual Ethics in a New Key

Powerful experiential testimony exists on both sides of the contemporary family planning discussion; listening to all of it is the first step toward a new sexual ethics. Though NFP "works" for far fewer couples than contraception, the testimonies of those who find it satisfying are numerous and enthusiastic enough to compel attention. Conversely, the relative paucity of testimonies and studies on the benefits of contraception is partially made up for by the large numbers of users and by the silence about contraception in most mainstream Christian sexual ethics. But what are moral theologians to make of the many divergent claims embedded in the discussion? Is it appropriate to make judgments about the relative worth of differing arguments? My hope is that bringing the distinctive experiential wisdom of both groups into relief and exploring the common ground that both sides share will make room both for respectful agreement and mutual correction, thus moving the dialogue on sexual ethics beyond the current impasse. I offer a few examples of the sort of critique that may be possible.

The foremost insight of NFP users, total self-giving, ought to be taken more seriously by those who accept contraception. John Paul II has said that total self-giving is the purpose of human existence. If so, NFP couples rightly place donation of the self at the center of their lives. Learning to embrace rather than become frustrated by abstinence and (perhaps) more children, they fully integrate their sexual and spiritual lives. Though proponents of contraception may be correct in their assertion that self-giving is not the whole of sexuality, it seems a crucial dimension, especially when distinguished from the classic norm of "paying the marriage debt." In sexuality, as in all things, human beings are tempted to selfishness or single-minded pursuit of their own pleasure, and though this is not the only sexual sin, it nonetheless remains significant. If a theological concept of self-giving allows couples to transcend individualist desires for pleasure and think more about what sex is really for, and what their partners truly need, perhaps more sexuality could aim toward, if not achieve, real union. In addition, if an ethic of self-giving encourages a greater openness to children and grants them a more significant place in the life of married couples, this may be beneficial. The generous testimonies of NFP couples who speak of their children and their sex lives as parts of a whole stand in contrast to pro-contraception sexual writing that, with few exceptions, fails to mention children. Centering on self-giving seems to open NFP couples in profound ways that cry out for imitation.

Second, NFP practitioners' praise of abstinence calls for serious consideration. In David McCarthy's reading of popular literature on sex, boredom is a recurring theme. Sexologists respond by encouraging couples to re-create the constraining conditions of the courtship period, by spending a weekend at a grandmother's house, having sex in a car, or going to luxury hotel. McCarthy rightly criticizes this attempt to make marriage more exciting by divorcing it from the home, and provocatively advocates a "sexier" reading of the ordinary.[91] But is it not also important to listen to the vast majority of couples (most of whom practice contraception) who find a need to increase sexual tension? According to one extensive study of satisfaction with family planning methods in West Germany, 22-28% of female NFP-users found that the method increased their sexual desire and pleasure. No other method made this large of a difference.[92] Taking regular sabbaths from sex seems to energize sexual relationships, especially in mature marriages. Perhaps women in particular (but not women alone) delight in having a space for non-sexual intimacy that is hard to find when sex is always a possibility. NFP couples may be right to contend that abstinence is "utterly sexual." The practice of NFP inspires many married couples to grow in self-giving and sexual intimacy; it ought not be dismissed.

Yet, writers who assume or argue for contraception have important insights to challenge those who practice NFP. Their insistence on the multiple meanings of sex, including the neglected good of pleasure, is crucial. Advocates of contraception have argued strongly that receiving pleasure is essential to good sex, just as essential as self-giving. While many NFP advocates already affirm that periodic abstinence increases sexual pleasure, most persist in emphasizing the giving over receiving and the need for self-mastery over uncontrollable desire. The reality is that most couples struggle not to contain desire, but to stir it up. Encouraging Christian spouses to enjoy the sexual gifts of their marriage and renew their rela-

91. McCarthy, *Sex and Love in the Home,* 34-44.

92. Oddens, 220. The discrepancy between this finding and pre-1968 surveys is likely due both to the greater reliability of modern NFP as well as strong formation for NFP users.

tionships through sex may be a more important project than reminding them to be chaste.

Second, advocates of contraception rightly recognize that Christians are called to self-giving in many areas of their lives and cannot always open themselves to receiving another child. The desire for some measure of control over how many children they have and when they have them is an expression of their desire to grow in self-giving, as they wish to come together in sexual intimacy without compromising their ability to parent their existing children (or prepare for future children) and to contribute to the broader common good. If the Catholic tradition points toward a dual vocation of family and work for Christian spouses,[93] those who practice contraception uniquely recognize that balancing these commitments requires limitation in both spheres.

Despite bringing distinct, corrective insights to the dialogue on sexual ethics, the two groups share significantly more common ground, including desires to encourage self-giving inside and outside the home, cultivate strong relationships, practice mutuality, grow in sexual intimacy, and discover the transcendent dimensions of sexuality. This common ground is most evident among a new generation of scholars and lay people who cannot be easily categorized as liberal or conservative. In their writing, a counter-cultural focus on self-giving in sexual relationships and beyond sharply contrasts with a cultural backdrop of promiscuous sex for personal pleasure. In addition, a shared relational focus (largely absent in traditional sexual ethics) can be found just as strongly in NFP advocates' frequent testimony that the practice increases communication, intimacy, and union as in contraceptive users' insistence that sex is a necessary glue that binds them together, a natural way for couples to grow in love. Sexual pleasure is a good identified both by NFP advocates who claim that abstinence is sexy and by contraception users who do not want to derail sexual desire when it arises. Both groups are also concerned with mutuality in marriage, and though NFP practitioners focus on shared responsibility for family planning, while those who use contraception emphasize the desires of both men and women for anxiety-free sex and the freedom to pursue multiple vocations, neither group is wedded to the gender-specific limitations of earlier generations of Catholic writers.

Perhaps most important, however, is the shared focus on the transcendent dimensions of sexuality. This is fully evident in writings on both sides, for NFP users, in the language of total self-giving, and for contraception advocates, in the language of passionate human desire connected to divine love. Moreover, theologians on both sides use sacramental language to talk about "the more" of sex. Sr. Mary Timothy Prokes, a passionate defender of John Paul II's theology of the body, claims that Eucharist and sex both "involve reverence for real presence or they are treated with shallow casualness. Sexuality is the possibility of true self-gift and genuine communion of persons: there is no greater realization of this than sacramental Self-Gift as food and drink. What better Common Ground in the Body of Christ than shared understanding of sexual reality and Eucharist?"[94] Similarly, radical Protestant theologian James Nelson quotes Molly in James Joyce's *Ulysses* ("yes I said yes I will Yes."), affirming, "We human beings know in our sexual experience something of Molly's yes. But Molly is not only us. Molly is also the hungering, passionate God who meets us bodily."[95] Even as they take from the secular culture promising commitments to relational growth and mutuality, advocates of different family planning methods are joined together in their rejection of secular tendencies to not take sex seriously enough and in a common understanding of sexual experience as sacramental.[96]

The most important task for both sides of this dialogue is to continue developing an experientially-based theological vision that can serve as a guide for the sexual relationships that are central in the lives of most Christians. The Papal birth control commission began this work some forty years ago when they listened to the experiences of married couples who were struggling with what the church asked of them. Although support for contraception did not find favor with Paul VI, there is no doubt that the CFM surveys influenced the development of a more personalist understanding of sex and marriage that was evident in *HV*. The dialogue that followed was valuable in laying out the defense of each side's positions on contraception, but it often failed in attentiveness to experience and in situating sexual ethics within the context of Christian discipleship. Now a new generation of scholars, which includes many more married theologians, many more women, and many more Catholics born after the second Vatican Council and raised out of Catholic subcultures, has come to the fore.[97] They share a desire to live distinctive Christian lives and know sex is a part of that. They will do well to continue to listen rightly to experience in all its diversity, not so they can prove one side right or wrong, but so that they might raise up for married Christians values worth pursuing in sexual relationships. If couples can then ask good questions (Are we giving as much of our selves as possible in our sexual relationship? Does sex contribute to our growth in mutuality? Are we honoring the goodness of sexual desire? Do we recognize the presence of grace when we have sex?), theologians will have made a valuable contribution.

93. See Julie Hanlon Rubio, "The Dual Vocation of Christian Parents," *Theological Studies* 63 (December 2002): 786-812.

94. Sr. Mary Timothy Prokes, "The Catholic Tradition and Sexual Teaching," unpublished paper, 2004.

95. Nelson, 32.

96. David McCarthy's critique of sexual theologies that place too much importance on individual sexual acts is important to keep in mind here. Sex may be sacramental in the context of a lifelong marriage, even if particular acts mean relatively little (see *Sex and Love in the Home*, 46-48).

97. See William Portier, "Here Come the Evangelical Catholics," *Communio* 31/1 (Spring 2004): 35-66.

113 Procreation, the Development of Peoples, and the Final Destiny of Humanity

David M. McCarthy

Why another article on *Humanae Vitae?* As exhaustive and interminable as the debate has been, prominent defenders and opponents have not presented the encyclical's arguments accurately. *HV* is a statement about the very meaning of our nature and the continuity of our natural life with our supernatural fulfillment. The encyclical is not an argument from nature as much as a proposal about our nature from the givens of our true end. To speak of nature in this way is to make a claim about what binds us in human solidarity, ultimately defined as our common life with God. *HV*'s appeal to nature is set before this backdrop of our eschatological communion, and this theological setting is the basis for *HV*'s teaching on contraception as a social teaching.

Opponents are apt to interpret Paul VI's reference to nature as vulgar physicalism, claiming that it binds human nature to biological functions in a way that is both irrational and inconsistent. First, they argue that a rejection of "artificial" contraception disregards the fundamental character of human thinking and doing as artistry, through which we impose form upon nature. Second, they hold that the Catholic tradition's supposedly physicalist orientation to sex is inconsistent with its personalist, historically conscious approach to other issues, particularly the tradition's social teaching.[1] Opponents are convinced that the encyclical marks a point where magisterial teaching has refused to develop. In their view, the teaching of *HV* resists not merely modern developments in the Church, but especially cultural, political, and scientific advancements.

Defenders of the teaching share a great deal with opponents, particularly their questions about rational arguments and natural law. Defenders debate among themselves whether *HV*'s arguments are inadequate, incomplete, or not arguments at all.[2] Some depart from the document entirely for the sake of what they take to be firmer rational principles. Others create or develop arguments by making selected sections of the document, say nos. 9-12, the context for the whole. The framework of *HV* is, however, at once social and theological, since it begins with a statement about our cooperation with God and repeatedly turns to concerns about human community. Either by design or by a simple shift in focus, defenders exclude Paul VI's social arguments and, in doing so, miss his eschatologically informed claims about our social nature.

This article challenges both opponents and notable defenders by assuming that *HV* does provide clear arguments, that the encyclical as a whole provides the context for these arguments, and that *HV* squares with Paul VI's other pronouncements and addresses, that is, with his persistent social, political, and economic themes. The first section of the article sets out the encyclical's themes in summary form: the procreative character of sexual acts must be defended if we seek true human development, and, in this regard, the very meaning and destiny of our created nature is at stake. The second section attends to *HV*'s introduction, where Paul VI articulates the theological significance of procreation and immediately turns to various social questions. This second section discusses Paul VI's critique of modern accounts of economic development, which ironically do not advance but rather diminish human life since they block a full theological understanding of human flourishing. It is not merely coincidental that reductionist proposals for economic progress depend upon contraceptive technology as a means for advancement, for the upward mobility of citizens, and for the development of nations. To this degree, *HV*'s opposition to artificial contraception parallels Paul VI's arguments in documents such as *Populorum Progressio* and *Octogesima Adveniens*. The teaching on contraception is a social teaching, and the social teaching is founded on theological claims about human solidarity and upon the continuity between our natural and supernatural, or eschatological, fulfillment.

Sections three and four proceed by showing both the ironies in contemporary arguments and Pope Paul VI's contrasting proposals for the dignity of women and the meaning of marital love. Sections five and six deal with arguments in support of *HV* that attempt to extract the teaching from its theological context and social concerns in favor of a phenomenology of the sexual act, on one hand, and a Kantian appeal to the will, on the other. In the first case, a certain kind of personalist philosophical approach neglects Paul VI's social arguments and shifts emphasis from his practical economic and political questions to the "private" act of nuptial self-giving. In the second case, Germain Grisez's philosophical defense, it is argued, fails in its attempt to secure the procreative character of sexual acts without an account of grace, without reference to the fullness of our nature in terms of our eschatological communion. In each case, the integrity of *HV*'s theological framework is diminished, and the

1. Charles E. Curran, "Official Catholic Social and Sexual Teachings: A Methodological Comparison," in *Tensions in Moral Theology* (Notre Dame: University of Notre Dame Press, 1988), 87-109.

2. Janet E. Smith, *Humanae Vitae: A Generation Later* (Washington, D.C.: The Catholic University of America Press, 1991), 68f, 98f.

From David Matzko McCarthy, "Procreation, the Development of Peoples, and the Final Destiny of Humanity," original publication and copyright by *Communio: International Catholic Review* 26 (Winter, 1999): 698-721.

teaching on contraception is weakened. Insofar as they disregard Paul VI's social concerns, these defenses of *HV* miss the necessity of his call to the Church to be a sign of human solidarity in the fullness of our creation.

1. A Truly Human Society

Paul VI proposes that we cannot make the world a better place by denying the procreative character of human sexuality. In *HV,* he relates the issue of contraception to contemporary social problems, to which contraception is considered by many to be a solution but, in fact, holds out only hollow promises for the goods of life. Contraceptive practices promise relief in a culture where child rearing is an economic liability and a risk to one's personal lifestyle, but Paul VI warns that we will undercut the basic structure of social life if we abdicate our common calling to bear and raise children. Modern development strategies promote advancement by means of eliminating the social and economic drag of having children. Paul VI, in contrast, is convinced that true development necessarily includes the basic human activities of child rearing. *HV* fits with his wider proposals for authentic human development. True human community cannot be attained at the cost of its own generative character, and true development is known through the flourishing of creation, of which this generative character is a part.

In strong terms, Paul VI asserts that procreation is fundamental to God's design, and, as such, the procreative character of sexual acts is not optional. The generative quality of sexuality, as a given of creation, does not determine that every sexual act produces a child, nor does it exclude scientific analysis, moral discernment, and "life-determining" decisions. On the contrary, *HV* holds that the givens of procreation and of human rationality mandate scientific artistry and reasoned choices. Such mastery, though, must accord with our proper dominion over nature and our role in the perfection of creation in cooperation with God's creative activity.[3] As we reason and act as creatures upon creation, human artistry and technological manipulations are excessive only insofar as we attempt to undermine God's providential order, which is to say, when we subvert our own good. We cross over into excess when we attempt to extricate sex from its own procreative character, even if we do so in an effort to make our lives better. When our answers to human need sever the link between our human good and the Creator, we cannot but fail.

The link between God's design, our nature, and our good end is the linchpin for the encyclical's arguments. The character of our nature as ordered creation underlies every point and sets the claims of *HV* within the framework of our participation in God's gracious activity and the fulfillment of our human nature through a supernatural end. Questions about our nature are always social because they refer to claims about human solidarity, and these claims are eschatological: true human community is precisely the meaning and mission of the Church.[4] By abiding in continuity with our supernatural end, we will see creation coming to fulfillment, which is the very possibility of authentic human community. *HV* says nothing less.

2. Population and Progress

"The transmission of human life," Paul VI begins, "is a most serious role [*munus*] in which married people collaborate freely and responsibly with God the Creator" (*HV,* 1).[5] Our *munus* has a definite theological character as participation in God's creative activity.[6] The second paragraph of *HV*'s introduction turns to social questions as a further account of this role of transmitting human life — as "intimately connected with the life and happiness of human beings" (no. 1). Part 1 of the encyclical outlines various social developments and the new questions that they bring (nos. 2-3). The substance and tenor of this section are repeated in what are supposed to be Paul VI's more "social" pronouncements. In *Octogesima Adveniens,* for instance, he explains that amid "present changes, which are so profound and so rapid . . . man discovers himself anew, and he questions himself about the meaning of his own being and of his own collective survival" (no. 7).[7] Paul VI sets contraception in this context of inquiry.

First in *HV*'s list of social concerns are the rapid increase in population, which creates hardships for families and developing countries, and modern economic conditions, which put an increasing burden on housing and raising large families. Faced with fears of overpopulation, public authorities, Paul VI worries, may attempt to relieve the strain by resorting to "drastic measures." To the World Food Conference in 1974, he holds that "it is inadmissible that those who have control of the wealth and resources of mankind should try to resolve the problem of hunger by forbidding the poor to be born, or by leaving to die of hunger children whose parents do not fit

3. Cf. *Summa Theologiae* I, qq. 90-102.

4. Henri de Lubac, *Catholicism: Christ and the Common Destiny of Man,* trans. Lancelot C. Sheppard and Sister Elizabeth Englund, OCD (San Francisco: Ignatius Press, 1988), 48-55.

5. *The Papal Encyclicals 1958-1981,* trans. Claudia Carlen (Wilmington, NC: McGrath Publishing Co., 1981), 223-33. The Latin text is in Peter Harris, et al., *On Human Life: An Examination of* Humanae Vitae (London: Burns and Oates, Ltd, 1968), 107-61.

6. Janet Smith argues that our *munus* is key to the document and is best rendered as our "mission" of transmitting new life — in order to highlight the term's meaning as a privilege and honor, a special assignment, a mark of human dignity, and a role corresponding to our supernatural destiny (*Humanae Vitae: A Generation Later,* 136-37, 297, 314). Smith, though, attempts an exhaustive treatment of our *munus* with virtually no reference to the social commentary at the beginning and end of *HV.*

7. Msgr. Joseph Gremillion, *The Gospel of Peace and Justice* (Maryknoll, NY: Orbis Press, 1976), 85-512.

into the framework of theoretical plans based on pure hypotheses about the future of mankind" (*Address to the World Food Conference* [= *WFC*], 6).[8] These pure hypotheses were, in the 60s and 70s, based on mere numbers.[9] Since then, Paul VI's objections have become an important part of the debate. Population is now understood to be a problem of economic justice, urbanization, and First World consumption.

Population and hunger, for Paul VI, are crises of human solidarity as well. "Is it not a new form of warfare to impose a restrictive demographic policy on nations, to ensure that they will not claim their just share of the earth's goods?" (*WFC*, 6). Ironically, the poor and hungry increase in number through so-called development programs. These programs reduce social life to economic value; they assume that "progress" means industrialization, and they place too much confidence in purely technological solutions (which ultimately serve already "advanced" nations) (*WFC*, 4). Six years before the World Food Conference, Paul VI articulates the same critique in reference to artificial regulation of births. Contraception is a false solution that diminishes the lives of those who purportedly will be helped the most.

After population and progress, *HV* lists other pertinent developments. Our new situation is characterized by new understandings of a woman's role in society, the value of conjugal love, and the relationship of sex to this love. We will treat these issues in the subsections that follow. At this point, in order to fit these matters in Paul VI's frame of reference, we will consider what he refers to as the most significant modern advance; i.e., the remarkable progress "in the domination and rational organization of the forces of nature to the point that he [man] is endeavoring to extend this control over every aspect of his own life. . . ." Paul VI's comments on population, economic change, and issues like the role of women culminate with this pressing concern. Humans are attaining control over the body, the mind, social life, "and even over the laws that regulate the transmission of life" (*HV*, 2).

Our increasing ability to manipulate human life coincides with contemporary assumptions about progress. Common sense formulae for economic growth pit money-making and childbearing against each other not only in terms of a global equation for developing countries, but also for the American middle-class couple who secure their own bit of economic and social advancement (along with their careers) with what has become a requisite access to contraceptives. Control and efficiency are fundamental to progress because children are inefficient (they are voracious time consumers). Controlling births is risk management. Bearing and raising children (and domestic life as a whole) is no longer considered a productive venture, but a practice of consumption that drains rather than accrues resources. Contraception allows women and men to shift energy, time, and talent from the domestic to the productive sphere, and to this degree controlling the procreative character of human life has become the necessary insurance required to bear and raise children properly. Contraception is as obvious to economic common sense as mutual funds and putting money in the bank.

Paul VI challenges this logic of contraception by objecting to its underlying assumptions about productivity and progress. In *Populorum Progressio* and *Octogesima Adveniens,* he argues that development and progress are false when defined primarily in economic terms. Such progress actually frustrates growth on both personal and social levels. Reductively economic development divides the rich from the poor both within and between nations. It causes injustices, civil unrest, and disenfranchisement. Economic progress, typically conceived, leaves much of the human being behind, sets humans against themselves, and destroys the earth. Reductively defined economic progress is nothing but human decline, while genuine development, in contrast, rejects the reduction of human life to merely economic terms. Here, Paul VI is merely elaborating the Church's social teaching, explicitly stated by Leo XIII, that economics is defined by relations that exceed economic terms. Rich and poor, employer and employee, governor and governed are bound together by a deeper, organic bond. True progress, then, embraces the whole human being and the whole of human community, and it is directed to our eschatological (rather than merely temporal) solidarity.

Because economic development, in the materialist sense, is progress only in the most narrow terms, it develops into a privation of human life. When a reductionist view of social life dominates public goods, so-called advancement diminishes us. Paul VI suggests this same irony in *HV* when he notes that working and housing conditions are posing increasing difficulties for families. While large families are usually understood as barriers to economic advancement, could the reverse be the case? Could so-called progress place a burden upon families because it is not real progress at all? Are technological solutions simply exacerbating the problem; i.e., encouraging "developments" that are, in fact, set against the progress of humanity? Put another way, is childbearing set against money-making because the system of money-making is itself set against human solidarity and true social development?

When pursued outside of God's design for human community, human advancement contradicts itself. To this degree, human nature "as we have it" is properly understood only against the backdrop of our eschatological end. Modern political and economic structures, in contrast, prescind from (and actually disavow) questions about common ends, but then, through assumptions about scientific inevitability, ends are defined technologically (and technology is shaped in large part by the market). More precisely, technology defines the meaning of

8. *The Gospel of Peace and Justice,* 599-600.

9. See *Limits to Growth* (New York: Universe Books, 1972); *The Gospel of Peace and Justice,* 91-96; Nicholas Eberstadt, "Population Policy: Ideology as Science," *First Things* 40 (January 1994): 30-38.

its own advancement as though it stood apart from human culture. Technology in this sense is inherently disordered, and contraceptive technology is likely to be a symptom of social problems rather than a real solution.

Contraceptive practices assume that our God-given nature inhibits our fulfillment, while *HV*, in contrast, assumes that our regulation of births must accord with the completion of our natures through participation in the life of God. For this reason, Paul VI states outright that the procreative character of human life is not an option. "[Couples] are not free to act as they choose in the service of transmitting life . . . [but] are bound to ensure that what they do corresponds to the will of God the Creator" (*HV*, 10). In *Populorum Progressio* as well, Paul VI situates human development within the context of the Creator's design. "Self-development is not left up to man's option. Just as the whole of creation is ordered toward its Creator, so too the rational creature should of his own accord direct his life to God, the first truth and the highest good. Thus human self-fulfillment may be said to sum up our obligations" (*Populorum Progressio* [= *PP*], 16). Both *Populorum Progressio* and *Humanae Vitae* hold economic and cultural progress up to the test of human fulfillment — earthly and eschatological. If "self-development" and the procreative character of human life are disregarded, then progress and human mastery are out of control. The abundance that comes in these reductionist terms is inauthentic, self-serving, and unjust.

3. The Role and Dignity of Women

Contemporary views about the dignity of women reveal the same irony of so-called progress. In the modern conception, reproductive rights (to abortion as well as contraception) have been hailed as guarantors of women's equality, autonomy, and bodily integrity. Paul VI proposes the contrary. Contraception, he holds, establishes habits (basic social practices) which disregard the dignity of women, disrupt their "physical and emotional equilibrium," and reduce them to instruments of desire (*HV*, 17). Contraception fosters a lack of reverence for women insofar as it frees up the arbitrary will of men and violates the limits of control set within creation. In *Octogesima Adveniens*, Paul VI rejects "that false equality [for women] which would deny the distinctions laid down by the Creator himself and which would be in contradiction with woman's proper role, which is of such capital importance, at the heart of family as well as society" (*OA*, 13). Contraceptive practices, Paul VI claims, diminish the dignity of women and the integrity of their bodies.

To many, such a claim is understood as discriminatory and patriarchal. To liberal feminist ears, Paul VI's notion of "a woman's proper role" rings of a tradition where men dominate women. Such control over women is, however, precisely Paul VI's fear. *HV* is not concerned with what women will do with contraceptives but what men will do to women. This focus on men will be considered by some to be merely a consequence of sexist assumptions; that is, the actions of men are at issue only because it is assumed that women are not moral agents and that society, perforce, is an audience of men. This interpretation of audience misses the radical implications of Paul VI's appeal to woman's dignity and his rejection of contraceptive control over a woman's body.

Contraceptive rights promise a measure of freedom, but the deeper irony is that they insure that procreation, parenting, and sexual pleasure continue to be defined according to the "arbitrary will of men." To expand a point made by Germaine Greer, "historically the only thing pro-abortion agitation achieved was to make an illiberal establishment look far more feminist than it was."[10] The same can be said for reproductive rights in general. From a trenchant feminist point of view, Greer argues that reproductive technology has liberated men — sexually, socially, and economically — far more than it has women.[11] Not Paul VI's ally by any means, she shares his concerns about modern technological control over fertility and childbirth. Like Paul VI, she points to a diminishing regard for a woman's role, the social role, of bearing and nurturing their infants. Greer advances her arguments by appealing to common economic and social practices.

Contemporary economic and cultural developments, she agrees, have shaped liberation for women such that motherhood is a liability in a way that fatherhood is not. Women have had to succeed in work through standards established for men who have been and remain free from the day-to-day burdens of raising children. Women, far more than men, are confronted with difficult decisions dividing career and parenting. The privatization of the domestic sphere promises liberation by leaving distinctions between women's and men's work a matter of personal preference, but this preference seems to be the prerogative of men. Mothers, more often than not, will schedule employment around the needs of their children. Fathers, on the other hand, will schedule their care for children around the dictates of work. Parenting for a father is, by and large, an option — on the occasions when he agrees to babysit the children. Men who raise children on their own are saints, but women who do so are regarded largely as a social and economic plague. Single mothers who work are considered inferior parents, and those who stay home are welfare queens. When all is said, it seems that women have been liberated except in spheres of life where they cannot help being women.[12]

10. G. Greer, *The Whole Woman* (New York: Alfred A. Knopf, 1999), 92.

11. Ibid., 39-48, 127-36.

12. Paula Allen-Meares and Eric M. Roberts, "Public Assistance as Family Policy: Closing off Options for Poor Families," *Social Work* 40 (July 1995) 4: 559-65; Susan L. Thomas, "Women, Welfare, Reform and the Preservation of a Myth," *The Social Science Journal* 34 (1997) 3: 351-68; Rosanna Hertz and Faith I. T. Ferguson, "Childcare Choice and the Constraints in the United States: Social Class, Race, and the Influence of Family Views," *Journal of Comparative Family Studies* 27 (Summer 1996): 249-80.

Economic and social equality for women is achieved by avoiding children or at least the practical burdens of bearing them. Parents who conceive a child (and are economically viable) begin to plot damage control — because the modern economy will not allow a place for children and child rearing. The modern economy does not make room for pregnancy, breast feeding, or "idling" about with youngsters. None of these are understood to be work at all — unless, of course, one is a surrogate mother or day care worker, unless one is contracted to raise someone else's child. Men, for their part, have successfully defined productivity in terms that belittle the private, domestic sphere and keep women's equality from increasing their own role in childcare. Dependable reproductive control has become a basic principle of economic freedom and advancement; it has become necessary for meaningful work and social equality for women in relation to this work. A distinctive woman's role has no economic currency, even if we give a modest description of this role as nine months of pregnancy and several more of breast feeding. Our economy is set against it, and contraception sustains the false promises of this so-called economic freedom.

The same can be said for sexual liberation. Contraception buttresses social practices that are inhospitable to children, so that women are burdened with child rearing but allowed to enter public and economic life only without their offspring. All the while, pornography, strip clubs, and other facets of the sex industry are an economic boon. Contraception has been indispensable in shaping liberation so that women continue to serve the sexual needs of men. In this way, sexual liberation has given a new meaning to "a woman's role." If the connection between sex and procreation is a problem for sexual liberation, it is a problem fundamentally for men, and severing the link is fundamentally liberation for men. Women are available to men without complications of children, and if conception does occur, men avoid the burden with the line, "whatever you decide, honey." If, in this culture of pleasure, the distinctiveness of being a woman were taken seriously, dependence on natural family planning would be the most decisive feminist step in taking the pleasure of women out of the control of men. It seems unimaginable in modern culture, even among the liberated, to ask a man to conform his desire to what is natural to a woman. The radical feminist should find an ally in Paul VI, who would see both pornography and contraceptive practices as giving women over to the desires of men. If we believe that our God-given nature directs us to genuine fulfillment, defending the natural generative process is speaking for the advancement of women. It is plausible that *HV* troubles liberal feminists not because it is retrograde but because it is too radically progressive, calling both men and women to the "mission" of raising children.

4. Love

In *HV* no. 2, Paul VI also points to new understandings of "the value of conjugal love in marriage and the relationship of conjugal acts to this love." Throughout the encyclical, he responds to the view that contraceptive acts might be permissible if they protect the good of raising existing children and strengthen love by serving the end of conjugal union.[13] In response, Paul VI does not allow procreative and unitive ends to be divided and set against one another. "The reason is that the fundamental nature of the marriage act, while uniting husband and wife in the closest intimacy, also renders them capable of generating new life — and this is the result of laws written into the actual nature of man and of woman" (no. 12). This statement raises topics which will be considered in sections that follow, particularly the issue of natural law. At this point, we will deal with the claim, which Paul VI rebuts, that sexual lovemaking is a separable good that can be sustained over against the procreative character of sexual intercourse.

Like so-called economic development, sexual lovemaking, in the modern sense, has an ironic result. Sexual notions and practices have shifted focus from "making babies" to "making love." Whether sex was considered a marital duty, a generative act (for the common good), or the prerogative of social status, only in the twentieth-century does intercourse become a producer of love. It is common in our culture to establish or verify love through sex. That is, either the sexual relationship precedes and creates the context for germinating love, or love is confirmed or invalidated according to criteria of sexual compatibility. Intimate relationships might be carried on "just for the sex," but it is unthinkable to sustain such a bond merely for the sake of progeny. The former is assumed to be filled with pleasure, while the latter is thought to be hollow — lacking true love. The logic of contraception is obvious here. In order to free sex for its lovemaking, procreation must be extracted from the essential possibilities of sexual events. Paul VI points to the irony. Contraceptive habits contribute to marital infidelity (no. 17). When sex is freed from procreation for the sake of love, our sexual practices are less able to sustain this love. When sexual lovemaking proliferates, there is no evidence that more love has been produced.[14]

Love is generative. Few would disagree, but it is striking that we, in the modern world, consider the non-procreative aspects of sex the lovemaking part, while our procreative capacities are considered impersonal — the realm of reproductive instincts that bring psychological satisfaction. Technological interventions promise better

13. Cf. *HV*, nos. 3, 7, 8-9, 12-14.

14. In a culture with a high divorce rate, proponents of natural family planning promote its relational and psychological benefits. They are quick to cite statistics about the enduring marriages among couples who use natural family planning. See Nona Aguilar, *No-Pill, No-Risk Birth Control* (New York: Rawson, Wade Publishers, Inc., 1980), 97-106.

children, and with modern know-how, it is assumed that anyone can have a child if he or she wants. The Catholic tradition, in contrast, assumes that marital sex is the requisite context for childbearing (but not always rearing: e.g., in the case of adoption). The tradition understands love as fecund, receptive, and hospitable — by its nature open to the stranger, to expanding community, to growth, and to life. When outlining the character of conjugal love (*HV*, 9), Paul VI holds that this love "is not confined wholly to the loving interchange of husband and wife; it also contrives to go beyond this to bring new life into being."[15] In an address two years later, he summarizes this section of the encyclical by making fruitfulness not only the last on his list of love's qualities (human, total, faithful, fecund), but also the completion of all. "The marriage act . . . supports and strengthens their love, and in the fruitfulness of this act the couple finds its total fulfillment: in the image of God the couple becomes a source of life" (*To the Teams of Our Lady*, 6).[16] When defining "the fruitfulness of this act," Paul VI speaks not of a couple's intentions (their openness to children) but of actually bearing and raising children. Bearing children turns love to hospitality and, in doing so, fulfills it. To this degree, it is couples who choose not to have children, rather than parents, who carry the heavy burden (*To the Teams of Our Lady*, 10-11). The fulfillment of their love does not take its usual concrete form. Childbearing, nevertheless, defines their bond, and they must seek other means to express love's generativity.

The fulfillment of love in childbearing is not an abstract theological point. In a contraceptive world, raising children is a set of practices that transforms our lives. We must accommodate the life of an utterly dependent infant who grows into a child whose personality and demands upon us we cannot anticipate. We are taken into a pilgrimage of love — often sitting down with a stranger at our own supper table. In a world obsessed with economic efficiency, children require time and attention, and in the process of opening to children, we learn the habits of community. Parents are active in their communities when they are engaged in the management of the household, when they extend the practices of parenthood to the front stoop and the neighborhood park. When a person cooks for one or two, he or she is not likely to make a full meal on a day to day basis, but parents who cook for four or five must make a banquet every night (hot dogs and macaroni and cheese perhaps). When a banquet is served guests are expected and appreciated — even neighboring children are a welcomed entertainment. Hospitality, Paul VI claims, is the special vocation of the family (*To the Teams of Our Lady*, 12).

Community and hospitality are undone, of course, when the modern economy and our social atomization dictate our practices of care, when both parents rush home at six o'clock every day to throw together a meal, or when parents, especially single parents, must struggle alone without the bonds of a neighborhood community. We make child-rearing a private matter, rather than a basic social bond, and openness to children likewise becomes a private gesture, rather than a practice of common life.

Modern lovemaking is sustained by restricting procreation; children are not and certainly cannot be a basic sign of nuptial love. Not only are the practices of raising children made relative to personal preferences, but the full meaning of a woman's body is disjoined from childbearing and defined fundamentally by her receptivity to men. In contrast, love, theologically understood, is prolific. In the greater part of the Catholic tradition, a man and a woman, it is believed, do not fully express their love in the complementarity of their binary intimacy. If, following Paul VI, bearing and raising children is understood as the concrete progression of love, the pregnant woman (not the conjugal act in itself) should be considered the full sign of our participation in the life of God (for both women and men).[17] It is the expanding womb that gives the most visible expression to the *munus* of marriage and the generative quality of love. The pregnant woman is not an image of oppression — unless a society conceives of a child as a woman's burden and offers (so-called) aid primarily through technological mastery and control over a woman's body. In a community of hospitality, a woman's distinctive role in childbirth could take the lead in expressing the human image of God, our cooperation in the life of the Creator, and our assent to grace — all in a profoundly mariological sense. Mary is our archetype, as our receptivity to God grounds all human agency and the activity of love.

5. Union and Procreation

The modern notion of lovemaking takes a different trajectory in Catholic theology, from the priority of procreation to, at least, an equality of the procreative and unitive ends of conjugal love. This development (as seen in *HV*) maintains that the two ends are inseparable. Subsequent defenses of the teaching have secured the connection by fitting the procreative end within the wider scope of unity and love; that is, the total self-giving of spouses, if authentic, must include the procreative qualities of their own sexuality.[18] It is arguable that this con-

15. From *Gaudium et Spes*, 50.

16. Janet E. Smith, ed., *Why Humanae Vitae Was Right: A Reader* (San Francisco: Ignatius Press, 1993), 85-104.

17. As an aside, it is interesting to note that some feminists now argue that modern political, economic, and legal structures will be set against women until the pregnant woman (rather than the wage earning man) conceptually represents the "individual" in politics and law. See Zillah R. Eisenstein, *The Female Body and the Law* (Berkeley: University of California Press, 1988). Cf. Carole Pateman, *The Sexual Contract* (Stanford: Stanford University Press, 1988).

18. The collection of essays in *Why Humanae Vitae Was Right*, edited by Janet E. Smith, is representative. Smith includes early de-

ceptual development is consistent with Paul VI's assertions regarding the indivisibility of unitive and procreative ends, but it is, nevertheless, an interpretive strategy with its own distinct philosophical background — a certain school of philosophical personalism. And while the consistency of this view with *HV* is plausible and well argued, I will suggest that, as often defended, it implies a subtle departure from the encyclical. There is no reason simply to reject personalist arguments; but often these arguments do not provide an adequate philosophical foundation, because they do not pay enough attention to the theological content of God's design.

A certain "personalist" argument situates procreation within the unitive end of marriage, but we have seen in the previous discussion of love that, if anything, Paul VI reverses this, arguing that conjugal union is given a procreative meaning. "To experience the gift of married love while respecting the laws of conception is to acknowledge that one is not the master of the sources of life but rather the minister of the design established by the Creator." Paul VI punctuates this claim, once again, by rejecting "unlimited dominion" over our own bodies and by asserting that our sexual faculties are "concerned by their very nature with the generation of life, of which God is the source" (no. 13). Therefore, although there is a school of philosophical personalism that presents our openness to children as necessary to our full personal union, Paul VI holds that our union has its full expression in the actual presence of children. This slight shift in emphasis makes a significant difference.

This philosophical personalism is concerned to answer contending personalist attempts to separate unitive and procreative ends so that contraceptive acts might be justified for the good of the nuptial bond. Such a philosophical view defends *HV* by showing that our subjective openness to the procreative character of our sexuality is necessary to expressing conjugal love. But like its opponents, this "conservative" personalism constructs an argument which tends to make actual children unnecessary to the full articulation of conjugal union. According to this view, artificial contraception differs from natural family planning to the degree that the former withholds an aspect of the self while the latter does not. In the latter case, true sexual expression, including its procreative quality, is not diminished, so that total self-giving is sustained. Sexual intercourse itself, when open to procreation, is the basic sign of love, and to this degree the philosophical personalists outpersonalize their liberal opponents. Contraceptive intercourse does not sustain nuptial unity, because it withholds part of the sexual self and therefore is a false self-giving (i.e., a lie).

Paul VI responds to opponents by referring directly to God's design and to the problems of our unlimited dominion over human life. Artificial contraception is false in relation to God and our *munus* of transmitting new life. It is first of all pride in relation to God. This distinction between Paul VI's claim and the personalist development is slight, but important. The latter approach has the personalist (and modern) advantage of putting intercourse during fertile and infertile periods on the same level; i.e., both are the same total self-giving. It is not obvious, however, that this is the case in *HV*. This is not to say, of course, that the two perspectives are mutually exclusive, but only that they need to be integrated in such a way that the concreteness of childbearing remains essential to the integrity of sexuality.

In *HV*, recourse to infertile periods and abstinence during fertility (no. 16) are understood as interim practices which have their meaning in reference to the birth of children. They involve a reasoned decision not to have *another child*, for a time or permanently (no. 10). The meaning of recourse to infertile periods, then, is dependent on preceding or subsequent intercourse during fertility. Infertile intercourse and abstinence are not self-sustained but have meaning only in subordinate relation to actual conception and childbirth. For Paul VI, conjugal love (whether fertile or not) has a natural movement toward fulfillment in childbirth and generative practices of hospitality. A personalist difficulty with this argument is that it puts modern lovemaking in a subordinate position, along with intercourse for post-menopausal and barren couples. The argument requires the childless couple to understand the fullness of their love as completed in the childbearing of others and in their own cooperation in the generative practices of a community — educating children or the works of mercy perhaps.[19] The advantage to Paul VI's argument is that he does not have to develop a separate set of arguments for having children at all.

In short, *HV* is more practically oriented toward children. A certain philosophical personalism is more abstract and "private," since openness to procreation is understood as an openness to our humanity and a full self-giving to another. *HV* does not simply contradict this,

fenses such as Dietrich Von Hildebrand's *The Encyclical* Humanae Vitae: *A Sign of Contradiction* (Chicago: Franciscan Herald Press, 1969), and elaborations of John Paul II's phenomenology of the body, such as Cormac Burke's "Marriage and Contraception," *Linacre Quarterly* 55 (1988): 44-55. See John Paul II's *Love and Responsibility* (New York: Farrar Straus, Giroux, 1981) and *Sacred in All Its Forms* (Boston: Daughters of St. Paul, 1984). It seems to me that those who use John Paul II's phenomenology do not give full account of his theological and social framework, found in *Familiaris Consortio* for instance (1981). In *Familiaris Consortio,* arguments against contraception are supported mainly by the ecclesiological structure of the document (including a theology of sacrament and vocation). In John Paul II's more recent *Letter of Families* (1994), his notion of culture, which animates his social teaching, provides the structure.

19. The point here is not that infertile couples are inferior, but like all couples, their love is not autonomous. Their sexual expression has the same status as infertile intercourse for all married. Sexual intercourse, whether leading to conception or not, is intelligible within the childbearing and rearing practices of common life (thus Paul VI's social concerns are essential to the argument).

but assumes that this openness is fully expressed only in the birth of a child. Children expand the concrete expression of a single sexual act over a lifetime — as bearing and raising children determine us through the role of parenting. We are called not only to union as spouses, but to openness as mother and father — in the concrete and particular presence of another (or third, fourth, fifth) human being. Bearing children is the primary sign of love because it is a practical and social expression of love's generativity. Our created nature determines that the intimacy of sexual union has an intrinsic relationship to the transmission of life.

6. Social Teaching, Eschatology, and "Every Act"

Paul VI argues against contraception on the same terms that he critiques global economic planning and reductively technological (impersonal) solutions to problems of human community. In each, he appeals to God's design for creation and the eschatological destiny of human life. Reductionist standards of progress and easy technological solutions do not promote nurture and human growth — whether in the areas of Third World development or of sexual freedom. Contraception is certainly a question about the beginning of life, but primarily it is an issue of human solidarity, in accord with the end of creation and our community with God. Elaborating this theme, Paul VI calls the Church a sign of contradiction (*HV*, 18). Contraception represents a set of social practices directed toward improving the conditions and fate of the world, and to be against such noble efforts is certainly foolishness. The Church's rejection of contraception resists the goals of modern progress for the sake of our end in God. The rejection of contraception, then, entails a set of practices as well, "contributing to the creation of a truly human civilization" (no. 18). The teaching against contraception is a call for instituting the practices of an authentically generative economy and a procreative way of life.

In response to this critique of our contraceptive economy and culture, many will nod in approval; yet, at the same time, many will continue to reject the notion that all contraceptive acts are illicit.[20] In fact, when a qualified use of contraceptives is justified, it is precisely the social and economic burdens of child rearing that count as good reasons. *HV*'s own social critique is used to reject its basic teaching that each and every conjugal act must be open to new life (*HV*, 11). In the context of this debate, the "every act" provision has become the dominant issue of the encyclical, and defenders of the teaching have shaped their moral arguments in order to diminish the importance of social and economic pressures. In their arguments, defenders have extracted the middle of the document (nos. 7-16) from its social and theological context — in order to establish a firmer, independent basis for the "every act" teaching. In the end, such defenses actually undercut the internal logic of *HV*'s "every act" qualification by disengaging it not only from its social framework but, at the same time, from its eschatological convictions about the social teleology of nature as well.

In the Catholic tradition, nature makes sense in relation to the Creator, and natural law makes sense insofar as we assume: (1) that the integrity of human reason is established by God for human good; and (2) that human goods and good actions are good because they accord with God's providential design (whether intentionally directed to God or not).[21] A typically modern misunderstanding of natural law assumes that its reasoning is generated from a disinterested, general point of view (in Kantian fashion). Such is not the case. Natural law is a distinctive account of human life generally. It is an account of human solidarity in terms of God as beginning and end, and because human community is not yet perfectly related, natural law depends (whether explicitly or not) upon an understanding of human unity in creation and our eschatological communion.

Paul VI appeals to creation and our supernatural kinship in *HV* and in all his social documents, but his statement about "natural law as illuminated and enriched by divine revelation" (*HV*, 4) is usually interpreted in a theologically weak sense. Contemporary natural lawyers (and their opponents) tend to define the integrity of nature through a Newtonian-like notion of nature's autonomy and, therefore, understand divine revelation's enrichment of natural law as a matter of facility rather than of substantive vision and knowledge. In their view, natural law need not involve theology, and best not, since theological claims are assertions of faith and less secure than what are believed to be more broadly (and distinctively) human, rational arguments. The point here is not to deny the consistency of human reason, but to stress that its integrity is, from the beginning, given within, not outside, intrinsic relation to eschatological communion with God.

The most ardent defenders of the Church's teaching on contraception have been, arguably, Germain Grisez, Joseph Boyle, John Finnis, and William E. May. Significantly, however, while Grisez and the others find *HV*'s central teaching sound (i.e., that contraception is illicit and natural family planning acceptable), they hold that "certain formulations" in the encyclical are inadequate and need to be buttressed by independent arguments.[22]

Contraception, they argue, is irrational (and therefore immoral) because the act comes to be through a "contralife" will: i.e., "It is wrong for those who engage in marital intercourse to attempt to impede the transmission of life which they think their act otherwise might bring

20. See "Contraception: A Symposium," *First Things* 88 (December 1998): 17-29.

21. G. E. M. Anscombe, *Contraception and Chastity* (London: Catholic Truth Society, 1975), 13.

22. G. Grisez, "Every Marital Act Ought to Be Open to New Life: Toward a Clearer Understanding," *The Thomist* 52 (1988) 3: 367-68.

about."[23] An act of sexual intercourse during the fertile period of a woman's cycle implies the prospect of a human-coming-to-be. Contraception is willing that this future not come to pass, and as such, it is a direct choice to reject the prospect of a human-coming-to-be (and therefore akin to deliberate homicide). Contraception is willing against life.

In the contemporary world, any argument against contraception will be subject to criticisms, justified or not, that it violates the self-conscious and rational nature of human beings by binding human action to biological processes. Moral "oughts," it is said, cannot be deduced from our sexual nature as if human beings reproduced like animals. This attempt to determine what we "ought" to do from what apparently "is," is referred to as the naturalistic fallacy — or "physicalism" when the apparent "is" is assumed to be that of our physical/biological nature.[24] Grisez et al. accept the moral divide between "is" and "ought" and preclude naturalist/physicalist fallacies by locating the question of contraception in the distinctive character of human choices.

The intention of the will, according to Grisez et al., determines the moral character of the act. By shifting their argument to the will, they appear to safeguard the Church's teaching. In the end, however, their argument assumes that the reproductive character of sexual acts is an uninterpreted natural fact, while the question of contraception is a matter of human choice. The moral "ought" is determined by human intentions in relation to the objective character of given acts; i.e. the given of intercourse during infertile periods is that it is not procreative and the given of fertile periods is the prospect of a human-coming-to-be. But where does this "givenness" come from if not from an "is" that implies an "ought"? Grisez et al. appear to reject contraception through a naturalist/physicalist sleight of hand: they presuppose an account of human choices tied to a "brute" or irrational nature. As a consequence, they can, in the end, only impose rational choices on such a nature.

The idea of "nature" in *HV*, in contrast, is not irrational but interpreted through our eschatological end. *HV*'s appeal to "the natural generative process" implies a social teleology: that is, the natural generative process, like other aspects of our nature, provides a framework for the satisfaction and flourishing of human activities, which coincide (although are not identical) with our supernatural perfection. Nature gives a form that directs human beings to a natural fulfillment which implies an eschatological fulfillment in God. The reverse is also the case, as it is for Thomas Aquinas; namely, grace not only elevates human nature, infusing a supernatural form, but also sets human, natural fulfillment in order.[25] Natural and supernatural ends are distinguished, but there is no sense that the human being, in the one real historical order, can adequately (successfully) attend to the activities of one without implying the other. Paul VI assumes this strong connection between nature and grace, or, we could say, between our temporal social life and our eschatological communion.

HV's "every act" provision is not framed in terms of a reductive understanding of the "givens" of sexual intercourse, which ironically concedes the fundamental premise of so-called "physicalism." Rather, it is framed in terms of our supernatural destiny. Nature, including human nature, is not a closed system. In a world divided against itself, the illumination and enrichment provided by revelation make a substantive difference to human reasoning about our nature (natural law). Elsewhere, Paul VI holds that "without reference to Christ's teaching handed on by the Church, it is not possible for man to pass judgment on himself and his own nature . . ." (*Ecclesiam Suam*, 41). In *HV*, the natural generative process is understood as God's design, and the integrity of our nature is understood in terms of human fulfillment and the faithfulness of God. As a law of God, the proper regulation of birth "cannot be observed unless God comes to their [individual's, families', society's] help with the grace by which the goodwill of men is sustained and strengthened. But to those who consider this matter diligently it will indeed be evident that this endurance enhances man's dignity and confers benefits on human society" (*HV*, 20).

To understand the "every act" provision, then, we will have to accept: (1) that our creation is in continuity with our communion with God; (2) that our sexual nature is social and that sexual practices have inherent economic and political implications (sections 1-3 above); and (3) that our distinctively human nature, as yet incomplete, finds fulfillment, even as nature, in grace — in a movement toward the fullness of creation. If a contraceptive economy and culture set economic advancement against childbearing, if the social and economic equality of women is defined in terms of the non-procreative activity of men, if "making love" is set over against "making children," then the procreative character of human sexuality has become detached from social and economic life. It is for this reason that it becomes necessary to insist upon the procreative goods of sexuality and of human life.

The "every act" provision is a claim about the unity of creation, social life, and our eschatological communion. Contraception perpetuates discontinuity, not because a prospect of a "human-life-coming-to-be" is avoided, but because our relationship to our created nature is altered. Our sharing in God's generativity and our procreative mission become accidental to our nature. Grisez et al. might respond that the social and theological proposal offered here, although interesting, is intellectually flimsy. Yet, these thinkers themselves have no consistent means to ask whether or not a couple or society has structured its life in such a way that it has become inhospitable to

23. Ibid., 365.

24. G. Grisez, "Practical Principles, Moral Truth, and Ultimate Ends," *The American Journal of Jurisprudence* 32 (1987): 115-20, 125.

25. *Summa Theologiae* I-II, qq. 109-14.

children.[26] They give us little means to judge reasons that are not so much discrete choices but assumptions about the needs of children and a general orientation toward economic and cultural goods. Because they systematically exclude social and theological arguments, they cannot, within their system, attend to the fact that the American way of life is set up to accommodate more cars than children.[27] The question, then, is not about rational arguments as such against contraception, but about whether an eschatological context or a division between nature and grace gives us a fuller and richer picture of rationality.

While Grisez et al. protect the teachings of *HV* through what amounts to a kind of abstraction, Paul VI looks to the Church as a sign of hope — as a sign of contradiction. In offering the Church as a sign of contradiction (*HV,* 18), Paul VI calls us to a renewed vision of our nature in light of true human solidarity and our participation in the life of God. The "every act" clause of *HV* is not so much a conclusion drawn from independent principles as a principle itself, which has its proof in the way that it coheres with an eschatological understanding of nature and implies certain conclusions about practical, common life. The "every act" provision is an assertion first of all about the very meaning of our social nature. The meaning and destiny of our nature, God's creation, is precisely what is at stake. The possibilities for human community coincide with either our rejection or our acceptance of God's design, and for this reason, God's design for creation is key both to *HV* and to Paul VI's other social documents. The openness of every marital act will make sense in relation to human solidarity, the goods of truly human community, and our supernatural end.

Conclusion

"[Man] must act according to his God-given nature, freely accepting its potentials and its claims upon him." This quotation is not from *Humanae Vitae* but *Populorum Progressio* (no. 34), yet the logic of each document is the same. The appeal to our nature is a social claim that implies an analysis of social, economic, and political practices. In *Populorum Progressio* nos. 33-34, Paul VI is setting guidelines for economic development. "It is not enough to develop technology so that the earth may become a more suitable living place for human beings" (*PP,* no. 34). He proposes that human beings are called to a certain fulfillment, both in human solidarity and life with God. For this reason, Paul VI holds that technology and economics must serve human nature — must complete and perfect God's creation (*PP,* nos. 22, 27), build authentic human community (no. 47), and fulfill human life in light of our supernatural destiny (nos. 14-18). This principle applies as much to the use of private property (nos. 23-24) as it does to procreation (no. 37).

When considering "the question of procreation" in *HV,* Paul VI holds that "it is the whole man and the whole mission to which he is called that must be considered: both its natural, earthly aspects and its supernatural, eternal aspects" (*HV,* 7). Our supernatural fulfillment through conformity to our creation is the basis of *HV*'s appeal to the natural generative process and its call for every conjugal act to sustain its intrinsic openness to life. "[L]ife together in human society will be enriched with fraternal charity and made more stable with true peace when God's design which He conceived for the world is faithfully followed" (*HV,* 30).

26. Grisez does not treat economics systematically, but he does treat cases which deal with economic matters in *The Way of the Lord Jesus,* vol. 3. Typically, the cases do not deal with systemic questions, but with possible conflicts of obligation, contractual matters, and applications of the golden rule. Economic questions are reduced to the duties of individuals.

27. In 1995, there were just about 76,000,000 children nineteen years old and under (U.S. Department of Commerce). There were close to 135,000,000 passenger cars and over 200,000,000 total vehicles (American Automobile Manufacturers Association).

114 The Pill Is Like . . . DDT? An Agrarian Perspective on Pharmaceutical Birth Control

Elizabeth Bahnson

I am convinced . . . that no satisfactory solution can come from considering marriage alone or agriculture alone. These are our basic connections to each other and to the earth, and they tend to relate analogically and to be reciprocally defining: our demands upon the earth are determined by our ways of living with one another; our regard for one another is brought to light in our ways of using the earth.

Wendell Berry, "The Body and the Earth"

I started taking the pill two months after our first son was born. It was a safety measure. After all, he was conceived while my husband and I were (incorrectly) using the natural method. I was only halfway through my master's degree program. How could I possibly graduate if I got pregnant again? So I started taking the "mini-pill" or progesterone-only-pill, which allowed me to continue breast-feeding.

I took the pill for a year and a half and didn't get pregnant, which was a relief. But, I wondered, should I be doing this? It made practical sense — I needed to finish my degree. As my husband, Fred, often reminds me, we moved to the Piedmont of North Carolina so that I could go to school, a decision that he supported but, as a native of Montana, was not entirely thrilled about. We are Christians, members of a community that has long had serious moral concerns about birth control — although our denomination does not have much to say about the matter. While the Catholic Church has an official statement against it (most notably articulated in the 1968 papal encyclical *Humanae vitae*), Protestant Christianity, at least in practice, has unofficially embraced the use of birth control. At the 1930 Lambeth Conference, the Anglican Church passed a resolution allowing the "restricted" use of birth control. The Anglican Church shared some of the Catholic concerns about birth control, such as the likelihood that it would encourage promiscuity, but maintained the value of sex apart from procreation, asserting that "motive, not method, is what made birth control good or bad."[1] The conference agreed that, "in those cases where there is such a clearly felt moral obligation to limit or avoid parenthood, and where there is a morally sound reason for avoiding complete abstinence," contraceptives "may be used . . . provided that this is done in the light of the same Christian principles."[2] Where the health of the mother or the family's financial situation was pressing, contraceptives were deemed morally acceptable. However, the use of birth control was not an option if it was merely a question of convenience, selfishness, or luxury. After 1930, most other Protestant churches followed the Anglican lead.

Yet, in the largely acculturated Protestant church in America, the question of motive has become an ambiguous one. Indeed, it seems that mainline Protestants today are motivated more by the prospect of convenience than by that of welcoming the stranger or the unplanned child. How can we challenge one another's motives for using birth control when we are not held accountable for career choices or home size? At the church I attend, birth control of any kind is rarely discussed and never challenged. We are an unusually young congregation, many of whom are graduate students. On average, there are about thirty people in attendance every week, most of whom are married. There are only two children.

Farmers and Fertility

Fred and I are organic farmers. One day, we got into an argument about birth control — specifically, whether I should be taking the pill. I had been reading up on the Catholic position and was staunchly defending it. Fred was on full attack against. Suddenly I blurted, "What if it's like putting chemicals on our garden?" That stopped him in his tracks. "You're right," he said, after thinking a moment. "I guess it's kind of a 'quick-fix' to control fertility, like the 'quick-fix' fertilizers we don't use to control the fertility of our land." The argument ended there, but I couldn't get away from the thought. How could we be passionate about organic, sustainable agriculture and use hormonal birth control? If we refuse to boost our fertility in the garden using chemical fertilizers or to reduce the numbers of bugs and weeds with pesticides and herbicides, how could we justify using a chemical to control our own fertility?

While there are a lot of good arguments against using birth control, this one had a strong hold on me. I was curious: Are other female farmers asking the same question? What I found was fascinating. None of the women

From Elizabeth Bahnson, "The Pill is Like . . . DDT? An Agrarian Perspective on Pharmaceutical Birth Control," in *Wendell Berry and Religion: Heaven's Earthly Home,* ed. Joel J. Shuman (Lexington: University Press of Kentucky, 2009), pp. 85-97. Used by permission of The University Press of Kentucky.

1. Jenell Williams Paris, *Making Wise Choices: Birth Control for Christians* (Grand Rapids, MI: Baker, 2003), 24.

2. 1930 Lambeth Conference of Anglican Bishops, "Resolution 15: The Life and Witness of the Christian Community — Sex and Marriage," available at http://www.lambethconference.org.

farmers I asked used hormonal birth control. Many of them had tried it at some point but were unhappy with the way it made them feel. Others refused to take it at all. And one friend, who had been taking the pill for years, just recently quit because she has been raising sheep for the last year. Now that she is in touch with nature's seasons and cycles of fertility, she can't justify taking a pill that tricks her body into thinking she's pregnant. I suggested to my sister, who is an organic vegetable farmer, that women who farm are more in touch with nature, including their own bodies. Perhaps that is why they complain about the side effects of the hormones. She laughed and said, "Well, I guess I am in touch with the cycles of the moon." This is because she plants by the moon. Her own cycles are connected to the lunar cycles through the soil she touches every day. It is no coincidence that these women refuse to use hormonal birth control. In every case, it was something inherent in each woman's agrarian way of life that informed her decision.

In his essay "The Body and the Earth," Wendell Berry — perhaps the preeminent agrarian thinker in America — makes a connection between human fertility and the fertility of the earth. He writes, "There is an uncanny *resemblance* between our behavior toward each other and our behavior toward the earth. Between our relation to our own sexuality and our relation to the reproductivity of the earth, for instance, the resemblance is plain and strong and apparently inescapable."[3] In this essay, I try to show how Berry makes that connection. I focus specifically on "The Body and the Earth" as it pulls together many strands of his thought and articulates well an agrarian vision of the world. Then I try to show how that vision is particularly biblical and important for the church to take seriously. Finally, I propose an agrarian perspective on birth control that might help frame the way Christians engage in this debate.

The Agrarian Vision

In "The Body and the Earth," Berry offers a sharp critique of our attitude toward the body in modern industrial society. The chief problem, as he sees it, is that we have forgotten the proper place of human beings within the order of creation. In contrast to preindustrial societies, where art and literature reveal an innate sense that humans are one small part of a much larger creation, Berry observes that, with the rise of industry, "we became less and less capable of sensing ourselves as small within Creation, partly because we thought we could comprehend it statistically, but also because we were becoming creators, ourselves, of a mechanical creation by which we felt ourselves greatly magnified" (100). Effectively thinking ourselves gods, we have created works that cut us off from the wilderness, forgetting that we are a small part of creation and dependent on the whole of creation to survive.

This forgetfulness leads to isolation because it allows us to live under the illusion that we are independent, disconnected beings who can and should pursue our individual self-interests at all costs. Thus our relationships are increasingly determined by competition, and this isolates us — from the earth and from one another. It is this isolation, Berry argues, that is the source of the disintegration of modern society. But, for Berry, the most fundamental and damaging isolation is that of the body. Not only have we divided ourselves from others, but we are also divided within the self: "At some point we began to assume that the life of the body would be the business of grocers and medical doctors, who need take no interest in the spirit, whereas the life of the spirit would be the business of churches, which would have at best a negative interest in the body" (104). Just as modernity sets one body against another, so it sets the body against the soul. The isolated body is, thus, set against the world, pursuing its satisfaction at the expense of other bodies, of the earth, and even of its own soul. Whether we set the soul against the body or indulge the body at the expense of the soul, we are destroying both.

These divisions between body and soul and world are destructive because, Berry argues, despite our efforts to deny it, everything is connected. We are dependent creatures. Our lives and all life, human and nonhuman, are caught up in a complex system of interdependence that constitutes the whole. Berry writes, "These things that appear to be distinct are nevertheless caught in a network of mutual dependence and influence that is the substantiation of their unity. Body, soul (or mind or spirit), community, and world are all susceptible to each other's influence, and they are all conductors of each other's influence" (110). Trying to divide what is inherently connected threatens the health of the whole. It is like severing the veins of a circulatory system. We are endangering our own lives by living in denial of our connections, to others and to the earth.

As Berry sees it, this begets the disintegration of modern culture, a pattern that is at once cultural and agricultural. Culture and agriculture are disintegrating precisely because we have divided them. We have forgotten that souls cannot thrive apart from healthy bodies, that bodies cannot thrive without healthy food, and that culture cannot thrive without healthy agriculture. Berry argues that healing is possible only by the restoration of these long-ignored connections. Body, soul, community, and world must be reconnected because the health of each is essential for the health of the whole. In a nutshell, this is the agrarian vision of the world. It is a vision in which humans are returned to the status of creature and, thus, reconnected to everything in creation. It is a vision in which care for the earth, care for bodies, and care for souls are all bound up in each other.

3. Wendell Berry, "The Body and the Earth," in *The Unsettling of America: Culture and Agriculture,* 3rd ed. (San Francisco: Sierra Club Books, 1977), 124. Page numbers for subsequent cites will be given parenthetically in the text.

From this framework, Berry considers how we might reconnect, find healing and wholeness, and overcome division. He begins by considering two core divisions in need of healing. He writes: "The divisions issuing from the division of body and soul are first sexual and then ecological. Many other divisions branch out from those, but those are the most important because they have to do with the fundamental relationships — with each other and with the earth — that we all have in common" (113). Berry brings these two relationships together in his concept of *household*. Far from our modern notions of home, the notion *household* suggests something more like a preindustrial family farm or a cottage industry. It is built on the practical bond of mutual dependence and work. It is the place where a husband and wife are joined in lifework together, where they learn to enact their marriage and practice their love in the midst of being bound together by necessity, not simply to each other, but also to other, similar households. But the household has been dismembered, and what was once a sexual difference — differences in particular tasks that were of equal importance for sustaining the household — became a sexual division. Just as body and soul have been divided, so have women and men, even husband and wife. Berry's critique, in this case, is a bit outdated but useful nonetheless. At the time of writing "The Body and the Earth" (the mid-1970s), he argued that, in modern industrial society, men have been cut off from their nurturing role, sent away from the home to the specialized work that is the lifeblood of the market economy, while a woman's nurture is regarded as being of little use economically. Woman is valued more for her potential buying power than for the complex discipline of housewifery. Berry writes: "In modern marriage, then, what was once a difference of work became a division of work. And in this division the household was destroyed as a practical bond between husband and wife. . . . It was no longer a circumstance that required, dignified, and rewarded the enactment of mutual dependence, but the site of mutual estrangement" (115). It could be argued that, in the twenty-first century, both husband and wife have been sent away from home, either to work as highly specialized, well-paid professionals or to be underpaid housekeepers and landscapers in the employ of those same professionals. Either way, households have been dismembered.

It is to the household that Berry says we must return in order to heal these divisions between men, women, and the earth. Here, he makes a vital connection. In the household, there is no sexual or ecological division. In the household, a husband and wife's work is bound to the cycles of fertility and the seasons that make human life possible: "The motive power of sexual love is thus joined directly to constructive work and is given communal and ecological value" (132). Household sex, then, is tied to the constructive work of making and sustaining one another, which is entirely dependent on the fertility of the earth. Thus, the household is the link "between human sexuality and its sources in the sexuality of Creation" (124). Our sexual relationship binds us together in the household; our household binds us to the earth. The way we treat one will invariably affect the other. This is how Berry is able to say that there is a strange "resemblance" between our relation to our sexuality and to the soil we live on.

It is at this point in his essay that Berry makes the connection between the way we treat our own fertility and the way we treat that of the earth. However, before we get into that particular discussion, we must first ask how this vision has any bearing for the church. Does Wendell Berry have anything relevant to say to Christians on this matter? In the next section of this essay, I try to show that he is not far from a biblical vision of the world. Many of the connections he makes are congruous with what the Bible tells us about humankind's relationship with soil. His critique of modern industrial capitalism is a prophetic call to righteousness — that is, right relationships with God, neighbor, and the earth.

In the Garden

We must begin with the creation account, for that is the story that tells us who we are and who God is. One of the primary functions of the creation story is to put us in our proper place in the order of creation. Central to the biblical vision is the notion that we are creatures and God alone is Creator. That essential truth should dispel any illusion we might have about ourselves as godlike. When we acknowledge ourselves as creatures, we discover ourselves connected to everything else in creation. The Old Testament scholar Ellen Davis writes: "The biblical writers . . . help us see the degree to which our relationship with God is bound up in our relationships with the other creatures whom God has made."[4] This complex relationship between God, humans, and the earth is established at the very beginning.

The two creation stories in Genesis, seen together, make clear that, while we have a share in divinity on one side, we are also connected to the fertile soil on the other. In the first creation story, humans are made in the image of God (Gen. 1:26-27). In the second, humans are made from humus; the Potter forms a human body out of clay and breathes life into it (Gen. 2:7). Thus, while humans are to rule the earth as God would (Gen. 1:26-30), representing God's interest in the world, they are also of the earth and dependent on it for life. God and the soil are the sources of human life — both at the beginning and for the rest of the story. Indeed, while humankind, as God's image on earth, has a unique place in the order of creation, the second creation story is a sober reminder of the claim that the soil finally has on us. After the disobedience in the garden, God said: "By the sweat of your face you shall eat bread until you return to the ground, for out of it you were taken; you are dust, and to dust you

4. Ellen Davis, *Getting Involved with God: Rediscovering the Old Testament* (Boston: Cowley, 2001), 183.

shall return" (Gen. 3:19 [NRSV]). In the biblical vision, Berry's dyad — body and earth — becomes a triad. God, humankind, and the soil are in relationship and — as we shall see — connected in a way that is very close to Berry's agrarian vision.

Davis argues that, while we are used to the idea that the Bible calls us to love God and neighbor, we may be surprised to discover that the Old Testament is especially interested in our relationship with soil. That relationship is first established in Eden. In the second creation story, God set the first humans in the garden to "watch and work" the land. Davis points out that these Hebrew words (*'avad* and *shamar*) are not common agricultural terms but are used more often to describe human activity toward God. When directed toward God, *'avad* means "worship" and *shamar* means "'to watch,' or 'watch over', 'observe,' 'keep' or 'preserve.'" Humans are, thus, called into a particular kind of relationship with the soil that goes beyond "till and keep." Humans are called to serve the land, to be subservient to that upon which we and all creatures depend for life. We are also called to observe the land as we would God's commands, learning from it as well as protecting it from harm. Davis writes: "Together, these two verbs outline humanity's complex relationship with the fertile soil, a relationship that is meant to be deferential, observant, and protective. We must serve *('avad)* the land, not worshipping it but showing it reverence as God's own creation, respecting it as one whose needs take priority over our immediate desires. We must watch it and watch over it *(shamar)* as one who has something to teach us and yet at the same time needs our vigilant care."[5] Thus, in the biblical vision, humans are members of a complex network of relationships, and the call to righteousness entails maintaining the integrity of all those relationships — to God, neighbors, and earth.

The interweaving of these relationships appears again and again throughout the Bible but is particularly vivid in the Song of Songs. In her commentary on the Song of Songs, Davis argues that, most centrally, "the Song is about repairing the damage done by the first disobedience in Eden, what Christian tradition calls 'the Fall.'" Adam and Eve's disobedience to God had the disastrous result of division: division between man and woman, humanity and nature, and humanity and God. The Song, through which we experience healing on all three levels, represents "the reversal of that primordial exile from Eden." This healing is a love story with two primary characters, a man and a woman, who speak passionately of their mutual desire. The Song shows us what pure love looks like, love as it once was in the Garden. Yet the language of love that dominates the Song not only speaks of two lovers in the heat of passion but is also about the love between God and humanity (Israel in particular). Moreover, some of the most striking imagery in the Song refers to the land, which is not only the setting for the lovers' encounter but "also becomes an object of love, especially as the perfumed mountains and lush fields of Israel are at times identified with the lovely 'topography' of the woman's body."[6] In fact, the image of the woman we get in the Song looks much more like the land of Israel than a female form. This is revealing. It suggests that God loves the beautiful earth and calls us into that same kind of relationship with creation. Indeed, it calls us back into the garden to reclaim intimacy that once existed: intimacy between God and humanity, between man and woman, and between humans and the earth.

As we have seen, the church has something to learn from the agrarian vision. The Bible makes clear that we are in relationships in which the health of each affects the health of the whole. The biblical vision is like a three-sided prism through which all those relationships are displayed in myriad colors. God, humanity, and the earth are in relationship, and that relationship was once defined by pure love. Yet those relationships have been disordered since the Fall. Division has ensued. But the reality of the Fall does not mean that the connections among God and creatures no longer exist. Indeed, God, humans, and the earth are so deeply connected that disorder in one area causes disorder in another, and these relationships, using Berry's language, are still "reciprocally defining" (131). The way we treat the earth is reflective of our relationship with God, which is reflected back into our relationships with our neighbor or spouse; it is all deeply interwoven.

Sex and Soil

To return to my original question regarding birth control: Does the way we treat our own fertility relate to the way we treat the earth's fertility? In Berry's account in "The Body and the Earth," the disintegration of the household has resulted in the division of sexuality from fertility. That division, of course, is made possible by the advent of hormonal birth control. Whereas natural forms of birth control certainly existed in preindustrial societies, they were determined by what Berry calls "a cultural response to an understood practical limit." Knowing that the land can produce only so much food, most agrarian and hunter-gatherer people used some form of birth control, but it was intimacy with the land that informed their sexual practice. Modern industrial societies, however, have severed the connections between sexuality and fertility. We have also, Berry observes, done the same with the earth's fertility. We have handed it over to the "farming experts" or agribusinessmen. We have allowed the "specialists" to take over our fertility, entrusting "the immense questions that surround the coming of life into the world" (133) to those who, in return, hand us the chemicals and devices to use without

5. Ibid., 186, 192 (first quote), 193, 194 (second quote).

6. Ellen Davis, *Proverbs, Ecclesiastes, and the Song of Songs,* Westminster Bible Companion (Louisville: Westminster/John Knox, 2000), 231, 232, 233.

restraint. We are now "free from fertility" — both our own and that of the earth — which, Berry writes, "is to short-circuit human culture at its source. It is, in effect, to remove from consciousness the two fundamental issues of human life. It permits two great powers to be regarded and used as if they were unimportant" (134).

There is danger in this "freedom," as Berry warns. As laid out in Genesis, there is a divinely ordained relationship between humans and the land that is marked by servanthood, observance, and protection. That is a stark contrast to the agricultural practices we find today on corporate farms across the world. Rather than "watching" the land and working within its natural limits, "the dominant practices of modern industrial agriculture are based on the idea that technology has given us the power to reinvent our human relationship to the soil."[7] As we dump massive quantities of pesticides and herbicides on our genetically modified corn and soybeans, as we pump stockyards of beef and cooped-up chickens full of growth hormones, as we watch soil erode and wash into the rivers along with thousands of gallons of animal waste, we are practicing agriculture in a way that threatens the health of our relationship to God and to all our neighbors with whom we share this earth. Can the same be said about the way we treat our own fertility? That we pump our own bodies full of hormones to prevent pregnancy — thus dividing sex from fertility — is a technological achievement that skews our very sexuality.

Wendell Berry published "The Body and the Earth" when pharmaceutical contraceptives were a relatively new phenomenon. He warned that our full embrace of something about which we knew so little, and that affected so significant a part of our lives, could have dire consequences — as the technology of land use already has. It could be said that his view about our treatment of fertility was prophetic. Last summer I was in England visiting my relatives. My cousin is a geneticist, and I asked him about his latest research. He was studying the negative effects of estrogen on fish in rivers in the United Kingdom. "How does estrogen get into the water?" I asked. "The pill," he replied. Berry was right. There is, in fact, a connection between the way we treat our bodies and the way we treat the earth, and scientists are just now stumbling on this.

It is now generally accepted in the scientific community that there is a worldwide decline in amphibian populations.[8] There have been a number of reasons suggested for this: habitat depletion, infectious diseases, and environmental pollution. Recent research suggests that estrogen in the water supply is affecting the reproductive systems of amphibians. There are two forms of estrogen found in amphibian habitats, natural and synthetic. These come from human waste (hormonal birth control, hormone replacement therapy, etc.) and certain types of plants. There are also estrogen mimics that have a different chemical structure but the same effects as estrogens. These come from man-made chemicals that are used for pesticides, such as DDT, and the production of plastic. All these estrogens or estrogen mimics seem to affect amphibian reproductive systems in similar ways, which suggests that this could be one cause of population decline. It is important to note here that "amphibian populations are excellent indicators of the general health of the environment because of their position near the top of the food chain and their significant biomass in many ecosystems" and the permeability of their skin, which allows them to be more sensitive to pollutants.[9] Indeed, there *is* a connection between our attitudes toward our own fertility and that of the earth, and it is found in the creeks and streams that surround us. Our attempt to control fertility threatens the fragile eco-systems in which we live.

Over the course of writing this essay, I stopped taking the pill. I had not worked out all the reasons yet, but it seemed the right thing to do (it also saved us thirty dollars a month). One direct result has been an actual change in my own makeup. Quite literally, I find myself a happier person. I had been taking the progesterone-only pill. Progesterone is the hormone that dominates a woman's cycle after she has ovulated, approximately fourteen days prior to menstruation. As progesterone levels rise, a woman often feels slightly depressed, tired, bloated — all symptoms of PMS. By ingesting progesterone, I was daily forcing PMS down my throat. Now, as my body is returning to its natural rhythm, I find that my mood has changed, and I follow its changes throughout my monthly cycles. Estrogen, the hormone that dominates the first part of the cycle, lifts my mood. I generally feel happy, energetic, confident. After I ovulate, I can feel myself slide downward until I menstruate. The beauty for me (and for my family) is that I *understand* these feelings. Instead of getting frustrated or blaming myself for mood swings, I can see that my own body often determines how I feel. It also helps in my relationship to my husband. I can warn him, "I may be more sensitive this week." Or I can apologize, "I'm sorry I reacted that way; I think I know why I was more defensive than usual."

Early in the process of writing this essay I contacted Norman Wirzba, then a philosophy professor at Georgetown College who is also an agrarian, a husband, and a father of four. I thought that he might have some insights on the subject of birth control and asked him to discuss my questions with his wife, Gretchen Ziegenhals — specifically, the parallels between chemicals put on a garden and chemicals put into our bodies. He replied: "My wife

7. Davis, *Getting Involved with God*, 195.

8. Edmund J. Clark, David O. Norris, and Richard E. Jones, "Interactions of Gonadal Steroids and Pesticides (DDT, DDE) on Gonaduct Growth in Larval Tiger Salamanders, *Ambystoma tigrinum*," *General and Comparative Endocrinology* 109 (1998): 94.

9. T. Rouhani Rankouhi et al., "Effects of Environmental and Natural Estrogens on Vitellogenin Production in Hepatocytes of the Brown Frog *(Rana temporaria)*," *Aquatic Toxicology* 71 (2005): 94 (quote), 97.

is concerned that women's bodies not be understood in a passive way, something like a garden upon which men can exact their wishes."[10] I agree. It is not women's bodies that we should think of as a garden. Both women and men have fertile bodies, and, when they become one flesh, their fertility is joined. It is not a singular but a plural concept — *our* fertility. But I think that the garden metaphor is still helpful here. Fred and I work the garden together. It is a mutual effort that requires both of us — he usually does the digging and planting, while I do the weeding and harvesting. We both do the cooking. But all that labor requires working together and working with nature. We have to plant cabbage and broccoli early in the spring — otherwise worms will eat it. We have to plant sweet potatoes in the heat of summer so that we can eat them over the winter. We compost our weeds and scraps and plant cover crops on our garden beds so that we will have good fertility next year. We are learning to "watch and work" the land on which God has placed us. All this helps us reimagine how we think about our own fertility. And we are learning to "watch and work" our bodies so that we do not divorce sexuality from fertility and, as Berry says in "The Body and the Earth," "pleasure from responsibility" (135).

As Christians, we are called to a particular kind of relationship with nature — the nature of the earth and that of our bodies. We are called to treat it respectfully, with holy reverence, as God's own creation. We are called to learn from it, to be amazed by it, and to work with it. And we are also called to protect it and keep it from harm. In treating the earth this way, in treating our own bodies that way, we will treat other bodies that way. This begins to approach the shalom, the peace and wholeness that God desires. Even so, we cannot plan for everything. God sends us surprises. After putting compost on my flower bed this year, a tomato plant sprouted. Instead of pulling it up, I let it grow in the middle of my perennials. To our surprise, that plant produced the first tomato of the year.

10. Norman Wirzba, e-mail message to author, June 17, 2006.

CHAPTER EIGHTEEN

Assisted Reproductive Technologies

ART (assisted reproductive technologies) is big business. It is a $3 billion annual market in the U.S. Worldwide; between 219,000 and 245,000 live births result annually from ART. In the U.S., a single cycle of IVF (*in vitro* fertilization) costs between $6,000 and $15,000, with the average cost of $35,000 per live delivery to women under the age of 35 and an average cost of $132,000 per live delivery to women over the age of 40. With approximately 12 percent of reproductive-age couples experiencing infertility, it is perhaps unsurprising that the utilization of these procedures keeps growing. Moreover, ART enables nontraditional parents, such as same-sex partners and women past menopause, to have genetically or biologically connected children.[1]

ART is variously defined. For example, the CDC (Centers for Disease Control and Prevention) includes only infertility treatments in which both egg and sperm are handled.[2] This definition is more restrictive than most and too narrow for our purposes. Instead, we include all those procedures in which reproduction is medically assisted, whether through medication, medical procedures, or surgery. ART most frequently addresses infertility but is also used to help fertile couples diminish the chances of passing on genetic defects or diseases and to enable nontraditional parents to have children.

The most common forms of ART are:

Medication. Various drugs are used to stimulate ovulation, increasing a woman's chance of conceiving. This is the least invasive, least "mechanical" form of ART, and is not even viewed as ART by some. One drawback is that these medications can also increase the likelihood of multiple births, which increases the risk to both woman and fetus. The long-term health consequences of these medications are also unknown.

***In Vitro* Fertilization (IVF)**. IVF has been with us since the birth in 1978 of Louise Brown, the first child born alive who was conceived in a petri dish or *in vitro* (Latin for "in glass"). With IVF, a woman takes fertility drugs to produce more eggs than are normally produced in a reproductive cycle. Eggs are removed by laparoscopy or by passing a needle through the vaginal wall. They are then fertilized with sperm *in vitro,* with some number of the resulting "pre-embryos"[3] being implanted in the uterus. In Louise Brown's case, the eggs were from her mother, the semen was from her father, and she was implanted in the womb of her mother. However, the technology can be used with donor eggs, donor sperm, and a surrogate mother for gestation.

1. Adrienne Asch and Rebecca Marmor, "Assisted Reproduction," in *From Birth to Death and Bench to Clinic: The Hastings Center Bioethics Briefing Book for Journalists, Policymakers, and Campaigns,* ed. Mary Crowley (Garrison, N.Y.: The Hastings Center, n.d.), pp. 5-10; International Committee for Monitoring Assisted Reproductive Technology (ICMART): Jacques de Mouzon, et al., "World Collaborative Report on Assisted Reproductive Technology, 2002," *Human Reproduction* 24, no. 9 (2009): 2310-20, accessed November 27, 2009, at http://humrep.oxfordjournals .org/cgi/reprint/24/9/2310; Debora L. Spar, *The Baby Business: How Money, Science, and Politics Drive the Commerce of Conception* (Boston: Harvard Business Press, 2006); Victoria Clay Wright, Jeani Chang, Gary Jeng, and Maurizio Macaluso, "Assisted Reproductive Technology Surveillance — United States, 2005," *Morbidity and Mortality Weekly Report* 57, no. SS-5 (June 20, 2008): 2-12, accessed on November 27, 2009, at http://www.cdc.gov/Mmwr/PDF/ss/ss5705.pdf.

2. Centers for Disease Control and Prevention, "Assisted Reproductive Technology: Home," web page, accessed November 28, 2009, at http://www.cdc.gov/ART/index.htm.

3. Naming is seldom, if ever, a morally neutral activity. This becomes especially apparent in debates about human reproduction. Many working in the infertility industry and many scientists refer to the conceptus before implantation or before the appearance of an inner cell mass or development of an embryonic disk (thus fourteen days or longer after conception) as a "pre-embryo." However, others, appealing to the organism's self-actuated activity, believe that the term "pre-embryo" is unnecessary, even deceptive, and prefer the term "embryo" to refer to the human organism from fertilization onward. In general, those favoring stem cell research and other potentially destructive uses of the zygote prefer the term "pre-embryo," while those opposed to stem cell research and those suspicious of certain ART practices tend to favor the term "embryo." "Embryo" suggests a new being that will eventually become a baby if given the proper support. "Pre-embryo" suggests an organism that is not yet one of us and therefore one that has less claim on us for support or protection. For more on this, see the essays by Thomas Shannon and Allan Wolter and by Michael Panicola earlier in this volume (Chapter Seven, selections 47 and 48). Naming is morally relevant, even decisive. The editors of this edition of *On Moral Medicine* prefer "embryo."

According to the CDC, IVF has been disproportionately associated with multiple births, which is tied to a significantly higher risk of premature birth and subsequent health problems for the infants. Because IVF is expensive and each cycle has a roughly one in four chance of success, many doctors implant multiple embryos at a time, in hopes that at least one of them will implant in the uterine wall and come to term. Often, however, more than one implants and comes to term, and thus the higher rate of multiple births. There is a recent trend toward the implantation of a single embryo, but as of 2005, nearly 50 percent of IVF babies came in multiple births.

Even beyond the issue of multiple births, studies correlate IVF utilization with multiple-times higher risks to the child of autism, cerebral palsy, cancer, and various other handicaps and neurological challenges.[4] The safety of IVF for the women involved is also unclear, since it is associated with higher rates of hospitalization for pregnancy complications. While the risk of these added adverse health outcomes for women and children is comparatively low, the risks are substantially higher than with natural conception. The reasons for the added risks are unclear.

Artificial Insemination (AI). Artificial insemination is an older and simpler technology than IVF, usually utilizing a needleless syringe to deposit sperm into a woman's uterus during ovulation. The sperm can come from the husband or partner or from a donor. It can be placed in the uterus of the wife or a surrogate mother. The sperm can be fresh or thawed after having been frozen. If the sperm is derived from a donor at a sperm bank, it is first frozen, quarantined, and tested for transmittable diseases. The modern practice of AI was originally developed by the dairy industry, so that multiple cows could be impregnated by a bull with desirable characteristics. AI is the prototype of ART in this respect — many forms of ART were first developed for use in animal husbandry and then transferred to use in human reproduction.

Intracytoplasmic sperm injection (ICSI). This procedure utilizes surgery on a minute scale to insert a single sperm into the egg. It is helpful in addressing male infertility due to very low sperm count or poor sperm motility. It is often used as an extension of IVF. If fertilization occurs, the embryo is allowed to develop for a few days *in vitro* before being implanted in the uterus.

The use of ICSI is increasing dramatically. Indeed, the use of ICSI in Europe now exceeds that of the standard IVF.[5] This increase is striking, especially given that ICSI is more complicated and more expensive than standard IVF and is no more effective at achieving pregnancy than standard IVF except in cases of diagnosed male infertility. Still, for many, ICSI is the preferred form of ART.

Signs of ART's acceptance are everywhere. ART is almost entirely unregulated in the U.S., seeming to suggest that the various procedures are both safe and morally unproblematic. Utilization is high and growing, with over 1 percent of all live births in the U.S. resulting from ART (over 3 percent of live births in Massachusetts). There are strong advocacy groups, such as Resolve, that urge legislators to make infertility treatment a legally required part of health insurance, as it already is in states such as Connecticut, Massachusetts, and Illinois. Surveys indicate high approval across industrialized nations of assisted reproduction to address infertility. Sperm and egg banks are easily located using the Web. Postmenopausal women having children has become relatively common, drawing media attention only when the women are in their late 60s or older. ART appears to be here to stay.

Perhaps another sign of ART's acceptance is the proliferation of ads recruiting egg donors. Such ads are readily found on the Web and in local newspapers. They are especially common in campus newspapers. Recruiters typically target college women, a demographic that often needs money, feels somewhat invulnerable about their own fertility, and are at a prime age for egg donation. Compensation for egg donation ranges from $3,000 to as much as $50,000, the latter for students attending Ivy League schools or with high SAT scores. Couples seeking egg donors can scan web sites that show current and childhood pictures of the donors, along with listings of physical characteristics, ethnicity, place of origin, and various accomplishments (especially academic). Many couples seeking donation are from Europe, where paying for such services is illegal and waits are often long. Donation is a complicated, time-consuming process involving multiple hormone injections, extensive medical monitoring, and the extraction of eggs with a needle through the vaginal wall. The long-term health risks to the donors are unknown. Even with the complications and unknown health risks, the financial compensation brings in many donors.[6]

Despite the wide acceptance of ART, vexing questions persist for many philosophers, feminists, and Christian thinkers. A helpful place to start reviewing thoughtful Christian responses to ART is with the "Instruction on Respect for Human Life in Its Origin and on the Dignity of Procreation" (available on the Vatican web site[7]) issued by the Roman Catholic Church's Congregation for the Doc-

4. Helen Pearson, "IVF Health Risks Pinpointed," *Nature News*, accessed November 28, 2009, at http://www.nature.com/news/2004/041018/full/news041018-9.html; Sari Koivurova et al., "Post-Neonatal Hospitalization and Health Care Costs Among IVF Children: A 7-Year Follow-up Study," *Human Reproduction* (June 21, 2007); Laura A. Scheive et al., "A Population-Based Study of Maternal and Perinatal Outcomes Associated with Assisted Reproductive Technology in Massachusetts," *Maternal and Child Health Journal* 11, no. 6 (2007).

5. European Society for Human Reproduction and Embryology, "Fertility Treatments: Researcher Says That ICSI May Be Over-Used in Some Countries," *ScienceDaily*, July 9, 2008, accessed November 29, 2009, at http://www.sciencedaily.com/releases/2008/07/080709083953.htm.

6. See, for example, Melinda Beck, "Ova Time: Women Line Up to Donate Eggs — for Money," *The Wall Street Journal* (December 9, 2009), accessed November 28, 2009, at http://online.wsj.com/article/SB122878524586490129.html.

7. http://www.vatican.va/roman_curia/congregations/cfaith/documents/rc_con_cfaith_doc_19870222_respect-for-human-life_en.html (accessed February 25, 2012).

trine of the Faith in 1987. The "Instruction" rejects all forms of "artificial fertilization," partially on the basis of the respect due to persons as embodied, partially on the basis of a specific understanding of marriage and the interconnection of marriage, sex, and children. The "Instruction" worries that these technologies commodify children, are an affront to the dignity of the embryo, disembody procreation, and draw third parties into the heart of the marriage/family relationship. However, recognizing the suffering caused by infertility in marriage and that children are a gift (but not a right), the "Instruction" urges scientists to continue work aimed at preventing and correcting causes of sterility.

The "Instruction" represents both a thoughtful Christian response to ART and official Roman Catholic teaching. As such, nearly every author included in this section engages the "Instruction" directly or wrestles with many of the same themes. For example, Paul Lauritzen's essay, "Whose Bodies? Which Selves? Appeals to Embodiment in Assessments of Reproductive Technology" (selection 115), compares the "Instruction" to certain feminists who have rejected reproductive technologies, noting that both groups share a concern for embodiment and worry that such technologies encourage us to disassociate from the body. However, while the "Instruction" worries about commodifying children and the disembodiment of procreation, some feminists worry that these technologies commodify women, reducing them to reproductive machines. Lauritzen goes on to argue that the differences between the groups show that the context of the appeal to embodiment matters. Thus, the Catholic appeal arises from a context that lacks sufficient commitment to women's equality, while the feminist appeal fails to take seriously enough the embodied value of pregnancy and parenthood. While Lauritzen shares some of both groups' concerns over embodiment, he suggests that for many infertile couples reproductive technologies facilitate embodiment, not the reverse. Indeed, he concludes his essay by observing that the failure of both official Catholic teaching and certain feminists to note "this fact demonstrates how important the context of appeals to embodiment can be."

In "The Ethical Challenge of the New Reproductive Technology" (selection 116), Sidney Callahan seems to have the "Instruction" (or something very much like it) in mind when she rejects a "conservative approach" that focuses on the "biological integrity of the marital sexual act," which she rejects in part because "mastery of nature through technological problem-solving is also completely natural to us." Calling reproductive technology a "wonderful" gift in overcoming the handicap of infertility for certain married couples, Callahan nevertheless argues that a fully permissive attitude toward these technologies is as problematic as those that forestall all uses of it. She contends that reproductive technology should be used "if, and only if, it makes it possible for a normal, socially well-adjusted heterosexual couple to have a child that they could not otherwise have owing to infertility," and she draws a clear line against employing third-party donors or surrogate mothers. Callahan maintains that many proposed uses of assisted reproductive technologies undermine cultural norms that are important for the well-being of children, women, and society. She is especially concerned with the way identity is challenged when we sever genetic ties, the way these technologies play into the commodification of children (a concern shared with the "Instruction"), and the way isolating sexual and reproductive acts from long-term personal responsibility exacerbates existing problems with divorce, illegitimate conception, and parental responsibility.

The "Instruction" mentions the suffering that accompanies infertility. Maura Ryan writes about the suffering that goes with "involuntary childlessness." In *Ethics and Economics of Assisted Reproduction: The Cost of Longing,* rooting her argument in a Catholic understanding of the common good, Ryan contends not only that certain limited uses of reproductive technology are justified but also that assisted reproduction belongs within a "comprehensive but temperate view of health and the obligation of societies to sustain it."[8] Addressing the "Instruction," Ryan draws extensively on Lisa Cahill in developing a position similar to Callahan's: procreation through ART should be tied to an exclusive sexual and marital relationship. This position allows the goods of marriage (sexual intimacy, fidelity, openness to new life, parenthood) to be experienced in the totality of the couple's life together. Ryan then uses Eric Cassell's work on suffering and Daniel Callahan's work on the goals of medicine to contend that infertility causes a kind of suffering that is an appropriate concern of medicine. Infertility challenges numerous dimensions of the self, including social roles; self-esteem; understanding of sexuality; relationship with self, body, and family; and major life goals. Moreover, having children is a normal part of human potential and is typically understood as part of a good life. Thus, says Ryan, there is reason to believe that infertility treatment belongs in an account of basic care. The essential claim is clear: assistant reproduction within specific limits is an appropriate medical response to a malady that causes significant suffering for many couples.

Ryan offers a different response, reprinted here, to the suffering of infertility in the essay "Faith and Infertility" (selection 117), which is a more recent version of a latter chapter in *Ethics and Economics of Assisted Reproduction.* Noting that infertility can be a personal and spiritual crisis that involves "a kind of 'dying,' a loss of both an envisioned future and a possible self, a potential role and a longed-for relationship," Ryan suggests that we need "a Christian spirituality for growth or transcendence through infertility." Infertility is highly visible in Scripture, but it is nearly invisible in most congregations, where parenting and reproduction are celebrated as completing marriage and

8. Maura A. Ryan, *Ethics and Economics of Assisted Reproduction: The Cost of Longing* (Washington, D.C.: Georgetown University Press, 2001), p. 10.

offering opportunities for ministry. Instead, says Ryan, the church needs to acknowledge those struggling with infertility and reframe generativity such that mutual self-giving is more central and all laity have a critical vocation within the church's ministry. For the individual, learning to re-narrate one's story, gaining self-acceptance, and nurturing the virtue of hope are all crucial to growth through infertility.

The reader can rightfully wonder if Ryan's medical and spiritual responses to the suffering of infertility are complementary, as she means them, or if they push in somewhat different directions *vis-à-vis* the appropriation of ART. Are these two sides of the same response to suffering? Or does the argument regarding health care push toward ART's utilization while the notion of a Christian spiritual journey through infertility incline us away from ART's usage?

This chapter's last essay, "A.R.T., Ethics, and the Bible," by Allen Verhey (selection 118), engages the "Instruction" throughout, both explicitly and implicitly. Verhey first talks about Scripture, focusing on the role of sex and marriage, but also about infertility, surrogacy, and the place of children. This focus signals Verhey's conviction that the proper context for considering ART is a Christian view of marriage, sex, and children. This conviction is shared by the "Instruction," although they use different resources in developing their views.

Verhey next argues that many ART practices easily fall into the commodification of reproduction and are at odds with understanding ourselves as embodied and communal. The surrogate mother, for example, is alienated from the embodied experience of pregnancy, and community is sundered because another who views genetic ties as important for himself or herself encourages the surrogate to ignore those ties for herself. We should, says Verhey, preserve a sense of ourselves as embodied and communal. Again, these basic concerns are shared with the "Instruction," although Verhey, with Lauritzen, contends that IVF and some other forms of ART enable a couple's embodied relationship.

The remainder of Verhey's essay engages the "Instruction" more directly by appreciatively noting five aspects of the document. First, Verhey applauds the "Instruction" for its balanced appraisal of technology, buying neither into the "Baconian project" nor into an anti-technological stance. Second, Verhey commends the "Instruction" for its embodied view of human sexuality. However, he argues that lovemaking and babymaking belong together as part of marriage rather than, as per the "Instruction," naturally joined to each other in every conjugal act. Third, Verhey believes we can be instructed by the "Instruction" in its concern that we do not sunder genetic relationships. Many ART practices essentially deny that a biological relationship with a child carries an obligation to care for him or her. Verhey worries that the specific language in the "Instruction" unintentionally devalues the hospitality of adoption, but it is right to value the connection between genetic parenthood and a vocation to nurture. Fourth, we can learn from the "Instruction" to view children as gift, rather than, as ART may tempt us, to see them as a human achievement. Fifth, we can join the "Instruction" in acknowledging the suffering of those struggling with infertility. For Verhey, this means that we should support many efforts to address infertility, but it also means that we must correct Christian rituals that are compounding their suffering, as well as insisting that there is no obligation to have children, nor are they our hope for the future.

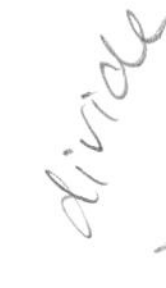

None of the included essays suggests the kind of open-ended acceptance of ART that we see throughout our society. The "Instruction" places the firmest boundaries, but every author here expresses reluctance about some form of ART.[9] You are invited to consider what boundaries we should draw. How should we talk about these matters within the church? And how should we engage our fellow citizens about them? What, moreover, are the implications for public policy? Should certain forms of ART be publicly funded or a mandated part of insurance coverage? Are there procedures we should legally prohibit? Of course, it is possible that to discuss public policy regarding ART is to get ahead of ourselves. Perhaps ART is an instance where the church first needs to witness to its convictions by its life together before further engaging in public policy debates.

SUGGESTIONS FOR FURTHER READING

Bouma, Hessel, III, Douglas Diekema, Edward Langerak, Theodore Rottman, and Allen Verhey. *Christian Faith, Health, and Medical Practice* (Grand Rapids: Eerdmans, 1989), pp. 176-204.

Braine, David. "The Human and Inhuman in Medicine: Review of Issues Concerning Reproductive Technology." In *Moral Truth and Moral Tradition: Essays in Honor of Peter Geach and Elizabeth Anscombe,* ed. Luke Gormally (Dublin: Four Courts Press, 1994).

Cahill, Lisa Sowle. *Sex, Gender, and Christian Ethics* (Cambridge: Cambridge University Press, 1996), pp. 217-57.

Cohen, Cynthia B. "'Give Me Children or I Shall Die!': New Reproductive Technologies and Harm to Children." *Hastings Center Report* 26, no. 2 (March-April 1996): 19-27.

Cohen, Cynthia B., ed. *New Ways of Making Babies: The Case of Egg Donation* (Bloomington: Indiana University Press, 1996).

Hall, Amy Laura. *Conceiving Parenthood: American Protestantism and the Spirit of Reproduction* (Grand Rapids: Eerdmans, 2007).

Kilner, John F., Paige C. Cunningham, and W. David Hager. *The Reproduction Revolution: A Christian Appraisal of Sexuality, Reproductive Technologies, and the Family* (Grand Rapids: Eerdmans, 1999), pp. 3-123.

Lauritzen, Paul. *Pursuing Parenthood: Ethical Issues in Assisted Reproduction* (Bloomington: Indiana University Press, 1993).

May, William F. *The Patient's Ordeal* (Bloomington: Indiana University Press, 1994), pp. 71-79.

9. Aside from the "Instruction," this reluctance is often expressed without significant attention to issues surrounding the creation, selection, and disposition of embryonic life. These contentious matters are largely treated elsewhere in this volume (for example, see Chapters Fourteen and Fifteen).

Meilaender, Gilbert C. *Bioethics,* 2nd ed. (Grand Rapids: Eerdmans, 2005), pp. 10-24.

Meilaender, Gilbert C. *Body, Soul, and Bioethics* (Notre Dame: University of Notre Dame Press, 1995), pp. 61-105.

Muers, Rachel. "It Takes at Least Two to Reproduce." *Cross Currents* 55, no. 2 (2005): 162-71.

Mundy, Liza. *Everything Conceivable: How Assisted Reproduction Is Changing Our World* (New York: Anchor Books, 2008).

Nikolaos, Metropolitan. "The Greek Orthodox Position on the Ethics of Assisted Reproduction." *Reproductive BioMedicine Online* 17, no. S3, Supplement (November 3, 2008): 25-33.

O'Donovan, Oliver. *Begotten or Made?* (Oxford: Clarendon Press, 1984), pp. 66-86.

Overall, Christine, ed. *The Future of Human Reproduction* (Toronto: Women's Press, 1989).

Ramsey, Paul. *Fabricated Man* (New Haven: Yale University Press, 1970).

Shannon, Thomas A., and Lisa Sowle Cahill. *Religion and Artificial Reproduction: An Inquiry into the Vatican "Instruction on Respect for Human Life in Its Origin and on the Dignity of Procreation"* (New York: Crossroad, 1988).

Smith, David H., and Judith A. Granbois. "New Technologies for Assisted Reproduction." In *The Crisis in Moral Teaching in the Episcopal Church,* ed. T. Sedgwick and P. Turner (Harrisburg, Pa.: Morehouse Publishing, 1992).

Smith, Harmon L., and Paul A. Lewis. "A Protestant View of New Reproductive Technologies." *Second Opinion* 14 (July 1990): 94-106.

"Symposium on the Warnock Report." *Ethics and Medicine* 1, no. 2 (1985).

Tiefel, Hans. "When Baby's Mother Is Also Grandma — and Sister," *Hastings Center Report* 15 (1985): 30-31.

Verhey, Allen. "Commodification, Commercialization, and Embodiment." *Women's Health Issues* 7, no. 3 (May/June 1997): 132-42.

115 Whose Bodies? Which Selves? Appeals to Embodiment in Assessments of Reproductive Technology

Paul Lauritzen

Now men are far beyond the stage at which they expressed their envy of women's procreative power through couvade, transvestism, subincision. They are beyond merely giving spiritual birth in their baptismal-font wombs, beyond giving physical birth with their electronic fetal monitors, their forceps, their knives. Now they have laboratories.

([3], p. 314)

This passage from Gena Corea's book *The Mother Machine* typifies the reaction of one important strand of feminist thought to the new technologies of reproduction and birth. It is fairly representative, for example, of the grave suspicion with which feminists associated with FINRRAGE (Feminists International Network of Resistance to Reproductive and Genetic Engineering) have greeted such possibilities as *in vitro* fertilization, embryo flushing and transfer, and gene therapy. According to this general line of thinking, the new reproductive technologies should be resisted because they concentrate power in the hands of a predominantly male and patriarchal medical establishment by disembodying procreation. By separating procreation from women's bodies, reproductive technology simultaneously reduces women to bodies, or body parts, and strips women of one traditional source of power, namely, the power to procreate. Hence Corea's warning. Previously men were denied direct control over the process of procreation; they might give birth symbolically or intervene medically in this process, but these were only simulacra of control. The existence of *in vitro* fertilization, however, and the distinct possibility of *in vitro* gestation turn resemblance into reality. Laboratory conception and gestation are a threat to women.

At the same time that FINRRAGE has mobilized to resist the new reproductive technologies, opposition has come from other quarters as well. The most substantial

From Lisa Sowle Cahill and Margaret A. Farley, eds., *Embodiment, Morality, and Medicine* (Dordrecht: Kluwer Academic Publishers, 1995), pp. 113-26. Used with kind permission of Kluwer Academic Publishers.

opposition has come from groups at the opposite end of the political spectrum, most notably the Roman Catholic Church. For example, the Catholic Church has also condemned *in vitro* fertilization, embryo flushing and transfer, and genetic engineering. Indeed, the Vatican has rejected virtually every application of the new reproductive technology (NRT), and, like FINRRAGE, the Vatican is worried about disembodiment. Thus, in the Vatican *Instruction* [2] on reproductive technology, we hear an echo of Corea's concern. We must take seriously the embodied nature of our existence, and failure to do so results in the reduction of a person to a product. So, for example, we find the Vatican insisting that "an intervention on the human body affects not only the tissues, the organs and their functions but also the person himself on different levels" ([2], p. 8).

This apparent convergence of two such different traditions of thought is interesting in itself. It is doubly so when, as in this volume [*Embodiment, Morality, and Medicine*], attention is focused on "how the realities of embodiment influence moral relationships in practical health care settings." Despite very serious differences between these traditions of thought — even on issues of embodiment — they agree in their rejection of reproductive technology, and they do so for reasons connected to worries about treating procreation as an out-of-the-body laboratory production. So examining how appeals to embodiment function in feminist and Vatican critiques of reproductive technology promises to be quite useful to the overall project of this volume. Moreover, if we attend to the similarities and differences between feminist appeals to embodiment and those of the Catholic Church, we may come to appreciate how the meaning of embodiment may vary from context to context. We may see, for example, how a religious appeal to embodiment in the Christian tradition takes quite a different form from an appeal to embodiment rooted in feminist thought, even if there are also substantial similarities between the two appeals.[1]

Feminist Opposition to Reproductive Technology

We can begin, then, with feminist opposition to reproductive technology. That one significant strand of feminist resistance is fueled by concerns about embodiment is clear. Yet, how precisely does the appeal to embodiment function in this particular feminist critique of reproductive technology? To answer that question, we can return to Gena Corea's work. According to Corea, reproductive technology is best understood in terms of two analogies that have implications for how we think about women's bodies and thus for how we think about, and treat, women. On the one hand, techniques for assisting human reproduction bear a striking resemblance to techniques used to facilitate reproduction in livestock. On the other hand, the commercial transactions frequently associated with reproductive technology bear a striking resemblance to those associated with sexual prostitution. Let us consider each of these analogies in turn.

Corea makes the comparison between reproductive technology in humans and scientific breeding of animals repeatedly and forcefully in her writings (see [3], [4], and [5]). Consider, she says, the techniques commonly used for breeding animals. Artificial insemination, superovulation, estrus synchronization, ova recovery, embryo evaluation, embryo transfer, and caesarean section are all available to animal breeders, just as they are to physicians of reproductive medicine [4]. Indeed, many applications of this technology used in infertility clinics have been adapted from their original use in the livestock breeding industry. This, says Corea, should give us pause because women have frequently been symbolically associated with animals in Western thought, as "parts of nature to be controlled and subjugated" ([3], p. 313).

The point of the comparison between reproductive medicine and animal breeding is to invite an inspection of the attitudes that stand behind the practice of animal breeding. Once we see the attitudes driving animal reproduction, we may come to ask whether similar attitudes do not also drive reproductive medicine. And, as Corea shows, there is no mistaking the attitudes of animal breeders.

> When reproductive engineers manipulate the bodies of female animals today, they are clear, blunt and unapologetic about why they are doing it. They want to turn the females into machines for producing "superior" animals or into incubators for the embryos of more "valuable" females. They want, as one entrepreneur told me, to "manufacture embryos at a reduced cost." They aim to create beef cows yielding "quality carcasses of high cutability," and dairy cows producing more milk on the same amount of feed ([3], p. 312).

Or as a manager for Wall's Meat Company put it, this time in relation to the production of pork, "[t]he breeding sow should be thought of, and treated as, a valuable piece of machinery whose function is to pump out baby pigs like a sausage machine" ([4], p. 41).

Corea's point is clear: When the bodies of animals are treated in this fashion, when the animal is essentially reduced to its reproductive parts, the animal ceases to have any individuality or spiritual worth ([4], p. 39). The upshot of reproductive technology is thus that the animal is reduced to a reproductive commodity and nothing more. The worry is that we may come to think of women and their bodies in precisely the same terms.

This worry informs Corea's second analogy as well. If comparing reproductive medicine to livestock production is meant to highlight the possibility that employing reproductive technology may lead us to think about women's bodies as commodities, comparing reproductive medicine to prostitution is meant to highlight the fact that our society already conceptualizes women's

1. For a fuller discussion of feminist and Catholic opposition to reproductive technology, see [8]. See also [14], [15].

bodies in market terms. Drawing on Andrea Dworkin's work, Corea shows that the reduction of women to commodities has already taken place. As Corea notes, our society already markets parts of women's bodies. Pornography is a thriving industry and sexual prostitution is widely perceived to be harmless and is thus tolerated as largely benign. But if women can sell vagina, rectum, and mouth, Corea asks, why not wombs, embryos, or eggs? Given how women are conceptualized in our society, the answer, of course, is that there is no reason to object to the marketing of women as reproductive commodities, and indeed, Corea says, that is precisely what we see with the development of a commercial surrogate mother industry and egg "donor" programs.

In fact, says Corea, we do not need to attend merely to the obvious comparison case, namely, surrogate motherhood. Talk to women who have been through *in vitro* fertilization programs. Quoting from an Australian study of women who had been treated in IVF programs, Corea draws attention to the dehumanizing aspects of the treatment.

> It [the IVF treatment] is embarrassing. You leave your pride on the hospital door when you walk in and pick it up when you leave. You feel like a piece of meat in a meat-works. But if you want a baby badly enough you'll do it ([5], p. 86).

Corea notes, for example, that many women report undergoing a process of emotional distancing during IVF. They attempt to separate mind from body and in fact come to feel disconnected from their bodies in ways that interfere with bodily lovemaking with their partners. Here, Corea says, the comparison to prostitution is direct and disturbing.

> What kind of spiritual damage does it do to women when they emotionally separate their minds and bodies? . . . We have heard some prostitutes say that during intercourse with strangers who have rented the use of their bodies, they too separate their minds from their bodies as a means of self-protection. We have heard some people with multiple personalities say that during extreme sexual abuse and torture in childhood, they split off into separate personalities in order to make what was happening to them endurable. In order to survive.
>
> What does it do to women in IVF "treatment" programs when, to varying extents, they separate their minds and bodies in order to make all the poking and prodding and embarrassments endurable? ([5], p. 86).

Corea is not the only feminist asking such questions, nor is she the only one to focus on the importance of embodiment to assessments of reproductive technology. Barbara Katz Rothman, for example, has made essentially the same point in her book, *Recreating Motherhood* [11].[2]

2. It is important to note, however, that Rothman does not reach the same conclusions about reproductive technology as Corea, even though she shares Corea's worries about disembodiment.

In a chapter on the ways in which technological ideology shapes how we think about ourselves, Rothman summarizes one important line of resistance to technological thinking in terms that are strikingly similar to those set out above. "It is an objection," Rothman says, "to the notion of the world as a machine, the body as a machine, everything subject to hierarchical control, the world, ourselves, our bodies and our souls, ourselves and our children, divided, systematized, reduced" ([11], p. 54). Rothman's earlier work also focused on the effects of technology on conceptions of selfhood. In *The Tentative Pregnancy* [12], for example, she documents the effects of technologies of prenatal diagnosis on the experience of pregnancy, demonstrating that the existence of amniocentesis generates the same sort of emotional distancing, the same sort of splitting of the self, as Corea documents in regard to *in vitro* fertilization.

In fact, a careful reading of feminist responses to the technologies of reproductive medicine shows this to be a pervasive theme: reproductive technology encourages women to separate their selves from their bodies, and the resulting fragmentation leaves women vulnerable. Women become vulnerable because, with fragmentation, comes a willingness to treat women's bodies as biological machines that can be manipulated and controlled. Reproductive technology thus alienates women from their bodies and thereby strips them of an important source of personal fulfillment and power. As Margaret Farley puts it, "For many feminists the sundering of the power and process of reproduction from bodies of women constitutes a loss of major proportions. Hence, the notion of moving the whole process to the laboratory (using not only *in vitro* fertilization but artificial placentas *et al.*) is not one that receives much enthusiasm" ([7], p. 301).

Catholic Opposition to Reproductive Technology

If we turn now to the Vatican's response to reproductive technology, we see that the Catholic Church is also concerned about issues of embodiment. Consider, for example, the *Instruction* on reproductive technology issued by the Congregation for the Doctrine of the Faith in 1987, in which the position of the Church is set out at length. For our purposes, the introduction and the first two sections of this document are of particular interest, because the introduction sets out the basic moral considerations that are then applied in sections one and two to arrive at particular conclusions about reproductive technology. A careful reading of these three sections reveals that Vatican opposition to reproductive technology is supported by two lines of argument, both of which are rooted in concerns about embodiment. The first line of argument is set out in the introduction in terms of what the Vatican describes as "a proper idea of the nature of the human person in his bodily dimension" ([2], p. 8). The Congregation asks: What moral criteria must be used to assess reproductive technology? The first answer it gives is that any adequate criteria must recognize the bodily and spiritual unity of the person. In the Vatican's view, a person is a "unified totality," and thus it is wrong to treat a person in a way that reduces that person either to mere body or mere spirit. It is particularly important to keep this principle in mind, the Vatican says, when addressing ethical issues in medicine because there is a tendency in medicine to treat the body as "a mere complex of tissues, organs, and functions." Indeed, this is one of the central difficulties with reproductive medicine: it approaches human reproduction as if it were nothing more than the union of bodily parts, namely, of gametes. So one of the most serious problems with reproductive technology, the Vatican concludes, is precisely that it fails to treat the person as a unified whole. Instead, it treats the body in just the way the Vatican says it must not be treated, as a mere complex of tissues and organs. In other words, this technology treats our bodies functionally, the consequence of which is that persons get objectified and treated merely as means to an end. When this happens, technology is not simply assisting, but dominating the process of reproduction.

The second line of argument used to oppose interventions in the reproductive process is less obviously rooted in a concern about embodiment, but, once again, a careful reading of the text highlights the relevance of considerations of embodiment. This second line of reasoning is related to what the Vatican calls "the special nature of the transmission of human life in marriage." In the Vatican's view, since human procreation is the fruit of a "personal and conscious act," it is irreconcilably different from the transmission of life in other animals. It is intentional and purposive and therefore governed by laws. What laws? Laws, says the Vatican, given by God and "inscribed in the very being of man and woman."

As the language here suggests, the appeal is to a natural law conception of human nature, according to which we must understand the telos of human sexual life, marriage, and the family in order to discern the range of acceptable reproductive interventions. Moreover, the appeal is to a particular understanding of this telos, one in which intercourse, love, procreation, marriage, and the family belong together. In the Vatican's view, procreation is properly undertaken in the context of a loving monogamous marriage through an act of sexual intercourse. Here, then, is a second standard by which to assess interventions in the reproductive process. Any type of assisted reproduction that conforms to the procreative norm just articulated, i.e., any procreative attempt that includes sexual intercourse between partners in a loving monogamous marriage, helps facilitate the natural process of procreation and is therefore acceptable. Any intervention that fails to conform to the norm is a departure from the natural law with respect to human sexuality and is therefore morally problematic.

Two points are worth noting at this juncture. First, in rejecting reproductive technology as a violation of natural law, the Vatican is invoking the "inseparability thesis" set out in *Humanae Vitae,* and which supports Catholic opposition to contraception. Just as the Catholic Church condemns contraception because it separates what is never permitted to be separated by allowing for sex without procreation, so it condemns reproductive technology because it provides for the possibility of procreation without sex. This is important to note because many critics of the inseparability thesis have argued that, by insisting that each and every act of sexual intercourse must be open to procreation, the Vatican itself accepts a sort of "physicalist" understanding of sexuality that is incompatible with the holistic picture of the person as a "unified totality" of body and spirit that grounds the first line of argument against reproductive technology discussed above.

This observation suggests a second one. To say that reproductive technology separates procreation from sex is not equivalent to saying that reproductive technology disembodies procreation. So opposition to reproductive technology is not just opposition to those techniques, like IVF, that actually disembody conception, but opposition to how the body is used and viewed by reproductive technology generally. To be sure, the Vatican objection is not merely reducible to the consequentialist concern that all forms of reproductive technology move us toward the objectionable endpoint of extracorporeal gestation. Nevertheless, whether emphasis is placed upon the bodily and spiritual unity of a person, or upon the importance of keeping sex and procreation together, the Vatican is concerned that reproductive technology leads us to treat our bodies merely as a source of gametes, and that so treating our bodies is the first step to disembodying procreation altogether. We already have extracorporeal conception; can extracorporeal gestation be far behind? Ultimately, then, one important source of Vatican resistance to reproductive technology is that it encourages the disembodiment of procreation.

At this point it is worth noting that Vatican opposition to reproductive technology appears strikingly similar to feminist opposition to this technology, and that both groups couch their opposition in terms of the unfortunate consequences of disembodying procreation. Indeed, the language of complaint is almost identical. Technological intervention in the process of procreation reduces reproduction to a production process in which humans are themselves reduced to products. Given the similarity of complaint, may we conclude that Vatican appeals to embodiment are essentially identical to feminist appeals to embodiment?

Janice Raymond [10] has argued that the answer to this question should be an emphatic and unequivocal "no!" The similarities, she says, are apparent only. In fact, according to Raymond, feminists should resist this equation, not only because it will be used by their opponents to discredit them as latter-day Luddites, but because it is offensive to women. Linking fetalists — the term she uses for conservative religious opponents of reproductive technology — and feminists, she writes, "is an insult of the first order to women. It's tantamount to saying that behind every female idea or movement is male impetus, that women cannot stand on our own and create a woman-defined opposition to the NRTs for autonomous feminist reasons . . . " ([10], p. 60). "Feminists and fetalists," she says flatly, "are not aligned in any way" ([10], p. 65).

Raymond's total rejection of the similarities between Vatican opposition and feminist opposition is too extreme, but her argument is instructive nonetheless, for it demonstrates how an appeal to embodiment is inextricably tied to the context in which it is made. We therefore do well to take up her argument in some detail.

Raymond begins by noting that there are essentially two groups that have mounted substantial opposition to reproductive technology, feminists and the Roman Catholic Church, and that supporters of reproductive technology have an interest in trying to link feminist opposition to Catholic opposition as a way of discrediting both. Not only will advocates of reproductive technology adopt this "politics of guilt by association," but some conservative religious groups may attempt "to co-opt feminist language, ethics, and politics for their own cause" ([10], p. 60). So there may be a variety of reasons why individuals or groups might seek to conflate feminist opposition and Catholic opposition. Nevertheless, there are philosophical and political differences that make these traditions irreconcilable.

Raymond acknowledges that both the Catholic Church and feminists appeal to the language of embodiment in their critique of reproductive technology, but she says they "are talking about different bodies" ([10], p. 61). Feminists locate their appeal to embodiment within a context of opposition to violence against women, "Feminists," Raymond writes:

> are concerned about the ways in which the NRTs destroy a woman's bodily integrity and the totality of her personal and political existence. Many feminists criticize the way in which the 'technodocs' sever the biological processes of pregnancy and reproduction from the female body while at the same time making ever more invasive incursions into the female body for eggs, for implantation, for embryo transfers, and the like. Through such incursions, women can only come to be distanced from their autonomous bodily processes. And the net result of this is that women's bodies are perceived by themselves and others as a reproductive resource, as a field to be seeded, ploughed and ultimately harvested for the fruit of the womb. The feminist value of 'embodiment' translates to bodily integrity and the control of one's body ([10], pp. 61-62).

By contrast, Raymond argues, Catholic opposition to disembodiment is located within a context of opposition to violence against fetuses. Consequently, in the Vatican *Instruction,* a document that, as we saw, appeals repeatedly to the language of embodiment, an entire section is devoted to a discussion of the effects of disembodied procreation on the fetus, but scarcely a word to the effects on women. "Nowhere," writes Raymonds about the Vatican *Instruction:*

> is there one mention of the 'disrespect' that is accorded to the woman's 'human life' by these technologies. One might expect that a document whose title purports to talk about the 'origin' of human life might at least mention women. But the so-called 'dignity of procreation' is applied in a general sense to the dignity of the human person and certainly not specifically to the dignity and integrity of the woman's body. . . . Nowhere is there any recognition that the body of the woman becomes an instrument in the technological procreative process and that this constitutes an assault against the dignity of women and a form of violence against women. The abstract inviolability of fetal life reigns supreme; the real and present violability of a woman's life, on which the new reproductive technologies depend for their very existence, is once more invisible ([10], pp. 63-64).

Moreover, Raymond argues, even when the Vatican is not focused exclusively on the bodies of fetuses, even when women's bodies come into view, the consequences of reproductive technology on women's bodies are seen against the backdrop of concern about sexuality, parenthood, or marriage, and not against a backdrop of concern about the bodily integrity of women, nor of concern that women have control of their bodies. So whereas feminist appeals to embodiment are rooted in a commitment to subverting "the entire fabric of sexual subordination and the ways in which that subordination has insured for men both sexual and reproductive access to women," Vatican appeals to embodiment are rooted in a pro-naturalist world view that embraces compulsory motherhood for women and thus subsumes ". . . the autonomy and independence of the woman to the 'interests' of the family . . ." ([10], p. 62).

Given the striking similarities that we noted above between feminist opposition to reproductive technology and Vatican opposition, is Raymond right? The answer is that Raymond is both partly right and partly wrong. Although Raymond is right to point out the very real differences between some of the feminist objections and some raised by the Catholic Church, she is wrong to dismiss as quickly as she does the mutual concern about disembodiment. To be sure, there are good reasons for feminists to be skeptical about Catholic opposition to reproductive technology. As we saw, the rather glaring omission of any explicit discussion of how reproductive technology affects women is one. Nevertheless, a healthy skepticism here does not justify Raymond's hasty dismissal of Vatican concerns about disembodiment.

For example, Raymond claims that while the Vatican uses the language of embodiment in criticizing reproductive technology, it is only concerned about women's bodies derivatively. That is, the Catholic Church is only concerned about women's bodies to the extent that these bodies serve the reproductive interest of men or are necessary to safeguarding the bodies of fetuses. She says, "for feminists, women are our bodies," and the unstated implication is that for the Catholic Church this is not true. If we look closely at the Vatican *Instruction,* however, we see nearly identical language, language that, I believe, is meant to express the same worry. Quoting Pope John Paul II, the Congregation for the Doctrine of the Faith endorses a claim that might well be summarized as, "touch the body, touch the person." "Each human person," we read, "in his absolutely unique singularity, is constituted not only by his spirit, but by his body as well. Thus, in the body and through the body, one touches the person himself in his concrete reality" ([2], p. 8). "Touch the body, touch the person" might well be substituted without loss of meaning for "women are our bodies."

Yet, if this comparison highlights the fact that Raymond states her case too strongly by claiming that the Vatican and feminists are not aligned in any way, it also reveals the truth of her observation that the context of appeals to embodiment is all important. Feminists apply the insight behind the aphorism "women are our bodies" from a context in which there is an explicit and unequivocal commitment to women's bodily integrity and to securing personal and political liberty for women. So feminists move directly from a concern about the disembodiment of procreation that appears to come with reproductive technology to an explicit discussion of how this technology affects women's bodies and thus women's hope for freedom and equality.

By contrast, the Catholic Church appeals to embodiment from within a context in which there has not traditionally been a significant commitment to women's equality. The upshot is that when the Vatican talks about embodiment, it is not typically speaking about women's bodies. So although "touch that person, touch the body" in fact articulates the same view of the human person as "women are our bodies," the former aphorism refers primarily to male bodies. Thus, when the Vatican turns to apply this insight in an assessment of reproductive technology, we should not be altogether surprised — though we may still be outraged — by the fact that it takes up the effects this technology has on the bodies of fetuses, but says nothing about its impact on the bodies of women.

Indeed, Raymond's emphatic repudiation of Vatican appeals to embodiment forces us to confront the fact that the Church's discussion of the effects of disembodiment takes place against the backdrop, not merely of an undistinguished record of commitment to the rights of women, but against a significant legacy of denigration of the body, women, and sexuality. Margaret Farley, for example, has pointed out that any appeal to embodiment within the Christian tradition must come to grips with the fact that the Christian tradition has frequently embraced a dualism that pits spirit against body, man against woman, reason against emotion, a dualism that has served to oppress women. "Body/spirit," Farley writes:

> is in many ways the basic dualism with which historical religions have struggled since late antiquity. Women, as we have already noted, have been associated with body, men with mind. Women's physiology has been interpreted as 'closer to nature' than men's in that many areas and functions of a woman's body seem to serve the human species as much or more than they serve the individual woman. Women's bodies, in this interpretation, are subject to a kind of fate — more so than men's. Women are immersed in 'matter,' in an inertness which has not its own agency. This is manifest not only in the determined rhythms of their bodily functions, but in a tendency to act from emotion rather than from reason, and in women's 'natural' work which is the caring for the bodies of children and men ([7], p. 291).

Has the Church come to grips with this legacy in its appeal to embodiment in the *Instruction* on Reproductive Technology? Raymond has shown decisively that the answer to this question is "no." The lesson to be drawn here is that the Church's own best insights have been undermined by a continuing legacy of sexism and dualistic thinking. If the Vatican was not in fact blinkered by the regrettable bifurcation of reality that runs deep in the tradition, if instead the Vatican took seriously an incarnational theology that, in Carolyn Walker Bynum's words, treats the "body as locus, not merely of pleasure but of personhood itself" ([1], p. 19), then the Vatican appeal to embodiment in the *Instruction* on Reproductive Technology would in fact commit it to attend seriously to women's bodily autonomy and to the threat posed to women's bodies by reproductive technology. It is regrettable that the *Instruction* does not do justice to the Church's own vision of the human person as "a unified totality" of body and spirit, but we should not dismiss the vision itself as sexist or misogynist for that reason.

If Raymond's juxtaposition of feminist criticism with Vatican criticism of reproductive technology helps us to see that any appeal to embodiment must be taken in context, and, if attending to the context of Vatican appeals to embodiment helps us to discern the shortcomings of Catholic opposition to reproductive technology, it is worth asking whether this juxtaposition does not also highlight the shortcomings of some feminist appeals to embodiment. I want in closing to suggest that it does and, indeed, to show how the Vatican *Instruction* might offer an important corrective to one strand of the feminist critique precisely at the point where the context of feminist appeals to embodiment undermines feminist insights.

To see once again that the comparison of feminist and Catholic opposition to reproductive technology is instructive, we may return to the analogy Gena Corea draws between sexual prostitution and the commodification of reproduction. We saw above that this comparison is made to highlight the dangers of an activity that appears to commodify women's bodies in a cultural context where women's bodies are already for sale in the marketplace. To explain the full force of this analogy, however, we must ask why sexual prostitution is morally problematic.[3] If feminism is committed to the bodily autonomy of women, why should women not be able to sell their bodies if they so choose? This is a difficult question for feminism, and it is instructive to see how one strand of feminist thought has answered this question. One answer to the question has essentially been to suggest that prostitution is so degrading and so dehumanizing that no woman would choose to be a prostitute unless she were coerced.

It is this line of reasoning, for example, that Catherine MacKinnon has in mind when she writes that the fact that ". . . prostitution and modeling are structurally women's best economic options should give pause to those who would consider women's presence there a true act of free choice" ([9], p. 180). As MacKinnon points out, in other contexts, we readily acknowledge that people do degrading work for lack of better economic options, and we neither deny that the work is degrading nor deceive ourselves by thinking that the work is freely chosen. Indeed, even where a woman "chooses" prostitution in a context where she is not doing so, say, to feed herself or her children, we have good reason to suspect that other forms of coercion are at work. Perhaps self-esteem has been so undermined by a society that systematically devalues women that there is not a sufficient sense of self-worth to recognize the degradation of prostitution.

Thus, whether we are talking about economic coercion or other, perhaps less obvious forms of coercion, the important point is that this approach to prostitution challenges the presumption that prostitution is freely chosen. What MacKinnon says of pornography could also be said of prostitution. "I will leave you wondering . . . ," MacKinnon writes, "why it is that when a woman spreads her legs for a camera, she is assumed to be exercising free will" ([9], p. 180). Why is it, critics of prostitution might ask, that when a woman sells her body for money, she is assumed to be exercising free will? To reverse the presumption here is to take the view that sexual prostitution in itself could not possibly fulfill any legitimate interest for a person of self-respect. Hence, if a woman is selling her body, there is reason to suspect coercion.

I have argued elsewhere that this is in fact a powerful argument and that the critique of "liberal" conceptions of autonomy implicit in it is also significant (see [8]). For our purposes, it is important to see how the logic of this argument must be extended to reproductive technology if the comparison of assisted reproduction to sexual prostitution is to carry any weight. Take, for example, the argument that IVF turns a woman into a sort of reproductive prostitute. Part of the force of this argument comes from the suggestion that women are coerced into IVF, just as they are coerced into becoming prostitutes. Yet, if we consider the claim that to offer IVF to a childless woman is coercive, we discover that for this claim to be plausible we require a conviction comparable to the belief that eliminating prostitution could not conflict with any legitimate interest a woman of self-respect might have.

In one sense, of course, this is not true even of prostitution. If a woman sells her body in order to feed herself or her children, she is obviously pursuing a legitimate interest. Nevertheless, the point opponents of prostitution and of reproductive technology wish to make is that there is nothing in the activity of selling one's body or in the procedures of assisted reproduction that is itself rewarding for women, and, consequently, if women choose either activity, the only explanation is that they have been coerced. The problem with pressing this line of argument, however, is that there is a more direct connection between assisted reproduction and the good of bearing and begetting a child than between prostitution and the good of feeding children. The upshot is that opponents of reproductive technology can only utilize this analogy with prostitution effectively, if they are simultaneously prepared to reject or devalue the importance of begetting and bearing children.

Unfortunately, when we examine the work of some who have opposed IVF on the grounds that it may be coercive, we see precisely this sort of skepticism about the value of children. For example, in an article entitled "'Women Want It': *In Vitro* Fertilization and Women's Motivations for Participation," Christine Crowe argues that women participate in IVF programs largely because they accept the dominant ideology of motherhood in Western culture, an ideology that includes the belief that biological motherhood is valuable. "IVF," Crowe writes, "relies upon women to perceive motherhood as desirable" ([6], pp. 547-48). Or consider Robyn Rowland's explanation of the pressures facing infertile women. Under the heading "pro-natalism and the experience of infertility," Rowland writes:

> To understand the impact of infertility, we need to understand that we live within a society which says that it is good to have children. That is, one which has pronatalist values. . . . The exclamations of wonder whenever we see something young, vulnerable, and cuddly such as a kitten are also reinforcing the desire for children ([13], p. 85).

Rowland is certainly correct that childless women face enormous pressure in Western societies, but does recognizing this fact, and the coercion that may come with it, also require rejecting any affirmation of children, as this passage appears to suggest?

Here we see how the context of feminist appeals to embodiment may also subvert the full significance of embodiment. To appeal to embodiment from within a context that emphasizes the way in which pregnancy,

3. In fact, I cannot hope to unpack this analogy fully here. To do so would require a complete analysis of the relationship between a prostitute and client, and an examination of that relationship compared to the relationship among infertile individuals, physicians, and gamete donors. I will focus only on the comparison between an infertile woman and a prostitute.

childbirth, and the care of children have been oppressive to women, poses the danger of neglecting the value of the decidedly embodied experience of pregnancy and the embodied goodness of children.

This is not to say that all, or even most, feminists who have opposed reproductive technology out of concerns over embodiment devalue children. Nor do I wish to deny that pregnancy is sometimes oppressive for women and perceived by women as such. Nor would I deny that having and rearing children can be unfulfilling or even disastrously burdensome. Still, those feminists who have categorically discounted the value to women of pregnancy and parenthood have not taken embodiment seriously enough. Given a preoccupation with combatting an ideology that sacralizes pregnancy and motherhood, it is easy to conflate the socially sanctioned belief that having children is desirable (and pregnancy uniquely fulfilling) with the very different proposition that women cannot be fulfilled unless they have children. Thus, in their eagerness to reject the latter claim, some feminists have been blinded to the fact that women may legitimately value carrying and caring for children. To celebrate is not to sacralize, and any view that fully embraced the importance of embodiment could not but celebrate the experiences of bearing and rearing children.

In the final analysis, careful attention to Vatican and to feminist appeals to embodiment reveals striking differences that in turn highlight the shortcomings of both Vatican and some feminist opposition to reproductive technology. At the same time, however, we can see striking similarities. Both traditions of thought draw our attention to the potential dangers of disembodying procreation, and in doing so, both traditions properly highlight the importance of attention to issues of embodiment when reflecting morally on medicine. It is perhaps ironic, therefore, that, in assessing reproductive technology in light of the embodied character of human life, critics in both traditions go so wrong. For, surely, no adequate account of embodiment and reproductive technology would conclude that this technology always or necessarily violates the embodied quality of human procreation. On the contrary, for many infertile individuals, reproductive technology mediates embodiment, not the reverse (see [7]). That both Catholic opposition and some feminist opposition to reproductive technology appear blind to this fact demonstrates how important the context of appeals to embodiment can be.

Bibliography

[1] Bynum, C. W.: 1991, *Fragmentation and Redemption,* Zone Books, New York.

[2] Congregation for the Doctrine of Faith: 1987, *Instruction on Respect for Human Life in Its Origin and on the Dignity of Procreation,* United States Catholic Conference, Washington.

[3] Corea, G.: 1985, *The Mother Machine,* Harper & Row, New York.

[4] Corea, G.: 1987, "The Reproductive Brothel," in G. Corea et al. (eds.), *Man-Made Women,* Indiana University Press, Bloomington, pp. 38-51.

[5] Corea, G.: 1988, "What the King Can Not See," in E. H. Baruch, A. F. D'Adamo, Jr. and J. Seager (eds.), *Embryos, Ethics, and Women's Rights,* Harrington Park Press, New York, pp. 77-93.

[6] Crowe, C.: 1985, "'Women Want It': *In Vitro* Fertilization and Women's Motivations for Participation," *Women Studies International Forum* 8(6): 547-52.

[7] Farley, M.: 1985, "Feminist Theology and Bioethics," in B. H. Andolson, C. E. Gudorf, and M. D. Pellauer (eds.), *Women's Consciousness, Women's Conscience,* Harper and Row, San Francisco, pp. 285-305.

[8] Lauritzen, P.: 1993, *Pursuing Parenthood,* Indiana University Press, Bloomington.

[9] MacKinnon, C.: 1987, *Feminism Unmodified,* Harvard University Press, Cambridge, Mass.

[10] Raymond, J.: 1987, "Fetalists and Feminists: They Are Not the Same," in P. Spallone and D. L. Steinberg (eds.), *Made to Order,* Pergamon, Oxford, pp. 58-66.

[11] Rothman, B. K.: 1989, *Recreating Motherhood,* W. W. Norton, New York.

[12] Rothman, B. K.: 1985, *The Tentative Pregnancy,* Viking Press, New York.

[13] Rowland, R.: 1987, "Women as Living Laboratories: The New Reproductive Technologies," in J. Figuerra-McDonough and R. C. Sarri (eds.), *The Trapped Woman,* Sage, Newbury Park, pp. 81-111.

[14] Ryan, M.: 1993, "Justice and Artificial Reproduction: A Catholic Feminist Analysis," Ph.D. dissertation, Yale University, New Haven, Conn.

[15] Ryan, M.: 1990, "The Argument for Unlimited Procreative Liberty: A Feminist Critique," *Hastings Center Report* 20(4): 6-12.

116 The Ethical Challenge of the New Reproductive Technology

Sidney Callahan

How should we ethically evaluate the new reproductive technologies developed to treat the increasing problem of human fertility? Our national debate over this troubling issue is just beginning. At this point, there are lacunae in law and regulatory procedures, while medical technological innovation and practice proceed without ethical consensus. This situation is due in part to the speed of recent developments, but we also find ourselves ethically perplexed because we, as a society, did not arrive at a consensus on the ethics of reproduction and responsible parenthood *before* the newest technologies appeared on the scene.

One obvious sign of the society's unresolved conflicts over the morality of reproduction can be found in the bitter debates over abortion and, to a lesser extent, contraception and contraceptive education in the schools. With no societal consensus on the ethical use of medical technology to plan, limit, or interrupt pregnancies, we are unprepared to evaluate the newest alternative reproductive technologies which *promote* conception and pregnancies. At the same time as we have seen rapid advances in regulating fertility, we have experienced an evolution in attitudes toward women, children, sexuality, and the family. These intersecting social developments have produced the pressing need to develop a new ethic of parenthood and responsible reproduction.[1] My focus here, however, is on the most recent challenge. How should we ethically assess the innovative array of techniques developed to overcome fertility — egg and sperm donations, surrogate mothers, in vitro fertilization, and embryo transplants?

Two Inadequate Approaches to Alternative Reproductive Technology

Two inadequate approaches to the ethical assessment of the new alternative reproductive technologies are mirror images of each other in the narrowness of their focus and the limitations of their analysis. On the one hand, a conservative approach adopts as a moral standard the biological integrity of the marital sexual act. The married couple's marital sexual and reproductive acts must not be tampered with for any reason, and sexual intercourse and procreation must remain united in each marital act so that "lovemaking and babymaking" are never separated. In this "act analysis," no technological intervention in the sexual act is countenanced or approved for any reason. Older arguments employed against artificial contraception are reiterated and applied to condemn any procedure separating functions which naturally occur together, and thus all reproduction by in vitro fertilization, artificial insemination, or third party surrogacy is deemed immoral. The only ethical stance toward new reproductive technologies would be to absolutely cease and desist; such procedures should come to a full stop.

At the other end of the ideological spectrum, another form of act analysis narrows its own focus to a person's desire for a child and the individual acts the person might perform in carrying out private arrangements for reproduction. As long as due process and informed consent by competent adults is guarded by proper contracts, any adult should be able to engage in any alternative reproductive procedure that technology can provide or that persons will sell or procure. This permissive stance is held to be justified on the basis of individual liberty, autonomy, reproductive privacy, and reproductive right. The burden of proof supposedly lies with those who would limit alternative reproductive technology, and in the name of liberty and individual autonomy, potential regulators are enjoined to show that concrete harmful consequences will result from a particular practice (if it is to be rejected). Of course, when there are as yet no existing consequences, it is impossible to *prove* harm will result. Indeed, even when there have been relevant cases (e.g., the AID children conceived by artificial insemination by donor), no long-term in-depth studies have been done. Therefore, the ethical response to alternative reproductive technologies is to proceed full steam ahead (with consideration given to due process and informed consent).

The premature ethical foreclosure implied in either of the above approaches to reproductive technologies is not adequate. An ethic based solely on the natural biological integrity of marital acts will not serve, because the mastery of nature through technological problem-solving is also completely natural to us — indeed, it is the glory of *homo sapiens*. Yet, because we are rational, we can also see that a fully permissive attitude toward reproductive technology presents serious problems as well. We are reminded that in the past, innovative uses of technology have resulted in ecological and ethical disasters. Abuses have been either fully intended, as with the Nazis, or inadvertent and accidental, as in countless innovative interventions, such as the use of diethylstilbestrol (DES) or thalidomide, which had bad side effects far outweighing

1. See Sidney Callahan, "An Ethical Analysis of Responsible Parenthood," in *Genetic Counseling: Facts, Values, and Norms*. Birth Defects: Original Article Series, vol. 15, no. 22 (New York: Alan R. Liss, 1979).

From Sidney Callahan, "The Ethical Challenge of the New Reproductive Technology," in John F. Monagle and David C. Thomasma, *Medical Ethics: A Guide for Health Professionals* (Rockville, Maryland: Aspen Publishers, Inc., 1988), pp. 26-37. Used by permission.

the supposed advantages. There is a grain of truth in the warning that "control of nature" often ends up producing increased control (or oppression) of some people by other more powerful people. Technology itself has to be ethically assessed and rationally controlled. Faced with new reproductive technologies, we should not let the technological imperative (what can be done should be done), fueled in this case by people's desires, decide the question whether a course of action is right or good.

The Basis for Developing an Ethical Position

In the case of reproductive technology, ethical positions should emerge from a consideration of what will further the good of the potential child and the family, as well as provide appropriate social conditions for childrearing and strengthening our commitment to moral principles concerning individual responsibility in reproduction. We should move beyond a narrow focus on either biology or people's desires for children. In this serious matter, which involves children's lives and the social structure of our society, it is more prudent to consider first the values and goods safeguarded and protected at present by the operating norms of reproduction and childrearing before countenancing radical alterations. In matters of such serious collective import, the burden of proof should rightly be upon those who wish to experiment with the lives of others. (An ethical problem also arises in an overpopulated, impoverished world. However, since the main issue here concerns the use of reproductive technology, I think the correct statement of the ethical question is whether, or how far, present norms should be altered.)

One troubling tactic used by those urging the permissive acceptance of all new reproductive technologies is to base their arguments upon analogies from adoption or other childrearing arrangements that arise from divorce, death, desertion, or parental inadequacy. Much is made of the cases in which persons cope with single parenthood or successfully adapt to less-than-ideal situations. But the adequacy of "after the fact" crisis management does not justify planning beforehand to voluntarily replicate similar childrearing situations. Emergency solutions make poor operating norms. Even a child conceived through rape or incest might adapt and be glad to have been born, but surely it would be wrong to plan such conceptions beforehand on the grounds that the future child would rather exist than not or that the sexual abuser had no other means to reproduce. Similarly, and more to the point, heretofore we have not ethically or legally countenanced the practice of deliberately conceiving a child in order to give it to others for adoption, with or without payment. We have forbidden the selling of babies or, for that matter, the purchasing of bribes, sexual intercourse, or bodily organs. Certain cultural goods, safeguards, and values have been preserved by these existing norms. How can ethical guidelines for employing alternative reproductive methods strengthen rather than threaten our basic cultural values?

A Proposed Ethical Standard

It is ethically appropriate to use an alternative reproductive technology if, and only if, it makes it possible for a normal, socially well-adjusted heterosexual married couple to have a child that they could not otherwise have owing to infertility. Infertility does not seem strictly classifiable as a disease, but for a married couple it is clearly an unfortunate dysfunction or handicap, one which medicine may sometimes remedy. It seems wonderful, almost miraculous, that medical technology can often overcome a couple's infertility to restore normal function with techniques such as artificial insemination by husband (AIH), in vitro fertilization (IVF), or tubal ovum transfer methods. But holding to a proposed ethical standard of medical remediation and restoration of a married couple's average expectable fertility implies that medical professionals should not aim to alter or contravene what would otherwise exist as the normal conditions for procreation and childrearing.

A remedial standard based upon operating cultural norms requires that the genetic parents, the gestational parents, and the rearing parents be identical and that the parents be presently alive and well, in an appropriate time in their life cycle, and possess average or adequate psychological and social resources for childrearing. Helping the severely retarded, the mentally ill, the genetically diseased, the destitute, the aged, or a widow with a dead spouse's sperm to have children they otherwise could not would be ethically unacceptable by this standard. It would also be unacceptable to alter average expectable conditions by efforts to produce multiple births or to select routinely for sex (the latter practice producing a whole host of other ethical problems which cannot be dealt with here). The power to intervene in such a crucial matter as the procreation of a new life makes the medical professionals or medical institutions involved into ethically responsible trustees of a potential child's future. As trustees, medical professionals would seem to have an ethical duty not to take risks on behalf of unconsenting others.

Medical professionals should be guided by a form of communal judgment influenced by cultural values and norms. What would most responsible would-be parents deem ethically appropriate reproductive behavior in a particular case? Physicians or other health care personnel can hardly, in good conscience, agree to and make possible irresponsible or ethically inappropriate reproductive acts affecting innocent new lives. Socially informed ethical judgments on behalf of the society are unavoidable. The fact that medical professionals and medical resources must be employed for remedial infertility treatments, which will produce direct social consequences, justifies using standards of judgment that take into account the general social good. Ethical standards which protect and strengthen positive outcomes for children, childrearing conditions, and cultural norms of responsible parenthood should be used to judge the appropriateness of a particular request for treatment of infertility.

The claim that an individual's right to reproduce would be violated if fertility treatments are not made available to any individual who requests them seems wrongheaded. A negative right not to be interfered with (e.g., the right to marry, which itself is not absolute) does not entail a positive right (e.g., that society is obligated to provide spouses). Moreover, as a society, we have already decided that when adequate childrearing conditions and the well-being of children are in the balance, social and professional intervention is justified. Adoption procedures, custodial decisions, and child abuse laws involve rights and duties of professionals to make judgments on the fitness of parents. And as child abuse and resulting deaths regularly attest, it is far better to err on the side of safety than take risks. Should not medical professionals be similarly responsible in carrying out the interventions which will in essence give to a couple a baby to rear? If a couple seems within the normal range of average expectable parents, then remedial techniques that maintain the identicalness of genetic, gestational, and rearing parentage, techniques such as AIH or IVF or tubal ovum transfer, would be ethically acceptable.

Employing third party donors or surrogate mothers is not, in my opinion, ever an ethically acceptable use of reproductive technologies. Procedures using donors or surrogates separate and variously recombine the source of sperm, eggs, embryos, gestational womb, and rearing parents. Such a separation — whether through artificial insemination by donor (AID), embryo transplants, or surrogate mothers — poses too many ethical and social risks to the dignity and well-being of the future child, the donor, individual spouses, the family as a whole, and our cultural ethos. To argue the case against third party donors, even for acceptable couples, we need to consider what values, goods, and safeguards have been inherent in the cultural norm: two heterosexual parents who are the genetic, gestational, and rearing parents of their child.

Many proponents of third party donors in alternative reproduction — for single men and women, homosexual couples, or infertile couples — ignore what happens *after* a baby is conceived, produced, or procured. Focusing on an individual or individual couples, the psychological and social dimensions of childrearing are separated from conception, gestation, and birth. Little account is taken of the fact that individuals live out their life span intergenerationally and in complex ecological and social systems.[2] No account is taken of the newest developments in family therapy and family system analysis. The assumption seems to be that why and how one gets a baby makes no difference in what happens afterwards. This may be true of hens or cows, but it is hardly true of complex, thinking, emoting, imaginative human beings functioning within social systems.

Another equally invalid line of argument cites the current trends toward the breakdown of the traditional family unit and jumps to the conclusion that since the nuclear family seems to be disintegrating anyway, and the society survives, why try to preserve the norms heretofore valued? Ominous cultural effects on children and women that correlate with the breakdown of the family are dismissed as having no application to individual cases.[3] But a growing body of psychological literature points to a less sanguine judgment. Having *two* rearing parents provides important advantages, and fathers play more of a role in the moral, social, and sexual-identity development of the child than has been recognized.[4]

Legitimizing and morally sanctioning third party or collaborative reproduction or assisting single or homosexual conceptions can contribute directly to the specific negative childrearing conditions in the culture which *do* harm individuals and the larger community. The culture's operating norms concerning the family provide irreplaceable goods and safeguards — particularly for women and their children — which we come to truly value as we see them attenuated. Arguments for limiting reproductive interventions to remediation with no third party interventions can best be made by considering what is at stake if we alter our norms. We put at risk the good of the family, the parents, the child, and the donor(s), as well as our sexual morality, with its focus on sexual responsibility.

The Family

The advantages and safeguards of having two heterosexual parents who are the genetic, gestational, and rearing parents are manifold and basic; this type of family was not accidentally selected for in biological and cultural evolution. Mammalian "in vivo" reproduction and primate parent-child bonding provide adaptive means for the protection, defense, and complex socialization of offspring. They far outperform reproduction by laying eggs that are then left floating in the sea or buried in the sand to take their chances with passing predators.[5] With the

2. Barbara M. Newman and Philip R. Newman, *Development Through Life: A Psychosocial Approach* (Homewood, Ill.: The Dorsey Press, 1979); Lynn Hoffman, *Foundations of Family Therapy: A Conceptual Framework for Systems Change* (New York: Basic Books, 1981).

3. Daniel P. Moynihan, *Family and Nation* (New York: Harcourt Brace Jovanovich, 1986); Lenore J. Weitzman, *The Divorce Revolution* (New York: The Free Press, 1986).

4. The role of the father has been seen as critically important in both the female and male child's intellectual development, moral development, sex role identity, and future parenting; for a summary of relevant research, see Ross D. Parke, *Father* (Cambridge, Mass.: Harvard University Press, 1981), and Shirley M. H. Hanson and Frederick W. Bonett, *Dimensions of Fatherhood* (Beverly Hills, Calif.: Sage Publications, 1985).

5. See Jeanne Altman, "Sociobiological Perspectives on Parent-

advent of long-living rational animals such as human beings, the basic primate models are broadened and deepened, with results in family units that include fathers and encompass additional kinship bonds.[6] Two heterosexual parents supported by kin and clan can engage in even more arduous parenting, including nurturing the young over an extended period. The nuclear family is founded on biology and may have originally evolved through natural selection, but it is as a cultural phenomenon, with its psychological and social effectiveness in generating responsibility, socialization, and deep altruistic bonds, that the family has achieved stability and universality.

Why has the nuclear family worked for so long and held first place in the cultural competition?[7] The Western cultural ideal, gradually becoming less patriarchic as it comes to recognize the equality of women and children, has ensured far more than law, order, and social continuity. As the heterosexual members of a couple freely choose each other, they make a loving commitment to share the vicissitudes of life. Bonded in love and legal contract, they mutually exchange exclusive rights, giving each other emotional and economic priority. Love and sexuality often result in procreation, and the children then have a claim to equal parental care from both their father and mother. In addition, the extended families of both parents are important as supplemental supports for the couple, especially in cases of death or disaster.

No act analysis of one procreative period of time in a marriage can do justice to the fact that the reproductive couple exists as a unit within a family extended in time and kinship. Grandparents, grandchildren, aunts, cousins, and other relatives are important in family life for both pragmatic and psychological reasons. Individual identity is rooted in biologically based kinship and in small cooperating social units. The family is one remaining institution where status is given by birth, not earned or achieved. The irreversible bonds of kinship over time and through space produce rootedness and a sense of identity. Psychologically and socially the family provides emotional connections, social purpose, and meaning to life. Those individuals who do not marry and found families or who achieve membership in larger communities are still strongly connected to others through their families.[8] Each human being exists within a social envelope and must do so to flourish; the family is one of the most important elements in a human life. But as a cultural invention, why must a family be based upon biological kinship? Cannot any persons who declare themselves a family be a family?

While the internalized psychological image of a family and the intention to belong to a family are part of the foundations of a family, there is no denying the bond created by genetic kinship. One definition of the family is that a family consists of people who share genes. Sociobiologists have not exaggerated the importance of gene-sharing in human bonding.[9] In fact, the unwillingness of infertile couples to adopt and their struggles to have their own baby is testimony to the existence of what appears to be a strong innate urge to reproduce oneself. Culturally this is understood as the fusion of two genetic heritages, with the child situated within two lineages. Members of both lineages may be supportive, or one set of kin may by choice or chance be more important than the other, but having both sets provides important social resources. The child is heir to more than money or property when situated in a rooted kinship community.

The search by adopted children for their biological parents and possible siblings reveals the psychological need of humans to be situated and to know their origins.[10] When there is one or more third party donors — of sperm, eggs, or embryo — the child is cut off from either half or all of its genetic heritage. If deception is practiced concerning the child's origins, then both the child and the extended family will be wronged. Since family secrets are rarely kept completely, the delayed revelations produce disillusionment and distrust among those deceived. When a child and relatives are not lied to, the identity of the donor (or donors) becomes an issue for all concerned.

Parents and Spouses

Psychology has come to see genetic factors as more and more important in parent-child interactions and child-rearing outcomes.[11] When rearing parents and genetic

hood," *Parenthood: A Psychodynamic Perspective* (New York: Guilford Press, 1984).

6. Kathleen Gough, "The Origin of the Family," *Journal of Marriage and the Family* (November 1971): 760-68. Peter J. Wilson, *Man the Promising Primate: The Conditions of Human Evolution* (New Haven, Conn.: Yale University Press, 1980).

7. George Peter Murdock, "The Universality of the Nuclear Family," in *A Modern Introduction to the Family,* ed. Norman W. Bell and Ezra F. Vogel (New York: The Free Press, 1968); Mary Jo Bane, *Here to Stay: American Families in the Twentieth Century* (New York: Basic Books, 1976).

8. Stephen P. Bank and Michael D. Kahn, *The Sibling Bond* (New York: Basic Books, 1982); Gunhild O. Hagestad, "The Aging Society as a Context for Family Life," *Daedalus: The Aging Society* (Winter 1986): 119-39.

9. E. O. Wilson, *Sociobiology* (Cambridge, Mass.: Harvard University Press, 1975).

10. Carol Nadelson, "The Absent Parent, Emotional Sequelae," in *Infertility: Medical, Emotional and Social Considerations,* ed. Miriam D. Mazor and Harriet F. Simons (New York: Human Sciences Press, 1984); Arthur D. Sorsky, Annette Baron, and Reuben Pannor, "Identity Conflicts in Adoptees," in *New Directions in Childhood Psychopathology,* vol. 1 (New York: International Universities Press, 1982).

11. Twin studies and the recognition of inherited temperamental traits have followed studies showing a genetic component to alcoholism, manic-depression, schizophrenia, antisocial behavior, and I.Q. For a popular discussion of the findings in regard to schizophrenia and criminal behavior, see Sarnoff Mednick, "Crime in the Family Tree," *Psychology Today,* 19 (March 1985): 58-61. For a more general discussion by an anthropologist, see Melvin Konner, *The Tangled Wing: Biological Constraints on the Human Spirit* (New York: Holt, Rinehart & Winston, 1982).

parents differ and the donor is unknown, there is a provocative void. If the donor is known and part of the rearing parents' family or social circle, there are other psychological problems and potential conflicts over who is the real parent and who has the primary rights and responsibilities. When the third party donor is also the surrogate mother, combining genetic and gestational parenthood, the social and legal problems can be profound. The much discussed Whitehead-Stern court struggle indicates the divisive chaos, struggle, and suffering that is possible in surrogate arrangements.

In the average expectable situation, two parents with equal genetic investment in the child are unified by their mutual relationship to the child. They are irreversibly connected and made kin to each other through the biological child they have procreated. Their love, commitment, and sexual bond have been made manifest in a new life. Their genetic link with the child, shared with their own family, produces a sense of family likeness and personal identification, leading to empathy and affective attunement. The child's genetic link to each spouse and his or her kin strengthens the marital bond. But the fact that the child is also a new and unique creation and a random fusion of the couple's genetic heritage gives enough distance to allow the child also to be seen as a separate other, with what has been called its "alien dignity as a human being" intact.[12] (Cloning oneself would be wrong for its egotistic intent and for the dehumanizing effects of trying to deny the uniqueness of identity.) The marital developments that occur during pregnancy also unite the couple and prepare them for the parental enterprise.[13] Since we are embodied creatures, the psychological bonds of caring and empathy are built upon the firm foundation of biological ties and bodily self-identity.

When technological intervention without donors, such as AIH or IVP or tubal ovum transfer, is used to correct infertility, the time, money, stress, and cooperative effort required to serve to test the unity of the couple and focus them upon their marital relationship and their mutual contribution to childbearing. The psychological bonding between them can transcend the stress caused by the less-than-ideal technological interventions in their sexual lives. The result of their joint effort will, as in natural pregnancy, be a baby they are equally invested in and equally related to. (In adoption, both parents also have an equal relationship to the child they are jointly rescuing.) Given the equal investment in their child, both parents are equally responsible for childrearing and support.

With third party genetic or gestational donors, however, the marital and biological unity is broken asunder. One parent will be related biologically to the child and the other parent will not. True, the nonrelated parent may give consent, but the consent, even if truly informed and uncoerced, can hardly equalize the imbalance. While there is certainly no real question of adultery in such a situation, nevertheless, the intruding third party donor, as in adultery, will inevitably have a psychological effect on the couple's life. Even if there is no jealousy or envy, the reproductive inadequacy of one partner has been made definite and reliance has been placed on an outsider's potency, genetic heritage, and superior reproductive capacity.[14]

Asymmetry in biological parental relationships within a family or household has always been problematic, from Cinderella to today's stepparents and reconstituted families. The most frequently cited cause of divorce in second marriages is the difficulty of dealing with another person's children.[15] Empathy, identification, a sense of kinship, and assurance of parental authority arise from family likeness and biological ties. In disturbed families under stress, one finds more incest, child abuse, and scapegoating when biological kinship is absent.[16] Biological ties become psychologically potent, because human beings fantasize in their intersubjective emotional interactions with one another and with their children. Parents' fantasies about a child's past and future do make a difference, as all students of child development or family dynamics will attest. Identical twins may even be treated very differently because parents project different fantasies upon them.[17] Third party donors and surrogates cannot be counted on to disappear from family consciousness even if legal contracts could control other ramifications or forbid actual interventions.

The Child

The most serious ethical problems in using third party donors in alternative reproduction concern the well-being of the potential child. A child conceived by new forms of collaborative reproduction is being made party to a social experiment without its consent. While no child is conceived by its own consent, a child not artificially produced is at least born in the same way as its par-

12. Helmut Thielicke, *The Ethics of Sex* (New York: Harper & Row, 1964), pp. 32ff.

13. Aidan Macfarlane, *The Psychology of Childbirth* (Cambridge, Mass.: Harvard University Press, 1977); M. Greenberg, *The Birth of a Father* (New York: Continuum, 1985).

14. The difficulties of undergoing AID are described in Sharon Gibbons Collotta, "The Role of the Nurse in AID," in *Infertility;* see also R. Snowden, G. D. Mitchel, and E. M. Snowden, "Stigma and Stress in AID," in *Artificial Reproduction: A Social Investigation,* (London: George Allen & Unwin, 1983).

15. Brenda Maddox, *The Half Parent: Living with Other People's Children* (New York: M. Evans and Company, 1975); Renato Espinoza and Yvonne Newman, *Stepparenting: With Annotated Bibliography* (Rockville Md.: National Institute of Mental Health, Center for Studies of Child and Family Mental Health, 1979).

16. See "Explaining the Differences between Biological Father and Stepfather Incest" and "Social Factors in the Occurrence of Incestuous Abuse," in Diana E. H. Russell, *The Secret Trauma: Incest in the Lives of Girls and Women* (New York: Basic Books, 1986).

17. Daniel N. Stern, *The Interpersonal World of the Infant: A View from Psychoanalysis and Developmental Psychology* (New York: Basic Books, 1985).

ents and other persons normally have been. A child who has a donor or donors among its parents will be cut off from at least part of its genetic heritage and its kin in new ways. Even if there is no danger of transmitting unknown genetic disease or causing physiological harm to the child, the psychological relationship of the child to its parents is endangered, whether or not there is deception or secrecy about its origins.

It should be clear that adoption (which rescues a child already in existence) is very different ethically from planning to involve third party donors in procuring a child. An adopted child, while perhaps harboring resentment against its birth parent, must look at its rescuing adopters differently than a child would look at parents who have had it made to order. Treating the child like a commodity — something to be created for the pleasure of the parents — infringes the child's dignity. When one is begotten (not made), then one shares equally with one's parents in the ongoing transmission of the gift of life from generation to generation. The child procreated in the expectable way is a subsidiary gift arising from the prior marital relationship, not a product or project of the parental will.

Alternative reproductive techniques made available to single men and women or to homosexual couples will further endanger the child's status. Why should a child, at its creation, be treated as a property, a product, or a means to satisfy the wishes of adults? Even in natural reproduction, we now consider it ethically suspect to attempt to have a child not for its own sake, but because an adult wants to satisfy some personal need or desire.

Unfortunately, we are still saddled with residual ideologies that view children as a kind of personal property. Only gradually have we welcomed children as gifts — new lives given in trusteeship — and treated them as equal to adult persons in human dignity despite their dependency and their powerlessness.[18] Having a child for some extrinsic reason is now as generally unacceptable as marrying for money or some motive besides love and a desire for mutual happiness. Unfortunately, in the past some persons have wanted children to secure an inheritance, to prove sexual prowess, to procure a scapegoat, to gain revenge, to increase marital power, to secure social prestige, or to have someone of their own to love. The motives for conception influence the future relationship of the child to the parents. A couple absolutely and obsessively driven to have a child (as some couples become when faced with infertility) may not be prepared to rear the actual child once it is born. Being wanted and being well reared are not identical. Parental overinvestment in "gourmet children" can be psychologically difficult for a child.[19] Every child must achieve independence and a separate identity. Adolescent problems of anorexia, depression, and suicide have been seen as related to the dynamics of parent control.[20] Growing up and leaving home becomes a problem for children who have been used to fulfill parents.[21] The child who was wanted for all the wrong reasons is pressured to live up to parental dreams of the optimal baby or perfect child. Outright rejection of imperfect or nonoptimal babies contracted for by alternative reproductive technology is possible and should be a matter of grave concern.

In the course of a child's development, psychologists note that thinking and fantasizing about one's origins seems to be inevitable. A child with a "clouded genetic heritage" has a more difficult time achieving a secure personal identity.[22] Yet a secure identity, self-esteem, and a sense of autonomy and self-control are crucial in children's growth.[23] Parental control is overwhelming to children. If they know or believe their parents contracted to fabricate them rather than merely received them, they feel more reduced in power.

In alternative reproduction, the questions "Whose baby am I?" becomes inevitable.[24] "Why was my biological parent not more concerned with what would happen to the new life he or she helped to create?" The need to know about possible half-siblings and other kin may become urgent at some point in later development. From the child's point of view, the asymmetry of the relationship with the rearing parents is also a factor. Even if the Freudian psychoanalytic account of Oedipal family relationships is not correct in all its details, there still exist extremely complex fantasies and psychological currents that arise in the family triangle of mother, father, and child. Having two parents with whom one can safely identify, love, and leave behind is a great advantage. One's sexual origins and one's kin are important psychological realities to a child.

Donors and the Cultural Ethos

Procuring donors of sperm, eggs, embryos, or wombs is an essential component of collaborative reproduction. Yet encouraging persons to give, or worse to sell, their

18. There is the beginning of a philosophical reassessment of the status of children in Jeffrey Blustein, *Parents & Children: The Ethics of the Family* (Oxford: Oxford University Press, 1982), and in Onoroa O'Neill and William Ruddick, eds., *Having Children: Philosophical and Legal Reflections on Parenthood* (New York: Oxford University Press, 1979).

19. See "The Child as Surrogate Self" and "The Child as Status Symbol," in David Elkind, *The Hurried Child* (Reading, Mass.: Addison-Wesley, 1981).

20. Salvador Minuchin, Bernice L. Rosman, and Walter Baker, *Psychosomatic Families: Anorexia Nervosa in Context* (Cambridge, Mass.: Harvard University Press, 1978).

21. Jay Haley, *Leaving Home: The Therapy of Disturbed Young People* (New York: McGraw-Hill, 1980).

22. Betty J. Lifton, *Lost and Found: The Adoption Experience* (New York: Dial Press, 1979).

23. See "The Sense of Self," in Eleanor E. Maccoby, *Social Development: Psychological Growth and the Parent-Child Relationship* (New York: Harcourt Brace Jovanovich, 1980).

24. Lori Andrews, "Yours, Mine and Theirs," *Psychology Today* 18 (December 1984): 20-29.

genetic or gestational capacity attacks a basic foundation of morality — that is, the taking of responsibility for the consequences of one's actions. Adult persons are held morally responsible for their words and deeds. In serious matters, such as sex and reproduction, which have irreversible lifetime consequences, we rightly hold persons to high standards of moral and legal responsibility. To counter the tendency or temptation toward sexual irresponsibility or parental neglect, Western culture has insisted that men and women be held accountable for their contribution to the creation of new life.

A donor, whether male or female, who takes part in collaborative reproduction does not assume personal responsibility for his or her momentous personal action engendering new life. In fact, the donor contracts (possibly with payment) to abdicate present and future personal responsibility. The donor is specifically enjoined not to carry through on what he or she initiates, but instead to hand over to physicians or others, often unknown others, the result of his or her reproductive capacity. The generative power to create a new life is by design ejected from consideration. This genetic generative capacity is not like a kidney (or any other organ), but is part of the basic identity that is received from one's own parents. When a person treats this capacity as trivial or sells the use of it, he or she breaks an implicit compact. Parental responsibility is an essential form of the natural responsibility human beings have to help each other, and it gives rise to moral claims not governed by specific contracts or commitments.[25]

Persons who abdicate parental responsibility also deprive their own parents of grandparenthood and any other of their descendants of knowledge of their kin. Future children from the donor, or other children of a surrogate mother, will never know their half brother or sister. To so disregard the reality of the biological integrity of our identity and allow donors to engage in contractual reproduction is to have a mistaken view of how human beings actually function — or should function.

If we succeed in isolating sexual and reproductive acts from long-term personal responsibility, this moral abdication will increase existing problems within the culture. Do we want to encourage women to be able to emotionally distance themselves from the child in their womb enough to give it up? Do we wish to sanction male detachment from their biological offspring? Already epidemics of divorce, illegitimate conceptions, and parental irresponsibility and failures are straining the family bonds and the firm commitment that are necessary for successful childrearing and the full development of individuals. If we legitimize the isolation of genetic, gestational, and social parentage and regularly allow reproduction to be governed by contract and purchase, our culture will become even more fragmented, rootless, and alienated.

25. Hans Jonas, *The Imperative of Responsibility: In Search of an Ethics for the Technological Age* (Chicago: University of Chicago Press, 1984).

One of the foundations of a responsible ethic concerning sexuality is to see sexual acts as personal acts involving the whole person. Lust is wrong because it disregards the whole person and his or her human dignity. Another person is reduced to a means of selfish pleasure, and if money is involved, exploitation of the needy can occur. So, too, it seems wrong to isolate and use a person's reproductive capacity apart from his or her personal life. When it is a woman donating her egg and gestational capacity, there is a grave danger of exploitation, as feminists have warned.[26] The physiological risks attending the drastic intervention in a woman's reproductive system needed for surrogacy or embryo transplants are considerable. But perhaps more important is that pregnancy is not simply a neutral organic experience, but a time of bonding of the mother to her child.

If a great deal of money is offered for surrogacy, needy women will be tempted to sell their bodies and suffer the emotional consequences — and the experience of prostitution leads one to expect that many of these women will then hand over the money to males. Feminists rightly protest that allowing women to be surrogates will in fact turn women into baby machines bought and regulated by those rich enough to pay.[27] From another perspective, a surrogate mother could also be seen as deliberately producing and selling her baby. What will these practices do to other children of the surrogate or, for that matter, other children in the society? Can children comprehend, without anxiety, the fact that mothers make babies and give them away for money? The great primordial reality of interdependency and mutual bonding represented by mother and child is attacked. Contracts and regulations can hardly stem the psychological and social harm alternative reproductive technologies make possible.

Conclusion

Our society faces a challenge to its traditional ethics of reproduction and family norms. The cultural norms, based upon biological predispositions, is for the genetic, gestational, and rearing parents to be identical and for the nuclear family to exist within an extended family kinship system. The family should be seen as an intergenerational institution having an ecological relationship with the larger society.

As the range of ethics has broadened to include a concern for the dignity, worth, and rights of women and children, so has our understanding of morally responsible parenthood been refined and developed. The parental enterprise is rightly seen as basically an altruistic one — children should not be viewed as a form of personal

26. Barbara Rothman, *The Tentative Pregnancy* (New York: Viking Press, 1986); H. Holmes, B. Hoskins, and M. Gross, *The Custom Made Child* (Clifton, N.J.: Humana Press, 1981).

27. Angela R. Holder, "Surrogate Motherhood: Babies for Fun and Profit," *Law, Medicine, and Health Care* 11 (June 1984): 115-17.

property or as a means to satisfy adult desires or fulfill adult needs. When making reproductive decisions, the good of the potential child, along with the general cultural conditions which further childrearing and family support systems, should take precedence over other considerations, such as biologically integral acts or individual desires.

I have argued for an ethical position that limits alternative reproductive techniques to remedying infertility in expectable parental conditions that preserve the cultural norm, which includes the identity of genetic, gestational, and rearing parents. Collaborative reproduction will not serve the good of the potential child or the family, nor will it meet the need of the culture for morally responsible reproductive behavior.

It seems a sign of cultural progress that children are highly valued and infertility is acknowledged as a misfortune. It is also wonderful that medical reproductive technology can remedy the handicap of infertility. But as medical professionals and people in general confront these innovative interventions, the ethical, psychological, and cultural dimensions of technological procedures cannot be discounted. For the good of the child, the donors, the family, and our society, certain ethical limits must be set. Not everything that can be done to satisfy individual reproductive desires should be done. As Gandhi said, "Means are ends in the making."[28] Collaborative reproduction using third parties comes at too high a price.

28. Mahatma Gandhi, *The Essential Gandhi* (New York: Random House, 1962).

117 Faith and Infertility

Maura A. Ryan

I recall hearing the influential Jesuit moral theologian Richard McCormick say more than once that the best reason to ban reproductive cloning was that there were no good reasons to do it. By the time of McCormick's death in 2000, Chicago entrepreneur Richard Seed had already announced his intentions to found a cloning clinic and the international debate over whether cloning should be permitted in any form loomed on the horizon.

Always a pastor, McCormick considered deeply the arguments marshaled by supporters in the name of compassion: reproductive cloning would extend the possibilities for overcoming infertility; allow gay and lesbian partners to have a genetically-related child; turn back the clock on aging; and make it possible for parents who suffered the loss of a child to see that child, in some measure, "raised from the dead." Yet, he would remind us, no technology is an unqualified good or suffering an absolute evil; "good reasons" for developing new reproductive technologies must acknowledge our creaturely status, weigh the social and individual risks against the benefits and, especially where fundamental human practices such as parenthood are threatened with radical reinterpretation, consider alternatives.

Although McCormick was not opposed to in vitro fertilization, he was never persuaded that the losses experienced because of infertility (or even the suffering occasioned by the loss of a child) outweighed the significance of reproduction as an "enfleshed partnership" between husband and wife nor the duty of science and public policy to respect certain "natural" boundaries of human agency. While I don't remember him addressing directly the use of cloning to "replace" a deceased child, I suspect that he would have echoed bioethicist Thomas Murray in cautioning against the illusion that technology can erase grief: "Life flows in only one direction. Science can't reverse the stream or reincarnate the dead."[1]

I think that McCormick was right about reproductive

1. R. W. Dellinger, "Cloning Can't Replace Lost Loved Ones, Says Bioethicist," *Tidings Online* (June 15, 2001) at www.the-tidings.com/2001/0615/cloning.htm. Thomas Murray is a member of the President's National Bioethics Advisory Commission and the father of a daughter who was abducted from her college dorm room and murdered.

From Maura A. Ryan, "Faith and Infertility," in Cloning, *Christian Reflection: A Series in Faith and Ethics,* 16 (Waco: The Center for Christian Ethics at Baylor University, 2005): 65-74. Reprinted by permission. Available online at www.ChristianEthics.ws.

cloning. Even if the serious safety concerns that currently attend cloning technologies could be overcome, it is not obvious that the ends served by reproductive cloning justify the potential social and individual costs of ushering in the practice of asexual reproduction. Widespread international resistance to reproductive cloning signals a deep and healthy concern that the advent of cloning is not simply an incremental addition to the arsenal of technologies for serving the desire to have a child, but a shift in our way of understanding the nature of reproduction that touches the very foundations of respect for human dignity.

However, there remains the question of how to take seriously the intense desire for a child that helps to drive the development of reproductive technologies and fuels the willingness of individuals, especially women, to assume great physical, relational, and economic burdens for an outside chance of a successful delivery. If we are to say that there are limits to what ought to be sanctioned in the pursuit of parenthood (either limits to the sort of technologies we allow or limits to the medical resources we commit to addressing infertility) how are we to respond to the very real losses experienced by those who are infertile or unable to carry a child to term?

Facing the fact that one will never conceive or bear children is not just an experience of profound disappointment. Rather, those who have gone through it describe it as a kind of "dying," a loss of both an envisioned future and a possible self, a potential role and a longed-for relationship. Infertility is rarely recognized as a personal crisis, however, and even when it is, it is treated largely as a medical or social crisis. It is seldom recognized as a spiritual crisis, a deep confrontation of meaning and belief. Yet, it is precisely when infertility is acknowledged as a question to one's very understanding of oneself and one's place in the universe that the pain and disappointment of infertility can become an opportunity for personal and spiritual growth. Indeed, it is only when infertility is seen as a spiritual crisis that it can initiate a *spiritual quest,* an occasion for "a blossoming of self far more rewarding than mere endurance."[2] In the same way, it is when the threat to the integrity of the self (posed by a diagnosis of infertility) is addressed that it becomes possible to say no to medical interventions that have become pointless or destructive to persons or relationships, and to explore other alternatives such as adoption in a healthy way.

How might we develop a Christian spirituality for growth or transcendence through infertility? What theological and liturgical resources exist for helping those who struggle with infertility to learn as well as to share the lessons it teaches about finitude and humility? What would it mean to see the liturgical and pastoral life of the churches as a context for acquiring the grace to live into involuntary childlessness with hope and dignity?

2. Jan Renner, *Infertility: Old Myths, New Meanings* (Toronto, ON: Second Story Press, 1989), 112.

Mixed Messages and Missed Opportunities

There are many references to infertility in Scripture.[3] The birth of a son to a long-infertile or "barren" wife is a familiar symbol of God's favor. Isaac is born to Abraham, signifying both Abraham's reward for his fidelity and Yahweh's guarantee of a viable future for Israel. Through the child, the covenant is established; Sarah (at the biblical age of ninety) becomes not only an improbable mother, but the "mother of nations" (Genesis 17:15-21). In turn, the Lord grants Isaac's prayer and the barren Rebekah gives birth to Esau and Jacob (Genesis 25:21). Vowing to dedicate her child to God if only God would grant her a son, Hannah is finally "remembered," and she bears Samuel (1 Samuel 1:9-11, 19-20). Like Abraham and Sarah, the righteous Zechariah and Elizabeth of the New Testament, well beyond childbearing years, are sent a son who is to be "great in the sight of the Lord," whose birth in joy and wonder is a foretaste of the redemptive events to come (Luke 1:5-25). The long-awaited child, born to this woman now at the "end" of her life, is testimony indeed that "nothing will be impossible with God" (Luke 1:36-37).

Although barrenness plays many different roles in biblical texts — sometimes standing as a sign of God's judgment, sometimes a pretext for miraculous intervention (as in the life-long infertility of Sarah and Elizabeth) — the individual or personal suffering associated with barrenness is clearly visible. Infertility is linked to illness and famine in the promises of Sinai: "You shall worship the LORD your God, and I will bless your bread and your water; and I will take sickness away from among you. No one shall miscarry or be barren in your land; I will fulfill the number of your days" (Exodus 23:25-26). The barren woman is an object of pity, because the inability to conceive and bear children, and in particular to bear sons, is assumed to lie with her. We get glimpses of the pain of infertility in Rachel's cry to Jacob: "Give me children, or I shall die!" (Genesis 30:1); in Isaac's plea to Yahweh on behalf of his wife (Genesis 25:21); and in the psalmist's identification of the barren woman with the poorest of the poor: "[Yahweh] raises the poor from the dust, and lifts the needy from the ash heap, to make them sit with princes. . . . He gives the barren woman a home, making her the joyous mother of children" (Psalm 113:7-8a, 4a). The most poignant glimpse is the picture of Hannah in the first book of Samuel. The second wife of Elkanah, she is taunted, year after year, by her rival because "the LORD had closed her womb" (1 Samuel 1:6). Rising in the temple, she prays to Yahweh "in the bitterness of her soul": "O LORD of Hosts, if only you will look on the misery of

3. I am using the terms "infertility" and "barrenness" interchangeably here, although, of course, the terms do not have exactly the same meaning. In the biblical texts, for example, it is not always clear whether "barrenness" refers simply to the state of not having borne children (i.e., "infertility") or also to the state of not having borne sons or descendents in the sense of followers in male lineage. However, both terms connote involuntary childlessness, and it is in that sense that I am using them.

your servant, and remember me, and not forget your servant, but will give to your servant a male child, then I will set him before you as a nazirite until the day of his death. He shall drink neither wine nor intoxicants, and no razor shall touch his head" (1 Samuel 1:11). So great is her distress that she is mistaken by the priest Eli for drunk.

It would seem that religious traditions shaped by sacred texts so rich in the imagery of fertility and infertility would provide a natural context in which to come to terms with the suffering occasioned by infertility. But Arthur Greil's study of American infertile couples showed instead that it is extremely difficult for believers to draw on their religious faith in trying to make sense of infertility. Some of the couples he interviewed reported drawing strength from the social relationships they enjoyed within their faith communities, but they were far outnumbered by those couples who viewed religious affiliation as one more obstacle to be overcome in their attempt to deal with their infertility. Overall, he concluded, "religion [did] not provide most couples . . . with resources upon which they can call to explain to themselves their experience of suffering."[4]

Why do many Christians who are dealing with infertility have difficulty finding solace and usable wisdom in religion? One reason is that for all its relative visibility in the Bible, infertility is an invisible reality in most congregations. I have attended countless liturgical celebrations on Mother's Day, Christmas, and the Feast of the Holy Family in my own Roman Catholic community. I cannot recall a single time in which, during these key celebrations of parenthood and rededication of family life, the pain of *longing for* parenthood was acknowledged liturgically alongside the joy and struggles of its realization.

Another reason why religion can be more of an obstacle than a pathway to healing for the infertile is the ambiguous and somewhat contradictory character of fertility in religious literature. In the Roman Catholic tradition, for example, procreation is treated as one of the primary goods of marriage. The tradition recognizes what many infertile couples come to believe passionately: that reproduction "completes" or "embodies" an intimate relationship. To bring forth a child who is "flesh of our flesh" symbolizes the joining of their separate lives in a concrete and living way. The act of reproducing moves the relationship to a new level, not only symbolically but practically, as the couple makes the transition to an all-encompassing, necessarily responsible or outwardly-focused intimacy. Despite long-standing disagreements about the ethics of contraception, it is nonetheless assumed in Catholic sexual ethics that reproduction is a primary, "essential" end of sexual expression and that the transmission of life is a central dimension of the vocation of marriage. Parenting is the most celebrated channel through which lay Catholics participate in the ministry of the church. Yet, the inability to have children is readily dismissed as merely a frustrated desire, easily redirected toward adoption or other forms of interaction with children. The problem for infertile believers is not in the suggestion that the longing for children of one's own can be tapped as an energy for service or fulfilled through adoption. It is in the dissonance between the high value placed on biological reproduction as a gift from God and the assumption that, being surrounded by and having taken in this interpretation of its significance, the infertile can simply reinterpret it.

Yet another reason why, for many people, religion provides little comfort in the journey through infertility is suggested in the brief survey of biblical references to barrenness above. The interwoven symbolisms of judgment, blessing, and mystery yield a confusing answer to the suffering occasioned by infertility. Infertile women, in particular, are tempted to blame themselves because of earlier failures of judgment or volition, or a previous shortsightedness or youthful self-centeredness, for their present inability to conceive or bear a child; some believe that they are being punished by God for their earlier ambivalence about having children. But efforts to levy blame (even self-blame) for conditions such as infertility are ultimately as unsatisfying as they are understandable. The nightly news is full of accounts of unwanted and badly cared for children, born to seemingly "undeserving" mothers and fathers. How is it that these infertile women and men, who understand as well as anyone how precious is the life of a child, are pointedly passed over when the blessing of children is elsewhere so freely and apparently indiscriminately bestowed? What exactly could they have done that warrants such a devastating punishment?

At the same time, to conclude that there is no theological answer for infertility, that we simply must regard it as a mystery to be lived obediently, is not much more helpful. Indeed, such an answer to suffering may play directly into the hands of contemporary "medical" or "scientific" theodicies. From the standpoint of reproductive medicine, impaired reproduction is not a mystery to be pondered but a technical problem in need of a technical solution. In such circumstances, argues Greil,

> traditional theodicies which counsel stoicism in the face of the inevitable [or unexplainable] may lose ground to the impatient theodicy implied by the medical model. According to the medical model, suffering is not something to be understood but rather something to be conquered. Explanations that rely on such concepts as 'God's will' cannot be convincing when we believe as strongly as we do in the human ability to pull ourselves out of our condition through technical knowledge.[5]

The difficulties infertile believers encounter in drawing a usable or healing wisdom from faith traditions stem both from how we treat infertility within communities of

4. Arthur L. Greil, *Not Yet Pregnant: Infertile Couples in Contemporary America* (New Brunswick, NJ: Rutgers University Press, 1991), 161ff.

5. Ibid., 173.

faith and the way we talk about infertility in theological terms. Constructing a healing spirituality, therefore, includes practical or pastoral strategies as well as theological reconstruction.

Creating a Context

If infertile believers find religious services "among the most painful times in their week"[6] in large part because they feel invisible or marginalized within faith communities that place a great deal of emphasis on families and family life, much could be done to create opportunities for healing simply by "attending to the moment." With sensitivity on the part of the celebrants, the same liturgical events that we now use for celebrating and supporting families could become opportunities for making the invisible struggle of the infertile visible. By including a prayer for all those who want to be mothers or fathers and are experiencing difficulty, for example, the liturgical celebrations of Mother's and Father's Day could be both a "teachable moment" for the congregation and an opportunity for the expression of solidarity.[7] Simply by acknowledging the varied experiences of family present in any faith community, our observances of the feast of the Holy Family could become occasions for inviting in those who feel on the margins rather than merely retracing the lines of inclusion and exclusion. Attention to the language and symbols we use in the public rituals and sermons marking religiously important moments of family life, such as baptisms, first communions, and confirmations, and an effort to listen from the perspective of those who are currently struggling with some aspect of family could go far in easing the pain of those who experience those events as excruciating.

It is also possible to create moments for reaching out to the infertile within the liturgical year. The Cedar Park Assemblies of God Church in Bothell, Washington, sets aside Presentation Sunday each year for a special blessing for infertile couples. In 1998, twenty parishes in Bothell joined Cedar Park in inviting those who were suffering infertility or pregnancy loss to come together to pray and to experience the support of the community.[8] Widely publicized, Presentation Sunday calls attention to the reality of infertility within congregations and gives public witness to the possibilities for encountering infertility as a spiritual journey. Although many people come to such a service to pray for a miracle, it also provides a context for exploring the challenge of living faithfully in the absence of miracles.

From Spiritual Crisis to Spiritual Quest

Jan Rehner argues that healing from infertility begins with a reconception of the self: "There needs to be, in short, a new story, the creation of an alternate vision of self that is not a negation, but a statement of the wholeness and fulfillment of other equally viable possibilities."[9] This "new naming" of the self is not a denial of infertility, nor is it merely a matter of throwing oneself into other projects, as infertile couples are often encouraged to do. Those who have resolved the infertility crisis (whether or not they ever became parents) have learned how to tap into the vital energy which all human beings possess and of which the ability to impregnate or give birth is only one small manifestation. They have come in touch with the deep life-giving forces outside themselves and have grown to see the many possibilities for generativity in the lives they are now living. From denying and hating a body that will not make babies, they come to embrace a body as rich as ever in capacities for love, recreation, passion, and courage, only grown wiser now through suffering. In some sense, those who successfully transcended the loss posed by infertility are those for whom the experience of infertility has become a kind of "spiritual pregnancy," an occasion for giving birth to a new understanding and appreciation of the self.[10]

Self-acceptance is a critical moment in the spiritual journey through infertility. So, too, is coming to a new relationship with God and with God's purposes for one's life. "The faith that will make us well" is not principally a relentless expectation of a miracle. Rather, it is the willingness to be touched in our infirmity by the God who is the source of all life and all energy. Feelings of anger at God are normal and even necessary to the process of healing. But equally necessary is the movement from asking "What is God doing to me/us?" to "Where is God leading me/us?"[11]

Edmund Pellegrino and David Thomasma argue that the virtue of hope is necessary for genuine healing to take place. Such a hope faces "the realities of the patient's predicament, but directs the mind and heart to something much larger, the reality of God's presence in history, his

6. See Hannah's Prayer Ministries at www.hannah.org. This ministry "provides Christian based support and encouragement to couples around the world who are struggling with the pain of '*fertility challenges*' including infertility, pregnancy loss, or early infant death."

7. The founders of Hannah's Prayer make the important point that Mother's Day and Father's Day are civic rather than religious holidays and need not be celebrated in church at all. It seems to me that these holidays provide an opportunity to highlight a primary feature of life for most members of the congregation and a valued set of relationships within religious traditions. I would argue that they should be celebrated liturgically, provided they can be celebrated with sensitivity to the various forms of family life within the congregation.

8. "Having Faith: Service Devoted to Infertile Couples," *Seattle Times* (January 26, 1998), C1.

9. Rehner, *Infertility,* 20-21, quoting Carol Christ, *Diving Deep and Surfacing* (Boston, MA: Beacon Press, 1980), 76.

10. Rehner, *Infertility,* 120.

11. Julie Kelemen, *Dealing With Infertility: A Guide for Catholics* (Liguori, MO: Liguori Publications, 1997), 18.

promises to humanity, and his unfailing love for every one of his creatures."[12] As this description suggests, a transformative spirituality in the face of infertility will not be built on the expectation of miracles (as important as it may be to the infertile not to lose confidence entirely in the possibility of an unexpected blessing) but on awareness of the constant companionship of God in the experience of infirmity, disappointment, or despair. The community of faith is called to embody this transcendent hope, not by piously "denying the realities" of infertility, but by becoming a site where the "something much larger" can be witnessed and the capacity to trust that all things, even our present sufferings, are working to good can be learned.

When hope is grasped as an awareness of God's redeeming work within our experiences of illness or loss or despair, when it is not mistaken simply for a commitment to a certain outcome, it becomes possible for infertility to be the catalyst for a new and deeper relationship with God and the community. It also becomes possible to bring realistic expectations to medicine. Stopping treatment is "abandoning hope" only when success or failure is measured as the achievement of a certain result. When the experience of infertility is lived as an invitation to experience the mystery of God's care for us, God's infinite "motherhood" and "fatherhood," God's desire for our flourishing, it is not necessary to pursue "success" at the expense of the self. Indeed, it does not even make sense.

Reframing Generativity

Finally, we can only hint here at the directions of a theological reconstruction of the place of procreation in a theology of marriage. Three observations are worthy of reflection.

A continued emphasis on procreation as the "fullness" or "flowering" of marital intimacy tends to render the childless marriage "second class." Raising up the theological significance of marriage as first and foremost the site for the mutual self-giving of the partners reflects more accurately the reality of married life and the place of procreation within it, as well as giving rise to a norm for reproduction that respects the conditions for healthy and responsible reproduction.

Second, while privileging the family as the primary place of ministry for laypersons lends valuable support to the work of family life, it has tended to eclipse the more fundamental call to ministry and service which all Christians share. It has the practical effect of making single Christians and childless couples invisible, not only liturgically, but as a force for effective witness in the world. What is needed is a way of talking seriously about the call to faithfulness and action that follows directly from our baptism, which we all share, and which can be lived out in a variety of equally viable forms of life. What is needed is a theology of lay vocation which treats single life or marriage without children as a unique and valuable context for ministry — not, as we tend to treat them now, simply as "holding patterns."

Finally, looking hard at what exactly we as Christians value in parenthood is necessary if we are to create a context in which we can commend adoption or other ways of relating to children as attractive paths to resolving the infertility crisis. Christian sexual ethics is in need of a shift from an emphasis on the generation of life, the acquisition of children, to an emphasis on the sustenance of life, the care of children.

What those struggling with infertility need, and what we as communities of faith owe to them, is an inviting witness to the "something more" that lies beyond the limits of their loss. It is only then that we can turn faith or religion from "one more painful obstacle to resolving infertility" to a genuine source and context for healing.[13]

12. Edmund D. Pellegrino and David C. Thomasma, *The Christian Virtues in Medical Practice* (Washington, DC: Georgetown University Press, 1996), 67-68.

13. An earlier version of this essay appears as chapter six in Maura A. Ryan, *Ethics and Economics of Assisted Reproduction: The Cost of Longing* (Washington, DC: Georgetown University Press, 2001), 150-170.

118 A.R.T., Ethics, and the Bible

Allen Verhey

Now the man knew his wife Eve, and she conceived and bore Cain, saying, "I have produced a man with the help of the Lord."

Genesis 4:1

Everyone has heard of new versions of the Bible — the New Revised Standard Version, the New International Version, the Jerusalem Bible, the Cottonpatch Version, to name only a few. Some time ago in *The Wittenberg Door* yet another version was announced — the Valley Bible, "a really tubular Bible, for sure."[1]

Everyone has also heard about the new versions of procreation, or assisted reproductive technologies (A.R.T.). In 1978 a new version was announced that went something like this:

> Now Gilbert Brown took his specimen bottle and filled it with sperm, and the sperm were placed in a little glass dish along with an ovum which had been surgically removed from his wife, Leslie Brown, and, behold, after the egg was fertilized, it was implanted into the wall of Leslie's uterus and grew. And she bore Louise Brown, saying, "I have produced a little girl with the help of Drs. Steptoe and Edwards and, oh yes, God" — "a really tubular" little girl, for sure.

The A.R.T. that Drs. Steptoe and Edwards used to help Gilbert and Leslie Brown was, of course, in vitro fertilization, and Louise Brown was the first child to be born after being conceived in a "test tube." In vitro fertilization, of course, was not the first new version of procreation — or the last!

Of the new versions of the Bible, some are good and some are appalling. The same can be said about the new versions of procreation: some of them are good, and some of them are appalling. But which ones, and why? We will return to that question shortly, but first consider the strange world of begetting in Scripture and the (still stranger) world of A.R.T.

1. "Totally Awesome: The Valley Bible," *The Wittenberg Door* (April-May 1982): 22.

From Allen Verhey, "A.R.T., Ethics, and the Bible," in *Reading the Bible in the Strange World of Medicine* (Grand Rapids: Wm. B. Eerdmans, 2003), 253-404.

The Strange World of Begetting in Scripture

Begetting is a part of the story from the very beginning. In the beginning it is promised in the blessing of God upon the man and the woman, "Be fruitful and multiply" (Gen. 1:28). As we observed in the last chapter, from the beginning children were regarded as a blessing of God. The verdict of God upon the creation, that it is "very good" (Gen. 1:31), was spoken over the promise of children — and over human sexuality.

The Story of Creation and Good Sex[2]

In the beginning, there was love. That's the story. It is a story, first, of God's love. In the beginning God so loved humanity that of the one two were made, so that the two might be one. The triune God said, "It is not good that the man should be alone" (Gen. 2:18),[3] and at the climax of creation God made community. In "the beginning" God created male and female (Gen. 1:26-28; Mark 10:6). Our creation as male and female is a gift of God's love.

It is a story of God's love, but it is also a story of human love, of Adam's love for Eve and Eve's for Adam. Indeed, it can be read as a romantic story of human love. In the romantic story we hear of a love evoked by a vision of the beloved as lovely, as wholly lovable; to that vision the romantic hero responds with affection and passion. Once upon a time Adam awakened from a deep sleep and saw . . . a vision. He probably pinched himself, thinking, "I must still be sleeping — and dreaming." "She is made for me," he said, or words to that effect. He looked upon this woman and said what God had said over the creation, "It is good, very good." And once upon a time Eve watched Adam wake from sleep, glad for his awakening. "Flesh of my flesh and bone of my bones," she said, "It is good, very good," or words to that effect.

There they stood, in the beginning, together: at home in their flesh, "naked, and . . . not ashamed" (Gen. 2:25); at home with each other, vulnerable and not anxious, the vulnerability of their nakedness an occasion for delight and mutuality, not shame and power; and at home with God, the giver of life and love and joy. The vision of the beloved, that romantic vision, called forth affection and passion — and also *commitment!* "Therefore," the story goes, "a man leaves his father and his mother and clings to his wife, and they become one flesh" (Gen. 2:24; cf. Mark 10:7-8). The vision prompted Adam not only to say, "Eve, I love you," but, "Eve, I *will* love you." Her delight prompted Eve not only to say, "Adam, I love you," but, "Adam, I *will* love you." Adam and Eve made commitments to each other, made love in celebration of those

2. For this section, see further my *Remembering Jesus* (Grand Rapids: Eerdmans, 2002), pp. 214-19, from which some of these paragraphs are taken.

3. It should be admitted, of course, that the original authors of Genesis did not have a notion of a *triune* God, but to read Scripture in Christian community, to read it according to the Rule of Faith, permits us to tell the story in this way.

commitments, and anticipated the blessing of children as an extension of their love. Marriage, like our creation as male and female, is a gift of God's love. And marriage — with its commitments — is from the beginning the context for both having sex and having children, the context for both lovemaking and begetting.

Sex is good in the creation, very good. It is a story of an embodied relationship, a "one flesh" union of male and female — begun in vows, carried out in fidelity, and blessed with children. Good sex "in the beginning" involves mutuality and equality, intimacy and continuity, and the blessing of children. Sex is good, and the promise of children is good, but neither sex nor children are God. Nothing God made is God. The story from the beginning cautions against idolatrously extravagant expectations of sexuality or of procreation. When human fulfillment is made dependent on sexual fulfillment, then we have failed to remember creation. And when human fulfillment is made dependent upon having children, then we have failed to remember creation. Sex is good, and from the beginning it involves whole persons, embodied selves. The story cautions against the dualism that drives a wedge between body and soul and against any reductionism that reduces persons to their sexual or reproductive capacities. Sexual intercourse itself may not be reduced to either a technology of pleasure or to an instrument of reproduction.

Sex is good, and from the beginning it requires commitment. That was the way God intended it. Love that is good offers itself fully and finally. Love that is good makes promises. So it is with God's love, and so it was with Adam and Eve. There at the beginning commitment was a way to love into the future, a way to give a future to their present love, binding not only Adam to Eve and Eve to Adam but binding present and future together. The romantic moment, the original vision, was not closed in upon itself but open to the future. Their love would have a history. Their relationship would endure — either as fidelity or as betrayal. Even in the beginning, evidently, they knew that the romantic moment, the original vision, would not last, could not last. Perhaps God had told Adam that there would be mornings when he would wake up and look over at Eve and wonder what he could have been thinking that morning long ago. Perhaps God had warned Eve that there would be times when she only delighted in Adam's awakening because it put a stop to his miserable snoring.

At any rate, things soon got much more difficult. Creation is, after all, only the beginning of the story of human sexuality. It continues under the shadow of human sin. Sin is a dreadful mystery, but this much is clear: the fault was not in God and not in nature. The fault was in human choice. Humanity's free grasping at freedom in the demand to be "autonomous," to be a law unto themselves, brought not freedom but bondage, a "voluntary bondage" to the powers of sin and death that usurp God's rule and resist God's cause. In the wake of sin came death and a curse.

Death fell heavy on the story of Adam and Eve, and heavy on their love. Death alienates us from our flesh, and Adam and Eve, once naked and not ashamed, at home in the flesh, felt the power of death in the shame of their nakedness. Death alienates us from each other, and Adam and Eve, once vulnerable and not anxious, confident of their mutuality and community, felt the sting of death in power and patriarchy. Death alienates us from God, and Adam and Eve, who had walked with God in the garden, now hid from God and felt the power of death in their hiding.

Because of human sin, the curse weighed down on them — and on good sex, too. The story of Genesis 3 itself identified the curse with patriarchy and with the pain of childbirth (Gen. 3:16). But the marks of the curse are legion. Other stories made it clear that not just pain in childbirth but barrenness bore the mark of the curse. The curse makes its power felt in the reduction of any to a sexual function and in the reduction of sexual relations to a technology of pleasure. Under the power of the curse sexuality becomes the occasion for lust and for shame, for license and for legislation, for the confounding of expectations of fecundity, for the breaking of covenant, for the betrayal of partners.

It's a sad story, and in the midst of it, that original vision, that romantic moment, must have seemed to Adam and to Eve long ago. And their commitment must have seemed wishful thinking. You can imagine it. Adam, irritated, complains that Eve seems not to understand how hard he has to work to get the miserable ground to yield a crop. And Eve, angered, complains in turn that Adam seems to think that patriarchy is the way it is meant to be, not a curse to be worked against just as vigorously as the stubborn ground. You can imagine it. Each complains to the other and to God — but mostly to themselves — that the original vision in that romantic moment long ago had simply been wrong: "I did not see these things before." "Now I know the other better than I did then." "How could I have missed what is now so obvious?" "How could I have been such a fool as to bind myself and my future so irrevocably?" "Now I see what the man is really like!" "Now I see what the woman is really like!"

So they grew suspicious of the original vision, and they were right in a way. Each had come to know more of the other than at the beginning: the flaws, the faults, the irritating oddities, the aggravating eccentricities, the wearying habits, the boring routines (even of the other's affection and passion). Such knowledge can make one suspicious of the original vision. A man waking from sleep is seldom entrancing, and the sight of a woman when one awakes is frequently less than enchanting. But they were wrong, too. That first vision was right, still. Eve was a gift of God to Adam. Adam was a gift of God to Eve. And in such gifts there was and remained the vocation of gratitude to God for the other and the calling of faithfulness to the other. In that first vision Adam and Eve saw the other well, for they saw the other as a gift of God. That moment contained a truth about the other that should not be forgotten, but they — like all their children — grew weary of the wonder of those who were near them. They grew tired of beholding beauty; they thought the beauty had faded when their vision had dimmed. It is, I think, a mark of the curse. Such knowledge of the other (and such forgetfulness of the other) made the task of living together with gratitude and fidelity harder still.

So they grew suspicious of commitment, too. And they were right in a way, for commitment, too, can be distorted by the power of death. Where death rules, commitment — when it still exists — can take the form of resisting time, because time leads to death. Commitment under the threat of death insists that some romantic moment last in spite of time, as if there were no time. But, of course, there is time, and it will not be resisted, and the effort to preserve some precious present by cutting it off from any future is futile (and boring). They were right in a way to be suspicious of commitment, but they were wrong, too. For death and the curse were not the end of the story of Adam and Eve. It is a story — not only first, but also finally — of God's love. The grace of God would not let death have the last word in God's creation, or the last word about Adam and Eve and their love. Commitment could be dared and done with hope in God. With hope in God Adam and Eve had courage for commitment, not in order to resist time or to deny it but to embrace time and to embrace each other into the future.

Far as the curse is found, so far the grace of God would reach to restore and to bless, even finally and hilariously to the grave. The grace of God made its power felt in a world now marked and marred by sin and death, by power and patriarchy, by lust and selfishness, but it made its power felt. The grace of God made its power felt when a child was born to Adam and Eve, a token of the promise of another child: that death would not have the last word. The grace of God made its power felt in the tender affection that remembered the first vision, in their forgiveness and faithfulness, in their mutuality and equality, and yes, in their passion, naked again and not ashamed again, vulnerable still, but entrusting themselves to the care of the other and to God. The grace of God made its power felt in the hope that gave their love a history again. It made its power felt in a commitment that celebrated God's love and signaled their confidence in God's future. They embraced time, embraced the future, cleaving to each other and to God, and they bore a child as a signal of their hope in God and of their love in spite of the curse. "Now the man knew his wife Eve, and she conceived and bore Cain, saying, 'I have produced a man with the help of the LORD'" (Gen. 4:1; see also Gen. 5:1).

The grace of God made its power against the curse felt in Sarah's "laughter" (in her Isaac; see Gen. 17:19; 21:6), in Joseph's fidelity against the temptations of Potiphar's wife (Gen. 39), in the tender affection of Boaz and Ruth and in their fecundity, in the forgiveness and faithfulness of Hosea to Gomer, in the mutual passion of the lovers of Solomon's song, and in the countless genealogies of Scripture. The signs of God's grace were in the midst of a fallen world, of patriarchy and polygamy, of barren wombs and broken promises, but there were signs of it. And the signs of it gave hope for the good future of God's unchallenged reign — for sexuality, too.

Christians marry in the presence of God because they know that their story is a part of the story of God's love. They commit to God their commitments to each other because they dare to bind themselves and their future irrevocably to each other only by faith in a God who loves and whose love makes and keeps promises. They dare to embrace each other and time and change only with hope in a God who will not allow death and the curse to have the last word. They dare to contemplate the blessing of children only because they trust in God, but because they trust in God they do dare to hope for children. There is some token of a new creation in Christian marriage, and together the community celebrates it, as Jesus did at a wedding at Cana of Galilee long ago (John 2:1-11). And there is some token of a new creation in the birth of a child, and we may and should delight in it.

The Strange, Sad World of Barrenness in the Bible

Barrenness was a mark of the curse, and strange measures were taken against it in the Bible. Assisted reproductive technologies are evidently a lot older than Louise Brown. Already in Genesis we read of mandrakes, the plant that was regarded as both an aphrodisiac and an aid to fertility (Gen. 30:14-16). And although there was no sophisticated technology involved, there were other arrangements in the Bible that "assisted" reproduction. Female slaves could evidently be treated as "animated tools" in reproduction (Gen. 16:1-6; 30:1-13), and brothers could be conscripted to produce an heir for the brother who died without an heir (Deut. 25:5-10). It was a strange world of begetting in Scripture.

In the unhappy story of Sarah's barrenness, "Sarai said to Abraham, 'You see that the LORD has prevented me from bearing children; go in to my slave-girl; it may be that I shall obtain children by her'" (Gen. 16:2). Hagar, Sarah's Egyptian slave, is given to Abraham "as a wife" (16:3), and she becomes pregnant. Hagar becomes a surrogate mother (without benefit of the A.R.T. of artificial insemination). If this story is taken as a precedent for surrogacy, however, it can only serve as a warning. The outcome is contempt, jealousy, abuse, and abandonment. Hagar evidently does not regard the child as Sarah's but as her own; she "looked with contempt on her mistress" (16:4). Sarah becomes jealous of this pregnant slave (and co-wife), and she complains to Abraham. Abraham's response is hardly a model of responsibility; he simply reduces Hagar, this woman who carried his child, his "wife," to her position as Sarah's slave: "Your slave-girl is in your power," he says to Sarah, "do to her as you please" (16:6). And it pleases the jealous Sarah to abuse Hagar. Hagar runs away; even "animated tools" have some self-respect. God visits her in the wilderness and tells her to return and to call her son "Ishmael" (16:7-12),[4] so Hagar returns and gives birth to Ishmael. But then Sarah herself gives birth to Isaac, and Sarah's Isaac, her "laughter," turns out to be Hagar's sorrow. Sarah — still jealous, now for her son's inheritance — sends Hagar and Ishmael away, back into the wilderness and to almost certain death (21:9-10). In the wilderness Hagar cannot bear to watch her child die, so she sets Ishmael under a bush and sits down some distance away to weep and grieve. But the boy's name, assigned by God, means "God hears," and God did; "God heard the voice of the boy" (21:17), and God provided a well of water in the wilderness and a blessing.[5]

In the story of Rachel's use of her slave as an "animated tool" in reproduction, jealousy comes first. She envies her sister Leah and her fertility. She despairs to Jacob, "Give me children, or I shall die!" (Gen. 30:1).[6] When Jacob responds, rather callously by my lights, "Am I in the place of God, who has withheld from you the fruit of the womb?" (30:2), she can think of nothing else than to instruct Jacob to have sexual intercourse with her slave Bilhah and to get her pregnant, "that she may bear upon my knees and that I too may have children through her" (30:3). The reader wonders how she could have forgotten the cautionary tale of her grandmother Sarah and her Egyptian slave. No good can come of this. It's another story of desperation and jealousy, but a little good did come of it; more boys were added to the clan. Bilhah had two sons (30:5-8), whom Rachel named Dan and Naphtali to claim that God had vindicated her and that she had finally defeated her sister in their fertility contest.[7] Not to be so easily defeated, Leah then gave her slave Zilpah to Jacob, and she bore two more sons, whom Leah named Gad and Asher (30:9-13) to reclaim her "good fortune" and "happiness."[8] It's a strange world of begetting in Genesis.

Patriarchy always risks reducing women to their reproductive capacities. And women in a patriarchal culture are not only at risk of both desperation about their barrenness and jealousy about a sister's fertility but also at risk of being co-opted into reducing other women to their reproductive capacities, to "animated tools" of their desire for children to call their own. The stories of Sarah and Rachel are hardly promising precedents for A.R.T.

Patriarchy is displayed not only in the stories of the matriarchs but also in the law about levirate marriage (Deut. 25:5-10), another assisted reproductive relationship in the Old Testament. If a man died without a son, the law required that his brother would marry the man's wife and that their firstborn son would "succeed to the name of the deceased brother, so that his name may not be blotted out of Israel" (25:6).[9]

The Sadducees, as we noted in the last chapter, cited this law about levirate marriage in their confrontation with Jesus (Mark 12:18-23). They hoped to dismiss the idea of the resurrection with their story of a widow who marries in succession seven brothers and with their question, "In the resurrection whose wife will she be?" (v. 23). But Jesus replied that in the good future of God, "they neither marry nor are given in marriage" (12:25). The "power of God" will make itself felt when the relations of men and women are not governed by patriarchal marriage laws nor by a man's need to secure for himself a name and an heir but by the mutuality and equality that belong to God's good future.[10]

Indeed, because that good future was already making its power felt, singleness and celibacy were already and suddenly an option, signaled by Jesus' own singleness. Already and suddenly marriage and procreation were no longer to be regarded as duties of Torah or as necessary conditions for human fulfillment and divine approval. Celibacy, however, was not a duty either (Matt. 19:12; 1 Cor. 7:1-7); it was a "gift," a *charisma,* of God. And marriage, too, was now a "gift" (1 Cor. 7:7), and it could provide a token of a good future of mutuality and equality, even in sexual relations (1 Cor. 7:3-5). Within marriage — and within the community — children remained the blessing of God. Jesus made God's good future felt by his hospitality to children (Mark 10:13-16). Children, too, were among those whom Christ exalted and blessed. Those who did not count for much counted with Jesus. And he made it clear that to welcome him was to welcome children, and that to welcome children was to welcome both Jesus and the reign of God made known in his delight in little ones (Mark 9:37; 10:13-16). Nevertheless, to have children was not a duty, nor a condition for human fulfillment and divine approval, and barrenness was surely not a reason for divorce.[11] The child had been born — and born "to you," as the angel said to some shepherds (Luke 2:11). This was tidings of great joy to all

4. It is the first of several annunciation scenes in Genesis.

5. That God hears the cries of the slaves when they are afflicted foreshadows, of course, the story of the exodus. The same attention to the voice of afflicted slaves that saved Ishmael would save Israel from Egyptian bondage.

6. Ironically, she dies in childbirth with her second son, whom she called Ben-oni, or "Son of my sorrow" (Gen. 35:16-19).

7. Dan means "judged," and Naphtali means "my wrestling."

8. Gad means "fortune" (judging from Gen. 30:11), and Asher means "happy."

9. Two passages suggest that other relatives of the deceased man could also bear the obligation of levirate marriage. In Genesis 38, after Onan refused to honor the law by spilling "his semen on the ground whenever he went in to his brother's wife, so that he would not give offspring to his brother" (v. 9), and after her father-in-law Judah refused to assign his son Shelah to the duties of levirate marriage (v. 11), Tamar tricked Judah into sexual intercourse with her so that she could have a son. She was regarded as "more in the right" than Judah was, for Judah did not give Shelah to the duty of the Law. The book of Ruth assumes that the duty of levirate marriage falls on the nearest kinsman. The passages differ, and so presumably did the requirement over time and in different regions.

10. See further Elisabeth Schüssler Fiorenza, *In Memory of Her: A Feminist Theological Reconstruction of Christian Origins* (New York: Crossroad, 1985), pp. 143-45.

11. Cf. *Yebamoth* 6:6.

the people; the child had been born "to you" — and to the childless, too. The genealogies had been fulfilled. It was no longer a fault to be infertile. Therefore, sexual relations in the Christian story are not simply *for* procreation; they perform the mutual delight of those who are "one flesh."

The Strange World of Begetting in A.R.T.

Until recently the story of human procreation was, for all of its wonder, a fairly commonplace story, reminiscent of the story in Genesis 4:1. A man knew his wife, and she conceived and bore a child. Sexual intercourse sometimes resulted in a child; nothing else human beings did or could do resulted in a child; and the child that resulted was (by necessity) received as given. Technology has changed all that. We are living in what John A. Robertson has called a "reproductive revolution."[12] The technological control over procreation is not revolutionary because large numbers of children are born with these technologies.[13] It is revolutionary because it requires a revisiting of some fundamental questions, questions about the significance of human sexual intercourse, about the responsibilities that attend human acts of begetting, about the meaning of becoming and being parents, about the appropriate disposition toward children. These are not easy questions, of course, nor questions about which we may presume a "rational" consensus.

One signal of the "reproductive revolution" was the birth of Louise Brown in 1978 following in vitro fertilization (IVF). IVF involves the removal of oocytes, or eggs, from a woman, their fertilization in vitro, and the implantation of the resulting pre-embryos into the uterus. Louise was born with oocytes from her mother, semen from her father, and after fertilization she was implanted into the womb of her mother. The technology, however, can utilize donor oocytes, donor sperm, and a surrogate mother for gestation. There could be, therefore, several parents: a genetic mother, a genetic father, a gestational mother, a rearing mother, and a rearing father. It's a strange world of begetting in A.R.T.

Even before the development of IVF, however, there was the simpler technology of artificial insemination (AI). Artificial insemination involves utilizing a syringe (or a turkey baster) to deposit sperm into a woman's uterus at the time of ovulation. AI can use the sperm of either the husband (AIH) or a donor (AID), depositing it either into the woman who will also rear the child or into a surrogate, who will be the genetic and gestational mother.

The strange world of A.R.T. grew stranger still with the development of cryopreservation techniques that allowed the freezing of sperm, ova, and embryos for later use. Cryopreservation permitted, for example, the development of sperm banks, including the famous sperm bank to which Nobel Prize–winning scientists were donors. It permitted the transfer of embryos not to the womb but to the freezer, awaiting possible future use. It's a strange world of begetting in A.R.T.

In the decades since 1978 a number of other assisted

12. John A. Robertson, *Children of Choice: Freedom and the New Reproductive Technologies* (Princeton, N.J.: Princeton University Press, 1994), pp. 4-5. The assessment of the risks of and hopes for this "reproductive revolution" is not a purely scientific matter; it depends in part upon a person's perspective on the future. Optimists are disposed to react to new versions of procreation with confidence and hope. Pessimists are disposed to react to the same new powers with anxiety and fear. Their perspectives on the future affect their assessments of the magnitude and the possibility of harms and benefits.

In 1978 those who celebrated the birth of Louise Brown, the world's first "test-tube baby," pointed to a healthy baby girl and envisioned many other childless couples being helped by this procedure to have the baby for which they longed and prayed. And it did seem wrong somehow not to rejoice with the Browns, not to join them in celebrating human ingenuity and divine goodness and a beautiful little girl, not to join them in the hope and vision of other childless couples having babies. On the other hand, those who reacted with horror and alarm shared a different vision, a vision of egg banks, surrogate mothers, classified ads announcing "eggs for sale" and "celebrity seed wanted" and "wombs for rent," sex choice, quality control, and the creation of a real London Hatchery and Conditioning Center to match the fictitious one in Aldous Huxley's *Brave New World.* And that vision has not lost its plausibility or its horror — especially for the pessimists.

We shall do best, however, to avoid the fateful script of either the optimists or the pessimists, as though either progress or catastrophe were inevitable. G. K. Chesterton once said "that the optimist thought everything good except the pessimist, and the pessimist thought everything bad, except himself" (*Orthodoxy* [Garden City, N.Y.: Image, 1959], p. 66). There is wisdom there, a wisdom borne out by many discussions of new versions of procreation; both optimistic proponents and pessimistic opponents have sometimes been guilty of moral and intellectual pride. There is also a marvelous — even if accidental — insight in the child's definition that an optimist is the person who looks after your eyes and a pessimist is the person who looks after your feet. That combination of vision and pedestrian realism, of hope and prudence, is the appropriate perspective on the future, especially for the Christian community, which knows both the common grace of God and the intransigence of human pride and sloth.

That said, it may be remarked that the American Christian community seems particularly tempted to a kind of optimism called "possibility thinking," which presumes the inevitability of success if people just put their minds to it instead of to negative thoughts. According to that perspective, people can "turn scars into stars," to quote one exponent. I think that view lacks realism, and I fear that it simply fuels our culture's confidence in technological progress and our society's notion of reproductive success. Thoughtless reproductive interventions may leave scars no one can turn into stars.

13. In 2000 there were 25,228 live births (and 35,025 babies) following 99,639 A.R.T. cycles. (The report did not include the number of births following artificial insemination.) That is about .9% of the total U.S. births. Over 75% of the A.R.T. cycles used fresh (non-frozen) non-donor eggs. About 13% used frozen non-donor eggs. About 10% used donated eggs or embryos. And 1% used a gestational carrier ("2000 Assisted Reproductive Technology Success Rates," CDC's Reproductive Health Information Source, www.cdc.gov.nccdphp/drh/ART).

reproduction technologies have been developed, including GIFT, ZIFT, and ICSI. In gamete intrafallopian transfer (GIFT), after the oocytes are removed, a catheter is used to transfer them along with sperm into a woman's fallopian tube, where it is hoped that they will produce a fertilized egg that will make its way down the fallopian tube and implant itself in the woman's uterus. In zygote intrafallopian transfer (ZIFT) the oocytes are inseminated in vitro but transferred as early pre-embryos into a woman's fallopian tube. ICSI, or intracytoplasmic sperm injection, utilizes surgery on a minute scale in order to insert a single sperm into the ooplasm of an oocyte and to achieve fertilization.[14]

This is only a partial list of current possibilities in A.R.T. It leaves aside the more conventional therapies that attempt to enable or preserve a pregnancy, as well as surgical fallopian tube repair. And it leaves aside the technologies on the horizon, like human reproductive cloning and artificial wombs that would provide for gestation from fertilization to viability. The list of human powers enabling us to intervene purposefully in procreative processes is sure to grow even more rapidly than the list of new versions of Scripture.[15]

Of the new versions of the Bible, some are good and some are appalling. The same can be said about new versions of procreation: some of them are good, and some of them are appalling. But which ones, and why? Granted that people can do a number of things in begetting children that they never could do before, the questions arise: Which of these new versions of procreation are worthy of the story Christians still love to tell and long to live? Which of them are good? And which are appalling? Let's begin with an appalling case.

Ron's Angels: Eggs for Sale on the Internet

Recently Ron Harris posted an Internet site offering the eggs of models to the highest bidder.* The site is called Ron's Angels (ronsangels.com/index2.html), and I visited it. The opening page invited me (or any visitor) to "come up to beauty." There was a picture of a very pretty woman smiling at me. And below the picture was a little text welcoming me to ronsangels.com, and proclaiming that it is "the only web site that provides . . . the unique opportunity to bid on eggs from beautiful, healthy, and intelligent women."

I clicked on the auction page and was greeted with a similar invitation, and here there were pictures of three models. They were presented as my "choices," and they were nameless. There was not even the sort of description *Playboy* provides of its centerfolds. For a fee you can get some information, including, I am told, the ages and measurements of these women. The page did inform me that the lowest acceptable bid for the ova of one of these models was $15,000 and that the bidding was expected to go up to $150,000.

There were five paragraphs of text on the auction page, but the five paragraphs did not display much evidence of critical thinking skills. We are told, for example, that there are six million infertile women in the United States. Fine so far, but then we are told that they are all looking for eggs so that they can have children. There are, however, many causes of infertility that will not be remedied by access to donor eggs. The largest single factor in infertility is low sperm count in the males with whom women are trying to have a baby. To give one other example, we are told, "All genetic modifications serve to improve the shape, color, and traits of the organism." One might wish that it were so, but of course it is not. I resisted the impulse to put a giant F on my computer screen just then. I could not resist the impulse to

14. Developments in genetic diagnosis have been joined to A.R.T. in order to make possible genetic screens for sperm and oocytes and the pre-implantation diagnosis of the pre-embryos awaiting transfer to a woman's womb. On such developments see pp. 165-66 of Chapter Five of *Reading the Bible in the Strange World of Medicine.*

15. But not perhaps any more rapidly than the list of reasons for developing and using these new powers. Again, it is necessary to be satisfied with a mere sampling. The "good" sought might be safeguarding the health and well-being of the child; enabling a childless couple to circumvent their infertility and to have a child conceived with their own seed; enabling a childless couple to have a child conceived with donors' seed; enabling a couple to have a particular sort of child — say, a boy or a "normal" child or a gifted child; enabling a single person to have a child; or enabling prospective parents to make an informed choice about whether to conceive when they may be at some genetic risk or to make an informed decision about therapy or abortion on the basis of a prenatal diagnosis. These could be called "personal" purposes (although they also have social dimensions simply because they involve the social roles of husband, wife, and parent), and they could be contrasted with an assortment of "societal" purposes. The societal "goods" sought might include the following: to enable society to avoid the genetic disaster some have predicted if we continue to treat those who would otherwise die from certain genetic diseases; to enable society to avoid the costly care of persons who are retarded or disabled when there are many other demands on our resources; to enable society to reproduce geniuses or good soldiers or short and strong people to work the mines; to enable society — to quote Joseph Fletcher — "to offset an elitist or tyrannical power plot by other clonors" by "cloning top-grade soldiers and scientists" ("Ethical Aspects of Genetic Controls," *New England Journal of Medicine* 285 [1971]: 776-83, at p. 779). (During the Cold War it had been seriously suggested that a "reproduction race" and a "cloning gap" might become as critical to national security as the "missile gap" and the "arms race" putatively were.) This list of purposes for revising the old version of procreation is, as previously noted, only partial. It does not include, for example, some of Joseph Fletcher's most imaginative hypothetica.

*[Editors' Note: The "Ron's Angels" website purporting to auction eggs of "supermodels" was likely a hoax to generate traffic for Ron Harris's various nude photography and pornography websites. See, for example, http://news.bbc.co.uk/2/hi/americas/488453.stm and http://jaydixit.com/writing/salon/eggs.htm (both accessed March 6, 2012). Despite the website being a hoax, reactions to "Ron's Angels" at least partially confirm Verhey's arguments about commodification. We do not recommend rewarding Mr. Harris by visiting his website.]

click the credentials link. I wanted to know a little more about this Ron Harris.

On that page I was told of Ron Harris's credentials for this venture. He is a fashion photographer. He is the creator of Aerobicise, an exercise video. He has produced thirteen one-hour specials for Playboy television. And, almost relevantly, he is a horse breeder. Later, thinking that perhaps I should be a little more generous in my judgment of Ron Harris, I decided to visit Aerobicise on the Internet. It might, after all, have some connection with medicine. I discovered, however, that it is connected, rather, with what is called euphemistically adult entertainment. It is linked on the Internet with several sites that you can only enter by promising that you are an adult and by paying a fee. Aerobicise, I gather, is closer to soft porn than it is to reproductive endocrinology.

At the end of my visit to ronsangels.com I learned that Ron Harris takes no remuneration from the donors. That sounded generous until I also learned that, for his fee, he adds a 20 percent surcharge to the bid. And he pays nothing. Donors (as Harris calls them, although they might more accurately be called "vendors") and bidders have to get their own doctors and their own attorneys. There is no mention on the site of the considerable health risks of being an egg donor and no mention of the success rate (or failure rate) for in vitro fertilization.

What's wrong with this? I will not pretend to give a complete answer to that question in a few pages. There are a whole bunch of things wrong with this:

First, it is sexist, reducing women to their reproductive utility. But I will leave that issue aside here.[16] Second, it panders to this society's focus on the young and beautiful. I will also leave this issue aside. Third, it is genetic foolishness. There is a story that Marilyn Monroe once told Albert Einstein that she would love to have his baby. "With my looks and your brain, our child would be a gift to the world." To which Albert Einstein is said to have replied, "But my dear, what if the child had my looks and your brain?" Fourth, it commodifies and commercializes what should not be commodified or commercialized. That is a modest and, I think, obvious claim with respect to ronsangels.com, but if it is true, then it is relevant not just to ronsangels.com but to many other things that go on under the umbrella of reproductive medicine. Attention to legitimate worries about commodification may be the best place to begin if we are to exercise discernment in the "reproductive revolution."

16. This important objection to ronsangels.com is emphasized in the objection of many feminists to A.R.T. more generally. See, for example, Gena Corea, *The Mother Machine* (New York: Harper and Row, 1985), and Barbara Katz Rothman, *Recreating Motherhood* (New York: W. W. Norton, 1989). There is even an organization called FINRRAGE (Feminists International Network of Resistance to Reproductive and Genetic Engineering). We will not leave this important issue altogether aside; it is obviously intimately connected with the issue of commodification, which we focus on below. See further the essay by Paul Lauritzen, "Whose Bodies? Which Selves? Appeals to Embodiment in Assessments of Reproductive Technology," in *Embodiment, Morality, and Medicine*, ed. Lisa Sowle Cahill and Margaret A. Farley (Dordrecht, Netherlands: Kluwer Academic, 1995), pp. 113-26; reprinted in Stephen E. Lammers and Allen Verhey, eds., *On Moral Medicine: Theological Perspectives in Medical Ethics*, second ed. (Grand Rapids: Eerdmans, 1998), pp. 486-95 [pp. 850-57 of the present volume]. Lauritzen compares and contrasts the objections made against commodification in A.R.T. by feminists and by the Roman Catholic document *Instruction on Respect for Human Life in Its Origin and on the Dignity of Procreation*, issued by the Congregation of the Doctrine of the Faith (and reprinted in the same edition of *On Moral Medicine*, pp. 469-85).

Commodification, Embodiment, and "Reproductive Liberty"

Ronsangels.com is an egregious example of commodification, but it is not the only one. Indeed, complaints about commodification are commonplace in conversations about A.R.T. The specific worry with respect to ronsangels.com, of course, is that ova, or human eggs, are being commodified, reduced to the status of vendible objects, like chicken eggs or caviar. But one might worry about the commodification of all sperm and ova when "donors" (or "vendors") are compensated. One might worry that the new reproductive technologies will turn children into "products." One might complain that the donors themselves are commodified, reduced to the status of the animated tools of reproductive technologies — and "animated tool," of course, was Aristotle's definition of a slave. One might complain that women have been — and still are — commodified, reduced to the status of baby-machines. Some complain that the technologies inevitably treat procreative behaviors, whether providing sperm or ova or gestating an embryo, as if these could be regarded merely as matters of physiology and as matters for contract. And one might worry about the integrity of medicine when a medical specialty looks for all the world like an industry, "the infertility industry," as it is sometimes called, and when the marketing of these technologies treats desperate couples as consumers and seems sometimes to follow that axiom of commerce, *caveat emptor*.

It is a daunting set of worries. What links these worries and complaints together, however, is the concern about the commodification and commercialization of begetting. But what is wrong with commodification and commercialization of begetting? To answer that question could be an important clue for our discernment in the midst of a "reproductive revolution."

Let me begin with an obvious but not unimportant point: The market is a good instrument for distributing many good things and for rewarding much good work.[17] While I am praising markets, moreover, it is important to observe that the market is not without morality. Commerce as a practice is not without rules. Commerce is

17. William F. May, *The Patient's Ordeal* (Bloomington: Indiana University Press, 1991), p. 72.

ruled by contract, and contracts require free and informed consent. Commerce itself prohibits not only coercion but also the sort of deception that I think one can find in the Ron's Angels site. Those who, like me, complain about commodification and commercialization in A.R.T. need not — and usually do not — deny the fact that the market is a good instrument for distributing many good things and for rewarding much good work. We do not claim that the market itself is immoral. We complain, rather, that the morality of the marketplace is *insufficient* for human procreation and for the practice of medicine. And we worry that, if we pretend the marketplace account *is* sufficient, then we risk distorting or demeaning or corrupting both parenting and health care.

The complaints and worries about commodification appeal to a point no less obvious and no less important than the one just made about markets. The point is this: that markets are not good instruments for distributing *everything*. The market's sphere is — and should be — limited.[18]

This society's enthusiasm for the market has not kept it from acknowledging that obvious point: some things are not to be regarded as marketable objects. We do not believe that anything and everything can be or should be sold. We do not believe that everything and anything "has a price." And even in our most cynical moments, when we think that perhaps, after all, everything or everyone does "have a price," we do not think it should be so!

It is not difficult to come up with examples of points at which we have limited the sphere of the market, points at which we have rejected commodification and commercialization. We have prohibited a market in persons, for example; we do not want slavery. We have prohibited a market in criminal justice; we do not want judges' decrees or juries' verdicts to be bought and sold. We do not want a market in political power and influence; we do not want citizens or their representatives to sell their votes. We do not want a market where people are desperate; we prohibit child labor and sweat shops. We do not want a market in body parts; we prohibit the sale of organs — even the organs of the dead. We do not want babies sold at auction. We do not want . . . , but you get the idea. Some things are not to be commodified and commercialized. There are some boundaries, some limits, to the sphere of the market.

Michael Walzer calls these limits, these boundaries, "blocked exchanges."[19] And he regards these limits on the sphere of the market as no less important to social justice than "blocked uses of power," or the limits on the sphere of the state.

Now, if we agree that the market is a good instrument for distributing many good things and for rewarding much good work and that, nevertheless, some things ought not be marketable, then some questions seem unavoidable: How will we draw the lines? And where? How will we set the boundaries? Or enforce them? What exchanges should be "blocked"? And how?

Those are not easy questions, but we will make little progress in answering them unless we think first about *why* we would draw such a line. Why should we "block" certain exchanges? What is wrong with the commodification of some things? What is wrong with the commercialization of some relationships? I promise to return to these questions in the context of human procreation, but I want to begin to address them by telling three stories taken from other contexts.

Three Stories of Commodification

The first story displays that, when some goods are commodified, they do not remain quite the same goods. The story is told in the New Testament, in the eighth chapter of Acts. There was a man named Simon who lived in Samaria and had a reputation as a great magician. When he witnessed the miracles done by those who had received the gift of the Spirit, he offered the disciple Peter money for the gift. He tried to *buy* the Spirit and its power. And Peter said, "It's a 'blocked exchange.'" Well, not quite in those words. He actually said, "May your silver perish with you, because you thought you could obtain God's gift with money!" (Acts 8:20). One way of taking Peter's remark, I suppose, is simply that one *cannot* buy God's favors. But I think Peter was not so much concerned with the impossibility of purchasing the Spirit as with the impropriety of it. The Spirit was not to be commodified. Commerce in the Spirit would have corrupted miracle into magic. The wrong done by commercialization was here — and sometimes still is — the corruption, the demeaning, the distortion of the good exchanged. Sometimes what is good cannot remain quite the same good if commodified and commercialized.

The second story displays a second problem, that commodification can corrupt community. This story is taken from American history.[20] It was 1863. President Lincoln had decided that a military draft was the only way to win the Civil War and to preserve the Union. It was the first military draft in American history, and it was not popular. One provision of the Enrollment and Conscription Act of 1863, however, was not only unpopular but thoroughly despised. This provision allowed for the exemption of any man whose name was drawn in the draft lottery if he was willing and able to put up three hundred dollars to pay a substitute. Throughout the Union the cry went up, "This should be a 'blocked exchange.'" Well, not exactly; but the impropriety of the provision was obvious to many. The danger of death was an incentive for some men to pay three hundred dollars to other men, and for these other men three hundred

18. May, *The Patient's Ordeal,* p. 72: "We live in different spheres, and different principles of distribution apply in different spheres."

19. Michael J. Walzer, *Spheres of Justice: A Defense of Pluralism and Equality* (New York: Basic, 1983), pp. 100-102.

20. It is told by Walzer, *Spheres of Justice,* pp. 98-99.

dollars was an incentive to accept the danger. The impropriety of it was not that three hundred dollars was *too cheap* a price; the impropriety was that there *was* a price. The impropriety was not, however, simply that a price was put on risk; the labor market included — and sometimes rewarded — risky work. Why, then, should this exchange have been blocked? What was the wrong in the commodification and commercialization of the draft? The provision expressed and nurtured a wrong account of the sort of society we were and wanted to become. It undercut and put at risk a sense of community — and ironically for the sake of the republic — turning public responsibility into a private transaction.[21] To our credit we never reenacted that provision. Sometimes the wrong done by commodification or commercialization is the damage done to relationships in community. Commodification can risk rupturing the fabric of the common life. If we do not block some exchanges, we may risk corrupting, demeaning, or distorting relations in community.[22]

The first story illustrated the risk of corrupting the good exchanged. The second illustrated the risk of corrupting the sort of community we are. There is a third risk, I think, a risk of distorting our rhetoric, the way we think of and talk of morality and ourselves. Let me illustrate it by a third story, a story that returns (finally) to some issues in reproductive medicine, a story of a conversation in my classroom a few years ago.

The scandal involving Dr. Ricardo Asch, then reproductive endocrinologist at the University of California, Irvine, had recently been in the news. In an effort to remind students that not all cases are hard cases I reported the allegations against Dr. Ricardo Asch. Suppose, I said, that the allegation is true that Dr. Asch took eggs from women in the course of their infertility treatment and — without the consent of those women — used their eggs in the infertility treatment of other women. Then I asked, how many of you would defend the behavior of Dr. Asch?

When no one raised a hand, I was pleased. I prepared to make my point that not all moral choices are ambiguous. I decided, however, to press my luck a little and to ask them to suppose that Asch was a compassionate human being who saw the suffering of the childless and wanted to put a stop to that suffering. No one said that they would change their minds even if Dr. Asch were known to be a compassionate human being. So I pressed my luck a little further still. What was the wrong in what he did? I asked.

One bright young man was quick to offer what he took to be the obvious answer. "He's a thief," he said. A young woman sitting nearby disagreed. "I don't think the wrong was theft," she said. "It feels more like kidnapping." She had evidently seen some report on the scandal, and she asked whether embryos had been taken too. I said that the allegations against Dr. Asch included that he had taken embryos as well as eggs, but I suggested that we stick with the allegation that eggs were taken, not embryos. She accepted the suggestion and said, "Okay, well, the wrong may not have been kidnapping exactly then — but not theft exactly either."

By this time I wanted to make my point and get back to the agenda for the day; so I said, "At least we all agree that there is something wrong with this behavior. Not all moral choices are ambiguous." The young woman, however, was not quite ready to move on. "But there does seem to be some ambiguity about how to name this wrong," she said, "and there still seems to me to be something wrong with calling the wrong theft," she repeated. And then she made a point that made me humble (and proud) to be her teacher. She said that what we call a thing is important, that the way we talk of how and why something is right or wrong is not a morally trivial thing.

I commended her for her point, and asked her what she thought was wrong about calling Dr. Asch's behavior theft. "It's like calling rape theft," she said. So I asked the Socratic question, "And what's wrong with calling rape theft?" She startled just a little, as if she could not quite believe either that I had asked such a question or that she had expected to learn anything from someone who would ask such a question.

Then she answered, "Rape is an attack on me, on my person; theft is an attack on my property. Both are wrong, but they are different wrongs. And to call rape theft suggests that my person, my self, my embodied integrity, is something that can be exchanged for cash."

The young man had had quite enough of this. "Oh, come on," he said, "prostitutes exchange their 'embodied integrity' for cash every day."

"But they shouldn't," the young woman replied, "and even if they are driven to prostitution because they have no other options, their 'pimps' and their 'Johns' shouldn't think of them or treat them like commodities."

"Look," the young man said, "I agree that prostitution is, well, 'unsavory,' but at least it's voluntary. If Asch had purchased the eggs instead of taking them, that might have been 'unsavory,' too, but no great wrong would have been committed; nobody's freedom would have been violated. The thing that makes what Asch did wrong was the same thing that makes theft wrong: He took something valuable from the victims without their consent. And, for that matter, the same thing can be said of rape; it *is* like theft."

The young woman paused for a moment, whether to control her temper or to gather her thoughts I was not sure. When finally she spoke, she said something like this: "That way of thinking and talking makes me angry — and anxious. Embodied integrity is not some object

21. Walzer, *Spheres of Justice*, p. 99: "It seemed to abolish the public thing and turn military service (even when the republic itself was at stake!) into a private transaction."

22. Even when we agree, however, that a certain exchange should be blocked and why, it will not always be easy to say exactly where and how the line should be drawn. During the Vietnam conflict there were draft deferments for college students, and there were questions about the practice. There was a sense that there was a boundary that ought not be crossed, but there was no clear sense about exactly where to draw it.

persons own. It is not some commodity people may sell if they choose. Persons are not just disembodied choice-makers, and they — in their embodiment — should not be treated as commodities. There are other ways to violate persons than just by violating their freedom. To think and talk about rape or about what Asch did as 'theft' is dangerously close to thinking and talking about embodied integrity as if it were a commodity. And to think or talk about embodied integrity as if it were a commodity is not far from treating embodied integrity as a commodity!"

Two Views of Commodification

There were clearly two different views in that class that day, but they simply echoed two different views that exist in the culture. The young woman echoed an essay by Margaret Jane Radin on "Market Inalienability."[23] For Radin — and for the young woman — "commodification" includes not only the actual buying and selling of something but also thinking and talking about things as if they were marketable objects. Our rhetoric — the way we think and talk about things — forms the sort of life we can live. Radin — and the young woman — insisted that things important to personhood should not be commodified. And they were suspicious of disembodied accounts of what is important to personhood; they were suspicious of the dualistic rhetoric that conceives of the person, the self, "as pure subjectivity standing wholly apart from an environment of pure objectivity."[24] In her search for a better view of personhood, Radin calls attention to the fact that we are human persons — and we flourish as human persons — always as embodied and communal selves. Such a view of personhood, she claims, would regard many sorts of things and experiences "as integral to the self."[25] And among these things "integral to the self" are sexuality and the experience of becoming a parent. If we commodify these things, we "do violence to our deepest understanding of what it is to be human."[26]

The wrong of commodification and commercialization, according to Radin, is that both the rhetoric and the practices consistent with them do violence to our personhood as embodied and communal selves. They create two kinds of alienation. The first kind of alienation is an alienation from our bodies, a disorientation in the self who makes the commodification her own. For example, the surrogate mother who has entered into a contract that commodifies both her pregnancy and the child who results is alienated from the daily embodied experience of pregnancy. (Or else the experience of pregnancy and birth — and the normal embodied experience of bonding — will alienate her from the contract.)[27] The second kind of alienation is an alienation from community, an alienation created, Radin says, "between those who use the discourse [of the market] and those they wrong in doing so." For example, the men who would use the eggs of a vendor regard some biological relationship to their child as important to their own flourishing, but for the sake of it, they encourage the "donor" to regard the biological relationship with a child as trivial.[28]

The young man in class provided a weak echo of a different view of commodification, a view that has been influential in the public moral discourse about A.R.T. His use of the term "unsavory" and his emphasis on freedom echoed an intriguing essay by Ruth Macklin.[29] "Commodification of human beings is 'unsavory,'" Macklin said, "yet 'unsavoriness' is not a category of moral disvalue strong enough to warrant prohibition."[30]

It is not that Macklin or the young man thought that there could *never* be a warrant to "block" or prohibit commerce. (They were not in favor of slavery, after all.) But they found such warrants only in a violation of "rights," only in a violation of fundamental ethical principles like respect for persons and justice. Macklin acknowledged, to her great credit, that those ethical principles are open to more than one interpretation. She distinguished between what she called a "broad interpretation" of these principles and a "narrow interpretation." The broad interpretation of the principle of respect for persons calls for respect for persons in the richness of their humanity; the narrow interpretation calls for respect for their freedom, for their voluntary and informed consent. She wanted, so she said, to "respect" what she calls the broad interpretation, but she insisted that only the narrow interpretation, only respect for autonomy, could be used to "block" or prohibit commerce. A richer account of personhood and a broader account of the respect due persons, she acknowledged, might prompt a community to prohibit commodification and commercialization and not simply regard them as "unsavory." But Macklin disqualifies "the broader interpretation" from public relevance because, so she claimed, it rests on "a religious or moral view of human dignity that is not universally shared."[31] Such "moralistic or symbolic reasons for prohibiting payment could not count as a suffi-

23. Margaret Jane Radin, "Market Inalienability," *Harvard Law Review* (1987): 1849-1937; an abridged version is found in Kenneth D. Alpern, ed., *The Ethics of Reproductive Technology* (New York: Oxford University Press, 1992), pp. 174-94.

24. Radin, "Market Inalienability," in Alpern, p. 178.

25. Radin, "Market Inalienability," in Alpern, p. 179.

26. Radin, "Market Inalienability," in Alpern, p. 179.

27. See further May, *The Patient's Ordeal*, pp. 74-77.

28. Moreover, commodification expresses and forms individualism. When we regard something personal as a commodity we form a society in which people finally "cannot freely give of themselves to others. At best they can bestow commodities. At worst . . . the gift is conceived of as a bargain" (Radin, "Market Inalienability," in Alpern, p. 180).

29. Ruth Macklin, "What Is Wrong with Commodification?" in *New Ways of Making Babies: The Case of Egg Donation*, ed. Cynthia Cohen (Bloomington: Indiana University Press, commissioned by the National Advisory Board on Ethics in Reproduction [NABER], 1996), pp. 106-21.

30. Macklin, "What Is Wrong with Commodification?" p. 106.

31. Macklin, "What Is Wrong with Commodification?" p. 114.

cient justification for interfering with a fundamental right, that is the infertile couple's right to form families noncoitally."[32] Here Macklin echoes — and cites — the influential work of John Robertson.[33]

Robertson emphasizes "the importance of procreative liberty."[34] A policy of "procreative liberty" affirms the right of people to reproduce (or not), and so it affirms the right to utilize technology to achieve personal reproductive goals. Moreover, this right is limited only by the duty not to harm others. Then, of course, the meaning of "harm" is critically important. Robertson seems to restrict the meaning of harm to the violation of another person's "procreative liberty," that is, to using another person in one's own reproductive project without his or her consent. To be sure, the offspring of reproductive technologies might also be harmed, but it counts as actual harm only if their lives are so full of suffering as to be worse than no life at all.[35] Most of the objections against the exercise of "procreative liberty" seem to Robertson to call attention not to actual harms but to "symbolic" concerns. And "symbolic" concerns, for Robertson as for Macklin, are insufficient to limit this right because reasonable people in a pluralistic society can reasonably differ on the "symbols."

As it turns out, there are few acts of reproduction that Robertson thinks may be blocked. He can even envision commercialization and commodification, "a widespread market in paid conception, pregnancies, and adoptions," and view that prospect with apparent equanimity.[36] To his credit, Robertson says toward the end of his book that "the invocation of procreative liberty as a dominant value is not intended to demolish opposition or end discussion."[37] Again and again, however, the invocation of the word "symbolic" *is* used to end discussion. For example, concerns about the payment of "donors" of sperm and ova and embryos are described as "symbolic";[38] the unwillingness of some to enforce surrogacy contracts is, he says, "based . . . on a symbolic view of maternal gestation";[39] and other objections to commodification and commercialization are said to express a "symbolic concern."[40] In all of these cases calling an objection "symbolic" is a way of discounting it.

Robertson is right in describing these positions as involving symbolic ways of thinking. But he is wrong in using such a description to close discussion. And he is wrong in supposing that his position is not itself based on a symbolic account of human life and parenting. We can make our arguments about commercialization and commodification of reproductive technologies boring, but we cannot make them nonsymbolic.[41]

32. Macklin, "What Is Wrong with Commodification?" p. 118.

33. She cites John A. Robertson, "Technology and Motherhood: Legal and Ethical Issues in Human Egg Donation," *Case Western Reserve Law Review* 39 (1988-1989): 30. He subsequently published the widely influential book cited earlier, *Children of Choice.*

34. Robertson, *Children of Choice,* p. 3.

35. On Robertson's account of weighing the harm to possible children see Cynthia Cohen, "'Give Me Children or I Shall Die!': New Reproductive Technologies and Harm to Children," *Hastings Center Report* 26 (1996): 19-27.

36. Robertson, *Children of Choice,* p. 143. To be sure, in 1994 at least, Robertson did rule out some procreative actions, including actions aimed at nontherapeutic enhancement, actions aimed at replicating (or cloning) other human genomes, and actions aimed at producing offspring who are less than normal (Bladerunner, for example; p. 167). The reason given for the judgment that such actions are not protected by reproductive liberty, moreover, is that "they deviate too far from the experiences that make reproduction a valued experience" (p. 167). Indeed, in this same context, when he attempts to "posit a core view of the goals and values of reproduction," he says, "on such a view, procreative liberty would protect only actions designed to enable a couple to have normal, healthy offspring whom they intend to rear" (p. 167).

There seems — to this reader, at least — to be some tension between these statements and some of his other views, including his view of commodification and commercialization. He does not elsewhere, for example, restrict the exercise of this right to a "couple." The right is fundamentally an individual right. Elsewhere he *does* include within reproductive liberty the use of measures to select the characteristics of one's offspring (e.g., pp. 152-53). And if Bladerunner would not have been born at all apart from the act aimed at offspring like Bladerunner, then — given Robertson's account of weighing the harm to possible children — it is hard to see how he could think any actual harm would have been done.

Usually, then, Robertson presents his readers with a thin account of human life and parenting, a *disembodied* and *individualistic* account. Individuals are presented as pure subjects, isolated wills, over-against nature, over-against their own bodies, which belong to the realm of objects and may be commodified without great cost. These individuals associate by contract when they choose to cooperate in the pursuit of their individual interests. Such an account of our humanity and of our begetting, however, should not be regarded as less "symbolic" because it is thin.

Upon occasion, however, Robertson presents his readers with a somewhat richer account of human life and parenting, a more embodied account, notably not only in the passage I cited but also in his account of *why* "procreative liberty deserves presumptive respect" (p. 16). There we hear, among other things, that "transmission of one's genes through reproduction" may be the "expression of a couple's love or unity" (p. 16). He even asks at one point whether a collaborator is "meaningfully procreating if he or she is merely providing gametes or gestation without any rearing role" (p. 120). He does not answer that question (not in my reading, at least). Nevertheless, when he thinks and talks about procreation in ways that honor embodiment as well as autonomy, then he can and does challenge the assumption that "procreative liberty" still "deserves presumptive respect" in those cases that depart significantly from the "goals and values" of parenting, or from the embodied significance of procreation.

I would like Robertson to admit the tension here — and to admit that the tension results from different *symbolic* accounts of persons and parenting. I fear, however, that if he admits the tension he may discount even his own attempt to "posit a core view of the goals and values of reproduction" as "symbolic" and as, therefore, irrelevant to public (or at least legal) restrictions on "procreative liberty." See further the review of Robertson's work in Gilbert Meilaender, *Body, Soul, and Bioethics* (Notre Dame, Ind.: University of Notre Dame Press, 1995), pp. 61-88.

37. Robertson, *Children of Choice,* p. 221.

38. Robertson, *Children of Choice,* p. 141.

39. Robertson, *Children of Choice,* p. 132.

40. Robertson, *Children of Choice,* p. 141.

41. Meilaender, *Body, Soul, and Bioethics,* pp. 85-88.

Given the fact that there are these two quite different views, how can we adjudicate them? How can we reasonably choose between them? Robertson and Macklin evidently think that their view is the rational, objective, and (at least potentially) universal one. Macklin's response to the article by Margaret Jane Radin is in that respect hardly surprising: "it is sufficient to note," Macklin said, "that not everyone is likely to buy into her analysis."[42] Radin might, however, respond in kind that "it is sufficient to note that not everyone is likely to buy into Macklin's or Robertson's analysis." None of these authors thinks, I suppose, that everyone will "buy into" their view, but the reasons they give for disagreement are interestingly and importantly different.

Macklin and Robertson evidently think that there is an "objective and rational" (if minimal) account of what is normatively human. Because this account is "objective and rational," it can claim also to be "universal." It may be only a minimal account, but that minimal account provides a foundation for moral discourse in a pluralistic community. In addition to this "objective and rational" account (that is, their account), there are a series of "symbolic" accounts about which reasonable people will, of course, disagree.

Radin, however, refuses to privilege their account — or any account of the normatively human — as "objective and rational," as free from the symbols and rhetoric which we inevitably use to describe and to reason and to exercise moral discernment. "Fact- and value-commitments are present in the language we use to reason and describe, and they shape our reasoning and description, and the shape (for us) of reality itself."[43]

From Macklin's perspective, Radin provides a "symbolic" view of personhood, and therefore its public relevance can be discounted. From Radin's perspective, Macklin and Robertson also provide a "symbolic" view of personhood, but the issue for Radin is not whether an account is "symbolic" or not. All accounts are "symbolic"! The issue for Radin is, rather, which symbols are more appropriate to the human condition. And she is suspicious of the philosophical and rhetorical tradition that has "shaped" the account of Macklin and Robertson. She is suspicious, that is, of dualism, of the philosophical and rhetorical tradition that divides the self into subject and object, that conceives of the true self as pure subjectivity standing over — and over-against — the body and the community and the environment.

I think Radin has it right: both accounts are "symbolic." No account of human procreation is unencumbered with metaphysical baggage. The thin account favored by Robertson and Macklin does not simply transcend particular traditions by its emphasis on freedom and rationality. It stands squarely within the tradition of dualism. An account more attentive to embodiment and community is also "symbolic," of course. If we are to choose between them, we will not get very far by asking which one is "rational" and which one is "symbolic." We will have to ask which symbols are more appropriate to human experience. And Christians will have to ask which symbols are more appropriate to Scripture.[44] When we view human beings chiefly as "choice-makers" characterized by their interests and capable of contracts, we see something important and true, but we miss much else that is also important and also true. Human beings are embodied creatures. They are not in the body the way a taxi-driver is in the cab, or the way Descartes's ghost is presumably in the machine. And human beings are communal creatures. They find themselves in relationships and with responsibilities not all of which are of their choosing. There are good reasons to prefer the symbolic account of human beings and of their begetting that acknowledges embodiment and community.

If there is no nonsymbolic account of humanity and its procreation, and if it is better to talk and to think about these issues in ways that honor human embodiment and community, then the justification for limiting the market will be larger than the protection of choice. If there are reasons to be suspicious of a symbolic account of persons and of their procreation that severs body and self, that reduces us to choice-makers and our bodies to vendible commodities, then the justifications for limiting the sphere of the market may well include the protection of persons as embodied and communal, the protection of the good exchanged against commodification, and the protection of the covenants that make community against being reduced to contract.

If we were to think and talk about procreation in ways that honored embodiment, I think we would be more likely to be suspicious of the commodification and commercialization of procreation. We would be readier to limit the sphere of the market as it abuts parenting. With the Canadian Royal Commission on New Reproductive Technologies and its final report, *Proceed with Care,* we would prohibit the buying and selling of fetuses, embryos, eggs, and sperm, and commercial surrogacy.[45] And to return to our "unsavory case," we would prohibit ronsangels.com. Commodification here demeans the "good" exchanged; it corrupts the community of parent and child; and it distorts the way we think and talk about children and about ourselves.

Of course, even if we were to agree *that* a line should be drawn somewhere, it is not always easy to say precisely *where* and *how* that line should be drawn. In "Market Inalienability," Margaret Jane Radin describes three different arguments that can justify limiting the sphere of the market or "blocking exchange."

The first argument or strategy for limiting the market, which she calls "the prophylactic argument," starts with

42. Macklin, "What Is Wrong with Commodification?" p. 117.

43. Radin, "Market Inalienability," in Alpern, p. 177.

44. See Chapter Three in this volume [*Reading the Bible in the Strange World of Medicine*].

45. See *Proceed with Care: Final Report of the Royal Commission on New Reproductive Technologies,* vol. 2 (1993): 718.

the observation that at least some commodifications of the self allow the inference that one has been coerced. She gives selling one's sexual services as an example. In such cases a "blocked exchange" may be the most reliable way to protect persons and their freedom. (This argument, of course, with its attention to freedom, could be utilized by Macklin and Robertson without their acknowledging the symbolic character of their account of persons and their procreation.) Where poverty is regarded as a form of coercion, however, this strategy runs into the problem of the "double bind"; that is, for the sake of protecting the freedom of some poor women we foreclose a choice to them which has (short-term) economic and personal gains. One strategy for mediating the "double bind" is what Radin calls "incomplete commodification." This strategy would, for example, permit prostitution in order to protect the women driven to it but prohibit brokerage, recruitment, and advertising.

The second strategy she calls "prohibition." It starts either with the assumption that commodification is bad in itself or with the observation that a commodified thing is never quite the same thing it was when it was not commodified. A problem with prohibition, however, is that it can lack discernment, failing to distinguish the commodification of six-penny nails from the commodification of sexuality and procreation.

The third strategy she calls "the domino theory." The assumption here is that for *some* things a noncommodified way of thinking and talking is morally preferable. Moreover, it assumes that a noncommodified way of thinking and talking about some things is put at risk by the presence of commodification and commercialization. The problem with "the domino theory," however, is that "the feared domino effect of market rhetoric need not be true."[46] It may be that there is no "slippery slope" leading to the domination of market rhetoric, and that commodified ways of thinking and talking about something can coexist with noncommodified ways of thinking and talking about the same thing. This would certainly seem to be true when people talk about their homes, for example.

These strategies, of course, are not mutually exclusive. We should make some use of all three, and recognize the problems of all three. There are *some* things that simply should not be commodified, some places where a market should be prohibited. Babies, for example, should not be commodified. Baby-selling should be prohibited. Even if it were not the case that selling one's child suggested the presence of coercion, baby-selling should be prohibited. Even if it were not the case that a domino effect of permitting the selling of children would lead to the measuring of all children in terms of their market value, a market in babies should be blocked. In spite of the problem of the "double bind" of poor women who might want to sell a child on the black market in order to provide for other children, baby-selling should be prohibited. The good of a "commodified child," a "marketable child," simply should not exist.

Of course, it is a matter of some dispute just how large the set of things that simply should not be commodified is, but I hope we have made some progress in thinking about how to engage in that dispute. It will not do to neglect prophylactic arguments, arguments attentive to the protection of freedom. It is also important, however, not to neglect the prohibitive argument where that is based on the wrong done by commodification to things important to persons as embodied and communal, or to dismiss such concerns about commodification as "symbolic." Finally, it is important to consider the possible "domino effect," the slippery slope to the domination of a commodified account of children and parenting or to baby-selling.

There are, of course, some things, indeed many things, many commodities, which can be included in the market without alienating people either from themselves or from their communities. And there are some things that can be included in the market while we preserve and protect a noncommercial account of them. In such cases we will not prohibit commercialization, but we may well be a little suspicious of it, attentive to the possible "domino effect" by which the rhetoric of the market overwhelms a noncommercial account of these things. And reproductive medicine is one such thing! Payment for medical services does not wrong anyone, but it is important to preserve and protect the relation of physician and patient from being distorted, corrupted, and demeaned into a relation of merchant and customer (or merchant and supplier).[47]

46. Radin, "Market Inalienability," in Alpern, p. 182.

47. Caution about commodification and commercialization is important in A.R.T. in part because of the desperation of patients. And there are certainly reasons to be anxious about the slippery slope in A.R.T. There is already a widespread perception of reproductive medicine as an industry, the "infertility industry." The slope has been greased by misleading information, for physicians have done little to discourage the belief that this is "a miracle technology" — and advertising frequently encourages such a belief — but many infertile couples still go home to an empty crib. One reason is that, as a 1992 study reported, in IVF the success rate drops with each attempt. There is evidence some dominoes have fallen when physicians fail to help patients say "no" to yet another attempt, when they fail to help patients to begin to write the next chapter of their lives without genetically related children. Commenting on the decreasing success rate for each successive attempt, Dr. Edward Kaplan of Yale made a simple and compassionate suggestion; "Don't encourage people to keep on trying," he said (quoted in S. Begley, "The Baby," *Newsweek*, September 4, 1995, p. 45).

The failure to follow such advice suggests that the commercialization of reproductive medicine has crowded out other ways of thinking and talking about medicine as a sphere of our lives. "When you make your money off couples who say, 'Do what's possible,' there's quite an incentive to encourage patients to do [still] more" (Michelle Oberman, as quoted by Begley, "The Baby," p. 45). There is more evidence that reproductive medicine has slipped when physicians fail to help women who "donate" their ova again and again to keep in mind the long-term effects of hyperstimulation and increased ovulation, and to say "no" to yet another donation. There is evidence of a domino effect when clinics charge for

The conclusions to our examination of this "unsavory" case of ronsangels.com, and to the dangers of commodification in the world of procreation, are, then, these: First, we may and should prohibit ronsangels.com — and, indeed, any buying and selling of ova and sperm and embryos and any renting of wombs. Second, and more generally, we should preserve in our rhetoric and in our practices of begetting a sense of ourselves as embodied and communal creatures. We should not pretend that "reproductive liberty," or freedom, or "choice" provides a sufficient account of what is morally at stake in our begetting.[48] It may, however, be equally important to state candidly what we have not concluded. We have not concluded that A.R.T. always violates the embodied and communal character of human begetting. Indeed, if the purpose of A.R.T., whether IVF or ICSI or another form of A.R.T., is to enable a couple who would otherwise be infertile to conceive and bear a child, it may well serve their embodied relationship.[49] We have not reached, that is to say, the conclusion of the Vatican's Congregation for the Doctrine of the Faith in its *Instruction on Respect for Human Life in Its Origin and on the Dignity of Procreation.*

Responding to the *Instruction*

The *Instruction* condemns all A.R.T. that achieves conception by means other than sexual intercourse. Why? Not because A.R.T. involves technology! Science and technology express the "dominion of man over creation" given with the creation.[50] Science and technology can serve the common good. Still, it is "illusory" to claim that science and technology are "morally neutral." They not only can but *must* be ordered toward the service of the "true and integral good according to the design and will of God." "Science without conscience can only lead to man's ruin."[51] Here we may all be instructed by the *Instruction,* by its measured approval of technology and by its refusal to accept the logic that, if we can, we may.[52]

Technology and the Mastery of Nature

An assessment of A.R.T. depends in part upon one's disposition toward nature and human control over it by means of technology. Some of those who celebrate the new procreative powers too confidently assume that scientific knowledge and its technological applications provide the control over nature that leads to human well-being. And some of those who resist the new powers too optimistically celebrate nature itself and demean the new powers as violations of the natural order and natural processes.

The celebration of technology in Western culture traces its pedigree at least to Francis Bacon (1561-1626). It was Francis Bacon who first construed knowledge as power over nature and who linked power over nature to human welfare. Since then "the Baconian project" has celebrated human mastery over nature.[53] From the perspective of the Baconian project, all dignity belongs to human persons, who are set over and against nature. The natural order and natural processes have no dignity of their own, and that which commands no respect may be mastered.

There can be no denying that the Baconian project has contributed to human well-being; we may and should celebrate the new possibilities that medical technology provides for intervening in the sad stories people tell with and of their bodies and for giving those stories (sometimes) happy endings. But there can also be no denying that science and technology do not always bring well-being in their train.

The close links forged by the Baconian project between knowledge, control over nature, and human welfare make intelligible the foolishness of otherwise brilliant people. No thoughtful person, for example, would accept the logic that "if we can, we may," for every reflec-

---

harvesting an ovary prior to cancer therapy without scientific evidence that the immature eggs will be able to be fertilized later. There is evidence of a slippery slope when clinics advertise "pregnancy suspension" without scientific evidence that the frozen fetal tissue can be revivified.

The best resistance to this slippery slope, and the best protection of a noncommodified account of reproductive medicine, is, of course, professional integrity. It is a hopeful sign that the ASRM (American Society of Reproductive Medicine) is publishing guidelines to help determine which procedures are best for certain infertility conditions (as related to me by Dr. Robert Visscher in personal correspondence). It is a hopeful sign that professionals talk together about "A.R.T., Ads, and Ethics," as they did in a conference sponsored by the National Advisory Board on Ethics in Reproduction (NABER) called "A.R.T., Ads, and Ethics" on October 19, 1997.

48. It is important to observe, however, that although freedom is an insufficient value, it is not insignificant (see pp. 153-55, 166 of Chapter 5 [of *Reading the Bible in the Strange World of Medicine*]) and that respect for freedom does warn us against *unwarranted* intrusions into the procreative decisions of others.

49. So, for example, both Margaret A. Farley, "Feminist Theology and Bioethics," in *Theology and Bioethics: Exploring the Foundations and Frontiers,* ed. Earl E. Shelp (Dordrecht, Netherlands: D. Reidel, 1985), pp. 163-86; reprinted in Lammers and Verhey, *On Moral Medicine,* second ed., pp. 90-103, at p. 100; and Lauritzen, "Whose Bodies? Which Selves?" in *On Moral Medicine,* ed. Lammers and Verhey, second ed., p. 495 [p. 857 of the present volume].

50. Point 2 of "Introduction" in *Instruction on Respect for Human Life,* in *On Moral Medicine,* ed. Lammers and Verhey, second ed., p. 470. Again, point 3 of the introduction: "These interventions are not to be rejected on the grounds that they are artificial" (p. 471).

51. Point 2 of "Introduction" in *Instruction on Respect for Human Life,* p. 470.

52. Point 4 of "Introduction" in *Instruction on Respect for Human Life,* p. 471: "But what is technically possible is not for that very reason morally admissible."

53. Ramsey, *Ethics at the Edges of Life: Medical and Legal Intersections* (New Haven: Yale University Press, 1978), pp. 139, 256. See further the account of the Baconian project in Chapter Five of this volume [*Reading the Bible in the Strange World of Medicine*].

tive person knows there are many things we can do that we ought never to do. But some brilliant scientists seem to follow this logic. The same Dr. Edwards who presided over the conception of Louise Brown had said in 1966, "If rabbit and fly eggs can be fertilized after maturation in culture, presumably human eggs grown in culture could also be fertilized, although obviously it would not be permissible to implant them in a human recipient. We have therefore tried to fertilize cultured human eggs in vitro."[54] He moved from *can* fertilize to *may* fertilize with apparent ease. And twelve years later, in spite of how obvious it had been in 1966 that it would not be permissible to implant the fertilized egg in a human recipient, he evidently moved from *can* implant to *may* implant. Such inferences from what we *can* do because of advances in science and technology to what we *may* do are intelligible if, and perhaps only if, the Baconian project is accepted — if, that is, we assume that knowledge is power over nature and that power over nature increases human welfare. Being able to implant an egg fertilized in vitro was not the end of the story, of course. As Dr. Edwards said of in vitro fertilization later, "The procedures . . . open the way to further work on human embryos in the laboratory."[55] Again he had some scruples about some of the "further work," especially about creating hybrids of human beings with other animals, but one could only wonder whether the scruples would dissolve again as scientists expanded what they *can* do. In the same article Edwards said, "Scientists must maintain their right to exercise their professional activities to the limit that is tolerable by society."[56] This sounds promising, as if Edwards recognized some limits besides the temporary and technical limits on what scientists can do, but it turns out not to be so. The attitudes of society, the limits on what it finds "tolerable," according to Edwards, simply lag a little behind the technological achievements of its scientists and "struggle to catch up with what scientists can do."[57] *Can* still evidently implies *may,* and the public morality needs to catch up. The tail wags the dog — and let the dog beware.

Even among those who reject the logic that if we can, we may (as all do, upon reflection), the Baconian project affects our culture's perspective on technology. It is popular to think of technology as society's "toolbox."[58] In this view, any new technology is just a new tool introduced as an option for people and society to use as they see fit. How the tool is used will depend on the values of the individual or society. We will make what we want with it. Indeed, if we master enough tools, we may yet learn to master the world, to achieve human well-being, to build a new world, a new age. The assumption is that the development and use of technology are simply functions of our values, simply a way to get what we already want. But such a view of technology is naive and, when applied to new versions of procreation, dangerous.

Against such a view of technology it seems clear, first of all, that although technologies are introduced as increasing our options, they can quickly become socially enforced. The automobile, for example, was introduced as an option, a possible alternative to the horse, but the horse is no longer an option; the automobile has become socially enforced. Genetic counseling was introduced as an option for prospective parents, but already some are insisting that parents have a *duty* to be informed and, given certain risks, a duty to avoid childbearing.[59]

Second and more important, against the view of technology as society's "toolbox" it may be observed that although technologies are introduced to get things people want, they seldom satisfy wants; at least, not for long. If people can travel faster by car than they can by horse, they want still faster cars. And if people can have a child when they could not have one before, they are tempted next to want a particular kind of child — say, a bright, blond boy, but surely no "mishap." Technology does not only attempt to satisfy wants; it also stimulates them.[60] Technology shapes our lives and our values as much as it is a function of them. The new versions of procreation will shape and form a view of becoming and being parents as much as they are a function of a desire to be parents.

But it is not just some scientists who have adopted the Baconian project as their own. There are philosophers and theologians who lead the cheers for technology, for knowledge as power over nature, and for power over nature as leading inevitably to human well-being. Joseph Fletcher, for example, frequently said, "Man is a maker and a selector and a designer, and the more rationally contrived and deliberate anything is, the more human it is."[61] The implication is obvious, but no less remarkable for all that: "Laboratory reproduction is radically human compared to conception by ordinary heterosexual intercourse. It is willed, chosen, purposed and controlled, and surely these are the traits that distinguish *Homo sapiens*. . . . Coital reproduction is, therefore, less human than laboratory reproduction."[62] Even the language used is significant. People used to beget children, or procreate; now, according to Fletcher (and, I fear, common usage), people reproduce children — like furniture manufacturers.

54. R. G. Edwards, "Mammalian Eggs in Laboratory," *Scientific American* 214 (1966): 73-81, at p. 80.

55. R. G. Edwards and D. J. Sharpe, "Social Values and Research in Human Embryology," *Nature* 231 (1971): 87; cited by Paul Ramsey, *On In Vitro Fertilization,* in Studies in Law and Medicine, no. 3 (Chicago: Americans United for Life, Inc., 1978), p. 13.

56. Edwards and Sharpe, "Social Values and Research," p. 90.

57. Edwards and Sharpe, "Social Values and Research," p. 90.

58. Emmanuel G. Mesthene, "Technology and Values," in *Who Shall Live? Medicine, Technology, Ethics,* ed. Kenneth Vaux (Philadelphia: Fortress, 1970), p. 26.

59. Daniel Callahan, "Science: Limits and Prohibitions," *Hastings Center Report* 3 (November 1973): 6; reprinted in Lammers and Verhey, eds., *On Moral Medicine,* second ed., pp. 283-86.

60. Callahan, "Science," p. 6.

61. Fletcher, "Ethical Aspects," p. 780.

62. Fletcher, "Ethical Aspects," p. 781.

But persons are children of nature as well as children of spirit. Persons are embodied, and for embodied persons to put hope in the Baconian project is presumptuous and foolish. It is presumptuous because embodied persons are plainly *part* of nature; persons transcend the natural order in certain important ways, but they can never live simply over-against nature; they can live only in the embodied state that depends on nature. It is foolish because, ironically, it makes people even more dependent upon external objects, even if these objects are of their own making and choosing and owning, and it does not entirely release them from their dependencies upon the natural world. We also reject the Baconian project with respect to new beginnings of life.

On the other hand, it will hardly do to adopt a casual anti-technological spirit, to be content with slogans about "playing God" when people intervene in natural processes,[63] to raise the cry that "It's not nice to fool with Mother Nature." Such a casual anti-technological spirit would be required to regard respirators, dialysis machines, insulin, and penicillin illicit. Embodied persons are children of spirit as well as children of nature, and it is slothful to suppress and refuse the dominion that has been given to humanity as a mandate and a blessing. The question should not be whether human beings will "play God" or not — God settled that issue by making us image bearers and stewards. The question should rather be whether or not persons are exercising their God-given dominion responsibly. It would be moral sloth and folly to reject medical technologies, including reproductive technologies, simply because they interfere with natural processes.

In summary, then, part of what is at stake in the new versions of procreation is the image that people have of themselves in relation to nature and to their own powers of mastery over nature. One perspective, the Baconian project, sets people *over and against* nature, as controllers and possessors of it for the sake of human well-being. Another perspective puts people *under* nature, making them obsequiously subservient to Mother Nature because it prohibits interference with the natural order and natural processes. But the Christian story puts human beings *in* nature, exercising stewardship over it, responsible to God in covenant faithfulness.

The sort of dominion that keeps faith with God the creator and provider will be more care-taking than conquering, more nurturing than controlling, more ready to suffer patiently with nature than to lord it over and against nature. A dominion that serves God will be prepared to acknowledge that human beings are only creatures themselves, as fallible as they are finite, ultimately dependent on God the creator and on the creation that God has put in their care. A dominion covenanted to God will not presume that the fault in the world is a part of creation to be remedied by human ingenuity. It will recognize that the fundamental problems of coping with human existence do not permit technological solution, that greed and pride and ennui are not technological problems awaiting a quick technological fix but human faults that can conscript technology into their service. Such a dominion will be able to recognize that the Baconian project's habit of looking for the quick technological fix is folly — and reproductive interventions can feed on that folly. It is God, not technology, who brings in the good future. Technology has brought real and significant benefits, but it is folly to be confident that it will always bring well-being in its train or that, if it doesn't, some new technology can correct the harm. For all its accomplishments and for all its promises, technology has yet to deliver people from their finitude or to the truly good — and it never will. Recognizing the limits of technology, people may be able to lower their expectations and demands of it and to respond in other ways to human problems. In all of this we are simply agreeing with the *Instruction,* with its measured approval of technology and its refusal to accept the logic that if we can, we may.

But if the condemnation of A.R.T. in the *Instruction* is not based on a condemnation of artifice, what reason does it have for condemning the technologies that achieve conception by means other than sexual intercourse? The *Instruction* appeals, as one would expect in a Roman Catholic argument, to "the natural moral law," but this seems in this document simply to represent the claim that the argument finds its basis not simply in revelation or in the reading of Scripture but in reason. The argument relies on a perspective accessible to all and on principles knowable by all rational persons.[64] The work of the argument is done, first, by attention to embodiment, to the "unified totality" of human persons as embodied souls or ensouled bodies,[65] and then by appealing to what it says are the two "fundamental values connected with the techniques of artificial human procreation."[66] These are "the inviolability of innocent human life 'from the moment of conception until death'"[67] and "the special character" of the transmission of human life.[68] We may leave aside the first point, having treated the disputed question of the status of the fetus in earlier chapters.[69] In any case, even if

63. See Allen Verhey, "'Playing God' and Invoking a Perspective," *The Journal of Medicine and Philosophy* 20 (1995): 347-64.

64. As Lisa Cahill points out, however, the *Instruction* comes to opposite conclusions about reproductive technologies and about the human values at stake in them than the Warnock Report and the Office of Technology Assessments report, *Infertility,* both of which also claim to base their argument on universal and rational principles. See Lisa Sowle Cahill, *Sex, Gender, and Christian Ethics* (Cambridge: Cambridge University Press, 1996), p. 230.

65. Point 3 of "Introduction" in *Instruction on Respect for Human Life,* p. 471, citing *Gaudium et Spes* 14.1: *"corpore et anima unus."*

66. Point 4 of "Introduction" in *Instruction on Respect for Human Life,* p. 471.

67. Point 4 of "Introduction" in *Instruction on Respect for Human Life,* p. 471, citing Pope John Paul II.

68. Point 4 of "Introduction" in *Instruction on Respect for Human Life,* p. 471.

69. See Chapters Three and Six [of *Reading the Bible in the*

A.R.T. could avoid the problems of the destruction of "spare" embryos, because of the "special character" of the transmission of human life the *Instruction* condemns the technologies that achieve conception by means other than sexual intercourse. It is that part of the *Instruction* that calls for some response.

Embodied Sexuality and Begetting

When the *Instruction* turns to sexuality and to the "special character" of the transmission of human life, it does not turn directly to Scripture, but it is nevertheless clear that the tradition has been formed and informed by reading Scripture. There is much here that revisits the story of good sex in the creation. The paradigm for good sex is the embodied, "one flesh" relationship between a man and a woman, marked by mutuality, begun in vows and carried out in fidelity, and open to children, who are "the fruit and the sign of [their] mutual self-giving."[70] One might wish, I suppose, for more attention to the marks of the curse upon our sexuality, including both patriarchy and infertility, and for more of a commitment to resist the power of the curse, but this account of embodied sexuality is a good place for Christians to begin to think about A.R.T. Then, however, the *Instruction* infers that the "special character" of human procreation requires an "inseparable connection . . . between the two meanings of the conjugal act: the unitive meaning and the procreative meaning."[71] This intimate link is regarded as an implication of embodiment, based on the unity of body and soul. "The conjugal act by which the couple mutually express their self-gift at the same time expresses openness to the gift of life. It is an act that is inseparably corporal and spiritual."[72] To separate the unitive and procreative ends of human sexual intercourse is "unnatural" and wrong. Thus, as contraception is wrong because it represses the procreative meaning in the act of human sexual intercourse,[73] so A.R.T. that achieves conception by means other than sexual intercourse is wrong because it takes procreation out of the context of the conjugal act with its unitive significance. Such a prohibition is not, according to the *Instruction*, obsequious subservience to Mother Nature; it is simply to call attention to the embodied significance of human sexual intercourse.

I mean to applaud the *Instruction*'s attention to the embodied character of human sexuality, but I do not think it gets this inference quite right. It should be noted, however, that it is not only Roman Catholics who have been concerned about sharply distinguishing the sexual act as a gesture of covenant fellowship in marriage from the sexual act as the generation of human life, or about separating "lovemaking" from "baby-making." Paul Ramsey[74] and Leon Kass,[75] for example, have claimed that moving generation into the laboratory is dangerous precisely because it suppresses the biological, sexual, bodily meaning of marital love. The child conceived in the laboratory may be the result of a loving decision and welcomed into a family to be sustained and nurtured, and so they grant that it is quite proper to say that such a child is a product of marital love. But the meaning of "marital love" in this context, they insist, has subtly shifted. It no longer has both natural and spiritual components; it no longer has its bodily connotation and, therefore, its full human connotations. It is the obverse of the way our culture trivializes sex. By suppressing the personal and spiritual dimensions of sexual intercourse our culture reduces sex to a technology of pleasure. But this suppression of the physical and biological dimensions of marital love is, according to Ramsey and Kass, no less dangerous. I applaud their attention to the embodied character of human sexuality, too, but I do not think they get the inference quite right either.[76]

In lovemaking and in baby-making, we are children of nature and children of spirit. Neither may be reduced to mere physiology or elevated to pure spirit. The *Instruction*, Ramsey, and Kass are all right to insist that they belong together — but not because they are essentially or "naturally" joined to each other in every conjugal act. They belong together because they both belong to marriage!

Marriage, with its vows and demands of covenant fidelity — "till death do us part" and "for better or worse" — is the appropriate context for both lovemaking and baby-making. When lovemaking takes place in a context other than marital fidelity, it is diminished and distorted, reduced to a biological urge, a natural necessity, a technology of pleasure governed only by the requirement that it take place between consenting adults, or, at best, a romantic quest for intimacy without a commitment to continuity. But there remains in every act of coitus, and perhaps in the vulnerability of nakedness and any clumsy gesture toward lovemaking, a sign of God's intention for

Strange World of Medicine]. Among the implications drawn by the *Instruction* in its section "Respect for Human Embryos" are prohibitions against prenatal diagnosis with the deliberate intention of an abortion (point 2), against nontherapeutic experimentation on embryos (4), including embryos obtained by fertilization in vitro (5), and against the freezing of embryos (6). See pp. 472-75 of the *Instruction* in *On Moral Medicine*, second edition.

70. Point 1 under "Interventions upon Human Procreation," in *Instruction on Respect for Human Life*, p. 476.

71. Point 4 under "Interventions upon Human Procreation," in *Instruction on Respect for Human Life*, p. 477.

72. Point 4 under "Interventions upon Human Procreation," in *Instruction on Respect for Human Life*, p. 478.

73. Paul VI, *Humanae Vitae*, in *The Pope Speaks* 13 (1968): 330-46; reprinted in Lammers and Verhey, eds., *On Moral Medicine*, second ed., pp. 434-38.

74. Paul Ramsey, *Fabricated Man: The Ethics of Genetic Control* (New Haven: Yale University Press, 1970), pp. 38-39.

75. Leon Kass, "New Beginnings in Life," in *The New Genetics and the Future of Man*, ed. Michael P. Hamilton (Grand Rapids: Eerdmans, 1972), pp. 15-63.

76. In fact, neither Ramsey nor Kass prohibited artificial insemination when the husband's sperm was used.

sex, for there remains an implicit exchange of trust and commitment. To ask during the intimacies of making love, "But will you love me tomorrow?" is to impugn the *committal* of the act.[77]

Lovemaking belongs to marriage; and so does baby-making. When baby-making takes place in a context other than marital fidelity, it too is diminished and distorted, reduced to mere physiology or to contract, to a marketable reproductive capacity or to a technology of producing children without a commitment to care for them when they are not what we want. But there remains in every act of parenting, even in the "mere" donation of gametes, and perhaps also in the very vulnerability of children and in their curiosity about their genetic parents, a sign of God's intention for sex, for there remain implicit responsibilities and commitments. Imagine a child asking a sperm donor or an ovum donor or a surrogate, "But will you care for me?" Acts of parenting may not be reduced to mere physiology or to mere contract. Children have a place in the fidelity of marriage, and they extend that fidelity to faithfulness in a family. Children have a secure place when there is a commitment to continuity in a marriage, and they extend that continuity to another generation.

Neither lovemaking nor baby-making may be reduced to nature or set over-against nature as purely spiritual and "free." Lovemaking and baby-making are not necessarily joined to each other, but both must be joined to the covenant fidelity of marriage and family. Not every act of lovemaking is — or need be — apt for procreation. And when a couple's legitimate desire for "the fruit and the sign of [their] mutual self-giving" is frustrated, their mutual self-giving can be enacted by the trouble each takes for the other in the context of A.R.T. The inference to be drawn from the "special character" of human sexuality is not that *every act* must be both unitive and procreative. The inference is rather that unitive acts and procreative acts — including procreative acts utilizing A.R.T. — belong within the context of the commitments of marriage.

Parenting: Begetting and the Vocation to Nurture

The new versions of procreation require attention not only to the questions about our relationship to nature and technology but also to the questions about our relationship to our own children. They require consideration not only of embodied sexuality and the relation of the unitive and procreative significance of sexuality but also of parenting and the relation of acts of begetting to the vocation to nurture. May parenting as an act of begetting be distinguished from parenting as a vocation to nurture? May the biological relation be separated from the social relation?

The *Instruction* prohibits "a rupture between genetic parenthood, gestational parenthood and responsibility for upbringing."[78] *"The fidelity of the spouses in the unity of marriage involves reciprocal respect of their right to become a father and a mother only through each other."*[79] Such conclusions, however, overreach the legitimate concern of the *Instruction* to cast suspicion on adoption. In adoption, too, after all, the relation of genetic parenthood and the vocation to nurture is sundered. In adoption the couple become a father and a mother not *"through"* each other but *with* each other. The language of the *Instruction* would seem to condemn the commendable work of Catholic adoption agencies. That is not, of course, what the *Instruction* intends. Catholics — and all Christians — quite properly celebrate the hospitality that adoptive parents show to children not biologically related to them. Indeed, the relationship of human beings to the heavenly Father is celebrated as an adoptive relationship.

What is celebrated, of course, is not the sundering of genetic and social relationships but the gracious character of the covenant relationship of adoption, the fact that adoptive parents perform something of the story of God's love. Adoptive parents love their adopted children, whom they were under no prior obligation to love, as though those children were theirs by birth. Biological parents, on the other hand, are — simply by virtue of being biological parents — under an obligation to love and nurture their children as their children. Sometimes that obligation can be impossible or very difficult to fulfill, as it is when parents die or when a parent is herself or himself still a child. Sometimes it may even be that the obligation to love and nurture the child is best fulfilled by giving the child up for adoption. But such situations are tragic cases, neither normal nor normative. Acts of begetting are normally and normatively not merely biological and physical; they are essentially parental, entailing obligations for nurturing the child.

Moreover, the very desire of many couples to have a child biologically "their own" suggests that parenting is not altogether abiological. Indeed, in vitro fertilization and artificial insemination were first defended in terms of a crucial relationship between biology and parenting. The phenomenon of bonding during pregnancy and at birth also suggests the embodied character of the relationship of parent and child. Bonding is not just an abstract moral and spiritual commitment; it is borne and nurtured by carrying and caressing, by the surprise and delight of "quickening," and by the patient endurance of sickness and pain for the sake of another. The point is not that bonding is simply physical or that a physical relationship (e.g., a newborn lying across the mother's warm abdomen) works automatically and magically to achieve a spiritual relationship. The point is rather that

77. See Stanley Hauerwas and Allen Verhey, "From Conduct to Character — A Guide to Sexual Adventure," *The Reformed Journal* (November 1986): 12-16.

78. Point 2 under "Interventions upon Human Procreation," in *Instruction on Respect for Human Life*, p. 477.

79. Point 1 under "Interventions upon Human Procreation," in *Instruction on Respect for Human Life*, p. 476.

the relationship is not purely spiritual and that the acts of begetting may not be treated (and dismissed) as merely physical.

The relationship of parent and child can begin adoptively, of course, in the voluntary consent of an adult or a couple to nurture and care for a child not biologically their own; such consent to care for a child, to be parent to a child, cannot be demanded or expected. Ordinarily, however, the relationship of parent and child begins biologically in the "physical" relationship of parents to children. Such a relationship is not simply created by the voluntary consent of independent adults to care for the child born to them; the relationship antedates the consent. When parents assent to care for a child born to them, they do what may be demanded and expected of them: they simply promise fidelity to an identity and a relationship already and "naturally" established.[80]

Again, therefore, we may be instructed by the *Instruction,* this time by its concern about the sundering of parenting as a genetic relationship from parenting as a vocation to nurture. To be sure, the language of the *Instruction* overreaches. Adoptive relationships should not be prohibited; indeed, they should be encouraged, also toward the "spare" embryos that are frozen in the process of the infertility programs. The problem is not the adoptive relationship of parents to children, even in in vitro fertilization and artificial insemination. The problem is, rather, that donors, even when they are not "vendors," even when they are not compensated for their donation of sperm or ova or gestation, engage in acts of begetting without any intention to care for the children who might result. If we would continue to insist that biological parents have a responsibility to care for their children, then this is the sundering of the connection between genetic parenthood and the vocation to nurture that we should prohibit. There is also a problem, of course, on the side of the adoptive parents if they encourage that rupture, and especially if, for the sake of some genetic relationship with their child, they encourage the donor to treat a biological relationship as trivial. We should remain morally suspicious of any act of begetting that is void of an intention to care for one's child, including acts like donating ova or sperm or lending a womb. And we should prohibit those practices, including those practices of A.R.T., that would encourage such actions and deny that a biological relationship with a child carries an obligation to care for that child.

The Child As Gift

We may be instructed by the *Instruction* on another point, that "a child is a gift."[81] Again, we may question the inference, that "for this reason, the child has the right . . . to be the fruit of the specific act of the conjugal love of his parents."[82] But it does well to remind us that a child is not an object to which one can have a right or over which one may exercise property rights. The question of the relationship of parents and children is itself at stake in the new versions of procreation. Human beings are seizing control of procreation, gaining power to intervene purposefully in the begetting of children, precisely when society is more confused about parenting than ever, and the new powers only add to our confusion.

Consider, for example, the possibilities of preimplantation diagnosis given with in vitro fertilization. Even apart from A.R.T., the possibilities of genetic diagnosis raised the question of the relation of parents and children. Many years ago now John Fletcher interviewed a number of parents who were undergoing amniocentesis and contemplating abortion. He found, he said, that even a responsible decision to undergo amniocentesis and to contemplate abortion "permanently altered" the relation of the parents with their children, even though it "does not lessen the affection they bear for their children."[83] It's a stunning point, but quite obvious in a way. Imagine trying to explain to a young child that Mommy is not going to have a baby after all because a test showed the baby was sick or not normal or defective. Even if the mother doesn't say, "So the doctor killed it," even if she just says, "So the doctor took it away," one can imagine the child's insecure questions: "What if I get sick? Do I measure up?" The relationship of uncalculating nurturance and basic trust has been threatened. And if amniocentesis can subtly threaten the relation of parent and child, how much more can the relation be threatened by pre-implantation diagnosis as a part of A.R.T.? The point is not that all reproductive interventions are immoral (or even that all abortions following amniocentesis are).[84] The point is rather that without greater communal wisdom about parenting, our culture may not be able to limit or guide such powers properly. And in the midst of public enthusiasm about reproductive technologies and genetics one may worry that our culture will not be able to learn — or relearn — that wisdom. The technology now commended as a way of becoming parents, a way that not too long ago did not exist, may well shape our way of being parents. A.R.T. may tempt us to view our children as human achievements rather than as a gift of God, and as the basis of hope rather than as a gesture of hope in God.

If the family is a microcosm of society, then the new versions of procreation confront us also with the question of the sort of society we want to be and to become. Our dispositions toward each other will affect and be affected by the new reproductive powers. If genetic

80. This is recognized legally, of course, in the obligations of paternity and prohibitions of abandonment.

81. Point 8 under "Interventions upon Human Procreation," in *Instruction on Respect for Human Life,* p. 480.

82. Point 8 under "Interventions upon Human Procreation," in *Instruction on Respect for Human Life,* p. 480.

83. Fletcher, "The Brink: The Parent-Child Bond in the Genetic Revolution," *Theological Studies* 33 (1972): 457-85.

84. Indeed, as I said in Chapter Six, pp. 246-49 [of *Reading the Bible in the Strange World of Medicine*], I do not think they are.

diagnosis joined to A.R.T. can affect the parent-child relationship, the same power can subtly affect our relation-ships with all weak and handicapped people, with retarded or unlovely people, with outcast and unacceptable people, and perhaps with new categories of people — unwanted, unchosen, and "carrier" people. God knows we find it comfortable and convenient to ignore and avoid them now. Our new reproductive powers promise (or threaten) not only to help us to ignore them but also to help us to eliminate them. And the reservoirs of affection — whether in parenting or in politics — that refuse to ignore them and insist on nurture for them are subtly undercut.[85] As reproductive technologies tempt us to think of our own children as products and to pin our hopes on them, society may encourage us to think about our children in terms of "quality control." The technologies introduced to increase the options of parents may easily lead to social expectations that parents exercise this "option" for genetic diagnosis when a mother is at risk of having a child with, say, Down's syndrome. Perhaps it is unnecessarily melodramatic to envision a society that refuses to share the burden of care for "reproductive products" who do not meet standards, but our dispositions toward children in our present society hardly make it implausible.[86] And if society refuses to care for the genetically retarded or diseased, then it will be unfair to ask parents to heroically bear the burden alone. The issue is not just what sort of parent we would like to be but also what kind of society we want to be and to become: a society that cares for and nurtures children, including its so-called "defective children," or a society that "produces" children and cannot tolerate the "defective" or allow them to exist.[87]

In this context we may and should be grateful for the reminder provided by the *Instruction* that "a child is a gift," not an "object of ownership."[88] The child is not chattel,[89] not a commodity. That, of course, is where we began, with the rejection of commodification. To be sure, few parents think any longer that children are parental property, to be disposed of as parents wish. Today the confusion stems — especially among the compassionate — from the view that parents have the awesome responsibility of making perfect children (through our reproducing) and of making children perfect (through our parenting), of assuring them a happy and successful life, or at least the capacity to attain and to conform to the American ideal of "the good life." But this account of parenting as the awesome responsibility to make perfect children and to make children perfect also turns our children into products, into human and technological achievements. It turns them into "objects" no less certainly than notions of property do. Such an account may encourage — and finally require — the discarding of embryos in vitro who do not match our specifications, the abortion of the unborn who do not meet our standards, the neglect of newborns with diminished capacities to achieve our ideal of "the good life," and the pursuit of technical possibilities of genetically improving our children. Such a view of parenting and of children may finally reduce our options to a perfect child or a dead child.

But children are begotten, not made.[90] They are gifts, not achievements. To the old assumption that children are the property of parents, to be disposed of as they choose, the Christian church has always said no, for our children are first of all God's, not ours. Children have a heavenly Father who would nurture them and who entrusts them to us as gifts. Today the Christian church must tell that story to contradict the idea that parenting is an awesome responsibility to make perfect children and to make children perfect.

The language of "gift" is important but tricky. It is not used in Christian discourse to confer ownership, as though children were a birthday present we could exchange or return for cash. It is used to confer stewardship: we receive children in trust from God, and with the gift always comes the claim of God. So we receive children with delight and sobriety, delighting in the loving hand of God which gives them, soberly responsible before the claims of God, who entrusts them to us.

Of course, Christians call many things "gifts of God": food, friends, recreation, life, work — indeed, all the good things of life. It would seem we so stretch the language of "gift" that we make it trivial, that we become powerless to speak of children as "gifts." But when we call anything "gift of God," we call ourselves to relate to it as it is related to God. To call so many things gifts does not diminish the power of the language; it acknowledges that we are indebted in many things and made stewards in many things, that we are to relate to many things — indeed, all things — as they are related to God. So the language of "gift" nurtures the disposition to relate to children as children related to God.

85. See Hans Reinders, *The Future of the Disabled in Liberal Society: An Ethical Analysis* (Notre Dame, Ind.: University of Notre Dame Press, 2000).

86. Hauerwas, *A Community of Character,* pp. 187-94.

87. The issue bears on questions of funding quite immediately. We should not allocate public funds for reproductive technologies — say, for in vitro clinics and in vitro research — before we have provided a minimal standard of prenatal and postnatal care for the poor and decent support services for families with disabled children. The children of the poor are gifts of God as well, even if the world regards them as no great human accomplishments, yet the infant mortality rates among the poor are scandalous for a society with the resources to develop in vitro fertilization clinics. Children with disabilities are gifts of God as well, even if they bring more pain and suffering with them than the children their parents wanted. For society the most precious gift of all may be the lesson to care for those who are not as we wish them to be.

88. Point 8 under "Interventions upon Human Procreation," in *Instruction on Respect for Human Life,* p. 480.

89. See the commentary on the *Instruction* by James Tunstead Burtchaell, "The Child As Chattel," in *The Giving and Taking of Life* (Notre Dame, Ind.: University of Notre Dame Press, 1989), pp. 119-52.

90. O'Donovan, *Begotten or Made?* (Oxford: Clarendon, 1984).

And no Christian may forget that Jesus, in whom God's good future already made its power known, took little children in his arms and blessed them (Mark 10:13-16). There must have been babies there, and more than one with a dirty diaper, yet Jesus took them in his arms. There must have been toddlers, curious and energetic, crying occasionally and interrupting often. "Women are meant to deal with them," the disciples must have thought, but Jesus blessed them. And there must have been boys and girls, taking an infrequent break from playing tag and catch, or standing on the sidelines because a limp or a disease or something else made them unwelcome in the game, and Jesus laid his hands on them. Other shocking behavior of this Galilean had hardly prepared people for this. Sure, he made the last first — but kids? Sure, he exalted the humble — but kids? Sure, those who didn't count for very much in other stories counted with him — but dirty-diapered, sweaty, silly, obnoxious kids? Yes, and he made it clear that to be his disciple, to welcome the kingdom, means to welcome, to serve, and to help little children.

No Christian may forget that when the Spirit works in our hearts, we cry "Abba! Father!" (Rom. 8:15; Gal. 4:6). And no Christian should forget (although some have) that God is like a mother, too: we are promised that as a mother comforts her child, so God will comfort us (Isa. 66:13). The images of God as mother can protect us from abusing the image of God the Father. We abuse that image when we think it means that God is literally male. In whatever ways God is like a father, God is not male. God transcends the human category of sex — and the image of God as mother can remind us of that. And we abuse the image of God the Father when we interpret it according to flawed and misleading models of fatherhood. From Roman to Puritan times a father was an authoritarian, totalitarian head of a family. Since industrialization, a father has been mostly absent, working outside the home to earn a living for the family. The modern father is alternately indulgent, the one to ask when mother says no, and demanding, the one whose affection is contingent on success. But none of these images of father is what Jesus had in mind when he called God "Abba" and taught his disciples to do the same. Abba might best be translated "Papa" or "Dada." It's the first word for father that a Hebrew child would learn to say. This image of father is the image of one who cares, one who carries, one who loves, one who can be trusted to provide uncalculating nurturance. It is, speaking culturally, a very motherly father whom Jesus taught us to trust and to love.

The language of "gift" calls upon us to relate to our children as little ones related to God, to the God invoked as "Abba" and known in Jesus, who blessed little children. It is no accident, then, that the language of "gift" involves acceptance of our children as given. We do not regard them as products, as achievements, and we may not beget them as though they were. Children are gifts, not products — they are not of our choosing, not under our control, not necessarily the children we want or expect or would choose if we could. Children are gifts, not products — and therefore they always have a measure of independence from us and from our rational choices. To regard children as gifts may be necessary if children are to be regarded as ends in themselves and not merely as instruments for achieving parental ends.

It is not because they always bring happiness that children are to be regarded as gifts. Sometimes children bring pain and suffering, but they are nevertheless always gifts from the loving hand of God. Indeed, even as parents endure the pain and suffering of having and caring for children as given, children are the most precious gift of all, for they teach us to love those who are not (and refuse to be) just as we wish. The language of being "entrusted" with children, then, points not toward the impossible responsibility of making perfect children and making children perfect but toward the duty and the surprising joy of nurturing those who are given. Parents are entrusted with children as gifts from the loving hand of the Father. And the Father's uncalculating nurturance is still the place to learn parenting, to learn to love the imperfect, the snotty-nosed, and the just plain snotty. Christians call God "Abba" and learn again and again in addressing God the sort of uncalculating nurturance and basic trust that should mark the relation of parents and children.

The tasks of nurturing children do not turn them into products, but they do involve support for the child as given. A parent covenanted to a child as given need not — and, indeed, may not — be altogether passive and "accepting." A parent may and should nurture the child so that the child as given can not only be but also flourish. And a parent may and should enlist the help of others to enable the child as given to be and to flourish within the limits of the world's finitude and the child's condition. A parent entrusted with the gift of a child must foster the excellence and well-being of the child as given, enlarging the capacities of the child as given and helping the child to fulfill the promise the child has as given.

But the "as given" prevents this parental activity from becoming demonic, from turning the child into a product and making acceptance and affection contingent upon the success of the interventions. Being entrusted with a child as a gift will require nurturing, but not nurturing undertaken as though all value rests on the success of making the child as given into something more or better, "as though the imperfect materials themselves had to be surpassed for anything good to come of the life."[91]

Another confusion about parenting today, mentioned earlier, is captured by the assertion that "Our children are our hope for the future." Christians can only regard such a view of children as blasphemous and foolish. It is blasphemous because Jesus is our hope for the future. It is foolish because our children are destined for suffering and death like the rest of us. The view that our children

91. William F. May, *The Patient's Ordeal*, p. 51.

are our hope for the future can only make more urgent the awesome responsibility to make perfect children and to make children perfect, for so much is at stake. And to deny that view takes a good deal of pressure off parents. Children are not the hope for the future — Jesus is. And because that is so, Christians are free to delight in children as gifts from God's gracious and nurturing hand. This world is not yet God's unchallenged realm, and we may not beget or rear our children in this world as though they can be spared suffering and death. There is wisdom about parenting in the Passover ritual that requires the children to eat bitter herbs with the rest of the family, reminding them of the suffering of the community of which they are a part. But God does reign — even over a world marked and marred by suffering — and God will reign. And Christians sign and seal their confidence in God's future by having and rearing and loving children. Children are not the basis for our hope; they are a gesture of our hope in God.

The inference to be drawn from celebrating a child as a gift of God is not a prohibition of all A.R.T. that achieves conception without "the specific act of the conjugal love of his parents." The inference is rather a limit on the conditions tested for in pre-implantation diagnosis to those conditions inconsistent with life or attached to a confident prognosis of a life subjectively indistinguishable from torture.[92] The inference is that we must protect and preserve the relationship of uncalculating nurture and basic trust between parents and children; that wisdom is learned in a story of God's parental care that evokes human faith.

Ministry to the Childless

Finally, we may be instructed by the *Instruction* when it acknowledges the suffering caused by infertility.[93] One may wish that the acknowledgment were stronger. One may wish that it were set earlier in the document. One may wish that the suffering were traced theologically to the power of the curse. One may wish that the acknowledgment were accompanied by a more generous attitude to A.R.T. But it is there, and we should be instructed by it!

The *Instruction* even encourages further research "in the fight against infertility" with the aim both of preventing the causes of sterility and of being able to remedy them in ways respectful of the child to be born and of the "special character" of human procreation.[94] Our response to the *Instruction* has permitted more forms of A.R.T. than the *Instruction* did; it has drawn the lines in a different place. But we should be instructed by its attention to ministry to the childless.

The first inference here is this: as long as Christians think of children as gifts of God and of having children as a gesture of our trust in God's future, they will welcome the ministry of physicians to infertile couples who long for a biological child as "the fruit and sign of [their] mutual self-giving." They will welcome the capacity to repair fallopian tubes, for example, or to regulate hormones, and — although here we disagree with the *Instruction,* of course — they will welcome artificial insemination or in vitro fertilization or ICSI, using the gametes of a married couple, to circumvent certain problems of infertility.

A second inference is this: as long as Christians delight in the adoptive love of God, they will welcome the ministry of adoption agencies to children in tragic circumstances and to the childless. They should welcome the extension of that ministry to "spare" embryos who might otherwise be left to die in the freezer. They will celebrate and delight in the inclusion of an adopted child in a family and in the community.

Ministry to the childless, however, must attend to other issues besides putting a stop to their suffering by providing a child, whether by A.R.T. or adoption. Again, compassion starts with attention to the suffering and may not be reduced to the effort to put a stop to it. The Christian community should be sensitive to the profound and sometimes desperate longing of some childless couples for a baby of their own. And ministry to them might start by attending to the ways in the common life of the church that people remind them of their childlessness and even subtly and unfairly rebuke them for it. Gatherings in which the topic of children dominates the conversation can be painful to the childless. Well-intentioned advice that it is time to begin a family or that a couple is "trying too hard" may tear at their sexuality and self-esteem. Ministry to the childless demands sensitivity and care, a readiness to listen, to appreciate the pain and suffering, to share the grief over the child of promise they lost by never having.

Ministry to the childless will not belittle their sense that their childlessness is a lack — children are, after all, a gift of God.

Nevertheless, the Christian community may and must say clearly, both to those with children and to those who are childless, that children are not the basis for hope, that children are not the hope of the world and not the hope of a person's or a couple's flourishing. The child on whom the world's hope — and theirs — depends has been born. The child has been born "unto us" (Luke 2:11) — whether we have children of our own or not. And since then, *post Christum natum,* childbearing is no longer the necessity and the duty it was in the old covenant.[95] In the church it cannot be a fault to be childless! Ministry to the childless will acknowledge and engage the gifts, including the gifts of nurturance and care, which the childless may have in abundance. Their child-

92. See Chapter Six, pp. 246-49 [of *Reading the Bible in the Strange World of Medicine*], on the genetic indications for abortion.

93. Point 8 under "Interventions upon Human Procreation," in *Instruction on Respect for Human Life,* pp. 480-81.

94. Point 8 under "Interventions upon Human Procreation," in *Instruction on Respect for Human Life,* p. 480.

95. Karl Barth, *Church Dogmatics,* III/4, p. 266.

lessness may be received as an opportunity to be hospitable to the children of others or as the opportunity to signal the good future of God in some other way. Such a suggestion may sound like stones for bread (Matt. 7:9), but *post Christum natum* the child born "unto us" calls us out of our grief and into God's good future. The Christian community, including those members with children, must work against aspects of a common life that force the childless to the margins, including the extravagant and idolatrous expectations that children bring human flourishing and make our lives and our marriages meaningful. No small part of this effort must be resistance to the residual patriarchalism of our culture. As Lisa Cahill notes,

> Women are presented from birth with images of mothering as crucial to their identity, with pregnancy and childbearing as the culmination both of their sexuality and of their relationships of intimacy, and of fertility as a sign of youthfulness, desirability, and worth. Men are taught to see virility and sexual potency as confirmed in the ability to "father" a child (i.e., to inseminate a woman), and both men and women are led to see the sexual and reproductive services of women as men's natural right and due.[96]

No wonder the childless suffer. No wonder they are sometimes desperate. Their childlessness threatens the identities formed in the community. And no wonder the rhetoric of "choice" does not adequately address or protect the childless. Attention to the suffering of the childless need not necessarily provide an A.R.T.ful remedy for their childlessness; it might help to reconstruct an identity and to begin the next chapter of their lives. In Christian community both those with children and those without may and must set their hope on God, not on children. Then the whole Christian community may avoid both excessive expectations of the children they have or still dream of and excessive anxiety about their flourishing if the children they have do not "measure up" or if the child of their dreams never comes.

Conclusions and Cautions

Of the new versions of the Bible some are excellent and some are appalling. And of the new versions of procreation some are excellent and some are appalling. The "reproductive revolution" has made some enduring moral questions urgent. The irony is that at the very time the issues are so urgent, we as a society are ill prepared to deal with them. We have magnificent tools, but we don't know what we're building or whether what we're building will be habitable. We're making great time, but we don't know where we're going.

If we lack the ultimate wisdom to be able to settle these enduring moral issues, then the best penultimate wisdom is caution. Nothing I have said requires installing a permanent red light against A.R.T. Almost everything I have said would argue against installing a green light. I guess I am an amber man. The signal set before A.R.T. is amber. Caution is called for. It is a caution born of humility rather than fear, but it is caution nevertheless.

Along the way in this chapter I have suggested something of the shape of that caution, the shadows cast by that amber light. I have suggested that the burden of proof be shifted, that it be borne not only by those who would restrict "procreative liberty" and restrain "progress" but also and equally by those who, in the name of "procreative liberty," establish a manipulative and calculating relationship with children and by those who presume that all technological innovation entails human well-being.

I have urged respect for persons not only as "choicemakers" but also as embodied and communal selves. I have urged a reticence to separate either lovemaking or baby-making from marriage and a reticence to sunder deliberately the "natural" (or bodily or genetic) relationship of parents and children from the social obligations and roles of parents and children.

I have insisted that children be regarded as gifts of God, not as human achievements, and that they not be regarded as our hope for the future. To regard children as gifts will affect our motivation for having children and may free us from inordinate anxiety about *whether* we have children and *what* children we have. Such conviction may sustain in our culture an otherwise unsustainable courage to be cautious, to say no to technology and its promises, and an otherwise unsustainable courage to assent to a covenant with the children we are given, to promise the sort of uncalculating nurturance that can evoke and confirm the trust of children.

I have urged hospitality to all children, including the children of the poor and children with disabilities. And I would urge social support for the children of the poor and for children with disabilities before public funding is allocated to research and development or clinical use of A.R.T.

I have flashed a few red lights along the way. We should signal a stop to the commodification and commercialization that marks and mars such sites as ronsangels.com and all vendoring of sperm, ova, and commercial contracts for surrogacy. We should also set a red light before A.R.T. outside of the context of a covenant of marriage and a red light before the use of donor sperm, donor ova, and surrogacy, where such procreative acts are void of an intention to care for the child who might result. I would also prohibit the creation of human embryos with the potential for life strictly for experimental purposes. What we learn from them may be important and useful, but it is wrong to begin human life without the intention to care for the child, with the intention of discarding it once we have used it.

The most important clue to discernment in the "reproductive revolution" is to attend to our embodiment

96. Cahill, *Sex, Gender, and Christian Ethics*, pp. 245-46.

and community. If we were more attentive to embodiment and community, we would be more suspicious of the pretense that freedom provides a sufficient account of what is morally at stake in begetting and more suspicious of regarding freedom as the capacity of a neutral agent to will what she will. If we were more attentive to embodiment, we would hesitate before reducing our bodies and our begetting to objects to be mastered by our technology. If our rhetoric were more appreciative of the embodied significance of procreation, we would be more likely to be suspicious of practices that deliberately separate procreation into something physiological and something contractual (or that separate procreation from the embodied "expression of a couple's love or unity"). If we were more attentive to community, we would be more likely to be suspicious of reproductive acts void of an intention to care for the children who might result.

All these cautionary words must finally be joined with an exhortation to preserve and to cherish some ancient wisdom. The wisdom about the future is hopeful realism. The wisdom about nature is that we are creaturely stewards. The wisdom about parenting is nurturance and trust. The wisdom about one another is the care and respect we owe each other, especially the weak, "the little ones." Such wisdom and the corollary dispositions it suggests will not tell us exactly what to do and what to leave undone with our new powers, but it will provide some guidance for and some limits to our powers, including the awesome new powers of reproductive technology, even when we cannot solve a quandary with a rule. A reproductive revolution — if such it is — will require wise people, not just clever ones.

CHAPTER NINETEEN

Abortion

Almost forty years after the January 22, 1973, U.S. Supreme Court decision *Roe v. Wade,* abortion remains one of the most divisive social issues on the U.S. public and political landscape, fomenting "bitter social discourse"[1] and increasingly militant rhetoric.

The structure of the public debate remains much the same as in 1973. For pro-life advocates, the central issue is that of the intentional taking of human life. Claims for the inviolability of prenatal life cite the genetic uniqueness and internal developmental directedness that characterize the fertilized human ovum from the moment of conception. Biological arguments are joined to longstanding Judeo-Christian convictions regarding the special status of human persons — as created in the image of God, as redeemed by the Word made flesh — as well as convictions regarding the special protections to be afforded to the least among us.

Both sides of the argument emphasize the issue of rights. In addition to the above arguments, pro-life positions often champion the rights of the fetus. Pro-choice advocates champion the rights of pregnant women to control their own bodies, free from government regulation or other forms of social control. Under the Enlightenment political philosophy that frames the U.S. Constitution and culture, only persons can be bearers of social and political rights. Prenatal life, though often admitted to be genetically human, is not considered by some to meet the criteria to be counted as full human persons.

Those who have been reading *On Moral Medicine* sequentially will find these positions familiar, for of course the arguments surrounding the question of abortion have been brought to bear on related issues — particularly those of embryonic research (stem cell and otherwise) as well as the issue of personhood. We recommend revisiting or taking up those chapters in conjunction with the following essays.

A few data points help to set the context for the debate. While documented abortion rates began to rise in the U.S. prior to *Roe v. Wade,* the number and rates of abortion nearly doubled in the seven years following the Supreme Court decision, peaking in 1980 at over 1.5 million abortions, with a rate of over twenty-nine abortions per one thousand women of childbearing age (15 to 44).[2] These figures have declined since 1980, falling to 1.2 million abortions in 2005, for a rate of nineteen per one thousand women of childbearing age. The Guttmacher Institute reported in July 2008 that nearly half the pregnancies in the U.S. are unintended, that 40 percent of these are terminated via abortion, and half of the abortions each year are obtained by girls and women under the age of 25.[3] It is estimated that in the U.S. only 1 percent of abortions occur annually owing to rape and only 6 percent owing to health reasons in the mother or the fetus.[4]

What has accounted for these trends? Certainly, the issue of abortion cannot be separated from social and economic questions. Still in the twenty-first century, women — even in the U.S. — live in a context of patriarchy and oppression, factors that are more apparent and powerfully operative for women in many developing countries yet certainly not absent from the U.S context. The U.S. is notable among developed countries for its lack of socioeconomic support for women and children, factors that are often cited in women's decisions to terminate their pregnancies.

Yet by any measure, 1.2 million abortions per year is an extraordinary number, as is the reported figure for annual abortions on a global basis, 42 million in 2005.[5] Equally extraordinary is the fact that almost half the pregnancies in

1. Beverly Wildung Harrison, "A Feminist-Liberation View of Abortion," in *On Moral Medicine,* 2nd ed., ed. Stephen E. Lammers and Allen Verhey (Grand Rapids: Eerdmans, 1998), p. 617.

2. "United States Abortion Rates 1960-2005," Robert Wood Johnson Foundation, available at: http://www.johnstonsarchive.net/policy/abortion/graphusabrate.html (accessed June 30, 2009).

3. "Facts on Induced Abortion," The Guttmacher Institute, available at: http://www.guttmacher.org/pubs/fb_induced_abortion.html (accessed June 30, 2009).

4. "Abortion Facts," The Center for Bio-Ethical Reform, available at: http://www.abortionno.org/Resources/fastfacts.html (accessed June 30, 2009).

5. "Abortion Facts," The Center for Bio-Ethical Reform, available at: http://www.abortionno.org/Resources/fastfacts.html (accessed June 30, 2009).

the U.S. are described as unintended. And while the pro-life side of the debate is characterized largely by Christian language and partisans, studies report that 43 percent of women obtaining abortions identify themselves as Protestant, and 27 percent as Catholic.[6] Apart from the question of the law, these facts should trouble the Christian conscience. Abortion is far from "legal, safe, and rare," as many of the more moderate pro-choice advocates would advise, even among those whose convictions generally counsel against the taking of innocent human life (questions of personhood aside).

Thus, it is particularly important for Christians to reflect on the question of abortion. Feminist theologian Beverly Wildung Harrison provides the classic argument for the pro-choice position in her essay "Theology and the Morality of Procreative Choice" (selection 119). For Harrison, social control of reproduction is control of power, a unique life-shaping power possessed by women, a power men seek to control, constrain, or usurp, often using theologically based arguments. Harrison takes equally to task both Protestant, Scripture-based arguments and Catholic natural law arguments against abortion (and, for the Catholics, against contraception). Central to Harrison's argument, as with other essays in this chapter, are questions of history, theory, and social context. How do we read history, especially in relation to the questions of abortion and human life? How do we understand the moral theory that shapes how we reason through a question? Which principles do we hold as fundamental and why? And finally, how do we understand the role of social context and social policy in moral deliberation? One does not have to ascribe to "situation ethics" to acknowledge that context is critical to moral discernment. But most fundamentally, how does one assess all of these questions particularly from the perspective of women? How do they construct women's identity and moral agency? How do particular principles, decisions, policies, and practices impact women and the flourishing of women?

Harrison believes that a feminist must be pro-choice. Sidney Callahan, nationally renowned author, professor, and licensed clinical psychologist, disagrees. Her piece "Abortion and the Sexual Agenda: A Case for Pro-Life Feminism" (selection 123) offers a direct response to Harrison and brings to the conversation the voice of the many women, in the U.S. and abroad, who would count themselves as both ardently feminist and ardently pro-life. Callahan clearly outlines the four central claims of the pro-choice argument — the moral right to control one's own body; the moral necessity of autonomy and choice; the contingent value of fetal life; and the goal of full social equality for women — and then responds to each of these claims from a feminist perspective.

Callahan is a Catholic, and her Catholic faith informs her arguments. But differences on the question of abortion transcend differences in Protestant and Roman Catholic perspectives. Officially, many evangelical Protestant positions side with the official Roman Catholic teaching on "life" questions, while some Catholics disagree with official church teaching. One example of the contours of the internal debate within the Catholic tradition is provided by Daniel Maguire and James Burtchaell in their piece "The Catholic Legacy and Abortion: A Debate" (selection 120).

Callahan is not the only woman and feminist to take issue with the kinds of arguments Harrison advances. Andy (Andrea) Smith addresses the question of abortion from the perspective of a Cherokee intellectual, feminist, and anti-violence activist in her essay "Women of Color and Reproductive Choice: Combating the Population Paradigm" (selection 122). As the essays by Harrison and by Maguire and Burtchaell make clear, a central concern of many pro-choice advocates is the question of overpopulation and the need for population control to avert an impending eco-human cataclysm. Smith, while clearly located in the pro-choice camp, makes starkly clear how the platform of abortion-rights-for-all women has become an overriding preoccupation for many Western feminists in a way that dismisses the more fundamental concerns of most women worldwide, and in fact erases women of color. She takes particular issue with the ideology of population control and outlines the history of that particular issue as seen from the perspective of non-Western women. For many from "the underside of history" the issue of population control is deeply intertwined with colonial subjugation of native peoples, and contemporary movements prove to be deeply enmeshed in neocolonial politics and neoliberal economics, which have had a clearly destructive and well-documented impact on Third World peoples. Smith then turns to a surprising finding: many First World feminist theologians have bought into the population control ideology to the detriment of Third World women.

While Callahan and Smith take issue with Harrison's feminist arguments, Michael Gorman takes issue with Harrison's and with Maguire and Burtchaell's reading of Scripture and Christian history in his essay "Ahead to Our Past: Abortion and Christian Texts" (selection 121). Here Gorman comments on the Durham Declaration, a statement of the Taskforce of United Methodists on Abortion and Sexuality, responding to it from the perspective of a scholar of Scripture and the early church.[7] Like Callahan, he challenges the notion of embodiment operative in Harrison's argument. He seeks to highlight the radically alternative vision of embodiment contained within the New Testament, one that was as countercultural in the first century as it is in the twenty-first. Rather than simply proof-texting, he seeks to locate early Christian claims about abortion within the broader context of beliefs about children, the body, nonviolence/justice (or better, *shalom*), and power.

6. "Facts on Induced Abortion," The Guttmacher Institute, available at: http://www.guttmacher.org/pubs/fb_induced_abortion.html (accessed June 30, 2009).

7. The Durham Declaration is available at: http://lifewatch.org/durham.html (accessed June 30, 2009).

The sort of scripturally informed vision outlined by Gorman is fleshed out in a sermon preached by Terry Hamilton-Poore. This sermon opens Stanley Hauerwas's essay "Abortion, Theologically Understood" (selection 124). Rev. Hamilton-Poore's sermon demonstrates how scriptural reasoning on abortion is not tied to particular texts that mention abortion (upon which the Christian Scriptures are silent). Rather, she demonstrates how the richness of Scripture ought to inform our moral reasoning more broadly. For Hamilton-Poore, as for Gorman and Hauerwas, the more pressing question on abortion is not the question about *Roe v. Wade,* not the question about the law, but the question about Christian identity: the question about "what kind of people we are to be as the Church and as Christians." As mentioned earlier, some 70 percent of women having an abortion identify as either Protestant or Catholic. Hamilton-Poore and Hauerwas locate the main issue not in the failure of particular Christians to be moral but in the failure of the church to be the kind of place that makes abortion a less reasonable or less imperative option for its women members. Hauerwas takes up Harrison's claims about moral theory and, like Callahan, demonstrates how problematic such theory is for those with Christian commitments. He demonstrates how U.S. Christians are far more deeply informed by our culture than by the Christian tradition. He pushes us to examine, in particular, the language within which we are immersed, especially regarding sexuality, bodies, and children — for example, the construct of the "wanted" child. Our very language contains formative assumptions, assumptions deeply at odds with theological convictions, yet deeply operative insofar as they drive us to act without our even knowing it. If the church, Protestant and Catholic, is concerned about abortion, how might it begin to change itself so that it becomes a place where new lives — anticipated and planned or not — are welcomed and nurtured? This for Hauerwas and Hamilton-Poore is the more fundamental question for Christians.

Joseph Kotva agrees. Yet in his essay "The Question of Abortion: Christian Virtue and Government Legislation" (selection 125), Kotva addresses directly the question of how Christians — or at least Anabaptist Christians — should position themselves relative to ongoing public efforts to make all or most abortions illegal. Kotva joins Gorman, Hamilton-Poore, and Hauerwas in seeing the fundamental issue for Christians as one about the identity of the church. For Kotva, the primary Christian response to abortion should be for the church to focus on becoming "a worshipping community that welcomes children, empowers women and accepts that burdens and suffering often accompany the moral life." His analysis complements and extends that offered by the selections by Gorman, Callahan, and Hauerwas. But he takes it one step further and offers a multilayered argument about why Christians ought not to support legislative efforts to make all or even most abortions illegal.

The above essays will not resolve the ongoing debate, but we do hope that they will contribute to a more careful, nuanced, and theological framing of the question of abortion, both practically and methodologically. We also hope that they help Christians on both sides of the debate to understand that the frontline of the issue — for Christians — ought not first to be the courtroom but the congregation. For while "pro-choice" language and anthropology constitute the currency of the public sphere, we hope these essays demonstrate how tenuously such reasoning fits with the best of the Christian tradition. Likewise, only insofar as Christians begin actively to treat all human beings as sacred — by addressing practically the social and economic factors driving abortion, by countering patriarchy and the oppression of women, by practicing hospitality toward life — will their arguments carry moral credibility.

SUGGESTIONS FOR FURTHER READING

Bauerschmidt, Frederick. "Being Baptized: Bodies and Abortion." In *The Blackwell Companion to Christian Ethics* (New York: Blackwell Publishers, 2006), pp. 250-62.

Cahill, Lisa Sowle. "Abortion, Sex, and Gender: The Church's Public Voice." *America* (May 2, 1993): 6-11.

Gustafson, James. "A Protestant Ethical Approach." In *On Moral Medicine,* 2nd ed., ed. Stephen E. Lammers and Allen Verhey (Grand Rapids: Eerdmans, 1998), pp. 600-611.

John Paul II. *Evangelium Vitae* (The Gospel of Life). 1995.

Jung, Patricia Beattie. "Abortion and Organ Donation: A Christian Reflection on Bodily Life-Support." *Journal of Religious Ethics* 16, no. 2 (Fall 1988): 273-305.

Jung, Patricia Beattie, and Thomas A. Shannon. *Abortion and Catholicism: The American Debate* (New York: Crossroads, 1988).

Meilaender, Gilbert. *Bioethics: A Primer for Christians* (Grand Rapids: Eerdmans, 1996), chapter 3.

Meilaender, Gilbert. "The Fetus as Parasite and Mushroom." In *On Moral Medicine,* 2nd ed., ed. Stephen E. Lammers and Allen Verhey (Grand Rapids: Eerdmans, 1998), pp. 612-15.

Rudy, Kathy. *Beyond Pro-Life and Pro-Choice: Moral Diversity in the Abortion Debate* (Boston: Beacon Press, 1995).

Tickle, Phyllis. *Confessing Conscience: Churched Women on Abortion* (Nashville: Abingdon Press, 1990).

119 Theology and the Morality of Procreative Choice

Beverly Wildung Harrison

Much discussion of abortion betrays the heavy hand of misogyny, the hatred of women. We all have a responsibility to recognize this bias — sometimes subtle — when ancient negative attitudes toward women intrude into the abortion debate. It is morally incumbent on us to convert the Christian position to a teaching more respectful of women's concrete history and experience.

My professional peers who are my opponents on this question feel they own the Christian tradition in this matter and recognize no need to rethink their positions in the light of this claim. As a feminist, I cannot sit in silence when women's right to shape the use of our own procreative power is denied. Women's competence as moral decision makers is once again challenged by the state even before the moral basis of women's right to procreative choice has been fully elaborated and recognized. Those who deny women control of procreative power claim that they do so in defense of moral sensibility, in the name of the sanctity of human life. We have a long way to go before the sanctity of human life will include genuine regard and concern for every female already born, and no social policy discussion that obscures this fact deserves to be called moral. We hope the day will come when it will not be called "Christian" either, for the Christian ethos is the generating source of the current moral crusade to prevent women from gaining control over the most life-shaping power we possess.

Although I am a Protestant, my own "moral theology"[1] has more in common with a Catholic approach than with much neoorthodox ethics of my own tradition. I want to stress this at the outset because in what follows I am highly critical of the reigning Roman Catholic social teaching on procreation and abortion. I believe that on most other issues of social justice, the Catholic tradition is often more substantive, morally serious, and less imbued with the dominant economic ideology than the brand of Protestant theological ethics that claims biblical warrants for its moral norms. I am no biblicist; I believe that the human wisdom that informs our ethics derives not from using the Bible alone but from reflecting in a manner that earlier Catholic moral theologians referred to as consonant with "natural law."[2] Unfortunately, however, all major strands of natural law reflection have been every bit as awful as Protestant biblicism on any matter involving human sexuality, including discussion of women's nature and women's divine vocation in relation to procreative power. And it is precisely because I recognize Catholic natural law tradition as having produced the most sophisticated type of moral reflection among Christians that I believe it must be challenged where it intersects negatively with women's lives.

Given the depth of my dissatisfaction with Protestant moral tradition, I take no pleasure in singling out Roman Catholic moral theology and the activity of the Catholic hierarchy on the abortion issue. The problem nevertheless remains that there is really only one set of moral claims involved in the Christian antiabortion argument. Protestants who oppose pro-creative choice[3] either tend to follow official Catholic moral theology on these matters or ground their positions in biblicist anti-intellectualism, claiming that God's "word" requires no justification other than their attestation that divine utterance says what it says. Against such irrationalism, no rational objections have a chance. When, however, Protestant fundamentalists actually specify the reasons why they believe abortion is evil, they invariably revert to traditional natural law assumptions about women, sexuality, and procreation. Hence, direct objection must be registered to the traditional natural law framework if we are serious about transforming Christian moral teaching on abortion.

To do a methodologically adequate analysis of any moral problem in religious social ethics it is necessary to

1. I use the traditional Roman Catholic term intentionally because my ethical method has greater affinity with the Roman Catholic model.

From Beverly Wildung Harrison, *Making the Connections: Essays in Feminist Social Ethics* (Boston: Beacon Press, 1985). Revised from an earlier version with the collaboration of Shirley Cloyes.

2. The Christian natural law tradition developed because many Christians understood that the power of moral reason inhered in human beings qua human beings, not merely in the understanding that comes from being Christian. Those who follow natural law methods address moral issues from the consideration of what options appear rationally compelling, given present reflection, rather than from theological claims alone. My own moral theological method is congenial to certain of these natural law assumptions. Roman Catholic natural law teaching, however, has become internally incoherent by its insistence that in some matters of morality the teaching authority of the hierarchy must be taken as the proper definition of what is rational. This replacement of reasoned reflection by ecclesiastical authority seems to me to offend against what we must mean by moral reasoning on best understanding. I would argue that a moral theology cannot forfeit final judgment or even penultimate judgment on moral matters to anything except fully deliberated communal consensus. On the abortion issue, this of course would mean women would be consulted in a degree that reflects their numbers in the Catholic church. No a priori claims to authoritative moral reason are ever possible, and if those affected are not consulted, the teaching cannot claim rationality.

3. For a critique of these positions, see Paul D. Simmons, "A Theological Response to Fundamentalism on the Abortion Issue," in *Abortion: The Moral Issues*, ed. Edward Batchelor, Jr. (New York: Pilgrim Press, 1982), pp. 175-187.

(1) situate the problem in the context of various religious communities' theologies or "generative" stories, (2) do a critical historical review of the problem as it appears in our religious traditions and in the concrete lives of human agents (so that we do not confuse the past and the present), (3) scrutinize the problem from the standpoint of various moral theories, and (4) analyze existing social policy and potential alternatives to determine our "normative moral sense" or best judgment of what ought to be done in contemporary society. Although these methodological basepoints must be addressed in any socio-ethical analysis, their treatment is crucial when abortion is under discussion because unexamined theological presumptions and misrepresentations of Christian history figure heavily in the current public policy debate. Given the brevity of this essay, I will address the theological, Christian historical, and moral theoretical problematics first and analyze the social policy dimensions of the abortion issue only at the end, even though optimum ethical methodology would reverse this procedure.

Abortion in Theological Context

In the history of Christian theology, a central metaphor for understanding life, including human life, is as a gift of God. Creation itself has been interpreted primarily under this metaphor. It follows that in this creational context procreation itself took on special significance as the central image for the divine blessing of human life. The elevation of procreation as the central symbol of divine benevolence happened over time, however. It did not, for instance, typify the very early, primitive Christian community. The synoptic gospels provide ample evidence that procreation played no such metaphorical role in early Christianity.[4] In later Christian history, an emergent powerful antisexual bias within Christianity made asceticism the primary spiritual ideal, although this ideal usually stood in tension with procreative power as a second sacred expression of divine blessing. But by the time of the Protestant Reformation, there was clear reaffirmation of the early Israelite theme of procreative blessing, and procreation has since become all but synonymous among Christians with the theological theme of creation as divine gift. It is important to observe that Roman Catholic theology actually followed on and adapted to Protestant teaching on this point.[5] Only in the last century, with the recognition of the danger of dramatic population growth in a world of finite resources, has any question been raised about the appropriateness of this unqualified theological sacralization of procreation.

The elevation of procreation as the central image for divine blessing is intimately connected to the rise of patriarchy. In patriarchal societies it is the male's power that is enhanced by the gift of new life. Throughout history, women's power of procreation has stood in definite tension with this male social control. In fact, what we feminists call patriarchy — that is, patterned or institutionalized legitimations of male superiority — derives from the need of men, through male-dominated political institutions such as tribes, states, and religious systems, to control women's power to procreate the species. We must assume, then, that many of these efforts at social control of procreation, including some church teaching on contraception and abortion, were part of this institutional system. The perpetuation of patriarchal control itself depended on wresting the power of procreation from women and shaping women's lives accordingly.

In the past four centuries, the entire Christian story has had to undergo dramatic accommodation to new and emergent world conditions and to the scientific revolution. As the older theological metaphors for creation encountered the rising power of science, a new self-understanding including our human capacity to affect nature had to be incorporated into Christian theology or its central theological story would have become obscurantist. Human agency had to be introjected into a dialectical understanding of creation.

The range of human freedom to shape and enhance creation is now celebrated theologically, but only up to the point of changes in our understanding of what is natural for women. Here a barrier has been drawn that declares, No Radical Freedom! The only difference between mainstream Protestant and Roman Catholic theologians on these matters is at the point of contraception, which Protestants more readily accept. However, Protestants like Karl Barth and Helmut Thielicke exhibit a subtle shift of mood when they turn to discussing issues regarding women. They follow the typical Protestant pattern: They have accepted contraception or family planning as part of the new freedom, granted by God, but both draw back from the idea that abortion could be morally acceptable. In *The Ethics of Sex,* Thielicke offers a romantic, ecstatic celebration of family planning on one page and then elaborates a total denunciation of abortion as unthinkable on the next.[6] Most Christian theological

4. Most biblical scholars agree that either the early Christians expected an imminent end to history and therefore had only an "interim ethic," or that Jesus' teaching, in its radical support for "the outcasts" of his society, did not aim to justify existing social institutions. See, for example, Luke 4 and 12; Mark 7, 9, 13, and 14; Matthew 25. See also Elisabeth Schüssler Fiorenza, "You Are Not to Be Called Father," *Cross Currents* (Fall 1979), pp. 301-323. See also her *Bread Not Stone: The Challenge of Feminist Biblical Interpretation* (Boston: Beacon Press, 1985).

5. Few Roman Catholic theologians seem to appreciate how much the recent enthusiastic endorsement of traditional family values implicates Catholicism in Protestant Reformational spirituality. Rosemary Ruether is an exception; she has stressed this point in her writings.

6. Helmut Thielicke, *The Ethics of Sex* (New York: Harper and Row, 1964), pp. 199-247. Compare pp. 210 and 226ff. Barth's position on abortion is a bit more complicated than I can elaborate here, which is why one will find him quoted on both sides of the debate. Barth's method allows him to argue that any given radical

opinion draws the line between contraception and abortion, whereas the *official* Catholic teaching still anathematizes contraception.

The problem, then, is that Christian theology celebrates the power of human freedom to shape and determine the quality of human life except when the issue of procreative choice arises. Abortion is anathema, while widespread sterilization abuse goes unnoticed. The power of man to shape creation radically is never rejected. When one stops to consider the awesome power over nature that males take for granted and celebrate, including the power to alter the conditions of human life in myriad ways, the suspicion dawns that the near hysteria that prevails about the immorality of women's right to choose abortion derives its force from the ancient power of misogyny rather than from any passion for the sacredness of human life. An index of the continuing misogyny in Christian tradition is male theologians' refusal to recognize the full range of human power to shape creation in those matters that pertain to women's power to affect the quality of our lives.

In contrast, a feminist theological approach recognizes that nothing is more urgent, in light of the changing circumstances of human beings on planet Earth, than to recognize that the entire natural-historical context of human procreative power has shifted.[7] We desperately need a desacralization of our biological power to reproduce[8] and at the same time a real concern for human dignity and the social conditions for personhood and the values of human relationship.[9] And note that desacralization does not mean complete devaluation of the worth of procreation. It means we must shift away from the notion that the central metaphors for divine blessing are expressed at the biological level to the recognition that our social relations bear the image of what is most holy. An excellent expression of this point comes from Marie Augusta Neal, a Roman Catholic feminist and a distinguished sociologist of religion:

> As long as the central human need called for was continued motivation to propagate the race, it was essential that religious symbols idealize that process above all others. Given the vicissitudes of life in a hostile environment, women had to be encouraged to bear children and men to support them: childbearing was central to the struggle for existence. Today, however, the size of the base population, together with knowledge already accumulated about artificial insemination, sperm banking, cloning, make more certain a peopled world.
>
> The more serious human problems now are who will live, who will die and who will decide.[10]

A Critical Historical Review of Abortion: An Alternative Perspective

Between persons who oppose all abortions on moral grounds and those who believe abortion is sometimes or frequently morally justifiable, there is no difference of moral principle. Pro-choice advocates and anti-abortion advocates share the ethical principle of respect for human life, which is probably why the debate is so acrimonious. I have already indicated that one major source of disagreement is the way in which the theological story is appropriated in relation to the changing circumstances of history. In addition, we should recognize that whenever strong moral disagreement is encountered, we simultaneously confront different readings of the history of a moral issue. The way we interpret the past is already laden with and shaped by our present sense of what the moral problem is.

For example, professional male Christian ethicists tend to assume that Christianity has an unbroken history of "all but absolute" prohibition of abortion and that the history of morality of abortion can best be traced by studying the teaching of the now best-remembered theologians. Looking at the matter this way, one can find numerous proof-texts to show that some of the "church fathers" condemned abortion and equated abortion with either homicide or murder. Whenever a "leading" churchman equated abortion with homicide or murder, he also *and simultaneously* equated *contraception* with homicide or murder. This reflects not only male chauvinist biology but also the then almost phobic antisexual bias of the Christian tradition. Claims that one can separate abortion teaching into an ethic of killing separate from an antisexual and antifemale ethic in the history of Christianity do not withstand critical scrutiny.[11]

---

human act could turn out to be "the will of God" in a given context or setting. We may at any time be given "permission" by God's radical freedom to do what was not before permissible. My point here is that Barth exposits this possible exception in such a traditional prohibitory context that I do not believe it appropriate to cite him on the pro-choice side of the debate. In my opinion, no woman could ever accept the convoluted way in which Barth's biblical exegesis opens the door (a slight crack) to woman's full humanity. His reasoning on these questions simply demonstrates what deep difficulty the Christian tradition's exegetical tradition is in with respect to the full humanity and moral agency of women. See Karl Barth, "The Protection of Life," in *Church Dogmatics,* part 3, vol. 4 (Edinburgh: T. and T. Clark, 1961), pp. 415-422.

7. Compare Beverly Wildung Harrison, "When Fruitfulness and Blessedness Diverge," *Religion and Life* (1972), vol. 41, no. 4, pp. 480-496. My views on the seriousness of misogyny as a historical force have deepened since I wrote this essay.

8. Marie Augusta Neal, "Sociology and Sexuality: A Feminist Perspective," *Christianity and Crisis* 39, no. 8 (14 May 1979), pp. 118-122.

9. For a feminist theology of relationship, see Carter Heyward, *Toward the Redemption of God: A Theology of Mutual Relation* (Washington, D.C.: University Press of America, 1982).

10. Neal, "Sociology and Sexuality." This article is of critical importance in discussions of the theology and morality of abortion.

11. Susan Teft Nicholson, *Abortion and the Roman Catholic Church,* JRE Studies in Religious Ethics II (Knoxville: Religious Ethics Inc., University of Tennessee, 1978). This carefully crafted study assumes that there has been a clear "antikilling" ethic separa-

The history of Christian natural law ethics is totally conditioned by the equation of any effort to control procreation with homicide. However, this antisexual, antiabortion tradition is not universal, even among theologians and canon lawyers. On the subject of sexuality and its abuse, many well-known theologians had nothing to say; abortion was not even mentioned in most moral theology. An important, untold chapter in Christian history is the great struggle that took place in the medieval period when clerical celibacy came to be imposed and the rules of sexual behavior rigidified.

My thesis is that there is a relative disinterest in the question of abortion overall in Christian history. Occasionally, Christian theologians picked up the issue, especially when these theologians were state-related, that is, were articulating policy not only for the church but for political authority. Demographer Jean Meyer, himself a Catholic, insists that the Christian tradition took over "expansion by population growth" from the Roman Empire.[12] Christians opposed abortion strongly only when Christianity was closely identified with imperial state policy or when theologians were inveighing against women and any sexuality except that expressed in the reluctant service of procreation.

The Holy Crusade quality of present teaching on abortion is quite new in Christianity and is related to cultural shifts that are requiring the Christian tradition to choose sides in the present ideological struggle under pressure to rethink its entire attitude toward women and sexuality. My research has led me to the tentative conclusion that, in Protestant cultures, except where Protestantism is the "established religion," merging church and state, one does not find a strong antiabortion theological-ethical teaching at all. At least in the United States, this is beyond historical debate.[13] No Protestant clergy or theologian gave early support for proposed nineteenth-century laws banning abortion in the United States. It is my impression that Protestant clergy, usually married and often poor, were aware that romanticizing nature's bounty with respect to procreation resulted in a great deal of human suffering. The Protestant clergy who finally did join the antiabortion crusade were racist, classist white clergy, who feared America's strength was being threatened because white, middle-class, respectable women had a lower birth rate than black and ethnic women. Such arguments are still with us.

One other historical point must be stressed. Until the late nineteenth century the natural law tradition, and biblicism following it, tended to define the act of abortion as interruption of pregnancy after ensoulment, which was understood to be the point at which the breath of God entered the fetus. The point at which ensoulment was said to occur varied, but most typically it was marked by quickening, when fetal movement began. Knowledge about embryology was primitive until the past half-century, so this commonsense understanding prevailed. As a result, when abortion was condemned in earlier Christian teaching it was understood to refer to the termination of a pregnancy well into the process of the pregnancy, after ensoulment. Until the late nineteenth century, when Pope Pius IX, intrigued with the new embryonic discoveries, brought the natural law tradition into consonance with "modern science," abortion in ecclesiastical teaching often applied only to termination of prenatal life in more advanced stages of pregnancy.

Another distortion in the male-generated history of this issue derives from failure to note that, until the development of safe, surgical, elective abortion, the act of abortion commonly referred to something done to the woman, with or without her consent (see Exodus 22), either as a wrong done a husband or for the better moral reasons that abortion was an act of violence against both a pregnant woman and fetal life. In recent discussion it is the woman who does the wrongful act. No one would deny that abortion, if it terminates a pregnancy against the woman's wishes, is morally wrong. And until recent decades, abortion endangered the woman's life as much as it did the prenatal life in her womb. Hence, one premodern moral reason for opposing abortion was that it threatened the life and well-being of the mother more than did carrying the pregnancy to term. Today abortion is statistically safer than childbearing. Consequently, no one has a right to discuss the morality of abortion today without recognizing that one of the traditional and appropriate moral reasons for objecting to abortion — concern for women's well-being — now inheres in the prochoice side of the debate. Anti-abortion proponents who accord the fetus full human standing without also assigning positive value to women's lives and well-being are not really pressing the full sense of Christian moral tradition in the abortion debate.

Beyond all this, the deepest moral flaw in the "prolife" position's historical view is that none of its proponents has attempted to reconstruct the concrete, lived-world context in which the abortion discussion belongs: the all but desperate struggle by sexually active women to gain some proximate control over nature's profligacy in conception. Under the most adverse conditions, women have had to try to control our fertility — everywhere, always. Women's relation to procreation irrevocably marks and shapes our lives. Even those of us who do not have sexual contact with males, because we are celibate or lesbian, have been potential, even probable, victims of male sexual violence or have had to bear heavy social stigma for refusing the centrality of dependence on men and of procreation in our lives. The lives of infertile

---

ble from any antisexual ethic in Christian abortion teaching. This is an assumption that my historical research does not sustain.

12. Jean Meyer, "Toward a Non-Malthusian Population Policy," in *The American Population Debate,* ed. Daniel Callahan (Garden City, N.Y.: Doubleday, 1971).

13. See James C. Mohr, *Abortion in America* (New York: Oxford University Press, 1978), and James Nelson, "Abortion: Protestant Perspectives," in *Encyclopedia of Bioethics,* vol. 1, ed. Warren T. Reich (New York: Free Press, 1978), pp. 13-17.

women, too, are shaped by our failure to meet procreative expectations. Women's lack of social power, in all recorded history, has made this struggle to control procreation a life-bending, often life-destroying one for a large percentage of females.

So most women have had to do whatever we could to prevent too-numerous pregnancies. In societies and cultures, except the most patriarchal, the processes of procreation have been transmitted through women's culture. Birth control techniques have been widely practiced, and some primitive ones have proved effective. Increasingly, anthropologists are gaining hints of how procreative control occurred in some premodern societies. Frequently women have had to choose to risk their lives in order not to have that extra child that would destroy the family's ability to cope or bring about an unmanageable crisis.

We have to concede that modern medicine, for all its misogyny, has replaced some dangerous contraceptive practices still widely used where surgical abortion is unavailable. In light of these gains, more privileged western women must not lose the ability to imagine the real-life pressures that lead women in other cultures to resort to ground-glass douches, reeds inserted in the uterus, and so on, to induce labor. The radical nature of methods women use bespeaks the desperation involved in unwanted pregnancy and reveals the real character of our struggle.

Nor should we suppress the fact that a major means of birth control now is, as it was in earlier times, infanticide. And let no one imagine that women have made decisions to expose or kill newborn infants casually. Women understand what many men cannot seem to grasp — that the birth of a child requires that some person must be prepared to care, without interruption, for this infant, provide material resources and energy-draining amounts of time and attention for it. The human infant is the most needy and dependent of all newborn creatures. It seems to me that men, especially celibate men, romanticize this total and uncompromising dependency of the infant on the already existing human community. Women bear the brunt of this reality and know its full implications. And this dependency is even greater in a fragmented, centralized urban-industrial modern culture than in a rural culture, where another pair of hands often increased an extended family unit's productive power. No historical interpretation of abortion as a moral issue that ignores these matters deserves moral standing in the present debate.

A treatment of any moral problem is inadequate if it fails to analyze the morality of a given act in a way that represents the concrete experience of the agent who faces a decision with respect to that act. Misogyny in Christian discussions of abortion is evidenced clearly in that the abortion decision is never treated in the way it arises as part of the female agent's life process. The decision at issue when the dilemma of choice arises for women is whether or not to be pregnant. In most discussions of the morality of abortion it is treated as an abstract act[14] rather than as a possible way to deal with a pregnancy that frequently is the result of circumstances beyond the woman's control. John Noonan, for instance, evades this fact by referring to the pregnant woman almost exclusively as "the gravida" (a Latin term meaning "pregnant one") or "the carrier" in his *A Private Choice: Abortion in America in the Seventies.*[15] In any pregnancy a woman's life is deeply, irrevocably affected. Those such as Noonan who uphold the unexceptional immorality of abortion are probably wise to obscure the fact that an unwanted pregnancy always involves a life-shaping consequence for a woman, because suppressing the identity of the moral agent and the reality of her dilemma greatly reduces the ability to recognize the moral complexity of abortion. When the question of abortion arises, it is usually because a woman finds herself facing an unwanted pregnancy. Consider the actual circumstances that may precipitate this. One is the situation in which a woman did not intend to be sexually active or did not enter into a sexual act voluntarily. Since women are frequently victims of sexual violence, numerous cases of this type arise because of rape, incest, or forced marital coitus. Many morally sensitive opponents of abortion concede that in such cases abortion may be morally justifiable. I insist that in such cases it is a moral good because it is not rational to treat a newly fertilized ovum as though it had the same value as the existent, pregnant female person and because it is morally wrong to make the victim of sexual violence suffer the further agonies of unwanted pregnancy and childbearing against her will. Enforced pregnancy would be viewed as a morally reprehensible violation of bodily integrity if women were recognized as fully human moral agents.

Another more frequent case results when a woman — or usually a young girl — participates in heterosexual activity without clear knowledge of how pregnancy occurs and without intention to conceive a child. A girl who became pregnant in this manner would, by traditional natural law morality, be held in a state of invincible ignorance and therefore not morally culpable. One scholarly Roman Catholic nun I met argued — quite appropriately, I believe — that her church should not consider the abortions of young Catholic girls as morally culpable because the Church overprotected them, which contributed to their lack of understanding of procreation and to their inability to cope with the sexual pressures girls experience in contemporary society. A social policy that pressures the sexually ill-informed child or young

14. H. Richard Niebuhr often warned his theological compatriots about abstracting acts from the life project in which they are embedded, but this warning is much neglected in the writings of Christian moralists. See "The Christian Church in the World Crises," *Christianity and Society* 6 (1941).

15. John T. Noonan, Jr., *A Private Choice: Abortion in America in the Seventies* (New York: Free Press, 1979). Noonan denies that the history of abortion is related to the history of male oppression of women.

woman into unintended or unaware motherhood would be morally dubious indeed.

A related type of pregnancy happens when a woman runs risks by not using contraceptives, perhaps because taking precaution in romantic affairs is not perceived as ladylike or requires her to be too unspontaneous about sex. Our society resents women's sexuality unless it is "innocent" and male-mediated, so many women, lest they be censured as "loose" and "promiscuous," are slow to assume adult responsibility for contraception. However, when pregnancies occur because women are skirting the edges of responsibility and running risks out of immaturity, is enforced motherhood a desirable solution? Such pregnancies could be minimized only by challenging precisely those childish myths of female socialization embedded in natural law teaching about female sexuality.

It is likely that most decisions about abortion arise because mature women who are sexually active with men and who understand the risk of pregnancy nevertheless experience contraceptive failure. Our moral schizophrenia in this matter is exhibited in that many people believe women have more responsibility than men to practice contraception and that family planning is always a moral good, but even so rule out abortion altogether. Such a split consciousness ignores the fact that no inexorable biological line exists between prevention of conception and abortion.[16] More important, such reasoning ignores the genuine risks involved in female contraceptive methods. Some women are at higher risk than others in using the most reliable means of birth control. Furthermore, the reason we do not have more concern for safer contraceptive methods for men and women is that matters relating to women's health and well-being are never urgent in this society. Moreover, many contraceptive failures are due to the irresponsibility of the producers of contraceptives rather than to bad luck.[17] Given these facts, should a woman who actively attempts to avoid pregnancy be punished for contraceptive failure when it occurs?

In concluding this historical section, I must stress that if present efforts to criminalize abortion succeed, we will need a state apparatus of massive proportions to enforce compulsory childbearing. In addition, withdrawal of legal abortion will create one more massively profitable underworld economy in which the Mafia and other sections of quasi-legal capitalism may and will profitably invest. The radical right promises to get the state out of regulation of people's lives, but what they really mean is that they will let economic activity go unrestrained. What their agenda signifies for the personal lives of women is quite another matter.

An adequate historical perspective on abortion recognizes the long struggle women have waged for some degree of control over fertility and their efforts to regain control of procreative power from patriarchal and state-imperial culture and institutions. Such a perspective also takes into account that more nearly adequate contraceptive methods and the existence of safe, surgical, elective abortion represent positive historic steps toward full human freedom and dignity for women. While the same gains in medical knowledge also open the way to new forms of sterilization abuse and to social pressures against some women's use of their power of procreation, I know of no women who would choose to return to a state of lesser knowledge about these matters.

There has been an objective gain in the quality of women's lives for those fortunate enough to have access to procreative choice. That millions upon millions of women as yet do not possess even the rudimentary conditions — moral or physical — for such choice is obvious. Our moral goal should be to struggle against those real barriers — poverty, racism, and antifemale cultural oppression — that prevent authentic choice from being a reality for every woman. In this process we will be able to minimize the need for abortions only insofar as we place the abortion debate in the real lived-world context of women's lives.

Abortion and Moral Theory

The greatest strategic problem of pro-choice advocates is the widespread assumption that pro-lifers have a monopoly on the moral factors that ought to enter into decisions about abortion. *Moral* here is defined as that which makes for the self-respect and well-being of human persons and their environment. Moral legitimacy seems to adhere to their position in part because traditionalists have an array of religiomoral terminology at their command that the sometimes more secular proponents of choice lack. But those who would displace women's power of choice by the power of the state and/or the medical profession do not deserve the aura of moral sanctity. We must do our homework if we are to dispel this myth of moral superiority. A major way in which Christian moral theologians and moral philosophers contribute to this monopoly of moral sanctity is by equating fetal or prenatal life with human personhood in a simplistic way and by failing to acknowledge changes regarding this issue in the history of Christianity.

We need to remember that even in Roman Catholic natural law ethics, the definition of the status of fetal life has shifted over time, and in all cases the status of prenatal life involves a moral judgment, not a scientific one. The question is properly posed this way: What status are

16. We know now that the birth control pill does not always work by preventing fertilization of the ovum by the sperm. Frequently, the pill causes the wall of the uterus to expel the newly fertilized ovum. From a biological point of view, there is no point in the procreative process that can be taken as a clear dividing line on which to pin neat moral distinctions.

17. The most conspicuous example of corporate involvement in contraceptive failure was the famous Dalkan Shield scandal. Note also that the manufacturer of the Dalkan Shield dumped its dangerous and ineffective product on family planning programs of third world (overexploited) countries.

we morally wise to predicate to prenatal human life, given that the fetus is not yet a fully existent human being? Those constrained under Catholic teaching have been required for the past ninety years to believe a human being exists from conception, when the ovum and sperm merge.[18] This answer from one tradition has had far wider impact on our culture than most people recognize. Other Christians come from traditions that do not offer (and could not offer, given their conception of the structure of the church as moral community) a definitive answer to this question.

Even so, some contemporary Protestant medical ethicists, fascinated by recent genetic discoveries and experiments with deoxyribonucleic acid (DNA), have all but sacralized the moment in which the genetic code is implanted as the moment of humanization, which leaves them close to the traditional Roman Catholic position. Protestant male theologians have long let their enthrallment with science lead to a sacralization of specific scientific discoveries, usually to the detriment of theological and moral clarity. In any case, there are two responses that must be made to the claim that the fetus in early stages of development is a human life or, more dubiously, a human person.

First, the historical struggle for women's personhood is far from won, owing chiefly to the opposition of organized religious groups to full equality for women. Those who proclaim that a zygote at the moment of conception is a person worthy of citizenship continue to deny full social and political rights to women. Whatever one's judgment about the moral status of the fetus, it cannot be argued that that assessment deserves greater moral standing in analysis than does the position of the pregnant woman. This matter of evaluating the meaning of prenatal life is where morally sensitive people's judgments diverge. I cannot believe that anyone, if truly morally sensitive, would value the woman's full, existent life less than they value early fetal life. Most women can become pregnant and carry fetal life to term many, many times in their lifetimes. The distinctly human power is not our biologic capacity to bear children, but our power to actively love, nurture, care for one another and shape one another's existence in cultural and social interaction.[19] To equate a biologic process with full normative humanity is crass biologic reductionism, and such reductionism is never practiced in religious ethics except where women's lives and well-being are involved.

Second, even though prenatal life, as it moves toward biologic individuation of human form, has value, the equation of abortion with murder is dubious. And the equation of abortion with homicide — the taking of human life — should be carefully weighed. We should also remember that we live in a world where men extend other men wide moral range in relation to justifiable homicide. For example, the just-war tradition has legitimated widespread forms of killing in war, and Christian ethicists have often extended great latitude to rulers and those in power in making choices about killing human beings.[20] Would that such moralists extended equal benefit of a doubt to women facing life-crushing psychological and politicoeconomic pressures in the face of childbearing! Men, daily, make life-determining decisions concerning nuclear power or chemical use in the environment, for example, that affect the well-being of fetuses, and our society expresses no significant opposition, even when such decisions do widespread genetic damage. When we argue for the appropriateness of legal abortion, moral outrage rises.

The so-called pro-life position also gains support by invoking the general principle of respect for human life as foundational to its morality in a way that suggests that the pro-choice advocates are unprincipled. I have already noted that pro-choice advocates have every right to claim the same moral principle, and that this debate, like most debates that are morally acrimonious, is in no sense about basic moral principles. I do not believe there is any clear-cut conflict of principle in this very deep, very bitter controversy.

It needs to be stressed that we all have an absolute obligation to honor any moral principle that seems, after rational deliberation, to be sound. This is the one absolutism appropriate to ethics. There are often several moral principles relevant to a decision and many ways to relate a given principle to a decisional context. For most right-to-lifers only one principle has moral standing in this argument. Admitting only one principle to one's process of moral reasoning means that a range of other moral values is slighted. Right-to-lifers are also moral absolutists in the sense that they admit only one possible meaning or application of the principle they invoke. Both these types of absolutism obscure moral debate and lead to less, not more, rational deliberation. The principle of respect for human life is one we should all honor, but we must also recognize that this principle often comes into conflict with other valid moral principles in the process of making real, lived-world decisions. Understood in an adequate way, this principle can be restated to mean that we should treat what falls under a reasonable definition of human life as having sanctity or intrinsic moral value. But even when this is clear, other principles are needed to help us choose between two intrinsic values, in this case between the prenatal life and the pregnant woman's life.

Another general moral principle from which we can-

18. Catholic moral theology opens up several ways for faithful Catholics to challenge the teaching office of the church on moral questions. However, I remain unsatisfied that these qualifications of inerrancy in moral matters stand up in situations of moral controversy. If freedom of conscience does not function *de jure*, should it be claimed as existent in principle?

19. I elaborate this point in greater detail in "The Power of Anger in the Work of Love" in my *Making the Connections*.

20. For example, Paul Ramsey gave unqualified support to U.S. military involvement in Southeast Asia in light of just-war considerations but finds abortion to be an unexceptional moral wrong.

not exempt our actions is the principle of justice, or right relations between persons and between groups of persons and communities. Another relevant principle is respect for all that supports human life, namely, the natural environment. As any person knows who thinks deeply about morality, genuine moral conflicts, as often as not, are due not to ignoring moral principles but to the fact that different principles lead to conflicting implications for action or are selectively related to decisions. For example, we live in a time when the principle of justice for women, aimed at transforming the social relations that damage women's lives, is historically urgent. For many of us this principle has greater moral urgency than the extension of the principle of respect for human life to include early fetal life, even though respect for fetal life is also a positive moral good. We should resist approaches to ethics that claim that one overriding principle always deserves to control morality. Clarification of principle, for that matter, is only a small part of moral reasoning. When we weigh moral principles and their potential application, we must also consider the implications of a given act for our present historical context and envision its long-term consequences.

One further proviso on this issue of principles in moral reasoning: There are several distinct theories among religious ethicists and moral philosophers as to what the function of principles ought to be. One group believes moral principles are for the purpose of terminating the process of moral reasoning. Hence, if this sort of moralist tells you always to honor the principle of respect for human life, what he or she means is for you to stop reflection and act in a certain way — in this case to accept one's pregnancy regardless of consequences. Others believe that it is better to refer to principles (broad, generalized moral criteria) than to apply rules (narrower, specific moral prescriptions) because principles function to open up processes of reasoning rather than close them off. The principle of respect for life, on this reading, is not invoked to prescribe action but to help locate and weigh values, to illuminate a range of values that always inhere in significant human decisions. A major difference in the moral debate on abortion, then, is that some believe that to invoke the principle of respect for human life settles the matter, stops debate, and precludes the single, simple act of abortion. By contrast, many of us believe the breadth of the principle opens up to reconsideration the question of what the essential moral quality of human life is all about and to increase moral seriousness about choosing whether or when to bear children.

Two other concerns related to our efforts to make a strong moral case for women's right to procreative choice need to be touched on. The first has to do with the problems our Christian tradition creates for any attempt to make clear why women's right to control our bodies is an urgent and substantive moral claim. One of Christianity's greatest weaknesses is its spiritualizing neglect of respect for the physical body and physical well-being. Tragically, women, more than men, are expected in Christian teaching never to honor their own well-being as a moral consideration. I want to stress, then, that we have no moral tradition in Christianity that starts with body-space, or body-right, as a basic condition of moral relations. (Judaism is far better in this regard, for it acknowledges that we all have a moral right to be concerned for our life and our survival.) Hence, many Christian ethicists simply do not get the point when we speak of women's right to bodily integrity. They blithely denounce such reasons as women's disguised self-indulgence or hysterical rhetoric.[21]

We must articulate our view that body-right is a basic moral claim and also remind our hearers that there is no unchallengeable analogy among other human activities to women's procreative power. Pregnancy is a distinctive human experience. In any social relation, body-space must be respected or nothing deeply human or moral can be created. The social institutions most similar to compulsory pregnancy in their moral violations of body-space are chattel slavery and peonage. These institutions distort the moral relations of a community and deform a community over time. (Witness racism in the United States.) Coercion of women, through enforced sterilization or enforced pregnancy, legitimates unjust power in intimate human relationships and cuts to the heart of our capacity for moral social relations. As we should recognize, given our violence-prone society, people learn violence at home and at an early age when women's lives are violated!

Even so, we must be careful, when we make the case for our right to bodily integrity, not to confuse moral rights with mere liberties.[22] To claim that we have a moral right to procreative choice does not mean we believe women can exercise this right free of all moral claims from the community. For example, we need to teach female children that childbearing is not a purely capricious, individualistic matter, and we need to challenge the assumption that a woman who enjoys motherhood should have as many children as she and her mate wish, regardless of its effects on others. Population self-control is a moral issue, although more so in high-consuming, afflu-

21. See Richard A. McCormick, S.J., "Rules for Abortion Debate," in Batchelor, *Abortion: The Moral Issues*, pp. 27-37.

22. One of the reasons why abortion-on-demand rhetoric — even when it is politically effective in the immediate moment — has had a backlash effect is that it seems to many to imply a lack of reciprocity between women's needs and society's needs. While I would not deny, in principle, a possible conflict of interest between women's well-being and the community's needs for reproduction, there is little or no historical evidence that suggests women are less responsible to the well-being of the community than are men. We need not fall into a liberal, individualistic trap in arguing the central importance of procreative choice to issues of women's well-being in society. The right in question is body-right, or freedom from coercion in childbearing. It is careless to say that the right in question is the right to an abortion. Morally, the right is bodily self-determination, a fundamental condition of personhood and a foundational moral right. See Beverly Wildung Harrison, *Our Right to Choose: Toward a New Ethic of Abortion* (Boston: Beacon Press, 1983).

ent societies like our own than in nations where a modest, simple, and less wasteful lifestyle obtains.

A second point is the need, as we work politically for a pro-choice social policy, to avoid the use of morally objectionable arguments to mobilize support for our side of the issue. One can get a lot of political mileage in U.S. society by using covert racist and classist appeals ("abortion lowers the cost of welfare rolls or reduces illegitimacy" or "paying for abortions saves the taxpayers money in the long run"). Sometimes it is argued that good politics is more important than good morality and that one should use whatever arguments work to gain political support. I do not believe that these crassly utilitarian[23] arguments turn out, in the long run, to be good politics, for they are costly to our sense of polis and of community. But even if they were effective in the short run, I am doubly sure that on the issue of the right to choose abortion, good morality doth a good political struggle make. I believe, deeply, that moral right is on the side of the struggle for the freedom and self-respect of women, especially poor and non-white women, and on the side of developing social policy that ensures that every child born can be certain to be a wanted child. Issues of justice are those that deserve the deepest moral caretaking as we develop a political strategy.

Only when people see that they cannot prohibit safe, legal, elective surgical abortion without violating the conditions of well-being for the vast majority of women — especially those most socially vulnerable because of historic patterns of oppression — will the effort to impose a selective, abstract morality of the sanctity of human life on all of us cease. This is a moral battle par excellence, and whenever we forget that we make it harder to reach the group most important to the cause of procreative choice — those women who have never suffered from childbearing pressures, who have not yet put this issue into a larger historical context, and who reverence women's historical commitment to childbearing. We will surely not reach them with pragmatic appeals to the taxpayer's wallet! To be sure, we cannot let such women go unchallenged as they support ruling-class ideology that the state should control procreation. But they will not change their politics until they see that pro-choice is grounded in a deeper, tougher, more caring moral vision than the political option they now endorse.

The Social Policy Dimensions of the Debate

Most people fail to understand that in ethics we need, provisionally, to separate our reflection on the morality of specific acts from questions about how we express our moral values within our social institutions and systems (that is, social policy). When we do this, the morality of abortion appears in a different light. Focusing attention away from the single act of abortion to the larger historical context thrusts into relief what "respect for human life" means in the pro-choice position. It also illuminates the common core of moral concern that unites pro-choice advocates to pro-lifers who have genuine concern for expanding the circle of who really counts as human in this society. Finally, placing abortion in a larger historical context enables proponents of pro-choice to clarify where we most differ from the pro-lifers, that is, in our total skepticism that a state-enforced anti-abortion policy could ever have the intended "pro-life" consequences they claim.

We must always insist that the objective social conditions that make women and children already born highly vulnerable can only be worsened by a social policy of compulsory pregnancy. However one judges the moral quality of the individual act of abortion (and here, differences among us do exist that are morally justifiable), it is still necessary to distinguish between how one judges the act of abortion morally and what one believes a societywide policy on abortion should be. We must not let those who have moral scruples against the personal act ignore the fact that a just social policy must also include active concern for enhancement of women's well-being and, for that, policies that would in fact make abortions less necessary. To anathematize abortion when the social and material conditions for control of procreation do not exist is to blame the victim, not to address the deep dilemmas of female existence in this society.

Even so, there is no reason for those of us who celebrate procreative choice as a great moral good to pretend that resort to abortion is ever a desirable means of expressing this choice. I know of no one on the pro-choice side who has confused the desirability of the availability of abortion with the celebration of the act itself. We all have every reason to hope that safer, more reliable means of contraception may be found and that violence against women will be reduced. Furthermore, we should be emphatic that our social policy demands include opposition to sterilization abuse, insistence on higher standards of health care for women and children, better prenatal care, reduction of unnecessary surgery on women's reproductive systems, increased research to improve contraception, and so on. Nor should we draw back from criticizing a health care delivery system that exploits women. An abortion industry thrives on the profitability of abortion, but women are not to blame for this.

A feminist position demands social conditions that support women's full, self-respecting right to procreative choice, including the right not to be sterilized against our wills, the right to choose abortion as a birth control means of last resort, and the right to a prenatal and postnatal health care system that will also reduce the now widespread trauma of having to deliver babies in

23. A theory is crassly utilitarian only if it fails to grant equal moral worth to all persons in the calculation of social consequences — as, for example, when some people's financial well-being is weighted more than someone else's basic physical existence. I do not mean to criticize any type of utilitarian moral theory that weighs the actual consequences of actions. In fact, I believe no moral theory is adequate if it does not have a strong utilitarian component.

rigid, impersonal health care settings. Pro-lifers do best politically when we allow them to keep the discussion narrowly focused on the morality of the act of abortion and on the moral value of the fetus. We do best politically when we make the deep connections between the full context of this issue in women's lives, including this society's systemic or patterned injustice toward women.

It is well to remember that it has been traditional Catholic natural law ethics that most clarified and stressed this distinction between the morality of an individual act on the one hand and the policies that produce the optional social morality on the other. The strength of this tradition is probably reflected in the fact that even now most polls show that slightly more Catholics than Protestants believe it unwise for the state to attempt to regulate abortion. In the past, Catholics, more than Protestants, have been wary of using the state as an instrument of moral crusade. Tragically, by taking their present approach to abortion, the Roman Catholic hierarchy may be risking the loss of the deepest wisdom of its own ethical tradition. By failing to acknowledge a distinction between the church's moral teaching on the act of abortion and the question of what is a desirable social policy to minimize abortion, as well as overemphasizing it to the neglect of other social justice concerns, the Roman Catholic church may well be dissipating the best of its moral tradition.[24]

The frenzy of the current pope and many Roman Catholic bishops in the United States on this issue has reached startling proportions. The United States bishops have equated nuclear war and the social practice of abortion as the most heinous social evils of our time.[25] While this appallingly misguided analogy has gained credibility because of the welcome if modest opposition of the bishops to nuclear escalation, I predict that the long-term result will be to further discredit Roman Catholic moral wisdom in the culture.

If we are to be a society genuinely concerned with enhancing women's well-being and minimizing the necessity of abortions, thereby avoiding the danger over time of becoming an abortion culture,[26] what kind of society must we become? It is here that the moral clarity of the feminist analysis becomes most obvious. How can we reduce the number of abortions due to contraceptive failure? By placing greater emphasis on medical research in this area, by requiring producers of contraceptives to behave more responsibly, and by developing patterns of institutional life that place as much emphasis on male responsibility for procreation and long-term care and nurturance of children as on female responsibility.

How can we reduce the number of abortions due to childish ignorance about sexuality among female children or adult women and our mates? By adopting a widespread program of sex education and by supporting institutional policies that teach male and female children alike that a girl is as fully capable as a boy of enjoying sex and that both must share moral responsibility for preventing pregnancy except when they have decided, as a deliberative moral act, to have a child.

How would we reduce the necessity of abortion due to sexual violence against women in and out of marriage? By challenging vicious male-generated myths that women exist primarily to meet the sexual needs of men, that women are, by nature, those who are really fulfilled only through our procreative powers. We would teach feminist history as the truthful history of the race, stressing that historic patterns of patriarchy were morally wrong and that a humane or moral society would be a fully nonsexist society.

Technological developments that may reduce the need for abortions are not entirely within our control, but the sociomoral ethos that makes abortion common is within our power to change. And we would begin to create such conditions by adopting a thoroughgoing feminist program for society. Nothing less, I submit, expresses genuine respect for all human life.

24. For a perceptive discussion of this danger by a distinguished Catholic priest, read George C. Higgins, "The Prolife Movement and the New Right," *America,* 13 Sept. 1980, pp. 107-110.

25. Philip J. Murnion, ed., *Catholics and Nuclear War: A Commentary on the Challenge of the U.S. Catholic Bishops' Pastoral Letter on War and Peace* (New York: Crossroads, 1983), p. 326.

26. I believe the single most valid concern raised by opponents of abortion is that the frequent practice of abortion, over time, may contribute to a cultural ethos of insensitivity to the value of human life, not because fetuses are being "murdered" but because surgical termination of pregnancy may further "technologize" our sensibilities about procreation. I trust that all of the foregoing makes clear my adamant objection to allowing this insight to justify yet more violence against women. However, I do believe we should be very clear that we stand ready to support — emphatically — any social policies that would lessen the need for abortion *without* jeopardizing women's right to control our own procreative power.

120 The Catholic Legacy and Abortion: A Debate

Daniel C. Maguire and James T. Burtchaell

In February of 1987 the theology department at the University of Notre Dame sponsored a major debate on abortion. The debaters in what was locally referred to as a "heavyweight bout" were James Tunstead Burtchaell, C.S.C., and Daniel C. Maguire. Father Burtchaell is a professor of theology at Notre Dame, a former provost of the university, and the author of *Rachel Weeping: The Case Against Abortion* and other books. Professor Maguire is a professor of theology at Marquette University, a past president of the Society of Christian Ethics, the author of *The Moral Choice* among other works, and an active critic of official Catholic teaching on abortion. The proposition Burtchaell and Maguire debated was: "*Recent developments and reflection provide authentic reasons to reconsider the virtually total Christian disapproval of abortion.*"

Daniel C. Maguire

In the 1980s, when the abortion issue has been most acrimonious and mischievous in church and state, honest debate is the only way to get this abortion bone out of the Catholic throat so that we can get on to more important pro-life issues.

There are more important pro-life issues. Forty-two thousand children die daily due to lack of basic nourishment and medicine. There are now some four tons of TNT stockpiled for every head on the planet. The number of heads on the planet may reach 8.5 billion by the year 2025, with 7 billion of them being in the third world. The problems of Ethiopia are but preview of the havoc of hunger to come unless reason and justice replace militarism and greed. Meanwhile, the arms race is poised to move into outer space, leaving the earth in a state of terminal peril.

Still, the abortion debate must get on. This debate between Burtchaell and myself is important, regardless of what Burtchaell and I say. This debate implies that the issue is debatable. If the absolute negative position on abortion were clear, there would be no need to debate it. There are no pro and con debates on the morality of rape. Abortion is an open question since, as John Connery, S.J., says, "not enough time has elapsed to provide a test of current opinions." Furthermore, Catholic bishops, while pressing for a no-abortion amendment to the Constitution, have said they are not trying to force Catholic dogma into law, but to appeal to the public on the basis of reason. It is precisely on the basis of reason that Protestants, Catholics, Jews, and others disagree, and so we must reason together about our agreements and disagreements. There is no one infallible view on abortion, and we do well to debate the fallible.

It may disappoint some who come to feast on conflict that Burtchaell and I are not in total disagreement on abortion. We agree in three ways: First, both Burtchaell and I are pro-moral-choice on abortion. In his book, *Rachel Weeping*, Burtchaell writes: "Save for the rare, rare instance when it is a moral threat to a mother's life to carry her child to birth, there is no abortion that is not the unjust taking of another's life because it is a burden to one's own." Pronouncing this exception "rare, rare" is, of course, an empirical, first-world judgment. Bishop Francis Simons, former bishop of Indore, India, says such cases are not at all rare in the third world. Thus Burtchaell is approving of a lot of direct abortions. He has admitted a class that has many members. In so doing, he departs from the Vatican theology of abortion as, of course, do I when the circumstances warrant it.

Second, neither Burtchaell nor I is pro-abortion. Indeed, only a sadist could be "pro-abortion." Abortion is a negative value at best. In Utopia, it would be almost uncalled for. This is a matter of common sense. One would not say of a woman who had a fulfilling family and professional life that it was a pity she had not had an abortion to lend a touch of completion.

Third, both Burtchaell and I object to the idea of "abortion on demand." I object because the term is a sexist ellipsis. The phrase implies a verb, *demand,* and an object, *abortion,* but it tellingly omits the subject, *woman.* This is significant because woman is often missing in the conservative analysis of abortion. I further object to the expression "abortion on demand" because a woman should not have to demand that to which she has a moral right. Burtchaell, it would seem, is for un-abortion on demand imposed on women. There we do not agree, and so there are grounds for debate. Basically, Burtchaell and I differ because he stakes out a definitive and apodictic position on abortion before the witness of women has been heard and evaluated in Catholic theology.

This is a major problem in conservative Catholic theology on abortion. By saying that all abortions are immoral, a stinging judgment is delivered on one to two million American women and forty to fifty million women worldwide who decide each year for abortions. The absolutist position allows for only three judgments

From Daniel C. Maguire and James T. Burtchaell, C.S.C., "The Catholic Legacy & Abortion: A Debate," *Commonweal* 126 (20 November 1987): 657-72. Abridged and edited from the original. Used by permission.

of these women: (1) They are evil since they knowingly choose objective evil. (2) They are ignorant, and are thus excused from subjective guilt. (3) They are excused by insanity. There is no gentle alternative. We should await the newly emerging witness of women on abortion before sealing off the issue in ways that indict all or most women who make these crisis choices. This is a call for modesty, not a call to justify all abortion decisions.

I also find Burtchaell ecumenically insensitive on this issue. He seems to take no account of the broad disagreement with his simplistic position found among mainstream Protestants. The General Board of the American Baptist churches, U.S.A., said in 1981 that the decision for abortion may be morally made "when all other possible alternatives will lead to greater destruction of human life and spirit." Abortion, they continued, must be a matter of "responsible, personal decision." The American Friends Service Committee said in 1970 that "it is far better to end an unwanted pregnancy than to encourage the evils resulting from forced pregnancy and childbirth." The General Convention of the Episcopal Church in 1982 listed serious threats to the mental or physical health of the woman, deformation of the fetus, and rape and incest as reasons making abortion "permissible." The General Assembly of the Presbyterian Church affirmed in 1983 the *Roe v. Wade* decision of the Supreme Court and said the "principle of inviolability can be applied" only when the fetus is viable. The General Synod of the United Church of Christ said "every woman must have the freedom of choice to follow her personal religious and moral convictions concerning the completion or termination of her pregnancy." They also called for public funding for abortion. The United Methodist Church in their General Conferences in both 1976 and 1984 listed a number of cases when "the path of a mature Christian judgment may indicate the advisability of abortion." The Lutheran Church in America, at its Biennial Convention in 1970, said that "on the basis of the evangelical ethic, a woman or couple may decide responsibly to seek an abortion."

A number of Jewish groups have offered similar witness, including the American Jewish Congress, B'nai B'rith Women, the Central Conference of American Rabbis, the Union of American Hebrew Congregations, and the National Council of Jewish Women. It is simplistic and arrogant to treat all of these relatives in faith as insensitive defenders of murder or irresponsible abortion. The Second Vatican Council said the ecumenical dialogue should "start with discussions concerning the application of the Gospel to moral questions." Such discussions have barely begun, and Burtchaell and others would bar the door by brandishing obnoxious analogies that compare persons with nuanced views of abortion to defenders of the Nazi Holocaust and racism.

THE HEART of this debate is the question: is the anti-moral-choice position on abortion *the* Christian and Catholic view? Are the Catholic bishops correct when they refer to the "clear and constant" teaching of the church on abortion? My answer is negative to both questions. There is no "clear and constant" teaching on abortion, and Catholic moral theology and Christian ethics generally have been pro-moral-choice ever since we started looking at the circumstances of abortion. Since, as Teilhard de Chardin said, nothing is intelligible outside its history, let us look to the history of abortion theology in the Christian church. In doing this, I will often refer to the work of John Connery. I do this for several reasons. To begin with, he holds the most conservative position on abortion since he, unlike Burtchaell and me, allows *no* exceptions. Thus I cannot be accused of bringing in a witness who shares my position. More importantly, Connery's book, *Abortion: The Development of the Roman Catholic Perspective* (Loyola, 1977), is the most important modern Catholic book on abortion. Since its publication ten years ago, it has not had the influence it deserves. I do not say Connery would agree with all my interpretations of his work. I also do not say his book is all one needs for a historical study of this issue. However, Connery's anti-moral-choice conclusions are based on his ecclesiology, not on his historical research, and that research has pro-moral-choice implications that have not been mined.

Before treating the Jewish prelude to Christian thought on abortion, Connery advises us that "the Christian attitude toward abortion will be in general continuity with the tradition of the Jews of the pre-Christian and early Christian era."

No text in the Bible discusses abortion in the terms of our debate today. The only reference in the Hebrew Bible to abortion is in Exodus 21:22, which speaks of accidental abortion. Connery says the text shows that "the fetus did not have the same status as the mother in Hebrew Law." That is certainly true. The text also suggests that the key issue was the rights of the father to progeny; he could fine you for the misdeed, but he could not claim "an eye for an eye" as he could if a person such as the woman had been killed. Thus the biblical witness on abortion.

The Roman and Stoic position, from which Christians would borrow freely, stressed the rights of the *paterfamilias* and that there was no soul until birth. The Jewish Talmud taught that the fetus was a part of the mother. The Mishnah says you can kill the fetus to save the mother since it is not a child until born. Josephus criticized abortion because it "diminishes the multitude." There is no evidence of a Christian revolution against these views or for them.

In the absence of scriptural support, the modern absolutists on abortion turn to the earliest Christian writers. What they find is that those few writers who mention abortion without elaboration were opposed to it, but not as homicide. No distinctively Christian position on abortion is in evidence. Indeed, there is no theology of abortion at all, according to Connery, since he says that does not begin on the subject until the thirteenth century. (I would place that beginning in the fifteenth century.) It violates historiography and the canons of literary criticism to say that *the* Christian viewpoint on abortion starts in the early church and floats clearly and constantly through the ages.

The Didache, discovered in 1875, was not a shaper of our tradition, but it is a favorite of the anti-moral-choice faction. It seems to be the product of an isolated Christian community in Syria and it draws on Jewish sources. It offers no textual evidence of discontinuity with Jewish views on abortion. Neither does *Pseudo-Barnabas,* which also had Jewish roots. Athenagoras brought up abortion in his defense against cannibalism. This is not the setting of our debate. Clement of Alexandria opposed abortion as a cover-up for fornication. We do not know what views he held on other cases since he did no theological ethics on the subject. Cyprian was concerned about the case of a man kicking a woman in the stomach until she aborted. That is a bad idea, but it is not our debate. It is text-proofing and patristic fundamentalism to pretend these texts contain, even in germ, the modern negative absolute position on abortion.

Most important of the early writers is Tertullian. In his *Apologetica,* he seems to take the Jewish position on animation at birth. Elsewhere, he inclines to the Greek view that the fetus is ensouled when sufficiently formed *in utero.* Again, eclecticism and variety. Tertullian is important on another count. He addressed what we would call craniotomy and called it a "necessary cruelty." Connery concedes that Tertullian "does use expressions which might imply a justification of the procedure in his mind." It seems that the first primitive theology on abortion is open to moral choice.

A number of fourth- and fifth-century writers adopted the Greek idea of delayed animation. Early abortion in this view would not be homicide. Augustine said that the early fetus will perish like the sperm does. It will not rise with us at the resurrection of the dead. (Neither, he assures us, will the sperm, for which we can all be grateful.) The Council of Elvira's oft-cited canons may not refer to abortion at all, and the Council of Ancyra gives lesser punishments for abortion than for homicide. These documents influenced the Penitentials which dominated the moral scene from the sixth to the eleventh centuries.

IN SUM, let it be said that the sparse references to abortion in the first twelve hundred years of the Christian era are set in this context: (1) All occurred before the beginning of any formal theology on abortion. (2) They rose from a period of ignorance of the processes of generation, the ovum having been discovered only in the nineteenth century. (3) They came at a time of underpopulation. (4) They came in a time of notable sexism and negativity to sexuality. (5) Abortion was often condemned as a violation of the procreative nature of sex and not as murder. As Susan Teft Nicholson says, it is "misleading" in the terms of our public debate "to maintain that the Roman Catholic church has always condemned abortion." Sometimes abortion is called homicide, but so too are contraception and sterilization, suggesting that a dominant concern was sex used nonprocreatively. It is fallacious and disingenuous to say that Christian teachers always condemned abortion without saying on what grounds they did so and without saying whether one accepts and argues from those same grounds today. At least the Vatican is consistent: it applies the natural law argument that sex is intrinsically procreative and rules out homosexuality, sterilization, and birth control.

The thirteenth was not the greatest of centuries for the theology of abortion. Small wonder Connery finds it "disappointing." Albert the Great revealed the central concern (which was for sex as necessarily procreative) by saying that sterilization is more damaging than abortion. Thomas Aquinas, in his entire *Summa,* has no articles on abortion at all. He only mentions the subject in answering two objections, one on accidental abortion and one on killing a woman to baptize her fetus. (Thomas said that was not to be done.) Elsewhere Thomas accepted the idea of delayed ensoulment. The thirteenth century did not share today's obsession with abortion.

Real analytical theological ethics of abortion began in the fifteenth century. Two Thomists set the tone for what would become common opinion into the eighteenth century. Antoninus, the archbishop of Florence, and John of Naples allowed early abortions of unanimated fetuses partly because of the perceived need for baptism and also for fear for the life of the woman from a late abortion, given the crude state of surgery then. These writers allowed probability as the basis for judgment whether or not the fetus was animated, giving the benefit of the doubt, in effect, to the woman. They did this even though they believed that baptism was necessary for salvation. This presaged the modern contention of scholars like Carole Tauer that the *dubium facti* of animation was equivalent to a *dubium juris,* in the language of later Probabilism, thus justifying some abortions as moral. The opinion approving direct early abortion became common in the church and was used in confessional practice.

The sixteenth century brought the influential Antoninus de Corduba into abortion theology. He said that if medicine of its nature is conducive to the health of the woman, even if it causes the abortion of an animated fetus, it may be used. The mother had a "prior right"; her health was more important than the life of the fetus. Thus bathing, bleeding, purgatives, or pain-killers could be used even though they were abortifacient. His language lacks the precision of early twentieth-century moral theology, but he clearly used a very broad reading of "saving the woman's life." It is hard to see the treatments he discusses as being a matter of life and death. Certainly, you could not kill a person just to save yourself from pain or to get your bowels moving. Corduba expanded the discussion.

Jesuit Thomas Sanchez, who died in the early seventeenth century, said all his contemporary theologians justified early abortions to save the woman. He introduced the idea which had much resonance that the fetus may be a quasi-aggressor. As Connery says: "Anyone who reads his text can hardly doubt that he is speaking of what later authors will call direct abortion." Catholic theology was struggling with the complexities of this issue and not succumbing to the panacea of a simplistic negative absolute.

After Sanchez, other theologians argued that the fetus is a kind of unjust aggressor at times . . . or that the fetus is not a formal but a material aggressor like an insane person, and that even causes like the woman's reputation might at times be enough to justify early, direct abortions. These Catholic theologians were allowed to debate the issue freely, and they did not believe like men (they were all men) who possessed a factotum principle that would solve all or almost all abortion questions.

In the mid-nineteenth century, *Revue Théologique* published an essay in which it was argued that an abortion could be performed to save a woman four or five months pregnant if she would bleed to death without the abortion. The Holy Office had already declined to solve such a case even though several of its members favored the abortion. The Jesuit Ballerini of the Roman College justified therapeutic abortions by using a novel distinction between the acceleration of the birth with the resultant death of the fetus, and direct attacks on the fetus. Another Jesuit, Augustine Lehmkuhl, who died in 1917, allowed the death of the animated fetus to save the life of the woman, and he called this a probable opinion. As was admitted at the time, this was direct abortion intended as a means. Lehmkuhl said the fetus could be assumed to have surrendered its right to life just as a person can give up a life jacket to a friend.

The nineteenth-century debates on craniotomy also showed more flexibility than the anti-moral-choice partisans today. In 1869 the Sacred Penitentiary referred a questioner on a craniotomy case to the "well-tested and reliable authors" (*auctores probati:* a term that is usually mistranslated "approved authors") for an answer. This, in effect, invoked the tradition of Probabilism for what is virtually infanticide. Even two editors of the Vatican's *Acta Sanctae Sedis* defended direct killing through craniotomy, as did a number of other theologians.

At the end of the nineteenth century, the Vatican changed its mind on these matters and tried to impose cloture on theological discussion. Here, of course, we leave moral theology and philosophy and enter ecclesiology. The ecclesiological question is: do the Vatican dicasteries possess a supernatural talent to see through and beyond the empirical complexities of these issues, and are they endowed with the exclusive power to reach beyond theology and philosophy to irrefragable absolutes that are immune to informed dissent? The primitive ecclesiology that affirms such tendentially magical power bears burdens of proof that cannot be met.

As these debates arrived into the twentieth century, we can see that they had not achieved a high level of clarity. Even the critical category "direct/indirect," which still dominates the conservative position today, was a greased pig that could not be tied down. In 1932, Gregorian University's Arthur Vermeersch marked out three different meanings of "direct/indirect," and the meanings have multiplied since Vermeersch. Those who say that the "clear and constant" Catholic teaching is that you may never directly terminate fetal life are standing on a loose philosophical plank. And it is a *philosophical* plank, not a given of faith.

The abortion debate in our day has taken on an intensity it never before had. It also has a new breadth for Catholics with Vatican II's recognition of the truly ecclesial nature of Protestant communions and with the arrival of laity and women into theology. It becomes even more inaccurate to speak of *the* Christian view. This is not to say that clerical theologians have not paid some dues on the issue. On the occasion of the Vatican attack on Charles Curran, hundreds of theologians internationally declared his work well within the perimeters of Catholic orthodoxy. He justifies abortion "to save human life" or for values "commensurate with human life." These commensurate values could be grave threats to the psychological health of the woman and extreme socioeconomic conditions. Richard McCormick, who is widely seen as a moderate in moral theology, finds Curran's position "very close" to his own and adds that abortion can be justified by other values "consistent with our assessment of the values justifying the taking of extrauterine life." Now, as ever, there is no one Christian view of the morality of abortion.

The negative absolutists on abortion say that the personhood question has been settled by modern embryology. This is a strange departure since the tradition has always maintained that there is something transcendent about personhood, something spiritual called a "soul" by the ancients. The mystery here cannot be settled by a materialistic and scientific analysis. The efforts to do so reveal the theological emptiness of the absolutists.

What comes close to being "clear and constant" in the tradition is the theory of what is called "delayed animation," or "ensoulment." For nineteen hundred years, the early conceptum was not seen as a person. Opinions have run the full gamut from conception to puberty! The Greek view of ensoulment in forty to ninety days was dominant, but the jurist Baldus and some of the Louvain theologians like John Marcus said the rational soul did not arrive until birth.

Significantly, there were and are no funerals for miscarriages. The Holy Office in 1713 forbade baptism of a fetus that was not well formed. St. Alphonsus Liguori spoke as a traditionalist when he said: "Some are mistaken who say that the fetus is ensouled from the first moment of its conception, since the fetus is certainly not animated before it is formed." The prestigious *Catechism of the Council of Trent* said that if Jesus was animated at conception it was a miracle because "in the natural order, no body can be informed by a human soul except after the prescribed space of time." Dominican H. M. Héring said in 1951 that the theory of delayed animation still had strong Catholic support "especially among the philosophers, who are wont to investigate the matter more profoundly than the moralists and the canonists." As Professor Carol Tauer says, if one were to argue for the presence of a rational soul, "there is better positive argument available for animals like mature dolphins than there is for human zygotes, morulae, and blastocysts."

THE MOST INTELLIGENT way to be anti-abortion is to look to the causes of unwanted pregnancies. Too often in the past we looked only at the woman with the crisis pregnancy, not to hear her, but to stone her, picket her, excommunicate her, and call our work pro-life. We should look rather to the causes that bring women to the clinic door and attack those rather than the woman.

I would list sexism as the first cause of unwanted pregnancies. Sexism is the belief that women are inferior, and how do you make love to an inferior? Carelessly and casually. This yields the hostile inseminator syndrome. It is hostility to enter a woman's body sexually, taking no account of the fact that you may thereby be entering the next century. In terms of Christian hope, the implications may be eternal.

Poverty brings women to the clinic door, since poverty breeds chaos and despair, and these breed unwanted pregnancies. In this light, the military budget can be seen as a major abortifacient in our society. The largely useless budget which sucks $35 million an hour, twenty-four hours a day out of our economic veins, causes social decay with its yield of unwanted pregnancies.

The surprised virgin syndrome leads to unwanted pregnancies. This is the inability to admit that the relationship is nearing the point where it could get sexual and that moral choices are called for. Counselors are told that "it just happened," but that is not candid since the onset of sexual ardor is noticeable.

The cult of romantic love produces unwanted pregnancies. The couple in the movie who tumble into bed for the final denouement are not to be interrupted for contraceptive indignities. The sacred exigencies of romantic love must be honored whatever the cost to the woman. And there are other social evils that contribute to unwanted pregnancies: the lack of sex education, the religious ban on contraception, and the negative attitudes toward sexuality that lead to eruptive sex.

Christians might best imitate the apostle Paul who, when he wrote to the sexually rambunctious Corinth, where abortion could have been no stranger, produced an epic song of love. The Judeo-Christian treasure houses a notion of love that could lead to more respectful relationships and more reverent sexual mores and fewer and fewer women at the clinic door.

As the abortion debate continues, I hope it would be freed from noxious and insulting analogies. The Holocaust imagery, used by Burtchaell and others, is repulsive in this context. It is offensive for Jewish people and other victims to be compared to blastocysts, embryos, and fetuses. It is especially galling when this is done by Catholics who, as a church, were not distinguished in their resistance to the real Holocaust. Slavery is another false analogue that equates pre-personal with personal life. And, once again, Catholics in this country were not in the forefront of the fight against slavery or for civil rights. Such analogies do not encourage the reasoned discourse that the problem of abortion needs.

James Tunstead Burtchaell

The men and women who first tried to follow the risen Jesus were Jews. They were not entirely unprepared for the moral demands this would make on them. The Christian road followed terrain already familiar to Jewish moral teaching. Infidelity was to be avoided in all its forms: adultery, incest, and idolatry. Believers were never to take crafty advantage of others, by perjury or sorcery or usury. And they were to restrain themselves from all violence, whether drunkenness, gossip, or murder. This ethical standard rests as firmly on rabbinical teaching as on the New Testament, which shows what a direct lineage there is from Hellenistic Judaism to early Christianity.

In the Sermon on the Mount Jesus invites his followers to go even further along this Way. It was not enough to spare your neighbor's life; you must not even hurl insults at him. If adultery was wrong, then so was lustful intent. And there was scant advantage from being a person of your sworn word if you were a chiseler whenever you were not under oath. Yet even this prophetic summons to a righteousness higher than that of the scribes and Pharisees would have found strong endorsement in many of the better synagogues around Judaea.

Christian moral doctrine showed its direct descent from Jewish ethics. It was ironic, then, that its great breakaway point of departure would be from one of the teachings Christians and Jews most closely shared. Both synagogue and church taught that authentic religion meant coming to the aid of women and children deprived of breadwinners, and of the indigent and the refugee aliens. Nothing could be more traditional for a Jew or more fundamental for a Christian than this ancient commitment to provide for the widow, the orphan, the pauper, the stranger. Yet it was precisely here that the young Christian community found a distinctive vigor and vision, and set forth from its mother's house on a moral journey of its own.

The alien and the pauper, the widow and the orphan, classic beneficiaries of preferential sustenance since Sinai, were suggestive to the Jesus people of four other forlorn categories that they must safeguard: the enemy and the slave, the wife and the infant — unborn or newborn.

The resident alien had to be guaranteed shelter, for he dwelt within the national enclosure of the land and trusted its people. But the Christian was bidden to go far beyond protecting the nearby alien. He was charged to cherish the distant enemy. He had heard it said that he must love his neighbor and hate his enemy. Jesus told him he must love his enemy even at the risk of receiving hatred from both his countrymen and his enemy. He was to set no more bounds to his bounty than the Father who lavished sunshine and rainfall on all fields alike. His pattern was the Lord Jesus, who had loved to the death those who betrayed and denied and deserted and condemned and crucified him.

The poor were always a special charge on the Christian's conscience. But their endless needs suggested another, even more vulnerable, group. For those "in the Lord," no one was any longer to be demeaned as mere property of another. Even slaves had to be dealt with as brothers and sisters in the Lord.

Every man was to join in supporting the wives his fellow believers had left behind as widows. But now he was startled to be told that he no longer had a male's freedom of choice to dismiss his own wife. Jesus' rejection of divorce affected men and women differently, since only husbands had previously been free to reject their partners. Now women could no longer be chosen and then discarded by their men. Both alike must now be faithful throughout life, if they loved and married in the Lord.

There were four radical, prophetic imperatives that the new Christian faith set before those who would live in the Spirit and fire of Christ: four disconcerting duties that would distance them from Jews and Romans alike. First, the command to love their enemies struck down forever their exclusionary allegiance to a single race or nation. Second, the command to acknowledge slaves and masters as brothers and sisters condemned slavery to a long and sullen retreat, and ultimately to extinction. Third, the command that husbands and wives were to pledge an equal fidelity was a first yet crucial rejection of the corruption of men and women by their respective domination and acquiescence. These were thunderclaps of moral exclamation that bound the small and scrappy new fellowship to make the purpose of their lives the liberation of those most at a loss.

And there was a fourth point of radical conversation, for there was a fourth group of victims they had to embrace: Beyond the children orphaned by their parents' deaths were those still more helpless children whom their parents slew themselves.

Early Jewish law seems to have regarded the unborn as paternal property. A monetary indemnity was due to the father from anyone who caused his wife to abort. By the time of Jesus some Jewish circles were ready to see the fully formed fetus as a protectable human being. But abortion law was scanty and ambiguous. Roman law in the same era offered no protection against either abortion or infanticide, both of which were within the prerogatives of the male head-of-household. Neither tradition offered a protection for infants reliable enough to suit the first Christians, and they soon stated their own conviction which was to the point.

The most ancient Christian document we possess, besides the New Testament, is called *The Didache, The Instruction of the Twelve Apostles.* Already in this first-century catechism, the obligation to protect the unborn and the infant was included within the roster of essential moral duties:

> You shall not commit murder, you shall not commit adultery; you shall not prey upon boys; you shall not fornicate; you shall not deal in magic; you shall not practice sorcery; you shall not murder a child by abortion, or kill a newborn; you shall not covet your neighbor's goods . . . (*Didache 2:2-3*).

In a later passage the instruction describes what it calls "the way of death":

> It is the path of those who persecute the innocent, despise the truth, find their ease in lying . . . those who have no generosity for the poor, nor concern for the oppressed, nor any knowledge of who it was who made them; they are killers of children, destroyers of God's handiwork; they turn their backs on the needy and take advantage of the afflicted; they are cozy with the affluent but ruthless judges of the poor; sinners to the core. Children, may you be kept safe from it all! (5:2).

The Greek is as straightforward as my translation, bluntly choosing works like "kill" (*apokteinein*) and "murder" (*phoneuein*). Its word for abortion, *phthora,* means, literally, "destruction," and the one destroyed is called "child," *teknon,* the same gentle word used in the final sentence to address the readers themselves.

Shortly before or after the turn of the second century, the *Letter of Barnabas* repeats the *Didache's* injunction against abortion and infanticide in virtually the same words, and laments that they destroy small images of God (*Barnabas* 19:5; 20:2).

Early in the second century the Christian movement had achieved momentum enough to arouse antagonism in Roman society. Some of the most articulate writers of that age were apologists defending their fellow Christians against libel. And one of the slanders that outraged them most was the rumor that Christians slew infants to obtain blood for their eucharistic rites. It was a particularly galling lie, precisely because protection of the young had become such a Christian priority. These apologists did not conceal their contempt for the surrounding pagan society which was willing to destroy its young by choice. Minucius Felix, a Roman attorney of African origin, states the contrast angrily.

> There is a man I should now like to address, and that is the one who claims, or believes, that our initiations take place by means of the slaughter and blood of a baby. Do you think it possible to inflict fatal wounds on a baby so tender and tiny? That there could be anyone who would butcher a newborn babe, hardly yet a human being, who would shed and drain its blood? The only people capable of believing this is one capable of actually

> perpetrating it. And, in fact, it is a practice of yours, I observe, to expose your own children to birds and wild beasts, or at times to smother and strangle them — a pitiful way to die; and there are women who swallow drugs to stifle in their womb the beginnings of a man on the way — committing infanticide even before they give birth to their infant (*Octavius* 30:1-2).

The same rumor was challenged by Athenagoras of Athens. How could Christians be accused of murder when they refused even to attend the circus events where humans perished as gladiators or as victims of wild beasts? Christians consider, he wrote, that even standing by and tolerating murder was much the same as murder itself. He then continues:

> We call it murder and say it will be accountable to God if women use instruments to procure abortion: how shall we be called murderers ourselves? The same person cannot regard that which a woman carries in her womb as a living creature, and therefore as an object of value to God, and then slay the creature that has come forth to the light of day (*Embassy for the Christians* 35).

Tertullian, perhaps the most eloquent of the second-century apologists, repeatedly opposed the teaching of the Stoics that children are not yet alive in the womb, and that their soul is given them at birth. Arguing from philosophical more than biological grounds, he insisted that the body and soul grow together from the beginning.

> We have established the principle that all the natural potentialities of the soul with regard to sensation and intelligence are inherent in its very substance, as a result of the intrinsic nature of the soul. As the various stages of life pass, these powers develop, each in its own way, under the influence of circumstances, whether of education, environment, or of the supreme powers (*De Anima* 38:1; see also 37).

Abortion, he said, was not only homicide, it was parricide: the slaying of one's own flesh and blood.

> With us, murder is forbidden once for all. We are not free to destroy anyone conceived in the womb, while the blood is still being absorbed to build up the human being. To prevent the birth of a child is simply a swifter way to murder. It makes no difference whether one destroys a soul already born or interferes with it on its way to birth. It is a human being and one who will be a human being, for every fruit is there present in the seed (*Apologeticum* 9:8; see also 9:4-7).

Even in the case of a child whose uterine position makes birth impossible, when Tertullian would accept dismemberment to save the mother's life, he bluntly says the child is being "butchered by unavoidable savagery" (*De Anima* 25:4).

These are statements Christian apologists were making to outsiders. Among themselves, abortion continued to be reviled as a procedure unthinkable for believers. Clement of Alexandria, perhaps the leading theologian of the second century, wrote:

> If we would only control our lusts at the start, and if we would refrain from killing off the human race born or developing according to the divine plan, then our entire lives would be lived in harmony with nature as well. But women who resort to some sort of deadly abortion drug slay not only the embryo but, along with it, all human love [*philanthropia*] (*The Pedagogue* 96).

Early in the next century Hippolytus of Rome condemned bishop Callistus for his readiness to encourage marriage, legal or otherwise, between affluent women and lower-class or slave-class men. Such unions, he observed, had only tended to encourage abortion.

> Women who pass for believers began to resort to drugs to induce sterility, and to bind their abdomens tightly so as to abort the conceptus, because they did not want to have a child by a slave or lower-class type, for the sake of their family pride and their excessive wealth. Look what abuse of duty this lawless man has encouraged, by inciting them both to adultery and to murder. And after such outrageous activity they have the nerve to call themselves a Catholic church! (*Refutation of All Heresies* 9:12:25).

These forthright voices from the first and formative Christian years all argued that the destruction of the child — unborn or newborn — is infamy for those who follow Christ.

Now I CALL your attention to five facts, five aspects of that early Christian conviction, which we should note and take to heart. First, the repudiation of abortion was not an isolated or esoteric doctrine. It formed part of an obligation by all believers to protect the four categories of people whom they now saw as peculiarly exposed to the whim and will of their fellow humans: the slave, the enemy, the wife, the infant — unborn or newborn. These were at great risk, as were the four traditional protégés: the poor, the alien, the widow, the orphan. And this fourfold obligation was preached across the full expanse of the church: from Carthage to Egypt and up into Syria, then across Greece and in Rome.

Second, this was not a program simply for the more strenuous. It was presented as the imperative agenda for the church, the test for all discipleship. Believers were warned away from abortion as they were from adultery, murder, greed, and theft. The four Christian innovations were offered as the classic new signs of authenticity. If theirs was not a community where Jew and Gentile, man and woman, slave and free could show forth as one, then it failed to be Christian. That was their test.

Third, though these exhortations show a sensitive and compassionate sympathy for the victims, their principal moral concern is for the oppressors. It is the husband that bullies his wife whose person dwindles even more sadly than hers. The master or mistress who abuses the slave sustains an injury even greater than what the slave experiences. It is the mother who eliminates her son that Clement cares about, because she must destroy her *philanthropia* as well, her love for humankind, in order to do it. The disease of character that follows from exploitation of others was seen, in Christian perspective, to be more hideously incapacitating than the worst that befell victims. It could be a death far worse than death. Even when they enter the contemporary dispute over the ensoulment of the unborn, these writers dismiss it as a quibble when it comes to abortion: it is the same ruthless willingness to eliminate unwelcome others that shows itself in the slaying of the unborn, the newborn, or the parent. In truest Christian perspective, it is the oppressor who is destroyed.

Fourth, these writers knew well that any true protection of the helpless and exploited calls for a stable empowerment, so that those same people will not continue to be victimized. This means that the Christian moral agenda demands a price. Oppressors must give up their advantage. It little matters whether the advantage was seized purposefully or inherited unwittingly. There is suffering to be accepted by those in power if the disadvantaged and helpless are to be afforded true protection.

But there is a further sacrifice to be made. The victims must accept suffering as well. The price they must pay — if they are to be Christians — is that they must forgo resentment and hatred. Empowerment cannot be grasped as the means to take revenge or, still worse, as the way to begin to be an exploiter oneself. The victims must gaze directly upon those who have taken advantage of them, and recognize them as brothers and sisters who themselves may have been pressed by distress of one kind or another. So there is no moral accomplishment possible unless reconciliation extends the hand of fellowship across the battle line of suffering. There will be heavy and sometimes bitter things to accept if hatred is to be extinguished, and not merely aimed in a new direction.

Fifth, we must note that this was a rigorous duty presented to our Christian ancestors. The light was dazzling, and they often preferred to draw back into the cover of darkness. They and we have sinned against that light. Christians continued to relish and even to justify hatred against their enemies. They did not set the slaves free. Women were not welcomed into full and equal status. And parents continued to destroy their young.

Every person interested enough to follow this debate is aware that we live in an extraordinary age. Four great movements have stirred us round the world: (1) a movement for world peace that is more than a weariness of war; it is making bold and positive ventures towards the reduction of enmity and distrust; (2) a movement for the relief of bondage of every sort; freedom from slavery and from racial subjection, dignity for the worker, status for the migrant; (3) a movement for equality of women and a more integrated companionship with men, so that family and work can be humanized for each and for both together, and (4) a movement to rescue children from abortion, infanticide, infant mortality, and every sort of neglect and predatory danger.

In the trough of some of the most genocidal carnage and oppressive bondage and degradation of women and slaughter of innocent children, our era may be unusual in the readiness of some to listen to that bold and visionary Christian age whose teaching I have held up to your minds and memories.

Each of these movements is bent on empowerment. If the exploited do arise and claim their rightful places, will they take power like Spartacus or Robespierre or Pol Pot? Or will they take power like Mahatma Gandhi and Nelson Mandela . . . like Jesus? Christians may make the difference. This fourfold phalanx of conscience on the march is only partly Christian in origin. But I say that Christians will mean much to these movements of grace, and these movements must mean much to us.

We, possibly more than others, must immediately recognize that these various struggles are in alliance with each other. None can be pitted against another. The United States, for instance, must never imagine that enmity between nations will be subdued if our neighbors are in bondage to us. Enslavement and enmity must both vanish. Likewise, the movement of enhancement for women will never be furthered by making their children expendable. In America today abortion is said to involve a conflict of rights, a conflict of interests between women and their children. A Christian must hold suspect any human right which must be guaranteed by another human's elimination.

Another Christian contribution will be to tell all those who stand to lose power that it is in their highest interest to do so. For they have truly withered under the weight of their exploitative advantages. To say this to them with any credibility, we must first be utterly persuaded that oppressors suffer an even more tragic injury than their victims. Are you really ready to believe that the staff of Auschwitz perished in a worse tragedy than those they exterminated? Do you mourn more for the two thousand or so abortionists in America than for the eighteen million or so infants they have efficiently butchered? Were you more dismayed about Bull Connor than about Martin Luther King, Jr.? Or if you do believe that, can you say believably that you care for the mothers who destroy their unborn children, for they stand to lose even more than do their tragically destroyed offspring.

There is another characteristic Christian insight needed in the abortion struggle. We must see and say how often it is that women who victimize their children are themselves handicapped by never having enjoyed control over their own lives. They are victims . . . even though they are victims who destroy others.

How often it is that some helpless group is savaged by aggressors who have themselves been victims. They are survivors of outrage, and they now seek to relieve their stress and suffering by turning on others who are weaker still. Victims exploiting victims.

What is the background of parents who abuse and batter their children? A childhood of violence, incest, contempt. Victims lashing out at victims.

And who are aborting their daughters and sons today? Women and men who are alienated, abused, poor, who are at a loss to manage their own lives or intimacies. Victims destroyed, destroying victims.

Hate them — hate any victimizers — and you are simply cheering on the cycle of abuse and violence. Suppress your rage well enough to look closely and humanely at drug dealers, at rapists, at pathological prison guards, and you may see it there too: the same pathetic look of the battered spirit, preying on others wantonly.

Women who are desperate or autistic enough to destroy their children are among society's most abused victims. We owe them every help. But a truly compassionate support could never invite them to assuage their own anger by exterminating those more helpless still. It is by breaking the savage cycle of violence that victimization is laid to rest.

When you grasp the uplifted hand to prevent one injured person from striking out at another, you must do so in love, not in anger, for you are asking that person to absorb suffering rather than pass it on to another. And, to be a peacemaker, you must be as ready to sustain as you are to restrain. One must be more than just to accept injustice, yet deal out justice.

Our belief is in a Lord who was the innocent victim of injustice. Yet he caught the impact of that injustice in his own body, his own self. He deadened it and refused to pass it on, he refused to let the hatred go on ricocheting through humankind. If we truly follow him we are committed to doing the same. And the truest test of that faith is whether we have the gumption to share it with others, with those who are treating others unjustly, but especially with people who are victims. We must prevail upon them to let us help them catch the impact of their distress in their own bodies, and in our own selves alongside theirs, without permitting the cycle of violence to carry on.

The fire of Pentecost rapidly enflamed the Christian community to a sense of what it was about. These Christians were in so many ways an observant Jewish movement: in their worship, their hopes, their moral way of life. But in two great matters they burst forth as men and women possessed by a new Spirit. They witnessed to the Resurrection: Jesus, at whose unjust execution they had been inert and disengaged, was risen to power as Messiah and Lord. That was the first great matter.

The second was like it. They too had been raised to unexpected power, and they stated with vehemence that they would no longer be passive before affliction. That determination was embodied in the entirely distinctive and innovative moral commitment to befriend the enemy, to embrother the slave, to raise up the wife, and to welcome the child. Their own lives were at stake, for these Christians believed that they would perish in their persons if they proved nonchalant about the suffering of any of these most vulnerable brothers and sisters. They rushed to their task, for many others' lives depended on them: the lives of those so powerful they could crush others without noticing; and the lives of their victims — unnoticed, undefended, even unnamed.

The revolt against abortion was no primitive and narrow dogma that a more sophisticated church has now outgrown. It was in the very center of the moral life by which the church first defined itself before the Lord and before the world. We have not yet approached it, and some speak of having surpassed it. Those first disciples who reverenced every unwanted child, born or unborn, would have been stupefied by the sight of their own children in the faith gainsaying this or any of that fourfold commitment. Were we to forswear the hated enemy, the enslaved laborer, the subjected woman, or the defenseless infant, and do that in his name, Christ would have died in vain.

In this debate we are asking whether recent developments and reflection give us authentic reasons to reconsider what the *Didache* and Athenagoras and Tertullian and our other ancestors in faith held to be essential. I say to you we have never had more reasons to reconsider their teaching. And I say that their teaching has never rung more defiantly as the prophetic call of Christ.

Maguire

John Courtney Murray used to say that disagreement is a rare achievement. We have achieved it in this debate. Burtchaell finds his position on abortion "in the very center of the moral life by which the church defined itself." The theological record does not support this simplistic contention.

Our differences are primarily methodological. Burtchaell designates the *Didache,* Athenagoras, Tertullian, and others as his "Scripture" since Scripture does not support his position. The difference is not that he goes to these texts and those of us who differ with him do not. The difference is that he finds in these texts what is not there. You cannot extract from words like *teknon* or *trucidatur* a revolution of consciousness on abortion. This kind of text-proofing and ignoring of the *Sitz im Leben* would not be tolerated in biblical exegesis.

What Burtchaell does is not good ethics. He wants to find an ideal in various disparate texts and leap from there to very practical conclusions in ethics that apply transculturally and transtemporally. James Gustafson and others have long warned of this temptation to avoid homework by rushing from perceived ideals to simple conclusions. Aquinas says that "human actions are good or bad according to their circumstances," and that moral life is marked by "*quasi infinitae diversitates.*" The tough part of ethics is the circumstantial analysis in which we confront these *diversitates.* Burtchaell would spare us this by claiming to find an ideal that solves all (or almost all) abortion cases for all time.

Moral meaning does not just come from ideals. It is also housed in principles, and it is incarnate in the circumstances of flesh and life. The moral decision is born at the interstices of all these sources of moral meaning. Burtchaell purveys a perceived ideal and then rushes to a conclusion that binds all kinds of people in all kinds of circumstances. I find in this approach the seeds of fanaticism. Even the old Penitentials that dominated Catholic thought for centuries were more capable of making distinctions where there were differences. They could allege that adultery was more serious than abortion. They tried for some sense of differentiation in their analysis of reality. Burtchaell fails here.

Burtchaell also assumes, what the Christian tradition did not, that the human embryo is a child, a baby, a person. Fifty-one percent of all abortions are done before the embryo has become a fetus. Even the Vatican, which is not shy in these matters, has not tried to settle the ensoulment question. Burtchaell is more dogmatic than the tradition, which recognized doubt and gave the woman the benefit thereof.

Burtchaell would put all abortions, except the ones he approves of, in the category of butchery and murder. That makes forty to fifty million women butchers and murderesses every year. That is a sweeping judgment of a huge part of humanity, the feminine part, and the implications of that judgment, as I have said, are sexist.

In his opening statement, Burtchaell said many beautiful things beautifully. At times, I wished I could be entirely on his side. Our paths part when we come to the thorns of conflict situations where I find him guilty of oversimplification. Burtchaell dismisses Probabilism, which theologians use to justify some abortions. The *doubt of fact* on embryonic and fetal personhood has been treated as a *doubt of law;* the basic assumptions of Probabilism were used even before the theory was formulated.

In conclusion, I return to my keynote positions that neither of us is pro-abortion. We would both like to see conditions which would make abortion less likely. We differ in our sense of the tragic possibility that those conditions are not always present.

Burtchaell

Professor Maguire points out that he does not read the Christian record as a constant support for the moral imperative against abortion. He is correct. The record of the church is no more honorable in its pursuit of that early commitment than it is in support of the early commitment to make slaves truly brothers and sisters. Nor would we want to use the history of the church to vindicate its failure to pursue its early insights regarding even companionship between women and men. On the contrary, there has been a great slumbering, denial, turning of the back on these convictions.

Professor Maguire also says that in Utopia abortion would be almost unnecessary. I do not think it is our task to frame ethics for Utopia. Nor do I think that Jesus was asking people to be just only when the world settled down to being just in return. Anyone who agrees to accept injustice without retaliating knows that she or he is not following a utopian ethic. *All* of these characteristically Christian moral imperatives require a readiness to do the good and life-giving thing because one is determined to *do* justice, not merely because one can count on *receiving* justice.

"Are the many women who have committed abortion evil?" Professor Maguire asks. Are the many men who bullied them into it evil? Are the many men who aborted them evil? Those who have recounted their experiences to me deplore beyond anything else in their entire lives the destruction of their own children. I have known them to have carried this sadness for weeks, months . . . as long as sixty years. It was I who found myself trying to draw them away from the conviction that they must be evil, trying to draw them into a resolve that now they must turn and offer their lives to other helpless people who needed them. It was not I who was pointing the finger at them, but they who seemed to have sensed that people who do evil things to others wither. We all carry around the scars and handicaps and disablements of the advantage we have taken of others from time to time. I think it is entirely specious and sentimental to say: "So many have done it." So many have done a lot of things.

Lastly, I must disallow my opponent's use of Probabilism. Professor Maguire knows very well, for he is a well enough trained professor of ethics, that the tradition which developed the theology of Probabilism absolutely vetoed its use in any matter like abortion. Probabilism says that where there is confusion — legitimate, objective confusion — among good-minded people without a conflict of interest about the requirements of moral obligation, then you may follow a lenient course except when that more permissive choice might do harm to another, in which case you may not follow a probable opinion but must pursue the safer course. You may not go out and fire off your 30.06 rifle in the woods at every sound behind a bush. Indeed, when there is doubt, and when injury might follow, all benefit of doubt accrues to the potential victim. Therefore the doctrine of Probabilism would say: until the question of personhood of the unborn at various stages is resolved, all benefit of doubt goes to the potential victim.

121 Ahead to Our Past: Abortion and Christian Texts

Michael J. Gorman

According to a sympathetic but critical reviewer, The Durham Declaration "makes a significant contribution to the church's reflection on the abortion issue . . . by attempting to address it from a distinctly biblical and theological perspective while avoiding the language of rights that dominates all political discourse in the United States and the abortion debate in particular."[1] This "distinctly biblical and theological perspective" is an effort to view the abortion issue in a broad, rather than a narrow, framework that is shaped by the ethics of the New Testament.[2] The Declaration is also a deliberate attempt to reappropriate historical Christian texts and practices within this New Testament framework.[3]

The aim of this essay is first to identify and explore the significance of the Declaration's New Testament foundations, then to examine specific early Christian attitudes and practices regarding abortion and closely related issues, and finally to suggest some ways in which the texts and practices discussed speak to the church today. Before pursuing those tasks, however, we must first acknowledge the New Testament's silence on abortion per se and determine the proper questions to ask in pursuing a perspective on abortion grounded in the New Testament.

A. Asking the Right Questions

The silence of the Bible generally, and the New Testament specifically, on abortion has been a source of distress for many Christians. It has led to a wide range of interpretations — from assertions of early Christian ignorance of or apathy toward the issue, to belief in divine apathy ("If the Bible is silent, can God care?"), to attempts at discovering prooftexts that demonstrate Christianity's (and God's) condemnation or approval.

As we will see below, there are historical reasons for the New Testament's silence on abortion. Ironically, when this silence is understood historically, it proves to speak quite loudly. For now, however, our task is to engage the New Testament in the discussion of a topic that it does not directly address.

To use the Bible in facing the abortion issue is no simple task. We must first recognize, however, that even if the canon spoke a clear No! on the abortion issue, the church would almost certainly still have a debate on its hands. In the face of the canon's silence and the likelihood of debate even if it spoke clearly, we must phrase our questions properly. Two appropriate questions are the following:

1. To what kind of ethical perspectives and moral life does the New Testament bear witness through its narratives and arguments, its claims and convictions, and how should that affect our view of abortion?

2. To what kind of moral lives and views of abortion have earlier generations of Christians been called through their reflection on scriptural, especially New Testament, texts and themes?

The first question reflects a particular view of the role of the New Testament in Christian moral thinking: it shapes our basic perspectives and molds our individual and corporate character (virtues actualized in deeds). The second reflects a belief in the Church universal and in the Holy Spirit as the one who has inspired the Church in other times and places. The focus of this paper will be on the early Church, which has a claim to unique importance because of its proximity to Jesus and the apostles and its pervasive influence on later Christian faith and practice.

The thesis of this paper, and the contention of The Durham Declaration, is that the New Testament, both in principle and as embodied in early Christian communities, leads us away from abortion, toward protecting and welcoming the unborn, and toward providing compassionate care to those in need.

1. Barry Penn Hollar, "Increasing the Burden on Women: An Appreciative, but Critical Response to the Durham Declaration, on the Abortion Issue," *Christian Social Action* (July/August 1991): 28.

2. It is, in Professor Hauerwas's words, a statement of "those deep [specifically Christian] convictions that make our rejection of abortion intelligible" (Stanley Hauerwas, "Abortion: Why the Arguments Fail," in James T. Burtchaell, ed., *Abortion Parley* [New York: Andrews and McMeel, 1980], p. 325).

3. Harvard historian George H. Williams once suggested that a long-standing general Protestant silence on fetal value and abortion is due to the general Protestant zeal for the principle of *sola Scriptura,* which has often led to ignorance of all early Christian beliefs and practices not specifically recorded in the canonical New Testament ("Religious Residues and Presuppositions in the American Debate on Abortion," *Theological Studies* 31 [1970]: 42). The United Methodist Church's Social Principles do refer to the Christian tradition about abortion, but only to the (implicitly common and most significant) instances of establishing criteria, for choosing abortion under certain circumstances. The text of the Social Principles (Paragraph 71G) reads, in part: "In continuity with past Christian teaching, we recognize tragic conflicts of life with life that may justify abortion, and in such cases support the legal option of abortion under medical procedures."

From Michael J. Gorman, "Ahead to Our Past: Abortion and Christian Texts," in Paul T. Stallsworth, ed., *The Church and Abortion: In Search of New Ground for Response* (Nashville: Abingdon Press, 1993).

B. The Framework of the Declaration: Fundamental Affirmations

The Durham Declaration rests on three fundamental New Testament convictions:

1. We are not our own, but God's.
2. We are members of Christ and of one another.
3. Welcoming children is an integral part of Christian discipleship.

In other words, the Declaration is built on basic New Testament teachings about the human body, the Christian body, and children. To these three, a fourth should be added that is necessary to complete a New Testament framework for viewing any moral concern:

4. The age of shalom (peace) has begun in the life of Jesus and his Church.

In its own way, each of these convictions was and is a radical challenge to normal perceptions of reality and morality.

1. The Human Body

The Declaration begins with an appeal to Paul's fundamental text on the nature of Christian freedom with respect to the body (I Cor. 6:12-20). In Paul's day, many Corinthian believers associated Christian faith with the realm of the spirit alone, not the body. They believed that no bodily action — not even sex with prostitutes, probably at pagan temples — could adversely affect their relationship to God and, therefore, that they had the right and freedom to do whatever they wished with their bodies.[4]

Paul counters these attitudes by asserting the importance of the physical body as an integral part of the self: the body — or the embodied self — will be raised on the last day, is a "member" of Christ's body, is a temple of the Holy Spirit, and — most importantly — has been purchased (a metaphor for the ransom of slaves) by God through the death of Christ. "You are not your own [lord]; you were bought with a price," says the apostle. For Paul, Christians do not belong to themselves; they have relinquished control of their lives and bodies to God who redeemed them, to Christ who died for them, and to the Spirit who indwells them. They no longer live for themselves, looking to assert their own rights, but for the God to whom they now belong.[5] Freedom consists not of asserting one's desires and rights — this is giving opportunity to the "flesh" (see Gal. 5) — but of yielding one's body, soul, and mind in service to God and others.

St. Paul's perspective, that Christians belong not to themselves but to Another, is at the core of his Christian ethics and is echoed in various ways throughout the entire New Testament. Such a vision is fundamentally at odds with the world, where individuals seek to exercise ultimate control over their own lives and bodies, using their bodies not for divine service but for self-service. Like the Corinthians, many contemporary Christians, both male and female, believe that they are their own masters, with the right to do as they please with their own bodies.

The New Testament perspective is completely antithetical to this notion. It is, therefore, completely antithetical to the claim that there is a divinely granted right to engage in whatever form of sexual activity one prefers, or to choose an abortion because there is a divinely given gift of freedom to do with one's body whatever one wishes to do. For Paul and the New Testament generally, that is not freedom but slavery. The Pauline/New Testament perspective, therefore, challenges two of the dominant cultural values of our day that have too often been absorbed and advocated by spokespersons for the church — virtually unlimited sexual and procreative freedom.[6] The Declaration begins with a direct assault on these two pillars of the case for abortion.

2. The Christian Body

The assertion of absolute choice in sexual and procreative matters is a manifestation of our culture's obsession with individual rights that impacts the Christian church in other ways, too. The Declaration continues with a statement of the nature and mission of the church in contrast to this rampant individualism. For many Christians, the church is still a voluntary association of individuals who convene weekly but who actually exist as individuals responsible for and to themselves alone. When serious emotional, financial, or other kinds of problems develop, many Christians look at best to the pastor or other church leaders, at worst to no one in the church at all. A woman's unplanned or crisis pregnancy is perhaps the most isolating and difficult of such experiences.

The New Testament, in such passages as I Corinthians 12 and Ephesians 4, depicts the church as a human body that consists of interdependent parts — connected people who are mutually supportive, responsible, and accountable; people who learn and practice the ways of Christ together in community. Moreover, the kind of love that exists in this fellowship extends to others in need. It was this kind of vision of community that motivated early Chris-

4. Furthermore, some Christians may have been attracted to this particular form of sex because of the frequent connection in pagan religion between sexual experience and experience of the divine. Certain recent understandings of sexuality that equate, or nearly equate, erotic love with divine love are more pagan than Christian.

5. Implicit in I Corinthians 6 and explicit elsewhere (e.g., Romans 6) is the Pauline conviction that prior to Christian faith people are slaves to sin and to self; afterwards they are "slaves" — willing servants — to righteousness and to God.

6. It is difficult to miss the similarity between some of the current theologies of sexual and procreative freedom and the errors described in II Peter 2:17-22, where certain leaders, "uttering loud boasts of folly, . . . entice with licentious passions of the flesh those who have barely escaped from those who live in error, promising them freedom while they themselves are slaves of corruption; for by whatever you are overcome, to that you are enslaved" (vv. 18-19 RSV [with alterations]).

tians to band together to serve one another and the world. In fact, the text of I Corinthians 12 inspired Basil of Caesarea, a monk of the late fourth century, to organize monasteries whose purpose was not merely to pray and study but to serve.[7] This led to the establishment of the first Christian hospitals, hospices, and orphanages.

3. *Children*

Few episodes in the life of Jesus had as much impact on the shape of early Christian morality and ministry as did the well-known encounters between Jesus and the children. When Jesus' disciples attempt to prevent children from approaching their master (Mark 10:13-16 and parallels), Jesus' reaction is startling: he is indignant.[8] It is only in historical perspective that Jesus' attitude and action, and its effect on the early Christians, can be fully understood.[9] Among the Jews, rabbis classified children along with the deaf, mute, and mentally deficient. Elsewhere in the Roman Empire children were thought of as no better. In Roman custom and law children were understood to be the property of their father. Furthermore, fathers had the legal right to discard or kill children who were of the "wrong" (i.e., female) gender or who were "imperfect" — deformed or handicapped.[10] If exposed at the local garbage heap, the children who survived would often be picked up to be made into slaves or prostitutes.

In this context it is very clear that the Kingdom of God reverses normal human values. People taken to be of no value by other people take on infinite value.[11] Jesus' treatment of children inaugurated nothing less than the elevation of their status from the marginalized, even the disposable, to full persons. Moreover, Jesus made it clear that one's reception of children is determinative of one's reception of Jesus, his Father, and the Kingdom: "whoever welcomes one such child in my name welcomes me, and whoever welcomes me, welcomes not me but him who sent me" (Mark 9:37).

7. See his *Longer Rules* 7.

8. The Greek word used in Mark's narrative (10:14) to describe Jesus' extreme anger at his disciples is used of Jesus nowhere in the New Testament.

9. For a readable account of the situation, see Hans-Ruedi Weber, *Jesus and the Children: Biblical Resources for Study and Preaching* (Geneva: World Council of Churches, 1979). See also Ian Stockton, "Children, Church, and Kingdom," *Scottish Journal of Theology* 36 (1983): 87-97.

10. A famous letter testifying to the common acceptance of such attitudes has been preserved from the first century B.C. In that letter a husband who is away on a military assignment writes to his wife, who is about to give birth to their child, as follows: "if it is a male child, let it live; if it is female, cast it out." (The text of this letter may be found in various sources, including C. K. Barrett, *The New Testament Background: Selected Documents* [New York: Harper & Row, 1961], p. 38.)

11. The infinite worth of children is finally revealed in the cross. As the Declaration, drawing on Karl Barth, affirms, even the unborn child "is one for whom the Son of God died" (see Karl Barth, *Church Dogmatics* III/4 [Edinburgh: T. & T. Clark, 1961], p. 416).

Jesus did not, however, limit his full humanization of the marginalized to children; he similarly elevated the status and value of women. Although the early Church did not always implement Jesus' example fully, it was extremely sensitive to the needs of women and children who most often were not otherwise treated as neighbors: widows and orphans. As the Declaration notes (footnote 1 in chapter 1 [of *The Church and Abortion*]), the early Church's commitment to the orphan and widow was universally recognized and exercised.

4. *Shalom*

The Durham Declaration is built primarily on the three New Testament themes discussed above. One additional biblical and early Christian theme that is absolutely essential to any description of Christian morality is that of shalom, which means "divine peace and justice" or "eschatological wholeness." The Hebrew Scriptures point forward to a time when violence will cease and when peace, security, and justice will reign. Jesus taught that this promised age of shalom, often referred to as the Kingdom (or Reign) of God, broke into history in his ministry and was to take effect in the common life of his followers: "Blessed are the makers of shalom" (Matthew 5:9). The New Testament and other early Christian writers share this conviction, too, believing that the age to come, the age of peace and justice, has begun in the life and mission of Jesus and in the community of his followers who are assured and empowered by the Resurrection and Spirit of Jesus.[12]

Beginning in the first century, Christians lived in peace by refraining from violence, fighting spiritual rather than military battles (see Ephesians 6), and engaging in concrete acts of peacemaking. This continued into the second century and beyond, when writers such as Justin Martyr (c. 150) expressed their conviction that the Christian community fulfilled the prophecies of a time of shalom in the following manner: "We who were full of war and murder of one another and all evil have everywhere changed our instruments of war — swords into plows and spears into farm tools."[13] This moral vision was articulated in a world that was, in the estimation of the early Church, engulfed in violence and bloodshed.

12. Professor Hauerwas summarizes this view and its relationship to the protection of human life as follows: "As members of such a kingdom [of peace], moreover, we are pledged to extend God's peace through the care and protection of his creation. . . . Therefore the Christian commitment to the protection of life is an eschatological commitment. Our concern to protect and enhance life is a sign of our confidence that in fact we live in a new age in which it is possible to see the other as God's creation. . . . The risk of so valuing life can only be taken on the basis of the resurrection of Jesus as God's decisive eschatological act. . . . Peace has been made possible by the resurrection" (*The Peaceable Kingdom: A Primer in Christian Ethics* [Notre Dame, Ind.: University of Notre Dame Press, 1983], pp. 88-89).

13. *Dialogue with Trypho* 110 (author's translation).

Early Christians perceived in their culture an "interlocking directorate of death,"[14] which stretched from abortions to gladiator spectacles to crucifixions. Their response was to forsake violence and to form a new army engaging in a new form of warfare: "an army without weapons, without warfare, without bloodshed . . . [supporting] old men, orphans dear to God, widows . . .";[15] "[our] warfare is justice itself."[16] One form of this "warfare" called shalom was opposition to abortion, and support of children left to die.[17]

C. Abortion and the Early Christian Moral Vision

The four basic New Testament perspectives we have examined — on the human body, the Christian body, children, and shalom (justice/non-violence) — helped create a moral vision that produced a distinctly Christian attitude toward abortion and related issues (e.g., exposure and infanticide), as well as a ministry to women and children in need that complemented their attitude.[18] The Christians' new perspectives confirmed and strengthened the opposition to abortion that already existed among their Jewish forebears, whose condemnation of induced abortion (with the exception of therapeutic abortion) is heard in Philo, Josephus, and popular early Jewish moralists.[19]

Building on its Jewish heritage, the early Church was, indeed, a vocal opponent of abortion. The unified voice of early Christian writings on the abortion issue includes some of the most important documents of the early Christian era. In fact, the three earliest documents that mention (and condemn) abortion were extraordinarily popular and widely distributed, considered by many of those who read and heard them to be inspired Scripture: the *Didache, The Instruction of the Twelve Apostles;* the *Epistle of Barnabas;* and the *Apocalypse of Peter.* These Jewish-Christian documents from the late first and early second centuries were included in many of the early Christian canons (lists of inspired Scripture) and were, therefore, functionally part of the New Testament for many Christians for many years.[20] Eventually these writings were found to be Post-apostolic and were therefore omitted from the final New Testament canon, henceforth categorized as "profitable," but not authoritative, texts.[21]

It is clear, therefore, that Christian leaders, who used the criterion of orthodoxy as one essential test of a document's claim to a place in the canon or in the Church's devotional life, considered opposition to abortion to be an orthodox Christian belief. It is important to recognize, then, that early Christianity saw rejection of abortion as consonant with the teachings of Jesus and the Christian gospel.[22]

The early Christian attitude toward abortion can be analyzed in several ways. One helpful way to approach the topic is to look at the Church's perspectives on four of its dimensions: the unborn child, the act of abortion, the moral agent who obtains or performs the abortion, and pastoral responses to abortion.

14. The term is from Daniel Berrigan, who decries this country's "interlocking directorate of death that binds our culture, stretching from the Pentagon to the abortion clinic" (interview, "The Dying and the Unborn," *Reflections* reprint, n.d.).

15. Clement of Alexandria, *Who Is the Rich Man That Is Saved?* (author's translation).

16. Lactantius *Divine Institutions* 6.20.10.15-17 (*The Ante-Nicene Fathers,* vol. VII, ed. Alexander Roberts and James Donaldson [New York: Charles Scribner's Sons, 1899]).

17. For further discussion of the meaning of shalom and its relation to abortion, see Michael J. Gorman, "Shalom and the Unborn," *Transformation* 3 (January-March 1986): 26-33.

18. For a more detailed description of this entire topic, see Michael J. Gorman, *Abortion and the Early Church: Christian, Jewish, and Pagan Attitudes in the Greco-Roman World* (InterVarsity and Paulist, 1982), and G. Bonner, "Abortion and Early Christian Thought," in ed. J. H. Channer, *Abortion and the Sanctity of Human Life* (Greenwood, S.C.: Attic Press, 1985), pp. 93-122.

19. No known ancient Jew supported abortion except to save the mother's life. For further discussion, see Gorman, *Abortion and the Early Church,* chapter 3.

20. The failure to recognize the widespread authority, canonicity, and use of early Christian documents condemning abortion is one of the chief reasons for erroneous conclusions like that of Beverly W. Harrison in *Our Right to Choose: Toward a New Ethic of Abortion* (Boston: Beacon, 1983), who argues for a "widespread silence about abortion in early Christian writings" (p. 134). She further contends that "apart from [the *Didache*], . . . explicit denunciations of abortion, separate from views on the irreducible responsibility to procreation, are rare in early Christianity. [Historian John] Noonan's claim . . . that 'by 450 [C.E.] the teaching on abortion East and West had been set out for four centuries with clarity and consistency' is doubtful at best, though the fragmentary evidence on the question makes dogmatism either way impossible" (p. 133). Ironically, by failing to recognize the role of the developing canon, Harrison is guilty of limiting herself to the "methods of intellectual history" rather than "the newer methodologies of social and cultural history" (p. 120) — the same error Harrison attributes to "traditional" historians of the Christian position on abortion.

21. These three works are completely unknown to most people today because they are not part of the New Testament canon we have inherited from Athanasius (A.D. 367). All three of these writings, however, were still frequently considered part of the New Testament even into the fourth century, and all were read for inspiration even after they were officially excluded from the canon in 367. When many people think of the New Testament, they think of a first-century collection of inspired Christian books. It is true that most, if not all, of the books that make up the New Testament were written in the second half of the first century. But these were not the only Christian writings considered by early Christian congregations to be inspired. Nor was the New Testament assembled and published all at once some time in the late first or early second century. Rather, its formation was gradual, beginning perhaps in the late first or early second century and ending (in most churches) in the late fourth. In other words, the 27-book New Testament as a whole, as a collection, is not really a first-century publication but a fourth-century publication of first-century writings.

22. It should also be noted that the eventual omission of the *Didache, Barnabas,* and *the Apocalypse of Peter* from the canon was not due in any way to their view of abortion, which was accepted throughout the Church.

1. The Unborn Child

It is clear from early Christian texts, first of all, that the early Christians lived under the conviction that newborn and unborn children were special creations of God and were, in fact, their neighbors. The two earliest (late first-century, and very early second-century) Christian texts on abortion, found in the *Didache* and the *Epistle of Barnabas,* discuss it in their exposition of the command to "love your neighbor as yourself" (or, as *Barnabas* has it, "more than yourself"). They say, "Thou shalt not murder a child by abortion, nor kill the newborn."[23] In the latter part of the second century, Athenagoras proclaimed that the fetus is the "object of God's care," while Clement of Alexandria argued that the unborn and newborn are the "designs of providence."[24] Tertullian, trained in rhetoric and probably law, challenged the Roman legal view of the fetus as an appendage of the mother,[25] arguing that the fetus is already a person "while as yet the human being derives blood from other parts of the [mother's] body for its sustenance."[26] In other words (despite Roman and even Jewish law[27]), dependence on the woman does not render the fetus merely a part of the woman.

This high view of the newborn and unborn was part of the general Christian "neighborization" of people who were deemed non-persons by much of the surrounding culture. Personhood and human value were determined in the Greco-Roman world by those in power: adult males who were heads of households. Christianity claimed that those under the power of a householder (wife; children, both born and unborn; and slaves) were "neighbors" — in philosophical language, "persons" — and, if members of the household of faith, even brothers and sisters.[28] Thus the unborn constituted one group among several whose status as "neighbor" was recognized and proclaimed in the Church.

It is clear, furthermore, that in the early Church the unborn's status as neighbor, or person, was independent of its biological development.[29] Greek concern about the time at which an embryo or fetus receives a soul (and thus becomes a "person" in some sense), and even Jewish concern about the legal status of the fetus, are completely absent from the earliest Christian discussions.[30] When the issue of fetal development is finally raised in the late fourth century, it is dismissed by Basil (the Great) of Caesarea as irrelevant to the abortion question: "She who has deliberately destroyed a fetus has to pay the penalty of murder. And there is no exact inquiry among us as to whether the fetus was formed or unformed."[31]

2. The Act of Abortion

Early Christianity, believing the embryo or fetus to be the special creation of God, a neighbor claiming the Christian community's love, could draw no other conclusion about abortion than this: that it is a violation of the commandment "Thou shall not kill."

In the above-cited earliest Christian texts, the *Didache* and *Epistle of Barnabas,* abortion is termed murder and prohibited categorically in the form of a commandment: "Thou shalt not. . . ." Other writers of the early Church echo this perspective:

> We say that women who induce abortions are murderers, and will have to give account of it to God. (Athenagoras, a great apologist of the late second century, *Plea* 35 in *Early Christian Fathers,* ed. Cyril C. Richardson et al. [New York: Macmillan, 1970])

> In our case, murder being once for all forbidden, we may not destroy even the fetus in the womb. To hinder a birth is merely a speedier homicide. (Tertullian, late

23. *Didache* 2:2 and *Epistle of Barnabas* 19:5 (author's translation).

24. Athenagoras, *A Plea Regarding Christians* 35 (*Early Christian Fathers,* ed. Cyril C. Richardson et al. [New York: Macmillan, 1970]); Clement of Alexandria *Tutor* 2.10.96.1 (author's translation).

25. Justinian *Digest* 25.4.1.1 and elsewhere.

26. *Apology* 9.6 (*The Ante-Nicene Fathers,* vol. III).

27. Although Jews opposed abortion and viewed the fetus as God's creation, they did not believe that one became a person legally until birth.

28. This is implied, for example, in the household tables of Ephesians 5–6 and Colossians 3–4.

29. People in antiquity believed that the unborn becomes truly human at a variety of stages in its development — conception, 40 or 90 days of gestation, birth, and perhaps even after birth. The criteria for determining humanity were also somewhat varied, with possession of a soul being the chief criterion. In other words, philosophical import was attributed to biological development; moral status was a function of psychological and biological status. But even the attainment of a certain stage of development was deemed insufficient for unborn, or even newborn, life to have value. Its value was determined primarily on a utilitarian basis, either individualistic or social. That is, the value of the fetus was assigned by a controlling power, either the father or the state, according to his or its own desires and needs.

30. The absence of such distinctions is especially remarkable because the early Christians Old Testament (the Greek Septuagint [LXX]), under the influence of Greek philosophy, had mistranslated the Hebrew of Exod. 21:22-23 and erroneously introduced the notion of formed and unformed fetuses into the text, implying by the different penalties assigned that only the abortion of a formed fetus is murder. (The Hebrew words "no harm . . . harm" were translated as "no Form . . . form.") Thus the LXX could easily have been used to distinguish human from nonhuman fetuses and homicidal from non-homicidal abortions, yet the early Christians, until the time of Augustine in the fifth century, did not do so.

31. *Letter* 188.2, written c. 374 (Saint Basil, *Letters,* vol. II, trans. Agnes Clare Way, Fathers of the Church, vol. 28 [New York: Fathers of the Church, 1955]). Basil, it should be noted, also stressed leniency and grace for the crime. In the twentieth century, Dietrich Bonhoeffer would echo the same sentiments in his *Ethics* (New York: Macmillan, 1955, pp. 175-76): "To raise the question whether we are here concerned already with a human being or not is merely to confuse the issue. The simple fact is that God certainly intended to create a human being and that this nascent human being has been deliberately deprived of his life. And that is nothing but murder." Bonhoeffer also emphasizes that "the guilt may often lie rather with the community than with the individual" (p. 176).

second–early third-century theologian and apologist, *Apology* 9.6 in *The Ante-Nicene Fathers,* vol. III, ed. Alexander Roberts and James Donaldson [New York: Charles Scribner's Sons, 1903])

There are women who . . . [are] committing infanticide before they give birth to the infant. (Minucius Felix, early third-century theologian, *Octavius* 30.2 in *The Octavius of Minucius Felix,* ed. G. W. Clarke, Ancient Christian Writers, vol. 339 [New York: Newman Press, 1974])

[Abortion is] murder before the birth . . . or rather . . . something even worse than murder. (John Chrysostom, *Homily 24 on Romans* in *Nicene and Post-Nicene Fathers,* vol. XI, ed. Philip Schaff [New York: Charles Scribner's Sons, 1899])

The early Church did not, however, see the act of abortion as a unique act, an act in isolation. Rather, it viewed abortion as a manifestation of the social injustice, drive to power over the powerless, and violence of its culture.[32] It was these things that Christ and thus the Christian community rejected; abortion was perceived as part of the "interlocking directorate of death" that was the antithesis of Christian existence. Furthermore, following the example and teachings of Jesus, Christians redefined power and greatness as love and service. They saw abortion and infanticide as acts of raw power by the powerful over the powerless.[33] In all early Christian texts about children — unborn, newborn, and others in the household — and in Christian dealings with children, there is a radical rejection of the Roman notion that the father owned his children and thus held the right to determine their fate — life or death.

3. The Moral Agent

What did early Christians say about those who obtain or perform abortions? Objectively, they held, the agent is guilty before God. Although some of the early texts specifically reproach only the woman who obtains an abortion, from the earliest times Christianity also condemned those who perform abortions. The prohibition "Thou shalt not murder a child by abortion" applied equally to those who obtain and perform abortions. Basil summarizes the Christian position: "Those, too, who give drugs causing abortion are murderers themselves, as well as those receiving the poison which kills the fetus."[34] For Origen and Hippolytus in the third century, obtaining (and, implicitly, performing) an abortion called into question the reality of one's Christian faith.[35] Shortly thereafter, when the penitential system developed, women who aborted were barred from communion and church life, at first until their death and then, as penalties were relaxed, for a period of ten years.

Subjectively, it was felt by some early Christians that the act of abortion had psychological and spiritual effects on the moral agents involved. According to Clement, "women who [abort] . . . abort at the same time their human feelings."[36]

4. Pastoral Responses

The early Christian pastoral responses to abortion have been hinted at in earlier sections of this paper. Broadly speaking, this response had three dimensions: (1) prophetic preaching and teaching; (2) administration of grace and penance; and (3) provision of assistance to the poor, including orphans. This last aspect, though not directly addressing abortion, is perhaps the most significant.

The earliest Christians did not open counseling centers to dissuade women from seeking abortion or men from exposing deformed children. The Christians did, however, feel compelled to "rescue the orphan" — the child abandoned on the dung heap — and to provide for the poor, especially poor women.[37] Although these ministries did not focus on "problem-pregnancy situations" in the modern sense, there can be little doubt that the Church's practices would remind the Church's poor and others in crisis situations that they were not alone in the world; that children mattered to the Christian community and therefore to God; and that their needs would be met, their children cared for. In all probability, this

32. Abortion is rejected along with other forms of social injustice in the *Didache* and the *Epistle of Barnabas.* In Tertullian's *Apology* and Athenagoras' *Plea* it is rejected as a form of lethal violence, to which Christians are consistently opposed in theory and practice.

33. Cf. John Calvin, in his commentary on Exodus 21:22-23: "if it seems more horrible to kill a man in his own house than in a field, it ought surely to be deemed more atrocious to destroy a fetus in the womb before it comes to light" *(Commentary on Exodus).*

34. *Letter* 188.8.

35. Origen refers to such people as "so-called Christians."

36. *Tutor* 2.10.96.1 (author's translation). This sentiment has been echoed by others in our own day, including Mother Teresa, who has said that those who cause abortions kill not only the child in the women but their own compassion. If it seems that some of the early texts put an undue amount of guilt and burden on women, we should perhaps respond not by condemning the early Christians but by recognizing the breadth of guilt and of negative effects in our own culture and churches. As both pro-life and pro-choice advocates have said, we do indeed live in an "abortifacient" (Paul Ramsey) or "abortion-conducive" (Virginia Ramey Mollenkott) culture, and the practice and acceptance of abortion in such overwhelming numbers for so long have undoubtedly desensitized us to human pain and human life and allowed us to continue accepting violence as a solution to problems.

37. The phrase "the orphan and the widow" was probably a generic term for all women and children left without a protector and provider, whether by death or abandonment. Of the many early Christian admonitions to and descriptions of care for the orphan and the widow, The Durham Declaration (footnote 1) notes seven. These, as well as other texts, claim that Christians "do not abandon their offspring" (*Epistle to Diognetus* 5) but do "save the orphan" (Aristides, *Apology* 15). They also exhort Christians to "uphold the rights of the orphan" (I *Clement* 8:4), never "neglecting the widow or orphan or one that is poor" (Polycarp, *Epistle to the Philippians* 6:1). (All quotations are author's translations.)

would provide encouragement and hope to those who might consider abortion. This kind of social ministry was, according to all historians of early Christianity, one of the chief reasons for its success in the ancient world. The Church's ministry to the poor and orphans, then, was a sign of life and of grace — a "sacrament." While the precise impact of this kind of ministry is impossible to measure, it is clear that the Church's protection and improvement of human life was both an essential part of its self-understanding and an influential presence in the pagan world.

D. Once Again: The New Testament's "Silence"

At the outset of this paper it was noted that the New Testament does not speak *about* the abortion issue. Nonetheless, in the early Church, the life and teachings of Jesus, the gospel message, and the Scriptures did speak *to* the abortion issue. Ironically, the former reality is largely the result of the latter. That is, the canonical New Testament is accidentally silent; there is abundant testimony to what the early Christians heard about abortion in the gospel message. Christian opposition to abortion was so universal and so integral to the Christian vision — as it had been to the Jewish — that its absence from the canon when it was "closed" in the late fourth century would be neither remarkable nor immediately noticeable. Indeed, long before the canon was finalized, Christian opposition to abortion had been institutionalized by being included in the Church's canon law.[38]

When we consider the New Testament, we must remember that it was not carefully planned and assembled by a committee attempting to prepare a comprehensive guide to the Christian way. It is an occasional collection of occasional documents. As in the case of certain other acts — most notably infant exposure and infanticide, which are not explicitly condemned in the New Testament either — early Christianity's natural rejection of endangering or taking human life sometimes found explicit expression in its literature, and sometimes did not. The New Testament's lack of a text on abortion may be surprising, but its meaning must not be misinterpreted. Understood in its historical context, it is evidence of early Christianity's clear and consistent rejection of abortion.

E. Conclusion and Directions

What the early Christians heard in their assemblies was a message of non-violence and compassion that spoke directly to the issue of abortion. The result was a church with a moral vision and character that may well be needed in the contemporary church. This can be summarized in the following list of the virtues found among the early Christians: holiness in sexual matters, horror of bloodshed, "neighborization" or "humanization" of nonpersons, and compassionate help to the needy.

Are these virtues not the essence of biblical ethics, the New Testament vision, and the Christian moral tradition? If they are, and if the Christian message is not to be ignored or distorted, then the contemporary church's mandate seems clear: to move away from abortion, toward protecting and welcoming the unborn, and toward providing compassionate care to those in need.

The greatest challenge to commonly held beliefs, both within and beyond the church, will be to convince both men and women that they have no absolute right over their own bodies, and absolutely no right over the lives and bodies of others. Many men still believe they have power over women and children, the power to use and abuse, even the power of life and death. It is often they — as fathers, boyfriends, husbands, employers — who urge unwilling women to choose them over a child *in utero*. At the same time, many women have learned to believe that they have absolute power over their bodies and thus also over the child within. In law, philosophy, theology, and custom, the ancient paternal power of life and death over the unborn has been transferred to women. Nothing short of radical conversion from these reincarnations of Roman power over women and the unborn will alter the current situation. This conversion, like divine judgment, must begin with the household of God.[39]

The greatest challenge to the moral life of the Church and its various institutions will be to find the imagination and will to become channels of life and grace, where the "orphan and widow" are welcome.[40] This life will be

38. At the Councils of Elvira (c. 309) and Ancyra (314).

39. Although space does not permit detailed discussion, it seems to me that recent feminist analysis of the Bible confirms rather than contradicts the thesis of this paragraph. Two of the main concerns of feminist analysis are (1) feminine images of God in the Bible; and (2) criticism of traditional biblical interpretations that find justification for power and domination. An understanding of God and Christ as our life-giving, protecting mother would logically lead to divine imitation in the form of compassion for, rather than destruction of, children. Similarly, criticism of male-generated justifications for power ought to lead to an ethic of all-inclusive compassion that would be critical of all, not just male, forms of power over the powerless. For pro-life feminism, see, among others: Denise Lardner Carmody, *The Double Cross: Ordination, Abortion and Catholic Feminism* (New York: Crossroad, 1986); Sidney Callahan, "Abortion and the Sexual Agenda," *Commonweal* (April 25, 1986): 232-38 and reprinted in Robert M. Baird and Stuart E. Rosenbaum, eds., *The Ethics of Abortion: Pro-Life vs. Pro-Choice* (Buffalo: Prometheus Books, 1989), pp. 131-42; and Gail Grenier Sweet, ed., *Pro-Life Feminism: Different Voices* (Toronto: Life Cycle Books, 1985).

40. In addition to the obvious forms of ministry — counseling centers, food and clothing assistance, shelters, orphanages, adoption, childcare — the Church will have to be creative to meet the overwhelming challenge. As an example, shortly before his death, Professor (and United Methodist layperson) Paul Ramsey suggested to me in a private conversation that churches initiate a new form of "godparenting" in which young, economically disadvantaged, or otherwise needy mothers/parents who could not adequately provide for children would temporarily (or even perma-

dedicated not only to rescuing the unborn from death but also to improving the quality of life for women and children. For, to paraphrase I John, how can we say that we love the unborn whom we have not seen, if we do not love the already born whom we have seen?[41]

nently) place them in the care of people within their church. Human life would be spared, contact between parent(s) and child would continue, and the church would function as the church. Ramsey discusses this idea briefly in (oddly enough) his *Speak Up for Just War or Pacifism* (University Park, Pa.: Pennsylvania State University Press, 1988), p. 146.

41. I wish to thank Rev. John Heinsohn, former colleague in ministry and pastor of Kingston (N.J.) Presbyterian Church, for suggesting the paraphrase of I John in a sermon.

122 Women of Color and Reproductive Choice: Combating the Population Paradigm

Andy Smith

Zero population growth may be all right for the white man, because he's crowding the continent. . . . But for the Indian, it's genocidal. Let's control our own reproduction, instead of meeting the demands of the white economic-social values.

Connie Uri, the doctor who discovered rampant sterilization abuse among American Indians in the 1970s[1]

A few years ago at a potluck for the United Council of Tribes in Chicago, two representatives of a local mainstream pro-choice organization asked the Indian women there about their top concerns. The women listed poverty, homelessness, cultural identity, substance abuse, and violence. The speakers then replied that the top priority for Indian women *should* be abortion rights. As they continued their lecture, one Native woman interrupted in exasperation, "Who cares about abortion rights? We don't have any rights, period!"

This woman's statement summarizes the relationship between Native women and the mainstream pro-choice movement. Native women, like many other women of color, are in fact predominantly pro-choice.[2] In my experience of organizing around reproductive health issues for communities of color, Native women are interested in reproductive rights, depending on how the issues are framed. There is a Native Women's Reproductive Rights coalition that meets annually, with numbers growing steadily each year. However, Native women (and women of color in general) are underrepresented in the mainstream pro-choice movement. I believe this is largely be-

1. "Oklahoma: Sterilization of Native Women Charged to I.H.S. [Indian Health Services]," *Akwesasne Notes* (Midwinter 1989): 30.

2. According to the 1991-1992 Women of Color Reproductive Health Poll, 80 percent of Native women agree with the statement that "the decision to have or not to have an abortion is one that every woman must make for herself." In addition, 80 percent of African American women, 55 percent of Latinas, and 81 percent of Asian women agree with this statement. Poll data from the National Council of Negro Women, Washington, D.C.

Andrea Smith, "Women of Color and Reproductive Choice: Combating the Population Paradigm," *Journal of Feminist Studies in Religions* 11.2 (Fall 1995): 39-66. Used by permission of the author.

cause the mainstream movement has yet to frame issues of reproductive rights in terms of larger issues of community health, sovereignty, and empowerment. The issue is still defined primarily in terms of a woman's personal choice. Consequently, the mainstream movement is ill prepared to deal with reactionary forces that co-opt its language for their own agendas. In particular, the mainstream movement has not sufficiently addressed the ideology of population control that is becoming widely popular among liberal Europeans and Euro-Americans but is having a devastating impact upon communities of color. For instance, when I was on the board of the Illinois affiliate of a national pro-choice organization, we were told by the national office to "cease and desist" from educating about informed consent regarding Norplant in communities of color. Another Native woman, who was working at a feminist health center, was advised by a Euro-American health worker not to tell young black women about the side effects of Norplant because it was imperative that she be prevented by any means necessary from having children. (Fortunately, this center later reversed its stance on this issue.) Examples of this kind are endless. It is not surprising, then, that women of color doubt that being "pro-choice" includes endorsing choice for women of color.

Unfortunately, this population control ideology has gripped European and Euro-American religious communities as well, particularly liberal Christian communities. Thus, even European and Euro-American Christian feminists who are committed to racial and economic justice needlessly risk alienating themselves from women of color when they do not question their own assumptions regarding population control. Before assessing the limitations of Christian feminist responses to population control ideologies, I analyze the prevailing population paradigm. In the second part of this essay, I assess Christian responses to this paradigm.

The Population Paradigm

The population paradigm holds that overpopulation, particularly overpopulation of people of color and/or of people in the Third World, explains any number of global trends, such as political instability, poverty, and environmental destruction. Because population growth is seen as a cause rather than a symptom of other global ills, controlling population growth is considered of paramount importance. Typically, populationists ignore the role of colonization and economic injustice in all of these global trends. As Hannah Creighton of the Urban Habitat Program states,

> [Populationists] begin with the fact of exploding fertility rates and increased migration in many less developed countries. The fact becomes, for them, the cause of the problem and they are unwilling to examine the real, hard-to-change economic and social causes of increased fertility . . . the destruction of family-based, subsistence agriculture by export farming and resource extraction. Once they've named the effect the cause, they treat as secondary the real cause of population growth, global migration and environmental degradation, which is over-consumption by the affluent.[3]

This section will analyze the inadequacy of the population paradigm to explain political instability, environmental destruction, and poverty, and will assess whose interests are served by maintaining this paradigm.

Population Control in the United States

Population control is not new to the United States. Since the beginning of the European conquest, colonizers have focused their destructive energies upon women because, as David Stannard points out, "No population can survive if its women and children are destroyed. . . . This slaughter of innocents [is nothing] . . . but intentional in design."[4] Since the destruction of women's capacity to reproduce is essential to destroying a people, the killing of women has long been a preferred tactic of would-be perpetrators of genocide. "It is because of a Native American woman's sex that she is hunted down and slaughtered," argues Inés Hernández-Ávila. "In fact, [she is] singled out, because she has the potential through childbirth to assure the continuance of the people."[5]

These policies continue in a more subtle form. In the

3. Hannah Creighton, "Not Thinking Globally: The Sierra Club Immigration Policy Wars," *Race, Poverty and the Environment* 4 (Summer 1993): 25.

4. David Stannard, *American Holocaust* (Oxford: Oxford University Press, 1992), 119. According to Stannard, despite the mass destruction of Hiroshima and Nagasaki, the population of Japan actually increased by 14 percent between 1940 and 1950. This is because a disproportionate number of men were killed. If the women of a nation are not disproportionately killed, then that nation's population will not be severely affected. This is why colonizers like Andrew Jackson recommended that troops systematically kill Indian women and children after massacres to complete the extermination. Similarly, Methodist minister Colonel John Chivington's policy was to "kill and scalp all little and big" because "nits make lice." Quoted in Stannard, 131.

Stannard also points out (140) that Spain was primarily interested in Indians as a labor force, whereas the British were interested in land. Consequently, the Spanish were often preoccupied with getting Native people to reproduce. When, through starvation and brutal working conditions, Native people were having fewer children on a Santa Cruz mission, one Franciscan priest forced an Indian couple to have sex in front of him.

According to Patricia Hill Collins, black women faced similar policies under slavery. Since slave owners wanted to increase their workforce, prolific women were often rewarded with bonuses whereas infertile women were treated "like barren sows" and passed off to the next unsuspecting buyer. *Black Feminist Thought* (New York: Routledge, 1991), 51.

5. Inés Hernández-Ávila, "In Praise of Insubordination, or What Makes a Good Woman Go Bad?" in *Transforming a Rape Culture*, ed. Emilie Buchwald, Pamela R. Fletcher, and Martha Roth (Minneapolis: Milkweed, 1993), 386.

1970s, Indian Health Services (IHS) sterilized over 25 percent of Indian women without their informed consent. Sterilization rates went as high as 80 percent in some tribes.[6] Other women of color faced similar situations. In 1979 it was discovered that seven in ten U.S. hospitals performing voluntary sterilizations for Medicaid recipients violated the 1974 Department of Health, Education, and Welfare guidelines by disregarding sterilization consent procedures and by sterilizing women through "elective" hysterectomies.[7] Patricia Hill Collins links these sterilization policies with the beginning of post–World War II welfare provisions that have allowed many people of color to leave exploitative jobs. As a result, the growing unemployment rate among people of color means that nonwhite America is no longer simply a reservoir of cheap labor; it is considered "surplus" population.[8] One recently declassified federal document, National Security Study Memorandum 200, revealed that in 1976 the U.S. government regarded the growth of nonwhite populations as a threat to national security. As one doctor stated in *Contemporary Ob/Gyn:*

> People pollute, and too many people crowded too close together cause many of our social and economic problems. These in turn are aggravated by involuntary and irresponsible parenthood. . . . We also have obligations to the society of which we are part. The welfare mess, as it has been called, cries out for solutions, one of which is fertility control.[9]

Although sterilization abuse in the United States has ebbed somewhat since the 1970s, for women of color, women on federal assistance, and women with disabilities, state control over reproductive freedom continues through the promotion of unsafe, long-acting hormonal contraceptives such as Depo-Provera and Norplant. Depo-Provera, a known carcinogen condemned as an inappropriate form of birth control by several national women's health organizations,[10] was routinely used on Indian women through IHS and on women with disabilities before the Food and Drug Administration (FDA) approved it in 1992.[11] And although there are no studies to date on the long-term effects of Norplant, which is supposed to remain implanted in the arm for five years, its known side effects: constant bleeding (sometimes for over ninety days), tumors, kidney problems, strokes, heart attacks, and sterility — just to name a few — are so extreme that approximately 30 percent of women on Norplant want it removed within one year, and a majority want it out within two.[12] So far, over twenty-five hundred women suffering from more than 125 Norplant-related side effects have joined a class-action suit against Norplant's manufacturer, Wyeth-Ayerst.[13]

As the population scare and the demonization of poverty have moved to the mainstream of the dominant culture in the United States, Norplant and Depo-Provera have become frontline weapons in the war against the poor and populations of color. The Native American Women's Health Education Resource Center (NAWHERC) conducted a survey of the Norplant and Depo-Provera policies of the IHS and found that Native women were not given adequate counseling regarding the drugs' side effects and contraindications.[14] State legislatures have been considering bills that would give bonuses to women on public assistance if they use Norplant. In California a black single mother convicted of child abuse was given the "choice" of using Norplant or being sentenced to four years in prison. In addition, the *Philadelphia Inquirer* ran an editorial suggesting that Norplant could be a useful tool in "reducing the underclass."[15]

Population Control as Foreign Policy

The population scare at home has its counterpart in U.S. and European policies abroad. During the colonial period, U.S. and European countries depleted their Third World colonies of natural resources while destroying any local industry that might compete with European and North American manufactured goods. As a consequence, since World War II, Third World countries have plunged into debt because they have had to pay more for imported goods than they have received in export reve-

6. See "The Threat of Life," *WARN Report* (n.d.), 13-16 (available through Women of All Red Nations [WARN], 4511 N. Hermitage, Chicago, Ill. 60640); Brint Dillingham, "Indian Women and IHS Sterilization Practices," *American Indian Journal* (January 1977): 27-28; Brint Dillingham, "Sterilization of Native Americans," *American Indian Journal* (July 1977): 16-19; Pat Bellanger, "Native American Women, Forced Sterilization, and the Family," in *Every Woman Has a Story,* ed. Gaya Wadnizak Ellis (Minneapolis: Midwest Villages & Voices, 1982), 30-35; and "Oklahoma" (cited above, n. 1), 30.

7. "Survey Finds Seven in 10 Hospitals Violate DHEW Guidelines on Informed Consent for Sterilization," *Family Planning Perspectives* 11 (November/December 1979): 366.

8. Hill Collins, 76.

9. Quoted in "Oklahoma," 11.

10. For a statement on Depo-Provera from the National Black Women's Health Project, the National Latina Health Organization, the Native American Women's Health Education Resource Center (NAWHERC), the National Women's Health Network, and the Women's Economic Agenda Project, contact NAWHERC, P.O. Box 572, Lake Andes, South Dakota 57356-0572.

11. "Taking the Shot," series of articles in the *Arizona Republic,* November 1986.

12. Debra Hanania-Freeman, "Norplant: Freedom of Choice or a Plan for Genocide?" *Executive Intelligence Review,* 14 May 1993, 20.

13. Kathleen Plant, "Mandatory Norplant Is Not the Answer," *Chicago Sun-Times,* 2 November 1994.

14. NAWHERC, "A Study of the Use of Depo-Provera and Norplant by the Indian Health Services," Lake Andes, South Dakota, 1993. Available from NAWHERC.

15. Quoted in Gretchen Long, "Norplant: A Victory, Not a Panacea for Poverty," *National Lawyers Guild Practitioner* 50, no. 1 (1991): 11.

nues.[16] Around 1980 the World Bank and the International Monetary Fund (IMF) began to address the debt crises by imposing "structural adjustments" on debtor nations, requiring them to develop cash crop export economies, reduce tariff protection for local industry, devalue currency, and cut social services.[17] But as Third World products have flooded the world market, their value has dropped dramatically, preventing Third World countries from ever being able to pay off their loans. Thus, even though the six years between 1984 and 1990 saw the net transfer of $178 billion in financial resources from the Third World to their industrialized creditor nations, increased interest rates nearly doubled the debt from $785 million to $1.3 billion.[18] Trying vainly to service their debts, Third World countries divert land and resources from meeting local needs, forcing them to spend even more on costly imports. Marcus Arrudo sums it up; "The more we pay, the more we owe."[19]

Not surprisingly, as many debtor nations have begun to rebel against the austerity policies imposed by the World Bank and the IMF, U.S. government and business interests have tried to blame the unrest on the Third World's "overpopulation problem." In 1977 R. T. Ravenholt from the U.S. Agency for International Development (AID) announced the plan to sterilize a quarter of the world's women because, as he put it,

> Population control is necessary to maintain the normal operation of US commercial interests around the world. Without our trying to help these countries with their economic and social development, the world would rebel against the strong US commercial presence.[20]

One national pressure group, the Population Institute, even went so far as to blame the Persian Gulf War on overpopulation rather than on U.S. military and economic imperialism and our ravenous appetite for foreign oil.[21]

Profits, Poverty and "Overpopulation"

Relying on Malthusian logic, population alarmists espouse the idea that overpopulation is the primary cause of poverty in the world. According to this logic, population grows geometrically while food production grows arithmetically; eventually the number of people on the earth must outstrip the earth's "carrying capacity."[22] Conveniently, because the birthrates of the industrialized world are stable at replacement levels, populationists are free to devote their time and energy to growth rates in the Third World and immigration rates in the United States. Ironically, birthrates are currently *decreasing* in the Third World. What concerns populationists is that the current populations are young; thus there is the potential for increased birthrates in the future.

The argument of Rosemary Radford Ruether and others that the rise in Third World population stems from lowered death rates and improved health care is erroneous, because it does not explain why these trends have not led to a leveling off of the birthrate to replacement levels, as has happened in the United States.[23] We must also question to what extent Western medicine has significantly improved the health of people in the Third World and of indigenous peoples. Bernadine Atcheson and Mary Ann Mills, Traditional Dena'ina, note that the health of Alaska Natives has deteriorated because of the imposition of Western diets, the invasion of Western pharmaceuticals, and the environmental degradation brought on by industrialization. Mills states, "Today we rely on our elders and our traditional healers. We have asked them if they were ever as sick as their grandchildren or great-grandchildren are today. Their reply was no; they are much healthier than their children are today."[24] Today American Indian women have a life expectancy of forty-seven years.[25]

Rather than investing dollars in healthcare for Third World Women and women of color, the "population establishment," as Betsy Hartmann calls it, spends billions of dollars each year on population programs, policy setting, and (mis)education.[26] Certainly, Third World

16. Walter Rodney, *How Europe Underdeveloped Africa* (London: Bogle L' Ouverture Publications, 1972), 154-73; and Gita Sen, *Development, Crises and Alternative Visions* (New York: Monthly Review Press, 1987), 32-33.

17. Tom Barry and Deb Preusch, *The Central America Fact Book* (New York: Grove Press, 1986), 32.

18. "Creating a Wasteland," *Food First Action Alert* (Winter 1993): 1-2; and "Structural Adjustment: Deadly Development," *The Global Advocates Bulletin* (October 1994): 1, 2, 5, 7, 9.

19. Marcos Arruda, "Brazil: Drowning in Debt," in *Fifty Years Is Enough*, ed. Kevin Danaher (Boston: South End Press, 1994), 45.

20. Quoted in the *WARN Report,* 15.

21. Population Institute, *Annual Report* (1991).

22. See, for example, Population Institute, *Annual Report* (1991); and the Sierra Club (Los Angeles chapter, population committee), "Population Stabilization: The Real Solution" (pamphlet, n.d.).

23. Rosemary Radford Ruether, *Gaia and God: An Ecofeminist Theology of Earth Healing* (San Francisco: HarperSanFrancisco, 1992), 91.

24. Mary Ann Mills (speech delivered at a WARN Forum, Chicago, Ill., September 1993).

25. Ward Churchill, *Struggle for the Land* (Monroe, Maine: Common Courage Press, 1993), 55. Dr. William Jordan of the U.S. Health Department has noted that virtually all field trials for new vaccines in the United States are first tested on indigenous people in Alaska, and most of the vaccines do absolutely nothing to prevent disease. See Traditional Dena'ina Health Committee, *Summary Packet on Hepatitis B Vaccinations,* Sterling, Alaska, 9 November 1992. Also, according to Linda Burhansstipanov of the National Cancer Institute, if Native people do not get healthcare through experimental programs, then they will not get any healthcare at all. Conversation with author, Phoenix, Ariz., February 1992.

26. Betsy Hartmann identifies the major players as the U.S. Agency for International Development (AID), the United Nations Fund for Population Activities, governments of other developed countries (particularly Japan), the World Bank (which has forced Third World countries to adopt population policies as a condition of its release of loans for structural adjustments), the International

women and women of color want family planning services, but many programs have been foisted upon them without concern for their health. Before Norplant was introduced in the United States, nearly half a million women in Indonesia received it from the Population Council, often without mention of its side effects. Moreover, many women were not told that it needed to be removed after five years to avoid an increased risk of ectopic pregnancy.[27] Thirty-five hundred women in India were implanted with Norplant without being warned about possible side effects or being screened to determine whether they were suitable candidates. Norplant trials had to be halted because of concerns about "teratogenicity and carcinogenicity."[28] In both cases, women who wanted their implants removed had great difficulty finding doctors to remove them. (Even in the United States many doctors who insert Norplant do not know how to take it out.) In the last six months of 1976, the Indian government sterilized 6.5 million people, many of them having been rounded up in police raids. Thousands died from infections caused by the unsanitary conditions of the operations. In one village all young men were sterilized.[29]

Population programs push "high-tech," long-acting contraceptives that do more to pad the profits of pharmaceutical companies than they do to improve choices for women. In fact, oral and injectable contraceptives are among the most lucrative of all pharmaceuticals.[30] These programs all but ignore "low-tech" methods, such as natural family planning (because of the Vatican's reliance upon it alone, this method is treated as a joke), indigenous herbal methods, barrier methods (despite the epidemic of AIDS), and insulated underwear for men.[31] In fact, AID pressured one agency to circulate a warning to its clinic to discourage the use of condoms and encourage more IUDs and pills.[32] Particularly for women of color, reproductive choice often means a choice among unsafe contraceptives. Farida Akhter states,

> The western woman was demanding the "right" to have more choices in contraceptives. But we are getting it free without even raising our voice. . . . We were inundated with devices to render our reproductive organs dysfunctional. . . . Here merges a different perception of the concept of the reproductive right. Many of us who are living at the margin of life in poverty, coercion and militarization, and living in a politico-economic system dictated by external coercion, feel that our immediate task is to achieve a democratic society where both men and women can be free. In the process of achieving that society we will achieve our reproductive right as well, but not vice versa.[33]

But while there are those who profit from coercive and high-tech reproductive technologies, the economics of colonialism actually work to sustain fertility rates. The problem with the Malthusian argument is that it assumes that "natural fertility rates" are always high and are checked only by the vicissitudes of famine, war, and disease. In fact, however, women have always had means of controlling reproduction. Ironically, colonial powers often tried to stamp out traditional means of birth control to ensure a large supply of cheap labor and a captive market for their finished goods.[34] In recent years Nestlé has discouraged breast-feeding, a natural birth spacer, to increase sales of its infant formula among Third World women; more babies means more formula, and more formula means more babies. Also, as Vandana Shiva notes, the population of India was stable *until* the advent of British colonialism.[35] As colonization forced women into cash economies, it became necessary for them to have more children to raise more cash crops. Also, increased mortality rates motivate women to have more children in the hope that some will survive. With cuts in social services resulting from the World Bank's imposed "structural adjustments," children are also needed to provide old-age security and to help with women's increased workloads.[36]

Planned Parenthood Federation, the Population Council, various consulting firms, academic centers, foundations (particularly Ted Turner and Pew Charitable Trusts), and pressure groups (including Zero Population Growth and Population Action International, as well as environmental organizations such as the Sierra Club). *Reproductive Rights and Wrongs — Revised* (Boston: South End Press, 1986), 113-24.

27. Ibid., 29-30.

28. Ammu Joseph, "India's 'Population Bomb' Explodes over Women," *Ms.*, November/December 1992, 12.

29. Hartmann, 254.

30. For a discussion of the close relationship between pharmaceutical companies and population agencies, see Hartmann, 177-79. She notes, for example, that Dr. William Hubbard, president of Upjohn Company (maker of Depo-Provera), was on the board of Family Health International (FHI), whose population research is heavily funded by AID, when FHI testified for approval of Depo-Provera before a U.S. board of inquiry.

31. Noninvasive contraceptives for men do exist. For example, soaking the testes in 116°F water for forty-five minutes daily for twenty-one days is believed to cause sterility for six months. Also, underwear that pushes the testes up into the body is also believed to have a contraceptive effect. See Elaine Lissner, "Eight New Nonhormonal Contraceptive Methods for Men," *Changing Men*, Summer/Fall 1992, 24.

32. Hartmann, 65.

33. Farida Akhter, "Issues of Women's Health" (paper presented at the Sixth International Women and Health Meeting, Philippines, November 1990).

34. Maria Mies and Vandana Shiva, *Ecofeminism* (London: Zed, 1993), 287-88. It is well known by Native women, for instance, that women, prior to colonization, controlled their births through herbs and other methods. However, this knowledge was destroyed by the colonizers' assault on Native cultures.

35. Mies and Shiva, 284.

36. By the age of fifteen, children in Bangladesh have repaid their parents' investment in their upbringing. In Java and Indonesia, children are net-income earners by the age of nine. Sons are important in some countries because daughters usually leave home when they marry and no longer contribute to their parents' income. In the Sahel, a couple has to bear ten children to be 95 percent certain of producing a son who will survive to the age of

Furthermore, there is actually enough food produced in the world to sustain every person on a diet of three thousand calories per day.[37] However, land is used inefficiently to support livestock for environmentally unsustainable Western meat-based diets.[38] In addition, food produced in the Third World is often exported to pay off debts to the World Bank rather than used to meet local needs. Consequently, even countries stricken by famine export food.[39]

Some populationists concede that poverty causes overpopulation, but they add that rapid population growth leads to greater poverty, creating a vicious circle. This, too, is not necessarily true, because increased population growth can lead to increased food production. Conversely, some of the most poverty-stricken areas do not experience mass population growth. Bangladesh's population policies, for instance, were designed to "prove that population growth can be reduced without any change in . . . health conditions, poverty or social justice,"[40] a fact which exposes the canard that populationists are primarily concerned with improving the lives of people in the Third World. This does not mean that population growth never causes problems for communities; however, the fundamental cause of poverty in the Third World is the extraction of resources from the South for consumption in the North. Without a restructuring of the global economy, we cannot ultimately alter the rates of poverty.

Environmental Degradation

Many populationists argue that, in addition to causing poverty and starvation, overpopulation is the primary cause of environmental degradation. Environmental organizations have been "educating" the public about the environmental degradation caused by overpopulation. In fact, according to much of the literature, overpopulation is "the single greatest threat to the health of the planet."[41] Actually, environmental damage is caused by environmentally destructive Western development projects, such as hydroelectric dams,[42] uranium development,[43] militarism,[44] and livestock production.[45] Projections of overpopulation ultimately benefit those in industrialized countries who are responsible for producing over 75 percent of the world's environmental pollution.[46] Over one-third of World Bank projects completed in 1993 were judged failures by World Bank staff, with

---

thirty-eight and thus provide the couple with old-age security. "Mythconceptions," *New Internationalist,* October 1987, 9.

37. Hartmann, 16.

38. The same land that is used to maintain livestock for 250 days could be used to cultivate soybeans for 2,200 days. Half of all water consumed in the United States is used on crops for feeding livestock. One-third of the value of all raw materials consumed in the United States is consumed in livestock foods. Carol Adams, *Neither Man nor Beast* (New York: Continuum, 1994), 92-93. Thirty-eight percent of the world's grain is fed to livestock, and in the United States 70 percent of grain use is for livestock. Alan B. Durning and Holly B. Brough, *Taking Stock: Animal Farming and the Environment* (Washington, D.C.: Worldwatch Institute, 1991), 14. By cycling grain through livestock, humans end up with only 10 percent of the calories that would be available if we ate the grain directly. John Robbins, *Diet for a New America* (Walpole, N.H.: Stillpoint Publishing, 1987), 351.

39. Hartmann (17) writes that during the Sahelian famine of the late 1960s and early 1970s, agricultural exports actually increased. She also cites A. K. Sen's observation that there has never been a large-scale famine in any country, rich or poor, that is a "democracy" with a relatively free press.

40. John Briscoe, of the Cholera Research Laboratory, quoted in Hartmann, 235.

41. Population Institute, *Annual Report* (1991).

42. The World Bank hydroelectric dam in Brazil, built to produce aluminum for export to the North, has destroyed native forests, forcing the removal of masses of native and rural people. Brazil will have to spend millions of dollars to clean up the organic matter that is now decomposing underwater; see Arruda (cited above, n. 19), 44.

43. One of the most polluted areas in the country, the Columbia River area where the Yakima people live, is near the Hanford nuclear reactor. Wastes from the reactor were placed in unstable containers that are now leaking, and the Yakima believe their water table has been contaminated. It will cost at least $150 billion to clean up these wastes. The U.S. government also failed to advise residents about the known dangers of radiation poisoning. Valerie Tallman, "Toxic Waste of Indian Lives," *Covert Action* 17 (Spring 1992): 16-22. The government plans to relocate all nuclear wastes in a permanent, high-level nuclear waste repository in Yucca Mountain on Shoshone land at a cost of $3.25 billion. Yucca Mountain is located in an active volcanic zone where kiloton bombs are exploded nearby, thus increasing the risks of radioactive leakage. In addition, if this plan is approved, for thirty years the proposed repository on Yucca Mountain would receive nuclear wastes produced throughout the United States. (Only five states would not be affected by the transportation of high-level radioactive wastes.) With up to four thousand shipments of radioactive waste crossing the United States annually, trucking industry statistics reveal that as many as fifty accidents per year could occur. Valerie Tallman, "Tribes Speak Out on Toxic Assault," *Lakota Times,* 18 December 1991.

After the Prairie Island nuclear generating plant was opened near the Prairie Island Reservation in Goodhue County, Minnesota, breast cancer deaths increased 43 percent in the area, compared with an increase of 1 percent in the rest of the state. A Pittsburgh School of Medicine study concluded that "Only 18 percent of all U.S. women live in those counties [near nuclear plants], but they account for 55 percent of all breast cancer." Since 100 percent of uranium mining and development takes place on or near Indian land, a disproportionate number of indigenous women are affected. "Expert Says Cancer Deaths Rise 43% Near Nuclear Plant," *St. Paul Pioneer Press,* 2 June 1994.

44. There have already been at least 650 nuclear explosions at a Nevada nuclear test site on western Shoshone land. Fifty percent of these underground tests have leaked radiation into the atmosphere. Tallman, "Tribes Speak Out."

45. More than 50 percent of water pollution is linked to the livestock industry. Cattle are responsible for 85 percent of topsoil erosion. Between 40 and 60 percent of U.S. imported oil requirements would be cut if the U.S. population switched to a vegetarian diet. Adams (cited above, n. 38), 92-93.

46. Patience Idemudia and Kole Shettima, "World Bank Takes Control of UNCED's Environment Fund," in Danaher (cited above, n. 19), 108.

some countries experiencing success rates of less than 50 percent.[47] Any damage done by peasants or indigenous people cannot compare to the damage done by multinationals and the World Bank. Moreover, the damage inflicted by these peoples generally results from their being driven off their lands. Furthermore, Fatima Mello of FASE (*Federacao de Orgaos para Assistencia Social Educacional,* a Brazilian environmental and development nongovernmental organization [NGO]) notes that in Brazil, a higher density of population in certain areas of the Amazon often helps to *stop* encroachment by the World Bank or multinationals and their environmentally disastrous projects.[48] Brazil is experiencing an increase in environmental destruction in an *inverse* relation to its population decline. The cutting of trees in the Amazon is not related to an excess of peasants cutting trees for survival but rather to the government policy of supporting commercial ranching for the benefit of those in the United States.[49] If the poorest 75 percent of the world's population were to completely disappear, the reduction in pollution would be only 10 percent.[50]

Population Control and the Anti-Immigration Movement

Neocolonial policies have resulted in mass immigration to the United States, a trend which has led environmental organizations such as Carrying Capacity Network (CCN), Population-Environment Balance, and Negative Population Growth to complain that the United States is now "overpopulated" by immigrants. Immigrants, Population-Environment Balance claims, cause "global warming, species extinction, acid rain, and deforestation. . . . Immigration . . . is threatening the carrying capacity limits of the natural environment." Because of their "excessive reproductive rates," immigrants cause mass environmental damage, "compete with our [*sic*] poor for jobs," and burden the taxpayer through "increased funding obligations in AFDC, Medicare, Food Stamps, School Lunch, Unemployment Compensation," and so on.[51] It would stand to reason that if these are the people who are "burdening the taxpayer" through federal assistance programs, then they are probably not the people causing the majority of environmental degradation in this country. Such organizations ignore the consumption patterns of the more well-to-do, as well as the role of U.S. businesses, in causing environmental degradation. Furthermore, immigrants contribute much more in taxes than they take in public services.[52]

Despite these facts, environmental organizations are increasingly urging a closing of the borders to "save the environment." Even more mainstream environmental organizations are becoming interested in this issue. Powerful members of the Sierra Club who also belong to the Federation of American Immigration Reform (FAIR) have attempted to get the Sierra Club to adopt an anti-immigration platform. Thanks primarily to the people of color on the Sierra Club's Cultural Diversity Task Force, they have not (yet) been successful.[53]

Not surprisingly, many far-right organizations are finding the xenophobic and racist policies of these organizations increasingly attractive. Tom Metzger, founder of the White Aryan Resistance, has declared his support for Earth First! because of its stand on overpopulation and statements in its newsletter claiming that AIDS is a positive trend for global birth control. Metzger has stated, "Don't you think, my Aryan comrades, that it's time to start using any and every means to put a stop to the . . . scum who are raping our mother earth to the point of her extinction?" Similarly, the Aryan Women's League has said that it can pursue its goal of preserving the pure Aryan race by "making ourselves known as environmentalists and wildlife advocates. There are many groups out there helping wildlife and the environment. They are not necessarily white power advocates like ourselves, but if we make contributions to these groups, we achieve two things, 1) we break out of our media stereotype . . . and 2) we gain recognition."[54]

Organizing against the Population Paradigm

Women of color and Third World women, as well as concerned European and Euro-American women, have

47. Pratap Chatterjee, "World Bank Failures Soar to 37.5% of Completed Projects in 1991," in Danaher, 137-38.

48. Fatima Mello, speech delivered at the Ninth Annual Conference of Hampshire College's "The Fight for Abortion Rights and Reproductive Freedom," Amherst, Mass., 1 April 1995.

49. Hartmann, 28.

50. Margot Kassmann, "Covenant, Praise and Justice in Creation," in *Ecotheology,* ed. David Hallman (Maryknoll, N.Y.: Orbis, 1994), 45.

51. Population-Environment Balance, "Why Excess Immigration Damages the Environment," *Carrying Capacity Network Focus* 2 (1992): 31-32.

52. "A Proposed Principled Policy Statement Based on Fact, Not Fear," *Race, Poverty and the Environment* 4 (Summer 1993): 39-40.

53. The Federation of American Immigration Reform (FAIR) was founded by John Tanton, formerly of Zero Population Growth, and receives funding from the Pioneer Fund. (The Pioneer Fund was started by a millionaire in 1887 who advocated sending American blacks back to Africa. It has also supported Nazi eugenic research, as well as most eugenic research in the United States, including Charles Murray's *Bell Curve* studies.) FAIR now works in cooperation with a number of environmental organizations. Paul Ehrlich of the Carrying Capacity Network (CCN) sits on the executive board of FAIR. Another member of both FAIR and the Sierra Club is Allan Weedem, who controls the multimillion-dollar Frank Weedem Foundation, which gives money to environmental and population/immigration groups, including FAIR. In 1990 Weedem gave $275,000 to the Sierra Club's population program, making it the best funded of all Sierra Club programs. He is now pressuring the Sierra Club to take stands opposing immigration. See Creighton; and Ruth Connif, "The War on Aliens," *Progressive,* October 1993, 22-29.

54. Metzger and the Aryan Women's League are both quoted in Michael Novick, *White Lies, White Power* (Monroe, Maine: Common Courage Press, 1995), 205.

been very active in combating the racism, sexism, and imperialism implicit in the population paradigm. The Women of All Red Nations (WARN) organized against sterilization abuse in the 1970s, producing the *WARN Report* on this issue. NAWHERC has organized around contraceptive abuse, as has the Black Women's Health Education Project. The women of color delegation to the United Nations International Conference on Population and Development (ICPD) in Cairo issued a statement calling for "a change of the present global development model [of] wasteful consumption [and] economic growth pitted against social progress."[55] A broad-based coalition of international women's organizations also signed a statement calling for "a new approach" to the population paradigm.[56]

Population control has been soundly condemned in national and international meetings of groups, including the International Women and Health organization. As Ananilea Nkya stated at the most recent meeting of the Tanzania Media Women's Association, "We question the views of population controllers who perpetuate the notion that rapid population growth is the major cause of poverty and environmental degradation in developing countries and that provision of family planning in those countries is the solution."[57] Grassroots women's groups have organized to end Norplant trials in Brazil, and FINRRAGE held a conference in Bangladesh in 1989 to organize against the abuses of long-acting hormonal contraceptives.[58] At the historic People of Color Environmental Summit held in Washington, D.C., in 1991, one woman echoed the concerns of many of the participants when she said to leaders of the mainstream environmental organizations who attended the conference, "We are not interested in controlling *our* population for the sake of *your* population."

Christian Responses to the Population Paradigm

Although many religious communities have been tackling population issues, I will focus on Christian communities because of their increased attention to this issue as a result of the Vatican's response to the Cairo conference on population and development. Liberal Protestant organizations have historically been supportive of population control. Dianne Moore notes that a relationship (albeit a complex one) exists between the eugenics movement of the 1930s and the first church statements supporting birth control.[59] In 1969 Reinhold Niebuhr of Union Theological Seminary, Henry Fosdick of Riverside Church, and Henry Knox Sherrill of the World Council of Churches signed a full-page ad in the *New York Times* calling for mass population control efforts in Latin America.[60] Most mainline denominations have issued statements supporting population control, and the writings of European and Euro-American liberal Christians concerned with environmental issues also tend to accept the population paradigm.[61]

Euro-American Christian feminists such as Sallie McFague, Rosemary Radford Ruether, Catherine Keller, and Christine Gudorf devote much of their writings on population to analyzing the relationships between overconsumption, socioeconomic injustice, and population growth. Even so, they do not sufficiently challenge the population paradigm. Consequently, although these authors are certainly concerned about racial and economic justice, many of their statements on overpopulation have unintended negative consequences for women of color and Third World women.

One reason these writers do not challenge the population paradigm may be that they do not base their analyses on work done by Third World women or women of color. In recent writings by each of these authors on this issue, they do not reference a single work by a person of color. It is ironic that, given their feminist commitments, they do not take as the starting point for their discussions the communities whose populations they advocate reducing. They do, however, approvingly quote individuals who have supported notoriously racist population programs, such as Paul Ehrlich of CCN, Margaret Catley-Carlson of the Population Council, and Werner Fournos of the Population Institute.[62] This gives the impression (mistaken, one hopes) that Ruether, Keller, and

55. United States Women of Color Delegation to the United Nations International Conference on Population and Development (ICPD), "Statement on Poverty, Development and Population Activities," in *Political Environments* 1 (Spring 1994): 28-29.

56. "A Call for a New Approach," reprinted in Hartmann, 311-13.

57. Quoted in Loretta Ross, "Why Women of Color Can't Talk about Population," *Amicus Journal* 15 (Winter 1994): 27.

58. Mello, speech (cited above, n. 48).

59. Dianne Moore, "Gender Essentialism and the Debate over Reproductive Control in Liberal Protestantism" (Ph.D. diss., Union Theological Seminary, 1995).

60. Reprinted in Dale Hathaway-Sunseed, "A Critical Look at the Population Crisis in Latin America" (unpublished paper, University of California at Santa Cruz, 1979). The efforts these men supported led to the sterilization of 30 percent of women in Puerto Rico and 44 percent of women in Brazil, despite the fact that sterilization was illegal in Brazil; see Hartmann, 248, 250.

61. For a discussion of population statements issued by the Lutheran, United Methodist, Southern Baptist, and United Presbyterian Churches, see Arthur Dyck, "Religious Views," in *Population and Ethics*, ed. Robert Veatch (New York: Halsted Press, 1977), 277-323. See also Jürgen Moltmann, "The Ecological Crisis: Peace with Nature," *Scottish Journal of Religious Studies* 9 (Spring 1988): 5-18; John Swomley, "Too Many People, Too Few Resources," *Christian Social Action* 5 (November 1992): 10-12; Nancy Wright and Donald Kill, *Ecological Healing: A Christian Vision* (Maryknoll, N.Y.: Orbis, 1993), 7-9, 119-21; Roger Shinn, *Forced Options* (San Francisco: Harper & Row, 1982), 85-105; James Nash, *Loving Nature* (Nashville: Abingdon, 1991), 44-50; and John Carmody, *Ecology and Religion* (New York: Paulist Press, 1983), 140-42.

62. See Ruether (cited above, n. 23), 88; Catherine Keller, "Chosen Persons and the Green Ecumancy: A Possible Christian Response to the Population Apocalypse," in Hallman (cited above, n. 50), 301; and Christine Gudorf, *Body, Sex and Pleasure* (Cleveland: Pilgrim Press, 1994), 43.

Gudorf consider these people to have greater expertise on the situations facing Third World women and women of color than do the women themselves. Keller, in particular, puzzlingly states that there is a "conspiracy of silence" on population, despite much work done on population by women of color and Third World women.[63] It is also interesting that Keller, and not a woman of color, was apparently asked to write the contribution on population control in *Ecotheology*.[64]

One reason for the omissions may be that these authors inadequately grapple with the racial aspect of the "overpopulation" issue. Ruether, for instance, states, "The challenge that humans face . . . is whether they will be able to visualize and organize their own reproduction, production, and consumption in such a way as to stabilize their relationship to the rest of the ecosphere and so avert massive social and planetary ecocide."[65] She seems to assume that all humans contribute equally to ecological disaster, that all are equally affected by population policies, and that all have the same access to power to organize their production and consumption.

This is not to say that all of these authors completely ignore the differing positions between Western women and Third World women. McFague, for instance, does say in her discussion on environmental degradation that "we are not all equally responsible, nor does deterioration affect us equally."[66] But then she says that ecology is a "people" issue in relationship to nonhuman creatures.[67] The problem, then, is "human overpopulation." However, because most industrialized countries have replacement-level fertility, with some even experiencing declining populations, clearly it is not these citizens who are considered to be "overpopulating" the earth and who are the targets of most population programs.[68] Keller and Gudorf further say that all women should make the commitment to have no more than one child.[69] Keller makes an exception for women from communities that have been targeted for genocide, implying that population policies are not in themselves genocidal in intent. (In fact, many population policies violate the UN Convention on Genocide.[70]) It would logically follow from Keller's analysis that only Europeans and Euro-Americans should reduce their population. In addition, this one-child recommendation implies that a Third World woman and a white woman are equally affected by having only one child. But a white middle-class woman stands to gain economically by having only one child, whereas a Third World woman stands to face tremendous economic hardship as a result of such a policy. Gudorf does acknowledge this point, but it does not seem to affect her policy recommendation in any way.[71]

Keller also erases the particularity of women of color by saying that "the rising global population rate is a catastrophic trend variously underplayed both by right-wing anti-abortionists and feminists combatting the misogyny implied by monofocal emphasis on population (often encouraging female infanticide and forced sterilization)."[72] She describes these population practices as "misogynist" but not racist as well, as though they significantly affect all women and not primarily women of color and Third World women. In addition, she implies that feminists are concerned only with "abuses" in population programs instead of with the fact that the programs are designed as a smoke screen for larger structures of socioeconomic injustice (from which European and Euro-American middle-class women gain many privileges). Also, given that it is women of color and Third World women who primarily suffer the brunt of environmental destruction, it might be helpful for Keller to consider what these women have identified as the real "catastrophic trends" — namely, colonization, Western overconsumption, and racism.

Each of these authors discusses the environmental destruction caused by Western consumption patterns. Each also analyzes how population growth is affected by colonialism. Keller, for instance, states, "Justice-centered Christians speaking on behalf of the world of the poor make the irrefutable point that . . . it is the exploitation of the resources of the Third World for the sake of the First World and its client elites — not overpopulation — which deprives those others of the resources they need. Is not the focus on population control thus dangerously akin to the genocidal policies which seek to rid the world of the troubling, potentially revolutionary masses of the poor?"[73] Keller then proceeds not to address this issue in the rest of her essay. If population is a symptom rather than a cause of other global trends, as these authors state, why do they value the population paradigm so highly? Ruether and Keller, in fact, describe overpopulation as one of the "four horsemen of doom," the others being economics, war, and environment.[74] Essentially they argue that the patterns of reproduction for Third World

63. Keller, "Chosen Persons," 301.

64. Ibid., 300. A similar experience happened at a conference on ecofeminism (sponsored by the Feminists for Animal Rights) that I attended in Washington, D.C., in April 1994. For a panel on overpopulation, a man from the right-wing Population-Environment Balance was asked to speak, but no women of color were asked to speak. The organizers claimed that they "couldn't find any women of color."

65. Ruether, 47.

66. Sallie McFague, *The Body of God* (Minneapolis: Fortress, 1993), 4.

67. Ibid., 5.

68. Hartmann, 6.

69. Keller, "Chosen Persons," 307; and Gudorf, *Body, Sex and Pleasure*, 48.

70. See United Nations, *Convention of the Prevention and Punishment of the Crime of Genocide*, II(d), which condemns imposing any measure intended to prevent births within a targeted group.

71. Gudorf, *Body, Sex and Pleasure*, 48.

72. Catherine Keller, "Talk About the Weather," in *Ecofeminism and the Sacred*, ed. Carol J. Adams (New York: Continuum, 1993), 31.

73. Keller, "Chosen Persons," 301.

74. Ruether, 111; and Keller, "Chosen Persons," 307.

women and women of color that have developed as a result of colonization are as bad as colonization itself. Ultimately, Christian feminists' claim — that population growth is as much a problem as are colonization and Western consumption patterns — is not really an improvement on the argument that overpopulation is wholly to blame for the world's problems. This claim still mitigates the responsibility of those in power.

Gudorf seems to let the rich off the hook when she prioritizes population stabilization over social justice by arguing that "getting the rich to agree to any standard significantly below what they now receive seems . . . doubtful."[75] The implication seems to be that we should focus on imperialistic population control policies because they will be easier to implement than economic justice. Further, she states that "combating hunger and . . . malnutrition must come primarily through population stabilization."[76] This seems to suggest that ending hunger through economic justice is not Gudorf's primary concern. Ruether does not say that population and overconsumption are equally to blame; rather, "the major cause of destruction of species comes *simply* from the expanding human population" [emphasis mine].[77] Furthermore, she says, it is overpopulation that leads to "war, famine, and disease," not the other way around.[78] Ruether then calls for "the promotion of birth control" instead of the provision of women's unmet needs for contraceptives. She seems to be oblivious to the devastating health effects that such "promotions" have had for women of color and Third World women.[79] Her vision of "a good society," outlined at the end of *Gaia and God,* entails population control, but it does not include redistribution of resources from the North to the South or anything that would significantly affect the privileges the North enjoys at the expense of the South.[80]

In addition, these writers uncritically espouse rather questionable ideas about population growth. Keller, Ruether, and McFague regard Malthusian orthodoxy as indisputably true.[81] As mentioned previously, Ruether describes population in the Third World as rising independently from patterns of colonization. She also uncritically employs Paul Ehrlich's formula: environmental impact = population × affluence × technology (I = PAT). Many feminists have argued that this formula is problematic because it assumes that all populations are the same, ignoring different peoples' different impacts on the environment. It also views "all humans as takers from, rather than enhancers of, the natural environment. This truncated, culture-bound view of humans in their environment originates from an industrial, urban, consumerist society."[82] Affluence is conceived only as per capita consumption. This view neglects the fact that the Third World sustains not only its own consumption but also the consumption of industrialized countries.[83] All technology is assumed to be equally harmful. In addition, the environmental impact of the military is lacking in this equation. As Hartmann states, "I = PAT obscures power relations at the global level, the precise dynamics of environmental degradation at the local, regional, and national levels are also hidden behind a Malthusian veil."[84] Also disturbing is Gudorf's approval of incentive and disincentive programs (such as paying women to use contraceptives) so long as they are as "voluntary" as possible.[85] Given the oppressive conditions most Third World women live in, it is unclear how incentives can be considered even remotely voluntary. If one is living hand-to-mouth, is the offer of financial resources in exchange for controlling one's reproductive capabilities any kind of a choice? The use of incentives in population programs has been devastating for Third World women and women of color.[86] Even the UN's ICPD *draft* proposal condemned the use of incentives and disincentives.[87]

Finally, these writers speak quite eloquently about the responsibilities of the Western world for addressing environmental degradation by targeting consumption patterns. But ultimately they say that the West should accomplish this so that Third World people will reduce their populations. McFague states, "Unless and until we drastically modify our life-style, we are not in a position to preach population control to others."[88] This is true, but it also suggests that if one is morally scrupulous in one's own "lifestyle," then one can excuse coercive control over others, and that the reason one should modify one's lifestyle is to be able to preach population control. This attitude motivates too many population program planners. Many policymakers attempt to determine the minimum amount of social and/or health reforms necessary to reduce population. For example, the International Center for Diarrheal Disease Research in Matlab, Bangladesh, determined that only a minimum amount of health care was necessary to induce women to accept contraceptives. Consequently, additional health care was withheld from them.[89] As Hartmann states, "Once social reforms, women's projects, and family planning pro-

75. Gudorf, *Body, Sex and Pleasure,* 42.

76. Ibid., 59.

77. Ruether, 101.

78. Ibid., 263.

79. Ibid., 264. Even the United Nations International Conference on Population and Development's (ICPD), *Report of the International Conference on Population and Development,* Cairo, 5-13 September 1994, calls for meeting unmet needs for contraceptives rather than promoting their use to women who do not want them.

80. Ruether, 258-68.

81. Keller, "Chosen Persons," 302; Ruether, 263; and McFague, 56.

82. H. Patricia Hynes, quoted in Hartmann, 24.

83. Mies and Shiva (cited above, n. 34), 283.

84. Hartmann, 26.

85. Gudorf, *Body, Sex and Pleasure,* 50.

86. See Hartmann, 66-72.

87. United Nations International Conference on Population and Development, *Draft Programme of Action,* 7.20.

88. McFague, 4-5. See also Keller, "Chosen Persons," 309.

89. Hartmann, 235-40.

grams are organized for the explicit goal of reducing population growth, they are subverted and ultimately fail. . . . These basic rights are worthy of pursuit in and of themselves; they have far more relevance to the general improvement of human welfare than reducing population growth alone ever will."[90]

Liberal Christians, particularly Christian feminists, focus their energies on countering claims made by the Vatican and other "pro-life" forces. Although this is important, it often fosters a false dichotomy between being pro-population control and anti-choice. Consequently, the experiences of Third World women and women of color become lost in these discussions. As Thais Corral, a Brazilian feminist, said about the proceedings at Cairo, population proponents insist that Third World women must join them in combating the fundamentalists and the Vatican.[91] Thus, as is typical of populationists, columnist Anna Quindlen argues, "It has become increasingly evident that Americans should not permit the Vatican to go unchallenged in its opposition to birth and population control. We can do this best by giving our own vocal support of US funding of family planning as an important measure that can deal with unintended pregnancies, burgeoning population, and poverty."[92] But the Vatican is a closer ally than Quindlen knows. Although the Vatican rejected abortion and all forms of birth control other than natural planning at Cairo, it did not necessarily reject the premises of overpopulation. Said Vatican Secretary of State Cardinal Angelo Dodana, "Everyone is aware of the problems that can come from a disproportionate growth of the world's population. The Church is aware of the complexity of the problem, but the urgency of the situation must not lead into error in proposing ways intervening."[93] In fact, it is because of population control that some Catholics are willing to oppose the Vatican's policy on birth control.[94]

Similarly, many "pro-life" Christians, including fundamentalists, wholeheartedly support population control policies.[95] In her book *Six Billion and More,* Susan Bratton, for instance, states that abortion is unethical. However, she sees no problem with population incentives. She also thinks coercive techniques are an option if all else fails to stabilize the population. In addition, she favors the use of long-acting hormonal contraceptives (such as Norplant and Depo-Provera), which she considers "safer," for some reason, than barrier methods. She does not address the AIDS crisis nor the devastating impact of emphasizing nonbarrier methods of birth control. Such is Bratton's "pro-life" position on population stabilization.[96]

Many conservative Christians who do not support population control are not motivated from a larger concern for social justice. Cindy Rollins argues against population policies for eugenic reasons; more Christian babies are needed to offset the growing numbers of non-Christians.[97] Similarly, in his exposé of Human Life International (HLI, founded by Father Paul Marx in 1981), Tom Burghardt claims that the Vatican supports HLI for racist reasons. HLI's purported goal is to stop the Jewish doctors who control the abortion industry and the Muslim conspirators who support their own large families by performing abortions on Christian women. HLI wants to "re-educate Western Europe to help fulfill Pope John Paul II's dream of a re-Christianized, united Europe from the Atlantic to the Urals."[98]

Other conservative Christians argue against population control because they think the world needs nothing but a free-market economy to thrive. They believe the earth has an endless capacity to sustain billions in Western-style comfort. Furthermore, Christians can trust God not to allow the earth to seriously deteriorate (as if it has not already done so).[99] Clearly, these "pro-life" positions are not pro-women's lives, particularly the lives of Third World women and women of color.

90. Ibid., 40.

91. Thais Corral, speech delivered at Hampshire College's "Fight for Abortion Rights," 1 April 1995.

92. Quoted in Swomley (cited above, n. 61), 12.

93. Quoted in Swomley, 11. For other papal statements on the urgency of population stabilization, see Dyck (cited above, n. 61), 316.

94. The Pontifical Academy of Sciences, for example, recommended that couples have only two children to help curb "the world population crisis." See "Vatican Contradiction on Population Control," *Christian Century,* 7-14 September 1994, 809.

95. Loren Wilkinson, "Are Ten Billion People a Blessing?" *Christianity Today,* 11 January 1993, 19; Wendy Steinberg, "The Population Problem," *Christianity Today,* 12 December 1994, 6; Nigel M. de S. Cameron, "Cairo's Wake-Up Call," *Christianity Today,* 24 October 1994, 20-21; Andrew Steer, "Why Christians Should Support Population Programs," *Christianity Today,* 3 October 1994, 51; Loren Wilkinson, ed., *Earthkeeping in the '90s* (Grand Rapids, Mich.: Eerdmans, 1992), 51-86; and Ronald J. Fasano, "A Biblical Perspective on Ecology," *Christianity Today,* 20 June 1994, 7-8.

96. Susan Bratton, *Six Billion and More* (Louisville, Ky.: Westminster, 1992), 178, 181, 193, 198. However, Bratton does not think Christians should advocate withholding funds from population programs that supply abortions, given the dire need to stabilize the population. She particularly supports the International Planned Parenthood Federation, which has a history of distributing hormonal contraceptives without providing follow-up care or properly educating users about contraindications and side effects. See Hartmann, 194, 204, regarding Depo-Provera and the pill.

97. Cindy Rollins, "Don't Limit the Size of the Family," *Alliance Life,* 23 November 1988, 21.

98. Tom Burghardt, "Neo-Nazis Salute the Anti-Abortion Zealots," *Covert Action* 52 (Spring 1995): 30.

99. See Michael Coffman, *Saviors of the Earth?* (Chicago: Northfield Publishing, 1994). See also Tim Stafford, "Are People the Problem?" *Christianity Today,* 3 October 1994, 45-60. Stafford suggests that there are two positions on the population issue: Ehrlich's radical Malthusianism and his oppressive population policies; and Julian Simon's cornucopianism, which holds that the earth is in better environmental shape than it has ever been. E. Calvin Beisner states, "From the Christian perspective of faith in a God of providence, we can be confident that human population will never present an insuperable problem." Quoted in John W. Klotz, review of *Prospects for Growth: A Biblical View of Population, Resources and the Future,* by E. Calvin Beisner, *Concordia Journal* 18 (April 1992): 218.

If the Christian pro-life position is not pro-women's lives, and particularly not the lives of women of color and Third World women, what of the Christian pro-choice movement? I argue that unless the Christian and secular pro-choice movements come to terms with the racial aspect of the population paradigm and its concomitant *lack of choice* for women of color and Third World women, Native women, like many other women of color and Third World women — although they are overwhelmingly pro-choice — will remain skeptical about the mainstream pro-choice movement. Although in many ways the "pro-choice" populationist movements and the "pro-life" movements seem very different, as Hartmann states, they "share one thing in common: they are both anti-woman," and, in particular, they are anti-woman of color.[100]

A Christian ethic that takes seriously the lives of women of color and Third World women must reject this false polarity and be truly pro-life *and* pro-choice for *all women.* To do so, such an ethic must reject the population paradigm completely. Some women choose to work within this paradigm in the hope that they can reform the system. Others are concerned about population but, like the Christian feminists previously described, are working toward social and economic justice as well. However, continuing to work within this paradigm is problematic, given the manner in which reactionary forces attempt (usually successfully) to co-opt the demands for social justice within the population movement, particularly within Christian churches.

Gudorf states in an article for *Second Opinion* that "There is a very real danger that religion . . . will decide that (1) there is a population crisis that threatens the whole society; (2) the birthrate must be lowered; and (3) controlling women's bodies is necessary to lower the birthrate."[101] Ironically, this article was funded by Pew Charitable Trusts, which is campaigning to get religious organizations to adopt these very attitudes. Pew, the largest environmental grant maker in the United States, spent over $13 million to increase public support for population control for the Cairo conference. Population control, one of Pew's top priorities, is organized through the Global Stewardship Initiative. The initiative's targeted constituencies are environmental organizations, internal affairs and foreign policy initiatives, and religious organizations.[102] In conjunction with the Park Ridge Center, Pew organized a forum on religious perspectives on population, consumption, and the environment in Chicago in February 1994. Then, in May 1994, it hosted a consultation that brought together thinkers from major world religions to deliberate population issues and to issue a statement contradicting the Vatican's anti-choice position.[103] Pew has also targeted evangelicals by funding a report and institutes on population control for *Christianity Today.*[104] Pew provides large amounts of denominational support for work on this issue, including all the funding for the National Council of Church's (NCC) ecojustice program.[105] The NCC general secretary sits on Pew's Global Stewardship advisory committee.

As part of its program to target religious communities, Pew organized focus groups with different constituencies, including religious constituencies. It identified as "problem" constituencies those who "accept overpopulation as a problem in terms of unequal distribution of resources and mismanagement of resources — not numbers of people."[106] According to its report, mainstream Protestants tend to fall into this category. Consequently, the best way to "convert" Protestants, as it were, was thought to be through an "environmental message."[107] The report then attempted to ascertain how messages could be crafted to reach different communities. It concluded that the most effective messages would have an emotional appeal, would emphasize how individuals will personally suffer from overpopulation, and would appeal to the specific concerns of different constituencies.[108] Pew planned to target the "elites" of the religious communities, i.e., those whom it thought would understand the problem of overpopulation.[109] It seems to have met with success; in 1993, a Pew survey of thirty U.S. denominations found that 43 percent had an official statement on population.[110]

Through this work, Pew has, in Hartmann's words, managed to "manufacture consensus" about the Cairo conference among Protestant denominations. Church leaders in both evangelical and liberal denominations came out in support of the Cairo conference, lauding its steps forward on women's reproductive health issues. However, as Carol Benson Holst states, the issue of reproductive rights at the Cairo conference was just a smoke screen concealing the fact that issues of economic injustice between northern and southern nations were barely addressed. Also, while claiming not to be number-centered, the conference "Programme of Action" calls for

100. Hartmann, xvii.

101. Christine Gudorf, "Population, Ecology, and Women," *Second Opinion* 20 (January 1995): 63.

102. Pew Global Stewardship Initiative, *White Paper* (July 1993): 12.

103. Amy L. Girst and Larry L. Greenfield, "Population and Development: Conflict and Consensus at Cairo," *Second Opinion* 20 (April 1995): 51-61. "Varied Religious Stands on Population," *Christian Century,* 27 July–3 August 1994, 714-15. "Morals and Human Numbers," *Christian Century,* 20 April 1994, 409-10.

104. Stafford, 45-60.

105. Carol Benson Hoist, conversation with author, 13 March 1995. All subsequent citations of Hoist will refer to this conversation.

106. Pew Charitable Trusts, *Report of Findings from Focus Groups on Population, Consumption and the Environment,* July 1993, 64.

107. Ibid., 67.

108. Ibid., 73; and GSA Focus Group Report Memorandum, 22 October 1993, 7.

109. Pew Charitable Trusts, *Report of Findings,* 73.

110. Pew Charitable Trusts, *Global Stewardship* 1 (March 1994): 1.

nations to stabilize the population at 9.8 billion by the year 2000. Although the program denounces incentives and coercive measures, it contains no safeguards against them. The program also covenanted the signer nations to increase funds to population programs from $5 billion to $17 billion per year. Jane Hull Harvey, the United Methodist Church's assistant general secretary of the General Board of Church and Society, argues that this increase is a blessing and speculates that perhaps "we will even be able to redirect some of the enormous amounts of military aid the United States pours into Egypt, and translate those dollars into work on sustainable development, consumption and family planning for men and women."[111] Of course, nothing in the Cairo "Programme of Action" addresses redirecting funding from the military; in fact, as Hartmann points out, money for population programs usually comes from money that might otherwise go for reproductive or general health care.[112] Finally, Harvey also does not mention that two-thirds of the money is supposed to come from *developing* nations.[113]

Hoist points out that, contrary to impressions manufactured by the media, many people were very critical of the Cairo program. For instance, Hoist's former organization, Ministry for Justice in Population Concerns (MJPC, which was funded by Pew), issued a statement that was not allowed to be read at the Cairo plenary even though the ICPD had requested a statement from the organization. The statement charged that the "Programme of Action" was "nothing but an insult to women, men and children of the South who will receive an ever-growing dose of population assistance, while their issues of life and death will await the Social Development Summit of 1995."[114] At the Pew–Park Ridge conference, Hoist also called for the "dominant culture to relinquish control of the economic infrastructure." Consequently, Pew (which had funded the MJPC knowing it was concerned primarily with the relationship between social justice and population growth) defunded the MJPC because it "was too accommodating to people of color."[115] Hoist says that, although Pew at first seemed concerned about justice issues, it became clear that Pew was interested only insofar as the MJPC furthered Pew's own population agenda. Other church-based organizations, Hoist says, have privately questioned Pew's slant on population but cannot do so publicly without jeopardizing their funding. As Stephen Greene reports, Pew, through its financial resources, has the clout to change the agendas of environmental organizations to suit its own interests.[116] Consequently, even Gudorf's Pew-funded article — which calls for the transfer of resources from the North to the South, denounces dangerous contraceptives, and cites many social justice concerns — participates in the Pew-engineered consensus by stating that "the Cairo Programme of Action is correct."[117]

Populationists are also becoming adept at appropriating feminist language of increasing women's status to increase contraceptive use. According to Zero Population Growth, for example, "In cultures where a woman's value often depends upon her fertility, she is subject to violence and abandonment if she does not produce the expected number of children. . . . Oftentimes, without her husband's approval, she cannot use contraceptives without fearing for her safety."[118] Setting aside for the moment that violence against women does not happen in just "those" cultures, what populationists generally refuse to acknowledge is the role of imperialism in perpetuating sexism in Third World communities and communities of color. For instance, as Paula Gunn Allen notes, violence against women was almost unheard of in most indigenous nations prior to colonization.[119] Similarly, colonial policies of overturning communal land systems to vest private ownership of land with the male "head of the household" in Africa and other parts of the world only exacerbated sexism in these societies.[120] Gita Sen further notes that Western domination can breed conservatism, particularly regarding women's status, as colonized societies attempt to resist assimilation and cultural erosion. Women, who are seen as the bearers of culture, are often blamed for cultural breakdown: "Historically, in unsettled economic and political times, attacks on women go hand in hand with reactionary tendencies and impulses."[121] Ending neocolonial practices against Third World nations would significantly improve the status of women in those countries. However,

111. Jane Hull Harvey, "Cairo — A Kairos Moment in History," *Christian Social Action* 7 (November 1994): 15.

112. Hartmann, 139.

113. Hoist, conversation.

114. Ramona Morgan Brown and Carol Benson Hoist, "ICPD's Suppressed Voices May Be Our Future Hope," *Ministry for Justice in Population Concerns* (October-December 1994): 1. For another critical view of Cairo, see Charon Asetoyer, "Whom to Target for the North's Profits," *Wicozanni Wowapi* (Fall 1994): 2-3. Asetoyer writes, "Early into the conference, it became obvious that the issues facing Third World countries such as development, structural adjustments, and capacity building were not high on the list of issues that the Super Powers wanted to address. It was clear that the issues facing world population were going to be addressed from the top down with little regard for how this may affect developing countries."

115. Ministry for Justice in Population Concerns, *Notice of Phase-Out*, 1 January 1995. Pew's March 1994 newsletter also dismissed as "rumor mongering" the concerns of women of color about the racist implications of population control. *Global Stewardship*, 3.

116. Stephen Greene, "Who's Driving the Environmental Movement?" *Chronicle of Philanthropy* 6 (25 January 1994): 6-10.

117. Gudorf, "Population, Ecology, and Women," 64.

118. Zero Population Growth, "Bearing the Burden" (fact sheet, Washington, D.C., Spring 1992), 2.

119. Allen writes, "The assault on the system of woman power requires the replacing of a peaceful, nonpunitive, nonauthoritarian social system wherein women wield power by making social life easy and gentle with one based on child terrorization, male dominance and submission of women to male authority." Paula Gunn Allen, *The Sacred Hoop* (Boston: Beacon Press, 1986), 40.

120. Isis, *Women in Development* (Geneva: Isis, 1983), 79.

121. Sen (cited above, n. 16), 75.

populationists are generally concerned neither with ending colonialism nor with raising women's status. At the NGO forum of the Fourth UN Conference on Women in Beijing, for example, a woman from Bangladesh complained that population planners were simply adopting "feminist" rhetoric without changing their coercive policies: "Now they [population planners] say after Cairo that we just have to start calling our programs 'women's health' rather than 'population planning,' but we don't need to change anything."[122]

Another example of how demands for social justice are being co-opted by the right wing is the anti-immigration movement's appropriation of the demand for curtailed Western consumption patterns. Anti-immigration groups note that the United States consumes far more resources than does the Third World, but they conclude from this fact that the answer is to restrict immigration into the United States. They reason that immigrants who come to this country imitate the consumption patterns of the well-to-do. Thus, while claiming to be concerned about overconsumption, the right wing employs anticonsumption rhetoric to protect the "desired way of life" — that is, the unsustainable consumption patterns — of the elite in the United States.[123] Challenging consumption patterns without questioning the population paradigm leaves us vulnerable to this kind of co-optation.

These trends suggest that as long as we retain the population paradigm when the term *population* operates as a code word to signify people of color and Third World people, these people will be seen as "the problem population." This is particularly problematic at present as people of color have reached new heights in organizing around environmental justice. Government and business interests recognize the potential power of the environmental justice movement and have taken measures to divide the potential collaboration between civil rights and environmental organizations. For example, an internal memo of the Environmental Protection Agency (EPA), leaked to the press by Rep. Henry Waxman (D-Calif.), announced its plan to drive a wedge between civil rights and environmental justice organizations.[124] The EPA was planning a public relations campaign, directed toward environmental organizations, that would hype the EPA's commitment to racial diversity so that environmental organizations would be less likely to join in coalition with civil rights organizations to target the EPA's historic racist policies. It is interesting that the hype over population growth seems to coincide with the growing strength of the environmental justice movement. Now millions of dollars are being used to support programs that will divide people of color and the mainstream environmental movement. Furthermore, anti-immigrant population control groups like CCN are targeting African Americans to disrupt organizing among people of color.[125] FAIR, for instance, attempted to appeal to the African American community by holding a conference in which it blamed immigrants for the Rodney King riots.[126]

Because it is the structures of global injustice that are decimating the earth and its inhabitants, we must target these structures rather than population growth. A focus on population only distracts us from the needed task of dismantling the "new world order." As Mary Mellor states, "The future of the planet [is] in the hands of a capitalist market economy united with other powerful forces — feudalism, patriarchy, colonialism, imperialism, militarism and racism — to form a monstrous global structure of economic, cultural and political power."[127] Reducing population without taking the fate of the earth out of these hands will not help us or the earth. And as long as communities of color continue to be subject to racist population policies, the banner of reproductive rights as defined by Europeans and Euro-Americans will not meaningfully address the needs of these communities.

122. Audience participant at the NGO Forum, Fourth UN Conference on Women, Beijing, China, 30 August–8 September 1995.

123. See the Carrying Capacity Network, *Clearinghouse Bulletin* 1 (June 1991): 4, 6; and 1 (October 1991): 2, 7, 8.

124. House Subcommittee on Health and the Environment, "Staff Report," 24 February 1992.

125. Carrying Capacity Network, fund-raising appeal, December 1994. In this appeal, CCN asks for lists of organizations representing minorities, particularly African Americans, so that it can send them complimentary copies of its Immigration Briefing Book.

126. Cathi Tactaquin, "Environmentalists and the Anti-Immigrant Agenda," *Race, Poverty and the Environment* 4 (Spring 1993): 6.

127. Mary Mellor, "Building a New Vision: Feminist, Green Socialism," in *Toxic Struggles*, ed. Richard Hofrichter (Philadelphia: New Society, 1993), 39.

123 Abortion and the Sexual Agenda: A Case for Pro-Life Feminism

Sidney Callahan

The abortion debate continues. In the latest and perhaps most crucial development, pro-life feminists are contesting pro-choice feminist claims that abortion rights are prerequisites for women's full development and social equality. The outcome of this debate may be decisive for the culture as a whole. Pro-life feminists, like myself, argue on good feminist principles that women can never achieve the fulfillment of feminist goals in a society permissive toward abortion.

These new arguments over abortion take place within liberal political circles. This round of intense intra-feminist conflict has spiraled beyond earlier right-versus-left abortion debates, which focused on "tragic choices," medical judgments, and legal compromises. Feminist theorists of the pro-choice position now put forth the demand for unrestricted abortion rights as a *moral imperative* and insist upon women's right to complete reproductive freedom. They morally justify the present situation and current abortion practices. Thus it is all the more important that pro-life feminists articulate their different feminist perspective.

These opposing arguments can best be seen when presented in turn. Perhaps the most highly developed feminist arguments for the morality and legality of abortion can be found in Beverly Wildung Harrison's *Our Right to Choose* (Beacon Press, 1983) and Rosalind Pollack Petchesky's *Abortion and Woman's Choice* (Longman, 1984). Obviously it is difficult to do justice to these complex arguments, which draw on diverse strands of philosophy and social theory and are often interwoven in pro-choice feminists' own version of a "seamless garment." Yet the fundamental feminist case for the morality of abortion, encompassing the views of Harrison and Petchesky, can be analyzed in terms of four central moral claims: (1) the moral right to control one's own body; (2) the moral necessity of autonomy and choice in personal responsibility; (3) the moral claim for the contingent value of fetal life; (4) the moral right of women to true social equality.

From *Commonweal* 123 (April 25, 1986): 232-38. Used by permission.

1. The moral right to control one's own body.

Pro-choice feminism argues that a woman choosing an abortion is exercising a basic right of bodily integrity granted in our common law tradition. If she does not choose to be physically involved in the demands of pregnancy and birth, she should not be compelled to be so against her will. Just because it is *her* body which is involved, a woman should have the right to terminate any pregnancy, which at this point in medical history is tantamount to terminating fetal life. No one can be forced to donate an organ or submit to other invasive physical procedures for however good a cause. Thus no woman should be subjected to "compulsory pregnancy." And it should be noted that in pregnancy much more than a passive biological process is at stake.

From one perspective, the fetus is, as Petchesky says, a "biological parasite" taking resources from the woman's body. During pregnancy, a woman's whole life and energies will be actively involved in the nine-month process. Gestation and childbirth involve physical and psychological risks. After childbirth a woman will either be a mother who must undertake a twenty-year responsibility for childrearing, or face giving up her child for adoption or institutionalization. Since hers is the body, hers the risk, hers the burden, it is only just that she alone should be free to decide on pregnancy or abortion.

This moral claim to abortion, according to the pro-choice feminists, is especially valid in an individualistic society in which women cannot count on medical care or social support in pregnancy, childbirth, or child rearing. A moral abortion decision is never made in a social vacuum, but in the real-life society which exists here and now.

2. The moral necessity of autonomy and choice in personal responsibility.

Beyond the claim for individual *bodily* integrity, the pro-choice feminists claim that to be a full adult *morally,* a woman must be able to make responsible life commitments. To plan, choose, and exercise personal responsibility, one must have control of reproduction. A woman must be able to make yes-or-no decisions about a specific pregnancy, according to her present situation, resources, prior commitments, and life plan. Only with such reproductive freedom can a woman have the moral autonomy necessary to make mature commitments, in the area of family, work, or education.

Contraception provides a measure of personal control, but contraceptive failure or other chance events can too easily result in involuntary pregnancy. Only free access to abortion can provide the necessary guarantee. The chance biological process of an involuntary pregnancy should not be allowed to override all the other personal commitments and responsibilities a woman has: to others, to family, to work, to education, to her future development, health, or well-being. Without reproductive freedom, women's personal moral agency and human consciousness are subjected to biology and chance.

3. The moral claim for the contingent value of fetal life.

Pro-choice feminist exponents like Harrison and Petchesky claim that the value of fetal life is contingent upon the woman's free consent and subjective acceptance. The fetus must be invested with maternal valuing in order to become human. This process of "humanization" through personal consciousness and "sociality" can only be bestowed by the woman in whose body and psychosocial system a new life must mature. The meaning and value of fetal life are constructed by the woman; without this personal conferral there only exists a biological, physiological process. Thus fetal interests or fetal rights can never outweigh the woman's prior interest and rights. If a woman does not consent to invest her pregnancy with meaning or value, then the merely biological process can be freely terminated. Prior to her own free choice and conscious investment, a woman cannot be described as a "mother" nor can a "child" be said to exist.

Moreover, in cases of voluntary pregnancy, a woman can withdraw consent if fetal genetic defects or some other problem emerges at any time before birth. Late abortion should thus be granted without legal restrictions. Even the minimal qualifications and limitations on women embedded in *Roe v. Wade* are unacceptable — repressive remnants of patriarchal unwillingness to give power to women.

4. The moral right of women to full social equality.

Women have a moral right to full social equality. They should not be restricted or subordinated because of their sex. But this morally required equality cannot be realized without abortion's certain control of reproduction. Female social equality depends upon being able to compete and participate as freely as males can in the structures of educational and economic life. If a woman cannot control when and how she will be pregnant or rear children, she is at a distinct disadvantage, especially in our male-dominated world.

Psychological equality and well-being is also at stake. Women must enjoy the basic right of a person to the free exercise of heterosexual intercourse and full sexual expression, separated from procreation. No less than males, women should be able to be sexually active without the constantly inhibiting fear of pregnancy. Abortion is necessary for women's sexual fulfillment and the growth of uninhibited feminine self-confidence and ownership of their sexual powers.

But true sexual and reproductive freedom means freedom to procreate as well as to inhibit fertility. Pro-choice feminists are also worried that women's freedom to reproduce will be curtailed through the abuse of sterilization and needless hysterectomies. Besides the punitive tendencies of a male-dominated health care system, especially in response to repeated abortions or welfare pregnancies, there are other economic and social pressures inhibiting reproduction. Genuine reproductive freedom implies that day care, medical care, and financial support would be provided mothers, while fathers would take the full share in the burden and delights of raising children.

Many pro-choice feminists identify feminist ideals with communitarian, ecologically sensitive approaches to reshaping society. Following theorists like Sara Ruddick and Carol Gilligan, they link abortion rights with the growth of "maternal thinking" in our heretofore patriarchal society. Maternal thinking is loosely defined as a responsible commitment to the loving nurture of specific human beings as they actually exist in socially embedded interpersonal contexts. It is a moral perspective very different from the abstract, competitive, isolated, and principled rigidity so characteristic of patriarchy.

How does a pro-life feminist respond to these arguments? Pro-life feminists grant the good intentions of their pro-choice counterparts but protest that the pro-choice position is flawed, morally inadequate, and inconsistent with feminism's basic demands for justice. Pro-life feminists champion a more encompassing moral ideal. They recognize the claims of fetal life and offer a different perspective on what is good for women. The feminist vision is expanded and refocused.

1. From the moral right to control one's own body to a more inclusive ideal of justice.

The moral right to control one's own body does apply to cases of organ transplants, mastectomies, contraception, and sterilization; but it is not a conceptualization adequate for abortion. The abortion dilemma is caused by the fact that 266 days following a conception in one body, another body will emerge. One's own body no longer exists as a single unit but is engendering another organism's life. This dynamic passage from conception to birth is genetically ordered and universally found in the human species. Pregnancy is not like the growth of cancer or infestation by a biological parasite; it is the way every human being enters the world. Strained philosophical analogies fail to apply: having a baby is not like rescuing a drowning person, being hooked up to a famous violinist's artificial life-support system, donating organs for transplant — or anything else.

As embryology and fetology advance, it becomes clear that human development is a continuum. Just as astronomers are studying the first three minutes in the genesis of the universe, so the first moments, days, and weeks at the beginning of human life are the subject of increasing scientific attention. While neonatology pushes the definition of viability ever earlier, ultrasound and fetology expand the concept of the patient *in utero*. Within such a continuous growth process, it is hard to defend logically any demarcation point after conception as the point at which an immature form of human life is so different from the day before or the day after, that it can be morally or legally discounted as a non-person. Even the moment of birth can hardly differentiate a nine-month fetus from a newborn. It is not surprising that those who countenance late abortions are logically led to endorse selective infanticide.

The same legal tradition which in our society guarantees the right to control one's own body firmly recognizes the wrongfulness of harming other bodies, however immature, dependent, different looking, or powerless. The handicapped, the retarded, and newborns are legally protected from deliberate harm. Pro-life feminists reject the suppositions that would except the unborn from this protection.

After all, debates similar to those about the fetus were once conducted about feminine personhood. Just as women, or blacks, were considered too different, too underdeveloped, too "biological," to have souls or to possess legal rights, so the fetus is now seen as "merely" biological life, subsidiary to a person. A woman was once viewed as incorporated into the "one flesh" of her husband's person; she too was a form of bodily property. In all patriarchal unjust systems, lesser orders of human life are granted rights only when wanted, chosen, or invested with value by the powerful.

Fortunately, in the course of civilization there has been a gradual realization that justice demands the powerless and dependent to be protected against the uses of power wielded unilaterally. No human can be treated as a means to an end without consent. The fetus is an immature, dependent form of human life which only needs time and protection to develop. Surely, immaturity and dependence are not crimes.

In an effort to think about the essential requirements of a just society, philosophers like John Rawls recommend imagining yourself in an "original position," in which your position in the society to be created is hidden by a "veil of ignorance." You will have to weigh the possibility that any inequalities inherent in that society's practices may rebound upon you in the worst, as well as in the best, conceivable way. This thought experiment helps ensure justice for all.

Beverly Harrison argues that in such an envisioning of society everyone would institute abortion rights in order to guarantee that if one turned out to be a woman one would have reproductive freedom. But surely in the original position and behind the "veil of ignorance," you would have to contemplate the possibility of being the particular fetus to be aborted. Since everyone has passed through the fetal stage of development, it is false to refuse to imagine oneself in this state when thinking about a potential world in which justice would govern. Would it be just that an embryonic life — in half the cases, of course, a female life — be sacrificed to the right of a woman's control over her own body? A woman may be pregnant without consent and experience a great many penalties, but a fetus killed without consent pays the ultimate penalty.

It does not matter (*The Silent Scream* notwithstanding) whether the fetus being killed is fully conscious or feels pain. We do not sanction killing the innocent if it can be done painlessly or without the victim's awareness. Consciousness becomes important to the abortion debate because it is used as a criterion for the "personhood" so often seen as the prerequisite for legal protection. Yet certain philosophers set the standard of personhood so high that half the human race could not meet the criteria during most of their waking hours (let alone their sleeping ones). Sentience, self-consciousness, rational decision-making, social participation? Surely no infant or child under two could qualify. Either our idea of person must be expanded or another criterion, such as human life itself, be employed to protect the weak in a just society. Pro-life feminists who defend the fetus empathetically identify with an immature state of growth passed through by themselves, their children, and everyone now alive.

It also seems a travesty of just procedures that a pregnant woman now, in effect, acts as sole judge of her own case, under the most stressful conditions. Yes, one can acknowledge that the pregnant woman will be subject to the potential burdens arising from a pregnancy, but it has never been thought right to have an interested party, especially the more powerful party, decide his or her own case when there may be a conflict of interest. If one considers the matter as a case of a powerful versus a powerless, silenced claimant, the pro-choice feminist argument can rightly be inverted: since hers is the body, hers the risk, and hers the greater burden, then how in fairness can a woman be the sole judge of the fetal right to life?

Human ambivalence, a bias toward self-interest, and emotional stress have always been recognized as endangering judgment. Freud declared that love and hate are so entwined that if instant thoughts could kill, we would all be dead in the bosom of our families. In the case of a woman's involuntary pregnancy, a complex, long-term solution requiring effort and energy has to compete with the immediate solution offered by a morning's visit to an abortion clinic. On the simple, perceptual plane, with imagination and thinking curtailed, the speed, ease, and privacy of abortion, combined with the small size of the embryo, tend to make early abortions seem less morally serious — even though speed, size, technical ease, and the private nature of an act have no moral standing.

As the most recent immigrants from non-personhood, feminists have traditionally fought for justice for themselves and the world. Women rally to feminism as a new and better way to live. Rejecting male aggression and destruction, feminists seek alternative, peaceful, ecologically sensitive means to resolve conflicts while respecting human potentiality. It is a chilling inconsistency to see pro-choice feminists demanding continued access to assembly-line, technological methods of fetal killing — the vacuum aspirator, prostaglandins, and dilation and evacuation. It is a betrayal of feminism, which has built the struggle for justice on the bedrock of women's empathy. After all, "maternal thinking" receives its name from a mother's unconditional acceptance and nurture of dependent, immature life. It is difficult to develop concern for women, children, the poor and the dispossessed — and to care about peace — and at the same time ignore fetal life.

2. From the necessity of autonomy and choice in personal responsibility to an expanded sense of responsibility.

A distorted idea of morality overemphasizes individual autonomy and active choice. Morality has often been viewed too exclusively as a matter of human agency and decisive action. In moral behavior persons must explicitly choose and aggressively exert their wills to intervene in the natural and social environments. The human will dominates the body, overcomes the given, breaks out of the material limits of nature. Thus if one does not choose to be pregnant or cannot rear a child, who must be given up for adoption, then better to abort the pregnancy. Willing, planning, choosing one's moral commitments through the contracting of one's individual resources becomes the premier model of moral responsibility.

But morality also consists of the good and worthy acceptance of the unexpected events that life presents. Responsiveness and response-ability to things unchosen are also instances of the highest human moral capacity. Morality is not confined to contracted agreements of isolated individuals. Yes, one is obligated by explicit contracts freely initiated, but human beings are also obligated by implicit compacts and involuntary relationships in which persons simply find themselves. To be embedded in a family, a neighborhood, a social system, brings moral obligations which were never entered into with informed consent.

Parent-child relationships are one instance of implicit moral obligations arising by virtue of our being part of the interdependent human community. A woman, involuntarily pregnant, has a moral obligation to the now-existing dependent fetus whether she explicitly consented to its existence or not. No pro-life feminist would dispute the forceful observations of pro-choice feminists about the extreme difficulties that bearing an unwanted child in our society can entail. But the stronger force of the fetal claim presses a woman to accept these burdens; the fetus possesses rights arising from its extreme need and the interdependency and unity of humankind. The woman's moral obligation arises both from her status as a human being embedded in the interdependent human community and her unique life-giving female reproductive power. To follow the pro-choice feminist ideology of insistent individualistic autonomy and control is to betray a fundamental basis of the moral life.

3. From the moral claim of the contingent value of fetal life to the moral claim for the intrinsic value of human life.

The feminist pro-choice position which claims that the value of the fetus is contingent upon the pregnant woman's bestowal — or willed, conscious "construction" — of humanhood is seriously flawed. The inadequacies of this position flow from the erroneous premises (1) that human value and rights can be granted by individual will; (2) that the individual woman's consciousness can exist and operate in an *a priori* isolated fashion; and (3) that "mere" biological, genetic human life has little meaning. Pro-life feminism takes a very different stance to life and nature.

Human life from the beginning to the end of development *has* intrinsic value, which does not depend on meeting the selective criteria or tests set up by powerful others. A fundamental humanist assumption is at stake here. Either we are going to value embodied human life and humanity as a good thing, or take some variant of the nihilist position that assumes human life is just one more random occurrence in the universe such that each instance of human life must explicitly be justified to prove itself worthy to continue. When faced with a new life, or an involuntary pregnancy, there is a world of difference in whether one first asks, "Why continue?" or "Why not?" Where is the burden of proof going to rest? The concept of "compulsory pregnancy" is as distorted as labeling life "compulsory aging."

In a sound moral tradition, human rights arise from human needs, and it is the very nature of a right, or valid claim upon another, that it cannot be denied, conditionally delayed, or rescinded by more powerful others at their behest. It seems fallacious to hold that in the case of the fetus it is the pregnant woman alone who gives or removes its right to life and human status solely through her subjective conscious investment or "humanization." Surely no pregnant woman (or any other individual member of the species) has created her own human nature by an individually willed act of consciousness, nor for that matter been able to guarantee her own human rights. An individual woman and the unique individual embryonic life within her can only exist because of their participation in the genetic inheritance of the human species as a whole. Biological life should never be discounted. Membership in the species, or collective human family, is the basis for human solidarity, equality, and natural human rights.

4. The moral right of women to full social equality from a pro-life feminist perspective.

Pro-life feminists and pro-choice feminists are totally agreed on the moral right of women to the full social equality so far denied them. The disagreement between them concerns the definition of the desired goal and the best means to get there. Permissive abortion laws do not bring women reproductive freedom, social equality, sexual fulfillment, or full personal development.

Pragmatic failures of a pro-choice feminist position combined with a lack of moral vision are, in fact, causing disaffection among young women. Middle-aged pro-choice feminists blamed the "big chill" on the general conservative backlash. But they should look rather to their own elitist acceptance of male models of sex and to the sad picture they present of women's lives. Pitting women against their own offspring is not only morally offensive, it is psychologically and politically destructive. Women will never climb to equality and social empowerment over mounds of dead fetuses, numbering now in the millions. As long as most women choose to bear children, they stand to gain from the same constellation of attitudes and institutions that will also protect the fetus in the woman's womb — and they stand to lose from the cultural assumptions that support permissive abortion. Despite temporary conflicts of interest, feminine and fetal liberation are ultimately one and the same cause.

Women's rights and liberation are pragmatically linked to fetal rights because to obtain true equality, women need (1) more social support and changes in the structure of society, and (2) increased self-confidence, self-expectations, and self-esteem. Society in general, and men in particular, have to provide women more support in rearing the next generation, or our devastating feminization of poverty will continue. But if a woman claims the right to decide by herself whether the fetus becomes a child or not, what does this do to parental and communal responsibility? Why should men share responsibility for child support or childrearing if they cannot share in what is asserted to be the woman's sole decision? Furthermore, if explicit intentions and consciously accepted contracts are necessary for moral obligations, why should men be held responsible for what *they* do not voluntarily choose to happen? By pro-choice reasoning, a man who does not want to have a child, or whose contraceptive fails, can be exempted from the responsibilities of fatherhood and child support. Traditionally, many men have been laggards in assuming parental responsibility and support for their children; ironically, ready abortions often advocated as a response to male dereliction legitimizes male irresponsibility and paves the way for even more male detatchment and lack of commitment.

For that matter, why should the state provide a system of day-care or child support, or require workplaces to accommodate women's maternity and the needs of childbearing? Permissive abortion, granted in the name of women's privacy and reproductive freedom, ratifies the view that pregnancies and children are a woman's private individual responsibility. More and more frequently, we hear some version of this old rationalization: if she refuses to get rid of it, it's her problem. A child becomes a product of the individual woman's freely chosen investment, a form of private property resulting from her own cost-benefit calculation. The larger community is relieved of moral responsibility.

With legal abortion freely available, a clear cultural message is given: conception and pregnancy are no longer serious moral matters. With abortion as an acceptable alternative, contraception is not as responsibly used; women take risks, often at the urging of male sexual partners. Repeat abortions increase, with all their psychological and medical repercussions. With more abortion there is more abortion. Behavior shapes thought as well as the other way around. One tends to justify morally what one has done; what becomes commonplace and institutionalized seems harmless. Habituation is a powerful psychological force. Psychologically it is also true that whatever is avoided becomes more threatening; in phobias it is the retreat from anxiety-producing events which reinforces future avoidance. Women begin to see themselves as too weak to cope with involuntary pregnancies. Finally, through the potency of social pressure and the force of inertia, it becomes more and more difficult, in fact almost unthinkable, *not* to use abortion to solve problem pregnancies. Abortion becomes no longer a choice but a "necessity."

But "necessity," beyond the organic failure and death of the body, is a dynamic social construction open to interpretation. The thrust of present feminist pro-choice arguments can only increase the justifiable indications for "necessary" abortion; every unwanted fetal handicap becomes more and more unacceptable. Repeatedly assured that in the name of reproductive freedom, women have a right to specify which pregnancies and which children they will accept, women justify sex selection, and abort unwanted females. Female infanticide, after all, is probably as old a custom as the human species possesses. Indeed, all kinds of selection of the fit and the favored for the good of the family and the tribe have always existed. Selective extinction is no new program.

THERE ARE far better goals for feminists to pursue. Pro-life feminists seek to expand and deepen the more communitarian, maternal elements of feminism — and move society from its male-dominated course. First and foremost, women have to insist upon a different, woman-centered approach to sex and reproduction. While Margaret Mead stressed the "womb envy" of males in other societies, it has been more or less repressed in our own. In our male-dominated world, what men don't do, doesn't count. Pregnancy, childbirth, and nursing have been characterized as passive, debilitating, animal-like. The disease model of pregnancy and birth has been entrenched. This female disease or impairment, with its attendant "female troubles," naturally handicaps women in the "real" world of hunting, war, and the corporate fast track. Many pro-choice feminists, deliberately childless, adopt the male perspective when they cite the "basic injustice that women have to bear the babies," instead of seeing the injustice in the fact that men cannot. Women's biologically unique capacity and privilege have been denied, despised, and suppressed under male domination; unfortunately, many women have fallen for the phallic fallacy.

Childbirth often appears in pro-choice literature as a painful, traumatic, life-threatening experience. Yet giving birth is accurately seen as an arduous but normal exercise of life-giving power, a violent and ecstatic peak experience, which men can never know. Ironically, some pro-choice men and women think and talk of pregnancy and childbirth with the same repugnance that ancient ascetics displayed toward orgasms and sexual intercourse. The similarity may not be accidental. The obstetrician Niles Newton, herself a mother, has written of the extended threefold sexuality of women, who can experience orgasm, birth, and nursing as passionate pleasure-giving experiences. All of these are involuntary processes of the female body. Only orgasm, which males share, has been glorified as an involuntary function that is nature's great gift; the involuntary feminine processes of childbirth and nursing have been seen as bondage to biology.

Fully accepting our bodies as ourselves, what should women want? I think women will only flourish when there is a feminization of sexuality, very different from the current cultural trend toward masculinizing female sexuality. Women can never have the self-confidence and self-esteem they need to achieve feminist goals in society until a more holistic, feminine model of sexuality becomes the dominant cultural ethos. To say this affirms the view that men and women differ in the domain of sexual functioning, although they are more alike than different in other personality characteristics and competencies. For those of us committed to achieving sexual equality in the culture, it may be hard to accept the fact that sexual differences make it imperative to talk of distinct male and female models of sexuality. But if one wants to change sexual roles, one has to recognize preexisting conditions. A great deal of evidence is accumulating which points to biological pressures for different male and female sexual functioning.

Males always and everywhere have been more physically aggressive and more likely to fuse sexuality with aggression and dominance. Females may be more variable in their sexuality, but since Masters and Johnson, we know that women have a greater capacity than men for repeated orgasm and a more tenuous path to arousal and orgasmic release. Most obviously, women also have a far greater sociobiological investment in the act of human reproduction. On the whole, women as compared to men possess a sexuality which is more complex, more intense, more extended in time, involving higher investment, risks, and psychosocial involvement.

Considering the differences in sexual functioning, it is not surprising that men and women in the same culture have often constructed different sexual ideals. In Western culture, since the nineteenth century at least, most women have espoused a version of sexual functioning in which sex acts are embedded within deep emotional bonds and secure long-term commitments. Within these committed "pair bonds" males assume parental obligation. In the idealized Victorian version of the Christian sexual ethic, culturally endorsed and maintained by women, the double standard was not countenanced. Men and women did not need to marry to be whole persons, but if they did engage in sexual functioning, they were to be equally chaste, faithful, responsible, loving, and parentally concerned. Many of the most influential women in the nineteenth-century women's movement preached and lived this sexual ethic, often by the side of exemplary feminist men. While the ideal has never been universally obtained, a culturally dominant demand for monogamy, self-control, and emotionally bonded and committed sex works well for women in every stage of their sexual life cycles. When love, chastity, fidelity, and commitment for better or worse are the ascendant cultural prerequisites for sexual functioning, young girls and women expect protection from rape and seduction, adult women justifiably demand male support in childrearing, and older women are more protected from abandonment as their biological attractions wane.

Of course, these feminine sexual ideals always coexisted in competition with another view. A more male-oriented model of erotic or amative sexuality endorses sexual permissiveness without long-term commitment or reproductive focus. Erotic sexuality emphasizes pleasure, play, passion, individual self-expression, and romantic games of courtship and conquest. It is assumed that a variety of partners and sexual experiences are necessary to stimulate romantic passion. This erotic model of the sexual life has often worked satisfactorily for men, both heterosexual and gay, and for certain cultural elites. But for the average woman, it is quite destructive. Women can only play the erotic game successfully when, like the "*Cosmopolitan* woman," they are young, physically attractive, economically powerful, and fulfilled enough in a career to be willing to sacrifice family life. Abortion is also required. As our society increasingly endorses this male-oriented, permissive view of sexuality, it is all too ready to give women abortion on demand. Abortion helps a woman's body be more like a man's. It has been observed that *Roe v. Wade* removed the last defense women possessed against male sexual demands.

Unfortunately, the modern feminist movement made a mistaken move at a critical juncture. Rightly rebelling against patriarchy, unequal education, restricted work opportunities, and women's downtrodden political status, feminists also rejected the nineteenth-century feminine sexual ethic. Amative, erotic, permissive sexuality (along with abortion rights) became symbolically identified with other struggles for social equality in education, work, and politics. This feminist mistake also turned off many potential recruits among women who could not deny the positive dimensions of their own traditional feminine roles, nor their allegiance to the older feminine sexual ethic of love and fidelity.

An ironic situation then arose in which many pro-choice feminists preach their own double standard. In the world of work and career, women are urged to grow up, to display mature self-discipline and self-control; they are told to persevere in long-term commitments, to cope with unexpected obstacles by learning to tough out the inevitable sufferings and setbacks entailed in life and work. But this mature ethic of commitment and self-discipline, recommended as the only way to progress in the world of work and personal achievement, is discounted in the domain of sexuality.

In pro-choice feminism, a permissive, erotic view of sexuality is assumed to be the only option. Sexual intercourse with a variety of partners is seen as "inevitable" from a young age and as a positive growth experience to be managed by access to contraception and abortion. Unfortunately, the pervasive cultural conviction that adolescents, or their elders, cannot exercise sexual self-control undermines the responsible use of contraception. When a pregnancy occurs, the first abortion is viewed by some pro-choice circles as a *rite de passage*. Responsibly choosing an abortion supposedly ensures that a young woman will take charge of her own life, make her own decisions, and carefully practice contraception. But the social dynamics of a permissive, erotic model of sexuality, coupled with permissive laws, work toward repeat abortions. Instead of being empowered by their abortion choices, young women having abortions are confronting the debilitating reality of *not* bringing a baby into the world; *not* being able to count on a committed male partner; *not* accounting oneself strong enough, or the master of enough resources, to avoid killing the fetus. Young women are hardly going to develop the self-esteem, self-discipline, and self-confidence necessary to confront a male-dominated society through abortion.

The male-oriented sexual orientation has been harmful to women and children. It has helped bring us epidemics of venereal disease, infertility, pornography, sexual abuse, adolescent pregnancy, divorce, displaced older women, and abortion. Will these signals of something amiss stimulate pro-choice feminists to rethink what kind of sex ideal really serves women's best interests? While the erotic model cannot encompass commitment, the committed model can happily encompass and encourage romance, passion, and playfulness. In fact, within the security of long-term commitments, women may be more likely to experience sexual pleasure and fulfillment.

THE PRO-LIFE feminist position is not a return to the old feminine mystique. The espousal of "the eternal feminine" erred by viewing sexuality as so sacred that it cannot be humanly shaped at all. Woman's *whole* nature was supposed to be opposite man's, necessitating complementary and radically different social roles. Followed to its logical conclusion, such a view presumes that reproductive and sexual experience is necessary for human fulfillment. But as the early feminists insisted, no woman has to marry or engage in sexual intercourse to be fulfilled, nor does a woman have to give birth and raise children to be complete, nor must she stay home and function as an earth mother. But female sexuality does need to be deeply respected as a unique potential and trust. Since most contraceptives and sterilization procedures really do involve only the woman's body rather than destroying new life, they can be an acceptable and responsible moral option.

With sterilization available to accelerate the inevitable natural ending of fertility and childbearing, a woman confronts only a limited number of years in which she exercises her reproductive trust and may have to respond to an unplanned pregnancy. Responsible use of contraception can lower the probabilities even more. Yet abortion is not decreasing. The reason is the current permissive attitude embodied in the law, not the "hard cases" which constitute 3 percent of today's abortions. Since attitudes, the law, and behavior interact, pro-life feminists conclude that unless there is an enforced limitation of abortion, which currently confirms the sexual and social status quo, alternatives will never be developed. For women to get what they need in order to combine childbearing, education, and careers, society has to recognize that female bodies come with wombs. Women and their reproductive power, and the children women have, must be supported in new ways. Another and different round of feminist consciousness-raising is needed in which all of women's potential is accorded respect. This time, instead of humbly buying entrée by conforming to male lifestyles, women will demand that society accommodate itself to them.

New feminist efforts to rethink the meaning of sexuality, femininity, and reproduction are all the more vital as new techniques for artificial reproduction, surrogate motherhood, and the like present a whole new set of dilemmas. In the long run, the very long run, the abortion debate may be merely the opening round in a series of far-reaching struggles over the role of human sexuality and the ethics of reproduction. Significant changes in the culture, both positive and negative in outcome, may begin as local storms of controversy. We may be at one of those vaguely realized thresholds when we had best come to full attention. What kind of people are we going to be? Pro-life feminists pursue a vision for their sisters, daughters, and granddaughters. Will their great-granddaughters be grateful?

124 Abortion, Theologically Understood

Stanley Hauerwas

I am going to start with a sermon. Every once in a while you get a wonderful gift. Recently a former student, who is now a Presbyterian minister, mailed to me a copy of a sermon on abortion. I could not do better than offer this sermon and an ethical commentary on it. The author of the following sermon is the Reverend Terry Hamilton-Poore, formerly the chaplain of Queens College, Charlotte, North Carolina, and now of Kansas City, Missouri.

Text and Sermon

The text for the sermon is Matthew 25:31-46, from the Revised Standard Version.

> "When the Son of man comes in his glory, and all the angels with him, then he will sit on his glorious throne. Before him will be gathered all the nations, and he will separate them one from another as a shepherd separates the sheep from the goats, and he will place the sheep at his right hand, but the goats at the left. Then the King will say to those at his right hand, 'Come, O blessed of my Father, inherit the kingdom prepared for you from the foundation of the world; for I was hungry and you gave me food, I was thirsty and you gave me drink, I was a stranger and you welcomed me, I was naked and you clothed me, I was sick and you visited me, I was in prison and you came to me.' Then the righteous will answer him, 'Lord, when did we see thee hungry and feed thee, or thirsty and give thee drink? And when did we see thee a stranger and welcome thee, or naked and clothe thee? And when did we see thee sick or in prison and visit thee?' And the King will answer them, 'Truly, I say to you, as you did it to one of the least of these my brethren, you did it to me.' Then he will say to those at his left hand, 'Depart from me, you cursed, into the eternal fire prepared for the devil and his angels; for I was hungry and you gave me no food, I was thirsty and you gave me no drink, I was a stranger and you did not welcome me, naked and you did not clothe me, sick and in prison and you did not visit me.' Then they also will answer, 'Lord, when did we see thee hungry or thirsty or a stranger or naked or sick or in prison, and did not minister to thee?' Then he will answer them, 'Truly, I say to you, as you did it not to one of the least of these, you did it not to me.' And they will go away into eternal punishment, but the righteous into eternal life."

"As a Christian and a woman, I find abortion a very difficult subject to address. Even so, I believe that it is essential that the Church face the issue of abortion in a distinctly Christian manner. Because of that, I am hereby addressing not society in general, but those of us who call ourselves Christians. I also want to be clear that I am not addressing abortion as a legal issue. I believe the issue, for the Church, must be framed not around the banners of 'pro-choice' or 'pro-life,' but around God's call to care for the least among us whom Jesus calls his sisters and brothers.

"So, in this sermon, I will make three points. The first point is that the gospel favors women and children. The second point is that the customary framing of the abortion issue by both pro-choice and pro-life groups is unbiblical because it assumes that the woman is ultimately responsible for both herself and for any child she might carry. The third point is that a Christian response must reframe the issue to focus on responsibility rather than rights."

Gospel, Women, and Children

"Point number one: the gospel favors women and children. The gospel is feminist. In Matthew, Mark, Luke, and John, Jesus treats women as thinking people who are worthy of respect. This was not, of course, the usual attitude of that time. In addition, it is to the women among Jesus' followers, not to the men, that he entrusts the initial proclamation of his resurrection. It is not only Jesus himself who sees the gospel making all people equal, for Saint Paul wrote, 'There is neither Jew nor Greek, there is neither slave nor free, there is neither male nor female; for you are all one in Christ Jesus' (Gal. 3:28 RSV).

"And yet, women have been oppressed through recorded history and continue to be oppressed today. So when Jesus says, 'as you did it to one of the least of these my brethren, you did it to me' (Matt. 25:40 RSV), I have to believe that Jesus includes women among 'the least of these.' Anything that helps women, therefore, helps Jesus. When Jesus says, 'as you did it to one of the least of these my brethren, you did it to me,' he is also talking about children, because children are literally 'the least of these.' Children lack the three things the world values most — power, wealth, and influence. If we concern ourselves with people who are powerless, then children should obviously be at the top of our list. One irony of the abortion debate, as it now stands in our church and

From Stanley Hauerwas, "Abortion, Theologically Understood," in *The Church & Abortion: In Search of New Ground for Response.* Ed. Paul T. Stallsworth (Nashville: Abingdon Press, 1993), 44-66. Used by permission of the editor.

society, is that it frames these two groups, women and children, as enemies of one another."

The Woman Alone

"This brings me to my second point. The usual framing of the abortion issue, by both pro-choice and pro-life groups, is unbiblical because it assumes that the woman is ultimately responsible both for herself and for any child she might carry. Why is it that women have abortions? Women I know, and those I know about, have had abortions for two basic reasons: the fear that they could not handle the financial and physical demands of the child, and the fear that having the child would destroy relationships that are important to them.

"An example of the first fear, the inability to handle the child financially or physically, is the divorced mother of two children, the younger of whom has Down syndrome. This woman recently discovered that she was pregnant. She believed abortion was wrong. However, the father of the child would not commit himself to help raise this child, and she was afraid she could not handle raising another child on her own.

"An example of the second fear, the fear of destroying relationships, is the woman who became pregnant and was told by her husband that he would leave her if she did not have an abortion. She did not want to lose her husband, so she had the abortion. Later, her husband left her anyway.

"In both of these cases, and in others I have known, the woman has had an abortion not because she was exercising her free choice but because she felt she had no choice. In each case the responsibility for caring for the child, had she had the child, would have rested squarely and solely on the woman."

Reframing With Responsibility

"Which brings me to my third point: the Christian response to abortion must reframe the issue to focus on responsibility rather than rights. The pro-choice/pro-life debate presently pits the right of the mother to choose against the right of the fetus to live. The Christian response, on the other hand, centers on the responsibility of the whole Christian community to care for 'the least of these.'

"According to the Presbyterian Church's *Book of Order* of 1983-1985, when a person is baptized, the congregation answers this question: 'Do you, the members of this congregation, in the name of the whole Church of Christ, undertake the responsibility for the continued Christian nurture of this person, promising to be an example of the new life in Christ and to pray for him or her in this new life?' We make this promise because we know that no adult belongs to himself or herself, and that no child belongs to his or her parents, but that every person is a child of God. Because of that, every young one is our child, the church's child to care for. This is not an option. It is a responsibility.

"Let me tell you two stories about what it is like when the Church takes this responsibility seriously. The first is a story that Will Willimon, the Dean of Duke University Chapel, tells about a black church. In this church, when a teenager has a baby that she cannot care for, the church baptizes the baby and gives him/her to an older couple in the church that has the time and wisdom to raise the child. That way, says the pastor, the couple can raise the teenage mother along with the baby. 'That,' the pastor says, 'is how we do it.'

"The second story involves something that happened to a woman named Deborah. A member of her church, a divorced woman, became pregnant, and the father dropped out of the picture. The woman decided to keep the child. But as the pregnancy progressed and began to show, she became upset because she felt she could not go to church anymore. After all, here she was, a Sunday School teacher, unmarried and pregnant. So she called Deborah. Deborah told her to come to church and sit in the pew with Deborah's family, and, no matter how the church reacted, the family would support her. Well, the church rallied around when the woman's doctor told her at her six-month checkup that she owed him the remaining balance of fifteen hundred dollars by the next month; otherwise, he would not deliver the baby. The church held a baby shower and raised the money. When the time came for her to deliver, Karen was her labor coach. When the woman's mother refused to come and help after the baby was born, the church brought food and helped clean her house while she recovered from the birth. Now the woman's little girl is the child of the parish.

"This is what the Church looks like when it takes seriously its call to care for 'the least of these.' These two churches differ in certain ways: one is Methodist, the other Roman Catholic; one has a carefully planned strategy for supporting women and babies, the other simply reacted spontaneously to a particular woman and her baby. But in each case the church acted with creativity and compassion to live out the gospel.

"In our Scripture lesson today, Jesus gives a preview of the Last Judgment":

> "Then the King will say to those at his right hand, 'Come O blessed of my Father, inherit the kingdom prepared for you from the foundation of the world; for I was hungry and you gave me food, I was thirsty and you gave me drink, I was a stranger and you welcomed me, I was naked and you clothed me, I was sick and you visited me, I was in prison and you came to me.' Then the righteous will answer him, 'Lord, when did we see thee hungry and feed thee, or thirsty and give thee drink? And when did we see thee a stranger and welcome thee, or naked and clothe thee? And when did we see thee sick or in prison and visit thee?' And the King will answer them, 'Truly, I say to you, as you did it to

one of the least of these my brethren, you did it to me.'" (Matthew 25:34-40)

"We cannot simply throw the issue of abortion in the faces of women and say, 'You decide and you bear the consequences of your decision.' As the Church, our response to the abortion issue must be to shoulder the responsibility to care for women and children. We cannot do otherwise and still be the Church. If we close our doors in the faces of women and children, then we close our doors in the face of Christ."

An Ethical Commentary

I begin with this sermon because I suspect that most ministers have not preached about abortion. Most ministers have not preached about abortion because they have not had the slightest idea about how to do it in a way that would not make everyone in their congregations mad. Most ministers considering a sermon on abortion have mistakenly thought that they would have to take up the terms that are given by the wider society.

Above you have a young minister cutting through the kind of pro-choice and pro-life rhetoric that is given in the wider society. She preached a sermon on abortion that derives directly from the gospel. Her sermon is a reminder about what the Church is to be about when addressing this issue in a Christian way. That is the primary thing that I want to underline: the Church's refusal to use society's terms for the abortion debate, and the churches' willingness to take on the abortion problem as Church. This sermon suggests that abortion is not a question about the law, but about what kind of people we are to be as the Church and as Christians.

Abortion forces the Church to recognize the fallacy of a key presumption of many Christians in this society — namely, that what Christians believe about the moral life is what any right-thinking person, whether he or she is Christian or not, also believes. Again, that presumption is false. We Christians have thought that when we address the issue of abortion and when we say "we," we are talking about anybody who is a good, decent American. But that is not who "we" Christians are. If any issue is going to help us discover that, it is going to be the issue of abortion.

Beyond Rights

Christians in America are tempted to think of issues like abortion primarily in legal terms such as "rights." This is because the legal mode, as Tocqueville pointed out long ago, provides the constituting morality in liberal societies. In other words, when you live in a liberal society like ours, the fundamental problem is how you can achieve cooperative agreements between individuals who share nothing in common other than their fear of death. In liberal society the law has the function of securing such agreements. That is the reason why lawyers are to America what priests were to the medieval world. The law is our way of negotiating safe agreements between autonomous individuals who have nothing else in common other than their fear of death and their mutual desire for protection.

Therefore, rights language is fundamental in our political and moral context. In America, we oftentimes pride ourselves, as Americans, on being pragmatic people who are not ideological. But that is absolutely false. No country has ever been more theory dependent on a public philosophy than America.

Indeed, I want to argue that America is the only country that has the misfortune of being founded on a philosophical mistake — namely, the notion of inalienable rights. We Christians do not believe that we have inalienable rights. That is the false presumption of Enlightenment individualism, and it opposes everything that Christians believe about what it means to be a creature. Notice that the issue is *inalienable* rights. Rights make a certain sense when they are correlative to duties and goods, but they are not inalienable. For example, when the barons protested against the king in the Magna Carta, they did so in the name of their duties to their underlings. Duties, not rights, were primary. The rights were simply ways of remembering what the duties were.

Christians, to be more specific, do not believe that we have a right to do with our bodies whatever we want. We do not believe that we have a right to our bodies because when we are baptized we become members of one another; then we can tell one another what it is that we should, and should not, do with our bodies. I had a colleague at the University of Notre Dame who taught Judaica. He was Jewish and always said that any religion that does not tell you what to do with your genitals and pots and pans cannot be interesting. That is exactly true. In the Church we tell you what you can and cannot do with your genitals. They are not your own. They are not private. That means that you cannot commit adultery. If you do, you are no longer a member of "us." Of course pots and pans are equally important.

I was recently giving a talk at a very conservative university, Houston Baptist University. Since its business school has an ethics program, I called my talk "Why Business Ethics Is a Bad Idea." When I had finished, one of the business-school people asked, "Well goodness, what then can we Christians do about business ethics?" I said, "A place to start would be the local church. It might be established that before anyone joins a Baptist church in Houston, he or she would have to declare in public what his or her annual income is." The only people whose incomes are known in The United Methodist Church today are ordained ministers. Why should we make the ministers' salaries public and not the laity's? Most people would rather tell you what they do in the bedroom than how much they make. With these things in mind, you can see how the Church is being destroyed by the privatization of individual lives, legitimated by the American ethos. If you want to know who or what is destroying the babies of this country through abortion, look at privatization, which is learned in the economic arena.

Under the veil of American privatization, we are encouraging people to believe in the same way that Andrew Carnegie believed. He thought that he had a right to his steel mills. In the same sense, people think that they have a right to their bodies. The body is then a piece of property in a capitalist sense. Unfortunately, that is antithetical to the way we Christians think that we have to share as members of the same body of Christ.

So, you cannot separate these issues. If you think that you can be very concerned about abortion and not concerned about the privatization of American life generally, you are making a mistake. So the problem is: how should we, as Christians, think about abortion without the rights rhetoric that we have been given — right to my body, right to life, pro-choice, pro-life, and so on? In this respect, we Christians must try to make the abortion issue our issue.

Learning the Language

We must remember that the first question is not, Is abortion right or wrong? or, Is this abortion right or wrong? Rather, the first question is, Why do Christians call abortion *abortion*? And with the first question goes a second, Why do Christians think that *abortion* is a morally problematic term? To call abortion by that name is already a moral achievement. The reason why people are pro-*choice* rather than pro-*abortion* is that nobody really wants to be pro-abortion. The use of *choice* rather than *abortion* is an attempt at a linguistic transformation that tries to avoid the reality of abortion, because most people do not want to use that description. So, instead of *abortion,* another term is used, something like *termination of pregnancy*. Now, the church can live more easily in a world with "terminated pregnancies," because in that world the Church no longer claims power, even linguistic power, over that medically described part of life; instead, doctors do.

One of the interesting cultural currents is the medicalization of abortion. It is one of the ways that the medical profession is continuing to secure power against the Church. Ordained ministers can sense this when they are in hospital situations. In a hospital today, the minister feels less power than the doctor, right?

My way of explaining medicine's power over the Church is to refer to the training of ministers and doctors. When someone goes to seminary today, he can say, "I'm not into Christology this year. I'm just into relating. After all, relating is what the ministry is really about, isn't it? Ministry is about helping people relate to one another, isn't it? So I want to take some more Clinical Pastoral Education (CPE) courses." And the seminary replies, "Go ahead and do it. Right, get your head straight, and so on." A kid can go to medical school and say, "I'm not into anatomy this year. I'm into relating. So I'd like to take a few more courses in psychology, because I need to know how to relate better to people." The medical school replies, "Who in the hell do you think you are, kid? We're not interested in your interests. You're going to take anatomy. If you don't like it, that's tough."

Now, what that shows you is that people believe incompetent physicians can hurt them. Therefore, people expect medical schools to hold their students responsible for the kind of training that's necessary to be competent physicians. On the other hand, few people believe an incompetent minister can damage their salvation. This helps you see that what people want today is not salvation, but health. And that helps you see why the medical profession has, as a matter of fact, so much power over the churches and their ministry. The medical establishment is the counter-salvation-promising group in our society today.

So, when you innocently say "termination of pregnancy," while it sounds like a neutral term, you are placing your thinking under the sway of the medical profession. In contrast to the medical profession, Christians maintain that the description "abortion" is more accurate and determinative than the description "termination of pregnancy." That is a most morally serious matter.

Morally speaking, the first issue is never what we are to do, but what we should see. Here is the way it works: You can only act in the world that you can see, and you must be taught to see by learning to say. Therefore, using the language of abortion is one way of training ourselves as Christians to see and to practice its opposite — hospitality, and particularly hospitality to children and the vulnerable. Therefore, *abortion* is a word that reminds us how Christians are to speak about, to envision, and to live life — and that is to be a baptizing people that is ready to welcome new life into our communities.

In that sense abortion is as much a moral description as suicide. Exactly why does a community maintain a description like suicide? Because it reminds the community of its practice of enhancing life, even under duress. The language of suicide also works as a way to remind you that even when you are in pain, even when you are sick, you have an obligation to remain with the People of God, vulnerable and yet present.

When we joined The United Methodist Church, we promised to uphold it with "our prayers, our presence, our gifts, and our service." We often think that "our presence" is the easy one. In fact, it is the hardest one. I can illustrate this by speaking about the church I belonged to in South Bend, Indiana. It was a small group of people that originally was an Evangelical United Brethren congregation. Every Sunday we had Eucharist, prayers from the congregation, and a noon meal for the neighborhood. When the usual congregation would pray, we would pray for the hungry in Ethiopia and for an end to the war in the Near East, and so on. Well, this bag lady started coming to church and she would pray things like, "Lord, I have a cold, and I would really like you to cure it." Or, "I've just had a horrible week and I'm depressed. Lord, would you please raise my spirits?" You never hear prayers like that in most of our churches. Why? Because the last thing that Christians want to do is show one another that they are vulnerable. People go to church because they are strong; they want to reinforce the presumption of strength.

One of the crucial issues here is how we learn to be a people dependent on one another. We must learn to confess that, as a hospitable people, we need one another because we are dependent on one another. The last thing that the Church wants is a bunch of autonomous, free individuals. We want people who know how to express authentic need, because that creates community.

So, the language of abortion is a reminder about the kind of community that we need to be. Abortion language reminds the Church to be ready to receive new life as Church.

The Church As True Family

We, as church, are ready to be challenged by the other. This has to do with the fact that in the Church, every adult, whether single or married, is called to be parent. All Christian adults have parental responsibility because of baptism. Biology does not make parents in the Church; baptism does. Baptism makes all adult Christians parents and gives them the obligation to help introduce these children to the gospel. Listen to the baptismal vows; in them the whole Church promises to be parent. In this regard the Church reinvents the family.

The assumption here is that the first enemy of the family is the Church. When I taught a marriage course at Notre Dame, I used to read to my students a letter. It went something like this, "Our son had done well. He had gone to good schools, had gone through the military, had gotten out, had looked like he had a very promising career ahead. Unfortunately, he has joined some eastern religious sect. Now he does not want to have anything to do with us because we are people of 'the world.' He is never going to marry because now his true family is this funny group of people he associates with. We are heartsick. We do not know what to do about this." Then I would ask the class, "Who wrote this letter?" The students would guess, "Probably some family whose kid became a Moonie or a Hare Krishna." In fact, this is a compilation of a fourth-century, Roman senatorial family about their son's conversion to Christianity.

From the beginning we Christians have made singleness as valid a way of life as marriage. This is how. What it means to be the Church is to be a group of people called out of the world, and back into the world, to embody the hope of the Kingdom of God. Children are not necessary for the growth of the Kingdom, because the Church can call the stranger into its midst. That makes both singleness and marriage possible vocations. If everybody has to marry, then marriage is a terrible burden. But the Church does not believe that everybody has to marry. Even so, those who do not marry are also parents within the Church, because the Church is now the true family. The Church is a family into which children are brought and received. It is only within that context that it makes sense for the Church to say, "We are always ready to receive children." The People of God know no enemy when it comes to children.

From the Pro-Life Side: When Life Begins

Against the background of the Church as family, you can see that the Christian language of abortion challenges the modern tendency to reduce morality to moral dilemmas and discrete units of behavior. If that tendency is followed, you get the questions, "What is really wrong with abortion?" and "Isn't abortion a separate problem that can be settled on its own grounds?" And then you get the termination-of-pregnancy language that wants to see abortion as solely a medical problem. At the same time, you get abortion framed in a legalistic way.

When many people start talking about abortion, what is the first thing they talk about? When life begins. And why do they get into the question of when life begins? Because they think that the abortion issue is determined primarily by the claims that life is sacred and that life is never to be taken. They assume that these claims let you know how it is that you ought to think about abortion.

Well, I want to know where Christians get the notion that life is sacred. That notion seems to have no reference at all to God. Any good secularist can think life is sacred. Of course what the secularist means by the word *sacred* is interesting, but the idea that Christians are about the maintenance of some principle separate from our understanding of God is just crazy. As a matter of fact, Christians do not believe that life is sacred. I often remind my right-to-life friends that Christians took their children with them to martyrdom rather than have them raised pagan. Christians believe there is much worth dying for. We do not believe that human life is an absolute good in and of itself. Of course our desire to protect human life is part of our seeing each human being as God's creature. But that does not mean that we believe that life is an overriding good.

To say that life is an overriding good is to underwrite the modern sentimentality that there is absolutely nothing in this world for which it is worth dying. Christians know that Christianity is simply extended training in dying early. That is what we have always been about. Listen to the gospel! I know that today we use the Church primarily as a means of safety, but life in the Church should actually involve extended training in learning to die early.

When you frame the abortion issue in sacredness-of-life language, you get into intractable debates about when life begins. Notice that is an issue for legalists. For the legalists, the fundamental question becomes, How do you avoid doing the wrong thing?

In contrast, the Christian approach is not one of deciding when has life begun, but hoping that it has. We hope that human life has begun! We are not the kind of people who ask, Does human life start at the blastocyst stage, or at implantation? Instead, we are the kind of people who hope life has started, because we are ready to believe that this new life will enrich our community. We believe this not because we have sentimental views about children. Honestly, I cannot imagine anything worse than people saying that they have children because their hope for the future is in their children. You would never have children if you had them for that reason. We are able to have children because our hope is in God, who makes it possible to do the absurd thing of having children. In a world of such terrible injustice, in a world of such terrible misery, in a world that may well be about the killing of our children, having children is an extraordinary act of faith and hope. But as Christians our hope is from the God who urges us to welcome children. When children are welcomed, it is an extraordinary testimony of faith.

From the Pro-Choice Side: When Personhood Begins

On the pro-choice side you also get the abortion issue framed in a non-communitarian way. On the pro-choice side you get the question about when the fetus becomes a "person," because only persons supposedly have citizenship rights. That is the issue of *Roe v. Wade.*

It is odd for Christians to take this approach since we believe that we are first of all citizens of a far different kingdom than something called the United States of America. If we end up identifying personhood with the ability to reason — which, I think, finally renders all of our lives deeply problematic — then we cannot tell why it is that we ought to care for the profoundly retarded. One of the most chilling aspects of the current abortion debate in the wider society is the general acceptance, even among pro-life people, of the legitimacy of aborting severely defective children. Where do people get that idea? Where do people get the idea that severely defective children are somehow less than God's creatures? People get that idea by privileging rationality. We privilege our ability to reason. I find that unbelievable.

We must remember that as Christians we do not believe in the inherent sacredness of life or in personhood. Instead we believe that there is much for which to die. Christians do not believe that life is a right or that we have inherent dignity. Instead we believe that life is the gift of a gracious God. That is our primary Christian language regarding abortion: Life is the gift of a gracious God. As part of the giftedness of life, we believe that we ought to live in a profound awe of the other's existence, knowing that in the other we find God. So abortion is a description maintained by Christians to remind us of the kind of community we must be to sustain the practice of hospitality to new life. That is related to everything else that we do and believe.

Slipping Down the Slope

There is the argument that if you let abortion start occurring for the late-developed fetus, sooner or later you cannot prohibit infanticide. Here you are entering the slippery slope argument. There is a prominent, well-respected philosopher in this country named H. Tristam Englehart who wrote a book called *Foundations of Bioethics.* In the book Englehart argues that as far as he can see, there is absolutely no reason at all that we should not kill children up to a year and a half old since they are not yet persons. *Foundations* is a text widely used in our universities today by people having to deal with all kinds of bioethical problems.

I have no doubt that bioethical problems exist. After all, today you can run into all kinds of anomalies. For example, in hospitals, on one side of the hall, doctors and nurses are working very hard to save a prematurely born, five-hundred-gram child — while, on the other side of the hall, they are aborting a similar child. There are many of these anomalies. There is no question that they are happening. You can build up a collection of such horror stories. But listen, people can get used to horror. Also, opposition to the horrible should not be the final, decisive ground on which Christians stand while tackling these kinds of issues. Instead, the issue is how we as a Christian community can live in positive affirmation of the kind of hospitality that will be a witness to the society we live in. That will open up a discourse that otherwise would be impossible.

One of the reasons why the Church's position about abortion has not been authentic is that the Church has not lived and witnessed as a community in a way that challenges the fundamental secular presuppositions of both the pro-life side and the pro-choice side. We are going to have to become that kind of community if our witness is to have the kind of integrity that makes a difference.

The Male Issue

When addressing abortion, we must engage the crucial question of the relationship between men and women, and thus sexual ethics. One of the things that the church has tried to do — and this is typical of the liberal social order in which we live — is to isolate the issue of abortion from the issue of sexual ethics. We cannot do that.

As the above sermon suggests, the legalization of abortion can be seen as the further abandonment of women by men. One of the cruelest things that has happened over the last few years is convincing women that Yes is as good as No. That gives great power to men, especially in societies like ours, where men continue domination. Women's greatest power is the power of the No. This simply has to be understood. The Church has to make it clear that we understand that sexual relations are relations of power.

Unfortunately, one of the worst things that Christians have done is to underwrite romantic presuppositions about marriage. Even Christians now think that we ought to marry people simply because they are "in love." Wrong, wrong, wrong! What could being in love possibly mean? The romantic view underwrites the presumption that, because people are in love, it is therefore legitimate for them to have sexual intercourse, whether they are married or not. Contrary to this is the Church's view of marriage. Marriage, according to the Church, is the public declaration that two people have pledged to live together faithfully for a lifetime.

One of the good things about the Church's understanding of marriage is that it helps us to get a handle on making men take responsibility for their progeny. It is a great challenge for any society to get its men to take up this responsibility. As far as today's Church is concerned, we must start condemning male promiscuity. A church will not have a valid voice on abortion until it attacks male promiscuity with the ferocity it deserves. And we have got to get over being afraid of appearing prudish. Male promiscuity is nothing but the exercise of wreckless power. It is injustice. And by God we have to go after it. There is no compromise on this. Men must pay their dues. There is absolutely no backing off from that.

Christians must challenge the romanticization of sex in our society. After all, the romanticization of sex ends up with high school kids having sexual intercourse because they think they love one another. To the contrary, we must often say that that is rape. Let us be clear about it. No unattractive, fourteen-year-old woman — who is not part of the social clique of a high school, who is suddenly dated by some male, who falls all over herself with the need for approval, and who ends up in bed with him — can be said to have had anything other than rape happen to her. Let the Church speak honestly about these matters and quit pussyfooting around. Until we speak clearly on male promiscuity, we will simply continue to make the problems of teenage pregnancy and abortion female problems. Males have to be put in their place. There is no way we as a church can have an authentic voice without this clear witness.

The "Wanted Child" Syndrome

There is one other issue that I think is worth highlighting. It concerns how abortion in our society has dramatically affected the practice of having children. In discussions about abortion, one often hears that "no unwanted child ought to be born." But I can think of no greater burden than having to be a wanted child.

When I taught the marriage course at Notre Dame, the parents of my students wanted me to teach their kids what the parents did not want them to do. The kids, on the other hand, approached the course from the perspective of whether or not they should feel guilty for what they had already done. Not wanting to privilege either approach, I started the course with the question, "What reason would you give for you or for someone else wanting to have a child?" I would get answers like, "Well, children are fun." In that case I would ask them to think about their brothers and/or sisters. Another answer was, "Children are a hedge against loneliness." Then I recommended getting a dog. Also I would note that if they really wanted to feel lonely, they should think about someone that they had raised turning out to be a stranger. Another common student reply to my question was, "Kids are a manifestation of our love." "Well," I responded, "what happens when your love changes and you are still stuck with them?" I would get all kinds of answers like these from my students. But, in effect, these answers show that people today do not know why they are having children.

It happened three or four times that someone in the class, usually a young woman, would raise her hand and say, "I do not want to talk about this anymore." What this meant is that she knew that she was going to have children, yet she did not have the slightest idea why; and she did not want it examined. You can talk in your classes about whether God exists all semester and no one cares, because it does not seem to make any difference. But having children makes a difference, and the students are frightened that they do not know about these matters.

Then my students would come up with that one big answer that sounds good. They would say, "We want to have children in order to make the world a better place." By that, they think that they ought to have a perfect child. And then you get into the notion that you can have a child only if you have everything set — that is, if you are in a good "relationship," if you have your finances in good shape, the house, and so on. As a result, of course, we absolutely destroy our children, so to speak, because we do not know how to appreciate them or their differences.

Now who knows what we could possibly want when we "want a child"? The idea of want in that context is about as silly as the idea that we can marry the right person. That just does not happen. Wanting a child is particularly troubling as it finally results in a deep distrust of children with physical and mental handicaps. The crucial issue for us, as Christians, is what kind of people we need to be to be capable of welcoming into this world children, some of whom may be born with disabilities and even die.

Too often we assume compassion means preventing suffering. Too often we think that we ought to prevent suffering even if it means eliminating the sufferer. In the abortion debate, the Church's fundamental challenge is to challenge this ethics of compassion. There is no more fundamental issue than that. People who defend abortion defend it in the name of compassion. "We do not want any unwanted children born into the world," they say. But Christians are people who believe that any compassion that is not formed by the truthful worship of the true God cannot help being accursed. Christians must challenge the misbegotten compassion of this world. That is not going to be easy.

Common Questions, Uncommon Answers

QUESTION ONE: What about abortion in American society at large? That is, in your opinion, what would be the best abortion law for our society?

HAUERWAS: The Church is not nearly at the point where it can concern itself with what kind of abortion law we should have in the United States or even in the state of North Carolina. Instead we should start thinking about what it means for Christians to be the kind of community that can make a witness to the wider society about these matters.

Once I was giving a lecture on medical ethics at the University of Chicago Medical School. During the week before the lecture, the school's students and faculty had been discussing abortion. They had decided that, if a woman asked them to perform an abortion, they would do it because a doctor ought to do whatever a patient asks. So I said, "Let's not talk about abortion. Let's talk about suicide. Imagine that you are a doctor in the Emergency Room (E.R.) at Cook County Hospital, here on the edge of Lake Michigan. It's winter; the patient they have pulled out of the lake is cold; and he is brought to the E.R. He has a note attached to his clothing. It says, 'I've been studying the literature of suicide for the past thirty years. I now agree completely with Seneca on these matters. After careful consideration, I've decided to end my life. If I am rescued prior to my complete death, please do not resuscitate.'"

I said, "What would you do?"

"We'd try to save him, of course," they answered.

So I followed, "On what grounds? If you are going to do whatever the consumer asks you to do, you have no reason at all to save him."

So they countered, "But it's our job as doctors to save life."

And I said, "Even if that is the case, why do you have the right to impose your role, your specific duties, on this man?"

After quite a bit of argument, they decided that the way to solve this problem would be to save this man the first time he came into the E.R. The second time they would let him die. My sense of the matter is that secular society, which assumes that you have a right to your body, has absolutely no basis for suicide prevention centers. In other words, the wider secular society has no public moral discourse about these matters.

In this kind of setting, Christians witness to wider society, first of all, not by lobbying for a law against abortion, but by welcoming the children that the wider society does not want. Part of that witness might be to say to our pro-choice friends, "You are absolutely right. I don't think that any poor woman ought to be forced to have a child that she cannot afford. So let's work hard for an adequate child allowance in this country." That may not be entirely satisfactory, but that is one approach.

QUESTION TWO: Should the Church be creating more abortion-prevention ministries, such as homes for children?

HAUERWAS: I think that would be fine.

Let me add that I have a lot of respect for the people in Operation Rescue. However, intervention in an abortion-clinic context is so humanly painful that I'm not sure what kind of witness Christians make there. But if we go to a rescue, one of the things that I think that we ought to be ready to say to a woman considering an abortion is, "Will you come home and live with me until you have your child? And, if you want me to raise the child, I will." I think that that kind of witness would make a very powerful statement. The children's homes are good, but also I think that Christians should be the kind of people who can open our homes to a mother and her child. A lot of single people are ready to do that.

QUESTION THREE: How should the Church assist a woman who was raped and is pregnant? Where is justice, in a Niebuhrian sense, for her?

HAUERWAS: First, I am not a Niebuhrian. One of the problems with Niebuhr's account of sin is that it gets you into a lesser-of-two-evils argument. Because I am a pacifist, I do not want to entertain lesser-of-two-evils arguments. As you know, Christians are not about compromise. We are about being faithful.

Second, I do know some women who have been raped and who have had their children and become remarkable mothers. I am profoundly humbled by their witness.

Now, stop and think. Why is it that The United Methodist Church has not had much of a witness about abortion, suicide, or other such matters? We must face it: moral discourse in most of our churches is but a pale reflection of what you find in *Time* magazine. For example, when the United Methodist bishops drafted their peace pastoral, they said that most Methodist people have been pacifists or just-war people. Well that was, quite frankly, not true. I sat in on a continuing-education session at Duke right after the peace pastoral came out. I asked how many of the ministers present had heard of just-war theory prior to the pastoral. Two-thirds of the approximately one hundred ministers indicated that they had never heard of just war. The United Methodist Church has not had disciplined discourse about any of these matters.

Does our church have disciplined discourse, even about marriage? No. We let our children grow up believing that what Christians believe about marriage is the same thing that the wider society believes about marriage — that is, if you are in love with someone, you probably ought to get married. It is a crazy idea. Being in love has nothing whatsoever to do with their vocation as Christians.

When was the last time you heard of a United Methodist minister who refused to marry a couple because they were new to the congregation? People should be married within our congregations if and only if they have lived in those congregations for at least a year. After all, those getting married are making serious promises.

Furthermore, when was the last time you preached or heard a sermon on abortion? When was the last time you preached or heard a sermon on war? When was the last time you preached or heard a sermon on the kind of care we ought to give to the ill? When was the last time you preached or heard a sermon about death and dying? When was the last time you preached or heard a sermon on the political responsibilities of Christians? The problem is that we feel at a loss about how to make these kinds of matters part of the whole Church. So, in effect, our preaching betrays the Church. I do not mean to put all the blame on preaching, but ministers do have a bully pulpit that almost no one else in this society has — except for television. It is not much, but it is something. At least preachers can enliven a discourse that is not alive anywhere else, and people are hungering to be led by people of courage.

One of the deepest problems about these kinds of issues is that ministers fear their own congregations. But as the Reverend Hamilton-Poore's sermon makes clear, this kind of sermon can be preached. And people will respond to it. And it will enhance a discourse that will make possible practices that otherwise would not be there.

This brings me to comment on how we conduct our annual conferences. I think that the lack of discussion of serious theological and moral matters at annual conferences is an outrage. It is an outrage! That is the one place where the United Methodist ministry comes together every year, and yet very little serious theological and moral challenge takes place there. Annual conference today is like any other gathering of people in a business organization. Of course we have Bible study and all of that, but it is pietistic. It is pietism. It is all individualism. It is about how I can find my soul's relationship with God. But God is not just interested in our little souls. God has bigger fish to fry. If all we are interested in is our little souls, we shortchange the extraordinary adventure that the gospel calls us to be part of.

You might wonder what this means in terms of supporting a constitutional amendment on abortion. More important than that is what Christians owe our fellow participants — I do not want to use the word *citizens* because I do not believe we are citizens — in this strange society in which we find ourselves.

125 The Question of Abortion: Christian Virtue and Government Legislation

Joseph J. Kotva Jr.

Most contemporary discussions of abortion argue along familiar lines: the moral status of embryonic and fetal life, and a woman's right to choose what happens within her own body. That these are the principal terms of debate makes sense given certain features of contemporary society, including a "liberal" moral/legal legacy that focuses on autonomy and individual rights.[1]

That debate along these lines seems to be intractable is discouraging. Even more discouraging is that such arguments miss the primary Christian convictions that make intelligible the claim that abortion is an unhappy and tragic practice. Arguments about whether a human fetus is a "person," or about "rights," "privacy" and "choice," fail to capture what is at stake when we consider abortion. The real issue, instead, is whether we truly believe ourselves called by God to be the type of people and communities described in our confessions and depicted in our worship.

The Christian *Telos* and the Practice of Abortion

I here highlight certain Christian convictions regarding (in the virtue language of Aristotle and St. Thomas) our *telos* — that is, convictions about the kind of community God is calling into existence, including notions concerning the community's good and the true nature of human flourishing. The particular convictions about our *telos* under consideration are widely affirmed within the broad stream of Anabaptists Christians. Specifically, our *telos* includes becoming a worshiping community that

1. By "liberal" I mean to indicate "a family of views concerning the person and the society resembling or rooted in the social contract theories of John Locke, Thomas Hobbes, and Jean-Jacques Rousseau, who have influenced, at least indirectly, Western democracy and the American constitutional tradition. In such views, persons are seen essentially as free and autonomous agents who come into society to protect self-interest by a series of mutually advantageous agreements." — Lisa Sowle Cahill, "Abortion, Autonomy, and Community," in *Abortion and Catholicism: The American Debate,* ed. Patricia Beattie Jung and Thomas A. Shannon (New York: Crossroad, 1988), 88.

From Joseph J. Kotva, "The Question of Abortion: Christian Virtue and Government Legislation," *Mennonite Quarterly Review* 79.4 (2005): 481-504. Used by permission.

welcomes children, empowers women, and accepts that burdens and suffering often accompany the moral life and fidelity to God.

Inseparable from our *telos* are those practices congruent with moving toward and sustaining that end; by contrast, other practices, such as abortion, move us away from and undermine that end. Consider, as an illustration, the notion that our *telos* includes peacemaking. One could reasonably contend that the practice of regularly praying for our enemies moves us toward that end of being peacemakers by reducing our own animosity and teaching us to see our enemy's humanity. By contrast, the seemingly innocuous practice of daily watching the evening news gradually moves us away from that end by teaching us both to be passive and to be suspicious of others. In a similar fashion, it is primarily when we consider which practices are consistent with Christian convictions about our *telos* that we see why abortion is such a deeply troubling activity.

The Worship of God

Consider the simple claim that central to the Christian life is the love and worship of God.[2] If the Christian life, in particular the gathered life of the Christian community, is about anything, it is about worship, about attending to God. We gather to offer prayers of gratitude and to sing songs of praise. We gather in the belief that life is for relationship to God, worship of God, and service to God, which includes our love and care of others. Moreover, we gather in the hope that others too will learn to love and worship God. Practices as different as "passing the peace," summer Bible school, and budget decisions or offerings designated for "missions" all reinforce the hope inherent in worship that the community of those who know and love God will grow.

One deeply troubling aspect of abortion is that it involves the intentional termination of a life that might one day have joined the church in the love and worship of God.[3] This is a troubling prospect irrespective of the actual moral status of a human embryo or fetus. When we view worship as central to the human *telos,* the concern with abortion is not whether the human fetus is a "person"; instead, the issue is that each abortion closes off the possibility, eliminates the hope, that this particular life might one day have joined us in the worship of God.

Consider by comparison the practice of child dedication, sometimes called "the consecration of parents and infants." During this dedication, parents and congregations give thanks for the new life entrusted to them, express the deep hope that the child will come to love and serve God, and commit themselves to nurture the child toward such love and service. Thus, our *Minister's Manual* includes questions to the parents such as: "Do you dedicate yourself/yourselves . . . [to] bring up your child in the nurture and admonition of the Lord, preparing him/her to come to an open confession of Christ?" and "Do you promise to gladly surrender your child to the ministry God has in mind for him/her, even if it might involve going to the ends of the earth?"[4] Similar questions are asked of the congregation. Then, during the consecration, the minister's prayer over the child includes the words "may this God watch over you, enabling you to seek, to find, and to know him."[5]

The familiar practice of child dedication points to an understanding of the Christian *telos* that is at odds with the practice of abortion. Granted that the dedication/consecration is of a fully formed infant rather than a human embryo or human fetus, there remains an important tension between this practice and abortion. Whatever the moral status of a human embryo or human fetus, it is alive; it is human, and given the right conditions, it will develop into a fully formed human infant who might someday serve and worship God. The dedication/consecration points to an understanding of our end that hopes that each new life will join us in the worship of God. Even the most justified abortions cannot point in this same direction. At a minimum, there is a tension here that suggests the tragedy involved in nearly every abortion: here ends a life that might one day have joined us in the worship of God. This tension also suggests that abortion as a common and readily accepted practice tends to undermine, tends to slowly shape us away from, a key aspect of the Christian *telos.* Each abortion slowly and gradually shapes us, making it less likely that we will greet each new life with the expectation that here is one who might join in the worship of God.

Welcoming Children

As already implied by the practice of child dedication/consecration, we are also called to be a community that welcomes and embraces children. The Old Testament admittedly expresses some ambivalence regarding children. Children are a divine blessing, and the community

2. Cf. Stanley Hauerwas's contention that for the contemporary North American church "nothing could be more salutary than being reminded that what makes Christians Christian is our worship of God. Of course, the praise of God cannot be limited to 'liturgy,' but it is nonetheless the case that Christians learn how to be praiseworthy people through worship." — Stanley Hauerwas, *In Good Company: The Church As Polis* (Notre Dame, Ind.: University of Notre Dame Press, 1995), 153-154.

3. Cf. ". . . there is traditional Christianity, which recognizes the status of humans as residing in their ability to worship God in this life and the next. It is for this reason that even infants are baptized, confirmed, and given Communion." — H. Tristram Engelhardt, "Moral Knowledge: Some Reflections on Moral Controversies, Incompatible Moral Epistemologies, and the Culture Wars," *Christian Bioethics* 10:1 (Jan.-Apr. 2004), 85.

4. John Rempel, ed., *Minister's Manual* (Scottdale, Pa.: Herald Press, 1998), 124-125.

5. Ibid., 126.

is called to instruct and protect them, but the discipline of children is harsh, and "compared to the adult and law-abiding Jew, children do not seem to count for much."[6]

The New Testament does not exhibit the same ambivalence. The implicit and sometimes explicit notion that the Christian community welcomes children appears throughout the New Testament. For example, the infancy narratives of Jesus in Matthew and Luke; Luke's story of the 12-year-old Jesus amazing the teachers in the temple; Jesus' reference to children as exemplifying greatness in the kingdom of God and his call for us to welcome children; Jesus' blessing the children against the disciples' instincts; the instructions to fathers in Ephesians and Colossians not to provoke their children; the Old Testament command reaffirmed in James to care for the orphan; even Paul's analogy that God's Spirit makes us the adopted children of God — all assume a high view of children and our need to welcome them.[7]

In truth, saying that we are to be a community that welcomes children is easier said than done. For all their wonderful qualities, children are expensive, vulnerable, dependent and often messy. We also do not get to choose our children; we simply get the ones that we get, and the ones that we get often do not behave according to our desires. Thus, the situation with children is comparable to that of various people on the margins, such as those who are mentally ill, homeless or elderly: learning to love and accept them as gifts, learning to truly welcome them, requires practice and training.[8] Welcoming them does not always come "naturally" and is readily undermined by our society's individualistic and consumption-driven priorities. If we are to be people capable of welcoming children, then we must engage in those practices that will inculcate and sustain that capacity. Conversely, we must eschew those activities that are likely to undermine our capacity to welcome children.

What types of activities are likely to improve our communities' abilities to welcome children? Several possibilities immediately suggest themselves. For example, a focus on the infancy narratives is especially appropriate during Advent and Christmas. During this time we can underline the joyful welcome offered by the wise men and the shepherds. We can similarly emphasize how Mary — a courageous, young, unmarried, pregnant woman whose future is at risk — chooses to serve God by welcoming her pregnancy and refusing to give up on her child.[9] Likewise, we can emphasize that Joseph is remembered because he did not abandon Mary or the developing infant.[10] Conversely, we can reflect on Herod's readiness to eliminate children in his effort to maintain power and control.[11]

Reflection on these and other biblical texts does not settle contemporary disputed questions surrounding abortion, such as the moral status of a human fetus. What such reflection can do, however, is play a role in shaping attitudes and convictions compatible with becoming the sort of people who welcome children.[12] Such reflection can teach us to be understanding and supportive of those like Mary and Joseph who find themselves caught in a difficult situation. Such reflection can help us see that greatness can come from the most unlikely of infants. Such reflection can prepare us to recognize when we are sacrificing the vulnerable to protect our own positions of power and prestige.[13]

Many additional practices are necessary if we are to become and remain people who welcome children. For example, when done well, the "children's story" or "children's time" that is a part of many worship services allows children to feel included, even special, and enables adults to think a bit *more* like children. Congregation-based day care is another possible practice in the right direction. When church members support such centers with their time and money, those centers provide members with practice in welcoming children and offer an important service to sometimes struggling parents, especially to single parents and those in low-income neighborhoods. A congregational ethos that encourages adoption is yet another promising practice. When a congregation emotionally and financially supports adoption — not limiting such encouragement to those couples struggling with infertility, and including support for adopting "special needs" children — we learn to welcome all children and learn that families are constituted in various ways.

All of these examples are illustrative of those practices that will likely encourage the attitudes, dispositions, convictions and skills necessary to being the kind of people who welcome children. Abortion is not among these practices. Indeed, under most circumstances abortion reinforces priorities deeply at odds with the welcoming of children — such as prizing economic or social status or

6. Allen Verhey, *Reading the Bible in the Strange World of Medicine* (Grand Rapids, Mich.: Wm. B. Eerdmans, 2003), 218. In highlighting this ambivalence, Verhey contrasts texts such as Gen. 1:28; 4:1; 13:16; 15:5; 21:6; Ex. 22:22-23; Deut. 6:7; Ps. 78:4, 7; 127:5 with texts such as Ex. 21:15; 2 Kings 2:23-24; Prov. 22:15.

7. Lk. 1:1–2:39; Mt. 1:18–2:15; Lk. 2:41-51; Mt. 18:1-5; 19:15-18; Mk. 10:13-15; Eph. 6:4; Col. 3:21; Jas. 1:27; Rom. 8:14-21; Gal. 4:1-6; cf. 1 Jn. 3:1-2. Also instructive is Paul's implicit understanding of Christian parenting when he compares himself to "a father with his children, urging and encouraging you and pleading that you lead a life worthy of God" (1 Thess. 2:11-12).

8. Stanley Hauerwas, *A Community of Character: Toward a Constructive Christian Social Ethic* (Notre Dame, Ind.: University of Notre Dame Press, 1981), 224-227.

9. Lk. 1:26-38, 46-56.

10. Mt. 1:18-25; 2:13-15; Lk. 2:4-7.

11. Mt. 2:13-18.

12. Verhey, *Reading the Bible in the Strange World of Medicine*, 222.

13. Obviously these are not the only biblical texts that should form and inform us on such issues. See, for example, the imaginative use of the "Good Samaritan" text in relation to the issue of abortion. — L. Gregory Jones, "Christian Communities and Biomedical Technologies," in *Bioethics and the Beginning of Life*, ed. Roman J. Miller and Burrell H. Brubaker (Scottdale, Pa.: Herald Press, 1990), 115.

thinking that we get to choose those to whom we have a duty or with whom we will be in relationship. Such notions, common in our society, are often associated with abortion but undermine the costly, messy, "givenness" of welcoming children.

To be sure, some women choose abortion as a mechanism for protecting their current children — having another child, for instance, would push the family into poverty. This protective instinct is both understandable and commendable. But choosing abortion to protect an existing family is hardly a practice likely to encourage the welcoming of children. Such reasoning is more akin to battlefield triage than something on par with "children's time," day care or adoption. Triage-type thinking might be the best we can do amidst the chaos and tragedy of the battlefield. But a church that is called to welcome children will strive to free women from "battlefield" choices and will seek imaginative, even if costly to the church, alternatives to this sort of triage mentality.

Given its acceptance of the status quo and the exclusionary character of the choice, even triage-type abortion seems likely to slowly undermine our capacity to welcome children. Other reasons and social forces promoting abortions, such as protecting economic status or social contract notions of obligation, are even more likely to undermine our capacity to welcome children. Seen in this light, one clear problem with abortion is its strong propensity to shape us into people other than those most equipped to welcome children.

Empowering Women

The Old Testament does not always regard women with due respect. Likewise, patriarchal attitudes dominated ancient Israel and first-century Palestine. Such attitudes remain visible in portions of the New Testament.[14] Still, it seems clear that our *telos* as Christian community involves the full equality and mutuality of the sexes and the empowerment of women to use their God-given gifts.

Think, for instance, of the role of women in the Gospels. Mary serves as a model of fidelity and servanthood; the courageous Syrophoenician woman teaches Jesus something about his own mission as Christ; Jesus' healing miracles, themselves manifestations of the coming rule of God, were done equally for women and men; Mary, Martha's sister, chooses the better way of listening to Jesus.[15] Moreover, in striking contrast to the twelve disciples, women follow Jesus to the crucifixion, visit the tomb, receive the message of resurrection and meet the resurrected Jesus.[16] Several important women leaders are also evident in Paul's letter to the Romans, including the deacon Phoebe of Cenchreae, Paul's "co-worker" Prisca or Priscilla, and the "apostle" Junia.[17] Of course, it is from Paul that we have the grand pronouncement of equality: "there is no longer male and female; for all of you are one in Christ Jesus."[18]

What types of practices will move us toward and sustain a community that fully recognizes women's gifts and the mutuality and the equality of the sexes? Perhaps the most important practice is the church analog of affirmative-action: intentionally, explicitly seeking out gifted women to fill roles of church leadership, ranging from congregational chair to pastoral leadership to key denominational and educational positions. Witnessing women in leadership provides younger women with models to emulate and provides readily available counterexamples to unflattering gender stereotypes.

More fundamentally, such practices are a means for us to start to act now like the people we want to become. Most often, changes in character, dispositions, and attitudes require us to initially act "out-of-character" — that is, act, not in the way that comes most naturally, but in a way that at least mimics the kind of character, dispositions, and attitudes we are trying to acquire. Usually, over time and with practice, the new way of acting becomes more "natural," more habitual, because we have begun to acquire the corresponding qualities of character. The way to become more generous or courageous is, at least in part, to start acting like those who are generous and courageous. So too, the way to become a community of equality is to start acting like one.

Of course, many other practices are necessary if we are to become communities of equality and mutuality. For example, our meetings and corporate discernment processes need to be structured so that everyone's voice is heard and genuinely considered. And, given the role that language plays in shaping our perception of reality, the use of inclusive language in sermons, hymns, church documents, and everyday conversation is an important practice. Role models, too, are important in shaping our dispositions and attitudes. Thus the various mechanisms of offering role models — sermons, hallway murals, biographies and children's picture books — must include numerous examples, ancient and modern, of Christian women whose character and actions we can aspire to emulate. Depending on a congregation's social location, other practices such as congregation-based child care, educational scholarships, and tutoring and mentoring programs might help shape and sustain communities that truly aspire to empower women.

While practices such as these will likely move us toward equality and mutuality, the same cannot be said of abortion. There is growing evidence that abortion as an unrestricted, widely accepted practice is not good for women and, indeed, undermines the type of empowerment, equality and mutuality affirmed in a Christian understanding of our *telos*. Abortion harms women at the

14. E.g., 1 Tim. 2:9-15.

15. Respectively: Lk. 1:38; Mk. 7:24-30; Mk. 1:30-31; 5:21-42; Lk. 13:10-17; Lk. 10:38-42.

16. Mt. 27:55–28:10.

17. Rom. 16:1-7; cf. Acts 18:2, 26; 1 Cor. 16:19; 2 Tim. 4:19.

18. Gal. 3:28.

physical, psychological and social levels. For example, while certainly much safer than earlier illegal, "back alley" abortions, today's legal, medically supervised abortion is not an entirely benign procedure. Complications range from minor infections, which are fairly common, to severe bleeding, uterine ruptures and even death, which are relatively rare.[19] Perhaps the most notable sign of physical harm is that an induced abortion significantly raises the risk of very premature delivery and low birthweight for future births.[20] Since premature delivery is associated with numerous neurological and developmental impairments,[21] there is a real sense in which a current abortion potentially harms the woman and her future children.

Less obvious but more frequent is the psychological harm to women associated with abortion. Women who abort unintended pregnancies subsequently show significantly higher rates of generalized anxiety and multiple symptoms of post-traumatic stress disorder.[22] Similarly, there appears to be an association between induced abortion and significantly higher rates of subsequent depression.[23] Admittedly, it is not entirely clear when and to what extent abortion is a causal factor for the subsequent generalized anxiety, post-traumatic stress and depression, and when these mental health issues and induced abortion share common risk factors. The correlation does suggest, however, that for many women: (1) abortion often takes place in emotional circumstances that they find deeply troubling; (2) abortion is not "empowering" enough to substantially mitigate subsequent mental health issues; and (3) a direct causal correlation between abortion and subsequent mental health issues often cannot be ruled out. What is absolutely clear is that for a substantial minority, if not the majority, of women an induced abortion is a deeply traumatic event that is accompanied by substantial anguish and grief.[24]

Beyond the potential physical and psychological harm, our society's open abortion policies contribute to a social ethos that is not good for women. For example, many women, perhaps even the majority of women, have an abortion in part because someone is pressuring them to do so.[25] The pressure can be relatively subtle, such as withholding emotional support or expressions of love until the woman agrees to have the abortion. Shockingly often, however, the pressure comes in the form of threats, such as threats that the male partner will leave the relationship or that the family will kick the woman out of the house unless she gets an abortion. This pressure, both in more subtle and in explicit forms, comes from parents, boyfriends, friends, employers and even health clinic workers.

When women face this type of pressure, at a time

19. The Alan Guttmacher Institute asserts that "less than 1 percent of all abortion patients experience a major complication." — The Alan Guttmacher Institute, "Facts in Brief: Induced Abortion in the United States" (2005), http://www.agi-usa.org/pubs/fb_induced_abortion.pdf. However, due in part to the way the Center for Disease Control and Prevention keeps such records, there are reasons to suspect that major complications, including death, occur at a higher rate. — Cf. David C. Reardon, "The Cover-Up: Why U.S. Abortion Mortality Statistics Are Meaningless," *The Post-Abortion Review* 8:2 (April-June 2000), http://www.afterabortion.org/PAR/V8/n2/abortiondeaths.html). "The Blackmun Wall" is a Web site listing some women who have died following complications from legal abortions, along with information regarding the circumstances of their death. The web site is strongly anti-abortion, but, as near as I can tell, the information is accurate. — "The Blackmun Wall," http://www.lifedynamics.com/Pro-life_Group/Pro-choice_Women/.

20. Brent Rooney and Byron C. Calhoun, "Induced Abortion and Risk of Later Premature Births," *Journal of American Physicians and Surgeons* 8:2 (Summer 2003), 46-49; Caroline Moreaua, et al., "Previous Induced Abortions and the Risk of Very Preterm Delivery: Results of the EPIPAGE Study," *British Journal of Obstetrics and Gynecology* 112:4 (2005), 430-437.

21. Neil Marlow, et al., "Neurologic and Developmental Disability at Six Years of Age After Extremely Preterm Birth," *The New England Journal of Medicine* 352 (Jan. 2005), 9-19, http://content.nejm.org/cgi/content/abstract/352/l/9.

22. Jesse R. Cougle, et al., "Generalized Anxiety Following Unintended Pregnancies Resolved Through Childbirth and Abortion: A Cohort Study of the 1995 National Survey of Family Growth," *Journal of Anxiety Disorders* 19 (2005), 137-142; Vincent M. Rue, et al., "Induced Abortion and Traumatic Stress: A Preliminary Comparison of American and Russian Women," *Medical Science Monitor* 10:10 (2004), SR 5-16, http://www.medscimonit.com/pub/vol_10/no_10/4923.pdf.

23. Jesse R. Cougle, David C. Reardon and Priscilla K. Coleman, "Depression Associated with Abortion and Childbirth: A Long Term Analysis of the NLSY Cohort," *Medical Science Monitor* 9:4 (2003), http://www.medscimonit.com/pub/vol_9/no_4/3074.pdf; David C. Reardon and Jesse R. Cougle, "Depression and Unintended Pregnancy in the National Longitudinal Survey of Youth: A Cohort Study," *British Medical Journal* 324 (2002), 151-152, http://bmj.bmjjournals.com/cgi/reprint/324/7330/151; Gissler Mika, Hemminki Elina and Lonnqvist Jouko, "Suicides After Pregnancy in Finland, 1987-94: Register Linkage Study," *British Medical Journal* 313 (1996), 1431-1434, http://bmj.bmjjournals.com/cgi/content/full/313/7070/1431.

24. Theresa Burke, *Forbidden Grief: The Unspoken Pain of Abortion* (Acorn Books, 2002); David C. Reardon, *Aborted Women: Silent No More* (Chicago: Loyola University Press, 1987). A more abortion-affirming study is Brenda Major, et al., "Psychological Responses of Women After First-Trimester Abortion," *Archives of General Psychiatry* (2000), 777-784. Even here, however, there is disturbing evidence regarding how women experience abortion. Specifically, two years after an abortion, 30 percent of women said they would not do it again if they had it to do over and 20 percent of women were depressed. Moreover, the high dropout rate from the study (50 percent at two years) raises questions of whether the women most adversely affected by their abortions were precisely the ones not being followed by the study. — Cf. Susan Wills, "Latest Abortion Research Proves Women Harmed," *Arlington Catholic Herald* (Sept. 28, 2000), http://www.catholicherald.com/articles/00articles/5wills.htm.

25. Frederica Mathewes-Green, *Real Choices: Listening to Women, Looking for Alternatives to Abortion* (Ben Lomond, Calif.: Conciliar Press, 1997); Amy Sobie and David C. Reardon, "A Generation at Risk: How Teens Are Manipulated Into Abortion," *The Post Abortion Review* 8:1 (Jan.-Mar. 2000), http://www.afterabortion.org/PAR/V8/nl/teensabortion.html; David C. Reardon, *Aborted Women*.

when they are often quite vulnerable, it is unclear what type of "choice" they are making. It certainly is not the empowering, autonomous choice implied by the pro-choice movement. Moreover, while women undoubtedly faced similar pressures in an earlier age, our society's permissive view of abortion as a "solution" to an unintended, untimely pregnancy lends itself to this type of pressure. After all, those exerting pressure can see themselves as encouraging a socially approved fix to a problem, even viewing the pregnant woman who refuses abortion as acting irresponsibly.

This pressure to abort is symptomatic of the kind of social ethos that permissive abortion attitudes or social policies encourage. Here, "pro-life feminist" arguments that abortion undermines the prospect of a social ethos of gender mutuality and equality are particularly persuasive.

Consider, for example, psychologist Sidney Callahan's observations relating current abortion practices to male and social responsibilities:

> Society in general, and men in particular, have to provide women more support in rearing the next generation, or our devastating feminization of poverty will continue. But if a woman claims the right to decide by herself whether the fetus becomes a child or not, what does this do to paternal and communal responsibility? Why should men share responsibility for child support or child rearing if they cannot share in what is asserted to be the woman's sole decision? Furthermore . . . why should men be held responsible for what they do not voluntary choose to happen? By prochoice reasoning, a man who does not want to have a child, or whose contraceptive fails, can be exempted from the responsibilities of fatherhood and child support. Traditionally, many men have been laggards in assuming parental responsibility and support for their children; ironically, ready abortion . . . legitimizes male irresponsibility and paves the way for even more male detachment and lack of commitment.
>
> For that matter, why should the state provide a system of day care or child support, or require workplaces to accommodate women's maternity and the needs of child rearing? Permissive abortion . . . ratifies the view that pregnancies and children are a woman's private individual responsibility. . . . If she refuses to get rid of it, it's her problem. . . . The larger community is relieved of moral responsibility.[26]

Callahan is right — interpersonal, emotional, and financial support, workplace accommodation, and broader social responsibility are all undermined by a context of ready abortion. In particular, we need to acknowledge that the incredible number of female-headed, single-parent households in poverty is in part the result of a cultural ethos that includes ready abortion as an important element.[27] Readily accepted and available abortion contributes to an ethos where broader society and government, employers and the individual sexual partners are relieved of financial and emotional responsibility to mother and child. Such an ethos is not good for women or their children.

In a similar way, readily available abortion plays an important role in sustaining a sexual ideal that suits many men but is not good for most women. Callahan observes:

> While the ideal has never been universally obtained, a culturally dominant demand for monogamy, self-control, and emotionally bonded and committed sex works well for women in every stage of their sexual life cycles. When love, chastity, fidelity, and commitment for better or worse are the ascendant cultural prerequisites for sexual functioning, young girls and women expect protection from rape and seduction, adult women justifiably demand male support in child rearing, and older women are more protected from abandonment as their biological attractions wane. A more male-oriented model of erotic or amative sexuality endorses sexual permissiveness without long-term commitment or reproductive focus. Erotic sexuality emphasizes pleasure, play, passion, individual self-expression, and romantic games of courtship and conquest. It is assumed that a variety of partners and sexual experiences are necessary to stimulate romantic passion. This erotic model of the sexual life has often worked satisfactorily for men, both heterosexual and gay, and for certain cultural elites. But for the average woman, it is quite destructive. Women can only play the erotic game successfully when, like the "*Cosmopolitan* woman," they are young, physically attractive, economically powerful, and fulfilled enough in a career to be willing to sacrifice family life. Abortion is also required. As our society increasingly endorses this male-oriented, permissive view of sexuality, it is all too ready to give women abortion on demand. Abortion helps a woman's body be more like a man's.[28]

Judging by nightly television and the popularity of Internet pornography, the more "male-oriented," erotic model of sexual life continues to gain ascendancy in our culture. If women are to play their role in this model, readily accepted and available abortion is an important prerequisite, especially since contraception is often eschewed and sometimes fails even when it is not.[29] It is

26. Sidney Callahan, "Abortion and the Sexual Agenda: A Case for Prolife Feminism," in *Abortion and Catholicism: The American Debate,* ed. Patricia Beattie Jung and Thomas A. Shannon (New York: Crossroad, 1988), 135-136.

27. For a brief discussion of the increase in female-headed, single-parent households as having a significant role in the increase of child poverty, see David Wood, "Effect of Child and Family Poverty on Child Health in the United States," *Pediatrics* 112 (Sept. 2003), 708, http://pediatrics.aappublications.org/content/112/Supplement_3/707.full.

28. Callahan, "Abortion and the Sexual Agenda," 138.

29. According to the Alan Guttmacher Institute, 47 percent of abortions occur among the 7 percent or 8 percent of women who do not use any contraceptive method. Roughly 41 percent of abor-

hard to see how such a model would be good for most women. It certainly does not fit with Christian ideals of love, fidelity, mutuality and equality.

In short, permissive attitudes toward abortion undermine a Christian *telos* that seeks to empower women and sustain relationships of equality and mutuality. Abortion physically, psychologically and socially directly harms some women. Moreover, abortion contributes to a social ethos that tends to impoverish women who have children by relieving men, employers and broader society of the moral responsibility of childrearing. It likewise contributes to a sexual ethic that is destructive for most women and at odds with Christian ideals.

Burdens and Suffering

A Christian understanding of the kind of people we are called to be includes an acceptance of burdens and suffering as often accompanying fidelity to God. This is not to affirm some type of masochism or self-depreciation. Christians know that we are of great worth because we are loved by God,[30] and Christian theology does not teach us to seek out humiliation and suffering. Yet, throughout the New Testament and church history, including much of our Anabaptist history, there is a fairly straightforward recognition that holding to Christian convictions will often entail significant inconvenience and outright suffering.

Admittedly, the Old Testament sometimes suggests a cosmic calculation in which misfortune follows the wicked and the righteous prosper.[31] However, Job's example explicitly denies that simple equation, and the dramatic stories of Joseph, Daniel and Esther remind us that faithfulness is often accompanied by great risk and suffering. Those stories also remind us that God often providentially uses those burdens and suffering to life-giving ends.

The New Testament is univocal in its witness that fidelity often involves inconvenience, risk and suffering. In Matthew's Gospel, for example, Joseph and Mary's flight to Egypt, Jesus' announcement of blessing on those who are persecuted and reviled for his sake, Jesus' demand that we must be willing to pick up the cross if we are to follow him and Jesus' own struggle in the garden of Gethsemane draw a clear connection between fidelity and suffering.[32] Similarly, the apostles are said to have actually "rejoiced that they were considered worthy to suffer dishonor for the sake of the name," and Paul goes so far as to "boast" of his many afflictions suffered for Christ's sake.[33] So too, the writers of 1 Peter and Hebrews assume that remaining faithful to Christ and doing the right thing sometimes entail hardship.[34] As with the Old Testament, God often providentially turns such hardship and suffering to kingdom ends. Thus, Mary and Joseph's sacrifice saves Jesus; Jesus' death saves humanity; and apostolic suffering spreads the Gospel. Accepting certain burdens and suffering as concomitant with faithfulness to Christ is part of the Christian *telos,* always with the hope that God may yet turn that suffering to some good purpose.[35]

What practices will best shape us toward an appropriate acceptance of inconvenience, risk and suffering as often concomitant with faithfulness to Christ and doing the right thing? Reflection on the relevant biblical material is a good start, as is reflection on Christian martyrs, ancient and modern. In a similar way, careful listening to our sisters and brothers who work and live in diverse international settings can challenge us to more costly understandings of Christian faithfulness.[36] Additional important practices likely include: communion services that force us to reflect on Christ's own suffering; fasting and other physical disciplines that teach our bodies to accept discomfort;[37] charitable giving "until it hurts" that teaches us to welcome inconvenience for the sake of another.

Some practices that teach us an appropriate acceptance of inconveniences and suffering revolve around the idea of bearing one another's burdens.[38] Practices of burden-sharing are diverse. They include "sharing time" during worship services, contributions to congregation and denomination-based "deacon's" or "mutual aid funds," providing meals for families who are grieving or ill, and respite services for those caring at home for

tions occur among the 76 percent of pill users and 49 percent of condom users who report inconsistent and improper use of the contraceptive methods. — The Alan Guttmacher Institute, "Facts in Brief: Induced Abortion in the United States." Even if contraception was perfectly used by everyone, the "male-oriented," erotic model of sexual life that Callahan discusses would result in numerous unintended pregnancies. That model assumes that women will be sexually active throughout their child-bearing years, including during their middle or late teens, irrespective of whether they are in committed, long-term relationships. Under those conditions, the sheer number of sexual encounters dramatically raises the statistical likelihood of unintended pregnancy, even when properly using contraception. This point is made by Teresa Wagner, "The Pro-Life View: 30 Years After Roe v. Wade," *The Connection (NPR Program from WBUR in Boston),* http://www.theconnection.org/shows/2003/01/20030114_a_main.asp.

30. E.g., Mt. 6:26-30.

31. E.g., Deut. 30:15-16; Prov. 13:2.

32. Mt. 2:13-15; 5:10-12; 10:37-39; 26:39.

33. Acts 5:41 (NRSV); 2 Cor. 6:4-5; 11:17-30.

34. 1 Pet. 2:19-25; Heb. 10:32-37.

35. Cf. Rom. 8:15-39.

36. Mennonite Central Committee, Mennonite Mission Network and Mennonite World Conference are model organizations that can help us listen to Christians around the world, many of whom sacrifice a great deal for their calling.

37. On the importance of training our bodies in moral formation, see M. Therese Lysaught, "Witnessing Christ in Their Bodies: Martyrs and Ascetics as Doxological Disciples," *The Annual of the Society of Christian Ethics* 20 (2000), 239-262; M. Therese Lysaught, "Eucharist as Basic Training: Liturgy, Ethics, and the Body," in *Theology and Lived Christianity,* ed. David M. Hammond (Mystic, Conn.: Twenty-Third Publications, 2000), 257-286.

38. Gal. 6:2.

chronically ill or elderly family members. While such practices do not make suffering immediately "meaningful," they are often remarkably effective at mitigating our perception of suffering. More importantly, such practices show us that we are not alone even in the midst of suffering. They are tangible signs of God's presence with us.

Recalling stories of martyrs, communion, fasting, mutual aid, meal preparation and respite services illustrate the types of practices that can help shape and sustain a people capable of appropriating certain risks, burdens, inconveniences and suffering. By contrast, abortion is a practice that belongs to a very different understanding of the human *telos*. Reflecting on the relationship between abortion and certain cultural values, Lisa Sowle Cahill notes, "Our culture has a low tolerance of the burdens and failures of life and tends to deny that life has value when conducted in irremediably painful conditions. There is an expectation of ready resort to the 'technological fix' and an inability to appropriate suffering in meaningful ways."[39] Abortion fits nicely in this context as a "fix" for circumstances that appear particularly burdensome or to involve significant suffering; it is an important component of a cultural context that teaches us the wrong things regarding burdens and suffering.[40]

Permissive attitudes regarding abortion teach us that burdens, even burdens that come as a direct result of our own actions, can be avoided or fixed.[41] Consider, for example, the top three reasons cited by the Alan Guttmacher Institute that women give for having an abortion: "¾ say that having a baby would interfere with work, school or other responsibilities; about ⅔ say they cannot afford a child; and ½ say they do not want to be a single parent or are having problems with their husband or partner."[42] These figures are particularly instructive since they are put forward by a strongly "pro-choice" organization.[43] As such, these figures represent what are assumed to be good reasons for having an abortion; but they focus on avoiding the burdens that come with having children.

39. Cahill, "Abortion, Autonomy, and Community," 91.

40. Cf. Callahan, "Abortion and the Sexual Agenda," 134; John Howard Yoder, "The Biblical Evaluation of Human Life," paper presented at a conference on A Theology of Life and Human Value, sponsored by the Mennonite Medical Association (Chicago, 1973), 10.

41. Although, as signaled in the section above, I suspect that in practice the real burden often being avoided by abortion is the burden of the woman's parents, male sexual partner, employer, etc.

42. The Alan Guttmacher Institute, "Facts in Brief: Induced Abortion in the United States."

43. The Alan Guttmacher Institute describes its mission as "to protect the reproductive choices of all women and men in the United States and throughout the world. It is to support their ability to obtain the information and services needed to achieve their full human rights, safeguard their health and exercise their individual responsibilities in regard to sexual behavior and relationships, reproduction and family formation." — http://www.agi-usa.org/about/index.html.

The institute does not suggest that most women have abortions due to the severe suffering that we might associate with rape, incest or compromised health. Indeed, by the institute's own figures, abortion due to rape or incest accounts for 1 percent of abortions.[44] Nor does the institute phrase the reasons in terms of women's aspirations to noble ends. Instead, the reasons given are about avoiding the significant inconveniences and burdens of bearing children, such as interfering with one's career or costing too much.

As Christians understand it, the moral life includes the worthy acceptance of the burdens, failures, and unexpected events that life presents. We do not get to choose all of our obligations or which burdens we would rather not bear — many obligations, burdens, risks and suffering come to us uninvited. Moreover, our choices and actions often have consequences that we may not avoid simply because they do not suit us. By contrast, permissive attitudes toward abortion teach us that we get to pick our obligations and avoid the burdens and suffering that we did not explicitly choose. Here, as with worship, welcoming children and empowering women, abortion undermines the Christian *telos* by teaching us the wrong things.

What Should We Do?

Focusing on a Christian understanding of our *telos* suggests a different framework for engaging the conversation about abortion than that generally assumed in the broader culture. By considering which practices are consistent with our convictions regarding our *telos* we see why Christians should view abortion as such a deeply troubling activity. Without attention to our *telos* and its concomitant practices, we are stuck framing the issue in terms ("rights," "privacy," "autonomy") that belong more to our culture's "liberal" heritage than to the Gospel. However, when we attend to Christian convictions about our *telos* and the corresponding practices, we begin to see the full extent to which abortion undermines our becoming the kind of people God calls us to be.

The argument could be extended with numerous additional examples. For instance, abortion undermines Christian understandings of parenthood by playing a key role in our culture's increasing tendency to see children as a parents' "project" or "product" rather than a gift entrusted to parents on behalf of God and the church. One could similarly argue that abortion undermines Christian understandings of hope, which are rooted in God's providence, or that it is contrary to Anabaptist Christian notions of nonviolence, or that it weakens Anabaptist Christian understandings of the support and accountability due each other within community.

44. The Alan Guttmacher Institute, "Facts in Brief: Induced Abortion in the United States." Abortion due to serious health concerns would be roughly comparable.

But where do such arguments leave us? How should we respond to abortion? What are the next steps?

Focus on Fitting Practices

Part of the answer is that we should not focus on "responding" to abortion; rather, we should focus on nurturing those practices that shape us in the right direction. That is, we should put our energy into the practices best associated with worship, welcoming children, empowering women, burden-bearing/burden-sharing and so on. If our calling is to become a particular sort of people — growing daily into conformity with Christ — then our energies should be in that direction.

Of course, this "nonresponse" is also a constructive response. If the Christian *telos* is indeed dramatically at odds with abortion as a practice, then people shaped well by the practices concomitant with the Christian *telos* will seldom view abortion as a live option for themselves and will be engaged in activities (such as providing day care and staffing pregnancy crisis centers, but also more general practices of welcome and respect) that help others avoid abortions.

Clearly, more congregational, regional and denominational efforts aimed at helping the "world" to be more hospitable to women and children are also in order. The church's own life is to provide a hint or foretaste of where God is taking the entire world.[45] We should therefore model that end for the world. We should also encourage the world's own incremental steps towards its true, though usually unacknowledged, *telos* — including welcoming children and empowering women. Moreover, if, as I have suggested, abortion is significantly at odds with these ends, we should work to help our neighbors avoid this practice.

Just as the Mennonite Church USA is currently engaged in addressing questions of health-care access, we would do well to have a period of concentrated effort aimed at improving the situation for children and women. For example, providing day care that is available on a sliding fee scale, staffing pregnancy crisis centers, working toward employment policies that provide for parental leave and child care, volunteering as tutors in our neighborhood schools, encouraging male neighbors and colleagues to emotionally and financially invest in their children, and sharing our respect of parenting as a vocation (perhaps in narrative book form or newspaper editorials) are a few ways we could help the world to be more affirming of women and children and less prone to the practice of abortion.

Community Discernment in Rare Cases

I have argued that abortion as a readily accepted practice is at odds with the Christian *telos*. This argument does not require the Christian community to rule out all possible cases of abortion. Although abortion will be extremely rare within a community committed to the practices concomitant with its end, highly unusual situations may arise in which an abortion might be justifiable.

Consider, for example, a fetus diagnosed as anencephalic (having only a brain stem) or as suffering from trisomy 18, or Edward's Syndrome — a terrible disease in which most die in utero, and 90 percent of those who are born die within the first year, and those who do survive the first year suffer from congenital heart disease, respiratory illnesses and severe retardation, and require significant medical interventions throughout their remaining days. In my estimation, these illnesses present significant reasons to at least consider an abortion.[46] These are not lives that we can justifiably hope will join us in worshiping God, at least not this side of the grave. It is far from clear what it means to welcome such children, except perhaps holding their hands as they die. It is equally unclear how we are empowering a woman by encouraging her to carry such a child to term. And, in terms of suffering, perhaps carrying such children to term asks those children to bear too much of the burden. In such rare and tragic instances, having an abortion does not reflect our society's permissive attitudes toward abortion and does not necessarily work against the Christian *telos*.[47]

If we are to avoid self-serving justifications and the atomistic tendency of "choice," community mechanisms of discernment, support and accountability are essential when such rare situations seemingly present themselves. New Testament emphases on mutual aid, burden-sharing, forgiveness and shared discernment suggest that such decisions and the subsequent responsibility (whether an abortion and its aftermath or raising the child) are partially shared tasks.[48] Because the pregnant

45. E.g., Mt. 5:14-16; Acts 2:41-47; Gal. 3:28; Eph. 2:13-22; Phil. 2:15; Jas. 1:18. This theme of church as first fruits is common in the work of Stanley Hauerwas and John Howard Yoder, for example: Stanley Hauerwas, *The Peaceable Kingdom: A Primer in Christian Ethics* (Notre Dame, Ind.: University of Notre Dame Press, 1983), 60-62; Hauerwas, *In Good Company,* 157; John Howard Yoder, *For the Nations: Essays Public and Evangelical* (Grand Rapids, Mich.: Wm. B. Eerdmans, 1997), 228; John Howard Yoder, *The Royal Priesthood: Essays Ecclesiological and Ecumenical* (Grand Rapids, Mich.: Wm. B. Eerdmans, 1994), 146, 151-56; John Howard Yoder, *The Christian Witness to the State* (Newton, Kan.: Faith and Life Process, 1964), 10.

46. Cf. Verhey, *Reading the Bible in the Strange World of Medicine,* 248.

47. Pregnancy due to violence (rape, incest), severe risks to the woman's health and other severe fetal diagnoses raise similar questions of potentially appropriate cases of abortion. I use anencephaly and Edward's Syndrome to illustrate the point because I believe they come the closest to providing an "ideal type" in which abortion likely does not undermine the Christian *telos*.

48. Mt. 18:15-20; Acts 2:41-45, 4:32-35, 15:1-30; Rom. 12:1-8; 1 Cor. 5:9–6:7, 14:26-31. As in the culture more broadly, abortion was rigorously debated within Mennonite circles in the early 1970s. In contrast to the broader culture, one theme repeatedly affirmed in those church settings was an emphasis on abortion as an interpersonal and social issue: the decision affects mother, child, other chil-

woman may be in a particularly vulnerable position, it is crucial that the mechanisms of shared discernment and responsibility occur within what the woman perceives to be a "safe space"; otherwise we risk new forms of coercion in the name of discernment.

The Limits of Legislation

It does not follow from the argument against abortion outlined above that Anabaptist Christians should support legislative efforts to make all or most abortions illegal.[49] My reservations regarding such legislative efforts are multilayered.

First, the physical, often life-threatening harm done to women from illegal, "back alley" abortions before Roe v. Wade was both real and common.[50] While there are no reliable statistics regarding this harm, many women died and many thousands of women were seriously injured. Since it is clear that many women will seek abortions irrespective of their legality, medically supervised, legal abortions are the safer, more prudent option.

Although the analogy is strained, the argument here is similar to that favoring needle exchange programs. Since most heroin addicts will use the drug despite the lack of clean needles, providing clean needles (or bleach kits) will help to prevent the spread of HIV and other illnesses. Support for needle exchange programs does not indicate a support for using heroin. Instead, support for such programs derives from a prudential evaluation of people's likely behavior and the desire that the individual and social harms inflicted by heroin not be compounded by the harm of dirty needles. So too, abortion inflicts individual and social harms, but that harm should not be compounded by illegal, higher risk abortions.

Second, to legislatively ban most abortions violates the conscience of those who believe that ready access to abortion is a moral requirement. Most Americans believe that most forms of abortion should be legal and available.[51] An unknown but significant percentage of these believe that ready access to abortion is a high moral priority, involving issues of social justice along with privacy and reproductive rights.

We should be concerned about the violence implied in using state power to impose too many limits on abortion at a time when society itself is far from a moral consensus on the issue. More specifically, we should be concerned about the violence implied in using state power against those who in good conscience believe that abortion is a fundamental right or essential matter of social justice.

Abortion is a flashpoint in the current culture wars that highlights the competing belief systems, ideologies and conceptual-linguistic frameworks at work in our society. Many Christian concerns about abortion are likely to be intelligible only in the context of specific practices, such as Christian worship, and specific Christian convictions, such as our value coming from our being loved by God.[52] The state and its laws seem ill-equipped to adjudicate such fundamental disputes. Using moral persuasion, through the example of our lives and the power of our words, to change people's minds about abortion is more in keeping with Anabaptist convictions regarding both violence and the state.

A closely related third point arises from John Howard Yoder's observation that Anabaptism recognizes a "distinction between discipleship standards which are incumbent upon those who have freely chosen and publicly pledged to follow Christ, and the moral life of the wider community."[53] According to Yoder, Christian groups that assume little difference between Christian morality and the civil order readily appeal to civil sanctions to support their judgment that a specific activity is wrong.

---

dren, father, church community and so on. Consequently, such questions should be answered in the context of safe, caring communities that also bear the responsibility for whatever decision is made, including providing care for the child or standing as a graceful presence with the one who has an abortion. — E.g., Ross T. Bender, "The Religious Perspectives," Conference on Life and Human Values, sponsored by Mennonite Medical Association (Chicago, 1973), 29-30; Willard Krabill, "Response to Ross Bender," Conference on Life and Human Values, sponsored by Mennonite Medical Association (Chicago, 1973), 35.

49. Most official and quasi-official statements from the larger Anabaptist groups in North America have voiced significant reservations about engaging in legislative efforts to ban most abortions, for example: Mennonite Church General Assembly, "Summary Statement on Abortion" (1975), http://www.mcusaarchives.org/library/resolutions/-abortion-1975.html; triennial sessions of the General Conference Mennonite Church, "Guidelines on Abortion" (Estes Park, Colo., 1980), http://www.mcusaarchives.org/library/resolutions/guidelinesonabortion-1980.html; 198th Annual Conference of the Church of the Brethren, "Statement on Abortion," *Messenger (Official Publication of the Church of the Brethren)*, Aug. 1984, 14; Kathy Shantz, comp. and ed., "MCC Canada Resource Packet on Abortion" (Available from Mennonite Central Committee, 21 South 12th St., PO Box 500, Akron, Pa., 17501 and MCC Canada, 134 Plaza Drive, Winnipeg, Man., R3T 5K9, 1991); Mennonite Church USA, "Mennonite Church USA Statement on Abortion," adopted by Delegate Assembly (Atlanta, 2003), http://www.mennoniteusa.org/-NewItems/delegates/statement_abortion.pdf Cf. "Statement on Abortion," Approved by the M.C.C. U.S. Board, Nov. 3, 2001, http://peace.mennolink.org/articles/mccabort.html; Joseph J. Kotva Jr, *The Anabaptist Tradition: Religious Beliefs and Healthcare Decisions,* Religious Traditions and Health Care Decisions Handbook Series (Park Ridge, Ill.: Park Ridge Center, 2002), 8. A statement more open to legislative action is General Conference of Mennonites in Canada, "Resolution on Abortion," reprinted in *A Theology of Life and Human Value* (Chicago: Mennonite Medical Association, 1973).

50. Dorothy Fadiman, prod., *From the Back Alleys to the Supreme Court & Beyond,* audio recordings (1999), http://www.albany.edu/history/FromTheBackAlleys.html.

51. E.g., see the ABC News/Washington Post poll of January, 2003 and the Public Agenda poll of July, 2003 available at http://www.publicagenda.org/issues/-pcc_detail.cfm?issue_type=abortion&list=9.

52. Cf. Engelhardt, "Moral Knowledge."

53. Yoder, "The Biblical Evaluation of Human Life," 11.

By contrast, the Anabaptist recognition of different moral levels produced a readiness "to abandon legislative control of the total culture" that is at the "very heart of the originality of the Anabaptists over against the state churches."[54] Our tradition's internal logic presumes that our moral stance will often differ significantly from that of the wider social order and explicitly eschews trying to bridge that gap with legislative control.[55]

Fourth, while assessments of fetal moral status are debatable, I cannot find a socially compelling argument that early abortion is equivalent to homicide. An assertion of that equivalency is behind most attempts to ban all or most abortions.[56] Yet, short of particular faith assertions about ensoulment at conception or Thomistic claims about "substance," the grounds for that equivalency are unclear.[57]

Sissela Bok correctly notes that because there is no "semblance of human form, no conscious life or capability to life independently, no knowledge of death . . . one cannot" meaningfully affix charges such as "murder" or "homicide" to early abortions.[58] This judgment is supported by our everyday moral intuitions regarding similar-stage miscarriages. While they are often sources of disappointment and grief, people do not typically mourn or ritualize early to mid-first trimester miscarriages in the same way they do postnatal life. The reality of miscarriages is not a justification for abortion. But our reaction to those miscarriages argues that we do not regard embryonic and early fetal life as having the kind of status that justifies referring to early abortions as murder or homicide.

Fifth, analogies to bodily life-support are sufficiently persuasive to reject severe legislative restrictions on abortion. Along these lines, Patricia Beattie Jung's argument comparing abortion to organ donation is especially helpful.[59] Just as we do not legally demand histocompatible parents to donate kidneys or bone marrow or even blood to their children, how could we legally demand a woman to carry her pregnancy to term? Surely a good father in even modestly good health will happily donate his kidney or bone marrow to his own child. Yet, we legally treat such donations as gift relationships that are socially honored but are not required or enforced by law. Indeed, should medical staff exert significant moral pressure on the father, that donation would likely be criticized as failing to meet standards of informed consent since the father did not fully understand the voluntary or discretionary character of the act.[60] We may rightly think less of a father who fails to make the needed donation, but we do not use the force of law to require him to do so. As a matter of consistency (and as a matter of political prudence), we should not legally require women to carry prenatal life against their will if we are unable or unwilling to make similar demands of fathers (and mothers) regarding postnatal life.

Despite these arguments against efforts to legislatively ban most forms of abortion, some more limited legislative efforts may be in order. Law can function in various ways, through regulation as well as punishment. Law can also serve a limited educative role, expressing society's moral judgments. Because law can serve this educative function and because there is fairly broad societal consensus that abortion ought not to be approached flippantly, legal measures such as mandating twenty-four-hour waiting periods, limiting easy access to abortion after the first trimester, and adding restrictions on dilation and extraction, or "partial-birth" abortions, all make good sense.

In practice, such legislation will directly prevent few abortions since it does not impose significant barriers to or restrictions on abortion. Moreover, because there is large social support for such measures and because the restrictions are minimal in practice, such measures do not constitute violence against those who view abortion as a matter of rights or social justice.[61] However, even

54. Ibid., 12.

55. Refraining from such legislative control regarding abortion is not analogous to other recent questions regarding the death penalty or health-care reform. With abortion, we would be asking the state to stop individuals from taking actions that we view as wrong. By contrast, appeals to eliminate the death penalty are attempts to persuade the state itself to refrain from specific wrongful actions that are done partially in our name. Questions of state involvement in health-care access are even more unlike abortion: here we are requesting that the state use its resources for the public good. However, the questions of abortion and health-care access are similar in that I do not favor the legislative imposition of a single-payer health-care system (even though I am convinced that it is the best way to control costs and provide access), precisely because many appear to have moral objections to such a system.

56. E.g., Teresa Wagner, "The Pro-Life View: 30 Years After Roe v. Wade," repeatedly refers to abortion as homicide.

57. Patrick Lee, "A Christian Philosopher's View of Recent Directions in the Abortion Debate," *Christian Bioethics* 10:1 (Jan-Apr. 2004), 7-31; Francis J. Beckwith, "The Explanatory Power of the Substance View of Persons," *Christian Bioethics* 10:1 (January-April 2004), 33-54 provide interesting accounts of personhood as "substance." If one accepts those accounts, the claim of abortion as homicide makes sense. However, as H. Tristram Engelhardt points out, those accounts fail to take seriously their own dependence on a specific (Thomistic) tradition and "pretend that all shared a common morality." — Engelhardt, "Moral Knowledge," 79. Moreover, if carried to its logical conclusion, their account of "substance" means that individuals who are brain-dead or in a persistent vegetative state remain "persons," which would be a highly contentious conclusion.

58. Sissela Bok, "Ethical Problems of Abortion," in *Bioethics,* 3rd ed., ed. Thomas A. Shannon (Mahwah, N.J.: Paulist Press, 1987), 32.

59. Patricia Beattie Jung, "Abortion and Organ Donation: Christian Reflections on Bodily Life Support," in *Abortion and Catholicism: The American Debate,* ed. Patricia Beattie Jung and Thomas A. Shannon (New York: Crossroad, 1988), 141-171.

60. Ibid., 143-145.

61. Cf. Kaiser, "Health Poll Search" at http://www.kaisernetwork.org/health_poll/hpoll_index.cfm. For example, depending on how the question is phrased, the percent of support for parental consent laws and twenty-four-hour waiting periods range from the low 60s to the mid-70s. — http://www.ropercenter.uconn.edu/cgibin/hsrun.exe/roperweb/-HPOLL/-HPOLL.htx;start=hpollsearchAM?sid=C19.

though the actual barriers are minimal, such legislation is substantial enough to educate by indicating that abortion is a serious matter not to be engaged in lightly.

Conclusion

The previous section on legislation should not unduly distract from the central argument that contemporary debates about abortion often miss the primary Christian convictions that make intelligible the claim that abortion is an unhappy and tragic practice that we should seek to minimize. Permissive abortion practices are at odds with the Christian *telos* and stand in stark contrast to those practices well-suited to becoming a worshiping community that welcomes children, empowers women and accepts that burdens and suffering often accompany the moral life. Our primary response to abortion should be to focus on becoming that sort of community by engaging in the appropriate practices, including practices of community support, accountability and discernment. We should also look for ways to help our society become more hospitable toward women and children, which may include some limited legislative efforts that signify abortion's seriousness.

CHAPTER TWENTY

Genetics

"Should George get a genetic test for Huntington's disease? May companies make a genetic diagnosis a condition for insurance or employment? Should Serena be tested to see if she is a carrier for sickle-cell disease before she marries Charles? Should Helen and Sam have prenatal diagnosis to indicate whether their fetus has the genetic mutation for cystic fibrosis? May they utilize IVF and preimplantation diagnosis? Should Marie and John have prenatal diagnosis to determine the sex of their fetus?"

Allen Verhey poses this list of questions in his essay "Mapping the Human Genome . . . Biblically."[1] This list could be expanded: Should Jane be tested for the main breast cancer mutation, BRCA1, and undergo prophylactic removal of her breasts to avoid the disease? If she tests positive, should she tell her sisters, daughters, and nieces? Should Peter and Alice have their children screened for Alzheimer's? Should insurance companies have access to that information? Should Matthew and Jenny allow their son Andrew to undergo gene therapy for cystic fibrosis? Should they prefer that the therapy affect Andrew's germline cells so that the correction to his CF mutation would be passed on to his children? What if the therapy was not for a disease, like cystic fibrosis, but sought to enhance his ability to play baseball?

And the list could continue. Such questions have long served as the major focus of ethical reflection on genetics. These are the questions that jump out from magazine covers at Target and at grocery stores as shoppers wait in the checkout line, that form the headlines on YahooNews, and that grace the science section and Sunday magazine of *The New York Times*. They form the table of contents of most books on the ethics of genetics, whether written from a secular or theological perspective. They structure the syllabi of hundreds of courses on medical ethics at colleges and universities across the U.S.

As the above list makes clear, these questions — and therefore the conversation on the ethics of genetics within scholarly and popular discourse — are shaped by two assumptions, identified helpfully by Bronislaw Szerszynski in his essay "That Deep Surface: The Human Genome Project and the Death of the Human" (selection 132). First, the questions assume that science and religion are complementary activities. Science addresses questions of reality (what is), how things work, and what can be done. Theology, on the other hand, addresses questions of meaning and ethics: What do these new technologies mean and should we use them? Second, they assume that the key questions pertain to specific technological advances: What should Christians think about technology X and how, if at all, should they use it?

These assumptions are both demonstrated and challenged by the selections in this chapter. For example, we see these assumptions at work in James Peterson's essay "Ethical Standards for Genetic Intervention" (selection 127). Genetic technologies provide benefits and risks, he argues, and the task of Christian reflection is to determine standards for intervention. Warned by the unfaithful steward in the New Testament parable who buries his talent, Peterson argues that Christians ought to be prudent and responsible with the gifts God has entrusted to us, even when those gifts come in the form of technology. Yet prudent stewardship requires recognizing limits as well, if harm will occur from overstepping these limits. The challenge is to determine standards for making such determinations; Peterson offers five criteria for making such determinations. With such criteria in hand, he argues, Christians can proceed responsibly.

Peterson is right that genetic knowledge can be put to good uses and that such uses should be affirmed. Advances in genetics have greatly enhanced the diagnostic capabilities of medicine, both in breadth and in specificity. At times, such diagnoses enable physicians to prescribe useful therapies — more frequent monitoring or prophylactic mastectomy for those with the BRCA1 gene, a modified diet for those with the PKU mutation, or even personally tailored pharmaceutical prescriptions based on individual genetic variations. At other times such diagnoses can allow persons or couples to engage in more realistic life-planning, if, for example, they discover they carry a gene for a late-onset disease (e.g., Huntington's or

1. Allen Verhey, "Mapping the Human Genome . . . Biblically," in *Reading the Bible in the Strange World of Medicine* (Grand Rapids: Eerdmans, 2003), p. 148.

Alzheimer's) or for genetic disorders that could be passed on to their children. And now, after almost two decades, human gene transfer (known popularly as "gene therapy") has proved therapeutically successful in a handful of cases.

Almost four decades after the advent of "genetic engineering," however, the diagnostic capabilities of genetics remain well ahead of therapeutic intervention. For most diseases diagnosed prenatally, no therapeutic intervention exists. Abortion in these cases remains the default presumption. For those with financial means, various reproductive technologies also offer an alternative path, but these raise their own complex questions (see Chapter Eighteen above). Likewise for many late-onset diseases, genetic diagnosis brings only the burden of knowledge — of the high probability or certainty that one's later years will be spent in affliction, in pain, in debilitation. For stigmatized conditions, such as mental illness, or even for chronic conditions, questions of confidentiality *vis-à-vis* the public, employers, or health insurers remain ongoing issues.

Broader questions of social justice push toward new ways of perceiving the ethical dimensions of genetics. Some questions are relevant in the U.S.: Is the current health care system in the U.S. capable of using genetic information without discrimination? Yet such questions transcend our borders. Maura Ryan, in "Justice and Genetics: Whose Holy Grail?" (selection 128), pulls back the lens not only to situate genetics within the U.S. cultural milieu but also to situate it within a framework of global economic disparity. How do we deliberate about a single diagnostic test for inherited susceptibility to breast cancer that costs $3,000 in a world in which per capita spending on health care in many countries figures in the range of $15-$50 per year? How do we assess the ethics of preimplantation diagnosis or the $3 billion price tag for the Human Genome Project in a world where millions of children die annually for lack of access to simple vaccinations? Ryan situates questions of genomics in the context of the "10/90 gap," the fact that "90% of the health research dollars are spent on the problems of 10% of the world's population." Ryan is concerned that with genetic diagnoses and interventions available only to the 10 percent, contemporary trends in genomics will only exacerbate this gap, creating a "genomics divide." She draws on the principles of Catholic social teaching to argue for a more just sharing of the benefits of genomic research. Readers may want to revisit the readings in Chapters Three and Four on the social responsibility of health care to further contextualize the questions Ryan raises.

But ought genetics or genomics be understood primarily as a "global public good"? As important as it is to contextualize genetics within the larger global context, does Ryan's analysis still presuppose Szerszynski's two assumptions? Several essays in this chapter challenge these assumptions, or at least seek to complicate the assumption that genetic technologies are, on the whole, best understood simply as public goods.

This critique comes from two directions. The first challenge emerged with the advent of the era of genetic engineering itself in the late 1960s, as is captured in the excerpt from Paul Ramsey's classic book *Fabricated Man: The Ethics of Genetic Control* (selection 129). Here Ramsey engages the arguments of geneticist H. J. Mueller and in doing so demonstrates that, although genetic technology has morphed radically from those early beginnings, the fundamental questions in many ways have not. Ramsey makes clear that what is at issue between him and Mueller is not the relationship between two complementary activities — genetics and theology — but rather the relationship between two different theologies. Mueller, he argues, offers a particular genetic eschatology or, more specifically, a genetic apocalypse. Accompanying this eschatology is a particular anthropology (understanding of what it means to be human), an account of "creation" (genetically construed), and, ultimately, a concept of salvation — all of which come in the form of genetic intervention.

The second challenge to the assumptions identified above is the challenge of history, particularly the history of eugenics. Given eugenics' historic relationship with Nazism, it was for many years considered somewhat bad form to raise the question of eugenics with regard to contemporary genetic technologies. Recent scholarship, however, makes clear the thick history of the eugenics movement and the continued power of eugenic reasoning. It also demonstrates the major role played by Christian pastors, lay leaders, theologians, and rhetoric in advancing eugenics in the U.S. and abroad. Amy Laura Hall's essay, "To Form a More Perfect Union: Mainline Protestantism and the Popularization of Eugenics" (selection 130), demonstrates in sobering detail how enthusiastically Protestant, Catholic, and Jewish leaders embraced the eugenics movement, particularly in the U.S., and how they became its major champions.[2]

The relationship between eugenics and religion, as Hall demonstrates, was complex. On the one hand, it was easy for the science of eugenics to "move effortlessly from laboratory to church" because, from its inception, eugenics was cast in religious terms and language, at least by its founder Francis Galton (cousin of Charles Darwin).[3] Galton advocated eugenics as "a new religion" and drew on Christian images, such as the parable of the talent, to argue for scientific reproduction. On the other hand, Galton's religious rhetoric resonated with religious leaders of the time who, in Christine Rosen's analysis, lacked a "coherent doctrinal vision."[4] Those religious leaders who championed eugenics, as she notes, "were preachers who embraced modern ideas first and adjusted their theolo-

2. Those interested in this history are encouraged to read Christine Rosen's excellent book *Preaching Eugenics: Religious Leaders and the American Eugenics Movement* (Oxford: Oxford University Press, 2004).

3. Rosen, *Preaching Eugenics,* p. 4.

4. Rosen, *Preaching Eugenics,* p. 4.

gies later."[5] Hall's chronicle of Christian enthusiasm for eugenics is not only of historical interest. The rhetoric of the early twentieth century with regard to eugenics finds striking parallels in the rhetoric of the late twentieth and early twenty-first centuries with regard to genetics and genomics. Contemporary Christians and religious leaders continue to uncritically embrace modern ideas of genetic science and technology, advocating for greater penetration of genetics into our lives and calling for the ongoing revision of theology.

The essays by Song, Szerszynski, and Shuman (selections 131-33) pick up the challenges outlined by Ramsey and Hall and broaden them. They expand on Ramsey's claim that genetics functions largely as a theology and push back further beyond Hall's history to the beginnings of the scientific revolution in the sixteenth and seventeenth centuries. Robert Song, in his essay "The Human Genome Project as Soteriological Project" (selection 131), expands on the last point above. Song is interested in the public obsession with genetics, particularly in the form of the Human Genome Project, and asks why the habits of genetic reductionism, biological determinism, and genetic essentialism should be so appealing to ordinary inhabitants of Western culture. With Shuman, Szerszynski, and Verhey, Song locates contemporary genetics within the longer history of science, tracing the roots of our assumptions to Francis Bacon. (For a more extensive discussion of Bacon, see Gerald McKenny's essay in Chapter Eight of this volume.) For Song, the Baconian project is a surrogate form of religion complete with a doctrine of creation, an anthropology, an eschatology, and a soteriology. He then demonstrates the soteriological — or salvific — claims of modern technological medicine, particularly genetic technologies, as they seek to redeem the world and the future of the human race through design and reconstruction of living creatures.

Bronislaw Szerszynski's essay (selection 132) supplements Song's historical account. He shows how modern science (and not genetics alone) has a theological character and locates the Human Genome Project as "a new and significant phase in a theologic-scientific project, originating in the early modern period." Joel Shuman, in his essay "Desperately Seeking Perfection: Christian Discipleship and Medical Genetics" (selection 133), augments Song's account of genetics' soteriology by adding to it an account of genetic and Christian sanctification. Shuman notes that both Christianity and genetics "have as their goal the *perfection* of the human being," particularly embodied perfection. But he demonstrates how different these accounts of embodied perfection are. In particular, Christian visions of perfection are shaped by the cross and resurrection, require the joyful, expectant embrace of our weaknesses and imperfections, and are sustained by communal bonds. The theology shaping a particular endeavor is best identified, he suggests, by asking whether it seeks to serve the weak and embrace difference or to eliminate weaknesses and differences from the individual and social body.

While the character of contemporary genetics has only recently been elucidated in such careful historical and theological terms, the public has long sensed that at issue were fundamental theological questions. For too long, this sense was captured in the slogan "playing God" — often used either to reject genetic technologies or to minimize theological concerns. Allen Verhey, in his essay "'Playing God' and Invoking a Perspective" (selection 134), demystifies this phrase, sorting through a number of ways the phrase has been used within discussions of genetics in particular as well as medical ethics more broadly. Verhey, again, traces many of the unhelpful and theologically suspect meanings of this phrase back to Bacon. But he also helps clarify the ways in which this phrase might be used appropriately, both as a caution in the face of technology and as a way of ordering our use of technology toward God's purposes.

Eugenics was, of course, about reproduction — the enhanced reproduction of the "fit" and the restricted reproduction of the "unfit and feebleminded," those who placed a burden on society. As the questions with which we opened this introduction make clear, the practice of genetics remains largely about reproduction and the quality and character of our children. Congregations played a key role in advancing the eugenics movement; Hall pushes us to rethink the role of congregations vis-à-vis these questions — no longer places of simple championing of genetics but as renewed places of moral discernment.

The questions posed at the opening of this introduction find no easy answers. In light of the following essays, the answers might seem even more complicated. But we hope that these essays will provide readers with a greater sense of the historical and theological underpinnings of contemporary genetic practices, a context that is necessary for those who wish to participate in genetic technologies in a way that is prudent rather than simply predetermined by the power of the market, the technological imperative, or both.

5. Rosen, *Preaching Eugenics*, p. 5.

Suggestions for Further Reading

Butler, Lee H. "Dreaming the Soul: African American Skepticism Encounters the Human Genome Project." In *Adam, Eve, and the Genome*, ed. Susan B. Thistlethwaite (Minneapolis: Fortress, 2003), pp. 129-44.

Byrnes, W. Malcolm. "Human Genetic Technology, Eugenics, and Social Justice." *National Catholic Bioethics Quarterly* 1, no. 4 (2001): 555-81.

Hall, Amy Laura. "Good Breeding: The Eugenics Temptation." *Christian Century* 121, no. 22 (November 2, 2004): 24-27, 29.

Hall, Amy Laura. "Public Bioethics and the Gratuity of Life: Joanna Jepson's Witness Against Negative Eugenics." *Studies in Christian Ethics* 18, no. 1 (2005): 15-32.

Lysaught, M. Therese. "From Clinic to Congregation: Religious Communities and Genetic Medicine." In *On Moral Medicine: Theological Perspectives in Medical Ethics*, 2nd ed., ed.

Stephen E. Lammers and Allen Verhey (Grand Rapids: Eerdmans, 1998), pp. 547-61.

McKenny, Gerald. "Technologies of Desire: Theology, Ethics, and the Enhancement of Human Traits." *Theology Today* 59, no. 1 (April 2002): 90-103.

Rahner, Karl. "The Problem of Genetic Manipulation." In *On Moral Medicine: Theological Perspectives in Medical Ethics,* 2nd ed., ed. Stephen E. Lammers and Allen Verhey (Grand Rapids: Eerdmans, 1998), pp. 542-46.

Rosen, Christine. *Preaching Eugenics: Religious Leaders and the American Eugenics Movement* (Oxford: Oxford University Press, 2004).

Verhey, Allen. "Mapping the Human Genome . . . Biblically." In *Reading the Bible in the Strange World of Medicine* (Grand Rapids: Eerdmans, 2003), pp. 145-93.

126 Mother and Father

David L. Schiedermayer

I inherited from you
the genes which promote easy tears
and crossing one's legs at the ankles
color blindness
(X-linked recessive)
male pattern baldness
(sex-influenced autosomal dominant)
early rising, myopia, shyness, high arches
(polygenetic multifactorial tendencies).

But I know I have 3 to 8 lethal genes
which if homozygous
would be fatal.
So believe me
I am thankful
for both of you.

127 Ethical Standards for Genetic Intervention

James C. Peterson

The Bedouin in the Negev desert traditionally live in tents and move from place to place with their camels. Some camels can be quite curious. It is not surprising to find a camel sniffing under the edge of a tent, trying to discern what smells so interesting inside. One learns quickly that even if one does not mind a pair of large nostrils sniffling nearby, one needs to strike the muzzle with a sandal or hand directly, lest the whole camel soon be inside the tent. Camels seem much larger inside the tent than outside of it.

A commonly raised concern in discussions of genetics and ethics may be referred to as the 'camel's nose under the tent argument'. Sometimes it is called the slippery slope or the thin edge of the wedge. The concern is that taking certain acceptable steps may lead to a camel in the tent (or a thick end of a wedge, or a bottom of a slope) that one never intended. In terms of human genetic intervention, how do we use it where it serves well, without allowing it where it does not belong? Is there a way that we can consistently distinguish appropriate from inappropriate use?

Consider the case of panic disorder. About two percent of Americans sometimes find their heart suddenly racing. Many first assume that they are having a heart attack. They are overwhelmed with a feeling of utter terror, but without being afraid of anything in particular. In ten to fifty minutes the terror subsides, only to return when people least expect it. The attacks are distributed through families in a way that implies inherited susceptibility. Would it not be helpful to diagnose genetically the condition before the first attack, so that people could be warned? Would it not be a positive contribution to limit the attacks by pharmaceutical or someday even genetic intervention, if that could be done without adverse side effects? What would make such treatments fall within or outside appropriate intervention?

A Christian Context

Chapter 25 of the biblical book of Matthew — in which Jesus instructs his disciples on what to do in the time between his resurrection and his return at the last day of judgment — contains several themes directly applicable to our question. Today is still the in-between time about which Jesus spoke. Matthew 25 contains three stories. Each one raises issues that the next one answers. The first story is of ten maidens watching into the night for the coming of the bridegroom. The wait was so long that five of them ran out of oil for their lamps. While they were away buying more, the bridegroom came and they missed the wedding feast. The story reminds us always to be ready for the return of Jesus Christ. It could be before the completion of this sentence. On the other hand, it may be a long time. It has now been almost 2,000 years since Jesus gave people this warning. One must have both the foresight to prepare for the long haul (bringing enough oil) and the perseverance to endure. So what then are we supposed to do in the meantime?

The story that immediately follows answers that question. It tells of a master who left five talents with one servant, two with another, and one with a third, to each according to his ability. When the master returned he was pleased to see that the first and second servants had doubled their talents. The master was outraged, however, to discover that the third servant had simply buried the entrusted resource in order to return exactly what he had received. He had failed in his responsibility to multiply the resources the master had given to him. The first story in Matthew 25 warns that we should always be ready, but we may have to wait some time before the second coming. The second story tells us that the intervening time should be spent wisely in God's service, producing fruit from what he has entrusted to us. We are responsible to employ and multiply our God-given resources. In other words, we are to have our suitcases packed and ready to go, but not merely hang out at the airport.

So how should we put our God-given talents to work? What goals would God have us pursue? The next and last story in the chapter answers that question. It is a description of the final day of judgment. Those who belong to God's kingdom are separated from those who are not according to how they treated their neighbours. Those who fed the hungry and clothed the poor, cared for those who were sick and visited those in prison, are welcomed into God's kingdom. Those who did not are cast away. Good works do not earn a place in God's family; rather, they are characteristic of people who are in God's family. Such actions do not achieve salvation but they do reflect it. In the second chapter of Ephesians we read that we are 'saved by grace through faith, lest anyone should boast'. Sometimes neglected, the next sentence reads 'for we are his workmanship, created in Christ Jesus for good works'. These good works are a result of reconciliation with God, not the cause of salvation. Reconciliation with God is a free gift that, if fully received, will affect how one treats others. If one is being shaped by God as a child of God, one will come to care about what God cares about. God cares deeply about people.

From James C. Peterson, "Ethical Standards for Genetic Intervention," in John F. Kilner, Rebecca D. Pentz, and Frank E. Young, eds., *Genetic Ethics: Do the Ends Justify the Genes?* The Center for Bioethics and Human Dignity.

The examples of expressing love for one's neighbour in these biblical passages address meeting physical and social needs such as feeding the hungry and caring for those who are sick. Apparently matter matters. In the first chapter of Genesis, Adam is described as made from the dust yet uniquely inbreathed with God's spirit. We human beings have a special calling, yet are of this earth. Being physical beings is not a bad thing. God created both this material world and our physical form and declared them 'good'. The physical is not our ultimate concern, but we should care about it because it is a part of God's creation and our stewardship.

Jesus lives this concern in his incarnation, teaching, and action. In the historic Christian tradition, Jesus is not only God among us but also the perfect example of what human beings are meant to be. Jesus came first and foremost to reconcile us with God, yet he also gave of himself in caring for people's physical concerns, sometimes to the point of utter physical exhaustion. In John he gives the commission that 'as the Father has sent him, so he now sends his disciples'.[1] We should actively care for people's physical concerns as he did.

Moreover, in all three of these sections of Matthew 25, errors of omission (not bringing enough oil, not multiplying talents, not caring for those in need) are treated as seriously as acts of commission. Pride is a serious danger, but so is sloth. Until the Lord returns, we are to do our best here. That includes our best effort to serve others, including addressing their physical needs.

This is only one chapter of the rich biblical tradition, but it is not an isolated one. Its themes are found throughout Scripture. They remind us to ask first, as we should of any potential tool, how human genetic intervention can best serve our neighbours. Asking that question is not trying to be God; it is following God's mandate to be of service.

Drawing the Line

Now remember the camel, which provides a great service to the Bedouin but does not belong in the tent. Usefulness in one context does not insure usefulness in another. Recognizing the potential service of human genetic intervention is not sufficient. We must ask under what circumstances it is possible to intervene without causing great harm. Thinking ahead is part of the mandate required of us, as illustrated in the story of the maidens and lamp oil in Matthew 25. How do we separate appropriate service of human genetic intervention from destructive use? The Parliamentary Assembly of the Council of Europe, the French National Ethics Committee, Canada's Royal Commission, and others have stated that genetic intervention is acceptable when it affects only the presenting patient. Such is called 'somatic cell therapy'. In contrast, 'germ-line therapy', a type of intervention which potentially affects future generations, would never be appropriate.[2] Others have argued that somatic therapy is the appropriate stopping point for pragmatic reasons. Germ-line intervention is not ruled out in principle; rather, it is ruled out until it is safe and reliable.[3]

However, the distinction between somatic and germ-line intervention is not the best place to draw the line between acceptable and harmful intervention. While the somatic/germ-line distinction is clear conceptually, in practice some somatic interventions will have germ-line effects. For example, a person who would not otherwise have been able to pass on a deleterious gene may be enabled to live to child-bearing age. The distinction misses the mark morally as well. If genetic surgery is safe and beneficial for one person, why not protect his or her children from having to endure the same genetic harm or repetitive somatic therapy?[4] The stakes of a mistake are greater, but so are the potential benefits. It is not possible to obtain informed consent from the future descendants, but neither is it for infants for whom we often act. When a child is born with a cleft palate, a largely inherited condition, we do not wait for the child to reach the age of eighteen for adult permission to do the needed surgery. Nor do we refuse to intervene because God sovereignly designed the child to be that way. We trust that God is pleased to work through us to improve the child's ability to speak and eat. If somatic therapy is warranted in some cases, germ-line extension of that change is probably so as well.[5]

The distinction between cure and enhancement does not provide a much better line.[6] First of all, it is a very dif-

1. John 17:18.

2. Parliamentary Assembly of the Council of Europe, "Recommendation 934 on genetic engineering," 1982. French National Ethics Committee, "Announcement on Gene Therapy," *Human Gene Therapy* 2 (1991): 329. Canadian Royal Commission, *"Proceed with Care: Final Report of the Royal Commission on New Reproductive Technologies,"* excerpted in *Human Gene Therapy* 5 (1994): 604. Wivel, Nelson A., and Walters, LeRoy, "Germ-line Gene Modification and Disease Prevention: Some Medical and Ethical Perspectives," *Science* 262 (22 October 1993): 533-38. Fletcher, John C., and Anderson, W. French, "Germ-line Gene Therapy: A New Stage of Debate," *Law, Medicine & Health Care* 20:1-2 (1992): 26-39.

3. Neel, James V., "Germ-Line Gene Therapy: Another View," *Human Gene Therapy* 4 (1993): 127-28.

4. Munro, Donald W., used the apt description of human genetic intervention as "microsurgery" in a speech entitled "Human Genetic Engineering, God's Gift?" at the Kepler Society, Boston, January 26, 1996.

5. Reichenbach, Bruce R., and Anderson, V. Elving, *On Behalf of God: A Christian Ethic for Biology* (Grand Rapids: Eerdmans, 1995), p. 186. Walters, LeRoy, "The Ethics of Human Germ-Line Genetic Intervention," in *Genes and Human Self-Knowledge: Historical and Philosophical Reflections on Modern Genetics,* ed. Weir, Robert F., Lawrence, Susan C., and Fales, Evan (Iowa City: University of Iowa Press, 1994), pp. 220-31.

6. For a detailed evaluation of the practical use and desirability of this distinction see Peterson, J., *An Ethical Analysis and Proposal for the Direction of Human Genetic Intervention* (Ann Arbor: UMI, 1992), order number 9237575 at 800-521-0600.

ficult line to discern.[7] The distinction seems to fade the more closely it is analysed. All correction involves enhancing capacity. One who was blind is now able to see. One who was crippled is now able to walk. The difference between the two is that correction is limited to achieving 'normal' levels.[8] But what are normal levels?[9] Human characteristics generally fall within a range. Some people's vision is 20/60; others' is 20/10. If we correct to average in that range there will still be people who have better sight than average. With the lower abilities eliminated from the calculation by correction to the average, the average will increase. What was beyond normal will become normal. If we define correction as rescinding disease or disorder, what is disease?[10] Do we define disease as that which produces pain and suffering? If so, then childbirth and teething are diseases, for they are certainly painful. If disease is departure from the statistical norm, red hair and AB blood type would be diseases. If disease is departure from the statistical norm that the individual does not want, personal values would define disease differently from one person to the next. The syndrome of 'Drapetomania' was described in great detail in the *New Orleans Medical and Surgical Journal* in 1851.[11] According to the article's author, physician Samuel A. Cartwright, it is the disease that causes a slave to want to run away.

If we tie correction to today's average, why such loyalty to our current state? If we tie the norm to our pre-sin state, how do we know what that was? How is removing 'the effects of sin' any clearer than removing 'disease'? Even if one could discern our physical pre-fall state, why make that the final standard? To do so would require the assumption that pre-sin Adam was God's final intent for human physical form. Do we actually know that? Why consider Adam the pinnacle and not the starting point? God has created a world where acorns take decades to become fifty-foot oaks. It would be a bit disconcerting for squirrels and hikers if acorns sprang to mature size upon first contact with the ground. Our physical and spiritual lives are characterized by birth followed by a lifetime of growth, rather than instant maturity. God has chosen to design a world that works that way. We can never 'out-design' God. Is it not possible that God might sovereignly choose to develop further our design through us? The point is not to try to be God; it is to listen, prayerfully and thoughtfully, to what the one and only God would have us to do.

7. Murray, Thomas, "Assessing Genetic Technologies: Two Ethical Issues," *International Journal of Technology Assessment in Health Care* 10:4 (1994): 573-82. Bouma III, Hessel, Diekema, Douglas, Langerak, Edward, Rottman, Theodore, and Verhey, Allen, *Christian Faith, Health, and Medical Practice* (Grand Rapids: Eerdmans, 1989), p. 266.

8. Anderson, W. French, "Genetic Engineering and Our Humanness," *Human Gene Therapy* 5 (1994): 755-60.

9. Pettersson, Berg K., Riis, P., Tranoy, K. E., "Genetics in Democratic Societies," *Clinical Genetics* 48 (1995): 202.

10. Juengst, Eric Thomas, *The Concept of Genetic Disease and Theories of Medical Progress* (Ann Arbor: UMI 1985). Caplan, Arthur L., Englehardt, H. Tristram Jr., and McCartney, James, eds., *Concepts of Health and Disease: Interdisciplinary Perspectives* (Reading, Mass.: Addison-Wesley, 1981).

11. Cartwright, Samuel A., "Report on the Diseases and Physical Peculiarities of the Negro Race," *The New Orleans Medical and Surgical Journal* 7 (May 1851): 707-9.

Five Standards

What would our Lord have us to do? It is much easier to raise questions than to make concrete proposals. However, as an alternative to the somatic/germ-line and cure/enhance criteria, I would propose the following five standards for recognizing if an intervention is appropriate. Any genetic intervention should be:

1. Incremental

Human genetic intervention should be incremental in degree and breadth of implementation. We are finite beings who do not begin to understand the interrelated complexity of our own bodies. The more I learn in genetic labs and clinics, the more I find myself humming the doxology. I am again and again awed at God's design in two senses. First I wonder at what I do see. One example is the 3,000 million base pairs of DNA in each cell of the human body, which would uncoil and stretch out to about two meters in a straight line. That is the proportional equivalent of stuffing thirty miles of fine fishing line into a plump blueberry, in such a way that the line could be unwound, copied, and restuffed at will. Secondly, I wonder at what I do not see or understand. At this point we do not even know what purpose most DNA serves. Only about ten percent of it is transcribed into mRNA for making proteins. What is the other ninety percent doing? It may be important for expression, structure, or some other function. At this point we do not know.

The pattern is consistent in human endeavours: more knowledge results in more awareness of what we do not know. One can learn a great deal about Thailand on a two-week visit, including some of its language, history, geography, and culture. Such new knowledge often reveals questions one would not have even thought of before. For that reason, growth in knowledge is not only fascinating and worthwhile. It is also humbling. When people as finite human beings are absolutely sure about anything, including genetics, they probably do not fully understand. The ones who most fully understand will rarely be absolutely sure (or at least so it seems). By pursuing genetic intervention incrementally, we can minimize the degree and extent of unexpected harms.

2. Choice-Expanding

We should also pursue only those interventions that enhance a person's options by freeing that individual from what is clearly destructive or by increasing the person's capability. Human development is immensely complex.

Genetic intervention will more often be able to influence formation than determine it. Using that influence to enhance a person's bodily defenses against cancer or to increase incrementally one's aptitude for memorizing vocabulary, would not predestine the individual to a particular life. It would contribute to the range of options available for the individual's pursuit and achievement. In contrast, interventions that would limit the recipient — attempting to predestine the individual to a narrow end — would claim an arrogant authority over the recipient and show a lack of respect for him or her as a person. For example, it would not be appropriate for deaf parents to choose deafness for their child even if they preferred deaf culture to hearing culture. Deafness limits options. C. S. Lewis made this point for entire generations in *The Abolition of Man*. He argued that the first generation that would have the power so deeply to shape the next generation should not use it in a way to predestine the next generation's choices.[12] Each generation should be able to further or undo the last generation's contribution as they learn from its effects.

3. *Parent-Directed*

Genetic intervention decisions should be made primarily by the persons to be affected, or if that is not possible, by their parents.[13] Decentralizing choice in this way would first of all help to protect valuable diversity. Second, it would take into account what some have called the only empirically verifiable doctrine of Christianity, original sin. Only a generation ago the horrible crimes of the Holocaust were committed under the claim and cover of racial hygiene and eugenics. People will abuse any powerful technology if they are not held accountable. When one prefers sight to retino-blastoma, a genetically-based disease involving blindness, one is valuing a particular genetic endowment over another. That judgment is not nefarious. It is better to be able to see than not to be able to see. In contrast, the Nazi Germany claim of eugenics was horrifying on the following two counts, among others. First, the preferred genetic endowment was defined in terms of race — a characteristic which, even if clearly definable, would be irrelevant to well-being.[14] If genetic intervention decisions were made primarily by parents, no racial group would be in a position to use such choices destructively against another. Second, having other than the desired genetic endowment (or politics, or IQ, or health history . . .) was grounds in Nazi Germany for taking that person's life. However, a person's ongoing life and worth does not depend on genetic heritage. Persons should be protected and nurtured from their beginning, regardless of genetic endowment.[15] Parents are central to meeting that need and so are particularly well-suited to make genetic intervention decisions for their children.

4. *Within Societal Boundaries*

What if parents intend to make abusive or even simply foolish choices to the detriment of their own children? A fourth standard is that society should set minimal, broad limits for intervention. An example of such a constraint would be the first standard above — that any genetic intervention should be incremental. Living within some minimal societal limits is how we currently deal with education and medical care. Clearly recognized minimums are required of all parents, although they are free to satisfy such minimums in a variety of ways. Parents may home school their child or choose a private or public school, but as parents they are required to provide a basic education for their child. Children may go to a chiropractor or Chinese herbalist, but life-threatening conditions must be addressed or parents will answer to the state. There is no end of conflict at these intersections, but that is the nature of accountability in a sinful world.

5. *By Acceptable Means*

Means are often as important as ends. First, the form of genetic intervention should be as non-invasive as possible for all involved.[16] This is a difficult goal to achieve in some cases; making a change that would multiply throughout the body would probably require intervention at the earliest stages of pregnancy. Second, zero risk is impossible. We cannot achieve zero risk at the dentist's or driving to school, but it is reasonable to limit the risks we take to those proportionate to the intended benefits. Such a criterion is as applicable to genetic interventions as to other aspects of life.

While these five standards can help keep the camel's nose out of the tent by providing criteria to distinguish acceptable from unacceptable interventions, another version of the camel's nose or slippery slope argument remains unanswered.[17] Even if there is a clear conceptual difference between acceptable and unacceptable inter-

12. Lewis, C. S., *The Abolition of Man* (New York: Macmillan, 1955).

13. Resnik, David, "Debunking the Slippery Slope Argument Against Human Germ-Line Gene Therapy," *The Journal of Medicine and Philosophy* 19 (1994): 35-37.

14. Hitler, Adolf, *Mein Kampf*, trans. Ludwig Lore (New York: Stackpole, 1939), p. 281. Seidelman, William E., "Mengele Medicus," *The Milbank Quarterly* 66:2 (1988): 223. Hohlfeld, Rainer, "Jenseits von Freiheit und Wurde: Kritische Anmerkungen zur gezielten genetischen Beeinflussung des Menschen," *Reformatio* 32 (May 1983): 220.

15. Jones, D. Gareth, and Telfer, Barbara, "Before I Was an Embryo, I Was a Pre-embryo: Or Was I?" *Bioethics* 9:1 (1995): 32-49.

16. Kass, Leon, *Toward a More Natural Science: Biology and Human Affairs* (New York: Free Press, 1985), p. 109. Ramsey, Paul, *Fabricated Man: The Ethics of Genetic Control* (New Haven: Yale University Press, 1970), pp. 89, 132-37.

17. Childress, James F., "Wedge Argument, Slippery Slope Argument, etc." in the *Westminster Dictionary of Christian Ethics*, ed. James F. Childress and John Macquarrie (Philadelphia: Westminster Press, 1986), p. 657.

ventions, this conceptual difference may not be honoured in the real world, either in the choices of individuals or in the formation of social guidelines. Once we head in a certain direction we may run roughshod over appropriate stopping points.[18] This danger is exacerbated by the pervasive self-deception and distortion of individual and corporate judgment characteristic of our sinful state. The most powerful motivators for intervention might even be defensive in nature. If countries or individual parents see children other than their own receiving enhancement safely and to their economic advantage — e.g., through improvement in some aspect of intelligence — they will have a strong incentive to intervene similarly in their own children in order to remain competitive.[19]

If a corporation has invested millions in developing a genetic technology, it will promote its use to gain a financial return.[20] A good illustration of this is the recent direct marketing of cystic fibrosis carrier screening on British television.[21] Not only do standards for genetic intervention need to be developed, but also warranted confidence that such standards will be honoured. Otherwise, the long-term results could be more harmful than beneficial.

Genetic intervention will never yield a utopia.[22] Genetics cannot solve all physical concerns, nor is human life only physical. Published hopes that genetic intervention might deliver us from homelessness, alcoholism, criminality, divorce, and more, expect more than physical change can provide by itself.[23] But genetic intervention within the five standards suggested above can make life somewhat better for many people. If such is possible, we are responsible to our Lord as faithful stewards to pursue it. Even some instances of germ-line enhancement — ruled out by some — may fall within that God-honouring mandate. Being 'bright in the corner where we are', doing what we can to serve our neighbors, is part of our God-given commission and responsibility. May we use the developing tool of genetic intervention wisely to that end.

18. Nelson, Hilde Lindemann, "Dethroning Choice: Analogy, Personhood, and the New Technologies," *Journal of Law, Medicine & Ethics* 23 (1995): 129-35.

19. Gardner, William, "Can Human Genetic Enhancement Be Prohibited?" *The Journal of Medicine and Philosophy* 20 (1995): 65-84.

20. Editorial, "Capitalizing on the Genome," *Nature Genetics* 13:1 (May 1995): 1-5.

21. Harper, Peter S., "Direct Marketing of Cystic Fibrosis Carrier Screening: Commercial Push or Population Need?" *Journal of Medical Genetics* 32 (1995): 249-50.

22. Passmore, John, *The Perfectibility of Man* (New York: Charles Scribner's Sons, 1970).

23. Holtzman, Neil A., "Policy Implications of Genetic Technologies," *International Journal of Technology Assessment* 10:4 (1994): 570-71. Proctor, Robert N., "Genomics and Eugenics: How Fair is the Comparison?" pp. 76-93 in *Gene Mapping: Using Law and Ethics as Guides,* ed. Annas, George J., and Elias, Sherman (New York: Oxford University Press, 1992).

128 Justice and Genetics: Whose Holy Grail?

Maura Ryan

A few years ago, I taught an undergraduate course in medical ethics in which one of the students was a young woman from Uganda. One day, the class became engaged in a heated debate about the right to terminate treatment. The discussion centered on a case involving a teenaged boy who had end-stage cystic fibrosis. The boy's mother argued vehemently for continued ventilator support, whereas the boy himself begged the medical team to let him die. The class disagreed passionately about who should be allowed to make the decision, the parent or the teenager.

I noticed that my Ugandan student (who had been fairly quiet in the class until then) was shaking her head, as if in amazement. When I asked her what she was thinking, she said, "In my country, if you had the treatment, you'd use it! How amazing it is to be in a country where the ethical debates are all about when to say too much is too much, and not about why some people have no treatment at all."

In *Bioethics and the Common Good,* her 2004 Pere Marquette Theology Lecture at Marquette University, Milwaukee, Lisa Sowle Cahill argues that what happened in my classroom that day has happened gradually in the field of Christian bioethics over the latter part of the 20th century.[1] As it has faced the challenges of globalization, bioethics has begun to shift its lens away from a narrow concern for the bedside — away, that is, from the morality of decisions made by individual patients and their physicians — to take seriously the multiple and unequal worlds of health care within which choices are made about how we will live and how we will die, what we will invest in, what ends medical science will seek, and how new technologies will he used.

Increasingly, the lens through which we view medical decision making presupposes the interdependence not only of individuals within families or communities but also the interdependence of communities, regions, nations, and continents. As a consequence, caregivers have begun to appreciate to a new degree the way in which

1. Lisa Sowle Cahill, *Bioethics and the Common Good,* Marquette University Press, Milwaukee, 2004, pp. 8-9.

health care choices are embedded, emerging within and responding to ever larger and more complex "webs of life."

Moreover, as Christian ethicists have confronted the complexity and enormity of the AIDS pandemic, they have become more attentive to the multiple factors that account for vastly differing vulnerabilities to infection and death, including deeply entrenched patterns of wealth and poverty, long-term political and social instabilities, global economic systems that favor the interests of Western industrial nations, and the role of cultural and religious norms concerning sexuality and gender. More than anything else, AIDS has made obvious the limits of bioethical approaches that privilege individual autonomy while ignoring the questions of social justice raised by persistent and, in some cases, growing disparities in access to health care and other basic human goods. Today, Christian bioethics is pressed not so much to abandon its foundational commitment to promoting the dignity of each human person but, rather, to ask what that commitment entails in the context of a global common good. In other words, bioethics has become ever more self-consciously *social* ethics.[2]

One way to explore the significance of this shift is to consider the development of generic technologies in light of the multiple and unequal worlds of health care that exist both here in the United States and around the world. Although progress from research to clinical application has been slow, few advances in science and medicine hold more promise for alleviating human suffering and advancing understanding of health and disease than the Human Genome Project (HGP), the 13-year effort funded by the U.S. Department of Energy and the National Institutes of Health (NIH) to map and sequence the human genome.[3]

Since publication of the complete sequence in April 2003, the human genome has been called the "code of codes," the "book of life," and "science's holy grail." Still, even though much has been written on the HGP's social and ethical implications, there has been relatively little reflection on the potential for a "genomic divide" between what the Princeton molecular biologist Lee Silver, PhD, calls the "genrich" (those who will have access to genetic breakthroughs) and the "gennaturals" (those who will live with the natural lottery) in the United States and, in the larger world, between nations that are rich in genomic technology and those that are not.[4]

Bioethics literature is full of debates concerning genetic privacy and the dissemination and use of genetic information. Rarely, however, have the questions pressed upon Christian bioethics by what we Catholics call the "option for the poor" been considered in a serious and sustained way. Such questions include:

- How will advances in genomics improve health in developing countries, particularly those areas already ravished by AIDS?
- How are genetic investments likely to affect health care for the more than 45 million people in the United States who are currently uninsured or underinsured?
- What values will govern our decisions concerning who will reap the benefits of the genetic revolution and who will bear the burdens?

When emerging genetic technologies are viewed through the lens of the Roman Catholic social tradition, it becomes clear not only why these questions are important but also why they deserve to be at the center — rather than at the margins — of our ministry's analysis.[5]

Genomics and the "10/90 Gap"

The HGP is likely to revolutionize the way medicine is practiced because it will allow for the identification of genetically based vulnerabilities (perhaps even before birth) and the use of information about individual genetic variations in prescribing drugs and choosing doses, and because it will eventually allow the development of therapeutic interventions on the genetic level.[6]

On the face of it, it may be hard to imagine what relevance such developments might have for areas of the world whose annual health care expenditures are, for example, less than the cost in U.S. dollars of a single diagnostic test for inherited susceptibility to breast cancer. What relevance would a test that currently costs between $300 and $3,000 have for countries like the Democratic Republic of the Congo, which in 2002 spent $15 per capita on health care; Sierra Leone, which spent $27 per capita; or Rwanda, which spent $48 per capita?[7] It is undeniable that, in many regions, access to basic health care, clean water, adequate nutrition, maternal and child care, and the means to prevent and treat HIV/AIDS are far more pressing problems than whether affordable genetic testing for osteoporosis will

2. Cahill, p. 8.

3. See National Human Genome Research Institute, *An Overview of the Human Genome Project,* Washington, DC, available as of January 10, 2006, at www.genome.gov/12011238.

4. See Lee Silver, *Remaking Eden: How Genetic Engineering and Cloning Will Transform the American Family,* Harper, New York City, 1998.

5. See Tikki Pang, "Equal Partnership to Ensure That Developing Countries Benefit from Genomics," *Nature Genetics,* vol. 33, no. 1, 2003, p. 18. See also Ted Peters, ed., *Genetics: Issues of Social Justice,* Pilgrim Press, Cleveland, 1998; and Cynthia Crysdale, "Christian Responses to the Human Genome Project," *Religious Studies Review,* vol. 26, 2000, pp. 236-242. For an example of an approach to bioethics that privileges issues of justice, see Lisa Sowle Cahill, *Theological Bioethics: Participation, Justice, Change,* Georgetown University Press, Washington, DC, 2005.

6. Lawrence Altman, "Genomic Chief Has High Hopes, and Great Fears, for Genetic Testing," *New York Times,* June 27, 2000, p. D6.

7. See the United Nations' *Human Development Report* for 2002, available at http://hdr.undp.org/statistics/data/indicators.cfm?x=52&y=2&z=2.

become available.[8] Yet emerging international voices, including voices from developing countries, suggest that assuming the irrelevance of genomics for low-income areas is dangerous in at least two ways:

- It overlooks the relation between the values that govern investments in medicine and public health generally and the values that will govern investments in genomics
- It underestimates the potential contribution of genomics to global public health goals

Genomics and World Health, a 2002 report published by the World Health Organization (WHO), begins by acknowledging what is often called the "10/90 gap," the fact that "90% of health research dollars are spent on the health problems of 10% of the world's population."[9] According to WHO, several features of genomics research reflect and potentially exacerbate this gap:

> Most genomics research was initially undertaken in the public sector of developed countries. But a recent survey reports that private-company spending on genomics has overtaken and is now substantially higher than government and not-for-profit spending. The concentration of research funding in developed countries as well as in the private sector has implications for setting research priorities and for accessing the products of research. . . . The private sector does not invest in research aimed at diagnostics or therapeutics for diseases that are predominant in developing countries because the populations that are afflicted and most likely to need them do not have purchasing power. In order to ensure high returns on their investments, companies tend to focus their research and development efforts on products aimed at diseases and health problems that are most prevalent among the populations of the developed countries.[10]

In 1997, WHO estimated that low- and medium-income countries accounted for only 20 percent of the global pharmaceutical market, even though they made up over 80 percent of the world's population.[11] In 2004, the United States continued to dominate the world pharmaceutical market, accounting for 35 percent of newly introduced products; Western European countries accounted for another 41 percent.[12] According to one industry forecaster, biotechnology drugs accounted in 2004 for 27 percent of those in the active research and development "pipeline" and for 10 percent of the global pharmaceutical market.

Even public research funding is driven in large part by market concerns through the increasingly common partnerships between government and private industry. As *Genomics and World Health* points out, "public research programs . . . tend to be focused on diseases such as cancer and cardiovascular diseases that are priorities in developed countries" whose economic interests drive global medical research agendas.[13] As WHO has said: "it has been estimated, for example, that pneumonia, diarrhea, tuberculosis and malaria, which together accounted for more than 20% of the disease burden of the world, receive less than 1% of the total public and private funds devoted to health research. . . . It was also estimated that in 1998, out of the US$ 70 billion global spending on health research, only US$ 300 million was directed to vaccines for HIV/AIDS and US$ 100 million to malarial research."[14]

A study by the Wellcome Trust in the United Kingdom estimated that malaria research in 1998 worldwide totaled $84 million. Since malaria killed between 1 and 2 million people that year, the total investment amounted to approximately $42 of research spending per malaria death.[15] Despite recent increases in international commitments to battle diseases that disproportionately affect the developing world, funding for diseases like malaria remains inadequate, said Jeffrey Sachs, director of the Earth Institute at Columbia University. Although lauding signs of progress, Sachs noted that, during its first round of funding in 2002, the UN Global Fund to Fight AIDS, TB, and Malaria committed only $22 million (out of a $616 million total) for malaria programs.[16]

Just as research priorities are heavily driven by the economic interests of nations in the world's industrial north, so also are the products of research. WHO noted that "of the 1,233 new drugs marketed between 1975 and 1999, only 13 were approved specifically for tropical diseases. Furthermore, of these, six were developed by WHO, United Nations Development Program (UNDP) and UNDP/World Bank/WHO-supported Special Program for Research and Training in Tropical Diseases."[17] Even a quick glance at the best-selling drugs in the world market for 2004 illustrates the predominance of "rich country" investments: Cholesterol-lowering drugs led the market, with sales of $30 billion (led by Lipitor, with sales totaling $12 billion), followed by anti-ulcerants, treatments for cardiovascular and central nervous system disorders, antidepressants, and antihypertensives.[18] Industry analysts

8. Cahill, p. 218.

9. *Genomics and World Health: Report of the Advisory Committee on Health Research,* World Health Organization, Geneva, Switzerland, 2002, p. 127.

10. *Genomics and World Health.*

11. *Genomics and World Health.*

12. "Looking to China and Cancer as Cost Containment Slows Growth," IMS Health, Inc., available at www.imshealth.com/web/content//0,3148,64576068_63872702_70260998_73052844,00.html.

13. *Genomics and World Health,* pp. 127-130.

14. *Genomics and World Health,* p. 130.

15. Quoted in Michael Kremer and Jeffrey Sachs, "A Cure for Indifference," *Financial Times,* May 5, 1999, available at www.brookings.edu/views/op-ed/kremer/19990505.htm.

16. Quoted in Tamar Kahn, "Fight Against Malaria Being Compromised," *Business Day,* November 5, 2002.

17. *Genomics and World Health,* pp. 130-131.

18. "Looking to China and Cancer." See also "IMS Reports 2004 Global Pharmaceutical Sales Grew 7 Percent to $550 Billion," available at www.imshealth.com/ims/portal/front/articleC/0,2777,6599_3665_71496463,00.html.

look to cancer drugs for the next big boom; according to IMS Health, "oncology projects accounted for almost 30% of the total industry R&D pipeline as of February 2005." IMS Health predicts that the "cancer market will be worth more than $40 billion by 2008."

Inequality Begins at Home

Some experts fear that concentration of investments in genomics in high-income, developed regions will skew genomic research disproportionately toward the development of potentially lucrative products. These concerns are at least initially borne out by present patterns of research activity. According to the U.S. Department of Energy, there were in 2002 600 clinical gene-therapy trials involving 3,500 patients going on worldwide. The vast majority of these trials were located in the United States (81 percent), followed by Europe (16 percent). Most trials focus on various types of cancers.[19]

Some critics have charged that the "10/90 gap" is a red herring. They argue that — given rising rates of obesity and obesity-related health problems worldwide, as well as rising rates of cancer in developing countries — distinctions between "rich country" and "poor country" diseases are misleading. They say, moreover, that the disease burden in developing countries is more a function of poverty and poor public health infrastructure than a lack of research and development efforts aimed at the diseases that predominate there. Diseases such as tuberculosis, malaria, and schistosomiasis, these critics argue, are both preventable and treatable with existing methods.[20]

But such objections miss the point of highlighting the gap between investments in rich countries, on one hand, and poor-country priorities, on the other. When profitability exclusively (or even overwhelmingly) drives research priorities, the products that are available are not only determined by market attractiveness but also are frequently priced beyond poor countries' means. Moreover, the prevailing market ethos presumes a producer/consumer posture toward genomics rather than an appreciation for genetic advances as public or "common" goods.

Such a posture results in multiple built-in disincentives to invest in public-health oriented or public-interest research. Following the publication of *Genomics and World Health,* 28 health research experts, either from developing countries or specialists in public health there, were asked to name the "top ten biotechnologies for improving health in the developing countries." At the top of their list were "modified molecular technologies for affordable, simple diagnosis of infectious diseases and recombinant technologies to develop vaccines against infectious diseases."[21] The respondents also mentioned technologies for more efficient drug and vaccine delivery systems and for environmental improvement, such as new approaches to sanitation and bioremediation.

However, existing market realities discourage investment in products such as the infectious disease vaccines that the developing world especially needs. Ruth Levine, of the Washington, DC–based Center for Global Development, has described some of the reasons why the development of such vaccines is unattractive to pharmaceutical companies. According to Levine, "vaccines make up less than two percent of the $340 billion global pharmaceutical market."[22] The "developing country vaccine market" is even smaller, "a mere $500 million or about one-tenth of a percent of annual global pharmaceutical sales." As a result, the number of big companies undertaking research on new vaccines has declined significantly over the past 20 years. Only three firms in the United States are licensed to produce childhood vaccines today (versus seven in the 1980s), and those three hesitate to invest in vaccines that would primarily be sold to customers in low-income countries.

Levine argues that limited research subsidies may work to hamper, rather than facilitate, development of solutions to medical problems that afflict the developing world. For example, a recent study by GlaxoSmithKline scientists, funded in part by the Bill and Melinda Gates Foundation, is showing some promise for the prevention of malaria. However, Levine notes, public and private donors must "pick a winner" early. As a result, other vaccine candidates, which in principle could prove to be even more effective, may never be developed.

Moreover, the introduction of new and highly sophisticated treatments risks simply exacerbating existing inequities. Audrey Chapman, PhD, a bioethicist with the American Association for the Advancement of Science, uses the case of inheritable genetic modifications — technologies allowing for the modification of a set of genes that can then be transmitted to one's offspring — as an illustration of the problem.[23] Although Chapman's topic is the introduction of genetic technologies into U.S. health care, the point she makes — about the relationship between factors conditioning access to highly sophisticated, high-cost treatment, on one hand, and factors likely to condition access to high-demand genetic technologies, on the other — is valid for thinking about access to genetic advances in general.

In asking whom technologies of this sort are likely to

19. U.S. Department of Energy, *Genomics and Its Impact on Science and Society: The Human Genome Project and Beyond,* Washington, DC, 2003, p. 7, available at www.ornl.gov/sci/techresources/Human_Genome/publicat/primer/.

20. See Philip Stevens, *Diseases of Poverty and the 10/90 Gap,* International Policy Network, London, 2004, available at www.fightingdiseases.org/pdf/diseases_of_poverty_final.pdf.

21. Abdallah S. Daar, et al., "Top Ten Biotechnologies for Improving Health in Developing Countries," *Nature Genetics,* vol. 32, October 2002, pp. 229-232.

22. Ruth Levine, "Solving the Real Vaccine Shortage," Center for Global Development, October 29, 2004, available at www.cgdev.org/content/opinion/detail/2963/.

23. Audrey Chapman, "Should We Design Our Descendants?" *Journal of the Society of Christian Ethics,* vol. 23, no. 2, Fall/Winter 2003, pp. 199-223.

benefit, Chapman suggests that the answer will be found by taking into account the interplay of four factors: longstanding patterns of inequalities of access to health care; a nonexistent system of universal health care; a projected scarcity of the availability of genetic services relative to demand; and the likely high cost of such interventions.[24]

Chapman notes the obvious facts about the current U.S. health care system:

> Problems in obtaining access to health care are unfairly distributed throughout our society. Blacks, Hispanics, and other minorities tend to receive lower quality health care than whites do . . . as a result of lower incomes, inadequate insurance coverage, and the absence of doctors in their areas of residence. Minorities are far more likely to be uninsured as compared to whites: Minorities comprised 46 percent of the uninsured in 2000, although these groups represented only 24 percent of the United States population. In 2001, 37.7 percent of the uninsured were Hispanic and 20.2 percent African American, compared to 14 percent who were white.[25]

Furthermore, various studies have documented a significant "therapeutic discrimination" in the type and quality of health care that U.S. minorities receive. A 1999 Institute of Medicine (IOM) report concluded that "racial and ethnic minorities in the United States receive notably lower-quality health care, even when they have the same incomes, insurance coverage, and medical conditions as whites."[26] The differences were especially significant for high-technology interventions, such as organ transplants and open heart surgery. An earlier IOM study *(The Unequal Burden of Cancer: An Assessment of NIH Research and Programs for Ethnic Minorities and the Medically Underserved)* had raised similar concerns about inequities in research priorities. It concluded that NIH funding for research targeting minority and medically underserved populations was both inadequate and unequal in comparison to research targeting nonminority populations.[27]

Considering these findings, it seems safe to assume that "current limitations on access to health care, particularly high technology interventions, will also likely operate with respect to genetic services."[28] High-demand genetic therapies, as well as enhancement interventions, are likely to be both very costly and (as in vitro fertilization and other reproductive technologies) available only to those who are willing and able to pay for them. Even if universal health coverage were to be adopted in the United States, underwriting access to some forms of genetic services (e.g., gene therapy for muscular dystrophy), current practice suggests that "the very groups who currently lack access to medical care, the poor and ethnic and racial minorities, are likely to still be disadvantaged."[29]

Unless our nation addresses underlying factors in disparities in access — such as the fact that both health care facilities and professionals tend to be located more often in areas where nonminority people live than in those where minority people do — claims made about the promises of genetics for advancing health for all are apt to be false, or at least only partially true.[30]

The factors accounting for disparities between high- and low-income nations in medical resources and research benefits differ from those accounting for disparities between high- and low-income groups in the United States. Still, they suggest that disparities in access to emerging genetic technologies are likely to have similar causes. Products have been developed and marketed to treat diseases, such as cancer and hypertension, long characteristic of developed nations. Today those illnesses are beginning to turn up in developing countries. Will those countries have access to new antihypertensive and anticancer products? Not if the conditions that made access to high-cost, high-demand therapies for HIV/AIDS virtually impossible in so many areas continue to prevail.

Genomics, Health, and the Common Good

Those who argue for equitable access to the benefits of genomic research make two crucial assumptions: first, that therapeutic advances in genetics are the fruit of a common human heritage; second, that access to health care is necessary for the protection of human dignity and the promotion of the common good. One can argue that the HGP is a "global public good" without referring to any particular religious tradition; and arguments defending equitable access to healthcare do not depend on religious convictions. Yet there is in Catholic social thought a rich tradition concerning the meanings of both *health* and *the common good* that provides an invaluable resource for reflecting on the challenges described above.

The Second Vatican Council defined the common good as "the sum of those conditions of social life which allow social groups and their members relatively thorough and ready access to their own fulfillment."[31] The common good is the "comprehensive human good of all who make up society," encompassing all the spiritual and material aspects that make possible a full and dignified human life. The common good concerns, in the words of the Catholic philosopher Jacques Maritain, the "common

24. Chapman, p. 210.

25. Chapman, p. 211.

26. Brian D. Smedley, Adrienne Y. Stith, and Alan R. Nelson, eds., *Unequal Treatment: Confronting Racial and Ethnic Disparities in Health Care,* National Academies Press, Washington, DC, 2003.

27. M. Alfred Haynes and Brian D. Smedley, eds., *The Unequal Burden of Cancer: An Assessment of NIH Research and Programs for Ethnic Minorities and the Medically Underserved,* National Academies Press, Washington, DC, 1999.

28. Chapman, p. 211.

29. Chapman.

30. Chapman.

31. "Gaudium et Spes," para. 26, quoted in National Conference of Catholic Bishops, *Economic Justice for All: Pastoral Letter on Catholic Social Teaching and the U.S. Economy,* U.S. Catholic Conference, Washington, DC, 1986, para. 79.

good of *human persons* . . . their communion in good living."[32] It is realized when prevailing social institutions function interdependently for the promotion of, among other things, "strong family life, strong educational institutions, rich cultural and artistic activity," and the "provision of material goods sufficient to meet the needs of all members of society and to allow participation in the civic community."[33]

Although St. Thomas Aquinas did not himself develop a full theory of the common good, the roots of this understanding of the relationship between civic participation and human flourishing come from his account of the natural orientation of the self toward community. As Susanne M. DeCrane has noted, "for Aquinas, morality emerges from and in a communal context. The inherent sociality of the human person results in some form of society or community being the context in which the person has the best hope of growing in her goodness and happiness. Human society exists (not as an end itself but) in order to facilitate and promote the common good of the group because in so doing the circumstances and necessities of full human life can be provided for all members."[34]

From this understanding of the human person as essentially communal, Catholic social thought advances a conception of justice as *relational* and *mutual*.[35] What is required of individuals, institutions, and the social order is specified by the concrete needs of individual persons as they seek to achieve fully human membership in various communities. For this reason, "basic justice demands the establishment of minimum levels of participation in the life of the human community for all persons."[36] As DeCrane puts it, "society is ordered toward an equity in the distribution of the goods of the group if it is to fulfill its reason for existence."[37] It is in this context that the right to adequate health care — as well as claims to a fair share of the benefits of genomics research — is to be understood. Adequate health care and protection from the threat of disease are human rights precisely because they are necessary for the full realization of human potential and for the fulfillment of social responsibilities.

When social institutions or policies fail to guarantee equitable access to the means for a dignified human life, justice will demand preferential treatment for those whose basic needs are not being met. Indeed, for Catholic social thought, the state of the least well-off stands as a challenge to and an indictment of all proposals for social organization. A preferential option for the poor entails a responsibility to examine social, economic, political, and cultural institutions and practices in light of the general requirements of human flourishing and to evaluate social policy from the perspective of those who are variously marginalized within the present order. What is at stake in "opting for the poor" is not simply trying to "change who is on top" but attending to the constellation of factors — poverty, geography, race, or gender — that systematically undermine full participation. The goal is to include those who have been marginalized in an order oriented toward human development in common.

If concerns about a growing "genomics divide" (domestically as well as globally) are at all well-founded, they join more general concerns — about growing gaps between rich and poor, between prosperous nations of the industrial northern hemisphere and sustenance-level nations of the south — that can be found in much Catholic social teaching, especially in contemporary social encyclicals such as *Sollicitudo Rei Socialis* and *Centesimus Annus*. It was in light of such growing divides that the U.S. Catholic bishops argued in their 1986 pastoral letter on the economy that "the obligation to provide justice for all means that the poor have the single most urgent economic claim on the conscience of the nation."[38]

But what exactly does it mean to provide "justice for all" in the context of genetic research and technology? What might "justice as participation" imply for how we value medical interventions or how we distribute medical goods, particularly as we are increasingly aware of a common good that is global in scope?

In *Harnessing the Praise of Genomics*, the Catholic Health Association has identified four key principles for reflecting on the obligations of justice with respect to genomic advances: respect for human dignity, relationality, solidarity, and subsidiarity.[39] These principles are not incompatible with the familiar principles of medical

32. Jacques Maritain, *The Person and the Common Good*, University of Notre Dame Press, Notre Dame, IN, 1966, p. 51.

33. David Hollenbach, "Liberalism, Communitarianism, and the Bishops' Pastoral Letter on the Economy," *Annual of the Society of Christian Ethics*, Georgetown University Press, Washington, DC, 1987, p. 27.

34. Susanne M. DeCrane, *Aquinas, Feminism, and the Common Good*, Georgetown University Press, Washington, DC, 2004, p. 75.

35. I am indebted here to the Interpretation of Fr. David Hollenbach, SJ, of justice in Roman Catholic social thought. See his *Justice, Peace, and Human Rights: American Catholic Social Ethics in a Pluralistic World*, Crossroad Publishing, New York City, 1988, pp. 16-33; "The Common Good Revisited," *Theologcal Studies*, vol. 50, 1989, pp. 83-84; and "Liberalism, Communitarianism, and the Bishops' Pastoral Letter on the Economy," pp. 19-53. For further commentary on the role of a relational anthropology in Roman Catholic social thought, see Jean-Yves Calvez and Jacques Perrin, *The Church and Social Justice: The Social Teaching of the Popes from Leo XIII to Pius XII*, Henry Regnery, Chicago, 1961, pp. 101-133; Daniel A. O'Connor, *Catholic Social Doctrine*, Newman Press, Westminster, 1956, pp. 149-159; Ernie Cortes, "Reflections on the Catholic Tradition of Family Rights," and Charles E. Curran, "Catholic Social Teaching and Human Morality," both in John A. Coleman, ed., *One Hundred Years of Catholic Social Thought: Celebration and Challenges*, Orbis Books, Maryknoll, NY, 1991, pp. 160-162; 74-80; and Michael J. Schuck, *That They Be One: The Social Teaching of the Papal Encyclicals, 1740-1989*, Georgetown University Press, Washington, DC, 1991, pp. 173-190.

36. National Conference of Catholic Bishops, para. 77.

37. DeCrane, p. 75.

38. National Conference of Catholic Bishops, para. 86.

39. Catholic Health Association, *Harnessing the Promise of Genomics: A Catholic Vision toward Genomic Advances*, St. Louis, 2004.

ethics. Respect for human dignity — for the fundamental equality of all human persons as *imago dei* (as representing the image and likeness of God) — presupposes that we respect every competent person's right to make health care choices in light of his or her own needs and values; it presupposes the right, when one is in the care of a trusted provider, to be neither harmed, exploited, manipulated, nor discriminated against on the basis of genetic or any other disease or disability; and it presupposes respect for privacy in the use of genetic information.

However, as we have seen, for the Catholic tradition, respect for persons as such is always expressed within a given set of communal relations. Thus, as one writer puts it, "justice requires that we see ourselves as bound in a covenant of life with life, in which human freedom and choice is always coupled with a sense of social responsibility."[40] The principle of *relationality* brings individual rights and duties into the conversation about the common good, asking how choices create conditions for the flourishing of all members of society. In the context of genetic technologies, a concern for relationality raises questions about our responsibilities to future generations; about how we set priorities for genetic research; about how we weigh the advantages to be gained through genetic technologies against other means for addressing disease, disability, and death; and about how we will distribute genetic services in light of the multiplicity of needs and limitations in resources.

The importance of ensuring the capacity for humane participation in society for all members calls for active *solidarity*. As noted, the "option for the poor" is not an adversarial slogan that pits one group or class against another. Rather, it expresses the recognition that the extent of suffering by some is a measure of how far we are from being a true community of persons.[41]

Solidarity captures the sense in which the claims of justice exerted by the poor enjoin not only our emotions but also our thinking about how we produce and use goods, as well as how we will organize our society. These are claims not simply to charity (sharing a surplus) but to justice — a rightful share of what is owed to all. Justice will require a reorientation of the use of goods as well as of the way society is organized to meet needs in light of the claims of the poor. Thus, in the context of genomics, the enduring commitment of Catholic health care "to the disadvantaged and our option for the poor requires a careful and delicate balancing — for example, balancing the pursuit of the goods of genomics with efforts to ensure that the basic human needs of all our citizens (and those most in need around the world) are adequately met; balancing the pursuit of genomics with meeting the health needs of the poor and effecting reform of an unjust health care system; and ensuring that the benefits of genomics are as available to the disadvantaged as they are to all other citizens."[42]

40. Karen Lebacqz, quoted in Chapman, p. 202.

41. Lebacqz.

42. Catholic Health Association, p. vii.

The principle of *subsidiarity* recognizes that the common good is best promoted and protected by enhancing the contribution and cooperation of various groups — in other words, by enabling various actors on different levels to act collaboratively. As in other areas, globalization presses us to imagine new ways of thinking about cooperation and governance as borders become more fluid and as we become more aware of the need for cooperative networks on a global scale. Subsidiarity pushes bioethics in two directions — toward the promotion of transnational participatory collaboration for equity, on one hand, and toward the further development of local capacity, on the other. These concerns encompass not only how partnerships might be forged between regions that are sophisticated about genomic technology and less sophisticated ones, but also how developments in biotechnology will interface with local and regional problems in health care delivery and infrastructure. *Genomics and World Health* makes the obvious but important point that "any benefits that result from genomics research will be irrelevant to countries that do not have a functioning health care system in place."[43]

Although one could say much more about the implications these principles have for decisions concerning access to genetic technologies (given existing global realities), the direction such an analysis would take should now be clear. As with efforts to bring affordable drugs to AIDS-ridden regions, strategies for mobilizing international cooperation for equitable access to biotechnologies must include assistance for developing nations in addressing such basic care delivery issues as training, education, and community organization. Needed also is support for the development of local capacity in bioethics, so that decisions about the conduct of research and the clinical application of developments in biotechnology incorporate and respect the religious and cultural values of those involved or affected. Some recognition on the part of the United States of the importance of this kind of empowerment can be seen in the NIH-funded "Communities of Color and Genetics Policy" program, which seeks to engage minorities in policy development to address issues of particular relevance for African-American and Latino communities.[44]

Discussing both the promises and the perils of global interdependence, Cahill argues that "a 'civic understanding of health,' not merely a consumerist one, [must emerge] at the global level if information and communication technologies are to be used not only to serve the market, but to envision and realize shared goods of health care in a newly integrated world."[45] One feature of

43. *Genomics and World Health*, p. 3.

44. Toby Citrin and Stephen M. Modell, "Genomics and Public Health: Clinical, Legal and Social Issues," in Marta Gwinn, et al., eds., *Genomics and Population Health: United States 2003*, Centers for Disease Control and Prevention, Atlanta, 2004, p. 55.

45. Lisa Sowle Cahill, "Biotech and Justice: Catching Up with the Real World Order," *Hastings Center Report*, vol. 33, no. 5, September-October 2003, p. 42.

such an understanding of health is a critique of what is often called "the culture of ownership" that dominates the research and regulation environment in biotechnology. Many people around the world have been sharply critical of current intellectual property laws that allow patenting of genetic material and control the rules under which drugs are produced and marketed. Such laws disregard the nature of genes (as naturally recurring information) and create monopolies on genetic information that are counter to the public interest.[46]

The most compelling arguments in this vein have significant overlap with Catholic social teaching on the universal destination of goods. Critics of the rush to patenting (and the overall inequities involved in access to the benefits of genomic research) argue that the character of the HGP, as a multinational cooperative effort aimed at identifying a common genetic code, makes its discoveries inherently "global public goods." Cahill and others have called for the creation of an "international or transnational forum for creating and implementing global policy" on the dissemination and use of genetic information, a forum that would be inclusive and participatory.[47] Some promising proposals are being offered as well for breaking the impasse between the claims of pharmaceutical corporations to protection against engaging in financially unsound research, on one hand, and the needs of developing countries for innovative approaches to the prevention and treatment of disease, on the other. Approaches such as patent regulations that encourage differential pricing for products developed for public health interests and government-guaranteed price packages for the development of vaccines aimed at underserved populations could encourage more companies to take the necessary risks.

A global option for the poor also encourages research collaboration between genetically advanced or more advanced countries (not all of which are developed nations) and genetically less advanced. According to Tikki Pang, PhD, WHO's director of Research Policy and Cooperation, asking ourselves how biotechnologies might serve public health in the developing world is a positive step, but doing so "must be accompanied by a genuine willingness on the part of developed countries and the pharmaceutical and biotechnology industries to share knowledge and help poorer countries apply such knowledge to solving their health problems."[48] Pang argues further that the "developed world must be prepared to invest more money in research in developing countries . . . in a spirit of helping developing countries ultimately to help themselves." Symbolizing its hopes, WHO released its report on genomics at a conference, hosted by the Africa Human Genome Initiative, that drew "world renowned super-scientists" along with leading African and South African scholars.[49] Pang and others endorsed the development of a Global Health Research Fund that would make resources for research available through peer-reviewed application to every country."[50]

It perhaps goes without saying that the big question concerning equity of access to genetic advances is: What can be done on behalf of the poor and the marginalized in the face of powerful counter values — profitability, self-interest, and market share — and in the face of such powerful actors as multinational corporations? How is interdependence to be transformed into solidarity? Although arguments for transnational or global governance structures appear compelling, there is no consensus about what such structures would look like or how exactly they would gain their authority.

Some experts — drawing on the interconnection of human rights, global public health, and biotechnology — argue for the formation of an international supervisory agency (perhaps as part of the United Nations Educational, Scientific, and Cultural Organization, UNESCO) to oversee research and development in genomics. Such an agency would possess regulatory power derived from documents such as UNESCO's *Universal Declaration on the Human Genome and Human Rights.*[51] The Catholic health ministry could take up the option for the poor by joining efforts to develop a workable vehicle for transnational solidarity around public health initiatives and working for its implementation.

However, Cahill has persuasively argued that the most important work religious groups can do on behalf of the poor may lie, not in the field of law and regulation, but rather in cooperation through global advocacy networks. Religion can and should be a powerful force for education, for joining parties in opposition to inequities and violations of human rights, and for consolidating an alternate vision in the face of the all-encompassing power of the market.[52]

As an example of the potential, Cahill points to international grassroots organizing in opposition to the imposition of genetically modified foods on developing countries, with its accompanying inattention to such foods' potential for displacing local crops. The effort she describes, involving religious groups, nongovernmental organizations, and episcopal conferences, has caught the attention of policy makers. Similar grassroots actions, in-

46. *Genomics and World Health,* p. 19.

47. Cahill, "Biotech and Justice," p. 36.

48. Pang, p. 18.

49. "Top Scientists to Attend Groundbreaking Human Genome Conference," press release, African Human Genome Initiative, March 2003.

50. "Genome Research Can Save Millions in Developing World," press release, World Health Organization, April 30, 2002.

51. United Nations Educational, Scientific, and Cultural Organization, "Universal Declaration on the Human Genome and Human Rights," New York City, November 11, 1997, available at http://portal.unesco.org/en/ev.php-url_id=13177&url_do=do_topic&url_section=201.html.

52. Lisa Sowle Cahill, "Bioethics, Theology, and Social Change," *Journal of Religious Ethics,* vol. 32, no. 3, December 2003, pp. 363-398.

volving both religious groups and secular advocacy groups, publicized the failure of U.S. and European pharmaceutical companies to make affordable drugs available for countries devastated by AIDS, especially in sub-Saharan Africa — and this publicity ultimately led to positive changes in pricing policies and to U.S. economic commitments to address AIDS.

The most recent report of the Global Forum for Health Research notes that "remarkable progress has been made in recent years in the development of international collaboration to solve major global health problems: between 1995 and 2003, more than 70 public-private partnerships and networks were created to address diseases such as HIV/AIDS, TB, malaria, and leishmaniasis. The challenge for the future will be to ensure their continued viability."[53]

A Bioethics of the Common Good

Christian bioethics is today inescapably bound up with social ethics; it is inescapably a bioethics of the common good. The risks of ignoring the social and global dimensions of health care choices, of overlooking the multiple worlds of health care that exist in this nation and around the world, are dramatically illustrated in the HGP and the genetic revolution now under way. Genomics promise to open new frontiers in the pursuit of health. But they also threaten to widen old gaps between developed and developing countries. There are many images used to describe the achievement of the HGP and its implications for our shared future. The philosopher Albert Jonsen has likened the genomics age to the beginning of the colonial period. He writes: "The ships that sailed from Europe five centuries ago not only mapped the world — they inaugurated social, political and economic events that radically changed humankind's view of itself and nations' views of their destinies. The rapidly redrawn map of discovery and colonization depicted areas of glorious achievement and areas of deplorable tragedy."[54]

The HGP represents a new kind of mapping. Whether it is used to chart areas of achievement or areas of continued tragedy will depend on choices made, for the most part, by those of us who live in the "90%" world. Will we choose profit, utility, and individual liberty — or respect for human dignity, solidarity, and concern for the common good?

53. Global Forum for Health Research, *10/90 Report on Health Research 2003-2004,* p. xi, available at www.globalforumhealth.org/site/002_what%20we%20do/005_publications/001_10%2090%20reports.php.

54. Albert Jonsen, "The Impact of Mapping the Human Genome on the Physician-Patient Relationship," in Thomas H. Murray, Mark A. Rothstein, and Robert F. Murray, Jr., eds., *The Human Genome and the Future of Health Care,* Indiana University Press, Bloomington, IN, 1996, p. 19.

129 Moral and Religious Implications of Genetic Control

Paul Ramsey

The Genetic Apocalypse and the End of Man

In order to analyze the moral implications of genetic control for western religions, it is necessary to lift up to view certain aspects of what it means to intend the world as a Christian or as a Jew. These also are modes of being human, and of how values are "otherwise known" in this world and ethical judgments made. On the assumption that it is a Christian *subject* who has come into the possession of all this genetic knowledge and who faces our genetic dilemma, what will be the attitude he takes toward eugenic proposals? Two ingredients are of chief importance. First, we have to contrast biblical or Christian eschatology with genetic eschatology, and observe how these practical proposals may change their hue when shifted from one ultimate philosophy of history to the other. This will be the matter of the present section of this chapter. Then, secondly (in the following section), we have to explore the bearing which the Christian understanding of the union between the personally unitive purpose and the procreative purpose of human sexual relations (sex as at once an act of love and an act of procreation) may have upon the question of the means to be used in genetic control.

The writings of H. J. Muller give the most vivid portrayal of the genetic cul-de-sac into which the human race is heading. He describes, in fact, a genetic apocalypse. His fellow geneticists can correct, if they must, the extremism of this vision. For the purpose of making clear, however, how one intends the world as a Christian, even in the face of such an apocalyptic account of the end toward which we are proceeding, or which is coming upon us, it is better to leave the vision unaltered and assume it to be a true account of the scientific facts.

Within a period of a few million years, according to Muller, provided that during this period our medical men have been able to continue to work with the kind of perfection they desire, "the then existing germ cells of what were once human beings would be a lot of hopeless, utterly diverse genetic monstrosities." Long before that, "the job of ministering to infirmities would come to con-

From Paul Ramsey, *Fabricated Man* (New Haven: Yale University Press, 1970), pp. 22-59.

sume all the energy that society could muster," leaving no surplus for general or higher cultural purposes.[1] People's time and energy would be mainly spent in an effort "to live carefully, to spare and prop up their own feebleness, to soothe their inner disharmonies and, in general, to doctor themselves as effectively as possible." Everyone will be an invalid, and everyone's accumulated internal disability would amount to lethality if he had to live under primitive conditions.[2] If any breakdown occurs in the complex hospital system that civilization will have become, mankind will be thrown back into a wretchedness with which his primitive beginnings cannot be compared.

> Our descendants' natural biological organization would in fact have disintegrated and have been replaced by complete disorder. Their only connection with mankind would then be the historical one that we ourselves had after all been their ancestors and sponsors, and the fact that their once-human material was still used for the purpose of converting it, artificially, into some semblance of man. However, it would in the end be far easier and more sensible to manufacture a complete man *de novo,* out of appropriately chosen raw materials, than to try to refashion into human form those pitiful relics which remained. For all of them would differ inordinately from one another, and each would present a whole series of most intricate research problems, before the treatments suitable for its own unique set of vagaries could be decided upon.[3]

It is unreasonable to expect medicine to keep up with the problem (especially because medical men themselves in that near, or distant, future will be subject to the same genetic decomposition); "at long last even the most sophisticated techniques available could no longer suffice to save men from their biological corruptions"[4] (and, again, I add to Muller's assumptions, medicine in that future could not be all that sophisticated, because of the genetic deterioration of the medical men who would be alive in the generation before the genetic *eschaton*).

Stripped of rhetoric, this means that, according to the genetic apocalypse, there shall come a time when *there will be none like us to come after us.* There have been other such scientific visions of the future. Whether this results from the pollution of our atmosphere and water by industrial refuse, or of the atmosphere by strontium 90, or from a collision of planets, the burning up of the earth, or the entropy of energy until our planet enters the eternal night of a universe run down, these scientific predictions — without exception — portray a planet no longer fit for human habitation, or a race of men no longer fit to live humanly. Because these are science-based apocalypses, the gruesome details of the "last days" can be filled in, and our imagination heightened in its apprehension of the truth concerning physical nature and the prospects of human history in the one dimension that is scientifically known to us. All these visions quite realistically teach that there will come a time when there will be none like us to come after us. It is as obvious as the ages are long that it is an infirm philosophy which teaches that "man can be courageous only so long as he knows he is survived by those who are like him, that [in *this* sense] he fulfils a role in something more permanent than himself."[5] Every scientific eschatology (with the single exception of the view that human history is eternal) places in jeopardy courage and all other values that are grounded in the future of the human generations. It does not matter whether the end comes early or late. Nor do the gruesome details do more than heighten the imagination. They do not add to the ultimate meaninglessness to which all human affairs were reduced when meaning came to rest in the temporal future (unless that future is foreknown to be eternal — and, if one thinks this through, it too is a melancholy prospect). All that can be said to the credit of the genetic apocalypse, or to the credit of any science-based eschatology, is that it makes *impressive* the truth that was already contained in the thought that men live in "one world."

Anyone who intends or perceives the world as a Christian will have to reply that he knew this all along, and that he has already taken into his system the idea that one day there will be none like us to come after us. Even gruesome details about what will happen in the "last days" are not missing from the Christian Apocalypse, even though admittedly these are not extrapolations from scientific facts or laws. The Revelation of St. John is still in the Bible; and even the so-called little apocalypse (Mark 13 and parallels) had this to say: "In those days shall be affliction, such as was not from the beginning of the creation which God created unto this time, neither shall be. . . . But in those days, after that tribulation, the sun shall be darkened, and the moon shall not give her light, and the stars of heaven shall fall, and the powers that are in heaven shall be shaken" (Mark 13:19, 24-25). Again, stripped of rhetoric, there will be none like us to come after us on this planet.

This means that Christian hope into, and through, the

1. H. J. Muller, "The Guidance of Human Evolution," in *Perspectives in Biology and Medicine* (Chicago: University of Chicago Press, 1959) 3 (Autumn 1959): 11.

2. H. J. Muller, "Our Load of Mutations," in *The American Journal of Human Genetics* 2 (June 1950): 146, 171.

3. Ibid., p. 146. Cf. also Muller, "Should We Strengthen or Weaken Our Genetic Heritage?" in Hudson Hoagland and Ralph W. Burhoe, eds., *Evolution and Man's Progress* (New York: Columbia University Press, 1962), p. 27. It does not seem a sufficient answer to all this to reply: "Norway rats . . . have been kept in laboratories since some time before 1840 and 1850. . . . But it does not follow that laboratory rats are decadent and unfit; nor does it follow that the 'welfare state' is making man decadent and unfit — to live in a welfare state!" (Theodosius Dobzhansky, *Mankind Evolving* [New Haven: Yale University Press, 1962], p. 326).

4. Muller, "Better Genes for Tomorrow," in Stuart Mudd, ed., *The Population Crisis and the Use of World Resources* (The Hague: Dr. W. Junk Publishers, 1964), p. 315.

5. Hannah Arendt, quoted in a *Worldview* editorial, Sept. 1958, p. 1.

future depends not at all on denying the number or seriousness of the accumulating lethal mutations which Muller finds to be the case (let his fellow geneticists argue with him however they will).

Where genetics teaches that we are made out of genes and unto genes return, Genesis teaches that we are made out of the dust of the ground and unto dust we and all our seed return. Never has biblical faith and hope depended on denying or refusing to face any facts — either of history, or of physical or biological nature. No natural or historical "theodicy" was ever required to establish the providence of God, for this providence was not confined to the one dimension within which modern thought finds its limits.

It is as easy (and as difficult) to believe in God after Auschwitz as it was after Sennacherib came down like a wolf on the fold to besiege and destroy the people of God. The Jews who chanted as they went to meet their cremation, "*Ani Ma'amin* . . ." — "I believe with unswerving faith in the coming of the Messiah" — uttered words appropriate to that earlier occasion, and to all temporal occasions. It is as easy (and as difficult) to believe in God after Mendel and Muller as it was after Darwin or the dust of Genesis. Religious people have never denied, indeed they affirm, that God means to kill us all in the end, and in the end He is going to succeed. Anyone who intends the world as a Jew or as a Christian — to the measure in which this is his mode of being in the world — goes forth to meet the collision of planets or the running down of suns, and he exists toward a future that may contain a genetic apocalypse with his eye fixed on another *eschaton: "Ani Ma'amin. . . .* " He may take the words literally, or they may imaginatively express his conviction that men live in "two cities" and not in one only. In no case need he deny whatever account science may give him of this city, this history, or this world, so long as science does not presume to turn itself into a theology by blitzing him into believing that it knows the one and only apocalypse.[6]

This does not mean a policy of inaction, or mere negative acceptance, of trends in history or in biology on the part of anyone who is a Christian knowing-*subject* of all that he knows about the world. Divine determination, properly understood, imposes no iron law of necessity, no more than does genetic determination. Only the ultimate *interpretation* of all the action that is going on is different, and significantly different. We shall have to ask what practical difference this makes as one man goes about responding (in all the action that comes upon him) to the action of the laws of genetics, while another goes about responding (in all the action coming upon mankind) to the action of God; or, as one gives answers to the ultimate untrustworthiness of the force behind genetic trends, while another answers with his life and choices to a trustworthiness beyond all real or seeming untrustworthy things.[7]

The differences are two — one pervasive and the other precise. In the first instance, one must notice the tone of assertive or declaratory optimism based on the ultimate and unrelieved pessimism that pervades the thought of some proponents of eugenics. The writings of H. J. Muller cannot be accounted for simply by the science of genetics, or even by the fact that his ethics is that of a man who intends the world as a scientist and who finds the whole dignity of man to consist in thought. As such, and in themselves, these things might be productive of more serenity, or serenity in action. But it is the whole creation, as it is known in genetics to be effectively present today and into the future, that Muller is fighting. No philosophy since Bertrand Russell's youthful essay[8] has been so self-consciously built upon the firm foundations of an unyielding despair. Mankind is doomed unless positive steps are taken to regulate our genetic endowment; and so horrendous is the genetic load that it often seems that Muller means to say that mankind is doomed no matter what steps are taken. Yet his optimism concerning the solutions he proposes is no less evident throughout; and all the more so, the more it is clear that his solutions (dependent as they are upon voluntary adoption) are unequal to the task. The author's language soars, he aspires higher, he challenges his contemporaries to nobler acts of genetic self-formation and improvement, all the more because of the abyss below. The abyss sets up such powerful wind currents that mankind seems destined to be drawn into it no matter how high we fly. These are some of the consequences of the fact that when all hope is gone, Muller hopes on *in despair.* An Abraham of genetic science, if one should arise, would be one who, when all hope is gone, hopes on *in faith,* and who therefore need neither fear the problem nor trust the solution of it too much.

The more precisely identifiable difference is the greater room there will be for an "ethics of means" in the outlook of anyone who is oriented upon the Christian *eschaton* and not upon the genetic cul-de-sac alone. Any-

6. In an article entitled, "Sex and People: A Critical Review" (*Religion and Life* 30 [Winter 1960-61]: 53-70), I sought to apply the edification found in Christian eschatology in refutation of certain genial viewpoints sometimes propounded by Christians on the basis of a doctrine of creation. These Christians hold that religious people *must* believe that God intends an abundant *earthly* life for every baby born, and that we would deny His providence if we doubt that world population control, combined with economic growthmanship, can finally succeed in fulfilling God's direction of human life to this end. Such a belief is secular progressivism with religious overtones. Taken seriously enough, it can lead, as easily as any other utopianism can, to the adoption of any means to that end, the control of the world's population. In essence, an independent morality of means, or righteousness in conduct, is collapsed into utilitarianism when the *eschaton* or man's supernatural end is replaced by any future *telos.*

7. The language of this paragraph reflects that of H. Richard Niebuhr, *The Responsible Self* (New York: Harper and Row, 1963).

8. "A Free Man's Worship." There is less posturing in Muller's despair, more in the optimism that floats over this despair, than in Russell.

one who intends the world as a Christian or as a Jew knows along his pulses that he is not bound *to succeed* in preventing genetic deterioration, any more than he would be bound to retard entropy, or prevent planets from colliding with this earth or the sun from cooling. He is not under the necessity of *ensuring* that those who come after us will be like us, any more than he is bound to *ensure* that there will be those like us to come after us. He knows no such *absolute* command of nature or of nature's God. This does not mean that he will do nothing. But it does mean that as he goes about the urgent business of doing his duty in regard to future generations, he will not begin with the desired *end* and deduce his obligation exclusively from this end. He will not define *right* merely in terms of conduciveness to the good end; nor will he decide what *ought to be done* simply by calculating what actions are most likely to succeed in achieving the *absolutely imperative end* of genetic control or improvement.

The Christian knows no such absolutely imperative end that would justify any means. Therefore, as he goes about the urgent business of bringing his duty to people now alive more into line with his genetic duty to future generations, he will always have in mind the premise that there may be a number of things that might succeed better but would be intrinsically wrong means for him to adopt. Therefore, he has a larger place for an ethics of means that is not wholly dependent on the ends of action. He knows that there may be a great many actions that would be wrong to put forth in this world, no matter what good consequences are expected to follow from them — especially if these consequences are thought of simply along the line of temporal history where, according to the Christian, success is not promised mankind by either Scripture or sound reason. He will approach the question of genetic control with a category of "cruel and unusual means" that he is prohibited to employ just as he knows there are "cruel and unusual punishments" that are not to be employed in the penal code. He will ask, What are right means? no less than he asks, What are the proper objectives? And he will know in advance that any person, or any society or age, expecting ultimate success where ultimate success is not to be reached, is peculiarly apt to devise extreme and morally illegitimate means for getting there. This, he will know, can easily be the case if men go about making themselves the lords and creators of the future race of men. He will say, of course, of any historical and future-facing action in which he is morally obliged to engage: "Only the end can justify the means" (as Dean Acheson once said of foreign policy). However, because he is not wholly engaged in future-facing action or oriented upon the future consequences with the entirety of his being, he will immediately add (as Acheson did): "This is not to say that the end justified any means, or that some ends can justify anything."[9] An ethics of means not derived from, or dependent upon, the objectives of action is the immediate fruit of knowing that men have another end than the receding future contains.

The ethics which, as we have seen, governs genetic proposals says as much. A fruit of intending the world as a geneticist is an ethics whose means are determined by the values of free will and thought. This puts a considerable limit upon the actions which can be proposed for the prevention of the genetic apocalypse (which, if a correct prediction, belongs only to the *contents* of the science of genetics). Still, this is not a sufficient substance for the morality of action, or at least not all the substance a Christian will find to be valid. One who intends the world as a Christian will know man's dignity consists not only in thought or in his freedom, and he will find more elements in the nature of man which are deserving of respect and should be withheld from human handling or trespass. Specifically in connection with genetic proposals, he will know that there are more ways to violate man-womanhood than to violate the *freedom* of the parties; and that something voluntarily adopted can still be wrong. He will pay attention to this as he goes about using indifferent, permitted, or not immoral means to secure the *relatively* imperative ends of genetic control or improvement. . . .

9. "Ethics in International Relations Today," an address delivered at Amherst College, Dec. 9, 1964; quoted from *The New York Times,* Dec. 10, 1964.

130 To Form a More Perfect Union: Mainline Protestantism and the Popularization of Eugenics

Amy Laura Hall

The first urgency is to know the axioms of eugenics. We are not even well educated nor modern if we have no bowing acquaintance with its larger truths.

Revd Phillips E. Osgood,
St Mark's Church, Minneapolis, 1926

Phillips Endecott Osgood's sermon 'The Refiner's Fire' won top honours in the first of a series of well-received sermon contests sponsored by the American Eugenics Society (AES). Using Malachi 3.3 as his text, Osgood admonished the 'temporary guardians of a miraculous gift' to respect their 'partnership with God to keep it pure'! 'The dross must be purged out' — and eugenics was the means for purging. The editors of the ecumenical journal the *Homiletic Review,* reprinting the sermon in 1929, registered their unequivocal assent: 'A contest is worthwhile which evokes so excellent a sermon. Eugenics is an approved thing. It is no longer on trial.'[1] Twenty years later, an avid Protestant eugenicist named Paul Popenoe would put the matter more subtly: the young Presbyterian, Methodist and Episcopal men and women reading the YMCA/YWCA-sponsored magazine needed to take on the civic responsibility of 'Surveying the Chances'. Citing his own study of children in the Sonoma State Home, he warned that 'feeble-minded' families were reproducing at a higher rate than those able to provide 'the best start'. Reminding his mobile, collegiate readers that 'cities always live as parasites on the rural areas', Popenoe emphasized their duty to consider patterns in 'the nation's birth-rate' when choosing their mates and planning their families.[2] Similar to Popenoe's article is one by Helen Southard entitled 'Planning Parenthood on Campus'. By the mid-twentieth century, the matter was largely settled among mainline Protestants: 'The Christian asks: how many; how healthy?'[3]

The history of the eugenics movement in the United States is seldom brought to the public eye. When popular historians do present the story, eugenicists are usually safely on the other side of a wide intellectual and cultural gap. Their science was faulty. Their ideas were blatantly racist. To quote one Public Broadcasting System (PBS) narration, the 'horrors of institutionalized eugenics revealed in Nazi Germany . . . doused [American eugenics] entirely as a movement' after the Second World War.[4] Arguably one of the trickiest tasks of narration is the one facing the writing staff at Cold Spring Harbor Laboratory. The lab recently celebrated '100 Years of Genetics' in 2004, reflecting a history that extends from Charles Davenport, lab director and mastermind of the Eugenics Record Office (ERO), to current chancellor James Watson, co-discoverer of the double-helix structure and advocate for 'making better human beings' through genetic engineering.[5] In May 2002 David Micklos, director of the lab's Dolan DNA Learning Center, marked the 75th anniversary of the landmark eugenic sterilization case, *Buck v. Bell,* with a special online article, 'None without Hope: Buck *vs.* Bell at 75'.[6] That original test of Virginia's sterilization laws went to the US Supreme Court in 1927, where Oliver Wendell Holmes, writing for the court, rendered the following:

> It is better for all the world, if instead of waiting to execute degenerate offspring for crime, or to let them starve for their imbecility, society can prevent those who are manifestly unfit from continuing their kind.

1. Phillips E. Osgood, 'The Refiner's Fire', in *Homiletic Review,* 97 (May 1929), pp. 405-409. Christine Rosen gives an account of Osgood's eugenic efforts in her *Preaching Eugenics: Religious Leaders and the American Eugenics Movement* (Oxford: Oxford University Press, 2004). See, in particular, pp. 3-4, 124-26.

2. Paul Popenoe, 'Surveying the Chances', *Intercollegian,* 65 (January 1948), p. 10.

3. An image of two children with a bicycle, with the caption 'The Christian asks: how many; how healthy?', appeared in 1948 in the YMCA/YWCA magazine, the *Intercollegian,* alongside two related articles: Paul Popenoe, 'Surveying the Chances', and Helen F. Southard, 'Planning Parenthood on Campus', *Intercollegian,* 65 (January 1948), pp. 9-10, 10-11. Popenoe was an active member of the American Eugenics Society (AES) and coauthor of the widely used textbook *Applied Eugenics.* Southard was an advocate for family planning. I am grateful to Rachel Maxson for finding these articles in the midst of her own research and for sharing the reference with me.

4. PBS, databank entry, 'Eugenics Movement Reaches its Height (1923)', A Science Odyssey, http:/www.pbs.org/wgbh/aso/databank/entries/dh23eu.html.

5. Watson has gone on record in support of genetic engineering to eliminate physical suffering. He has also grown increasingly blunt in his support of inheritable genetic engineering to avoid people who 'really are stupid' and to make 'all girls pretty'. The relevant sentences, as reported by *The Times:* 'People say it would be terrible if we made all girls pretty. I think it would be great', and 'If you really are stupid, I would call that a disease.' Mark Henderson, 'Let's cure stupidity, says DNA pioneer', *The Times,* 28 February 2003.

6. David Micklos, 'None without Hope: Buck *vs.* Bell at 75', Dolan DNA Learning Center, http://www.dnalc.org/resources/buckvbell.html.

From Amy Laura Hall, "To Form a More Perfect Union: Mainline Protestantism and the Popularization of Eugenics," in *Theology, Disability and the New Genetics,* edited by John Swinton and Brian Brock (T&T Clark, 2007), 76-95. Reproduced by kind permission of Continuum International Publishing Group. Slightly revised.

> The principle that sustains compulsory vaccination is broad enough to cover cutting the Fallopian tubes. Three generations of imbeciles are enough.[7]

With characteristic clarity, Justice Holmes thus linked several key eugenic concepts. In order to prevent individual suffering, the state may compel the prevention of certain 'kinds' of individuals. As an effective inoculation against degeneration, crime and imbecility, the social body may 'vaccinate' itself against the deleterious or parasitic 'unfit'.

Using subtle rhetorical cues, Micklos embeds this egregious story within the longer history of genetics at Cold Spring, distinguishing between the lab's dubious past and its promising present. Although Cold Spring's home team, led by Davenport, paved the way for the sterilization of Carrie Buck after the birth of her daughter, Vivian, their science was sullied by the 'biblical concept that "like breeds like"'. Impure, their scientific methods were eventually discredited by a more accurate strand of genetics; coercive, their political methods were untenable after the Nazi atrocities. As evidence of the state's mistake, the site features a link to Vivian Buck's first-grade report card, telling us that this supposed third-generation imbecile eventually made the elementary school honour roll. Micklos here brings the reader back to the point of his title. As it turns out, no lineage is 'without hope', because the new science of genetics is revealing a complicated combination of factors — factors that might 'predispose a person to autism' or 'predispose to genius' so that 'one can never predict where genius will arise'. Micklos situates the eugenics of the past on the other side of a chasm, distant from now-chastened politics and a science whose backward, biblical myopia has been duly corrected. The piece concludes that the Buck girls would likely wish us to take this lesson of 'hope' with us into our 'Brave New World'.[8]

This chapter is in part my attempt to tell a different story. One sign from the American Eugenics Society's Fitter Family fairs from the first half of the last century names a core assessment that still holds purchase: 'Some people are born to be a burden on the rest'. This gauge applied then to many kinds of difference; those who would judge scanned the horizon for those who variously did not 'fit'. Depending on the region, the signs of unfitness included poverty, disability, race and religion. I hope to complicate the standard narration of eugenics past and present by suggesting that this core assessment led to an arsenal of biotechnological tools to plan, evaluate and enhance children and to measure the worth of a given family, tools that today have become standard parental and political equipment. I will also suggest links between current hopes for genius and past attempts to vaccinate the social body against the menace of poverty, disability and deviance. As individual parents navigate the strand of genetics that supplanted the science of Davenport and his ilk, they are choosing in rising numbers to terminate pregnancies that show signs of genetic difference — choosing, in the majority of cases, to terminate for conditions ranging from physical disease to mental disability to gender ambiguity. At the same time, citizens in the United States view with increasing scepticism public spending on the supposedly indiscriminately bred children of poor African-American mothers as well as on the 'huge' families of recent Latino immigrants.[9] The cultural context in which individuals make what are increasingly seen as purely 'personal' decisions and in which a society makes what are often deemed purely pragmatic decisions is shaped by the powerful rhetoric of eugenics.

The pregnant body, the social body, and the burden of certain 'types' of babies are all culturally loaded in ways that reflect the vast movement in the past century in the United States to popularize eugenics. The quest to craft a more perfect union through 'fewer and better babies' is alive and well.[10] *Pace* Micklos, *pace* PBS, *pace* the tale often told, many eugenic ideas have jumped the gap from yesterday to today, bridging the chasm between overtly coercive eugenics and purportedly voluntary parental and social responsibility in the land of the free.[11]

The hypothesis of my narration is that eugenics gained popular support in large part through the endorsement of those mainstream and progressive Protestant spokesmen and women. Well after Henry Ward Beecher, self-declared 'cordial Christian evolutionist', endorsed from his pen and pulpit the social use of Charles Darwin and the social Darwinism of Herbert Spencer, mainline Protestantism continued to accept the thoroughgoing relevance of eugenic ideas.[12] From Paul Popenoe's *Intercollegian* and *Ladies' Home Journal* articles encouraging white middle-class men and women to replenish the race to the current United Methodist endorsement of 'responsible' parenthood in the UMC Social Principles, mainstream Protestantism has lent legitimacy to a trajectory of discriminating reproduction.

7. *Buck v. Bell,* 274 US. at 200, 207 (1927).

8. Micklos, 'None without Hope'.

9. The language is from the cover story of the 15 March 2004 issue of *Business Week,* featuring a photograph of two parents with their five sons. The article, by Brian Grow, is entitled 'Hispanic Nation', and the cover warns: 'Hispanics are an immigrant group like no other. Their huge numbers are changing old ideas about assimilation. Is America ready?' A graphic that accompanies the story charts 'America's *Bebé* Boom'.

10. The phrase is from the title of a book by William J. Robinson, MD, *Fewer and Better Babies,* published in multiple editions from 1915 to 1938.

11. I have found when presenting this material to non-Southerners that they are shocked to hear that the ERO was based on Long Island, New York, and that the AES had its headquarters in New Haven, Connecticut. The South has functioned in some ways to provide a second rhetorical chasm, allowing people from elsewhere mentally to dump most American ills in the supposed backwater of Southern culture.

12. See Richard Hofstadter, *Social Darwinism in American Thought* (New York: Braziller, 1959), pp. 29-30, 48.

Leading eugenicists in the United States used their own white, middle-class, literate, wholesome, productive, patriotic, native-born Protestant families as the standard by which other families would be measured and judged. The eugenics movement was germinated in a relatively elite, academic version of scientific racism from the previous century, but it took root in the heartland of America, arguably as a result of two primary forces: clergy eager to remain relevant in an era when other professionals, and scientists in particular, were gaining ascendancy; and middle-class laity eager to establish themselves as good, wholesome parents and productive, responsible citizens.

The 'born to be a burden' sign from the AES Fitter Family fairs warned with two intermittently flashing lights that of all persons born in the United States — that is, one 'every 16 seconds' — a mere 4 per cent, or one 'every 71/2 minutes,' is 'high-grade', able to 'do creative work and be fit for leadership'. A third flashing light underscored the associated economic toll: 'Every 15 seconds $100 of your money goes for the care of persons with bad heredity. . . .' That this display carried such rhetorical weight — that across the north-east and the heartland, farmers and shopkeepers and homemakers and minister's wives had their own and their children's heads and limbs measured and their extended family-trees mapped for taint or purity in order to be identified among the 4 percent of 'high-grade' people — is a sign that the AES knew well their constituency. That this display evoked among mainline Protestants hopeful aspirations rather than holy offence is an important part of the story of American eugenics.

Holy Husbandmen — 'Interpreting the Historic Faith in a Modern World'

One symbol of the eugenics movement in the 1920s and 30s was a 'Eugenics' tree, with roots branching out to tap the 'many sources' from which the eugenics movement drew in order to become a 'harmonious entity'. Through the 'self-direction of human evolution', eugenicists hoped to cultivate a tree that would flourish, bearing only good fruit for the future. It is worth noting that 'religion' was relegated to a root well off to the far right, one of the furthest roots from the main trunk of the tree. Biology, psychology, statistics, mental testing, history, geology, law and politics all had roles to play, with religion seemingly squeezed in almost as an afterthought — after sociology, to be precise. Yet the imagery of human advancement, hope and flourishing fruit was rhetorically potent, owing in part to echoes of the same biblical faith preached by Davenport's Congregationalist father, and the movement needed clergy to keep the echoes resonant.[13] Through the formation of the AES, eugenics leaders signalled that it would not be sufficient merely to keep careful measurements and records of the unfit and the fit, the impure and the pure, through the ERO. They needed to capture the imaginations of the citizenry. Religion was perhaps the root closest to the ground, and the AES found there clergy eager to prove that they were on the modernist side of the modernist/fundamentalist rift. Through cooperation with the AES, the YMCA and the ASHA, through thoughtful reviews and provocative sermons, clergy took up their calling in that 'great field of usefulness' that supported Protestant eugenics.[14] The sociologist, the psychologist, the anthropologist and the social worker were on the ascendancy, and mainline pastors throughout America were determined not to seem obsolete or, even worse, backward. As one reads the 'modern' attempts to prove a bowing acquaintance with eugenics, it is not difficult to surmise why mainline laity were unable to resist the allure of proving their own families fit at the expense of others. Faced with the challenge of remaining relevant and seeming well-educated in a modern world, many mainline Protestant clergy serving parishes and academe, in cities and in the country, did nothing less than capitulate.

In her meticulous treatment of the key religious players in the popularization of eugenics, Christine Rosen detects this as a 'clear pattern': 'The liberals and modernists in their respective faiths — those who challenged their churches to conform to modern circumstances — became the eugenics movement's most enthusiastic supporters'.[15] Rosen's conclusion is irrefutable. To cite one contrast, the Roman Catholic Church — with marked consistency from the grassroots to the Vatican — resisted laws against sterilization as well as the mind-set behind the movement, while some of the most hearty supporters of the AES found happy soil in the Anglican and Episcopal churches. The transatlantic links between the latter church allowed eugenic theologians such as Canon Charles Kingsley to influence priests such as Karl Reiland (in New York City) and Walter Taylor Sumner (in Chicago), who were eager to prove themselves legitimate fruit of the *forward*-thinking branch of the Apostolic Church. One article in the *Christian Century* from 1924 is telling. Reporting on a conference on the Church and science held by the aptly named 'British Churchmen's Union for the Advancement of Liberal Religious Thought', the piece relates at length the words of Oxford University professor and lay Anglican J. S. Haldane. In the quotation, Professor Haldane insists that people of

13. Harry Laughlin, who worked as superintendent of the ERO under Davenport, was the son of a minister.

14. The reference is to Leland Foster Wood, 'The Church and Education for the Family', in *Religion in Life*, 3 (1934), pp. 420-31. Arguing for 'premarital interviews' to promote emotional and social fitness, Wood declared: 'As rapidly as the clergy can be trained for this work, they will enter into a great field of usefulness'. Further: 'While the psychiatrist, the social worker, the judge of the court of domestic relations, the family physician and others render a great service to families, the minister of religion, whose business it is to interpret life as a whole, has his own unique place of service' (ibid., p. 431).

15. Rosen, *Preaching Eugenics*, p. 184.

faith 'cannot afford to be hampered by unintelligible beliefs which are mainly materialistic accretions of Christianity and which greatly weaken its influence on those who are worth influencing'. Distinguishing 'religion itself' from these accretions, Haldane warns that 'any shirking of the questions involved or cowardly sheltering behind mere traditional authority is fatal'.[16] The desire to remain in the good graces of 'those who are worth influencing', namely, (apparently) those well-educated citizens who had made the scientific turn, was clearly a part of the story.

Yet there are other salient patterns in Rosen's research. The 'modern circumstances' to which eugenics enthusiasts compelled their brethren to conform were the 'modern circumstances' of a significantly growing and noticeably changing populace — a populace that seemed out of ecclesial and civic reach. During a time when various 'helping' professions were on the rise among middle-class Protestants, there were regions, neighbourhoods and families who seemed out of 'charitable' control. Those who would not be assimilated into the organizational plans of progressives seemed not only extraneous but dangerously chaotic. One facet of the popular appeal of eugenics was its tidy promise to justify those margins. The right algorithms and tools helped those called to tend the boundaries of civic life to conceive of and perform their tasks. Variously unfit people played also, simultaneously, the necessary role of 'the problem'.

The sense that those gifted to do so should take up their civic duty to form a more perfect union was also pervasive. For many mainline Protestants, the call to be a 'good citizen' was tied up with the active formation of civic order. This perhaps puts a different spin on Rosen's well-drawn conclusion. The Protestants most accustomed to their role as well-educated *citizens* had the fewest theological resources to resist the messages of eugenics. The oldest and most unquestionably *American* of the Protestant churches were the first to jump on the eugenics bandwagon.

Is Christianity Dysgenic?

An active part of the eugenics conversation was the concern that Christianity itself was dysgenic, inasmuch as charitable giving took from the presumably productive and gave to the presumably parasitic. For those directly serving food and clothing, whether informally or professionally, the question was a practical one. To quote again the Revd Oscar McCulloch (who served many free hot meals through his Congregationalist parish in Indianapolis), the 'benevolent public' insisted on merely 'encouraging' those who lived an 'idle, wandering' existence. For those who were asked indirectly to give, the question was differently practical. They had worked hard for their money, and it was part of Christian stewardship to be responsible givers. A pithy piece in *Eugenics: A Journal of Race Betterment* addressed the question head-on. Asking, 'Is Christianity dysgenic?' and 'Is Christian morality harmful? Over-charitable to the unfit?' the 1928 report included responses from one rabbi and three clergymen serving in New York City.[17] The answers of the three Christian clerics warrant careful reading, for each explicates differently the relationship between traditional faith and science to draw conclusions about Christianity and eugenics.

'Evolution is a term that applies to religion as well as biology', explained the Revd Dr Karl Reiland of St George's Protestant Episcopal Church. The 'early Christian concept that the world should be despised' is 'footbinding', a 'drag on the progress of religious thought' that 'keeps the church from "stepping out"'. Those who were willing to embrace an aptly evolved religion would recognize that 'the first and foremost salvation of man individually, collectively and universally is the here and now salvation of a healthy heritage'. As Reiland read the relation between 'science and religion', the more conventional form of salvation — of one's soul and body through a saviour — is dependent on the securing of 'sound, safe and sane human beings'; indeed, 'the more we get of these salvations the more likely is any other, and the surer is the kind of religion that can help mankind'. Reiland understood his challenge as a clerical spokesman for eugenics — 'with inexorable certainty of perspective' — to be threefold: 'to revive and accelerate progress along the higher levels of thinking . . . to convince the religious conscience that whatever our creed, we are dealing with nature for the fundamental welfare of human nature; and lastly, to be prepared to discover that God was the God of biology before the Bible came on the scene'.

Reiland did not directly answer the immediate, practical question posed by the journal. He went well beyond such service, defining religion within the purview of human evolution and social utility. Situated in this way, Christianity could be cleared of the charge of practising dysgenics. But what is more, Christianity, 'whatever our creed', could be squarely in service to the eugenic aim 'to produce sound, safe and sane human beings'. Evolution applied to religion necessitated boldly taking one's place as a vanguard, eschewing when necessary both traditional doctrine and institutional polity in order to lead. As a final gesture of obeisance to the sponsors of the journal, Reiland suggested that evolved Christians concede the primary, revelatory power of biology.

16. J. S. Haldane, cited in a *Century* report, 'Churchmen and Scientists Discuss Mutual Problems' (25 September 1924), pp. 1244, 1250, 1252. See also J. S. Haldane, *The Sciences and Philosophy* (Garden City, NY: Doubleday, 1929), and Haldane, *The Philosophical Basis of Life* (Garden City, NY: Doubleday, 1931).

17. 'Is Christian Morality Harmful? Over-charitable to the Unfit? Four Religious Leaders Discuss a Charge Sometimes Made', in *Eugenics: A Journal of Race Betterment*, 1 (December 1928), pp. 20-21.

It is in the implied conversation between Ward and Ryan that Reiland's rather elastic theology hit the road. Harry F. Ward was professor of Christian ethics at Union Theological Seminary (1918-41) and was also a founder of the Methodist Federation for Social Service (1907). In 1928 John A. Ryan was a professor of both political science and moral theology at the Catholic University of America and director of the National Catholic Welfare Council's Social Action Department. Their roles in their respective denominations were parallel, each serving as a professor at his church's premier institution of higher education and as a national spokesman for the progressive wing of his church. Yet their answers were strikingly different.

Ward argued that 'the principles of Jesus' would not necessarily 'weaken and destroy society' unless one was overly 'shortsighted' in the interpretation of those principles. The true answer to the question posed by the journal would not overlook the 'vital fact' that 'the principles of Jesus' call for the 'transformation' of the weak. 'In seeking this goal', Ward argued, Christians with a properly broad vision would accept 'the challenge of removing the causes that produce the weak, including the hereditary factor'. And here Ward was blunt. The 'aim' of proper Christianity is 'a healthy society where all are strong'. The faithful are thus not only allowed but 'compelled' to be 'eugenic'. A 'social ethic based on the principles of Jesus' no less than requires 'the elimination of the weak, not their perpetuation, and this it accomplishes by making them strong and by preventing their production, through both breeding and environment'. By Ward's estimation, Christians had a crucial role to play in a 'coordinated world-wide effort to control population' and 'to the attainment of the highest standards of health and development by all the population'. While Reiland suggested that Christianity should be involved in securing 'sound, safe and sane human beings', Ward cut to the chase. The true goal of Christianity, as Ward read it, is to perpetuate strength and eliminate weakness. That the elimination of weakness would involve the sterilization of the weak was but part of a larger project of forming a 'healthy society'. With this trickled-down brew of Hegel, Darwin and American progressivism, Ward defended Christianity of the charge that it coddles the weak. Between Reiland and Ward, the answer was clear: Christianity would not prevent the social body from vaccinating itself against the unsafe, the unsound and the insane. Quite the contrary — the Christianity of their day was to participate in the process of inoculation.

John Ryan is the figure who most clearly complicates Christine Rosen's suggestion that progressivism and eugenics were inextricably linked. Here was a bona fide progressive, a tireless advocate for the working class and the unemployed poor who helped move his church to heed a radical strand of social thought all but buried in the nineteenth century. Yet Ryan answered the question of the relation between eugenics and Christianity with two points that cut to the heart of the eugenic presumption. First, he reminded his interlocutors that 'society, apart from the human beings composing it, is a mere abstraction' — that is, the social body exists only in and through real, embodied human beings. 'Therefore', Ryan patiently prodded, 'to subordinate the weaker groups to the welfare of society means simply that some human beings are to be made instruments to the welfare of other human beings.' This is all well and good, Ryan warned, for 'one who believes that morality is identical with physical force'. However, 'one who does not identify right with might' will be unable to make an argument for 'treating the weak as of less intrinsic worth than the strong, even though the former may be in the minority'. Ryan left unspoken that the 'one' who identified right with might and considered the weak to be of less intrinsic worth could hardly call him- or herself a Christian.

Then, with a rhetorical twist, Ryan reminded the eugenic readers, and presumably his fellow clergy, that they would do well to consider another, more practical problem. Reiland, Ward and other like-minded Christians might hope to find a hearing now by proving their solidarity with the strong. But if the eugenic programme succeeded, they might eventually find themselves on the receiving end:

> The practical argument against this theory is that once society decides that the weak may rightfully be left to perish, it will extend the principle to all of the so-called inferior classes, so that in the end the 'welfare of society' will come to mean the welfare of a few supermen, namely those who have been powerful enough to get themselves accepted at their own valuation.

As Ryan narrated the movement, eugenics was primarily about the power of the currently strong to use the apparently weak for the purposes of securing something as nebulous as a 'higher average welfare'. Faced with the temptation of siding with the worthy against the unworthy, the other two clergy had succumbed. Sacrifice your faith, Ryan warned, and tomorrow you may find yourself counted among the weak.

Purge the Dross

Many sermons inspired by the AES sermon contests reveal a tragically shortsighted tendency on the part of Protestant clergy to align with the strong against the vulnerable. Three sermons published during the same *year* (1929) in three different journals by men representing three different denominations may serve as characteristic examples. Edwin Bishop preached 'Eugenics and the Church' at Plymouth Congregational Church in Lansing, Michigan; like the dysgenic/eugenic debate above, the sermon appeared in the official ERO publication from New Haven, *Eugenics: A Journal of Race Betterment.*[18] A second, 'The Refiner's Fire', appeared in the *Homiletic*

18. Edwin Bishop, 'Eugenics and the Church', in *Eugenics: A Journal of Race Betterment,* 2 (August 1929), pp. 14-19.

Review. The Revd Phillips Endecott Osgood, rector of St Mark's Unitarian Church in Minneapolis, had won the 1926 AES eugenics sermon contest with his rousing demand to purge 'the dross' of humanity through eugenics, and the publishers of the ecumenical journal not only found the sermon worthy of print but endorsed the AES contest, declaring with editorial authority: 'Eugenics is an approved thing'.[19] The *Methodist Review* chose 'Eugenics: A Lay Sermon' by George Huntingdon Donaldson, published also in 1929.[20] The three sermons suggest that the popularizing efforts of the scientific eugenicists were quite effective. From an ERO journal to an ecumenical Protestant review to a focused, denominational publication, the message was taking hold. A Congregationalist in Michigan, a Unitarian in Minnesota and a Methodist in New York City each took to the pulpit to affirm (quoting Donaldson) that 'the strongest and best are selected for propagating the likeness of God and carrying on his work of improving the race'.[21]

In an ironic use of anti-Catholic dialect, the Congregationalist in the group noted that the science of heredity was confirming 'Irish Pat's sage dictum that "a family tree is a foine thing if it ben't too shady"'. Science had proven that everything from 'night blindness' to 'a tendency to health and longevity' was 'heritable', and, according to Edwin Bishop, it was through these scientific advances that God called humans to 'participate with him in *conscious* evolution' (emphasis original). Appealing, as did so many eugenicists, to old-fashioned animal husbandry, Bishop argued that 'if we used as much intelligence in human mating as we use in breeding horses and cows' we could prevent 'ills' and encourage 'excellencies'. Would not Jesus himself, Bishop asked, encourage 'any program that would aid children to be physically well-born?' Again, in a characteristic eugenic move, Bishop referred to the rock-solid proof of numbers. A quantitative study had shown that 'of 476 children born to 144 marriages among feeble-minded folk only six were normal', indicating that 'native ability furnishes the bulk of the basis of achievement'. Those who follow Jesus needed therefore to see eugenics as 'a potential ally' in the holy pursuit of 'racial self-fulfilment'. 'Through neglect of eugenic knowledge and practice', Bishop warned, 'tares are sprouting widely through the wheat.' By forming a prudent alliance with eugenics organizations, Christians could reverse the growing imbalance of the 'well-born' and the 'less favourably born' — a menacing imbalance proven by 'carefully assembled data' (probably provided by the AES in their letter of invitation to the sermon contest).[22]

It is for very good reason that Christine Rosen begins *Preaching Eugenics* with the example of Phillips Osgood's 'The Refiner's Fire'. His call, with which we began this chapter, to prove one's 'bowing acquaintance' with the 'larger truths' of eugenics was a rhetorically masterful use of his homiletic gifts.[23] Opening with Malachi 3.3, 'He shall sit as a refiner and purifier of silver', Osgood called God the 'Refiner of the generations', for whom Christians should 'count themselves the agents of his purposes'. Lest any of his hearers or readers ask inconvenient questions about Jesus and the meek or poor, Osgood reminded them: 'Jesus sometimes said ruthless things' if 'men deserved them'. Such was the time again. Jesus 'was superlatively concerned to better the qualities of human living' and testified that 'grapes cannot be gathered from thorns nor figs from thistles'. Citing children's 'inalienable right to life more abundant', Christians were to take up 'the refining responsibility', recognize that 'the future is in our hands', and secure by 'creative forethought' the purity of future generations. Loath to limit himself to Scripture, the Unitarian clergyman reminded his hearers that 'Xenophon, long ago, recommended that slaves should be allowed the reward of children for good conduct'. 'The recommendation', Osgood suggested, 'has merit also for those not slaves.'[24]

From sterilizing 'the criminal' to stigmatizing the 'victim of inheritable malady', Osgood argued with exegetical flourish for the basic tenet of eugenics — the excellent must prevent the propagation of the reprehensible and the pitiable. The present generation had a responsibility to act as 'redemptive helper of the next generation'. If one but compared the Jukes family to the family of Jonathan Edwards (a move first made by A. E. Winship)[25] one might see that heredity is the 'major factor' in 'our cooperation with the Refiner's work'.[26] Here Osgood played on the metallurgy metaphor in two ways. In order to determine who among the Refiner's creatures were called to do the cooperative refining, one needed to look primarily at heritage. In order to determine the proper tools to be used by the refined, one needed only to look at the heredity studies. Osgood's conclusion is horrifically clear:

> God will provide his Spirit to our children's children; why handicap its incarnation? It will be the finer in its manifesting if it need not labor under handicap. The kingdom of God on earth is not an end of growth, but the beginning of true destiny. Until sin and weakness and disease and pain are done away, we are only starting to commence to get ready to enter into life as it may be. Until the impurities of dross and alloy are purified out of our silver it can not be taken in the hands of the craftsman for whom the refining was done. God the Refiner we know: do we yet dream of the skill or the beauty of purpose of God the Craftsman with his once purified

19. Osgood, 'Refiner's Fire', pp. 405-406.

20. George Huntington Donaldson, 'Eugenics: A Lay Sermon', in *Methodist Review*, 112 (1929), pp. 59-68.

21. Donaldson, 'Eugenics,' p. 60.

22. Bishop, 'Eugenics and the Church', pp. 16-17.

23. Osgood, 'Refiner's Fire', p. 406.

24. Osgood, 'Refiner's Fire', pp. 405-406.

25. Albert E. Winship, *Jukes — Edwards: A Study in Education and Heredity* (Harrisburg, PA: R. L. Myers, 1900).

26. Osgood, 'Refiner's Fire', pp. 406-407.

> silver? May the time soon come when in refined humanity he can see his own face, clear and unsullied.[27]

Invoking no less than 'the name of God who is Love', Osgood suggested that the culmination of God's creation was dependent on the elimination of suffering. This involved not acts of mercy toward the sick and the poor but acts to secure a future free of those who would 'handicap [the Spirit's] incarnation.'[28] Twice referring to the *'saecula saeculorum'*, Osgood places the 'refining responsibility' within the Latin liturgy. The 'forever and ever', 'the ages of ages', becomes, in his sermon, a future dependent on eugenic resolve.[29]

From the husbandman to the blacksmith and, now, to the gardener: George Huntington Donaldson, in his sermon for the *Methodist Review*, used a botanical metaphor to extol the virtues of Christian eugenics. He urged Methodists and fellow humanists to see the 'beautiful and efficient answers' that emerge when one envisions God as akin to the nation's most beloved gardener, California plant-breeder and eugenicist Luther Burbank. 'When we contemplate this patient toiler in his wonderful garden, in fellowship with and conformity to that trinity of creative laws, namely: *heredity, variation,* and *selection*', we may understand 'the progressive creation of better life on this earth.' By reading Genesis with eugenic science in view, one can see that 'the whole creative process described [in the creation story] had been progressive'. Using Unitarian poet William Herbert Carruth's line 'Some call it Evolution, / And [others] call it God', Donaldson himself waxed poetic on the 'third law' of creation. Through selection, God continued to use 'the strongest and best' for 'propagating the likeness of God and carrying on his work of improving the race'. If one reads Scripture carefully, one may detect a pattern: from the story of Joseph's rise over his 'mongrel' brothers to the desert wandering (which 'purged' the weak) to the 'choicest souls' who followed Ezra and Nehemiah, 'those who have been purified' are able to 'see God'.[30]

Exegetes, sociologists, biologists and theologians heartily agreed on this point: 'there is but one fixed and unchangeable thing, and that is heredity'. To bring this point home to his congregation, the preacher sounded a liturgically resonant theme. For Methodists, hymnody was (and remains) a significant part of weekly worship. Donaldson's use of language from Matthew 7.24-25 played effectively upon echoes with the beloved Methodist hymn by Edward Mote, 'My Hope Is Built'. While the hymn intones, 'My hope is built on nothing less than Jesus' blood and righteousness', Donaldson proclaimed, 'Heredity is a rock on which we can build with unfailing certainty'. By setting the initial creation within the story of evolution, Donaldson was able to set the new creation through Jesus within the larger story of 'improving the race'. Those who were baptized into Christ became partners in the work of selecting, yanking out and cultivating. With 'proper selections and combinations all good can be produced and all evil eliminated'; the one following Jesus needed to cut down the 'crop of defectives' who 'weaken and burden the race'.[31]

Donaldson showed a characteristic familiarity with the big names of scientific eugenics. By alluding to the founder of British eugenics, Francis Galton, and quoting Henry Fairfield Osborn, president of the American Museum of Natural History in New York (1908-33) and of the Second Eugenics Congress (in 1921), he gave evidence of his own knowledge of the field as well as obeisance to those who were developing the proper gardening tools. His sermon came back to holy horticulture, employing the Johannine Jesus's imagery of vine and branches to link God the Father with God the Selective Gardener:

> So, returning to our Bible account, we read the words of Jesus, I am the vine, ye are the branches, and my Father is the gardener,' or husbandman. And just as at the beginning we saw Luther Burbank watching over his gardens, selecting here a fine strain, there another, and taking the pollen of one to unite with the egg cell of the other and so produce a finer fruit or flower, so in this wonderful book, God as Gardener has been watching over humanity.[32]

As the rousing conclusion of his sermon, Donaldson asked whether Christians would have the courage to 'Make democracy safe for the world' by ensuring 'progressive betterment'. In the hymn on which Donaldson relied for a potent echo, it was Jesus's blood that secured the future. Layering metaphor on metaphor, Donaldson suggested that those made 'perfect' by Jesus's 'death upon the cross' were called to make democracy safe by ensuring the 'pure and undefiled' transmission of human blood 'to the coming generations'.[33] The Christian hope is thus *rebuilt* on nothing less than Jesus's blood and Galton's best.

The subtitle for the 'Holy husbandmen' section above, 'Interpreting the historic faith in a modern world', plays on the current motto of the *Quarterly Review*, the United Methodist journal of 'theological resources for ministry'. Rather than a 'modern world', the journal aims to interpret 'the historic faith' in a 'postmodern' one. The editors explain that the journal will 'forthrightly engage the challenges of ministry by bringing the resources of the Christian faith in mutually critical conversation with the issues of our present reality'. In this quest, the articles emerge from 'the context of a distinctively United Methodist and Wesleyan perspective — without ever becoming parochial or narrow-minded'.[34] This promise — to

27. Osgood, 'Refiner's Fire', p. 409.
28. Osgood, 'Refiner's Fire', pp. 408-409.
29. Osgood, 'Refiner's Fire', pp. 405, 407.
30. Donaldson, 'Eugenics', pp. 59, 60, 63 (emphasis original).
31. Donaldson, 'Eugenics', pp. 63, 65.
32. Donaldson, 'Eugenics', pp. 65-66.
33. Donaldson, 'Eugenics', pp. 67-68.
34. 'About *Quarterly Review*', http://www.quarterlyreview.org/aboutqr.html.

avoid parochialism and narrow-minded thought — seems to most mainline and liberal Protestants today to be a key ingredient of truly *relevant* theology. The editors of the *Methodist Review* issue of 1929 may very well have chosen Donaldson's sermon using primarily that criterion. Donaldson more than amply proved his allegiance to what the editors of the *Homiletic Review* called the 'approved thing' of eugenics. Yet the editors of the current *Quarterly Review* also signal that essays 'interpreting the historic faith in a postmodern world' should emerge from within the Wesleyan tradition. Presumably, the call to remain relevant, to attempt to eschew parochialism or narrow-minded thought, does not trump the call to remain within the range of Wesleyan thought represented by the various Methodist traditions. Striking in the sermons above is the facility with which each of the preachers was able to bend Scripture to suit the eugenic project. Many mainline Protestants had come to believe that, as the pro-eugenics editor of the *Methodist Quarterly Review* put it, because 'the Bible nowhere undertakes to give a detailed account of the process of creation . . . it leaves ample room for any theory to which careful scientific investigation may lead'.[35] The scriptural story of salvation in the Old Testament all too swiftly became a story of God's refining, purifying and selecting in order to produce a stronger, heartier stock of humans. Jesus's parables regarding the kingdom of God swiftly became parables for the eugenic separation of human wheat from human chaff. Both Osgood and Donaldson also employed liturgical cues, setting the practices of sterilization and selective mating within the context of worship.

All three preachers were able to interpret 'the historic faith' in a 'modern' (i.e. Darwinian) way: defining Christians as cooperative agents in bringing to fruition God's purposes, which primarily meant the strengthening of the assumedly dominant race in the assumedly Promised Land of the United States. Having gone the way of the modernists in accepting evolutionary science, the mainline denominations represented in these published sermons were able to distinguish themselves from the 'backward' Christian creationists. In the words of Gilbert T. Rowe, editor of the *Methodist Quarterly Review* (1921-28), mainline readers were particularly interested when they found a 'thoroughly Christian' writer who could prove himself 'no hard and fast dogmatist'.[36] One who could so 'thoroughly' narrate the tradition in a way consonant with evolution was a particularly reliable guide to the present and future. But in the process of renarration, these preachers, and the theologians upon whom they drew, arguably left few theological barriers to the all-encompassing narrative of eugenics. And having accepted as their primary duty that of civic leadership, they left few theological barriers to the racist nationalism of eugenics. Determined to think in modern, patriotic and well-educated ways about the role of the faithful in America, these preachers attained their sophistication at the expense of the vulnerable. They used the lives of others in order to establish their own strength.

Safeguarding the Future

Another way to detect the theological moves made by mainline churches during the eugenic era is to read the distillation of eugenic thought in journals aimed at clergy and learned laity. Journals such as the *Methodist Quarterly Review* and *Religion in Life* sought to offer their readers essays relevant for the church's engagement with theological as well as secular disciplines. The volumes of journals from the 1920s and 30s reveal significant interest in the application of evolutionary thought to Christian theology. One *Methodist Quarterly Review* piece, a review essay by Rowe, is characteristic. Rowe sorted through the implications of three books from three different authors, attempting to forge a pathway *To Christ through Evolution* and to make a new theological language that combined *Evolution and Redemption*.[37] A *Religion in Life* piece considered *The Doctrine of Redemption in the Light of Modern Knowledge*, and yet another, by the author of *Do the Ten Commandments Stand Today?* and *Evolution for Christians*, asked, 'Has the concept of humanity a scientific basis?'[38] The journals served to give a particularly Christian (and particularly mainline Protestant) interpretation of the biology and sociology filtering through the university classrooms and over the radio airwaves. Mainline clergy and laity across the country faced the task of thinking at the intersection of evolutionary biology and practical theology. Their efforts are important for understanding the sense that 'Eugenics is an approved thing', again to quote the editors of the *Homiletic Review*.

One local pastor in Missouri, a Revd C. L. Dorris, wrote an extensive essay inspired by Philip Archibald Parsons's *An Introduction to Modern Social Problems* for the 1926 *Methodist Quarterly Review*.[39] This young pastor, trained at Central (Methodist) College and the University of Missouri, was serving in the Methodist Episco-

35. Gilbert T. Rowe, 'Christianity and Evolution', in *Methodist Quarterly Review*, 75 (1926), p. 138.

36. Rowe, 'Christianity and Evolution', p. 140.

37. Rowe, 'Christianity and Evolution', pp. 138-41. The essay involves a review of *To Christ through Evolution*, by Professor Louis Matthews Sweet (1925); *Nineteenth-Century Evolution and After*, by Revd Marshall Dawson (1923); and *Evolution and Redemption*, by Revd John Gardner, DD (1925).

38. Ismar J. Peritz, 'Christ and Evolution', review of *The Doctrine of Redemption in the Light of Modern Knowledge*, by George A. Barton, in *Religion in Life*, 4 (1935), pp. 462-64; J. Parton Milum, 'Has the Concept of Humanity a Scientific Basis?', in *Religion in Life*, 5 (1936), pp. 52-63. Milum is also author of *Do the Ten Commandments Stand Today?* (London: Epworth, 1936); *Man and his Meaning* (London: Skeffington, 1945); and *Evolution for Christians* (London: Skeffington, 1933).

39. C. L. Dorris, 'The Impending Disaster', in *Methodist Quarterly Review*, 75 (1926), pp. 720-24, citing Philip Archibald Parsons, *An Introduction to Modern Social Problems* (1924).

pal Church South in the small town of Milan, Missouri, when he felt compelled to write of 'The Impending Disaster', adding 'his voice to the voices in the wilderness warning that unless something is done disaster will soon befall us'. This, the last line of the essay, indicates the exigency of the effort. The sense of moral urgency, of peril and promise, registered even in a town of around 2,000 people, several days' travel from the nearest city.[40] The records of Dorris's training and travels do not indicate that he came to his conclusions after encountering the throngs of immigrants on either shore. Rather, they suggest that the message of eugenics came to him perhaps through his reading at the public library or through a teacher in his congregation. He, in turn, published an essay to be read by local Methodist ministers eager to bring the latest in sociological discernment to their parishes. In it, the rural pastor took in a considerable amount of intellectual territory, borrowing clout from Englishman Henry Havelock Ellis (author of the six-volume *Studies in the Psychology of Sex*), Professor James Quayle Dealey (tenth president of the American Sociological Society), the Reverend Josiah Strong (prominent Congregationalist pastor and author of the anti-urban tract *Our Country*), professor and sociologist Charles A. Ellwood and Harvard president Charles W. Eliot. The essay reads as a pithy, authoritative call to attention and action.

Beginning with the sin of sloth, Dorris admonished readers that 'one of the gravest dangers' among Methodist congregants was 'a lack of pride in providing capable offspring for future generations'. Clearly, there were 'too many physically, mentally, and morally defective' gaining way in society, and Christians needed to relinquish 'the individualistic theory of marriage for personal pleasure'. Quite the contrary — marriages needed to be planned with 'racial consequences' in view. Without such prudence, Dorris warned, 'we are going to continue to produce a crop of defectives'. Here Dorris returned to a practical strategy commonly enjoined in eugenic texts of the time — the sacrifice of romantic sentiment for the sake of society. Quoting Ellis's *Psychology of Sex,* Dorris affirmed that 'the birth of a child is a social act' and that the 'community', in being 'invited to receive a new citizen', is 'entitled to demand that that citizen shall be worthy of a place in its midst'. Dorris repeated this crucial point: 'We should demand that each child born is worthy a place in our midst'. The demand required the full arsenal of 'public sentiment in favour of safeguarding the future', for 'public sentiment is one of the most powerful weapons of defence'. In this way, Dorris defined the primary task of his clerical and lay readers: to bring the 'American people' to 'see the dangers threatening us', so that 'they will demand the raising of proper safeguards'. A local pastor from rural Missouri gave an effective populist appeal for the work of eugenics, bringing the civic role of 'safeguarding the future' down from New Haven and Cold Spring and Boston and Manhattan to the grassroots of the heartland. Methodists were to do their considerable part to enforce proper marital standards based on 'the law of the survival of the fittest'.[41]

There were multiple means for averting 'the disaster', ranging from the legal and institutional, to address the inferior, to the more nuanced propaganda necessary to encourage the 'truly better elements of society' to see their civic duty to replenish 'the stock'.[42] Regarding the former, there were laws 'to prohibit the marriage of the unfit', intended to 'eliminate the weaker stock' and 'build up the race through its stronger elements.' There was also the prospect of widespread sterilization. But Dorris argued that sterilization would be insufficient for the 'hopeless types of defectives'. For them, the public should seek means for 'permanent segregation' that would force these otherwise 'expensive' individuals 'to support themselves in properly conducted institutions and colonies'. Yet even with these concerted measures, leaders needed to be vigilant to encourage the reproduction of those representing 'the higher forms of life'. Quoting sociologist James Dealey, Dorris explained that only 'when [society] frowns alike on the large family of the poor and the childless family of leisure' will 'rapid advance' ensue. The 'future civilization' depended as much on the breeding of the 'leadership' class as it did on the institutionalization of the 'defectives'. And while he was on the topic, Dorris reminded the 'leisure class' not to 'confide their children to the care of ignorant and incapable servants'.[43]

Again, this from a local pastor in Milan, Missouri. It is a testimony to the brilliance of those in the eugenics movement that they were able to direct the mainline Protestant desire for class superiority toward the popularization of such notions. Dorris's essay thus reveals a crucial part of the tale. Recall the AES Fitter Family poster warning that a mere 4 per cent of Americans were born with the 'ability to do creative work and be fit for leadership'. The fact that the AES could display this sign at county fairs in Missouri, Michigan and Minnesota without engendering moral outrage is at first glance unfathomable. While it makes some intuitive sense that a Charles Davenport could appeal to the vanity of railroad tycoon-widow Mrs E. H. Harriman with such 'AES calculations', the fact that the *hoi polloi* in places such as rural Missouri found themselves in the 4 percent rather than the 95 percent begs for explanation. By writing of the 'impending disaster' from his unassuming Methodist parsonage, Dorris left behind evidence — a vital clue to the eugenics puzzle. He assumed that he and the people who read the *Methodist Quarterly Review* had as central a role to play in civic leadership as did Mr and Mrs Rockefeller. Quoting Professor Charles A. Ellwood, Dorris explained that 'the growing complexity of social

40. In 1920 the population of Milan was 2,395; in 1930 it was 2,002. (My thanks to Jason D. Stratman at the Missouri Historical Society for this statistic.)

41. Dorris, 'Impending Disaster', pp. 720-21.

42. Dorris, 'Impending Disaster', pp. 722-23.

43. Dorris, 'Impending Disaster', pp. 721-22.

life, as social evolution advances, calls for an ever-increasing means of control over individual character and conduct'. As good Christian citizens, Methodists needed to address 'the woes of the world' with 'religion of the right kind' — a religion with proven influence 'in elevating character, in diffusing peace and good will, in fitting men to labour and to endure', and, indeed, 'in lifting mankind to a higher sphere morally and spiritually'. It was a crucial time for the country, with aspirations as high as the sense of economic and demographic vulnerability. With progress, Dorris warned, also comes 'degeneration', and the mainliners of the heartland had a role to play in safeguarding against it.[44] And here Dorris was arguably dead-on. Religious and secular historians alike could have relegated the AES and ERO and the American Breeders Association to mad-scientist status had those organizations not made such headway on everything from state sterilization laws to the popularization of eugenic aspirations among the middle class. The movement *won* with the considerable aid of men such as Dorris and the women and men who heard his call to *'demand that each child born, is worthy a place in our midst'*.[45]

The Future of the Disabled

The residual logic of taint and purity underwrote much that passed for normative parenthood in the twentieth century. Dorris's cold assessment had arguably won the day by the time of the Second World War. The responsible citizenry had a right to demand that each child born was 'worthy a place in our midst'. The turn from overt, coercive eugenics to implicit, voluntary eugenics may be less a sign of the failure of eugenic ideology than a sign of its success. The 'modern', Darwinian, sense of a division between the 'highest' and the 'lowest' in humanity lent scientific legitimacy to the fears at play in the middle-class neighbourhoods that began to flourish in the post-war period. There were some children meant to flourish and others whose lives were insufficiently ordered and wholesome. Distinguishing the one group from the other was a whole set of signals from the shoes on a little boy's feet to the number of braids in a daughter's hair, from the marks on a second-grader's report-card to, eventually, the APGAR score assigned to his newborn sister. This is not even to mention the clear, blatant and often deadly markers of race. The same Methodists Dorris called upon to address the 'impending disaster' of America's degeneration were ready to lead again by way of voluntary eugenics. Promoting the medical tools of 'responsible parenthood', mainline Protestants endorsed family planning and orderly hygiene as practices integral to civic duty. Taking their cues from *Ladies' Home Journal* ('The Magazine Women Believe In'), mainline Protestant mothers employed Ivory Soap and the principles of discriminating reproduction to make sure that their offspring were legitimate inheritors of the Promised Land.

In *The Future of the Disabled in a Liberal Society,* Hans Reinders, Willem van den Bergh Professor of Ethics and Mental Disability at Vrije University in Amsterdam, suggests that the future looks considerably less excellent for those who do not follow the expert advice of such counsellors. Reinders was asked in 1996 to write on genetics and disability for the Dutch Association of Bioethics. His book is an extended moral reflection on the subject, and it directly counters the usual argument that the overriding ethical concern attending prenatal testing is that of simple distributive justice. Indeed, Reinders suggests, the ever-widening distribution of such technologies may in fact weaken the already tenuous commitment of liberal nations to funding disability services:

> Assuming that disabled people will always be among us, that the proliferation of genetic testing will strengthen the perception that the prevention of disability is a matter of responsible reproductive behavior, and that society is therefore entitled to hold people personally responsible for having a disabled child, it is not unlikely that political support for the provision of their special needs will erode.[46]

According to Reinders, the question of civic and social hospitality is key, but political liberalism is not ultimately capable of engendering and fostering hospitality toward people with overt, recalcitrant needs. The norms encircling the liberal axis of individual autonomy cannot easily accommodate lives dedicated to the care of perpetually dependent individuals, or admit the intrinsic value of these individuals. Meticulously considering the policy implications of this tension, Reinders concludes that it is neither within the liberal purview nor within the limits of the practical to address it through legal restrictions on procreative technology and abortion. The predicament facing liberal society, then, is 'cultural', not 'political'.

> The benefits bestowed by love and friendship are consequential rather than conditional, which explains why human life that is constituted by these relationships is appropriately experienced as a gift. A society that accepts responsibility for dependent others such as the mentally disabled will do so because there are sufficient people who accept [this] account as true.[47]

The sense that a life may be rightly mapped on a grid of social use, productivity or beauty begs for an account that can see life otherwise. Mainline Protestants in the United States failed to offer such an account in the past. The efficiently eugenic future now beckons.

44. Dorris, 'Impending Disaster', p. 723.

45. Dorris, 'Impending Disaster', p. 720.

46. Hans Reinders, *The Future of the Disabled in Liberal Society: An Ethical Analysis* (Notre Dame, IL: University of Notre Dame Press, 2000), p. 14.

47. Reinders, *Future of the Disabled,* p. 17.

131 The Human Genome Project as Soteriological Project

Robert Song

Introduction

A number of common themes recur in standard critiques of the new molecular genetics as applied to human beings. These centre on its propensity, or at least the propensity of the philosophy often associated with it, towards reductionism, biological determinism, and the geneticization of human identity.[1] Critics who pursue this line have in their sights ideas such as the following: that all traits and behaviour can be explained largely or even solely in genetic terms, and do not require much, if any, reference to environmental explanations; that an individual's behaviour can be understood as a product of his or her genes; that the behaviour of a group or collectivity can be interpreted by reference to the genes of the individuals that comprise it; that if a trait or behaviour can be described as genetic, it is therefore immutable; and that the role of DNA in the make-up of a person can be depicted as a 'blueprint', 'master molecule', or through other implicitly deterministic metaphors. Ideas like these, the critics note, reinforce the ideological power of genetic categories within a technological-scientific culture. In medicine, for example, they contribute to the expanding notion of genetic disease, in which the genetic component is singled out for especial prominence. In terms of personal self-understanding, they underwrite the increasing emphasis on genetic identity as the key to people's interpretation of their psychology and physiology, their successes and failures, their past and future. Socially, they emerge in the sociobiological legitimation of patriarchal gender relations, racial discrimination, and opposition to welfare handouts or egalitarian approaches to education.

These misgivings are surely justified. As Evelyn Fox Keller has written, 'Most responsible advocates are of course careful to acknowledge the role of *both* nature and nurture, but rhetorically, as well as in scientific practice, it is "nature" that emerges as the decisive victor.'[2] The reductionist tendency of the programme always appears to end up giving biology the explanatory priority. The potency of the gene as a cultural symbol has reinforced leanings towards a genetic essentialism that equates people with their genetic make-up, thereby squeezing out the manifold historical and cultural complexities of their formation. Under the spell of such a mentality it is easy for biological difference to become definitive of social identity, in relation to gender, class, race, intelligence, bodily health, sexuality, and the various traits and behaviours putatively associated with genetic influence. Equally, in such a context recognition of genetic factors runs the risk of a fatalist mind-set which forgets that it is the degree of malleability of traits which is critical, not the fact of their genetic inheritance. And such determinism consorts well with the social and political pressures towards programmes of genetic improvement that reached their nadir in Nazi Germany, only to reappear in a very different form in subsequent decades in the consumerist eugenics that is exemplified by pre-natal testing leading to abortion.[3]

I entirely concur with these critics, therefore. Indeed, in what follows I will take the general thrust of their criticisms for granted. However, in my view their understanding of the phenomenon of the new genetics is incomplete. They fail to give a sufficiently plausible account of its appeal not only to scientists and corporate biotechnology interests, but to the ordinary inhabitants of modern Western culture as a whole. They do not explain why anybody should be attracted to the reductionist project or should be inclined towards understanding human beings in these etiolated terms. In this chapter I want to explore some of the cultural commitments that have given rise to the new genetics, and ultimately to the Human Genome Project. In particular I will attempt to draw some connections between its roots on the one hand in seventeenth-century scientific and technological aspirations, and an underlying quality of motivation on the other which I will

1. For such criticisms see, for example, Steven Rose, R. C. Lewontin and Leon J. Kamin, *Not in Our Genes: Biology, Ideology and Human Nature* (Harmondsworth: Penguin, 1984) ('the twin philosophical stances with which this book is concerned' are 'reductionism' and 'biological determinism' [pp. 5-6]); Ruth Hubbard and Elijah Wald, *Exploding the Gene Myth: How Genetic Information Is Produced and Manipulated by Scientists, Physicians, Employers, Insurance Companies, Educators, and Law Enforcers* (Boston, MA: Beacon Press, 1993) (focuses on 'geneticization' and 'reductionism' [pp. 2-3]); R. C. Lewontin, *The Doctrine of DNA: Biology as Ideology* (London: Penguin, 1993) (criticizes 'the ideology of biological determinism' [p. 23]); and Dorothy Nelkin and M. Susan Lindee, *The DNA Mystique: The Gene as a Cultural Icon* (New York: Freeman, 1995) (argues that popular culture conveys 'genetic essentialism' [p. 2]). For a theological critique of the 'gene myth', see Ted Peters, *Playing God? Genetic Determinism and Human Freedom* (New York: Routledge, 1997).

From Robert Song, "The Human Genome Project as Soteriological Project," in *Brave New World? Theology, Ethics and the Human Genome.* Ed. Celia Deane-Drummond (New York: T. & T. Clark, 2003), 164-84. Reproduced by kind permission of Continuum International Publishing Group.

2. Evelyn Fox Keller, 'Nature, Nurture, and the Human Genome Project', in Daniel J. Kevies and Leroy Hood (eds.), *The Code of Codes: Scientific and Social Issues in the Human Genome Project* (Cambridge, MA: Harvard University Press, 1992), pp. 281-99 at p. 282.

3. Robert Song, *Human Genetics: Fabricating the Future* (London: Darton, Longman & Todd, 2002), pp. 41-50, 81-95.

argue should be seen as quasi-religious in nature. Only once this has been acknowledged, I shall claim, will we be free to ask the question whether the Human Genome Project is a project which human beings might properly embark on.

The Reductionist Project

According to the critics we are considering, the programme of the new genetics which has given birth to the Human Genome Project should be criticized for its reductive philosophical stance: it understands human beings solely, or at least predominantly, in terms of their genetic inheritance. As I have indicated, I share these concerns, and think that it is open to criticism at least to the extent that it shares in such a stance. However, of itself such a style of critique is inadequate, for a variety of reasons. By appreciating these, I hope that we may work towards a fuller understanding and perhaps more adequate critique of the new genetics.

The first problem with the critique of the new genetics as reductive is that the new genetics is not necessarily committed to this philosophical stance. While the science may often have proceeded under the impress of a reductive imperative, for reasons we shall discuss later, there is a plausible case for saying that the new genetics is not itself intrinsically reductive. It would be quite possible for a researcher to argue that the only way of understanding the relative contributions and mutual implications of genetic and environmental factors is to obtain a more precise comprehension of each, and that on the genetic side this requires the detailed knowledge that is being provided by gene mapping and sequencing that has been undertaken by the Human Genome Project, together with the exploration of protein structure and interaction and all the other developments in understanding which it is hoped will emerge during the next decades and beyond. Greater knowledge here would imply no prejudgement in favour of genetic explanations; indeed it might thwart the pretensions of reductive approaches by showing precisely what genetics is incapable of accounting for. In other words, to the extent that the philosophical commitments and broader cultural representations of the new genetics are guilty of reductionism or determinist essentialism, they should be rejected, but it should not be presumed that these errors are somehow intrinsic to the science itself.

The second problem with the critique is that by itself it does not complete the critical task. It is one thing to show the intellectual and moral errors of reductionism as a philosophical stance, another to give an account of what gave rise to it in the first place. To criticize a philosophy of genetics simply for being reductive leaves unexplained why anybody should be attracted to such a view, a difficulty which is made the more severe, the more obviously absurd the reductionist position can be shown to be. We can elucidate this point by developing the critique in a little more depth.

The reductionist approach to genetics, we might elaborate the critics' argument, compromises a true understanding of human persons. This is achieved by downplaying or even analysing out the role of environmental factors, or by neglecting the inward, self-constituting nature of agents, or both. In doing so, it aligns the study of human genetics with the modernist project of attempting to explain the properties of larger and more complex entities in terms of the properties of the units out of which they are composed. This project can in turn be seen as a consequence of the new approach to the science of nature that was articulated in the seventeenth century,[4] an account which (in Amos Funkenstein's portrayal) united four previously separate ideals: the drive for unequivocation in language, which required the abandonment of the picture of the natural world as itself symbolic and referential, with a view to ensuring that only language could designate; the drive to regard nature as homogeneous, such that the laws of nature should be presumed to apply uniformly throughout the universe; mathematization, that nature could be understood in the language of mathematics; and mechanization, that final causes should be discarded in favour of the complete explanatory adequacy of efficient causes alone.[5] These ideals paved the way for the considerable success of the physical sciences from the seventeenth century. But they were also increasingly applied to the study of human beings, and formed a framework of thought which has given rise to a family of theories that have recurred in a variety of forms, from mechanistic approaches to anatomy in the late eighteenth century to psychological behaviourism and attempts to create artificial intelligence in the twentieth century and beyond.

The specific ebbs and flows of this process of applying the methods and assumptions of the natural sciences to the study of human beings are of less concern to me here[6] than the question of the motivation of this naturalist programme. We need to uncover the nature of the appeal it has had.

In answer to this it is of course possible to see a number of intellectual attractions: it would be disingenuous to deny the enormous advances in scientific understanding made on the basis of such an approach, not just in relation to the ostensibly 'hard' sciences of the physical body, but also in relation to 'softer' sciences such as psychology.[7] But given the manifest unpersuasiveness of the

4. Rose *et al.* refer the origins of the reductive view of human nature to the emergence of bourgeois society in the seventeenth century and Hobbes's view that (in their words) 'it was biological inevitability that made humans what they were' (*Not in Our Genes*, p. 5).

5. Amos Funkenstein, *Theology and the Scientific Imagination from the Middle Ages to the Seventeenth Century* (Princeton: Princeton University Press, 1986), pp. 28-81.

6. Though for some insightful elaboration of this see Bronislaw Szerszynski's piece in [*Brave New World?*; also included as article 132 in the present volume].

7. For an account of what mechanistic models can and cannot

thoroughgoing reductive project, even starker in some fields than it is in genetics, the question arises compellingly for all but true believers how such an approach could ever have come to seem plausible.

In searching for the motivations behind reductive accounts of the human sciences, we might take a cue from conventional explanations for the appeal of their equivalents in the physical sciences, namely the search for a certain kind of knowledge. This might be expressed in terms of the increased powers of prediction and control over nature. If this were applied by analogy to the social sciences, it might illuminate how their naturalist desire for overarching laws of the social world could be explained by reference to greater capacities for organization and administration of populations. But it could also throw some light on the case we are concerned with, that of human genetics. For the early history of the attraction towards genetic determinism is inseparable from the rise of eugenic ambitions. Most geneticists in the early decades of the twentieth century regarded it as the proper role of science to improve the human race, and the prevalence of eugenic beliefs among those working in the field both informed and was informed by their belief in the decisive role of heredity in the formation of intellectual and moral traits.[8] Their confidence in eugenics grew because their belief in determinism made it possible; their confidence in determinism grew because their eugenic ideals made it desirable.

Yet even this kind of explanation only takes us so far. In relation to genetics, it does not account for the continuing appeal of genetic essentialism in an era which has repudiated all overt eugenic intentions. Nor does it explain the continuing presence of the reductive mentality even in areas such as the geneticization of identity — which have prima facie rather little to do with eugenics, even in its new consumerist form. There is an element in the explanation which is missing.

What we are searching for, therefore, is a critical explanatory account of the phenomenon of the new genetics as a whole which will do justice to the critique of the reductive tendencies that we have been discussing, but will also set it in a broader framework. More specifically, we may conclude from our discussion so far, such an account will do at least four things. First, it should be able to furnish an explanation of the coming-to-be of the new genetics, and not just assume its facticity as something to be subject to a posteriori criticism. Rather than taking the genetic phenomenon as a brute given, it should be able to provide a narrative of the causal dynamics that have given rise to the new genetics in such a way that some light will be shed on its possible future trajectories. This is not the same as asking it to predict the future, of course, but merely to give a deeper understanding of the forces that have created the present and will shape the future.

Second, this critique will not presume that the genetic phenomenon is necessarily reductive in nature. It will not lose all critical power if it were to be shown that the Human Genome Project is not inherently committed to a reductive programme. Third, on the other hand, it must be able to explain the temptation to reductionism with which genetics has rightly been connected. If the relation between genetics and reductionism is contingent, as I have suggested, the two still display a mutual affinity, and this needs illumination. Fourth, it must be able to give a full account of the motivations which might be associated with the reductive tendencies of the new genetics which goes beyond those which we have examined so far. In particular, we need to consider not merely the intellectual and socio-political attractions of determinism in genetics, but also the moral and even existential appeal of it.

The Seventeenth-Century Project

As a first step towards this account, we should note something insufficiently recognized by commentators on the Human Genome Project, namely that it is a public, social act. At one level it is a highly complex endeavour of scientific research, for which spending has had to be argued over against other funding priorities, but at another level it is also a social act with a high degree of ownership by the wider public. Evidence of this public interest can be found in the massively disproportionate media coverage devoted to new discoveries in genetics compared with other areas of science, as well as in the active support and vociferous advocacy of genetic research by interest groups and others. While those who undertake or fund genome research may do so for their own scientific or commercial (or charitable) reasons, they do so to a significant extent on behalf of society as a whole. No doubt there is a process of legitimation at work in order to render publicly plausible the genetics project as a whole (through rhetorical expansion of the notion of genetic disease, of the potential of genomic research, and so on), but even so the role of the public is still better depicted as knowing complicity rather than passive or innocent acquiescence.[9]

What then is the cause of the public obsession with the new genetics? At least at the level of presenting reasons, the most palpable attraction is of course the prom-

explain in psychology, see Charles Taylor, 'Peaceful Coexistence in Psychology', in *Philosophical Papers,* 2 vols. (Cambridge: Cambridge University Press, 1985), vol. 1: *Human Agency and Language,* pp. 117-88. Much of Taylor's *oeuvre* has been devoted to explaining the appeal of reductive naturalisms in the human sciences. In addition to both volumes of *Philosophical Papers,* see also esp. *Sources of the Self: The Making of the Modern Identity* (Cambridge: Cambridge University Press, 1989).

8. Diane Paul, *Controlling Human Heredity: 1865 to the Present* (Atlantic Heights, NY: Humanities Press, 1995), pp. 121-5.

9. David F. Noble assumes wrongly that the religion of technology was always 'in essence an elitist expectation, reserved only for the elect' (*The Religion of Technology: The Divinity of Man and the Spirit of Invention* [New York: Knopf, 1997], p. 201).

ise of benefits. These benefits include increased human self-understanding — the role of genes in behaviour, for example. But their main appeal is surely in relation to health and the potential they are perceived to hold for improved diagnosis and ultimately treatment of disease, from highly penetrant single-gene disorders such as Huntington's disease in which environmental factors play a minimal role, to cancers at the other extreme where the presence even of several alleles acting in concert may contribute only an incremental increase in susceptibility. Indeed, so intuitively plausible is the notion that human medical benefit is outstandingly the most compelling reason for undertaking genomic research that an official HGP website courts absurdity when it lists molecular medicine as just one of six potential benefits of human genome research, of which the others are 'microbial genomics; risk assessment; bioarchaeology, anthropology, evolution, and human migration; DNA forensics (identification); agriculture, livestock breeding, and bioprocessing' — as if bioarchaeology were on a par in the public mind with a cure for cancer.[10]

Scientists also have a fundamental interest in the medical benefits of genetic research, whatever else may motivate them. Even if individual researchers may be moved by the joy of knowledge alone, effective arguments for funding the Human Genome Project have been very largely based on the putative clinical outcomes. Thus Nancy Wexler, as chair of the working group on the Ethical, Legal and Social Implications of the Project: 'those of us who have been working in the field of genetic disease for a long time and who are engrossed in efforts towards finding treatments and cures, feel strongly that the question is not whether we can afford to do this project but whether we can afford *not* to do this project'.[11] Or James D. Watson, as co-discoverer of the structure of DNA and first director of the Human Genome Project: '[w]hen you ask a supporter of the project "Why do you want to do it?" the overriding reason is that it will let us get handles on genetic disease much more efficiently'.[12] The interests of corporate pharmaceutical and biotechnological interests likewise are not far removed from diagnostic and therapeutic success. While of course they may benefit from creating medical needs where none had existed previously (for example — in a currently nongenetic field — in the case of aesthetic surgery), in the vast majority of cases long-term commercial success will be dependent on satisfactorily meeting human medical need. At least in relation to human genomic research, therefore, there is a case for seeing the attractions of pure research and the pressures of the market economy as secondary levels of explanation compared with the potential for medical benefit.

Any reasonable interpretation of the whole phenomenon of the new genetics will therefore give a prima facie priority to the motivation of freedom from disease. How might this fit into the broader account we are attempting to construct? To answer this, we need to revisit the seventeenth century, this time interested in the period not just as the origin of mechanizing and reductivist motifs in the human sciences, but as the source of a particular kind of motivation.

The Human Genome Project is best seen, I suggest, as the latest avatar of a set of aspirations which were most influentially formulated in their distinctively modern form in seventeenth-century England. These ambitions, which I shall term 'the Baconian project', following Gerald McKenny,[13] centre on the effort to deny the necessity of suffering, achieved by the instrumental control of nature. Francis Bacon's project centred on the reconstruction of philosophy with a view to the discovery of nature's secrets and improvements in the conditions of human life. At his most visionary, these improvements included 'the prolongation of life, the restitution of youth in some degree, the retardation of age, the curing of diseases counted incurable, the mitigation of pain'.[14] Although he was not a Puritan, his emphasis on practical betterment over against sterile scholasticism ('the knowledge that we now possess will not teach a man even what to *wish*'),[15] set within a biblical framework, rendered him an instinctively congenial philosopher in Puritan eyes. They in turn busied themselves with exploitation of the fruits of the earth in the service of God, a process that would be eased by the mechanistic rejection of the teleological ordering of nature and the adoption of reductive modes of explanation.[16]

10. 'Potential Benefits of Human Genome Project Research', ttp://www.ornl.gov/hgmis/project/benefits.html (accessed 28 June 2002).

11. In a round-table discussion held in 1990, 'An Invitation to Genetics in the Twenty-First Century', in Necia Grant Cooper (ed.), *The Human Genome Project: Deciphering the Blueprint of Heredity* (Mill Valley, CA: University Science Books, 1994), pp. 314-29 at p. 318.

12. James D. Watson, 'The Human Genome Initiative', in Barry Holland and Charalambos Kyriacou (eds.), *Genetics and Society* (Wokingham: Addison-Wesley, 1993), pp. 13-26 at p. 19. Watson opines that this is the majority position of older scientists who find their minds turning to questions of disease; younger scientists by contrast are more fascinated by the HGP's 'intrinsic benefits to pure science' (ibid.).

13. Gerald P. McKenny, *To Relieve the Human Condition: Bioethics, Technology and the Body* (Albany, NY: State University of New York Press, 1997), pp. 17-21, drawing on the work of Charles Taylor. The term is used by synecdoche, and should not be taken to imply that Bacon himself was responsible for the larger project to which I have attached his name.

14. Francis Bacon, 'Magnalia Naturae', in *The Advancement of Learning and New Atlantis*, ed. Arthur Johnston (Oxford: Clarendon Press, 1974), p. 249. Strikingly, in view of the new genetics, the list also includes 'The altering of statures; The altering of features . . . Making of new species; Transplanting of one species into another'.

15. Preface to *De Interpretatione Naturae*, quoted by Johnston, p. x.

16. For the influence of the Puritans on the development of early modern science and medicine, see Charles Webster, *The Great Instauration: Science, Medicine and Reform, 1626-60* (London: Duckworth, 1975), esp. pp. 1-31, 324-42, 484-520. Note, how-

Mill

In subsequent centuries the goals would be furthered while the thought was slowly secularized. The early utilitarians of the radical Enlightenment reduced moral value to the net utility of pleasure over pain, thereby reducing suffering to a mere negative in a felicific calculus. Similarly, deist questioning of God's action in the world turned providence into impersonal fate, making unnecessary the spiritual discipline of finding meaning in suffering. Combined with an Enlightenment and Romantic emphasis on individual autonomy, and the increased mastery of nature afforded by nineteenth- and twentieth-century technological developments, the Baconian project has consequently bequeathed to modern medicine its animating ideals: namely, the elimination of suffering and the maximization of individual choice.

It is important to note that these twin ideals do not merely address the infirmities of bodily existence. They also implicitly raise the hope of freedom from subjection to the necessities of the human condition. Shorn of the limitations imposed by religion, the promise of modern medicine is not just of therapy for disease, but of therapy for the existential anxieties of finitude and mortality. The conquest of nature has become the conquest of fate, and it is this desire for domination which we should see as motivating the project of modern technological medicine, of which the Human Genome Project itself is but one part. The quest for an instrumentalized, reductive understanding of human beings is in other words the outworking of a desire for freedom from necessity.

This gives us in brief compass the elements of a theory in which reductionism has a role, but one that is secondary to a certain kind of motivation. Support for this interpretation of the direction of seventeenth-century thinking might also be argued from the case of Descartes. It is tempting to portray his philosophy as fundamentally motivated by epistemological concerns about the possibility of certainty, which in turn carried implications for his dualist metaphysics of mind-body relations. But, as Drew Leder has suggested,[17] it is at least arguable that his metaphysics was driven by existential concerns about disease and death. This may be seen from his own discussions about the motivations for his philosophy. Towards the end of the *Discourse on Method* he talks of 'the possibility of gaining knowledge which would be very useful in life, and of discovering a practical philosophy which might replace the speculative philosophy taught in the schools', through which we might 'make ourselves, as it were, the lords and masters of nature'. The most important reason he gives for this is 'the maintenance of health, which is undoubtedly the chief good and the foundation of all the other goods in this life', and includes freedom from 'innumerable diseases, both of the body and of the mind, and perhaps even from the infirmity of old age, if we had sufficient knowledge of their causes and of all the remedies that nature has provided'.[18] And beyond this, he claims, arguments for the distinct substances of body and mind are needed 'to show that the decay of the body does not imply the destruction of the mind' and 'to give mortals the hope of an after-life', such that 'while the body can very easily perish, the mind is immortal by its very nature'.[19] The mechanization of the body is therefore not just a propaedeutic to its yielding physiological knowledge, but part of a strategy of evading existential threats to the self by ensuring that the pure substance of the soul can never be contaminated by the accidents of the body.

The Baconian project, echoed by Descartes, provides us with the elements of a theory of modern technological medicine as a whole. But in relation to the Human Genome Project, we can go a step further in learning from the seventeenth century by looking further at Bacon's own philosophy of science. Antonio Pérez-Ramos, in an influential study, has argued that Bacon should not be understood in broad categories such as 'inductivism', 'utilitarianism', and the like.[20] Rather, underlying his thought is the notion of 'maker's knowledge', that knowledge of the truth of the thing is knowledge of the way it is constructed and could be reconstructed. The epistemological guarantee of one's understanding of nature is the ability to produce it and the interiorization of the skills to enable one to reproduce it. This analysis of the nature of knowledge cuts across the categories of pure/applied and theory/practice: since maker's knowledge is not simply knowledge as the capacity for making but also knowledge as the ability to conceptualize the practice, it reconfigures the terms.

One implication of this is that we should distinguish the broader 'Baconian project', extending over centuries, from the more precise understanding of Bacon's own philosophy of science. In the strict sense, Pérez-Ramos maintains, 'no recognizable artefact or technique can be identified as approximately bespeaking Baconian desiderata in the sense advanced here until, say, the development of the chemical or pharmaceutical industry in the nineteenth century, or the rise of genetic engineering in our own'.[21] Appreciating this enables us to refine our understanding of the Human Genome Project in relation to the broader account of technological medicine. Not only

ever, that the millenarianism and this-worldly utopianism that Webster sees as motivating technological development was relatively uncommon compared with more conventional eschatological beliefs: see John Henry, 'Atomism and Eschatology: Catholicism and Natural Philosophy in the Interregnum', *British Journal for the History of Science* (1982), pp. 211-39.

17. Drew Leder, *The Absent Body* (Chicago: University of Chicago Press, 1990), pp. 138-41, as discussed by McKenny, *To Relieve the Human Condition*, pp. 190-2.

18. René Descartes, *Discourse on Method* (1637), Part Six, in *The Philosophical Writings of Descartes*, trans. John Cottingham, Robert Stoothoff and Dugald Murdoch, 3 vols. (Cambridge: Cambridge University Press, 1985-91), vol. i, pp. 142-3.

19. Descartes, *Meditations on First Philosophy* (1641), Synopsis, in *The Philosophical Writings of Descartes*, vol. ii, p. 10.

20. Antonio Pérez-Ramos, *Francis Bacon's Idea of Science and the Maker's Knowledge Tradition* (Oxford: Clarendon Press, 1988).

21. Ibid., pp. 294-5.

does the HGP share in all the broader features of the project of eliminating suffering and maximizing choice, it does so in a particular way. It radicalizes the search for causes, not just by driving them back to their molecular basis, but by implicitly thinking of true knowledge of the body as the ability to construct it. And in this model, knowledge of the 'basic building blocks' of the body is not just knowledge of how it is constructed, but at once also knowledge of how it might be reconstructed.

The Soteriological Project

I have suggested therefore that the desire for reductionist explanations and for instrumental approaches to the body should be seen as secondary to and derivative from the motivation of freedom from necessity. But it has also been evident that this motivation cannot be divested of an existential dimension: the Baconian project has been not just a matter of healing of particular infirmities, but a more radical freedom from the burdens of finitude. This quasi-religious dimension needs to be explored more directly.

The Puritans of course handled their thinking about science and medicine within the matrix of the biblical narrative. It was not possible, they agreed, to be too well studied in the book of God's word or the book of God's works. 'To know the secrets of nature, is to know the works of God' was a common tag of the period, while a particular favourite of Bacon's had been Proverbs 25.2: 'The glory of God is to conceal a thing: the glory of the King to search it out.'[22] This knowledge of the workings of nature was interpreted as a restoration of Adam's former knowledge, a recapitulation of the lost condition of creation.

However, for them such knowledge was always bounded by religion. In answer to the question how knowledge could be a godly pursuit if the fall itself was the result of the desire for knowledge, Bacon had answered that 'all knowledge is to be limited by religion, and to be referred to use and action'.[23] And so the Puritans had guarded against the potential for moral corruption and social exploitation through the discipline afforded by the virtues and precepts of Christian morality, and had sought to control the distribution of the fruits of knowledge through careful oversight by the godly parliament.[24] Far from detracting from their service of God, the investigation of nature to advance learning and provide benefit for humankind was one of its highest expressions.

But it was not clear that the quest for knowledge of nature could always be limited in this way. This can be seen from Funkenstein's commentary on the seventeenth-century project. He argues that the constructivist understanding of knowledge, the theory which I earlier attributed to Bacon as 'maker's knowledge', was in fact characteristic of the new epistemological project of the seventeenth century as a whole.[25] In the medieval period, he suggests, the identity of truth with doing had been a characteristic mark of the divine knowledge of the Creator alone. In so far as it was a property of human knowledge, it was confined to machines and other human artefacts. Human knowledge of the universe as a whole, by contrast, whether it was conceived as a matter of illumination, introspection or abstraction from sense impressions, was fundamentally a passive or receptive knowledge. However, in the seventeenth century the active, constructionist epistemology was extended to human knowledge of the universe as well, threatening a disintegration of the barrier between divine and human knowledge so radical that many baulked at its implications. As Funkenstein writes: 'applying knowledge-through-construction to the whole world was as inevitable as it was dangerous. It was dangerous because it makes mankind be "like God, knowing good and evil".'[26] The new epistemology had a transgressive potential that could breach the ultimate of boundaries.

If the new epistemological commitments of the seventeenth century were to give human beings access to previously forbidden divine knowledge, so the trajectory of the Baconian project was to take the new learning far beyond the bounds placed on it by the Puritans. As millenarianism waned in the latter part of the century and gave way to a secularized faith in progress, so the theological framework for addressing the issues was also gradually dismantled. But the repudiation of the explicit theology did not mean the disappearance of religious functions or the loss of religious needs. Rather, as God was first made a function of the new scientific knowledge and then abandoned as unnecessary, so the existential nature of suffering changed, and the effort to eliminate it began to absorb the weight of soteriological expectation. Instead of suffering being an opportunity for receiving God's grace, through which endurance, character, and hope might come, in which one might participate in the sufferings of Christ, it began to be interpreted as brute, unreferential pain whose only value lay in being eradicated. In this new religious project, behind the relief of individual bodily infirmities lay the hope of freedom from the burdens and randomness of finitude and mortality.

So the Baconian project becomes a surrogate form of salvation, its religious significance and doctrinal commitments occluded from many of its proponents because of their self-conscious secularism. It develops, for example, a doctrine of creation, which conceives nature as raw material available for technological manipulation, while its anthropology defines human beings in terms of self-defining freedom above the contingencies of bodily life.

22. Webster, *The Great Instauration*, pp. 105, 329.

23. Ibid., p. 22.

24. Ibid., pp. 517-18.

25. Funkenstein, *Theology and the Scientific Imagination*, pp. 290-9.

26. Ibid., p. 327.

It espouses an eschatological hope, which lies in the dream of escape from finitude, and locates the means of salvation to that end in the application of technical reason and the 'power of modern science'. It has generated its own ethics, in which both utilitarian and Kantian lineages of standard philosophical bioethics share an allegiance to the instrumentalization of the nature and alienation of the self from the body.

Modern technological medicine, in its obsession with the elimination of suffering and its fetishization of health, can therefore be seen as soteriological in nature. But this dimension is most pointed in the case of molecular genomics, not just because of its potentially central role in the medicine of the future, nor because it requires the intensive application of high technology, but because of the conception of knowledge that it embodies: knowledge of construction which, as we have seen, is at once also knowledge of reconstruction and therefore of transformation. 'For the first time in all time,' as Robert Sinsheimer declared after an initial conference about launching a genome-sequencing project, 'a living creature understands its origin and can undertake to design its future.'[27] And at least something of the same goal is implied in James Watson's talk of the need for 'the courage to make less random the sometimes most unfair courses of human evolution'.[28]

We have become familiar with the religious resonances of many of the pronouncements about the potential of the Human Genome Project, from Walter Gilbert's early talk of the Grail,[29] to President Clinton's statement on announcing the completion of the first draft of the human genome: 'Today we are learning the language in which God created life.'[30] But their soteriological nature stems not from the fact that their authors felt compelled to reach for religious language to describe their feelings of awe at what might be and (partly) has been achieved, as that they represent the tip of the iceberg of a much profounder set of allegiances which are often only partly acknowledged, and which it is certainly blasphemous to question. And at this altar many comments which do not use religious language — 'the most important and the most significant project that humankind has ever mounted',[31] comparisons to the invention of the wheel,[32] and so on — are equally pinches of incense.

Because this allegiance to the elimination of suffering and the escape from the toils of finitude through the application of technological reason is a soteriological quest which is never quite acknowledged as such, a large number of questions which could be put to the Human Genome Project are hidden from sight and never receive the attention they deserve. Some of these are questions of priorities. For example, can money spent on this project finally be justified in a world where many are suffering and dying of diseases or other causes which are already much more easily treatable? Who is likely to benefit most in the short, medium and long terms — and how should we ensure equitable distribution of the benefits of the research?

Other questions focus on the idolatry of the technological fix. Should we be committing ourselves to a medicine of heavily technological intervention and cure when other kinds of medical practice might be more appropriate? Does the mentality behind the project not end up marginalizing even those with genetic diseases who might be expected to be among the first to benefit, reducing their needs merely to a cure at all costs?[33] Indeed, given the time span between the discovery of diagnostic techniques and possible clinical therapies (which may in many cases extend to several decades), as well as the daunting sense of the tiers of complexity in functional genomics that are now emerging subsequent to the sequencing of the genome, are we allowed to ask whether it was ever responsible to promote this entire line of research?

Following on from this, there are questions about esteeming technological enterprises above other valuable human undertakings. For example, why is this so much greater a project for human beings to embark on than concerted efforts to address global poverty or seek for reconciliation in situations of conflict? Should we really be so proud to belong to a culture which has prized all of this but has not had the wit or political will to address the threat of global warming?

And there are many other questions in different areas. In relation to the 'yuck factor' and talk of 'playing God', does the earlier discussion about knowledge by construction not suggest that concerns about these have a rather more illustrious pedigree and greater intellectual integrity than dismissing them as merely vacuous emotionalism would suggest? In relation to the only 'therapy' available now in the case of most genetic diseases, namely abortion, should we be happy to endorse James Watson's blithe expectation that 'over the next several decades we shall witness an ever-growing consensus that humans have the right to terminate the lives of genetically unhealthy fetuses'?[34] (One might also ask how our technical capacities influence our moral judgements here.) And

27. Quoted in Noble, *The Religion of Technology*, p. 189.

28. James D. Watson, 'Viewpoint: All for the Good — Why Genetic Engineering Must Soldier On' (1999), in *A Passion for DNA: Genes, Genomes and Society* (Oxford: Oxford University Press, 2000), pp. 227-9 at p. 229.

29. Cf. Walter Gilbert, 'A Vision of the Grail', in Kevles and Hood, *The Code of Codes*, pp. 83-97.

30. *The Times*, 27 June 2000, p. 1.

31. Francis Collins, quoted in Noble, *The Religion of Technology*, p. 191.

32. Mike Dexter, Director of the Wellcome Trust, quoted in *New Scientist*, 1 July 2000, p. 4. Cf. also John Sulston and Georgina Ferry, *The Common Thread: A Story of Science, Politics, Ethics and the Human Genome* (London: Bantam Press, 2002), p. 202.

33. See Alan Stockdale's discussion of cystic fibrosis research: 'Waiting for the Cure: Mapping the Social Relations of Human Gene Therapy Research', in Peter Conrad and Jonathan Gabe (eds.), *Sociological Perspectives on the New Genetics* (Oxford: Blackwell, 1999), pp. 79-96.

34. James D. Watson, 'Ethical Implications of the Human Genome Project' (1994), in *A Passion for DNA*, pp. 169-77 at p. 176.

with regard to suffering, do we not have to agree with Ivan Illich that the technological mentality is removing one of the functions of traditional cultures, namely to 'equip the individual with the means for making pain tolerable, sickness or impairment understandable, and the shadow of death meaningful'?[35]

Conclusion

These are not the only questions which could be put to the Human Genome Project or the broader project of the new genetics, but they give an indication. In putting them, I am not suggesting that the anti-reductivist critics I discussed earlier could not make them; on the contrary, they could — and many do. But they do so in separation from their views on the reductivist nature of modern genetics, whereas I have argued that the questions point to an overarching pattern of thought, only part of which is correctly diagnosed by the critique of reductionism.

This pattern of thought, which for shorthand I have labelled the Baconian project, answers the four criteria I laid down earlier. It gives an explanation of the coming-to-be of the new genetics in terms of the desire to eliminate suffering and address the condition of human disease and death, an explanation which (in the fuller setting I have pointed to) should not be neglected in any understanding of likely future trajectories. Since it shows that reductionism is secondary to this primary motivation, it allows the reductive tendencies of the new genetics to be a contingent part of its identity. But on the other hand, the desire to escape the burdens of finitude does go naturally with an objectifying mentality, which suggests an explanation for the natural affinity genetics has for reductive approaches. And in talking about a quality of motivation that is quasi-religious in nature, it gives a fuller account of the appeal of the new genetics which does not exclude or diminish the significance of socio-political and other factors.

It should not, however, be taken as another totalizing narrative which in one neat theory encapsulates the reality behind all the phenomena. The world is too complex to be hospitable to such accounts. Not all medicine currently practised bears the marks of the Baconian technological medicine that I have criticized: many doctors, patients and scientists have more limited and sober expectations, and have learned to place their ultimate hopes elsewhere. Rather, this is intended to delineate a pattern of thought, a characteristic quality of motivation that has taken up residence in the modern world and which leads us to ignore or misunderstand important questions.

Nor do these questions, some of which I have just mentioned, form part of an effort to demonstrate the wrongness of the Human Genome Project or the new genetics as a whole. They arise because we have invested hopes in a set of aspirations whose quasi-religious nature we dare not avow. It is only when we acknowledge these that we will be able to answer the questions truthfully and freely. And it is only when we are genuinely free to answer that the Human Genome Project might after all be wrong that we will be free to think that it might after all be right.

35. Ivan Illich, *Limits to Medicine: Medical Nemesis — The Expropriation of Health* (London: Marion Boyars, 1976), pp. 127-8. See in general his discussion of cultural iatro-genesis, according to which professionalized medicine leads people no longer to have the will to 'suffer their reality' (pp. 127-54).

132 That Deep Surface: The Human Genome Project and the Death of the Human

Bronislaw Szerszynski

Introduction

In the development and application of new technologies such as agricultural and human biotechnology it is becoming increasingly common for policy-makers to turn to philosophers, theologians and religious leaders to make ethical judgements on specific developments. There seem to be two assumptions underlying this kind of approach. The first assumption is that science and religion can be regarded as complementary activities, whose truth claims cannot directly conflict with each other. According to this widely held view, science is the arbiter over questions of ontology and causality — over what *is,* and how it came to *be* what it is — whereas religion can answer questions of meaning and purpose about the reality that is determined by science. Similarly, whereas technology determines what it is possible to do, and how it might be achieved, religious values and ethical reasoning can determine whether it is permissible or desirable. Put crudely, once science and technology have determined what we *could* do, religion can serve as an ethical resource that can help us determine whether we *should* do it or not. The second, related assumption in this approach is that the key questions that should be asked are ones about specific technological advances, about specific applications of such new technologies, or about specific consequences of their application.

In this chapter I want to suggest that at least *some* of the questions we might want to ask about the Human Genome Project (HGP) are ones that require us to set aside both of these assumptions. I do not want to deny that at certain times it is entirely appropriate for policy-makers to turn to religious and other experts for their judgements about specific proposals. Nevertheless, there is a danger that some more fundamental issues raised by technological development are thereby neglected. I will spend most of the chapter developing an argument against the first assumption mentioned above, suggesting that modern science, conceived as the theoretical and practical mastery of nature, is itself a partly theological project, one with a specific religious construal of the world and of the human place in it. If I am right, approaching human genetics as posing a series of discrete challenges, to be judged one at a time against ethical and religious criteria, risks obscuring a deeper challenge posed by genetic science to the language we use to describe the human — and thus to the human itself.

In questioning both of these assumptions I am seeking to develop a more specific argument that the HGP[1] can be seen as a new and significant phase in a theologico-scientific project, originating in the early modern period, to render existence according to a *mathesis universalis,* a universal formalized reference language. In particular, I suggest that the HGP is an attempt to complete this rendering, through the extension to *humanity* of certain theological moves made in that earlier period in relation to *God.* And just as this rendering of God in embodied and univocal terms rendered him[2] ultimately expendable — as famously captured by Laplace's purported comment to Napoleon that he had no need of that particular hypothesis — so too does the HGP threaten the future of the human person as we understand it.

This might be seen as a rather paradoxical claim: at most, the HGP might be seen as a project to *map* the human being. How could mapping something thereby threaten it? Of course, in relation to many episodes of world history, mapping places and things has indeed been a prelude to their destruction — wilderness areas, for example. Reassuringly, I do not think that the human being is the kind of thing whose mapping lends it to being threatened in *this* way.[3] However, the very features of the human being that make it *less* vulnerable to destruction by mapping in this sense make it *more* vulnerable in another, because of the way that our subjectivity is constitutively shaped by the languages we use to understand it.[4] As Hannah Arendt wrote of theories of behaviourism, which stand in the same tradition of attempts to theoretically reduce the human, the trouble 'is not that they are wrong but that they could become true'.[5] The worry I am focusing on in this chapter, then, is less about the material effects of human genetics, and more about the effects

From Bronislaw Szerszynski, "That Deep Surface: The Human Genome Project and the Death of the Human," in *Brave New World? Theology, Ethics and the Human Genome.* Ed. Celia Deane-Drummond (New York: T. & T. Clark, 2003), 145-63. Reproduced by kind permission of Continuum International Publishing Group.

1. At least as it is interpreted by some of its key commentators and advocates.

2. I have chosen to use the masculine pronoun for God in this chapter not for theological reasons, but in order to be consistent with the usage in the period about which I am writing.

3. Though of course there are many issues of ownership and patenting in human genetics that at least threaten people's possession over themselves and their powers, in the sense that Macpherson described as 'possessive individualism' — see C. B. Macpherson, *The Political Theory of Possessive Individualism: Hobbes to Locke* (Oxford: Clarendon Press, 1962).

4. P. Heelas and A. Lock (eds.), *Indigenous Psychologies: The Anthropology of the Self* (London: Academic Press, 1981).

5. H. Arendt, *The Human Condition* (Chicago: University of Chicago Press, 1998), p. 322.

such technologies might have on our language about human beings and thus on ourselves.[6]

But as well as being counterintuitive, my claim is also a rather apocalyptic one. While it is also possible that the ideas and practices of human genetics may simply provide additional conceptual and explanatory resources to add to the rich panoply of ways that modern humans have of talking about themselves and others,[7] this more positive outcome cannot be assumed. There are real signs of a kind of genetic reductionism starting to invade the way that we talk about human persons, a change that might start to alter fundamentally our conception of the human, to the point at which the connection becomes attenuated to breaking point. It is not necessary to posit an essential 'human nature' in the way that Francis Fukuyama does in his own apocalyptic account of genomics in order to be deeply concerned about what might be happening to our language of human persons.[8]

I will develop my argument by way of a three-part narrative: the death of nature; the death of God; the death of the human. First, in the development of modern science nature was 'killed' in the sense of being known in a new kind of way, one which stripped it of active power and meaning. Second, in the reordering of the concept of knowledge and truth which this involved, divine attributes were de-metaphorized and mapped on to specific aspects of reality as it was coming to be understood by natural philosophers, thus laying the ground for God's eventual dismissal as unnecessary. Third, by situating the HGP in this larger historical narrative I hope to illuminate ways in which genomic science might similarly threaten the existence of the human person, through its reordering of the language of 'depth' in relation to the human, and the reduction of the opacity and open-endedness of human identity to a spatialized genetic coding.[9]

The Death of Nature[10]

According to many accounts of the scientific revolution of the sixteenth and seventeenth centuries, this period was a crucial stage in the separation of science from religion. In terms of institutions and practices, this is indeed the case, with the birth pangs of this separation perhaps most graphically dramatized in the persecution by the Church of Galileo for his public support of the Copernican, heliocentric model of the cosmos.[11] However, as the historian Amos Funkenstein has convincingly argued, the work of Galileo and Descartes, Newton and Leibniz, Hobbes and Vico may in other ways be seen as a high point of *convergence* between science, philosophy and theology.[12] Funkenstein describes the activity of many natural philosophers of the time as a 'secular theology', and this in two senses. First, theirs was a theology practised by the laity rather than by clergymen, and by those without advanced degrees in divinity. Secularization of theology in this sense, its appropriation by laymen, had of course been encouraged by the Reformation. But, second, this was a theology oriented to the 'world' in a way that had not been the case before, a world increasingly seen not as a transient stage for the development of human souls, but as having its own religious value, both as a dwelling place and as a creation whose study can reveal the mind of its creator. As Funkenstein puts it, '[t]he world turned into God's temple, and the layman into its priests'. Theology was increasingly expected to import ideas and forms of reasoning from other disciplines, such as mathematics, and in turn 'God ceased to be the monopoly of theologians'.[13] In a related development,

---

6. In this way I am drawing on the *substantive* approach to the philosophy of science and technology, as contrasted with the *instrumental* approach. Rather than understanding technologies as neutral instruments or means that can be used for the pursuit of different (and morally assessable) ends, the substantive approach sees a specific technology or technology itself as having an essential framing quality that tends to gather the world around it in a particular way. It is in this way that I am approaching the Human Genome Project.

7. C. Taylor, *Sources of the Self: The Making of the Modern Identity* (Cambridge: Cambridge University Press, 1989).

8. F. Fukuyama, *Our Posthuman Future: Consequences of the Biotechnology Revolution* (London: Profile Books, 2002). By being apocalyptic, of course, I am assuming that it is worth being so at this stage in the hope of being proved wrong later.

9. I am focusing here on the fate of the human as an *object* of knowledge in genetic science. There are other theological questions raised by the new role of (some) human beings as *subjects* and wielders of genetic knowledge and technology. Robert Song (Chapter 8 in [*Brave New World?;* also included as article 131 of the present volume]) traces the roots of the activist and ameliorative construal of science and technology that he sees as animating the Human Genome Project back to a set of beliefs and attitudes initially assembled in the seventeenth century. Others, notably T. Peters, *Playing God* (London: Routledge, 1997), take this line of thought further in their construal of the genetic scientist as co-creator with God. An exploration of these and other rather different and non-reductive conceptions of the human in genetic science is outside the scope of this paper. Nevertheless, as John Brooke points out in a personal communication, there is an irony if we become more like God and erase ourselves with the same gesture — or, to use Song's more cautious language, if in the name of humanitarianism we erase the human.

10. My argument in this section is broadly compatible with that made by Carolyn Merchant in her book of the same name. However, while her account prioritizes the shift from organic to mechanical metaphors for nature as the key move in the death of nature, I follow Foucault and Funkenstein in seeing this as merely part of a more general epistemic shift. See C. Merchant, *The Death of Nature: Women, Ecology, and the Scientific Revolution* (San Francisco: Harper and Row, 1980).

11. W. R. Shea, 'Galileo and the Church', in D. C. Lindberg and R. L. Numbers (eds.), *God and Nature: Historical Essays on the Encounter between Christianity and Science* (Berkeley: University of California Press, 1986), pp. 114-35.

12. For a less controversialist account of the scientific revolution than Funkenstein's, but one that nevertheless also argues for a far more complex relationship between science and religion than that of separation and conflict, see J. H. Brooke, *Science and Religion: Some Historical Perspectives* (Cambridge: Cambridge University Press, 1991).

13. A. Funkenstein, *Theology and the Scientific Imagination from the Middle Ages to the Seventeenth Century* (Princeton, NJ: Princeton University Press, 1986), p. 6.

from the fourteenth century onwards, barriers between disciplines had been progressively eroded, not least with the rise of the peripatetic programme transmission as a model competing with the medieval university. Even as new disciplines emerged through this erosion of boundaries, the idea of a unified 'system' of thought and knowledge, conceived as 'a set of interdependent propositions' and based on one method, gained increasing currency, especially from the seventeenth century.

These changes were accompanied by another, related change in the understanding of nature which rendered it available for reinterpretation by modern science. According to the earlier, symbolist mentality of the Middle Ages, objects, plants and animals have been understood as signs, implicated in endless chains of resemblance.[14] As codified by Origen and Augustine, the medieval *Quadriga* gave rules for the interpretation of both scripture and nature, in terms of literal, allegorical, moral and supernatural levels of meaning. Through this method of interpretation, which formalized and to some extent attempted to 'tame' a broader symbolic approach to the natural world,[15] natural objects and not just words were seen as referring, either to other objects and events in nature and history, or to moral and spiritual truths as laid out in scripture.[16]

However, the Protestant Reformation saw a profound transition in Europe, one which included a shift of emphasis from image to word,[17] and from allegorical to literal meaning. As Peter Harrison argues, the search by Protestant reformers for a stable, unambiguous religious authority in the Bible led to an insistence that it should be interpreted literally, withdrawing intelligibility and meaning away from objects themselves and reserving such properties for words alone:

> The sacred rite which had lain at the heart of medieval culture was replaced by a text, symbolic objects gave way to words, ritual practices were eclipsed by propositional beliefs and dogmas. In the course of this process, that unified interpretive endeavour which had given meanings to both natural world and sacred text began to disintegrate. Meaning and intelligibility were ascribed to words and texts, but denied to living things and inanimate objects. The natural world, once the indispensable medium between words and eternal truths, lost its meanings, and became opaque to those hermeneutical procedures which had once elucidated it.[18]

Harrison can be accused of making this shift appear too stark — as if there were no proponents of literal truth in the Middle Ages, and there were no symbolic interpreters of nature in the seventeenth century. Nevertheless, the move away from symbolic interpretation — sometimes hesitant, sometimes robustly asserted — laid nature increasingly open to the radically new modes of ordering offered by the emergent natural sciences. These orderings were based not on similitude and analogy but on the precise comparison of sameness and difference — either through mathematics, an approach that reached its epitome in Galileo, or through taxonomy, for example, in the work of John Ray.

It is important to try to grasp the distinctiveness of this emergent theologico-scientific project of the theoretical mastery of nature. It was the quest for a *mathesis universalis* — an unequivocal, universal, coherent, yet artificial language in which could be formulated the clear and distinct ideas of science.[19] The search for this purified, formalized language played a crucial role in the idea of truth which science assumed, whereby '[w]ord and thing are brought to coincide in the sense that the former is a completely adequate and transparent representation of the latter'.[20] According to Michel Foucault, the Classical *episteme* of the scientific revolution was characterized by the use of this artificial, precise but arbitrary reference language to analyse the world into elementary elements, and at the same time to specify how they combine to form more complex phenomena:

> In the Classical age, to make use of signs is not, as it was in preceding centuries, to attempt to rediscover beneath them the primitive text of a discourse sustained, and retained, forever; it is an attempt to discover the arbitrary language that will authorize the deployment of nature within its space, the final terms of its analysis and the laws of its composition. It is no longer the task of knowledge to dig out the ancient Word from the unknown places where it may be hidden; its job now is to fabricate a language . . . as an instrument of analysis and combination.[21]

The whole Classical *episteme,* for Foucault, ultimately conceives of knowledge in the form of a unified table — a spatialized grid of interdependent but unequivocal propositions. In a complementary account Funkenstein describes modern science as the convergence of four ideals — homogeneity, univocity, mechanization and mathematization.[22] Each of these ideals has an often long history prior to the seventeenth century, but in the episteme of modern science they come together in a distinctive and powerful way. The ideal of homogeneity assumes

14. M. Foucault, *The Order of Things: An Archaeology of the Human Sciences* (London: Tavistock, 1970).

15. K. Thomas, *Man and the Natural World: Changing Attitudes in England 1500-1800* (Harmondsworth: Penguin, 1984).

16. P. Harrison, *The Bible, Protestantism, and the Rise of Natural Science* (Cambridge: Cambridge University Press, 1998), p. 15.

17. E. Duffy, *The Stripping of the Altars: Traditional Religion in England, c. 1400–c. 1580* (New Haven: Yale University Press, 1992), p. 591.

18. Harrison, *The Bible, Protestantism, and the Rise of Natural Science*, p. 120.

19. Funkenstein, *Theology and the Scientific Imagination,* pp. 28-9.

20. T. J. Reiss, *The Discourse of Modernism* (Ithaca, NY: Cornell University Press, 1982), p. 36.

21. Foucault, *The Order of Things,* pp. 62-3.

22. Funkenstein, *Theology and the Scientific Imagination,* pp. 28-42.

simplicity in *things*, that the universe is the same everywhere — the same matter, the same kinds of motion, ultimately the same laws. Univocity requires simplicity in *language* — that terms unambiguously denote their referent in terms of relations of identity and non-identity, rather than through similitude, analogy and metaphor. Mathematization involves not as it had for Plato and Pythagoras that *things* were mathematical, in the sense that nature takes simple, geometric forms, but that scientific *language* should be mathematical in order to perform its analytic and combinatory functions. Finally, mechanization required the expulsion of teleology, final causes and intentions from nature; matter was conceived as passive, its behaviour determined by causal relations and natural laws.[23] Nature in this *episteme* is no longer alive with agency, *telos*, meaning and mystery. Its death in this sense was necessitated by the very project of analysing and mapping it.

The Death of God

However, in this secular theology God was still alive and needed, but needed in new ways — ways which would easily render him just as unnecessary as at this point he was necessary. What was different about the secular theologians' discourse of God? In medieval thought God had characteristically been seen as the ground of language and meaning itself, rather than as an object of language.[24] Similarly, in liturgical understandings of language, God is more than an object of speech; he is an addressee or a speaker, an I or a Thou.[25] But in the secular theology of Descartes, Galileo and Newton, God was made necessary in a different way, by making him perform specific functions within the emergent scientific understanding of the world. While many natural philosophers were concerned to emphasize the transcendence of God from his creation, they did so in ways that actually made him vulnerable to being cut adrift altogether.

This was partly to do with the way that these thinkers brought theology within the systematization of thought mentioned above, and thus subject to the drive towards unambiguous speech that was occurring in science and elsewhere. For, whatever their differences, the progenitors of modern science agreed that what was crucial for the securing of truth about the world was the purification and formalization of language. The advocates of this perspective argued like Hobbes that knowledge depends on 'Perspicuous words . . . purged from ambiguity', rather than 'Metaphors, and senselesse and ambiguous words', relying upon which 'is wandering amongst innumerable absurdities'.[26] Some, such as Francis Bacon and John Wilkins, broadly following the classical distinction of logic and rhetoric, distinguished the precise, artificial, universal language required for scientific work from the rhetoric of common speech, ethics, and poetry. But others such as John Locke wanted all speech to be purified of ambiguity, part of a trend which at this time saw history and law, and even religion and morality, experiencing new fashions for 'plain speech'.[27]

For our secular theologians this desire for univocity involved the refiguring of theological discourse along the same lines, stripped of the analogical and symbolic relations between signs, ideas and things that had been central to the main currents of theological reasoning for centuries. Whereas for Thomas Aquinas all talk of God's attributes — even concerning his very existence — could only be analogical, Descartes, Newton, More and Leibniz aspired for a clarity and distinctness in their ideas about God which paralleled that which they sought in relation to nature. Language about God's attributes — about his very being — had to be stripped of its analogical character and rendered univocal; similarly, talk of the relation between God and his creation had to be clarified and purged of mystery. 'The medieval sense of God's symbolic presence in his creation, and the sense of a universe replete with transcendent meanings and hints, had to recede if not to give way totally to the postulates of univocation and homogeneity in the seventeenth century. God's relation to the world had to be given a concrete physical meaning.'[28]

Thus, rather than God holding meaning in place, meaning came to hold God in place. God's being was made the prisoner of a language that was understood as immanent, transparent, given and univocal. For example, it was necessary for the secular theologians to reject medieval ideas of God cooperating with vital principles immanent within nature. One of the preconditions of their project of the mechanical description of the world according to mathematical laws was that matter had to be seen as wholly passive, containing no vital force or *nisus*. Mechanical philosophers such as Boyle and Newton thus stressed the absolute sovereignty of God and the dependency of matter on him for its continued existence and movement. For Newton, for example, lifeless nature

23. G. B. Deason, 'Reformation Theology and the Mechanistic Conception of Nature', in D. C. Lindberg and R. L. Numbers (eds.), *God and Nature: Historical Essays on the Encounter between Christianity and Science* (Berkeley: University of California Press, 1986), pp. 167-91. For Foucault, mechanization and mathematization were not constant features in the origin of all sciences; what the latter did have in common, nevertheless, was the ideal of generating an ordered system of knowledge based on an artificial reference language, analysis and recombination — see Foucault, *The Order of Things*, p. 57.

24. N. Frye, *The Great Code: The Bible and Literature* (London: Ark, 1983).

25. C. Pickstock, *After Writing: On the Liturgical Consummation of Philosophy* (Oxford: Blackwell, 1998).

26. T. Hobbes, *Leviathan* (London: Dent, 1914), p. 22.

27. B. J. Shapiro, *Probability and Certainty in Seventeenth-Century England: A Study of the Relationships between Natural Science, Religion, History, Law, and Literature* (Princeton, NJ: Princeton University Press, 1983), pp. 242-3.

28. Funkenstein, *Theology and the Scientific Imagination*, p. 116.

was only animated by God's continuing intimate, active but predictable involvement in the world, as manifest in the operation of forces such as gravity.[29]

In different ways, then, God's attributes were stripped of metaphor and allegory and allotted specific functions in the emerging scientific understanding of the world. Ironically, this disambiguation of theological talk was associated sometimes with an emphasis on Divine transcendence, sometimes with a radical immanence; but either way the end result was similar. The de-metaphorization of God's attributes and being directly laid the grounds for his disappearance from Western science. As Funkenstein graphically puts it, '[i]t is clear why a God described in unequivocal terms, or even given physical features and functions, eventually became all the easier to discard . . . all the easier to identify and kill'.[30]

The fusion of science and theology thus ultimately led to a science that refuses to speak of God. Yet if this science is atheological, it is so not in the sense of not having a theology, but in the sense of having a theology without God. Furthermore, the period of 'secular theology' that Funkenstein describes was more than simply a transitional period, a not-yet-complete separation of science from religion. The theological elements in the thought of Descartes and Newton played an important role in the formulation of their scientific concepts. And, more importantly, rather than their talk of God representing merely a temporary resistance to the arrival of an atheological science, it was their very disambiguating of theological language in order to fit it for their project that laid the grounds for the later disappearance of God. This irony will become particularly relevant later when I turn to the possible irony that the Human Genome Project might destroy the human by mapping it. One might say that God was killed on the scientists' table — by his incorporation into the *mathetic* project of separating signs into words and things, rendering language arbitrary and unequivocal, banishing allegory and symbol, and construing knowledge as a spatialized grid of statements.[31]

The Death of the Human

Could the human ever suffer its own obsolescence in a similar way? The final stage of my narrative is indeed to ask this question, to wonder whether the human might suffer a parallel fate to that suffered by God. But what might it *mean* for the human to die as God has in mainstream Western culture? In my use of the term 'human' here I am not referring to the biological human species,[32] but to a specific, contingent, historically situated phenomenon, one that came into being at a particular historical moment and could perhaps as accidentally depart. Foucault uses 'man' in this kind of way when, inspired by Nietzsche, he suggests that man, who has killed God, might himself be in the process of being erased — 'that man is in the process of perishing as the being of language continues to shine ever brighter upon our horizon'.[33] However, although Foucault is here using 'man' in a formally similar sense, as a historically specific formation rather than a biological species, there are also significant differences in our prophecies — and not just in terms of Foucault's apparent lack of alarm at the prospect he describes.

Foucault is using 'man' to refer to the object studied in and constituted by the human sciences, such as sociology, psychology and linguistics. 'Man' in this sense is that being which lives through representations — of itself, of the world, and of its actions — and was only constituted as a potential object of knowledge with the rise of the human sciences in the nineteenth century. In fact, Foucault's 'man' only appears when the *mathetic* project stumbles. In the Classical *episteme* of the seventeenth and eighteenth centuries that we were exploring above, in which knowledge was understood as transparent and objective, 'man' as a subject which represents and posits knowledge had to remain invisible, outside the table of knowledge which he drew. 'The personage for whom the representation exists . . . is never to be found in the table himself.'[34] Within this episteme, the human could only appear as a material object but not as a knowing, representing subject.

In the nineteenth century this human-as-subject *was* incorporated into scientific knowledge. However, this incorporation, rather than reducing and destroying the human, in many ways has added to and enhanced the vocabularies of the 'self' available to modern subjects.[35] What had happened to science — to the theologico-scientific project of the theoretical mastery of nature — that allowed the human-as-subject to survive its incorporation in a way that God-as-subject had not? I want to suggest that a precondition for this safe incorporation was not just the rise of the specifically human sciences, but also a

29. Deason, 'Reformation Theology and the Mechanistic Conception of Nature'. Other accounts of Newton's work put greater stress on the diversity in his treatment of gravity — see, for example, E. McMullin, *Newton on Matter and Activity* (Notre Dame: University of Notre Dame Press, 1978), and B. J. T. Dobbs, *The Janus Face of Genius: The Role of Alchemy in Newton's Thought* (Cambridge: Cambridge University Press, 1992). Nevertheless, the particular version I am stressing here is the one which is closest to the *mathetic* project.

30. Funkenstein, *Theology and the Scientific Imagination,* p. 116.

31. Dobbs poignantly describes the irony of this outcome in respect of Isaac Newton, whom she presents as attempting to prove divine activity in nature, in order to stem the tides of mechanism and atheism. Far from the rise of atheological science representing Newton's triumph, Dobbs makes us see it as Newton's failure — see B. J. T. Dobbs, 'Newton as Final Cause and First Mover', in M. J. Osler (ed.), *Rethinking the Scientific Revolution* (Cambridge: Cambridge University Press, 2000), pp. 25-39. The deeper irony, of course, lies not in the dominant misrepresentation of Newton as a scientist who was only accidentally a theologian, but in the fact that Newton's secular theology in the long run had the opposite effect to that which he had hoped.

32. Although the future of the human in this sense too might be in question — see Fukuyama, *Our Posthuman Future.*

33. Foucault, *The Order of Things,* p. 386.

34. Ibid., p. 308.

35. Taylor, *Sources of the Self.*

transformation of the natural sciences, and of the relationship between the sciences — a precondition which might be threatened by the development of genomics.

As Foucault recounts, many sciences underwent a transformation in the nineteenth century, departing from the methods of analysis and recombination that had characterized the *mathetic* project of the seventeenth and eighteenth centuries. Rather than areas of knowledge being organized in terms of a horizontal table of similarities and differences, many of them thus started to be reorganized according to a new spatial metaphor — one of hidden unities lying underneath a surface of differences.[36] Take, for example, the shift from Linnaeus's natural history to Cuvier's biology. Linnaeus approached the study of living beings by analysing and measuring their visible similarities and differences — in an explicit rejection of the medieval search for analogies and similitudes, he wrote that the natural historian 'distinguishes the parts of natural bodies with his eyes, describes them appropriately according to their number, form, position, and proportion'.[37] Cuvier, by contrast, looked at the organs of the body in a very different way, prioritizing function over physical arrangement in what amounts to a return to Aristotelian ways of thinking about organisms. As Foucault puts it, 'from Cuvier onward, function . . . is to serve as a constant middle term and to make it possible to relate together totalities of elements without the slightest visible identity'.[38] Thus beneath the surface of the differences between species and species, and between organisms and their environment, lie the great unities of function — respiration, digestion, sensation and so on — not reducible to constituent material elements or visible to the senses, but nevertheless in many ways more ontologically fundamental.

In biology as elsewhere thus arose a language of surfaces and depths in a shift which amounted to the abandonment of the narrowly referential understanding of language that had dominated the last two centuries. Instead, there was a growing recognition of the enigmatic profusion of language as an evolving and complex human creation, and a return of exegesis and interpretation — the analogies binding objects together, the forces operating under the surface, were not visible to the eye but had to be discerned. Similarly, as the human sciences emerged they adopted similar metaphors of surfaces and depths. This was true of economics and sociology, but also psychology and wider culture, which saw the articulation of the psyche, 'a psychological space . . . between the body and its organs and the person and his or her conduct' that added a new language of 'depth' to our understanding of the human person.[39] This articulation was noticeable in the rise of 'literature', a use of language oriented to its own sheer power of disclosure and expression in relation to this psychological space, but also in that of the human sciences, which sought to know in a more systematic way the human being as a representing and knowing subject. It was these depths that at once reformulated the concept of the human, and gave it a safe place in which to dwell within the realm of positive knowledge. The non-reductive spatial metaphor of surface and depth, and the giving way of the idea of a unified system of thought to a more decentred system of ordering within and across disciplines, made space for the human as subject in a way that was not possible before.

Unlike Foucault I am less interested in 'man' as an object of various forms of knowledge that emerged in the nineteenth century than I am in the way that these new knowledges became extra 'sources of the self' — new resources for the way that human persons can talk about themselves and each other.[40] The surface-depth metaphor and the lack of unified tabular ordering across disciplines meant that social scientific and psychological knowledge did not successfully locate and pin down the human in the way that had happened to God. But now we have genomic science, which seeks to unravel the code that makes us human, and that makes us who we uniquely are, and to do so in a way that signals a robust return to *mathesis* — to the visible and measurable, to the method of analysis and recombination and to the aspiration to unify the sciences. The dominance of molecular biology, with its strongly reductionistic aspirations, threatens a reordering of the sciences, as human behaviour is seen as reducible to biology, and biology to physics and chemistry.[41]

In a genetic science dominated by molecular biology, the surface of the DNA molecule and its sequences now becomes the real, a 'deep surface' which can be mapped and measured. The ambiguities of human action and identity become by contrast a 'superficial depth', a vague and disordered space of forces and conations which can only be given determinate meaning by being mapped and flattened on to that deep surface. DNA has become the 'Book of Man'[42] in terms of which human behaviour, predispositions and competences should be interpreted. Rather as natural objects were interpreted in the Middle Ages as signs that allegorically or symbolically refer to spiritual truths laid out in the Bible, human behaviour is now increasingly interpreted in terms of the meanings inscribed in the sacred text of the human genome. Forms of

36. Foucault, *The Order of Things*, p. 251.

37. Ibid., p. 161.

38. Ibid., p. 265.

39. C. Novas and N. Rose, 'Genetic Risk and the Birth of the Somatic Individual', *Economy and Society* 29.4 (2000), pp. 485-513, p. 508.

40. Taylor, *Sources of the Self*; A. Giddens, *The Consequences of Modernity* (Cambridge: Polity Press, 1990).

41. P. R. Sloan, 'Introductory Essay: Completing the Tree of Descartes', in P. R. Sloan (ed.), *Controlling Our Destinies: Historical, Philosophical, Ethical and Theological Perspectives on the Human Genome Project* (Notre Dame: University of Notre Dame Press, 2000), pp. 1-28.

42. D. Nelkin and M. S. Lindee, *The DNA Mystique: The Gene as a Cultural Icon* (New York: W. H. Freeman, 1995), pp. 52-3; W. Bodmer and R. McKie, *The Book of Man: The Quest to Discover Our Genetic Heritage* (London: Abacus, 1994).

human action such as criminal behaviour, promiscuousness or alcoholism, for example, are interpreted as the working out of various genetic predispositions,[43] as 'natural signs' of deeper, molecular-biological arrangements.[44]

For two centuries the human person has had a place to dwell in knowledge. The human has inhabited the depths — spaces ordered not by a horizontal grid of similarities and differences but by a contrast between surface differences and deep unities, not by the visible but by the invisible, not by identity and nonidentity but by analogy and function. The human has also been able to slip through the gaps *between* disciplines, to avoid capture and redundancy by virtue of the impossibility of a unified *mathetic* method and language for the sciences. In the new genomic future, with a colonization of these depths by the *mathetic* grid and a new spatial metaphor of deep surface, and a renewed attempt to reductionistically unify the sciences, the human's ability to escape the fate of God in Western knowledge — our ability to retain a fully humanistic language of the human person — seems less certain.

I have suggested above that the HGP should be engaged with as a species of what Funkenstein calls 'secular theology', and thus that theological engagement should not just be with its technical and social ramifications, but with its *own* buried or not-so-buried theology.[45] I argued that the notion of the genetic code represents an attempt to complete a *mathesis* of the human — an ordered system of knowledge which attempts to analyse its subject matter into basic elements and to identify the logic and mechanism of their combination — by attempting to materialize the human essence on to the chromosomes in a way that parallels the embodiment of God in the seventeenth century. By trying to reduce the human to a *mathesis* the HGP can only accept features of the human that are describable in an unequivocal reference language referring to a self-identical referent. By giving the human essence a location, by stretching it out on the chromosomes, by mapping and plotting it, it may be all the more easy to destroy it.

43. R. C. Lewontin, *The Doctrine of DNA: Biology as Ideology* (Harmondsworth: Penguin, 1993).

44. Novas and Rose, 'Genetic Risk and the Birth of the Somatic Individual', remind us that 'one should not mistake the spontaneous philosophy of the scientist for the operative epistemology or ontology of scientific activity' (p. 508), and argue that the notion of the genetic code as a deep inner truth is only to be found in popular science writings, and is not characteristic of the practice of genetic science. They suggest that genetic practices such as screening and counselling *do* transform the self, but in a way in which genetic, somatized forms of personhood are hybridized with constructions of the self as autonomous, prudent and responsible, and are also embedded in networks of family members, experts and others. While their points are well made, and have helped the argument in the present chapter, nevertheless I think they underestimate the dangers posed by reductionistic genetic discourses of the human.

45. In the chapter I have specifically focused on worries I have about the HGP; however, theological engagements of the kind I am advocating need not be solely negative.

133 Desperately Seeking Perfection: Christian Discipleship and Medical Genetics

Joel Shuman

"Be perfect, therefore, as your heavenly Father is perfect."

Matthew 5:48

The great question . . . one that we have dealt with mainly by indifference, is the question of what people are for.

Wendell Berry, *What Are People For?*

Human beings must become what they copy.

St. Gregory of Nyssa, *On the Lord's Prayer*

Beloved, we are God's children now; what we will be has not yet been revealed. What we do know is this: when he is revealed, we will be like him, for we shall see him as he is.

1 John 3:2, 3

The "genetic revolution" has become, for better or worse, an apparently permanent fixture on the medical, cultural and moral landscape of our world, a development that has led to a decidedly mixed popular response. On the one hand, ours is a culture that has become quite enamored with the possibilities afforded by biotechnologies such as these; we cling stubbornly to the hope that, given sufficient time and resources, various technological advances may be able to forestall *ad infinitum* our eventual demise. On the other hand, however, our acquaintance with apocalyptic science fiction literature like Huxley's *Brave New World*, along with our memories of the horrors produced by the eugenics movements of earlier this century, are sufficient to give us some pause before we rush headlong to embrace the new genetics.

These conflicting sentiments have led to a widespread call for a public conversation about the "ethical issues" pertaining to that cluster of disciplines I conveniently refer to here as "medical genetics." Christian theologians have been among those who have been called upon to participate in that conversation and have responded with

From Joel Shuman, "Desperately Seeking Perfection: Christian Discipleship and Medical Genetics," *Christian Bioethics* 5.2 (Aug. 1999): 139-53. Used by permission.

great enthusiasm. The question with which Christians have been faced is not whether, but how, to enter into existing debates about whether or how these technologies are to be employed.

A good deal of Christian moral discourse about appropriate or inappropriate uses of biotechnologies such as those pertaining to medical genetics proceeds (and this for a variety of reasons) from the presumption that there exists at least a minimal "common morality," certain commitments (or at least sentiments) that are shared by all rational persons of goodwill. Typically these accounts are based in some supposedly perspicuous account of human nature or of creatures and creator and their respective appropriate roles. James Gustafson, for example, correctly noted as early as 1978 that although

> persons with theological training are writing a great deal about technology and the life sciences. . . . Whether theology is thereby in interaction with these areas, however, is less clear. For some writers the theological authorization for the principles and procedures they use is explicit. . . . For others, writing as "ethicists," the relation of their moral discourse to any specific theological principles, or even to a definable religious outlook is opaque (1978, p. 386).

The problem with arguments such as those to which Gustafson alludes, however, is that in their quest for relevance, they frequently obscure rather than illuminate the particular substantive moral commitments of Christianity. By failing to ask what Christianity might have to say in its own language about the morality of various sorts of medical genetics, they become participants in a moral project that is in many respects fundamentally unintelligible.[1]

The answer to the question of what, if anything, Christian theology *as theology* might contribute to ethical debates about appropriate uses of medical genetics is a complex one, which I believe can be best characterized by an explication of the common (or more properly the *analogous*) aspirations of the two. Both Christianity and medical genetics — or more accurately, the utopian project of modernity driving much of the work in medical genetics — have as their goal the *perfection* of the human being. Both Christianity and the world view underwriting research and practice in medical genetics assert that the present disposition of the human body is on a fundamental level more often than not other than it ought to be. Both aspire to transform the present state of the body, through one version or another of what Paul refers to in Philippians 3 as *epiktasis,* a kind of "straining ahead" toward a future state in which present imperfections will no longer exist.[2] Given these analogous concerns, it would seem that one of the primary *moral* contributions that Christianity can make to debates about medical genetics is to ask whether and to what extent the Christian vision of embodied human perfection is compatible with the vision of perfection offered by the sciences pertaining to medical genetics.

That Christianity is in any clear way concerned with the pursuit of human perfection — particularly with the perfection of the human *body* — is probably not immediately evident to most contemporary Christians. Our failure in this regard is largely related to the fact that the wider culture in which we find ourselves is so conducive to the promulgation of a version of gnosticism.[3] The contemporary United States is in this sense a culture of paradox: there is on the one hand in our culture a prevailing popular scientific positivism that gives rise to a widespread skepticism concerning the most substantive claims of Christianity and other religions making strong historical claims. Yet this skepticism has not led to the abandonment of religious belief, as some have predicted, but to its multiplication. Contemporary Christians are especially susceptible to this: as inheritors of the "radical monotheism" of liberal Protestantism, we find ourselves increasingly unable to think of Christianity except as a variety among others of a private, inward "spirituality" that has at best an oblique relationship to our day-to-day lives. In this sense we bear an uncanny resemblance to the ancient gnostics, who understood life in the body to be insignificant, if not fundamentally illusory, and who believed salvation to be primarily a matter of possessing certain esoteric information that enabled the "manipulation of words and ideas in order to find a safe path through the cosmic maze" (Williams, 1998, p. 24). Yet contrary to how we have been conditioned by the wider culture to think about it, Christianity is not concerned with the salvation of our immaterial, immortal souls without regard for our material, temporal bodies. As Irenaeus of Lyons remarked in his second century anti-gnostic tract *Adversus Haeresis,* "the things which are proper to righteousness are brought to completion in the body" (Williams, 1998, p. 25). Indeed, he says elsewhere in the same tract, the "fruit of the work of the Spirit is the *salvation of the flesh*" (Donovan, 1997, p. 141).[4] Thus any properly Christian account of human perfection must be an account of human perfection *embodied.* This is among the fundamental implications of the doctrine of the incarnation, that in becoming a perfect body of flesh, God has indicated to the world the desirability of redeeming and perfecting our bodies of flesh; moral perfection is irreducibly linked eschatologically to the perfection of the body. This assertion brings us once again to the question of whether and to what extent the Christian vision of bodily perfection is compatible with that vision of perfection provided by the utopian project of moder-

1. So suggests Alasdair MacIntyre in the closing pages of *After Virtue.* There, MacIntyre notes that many traditional-bearing communities with strong, particular accounts of the human good are "constantly in danger of being eroded, and this in search of . . . a chimera" (1984, p. 252).

2. See Williams, 1998, p. 52.

3. For an especially compelling account of this development, see Bloom, 1992.

4. From *Adversus Haereses* V.12.4, quoted in Donovan, 1997; emphasis added.

nity that seems to drive so much contemporary work in medical genetics.[5]

Establishing and characterizing the modern vision of human perfection is by no means a simple task.[6] For the purposes of this essay, I shall refer to modernity as that *ethos* — that way of seeing and speaking about and living in the world — that characterizes life in contemporary, technocentric societies such as our own. According to one quite convincing account, this *ethos* has its origins in fourteenth-century nominalist philosophy and the subsequent emergence of modern scientific thought during the Renaissance. With the rise of nominalism came a fundamentally new understanding of the proper place of women and men in the created order. The classical Christian understanding of human *dominium* as "the rational mastery of the passions and . . . the basis for one's legitimate control and possession of external objects" was abandoned and subsequently "redefined as power, property, active right, and absolute sovereignty" (Milbank, 1990, p. 12).

The redefinition of human *dominium* as the exercise of will and control of the created order creates a space for the emergence of the secular realm, the domain of the essentially private, isolated individual whose nearly unrestricted exercise of power is legitimated on both sociopolitical and theological grounds:

> *Dominium,* as power, could only become the human essence, because it was seen as reflecting the divine essence, a radical divine simplicity without real or formal differentiation, in which, most commonly, a proposing 'will' is taken to stand for the substantial identity of will, essence and understanding. . . . The later middle ages retrieved in a new and more drastic guise the antique connection between monotheism and monarchic unity. . . . In the thought of the nominalists, following Duns Scotus, the Trinity loses its significance as a prime locus for discussing will and understanding in God and the relationship of God to the world. No longer is the world participatorily enfolded within the expressive divine *logos,* but instead a bare divinity starkly confronts the other distinct unities which he has ordained (Milbank, 1990, p. 14).

In the nominalist understanding, power — understood as the capacity to manipulate and control everything created comes to be regarded as the defining human attribute. This understanding finds its practical scientific expression first of all in the work of the alchemists and magicians of the early Renaissance, and then, more significantly, in the work of the earliest modern philosophers, especially Sir Francis Bacon (Rossi, 1968, pp. 1-35).[7] Bacon took from the nominalists the idea that the scientist was "the servant of nature assisting its operations and, by stealth and cunning, forcing it to yield to man's domination" (Rossi, 1968, p. 21). This ideal is most clearly expressed in Bacon's *Novum Organum,* in which he argues that science would make possible "the 'dominion of man,' the *regnum hominis,* over all things, so that the wants of Man's life might be satisfied, his pleasure multiplied, and his power increased. The dominion of Man over things, Bacon urged, is the highest and indeed the sole end of science" (Galdston, 1981, p. 32).

Bacon held that the new approach to knowledge he advocated required the abandonment of traditional modes of reason, which he maintained were fundamentally flawed.[8] At the center of this shift in thinking lay Bacon's insistence that the reasoning of earlier thinkers was wrongheaded because they operated from the premise — which he attributed largely to theology and dismissed as "superstition" — that women and men had a properly fixed place *within* the order of creation and that there were certain predetermined ends toward which their lives and their knowledges ought to be directed (*Novum Organum* 1.54 in Creighton, 1900, p. 328).

Modernity's abandonment of such traditional modes of reason, useful as it was for the advancement of the sciences, had far-reaching long-term sociopolitical consequences. Chief among these was the fundamental alienation of what could be regarded as "real" human knowledge from substantive moral discourse. After Bacon, the fundamental moral question of antiquity and the Middle Ages, "What are people for?" (Berry, 1990, p. 125), could no longer be asked; for insofar as the modern world had become one in which true knowledge could be attained only scientifically, moral precepts had been reduced to the secondary status of values, which in the end came to be regarded merely as subjective preferences. At the same time the physical world — a world that included a human body now largely divorced from human agency — was being described by science in increasingly mechanistic terms, morality was being described in language that was increasingly individual and subjective; witness the moral philosophy of Immanuel Kant. Alasdair MacIntyre offers an excellent summary description of the situation at the time of Kant:

5. I am of course well aware that there are strands of the historical Christian tradition that do not share my Wesleyan sensibilities that are quite wary of any talk about perfection *except* as an altogether future eschatalogical occurrence. The reasons for my disagreements with those strands of the tradition will hopefully become evident below.

6. My use of the term "modern" in this context is chastened by Jeff Stout's warning in a recent article in the *Journal of Religious Ethics,* where he reminds readers of the dangers of oversimplifying a complex phenomenon like 'modernity.' In spite of Stout's warnings, however, I believe it is possible to identify certain social, cultural and political trajectories as modern and to juxtapose those to the account of historical, orthodox Christianity I am trying to explicate here.

7. For an especially strong account of the ways Bacon's works are displayed in contemporary medicine, see McKenny, 1997.

8. In *Novum Organum* 1.21-65, Bacon called these traditional modes of thought "idols" (implying their falseness), and said they were four in number: the "idols of the tribe," the "idols of the den," the "idols of the marketplace," and the "idols of the theater" (Creighton, 1900, pp. 317-328).

> The explanation of action is increasingly held to be a matter of laying bare the physiological and physical mechanisms which underlie action; and, when Kant recognizes that there is a deep incompatibility between any account of action which recognizes the role of moral imperatives in governing action and any such mechanical type of explanation, he is compelled to the conclusion that actions obeying and embodying moral imperatives must be from the standpoint of science inexplicable and unintelligible. After Kant the question of the relationship between such notions as those of intention, purpose, reason for action and the like on the one hand and concepts which specify the notion of mechanical explanation on the other becomes part of the permanent repertoire of philosophy (1984, p. 82).

In this latter world, in which human understanding of physical objects is governed by mechanical explanation, one can no longer speak intelligibly about what it might mean for someone to be a "good" person. Gone from moral discourse is any notion of women and men as what MacIntyre refers to as "functional concepts, in which 'man' stands to 'good man' as 'watch' stands to 'good watch.'" This disconnection stands in direct contrast to much moral discourse prior to modernity, in which "the concept of man [was] understood as having an essential nature and an essential purpose or function" (MacIntyre, 1984, p. 58).

> Within that teleological scheme there is a fundamental contrast between man-as-he-happens-to-be and man-as-he-could-be-if-he-realized-his-essential-nature. Ethics is the science which is to enable men to move from the former state to the latter. Ethics therefore in this view presupposes some account of potentiality and act, some account of the essence of man as a rational animal and above all some account of the human *telos* (MacIntyre, 1984, p. 52).

Yet it is the very notion that humans have a *telos* that the instrumental reason of modernity not only calls into question, but dismisses as superstition. Thus at the heart of the modern project is the unassailable belief that the proper goal of human life and therefore the proper application of human knowledge is the maximization of human freedom through an ever-increasing attainment of control over the effects of various kinds of freedom-robbing contingency. Consequently, says Hannah Arendt, in spite of the fact that the "earth is the very quintessence of the human condition. . . . For some time now a great many scientific endeavors have been directed toward making life also 'artificial,' toward cutting the last tie through which even man belongs among the children of nature" (Arendt, 1998, p. 2).[9] It is in this striving to escape the bonds of contingency that human perfection in modernity finally seems to exist.

If the assertion is true that at the center of the modern project rests an enthusiastic affirmation of the limitless capacity of the human agent to escape or to avoid contingency, then it at least suggests the possibility that the account of human perfection offered by the modern project is not an account of human perfection at all; for perfection in modernity seems to have been replaced by the notion of human *progress.* According to most modern, "scientific" accounts of the human situation, constituted as they are by the absolute rejection of teleology and the closely related view that human reason is properly autonomous and instrumental, human life is on the one hand almost *absolutely* contingent in nature. Consequently any attempt to alter the circumstances of human life will be characterized by paradox; for if human life is, apart from the autonomous exercise of the individual will, fundamentally contingent, then that project which has as its goal the *elimination* of contingency by willful human manipulation of the natural world can never really offer an account of precisely how much freedom from contingency might finally constitute human perfection. Hence an endless striving toward progress, which Christopher Lasch argues is modernity's "true and only heaven," becomes the one universally accepted goal of human existence and its one remaining hedge against human despair (Lasch, 1991, pp. 40-81).[10]

It is thus ironic that the flight from enslavement to circumstance, modernity's one nearly universally accepted hedge against despair, becomes itself an homogenizing and even enslaving modality of power. Václav Havel saw this some time ago when he claimed that:

> Technology — that child of modern science, which in turn is a child of modern metaphysics — is out of humanity's control, has ceased to serve us, has enslaved us and compelled us to participate in the preparation of our own destruction. And humanity can find no way out. . . . We look on helplessly as that coldly functioning machine we have created inevitably engulfs us, tearing us away from our natural affiliations . . . just as it removes us from the experience of 'being' and casts us into the world of 'existences' (Havel, 1987, p. 114).

Arendt's *The Human Condition* is a helpful resource for understanding this so-called enslavement. She argues there that in the modern world, many of those artifacts of technology produced in the name of progress "immediately assume the character of a condition of human existence" (1998, p. 9).[11] Such artifacts are thus assumed to be normal and even "natural" aspects of a way of life that, having been "deprived of those permanent measures that precede and outlast the fabrication process and form an authentic and reliable absolute with respect to the fabri-

9. Writing in 1998, Arendt counted among those efforts to make human life 'artificial' attempts to technologically alter the characteristics of human offspring.

10. Of particular relevance here is Lasch's comparison of the modern account of history to the Christian account which it supplanted. See also Arendt, 1998, pp. 105, 295.

11. Elsewhere Arendt says of these artifacts that "as we use them, we become used and accustomed" to them (1998, p. 94).

cating activity," cannot know when to say "enough!" to an infinite policing of life and of the body by a world that assumes the normativity and the unlimited goodness of technological development (Arendt, 1998, p. 307).

The vast financial and intellectual resources currently being expended on genetic research, together with what is in balance an overwhelmingly favorable depiction of that work by the popular mass media, suggests that medical genetics is on the verge of becoming a primary locus for such thinking.[12] Yet what is typically overlooked in the ethical discourse surrounding medical genetics (or at best simply mentioned in passing) is the fact that the very *ethos* that produces these knowledges and technologies, which afford so profound a capacity to manipulate the circumstances of human life, also renders problematic, if not impossible, any constraints on their application. Consequently we are at once reaffirmed in the desire to live lives free from the effects of all sorts of unhappy contingencies with virtually no consideration to the source, propriety, or appropriate limitations of those desires. It remains to be seen whether the enthusiasm of those who advocate the widespread implementation of these technologies will be vindicated from a strictly technical standpoint; what is relatively more certain is that such an implementation is from a theological perspective problematic.

The difference a theological account of human perfection might make for all this begins with the Christian claim to have at least a provisional understanding of the proper ends of human life. The possession of this understanding offers a way to begin delineating what we may or may not do to escape those contingencies we regard as unhappy. It is by no means the case that Christianity requires its adherents to remain passive in the face of suffering or to regard all suffering as inevitable; nor is it correct to say that a medicine shaped by the Christian tradition must always reject technically sophisticated therapies. Two well-established strands of the Christian tradition speak to this point: first, the Christian tradition reminds us that humans are charged with the responsible stewardship of creation, called to be workers who are to strain forward in a variety of ways to improve the circumstances of our lives. And second, we understand that the final *telos* of our lives, one toward which we are called to work, is a kingdom characterized by the absence of suffering, pain and death.

Yet these two strands of the tradition are relativized by a third strand that calls for us to wait patiently for the redemption of our bodies and to do the work of improving our lives only in ways that allow us to remain in proper relationship to God, to one another, and to the rest of the creation. The perfection we are called to seek, in other words, must be *theologically determined*. This determination begins and ends with the understanding that the full and final meaning of human history, and indeed the history of all creation, is found in and determined by the cross and resurrection of Jesus of Nazareth, and that only through participation by baptism into that event can human perfection rightly be pursued.[13] Eschatology in this sense rules and norms *all* Christian accounts of progress and perfection; for human perfection *in this age* cannot be known apart from the cross and resurrection of Christ. Hence Paul explains in his letter to the Philippians that those forms of perfection he considered desirable prior to his baptism he now regards "as loss because of the surpassing value of knowing Christ Jesus." Discipleship is the means by which the body's perfection is attained, and this discipleship is shaped by Christ's own life, by:

> the power of his resurrection and the sharing of his sufferings by becoming like him in his death, if somehow I may attain the resurrection from the dead.
>
> Not that I have already obtained this or have already reached the goal; but I press on to make it my own because Christ Jesus has made me his own. Beloved, I do not consider that I have made it my own; but this one thing I do: forgetting what lies behind and straining forward to what lies ahead, I press on toward the goal for the prize of the heavenly call of God in Christ Jesus (Philippians 3:10-14, NRSV).

At the center of Paul's thinking about perfection in this passage is a conviction central to all Christian moral reflection, and especially to reflection having to do with the human body: those who are baptized into Christ can no longer claim their bodies as their own; for being baptized into Christ means being buried with him in that baptism and rising into life as a member of the new creation that is his body, the Church. Membership in Christ's body and the perfection to which its members are called to aspire is constituted by three tightly interwoven moral commitments that are particularly relevant for determining whether and to what extent Christians should participate in the projects of medical genetics.

First, life in the Christian body is to be characterized by a fundamental interdependence of the body's members and an irreducible respect for the differences among them. This interdependence seeks neither to destroy the other by colonizing normalization nor to isolate it by mere tolerance; for difference in the Christian body is difference established by God for the sake of the body. In being made members of the body of Christ, Christians understand themselves to have been made part of a body in which there are

> varieties of gifts, but the same Spirit; and there are varieties of services, but the same Lord; and there are vari-

12. Gerald McKenny shows quite convincingly that the kinds of distinctions commonly made in conversations about medical genetics, such as those between therapy and enhancement, are on their own grounds problematic (McKenny, 1997, pp. 32-37).

13. On this point John Howard Yoder offers the following summary observation: "The relationship between the obedience of God's people and the triumph of God's cause is not a relationship of cause and effect but one of cross and resurrection" (Yoder, 1972, p. 238).

> eties of activities, but it is the same God who activates them in everyone. To each is given the manifestation of the Spirit for the common good. . . . All these are activated by one and the same Spirit, who allots to each one individually just as the Spirit chooses (1 Corinthians 12:4-11, NRSV).

The work of the Orthodox theologian John Zizioulas offers Protestants a helpful perspective on these matters. He suggests that the Christian body's constitution of unity-from-difference is rooted first of all in the fact of the fundamental diversity of the triune godhead of which the body's head (Christ) is the second person. Hence, because "God is not first one and then two and then three, but simultaneously One and Three," then, "otherness is not a threat to unity, but *a sine qua non* condition of it." Without difference, there can be no Christian body (Zizioulas, 1994, p. 12).[14]

In the face of a rush to name and create a "normal" humanity based on a particular, uniform genotype, Christians must remind themselves continually that their body is called not simply to tolerate nor even to appreciate difference, but (in this age at least) to be *comprised* by difference. "Indeed," says Paul, in an admonition that seems to speak directly to the homogenizing efficiency of the contemporary culture, "the body does not just consist of one member but of many. If the foot would say, 'Because I am not a hand, I do not belong to the body,' that would not make it any less a part of the body. If all were a single member, where would the body be?" (1 Corinthians 12:14-15, 19, NRSV).

A second moral commitment pertaining to life in the Christian body is the commitment to be present as servants to weakness and suffering within and beyond the body. The community addressed by Paul as the body of Christ is theologically continuous with the community called into existence by Jesus of Nazareth, a community shaped by the imitation of Jesus himself, who washed the feet of his disciples and exhorted them to follow him in the way of suffering. Which is to suggest that Jesus' entire life and especially his passion is for Christians morally normative, not simply because we are to imitate Jesus, but because, as Paul reminded the Philippians in the text cited above, we have been made part of a body whose perfection is achieved by way of sharing in the fellowship of his suffering.

This is not to suggest that suffering is in itself a good thing or that Christians should do nothing to avoid or to remedy suffering among the members of the body. Rather, it is to say that for those baptized into Christ, suffering is transformed along with the rest of our existence, and now carries with it the possibility of redemption for the entire body (Williams, 1998, p. 57). This point offers at least the beginnings of a way to make adjudications about using technologies like medical genetics; for among the basic assumptions surrounding these technologies seems to be that they have the capacity to eliminate suffering by eliminating those who suffer, since, after all, such persons would be better off having never been born, an assumption that is theologically, and hence morally, problematic.[15]

Which leads finally to the third characteristic of life in the Christian body, which is that it is a life which understands a particular, irreducible authority to belong to its weakest and most dependent members. This commitment is a call to understand that the perfection of the Christian body can be reached only as the body engages and embraces the weaknesses of its members. Again, we can turn to Paul for an explication of this point. He reminds his readers in Corinth that:

> the members of the body that seem weaker are indispensable, and those members of the body that we think less honorable we clothe with greater honor, and our less respectable members are treated with more respect; whereas our more respectable members do not need this. But God has so arranged the body, giving greater honor to the inferior member, that there may be no dissension within the body, but that the members may have the same care for one another. If one member suffers, all suffer together with it; if one member is honored, all rejoice together with it (1 Corinthians 12:22-25, NRSV).

And this point perhaps becomes the crux for Christian reflection on these matters: the perfection of the body toward which Christians are to strain, because it is shaped finally by the cross and resurrection of Christ, is a perfection that requires the joyful, expectant embrace of certain of our weaknesses and imperfections. Christian perfection is thus by the standards of contemporary medical science altogether *imperfect*. By making this qualification I am at once arguing for a profound Christian skepticism about the widespread employment of medical genetics and at the same time suggesting that it may indeed be possible, on theological grounds, for Christians to make certain kinds of discriminating judgments about their limited use. Yet just to the extent that certain approaches to medical genetics seek not to serve the weak or embrace difference, but to eliminate them from the body, those particular approaches must be rejected by Christians.

The fact that I have been addressing questions concerning the Christian use of biotechnologies in the context of the perfection of the body suggests that these sorts of adjudications need ultimately to be made by well-formed Christian communities in light of those specific social practices that constitute them as the body of Christ.[16] The answers to these sorts of questions will be

14. Interestingly, the Evangelical Protestant Biblical scholar Gordon Fee makes a complementary point in his commentary on this passage. See Fee, 1987, p. 565. For a more fully developed account of this point, see my 1999, pp. 103-109.

15. See McKenny, 1997, pp. 32-33.

16. John Howard Yoder has written what I regard as a definitive essay on moral discernment in the Christian community. See Yoder, 1984, pp. 15-45.

matters for communal discernment, with the primary question asked always being whether and how the anticipated ends of proposed uses of various modalities can be fit into what the community understands to be its hierarchy of ends.

Such discernment might proceed on two distinct levels. In order to begin at a more conceptual, level, let me propose a thought experiment: As Christians attempting to live faithfully in an age thoroughly immersed in scientific enquiry, we must imagine a mode of scientific enquiry that is and has always been properly conceived and conducted within a theologically determined hierarchy of ends.[17] Such a mode of enquiry is necessarily structured, suggests MacIntyre, not simply by technical proficiency at the science in consideration, but also by possession of those intellectual, moral and theological virtues that predispose one to the achievement of the Good (1990, p. 41). The conduct of this science would always be ruled hypothetically by the determination to produce only those knowledges that can be used in the service of Christian faithfulness.

Having proceeded to this point, we can then attempt to say whether and to what extent such enquiry would be concerned to discover, understand and map the human genome and how it would or would not apply clinically the results of those enterprises. Without attempting the daunting (if not impossible) task of answering each of these questions here, we can say at least this: Every step in the enquiry would proceed by way of a kind of dialectic (MacIntyre, 1990, pp. 34-35), and would require the participation of several members of the community, each bringing to the conversation his or her respective particular gifts or contributions to the rationality of the community. Each would ask finally whether and how what has to this point been discovered might serve the final end of the proper worship of God by all of creation.

Discernment will also take place on a second, more practical level. This level presumes the present existence of medical genetics in the world and seeks to determine whether and how Christians can make faithful use of that discipline. Because this level of discernment is engaging a discipline formed without due consideration of the proper relationship of creatures to God or to one another, it would proceed carefully and even a bit skeptically, but would not dismiss medical genetics out of hand. Thus therapies for a variety of illnesses which have been developed because of the knowledge afforded to medicine by the genome project might well be welcomed. Similarly, it might be seen as appropriate for a couple with a family history of genetically linked diseases to seek genetic counseling in the process of discerning whether they should have children. On the other hand, it might be more difficult for a couple to justify aborting a genetically "problematic" fetus or undergoing expensive somatic cell genetic therapies (assuming those will in the future be widely available) in order to have "normal" children. The question to be asked in all cases would be "does taking this or that action threaten to divide or disrupt the witness of this community to the perfection of human being established in the life, death and resurrection of Jesus of Nazareth?"

The Christian expectation that we shall one day be made perfect is an expectation that requires us to accept the finally contingent nature of our lives and to acknowledge that we are dependent in the end upon the work of Another. Christians are, in the words of Wesley, "going on to perfection," a perfection that is achieved not by the elimination of contingency or the maximization of individual freedom, but by our being made part of Christ's body. It is in that membership, where we share our bodies and our sufferings with one another, that we may finally discover that perfection we so desperately seek.

17. For a more fully developed account of this kind of enquiry, see MacIntyre, 1990.

References

Arendt, H. (1998). *The Human Condition,* second edition, University of Chicago Press, Chicago.

Berry, W. (1990). *What Are People For?* North Point Press, New York.

Bloom, H. (1992). *The American Religion: The Emergence of a Post-Christian Nation,* Simon and Schuster, New York.

Creighton, J. (ed.) (1900). *The Advancement of Learning and Novum Organum,* Colonial Press, New York.

Donovan, M. A. (1997). *One Right Reading?: A Guide to Irenaeus,* Michael Glazier, Collegeville, Minnesota.

Fee, G. (1987). *The First Epistle to the Corinthians,* Eerdmans, Grand Rapids, Michigan.

Galdston, I. (1981). *The Social and Historical Foundations of Modern Medicine,* Bruner/Mazel, New York.

Gustafson, J. (1978). 'Theology confronts technology and the life sciences,' *Commonweal* 105 (June 16), 386-392.

Havel, V. (1987). 'The Power of the powerless,' in *Living in Truth,* J. Vladislav (ed.), Faber and Faber, Boston.

Lasch, C. (1991). *The True and Only Heaven: Progress and its Critics,* W. W. Norton, New York.

MacIntyre, A. (1984). *After Virtue,* University of Notre Dame Press, Notre Dame, Indiana.

MacIntyre, A. (1990). *FRB Principles, Final Ends, and Contemporary Philosophical Issues,* Marquette University Press, Milwaukee, Wisconsin.

McKenny, G. (1997). *To Relieve the Human Condition,* SUNY Press, Albany, New York.

Milbank, J. (1990). *Theology and Social Theory,* Basil Blackwell, Cambridge, Massachusetts.

Rossi, P. (1968). *Francis Bacon: From Magic to Science,* S. Rabinowitz (trans.), University of Chicago Press, Chicago.

Shuman, J. (1999). *The Body of Compassion: Ethics, Medicine and the Church,* Westview Press, Boulder, Colorado.

Stout, J. 'Commitments and traditions in the study of religious ethics,' *Journal of Religious Ethics* 25 (3), 23-56.

Williams, R. (1998). *The Wound of Knowledge,* Wipf and Stock, Eugene, Oregon.

Yoder, J. H. (1972). *The Politics of Jesus,* Eerdmans, Grand Rapids, Michigan.

Yoder, J. H. (1984). 'The hermeneutics of peoplehood,' in *The Priestly Kingdom,* University of Notre Dame Press, Notre Dame, Indiana, pp. 15-45.

Zizioulas, J. (1994). 'Communion and otherness,' *Sobornost: The Journal of the Fellowship of St. Alban and St. Sergius* 16 (1).

134 "Playing God" and Invoking a Perspective

Allen Verhey

Should human beings play God? It is a question frequently raised in discussions of bioethics and of genetics. The question is sometimes asked rhetorically, as though the answer is obvious: "Human beings should not play God!"[1] Sometimes the question is set aside as if it were not a serious question, as though human beings have no choice but to play God, as though it is what human beings do. "The question is not whether we will play God or not, but whether [we will play God responsibly or not]" (Augenstein, 1969, p. 145).

We are sometimes invited to play God, and we are sometimes warned against it, but before we decide whether to accept the invitation or to heed the warning, it would be good to know what it means to "play God."

When my daughter, Kate, was very young, she once invited the rest of the family to play "52-semi." She was holding a deck of cards, obviously eager to play. But when we asked for an explanation of this game, she would give none, only repeating her invitation to play "52-semi." Finally we said, "OK, Katie, let's play '52-semi'." She threw the cards up into the air and, when they had fallen back to the floor, commanded triumphantly, "Now pick 'em up." She had gotten her trucks mixed up, confusing "52-semi" with "52 pickup" but suddenly — too late — we knew what she meant. Should human beings "play God"? It depends, you see, on what it means to "play God."

Unfortunately, the phrase does not mean just one thing; it means different things to different people in different contexts. That is hardly surprising, I suppose, given the fact that neither "play" nor "God" is a simple term. Moreover, sometimes the phrase is used in ways that have nothing to do with either "play" or "God."

In one recent survey of the uses of the phrase, Edmund Erde decided that the phrase is meaningless. Using the phrase as though it meant something, he said, ". . . is muddle-headed" (Erde, 1989, p. 594); moreover, he

1. Ted Howard and Jeremy Rifkin, for example, ask their readers *Who Should Play God?* in the title of their book (1977), but a reader who expects an extended discussion of the question or a reasoned defense of an answer will be disappointed. The question is evidently rhetorical and the answer is "no one."

From Allen Verhey, "'Playing God' and Invoking a Perspective," *The Journal of Medicine and Philosophy* 20 (1995): 347-64. Used with kind permission from Kluwer Academic Publishers.

regarded the phrase not only as "non-sensical," but also as "unconstitutional or blasphemous" (Erde, 1989, p. 599), even "immoral" (Erde, 1989, p. 594). Erde demanded that, for the phrase to be meaningful, it must mean a single moral principle, and a universal moral principle at that. That seems a bit much to ask.

This article undertakes to sort through at least some of the uses of this phrase. I hope to indicate that the phrase does not so much state a principle as invoke a perspective on the world; a perspective from which other things, including scientific and technological innovations in genetics — and the phrase itself — are meaningful. I hope to indicate that we must be attentive not only to particular moral problems raised by genetic engineering but also to the perspective from which we examine and evaluate these new powers and problems. And I hope to suggest, finally, the relevance of a perspective in which "God" is taken seriously and "play" playfully.

The President's Commission report on *Splicing Life* (1982) would seem a good place to begin. The commission noted the concerns voiced about "playing God" in genetics and, to their credit, undertook to make some sense of the phrase. It even invited theologians to comment on the phrase and its relevance to genetic engineering. The "view of the theologians" is summarized in a single paragraph.

> [C]ontemporary developments in molecular biology raise issues of responsibility rather than being matters to be prohibited because they usurp powers that human beings should not possess. . . . Endorsement of genetic engineering, which is praised for its potential to improve the human estate, is linked with the recognition that the misuse of human freedom creates evil and that human knowledge and power can result in harm (President's Commission, 1982, pp. 53-54).

There is much here that could reward a closer analysis. It is clear that the theologians rejected the warnings against "playing God" when those warnings were understood as warnings against usurping powers that are properly God's — but how else might they be understood? The theologians evidently thought that the notion of "responsibility" might be suggestive. It is indeed suggestive, and I will return to it. The President's Commission, however, decided to leave the notion of responsibility to God aside. It decided that the phrase "playing God" does not have "a specific religious meaning" (President's Commission, 1982, p. 54).

If, in stating this, the Commission had meant simply that the phrase does not mean one thing, and that the meaning of the phrase varies with the particular religious tradition and perspective within which it might be used, then one could hardly object. However, the Commission proceeded to assert that "at its heart" the phrase was "an expression of a sense of awe [in response to extraordinary *human* powers] — and concern [about the possible consequences of these vast new powers]" (President's Commission, 1982, p. 54). The Commission simply translated the warnings against "playing God" into a concern about the consequences of exercising great human powers (Lebacqz, 1984, p. 33).

The Commission reduced the meaning of the phrase to secular terms and made "God" superfluous. "At its heart," according to the Commission, the phrase "playing God" has nothing to do with "God." Moreover, there is nothing very playful about "playing God" either. The human powers in genetics and their possible consequences are too serious for playfulness.

"Playing God" might mean what the Commission interpreted it to mean, something like, "Wow! Human powers are awesome. Let's not play around!" It evidently does mean something like that to many who use the phrase. Such an interpretation of the phrase is hardly trivial, but it is also not very useful to guide or limit human powers. Moreover, it is worth pointing out that the President's Commission invoked a particular perspective in interpreting the phrase, and it then used the phrase as shorthand to invoke that perspective when interpreting developments in genetics.

The President's Commission highlighted one very important feature of contemporary culture, the hegemony of scientific knowledge. "Since the Enlightenment," it said, "Western societies have exalted the search for greater knowledge" (President's Commission, 1982, p. 54). Scientific knowledge, beginning with Copernicus, has both "dethrone[d] human beings as the unique center of the world" and delivered "vast powers for action" into their hands (President's Commission, 1982, pp. 54-55).

Leroy Augenstein had made the same point in *Come, Let Us Play God.* Science has taught us the hard lesson that human beings and their earth are not "the center of the universe" (Augenstein, 1969, p. 11), but it is now putting into human hands powers and responsibilities "to make decisions which we formerly left to God" (Augenstein, 1969, p. 142). Borrowing the phrase of Dietrich Bonhoeffer, Augenstein described this situation as humanity's "coming of age" (Augenstein, 1969, p. 143).

Where this is the context for talk of "playing God," it is not surprising that "God" is superfluous, that "God" is not taken seriously when we try to make sense of the phrase. Bonhoeffer, after all, described humanity's "coming of age" as an effort to think the world "*etsi deus non daretur*" ("as though God were not a given") (Bonhoeffer, 1953, p. 218). Science has no need of God "as a working hypothesis" (Bonhoeffer, 1953, p. 218); in fact, it is not even permitted for science *qua* science to make use of "God." There are assumptions operative in this perspective, however, not only about "God" but about humanity, knowledge, and nature as well. With respect to humanity, science has taught us that we are not "the center of the universe." However, science has not taught us where we do belong. As Nietzsche aptly put it, "since Copernicus man has been rolling from the center into x" (cited in Jüngel, 1983, p. 15). Once human beings and their earth were at the center. They did not put themselves there; God put them there, and it was simply accepted as a matter of course that they *were* there. After Copernicus had shown that they were not at the center, humanity was left to fend for itself (or simply to continue "rolling"). This positionlessness was the new assumption, and it entailed that humanity had to attempt to secure (if somewhat anxiously) a place for itself — and what better place than at the center. After Copernicus, humanity was not simply at the center, it had to *put* itself at the center, make itself *into* the center. Fortunately, the very science that destroyed the illusion that humanity was at the center gave to humanity power in the world and over the world. Such mastery, however, has not eliminated human insecurity and anxiety; in fact, the new powers and their unintended consequences evoke new anxieties.

In this context "playing God" *etsi deus non daretur* might well be interpreted as "an expression of a sense of awe [before human powers] — and concern [about unanticipated consequences]" (President's Commission, 1982, p. 54).

There are assumptions concerning knowledge, too. The comment of the President's Commission that "[s]ince the Enlightenment, Western societies have exalted the search for greater knowledge" (President's Commission, 1982, p. 54) requires a gloss. They have exalted a particular kind of knowledge, the knowledge for which they reserve the honorific term "science."

It is simply not the case that the search for knowledge only began to be exalted with the Enlightenment. Thomas Aquinas, for example, had exalted the search for knowledge long before the Enlightenment, affirming "all knowledge" as "good." He distinguished, however, "practical" from "speculative" (or theoretical) sciences, the difference being that the practical sciences are for the sake of some work to be done, while the speculative sciences are for their own sake (Aquinas, Commentary on Aristotle's *On the Soul,* I, 3; cited in Jonas, 1966, p. 188).

That classical account (and celebration) of knowledge must be contrasted with the modern account epitomized in Francis Bacon's *The Great Instauration* and "exalted" in Western societies. In Bacon all knowledge is sought for its utility, "for the benefit and use of life" (Bacon, [1620] 1960, p. 15). The knowledge to be sought is "no mere felicity of speculation" (Bacon, [1620] 1960, p. 29), which is but the "boyhood of knowledge" and "barren of works" (Bacon, [1620] 1960, p. 8). The knowledge to be sought is the practical knowledge that will make humanity "capable of overcoming the difficulties and obscurities of nature" (Bacon, [1620] 1960, p. 19), able to subdue and overcome its vexations and miseries. "And so those twin objects, human knowledge and human power, do really meet in one" (Bacon, [1620] 1960, p. 29). The knowledge "exalted" in Western societies is this power over nature which presumably brings human well-being in its train.

In the classical account, theory (or the speculative sciences) provided the wisdom to use the practical sciences appropriately. The modern account may admit, as Bacon did, that for knowledge to be beneficial humanity must "perfect and govern it in charity" (Bacon, [1620] 1960, p. 15), but science is "not self-sufficiently the source of that human quality that makes it beneficial" (Jonas, 1966, p. 195). Moreover, the compassion (or "charity") that responds viscerally to the vexations and miseries of humanity will urge us to *do something* to relieve those miseries, but it will not tell us *what thing* to do. Bacon's account of knowledge simply arms compassion with artifice, not with wisdom (O'Donovan, 1984, pp. 10-12). For the charity to "perfect and govern" human powers and for the wisdom to guide charity, science must call upon something else. But upon what? And how can humanity have "knowledge" of it? Knowledge of that which transcends "use" — and transcends "nature" known scientifically, even "human nature" known scientifically — has no place in Bacon's theory.[2]

Knowledge of that which might guide and limit the human use of human powers was the subject of classical theory, but not of the Enlightenment "search for greater knowledge." In this context there is no place for either "play" (because play is not "useful"[3]) or "God" (because God is transcendent and will not be used).

With the different assumptions concerning knowledge come different assumptions concerning nature, too. The Baconian project sets humanity not only over nature but against it. The natural order and natural processes have no dignity of their own; their value is reduced to their utility to humanity — and nature does not serve humanity "naturally." Nature threatens to rule and to ruin humanity. Against the powers of nature, knowledge promises the power to relieve humanity's miseries and "to endow the human family with new mercies" (Bacon, [1620] 1960, p. 29). The fault that runs through our world and through our lives must finally be located in nature. Nature may be — and must be — mastered (Jonas, 1966, p. 192).

This is the perspective invoked by the President's Commission. From this perspective "playing God" has nothing to do with either "play" or "God." Rather, it is concerned with human scientific knowledge and power over nature and it raises doubts about the taken-for-granted assumption that human well-being will come in the train of such knowledge and power.

2. To be sure, Bacon recommended his "great instauration" as a form of obedience to God, as a restoration to humanity of the power over nature which was given at creation but lost through the fall. Indeed, he prays "that things human may not interfere with things divine, and that . . . there may arise in our minds no incredulity or darkness with regard to the divine mysteries" (Bacon, [1620] 1960, pp. 14-15). Even so, such mysteries have no theoretical place in Bacon's account of knowledge.

3. Jonas (1966, p. 194) contrasts the relations of leisure to theory in the classical and modern traditions. In the classical account leisure was an antecedent condition for speculative knowledge, for contemplation; in modern theory leisure is an effect of knowledge (as power), one of the benefits of that knowledge that provides relief from the miseries of humanity, including toil. "Wherefore," Bacon says ([1620] 1960, p. 29), "if we labor in thy works with the sweat of our brows, thou wilt make us partakers of . . . thy sabbath."

Religious people have sometimes celebrated this Baconian perspective and its quest for scientific knowledge and technical power — and have sometimes lamented it. Some who have lamented it have raised their voices in protest against almost every new scientific hypothesis (witness Galileo and Darwin) and against almost all technological developments (for example, anesthesia during childbirth). These evidently regard scientific inquiry as a threat to faith in God and technical innovation as an offense to God. These lament a "humanity come of age" and long to go back to a former time, a time of our childhood (if only we knew the way!). They regret a world *etsi deus non daretur* and wish to preserve the necessity of "God" in human ignorance and powerlessness. But such a "God" can only ever be a "God of the Gaps" and can only ever be in retreat to the margins.

It is an old and unhappy story in Christian apologetics that locates God's presence and power where human knowledge and strength have reached their (temporary) limit. Newton, for example, saw certain irregularities in the motion of the planets, movements which he could not explain by his theory of gravity, and in those irregularities he saw, he said, the direct intervention of God. When later astronomers and physicists provided a natural explanation for what had puzzled Newton, "God" was no longer necessary. And there is the old joke of the patient who, when told that the only thing left to do was to pray, said, "Oh, my! And I didn't even think it was serious." The God of the Gaps is only invoked, after all, where doctors are powerless.

In the context of such a piety, when there is a defensive faith in the God of the Gaps, "playing God" means to encroach on those areas of human life where human beings have been ignorant or powerless, for there God rules, there only God has the authority to act. In this context "playing God" means to seize God's place at the boundaries of human knowledge and power, to usurp God's authority and dominion. In this context it is understandable that humanity should be warned, "Thou shalt not play God."

Once again the phrase is used not so much to state a principle as to invoke a perspective. To be sure, such warnings serve to remind humanity of its fallibility and finitude, and such warnings are salutary. There are, however, at least two problems with this perspective and with such warnings against "playing God."[4]

The first and fundamental problem with this perspective is that the God of the Gaps is not the God who is made known in creation and in scripture. The God of creation and scripture made and sustains the order we observe and rely upon. To describe that order in terms of scientific understanding does not explain God away; it is to give an account of the way God orders God's world. The order of the world comes to us no less from the gracious hand of God than the extraordinary events humans call "miracles." "Nature" is no less the work of God than "grace." The world and its order are not God, but they are God's. They are the work of God. And, to understand the world and its order as God's is not to understand it in a way that prohibits "natural scientific" explanations. It is to be called to serve God's cause, to be responsible to God in the midst of it.

The second problem with this perspective and with such warnings against "playing God" is that they are indiscriminate; they do not permit discriminating judgments. There are some things which we already know how to do (and so can hardly be said to trespass the boundaries of human ignorance and powerlessness), but which we surely ought never to do. And there are some things (including some things in genetics) which we cannot yet do, but which we must make an effort to learn to do if God is God and we are called to "follow" one who heals the sick and feeds the hungry. The warning against "playing God" in this perspective reduces to the slogan "It's not nice to fool with Mother Nature (at least not any more than we are currently comfortable with)." Ironically, then, the warning enthrones "nature" as god rather than the One who transcends it and our knowledge of it.

Some other religious people celebrate the advances of science and the innovations of technology, urging humanity bravely to go forward, uttering a priestly benediction over the Baconian project. These sometimes use the phrase "playing God," too, usually in inviting humanity to "play God." Joseph Fletcher, for example, responded provocatively to the charge that his enthusiasm for genetic technology amounted to a license to "play God" by admitting the charge (Fletcher, 1970, p. 131) and by making the invitation explicit; "Let's play God," he said (Fletcher, 1974, p. 126).

The "God" Fletcher invited us to "play" was still the God of the Gaps (Fletcher, 1970, p. 132), the God at the edges of human knowledge and power. For Fletcher, however, "that old, primitive God is dead" (Fletcher, 1970, p. 132; 1974, p. 200). Dead also are the "taboos" which prohibited trespass on the territory of that God's rule (Fletcher, 1974, p. 127), the "fatalism" that passively accepted the will of that God (Fletcher, 1974, p. 128), and the "obsolete theodicy" (Fletcher, 1970, p. 132) that attempted to defend that God. "What we need," he said, "is a new God" (Fletcher, 1970, p. 132), but Fletcher's "new God" bore a striking resemblance to the God of the eighteenth-century deist, and indifference to a God so conceived is inevitable; life may proceed — and "playing God" may proceed — *etsi deus non daretur*.

Although Fletcher said little more about this "new God," he did say that "any God worth believing in wills the best possible well-being for human beings" (Fletcher, 1974, p. xix). Fletcher's "new God" turns out to be a heavenly utilitarian, and this God, too, humanity must "play."

So, the invitation to "play God" comes to this: humanity should use its new powers to achieve the greatest good of the greatest number of people (not intimidated by "taboos"), to take control over "nature" (not ener-

4. This account of "playing God" was the one rejected by the theologians consulted by the President's Commission (1982, p. 53).

vated by "fatalism"), to take responsibility, to design and make a new and better world, to substitute for an absent God. "It was *easier* in the old days," Fletcher said (1974, p. 200),

> to attribute at least some of what happened to God's will — we could say with a moral shrug that we weren't responsible. Now we have to shoulder it all. The moral tab is ours and we have to pick it up. The excuses of ignorance and helplessness are growing thin.

Notice what has happened to responsibility. Fletcher underscores human responsibility, but we are responsible not so much *to* God as *instead of* God.[5] That shift puts an enormous (and messianic) burden on genetics, a burden which leaves little time for "play."

The phrase "playing God" here does state a principle, namely, utility, but it also does more than that — it invokes a perspective, a perspective in which the God of the Gaps is superfluous, in which humanity is maker and designer, in which knowledge is power, and in which nature must be mastered to maximize human well-being. Such a perspective makes the invitation to "play God" — and much else in Fletcher's discussion of genetics — meaningful.

Christians may welcome Fletcher's burial of the God of the Gaps, but they still wait and watch and pray not for the invention of some "new God" but for the appearance of the one God who continues to create, preserve, and redeem humanity and its world. Moreover, Fletcher's invitation to "play God" need not seem blasphemous to those trained to "imitate God," to "follow" God, to be disciples of the one who made God present among us. But, to map the path of discipleship and imitation as "the utilitarian way" must seem strange to those who know the law and the prophets, and the gospels.

It seemed strange, at least, to Paul Ramsey. In Ramsey's usage, although we are usually warned against "playing God," we are sometimes encouraged to "'play God' in the correct way" (Ramsey, 1978, p. 203) — and God is no utilitarian. "God," Ramsey said (1978, p. 205),

> is not a rationalist whose care is a function of indicators of our personhood, or of our achievement within those capacities. He makes his rain fall upon the just and the unjust alike, and his sun to rise on the abnormal as well as the normal. Indeed, he has special care for the weak and the vulnerable among us earth people. He cares according to need, not capacity or merit.

These divine patterns and images are, according to Ramsey, at "the foundation of Western medical care" (Ramsey, 1978, p. 205).

One might expect Ramsey, then, simply to echo Fletcher's invitation to "play God" while engaging him and others in conversation concerning who this God is whom we are invited to "play." However, he also (and more frequently) warned against "playing God." The phrase itself, he admitted, is "not [a] very helpful characterization" (Ramsey, 1970b, p. 90), but he used it to name — and to warn against — an "attitude," an "outlook," certain "operating, unspoken premises" at work in western scientific culture (Ramsey, 1970b, p. 91), and to invite a different perspective on the world.

The fundamental premise of the perspective Ramsey warns against is that "God" is superfluous. "Where there is no God . . . ," he said (Ramsey, 1970b, p. 93), there humanity is creator, maker, the engineer of the future (Ramsey, 1970b, pp. 91-92), and there nature, even human nature, may be and must be controlled and managed with messianic ambition (Ramsey, 1970b, pp. 92-96). Where "God" is superfluous and human beings are cast in this role of "the maker," there morality is reduced to the consideration of consequences, knowledge is construed simply as power, and nature — including the human nature given to humanity as embodied and communal — is left with no dignity of its own.

Ramsey's warnings against "playing God" are not immediately identified with a particular moral rule or principle; rather, they challenge the wisdom and the sufficiency of the assumptions too much at work in Western culture. It is not that some "God of the Gaps" is threatened. It is not simply that human powers are awesome or that the consequences of "interfering with nature" are worrisome, as the President's Commission suggested. It is rather that the fundamental perspective from which we interpret our responsibilities is critically important to seeing what those responsibilities are (Ramsey, 1970b, pp. 28, 143).

The fundamental perspective which Ramsey recommends and to which he contrasts "playing God" is "to intend the world as a Christian or as a Jew" (Ramsey, 1970b, p. 22), i.e., *etsi deus daretur* — and not just any old *deus* (nor Fletcher's "new God") but the God who creates and keeps a world and a covenant. That means, among other things, that the end of all things may be left to God. Where God is God and not us, there can be a certain eschatological nonchalance. From this perspective, our responsibilities, while great, will not be regarded as being of messianic proportion. There will be some room, then, for an ethic of means as well as the consideration of consequences (Ramsey, 1970b, pp. 23-32), for reflection about the kind of behavior which is worthy of human nature as created by God, as embodied and interdependent, for example.

When joined with such reflection, Ramsey's warnings that we should not play God do provide some prohibitions. When joined with an interpretation of human procreation, for example, the warning against "playing God" bears the prohibition against putting "entirely asunder what God joined together," against separating "*in principle*" the unitive and procreative goods of human sexuality, against reducing procreation either to biology or to contract (Ramsey, 1970b, pp. 32-33), and that prohibition supports in turn a series of more particular prohibitions,

5. On the shift from theodicy to "anthropodicy" see Becker (1968, p. 18) and Hauerwas (1990, pp. 59-64).

for example, a prohibition against artificial insemination using the sperm of a donor (Ramsey, 1970b, pp. 47-52).

When joined with an interpretation of the patient as "*a sacredness in the natural, biological order*" (Ramsey, 1970a, xiii), the "edification" drawn from the warning against "playing God" includes prohibitions against deliberately killing patients, including very little patients, for the sake of relieving their (or another's) suffering, against using one without consent, even a very little one, even one created in a petri dish, to learn to help others.

Ramsey warns against "playing God," against trying to substitute for an absent God, against trying to "be" God, but there remains room for "playing God" *etsi deus daretur*. Indeed, as we have seen, Ramsey can invite people to "'play God' in the correct way" (Ramsey, 1970a, p. 256). Such "playing" is not to substitute for an absent God, not to "be" God, but to "imitate" God (Ramsey, 1970a, p. 259), to follow in God's way like a child "playing" a parent.

In both the warning and the invitation a perspective is invoked, an outlook which assumes that God is God and not us, that humanity is called to honor and to nurture the nature God gave, that knowledge of that which transcends use is possible, and that the fault that runs through our lives and our world is not simply located in nature but in human pride or sloth.

One who — like me — shares this perspective will make sense of the phrase "playing God" in the light of this perspective. Sometimes it will be appropriate to sound a warning against "playing God," and sometimes it will be appropriate to issue an invitation to "play God" in imitation of God's care and grace. Permit me to focus on the invitation to "play God" — and first to underscore the invitation to "play."[6] Many have complained that "playing God" is serious stuff and regretted the implication of "playfulness" in the phrase (e.g., Lebacqz, 1984, p. 40, n. 19). Some "play," however, can be very serious indeed — as anyone who plays noon-hour basketball knows quite well. "Playfulness" is quite capable of being serious, but it is not capable of being purely instrumental.

When Teilhard de Chardin said that "in the great game that is being played, we are the players as well as . . . the stakes" (1961, p. 230), he created a powerful image to call attention both to the extraordinary powers of human beings and to the awesome consequences of exercising those powers. No wonder playfulness seems inappropriate. Precisely because the stakes are high, however, it may be apt to set alongside Teilhard's image a Dutch proverb: "It is not the marbles that matter but the game" (quoted in Huizinga, 1950, p. 49). When the stakes are high, or even when the stakes alone are taken seriously, then one is tempted to cheat in order to win. And when one cheats, then one only pretends to play; the cheat plays neither fair nor seriously.

Play, even marbles, can be serious, but it cannot be purely instrumental; it cannot allow attention to be monopolized by the stakes, by the consequences of winning or losing. When our attention is riveted by Teilhard's image that we are "the stakes," it may well be important to allow our imagination to be captured by his image that we are "the players," too. Then we may be able to avoid reducing the moral life to a concern about consequences, even where the stakes are high. We may be able to avoid reducing ourselves to makers and designers and our existence to joyless and incessant work. We may see that we are at stake, not just in the sense of some plastic destiny our powers may make but already in the imagination, in the image of ourselves with which human creativity begins (Hartt, 1975, pp. 117-134).

The invitation is an invitation to "play," but it is more specifically an invitation to "play God," and that invitation requires attention to the God whom we are invited to play. In the foreword to *Should Doctors Play God?* Mrs. Billy Graham wrote (1971, p. vii),

> [i]f I were an actress who was going to play, let's say, Joan of Arc, I would learn all there is to learn about Joan of Arc. And, if I were a doctor or anyone else trying to play God, I would learn all I could about God.

That seems a prudent strategy for an actress — and good advice for people called to imitate God. The invitation to "play God," to cast ourselves playfully in the role of God, invites theological reflection; it invites reflection about "God."

The invitation goes out to all, not just to Christians. When ancient Greek physicians swore the Hippocratic Oath by Apollos, Aesclepius, Hygiea, Panacea and all the gods and goddesses, they invoked a story. Healing had its beginnings among the gods, and the Hippocratic physicians swore to make that story their own. And when the temple to Aesclepius in the Areopagus was inscribed with the message that, like a god, Aesclepius healed both rich and poor without discrimination, a path was laid out for physicians to follow.

The invitation goes out to all, but reflection about God is always formed and informed by the particular stories and communities within which it is undertaken, and Christians will heed this invitation in the light of their own tradition and its talk of God. We play God in response to God, imitating God's ways and providing human service to God's cause. Our responsibility to God limits and shapes an account of what we are responsible for in God's good world — and its genetics.

Permit me, then, simply to select a few images of God in the Jewish and Christian tradition and to suggest something of their relevance to "playing God" in genetics. Two of these images are regularly invoked in these discussions: creator and healer — and the third is often overlooked: God is the one who takes the side of the poor.

6. A delightful essay by Jan van Eys (1982) also underscores the invitation to "play" in the phrase "play God"; unfortunately, van Eys treats "play" as a kind of psychological therapy and so renders it instrumental finally.

First, then, what might it mean playfully to cast ourselves in the role of the creator? This, of course, has been the topic of much discussion. If I read the story right, however, to cast ourselves in the role of the creator might mean something too much overlooked. It might mean that we look at the creation and at its genetics and say to ourselves, "God, that's good." It might mean, that is, first of all, to wonder, to stand in awe, to delight in the elegant structure of the creation and its DNA. It would mean a celebration of knowledge which was not simply mastery. It would mean an appreciation of nature — and of human nature — as given, rather than a suspicion of it as threatening and requiring human mastery.

And if I read the story right, it might mean a second thing too much overlooked. It might mean to take a day off, to rest, to play. But we have already talked of that.

It also means, of course, a third thing, a thing seldom overlooked in these discussions — that human creativity is given with the creation. Human beings are created and called to exercise dominion in the world — and I see no reason to suppose that such creativity and control does not extend to genetics. It is not "Mother Nature" who is God, after all, in the Christian story. Human creativity and control, however, are to be exercised in response to God, in imitation of God's ways, and in service to God's cause. That's a part of the Christian story, too, a part of the store usually captured in describing ourselves as stewards and our responsibility as stewardship.

We can discover something of God's cause, the cause stewards serve, in a second feature of the story. God is the healer. Jesus, the one in whom God and the cause of God were made known, was a healer. We discover there that the cause of God is life, not death; the cause of God is human flourishing, including the human flourishing we call health, not disease. What does it mean to cast ourselves playfully in the role of God the healer? It means to intend life and its flourishing, not death or human suffering. Therefore, genetic therapy, like other therapeutic interventions which aim at health, may be celebrated. Healing is "playing God" the way God plays God. Genetic therapies, however, are still mostly (but not completely) a distant hope. The more immediate contributions of genetics to medicine are in genetic diagnosis. And where there are therapeutic options, these too may be celebrated. However, genetic diagnoses without therapeutic options are sometimes deeply ambiguous.

Prenatal diagnoses, for example, are frequently ambiguous. Already we can diagnose a number of genetic conditions in a fetus, and the number is constantly growing. For most of these there is no therapy. The tests allow parents to make a decision about whether to give birth or to abort. How shall we "play God" here in ways responsible to God? If God's cause is life rather than death, then those who would "play God" in imitation of God will not be disposed to abort; they will not celebrate abortion as a "therapeutic option."

There are, I think, genetic conditions which justify abortion. There are conditions like Tay-Sachs which consign a child not only to an abbreviated life but to a life subjectively indistinguishable from torture. And there are conditions like Trisomy 18 which are inconsistent not only with life but with the minimal conditions for human communication. Prenatal diagnosis — and abortion — can be used responsibly. However, when some children with Down's Syndrome are aborted because they have Down's, there seems to exist a reasonable possibility that prenatal diagnoses have been — and will be — used irresponsibly. When the slogan about "preventing birth defects" is taken to justify preventing the birth of "defectives," those who do not measure up to the standards or match the preferences of parents, then there are reasons to worry a little, to worry that the disposition of a good "parent" will change from the sort of uncalculating nurturance that can evoke and sustain trust from children to the sort of calculating nurturance that is prepared to abandon or abort the offspring who do not match specifications. "Playing God" the way God plays God — or, if you will, the way God plays "parent" — would sustain care for the weak and the helpless, and for the little ones who do not measure up.

Genetic therapy, I said, may be celebrated as service to God's cause of health. It is to "play God" as God plays God. However, to use this knowledge and technology responsibly it must be aimed at "health," not genetic enhancement. The distinction between intervening for health and intervening for genetic enhancement may be a slippery one, but casting ourselves playfully in the role of God the healer will encourage us to make such a distinction and to abide by it. Eugenics is not the way to "play God" the way God plays God.

Consider, finally, this third image: God is one who takes the side of the poor. What would it mean to cast ourselves in the role of one who takes the side of the poor? It would mean, at the very least, I think, a concern for social justice. It would mean, for example, to ask about the allocation of resources to the human genome project. When cities are crumbling, when schools are deteriorating, when we complain about not having sufficient resources to help the poor or the homeless, when we do not have the resources to provide care for all the sick, is this a just and fair use of our society's resources? Is it an allocation of social resources that can claim to imitate God's care and concern for the poor?

Having raised that question, let me focus instead on the sharing of the burdens and benefits of the human genome project itself. Who bears the burdens? Who will benefit? And is the distribution fair? Does it fit the story of one who takes the side of the poor and powerless?

If we cast ourselves in this role, if we attempt to mirror God's justice and care of the poor and powerless, we will not be eager to create human life in order to learn from it with the intention of destroying it after we have learned what we can from it. We will not be eager to use the unborn for experiments to learn some things that would benefit others, even if it were a great benefit, even if it would benefit a great number of others. And we would be cautious about stigmatizing some as diseased and others as carriers.

But consider also the sharing of benefits. Who stands to benefit from the human genome initiative? Will genetic powers be marketed? Presumably they will, given the patenting of micro-organisms. And so the rich may get richer while the poor still watch and pray. Will the poor have access to health care benefits that their taxes helped develop? Since health care reform has died in Congress again, can we have any confidence that genetic technology will be available to the uninsured or to those with public insurance? Or will insurance companies use genetic information to screen candidates for insurance? Will the category of "preexisting condition" be redefined to make it easier for insurance companies to make a still larger profit? Will genetic information be included in actuarial tables? Will corporations use genetic information to screen applicants in order to hire those with greatest promise of long-term productivity? The point of these questions is not simply to lament our failure to accomplish health care reform. It is to suggest that "playing God" as God plays God will be attentive not only to intriguing questions about the frontiers of technology and science but also to mundane questions about fairness, about the effect of such innovations on the poor. If we are to "play God" as God plays God, then we have a pattern for imitation in God's hospitality to the poor and to the stranger, to the powerless and to the voiceless, to those who are different from both us and the norm, including some genetic norm. If we are to "play God" as God plays God, then we will work for a society where human beings — each of them, even the least of them — are treated as worthy of God's care and affection.

This has been just a selection of images of God, and I admit that the moves to claims about genetic interventions were made far too quickly. But enough has been said, I hope, to suggest the importance of the invitation to play God as God plays God. Enough has been said, I hope, to suggest the importance of the perspective in terms of which we think about genetics and in terms of which we make sense not only of our powers but of the phrase "playing God."

References

Augenstein, L.: 1969, *Come, Let Us Play God,* Harper & Row, New York.

Bacon, F.: 1960 [1620], *The New Organon and Related Writings,* F. H. Anderson (ed.), The Liberal Arts Press, Bobbs-Merrill Co., Indianapolis.

Becker, E.: 1968, *The Structure of Evil,* George Braziller, New York.

Bonhoeffer, D.: 1953, *Letters and Papers from Prison,* E. Bethge (ed.), R. H. Fuller (trans.), Macmillan Company, New York.

Erde, E.: 1989, "Studies in the Explanation of Issues in Biomedical Ethics: (II) On 'On Play[ing] God,' Etc.," *The Journal of Medicine and Philosophy,* 14: 593-615.

Fletcher, J.: 1970, "Technological devices in medical care," in K. Vaux (ed.), *Who Shall Live? Medicine, Technology, Ethics,* Fortress Press, Philadelphia, pp. 115-42.

Fletcher, J.: 1974, *The Ethics of Genetic Control: Ending Reproductive Roulette,* Anchor Books, Garden City, New York.

Graham, R.: 1971, "Foreword," in C. A. Frazier (ed.), *Should Doctors Play God?,* Broadman, Nashville.

Hartt, J.: 1975, *The Restless Quest,* United Church Press, Philadelphia.

Hauerwas, S.: 1990, *Naming the Silences: God, Medicine, and the Problem of Suffering,* William B. Eerdmans, Grand Rapids.

Howard, T., and Rifkin, J.: 1977, *Who Should Play God?,* Dell Publishing Co., New York.

Huizinga, J.: 1950, *Homo Ludens: A Study of the Play-Element in Culture,* Beacon Press, Boston.

Jonas, H.: 1966, *The Phenomenon of Life: Toward a Philosophical Biology,* Dell Publishing Co., New York.

Jüngel, E.: 1983, *God as the Mystery of the World,* D. Guder (trans.), William B. Eerdmans Publishing Company, Grand Rapids.

Lebacqz, K.: 1984, "The ghosts are on the wall: a parable for manipulating life," in R. Esbjornson (ed.), *The Manipulation of Life,* Harper & Row, San Francisco, pp. 22-41.

O'Donovan, O.: 1984, *Begotten or Made?,* Oxford University Press, Oxford.

President's Commission for the Study of Ethical Problems in Medicine and Biomedical and Behavioral Research: 1982, *Splicing Life: A Report on the Social and Ethical Issues of Genetic Engineering with Human Beings,* U.S. Government Printing Office, Washington, D.C.

Ramsey, P.: 1970a, *The Patient as Person: Explorations in Medical Ethics,* Yale University Press, New Haven.

Ramsey, P.: 1970b, *Fabricated Man: The Ethics of Genetic Control,* Yale University Press, New Haven.

Ramsey, P.: 1978, *Ethics at the Edges of Life: Medical and Legal Intersections,* Yale University Press, New Haven.

Teilhard de Chardin: 1961, *The Phenomenon of Man,* B. Wall (trans.), Harper and Row, New York.

van Eys, J.: 1982, "Should doctors play God?," *Perspectives in Biology and Medicine,* 25: 481-85.

VI. The End of Life

CHAPTER TWENTY-ONE

Death and Its (In)dignity

If life has "sanctity," what of death? How is death to be understood or imagined? What posture should we take toward it? What attitudes or dispositions are appropriate? These are not simple questions, but our answers to them will shape how we die and how we care for the dying. Indeed, according to Christopher Vogt and Vigen Guroian, those answers will also help shape how we live, for dying well requires lifelong preparation.

Our culture's response to death is at best confused. William May contends that we have two basic responses: concealment and obsession. An earlier edition of *On Moral Medicine* puts it somewhat differently: we endeavor either to deny or to domesticate death. There is evidence that we respond to death in all of these ways. For example, Mary Baker Eddy, founder of Christian Science, likely denied death when she called it part of the illusion that existence is material. Popular notions of the immortality of the soul — "she has simply gone to a better place" — arguably do the same. Even the common funeral practice of making the body look "natural" — that is, look as if the person were still alive — may be a denial or concealment of death's real power, as is our euphemistic suggestion that the "loved one" has "passed on." Denial of death is also sometimes visible when families combine the demand that doctors "do everything possible" with their expectation of "a miracle," no matter the medical prognosis.

Evidence of obsession is found in big-budget movies, video games, the evening news, and even some popular music. Our movies are filled with violence and death. The body count goes ever higher, with ever more technologically sophisticated means of killing and ever more visually graphic depictions of bodies torn asunder. Many popular video games do likewise, except that in them we get to be the killers. The evening news tallies up the dead from local murderers and far-off wars. And for a few rappers, a near endless focus on violence and death means higher music sales.

Efforts to domesticate death can look very different from each other. For instance, some claim that we should simply accept death as a "natural" event, as a "fact of life," and as part of the "cycle of life" for all mortal creatures. Accepting death is seen as the realistic and rational thing to do since all things die.[1] But do such accounts of death come too close to treating the human person as a mere biological organism? Do such accounts grapple with the rupture that constitutes death? Do such naturalistic accounts, which have been with us at least since the ancient Stoics, take seriously that neither the psalmists nor Jesus confronted death as simply a "fact of life" (Psalms 22; 88; Mark 15:34; Hebrews 5:7)? Moreover, are "natural" accounts of death fully compatible with St. Paul's linking of sin with death (Romans 5:12-21; 6:23; 1 Corinthians 15:21-22)?

A different kind of domestication of death may be emerging among a select group of scientists who are struggling to push off aging by decades or even centuries.[2] For this group, aging and subsequent death are not necessarily "natural," but rather forms of suffering that can be technologically overcome. An example of this perspective is Aubrey D. N. J. de Grey's "The Urgency Dilemma: Is Life Extension Research a Temptation or a Test?" (selection 73), found in our Chapter Eleven, "Aging and the Elderly." It is at least plausible to read such efforts to master aging and death as a form of domestication, not because death is "natural," but because it is within our control.

If our society deals with death largely by concealment, denial, obsession, and domestication, the readings here invite us to consider how Christians ought to approach death. Scripture provides a vital starting place for this conversation (selection 135). Psalm 88 is the saddest of the laments. The speaker, apparently sick since childhood, is suffering toward death. The last word of the psalm is "darkness." Death and darkness have the last word. The terror of death goes beyond the termination of existence; death threatens to unravel meaning, to destroy relationships, to bring chaos.[3] By contrast, Psalm 22, the words ut-

1. Roy Branson, "Is Acceptance a Denial of Death? Another Look at Kübler-Ross," *Christian Century* 92, no. 17 (May 7, 1975): 464-68.

2. See Ben C. Mitchell, "The Quest for Immortality," in *Aging, Death, and the Quest for Immortality*, ed. C. Ben Mitchell, D. Robert Orr, and A. Susan Salladay (Grand Rapids: Eerdmans, 2004), pp. 153-62.

3. See further Allen Verhey, "Meditation: Is the Last Word 'Darkness'?" in *Religion and Medical Ethics: Looking Back, Looking Forward*, ed. Allen Verhey (Grand Rapids: Eerdmans, 1996), pp. 146-50.

tered by Jesus on the cross, is more typical of biblical lament. The speaker gives eloquent expression to fear, suffering, abandonment, and possible death: "My God, my God, why have you forsaken me?" But the psalm oscillates between a sense of loss, grief, brokenness, and expressions of confidence in God, ending with an assurance that God rules and can be counted on to deliver God's people.

In the two New Testament texts included here (Romans 8:18-39; 1 Corinthians 15:20-26, 36-57), the apostle Paul frames suffering and death with confidence in God's love and an expectation of resurrection. Paul assumes that fidelity to Christ may include pain, suffering, and death, and he talks about the groaning of creation. As with the Psalms, the power of death is acknowledged upfront. But there is a confidence that God through Christ is able to hold us even through death. There is, moreover, an anticipation of resurrection. Paul does not deny death by asserting an immortal soul. His confidence is not in our immortality but in the power of God. We remain embodied selves, and the power of death is finally conquered by God through Christ in resurrection.

Selection 136 from Nicholas Wolterstorff's *Lament for a Son* does not conceal, deny, domesticate, or obsess about death. Instead, like Paul, Wolterstorff is confident that the last word belongs to God, a conviction that allows him to face the reality and horror of the death of his son. According to Wolterstorff, a certain kind of mourning reflects a quality of character in keeping with God's reign. Such people have caught a glimpse of God's kingdom and therefore "ache with all their being for that day's coming, and . . . break out into tears when confronted with its absence." Wolterstorff sees Jesus as praising those who have the character to feel and mourn humanity's wounds, but this mourning is framed by an assurance that God's good day is coming.

In "The Sacral Power of Death in Contemporary Experience" (selection 137), William F. May underlines the poverty of both evading and obsessing about death. May discerns in both tendencies the religious character of death since both tendencies are reactions to the fact that death confounds human effort to master it. Unfortunately, the Christian church has sometimes conspired with the culture in its attempt to deny, domesticate, or master death. However, in attending to the death and resurrection of Jesus, May finds resources for the church to deal honestly with the threatening and real power of death and to develop appropriate conduct toward the dying.

Paul Ramsey's now-classic essay, "The Indignity of 'Death with Dignity'" (selection 138), especially confronts the tendency to domesticate death as "natural." Behind the slogan "Death with Dignity," Ramsey finds ideologies suspiciously hospitable to death. Ramsey insists that death is to be regarded as an enemy. Death is evil. It can be "a good evil" if it teaches us to spend our days with some point and purpose, but it remains an evil. In addition, death has no dignity of its own; rather, it is precisely because death is an indignity that someone might bring dignity to the dying process. Even then death remains an enemy, an insult to the embodied and irreplaceable character of human persons and their lives. To forget that death is an enemy is to diminish the value of each person.

One potential criticism of Ramsey is that such an understanding of death lends support to preserving life as long as technologically possible. That is, Ramsey's emphasis on death as an indignity might lend support to efforts to master or domesticate death through medical technology. Oliver O'Donovan addresses this question in "Keeping Body and Soul Together" (selection 139). O'Donovan's argument is complex, but central to his claim is that Ramsey's apologetic strategy of refraining from explicit theological content "deprived his contentions of the full range of their interpretative force." O'Donovan suggests that this apologetic strategy results in inadequate attention to the relationship between sin and death and cannot properly situate the coherence of body and soul within the Christian affirmation of resurrection. Ramsey, says O'Donovan, is susceptible to being misread; one might believe that Ramsey supports trying to master death because he avoids the theological language — especially that of the death and resurrection of Christ — necessary to make his argument fully intelligible and compelling. Of course, one can then turn the question back to O'Donovan, asking whether we sacrifice our ability to talk with our non-Christian neighbors about the meaning of death if we frame the issue in such explicitly Christian terms.

While sharing the theological language especially evident in May and O'Donovan, the excerpt from Christopher Vogt's "Dying Well in Historical Perspective" (selection 140) broadens the frame of this discussion by asking "how to live one's entire life so as to be ready for death." Reviewing the *Ars Moriendi* ("The Art of Dying," how to die well) tradition of the sixteenth and seventeenth centuries, Vogt focuses on the lifelong development of several virtues. He is particularly attentive to the crucial roles of hope, compassion, and patience in dying well. Vogt is equally attentive to the convictions (such as a focus on God's mercy) and the practices (such as forgiving the sins of others, being present to the dying, and remembering one's mortality) that help form those virtues. Through historical survey, Vogt thus invites us to consider a Christian approach to death that assumes deep interconnections among how we live, what we believe, who we become, and how we die.

Vigen Guroian's essay, "Learning How to Die Well: Lessons from the Ancient Church" (selection 141), echoes the concern for the lifelong formation of virtue in meeting suffering and death. Guroian observes that medical ethics seldom discusses character formation, and when it does, the focus is usually on medical personnel. But much of what constitutes dying well — in freedom, faith, fortitude, courage, patience, and hope — depends on the religious and moral resources of the patient, not merely the health care setting or skills of the providers. Through the sacraments, prayer, and preaching, the church can help people acquire the convictions and virtues that enable them to die a good death.

Guroian adds an intriguing element to the discussion: "Eastern Christian writers employ medicinal metaphors to explain salvation." According to Guroian, the utilization of the medical metaphor for redemption has the effect of both affirming and limiting medicine. Thinking of God's redemptive act in Christ as a kind of "divine therapy" that remedies the effects of sin and cures mortal sickness affirms medical science as having a limited place contributing to a healthy and meaningful life. The metaphor implicitly affirms medicine's role in sustaining our earthly existence, but the metaphor also reminds us that it is God who provides the ultimate cure through cross and resurrection and that even death can be "a medicine of salvation."[4]

The readings in this section provoke many practical questions: How do we see death? How should we treat the dying? And what sort of medicine best serves them? But even beyond provoking such questions, the readings invite us to think theologically as Christians about death and to recognize the deep relationship between how we live and how we die. Still further, the readings challenge us to face death's real threats of alienation from flesh, community, and God without resorting to concealment, denial, domestication, or obsession about death. And they urge a renewed understanding of the church's role both in caring for the dying and in shaping people who are prepared to die well.

SUGGESTIONS FOR FURTHER READING

Aries, Philippe. *Western Attitudes toward Death: From the Middle Ages to the Present,* trans. Patricia M. Ranum (Baltimore: Johns Hopkins University Press, 1974).

Bailey, Lloyd R., Sr. *Biblical Perspectives on Death* (Philadelphia: Fortress, 1979).

Bottum, Joseph. "All That Lives Must Die." *First Things* 63 (May 1996): 28-32.

Bresnahan, Jim. "Catholic Spirituality and Medical Interventions in Dying." *America* 164 (June 22-29, 1991): 670-75.

Cullmann, Oscar. "Immortality of the Soul or Resurrection of the Dead." In *Immortality and Resurrection,* ed. Krister Stendahl (New York: Macmillan, 1965).

Gunderman, Richard B. "What Can Medical Science Contribute to Theological Ethics? Musings on Mortality." In *Christian Ethics: Problems and Prospects,* ed. Lisa Sowle Cahill and James F. Childress (Cleveland: Pilgrim Press, 1996), pp. 152-65.

Guroian, Vigen. *Life's Living Toward Dying: A Theological and Medical-Ethical Study* (Grand Rapids: Eerdmans, 1996).

Jüngel, Eberhard. *Death: The Riddle and the Mystery* (Philadelphia: Westminster, 1974).

Kilner, John F., Arlene B. Miller, and Edmund D. Pellegrino, eds. *Dignity and Dying: A Christian Appraisal* (Grand Rapids: Eerdmans, 1996).

Meilaender, Gilbert. "'Apart and Not a Part': Death and Dignity." In *Caring Well,* ed. David H. Smith (Louisville: Westminster John Knox Press, 2000), pp. 239-54.

Oden, Thomas C. *Life in the Spirit,* vol. 3 of his *Systematic Theology* (Peabody: Prince Press; reprint by arrangement with HarperSanFrancisco, 1992, 1998), pp. 369-96.

Pannenberg, Wolfhart. *Systematic Theology* (Grand Rapids: Eerdmans, 1998), pp. 555-79.

Steinfels, Peter, and Robert M. Veatch, eds. *Death Inside Out* (New York: Harper & Row, 1975).

Swinton, John, and Richard Payne, eds., with a foreword by Stanley Hauerwas. *Living Well and Dying Faithfully: Christian Practices for End-of-Life Care* (Grand Rapids: Eerdmans, 2009).

Tolstoy, Leo. *The Death of Ivan Ilyich,* trans. Lynn Solotaroff (New York: Bantam, 1981).

Verhey, Allen. *The Christian Art of Dying: Learning from Jesus* (Grand Rapids: Eerdmans, 2011).

Westphal, Merold. *God, Guilt, and Death* (Bloomington: Indiana University Press, 1984).

4. Compare Guroian's metaphorical appeal to medicine here with George Khushf's discussion in Chapter One above of the analogical connection between medicine and Christian claims — "Illness, the Problem of Evil, and the Analogical Structure of Healing" (selection 3).

135 Psalm 88; Psalm 22; Romans 8:18-39; 1 Corinthians 15:20-26, 36-57

Psalm 88

A Song. A Psalm of the Korahites. To the leader: according to Mahalath Leannoth. A Maskil of Heman the Ezrahite.

O Lord, God of my salvation,
 when, at night, I cry out in your presence,
let my prayer come before you;
 incline your ear to my cry.

For my soul is full of troubles,
 and my life draws near to Sheol.
I am counted among those who go down to the Pit;
 I am like those who have no help,
like those forsaken among the dead,
 like the slain that lie in the grave,
like those whom you remember no more,
 for they are cut off from your hand.
You have put me in the depths of the Pit,
 in the regions dark and deep.
Your wrath lies heavy upon me,
 and you overwhelm me with all your waves.
  Selah

You have caused my companions to shun me;
 you have made me a thing of horror to them.
I am shut in so that I cannot escape;
 my eye grows dim through sorrow.
Every day I call on you, O Lord;
 I spread out my hands to you.
Do you work wonders for the dead?
 Do the shades rise up to praise you?
  Selah

Is your steadfast love declared in the grave,
 or your faithfulness in Abaddon?
Are your wonders known in the darkness,
 or your saving help in the land of forgetfulness?

But I, O Lord, cry out to you;
 in the morning my prayer comes before you.
O Lord, why do you cast me off?
 Why do you hide your face from me?
Wretched and close to death from my youth up,
 I suffer your terrors; I am desperate.
Your wrath has swept over me;
 your dread assaults destroy me.

They surround me like a flood all day long;
 from all sides they close in on me.
You have caused friend and neighbor to shun me;
 my companions are in darkness.

Psalm 22

To the leader: according to The Deer of the Dawn. A Psalm of David.

My God, my God, why have you forsaken me?
 Why are you so far from helping me, from the words
  of my groaning?
O my God, I cry by day, but you do not answer;
 and by night, but find no rest.

Yet you are holy,
 enthroned on the praises of Israel.
In you our ancestors trusted;
 they trusted, and you delivered them.
To you they cried, and were saved;
 in you they trusted, and were not put to shame.

But I am a worm, and not human;
 scorned by others, and despised by the people.
All who see me mock at me;
 they make mouths at me, they shake their heads;
"Commit your cause to the Lord; let him deliver —
 let him rescue the one in whom he delights!"

Yet it was you who took me from the womb;
 you kept me safe on my mother's breast.
On you I was cast from my birth,
 and since my mother bore me you have been
  my God.
Do not be far from me,
 for trouble is near
 and there is no one to help.

Many bulls encircle me,
 strong bulls of Bashan surround me;
they open wide their mouths at me,
 like a ravening and roaring lion.

I am poured out like water,
 and all my bones are out of joint;
my heart is like wax;
 it is melted within my breast;

my mouth is dried up like a potsherd,
and my tongue sticks to my jaws;
you lay me in the dust of death.

For dogs are all around me;
a company of evildoers encircles me.
My hands and feet have shriveled;
I can count all my bones.
They stare and gloat over me;
they divide my clothes among themselves,
and for my clothing they cast lots.

But you, O Lord, do not be far away!
O my help, come quickly to my aid!
Deliver my soul from the sword,
my life from the power of the dog!
Save me from the mouth of the lion!

From the horns of the wild oxen you have rescued me.
I will tell of your name to my brothers and sisters;
in the midst of the congregation I will praise you:
You who fear the Lord, praise him!
All you offspring of Jacob, glorify him;
stand in awe of him, all you offspring of Israel!
For he did not despise or abhor
the affliction of the afflicted;
he did not hide his face from me,
but heard when I cried to him.

From you comes my praise in the great congregation;
my vows I will pay before those who fear him.
The poor shall eat and be satisfied;
those who seek him shall praise the Lord.
May your hearts live forever!

All the ends of the earth shall remember
and turn to the Lord;
and all the families of the nations
shall worship before him.
For dominion belongs to the Lord,
and he rules over the nations.

To him, indeed, shall all who sleep in the earth bow down;
before him shall bow all who go down to the dust,
and I shall live for him.
Posterity will serve him;
future generations will be told about the Lord,
and proclaim his deliverance to a people yet unborn,
saying that he has done it.

Romans 8:18-39

I consider that the sufferings of this present time are not worth comparing with the glory about to be revealed to us. For the creation waits with eager longing for the revealing of the children of God; for the creation was subjected to futility, not of its own will but by the will of the one who subjected it, in hope that the creation itself will be set free from its bondage to decay and will obtain the freedom of the glory of the children of God. We know that the whole creation has been groaning in labor pains until now; and not only the creation, but we ourselves, who have the first fruits of the Spirit, groan inwardly while we wait for adoption, the redemption of our bodies. For in hope we were saved. Now hope that is seen is not hope. For who hopes for what is seen? But if we hope for what we do not see, we wait for it with patience.

Likewise the Spirit helps us in our weakness; for we do not know how to pray as we ought, but that very Spirit intercedes with sighs too deep for words. And God, who searches the heart, knows what is the mind of the Spirit, because the Spirit intercedes for the saints according to the will of God.

We know that all things work together for good for those who love God, who are called according to his purpose. For those whom he foreknew he also predestined to be conformed to the image of his Son, in order that he might be the firstborn within a large family. And those whom he predestined he also called; and those whom he called he also justified; and those whom he justified he also glorified.

What then are we to say about these things? If God is for us, who is against us? He who did not withhold his own Son, but gave him up for all of us, will he not with him also give us everything else? Who will bring any charge against God's elect? It is God who justifies. Who is to condemn? It is Christ Jesus, who died, yes, who was raised, who is at the right hand of God, who indeed intercedes for us. Who will separate us from the love of Christ? Will hardship, or distress, or persecution, or famine, or nakedness, or peril, or sword? As it is written,

"For your sake we are being killed all day long;
we are accounted as sheep to be slaughtered."

No, in all these things we are more than conquerors through him who loved us. For I am convinced that neither death, nor life, nor angels, nor rulers, nor things present, nor things to come, nor powers, nor height, nor depth, nor anything else in all creation, will be able to separate us from the love of God in Christ Jesus our Lord.

1 Corinthians 15:20-26, 36-57

But in fact Christ has been raised from the dead, the first fruits of those who have died. For since death came through a human being, the resurrection of the dead has also come through a human being; for as all die in Adam, so all will be made alive in Christ. But each in his own order: Christ the first fruits, then at his coming those who belong to Christ. Then comes the end, when he hands over the kingdom to God the Father, after he has destroyed every ruler and every authority and power. For he must reign until he has put all his enemies under his feet. The last enemy to be destroyed is death.

Fool! What you sow does not come to life unless it dies. And as for what you sow, you do not sow the body that is to be, but a bare seed, perhaps of wheat or of some other grain. But God gives it a body as he has chosen, and to each kind of seed its own body. Not all flesh is alike, but there is one flesh for human beings, another for animals, another for birds, and another for fish. There are both heavenly bodies and earthly bodies, but the glory of the heavenly is one thing, and that of the earthly is another. There is one glory of the sun, and another glory of the moon, and another glory of the stars; indeed, star differs from star in glory.

So it is with the resurrection of the dead. What is sown is perishable, what is raised is imperishable. It is sown in dishonor, it is raised in glory. It is sown in weakness, it is raised in power. It is sown a physical body, it is raised a spiritual body. If there is a physical body, there is also a spiritual body. Thus it is written, "The first man, Adam, became a living being"; the last Adam became a life-giving spirit. But it is not the spiritual that is first, but the physical, and then the spiritual. The first man was from the earth, a man of dust; the second man is from heaven. As was the man of dust, so are those who are of the dust; and as is the man of heaven, so are those who are of heaven. Just as we have borne the image of the man of dust, we will also bear the image of the man of heaven.

What I am saying, brothers and sisters, is this: flesh and blood cannot inherit the kingdom of God, nor does the perishable inherit the imperishable. Listen, I will tell you a mystery! We will not all die, but we will all be changed, in a moment, in the twinkling of an eye, at the last trumpet. For the trumpet will sound, and the dead will be raised imperishable, and we will be changed. For this perishable body must put on imperishability, and this mortal body must put on immortality. When this perishable body puts on imperishability, and this mortal body puts on immortality, then the saying that is written will be fulfilled:

> "Death has been swallowed up in victory."
> "Where, O death, is your victory?
> Where, O death, is your sting?"

The sting of death is sin, and the power of sin is the law. But thanks be to God, who gives us the victory through our Lord Jesus Christ.

136 Lament for a Son

Nicholas Wolterstorff

Standing on a hill in Galilee Jesus said to his disciples:

> Blessed are those who mourn,
> for they shall be comforted.

Blessings to those who mourn, cheers to those who weep, hail to those whose eyes are filled with tears, hats off to those who suffer, bottoms up to the grieving! How strange, how incredibly strange!

When you and I are left to our own devices, it's the smiling, successful ones of the world that we cheer. "Hail to the victors." The histories we write of the odyssey of humanity on earth are the stories of the exulting ones — the nations that won in battle, the businesses that defeated their competition, the explorers who found a pass to the Pacific, the scientists whose theories proved correct, the athletes who came in first, the politicians who won their campaigns. We turn away from the crying ones of the world. Our photographers tell us to smile.

"Blessed are those who mourn." What can it mean? One can understand why Jesus hails those who hunger and thirst for righteousness, why he hails the merciful, why he hails the pure in heart, why he hails the peacemakers, why he hails those who endure under persecution. These are qualities of character which belong to the life of the kingdom. But why does he hail the mourners of the world? Why cheer tears? It must be that mourning is also a quality of character that belongs to the life of his realm.

Who then are the mourners? The mourners are those who have caught a glimpse of God's new day, who ache with all their being for that day's coming, and who break out into tears when confronted with its absence. They are the ones who realize that in God's realm of peace there is no one blind and who ache whenever they see someone unseeing. They are the ones who realize that in God's realm there is no one hungry and who ache whenever they see someone starving. They are the ones who realize that in God's realm there is no one falsely accused and who ache whenever they see someone imprisoned unjustly. They are the ones who realize that in God's realm there is no one who fails to see God and who ache whenever they see someone unbelieving. They are the ones who realize that in God's realm there is no one who suffers oppression and who ache whenever they see some-

From Nicholas Wolterstorff, *Lament for a Son* (Grand Rapids: Eerdmans, 1987), pp. 84-86.

one beat down. They are the ones who realize that in God's realm there is no one without dignity and who ache whenever they see someone treated with indignity. They are the ones who realize that in God's realm of peace there is neither death nor tears and who ache whenever they see someone crying tears over death. The mourners are aching visionaries.

Such people Jesus blesses; he hails them, he praises them, he salutes them. And he gives them the promise that the new day for whose absence they ache will come. They will be comforted.

The Stoics of antiquity said: Be calm. Disengage yourself. Neither laugh nor weep. Jesus says: Be open to the wounds of the world. Mourn humanity's mourning, weep over humanity's weeping, be wounded by humanity's wounds, be in agony over humanity's agony. But do so in the good cheer that a day of peace is coming.

137 The Sacral Power of Death in Contemporary Experience

William F. May

Theological reflection on the subject of death usually has an air of unreality because it has no contact with death as it is actually experienced by men in its sacral power. This is especially true of theology in an age that likes to think of itself as secular without remainder. Presumably there are no religious realities left to contend with. Men are relatively self-sufficient and autonomous, blessedly free of the incubus of religion in all its forms. The gospel has only to address itself to a world-come-of-age, commanded and populated by secular men.

Theologians of the secular persuasion may be right when they attempt to free the gospel from its earlier, uncritical ties with religion, but they are wrong when they assume that religion is dead. While religions, in the sense of official historical traditions, may indeed have entered a period of decline, the experience of the sacred is still very much with us. Nowhere is this more apparent than in the contemporary experience of death. . . .

Death in Its Religious Reality

Pastors rarely approach the gravely ill without noticing immediately the evasions and the brave lies that encircle the dying. Doctors often refuse to inform the patient of his true condition in the case of a terminal illness. Needless to say, most families cooperate readily with the doctor and his instructions.

A heavy silence surrounds death. I believe that this painful reticence has a source more profound than our childlike submission to the advice of a doctor. For the instructions of a doctor would not hold for a minute if men felt they had recourse in their words and actions against death. In fact, where else except from the dying has the doctor himself learned his reticence? He has seen too many men avoid asking the big question about their illness. Or he has heard them ask the question without being certain that they really wanted an answer.

Despite some charges to the contrary (which I will discuss later), I do not think of the doctor as the villain of the piece in this conspiracy of silence. Silence has its origin in the awesomeness of death itself. Just as the Jew, out of re-

From *Social Research* 39 (Autumn 1972). Used by permission of the publisher and the author.

spect for the awesomeness of God, would not pronounce the name of Yahweh, so we find it difficult to bring the word *death* to our lips in the presence of its power. This is so because we are at a loss as to how to proceed on the far side of this word. Our philosophies and our moralities desert us. They retreat and leave us wordless. Their rhetoric, which seemed so suitable on other occasions, suddenly loses its power, and we may well wonder whether our words themselves are not caught up in a massive, verbose, uneasy flight from death, while we are left with nothing to say, except to "say it with flowers."

Without provision against death, our rituals and ceremonies are characterized by a powerful flight from its presence. This is a phenomenon that has already received savage treatment at the hands of satirists in the Anglo-Saxon world: Aldous Huxley, *After Many a Summer;* Muriel Spark, *Memento Mori;* Evelyn Waugh, *The Loved One;* and most recently, Jessica Mitford, *The American Way of Death.* Interestingly enough, all are English writers, and three of the four focus on the American attitude toward death. They are wrong, however, when they suggest that Americans believe in a triumph of technology over death by virtue of which they reduce death to the incidental or the unreal. Rites are evasive not because Americans react to death as trivial or incidental but because they feel an inner sense of bankruptcy before it. The attempts at evasion and concealment are pathetic rather than casual. The doctor's substitute diagnoses and vague replies and the undertaker's allusions to the "loved one" or to the "beautiful memory picture" reflect a culture in which men sense their own poverty before this event.

Men evade death because they recognize in the event an immensity that towers above their resources for handling it. In effect, death (or the reality that brings it) is recognized as some sort of sacred power that confounds the efforts of man to master it. James Joyce uses a particularly gloomy expression to convey this sense of death as sacred power in *Ulysses* — *"Dio Boia"* — the "Hangman God." Joyce happens to import the phrase into English literature from the Italian, but the reality of which he speaks crosses national boundaries — death recognized as the power before which all human efforts are ineffectual longings to no avail; death admitted as the reality that may have inspired philosophers to meditate but brings these meditations to their conclusion, that may have crowned the hero or martyr with renown but eventually drags into oblivion even those whom it has lifted up; death honored as the power that unravels every human community, taking those fervent little intersections of human want — husband and wife, lovers, father and son — and eventually forcing all these intersecting lines to honor its presence with the rigid parallels of the graveyard.

So understood, death is not merely a biological incident that ends human life. It reaches into the course of life, gripping the human heart with love, fear, hope, worry, and flight, long before the end itself is reached. Whenever the concert is over, the meal is digested, or the career turns barren in one's hands, a man experiences the quiet, disturbing fall from life to death. Because death is more than the incident of biological demise, it is difficult to do justice to its scope without falling into parody of the psalmist's sense of the omnipresence of God. For the power that brings death besets men on every side. It drives men from behind as they flee into frenetic activities — the pursuit of career, virtuosity, or the display of some glory — hoping to escape their metaphysical solitude by outlining themselves against a dark background. It confronts men frontally as they mount their battles against their threatening enemies, whether that enemy happens to be soldier, competition, or sibling. It lies in wait and ambushes from the side — the young, the high-minded, and the frivolous — with the unexpectedness of a clipping at a football game. It stirs beneath human life in the profoundest of pleasures, as it touches with melancholy the marriage bed or as it ladens with guilt the relations between the generations. And at night, it settles down from above and breathes gently within men who are weary with all other forms of fleeting, fighting, and sidestepping death and who long now for sleep and the surcease of care.

If, in some such fashion, men experience death as a religious reality, then one might expect the language of religion to describe most appropriately man's primordial attitude toward the onslaught of the event. This is in fact the language that Joyce chooses in the opening passage of the *Dubliners.* A young boy — friend to a dying priest — muses on the word "paralysis," and offers therein a fine description of religious awe. "Paralysis. . . . It sounded to me like the name of some maleficent and sinful being. It filled me with fear and yet I longed to be near it and to look upon its deadly work."[1] Joyce's description captures beautifully that ambivalence of spirit that the phenomenologists of religion have recognized in all religious feeling and which they have variously termed: "awe," "dread," "astonishment," "wonder," or "amazement." A peculiar ambivalence, a strange vibration, a sort of motionless motion obtains in the religious man, an attentiveness somewhat akin to the attention that a hummingbird gives to a flower, when its wings beat furiously and yet it hovers at the spot. This is the way men relate to death in its dreadful reality.

The analysis has uncovered so far two basic responses to the event of death in contemporary culture: concealment and obsession. Only the category of the sacred explains their connection. Men are tempted to conceal death or to hold themselves enthralled before it only because they recognize death as an overmastering power before which all other responses are unavailing.

Geoffrey Gorer, the English sociologist, in his essay "The Pornography of Death,"[2] brings together the phe-

1. James Joyce, *The Dubliners* (New York: The Modern Library, [1967]), p. 7.

2. Reprinted as an appendix in his book, *Death, Grief, and Mourning* (Garden City, N.Y.: Doubleday & Co., 1965).

nomena of obsession and concealment by appeal to the religious category of *taboo.* On the one hand, death is a taboo subject, the unmentionable event; on the other hand, death (and violence) is an obsession at every level of our culture. Gorer finds the solution to this oddity in a comparison with the Victorian attitude toward sex. A prudish culture in which personal sexual life is a taboo subject is also likely to develop simultaneously a pornographic obsession with sex. In contemporary culture, argues Gorer, the personal event of death has replaced sex as a taboo subject: Death has replaced copulation and birth as the unmentionable. At the same time, an obsession with violence has dominated our age. Concealment and obsession go together in the same culture.

The chief feature of pornography, of course, is an obsession with the sex-act abstracted from its normal human emotion which is love; the pornography of death therefore is an obsession with death abstracted from its natural human emotion which is grief. For the sake of his thesis Gorer might be altogether satisfied with the development of the James Bond movie. When the sexual act is abstracted from love it becomes somewhat repetitive and dull; therefore, pornographic literature rescues its readers from boredom by filling the fantasy with the sex-act performed in an endless variety of ways, each more elaborate or intense than the last. Interest is removed altogether from love to the technology of the act itself. Correspondingly, when death is abstracted from grief the same restless elaboration of technology occurs. It is difficult to maintain interest in the subject of death unless violence is done in a variety of ways. Thus technicians in violence have to equip James Bond with the ultimate in a death-dealing car that surpasses with exquisite ingenuity the death-dealing instruments that General Motors has already put on the road. And the makers of the movie *Thunderball* bring both lines of pornography to their absurd conclusion, inasmuch as lovemaking and murdering are somehow managed underwater.

The fascination with death in pornography and the concealment of death in the liturgies of polite society are both rooted in religious feeling. It is a religious enthrallment with death that eventuates in the strategies of helpless evasion in the homelike atmosphere of the funeral parlor and in the pornographic experimentations of the entertainment industry.

The traditional belief in the immortality of the soul does not seem to provide men with a sense of resource against the threat of death. In this respect the consciousness of the twentieth century has undergone a radical break with the recent Western past. Christian theologians from the Church Fathers through the Reformers of the sixteenth century held to a doctrine of the immorality of the soul. This doctrine was continued in an altered form by many theologians and philosophers (particularly those of idealist persuasion) in the eighteenth through the late nineteenth century. But today the situation has changed. Naturalists among the philosophers dismiss the doctrine of the immortality of the soul as just so much idealistic vaporing. Psychoanalysts interpret the longing for immortality as a perpetuation of infantile desires. Social critics have condemned the doctrine for its encouragement of an attitude of otherworldly indifference to social ills. Existentialists have opposed the doctrine because it distracts a man from his most essential task as an authentic human being: the appropriation of his own finitude and morality. Even modern biblical scholars have rejected the doctrine as they usually distinguish today between the primitive Christian hope of the resurrection of the body and the Hellenic-idealist doctrine of the immortality of the soul.

This is not to say that a belief in the immortality of the soul has had its defenders in Germany, England, America, and France. Dualists of the stripe of Unamuno have tried to reckon with the heart's longing for eternal life, along with the mind's crushing sense of death. Even existentialists, such as Marcel, have made appeal to the existence of a beloved community that transcends the empirical order of death. Finally, and somewhat less grandly, the ordinary man likes to think of himself as immortal, or at least, invulnerable. Tolstoy has observed[3] that the passion for finding out the "cause" of someone else's death is a way of satisfying oneself that the other fellow died accidentally or fortuitously by virtue of special circumstances affecting him (but not me). This shabby impulse, however, is hardly a serious expression of the traditional confidence in the immortality of the soul. Rather, it is the hedonist's inveterate bargaining for a little more time in which to dawdle over just one more last cigarette.

Despite traces of contemporary belief in the immortality of the soul, the minister is ill advised to rely on it in the presence of death. Nowhere is the bankruptcy of the doctrine so evident as in a certain type of Protestant funeral service in which the minister strains to give the impression that the person "lives on" in the trappings of the service itself. The minister disastrously seeks to "personalize" the service, not by simple reference to the name and biography of the deceased, but by including his alleged favorite hymns, poems, prayers, and songs. We are supposed to have the impression that we are in the presence of a kind of *aurora borealis* of the dead man's personality, shimmering miraculously in the darkest hour of grief. Instead, however, the minister gives the sad impression that he has a repertory of three or four such "personalized" services, designed like Sears Roebuck seat covers to fit any and all makes and models of cars. Its ill-fitting imposition upon the dead man only reminds us ever so forcibly and comfortlessly that he is, indeed, dead.

3. Leo Tolstoy, *The Death of Ivan Ilyich* (New York: Boni and Liveright), p. 8. See also Sigmund Freud, "Thoughts for the Times on War and Death," *Collected Papers,* Vol. IV, 1915, trans. Joan Riviere (London: The Hogarth Press, 1925), p. 305.

Theological Reflection on Death

The attempt to cover up death in the funeral service is an unmitigated disaster for the church, preceded and prepared for by the church's failure to reckon with death in its own preaching and pastoral life. Many persons have said that they have never heard their minister take up frontally in a sermon the question of their own dying. This state of affairs, once again, is not entirely the fault of the professional. People tend to expect from the church service an hour's relief from the demons that plague them in the course of the week. In this atmosphere sermons on death would seem intrusive and unsettling. Better to avoid them and protect this hour from everything that jangles the nerves — even though the service comes to an end and the demons must be faced once again on Monday, fully intact, unexorcized, and screeching. The melancholic effect of this arrangement is that the church offers a temporary sanctuary, a momentary respite, from one's secret apprehensions about death, but inevitably they take over once again, without so much as a candid word of comfort intervening.

To preach about death is absolutely essential if Christians are to preach with joy. Otherwise they speak with profound melancholy of men who have separated the church from the graveyard. They make the practical assumption that there are two Lords. First, there is the Lord of the Sabbath, the God who presides over the affairs of cheerful Philistines while they are still thriving and in good health. Then there is a second Lord, a Dark Power about whom one never speaks, the Lord of highways, wrecks, hospitals, and graveyards who handles everything in the end. Under the circumstances, there can be no doubt as to which of the two Lords is the more commanding power. The death-bringer God already encroaches upon the sanctuary itself, inasmuch as people gathered there are so unsettled as to refuse to hear of his name.

The Christian faith, however, does not speak of two parallel Lords. The Lord of the church is not ruler of a surface kingdom. His dominion is nothing if it does not go at least six feet deep. The church affirms the one Lord who went down into the grave, fought a battle with the power of death, and by his own death brought death to an end. For this reason the church must be unafraid to speak of death. It is compelled to speak of death as the servant of Jesus Christ, the Crucified and Risen Savior, who has freed men from the power of the Unmentionable One.

But even when the church speaks about the subject, does the church evade it? Is theological reflection on the subject of death itself a method of circumlocution? Existentialism, after all, from Kierkegaard to Heidegger, has made men sensitive to the way in which objective discourse on the subject of death may be a way of escaping from one's own personal destiny as a creature who dies. Camus has condemned Christian thought on the subject of death for placing, in effect, theological screens before the eyes of the condemned.[4] Apparently the Christian hope of eternal life only serves to divert attention from the stark condition of life in the flesh. "The order of the world is shaped by death," says one of the heroes of *The Plague*.[5]

At the outset, then, by way of reply, it must be argued that Christian reflection, far from screening death from view, actually tears away the screens and forces men to look at death and to look toward their own dying. This is an unavoidable focus of a faith that has to reckon with the factual dying of its Savior. Even if men wanted to avoid death, they cannot if they look toward such a savior. In fact, he exposes the flimsiness of the partitions that men raise in order not to have to consider death. The purpose of this comment is not to outdo the existentialist in pessimism but to lay the only sure basis for Christian hope, a hope that is not based on screens, mirrors, or sentiment. It is based on the good news that men do not have to go beyond Jesus for a knowledge of death in its fullest scope; death is not an additional realm alongside of Jesus terrorizing men from the side.

Death in Jesus

In the light of Jesus Christ it is possible to explore the scope of death as it threatens a man in his three most fundamental identities as a human being. Death threatens a man's identity with his flesh, with his community, and with his God. (Insofar as the doctrine of the immortality of the soul abstracted the question of future life from these three fundamental identities, it tended to offer an impoverished if not ghostly sense of future existence.)

A man is clearly identified with his flesh. He is not a ghost. The body is more important to his identity than words to a poet. He both controls his world and savors his world, and reveals himself to others, in and through the living flesh. Part of the terror of death is that it threatens a man with a loss of identity with his flesh, an identity which is essential to him in at least these three ways.

First, man's flesh is the means to his control of his world. Except as he uses his flesh instrumentally (feet for walking, hands for working, tongue for talking) he could not relate to the world by way of mastery and control. When death therefore threatens to separate him from his flesh, it threatens him first with a comprehensive loss of possession and control of his universe. Death meets him as the dispossessor (Luke 12:15-21), even though he retaliates as best he can against his loss of control with an assortment of insurance policies. Quite shrewdly the medieval moralists saw a special connection between the

4. "In Italian museums are sometimes found little painted screens that the priest used to hold in front of the face of condemned men to hide the scaffold from them." Albert Camus, *The Myth of Sisyphus and Other Essays.*

5. Albert Camus, *The Plague,* trans. Stewart Gilbert (London: Hamish Hamilton, 1948), p. 123.

capital sin of avarice and old age. Avarice is the special sin in which a man focuses his life on his possessions. The closer a man gets to the time of his dispossession, the more fiercely he clings to what he has and the more suspicion he feels toward all those who would dispossess him with indecorous haste.

Second, a man's flesh is more than instrumental, it is also the site for the disclosure of the world to him, the world which he will never be able to reduce to property but which is there for the savoring. Except that flesh is sensitive, susceptible, and vulnerable, a man could not be open to the world as it pours in upon him in a wild profusion of colors, sounds, and feelings. He could not fall under the spell of powers that both enchant and terrify him. When death therefore threatens to separate him from flesh, it threatens also to separate him from the propertyless creation, the world which he may not control but which is his for the beholding in ritual, art, and daily routine.[6]

Third, flesh is more instrumental than and more sensitive to the world; it is also revelatory. A man reveals himself to his neighbor in and through the living flesh. He is inseparable from his countenance, gestures, and the physical details of his speech. Part of the terror of death, then, is that it threatens him with a loss of his revelatory power. The dreadfulness of the corpse lies in its claim to be the body of the person, while it is wholly unrevealing of the person. What was once so expressive of the human soul has suddenly become a mask.

We have referred to the *threat* of separation from the flesh in each case not only because a man can anticipate it before it occurs, but also because this separation does not occur all at once. It is shocking to encounter a young man who is dying and recognize a spirit that is still alive with its original power and promise while the flesh abandons it. Or again it is possible to look upon the aged whose spirits have long since absented themselves while their bodies persist so mindlessly alive.

Part of the melancholy of this loss of identity is no frontal assault can be launched against it. The fear of death only intensifies insofar as a man plunges deeper into his possessions as a way of securing himself against the day of his dispossession, or gives himself over to the frenetic carnivals of a death-ridden age as a way of savoring his world, or takes daily inventory of his physical appearance in the quest ceremonies before the morning mirror.

Death not only threatens a man with separation from the flesh; it also tears him away from his community. This threat has already been anticipated in the discussion of the revelatory power of the flesh. Death means the unraveling of human community. It divides husband and wife, father and son, and lovers from one another. Not even the child is exempt from this threat. In demanding the reassurance of a voice, the touch of a hand at bedtime, he shows that he knows all the essential issues involved in a sleep that is early practice in dying. Death threatens all men with final separation, exclusion, and oblivion. And again, this threat is operative beforehand, as the fear of oblivion can prompt men to force their way into the society of others in ways which are ultimately self-isolating.

But death also threatens men with separation from God. This is the terror of death that men have never fully faced because they have never wholly honored the presence of God. But it is the terror of which all others are but prologue and sign. Men fear separation from their flesh because they know life in and through their flesh. They fear separation from community because they know life in and through their community. But what are these compared with separation from God, who is the source of life in the flesh and life in the community? This question remains partly rhetorical for all men inasmuch as they do not know fully what they ask. But it was the last question on the lips of the One whom Christians worship and adore in his cry of abandonment from the cross.

Jesus knew death in all its dimensions. The creed puts it: He "suffered under Pontius Pilate, was crucified, dead and buried; he descended into Hell." His death, like others, meant separation from the flesh. The narratives are utterly factual in detail about his ordeal in the flesh. He suffered dispossession: the king with no subjects, the teacher with no pupils, the healer who bleeds. He suffered severance from the world, reduced as it was to a sop of vinegar, the darkness of the sixth hour, and a spear in his side; and he, like all other men before and after him, suffered the final conclusion of his life in the unrevealing corpse.

His death meant also separation from community. One can see this separation at work beforehand in the persecution of the high priest, the ambiguities of the Roman governor, the fickleness of the crowds, the betrayal of Judas, the cowardice of Peter, and the sleepiness of followers in Gethsemane. It was consummated in his burial when he, like all other men, was removed from sight.

Finally Jesus experienced what men know only through him: separation from God. The Son of God cries out, "My God, my God, why hast thou forsaken me?" The Son of God descends into the region that stands under the naked terror of the absence of God and stands fast there for every man.

Because the Son of God has done this, the Christian cannot be content simply to tell horror stories about the ravaging power of death. If in looking toward Jesus, he looks toward death in its full terror and power, so also he

6. Karl Rahner has argued that the severance of a man from his flesh may mean not the loss of a world but rather a release of the soul from the more restricted world it knows in the flesh to an all-cosmic relationship that transcends the limitations of life within the province of a body. Even so Rahner must admit that this eventuality, if it be our destiny, is precisely the future which death, in its darkness, obscures. As we know it now, death threatens to separate us from the flesh and so banish us from that sight through which the world is disclosed. See Karl Rahner, *On the Theology of Death,* pp. 29ff.

looks toward the Savior who exposes death in its ultimate powerlessness. No final power remains to death, if death itself has become the event in which Jesus exposes the powerfulness of God's love. Death can still menace, but it can no longer make good on its threats. In Jesus' death, God, flesh, and community are indissolubly met in self-expending love. For this reason, it is no longer necessary to stare in the mirror, worrying about the defeat of one's flesh, or to plunge into communities, worried about exclusion at their hands, or to lift up one's eyes to heaven, attempting in a blind fury of good works to force the presence of God. For the Savior who is identified, soul and body, with men in his descent is the one who remains their Lord in his ascent, to bring men new life — bodily, together, in the presence of God.

Life in Jesus

Usually when a man asks the question of eternal life, he wonders simply whether he will continue to live beyond the grave. Putting the question this way, he assumes that a human being can be separated from his ties with his flesh, community, and God. This is the assumption by virtue of which the doctrine of the immortality of the soul, in some of its versions, actually led to an impoverishment of the notion of eternal life. Eternal life, in effect, became an eternalization of death, as the soul projected itself endlessly into the future — deprived of everything that formerly made it jubilant with life. Cut off from its ties with its flesh, community, and God, the soul so imagined is spectral and wraith-like. Its daydreams about the future have turned into ghoul-ridden nightmares.

The Risen Christ, however, cuts through the nonsense of these daydreams about eternity with the sharp actuality of his life. He is not ghoulishly divested of a body; on the contrary, he shows himself to his disciples, his flesh still bearing the marks of his crucifixion. He is not banished from community like a spook (whose appearance always causes men to scatter and run); on the contrary, his appearance among men is such as to establish and nourish human community. Neither is he grievously separated from God; the account of his resurrection is followed by the acknowledgment of his ascension. This testimony to the ascension of Christ excludes the fantasy of a ghostly Savior drifting in the netherworld between God and men. His proximity to God, in turn ("at the right hand of the Father"), is at the basis of his power to create a full-bodied life for his community among men.

Correspondingly, the eternal life that Jesus imparts to men is neither spectral nor rootless. Jesus extends to men the specific hope of future life in the body. "We wait for adoption as sons, the redemption of our bodies" (Rom. 8:23). Wholly consistent with this promise of a glorified body is the apostolic assurance of a new heaven and a new earth to which the body gives access. Man is not destined to live on perpetually in the tedium of a worldless "I." Neither however will he live on in isolation from his fellow. Jesus imparts eternal life to him through a community. As Ephesians puts it, "God . . . made us alive together in Christ" (2:4, 5). The word "together" in the passage does not convey the incidental bit of intelligence that others beside oneself are involved in the resurrection, as though men were like strangers, temporarily herded together to receive a fortune from a benefactor whom each knew in his private way. Rather God creates in the community of disciples a freedom for each other that would not be there except through participation in his life.

Finally eternal life means bodily life, together, in the *presence* of God. Resurrection means intimacy with God. Jesus says to the thief on the cross, "Today you will be with me in paradise" (Luke 23:43). The Christian hope is not simply for a deathless, endless life in which relations between a man, his body, and his neighbor have been set in order. To center hope on a perfected world alone is eschatological atheism. If God exists, eternal life cannot be defined apart from his presence. Without him the perfection of this world would be like the sterile order of a house that a woman kept immaculate for no other end than its own tidiness, as though she did not desire the presence of her husband. As in the humblest of marriages the vital presence of the husband belongs to the joy of the house, so the presence of God fills out the joy of heaven.

Eternal life is the future destiny of man, but participation in this life is not reserved to the future alone. Just as death is not simply an event at the end of life but overtakes men by way of fear, worry, and disease in the present moment, so also the resurrection is not an event wholly reserved for the other side of the grave. Men can live now in the power of the resurrection. Surely the martyr faced death with hope in his heart for the future glory, yet he did so in the present enabling power of the resurrection. Otherwise the fullness of God fills only the future, fills only the far side, powerless finally to redeem the present and powerless to sustain men in the agony of dying itself. Men can look forward to the coming ages of his kindness toward them because he stands with them already on this side of the grave.

The fact of the resurrection of Christ, however, does not mean that the Christian is altogether removed from the experience of natural grief and sorrow. Were it otherwise, the Christian should be able to face his own death without a tremor, and he should be able to walk confidently into the sickroom, contending with its silence by "talking up" a victory that has not yet, apparently, reached the ears of those who await an imminent defeat. This is a professional Christian cheerfulness, a grisly boy-scoutism, for which there is no justification in Scripture. The apostle Paul expressed himself carefully: Only "when this corruptible *shall* have put on incorruption . . . *shall* there come to pass the saying that is written, Death is swallowed up in victory" (I Cor. 15:54, italics added). The Christian knows grief in this life. He is not granted on this side of the grave a pure, steadfast, confident, and transparent sense of his limits — or the limits of his neighbor — before God. He tastes of eternal life in Christ, but not a life that removes him from death and the sting of death. The work of death is still very much evident in the inner and the outer man. Death remains the last enemy. Not until the gift of life beyond the limit has been granted to man is it possible for him to say wholeheartedly:

> "O Death, where is thy victory?
> O Death, where is thy sting?"

This death does not mean, however, that nothing of importance has occurred. Although the Christian does not yet know an eternal life without death, he has reckoned in Christ with an eternal life under the conditions of death, that permits him to live hopefully in the crisis of his neighbor's death and his own. This is the basis for the witness of the church to the dying.

The Church's Behavior Toward the Dying

Let it be said at the outset that the church cannot act as though it possesses something that the dying lack. A demoralizing feature of illness for any patient is the condescending cheerfulness of nurses and friends, whose very display of good health reminds the mortally ill that they are about to be dispossessed of their world. The church cannot behave in such a way as to add yet another possession, i.e., Christian hope, that distinguishes the Christian from the unbeliever or the sorely tried believer who is mortally ill.

This consideration, however, produces an oddity. Does the Christian somehow have to assume the *unreality* of the resurrection in order to avoid removing himself from his fellowman? Must he ignore the resurrection so as not to appear like a self-assured Christ-dispenser in the sickroom? Does he find himself saying, in effect, that the resurrection has taken place but that its fruits are a long way off for all of us and therefore nothing has occurred that need disturb the humanity of my response to your illness and imminent death?

Actually, the reverse is the case. It is precisely in the absence of a sense of the resurrection that the Christian is tempted to think solely in terms of those possessions he has to offer the sick. He makes the painful assumption that he must be a God-producer, a Christ-dispenser, or a religious magician in the sickroom. Failing miserably, of course, at all these roles, he feels keenly his poverty. He makes a lame effort to produce the decisive and healing word, only to stutter and to fall silent. In the absence of a sense of resurrection he feels the terrifying lack of a gift between himself and the dying, a frightening guilt of silence between them. He is inclined therefore with every healthy fiber of his being to shy away from the dying to avoid his own poverty.

The resurrection of Christ frees a man for approach to the dying not because it arms him with a possession to give, but because it frees him from all this worry and confusion about possessions. Christ is already the decisive gift between the living and the dying, the mediator between them. There is no need to produce Christ in the sickroom when he is already there in advance of a man's approach. The Christian is mercifully free, therefore, to offer whatever secondary gifts he can — of anxiety, suffering, money, words, friendship, and hope — letting them be, whenever possible, signs of a divine love which they do not produce.

The Church's Witness and Separation from the Flesh

It is angelism to assume that the sole witness of the church to the dying and the bereaved is the testimony of theology alone. A ministry to the flesh is a true and valid ministry. It need not be supposed that Christian witness is invariably something more than this. Admittedly the apparatus of medicine — doctors, nurses, and sanitary hospitals — can function as a shield behind which the larger community of health protects itself from contact with the dying. But this need not be the case. There is no reason why the machinery of modern medicine — awesome and impersonal though it is — may not yet serve human purposes and therefore function as a sign of a life that exceeds its own powers to heal. To do this, however, some sensitivity must be shown toward the several crises that a man experiences in his flesh.

It was noted earlier that sickness and death involve a traumatic loss of control over one's world. A man who has brutally exploited his body as an instrument of aggression against his world suddenly suffers a heart attack. The very flesh through which he exercised mastery suddenly explodes from within. He is helpless in the hands of others, unable even to control disturbing noises down the hall. Under these circumstances the apparatus of medicine can be frightening; it demonstrates to him his helplessness and therefore reminds him of the poverty of all his attempts to solve the problem of his existence through mastery alone. The machinery of medicine thus assumes the terrifying shape of a parable of judgment. It brings his past life to naught. At the same time, however, the apparatus of medicine can be a testimony to grace. It does after all serve the body; and in this it can be a mute sign of the Lord whose mastery took the form of life-giving and life-comforting service. Seen in this light, it is the special task of the church not to ignore the work of medicine as a sub-Christian activity but to accompany and to criticize it in such a way as to help it to serve this end of service.

The second crisis for the flesh is the loss of the world in its uncontrolled splendor and diversity. A toothache has a way of reducing the world to itself. Unfortunately, the apparatus of medicine, dedicated as it is to the medical recovery of the patient, presents the hospitalized patient with a functional but blank and abstract environment, devoid of the irrelevant details that make up a truly human existence. (Yeats once registered his complaint against the scientific formula H_2O by observing, "I like a little seaweed in my definition of water.") Many European hospitals admirably manage to maintain gardens as part of their grounds. A functionally irrelevant expense, perhaps, in an institution dedicated to treating and discharging people as fast as it can, but some patients, after all, are discharged for burial, and it is well to maintain a sign for them of a world that has not shrunk to the final abstraction of their irremediable pain.

The third crisis for the flesh is the imminent loss of its revelatory power. The falterings of the body in old age increasingly prevent it from being expressive of the soul in its full dignity. There is warrant here for a sensitive ministry to the body in its infirmities which extends to the humblest of details in the daily routines of eating and cleansing. Upon death, moreover, there is warrant for a funeral service in which the body is not treated as a disposable cartridge to be thrown away like garbage. This argument for a fitting disposal of the remains, however, is hardly an apology for present-day funeral practice. Quite the contrary, it opens the way for an even more savage criticism of these practices. Precisely because the body has been (and will be) what it is only by the power of God to glorify it, it cannot become in Christian practice a lewd object of the mortician's craft. It is one thing for the mortician to minimize the violence done to the body by death, but it is quite another thing for him to impose upon the deceased the suggestion of a character other than its own. Only too often today Uncle John is not allowed to die. He must be prettied up with rouge on his cheeks and his casket opened so that his friends can see his face forced into a smile. Poor Uncle John never smiled in his life, but now he does — beatifically. It is not only the beautification of Uncle John, but his beatification that one attempts to achieve. The church won't canonize him but the mortician will. One is supposed to go to the funeral parlor, look on the face of the corpse, and say about Uncle John, "Doesn't he look natural?" which, of course, is the one thing he does not look. Let death be death. There is no reason to add to its hideousness by mocking the inability of the dead to reveal themselves.

The Witness of the Church and Separation from Community

One of the most devastating features of terminal illness is the fear of abandonment.[7] Sickness has already isolated the patient from his normal identity in the community. Strong and authoritative, he is now relatively helpless; gregarious by nature, he suddenly finds friends exhausting. Ironically the very apparatus by which the community ministers to his physical need isolates him further. The modern hospital segregates the sick and the dying from their normal human resources. One doctor has observed that in an Arabian village a grandmother dies in the midst of her children and grandchildren, cows and donkeys. But our high level of technological developments leads simply to dying a death appropriate to one's disease — in the heart ward or the cancer ward.[8]

Most desolating of all is the breakdown of communication between the dying patient, the doctor, and the nearest of kin. Substitute diagnoses are sometimes justified on the grounds that they establish an emotional equilibrium (homeostasis) essential to the health and comfort of the patient, but this justification ignores the fact that evasiveness can itself be emotionally disturbing. It is demoralizing for everybody concerned to get stuck with a lie, because, once told, life tends to organize itself around it. Even when the lie isn't working, even when it produces the anguish of suspicion, isolation, and uncertainty, the doctor may rely on it to keep his own relation to the patient in a state of equilibrium. Homeostasis, in other words, is a problem not only for the patient but also for the doctor and for the family. The family also grows accustomed to the explanation and enmeshes itself more deeply in the demands of make-believe. It seems too late for everybody concerned to recover an authentic relationship to the event. Isolated by evasion and lies, the patient is driven out of community before his time. He has forced upon him a premature burial. While trying to avoid the fact of death, the community actually reeks of death, for it has already excluded him.

It would be wrong, however, to make the doctor the scapegoat here and therefore to underestimate woefully the problems of sharing the truth. This was the mistake of a group of psychiatrists in the previously referred to study of *Death and Dying: Attitudes of Patient and Doctor*.[9] The psychiatrists reported that 69 to 90 percent of physicians (depending on the specific study) were not in favor of informing the patient in cases of mortal illness. Meanwhile on the basis of their own interviews with patients, the psychiatrists reported that approximately 82 percent of patients in terminal cases actually wanted to be informed of their true condition. Several psychiatrists explained this discrepancy between the apparent desire of patients and the actual performance of doctors by appeal to the psychological defects of doctors or to faults in their training: (1) they are more afraid of death than other professional groups; (2) they shy away from dealing with chronic and terminal cases because such cases are a blow to the doctor's professional self-esteem; (3) they receive inadequate preparation in medical school for coping with the problem of handling terminal cases.

7. "The dying patient faces emotional problems of great magnitude, including fear of death itself, fear of the ordeal of dying and the devastating fear of abandonment." See Ruth D. Abrams, M.S., "The Patient with Cancer — His Changing Pattern of Communication," *New England Journal of Medicine,* Vol. 274, No. 6, p. 320.

8. Bryant M. Wedge, in discussion at the conclusion of a symposium on *Death and Dying: Attitudes of Patient and Doctor,* sponsored by the Group for the Advancement of Psychiatry, Symposium No. 11, Vol. V.

9. See especially the essay by Herman Feifel, "The Function of Attitudes Toward Death," Ch. V in *Death and Dying: Attitudes of Patient and Doctor,* pp. 633-37.

Doubtless, all these observations are valid in given instances, but I found the psychiatrists breathtakingly naïve in the evidence they accepted as proof that patients really want to know the truth. First, it is not clear that patients are so willing to talk about the possibility — or the inevitability — of their own death *with their own doctor*, as the percentages reported by the psychiatrists in their interviews with patients would indicate. Dr. Samuel Feder indirectly admitted this fact when he observed that "all . . . patients, when they were asked to see me as a 'new doctor,' reacted with great anxiety."[10] All but two of the patients, however, were delighted to discover that he was "only" a psychiatrist. He admits that this was a unique experience for him as a psychiatrist. Obviously patients were glad that "he was not one of those other doctors — those other doctors being the bearers of bad tidings."

Dr. Feder interpreted these anxiety reactions as proof that people knew that they were going to die. Therefore the doctors had no excuse for avoiding the subject. I interpret them, however, as proof that these people were frightened of hearing just this verdict from their own doctors. The doctor in charge is less approachable on this subject precisely because he is the keeper of desolate truths. By the same token, the psychiatrist is more accessible since he brings no final verdict. If this analysis is correct, then the doctor's reticence to discuss the subject cannot be written off solely as a question of his own fear of death or his oversensitive, professional self-esteem. The sacral dimensions of death are too awesome to admit of easy professional solution. The problem of isolation cannot be solved by handing out truth like pills since the truth itself can have a disturbing and an isolating effect.

Yet there are ways in which people can reach out to one another in word and actions and maintain some measure of solidarity before the overwhelming event of death. It would be pretentious to outline these ways since they are not fully given to men except in the concrete case. Nevertheless it is possible to clarify (and perhaps even to clear the way of) certain obstacles that men face in their behavior toward the dying. They divide very simply into those of word and deed.

The Problem of Words

Perhaps we are especially inhibited in our talk with the dying because the alternatives in language seem so poor. There are several types of discourse available to us: (1) direct, immediate, blunt talk; (2) circumlocution or double-talk; (3) silence (which can be, of course, a mode of sharing, but oftentimes, is a way of evading); and (4) discourse that proceeds by way of indirection.

Too often we assume (especially as Americans) that the only form of truth-telling is direct, immediate, blunt talk. Such talk seems to be the only alternative to evasive silence or circumlocution On the subject of sex, for example, we assume that the only alternative to the repressions of a Victorian age is the tiresome, gabby explicit discussion of sex we impose upon the adolescent from junior high forward. So also on the subject of death we assume that truth-telling requires something approaching the seminar in loquacity. But obviously gabby bluntness in the presence of one dying is wholly inappropriate. It reckons in no way with the solemnity of the event. To plead for the explicit discussion of diagnosis or prognosis with every patient in clinical detail would be foolhardy. But the alternative to blunt talk need not be double-talk, a condescending cheerfulness, or a frightening silence. There is such a thing as *indirect* discourse in both love and death.

Perhaps examples of what I mean by indirection will suffice. One doctor reports that many patients instinctively brought up the question of their own death in an indirect form. Some asked him, for example, whether he thought they should buy a house, marry, or have plastic surgery done to their face. The doctor realized that the answer, "Yes, surely, go ahead — " in a big, cheerful voice was an evasion. Meanwhile the answer, "No," was a summary reply which would have made further discussion impossible. He found it important, however, to convey to them somehow that he recognized the importance of the question. From that point on, it was possible to discuss their uncertainties, anxieties, and fears. Some kind of sharing could take place. It was not necessary to dwell on the subject for long; after its acknowledgment it was possible to proceed to the details of daily life without the change of subject seeming an evasion.

Indirection may be achieved in another way. Although it may be too overbearing to approach the subject of death frontally under the immediate pressure of its presence, a kind of indirection can be achieved if death is discussed in advance of a crisis. The minister who suddenly feels like a tongue-tied irrelevancy in the sickroom gets what he deserves if he has not worked through the problem with his people in a series of sermons or in work sessions with lay groups. Words too blunt and inappropriate in the crisis itself may, if spoken earlier, provide an indirect basis for sharing burdens.

The language of indirection is appropriate behavior because, as it has been argued throughout, death is a sacred event. For the most part, toward the sacred the most fitting relation is indirect. The Jew did not attempt to look straight on Yahweh's face. A direct, immediate, casual confrontation was impossible. But avoidance of God's presence was not the only alternative. It was given to the Jew to hold his ground before his Lord in a relation that was genuine but indirect. So also, it is not necessary to dwell directly on the subject of death interminably or to avoid it by a condescending cheerfulness wholly inappropriate to the event. It is possible for two human beings to acknowledge death, be it ever so indirectly, and to hold their ground before it until they are parted.

10. Samuel L. Feder, "Attitudes of Patients with Advanced Malignancy," Chap. III in *Death and Dying: Attitudes of Patient and Doctor*, pp. 614-20.

The Problem of Action

Deeds are no easier to come by than words in extremity. Everyone grows uneasy. When nothing is left to be done toward the dying, a man is inclined to pay his respects, look at his watch, and fish out an excuse that fetches him home. Perhaps, however, our discomfort stems partly from a view of action somewhat inappropriate to overwhelming events. T. S. Eliot once said that there are two types of problems we face in life. In one case, the appropriate question is: what are we going to do about it? In the other case: how do we behave toward it? The deeper problems in life are of the latter kind.

But unfortunately as Americans, and especially as Americans in those professions that get tinged with a slight messianic pretension — medicine and the minister — we are used to tackling problems in terms of the first question, and are left somewhat bereft, therefore, when that question is inappropriate to the crisis. If all we can say is, What are we going to do about it?, then the dying indeed (and our own death) is a fatal blow to professional self-esteem. But this is not the only question we can ask ourselves in crisis. In extremity it may not be possible to do something about a tragedy, but this inability need not altogether disable our behavior toward it.

The Witness of the Church and the Threat of Separation from God

Since this is the threat in which the name of God appears, it is assumed that the special witness of the church in this case is theology. It may indeed be theology — but neither invariably nor exclusively so and certainly not theology conceived as a series of truths that provide men with access to God while putting them at a comforting distance from the sting of death. Such a theology, while trying to screen death from view, would only succeed in shielding men from the presence of God. For who is God as the Christian knows him? He is the God and Father of Jesus Christ, crucified and risen from the dead. Possessed by Jesus Christ, the church is not removed from the sting of existence come to an end. Rather it lives by a concrete existence that cuts into death with all the power of God's love to make death itself the very instance of that love. Because this is the case, the church cannot shield death from view without seeking — foolishly — to place theological screens before the eyes of the redeemed.

The witness of the church to the presence of God is not always direct and verbal. This fact has already been anticipated in our discussion of death. Just as an authentic acknowledgment of death can take place within the limits of indirect discourse, so also an authentic witness to Jesus Christ can occur without the inevitable footnote giving reference to his name. The Christian sense of the presence of God can express itself indirectly in the way in which the Christian responds to other levels of crisis. The calm with which he offers friendship in crisis may count for more than theological virtuosity in testifying to God's presence. The worry with which he offers advice will reveal more than the advice itself when he is really stricken with a sense of God's absence. But even in the case of failure he cannot, with Christian consistency, take his failure too seriously. God is the ultimate presence in death, whether men succeed in testifying to him or not. Neither life, nor death, nor the failure of Christians, will be able to separate men from the love of God. This is the message of Rom. 8 and the substance of Christian witness. When the church fails by its words and deeds to make this witness to the dying, let the dying among her members be brave enough to make this witness to the church.

138 The Indignity of "Death with Dignity"

Paul Ramsey

Never one am I to use an ordinary title when an extraordinary one will do as well! Besides, I mean to suggest that there is an additional insult besides death itself heaped upon the dying by our ordinary talk about "death with dignity." Sometimes that is said even to be a human "right"; and what should a decent citizen do but insist on enjoying his rights? That might be his duty (if there is any such right) to the commonwealth, to the human race or some other collective entity; or at least, embracing that "right" and dying rationally would exhibit a proper respect for the going concept of a rational man. So "The Indignity of Death" would not suffice for my purposes, even though all I shall say depends on understanding the contradiction death poses to the unique worth of an individual human life.

The genesis of the following reflections may be worth noting. A few years ago,[1] I embraced what I characterized as the oldest morality there is (no "new morality") concerning responsibility toward the dying: the acceptance of death, stopping our medical interventions for all sorts of good, human reasons, *only* companying with the dying in their final passage. Then suddenly it appeared that altogether too many people were agreeing with me. That caused qualms. As a Southerner born addicted to lost causes, it seemed I now was caught up in a triumphal social trend. As a controversialist in ethics, I found agreement from too many sides. As a generally happy prophet of the doom facing the modern age, unless there is a sea change in norms of action, it was clear from these premises that anything divers people agree to must necessarily be superficial if not wrong.

Today, when divers people draw the same warm blanket of "allowing to die" or "death with dignity" close up around their shoulders against the dread of that cold night, their various feet are showing. Exposed beneath our growing agreement to that "philosophy of death and dying" may be significantly different "philosophies of life"; and in the present age that agreement may reveal that these interpretations of human life are increasingly mundane, naturalistic, and antihumanistic when measured by *any* genuinely "humanistic" esteem for the individual human being.

These "philosophical" ingredients of any view of death and dying I want to make prominent by speaking of "The Indignity of 'Death with Dignity.'" Whatever practical agreement there may be, or "guidelines" proposed to govern contemporary choice or practice, these are bound to be dehumanizing unless at the same time we bring to bear great summit points and sources of insight in mankind's understanding of mankind (be it Christian or other religious humanism, or religiously-dependent but not explicitly religious humanism, or, if it is possible, a true humanism that is neither systematically nor historically dependent on any religious outlook).

Death with Dignity Ideologies

There is nobility and dignity in caring for the dying, but not in dying itself. "To be a therapist to a dying patient makes us aware of the uniqueness of each individual in this vast sea of humanity."[2] It is more correct to say that a therapist brings to the event, from some other source, an awareness of the uniqueness, the one-for-allness of an individual life-span as part of an "outlook" and "onlook" upon the vast sea of humanity. In any case, that is the reflected glory and dignity of caring for the dying, that we are or become aware of the unique life here ending. The humanity of such human caring is apt to be more sensitive and mature if we do not lightly suppose that it is an easy thing to convey dignity to the dying. That certainly cannot be done simply by withdrawing tubes and stopping respirators or not thumping hearts. At most, those omissions can only be prelude to companying with the dying in their final passage, if we are fortunate enough to share with them — they in moderate comfort — those interchanges that are in accord with the dignity and nobility of mankind. Still, however noble the manifestations of caring called for, however unique the individual life, we finally must come to the reality of death, and must ask, what can possibly be the meaning of "death with dignity"?

At most we convey only the liberty to die with human dignity; we can provide some of the necessary but not sufficient conditions. If the dying die with a degree of nobility, it will be mostly their doing in doing their own dying. I fancy their task was easier when death as a human event meant that special note was taken of the last words of the dying — even humorous ones, as in the case of the Roman Emperor who said as he expired, "I Deify." A human countenance may be discerned in death accepted with serenity. So also there is a human countenance behind death with defiance. "Do not go gently into that good night," wrote Dylan Thomas. "Old age should rage and burn against the close of day; Rage Rage against

1. Paul Ramsey, "On (Only) Caring for the Dying," *The Patient as Person* (New Haven: Yale University Press, 1971).

From the *Hastings Center Studies* 2 (May 1974): 47-62. © The Hastings Center. Used by permission.

2. Elisabeth Kübler-Ross, *On Death and Dying* (New York: Macmillan, 1969), p. 247.

the dying of the light." But the human countenance has been removed from most modern understandings of death.

We do not begin to keep human community with the dying if we interpose between them and us most of the current notions of "death with dignity." Rather do we draw closer to them if and only if our conception of "dying with dignity" encompasses — nakedly and without dilution — the final indignity of death itself, whether accepted or raged against. So I think it may be more profitable to explore "the indignity of 'death with dignity.'" "Good death" (euthanasia) like "Good grief?" is ultimately a contradiction in terms, even if superficially, and before we reach the heart of the matter, there are distinctions to be made; even if, that is to say, the predicate "good" still is applicable in both cases in contrast to worse ways to die and worse ways to grieve or not to grieve.

"Death is simply a part of life," we are told, as a first move to persuade us to accept the ideology of the entire dignity of dying with dignity. A singularly unpersuasive proposition, since we are not told what sort or part of life death is. Disease, injury, congenital defects are also a part of life, and as well murder, rapine, and pillage.[3] Yet there is no campaign for accepting or doing those things with dignity. Nor, for that matter, for the contemporary mentality which would enshrine "death with dignity" is there an equal emphasis on "suffering with dignity," suffering as a "natural" part of life, etc. All those things, it seems, are enemies and violations of human nobility while death is not, or (with a few changes) need not be. Doctors did not invent the fact that death is an enemy, although they may sometimes use disproportionate means to avoid final surrender. Neither did they invent the fact that pain and suffering are enemies and often indignities, although suffering accepted may also be ennobling or may manifest the nobility of the human spirit of any ordinary person.

But, then, it is said, death is an evolutionary necessity and in that further sense a part of life not to be denied. Socially and biologically, one generation follows another. So there must be death, else social history would have no room for creative novelty and planet earth would be glutted with humankind. True enough, no doubt, from the point of view of evolution (which — so far — never dies). But the man who is dying happens not to be evolution. He is part of evolution, no doubt; but not to the whole extent of his being or his dying. A crucial testimony to the individual's transcendence over the species is man's problem and his dis-ease in dying. Death is a natural fact of life, yet no man dies "naturally" nor do we have occasions in which to practice doing so in order to learn how. Not unless the pursuit of philosophy is a practice of dying (as Plato's *Phaedo* teaches), and that I take to be an understanding of the human being we moderns do not mean to embrace when we embrace "death with dignity."

3. Schopenhauer's characterization of human history: if you've read one page, you've read it all.

It is small consolation to tell mortal men that as long as you are, the death you contribute to evolution is not yet; and when death is, you are not — so why fear death? That is the modern equivalent to the recipe offered by the ancient Epicureans (and some Stoics) to undercut fear of death and devotion to the gods: as long as you are, death is not; when death is, you are not; there's never a direct encounter between you and death; so why dread death? Indeed, contrary to modern parlance, those ancient philosophers declared that death is *not a part of life;* so, why worry?

So "death is not a part of life" is another declaration designed to quiet fear of death. This can be better understood in terms of a terse comment by Wittgenstein: "Our life has no limit in just the way in which our visual field has no limit."[4] We cannot see beyond the boundary of our visual field; it is more correct to say that beyond the boundary of our visual field *we do not see.* Not only so. Also, we do not see the boundary, the limit itself. There is no seeable bound to the visual field. *Death is not a part of life* in the same way that the boundary is not a part of our visual field. Commenting on this remark by Wittgenstein, James Van Evra writes: "Pressing the analogy, then, if my life has no end in *just the way* that my visual field has no limit, then it must be in the sense that I can have no experience of death, conceived as the complete cessation of experience and thought. That is, if life is considered to be a series of experiences and thoughts, then it is impossible for me to experience death, for to experience something is to be alive, and hence is to be inside the bound formed by death."[5] This is why death itself steadfastly resists conceptualization.

Still, I think the disanalogy ought also to be pressed, against both ancient and contemporary analytical philosophers. That notion of death as a limit makes use of a visual or spatial metaphor. Good basketball players are often men naturally endowed with an unusually wide visual field; this is true, for example, of Bill Bradley. Perhaps basketball players, among other things, strive to enlarge their visual fields, or their habitual use of what powers of sight they have, if that is possible. But ordinarily, everyone of us is perfectly happy within the unseeable limits of sight's reach.

Transfer this notion of death as a limit from space to time as the form of human perception, from sight to an individual's inward desire, effort and hope, and I suggest that one gets a different result. Then death as the temporal limit of a life span is something we live toward. That limit still can never be experienced or conceptualized; indeed, death is *never* a part of life. Moreover, neither is the boundary. Still it is a limit we conative human beings know we live *up against* during our life spans. We do not live toward or up against the side-limits of our visual span. Instead, within that acceptable visual limit (and

4. Wittgenstein, *Tractatus,* 6.4311.

5. James Van Evra, "On Death as a Limit," *Analysis* 31 [5] (April, 1971): 170-76.

other limits as well) as channels we live toward yet another limit which is death.

Nor is the following analogy for death as a limit of much help in deepening understanding. ". . . The importance of the limit and virtually *all* of its significance," writes Van Evra, "derives from the fact that the limit serves as an ordering device" — just as absolute zero serves for ordering a series; it is not *just* a limit, although nothing can exist at such a temperature. The analogy is valid so far as it suggests that we conceive of death not in itself but as it bears on us while still alive. As I shall suggest below, death teaches us to "number our days."

But that may not be its only ordering function for conative creatures. Having placed death "out of our league" by showing that it is not a "something," or never a part of life, and while understanding awareness of death as awareness of a limit bearing upon us only while still alive, one ought not forthwith to conclude that this understanding of it "exonerates death as the purported snake in our garden." Death as a limit can disorder no less than order the series. Only a disembodied reason can say, as Van Evra does, that "the bound, not being a member of the series, cannot defile it. The series is what it is, happy or unhappy, good or bad, quite independently of any bound as such." An Erik Erikson knows better than that when writing of the "despair and often unconscious fear of death" which results when "the one and only life cycle is not accepted as the ultimate life." Despair, he observes, "expresses the feeling that the time is short, too short for the attempt to start another life and to try out alternate roads to integrity."[6]

It is the temporal flight of the series that is grievous (not death as an evil "something" within life's span to be balanced, optimistically or pessimistically, against other things that are good). The reminder that death is *not a part of life,* that it is only a boundary never encountered, is an ancient recipe that can only increase the threat of death on any profound understanding of human life. The dread of death is the dread of oblivion, of there being only empty room in one's stead. Kübler-Ross writes that for the dying, death means the loss of every loved one, total loss of everything that constituted the self in its world, separation from every experience, even from future possible, replacing experiences — nothingness beyond. Therefore, life is a time-intensive activity and not only a goods-intensive or quality-intensive activity. No matter how many "goods" we store up in barns, like the man in Jesus' parable we know that this night our soul may be required of us (Luke 12:13-21). No matter what "quality of life" our lives have, we must take into account the opportunity-costs of used time. Death means the conquest of the time of our lives — even though we never undergo the experience of the nothingness which is natural death.

"Awareness of dying" means awareness of *that;* and awareness of that constitutes an experience of ultimate indignity in and to the awareness of the self who is dying.

We are often reminded of Koheleth's litany: "For everything there is a season, and a time for every matter under heaven: a time to be born and a time to die; a time to plant, and a time to pluck up what is planted," etc. (Eccles. 3:1, 2). Across those words of the narrator of Ecclesiastes the view gains entrance that only an "untimely" death should be regretted or mourned. Yet we know better how to specify an untimely death than to define or describe a "timely" one. The author of Genesis tells us that, at 180 years of age, the patriarch Isaac "breathed his last; and he died and was gathered to his people, old and full of years . . ." (Gen. 35:29). Even in face of sacred Scripture, we are permitted to wonder what Isaac thought about it; whether he too knew how to apply the category "fullness of years" *to himself* and agreed his death was nothing but timely.

We do Koheleth one better and say that death cannot only be timely; it may also be "beautiful." Whether such an opinion is to be ascribed to David Hendin or not (a "fact of life" man he surely is, who also unambiguously subtitled his chapter on euthanasia "Let There Be Death"),[7] that opinion seems to be the outlook of the legislator and physician, Walter Sackett, Jr., who proposed the Florida "Death with Dignity" Statute. All his mature life his philosophy has been, "Death, like birth, is glorious — let it come easy."[8] Such was by no means Koheleth's opinion when he wrote (and *wrote* beautifully) about a time to be born and a time to die. Dr. Sackett also suggests that up to 90 percent of the 1,800 patients in state hospitals for the mentally retarded should be allowed to die. Five billion dollars could be saved in the next half century if the state's mongoloids were permitted to succumb to pneumonia, a disease to which they are highly susceptible.[9] I suggest that the physician in Dr. Sackett has atrophied. He has become a public functionary, treating taxpayers' pocketbooks under the general anesthesia of a continuous daytime soap opera entitled "Death Can Be Beautiful!"

"Death for an older person should be a beautiful event. There is beauty in birth, growth, fullness of life and then, equally so, in the tapering off and final end. There are analogies all about us. What is more beautiful than the spring budding of small leaves; then the fully-leaved tree in summer; and then in the beautiful brightly colored autumn leaves gliding gracefully to the ground? So it is with humans." These are words from a study document on Euthanasia drafted by the Council for Christian Social Action of the United Church of Christ in 1972. An astonishing footnote at this point states that "the naturalness of dying" is suggested in funeral services when the minister says "God has called" the deceased, or says

6. Erik Erikson, "Identity and the Life Cycle," *Psychological Issues,* I, [1] (New York: International University Press, 1959).

7. David Hendin, *Death as a Fact of Life* (New York: W. W. Norton, 1973).

8. Reported in *ibid.,* p. 89.

9. The *Florida Times-Union,* Jacksonville, Fla., Jan. 11, 1973.

he has "gone to his reward," recites the "dust to dust" passage, or notes that the deceased led a full life or ran a full course!

Before this statement was adopted by that Council on Feb. 17, 1973, more orthodox wording was inserted: "Transformation from life on earth to life in the hereafter of the Lord is a fulfillment. The acceptance of death is our witness to faith in the resurrection of Jesus Christ (Rom. 8). We can rejoice." The subdued words "we can rejoice" indicate a conviction that *something* has been subdued. The words "acceptance of death" takes the whole matter out of the context of romantic naturalism and sets it in a proper religious context — based on the particular Christian tenet that death is a conquered enemy, to be accepted in the name of its Conqueror. More than a relic of the nature mysticism that was so luxuriant in the original paragraph, however, remain in the words, "Death for an older person should be a beautiful event. There is beauty in birth, growth, fullness of life and then, *equally so,* in the tapering off and final end." (Italics added.) I know no Christian teaching that assures us that our "final end" is "equally" beautiful as birth, growth, and fullness of life. Moreover, if revelation disclosed any such thing, it would be contrary to reason and to the human reality and experience of death. The views of our "pre-death morticians" are simply discordant with the experienced reality they attempt to beautify. So, in her recent book, Marya Mannes writes "the name of the oratorio is euthanasia." And her statement, "dying is merely suspension within a mystery," seems calculated to induce vertigo in face of a fascinating abyss in prospect.[10]

No exception can be taken to one line in the letter people are being encouraged to write and sign by the Euthanasia Societies of Great Britain and America. That line states: "I do not fear death as much as I fear the indignity of deterioration, dependence and hopeless pain." Such an exercise in analyzing *comparative indignities* should be given approval. But in the preceding sentence the letter states: "Death is as much a reality as birth, growth, maturity, and old age — it is the one certainty." That logically leaves open the question what sort of "reality," what sort of "certainty," death is. But by placing death on a parity with birth, growth, maturity — and old age in many of its aspects — the letter beautifies death by association. To be written long before death when one is thinking "generally" (i.e. "rationally"?) about the topic, the letter tempts us to suppose that men can think generally about their own deaths. Hendin observes in another connection that "there is barely any relation between what people think that they think about death and the way they actually feel about it when it must be faced."[11] Then it may be that "the heart has its reasons that reason cannot know" (Pascal) — beforehand — and among those "reasons," I suggest, will be an apprehension of the ultimate (noncomparative) indignity of death. Talk about death as a fact or a reality seasonally recurring in line with birth or planting, maturity and growth, may after all not be very rational. It smacks more of whistling before the darkness descends, and an attempt to brainwash one's contemporaries to accept a very feeble philosophy of life and death.

Birth and death (our *terminus a quo* and our *terminus ad quem*) are not to be equated with any of the qualities or experiences, the grandeur and the misery, in between, which constitute "parts" of our lives. While we live toward death and can encompass our own dying in awareness, no one in the same way is aware of his own birth. We know that we were born in the same way that we know *that* we die. Explanations of whence we came do not establish conscious contact with our individual origin; and among explanations, that God called us from the womb out of nothing is as good as any other; and better than most. But awareness of dying is quite another matter. That we may have, but not awareness of our births. And while awareness of birth might conceivably be the great original individuating experience (if we had it), among the race of men it is awareness of dying that is uniquely individuating. To encompass one's own death in the living and dying of one's life is more of a task than it is a part of life. And there is something of indignity to be faced when engaging in the final act of life. Members of the caring human community (doctors, nurses, family) are apt to keep closer company with the dying if we acknowledge the loss of all worth by the loss of him in whom inhered all worth in his world. Yet ordinary men may sometimes nobly suffer the ignobility of death.

By way of contrast with the "A Living Will" framed by the Euthanasia Society, the Judicial Council of the AMA in its recent action on the physician and the dying patient had before it two similar letters. One was composed by the Connecticut Delegation:

> ***To my Family, my Physician, my Clergyman, my Lawyer —***
>
> If the time comes when I can no longer actively take part in decisions for my own future, I wish this statement to stand as the testament of my wishes. If there is no reasonable expectation of my recovery from physical or mental and spiritual disability, I, ____________, request that I be allowed to die and not be kept alive by artificial means or heroic measures. I ask also that drugs be mercifully administered to me for terminal suffering even if in relieving pain they may hasten the moment of death. I value life and the dignity of life, so that I am not asking that my life be directly taken, but that my dying not be unreasonably prolonged nor the dignity of life be destroyed. This request is made, after careful reflection, while I am in good health and spirits. Although this document is not legally binding, you who care for me will, I hope, feel morally bound to take it into account. I recognize that it places a heavy burden

10. Marya Mannes, *Last Rights* (New York: William Morrow, 1973), p. 6 (cf. 80, 133).

11. Hendin, *Death as a Fact of Life,* p. 103.

> of responsibility upon you, and it is with the intention of sharing this responsibility that this statement is made.

A second letter had been composed by a physician to express his own wishes, in quite simple language:

> ***To my Family, To my Physician —***
>
> Should the occasion arise in my lifetime when death is imminent and a decision is to be made about the nature and the extent of the care to be given to me and I am not able at the time to express my desires, let this statement serve to express my deep, sincere, and considered wish and hope that my physician will administer to me simple, ordinary medical treatment. I ask that he not administer heroic, extraordinary, expensive, or useless medical care or treatment which in the final analysis will merely delay, not change, the ultimate outcome of my terminal condition.

A comparison of these declarations with "A Living Will" circulated by the Euthanasia Society reveals the following signal differences: neither of the AMA submissions engages in any superfluous calculus of "comparative indignities";[12] neither associates the reality of death with such things as birth or maturation; both allow death to be simply what it is in human experience; both are in a general sense "pro-life" statements, in that death is neither reified as one fact among others nor beautified even comparatively.[13]

Everyone concerned takes the wrong turn in trying to "thing-ify" death or to beautify it. The dying have at least this advantage, that in these projects for dehumanizing death by naturalizing it the dying finally cannot succeed, and death makes its threatening visage known to them before ever there are any societal or evolutionary replacement values or the everlasting arms or Abraham's bosom to rest on. Death means *finis,* not in itself *telos.* Certainly not a telos to be engineered, or to be accomplished by reducing both human life and death to the level of natural events.

"Thing-ifying" death reaches its highest pitch in the stated preference of many people in the present age for *sudden* death,[14] for death from unanticipated internal collapse, from the abrupt intrusion of violent outside forces, from some chance occurrence due to the natural law governing the operation of automobiles. While for a comparative calculus of indignities sudden *unknowing* death may be preferred to suffering knowingly or unknowingly the indignity of deterioration, abject dependence, and hopeless pain, how ought we to assess in human terms the present-day absolute (noncomparative) preference for sudden death? Nothing reveals more the meaning we assign to human "dignity" than the view that sudden death, death as an eruptive natural event, could be a prismatic case of death with dignity or at least one without indignity. Human society seems about to rise to the moral level of the "humane" societies in their treatment of animals. What is the principled difference between their view and ours about the meaning of dying "humanely"? By way of contrast, consider the prayer in the Anglican prayer book: "From perils by night and perils by day, perils by land and perils by sea, and *from sudden death,* Lord, deliver us." Such a petition bespeaks an age in which dying with dignity was a gift and a task (*Gabe und Aufgabe*), a liberty to encompass dying as a final act among the actions of life, to enfold awareness of dying as an ingredient into awareness of one's self dying as the finale of the self's relationships in this life to God or to fellowman — in any case to everything that was worthy.

Man Knows that He Dies

Before letting Koheleth's "a time to be born and a time to die" creep as a gloss into *our* texts, perhaps we ought to pay more attention to the outlook on life and death as expressed in the enchantment and frail beauty of those words,[15] and ask whether that philosophy can possibly be

12. What, after all, is the point of promoting, as if it were a line of reasoning, observations such as that said to be inscribed on W. C. Field's tombstone: "On the whole I'd rather be here than in Philadelphia"?

13. I may add that while the House of Delegates did not endorse any particular form to express an individual's wishes relating prospectively to his final illness, it recognized that individuals have a right to express them. While it encouraged physicians to discuss such matters with patients and attend to their wishes, the House nevertheless maintained a place for the conscience and judgment of a physician in determining indicated treatment. It did not subsume every consideration under the rubric of the patient's right to refuse treatment (or to have refused treatment). That sole action-guide can find no medical or logical reason for distinguishing, in physicians' actions, between the dying and those who simply have a terminal illness (or have this "dying life," Augustine's description of all of us). It would also entail a belief that wishing or autonomous choice makes the moral difference between life and death decisions which then are to be imposed on the physician-technician; and that, to say the least, is an ethics that can find no place for either reason or sensibility.

14. Cf. the report of a Swedish survey by Gunnar Biörck, M.D., in *Archives of Internal Medicine,* October, 1973; news report in the *New York Times,* Oct. 31, 1973.

15. In the whole literature on death and dying, there is no more misquoted sentence, or statement taken out of context, than Koheleth's "time to be born and a time to die" — unless it be "Nor strive officiously to keep alive." The latter line is from an ironic poem by the nineteenth-century poet Arthur Hugh Clough, entitled, "The Latest Decalogue":

> Thou shalt not kill; but need'st not strive
> Officiously to keep alive,
> Do not adultery commit;
> Advantage rarely comes of it:
> Thou shalt not steal; an empty feat,
> When it's so lucrative to cheat:
> Bear not false witness; let the lie

a proper foundation for the practice of medicine or for the exercise of the most sensitive care for the dying.

That litany on the times for every matter under heaven concludes with the words, "What gain has the worker from his toil?" (Eccles. 3:9). In general, the author of Ecclesiastes voices an unrelieved pessimism. He has "seen everything that is done under the sun," in season and out of season. It is altogether "an unhappy business that God has given to the sons of men to be busy with" — this birthing and dying, planting and uprooting; "all is vanity and seeking after wind" (Eccles. 1:3b, 14). So, he writes with words of strongest revulsion, "I hated life, because what is done under the sun was grievous to me"; "I hated all my toil and gave myself up to despair . . ." (Eccles. 2:17, 18a, 20).

After that comes the litany "for everything there is a season" — proving, as Kierkegaard said, that a poet is a man whose heart is full of pain but whose lips are so formed that when he gives utterance to that pain he makes beautiful sounds. Koheleth knew, as later did Nietzsche, that the eternal recurrence of birth and death and all things else was simply "the spirit of melancholy" unrelieved, even though there is nothing else to believe since God died.[16] (The Pope knows; he was at the bedside.)

"Death with dignity" because death is a "part" of life, one only of its seasonal realities? If so, then the acceptable death of all flesh means death with the same signal indignity that brackets the whole of life and its striving. Dying is worth as much as the rest; it is not more fruitless.

"For the fate of the sons of men and the fate of the beasts is the same; as one dies, so dies the other. They all have the same breath, and man has no advantage over the beasts; for all is vanity" (Eccles. 3:19). "Death with dignity" or death a part of life based on an equilibration of the death of a man with the death of a dog? I think that is not a concept to be chosen as the foundation of modern medicine, even though both dogs and men are enabled to die "humanely."

Or to go deeper still: "death with dignity" because the dead are better off than the living? "I thought the dead who are already dead," Koheleth writes in unrelieved sorrow over existence, "more fortunate than the living who are still alive; and better than both is he who has not yet been, and has not seen the evil deeds that are done under the sun" (Eccles. 4:2, 3). Thus the book of Ecclesiastes is the source of the famous interchange between two pessimistic philosophers, each trying to exceed the other in gloom: First philosopher: More blessed are the dead than the living. Second philosopher: Yes, what you say is true; but more blessed still are those who have never been born. First philosopher: Yes, wretched life; but few there be who attain to that condition!

But Koheleth thinks he knows some who have attained to the blessed goal of disentrapment from the cycles in which there is a time for every matter under heaven. ". . . An untimely birth [a miscarriage] is better off [than a living man], for it [a miscarriage] comes into vanity and goes into darkness, and in darkness its name is covered; moreover it has not seen the sun or known anything; yet it finds rest rather than he [the living]" (Eccles. 6:3b, 4, 5). So we might say that death can have its cosmic dignity if untormented by officious physicians, because the dying go to the darkness, to Limbo where nameless miscarriages dwell, having never seen the sun or known anything. Thus, if dying with dignity as a part of life's natural, undulating seasons seems not to be a thought with much consolation in it (being roughly equivalent to the indignity besetting everything men do and every other natural time), still the dying may find rest as part of cosmic order, from which, once upon a time, the race of men arose to do the unhappy business God has given them to be busy with, and to which peaceful darkness the dying return.

Hardly a conception that explains the rise of Western medicine, the energy of its care of the dying or its war against the indignity of suffering and death — or a conception on which to base its reformation! Dylan Thomas's words were directed against such notions: "The wise men at their end know dark is right, / Because their words had forked no lightning."

There is finally in Ecclesiastes, however, a deeper strand than those which locate men living and dying as simply parts of some malignly or benignly neglectful natural or cosmic order. From these more surface outlooks, the unambiguous injunction follows: Be a part; let there be death — in its time and place, of course (whatever that means). Expressing a deeper strand, however, Koheleth seems to say: Let the natural or cosmic order be whatever it is; men are different. His practical advice is: Be what you are, in human awareness apart and not a part. Within this deeper understanding of the transcendent, threatened nobility of a human life, the uniqueness of the individual human subject, there is ground for awareness of death as an indignity yet freedom to encompass it with dignity.

Now it is that Koheleth reverses the previous judgments he decreed over all he had seen under the sun. Before, the vale of the sunless not-knowing of a miscarriage having its name covered by darkness seemed preferable to living; and all man's works a seeking after wind. So, of course, there was "a time for dying." But now Koheleth writes, ". . . There is no work or thought or knowledge or wisdom in Sheol, to which you are going" (Eccles. 9:10b). While the fate of the sons of men and the fate of the beasts are the same, still "a living dog is better than a dead lion"; and to be a living man is better than either,

---

Have time on its own wings to fly:
Thou shall not covet; but tradition
Approves all forms of competition.
The sum of all is, thou shalt love
If anybody, God above:
At any rate, shalt never labor
More than thyself to love thy neighbor.

16. Nietzsche, *Thus Spake Zarathustra,* especially XLVI and LXVI.

because of what Koheleth means by "living." "He who is joined with all the living has hope" (Eccles. 9:4), and that is hardly a way to describe dogs or lions. Koheleth, however, identifies the grandeur of man not so much with hope as with awareness, even awareness of dying, and the misery of man with the indignity of dying of which he, in his nobility, is aware. "For the living know that they will die," he writes, "but the dead know nothing. . ." (Eccles. 9:5). Before, the dead or those who never lived had superiority; now, it is the living who are superior precisely by virtue of their awareness of dying and its indignity to the knowing human spirit.

Therefore, I suggest that Koheleth probed the human condition to a depth to which more than twenty centuries later Blaise Pascal came. "Man is but a reed, the feeblest in nature, but he is a thinking reed. . . . A vapor, a drop of water, is sufficient to slay him. But were the universe to crush him, man would still be nobler than that which kills him, for *he knows that he dies,* while the universe knows nothing of the advantage it has over him. Thus our whole dignity consists in thought."[17] (Italics added.)

So the grandeur and misery of man are fused together in the human reality and experience of death. To deny the indignity of death requires that the dignity of man be refused also. The more acceptable in itself death is, the less the worth or uniqueness ascribed to the dying life.

True Humanism and the Dread of Death

I always write as the ethicist I am, namely, a Christian ethicist, and not as some hypothetical common denominator. On common concrete problems I, of course, try to elaborate analysis at the point or on a terrain where there may be convergence of vectors that began in our ethical outlooks and onlooks. Still one should not pant for agreement as the hart pants for the waterbrooks, lest the substance of one's ethics dissolve into vapidity. So in this section I want, among other things, to exhibit some of the meaning of "Christian humanism" in regard to death and dying, in the confidence that this will prove tolerable to my colleagues for a time, if not finally instructive to them.

In this connection, there are two counterpoised verses in the First Epistle of St. John that are worth pondering. The first reads: "Perfect love casts out fear" (which, being interpreted, means: Perfect care of the dying casts out fear of one's own death or rejection of their dying because of fear of ours). The second verse reads: "Where fear is, love is not perfected" (which, being interpreted, means: Where fear of death and dying remains, medical and human care of the dying is not perfected). That states nothing so much as the enduring dubiety and ambiguity of any mortal man's care of another through his dying. At the same time there is here applied without modification a standard for unflinching care of a dying fellowman, or short of that of any fellow mortal any time. That standard is cut to the measure of the perfection in benevolence believed to be that of our Father in Heaven in his dealings with mankind. So there is "faith-ing" in an ultimate righteousness beyond the perceptible human condition presupposed by those verses that immediately have to do simply with loving and caring.

Whatever non-Christians may think about the *theology* here entailed, or about similar foundations in any religious ethics, I ask that the notation upon or penetration of the human condition be attended to. Where and insofar as fear is, love and care for the dying cannot be perfected in moral agents or the helping professions. The religious traditions have one way of addressing that problematic. In the modern age the problematic itself is avoided by various forms and degrees of denial of the tragedy of death which proceeds first to reduce the unique worth and once-for-all-ness of the individual lifespan that dies.

Perhaps one can apprehend the threat posed to the dignity of man (i.e. in an easy and ready dignifying of death) by many modern viewpoints, especially those dominating the scientific community, and their superficial equivalents in our culture generally, by bringing into view three states of consciousness in the Western past.

The burden of the Hebrew Scriptures was man's obedience or disobedience to covenant, to Torah. Thus sin was the problem, and death came in only as a subordinate theme; and, as one focus for the problematic of the human condition, this was a late development. In contrast, righteousness and disobedience (sin) was a subordinate theme in Greek religion. The central theme of Greek religious thought and practice was the problem of death — a problem whose solution was found either by initiation into religious cults that promised to extricate the soul from its corruptible shroud or by belief in the native power of the soul to outlast any number of bodies. Alongside these, death was at the heart of the pathos of life depicted in Greek tragical drama, against which, and against the flaws of finitude in general, the major character manifested his heroic transcendence. So sin was determinative for the Hebrew consciousness; death for the Greek consciousness.

Consciousness III was Christianity, and by this, sin and death were tied together in Western man's awareness of personal existence. These two foci of man's misery and of his need for redemption — sin and death — were inseparably fused. This new dimension of man's awareness of himself was originally probed most profoundly by St. Paul's Letter to the Romans (5–7). Those opaque reflections, I opine, were once understood not so much by the intellect as along the pulses of ordinary people in great numbers, in taverns and marketplaces; and it represents a cultural breakdown without parallel that these reflections are scarcely understandable to the greatest intelligences today. A simple night school lesson in them may be gained by simply pondering a while the two verses quoted above from St. John's Epistle.

17. Pascal, *Pensées,* p. 347.

The point is that according to the Christian saga the Messiah did not come to bring boors into culture. Nor did he bear epilepsy or psychosomatic disorders to gain victory over them in the flesh before the interventions of psychoneurosurgery. Rather is he said to have been born *mortal* flesh to gain for us a foretaste of victory over sin and death where those twin enemies had taken up apparently secure citadel.

Again, the point for our purposes is not to be drawn into agreement or disagreement with those theological affirmations, and it is certainly not to be tempted into endless speculation about an afterlife. Crucial instead is to attend to the notation on the human condition implied in all that. Death is an enemy even if it is the last enemy to be fully conquered in the Fulfillment, the eschaton; meanwhile, the sting of death is sin. Such was the new consciousness-raising that Christianity brought into the Western world. And the question is whether in doing so it has not grasped some important experiential human realities better than most philosophies, whether it was not attuned to essential ingredients of the human condition vis-à-vis death — whatever the truth or falsity of its theological address to the condition.

The foregoing, I grant, may be an oversimplification; and I am aware of needed corrections more in the case of Hebrew humanism than in the case of Greek humanism. The New Testament word, "He will wipe away every tear from their eyes, and death shall be no more, neither shall there be mourning nor crying nor pain any more, for the former things have passed away" (Rev. 21:3, 4), has its parallel in the Hebrew Bible: "He will swallow up death forever, and the LORD God will wipe away tears from all faces . . ." (Isa. 25:8). Again, since contemplating the Lord God may be too much for us, I ask only that we attend to the doctrine of death implied in these passages: it is an enemy, surely, and not simply an acceptable part of the natural order of things. And the connection between dread of death and sin, made most prominent in Christian consciousness, was nowhere better stated than in Ecclesiastes: "This is the root of the evil in all that happens under the sun, that one fate comes to all. Therefore, men's minds are filled with evil and there is madness in their hearts while they live, for they know that afterward — they are off to the dead!"

One can, indeed, ponder that verse about the source of all evil in the apprehended evil of death together with another verse in Ecclesiastes which reads: "Teach us so to number our days that we may apply our hearts unto wisdom." The first says that death is an evil evil: it is experienced as a threatening limit that begets evil. The second says that death is a good evil: that experience also begets good. Without death, and death perceived as a threat, we would also have no reason to "number our days" so as to ransom the time allotted us, to receive life as a precious gift, to drink the wine of gladness in toast to every successive present moment. Instead, life would be an endless boredom and boring because endless; there would be no reason to probe its depths while there is still time. Some there are who number their days so as to apply their hearts unto eating, drinking and being merry — for tomorrow we die. Some there are who number their days so as to apply their hearts unto wisdom — for tomorrow we die. Both are life spans enhanced in importance and in individuation under the stimulus of the perceived evil of death. Knowledge of human good or of human evil that is in the slightest degree above the level of the wild beasts of the field is enhanced because of death, the horizon of human existence. So, debarment from access to the tree of life was on the horizon and a sequence of the events in the Garden of Paradise; the temptation in eating the fruit of the tree of knowledge of good and evil was that that seemed a way for mortal creatures to become like gods. The punishment of that is said to have been death; and no governor uses as a penalty something that anyone can simply choose to believe to be a good or simply receive as a neutral or dignified, even ennobling, part of life. So I say death may be a good evil or an evil evil, but it is perceived as an evil or experienced indignity in either case. Existential anxiety or general anxiety (distinguishable from particular fears or removable anxieties) means anxiety over death toward which we live. That paradoxically, as Reinhold Niebuhr said, is the source of all human creativity and of all human sinfulness.

Of course, the sages of old could and did engage in a calculus of comparative indignities. "O death, your sentence is welcome," wrote Ben Sira, "to a man worn out with age, worried about everything, disaffected and beyond endurance" (Ecclus. 41:2, 3). Still death was a "sentence," not a natural event acceptable in itself. Moreover, not every man grows old gracefully in the Psalms; instead, one complains:

> Take pity on me, Yahweh,
> I am in trouble now.
> Grief wastes away my eye,
> My throat, my inmost parts.
> For my life is worn out with sorrow,
> My years with sighs;
> My strength yields under misery,
> My bones are wasting away.
> To every one of my oppressors
> I am contemptible,
> Loathsome to my neighbors,
> To my friends a thing of fear.
> Those who see me in the street
> Hurry past me.
> I am forgotten, as good as dead, in their hearts,
> Something discarded. (Ps. 31:9-12)

What else is to be expected if it be true that the madness in men's hearts while they live, and the root of all evil in all that happens under the sun, lies in the simple fact that every man consciously lives toward his own death, knowing that afterward he too is off to the dead? Where fear is — fear of the properly dreadful — love and care for the dying cannot be perfected.

Unless one has some grounds for respecting the

shadow of death upon every human countenance — grounds more ultimate than perceptible realities — then it makes good sense as a policy of life simply to try to outlast one's neighbors. One can, for example, *generalize,* and so attenuate our neighbors' irreplaceability. "If I must grieve whenever the bell tolls," writes Carey McWilliams, "I am never bereft: some of my kinsmen will remain. Indeed, I need not grieve much — even, lest I suggest some preference among my brethren, should not grieve much — for each loss is small compared to what remains."[18] But the solace, we know, is denied the dead who have lost everything making for worth in their world. Realistic love for another irreplaceable, noninterchangeable individual human being means, as Unamuno wrote, care for another "doomed soul."

In this setting, let us now bring into consideration some empirical findings that in this day are commonly supposed to be more confirmatory than wisdom mediated from the heart.

In the second year anatomy course, medical students clothe with "gallows humor" their encounter with the cadaver which once was a human being alive. That defense is not to be despised; nor does it necessarily indicate socialization in shallowness on the students' part. Even when dealing with the remains of the long since dead, there is special tension involved — if I mistook not a recent address by Renée Fox — when performing investigatory medical actions involving the face, the hands, and the genitalia. This thing-in-the-world that was once a man alive we still encounter as once a communicating being, not quite as an object of research or instruction. Face and hands, yes; but why the genitalia? Those reactions must seem incongruous to a resolutely biologizing age. For a beginning of an explanation, one might take up the expression "carnal knowledge" — which was the best thing about the movie bearing that title — and behind that go to the expression "carnal *conversation,*" an old, legal term for adultery, and back of both to the Biblical word "knew" in "And Adam *knew* his wife and begat. . . ." Here we have an entire anthropology impacted in a word, not a squeamish euphemism. In short, in those reactions of medical students can be discerned a sensed relic of the human being bodily experiencing and communicating, and the body itself uniquely speaking.

Notably, however, there's no "gallows humor" used when doing or observing one's first autopsy, or in the emergency room when a D.O.A. (Dead on Arrival) is brought in with his skull cleaved open. With regard to the "newly dead" we come as close as we possibly can to experiencing the incommensurable contrast between life and death. Yet those sequential realities — life and death — here juxtaposed never *meet* in direct encounter. So we never have an impression or experience of the measure and meaning of the two different worlds before which we stand in the autopsy and the emergency room. A cadaver has over time become almost a thing-in-the-world from which to gain knowledge of the human body. While *there* a little humor helps, to go about acquiring medical knowledge from autopsies requires a different sort of inward effort to face down or live with our near-experience of the boundary of life and death. The cleavage in the brain may be quite enough and more than enough to *explain* rationally why this man was D.O.A. But, I suggest, there can be no gash deep enough, no physical event destructive enough to account for the felt difference between life and death that we face here. The physician or medical student may be a confirmed materialist. For him the material explanation of this death may be quite sufficient rationally. Still the heart has its reasons that the reason knows not of; and, I suggest, the awakening of these feelings of awe and dread should not be repressed in anyone whose calling is to the human dignity of caring for the dying.

In any case, from these empirical observations, if they be true, let us return to a great example of theological anthropology in order to try to comprehend why death was thought to be the assault of an enemy. According to some readings, Christians in all ages should be going about bestowing the gift of immortality on one another posthaste. A distinguished Catholic physician, beset by what he regarded as the incorrigible problems of medical ethics today, once shook his head in my presence and wondered out loud why the people who most believe in an afterlife should have established so many hospitals! That seems to require explanation, at least as against silly interpretations of "otherworldliness." The answer is that none of the facts or outlooks cited ever denied the reality of death, or affirmed that death ever presents a friendly face (except comparatively). The explanation lies in the vicinity of Christian anthropology and the Biblical view that death is an enemy. That foundation of Western medicine ought not lightly to be discarded, even if we need to enliven again the sense that there are limits to man's struggle against that alien power.

Far from the otherworldliness or body-soul dualism with which he is often charged, St. Augustine went so far as to say that "the body is not an extraneous ornament or aid, but a part of man's very nature."[19] Upon that understanding of the human being, Augustine could then express a quite realistic account of "the dying process":

> Wherefore, as regards bodily death, that is, the separation of the soul from the body, it is good to none while it is being endured by those whom we say are in the article of death [dying]. For the very violence with which the body and soul are wrenched asunder, which in the living are conjoined and closely intertwined, brings with it a harsh experience, jarring horribly on nature as long as it continues, till there comes a total loss of sensation, which arose from the very interpenetration of flesh and spirit.[20]

18. Wilson Carey McWilliams, *The Idea of Fraternity in America* (Berkeley: University of California Press, 1973), p. 48.

19. Augustine, *City of God,* Book I, Chapter XIII.

20. Ibid., Book XIII, Chapter VI.

From this Augustine correctly concludes: "Wherefore death is indeed . . . good to none while it is actually suffered, and while it is subduing the dying to its power. . . ." His ultimate justifications attenuate not at all the harshness of that alien power's triumph. Death, he only says, is "meritoriously endured for the sake of winning what *is* good. And regarding what happens after death, it is no absurdity to say that death is good to the good, and evil to the evil."[21] But that is not to say that death as endured in this life, or as life's terminus, is itself in any way good. He even goes so far as to say:

> For though there can be no manner of doubt that the souls of the just and holy lead lives in peaceful rest, yet so much better would it be for them to be alive in healthy, well-conditioned bodies, that even those who hold the tenet that it is most blessed to be quit of every kind of body, condemn this opinion in spite of themselves.[22]

Thus, for Biblical or later Christian anthropology, the only possible form which human life in any true and proper sense can take here or hereafter is "somatic." That is the Pauline word; we today say "psychosomatic." Therefore, for Christian theology death may be a "conquered enemy"; still it was in the natural order — and as long as the generations of mankind endure will remain — an enemy still. To pretend otherwise adds insult to injury — or, at least, carelessness.

There are two ways, so far as I can see, to reduce the dreadful visage of death to a level of inherently acceptable indifference. One way is to subscribe to an interpretation of "bodily life" that reduces it to an acceptable level of indifference to the person long before his dying. That — if anyone can believe it today, or if it is not a false account of human nature — was the way taken by Plato in his idealized account of the death of Socrates. (It should be remembered that we know not whether Socrates' hands trembled as he yet bravely drank the hemlock, no more than we know how Isaac experienced dying when "fullness of years" came upon him. Secondary accounts of these matters are fairly untrustworthy.)

Plato's dialogue *The Phaedo* may not "work" as a proof of the immortality of the soul. Still it decisively raises the question of immortality by its thorough representation of the incommensurability between mental processes and bodily processes. Few philosophers today accept the demonstration of the mind's power to outlast bodies because the mind itself is not material, or because the mind "plays" the body like a musician the lyre. But most of them are still wrestling with the mind-body problem, and many speak of two separate languages, a language for mental events isomorphic with our language for brain events. That's rather like saying the same thing as Socrates (Plato) while claiming to have gone beyond him (Søren Kierkegaard).

21. Ibid., Book XIII, Chapter VIII.
22. Ibid., Book XIII, Chapter XIX.

I cite *The Phaedo* for another purpose: to manifest one way to render death incomparably welcomed. Those who most have mature manhood in exercise — the lovers of wisdom — have desired death and dying all their life long, in the sense that they seek "in every sort of way to dissever the soul from the communion of the body"; "thought is best when the mind is gathered into herself and none of these things trouble her — neither sounds nor sights nor pain nor any pleasure — when she takes leave of the body. . . ." That life is best and has nothing to fear that has "the habit of the soul gathering and collecting herself into herself from all sides out of the body." (Feminists, note the pronouns.)

Granted, Socrates' insight is valid concerning the self's transcendence, when he says: "I am inclined to think that these muscles and bones of mine would have gone off long ago to Megara and Boeotia — by the dog, they would, if they had been moved only by their own idea of what was best. . . ." Still Crito had a point, when he feared that the impending dread event had to do with "the same Socrates who has been talking and conducting the argument" than Socrates is represented to have believed. To fear the loss of Socrates, Crito had not to fancy, as Socrates charged, "that I am the other Socrates whom he will soon see, a dead body." Crito had only to apprehend, however faintly, that there is not an entire otherness between those two Socrates *now,* in this living being; that there was unity between, let us say, Socrates the conductor of arguments and Socrates the gesticulator or the man who stretched *himself* because his muscles and bones grew weary from confinement.

The other way to reduce the dreadful visage of death is to subscribe to a philosophy of "human life" that reduces the stature, the worth, and the irreplaceable uniqueness of the individual person (long before his dying) to a level of acceptable transiency or interchangeability. True, modern culture is going this way. But there have been other and better ways of stipulating that the image of death across the human countenance is no shadow. One was that of Aristotelian philosophy. According to its form-matter distinction, reason, the formal principle, is definitive of essential humanity. That is universal, eternal as logic. Matter, however, is the individuating factor. So when a man who bears a particular name dies, only the individuation disintegrates — to provide matter for other forms. Humanity goes on in other instances. Anything unique or precious about mankind is not individual. There are parallels to this outlook in Eastern religions and philosophies, in which the individual has only transiency, and should seek only that, disappearing in the Fulfillment into the Divine pool.

These then are two ways of denying the dread of death. Whenever these two escapes are *simultaneously* rejected — i.e., if the "bodily life" is neither an ornament nor a drag but a part of man's very nature; and if the "personal life" of an individual in his unique life span is accorded unrepeatable, noninterchangeable value — then it is that Death the Enemy again comes into view.

Conquered or Unconquerable. A true humanism and the dread of death seem to be dependent variables. I suggest that it is better to have the indignity of death on our hands and in our outlooks than to "dignify" it in either of these two possible ways. Then we ought to be much more circumspect in speaking of death with dignity, and hesitant to — I almost said — thrust that upon the dying! Surely, a proper care for them needs not only to know the pain of dying which human agency may hold at bay, but also care needs to acknowledge that there is grief over death which no human agency can alleviate.

139 Keeping Body and Soul Together

Oliver O'Donovan

An admirer of Paul Ramsey's work has recently complained that in his later writing, and specifically in his writing on medical ethics since "The Patient as Person" in 1970, there is "much less direct appeal to theological warrants."[1] Whether or not this will stand as a generalization, there appears to be one striking counter-example, Ramsey's contribution to the *Hastings Center Studies* feature on "Facing Death" in 1974, an article entitled "The Indignity of 'Death with Dignity.'"[2] The occasion for that article, the author tells us, was his alarm at the sudden popularity of the view (his own, as well as that of many others) that the use of officious medical technique in the care of the dying should be discouraged (p. 47). In it he set out, in the first place, to chart the "'philosophical' ingredients of any view of death and dying," and, in the second "to exhibit some of the meaning of 'Christian humanism' in regard to death and dying" (p. 56). The result was a discussion so steeped in theological warrants that the two respondents, Robert S. Morison and Leon Kass, while acknowledging extensive practical agreement with Ramsey, hardly knew what to make of parts of it. Their three-cornered discussion has always seemed to me to be of especial interest, and that for three reasons. First, it succeeds in demonstrating what Ramsey set out to demonstrate: that the agreement about the unofficious care of the dying was a contingent coalition of divergent spiritual and intellectual viewpoints. Secondly, Ramsey's own article provides a striking example of his appeal to theological warrants in medical ethics, as well as of the ambiguities which make that appeal less decisive than it might be. And yet, thirdly, I would judge that it is something more than a personal declaration of sombre grandeur, but has integrity as an articulation of the Christian view of death.

My purpose in this essay is to concentrate on one particular theological theme of which Ramsey makes use in that article, as frequently in his other writings: the appeal to a unitary view of human nature, that is, to the mutual coinherence of body and soul. It is a familiar enough con-

1. Stanley Hauerwas, *Against the Nations* (Minneapolis: Winston Press, 1985), p. 49.

2. *Hastings Center Studies* 2:2 (May 1974): 47-62. Despite the author's insistence on every word of his title, I shall abbreviate as ". . . Death with Dignity."

Published as "Ne pas séparer l'âme du corps," trans. M.-B. Mesnet, *Ethique* xi (1994): 64-89. The English version is published here with permission of the author.

tention to anyone who has read Ramsey at all widely, that the chief errors of contemporary moral thought, whether about sexual freedom, nuclear deterrence, or euthanasia, are attributable to an over-spiritualisation of human action.[3] The only surprising thing about the appearance of this contention in ". . . Death with Dignity" might seem to be the lateness of its arrival there (p. 59, at the foot of the thirteenth of sixteen pages)! I shall, however, be drawing attention to some other surprising features. For Ramsey's use of this and other theological warrants in this article is strangely difficult to pin down. Not only did the argument prove difficult for sympathetic respondents from outside the Christian tradition to understand, let alone sympathise with; but it also involved Ramsey in some surprisingly evasive moves from the point of view of Christian theology itself. I take this fine piece of writing, then, as my starting-point for what will be at once a defense, an interpretation and, I hope, a refinement of a central thesis in theological anthropology, from which Ramsey launches his medical ethics as well as much else.[4]

Given the complexity of the article it may not be officious to offer an analytic summary of it, illuminating its structure, which, while thoroughly and soundly built, has been obscured both by the author's own use of art to conceal art and by an editorial disposition of sub-headings which savours of despair.[5] As I have indicated, the article falls into two parts: the first concerned with the "'philosophical' ingredients of any view of death and dying," the second with the "Christian humanism" which Ramsey himself, unwilling to speak as "some hypothetical common denominator," intends to profess. The word "philosophical" is placed by Ramsey himself in quotation marks. And that is because this first part of the article constitutes, in effect, a sustained *criticism* of traditional philosophical wisdom about death, a criticism summed up in a mocking misquotation from Dylan Thomas: "The wise men at their end know dark is right, because their words had forked no lightning."[6] Philosophy, in attempting to reconcile human beings to their death, has sold life short. The criticism embraces Aristotle and Plato (though the *Phaedo* is discussed in a tone of deep appreciation) and a horde of popular modern philosophers for which Ramsey does not attempt to disguise his scorn. It must also, by implication, embrace the Jewish wise men, Rabbi Meir and Maimonides, whom Kass holds out as examples. For Kass and Ramsey see the task of the philosopher differently. Kass, though he admits the dangers in judging doctrines by their moral "usefulness," understands the philosopher's duty as exhortation: "how *should* Socrates or Isaac or Ramsey or Kass or any human being regard . . . the fact that we must each and all die?"[7] For Ramsey it is interpretation: what is the truth about human dignity in the face of death? And Ramsey, at the very beginning of his article, does not conceal from us what he thinks the truth is, which philosophers, simply by attending to their own business, ought to have been able to see: it is that human dignity is not found *in* dying, but is brought *to* dying. Ramsey's standard of philosophical truth is found in the famous Pascal *Pensée,* which designates man as "a thinking reed" who "knows that he dies. . . . All our dignity, then, consists in thought."[8]

---

3. See, for example, *Christian Ethics and the Sit-In* (New York: Association Press, 1961), pp. 37f.; *Nine Modern Moralists* (Englewood Cliffs, N.J.: Prentice-Hall, 1962), pp. 105-9; "A Christian Approach to the Question of Sexual Relations Outside Marriage," *Journal of Religion* (1965): 102; *The Just War* (New York: Scribner's, 1968), pp. 49f., 221-25; *Fabricated Man* (New Haven: Yale University Press, 1970), pp. 36-38, 86-90, 130-38; *The Patient as Person* (New Haven: Yale University Press, 1970), pp. xiii, 187-88, 193; *Ethics at the Edges of Life* (New Haven: Yale University Press, 1978), pp. 139, 180. I am grateful for the assistance of David Attwood in locating these references.

4. I shall confine my use of the two responses, interesting as each is, to illuminating Ramsey's position. This means, in effect, making use only of Kass ("Averting one's eyes, or facing the music? — On dignity in death," *loc. cit.,* pp. 67-80), who has succeeded in putting into sharp focus the issues between Ramsey and his own position, shaped by the Jewish tradition. The interest of Morison's briefer response ("The last poem: the dignity of the inevitable and necessary," ibid., pp. 63-66) lies chiefly in the unsuspected convergences which appear between its professed neo-paganism and some of the existentialist positions viewed with sympathy by the Christian writer. As a criticism of Ramsey it is weakened by a failure to grasp his meaning at crucial points. But does Morison's use of a quotation from Alfred Kazin (p. 66) that "art is the fusion of suffering with form" leave him very far removed from Niebuhr's opinion that the fear of death is the source of all human creativity? And does not the point of unconscious sympathy sharpen the suspicion, which Ramsey himself articulated on an earlier occasion, that existential anxiety leads us back to the pagan consciousness?

5. The bare bones of the analysis on which my exposition is based are as follows:

Introduction: a defence of the title (pp. 47-48 col. 1).

- I. Philosophical ingredients of a view of death:
  - A. Statement of position (p. 48 col. 1: "There is nobility . . ." — col. 2: ". . . to grieve or not to grieve")
  - B. The meaning of death as a limit (p. 48 col. 2: "'Death is simply a part . . .'" — p. 50 col. 2: ". . . awareness of the self who is dying.")
  - C. The alleged fittingness of death (p. 50 col. 2: "We are often reminded . . ." — p. 56 col. 1: ". . . the worth or uniqueness ascribed to the dying life.")
- II. Christian humanism:
  - A. Love and fear (p. 56 col. 1: "I always write . . ." — p. 59 col. 2: ". . . the human dignity of caring for the dying.")
  - B. The anthropological alternatives (p. 59 col. 2: "In any case, from these empirical . . ." — p. 62)

6. Thus Ramsey, p. 55, attributing philosophical resignation to the failure of philosophical vitality. What Thomas wrote, however, was:

> Though wise men at their end know dark is right,
> Because their words had forked no lightning they
> Do not go gentle into that good night.

That is, the philosophers do not match their acceptance of death in theory with an acceptance in practice. Their words have forked no lightning for *them* to see their way by (*Collected Poems 1934-52* [London: Dart, 1966], p. 159)! Ramsey picks up this hint on p. 60, somewhat mischievously suggesting that Plato's account of Socrates' fortitude in death may not be trustworthy.

7. Kass, p. 71.

8. B. Pascal, *Pensées,* no. 347.

Kass, too, of course, assents to a version of this thesis. He, too, does not look to death itself as the source of man's dignity in dying. He contends that death is "neutral with respect to dignity"; for dignity is "something that belongs to a human being and is displayed in the way he lives, and hence something not easily taken away from him."[9] But Ramsey means, and understands Pascal to mean, something more negative about death than Kass could stomach. The very occasion for dignity is afforded by the fact that death is itself an *indignity,* in response to which the "human countenance" must be made to appear. On the one hand the therapist, and on the other the dying patient must bring to the event from outside it that sense of human worth which will enable it to appear. And this means encompassing "nakedly and without dilution" the fact that death is an indignity. What the philosophers should have grasped, as the fundamental ingredient of any view of death and dying, is that human mortality and human dignity are in dialectical contradiction. If the one evokes the other, it is not by sympathy but by antithesis.

The objection to received philosophical wisdom is then pursued in two stages. In the first Ramsey knocks together two characteristic consolations which attempt to accommodate human mortality to the life-projects of human agents. On the one hand, there is the claim that death is part of life; on the other, the claim that death is not part of life; either of which, if it were the whole truth, would be consoling. For we could be reconciled to the naturalness of death in the one case; or in the other we could dismiss it as something which, by definition, lies outside our ken. But neither is true. Or, perhaps we should say, neither is true except in such a way that the other is equally true. Death is not a part of life in such a way that it can be encompassed within our life-projects and so made comfortable; neither is it beyond our ken in such a way that it does not in fact impinge upon our life-projects and trouble them. It is a boundary; and a boundary is neither simply within the field nor simply beyond it. We live "up against" this limit during our life-spans. And whatever good may come to us from the fact that the limit is there, whatever creativity or virtue it may evoke, it does so because it is dreaded. Refusing to be accommodated within, and refusing to absent itself beyond our scope as human agents, it confronts us as the ultimate No to all that we aspire to be and do.

The second stage of the argument takes its cue from the saying of Koheleth (Ecclesiastes) that there is "a time to die" (3:2), and examines the grounds that philosophers have found for denying the character of death as the negation of the human. Koheleth himself, as Ramsey argues at the end of this section, knew better than those who had torn this thread out of the fabric of his thought. "Koheleth seems to say: Let the natural or cosmic order be whatever it is; men are different" (p. 55). And what Koheleth seems to say is, in Ramsey's view, what all philosophers ought to say instead of attempting to accommodate death within the sequence of life-experiences, and praising it for its fittingness. Philosophical "morticians" falsely ascribe to death the capacity to carry its own immanent meaningfulness, to be a *telos* when it is in fact no more than a *finis.* There is, to be sure, a legitimate way in which we can reach the conclusion that death is, on this or that occasion, *to be chosen:* that is, when it appears as the least of a number of possible indignities which the sufferer is compelled to choose among. But such an analysis of "comparative indignities" cannot justify talk of death's "beauty." Philosophy has struck an abstract posture which overlooks our human horror of death in order to think "generally." Against it Ramsey quotes another Pascal saying: "The heart has its reasons which reason does not know."[10] But he quotes it without entirely accepting the opposition of reason and heart which Pascal suggests. For the heart's reasons are genuine reasons; and philosophy which refuses to listen to the heart's reasons in its dread of death simply makes itself less than fully rational. Koheleth, when properly read, affords an example of what philosophy can say truly in the face of man's mortality; and so does Pascal.

All of which, as is evident enough, is Ramsey's way of making philosophy rebuke philosophy. He has allied himself (and not for the first time) with the existentialist philosophers in their contest with idealist metaphysics.[11] One of the questions he must face is how far "Christian humanism" can walk in this company without being consumed by it. For the moment it is enough to observe that in one feature of his exposition he is self-consciously dependent upon them. Kass complains of "Ramsey's frequent weaving back and forth between a subjective perspective on a particular death in its individuality . . . and an objective perspective on human mortality itself."[12] Such weaving, Ramsey would reply, is precisely what philosophy must do if it is to attend to its business. The dialectic between subjective dread, on the one hand, and objective recognition of the harmony of death and nature on the other, provides philosophers with the agenda for their thinking. If philosophy (as Plato, or Maimonides) refuses to attend to the dialectic, what has it left to think about? But if (as Koheleth, or Pascal) it does attend to it, then a further question arises: where, if anywhere, is it to turn for a resolution? Ramsey, for his part, turns to "Christian humanism."

Where, we may ask, is this turn meant to bring us? For there is more than one kind of resolution to the antinomy which we might envisage as the proper goal of our thought. Does Ramsey have in mind an evangelical rec-

9. Kass, pp. 68f.

10. Pascal, *Pensées,* no. 277.

11. See especially the use he makes of existentialist inspiration in his writing on sexual morality, "Jean-Paul Sartre: Sex in Being" in *Nine Modern Moralists* (Englewood Cliffs, N.J.: Prentice-Hall, 1962), and "A Christian Approach to the Question of Sexual Relations Outside of Marriage," *Journal of Religion,* 1965 (published in Britain as: *On Flesh* [Nottingham: Grove Books, 1975]).

12. Kass, p. 70.

onciliation, in which biological homogeneity and humane distinctiveness will embrace and kiss each other? Or does he envisage a resolution in thought alone, which will ground their opposition in metaphysics and show why it must always arise? This question is connected with another. When Ramsey turns to "Christian humanism," is that phrase meant to introduce a *theological* interpretation of human nature, a moment in the proclamation of the Christian Gospel? Or is he pointing us to something that is less decisively of faith, to a Christian wisdom that can prescind from evangelical proclamation and proceed on its own? On two occasions in what follows he invites non-Christians, "whatever [they] may think about the *theology* here entailed, . . ." to attend to the "penetration of [the] human condition" (56, 57). Yet those who know Ramsey's theoretical explorations of how Christ "transforms" the law of nature, will not expect to find him advancing an unambiguously "natural" account of human existence as that which properly belongs to Christendom.[13] If it is true that the argument of this second major section of Ramsey's article is not theological, it is also true that it is shaped by theology, and that evangelical proclamation lurks in its shadows. In order to illustrate this, I propose to read the first part of it (IIA) twice: once in order to trace its most obvious course, which seems to allow no place for evangelical reconciliation, and then a second time in order to notice the indications which point us towards one. Both readings are facilitated by a comparison with a published sermon of thirteen years before, entitled (after Donne) *Deaths Duell,* on which Ramsey drew heavily for this part of his article.[14]

The section begins with a twofold quotation from 1 John 4:18: "Perfect love casts out fear," and "Where fear is, love is not perfected." The same pair of sayings had served as a text for *Deaths Duell.* In what follows most of Ramsey's attention is directed to the second member of this pair, which he applies to the question of dying in the following paraphrase: "Where fear of death and dying remains, medical and human care of the dying is not perfected" (56). Fear, in other words, is the source of that medical officiousness which troubles the dying unnecessarily, as well as of other attempts to remove the human countenance from death, some of them masquerading under the slogan "death with dignity." One or another species of the denial of death operates to prevent that humane keeping-of-company which ought to be the truest form of care. It is in support of this thesis that Ramsey then turns to the assertion of Saint Paul that sin and death are connected — an assertion which differentiates Christianity, in his view, both from the Hebrew concern with sin and the Hellenistic concern with death. Death brings sin after it. And with this claim Christianity "has grasped some important experiential human realities" better than most philosophies (57). Not that it was not anticipated in the Old Testament: again, Koheleth can be quoted. Nor can we say that this "existential anxiety" is without possibilities for good; for the Psalmist was able to pray "Teach us to number our days that we may apply our hearts to wisdom."[15] The point is simply that such wisdom as springs from the knowledge of our mortality arises from *dread.* And in recognising the fact, and the equally striking fact that dread lies behind our refusal of love because it generates self-protection, Christianity has unmasked the pretensions of philosophy to accommodate death within the scheme of things. It has also made sense, as philosophy cannot otherwise do, of such instinctual responses to death as the "gallows humour" by which medical students negotiate their earliest engagements with the dissection of a corpse.

On this first reading of section IIA, then, which is the more straightforward reading, it contains no evangelical reconciliation, but merely points to elements of a theological anthropology which will ground the antinomy of mortality and human aspiration. The link between sin and death, in which death brings sin after it, highlights the fact that we cannot ignore the dread of death nor regard it as merely circumstantial weakness of mind; for it lies at the root of that universal failure of love which is the core of the human tragedy. There is no doubt from which source Ramsey derived this train of thought: it is from Reinhold Niebuhr, quoted at a significant moment as saying that anxiety over death is the source of all human creativity and of all human sinfulness.[16] The same

13. See *Nine Modern Moralists,* chs. 5-9 inclusive.

14. University Park: Pennsylvania State University, 1961. The sermon contains a number of passages on which Ramsey has drawn for his 1974 article: — on p. 1, the relation of Christianity to Greek and Hebrew views of death (cf. ". . . Death with Dignity," p. 57 col. 1); on p. 3 the two parts of the text 1 John 4:18 (cf. p. 56 col. 1), the reference to Ecclesiastes 9:3 (cf. p. 57 col. 2, but with the reference not given), and the use of Pascal's *Pensée* 347 (cf. p. 55 col. 2); on p. 5 love as respect for the shadow of death upon the face of another (cf. p. 58 col. 2). These are the obvious debts. In addition there are places where the thought of ". . . Death with Dignity" becomes clearer when it is seen to carry an allusion to an argument which was developed in *Deaths Duell:* such is the reference to "'faith-ing' in an ultimate righteousness" (p. 56 col. 2), which demands to be read in the light of p. 6 of the sermon.

15. Psalm 90:12, curiously misattributed by Ramsey to Ecclesiastes.

16. I have not traced the source of the quotation, though the sentiment is common enough in Niebuhr's writings. A more comprehensive treatment of Ramsey's theological debt to Niebuhr would illuminate a good deal. We find in *The Nature and Destiny of Man* sources for several observations in ". . . Death with Dignity": the criticism of Epicurus (I p. 98, II p. 9); the preoccupation of Hellenistic thought with finitude (II p. 58), *finis* and *telos* (II p. 293); the "testimony of the heart" (II p. 294); and in *Faith and History* (p. 170) the alternative strategies of the "worldly" and "other-worldly religions." All of which may conceal from us how Ramsey has, without naming him, turned against Niebuhr at a critical point. Take the crucial passage, *The Nature and Destiny of Man* (I pp. 173-76) (New York: Scribner Library edition, 1964). Niebuhr first distinguishes two ways of connecting sin and death, using Augustine's saying "It is by sin that we die and not by death that we sin." The latter connexion is purely pagan; the former is rabbinic, Pauline and preferable. However, even the rabbinic-Pauline view has the odour of dualism lingering over it, and obscures the organic relation of death and nature. There is another Pauline view,

train of thought featured prominently in *Deaths Duell.* But comparison of the two writings turns up a startling contrast. In the earlier essay Ramsey treated the thesis *death brings sin after it* merely as the preparation for a more important antithesis, and criticised any one-sided affirmation of it as "a return to the Greek religious consciousness and a breakdown of the Biblical tradition that is without parallel."[17] And he named "present-day existentialism" as one of the factors in that breakdown. The more profoundly Christian connexion between sin and death, Ramsey then argued, is found in the contrary assertion that *sin brings death after it.* The importance of this assertion lay in the fact that it constituted a "redefinition" of life and death, determining the locus of each in relation to the object of our human love and belief: "We *live* by faith; or else in lack of faith living according to the flesh we die."[18] The Christian Gospel, therefore, proclaims a reconciliation of humanity with mortality, for it proclaims that eternal life is present here and now, even under the conditions of mortality. Thus, Ramsey concluded, "perfect love casts out any fear over the loss of life," and this, the first member of the pair of sayings, proves (despite an early impression to the contrary) to be the more Christian because it is the more evangelical statement.[19]

We are struck, first of all, by the simple absence of this material from ". . . Death with Dignity." At first reading, Ramsey has turned his back on the evangelical emphasis which he was previously at pains to give — the connexion between sin and death in Christian thought. But a second reading does something to qualify this impression. He paraphrases the first part of his text as follows: "Perfect care of the dying casts out fear of one's own death or rejection of their dying because of fear of ours." The standard for care of the dying, he adds, is "cut to the measure of the perfection in benevolence believed to be that of our Father in Heaven"; and then, seizing on the word "believed" (which gives the impression of having been dragged in), he adds: "So there is 'faith-ing' in an ultimate righteousness beyond the perceptible human condition." Behind the perception that death brings lovelessness after it, there lies the proclamation that by faith in divine love we may overcome the lovelessness that death brings. All that is said in a moment, before the unbeliever is invited to prescind from theology and attend to the "notation upon" the human condition. In no more than a moment, too, Ramsey reminds us (in a passage which did not come ready-made from *Deaths Duell!*) that the Messiah was born as mortal flesh "to gain for us a foretaste of victory over sin and death." It becomes clear, then, that we are not meant to forget that Christianity has an evangelical proclamation to make, arising from the connexion of death and sin; but still there is no hint of the conclusion in the earlier piece, that a one-sided emphasis on existential anxiety is in danger of reverting to paganism, and that the Christian connexion between death and sin is better expressed as "sin draws death after." The implied criticism of Niebuhr has now been withdrawn. In 1974 Ramsey, writing with more explicitly apologetic motives perhaps, does not want to distance himself from Niebuhr, but simply to recall what he once taught us.

Thus we turn to the final section (IIB), which is the climax of the argument. It begins with the assertion of body-soul unity, the theological goal, as we may now see, to which the article has been tending. Ramsey has expounded this principle from many sources on many different occasions. Here he takes his lead from Augustine's *City of God,* with no more than a passing allusion to Saint Paul, which, however, I quote in order to comment later on what it omits: "Thus for Biblical or later Christian anthropology, the only possible form which human life in any true and proper sense can take here or hereafter is 'somatic.' That is the Pauline word; today we say psychosomatic" (60). The natural conclusion from this anthropology is that death (though theologically it may be a *conquered* enemy) is, in the natural order, an enemy still. Ramsey then outlines two alternative strategies of thought for reducing "the dreadful visage of death." If we are not prepared to follow either of these "escapes," he will conclude, then "Death the Enemy again comes into view" (62). One of these strategies is Plato's, the other Aristotle's. Plato reduces *bodily life to indifference* by arguing for the self-sufficient immortality of the dissevered soul, "gathering and collecting herself into herself . . . out

---

expressed in 1 Cor. 15:56, "The sting of death is sin," which is much better. It attributes no evil to death, but only to the fear of death (which is pride concealing its own mortality). This is the "general biblical view." This "general biblical view" which Niebuhr favours is the view which Ramsey thinks in danger of reverting to paganism if it is not balanced out, that "death brings sin after." The "rabbinic-Pauline view," which Niebuhr damns with faint praise, is Ramsey's own preferred view, that "sin brings death after." Niebuhr and Ramsey (in *Deaths Duell*) would each incline to accuse the other of temporising with paganism. In ". . . Death with Dignity" the qualified criticism of Niebuhr's preferred emphasis is suppressed; but only by an implicit denial of the distinction between that and the rabbinic-Pauline view. Paul's teaching that sin brings death after is made the theological chapter-heading for the exposition of Niebuhr's view! Ramsey will never, in fact, assert with Niebuhr that "death is no evil though it is an occasion for evil, namely the fear of death" (I p. 167). And that is because Ramsey has not accepted the starting-point of Niebuhr's anthropology, which is the dialectic of nature and freedom. Kass accuses Ramsey of failing "to give nature her due" (p. 76), and would, no doubt, be much happier with the generous concessions that Niebuhr will make to the mutual implication of nature and death. But it is at least arguable that Ramsey has understood better what a theology of the natural order requires when he refuses to follow Niebuhr's example of giving everything to nature with one hand, only to take it away with the other.

17. *Deaths Duell,* p. 5.

18. *Deaths Duell,* p. 6.

19. "This is the more basic direction of things . . . than that expressed by those other statements (which are also true), that death draws sin after, and where fear is, love is not perfected," p. 7. Contrast the impression given on p. 3: "The truth of this (i.e. where fear is love is not perfected) we have to discover by more profound insight. . . ."

of the body." Aristotle reduces the *uniqueness of individual life to interchangeability,* vesting all the value and worth of humankind in the species rather than the individual.

Ramsey's pincer-movement appears to be a fairly simple one. Either the soul is immortal and self-sufficient (and so the individual is unarmed by death); or the value of humanity resides in the species (and so the death of individuals is of little moment); or, the value of humanity residing in individuals and the soul being bound up in the death of the body, death is dreadful. The dreadfulness of death is thus argued as an implication of some fundamental Christian postures over against classical paganism; and that is why Christians should find themselves at one with existentialists in calling the bluff of idealist or naturalist evasions. But on inspection the argument appears to face at least two difficulties. Does the Christian affirmation of "somatic" existence imply the affirmation of *both* the arms of Ramsey's pincer, the one rejecting Plato and the other Aristotle? If we are to say so, then we need to lay a better foundation than is afforded by the simple assertion of body-soul unity. For psychosomatic unity, as it stands, also describes Aristotle's position; and if Ramsey wishes to differentiate Christian anthropology from the Aristotelian alternative, he will have to say more than he has done to characterise it as a view which conceives human value as not only bodily but individual.[20] The second difficulty we may allow Kass to express: "He should . . . be willing *in principle* to embrace current biochemical research which aims to retard the process of aging and greatly extend our life expectancy. . . . I suspect he would, on principle, refuse. His heart may know the reasons why . . . but his reason's reasons — at least those given in this paper — would not tell him or us why not."[21]

The programme of Ramsey's discussion has been to move from a disagreement internal to philosophy, in which existential anxiety in the face of death demands to be taken more seriously than palliating naturalist and idealist philosophies have taken it, to a Christian anthropology which grounds existential anxiety in two metaphysical assertions, the connexion of sin and death and the unity of body and soul. It appears, however, that the second of these two assertions, the principle of body-soul unity, is not strong enough to bear the weight which Ramsey puts on it. It will not rule out, on the one hand, an Aristotelian settlement which accepts individual perishability for the sake of species-survival; and it will not rule out, on the other, a defiance of natural mortality (by technique, if it can be done) which might seem to be the inevitable implication of the existential struggle which Ramsey admires. My argument will be that this undeniable weakness in Ramsey's anthropological foundations is not systemic, but that it arises from the apologetic strategy of the article, by which he encouraged his readers too readily to prescind from the theological context and so deprived his contentions of the full range of their interpretative force. We have already shown how, in his handling of the first assertion, he suppressed what had seemed to him elsewhere to be the more important aspect of the Christian association of sin and death, and how with it he surrendered the ground from which he could criticise the existentialist philosophies with which he was strategically allied. We must proceed by showing how he has done the same with the second assertion, the most persistently Ramseyan of the two and the one with which our own chief interest on this occasion lies. By positing the principle of body-soul unity in isolation from its context in the Christian gospel, Ramsey has left it weaker in explanatory force than it should be, and has accordingly failed to display the full intelligibility of his own position.

Leon Kass might have found an answer, had he come across *Deaths Duell,* to the challenge he threw down about research to avert aging. The reasons Ramsey would adduce for refusing such research emerge clearly enough there, from an elegant quotation of Donne: "When thou thinkest thyself swallowed, and buried in affliction . . . Christ Jesus shall remove thy grave stone, and give thee a resurrection; but if thou thinkest to remove it by thine own wit, thine own power, or favour of potent friends, *Digitus Dei non est hic,* the hand of God is not in all this, and the stone will lie upon thee, till thou putrefy into desperation, and thou shalt have no part in this . . . resurrection."[22] Expressed in a plainer style, the same answer can be found in some words of Niebuhr: "The hope of the resurrection . . . implies that the condition of finiteness and freedom, which lies at the basis of human existence, is a problem for which there is no solution by any human power. Only God can solve this problem."[23]

The road which leads from psychosomatic unity to an endeavour of technique to keep body and soul together, is blocked by an act of God. The decisive intervention of divine power is the warning that we must not (even if we could) secure the unity of body and soul by the strivings of practical ingenuity. But in ". . . *Death with Dignity* the resurrection is scarcely mentioned."[24] Denying himself an appeal to this central affirmation of

20. He has, of course, said that according to Aristotelian philosophy, "reason, the formal principle, is definitive of essential humanity. That is universal, eternal as logic. Matter, however, is the individuating factor" (61). But this is not sufficient. For Aristotle believes (in contradistinction to Plato) that the universal is not "separable" from the particular, but exists only as it is instantiated particularly. He therefore fulfils the formal requirement of believing that the particular body and the universal reason are inseparably united. Ramsey needs a criterion that goes beyond that formal requirement.

21. Kass, p. 79.

22. Once again Ramsey's commonplace book defeats the commentator. The quotation does not appear to be from Donne's *Deaths Duell.*

23. *The Nature and Destiny of Man* II, p. 295.

24. It appears, as though by reflection in a mirror, when Ramsey praises the "more orthodox wording" of a church statement on p. 51.

the Christian creed, Ramsey has denied himself the means of delimiting his position effectively and of refusing the unwelcome inference which Kass would make him draw from it.

The resurrection, however, plays more than a merely limiting role in relation to psychosomatic unity. It is, in fact, the intellectual foundation of it in Christian thought. It is the resurrection, rather than the principle of body-soul unity *in abstracto,* which performs the crucial task of criticising the idealist "over-spiritualisation" of human action in modern thought. And at this point we may have to acknowledge another coalition of otherwise divergent viewpoints; for there are, of course, other critiques of idealism, other assertions of the materialist affirmation of the human body, than that which a Christian will feel bound to make.[25] But in *Deaths Duell* Ramsey made clear enough the theological roots of his own materialism. The first page of that sermon proceeds tightly by the following steps: (i) Christianity (speaking through the mouth of Saint Paul) improved upon both Hebrew and Hellenistic thought by tying sin and death together. (ii) It is implied in this conjunction that death is an act of divine judgment, in which "God withdrew his perduring power." (iii) And it is implied in that view of death that there is no inherent immortality of the soul, which would be, in effect, a "robbery of God." Conversely, the denial of the authentic Christian belief in the resurrection of the body is grounded in an "ultra-spiritual estimate of man." Conclusion: Christian belief in resurrection and Hellenistic belief in the immortal soul are, therefore, opposed to each other.

This argument places Ramsey in the mainstream of an almost twentieth-century theological consensus, and in order to demonstrate the character of this consensus, I beg indulgence for a brief and sketchy historical excursus. It could almost be said that an opposition between idealist "spiritualisation" and Christian "materialism," based on belief in the resurrection, is the hallmark of all Western theology which postdates the great theological upheaval of the 1920s. It is common to all the diverse schools of Protestant theology, however differently they relate the resurrection to history.[26] It is proclaimed as a datum of Biblical research by the "Biblical theology" school.[27] Historical New Testament criticism plunges into the task of separating the "pre-Easter" from the "post-Easter" elements of the Gospel tradition. Thomists claim for St. Thomas the decisive articulation of a materialist Christian anthropology.[28] Reform-minded Roman Catholics challenge the Western Catholic tradition over the "shrinkage" of Easter.[29] Eastern Orthodox theologians recall that resurrection was central to the theology of the Greek fathers.[30] "Christian materialism" then survives the collapse and demise of all the leading mid-century schools of theology, and emerges, fresh and as though new-minted, in the historical dialectics of the neo-Hegelians.[31]

I take as an early manifesto for this twentieth-century consensus a small book by Karl Barth dating from 1926, *The Resurrection of the Dead.*[32] In it Barth addresses the fifteenth chapter of 1 Corinthians, the chapter about the resurrection, and argues that it is the key to the whole epistle and, more sweepingly, to the whole of Saint Paul's proclamation of the Gospel. In light of the resurrection all the issues of life and death are seen clearly and judged (p. 107). In this context Barth advances his criticism of romantic idealism, in which the main outline of what Ramsey will later want to say is already apparent. The Last Things of Christian proclamation are not the ultimate possibilities of human life; they are the end of all things — not in the sense of being their goal but as their termination (pp. 109f.). Death relativises all the abundant possibilities of life by putting a close to them (p. 113). Human aspirations cannot include death within their purposes, however spiritual. Life after death is not a possibility *within* a uniform cosmos which we can comprehend. The Gospel proclaims a *bodily* resurrection in order to reprove our "wanton play of imagination with respect to the invisible," and this challenges at its root all ideas of an immanent human fitness for immortality. The overcoming of death is a new world, unbelievable, inaccessible apart from the fact that God has simply confronted us with it (p. 157). Paul's opponents at Corinth, says Barth (and makes no secret of thinking that nineteenth-century idealism was their natural intellectual milieu), played down the general resurrection because it confronted them with the alien "other" of divine activity. But without the general resurrection, the resurrection of Christ could be only a meaningless isolated

25. It would appear that both Morison and Kass would give assent to some form of the body-soul unity principle. A striking example of its use outside a Christian context is given by Hans Jonas, in his article about the 1968 Harvard report advocating criteria for "brain-death": "I see lurking behind the proposed definition of death . . . a curious revenant of the old soul-body dualism. Its new apparition is the dualism of brain and body. In a certain analogy to the former it holds that the true human person rests in (or is represented by) the brain, of which the rest of the body is a mere subservient tool" (*Philosophical Essays* [University of Chicago Press, 1974], p. 139).

26. Thus it is held by Barth (reference below), Niebuhr (*Nature and Destiny of Man* II, pp. 294-98), Bultmann (*Theology of the New Testament,* London: SCM, 1955, I, pp. 192-203) and Tillich (*Systematic Theology* III [Chicago: University of Chicago Press, 1963], pp. 409-14).

27. See, for example, Oscar Cullmann, *Immortality of the Soul or Resurrection of the Dead?* (London: Epworth Press, 1958).

28. See Etienne Gilson, *The Spirit of Mediaeval Philosophy* (New York: Scribner's, 1936), pp. 168-88.

29. See Karl Rahner, "Dogmatic Questions on Easter," *Theological Investigations* IV (London: Darton, Longman & Todd, 1966), pp. 121-33.

30. See Georges Florovsky, "The 'Immortality' of the Soul," *Creation and Redemption* (Belmont, Mass.: Nordland, 1976), pp. 213-40.

31. See J. Moltmann, *God in Creation* (London: SCM, 1985), pp. 244-75.

32. Karl Barth, *The Resurrection of the Dead,* tr. H. J. Stenning (London: Hodder & Stoughton, 1933).

miracle (p. 122), not a true appearance of the divine horizon (p. 162). The "parousia" of Christ at the end of history is the surfacing of the subterranean stream which has run from the resurrection of Christ (p. 176). The resurrection is, therefore, already the decisive conquest of death and the inauguration of the new world.

Sixty years ago this was revolutionary. It is hard to find any eighteenth- or nineteenth-century voices which would assert the centrality of the resurrection of Christ as almost all twentieth-century voices have agreed in asserting it. The mood of the nineteenth century is set by Schleiermacher's cool estimate that "the disciples recognised in Jesus the Son of God without having the faintest premonition of his resurrection and ascension, and we too may say the same of ourselves; moreover, neither the spiritual presence which he promised, nor all that he said about his enduring influence upon those who remained behind, is mediated through either of these two facts."[33] But, of course, it was not original to the nineteenth century romantics to suggest that the salvific meaning of Christ's death could be explained on its own, without reference to the resurrection. In Western theology this assumption can be traced back at least as far as Anselm's *Cur Deus Homo*. And the corollary of it was a view of death which vested the hope of the believer in the immortality of the soul, and, at its worst, repudiated the body. We may observe this tradition at its most marked in the popular Lutheran piety of the early eighteenth century, as represented to us in the texts used by J. S. Bach for his church cantatas, with their constantly recurring prayers of longing for death.[34] Nobody ever told Bach or his contemporaries that "the only possible form which human life in any true and proper sense can take here or hereafter is 'somatic'."[35]

The Christian anthropology, then, to which Ramsey appeals to insistently is hardly the anthropology of the whole Christian tradition. If we are to affirm (as I, with him, would do) that this is authentic Christian anthropology, then we have to support our claim with another: that the revolution which swept the body to the centre of Christian thought earlier this century was a genuine rediscovery of elements of an original Christian understanding.

Where did the twentieth-century revolution spring from? Its sources are complex. On the philosophical side it is part of the general repudiation of idealism in the inter-war period, and so has negative affinities with the philosophical turn to materialism which occurred at the same time. More profoundly, however, it is the fruit of an accumulating weight of biblical and historical scholarship in at least three areas. It reflects the development in patristic scholarship which made theologians aware of the central place played by the resurrection of the body in early Christian anti-Platonist polemic. This is the more impressive as it occurs in a theological milieu which, as some modern objectors are inclined to feel, had already made dangerously extensive concessions to Platonic dualism; yet however great the concessions may have been, the Fathers characteristically viewed the resurrection of the body as a battle line which could not be abandoned. It reflects also the discovery of late Jewish apocalyptic and its role in shaping the categories of the New Testament. It reflects, in the third place, a new appreciation of the materialist character of psychological terms in Biblical Hebrew, and the disembarrassment of such words as *nephesh* and *leb* of the irrelevant overtones which "soul" and "heart" had acquired from other sources. The assertion that body-soul unity is the "Biblical" anthropology is based on a study of *Hebrew* words; though the Greek New Testament, it is true, often reflects Hebrew word-usage, as in the famous text about "losing one's soul" and "saving it," where *psyche* is properly the equivalent of the Hebrew *nephesh*.

But the claim for a "Biblical" concept of man as a unitary psychosomatic being cannot be sustained on the basis of Hebrew lexicography alone. It is quite clear that Jewish writers of the New Testament era allowed themselves a much greater eclecticism, of terminology and conceptualisation, than would ever be encountered in the Psalms. Compare the entirely "materialist" cry of Psalm 30:9, "Will the dust praise thee? Will it tell of thy faithfulness?," with the famous passage from the Book of Wisdom (3:1ff.) which declares that "the souls of the righteous are in the hand of God," and adds that "in the eyes of the foolish they *seem* to have died, and their departure was *thought* to be an affliction . . . but they are at peace" (emphasis added). And before we dismiss this as an aberration in a work deeply influenced by Hellenism, we have to account for a saying of Jesus himself, as we

33. F. Schleiermacher, "The Christian Faith," ed. H. J. Mackintosh and J. S. Stewart (Edinburgh: T&T Clark, 1928), p. 418.

34. This feature was highlighted by Albert Schweitzer (*J. S. Bach*, vol. I, tr. E. Newman [New York: Dover, 1966; 1st ed. 1911], pp. 169f.), who, however, misunderstood it as a personally distinctive feature of Bach's own outlook rather than as a cultural commonplace. Though universally exemplified in the Bach corpus, it is most striking in the Easter cantatas, where we might have expected the theme of resurrection to prevail. Thus in BWV 31 the librettist (S. Franck) prays: "Letzte Stunde, brich herein, mir die Augen zuzudrücken!," and in BWV 158 we take up the words of a hymn by J. G. Albinus, "Welt, ade, ich bin dein müde." In BWV 6 the theme is set by a metaphorical treatment of the words of Luke 24:29, "the day is far spent." The most notable exception is BWV 4, which has a text drawn throughout from Luther's hymn, "Christ lag in Todesbanden." The Reformation had, indeed, given a sharper definition to the resurrection than either the late-mediaeval inwardness which preceded it or the age of science and sensibility which succeeded it. It was never, therefore, banished from the edges of Christian consciousness, and in some traditions maintained a stronger presence throughout the seventeenth and into the eighteenth century. Handel's "Messiah," which does altogether more justice to the resurrection than we will usually find in Bach, has as its text an Anglican catena of Scripture quotations supplied by C. Jennens. And it was in the preaching of an Anglican seventeenth-century divine, John Donne, that Ramsey found a congenial model for his own proclamation of the resurrection in *Deaths Duell*.

35. Ramsey, ". . . Death with Dignity," p. 60.

find it in St. Matthew's Gospel (10:28), hardly the most Hellenistic of Jewish writings: "And do not fear those who kill the body but cannot kill the soul."[36] Even Saint Paul compares the body to a tent in which we conduct our pilgrimage, to be replaced after death by a more permanent dwelling (2 Cor. 5:1ff.). However true it may be that *psyche* in the New Testament does not mean what it means in Plato's *Phaedo,* it is clear that the New Testament writers are quite at home with the concept of an "inner man" — the phrase itself comes from Ephesians (3:16) — and are prepared to evoke this hidden level of human existence to give support to the believer's hope in the face of death. There is, of course, a great difference between the way they handle it and the way that it is handled in the Platonic tradition. But the point is that it is not the conceptual structure *itself* which differentiates New Treatment anthropology from Platonic. The conceptual structure is plastic and adaptable, responding to the ideas that the writers had to express, which are not exactly those which the Psalmists had to express.

The difference lies in the fact that the apostles of the earliest church made the resurrection of Jesus the centre of their proclamation, and it was this that forbade them to *develop* a dual conception of man as body and soul (which they could perfectly well *admit*) in the direction of an objectifying alienation of the body. Thus we find in their writings, too, something that can be called, not inappropriately, "body-soul unity" — though we might be wiser to find ourselves another term, since the effect of the words "unity" and "dualism" is to reduce all the options inflexibly to two. I prefer to speak of a Christian *identification* with the body, as opposed to an *objectification* of the body which marks the idealist tradition. Even where the discussion has not to do with death — notably at 1 Corinthians 6:12ff., where the theme is sexual morality — the ground of identification with the body is the claim that God has made upon the bodily life of a man by the resurrection of Christ. "The body is not meant for immorality but for the Lord, and the Lord for the body. And God raised the Lord, and will also raise us up by his power. Do you know that your bodies are members of Christ?"

The principle of psychosomatic unity, then, has no *free-standing* authority for Christian thought, but rides on the principle that the resurrection of Christ is central to Christian faith and the resurrection of all mankind to Christian hope. It is in this context that the Christian will wish to give his assent to the saying, "Embodiment is the end of all God's works."[37]

IT REMAINS for me to plead that the positions which Ramsey maintained in ". . . Death with Dignity" cohere around this central theological affirmation. This part of my argument can only be effected by a doctrinal sketch, which will be as unsatisfactory as such sketches always are — for it is the cartoonist's fate that his pencil-lines must seem too sweeping and dogmatic.

At the root of idealism, and therefore of the idealist view of human nature which Ramsey, with the majority of twentieth-century theologians, wishes to contest, is the contrast between appearance and reality. Idealism takes its bearings from the sharp difference between what it is to *be* a human being and what it is to *observe* one; and in its attempt to discern what is real, it follows those clues which are given by the hidden subjectivity of human existence, that which we know only in ourselves and not in other people. To speak, with Plato, of "the soul" is to use only one of the terms by which idealist philosophies have identified the hidden reality of what it is to be a human being. One may speak equally of "spirit" or of "mind" — the latter term drawing attention to the common conviction that the hidden reality is connected with the phenomenon of mental awareness, of world and of self.

To think of reality as hidden, is not, of course, to think of it as beyond knowledge — with such a contention philosophy would merely rule itself out. We know the hidden world because it is the source of the intelligible form with which appearances are presented to us; it is the intelligible principle behind their intelligibility. But knowledge can only be acquired by a philosophical askesis, by stripping away appearances and unmasking their pretensions to be the reality which they present. Idealism embodies the suspicion of appearances, the conviction that they create delusions which must be overcome. And so it is with its treatment of death. When Ramsey criticises idealist philosophers for not taking existential anxiety about death seriously enough, the truth probably is (as Kass hints) that they *have* taken it seriously — as a delusion! They have treated it as a form of the vulgar acceptance of what merely seems to be. Thus the *Phaedo* takes the form of a dialogue, in which the distress of Socrates' friends is overcome by his own philosophic calm. A dialogue, too, the most striking of the romantic expressions of calm before death, Matthias Claudius's "Der Tod und das Mädchen," famous from Schubert's unforgettable setting:

> 'Vorüber! ach, vorüber
> Geh, wilder Knochenmann!
> Ich bin noch jung, geh, Lieber!
> Und rühre mich nicht an.'
>
> 'Gib deine Hand, du schon und zart Gebild,
> Bin Freund und komme nicht zu strafen.
> Sei gutes Muts! Ich bin nicht wild,
> Sollst sanft in meinen Armen schlafen.'[48]

36. The parallel in St. Luke's Gospel (12:4) conforms much more closely to our expectations of a "Hebraic" anthropology: "Do not fear those who kill the body, and after that have no more that they can do."

37. A saying of the eighteenth-century theologian F. C. Oetinger, taken up by Moltmann (op. cit., p. 244).

38. "'Pass me by, pass me by, Go away, wild skeleton! I am still young — go, dear Death, and do not touch me.' 'Give me your hand, you lovely and tender creature; I am your friend and do not

Christian opposition to idealism is based on a different view of the relation of appearance to reality. The distinction between them is, of course, recognised in the biblical depiction of human nature: "Man looks on the outward appearance, but the LORD looks on the heart" (1 Sam. 16:7). Yet the distinction is developed differently. If in Platonism the essence of the inner man is self-conscious awareness (or "Mind"), with the biblical "heart" we encounter a conception of inwardness as a source of practical agency. The hidden man deliberates and originates action; it is not the philosopher who demonstrates our need to reckon with him, but the schemer, whose impassive face conceals elaborate plans for the downfall of the righteous. And that means that the hidden reality will not remain hidden, but will burst into appearance and manifest itself, as the intentions of the heart finally bear fruit in action. In the teaching of Jesus in the synoptic Gospels it is constantly repeated that the hidden must eventually publish itself: "Either make the tree good and its fruit good, or make the tree bad and its fruit bad; for the tree is known by its fruit. You brood of vipers! how can you speak good, when you are evil? For out of the abundance of the heart the mouth speaks. The good man out of his good treasure brings forth good, and the evil man out of his evil treasure brings forth evil" (Matt. 12:33-5). Appearances are not insulated against the hidden reality; there is no stable distance between them which will allow illusion to be indefinitely sustained. The appearance of ultimate annihilation which death presents is to be overcome, then, not by being seen through by the wise, but by being abolished and replaced with a truer appearance. The difference between the immortality of the soul and the resurrection of the dead is the difference between an esoteric reconciliation and a public one.

The resurrection was not named among the traditional Four Last Things of Christian thought — an arbitrary list, deservedly toppled long since from its place in the doctrinal textbooks. One might say that resurrection unmasks the pretensions of death to be a Last Thing, by superseding it as a Later-than-last Thing, and so demonstrating that it was never more than a penultimate thing. But from this it follows that death can no longer be regarded (though ever so philosophically, and in despite of appearances) as the goal towards which life in the body is ordered, the *telos* which sets the coping stone on its achievement. In the sonorous Coverdale version of the ninetieth Psalm we are accustomed to say that "we bring our years to an end as a tale that is told," a claim that seems to be false on at least two points. For, by whatever means our years come to their end, it is not we who bring them to it, unless we are in that small and unhappy group of those who end their own lives by violence. And when, however, our years come to their end, their end gives them no perceptible narrative coherence; rather, death comes bounding into them to disrupt whatever narrative coherence they might have been in course of achieving. Think of the difficulty which confronts every biographer in attempting to include the subject's death in the story of his life! Only fiction-writers can integrate death pleasingly into a narrative wholeness; and that is because characters who die in fiction exist only to die, whereas characters who die in life have existed to live. We would do better to choose a less sonorous but more truthful modern translation of the Psalmist's words: "Our years peter out in a whimper."

Behind the pretension of death to provide a *telos* for life there lies a way of looking at life itself. Or perhaps we should say, there lie several ways of looking at it; for not every philosophy that can be grouped under the umbrella-title of "idealism" will look at life in precisely the same way. Yet every way of looking at life that tries to find in it a thread of meaning which will make death its climax will seem to the Christian perspective to have sold life short. Of the tendency of Platonism to engender a suspicion of the body, and to ally itself with a Manichaean dread of sexuality and sense, more than enough has been said in this century by the voices of robust materialism, Jewish, Christian and unbelieving. We need not pursue that side of things further here. Less has been said (though some of it has been very memorable) of the life-renouncing character of modern romanticism.[39] In the Claudius poem we find an epitome not merely of the romantic view of death but of the romantic spirit as such, which trades heavily on death in order to project its vision of life. The secret meaningfulness of death which it uncovers is that the true goal of life is exhaustion. To live as though to become a pile of embers, burnt out in a momentary blaze of brilliant and unearthly luminosity, such is the aspiration which romanticism, in many forms, commends to us. And against that aspiration authentic Christianity will find itself forced to contend for all that is represented by the empty tomb of Easter. Bodily life is not given us in order for it to collapse spectacularly under the weight of the spirit; it is given to sustain spiritual life, and in turn to be renewed by it. Life is for life, not for the abnegation of life.

In this context we may take up a crucial charge that Kass has made against Ramsey: that he has not given nature its due (p. 76). Let us try to meet it, on Ramsey's behalf, by turning it round against Kass himself. He writes that "decline and death are a part of life, an integral part which cannot be extruded without destroying the whole" (p. 76). At the level of a purely biological teleology, that is obviously undeniable. But does it raise no difficulties for the wider concept of "nature" to which Kass would recall us, that is, the concept of an ordered teleological

come to punish. Be comforted! I am not wild. You will sleep gently in my arms.'" Text and translation from *The Penguin Book of Lieder*, ed. and tr. S. S. Prawer (Harmondsworth, Middlesex: Penguin, 1964), pp. 38f.

39. See, for example, the classic analysis of romanticism in D. de Rougemont, *Passion and Society*, tr. M. Belgion (London: Faber, 1956 rev.).

system which embraces the whole? When he describes life as a "bitter-sweet bargain" (p. 79), ought he not to sense an element of tension between this and the confident "very good" of Rabbi Meir and Maimonides? Whether he ought or no, it is a matter of simple intellectual history that the majority of moderns have claimed to find here such a sharp conflict between the biological and the humane, between *bios* and *zōē,* that they have declared the idea of an overarching natural order simply untenable. The would-be vindicator of nature has something more to do than simply read natural purposes off biology.[40] I would think that Ramsey has grasped more subtly what kind of teleological vindication the concept of "nature's due" requires. Yet he has failed to point us to the fulcrum on which Christian thought has believed it could comprehend a harmonious balance of *bios* and *zōē:* the new act of God which transforms the one to be the adequate vehicle of the other.

I think it was an error of exposition on Ramsey's part to embark on his account of "Christian humanism" from the connexion between sin and death. In the internal logic of Christian thinking such a connexion is reached only in the second place, from the way death is understood in the light of the vindication of life. To see death as the emblem of divine judgment requires that we have first seen life as an emblem of divine acquittal. Because God has said his final "Yes" to the world, we may understand the mysterious and world-denying absurdity of death as God's penultimate "No," the No which supports the Yes by refusing all forms of uncreation and destruction in the human will. The assertion that Christ's *death* is redemptive comes second (*pace* Anselm and Schleiermacher) to the assertion that his *resurrection* is redemptive.[41] Deutero-Isaiah's suffering servant, who bore the sin of many (Isa. 52:13–53:12), depends for intelligibility upon the prophet's message of divine liberation through the conquests of Cyrus. Even the Yahwist's picture of the encroachment of mortality in the wake of human disobedience is not self-standing; for the primaeval history of Genesis 1–11 could be no part of faith otherwise than as a preface to the story of God's blessing of the nations through Abraham's seed. The purposiveness of condemnation is never perspicuous in itself. It gains its perspicuity only in the light of the purposiveness of vindication.

I do not wish to underestimate the difficulty which thought encounters in handling the connexion of physical death with moral condemnation. No thinker of any sophistication (and least of all one who had learned from Jesus' words in John 9:3) could allow a simple concept of equivalence or desert between the two. Yet in ruling out the crudely superstitious ways in which the connexion might be made, we should not fail to recognise it as an inescapable task for any theism — even, perhaps, for any metaphysic. If we cannot discern moral purposiveness in what merely "happens," then events and meaning will simply fall apart. It is open to Morison to think of meaning as *imposed* upon the raw material of fate by human form-giving — though even he may one day have to explain how *such* a material is susceptible of *such* a form![42] But if anything more is to be said about nature than that it is "inevitable," then the task of discerning moral purpose is already upon us. The Christian view of death as the emblem of divine judgment is one way in which that task may be approached. Maimonides approaches it no less resolutely in another way. The argument is not whether, but only how our connexions between the physical and the moral are to be drawn.

The resurrection can thus be seen to undergird Paul Ramsey's assertions about the natural teleology of life and death: that death is not the fitting *telos* of human life taken as a whole, but only of one aspect of human life, its aspect as wilful rebellion against the created order. There remains to be considered another assertion, standing somewhat apart from these, which plays an important part in the argument of ". . . Death with Dignity," and is contested by Leon Kass: the importance of the individual as an irreplaceable bearer of human value. This, too, has to be seen as an implication of the resurrection; and in order to show how this is so, I shall analyse it as a contention about the *historical teleology* of human life.

The question has engaged the participants in contemporary Christian-Marxist dialogue as to whether the historical teleology on which the Marxist hope for the future is founded is inevitably totalitarian in structure, in that it sacrifices the interests of every prior generation that the later generations may enjoy true communism.[43] Where, it has been asked, is the justice of a final order which cannot reconcile the well-being of present members with the sacrifices of those who made it possible? The bald assertion that the sacrifices of preceding generations are compensated for by the achievement of the common goal seems to be formally totalitarian — which is to say that it does not permit the question of justice between generations to be raised, but makes the rights of the future stipulatively determinative of the duties of each present generation. One could, of course, soften the formal rigour of this position. Without denying that the question of justice could in principle be raised, one might appeal to the natural generosity of any generation to its successors (who are, after all, dependent upon it for the world they are to inherit) and urge that the question of justice should not dominate our thinking about the humanity of the future. That is excellent counsel, just so long as the question is posed that way round, in terms of the duties of present generations to the future. But what

40. As Kass himself will elsewhere acknowledge. See his *Toward a More Natural Science* (New York: Free Press, 1985), pp. 346ff.

41. Following Karl Barth (*Church Dogmatics* IV/1 [Edinburgh: T&T Clark, 1956], p. 313) and Jürgen Moltmann (*The Crucified God* [London: SCM, 1974], pp. 178-87).

42. Morison, p. 66: ". . . the whole business of life (is) the study of how to give form and dignity to suffering."

43. See C. Davis, *Theology and Political Science* (Cambridge: Cambridge University Press, 1980).

of the recipients of such generosity? Do they find themselves in a position in which their preferred status as inheritors of the goal of history makes them guilty, self-accusing, and therefore ill at ease with the welfare which their predecessors laboured to give them? That this is not entirely an idle worry may be judged from the characteristic demoralisation of every "post-war" generation, which confronts the task of living up to an infinite sacrifice made on its behalf and finds that the terms of daily existence do not permit it to discharge its debt.

Present generations have no monopoly on generosity, and they can hardly so determine to be generous to their successors that their successors will be deprived of any possibility of being generous in return. Yet the generation which inherits the goal of history has no comparable opportunity for sacrificing itself for its successors. In the earliest Christian church there was a group of believers who were sufficiently troubled by the prospect of a preferred status as to think that if the Lord were to return in their day, they could hardly welcome him if the Christian dead (who at this stage cannot have been numerous) were to be excluded. It was not that the Lord was insufficient to make his people happy; it was that the people lacked the conditions for being made happy if they were not to meet the Lord together. One answer to this anxiety would have been to say that the Lord would never come, but that each succeeding generation would live its life on the same terms as each preceding one. The answer which Saint Paul actually gave that anxious group was different: — "We who are left alive until the Lord comes shall not forestall those who have died. . . . the Christian dead will rise. Then we who are left alive shall join them" (1 Thess. 4:15-17).

The resurrection promises a reconciliation of the diastasis of history, and so makes historical teleology possible. This, in my view, is the heart of the difference between Ramsey and Aristotle. Aristotle makes no claims for history; it is that conclusion, rather than the form-matter distinction, which allows him to seek consolation for individual death in the succession of generations and the perpetuation of the human race. He has no problem of justice in the diastasis of history; for if no generation inherits the goal of humanity's striving, the balance of justice between generations has never been upset. Each generation participates equally in the ongoing life of the race; each, as its moment comes, relinquishes its place to another. But Messianic faith of any description, Jewish, Christian or Marxist, is debarred from Aristotle's settlement; for its hope for history has upset the balance and has made the later generations more completely human than the earlier — which lies uneasily with another aspect of Messianic faith, that the goal of history can effect the just reconciliation of all claims. The question is whether historical teleology can be made consistent with itself; and to that question the hope of resurrection offers a positive answer.

Kass has accused Ramsey, very effectively, of being too closely identified with "the stress on 'the unique worth of the individual'," which "connects together the mainstream of today's secular thought and its severed theological source, from which Paul Ramsey still takes his watering."[44] In reply to that accusation we first of all draw attention to what Kass concedes, that Ramsey's affirmation of the non-exchangeability of individual human beings is not free-standing. He has not posited the individual *in abstracto,* as the seat of consciousness or self-awareness or reason, and declared that he has discovered where the good of human existence lies. That is precisely the Cartesian move which his principle of psychosomatic unity is intended to reject. His affirmation of the individual springs from the eschatological affirmation that each person is to be recalled to an irreplaceable presence before the judgment seat of God. But from there we may take a further step: this eschatological affirmation is not "individualist" in the sense in which that term is used as a reproof. For the irreplaceable presence of the individual at the end of time is itself an aspect of the presence of the whole human community. It is true that the resurrection grounds the eternal value of the individual. But it does so, not by backing the claim of the individual against the community, but by doing away with the notion of *replacement* as applied to any part of the human community — which is why we could approach the question as well by way of the replacement of earlier by later generations. In the context of a historical *telos,* replacement is injustice; and the fundamental point behind Ramsey's contention for the individual is justice as a feature of perfected humanity.

We may never forget, indeed, that in Paul Ramsey we have to do with a thinker who has attempted more thoroughly than most to articulate the meaning of justice as a feature of the good of society. He can hardly be mistaken for an atomistic contractarian, reducing the whole social good to a list of individual rights, nor for an anti-social subjectivist, elevating inward integrity in defiance of community claims. If, in ". . . Death with Dignity" as occasionally elsewhere, he has found it possible to shed a few sympathetic tears for the late blooms on the Cartesian rosebush (all the while hacking vigorously at the roots), we may treat it as a characteristically dialectical moment of self-concealment in self-disclosure.

44. Kass, p. 69.

140 Dying Well in Historical Perspective: The *Ars Moriendi* Tradition of the Sixteenth and Seventeenth Centuries

Christopher P. Vogt

An important reason to begin this investigation by turning to history can be found in the widely held opinion that contemporary approaches to dying are seriously adrift.[1] Even some experts whose lives have been dedicated to offering insight into medical moral quandaries admit that many in the field have fallen short when it comes to offering contemporary people the intellectual resources they need to come to terms with mortality. For example, Daniel Callahan, a leading bioethicist, has written that bioethicists have neglected a discussion of the meaning of death and people's experience of dying.[2]

As a theologian, my task differs from that of most historians. For example, David Stannard undertakes a vigorous and careful attempt to understand the Puritan worldview and how the Puritan approach to death fit into it, but in the end he places a chasm between contemporary readers and the Puritans. In Stannard's view, concepts such as Providence and belief in God (key aspects of the Puritan approach to dying) are incompatible with contemporary sensibilities. On the basis of this assumption, he dismissed the traditions and beliefs that gave the Puritans comfort as being of exclusively historical interest.[3] In contrast, as a theologian I seek to entertain more seriously the possibility that the theological and ethical tradition that deeply informed the lives of the Puritans and other religious communities in the sixteenth and seventeenth centuries retains some credibility today.[4] Understanding the teaching of the religious writers of centuries past on death and dying can enrich contemporary theological thought and religious practice. To put the matter differently, the turn to history can be seen as a wise practical move at a time when current ways of approaching death are less than satisfying.

Once we have some sense of the logic of turning to history, the next question to be answered is what specific texts or tradition should be examined. I have chosen to focus upon the *ars moriendi* ("art of dying") tradition of the sixteenth and seventeenth century. This is a genre of devotional literature written for the laity with the primary aim of preparing faithful Christians for the difficult experience of dying.[5]

Although the tradition does have medieval precursors, the genre, as developed by the authors I will examine, has its origin more properly in the work of Erasmus.[6] His *Preparing for Death* is regarded as the seminal work in this area, decisively shaping the genre as a whole.[7] Building upon Erasmus's work were countless others.

1. Arthur E. Imhof sees the medicalization of dying as the fundamental problem with the contemporary approach to death. He also calls for a renewal of the historical understanding of death as an art to be learned. See Arthur E. Imhof, "An *Ars Moriendi* for Our Time: To Live a Fulfilled Life; to Die a Peaceful Death," in *Facing Death: Where Culture, Religion and Medicine Meet,* ed. Howard M. Spiro, Mary G. McCrea Curnen and Lee Palmet Wandel (New Haven: Yale University Press, 1996), 114-20. See Vigen Guroian, *Life's Living Toward Dying: A Theological and Medical-Ethical Study* (Grand Rapids, Mich.: Eerdmans, 1996).

2. Daniel Callahan, *The Troubled Dream of Life: In Search of a Peaceful Death* (New York: Simon & Schuster, 1993), 13.

3. History is not a matter of trivia for Stannard, but the conclusions he reaches are at the level of sociological patterns (e.g., how cultural changes that the Puritans found alarming affected their ways of dying, funeral customs). This is not the same task as engaging the beliefs and traditions of the period as a possible source for our own contemporary understanding of death and the way humans should approach it.

4. I am not suggesting the historically naïve position that such traditions can simply be appropriated without interpretation or modification. Rather, I am suggesting that the historical particularity of these texts does not preclude the possibility that they might remain meaningful in our own unique circumstances. To use the hermeneutical language of Hans-Georg Gadamer, a fusion of perspectives or worldviews is possible. For more on this hermeneutical question, see Hans-Georg Gadamer, *Truth and Method* (New York: Crossroad, 1991), especially 306-7 and 374-75.

5. For an excellent, concise introduction to the *ars moriendi,* see Carlos M. N. Eire, *"Ars Moriendi,"* in *Westminster Dictionary of Christian Spirituality,* ed. Gordon S. Wakefield (Philadelphia: Westminster Press, 1983), 21-22.

6. The origins of the *ars moriendi* can be traced to two late medieval tracts on dying which serve as a common source for this genre of literature. These two tracts are actually different versions of a single text. One version is a lengthier five-part text focusing on the temptations one faces on one's deathbed. The other version has the same focus, but consists primarily of woodcut illustrations with only an abbreviated supplemental text. Mary Catherine O'Connor's work remains a valuable study on the development of the *ars moriendi.* She not only describes the germinal works of the tradition, but also briefly examines how a wide array of authors over time developed their own version of it. See Mary Catherine O'Connor, *The Art of Dying Well: The Development of the Ars moriendi* (New York: Columbia University Press, 1942). A shorter, but helpful introduction to this genre focusing on its development in the English language can be found in David W. Atkinson's introduction to his collection of primary texts in the *ars moriendi* tradition. See David W. Atkinson, *The English Ars Moriendi* (New York: Lang, 1992), xi-xxxiv.

7. John W. O'Malley makes this assertion in his introduction to the volume of the collected works of Erasmus that includes *Pre-*

Excerpted and slightly edited from Christopher P. Vogt, "Dying Well in Historical Perspective: The *Ars Moriendi* Tradition of the Sixteenth and Seventeenth Centuries," in *Patience, Compassion, Hope, and the Christian Art of Dying Well* (Lanham: Rowman & Littlefield Publishers, 2004), 15-51.

The *ars moriendi* tradition is significant for several reasons. First, it was widely read in both Catholic and Protestant lands, and thus is not particular to any one denominational mode of piety. Furthermore, some of the most prominent theologians of this period are among the authors of the *ars moriendi* literature. These works not only enjoyed a wide geographical distribution, but were also widely read. Erasmus's *Preparing for Death* ran through twenty Latin editions in six years as well as four in French, two in Dutch and Spanish, one in German, and one in English.[8] The popularity of these works was such that their influence was widespread; the *ars moriendi* literature not only affected intellectual reflection on death, but also had a profound impact on the practices people undertook in the face of death.[9]

Another important reason to examine this historical tradition is that it seeks to locate discussion of the subject of dying within the context of the whole of the Christian life. In *Preparing for Death* and in one of his earlier Colloquies *(The Funeral),* Erasmus makes clear his view that it is too late to prepare for death when one has already reached one's deathbed.[10] In other words, beginning with Erasmus this body of literature focuses on how to live one's entire life so as to be ready for death; it is in many ways about the art of living as much as it is about the art of dying.[11] To give a more contemporary frame of reference, this tradition falls in the category of virtue ethics with its focus upon the questions of character ("Who am I becoming?") and the development of good habits and dispositions necessary for living a moral life — and dying a good death.[12]

A Puritan *Ars Moriendi:* William Perkins's *Salve for a Sicke Man* (1595)

A Salve for a Sicke Man was one of the most popular works on dying well written in English, appearing in at least six editions between 1595 and 1632. It was also included in many of the editions of William Perkins's *Workes* that were published during the same period.[13] Perkins was very influential and prolific in areas beyond the subject of dying well, most notably as a moral theologian and preacher. He is indisputably the father of British reformed casuistry, and he is widely regarded as the most popular English preacher of the late sixteenth century.[14]

Like the work of Erasmus, Perkins's tract is intended for a wide audience, directed to all the faithful.[15] Although his inclusion of some condemnatory material on what he saw as erroneous Roman Catholic approaches to dying makes this a less ecumenical work than that of Erasmus, its tone is not generally polemical.[16] Rather, it focuses how one should approach death in light of a very fundamental understanding of Christian faith.

Faith is the virtue at the center of Perkins's work. One of the distinguishing marks of *A Salve for a Sicke Man* in relation to the *ars moriendi* tradition as a whole can be found in Perkins's decision to avoid discussion of the specific deathbed temptations as found in the medieval tract in favor of emphasizing the vital importance of faith and God's mercy.[17] Perkins writes that the most important disposition at the time of death is to die in or by

paring for Death. Erasmus shaped the genre and the work of subsequent authors by shifting the focus of the *ars moriendi* from deathbed temptations to the importance of living a good life. The importance of this fact will be examined and developed below. See John W. O'Malley, ed., *Spiritualia and Pastoralia,* vol. 70, *Collected Works of Erasmus* (Toronto: University of Toronto Press, 1998), xxix. David Atkinson and Peter G. Bietenholz agree with O'Malley on the importance of Erasmus's tract in shifting the nature of the genre as a whole. See David W. Atkinson, "Erasmus on Preparing to Die," *Wascana Review* 15, no. 2 (1980): 3. Peter G. Bietenholz, "Ludwig Baer, Erasmus, and the Tradition of the 'Ars bene moriendi,'" *Revue de littérature comparée* 52 (1978): 159.

8. O'Malley, Introduction to vol. 70, xxvi.

9. Carlos Eire makes this argument that a sharp division between intellectual and social history (e.g., theology over and against faith and piety or practice) or between the practices and beliefs of the elite vs. the masses is a false dichotomy. See the prologue to his book, *From Madrid to Purgatory: The Art and Craft of Dying in Sixteenth-Century Spain* (New York: Cambridge University Press, 1995), 5.

10. Desiderius Erasmus, "The Funeral *(Funus),*" trans. Craig R. Thompson, in *Colloquies,* vol. 40, *Collected Works of Erasmus,* ed. John W. O'Malley (Toronto: University of Toronto Press, 1997), 763-95.

11. O'Malley, Introduction to vol. 70, xxviii. See also Carlos M. N. Eire, *"Ars Moriendi,"* 21.

12. See Joseph J. Kotva, *The Christian Case for Virtue Ethics* (Washington, D.C.: Georgetown University Press, 1996), especially chapter two where the teleological nature of virtue ethics and the priority of character ("Who are we morally?") are discussed.

13. David W. Atkinson, "*A Salve for a Sicke Man:* William Perkins's Contribution to the *ars moriendi.*" *Historical Magazine of the Protestant Episcopal Church* 46, no. 4 (December 1977): 409.

14. James F. Keenan, "William Perkins (1558-1602) and the Birth of British Casuistry," in *The Context of Casuistry,* ed. James F. Keenan and Thomas A. Shannon (Washington, D.C.: Georgetown, 1995), 114. Gordon Wakefield refers to Perkins as "the greatest Puritan theologian of all." See Gordon S. Wakefield, *Puritan Devotion: Its Place in the Development of Christian Piety* (London: Epworth Press, 1957), 3.

15. His emphasis of the duty of all Christians to play a part in giving comfort to the dying and being present at the bedside of the dying makes it particularly clear that this is not a book written for ministers in the pastoral care of the dying, but rather one written for pastors and lay people alike. The unity of moral, pastoral, and devotional theology in Perkins's work and in this genre as a whole is significant (especially as a contrast to most contemporary work in this area) and should be noted. Some attention to this quality of the *ars moriendi* literature as a whole will be taken up in the conclusion of this chapter.

16. For example, Perkins attacked the idea that auricular confession was necessary for the forgiveness of sins. He also questioned the validity of the sacrament of anointing the sick and the value of bringing the Eucharist to the homebound.

17. Erasmus makes this move to a certain extent, but simultaneously addresses some of the specific temptations believed to be visited upon the dying by Satan (e.g., his somewhat lengthy treatment of the temptation to heresy). Perkins makes no mention of a diabolical visit to the deathbed, nor of the temptations traditionally held to be specific to that venue. Atkinson concurs with the view that Perkins's work marks a noticeable shift in this regard. See Atkinson, "William Perkins's Contribution," 415.

faith.[18] He explains his meaning as follows: "To die by faith is when a man in the time of death doth, with all his heart, rely himselfe wholly on God's speciall loue and fauour and mercie in Christ, as it is reuealed in the word."[19] As was the case in Erasmus's work, faith, hope, and the mercy of God are closely connected and mutually interdependent in Perkins's understanding as well. One develops hope for salvation through faith in the promise of God through Jesus Christ to have mercy upon sinners.

Two characteristics of faith as understood by Perkins are important to recognize here. First, faith in Christ is not rooted in an egocentric concern for one's eternal fate, but rather is a fundamentally relational virtue rooted in love. On the side of the human being, the relationship of faith rooted in love is characterized by devotion and a deep attachment to the figure of Christ.[20] This fact is apparent in the following lines from the *Salve* where Perkins writes that the foundation of our very comfort is that

> Although the body be seuered from the soule in death, yet neither body nor soule are seuered from Christ, but the very body rotting in the graue . . . abides still united to him, and is as truly a member of Christ then as before. . . . Now, then, considering our coniunction with Christ is the foundation of all our joy and comfort in life and death, we are in the feare of God to learne this one lesson, namely that while we haue time in this world, we must labour to be vnited unto Christ that we may bee bone of his bone and flesh of his flesh.[21]

The language used here calls to mind the grief one might experience at the separation from one's beloved at death. Similarly, the image of "bone of his bone and flesh of his flesh" derives from Christian marital imagery, suggesting that the proper relationship to Christ in faith is not simply a matter of confidence in Christ's willingness and power to save one's soul, but also a matter of love and attachment to Christ. Thus, although Perkins does not explicitly connect faith to charity (the virtue of love for God), his emphasis on the importance of loving God makes such a connection implicit.

The second important characteristic of faith as understood by Perkins is its fundamentally active quality. Genuine faith in Jesus Christ leads inevitably to action, for as Perkins writes, "true faith is no dead thing."[22] In the Puritan view, one finds assurance that faith is genuine through the examination of the fruit it produces in one's mode of living.[23] Perkins writes,

> We must shewe our selues to be members of his mystical body by the daily fruits of righteousnesse and true repentance. And being once certainly assured in conscience of our being in Christ, let death come when it will, and let it cruelly part asunder both body and soule, yet shall they both remaine in the couenant, and by meanes thereof be reunited and taken up into life eternall. . . . Labour that your consciences by the Holy Ghost may testifie that ye are liuing stones in the temple of God and branches bearing fruite in the true vine.[24]

The importance of bearing fruit for faith points to a corresponding importance of particular practices geared toward nurturing and developing it.

Perkins highlights frequent examination of conscience and continual repentance as crucial for the development of faith, and as a preparation for death. He writes that death derives its strength and power from our own sinfulness. Were it not for our sins, death would have no sting because human beings would pass always into eternal life with God at the time of their death, making it a moment of joy rather than pain and sorrow.[25] This being the case, it is the duty of every Christian to endeavor to remove the sting and power of death as much as possible by frequently and humbly confessing one's sins before God, and "to carry a purpose, resolution and endeavor in all things to reform both heart and life according to God's word."[26] This duty of repenting for sins is joined by Perkins to the positive exhortation to endeavor to follow always the will of Christ in ordering one's own life rather than one's own will; he urges his readers to be able to echo Paul's words (Gal 2:20) that "I live not, but Christ lives in me." These exhortations to action under the heading of building up faith make clear the fact that Perkins understands faith not strictly as belief in a set of propositions so much as a habitual activity — a virtue. Faith is indeed right belief, but it is equally an activity characterized by striving to reform one's life according to God's will and God's word, and to become more closely attached to Jesus Christ in charity (to become "bone of his bone and flesh of his flesh"). Faith and repentance are inseparable for Perkins.[27]

18. Perkins, *Salve,* 157.

19. Perkins, *Salve,* 157.

20. Richard C. Lovelace has argued that in the view of early-modern Protestants, a deep union with Christ in conversion is central to Christian faith. Any outward signs of faith or practices were seen as useless without giving one's whole self over to Christ in devotion. See Richard C. Lovelace, "The Anatomy of Puritan Piety: English Puritan Devotional Literature," in *Post-Reformation and Modern,* vol. 3, *Christian Spirituality,* ed. Louis Dupré and Don E. Saliers (New York: Crossroad, 1989), 302.

21. Perkins, *Salve,* 135.

22. Perkins, *Salve,* 157. Charles Lloyd Cohen argues that Puritans saw love of God as always calling Christians to devote all aspects of their lives toward God. See Charles Lloyd Cohen, *God's Caress: The Psychology of Puritan Religious Experience* (New York: Oxford University Press, 1986), 129.

23. One's mode of living was indeed essential, but must also always be connected to a more emotional level at which the believer had a deep sense of being loved by God and loving God in return. Activity and attachment are equally important. See Cohen, *God's Caress,* 122-24.

24. Perkins, *Salve,* 135-36.

25. Perkins, *Salve,* 139.

26. Perkins, *Salve,* 139.

27. Note that even in his brief lament over the commonly

The tension between divine mercy and human initiative that was evident in Erasmus's work can also be found here in Perkins's writing. On the one hand, it is clear that Perkins was a devoted Puritan who sought to affirm Calvin's view that human beings are saved only by faith and grace. This perspective underlies Perkins's assertion that the dying must put their confidence in the "pure mercy of God."[28] At the same time, Perkins's awareness of the importance of practices and habituation for the development of virtue (even virtues such as faith and hope) lead him simultaneously to recommend that readers should pursue conscious activities in order to grow in virtue and prepare for death (e.g., learning to bear life's little crosses so as to patiently bear their ultimate demise).[29] Erasmus and Perkins are in agreement that neither divine mercy nor human initiative can be removed from the formula guiding Christian preparation for dying well.

A final virtue that Perkins emphasizes in his work is compassion. Erasmus makes note of the consolation that can come to the dying through the prayers of the full communion of the church, and also asserts that all Christians should be frequently at the bedside of the dying. However, whereas Erasmus encourages Christians to visit the dying for their own moral education, Perkins links the importance of this duty to development of the virtue of compassion.[30]

According to Perkins's understanding, compassion is a virtue that ought to be developed as a preparation for dying. However, developing compassion is a mode of preparation undertaken not primarily for oneself, but for one's family, friends, and neighbors. The context of dying here is unmistakably social.[31] This fact is made clear in Perkins's articulation of two related duties: the duty of the dying to invoke the help of others in renewing their own faith and repentance, and the duty of all Christians to come to the aid of the dying.[32] The purpose of both of these duties is to bring comfort to the dying, and to move them toward greater depths of faith and repentance.

Whereas Erasmus encouraged visiting the dying to learn the art for oneself, Perkins stresses that such visits have as their primary purpose to show compassion to the dying — to be with them in their suffering and to bolster their faith.[33] Here the connection between faith and compassion becomes clearer. Compassion — the activity of "suffering with" the suffering and seeking to bring them comfort — ultimately finds itself redirected toward the renewal of faith. This is so because the only true comfort to the dying is the hope of salvation, which in turn can only be derived from the assurance of true faith and repentance. Perkins writes, "Death joined with reformed life hath a promise of blessedness as adjoined unto it, and it alone will be sufficient means to stay the rage of our affections, and all inordinate fear of death."[34] It is for this reason that Perkins describes the duties of visitors to the dying as bolstering their faith through the use of appropriate prayers and reference to God's word. The exercise of compassion toward the dying thus not only requires the development of dispositions of concern and attachment toward the suffering, but also requires the very concrete preparation of nurturing one's own faith so that one is able to provide comfort through appropriate prayers and reference to scripture. This preparation is also essential for one to be able to communicate a deep personal sense of hope in God's mercy. Thus, the visitation of the dying is a key practice because it illustrates the deep interrelationship of faith, hope, and compassion, and because it points to the necessity of conscious, concrete activity to nurture those virtues and make them of value in the context of dying.

An Anglican *Ars Moriendi:* Jeremy Taylor's *Rule and Exercises of Holy Dying* (1651)

Jeremy Taylor's *Rule and Exercises of Holy Dying* was one of the most popular tracts published in English in the *ars moriendi* tradition. By 1710, the book was in its twenty-first English edition, and enjoyed considerable popularity well into the eighteenth century. A revival of interest in *Holy Dying* also came during the Victorian period when conduct books regained their popularity.[35] In addition to achieving high popularity in its own time, Taylor's work has enjoyed some acclaim in literary circles up to the present day, being regarded by many as the most so-

uncatechized state of persons as they approach death Perkins wonders how so many can live as upright Christians attending church and so forth, without regularly coming to renew "their faith *and repentance*" and wonders why people delay until their deathbed to "be catechized in the doctrine of faith *and repentance*" (*Salve*, 145). Faith and repentance are closely joined.

28. Perkins, *Salve*, 157.

29. Perkins, *Salve*, 141.

30. Perkins concurs with Erasmus on the point that being at the bedside of the dying can be morally educational, but places more emphasis in this regard on the preparation that one must undertake in order to be a useful helper to the dying. He admonishes those who make their visits to the sick and dying without the slightest notion of what it might be appropriate to say, or what prayers might be appropriate for such a circumstance. See *Salve*, 146.

31. This is also true in Erasmus, where the support of friends and a priest is assumed. Philippe Ariès provides a helpful discussion of the public nature of dying during this period. He observes that the bedchamber of the dying was considered a place to be entered freely. He writes that even as late as the early nineteenth century passers-by encountering the priest bearing the holy viaticum would form a small procession and accompany him to the sickroom. The presence of family, including children, was also customary and expected. See Ariès, *Western Attitudes*, 11-13.

32. Perkins, *Salve*, 146.

33. Despite the fact that these two authors emphasize different aspects of this one practice, I see no reason why one purpose necessarily excludes the other. Rather, these two perspectives on the importance of visiting the sick should be combined.

34. Perkins, *Salve*, 149.

35. Robert Nossen, "A Critical Study of the Holy Dying of Jeremy Taylor" (Ph.D. diss., Northwestern University, 1951), 206.

phisticated work (from an artistic and literary perspective) of the *ars moriendi* tradition.[36]

The guiding theme underlying Taylor's work is the metaphor of the way of the cross as the proper model for Christian life. A broad sense of Taylor's understanding of the shape of a life lived in the way of the cross is captured in the following quotation:

> He that desires to die well and happily, above all things must be careful, that he do not live a soft, a delicate and a voluptuous life; but a life severe, holy and under the discipline of the cross. . . . Let him confesse his sin and chastise it; let him bear his crosse patiently and his persecutions nobly, and his repentances willingly and constantly. . . . He that would die holily and happily, must in this world love tears, humility, solitude and repentance.[37]

Given the fact that such a life is marked by difficulty and (more than) its share of suffering, the central virtue that emerges in Taylor's *Holy Dying* is patience.[38]

Taylor's understanding of patience is not unlike that of William Perkins. That is to say that he sees it as a virtue that is crucial both for enabling a person to withstand the suffering associated with dying, and also as a virtue closely associated with growing in obedience to the will of God. In a section entitled "Constituent or integrall parts of patience" (chapter 3, section 3), Taylor explicitly includes obedience. Toward the end of this section, he writes:

> He is patient that calls upon God, that hopes for health or heaven, that believes God is wise and just in sending him afflictions; that confesses his sins and accuses himself, and justifies God; that expects God will turne this into good; that is civil to his Physitians and his servants; that converses with the guides of souls, the ministers of religion; *and in all things submits to God's will;* and would use no indirect means for his recovery; but had rather be sick and die, than enter at all into Gods displeasure.[39]

The theme of obedience is reprised in a later section on prayer as it relates to patience (chapter 4, section 2) where Taylor advises that those suffering should behave "as sons under discipline" and exhorts his readers to "humbly lie down under [God's] rod."[40]

Taylor's account of patience is distinguished from that of Perkins by his use of the way of the cross as the central metaphor for the practice of patience and the use he makes of the suffering of Jesus (i.e., portraying the suffering of Jesus as something to be imitated).[41] Here patient suffering takes on a dual function. Not only does one demonstrate a willingness to submit obediently to the will of God (out of recognition of God's status as divine, and out of an attempt to rightly order one's will). Patient suffering takes on additional soteriological significance as an imitation of Jesus Christ; in Taylor's view, any part in suffering sent by God implies a share in Jesus' suffering and therefore in his glory.[42] By seeking to see one's own sufferings as an occasion for imitation of Jesus Christ in his suffering, Taylor believes that one can make affliction a "school of virtue" and an opportunity to grow in holiness.[43]

Taylor is particularly effective in indicating the fundamental importance of God's mercy as the basis for hope. It is in Taylor's section on exercises against despair that it is most apparent that God's mercy is the foundation of Christian hope. Taylor writes that hope rises up in proportion to an awareness of God's great mercy, and that hope should always be sustained by the awareness that God's mercy exceeds one's own sinfulness.[44] Of equal importance is the way in which Taylor ultimately makes patience subordinate to the mercy of God. Despite the fact that Taylor's work focuses on what human beings can do to prepare themselves for holy dying (especially the importance of developing patience and embracing a way of life marked by the cross), he does remind readers that no effort can bear fruit in the absence of God's mercy. Even devout Christians cannot trust in the worthiness of their life for salvation or in their own strength in the face of the agony of death. Taylor writes, "But all that I can do, and all that I am, and all that I know of my self is nothing but sin, and infirmity, and misery; therefore I go forth of my self, and throw my self wholly into the arms of thy mercy, through Jesus Christ."[45]

Rather than point to the futility of one's own efforts, this reminder of the centrality of God's abundant mercy for salvation instead serves as a reminder of the proper

36. David Atkinson writes that "there is little question that Jeremy Taylor's [work] constitutes the artistic zenith of the *ars* tradition, despite its polemical overtones in criticizing Catholic 'how to die' books." See Atkinson, *English Ars Moriendi,* xxiii. Nancy Lee Beaty concurs, calling Taylor's *Holy Dying* "the artistic climax of the tradition." See Beaty, *Craft of Dying,* 197.

37. Taylor, *Holy Dying,* 52-53.

38. Six sections are devoted to patience, two times more than to any other virtue.

39. Taylor, *Holy Dying,* 74. Emphasis mine.

40. Taylor, *Holy Dying,* 132-33.

41. In Perkins, the focus is always upon the Christ of faith. Here, there is more emphasis on the human Jesus. See Beaty, *Craft of Dying,* 217.

42. Taylor, *Holy Dying,* 121.

43. Living through affliction properly not only promotes patience, according to Taylor; he writes that faith, hope and mercy all arise from "fellowship of sufferings" (see *Holy Dying,* 131). Such heavy emphasis upon the free endurance of suffering is a potentially problematic aspect of Taylor's spirituality. The model of selfless suffering as the keystone of the Christian life has been heavily critiqued by feminist scholars, among others. However, I would prefer to forego discussion of the potential problems of appropriating the *ars moriendi* literature to the concluding chapter [of *Patience, Compassion, Hope, and the Christian Art of Dying Well*], where I shall undertake to bring the historical tradition into productive dialogue with the contemporary theological and death and dying literature, and to move toward a synthesis of these together with my investigation of Biblical resources.

44. Taylor, *Holy Dying,* 155 and 210.

45. Taylor, *Holy Dying,* 156.

ordering of the virtues important for dying well (i.e., that faith and hope are primary). In addition, the centrality of mercy serves as a consolation to those who find themselves failing the test of patience put before them by God despite their sincere, even lifelong effort. In a simple, but moving prayer, Taylor writes, "If I suffer and am broken here, in your mercy gather me up in eternity."[46] Thus, the priority of faith and hope and the abundance of God's mercy have pastoral as well as theological importance.

Recovering the Tradition for Today

In the works examined in this chapter, hope emerged as a centrally important virtue for dying well. Furthermore, all pointed to the importance of a particular type of hope, namely one rooted deeply in faith. Indeed, the hope described by these authors is one that draws its strength from faith that God's compassion and mercy are more powerful than human sinfulness, and from faith that neither sinfulness nor death itself is enough to cut us off from the love of God through Christ.[47] This connection of hope to faith is perhaps its most salient feature to keep in mind for comparison as we move forward in this study and take up contemporary understandings of hope in the context of death and dying (in the next chapter [of *Patience, Compassion, Hope, and the Christian Art of Dying Well*]). There is a marked difference between hope rooted in the expectation of some kind of eschatological salvation and hope rooted in a sense of the worthiness of the life one has lived, for example.[48]

Compassion figures most prominently in the *ars moriendi* tradition as an activity of God in the context of discussion of the dependence of Christian hope upon God's compassionate forgiveness of sinners. However, it also emerges in this tradition as an important virtue both for the dying and those who care for them. For the one who is dying, these authors indicate the importance of forgiving the sins of others (an act of compassion) throughout life and in preparation for death.[49] The ongoing practice of compassion toward others is significant as a way in which one comes to know the compassion God shows unto oneself. The practice of compassion not only transforms one into a compassionate person, but also serves as a means of growth in the knowledge of God's compassion for us, which in turn supports our development of Christian hope.

The practice of compassion is also important for those who attend to the dying. Since Christian hope is rooted ultimately in God's mercy, it is imperative that caregivers bring God's compassion to the minds of the dying. Erasmus and Perkins suggest that caregivers and visitors recount appropriate passages from scripture that testify to God's enduring compassion. I would add that in their very manner of caring, family and friends should try to embody (however imperfectly) God's own compassion and care for the dying.

Finally, all of these authors saw a strong need for the development of patience as a lifelong preparation for dying well. As Perkins aptly puts it, those who would endure well the greatest loss of death must first become adept at enduring lesser suffering and loss.[50] Furthermore, these authors all highlighted the importance of finding meaning in suffering as a component of developing the ability to endure suffering patiently. Contemporary theologians may disagree morally and theologically with these authors in their advocacy of taking the obedient stance of a child under the correction of a stern but loving parent; however, this component of finding meaning in suffering as a step toward patiently enduring it cannot be overlooked. Indeed, either embracing this explanation for suffering or finding a viable substitute for it in support of patience will be one of the more urgent issues faced in subsequent chapters [of *Patience, Compassion, Hope, and the Christian Art of Dying Well*].

A full discussion of how this tradition might be appropriated will be postponed to the concluding chapter. . . . For now, I will merely highlight some of the features of these texts that I suspect will prove to be a valuable resource for articulating a contemporary Christian approach to dying well.

Among the key practices put forward by these authors is the discipline of "*memento mori*" or remembering the fact of one's mortality. Perkins and Taylor were particularly emphatic on the importance of this practice.[51] At a strategic level, these authors saw the constant remembrance of mortality as a way of highlighting the uncertainty of one's days and the corresponding need to waste no time in turning to a life of virtue and repentance. Along these same (strategic) lines, remembering one's mortality was seen as a fundamental prerequisite for a conscious, lifelong preparation for death. As Philippe Ariès has observed, many in the contemporary Western world live as though they were immortal, taking some practical precautions against dying (e.g., buying life insurance), but not acknowledging the reality of death existentially.[52] The effort by these authors to integrate a deep awareness of death into their articulation of basic Christian spirituality is something for which a contemporary equivalent is needed. A third theme highlighted by three of the authors examined here is the importance of being present at the death of others. The practice of

46. Taylor, *Holy Dying,* 133.

47. Taylor, *Holy Dying,* 156; Erasmus, *Preparing for Death,* 408; Perkins, *Salve,* 135; Bellarmine, *Art of Dying,* 346.

48. Ellen Carni suggests this understanding of hope as rooted in a faith in one's own sense of worth or in a life well lived. See "Issues of Hope and Faith in the Cancer Patient," *Journal of Religion and Health* 27, no. 4 (winter 1988): 285-90.

49. Erasmus, *Preparing for Death,* 416 and 433; Perkins, *Salve,* 154; Taylor, *Holy Dying,* 61.

50. Perkins, *Salve,* 141.

51. See especially Perkins, *Salve,* 137-41, and Jeremy Taylor, *Holy Dying,* 49-50.

52. Ariès, *Western Attitudes,* 106.

visiting the dying serves many functions. It is an important act of compassion in support of one's friends, family, and acquaintances.[53] It is a means by which the visitors can be reminded of their own mortality, and also an opportunity to be witness to the holy death of others that they might be role models to be remembered when we later find ourselves engaged in the dying process.[54] All of these factors point to the importance of exploring the social and interpersonal aspects of dying in a contemporary context, and how that social dimension is to be logically and practically integrated into a comprehensive contemporary Christian spirituality and approach to dying well.

53. See especially Perkins, *Salve,* 146-49, and Taylor, *Holy Dying,* 236.

54. See especially Erasmus, *Preparing for Death,* 447-48.

141 Learning How to Die Well: Lessons from the Ancient Church

Vigen Guroian

With the advent of a new millennium we on the North American continent are anticipating an increase of the average human life span to fourscore or more years. In this century the accomplishments of scientific medicine have been truly astonishing, and there are many reasons why we all should be grateful for these advances. But with these marvelous achievements come technologies that give us the capacity to control and manipulate life and death processes beyond the wildest dreams of our ancestors. It is no exaggeration to say that a society resembling Aldous Huxley's *Brave New World* may soon be within our reach and might even suit our desire. In such a society reproductive technologies and eugenics could ensure that every human being is "predestined" to be "useful" to society. And what Dr. Kevorkian has named obitiatric and thanatologic medicine might be carried on in hospitals as human being are exited from life the way we now put dogs and cats to "sleep."

In addition to the available technologies, ideological currents that challenge traditional religious prohibitions against radically altering human nature or medically ending human life are swirling all about in the culture. Today's medicine is not yet consciously antagonistic toward biblical faith, nor does it deliberately seek to subvert or contravene religiously inspired moral and legal limitations on what humans do with their bodies and biology. Nevertheless, the medical profession is under increasing pressure to use the new technologies in ways that challenge these limits.

In his hilarious but deeply troubling short story "The Death of Justina," John Cheever introduces his readers to a character named Moses, who rebels against our culture's aversion to death and disrespect of the dead. Moses makes this stunning comment at Justina's funeral: "How can a people who do not mean to understand death hope to understand love, and who will sound the alarm?"[1] Moses' unsettling statement is reminiscent of that chilling

1. John Cheever, "The Death of Justina," in *Stories of John Cheever* (New York: Ballantine, 1980), p. 515.

From Vigen Guroian, "Learning How to Die Well: Lessons from the Ancient Church," in *Ancient and Postmodern Christianity: Paleo-Orthodoxy in the 21st Century: Essays in Honor of Thomas C. Oden,* ed. Kenneth Tanner and Christopher A. Hall (2002). Used by permission of InterVarsity Press, PO Box 1400, Downers Grove, IL, 60515. www.ivpress.com.

scene in Aldous Huxley's novel when John, the so-called Savage, is called to the Park Lane Hospital for the Dying to visit his dying mother, Linda. In this facility, the "patients" are put out of their misery in the pleasantest way possible, with plenty of soma, canned music, perfume mists, television and other amenities. In *Brave New World,* care for the dying has been perfected into a clinical and sanitized form of warehousing bodies until they may be utilized by society one last time — as phosphorous extracted by cremation. Love and attachment and feelings of loss are discouraged in *Brave New World,* and marriage and parenthood have been abolished. Suffering has been isolated and death is not mourned; both are sequestered to places where, apart from the attendants, the living needn't be.

The Culture of Death

I think Moses is right. At the heart of our culture's moral sickness is a growing aversion to death and the dying, and this may be traced to a commensurate diminishment of abiding love in human relations. There spreads through society a willingness to impose death on the sick and dying in order to cause the least discomfort and distraction to the healthy and the living. With such attitudes in mind, Pope John Paul II has rightly warned that ours is becoming a culture of death. There is a compelling need for Christians to be far better educated about what the faith says about the meanings of sickness and death.

From the beginning the Christian church has understood death as the counterpoint of life within the broad scope of God's providence. God's unbounded and steadfast love in Jesus Christ remedies our mortality. In our day, however, the church has not said enough about death and is failing to persuade society to guard life and love adequately in the medical environment.

I will present, first, a religious view on the meaning of death that draws especially from Eastern Christian theology and liturgy. Second, I will examine the ancient sources of the church's long-standing interest in the healing arts. Third, I will illustrate with a true story how this theology of death and care for the dying applies to our own day, urging the Christian churches to assume a much greater role and responsibility for preparing people to die well.

Death and Christian Belief

Not according to God's will but by sin has sickness unto death come to define the human condition, says the ancient tradition. Because of sin the entire race of Adam and Eve has been disconnected from God's immediate life-giving energies. We are like rundown batteries that finally lose their charge. All humanity is under this condition of mortality: no one is exempt. Original sin is the intractable habit of making the wrong moral choices and doing damage to the human environment. It is passed on from generation to generation, much like alcoholism, and its effects are deadly. St. Paul writes in his epistle to the Romans: "Sin came to life, but I died" (7:9 NKJV).

The fear of death threads through the entire fabric of human life. It drives human beings to desperate and often selfish acts. Sometimes it moves them to end their own lives so that they do not suffer the agony of death's onset. The ancient fathers of the church named the death that we die due to sin "corruptible death." They often cite the Wisdom of Solomon, a Greek intertestamental text included among the so-called Apocrypha of the Old Testament. "God created us for incorruption, and made us in the image of his own eternity, but through the devil's envy death entered the world," says the Wisdom of Solomon (2:23-24 RSV). Drawing on this, St. Athanasius recounts the story of the advent of corruptible death in his tract titled *On the Incarnation.*

> God set them [Adam and Eve] in His own paradise, and laid upon them a single prohibition. If they guarded the grace and retained the loveliness of their original innocence, then the life of paradise should be theirs without sorrow, pain or care and after it the assurance of immortality in heaven. But if they went astray and became vile, throwing away their birthright of beauty, then they would come under the natural law of death and live no longer in paradise, but, dying outside of it, continue in death and corruption.[2]

Thus, because of sin human existence comes under the strict determinism of nature's law. In other words, sin throws human existence into nature's cycle of life and death, into the entropy of natural existence that draws every living thing toward extinction. Sin activates our creaturely proclivity to fall into the darkness and nothingness out of which we were lifted into light and life by God's creative doing. Corruptible death, therefore, is a profound tragedy that has befallen the image of God. A hymn of the Byzantine Burial Rite lends powerful expression to this: "I weep and I wail when I think upon death, and behold our beauty, fashioned in the image of God, lying in the tomb disfigured, dishonored, bereft of form. O marvel! What is this mystery which doth befall us? Why have we been given over unto corruption, and why have we been wedded to death?"[3]

Only for the human being is death contrary to nature because in man's case mortality is a consequence of sin. At the close of the Armenian Church Service for Burial of the Dead, the priest gives voice to the deceased as the coffin is carried in procession out through the doors of the sanctuary. The deceased laments his fallen and cor-

2. *St. Athanasius on the Incarnation:* The Treatise *De Incarnatione Verbi Dei,* trans. a Religious of C.S.M.V. (Crestwood, N.Y.: St. Vladimir's Seminary Press, 1982), pp. 28-29.

3. Service Book of the Holy Orthodox-Catholic Apostolic Church, ed. and trans. Isabel Florence Hapgood (Englewood, N.J.: Antiochian Orthodox Christian Archdiocese, 1975), p. 386.

ruptible state and prepares to meet "the Righteous Judge," adding the inevitable and strong penitential note in all Eastern Christian funeral and burial rites.

> Let the whole world look upon me and witness
> my woes. . . .
> I have sinned and am condemned to oblivion.
> I have dug my own grave. I have plotted
> against myself.
> I have betrayed, I cheated. . . .
>
> Once I was light, and now I am in darkness and
> the shadow of death.
> How shall I recount my sins, they are so
> numerous. . . .
>
> Hurry, O my person, flee from evil, desire goodness.
> Collect yourself, before Death's sleep overcomes you.
> Commit yourself to the Righteous Judge.
> Lord, have mercy. Lord, have mercy. Lord,
> have mercy.[4]

As reflected so poignantly in this Armenian hymn, the ancient tradition is quite clear that the death we know in a fallen world is not what God intended for human beings. St. Gregory of Nyssa writes: "From the nature of the dumb animals, mortality is transferred to a nature created for immortality."[5] God created Adam and Eve for eternal life, not to endure personal extinction, insists Gregory. Had the first couple not sinned, the parents of the race would have passed on to eternal life with God after the duration of their temporal lives. This passage into eternal life would not have entailed the radical rupture of body and soul and the demise of the person that we see in death. However, Jesus Christ, the only begotten Son and express image of the Father, reversed the entropy and corruption that sin activated in humankind. Only the incarnate Son of God, who lived and died in our human flesh, was capable of renewing human nature by restoring the image of God within us through his sinless life and freely-willing death on the Cross. By these things Christ healed humankind so that all might be whole and inherit eternal life. Christ by his good death transformed death back into a passage to eternal life. This is the sure conviction of the ancient tradition.

4. Canon for the Burial of Laypersons according to the Sacred Rites of the Armenian Orthodox Church, trans. Very Rev. Ghevont Samoourian, Armenian Orthodox Theological Research Institute, unpublished. A portion of this recessional hymn may be found in *The Ritual of the Armenian Apostolic Church* (New York: Armenian Prelacy, 1992), p. 145.

5. I am using Georges Florovsky's translation here as it appears in *The Collected Works of Georges Florovsky*, vol. 3: *Creation and Redemption* (Belmont, Mass.: Nordland, 1976), p. 106. This may be found in English translation also in *The Great Catechism* (chap. 3) in *Gregory of Nyssa: Selected Works*, Nicene and Post-Nicene Father of the Christian Church, 2nd ser. (Grand Rapids, Mich.: Eerdmans,1979), 5:483.

The Medicinal Metaphor in the Ancient Tradition

From this theological perspective we are invited to think of the redemptive act of God in Jesus Christ as a kind of divine therapy. God's love and compassionate care have cured our diseased and mortally sickened human nature. In Fr. Georges Florovsky's words: "Redemption is not just man's reconciliation with God. Redemption is the abolition of sin altogether, the deliverance from sin and death. . . . The death of Our Lord was the victory over death and mortality, not just the remission of sins, nor merely justification of man, nor again a satisfaction of an abstract justice."[6] Florovsky's view is rooted deep within the ancient tradition and is forcefully reflected especially in the liturgies of the Orthodox Church. Salvation is understood as healing and also growth toward perfection. God's medicinal prescription of salvation in Christ remedies the carcinogenic effects of sin and cures the mortal sickness that corrupts our whole being. The fourteenth-century Byzantine theologian Nicholas Cabasilas evokes this meaning of healing in his great work of sacramental theology, *The Life in Christ*. There he explains:

> Many are the remedies which down through the ages have been devised for this sick race; it was Christ's death alone which was able to bring true life and health. For this reason, to be born by this new birth [of baptism] and live the blessed life and be disposed to health and, as far as lies in man, to confess the faith and take on oneself the passion and die the death of Christ, is nothing less than to drink of this medicine.[7]

This is a wonderful image of salvation in Christ through faith and baptism by water and the Spirit. Cabasilas plumbs the deep etymology of salvation. Its Greek root is *sozo* from *saos*, which literally means "healthy." The Hebrew equivalent is *yasha*, which is to rescue from danger. The second-century church father Clement of Alexandria leads us in this same direction when he states: "The Word of the Father, who made man, cares for the whole nature of His creature; the all-sufficient Physician of humanity, the savior, heals both body and spirit."[8] Clement maintains that "the whole nature of His [God's] [human] creature" needs to be healed. Gregory of Nyssa may exceed all of the Greek fathers in his vivid description of the Christian Eucharist as medicine for a mortally sickened human nature, a remedy for corruptible death. In his Great Catechism St. Gregory states:

> Those who have been deceived into taking a poison use another drug to counter its harmful effects. Moreover, the antidote, just like the poison, must enter a man's

6. Florovsky, *Creation and Redemption*, pp. 103, 104.

7. Nicholas Cabasilas, *The Life in Christ*, trans. Carmino J. deCatanzaro (Crestwood. N.Y.: St. Vladimir's Seminary Press, 1974), p. 94.

8. Clement of Alexandria, *The Instructor* 1.2, in *Fathers of the Second Century, Ante-Nicene Fathers* (Peabody, Mass.: Hendrickson, 1994), 2:210.

system, so that its healing effect may be thereby spread throughout his whole body. Such was our case. We had eaten something that was disintegrating our nature. It follows, therefore, that we were in need of something to restore what had been disintegrated; we needed an antidote which would enter into us and so by its counteraction undo the harm already introduced into the body by the poison.

And what is the remedy? It is that body which proved mightier than death and became the source of our life. For, as the apostle says, a little yeast makes the whole lump of dough like itself [see 1 Cor 5:6]. In the same way, when the body that God made immortal enters ours, it transforms it entirely and makes it like itself. It is just like mixing poison with something wholesome, where everything in the mixture is rendered as worthless as the poison. Similarly the entry of the immortal body into the body that receives it transforms it in its entirety into its own immortal nature.[9]

If we venture to say that medicine has gained inspiration from the Christian ethos, it is equally true that Christian theology has taken from medicine metaphors that help to identify the mystery of salvation in Christ. And these in turn imprint deep within the Christian imagination a value to medicine. In contrast to the juridical and forensic metaphors that are dominant in Roman Catholicism and Protestantism, Eastern Christian writers employ medicinal metaphors to explain salvation; true faith brings about an inner change, or cure, that enables persons to pursue perfection. This perfection is no mere moralism. While it includes good works, it is primarily a process of inner transformation and healing of the sinful self. This process is engendered by faith, so that the human person may increase in divine similitude.

Ancient Christian Anthropology and Medicine

This medicinal interpretation of redemption is rooted in a Christian anthropology that will not make a sharp distinction between body and soul. Rather, the ancient tradition emphasizes that the unity of the two constitutes the whole person: God breathed the breath of life into the man whom he made from dust, and the man became a living soul (see Gen 2:7). The body without a soul is a corpse, and the soul without a body is a ghost. Only when they are perfectly one is the person alive and present. This notion of the human person as a psychosomatic unity was alien to the Hellenic mind. And my experience in the college classroom and in church parishes leads me to conclude that it is nearly as strange to many modern people, including Christians. Many in the churches embrace the Hellenic dualism that the soul is immortal but the body perishes. My undergraduate students at Loyola College — the vast majority of whom have attended Catholic parochial schools — are surprised to hear that the soul is by nature no more immortal than the body, and in the living person indistinguishable from the body. They have a hard time believing that Christianity defines personal identity as a unity of body and soul.

The earliest Christian creeds boldly insist that the final resurrection is a bodily resurrection. And it is precisely because the ancient church understood that salvation pertains to the whole human being, body and soul as one, that it was interested early in scientific medicine and valued it as an important human art aiding the process of our temporal journey to God. In the fourth century St. Basil the Great commented at length on the important place of medicine among the other arts and sciences that God uses to help us sustain our earthly existence and advance toward our heavenly home. In his *Long Rules* for monastic living, Basil declares:

> Each of the arts is God's gift to us, remedying the deficiencies of nature, as, for example, agriculture, since the produce which the earth bears of itself would not suffice to provide for our needs; the art of weaving, since the use of clothing is necessary for decency sake, and for protection from the wind; and similarly for the art of building. The same is true, also, of the medical art. In as much as our body is susceptible to various hurts, some attacking from without and some from within by reason of the food we eat, and since the body suffers affliction from both excess and deficiency, the medical art has been vouchsafed us by God, who directs our whole life, as a model for the cure of the soul, to guide us in the removal of what is superfluous and in the addition of what is lacking. Just as we would have no need of the farmer's labor and toil if we were living amid the delights of paradise, so also we would not require the medical art for relief if we were immune to disease, as was the case, by God's gift, at the time of Creation before the Fall.[10]

According to St. Basil, medicine functions within the catastrophic effects of the Fall and is a partial remedy for those effects. Rational or scientific medicine cannot save the human being from death, but it can contribute to a healthy and meaningful life, so long as human beings do not put their whole hope in it. St. Basil's advice is especially pertinent in our day when so may people mistakenly make an idol of medicine and expect their physicians to be priests and shamans also. He continues:

> So then, we should neither repudiate this art [of medicine] altogether nor does it behoove us to repose all our confidence in it but, just as in practicing the art of agriculture we pray God for fruits, and as we entrust the helm to the pilot in the art of navigation, but implore God that we may end our voyage unharmed by the per-

9. Gregory of Nyssa, *Catechetical Oration* 37, in *Documents in Early Christian Thought*, ed. Maurice Wiles and Mark Santer (Cambridge: Cambridge University Press, 1975), p. 194.

10. Basil of Caesarea, *The Long Rules* Q.55, in *Saint Basil: Ascetical Works*, trans. M. Monica Wagner, *The Fathers of the Church* (New York: Fathers of the Church, Inc., 1950), 9:330-31.

ils of the sea, so also, when reason allows, we call in the doctor, but not leave off hoping in God.[11]

How Even Death Becomes a Prescription for Life

The ancient tradition is able to guard against inflated expectations in the curative power of scientific medicine because it finds reason for hope even in death. The Cross and Resurrection have transformed even death into a medicine of salvation. Nowhere that I know of in Christian liturgy is this more movingly portrayed than in the central part of the Armenian funeral service for the home. We first encounter a series of penitential and intercessory hymns that are dialogical in character. Both the deceased and the congregation are lent voices. The deceased pleads with God for healing because sin — which is the infective source of all sickness and of mortality itself — requires supernatural cure even after death. By willing submission to the judgment and mercy of Christ, the sins of the deceased may be washed away forever.

> When my days are consumed, help me, O Lord, lover of mankind.
>
> You, who have assumed the tortures and death on the cross, help me, O Lord, lover of mankind.
>
> Through the intercession of the ever-virgin Holy Mother of God, help me, O Lord, Lover of mankind. . . .
>
> As a sinful person, I cry to you, O Heavenly Father, help me in my distress. I, who am dead in my sins, help me.
>
> I have been wounded by the invisible enemy, O Healer of the sick, cure my malady. I, who am dead in my sins, help me.
>
> I have gone astray like the lost sheep, O seeker of the enslaved seek me, the wandered. I, who am dead in my sins, help me. . . .
>
> O Lord, open the door of your mercy for us, and make us worthy of your luminous lodgers with your Saints.
>
> In the abode that you prepared for your Saints, O Savior, accept us also as adopted children into the discipleship of life.
>
> When you sit in your judgment, O formidable judge, have mercy upon your creatures, through the intercession and prayer of Holy ascetics.[12]

These hymns embrace the entire meaning of salvation understood both as rescue from danger and healing of the whole person. After several more hymns, a litany and prayers, the deacon chants the following verses from Psalm 39 as the mourners are reminded that they share the fate of the deceased under a common condition of mortality.

> Behold, Thou who has made my days a few handbreadths, and my lifetime is as nothing in Thy sight. Surely every man stands as a mere breath! Surely man goes about as a shadow! Surely for naught are they in turmoil; man heaps up, and knows not who will gather. (vv. 5-6)[13]

A reading from St. Paul's second epistle to the Corinthians follows immediately and complements the psalmist's meditation on the brevity of our lives. The apostle invokes God the Father who is merciful and comforts us in our afflictions so that we may comfort others. He reminds his reader of the Son, Jesus Christ, who has shared in human suffering and by his death and resurrection heals humanity of the sickness and mortality of sin.

> Blessed be the God and Father of our Lord Jesus Christ, the Father of mercies and God of all comfort, who comforts us in all affliction, so that we may be able to comfort those who are in any affliction, with the comfort with which we ourselves are comforted by God . . . rely[ing] not on ourselves but on God who raises the dead. . . . (2 Cor 1:3-11)[14]

These three elements of the Armenian Funeral Rite — penitential and intercessory hymns, psalm, and Pauline blessing — exemplify the three principal steps of the ancient Christian church's pedagogy of dying well in Christ. The first recalls our mortality in the light of God's enduring love. The second seeks meaning in our suffering in light of the crucifixion and resurrection of Christ. The third envisions salvation as cure of sin and healing of body and soul leading to eternal life. If this simple pedagogy were practiced more often and consistently in the Christian churches, medicine might be infused anew with an ethos of healing and life.

A Modern Story of Death and Dying

Medicine needs better patients, and the church can and should help provide them. In contemporary medical ethics the character of the patient often is ignored. All too frequently medical ethics is fixed in quandary ethics that focus on the decisions, agency and acts of the physician. Even when issues of character are taken up, the profes-

11. Ibid., p. 336.

12. *The Rituals of the Armenian Apostolic Church* (New York: Armenian Prelacy, 1992), pp. 123-24. This text is abbreviated and misleadingly lists this text as a single hymn. I have introduced ellipses and additional spacing where there is more text that is left out of this translation but which may be found in the recent translation of the complete Canon and Services that I have listed under footnote 4.

13. *Rituals of the Armenian Apostolic Church,* p. 124. This text leaves the impression that this reading of the psalm follows immediately. Once again *Canon for the Burial of Laypersons* cited in footnote 4 should be consulted for the full text of the service for the home.

14. *Rituals of the Armenian Apostolic Church,* p. 125. I have abbreviated the rite, which actually includes the entire text of 2 Cor 13:3-11.

sional care provider is the focus of attention, not the patient. But much good could be accomplished if the church were to attend to the rest of us who may never be professional care providers but will be patients at some point, at least when we are dying.

In a recent book *The Measure of Our Days: New Beginnings at Life's End,* physician Jerome Groopman tells a disturbing story that illustrates the importance of character and internal resources when facing the prospect of personal demise.

Kirk Bains was a highly successful businessman who made a small fortune in speculative investment ventures. Before coming to Dr. Groopman, Bains had been to the top hospitals in cancer treatment and was told repeatedly that nothing could be done for him. But Bains was a fighter. He told Groopman on their first meeting: "You've seen my records from Yale and Sloan-Kettering. . . . They think I'm too sick for their research studies. So you cook up some new magic. Make me a guinea pig, I take risks all the time. That's my business. I won't sue you."[15]

Groopman decided to run the standard tests. But he also trusted his intuition, believing that it is at least as important to know the story of the patient as to know clinically what he suffers from. The test results were as grim as the reports said. He explained to Kirk Bains the difficulty of his case. And the conversation turned in this direction:

> "I had hoped it would be a replay of *The Exorcist,"* Kirk painfully quipped. "Remember how the priest took the demon out of the child, a bloody, ugly creature? I thought the surgeon would do the same. Maybe I'd have been better off with a priest than a doctor. Never thought I'd need the clergy. But that's what everyone is recommending now."
>
> "Are you affiliated with a church?" I always try to learn the scope of religious feeling, the ties of the patient and his family to faith. God, whether positive, negative, or null, is an essential factor in the equation of dying.
>
> "Episcopalian. I celebrate Christmas. The food. The music. Decorating the tree. Giving gifts. That's fun. But the religion — I can't take much stock in a church founded because Henry VIII wanted a younger wife."
>
> My response was a skeptical look.
>
> "Let me put it in my own terms. I'm not a long-term investor. I like quick returns. I don't believe in working for dividends paid in heaven."[16]

Dr. Groopman decided to try a radical and unorthodox combination of treatments. The night before the surgery, Groopman visited Bains in his hospital bed. He noticed that Bains was troubled and agitated.

> "Are you thinking you could die tonight?" . . . "You won't, Kirk," I said confidently.
>
> "So you're a prophet, not a wizard. Shall I call you St. Jerome?" . . . "I didn't expect to be so afraid, Jerry," Kirk paused, reaching for his thoughts. . . . "Maybe it's because I know this is my last chance and I'll probably die, and after death . . . it's just nothingness."
>
> I absorbed his words and tightened my grip on his hand. I now understood why he had insisted on treatment, and I realized it would be wrong to readdress that decision tonight.
>
> "So then it would be the same as before we were born?" I softly replied. "Is that terrifying, to be unborn? That's what my father used to say to comfort me as a child when I asked him about death."
>
> "See if you still find that enough comfort when you're the one in this bed. Nothingness. No time. No place. No form. I don't ask for heaven. I'd take hell. Just to *be*."[17]

Kirk Bains's imagination is strong and vivid, and it terrorizes him. The church he neglected or which neglected him might have helped form in him a religious imagination better equipped to cope with the futility of his physical condition. Dr. Groopman himself is not unaware of the importance of imagination and how it is formed. He comments:

> "I thought about how we all develop our inner pictures of death and an afterlife, from stories and words we hear as children, which form our first image. As we pass through life, we redraw these images, hoping that at the end we will be prepared for what awaits."[18]

My friend Rev. Charles Kratz, an Episcopal priest, first brought Dr. Groopman's story to my attention. Rev. Kratz commented that he has seen many Kirk Bainses in his fifty-plus years as a priest, and he also knows how miserably his church has failed to address these matters of mortality and personal demise in the pulpit or at the bedside. "I couldn't help thinking," said Fr. Kratz, "that we clergy are to blame. Look at what kind of person and patient we left for this doctor to deal with."

The conversation Dr. Groopman cites constitutes a crucial moment in the life and death of Kirk Bains: he is open to counsel, but Dr. Groopman's father's religious views do not allay Bains's fears or satisfy his needs. Of this scene Rev. Kratz said: "Maybe something might have been accomplished with the right religious counsel at that moment. But we rarely get to be there at those moments. And by this time, it is almost too late for people like Kirk Bains, short of a divine act of grace."

Dr. Groopman is himself shaken by this conversation with Bains. He spends several paragraphs ruminating over it. He recalls his father's death. And he acknowledges that is probably why he rarely visits that memory; it is a nearly unbearable reminder of the personal nature of death.

> After he died, it was impossible for me to imagine my father as disintegrated into nothingness. . . . It was too

15. Jerome Groopman, *The Measure of Our Days* (New York: Penguin, 1998), p. 7.

16. Ibid., pp. 13-14.

17. Ibid., pp. 23-24.

18. Ibid., p. 25.

> painful, to stark an image in my mind, that his body, the warm expansive body that had snuggled me in bed when I was fearing the shadows of the night, held me in the water when I learned to swim, embraced me with surprising strength when I succeeded, and embraced me with even greater strength when I had failed. That that body was now inanimate matter. . . . And nothing more. . . . I hoped I would not lie terrified in bed, like Kirk.[19]

The radical treatment prescribed by Dr. Groopman worked for a time, the tumors shrank and the cancer went into remission. Kirk Bains was given four months of relatively comfortable living. But did he use this gift? Dr. Groopman stayed in touch with Bains and his wife during this time. When the cancer came back, he visited Bains in the hospital just after an initial radiation treatment.

> "I'm sorry the magic didn't work longer," I finally offered to Kirk.
>
> "It did more than anyone expected, Jerry. But you shouldn't feel sorry. There was no reason to live anyway. . . . You read newspapers?" Kirk asked abruptly. . . . "I don't read newspapers anymore. I don't know how to. Or why I should," Kirk paused and his voice lowered. "Newspapers used to be a gold mine for me. They're filled with what to you look like disconnected bits of information. A blizzard in the Midwest, the immigration debate in California. . . . For you, Jerry, those articles are about the lives and fortunes of individuals and nations. For me, they mean nothing beyond information for deals and commodity trading. I never really cared about the world's events or its people. Not deep down inside. . . .
>
> "And when I went into remission I couldn't read the papers because my deals and trades seemed pointless. Pointless because I was a short-term investor. Like I told you Jerry, I had no patience for the long term. I had no interest in creating something, not a product in business or a partnership with a person. And now I have no equity. No dividends coming in. Nothing to show in my portfolio," Kirk grimaced with pain.
>
> "How do you like my great epiphany? No voice of God or holy star but a newspaper left unread in its wrapper." . . .
>
> "Jerry, you realize I'm right. The remission meant nothing because it was too late to relive my life. I once asked for hell. Maybe God made this miracle to have me know what it will feel like."[20]

Groopman says he felt "the crushing weight of Kirk's burden." He continues pensively, "There is no more awful death than to die with regret, feeling that you have lived a wasted life — death delivering this shattering final sentence on your empty soul."[21]

It's a terrifying tale of modern death. The story is a challenge, not primarily to medicine but to the Christian faith. There will always be patients like Kirk Bains who believe in nothing or very little and who come to the medical practitioner with the demand, "Save me! Save me in whatever way you can!" But in the future there will be increasing numbers of others who will come to physicians with the equally ferocious demand, "If you can't fix me, then put me out of my misery!"

So much of what constitutes dying a good death depends not on the health care setting or the medical skills of the care providers but the religious and moral resources of the dying. My good friend Sr. Sharon Burns, R.S.M., taught theology for many years, but for the past fifteen years has worked as a chaplain at Stella Maris Hospice in Towson, Maryland. She told me how much it helps when her patients have religious formation equipping them with beliefs that can carry them through. She says these people can be healed deeply during their dying. At Stella Maris the stories, symbols and rituals of the Christian faith are brought to a prominence in the daily routine that the secular culture does not permit. Much in the way of penance and forgiveness, reunion and reconciliation can be accomplished in the lives of Stella Maris patients in a relatively brief period of time. Love, so often hindered and sometimes discouraged in more typical health care environments, is given and returned by staff and family at Stella Maris. Suffering is not isolated but shared in a manner that reflects the great pastoral counsel of St. Paul in 2 Corinthians.

Churches also need to more conscientiously prepare people for dying. Indeed, the ancient fathers of the church valued and commended an unremitting remembrance of death as one of the principal virtues of the Christian life. This is a virtue long neglected in Christian teaching and sorely needed today. "The unremitting remembrance of death is a powerful trainer of body and soul," wrote St. Hesychios of Sinai. "Vaulting over all that lies between ourselves and death, we should always visualize it, and even the very bed on which we shall breathe our last, and everything connected with it."[22] While a secular world might view this as a call to morbidity, Christians should receive this advice in the joyful light of their resurrection faith. Death and resurrection are inevitably and necessarily woven together in the Christian imagination. This pedagogy of the remembrance of death is already present in the liturgies of the church. I mean especially the theology and spirituality communicated through baptism, the Eucharist and the rites of burial. Thus, for example, near the conclusion of the Byzantine rite of burial, the mourners are asked specifically to exercise this remembrance of death. "As we gaze on the dead who lieth before us, let us all accept the example of our own last hour."[23]

Care of the dying has been a deep concern of the

19. Ibid., pp. 25, 26.
20. Ibid., pp. 35-37.
21. Ibid., p. 37.

22. St. Hesychios, "Watchfulness and Holiness," in *The Philokalia,* ed. and trans. G. E. Palmer, Philip Sherrard, and Kallistos Ware (London: Faber & Faber, 1970), 1:178.

23. Service Book of the Holy Orthodox-Catholic Apostolic Church, p. 390.

church from the earliest centuries, but so too has the preparation of Christians to meet their deaths. Much has been written in the annals of medical ethics about virtues that physicians and health care professionals need in order to care properly for the terminally ill and dying. Yet surprisingly little has been said about the character that the church must cultivate in persons so that they make good patients.[24] If there is a lesson to be learned from the story of Kirk Bains, it is that medicine cannot cure our mortality and we must be prepared to accept this truth with courage and hope in order to be best served by our physicians. The resources the Christian faith has to help people live toward their dying in freedom, courage, patience and hope cannot be instantaneously transmitted to the sick person whose flesh is already ravaged and whose mind is tormented by disease. The meaning that faith supplies for living and dying must be claimed over a lifetime.

Physicians have always needed good patients to be good healers. The situation has not changed in our day. In fact, this may be more necessary than ever before. How else will physicians be able to shift their goals at the appropriate time from cure to being present for their patients as death approaches? The physician's most important obligation is to be present throughout for the sick or dying person, to never abandon the patient. This can be accomplished successfully only if doctor and patient collaborate. As Christian ethicist Stanley Hauerwas has wisely said in *Suffering Presence:* "It is important, then, that the one who is dying exercise the responsibility to die well. That is, the person should die in a manner that is morally commensurate with the kind of trust that has sustained him or her in life. . . . A good death is a death that we prepare for through living because we are able to see that death is but the necessary correlative to a good life."[25]

Good care for the terminally ill and dying begins with care for the healthy and living. Through the church's own best standards, that care is the fundamental responsibility of the church, not of medicine. By the example of Christ and all the martyrs and saints, it is the responsibility of the church to prepare people to die well, while they are still living, through the sacraments, prayer and preaching. If the church and those of us who are its living members could look to this pedagogy and preparation more conscientiously, then we might stand to make a great contribution toward strengthening the humane ethos of medicine.

24. By "good patient" I do not mean a simply cooperative or compliant patient, as the term has come to mean in common medical parlance. I mean a patient that is formed and habituated in patience, fortitude and faith among other virtues valued and invoked in the Christian sacraments.

25. Stanley Hauerwas, *Suffering Presence* (Notre Dame, Ind.: University of Notre Dame Press, 1986), pp. 96, 98.

CHAPTER TWENTY-TWO

Choosing Death

Few issues in medical ethics are as contentious as that of physician assisted suicide (PAS) and euthanasia.[1] According to the Pew Forum on Religion & Public Life, the American public is evenly split on the issue of PAS, with a slight majority in favor of or opposed to it depending on how the question is phrased. Thus, for instance, when polled, the public responded less favorably to the notion of physicians offering the terminally ill assistance to commit "suicide" than to that of physicians providing the terminally ill with "the means to end their lives."[2] Similarly, another study concluded that public opinion shifted according to whether the issue was framed as a matter of "individual choice" or of "sanctity of life."[3]

Proponents of PAS rely most often on two arguments: autonomy and compassion. The commitment to autonomy means that each individual is free to set his or her own life direction, free to dispose of himself or herself as he or she sees fit. Given this commitment, we should respect a competent person's wishes to terminate his or her life, especially if that person is terminally ill and suffering greatly. Indeed, the right to autonomy is sometimes claimed to include the right to die.

It is unclear what this right to die might entail. For example, is it limited to a negative right not to have others interfere with one's dying? Or does it mean a positive right to have assistance in becoming dead? Others contend that there is no such right. How can one have a right to terminate one's life, that upon which all their other rights depend? Still others question autonomy as the overriding value in such circumstances. Might values concerning the sacredness of human life, the individual's place before God, or our commitment to each other in community be of equal or greater weight here than autonomy?

The appeal to compassion relies on a certain understanding of how we should respond to human suffering. Proponents of PAS view compassion as a commitment to eliminate suffering, even if that finally means eliminating the sufferer. Persons who are terminally ill and who are suffering should have their suffering relieved, up to and including aiding them in taking their own lives. Compassion demands that we aid them in this way in ending their suffering.

Others contend that this approach misunderstands compassion. They argue that compassion is first and foremost a commitment to be with the sufferer, a commitment to share in the burden of suffering. While compassion rightly strives to mitigate human suffering, engaging in euthanasia or assisting someone to commit suicide is abandonment, not compassion. Under this view, compassion is an assertion of interdependence that fights the tendency of suffering to isolate the sufferer.

The rhetoric surrounding PAS is often inflamed. For example, Barbara Coombs Lee, president ex officio of Compassion and Choices (formally the Hemlock Society), describes typical end-of-life care as "medical torture" that is foisted on us by a "medical-industrial complex." According to Ms. Lee, the "standard routine is to torture those in the process of dying by inflicting upon them a host of toxic chemicals, invasive machinery and painful surgeries."[4] To add to the insult, we spend huge sums of money at the

1. In antiquity, "euthanasia" meant an easy death, one free from serious pain. In contemporary language, it often means "mercy killing." For our purposes, "physician assisted suicide" is the more narrow term, referring to a physician providing some type of assistance, most often medication, to someone who has decided to terminate his or her own life. "Euthanasia" is used here as a broader term to indicate medical intervention to terminate life, not necessarily at the direction of the person being killed. Thus, "euthanasia" is an appropriate term for the termination of defective newborn children or of someone in a persistent vegetative state lacking end-of-life documents. Many who argue for PAS do not condone other nonconsensual forms of "mercy killing" often associated with the broader term "euthanasia."

2. David Masci, "The Right-to-Die Debate and the Tenth Anniversary of Oregon's Death with Dignity Act," *Pew Forum on Religion & Public Life,* October 9, 2007, accessed July 28, 2009, from http://pewforum.org/docs/?DocID=251.

3. Donald P. Haider-Markel and Mark R. Joslyn, "Just How Important Is the Messenger Versus the Message? The Case of Framing Physician Assisted Suicide," *Death Studies* 28, no. 3 (2004): 243-62.

4. Barbara Coombs Lee, "Healthcare Reform and the Price of Torture," *The Huffington Post,* July 14, 2009, accessed July 28, 2009, from http://www.huffingtonpost.com/barbara-coombs-lee/healthcare-reform-and-the_b_231720.html?view=print.

end of life with little to show for it in terms of survival outcomes. This is a "cultural paradigm" for dying that robs people of their dignity. We need, says Ms. Lee, a cultural shift in how we die, and we need a health care system that pays physicians "to talk with you about peaceful endings when death is imminent" — that is, we need legal, financially compensated PAS.

Not surprisingly, Lee's description of end-of-life care as "torture" brings a heated response. For example, Wesley J. Smith accuses Lee of "fear mongering," misrepresenting public policy concerns, and slandering physicians. According to Smith, Compassion and Choices — and Lee in particular — denies any standards for determining when someone is in "unbearable agony" and semi-secretly rejects the already-inadequate PAS guidelines established in Washington state and Oregon.[5] Here, too, the rhetoric around euthanasia and PAS is passionate and inflamed.

How should Christians think about these issues? Christians have commonly made a distinction between killing and allowing to die, between expediting death and no longer fighting its coming (see the next chapter in this volume, "Accepting Death"). Under this distinction, withdrawing or withholding treatment is sometimes permissible as an acknowledgment that death is approaching, but aiming at death, perhaps by giving more narcotics than is necessary to control pain, is illicit. Often, especially in Catholic circles, this distinction concerns the difference between "ordinary" and "extraordinary" treatment. One is obliged to utilize "ordinary" treatment, but treatment that is inordinately burdensome is deemed "extraordinary" and thus not obligatory. Pope John Paul II's "Declaration on Euthanasia" (available on the Vatican web site[6]) fits this basic paradigm.

If the rejection of assisted suicide and euthanasia has been typical for Christians, Richard McCormick's prescient essay, "Physician-Assisted Suicide: Flight from Compassion" (selection 142), suggests five cultural trends pushing in the other direction. Specifically, McCormick points to the ascendancy of autonomy, medicine becoming more like a business or service that can be hired out, inadequate pain management, public debates maintaining that nutrition/hydration must always be continued, and the financial pressures of caring for the elderly and chronically ill. Given these trends, it is unsurprising that many view physician assisted suicide as a preferable option, says McCormick. These trends are, if anything, more prominent than they were when McCormick wrote his essay in 1991.

In "The Case for Physician-Assisted Suicide?" (selection 143), James F. Keenan helps us consider another factor pushing toward PAS: the cases. Keenan looks at a typical case used to argue for PAS, that of "Uncle Louis." Keenan shows that cases like "Uncle Louis" are not representative of the typical person most likely to be seeking PAS. Rather than a terminally ill man with unmitigated pain who is making a fully informed, free decision for PAS with his long-standing physician, the typical candidate for PAS is "an isolated and depressed woman who does not want to be a burden and who has at best uncertain access to adequate health care and whose own wishes are rarely elicited or heeded."

Which case is more typical makes all the difference in the world. Looking at the case of "Uncle Louis," one easily conceives the question of PAS as being primarily about autonomy and compassion. But if Keenan is right about the typical candidates for PAS, then the question looks very different. PAS is then more about gender inequality and social failures relative to those already on the margins of society, such as the elderly, the poor, and people of color. Keenan admits that there are hard cases like that of "Uncle Louis." But, he argues, when those rare cases are held up as normative they distort our perception of what is really going on behind the debate.

Keenan's essay also suggests a distinction between a moral exception to the law and good public policy. Without granting that the "Uncle Louis" case would be a morally appropriate instance of PAS, Keenan suggests that such questions are better handled through the court system than through legislation. Precisely because "Uncle Louis" is atypical, the case does not make for good law. That answer leaves open a possible gap between good public policy and rare but morally legitimate instances of PAS.

Karen Lebacqz's short essay, "Reflection" (selection 144), comes to a similar conclusion from the opposite direction. Lebacqz contends that in circumstances where the patient is terminally ill, has requested that her life be terminated, and is in enduring and intractable pain, then not to admit the moral permissibility of "active euthanasia" is "a bit absurd, if not obscene." But, because the request for euthanasia can be the result of temporary depression, because of the possibility that the patient is not terminally ill, and because a social policy "supporting voluntary euthanasia would too easily turn into involuntary euthanasia," Lebacqz expresses significant reservations about legalizing PAS. Thus, although starting from the premise that there are legitimate instances of PAS, Lebacqz ends up questioning its legalization.

Keenan's question about the typical case is perhaps important in evaluating the excerpt from Hans Küng's argument for PAS. In "A Dignified Dying" (selection 145), Küng readily admits that his view is shaped by having watched his brother die in terrible pain from a brain tumor. The case here at least partially shapes the conclu-

5. Wesley J. Smith, "Assisted Suicide Advocate Slanders Physicians as Torturers," *Secondhand Smoke*, July 15, 2009, accessed July 28, 2009, from http://www.firstthings.com/blogs/secondhandsmoke/2009/07/15/assisted-suicide-advocate-slanders-physicians-as-torturers/; Wesley J. Smith, "Fear Mongering for Assisted Suicide," *Secondhand Smoke*, February 28, 2009, accessed July 28, 2009, at http://www.firstthings.com/blogs/secondhandsmoke/2009/02/28/fear-mongering-for-assisted-suicide/.

6. Sacred Congregation for the Doctrine of the Faith, *Declaration on Euthanasia:* http://www.vatican.va/roman_curia/congregations/cfaith/documents/rc_con_cfaith_doc_19800505_euthanasia_en.html.

sion. Yet, Küng also marshals a theological argument in favor of PAS that goes beyond personal experience or general appeals for compassion. Küng highlights various theologians and an ambivalent biblical record to suggest that PAS is not outside Christian consideration. In arguing for PAS, Küng primarily appeals to our divinely given freedom and responsibility for our lives, which he believes extends to our dying, but he also draws on notions of God's mercy and the Christian conviction that death is not the end. Thus, "Precisely because I am convinced that another new life is intended for me, as a Christian I see myself given freedom by God to have a say in my dying . . . out of unshakable trust in . . . the merciful God whose grace proves eternal."

Interestingly, Küng takes a position directly opposite that of Keenan regarding public policy. That is, he thinks PAS needs to be legalized and regulated. Not only is PAS sometimes morally appropriate, but legalization is more honest to what is actually going on, and regulation provides protection for the vulnerable. Moreover, says Küng, depending on moral exceptions to the law hands the patient's divinely given freedom to the physician and risks cases of intractable pain being left unaddressed. It is worth wondering if the case of Küng's brother is also evident in this conclusion about legislation.

Unlike Küng, who emphasizes freedom, Stanley Hauerwas stresses community in "Rational Suicide and Reasons for Living" (selection 146). For Hauerwas, our lives are not our own. The gift of life means that we have obligations to God and to one another. The notion of life as a gift that necessarily entails obligations already raises questions of suicide as self-disposal. But, for Hauerwas, the question is also about the kind of life we are to lead. The best life, the life to which we are called, involves being part of community that seeks friendship with God and is learning to care for each other. Such care involves bearing each other's burdens, including a willingness to be a burden. Suicide breaks fidelity to the community: the individual rejects care and/or the community fails to provide or teach care. Hauerwas's starting point, life as gift in community, is a fundamentally different point of departure than Küng's emphasis on divinely given freedom.

By stressing community, Hauerwas's essay questions the ascendancy of autonomy in discussions of PAS. He also implicitly questions certain notions of compassion by asking about the purposes of medicine. It is often said that medicine has two goals, to cure disease and to relieve suffering. In contrast, Hauerwas suggests that medicine is for "caring when we cannot cure." Compassion will sometimes surely look different depending on whether the focus is cure or caring when cure is beyond our reach.

In discussing cultural trends, Richard McCormick worries that the near-exclusive focus on autonomy makes an idol of independence and will make us far less tolerant of dependence. Gloria Maxson ("'Whose Life Is It Anyway?' Ours, That's Whose!") sees that threat as very real for persons with disabilities. Maxson (selection 147) not only sees the specific film — *Whose Life Is It, Anyway?* — as denying the value of the lives lived by persons with disabilities; she also sees a culture that is intolerant of dependence and vulnerability, where antagonism toward the disabled runs just below the surface. By contrast, Maxson affirms the creative and adaptive possibilities open to persons with disabilities and asserts the value in her own life of relationships, beauty, and the presence of God. Maxson reminds us that discussions of PAS have potential implications beyond the terminally ill with uncontrollable pain.

As you reflect on these matters, consider how we should weigh autonomy and community and what constitutes a proper account of compassion. Consider, too, the difference that cases make and what kind of case should be reflected in public policy. Finally, consider both what constitutes a meaningful life and what it means to stand, in life and in death, before a merciful God.

SUGGESTIONS FOR FURTHER READING

Biggar, Nigel. *Aiming to Kill: The Ethics of Suicide and Euthanasia* (Cleveland: Pilgrim Press, 2004).

Bresnahan, James F. "Observations on the Rejection of Physician-Assisted Suicide: A Roman Catholic Perspective." *Christian Bioethics* 1, no. 3 (1995): 256-84.

Campbell, Courtney S., Jan Hare, and Pam Matthews. "Conflicts of Conscience: Hospice and Assisted Suicide." *Hastings Center Report* 25 (May-June 1995): 36-43.

Cohen, Cynthia B. "Christian Perspectives on Assisted Suicide and Euthanasia: The Anglican Tradition." *Journal of Law, Medicine, and Ethics* 24, no. 4 (Winter 1996): 369-80.

Delkeskamp-Hays, Corinna, issue ed. "Euthanasia and Physician Assisted Suicide: Essays in Christianity's Positive Relationship to the World." *Christian Bioethics* 9, nos. 2-3 (August-December 2003): Entire Issue (Netherlands: Taylor & Francis Group).

Dowbiggin, Ian. *A Concise History of Euthanasia: Life, Death, God, and Medicine* (Lanham: Rowman & Littlefield, 2007).

Dyck, Arthur J. *Life's Worth: The Case Against Assisted Suicide*, Critical Issues in Bioethics Series (Grand Rapids: Eerdmans, 2002).

Engelhardt, H. Tristram, issue ed. "Physician-Assisted Suicide and Euthanasia: At the Front in the Culture Wars." *Christian Bioethics* 4, no. 2 (August 1998): Entire Issue (Netherlands: Swets & Zeitlinger).

Geis, Sally B., and Donald E. Messer, eds. *How Shall We Die? Helping Christians Debate Assisted Suicide* (Nashville: Abingdon Press, 1997), pp. 75-182.

Hamel, Ronald P., and Edwin R. DuBose, eds. *Must We Suffer Our Way to Death? Cultural and Theological Perspectives on Death by Choice* (Dallas: Southern Methodist University Press, 1996).

Hare, R. M. "Euthanasia: A Christian View," *Philosophical Exchange* 2 (Summer 1975): 43-52.

Jones, Robert P. *Liberalism's Troubled Search for Equality: Religion and Cultural Bias in the Oregon Physician-Assisted Suicide Debates* (Notre Dame: University of Notre Dame Press, 2007).

Kilner, John F., Arlene B. Miller, and Edmund D. Pellegrino, eds. *Dignity and Dying: A Christian Appraisal* (Grand Rapids: Eerdmans, 1996).

Larson, Edward J., and Darrel W. Amundsen. *A Different Death:*

Euthanasia and the Christian Tradition (Downers Grove: InterVarsity Press, 1998).
Maguire, Daniel. *Death by Choice* (New York: Schocken, 1975).
May, William F. *Testing the Medical Covenant: Active Euthanasia and Health Care Reform* (Grand Rapids: Eerdmans, 1996).
Meilaender, Gilbert. "Euthanasia and Christian Vision." *Thought* (Fordham University Press) 57 (December 1982): 465-75.
Quill, Timothy F. "Doctor, I Want to Die. Will You Help Me?" *Journal of the American Medical Association* 270, no. 7 (August 18, 1993): 870-73.
Ramsey, Paul. *Ethics at the Edges of Life* (New Haven: Yale University Press, 1978), pp. 143-335.
Spong, John Shelby. "Death: A Friend to Be Welcomed, Not an Enemy to Be Defeated." In *Physician-Assisted Dying: The Case for Palliative Care and Patient Choice,* ed. Timothy E. Quill and M. Pabst Battin (Baltimore: Johns Hopkins University Press), pp. 150-63.
Sulmasy, Daniel P. "Managed Care and Managed Death." *Archives of Internal Medicine* 155 (January 23, 1995): 133-36.
Vaux, Kenneth. *Death Ethics: Religious and Cultural Values in Prolonging and Ending Life* (Philadelphia: Trinity University Press, 1992).
Verhey, Allen. *Reading the Bible in the Strange World of Medicine* (Grand Rapids: Eerdmans, 2003), pp. 304-44.

142 Physician-Assisted Suicide: Flight from Compassion

Richard A. McCormick

Most Americans (64 percent of those questioned this year by the *Boston Globe* and the Harvard School of Public Health) approve of physician-assisted suicide. It was somewhat surprising, therefore, that an initiative to legalize it was defeated in Washington State on November 5. The American Medical Association opposed Initiative 119, and its senior vice-president of medical education and science, M. Roy Schwarz, stated that the profession would not soon change its position. "Maybe in five or ten years, but not soon." Five or ten decades would be too soon, in my judgment. But Schwarz's prediction may be close to the mark. The medical profession is usually, and often enough properly, conservative on these matters, but one wonders how long it will hold out against proposals like Initiative 119, especially if these represent shifts in public opinion. Not long, I fear.

Initiative 119 was no surprise apparition. It represents the convergence and culmination of at least five cultural trends. If we understand these trends we should be much better able to deal with clones of 119 in the years ahead.

The Absolutization of Autonomy

The past 20 years or so have witnessed the flowering of patient autonomy as over against an earlier medical paternalism. Paternalism refers to a system in which treatment decisions are made against the patient's preferences or without the patient's knowledge and consent. It is now all but universally admitted, at least in Western circles, that individual decision-making regarding medical treatment is a necessary part of individual dignity. What is not so widely realized is that the current heavy emphasis on autonomy represents a reaction, and reactions have a way of becoming overreaction. In the religious sphere, a reaction against legalism can lead us into the dangers of antinomianism. When we try to stop being overly authoritarian, we risk becoming anarchists.

I see two noxious offshoots of absolutizing autonomy. First, very little thought is then given to the values that ought to inform and guide the use of autonomy. Given

From Richard McCormick, "Physician-Assisted Suicide: Flight from Compassion," *The Christian Century* 108 (December 4, 1991): 1132-34. Used by permission.

such a vacuum, the sheer fact that a choice is the patient's tends to be viewed as the sole right-making characteristic of the choice. I call that absolutization. We have seen this approach in the way the pro-choice position on abortion is frequently presented. The fact that the choice is the woman's is regarded as the only right-making characteristic. But as Daniel Callahan notes, "There are good choices and there are bad choices." Unless we confront the features that make choices good or bad, autonomy alone tends to usurp that role. When it does, autonomy has become overstated and distorted. That overstatement translates into a total accommodation to the patient's values and wishes. If physician-assisted suicide is one of those wishes, well. . . .

The second concomitant of absolutizing autonomy is an intolerance of dependence on others. People abhor being dependent. Given the canonization of independence in our consciousness, "death with dignity" means: to die in *my way,* at *my time,* by *my hand.* Yet the Anglican Study Group was surely correct when it wrote in 1975:

> There is a movement of giving and receiving. At the beginning and at the end of life receiving predominates over and even excludes giving. But the value of human life does not depend only on its capacity to give. Love, *agape,* is the equal and unalterable regard for the value of other human beings independent of their particular characteristics. It extends to the helpless and hopeless, to those who have no value in their own eyes and seemingly none for society. Such neighbor-love is costly and sacrificial. It is easily destroyed. In the giver it demands unlimited caring, in the recipient absolute trust. The question must be asked whether the practice of voluntary euthanasia is consistent with the fostering of such care and trust [*On Dying Well,* p. 22].

Have we forgotten this? I think so. Assisted suicide is a flight from compassion, not an expression of it. It should be suspect not because it is too hard, but because it is too easy. Have we forgotten that dependent old age is a call to cling to a power (God) beyond our control? I think so. Rejection of our own dependence means ultimately rejection of our interdependence and eventually of our very mortality. Once we have achieved that, we fail to see physician-assisted suicide for what it so often is: an act of isolation and abandonment.

The Secularization of Medicine

By "secularization" I mean the divorce of the profession of medicine from a moral tradition. Negatively, this refers to the fact that medicine is increasingly independent of the values that make health care a human service. Positively, it refers to the profession's growing preoccupation with factors that are peripheral to and distract from care (insurance premiums, business atmosphere, competition, accountability, structures, government controls, questions of liability and so on).

Quite practically, the secularization of the medical profession means that it is reduced to a business and physicians begin acting like businesspeople. As Dr. Edmund Pellegrino has observed, they claim the same rights as the businessperson — that is, to do business with whom they choose to. Medical knowledge is viewed as something that "belongs" to the physician and that can be dispensed on her own terms in the marketplace, and illness is seen as no different from any other need that requires a service.

WHEN THE medical profession is fully secularized, clinical judgments will also become secularized. And one important outcome of the secularization of clinical judgments is an overemphasis on autonomy. In this sense the absolutization of autonomy and the secularization of the medical profession are twin sisters.

The Inadequate Management of Pain

Many people fear not death, but dying. And one thing they fear most about dying (we shall mention another below) is pain. Unfortunately, just about everything about physicians' treatment of pain is, well, painful. In a 1989 study conducted by Dr. Jamie H. Von Roenn of Northwestern University, some unsettling facts stood out. First, only one in ten physicians said they received good training in managing pain. A sign of this is that the National Cancer Institute spends only about one-fifth of 1 percent of its billion-dollar budget on pain research. Eighty-five percent of doctors surveyed stated that the majority of cancer patients are undermedicated. But Von Roenn estimated that if competently used, pain medicines could relieve the agony of 80 to 90 percent of cancer patients. Before pain can be controlled, it must be recognized. Yet in Von Roenn's findings, 60 percent of physicians admitted that the inability to assess pain remains a significant barrier to controlling pain. In brief, we have poor education, poor assessment and poor management.

Dr. Steven A. King, director of pain service in the department of psychiatry at the Maine Medical Center, put it forcefully:

> The pain associated with cancer can be managed successfully in the overwhelming majority of patients. Unfortunately, few medical schools and residency programs provide teaching on pain and its management and therefore many physicians are unaware of the wide array of treatment for cancer pain [*New York Times,* March 25, 1991].

If we had better education and better pain control, much of the perceived need for euthanasia would disappear.

The Nutrition-Hydration Debate

Several prominent cases (such as those involving Paul Brophy in Massachusetts and Clarence Herbert in California) have propelled this problem onto center stage. This was especially true in the Nancy Cruzan case. People can now be maintained in a persistent vegetative state (PVS) for years by use of nasogastric tubes or gastrostomy tubes. But must or ought we do so? Few would argue for doing so when the patient has expressly declined such treatment while competent. But what about those who have not so expressed themselves? Here controversy has swirled around cases like that of Nancy Cruzan. Many ethicists and physicians are convinced that artificial nutrition and hydration are not required for persons diagnosed as irreversibly in a PVS. They base this view on the judgment that continuing in a PVS is not a benefit to the patient and therefore is not in the patient's best interests. This is my own conviction, and I wrote as much in support of Lester and Joyce Cruzan's decision to stop Nancy's gastrostomy feedings.

Others, however — a minority, I believe — view this decision in much more sinister terms. For example, some saw continuance in a PVS as a "great benefit" to Nancy Cruzan. A group of authors writing in *Issues of Law and Medicine* in 1987 stated: "In our judgment, feeding such [permanently unconscious] patients and providing them with fluids by means of tubes is *not* useless in the strict sense because it does bring to these patients a great benefit, namely, the preservation of their lives." The most recent statement espousing this view is by Bishop John J. Myers of Peoria, Illinois, in his Pastoral Instructions to health-care administrators. He argues that artificial nutrition-hydration efforts are not useless, since they "effectively deliver nutrients" to these patients, even though they do not reverse their vegetative state. To me, that judgment defines usefulness to the patient so narrowly that personal benefit is reduced to the maintenance of physiological functioning. Patient benefit is exhaustively defined by medical effectiveness alone. Other authors (such as Gilbert Meilaender of Oberlin) view the cessation of artificial nutrition-hydration from PVS patients as direct killing.

I CANNOT ARGUE the case further here. My purpose is to note that the overwhelming majority of people I have polled on this matter do not want to be maintained indefinitely in a PVS because they do not regard this as a benefit to them. Indeed, they are appalled at the prospect. This is the second thing people fear about dying: the needless, heedless and aimless (as they see it) prolongation of the process. And this is where the nutrition-hydration question directly touches the issue of physician-assisted suicide. If our public policies are going to mandate nutrition-hydration treatments and prevent the discontinuance of them, people will easily view physician-assisted suicide as a preferable alternative. I am compelled to note here that certain fanatical fringes of the pro-life movement are counterproductive. By saying that Nancy Cruzan was "starved" and "killed" they will drive people to embrace physician-assisted suicide.

Closely connected with the nutrition-hydration discussion, indeed a part of it, is the distinction between killing and allowing to die. I realize that certain instances of allowing to die are irresponsible (and equivalent to killing); in some cases the distinction is hard to apply persuasively. But the distinction has served us well for many decades, and it would be irresponsible to abandon it. Yet it is being fudged, not least by some courts that threaten with murder charges those who withdraw hopeless and dying patients from ventilators or other life supports. Judge Robert Muir did this at one point in the Karen Quinlan case. Those who removed Karen from the respirator, he said, would be subject to New Jersey's homicide laws. When judges confuse the removal of life supports with homicide, they make homicide look all the more acceptable. One way to soften resistance to the unacceptable is to confuse it with the acceptable.

The Financial Pressures of Health Care

No one needs to be told that there is great pressure on everyone, especially hospitals, to cut health-care costs. We are now spending 12 percent of the GNP for health care, more than any other nation in the world. Hospitals are pressured to cut costs by Health Maintenance Organizations and by Diagnostic Related Groups. Between 1980 and 1986, 414 hospitals closed, and an Arthur Anderson study predicts conservatively that 700 more will close by 1995. Acquisition decisions, hiring practices and incentive proposals are often closely tied to market forces.

Such economic pressures constitute a coercive atmosphere for the debilitated elderly and chronically ill. "Why must I hang on like this? Am I not a drain on my family and limited resources?" As Dr. Robert Bernhoft, a surgeon and president of Washington Physicians Against Initiative 119, put it: "These people [the elderly of limited means] are already under tremendous pressure to get out of the way." The next step is not a huge leap.

Dr. Peter McGough, an opponent of Initiative 119, stated after the vote: "Saying No to assisted death is not enough. Now we have a responsibility to deal with the problems that brought out this concern." The five cultural trends described above indicate (even if they do not exhaust) the problems McGough was referring to. Failure to deal with them would invite a replay of Initiative 119 both in Washington and in other places.

143 The Case for Physician-Assisted Suicide?

James F. Keenan

The Case of 'Uncle Louis,' Which Is Presented as a Typical Case, Is Misleading in Eight Important Ways

Americans love cases. Television shows few debates about major moral issues. Instead it offers us police, legal and hospital dramas dealing with specific cases. "E.R.," "Homicide," "Chicago Hope" and "N.Y.P.D. Blue" combine a narrative with a moral quandary, making the ethical entertaining. Rather than hosting discussions about abortion, nuclear war or civil strife, pragmatic American television captures the moral imagination of its viewers through hard-hitting cases. We love not only fictional cases but also story-telling guests on daytime television and real-life trials (from Alger Hiss to O. J. Simpson to Bill Clinton). Cases are our preferred approach for the consideration of ethical issues. Whether this interest is due to our love for drama, the practical or the law, we understand and communicate our particular values and interests through cases.

We do not use cases only to understand; we also construct them in order to persuade, just as Jesus did in his parables. The parables of the prodigal son and the good Samaritan present cases as a way of teaching Jesus' values.

The discussion about physician-assisted suicide (P.A.S.) is likewise dominated by cases. Nearly every essay advocating it proposes a story to convince the listener of the proponent's point of view. James Vorenberg and Sidney Wanzer, for example, in "Assisting Suicide" (*Harvard Magazine,* March/April 1997) present the following case:

> Uncle Louis is in unmitigated pain. He has no relief because his cancer has no good pain management. His condition is clearly terminal; he has tried all sorts of therapies and even surgery. He has discussed P.A.S. as a final option with his physician with whom he has had a long relationship. He now wants P.A.S.

Proponents conclude the case by asking whether Uncle Louis should be left to suffer. The implication is that Uncle Louis has a right to die.

Reprinted with permission of James F. Keenan, S.J., and America Press, Inc., 106 West 56th Street, New York, NY 10019. Originally published in *America,* November 14, 1998 issue.

Is This a Representative Case?

How common is the case of Uncle Louis? If proponents argue that P.A.S. ought to be legalized because of people like Uncle Louis, it is important to know whether Uncle Louis really is representative of the people asking for P.A.S.

The case of Uncle Louis is, at best, misleading. In eight important ways the probable candidate for P.A.S. is unlike Uncle Louis. First, the person applying for P.A.S. would probably be a woman, not a man. Anyone familiar with Jack Kevorkian, M.D., who travels around the Michigan area providing P.A.S., ought not be surprised at the number of women he has helped die. Out of 43 deaths, 15 of his "patients" were men, 28 were women. As M. Cathleen Kaveny, M.D., has shown, women are more likely to be candidates for P.A.S. than men. Sixty percent of people over 65 years of age and 75 percent of people over 80 are women. But longevity is not the only reason why women are more typical; it is also because they are poorer. Seventy-five percent of all poor people over 65 are women. In a country where the poor are left without health care, elderly poor women are the most likely candidates for P.A.S. Finally, women are twice as likely to suffer from depression than men, and depression is among the leading reasons for P.A.S.

Changing the gender of the person in the case is significant. In our economy, women have been forced to accept inequities in income, available health care and promotion. When the case for P.A.S. becomes more gender specific, women grow suspicious of a program that "accommodates" them more than men. The feminist Susan Wolf notes: "The analogy to other forms of violence against women behind closed doors demands that we ask why the woman is there, what features of her context brought her there and why she may feel that there is no better place to be."

Gender Inequality

Since the person considering P.A.S. is more likely to be a woman, we are dealing here not with autonomy or rights, but with social failure. Social failure is evident when a woman, who has cared for her husband through his decline and death, elects P.A.S. so as not to be a burden to her children and society. Instructed by our society that she ought not to expect equal treatment, the elderly widow realizes that her options are fewer than her husband's.

The first eight persons Dr. Kevorkian helped to die were women. When insinuations were made of misogyny, he then assisted male patients. Curiously, these men were the first terminally ill patients he treated. As a writer in *The New Republic* discovered, the condition of the patient changed when the gender changed:

> Most of Kevorkian's men were declared terminally ill by their own doctors; they were in constant, severe pain

from medically diagnosed causes and were often physically incapacitated. . . . We see that most of the Kevorkian women were not diagnosed terminal and had not been complaining of severe or constant pain. We see conditions like breast cancer (for which there is now great hope), emphysema, rheumatoid arthritis and Alzheimer's (a condition that usually burdens relatives more than the people who have it). . . . In all-too-typical female fashion, the patient often seems to have been most worried about the disease's impact on others. Is it possible that a certain type of woman — depressive, self-effacing, near the end of a life largely spent serving others — is particularly vulnerable to the "rational," "heroic" solution so forcefully proposed by Dr. Death?

The failures in medicine intersect with our social failures regarding gender equality precisely in the case of P.A.S.

Gender inequality is found elsewhere. In legitimate end-of-life issues, women's wishes are not as well respected as men's are. A study of the records of incompetent patients found that after hearing families testify about a patient's wishes to be removed from life support, judges ruled in favor of the patient in 75 percent of the cases if the patient was a man. If the patient was a woman, the percentage dropped to less than 15. The court opinions show that judges regarded men's decisions as rational but women's as unreflective, emotional and immature. When cases concerning P.A.S. focus on gender differences, the debate over P.A.S. exposes a number of harmful practices against women, and P.A.S. is itself exposed as another such practice.

Pain Relief

A second misleading aspect of the Uncle Louis case is the absence of pain relief medication. Pain relief is probably available, but is it provided? *Time* magazine noted, "Look behind today's headlines about physician-assisted suicide and the right to die, and you'll find that what people are really talking about is the management of pain. Or rather, the mismanagement of pain."

A recent study of 4,000 patients who died after hospital interventions showed that 40 percent were in severe pain most of the time. Pain relief is available, but, as nearly every U.S. medical organization recognizes, it is all too frequently not provided. In 1994 the New York State Task Force on Life and the Law reported: "Taken together, modern pain relief techniques can alleviate pain in all but extremely rare cases. Effective techniques have been developed to treat pain for patients in diverse conditions."

It is deceptive to argue that a patient would pursue P.A.S. because of the lack of pain relief. This lack is another sign of failure in the medical community. Yet many believe that pain relief is not actually available, and the case of Uncle Louis exploits this ignorance.

A third misleading aspect of the Uncle Louis case is that pain relief is in fact a minor factor in the motivation of people who seek P.A.S., according to the medical ethicist Ezekiel Emanuel. Holland's Remmelink Report, he notes, states that pain relief played a role in only 32 percent of the requests for P.A.S. in the Netherlands, where P.A.S. has been legal since 1984. Another study — of Dutch nursing home patients — found that pain relief was the primary reason for P.A.S. in only 11 percent of the cases. In the state of Washington (which, with Oregon, has the strongest P.A.S. constituency) a survey found fewer than a third of terminally ill patients cited pain relief as a reason for pursuing P.A.S. One study of cancer patients in Boston even found that patients with pain were more likely to oppose P.A.S. than others. They were also more likely to change doctors if they learned that their physician had performed P.A.S. Emanuel concludes: "No study has ever shown that pain plays a major role in motivating patient requests for physician-assisted suicide or euthanasia."

The fourth misleading aspect of the Uncle Louis case is that P.A.S. candidates probably will not be clear-headed people, but rather persons suffering from depression. The overriding reason for pursuing P.A.S. seems to be the fear of being a burden to others, as 93 percent of Oregon physicians thought. In the Washington survey, 75 percent of terminally ill patients cited concern about being a burden as grounds for P.A.S. Distress and dependency are the primary concerns of P.A.S. candidates.

Here the case of Uncle Louis is again harmful and manipulative of already marginalized people. The case is about one man who has tried every possible option, has consulted physician and family and probably faces unmanageable pain; he is confident of the rightness of his decision, but he is unable to carry it out because our laws prohibit it. The case leads us to believe that the move toward P.A.S. is an advance in our understanding of individual human rights. But the more likely case is that of a woman who, if she fears pain, fears it because her health care system does not properly manage it; she opts for P.A.S. because she does not want to burden her family and because her experience with the health care industry is much more problematic than Uncle Louis's. The irony of a case like Uncle Louis's is that it persuades us to be mistakenly compassionate toward a rather small number of already empowered persons at the cost of doing away with those persons who already find themselves isolated from society, family and the health care industry.

Fully Voluntary?

The fifth misleading aspect of the case is that likely candidates will not enjoy the degree of personal freedom that Uncle Louis does. The Remmelink Report acknowledges that none of the initial euthanasia guidelines established by the Royal Dutch Medical Society are any longer being adhered to. Annually, 3,600 deaths, a startling 2 percent of all deaths, are reported as P.A.S.'s. The true number is higher, since over half of all cases of P.A.S. and euthanasia go unreported. Of the reported cases, about 1,000 are non-voluntary (the physician took the patient's life without an explicit request from family or patient) — a clear violation of Dutch policies.

Other developments are more disturbing. In 1993 a commission of the Royal Dutch Medical Society recommended that mercy killing should be made available to psychiatric patients. In 1995 the Dutch courts vindicated the mercy killing of an infant suffering from spina bifida. Three of the eight Dutch neonatal units now have active euthanasia policies. So striking are the statistics that two noted Dutch lawyers commented: "The creep towards involuntary euthanasia and mercy killing in the Netherlands has gone unchecked, despite legal conditions designed to guarantee voluntariness."

The two U.S. circuit courts of appeals that ruled favorably on P.A.S. viewed the Dutch experiment as irrelevant. Behind that assumption might be American arrogance — that what others are unable to regulate, the United States can. But when we compare the Netherlands with the United States we should be alarmed at the Dutch results. Since the Netherlands is a fairly homogenous society that provides universal health care and "a more advanced network of social services," Kaveny notes, the potential for abuse of P.A.S. is "exponentially greater in the American context." She asks, "What will the practice of assisted suicide look like in our racially fragmented and economically stratified United States?"

Sixth, the literature proposing P.A.S. depicts cases like Uncle Louis's as rare and exceptional. That presupposition goes against legitimate predictions. In the Netherlands, more than 5 percent of the population request P.A.S.; at least 2 percent are granted their requests. If we manage to keep P.A.S. to 2 percent, that would mean annually 43,500 American deaths assisted by physicians. The American underestimation of the impact of a law like this has happened before. Professor Stephen Carter of Yale Law School reminds us that the members of the Supreme Court never imagined, when they voted to legalize abortion in 1973, that "the United States would be home to 1.5 million abortions a year." Though proponents of the Uncle Louis case emphasize an individual's rights, they hide the enormous number of depressed individuals who would probably pursue P.A.S. if the law were changed.

Seventh, the Uncle Louis case claims that P.A.S. is a matter of last resort. That claim is fictive. Certainly, while P.A.S. is illegal, few consider recourse to it until all other options are tried. If it were made legal, however, why would a patient be constrained to consider it only as a last option? The ethicist Daniel Callahan, co-founder and president of the Hastings Center, suggests: "If this is so humane, it will become a legitimate medical option. People with a terminal diagnosis will find themselves facing a doctor who may not only pose it as an option, but even the first option, the most sensible, the most humane."

More importantly, since there is no guarantee of health care in the United States, would not P.A.S. become the only option available to depressed persons without insurance who, facing chronic illness, fear dependency? The bioethicist Arthur Caplan puts it succinctly: "With 30 million people uninsured under our current system, it scares the bejeebers out of me. You don't find many poor people's organizations lobbying for legalization of assisted suicide."

Dr. Caplan's concerns are shared by those who are most vulnerable in our society. In March 1996 the *Washington Post* reported that 51 percent of Americans favor P.A.S. (among men, 54 percent polled favored it; among women, 47 percent favored it). While 55 percent of the white respondents supported it, only 20 percent of African-American respondents did. While 57 percent between ages 40 and 49 approved, only 35 percent of those over 70 did. While 58 percent of people whose income is over $75,000 favored it, only 37 percent of those whose income is under $15,000 did. Does this disparity exist because African Americans, the elderly and the poor lack the strong sense of individual rights that those in other demographic categories have? Or is it due to a realistic suspicion on the part of those on the margins of our health system about the way the American health industry resolves its inability to serve all Americans?

Finally, one of the elements in the Uncle Louis case is the patient's long-standing relationship with a physician. Some physicians have provided P.A.S. to a familiar patient; probably a long-standing relationship prompted them to break the law willingly. This detail appears often in confessional narratives that depict the willingness of physicians to disobey the law in extreme cases. These narratives are rare, intimate and, for many, understandable.

It would be helpful, however, to recall the "compassionate physician" who appeared in the abortion stories before Roe v. Wade became law. What became of the sympathetic and compassionate doctors who in those stories accompanied women seeking abortions? Why did legalized abortions never really find a place in hospitals and why were women seeking abortions marginalized to clinics?

If 2 percent or even 5 percent of the population seek P.A.S., who will be the physicians practicing P.A.S.? If we remand our abortions to clinics and to those who are willing to perform them, why will not the same delegation occur in P.A.S.? After legalization of P.A.S., who will be the P.A.S. physicians for the 30 million persons who are uninsured? The narrative detail of Uncle Louis's long-standing relationship with a physician is clever but misleading.

The Hard Case

There are real cases like that of Uncle Louis. But in the field of ethics, such cases are called "hard cases," that is, cases that force us to reexamine whether a particular prohibition is absolute. Thirty years ago, for instance, many moral theologians did not believe that the encyclical *Humanae Vitae* was right in its claim that every instance of artificial birth control was wrong. Not having to prove that each instance was right, many were only interested in challenging the claim that birth control was always wrong. They proposed, therefore, the case of the mother of eight who could not survive another pregnancy, whose husband scorned sexual abstinence; they never proposed the case of a 22-year-old single woman who was dating and simply wanted to avoid conception.

Hard cases are cases crafted to convince readers that, contrary to shared assumptions, there are moral exceptions to a particular rule. They are rhetorical devices that move us to understand compassionately another's moral dilemma; while acknowledging that a moral rule prohibits a particular course of conduct, the hard case points us to the exceptions.

The hard case, then, breaks down a bias that refuses to entertain moral exceptions to a standing, absolute moral rule. Yet, just as the mother of eight is different from the 22-year-old woman, the hard case is different from the representative case that establishes a new law. The legitimacy of a hard case does not in itself negate the force of the law. Daniel Callahan notes: "Yes, there are cases where the termination of life might be merciful. But those are the exception and cannot be made the rule. It is no different from the woman whose husband has abused her for years and she finally shoots him. Perhaps she is justified. But do we then have a law that says if you can check off 12 of 15 things your husband does, you can kill him?" Thus the hard case of this abusive husband may persuade us that the wife is morally excusable or even morally right in her action, and a judge and jury may be persuaded to concur. But systematically condoning and legalizing that action would make it a suitable alternative and jeopardize other, more civil methods for resolving domestic conflict. A hard case like the abused wife, as an exception to the rule, does not create a new law. It likewise does not negate an existing one.

Whether the case of Uncle Louis is a morally legitimate exception to the rule is debatable. Certainly enough teachings in Catholic moral theology oppose Uncle Louis's claim. The familiar ones are found, for instance, in Thomas Aquinas's question on suicide (*Summa Theologiae,* II-II, 64.5). More recently both the *Catechism of the Catholic Church* and Pope John Paul II's encyclical *Evangelium Vitae* provide ample argument for opposing P.A.S.

The Case of Mary X

These teachings are valid, but we cannot underestimate the persuasive power of contemporary cases. In virtue of their apparent familiarity and humanity, they often have a greater impact on our culture than do our long-held, well-stated general principles. Thus, in the debate about P.A.S. legislation, we need to ask whether these cases are representative cases or hard cases. Whether Uncle Louis's case is a moral exception to the law is beside the point. The question is whether Uncle Louis's is a typical case. Does he significantly represent a group of persons for whom the law should be changed? If the answer is yes, then certainly his case is not exceptional. But if it is not representative, then it is exactly like the case of the abused housewife. Hard cases, like the case of the abused wife, depend not on legislators making new laws, but on judges and juries who interpret existing laws and precedents.

The case of Uncle Louis is touching, but its main claim is that an extension of individual autonomy by means of P.A.S. is the only solution. The strong American sympathy for autonomy is easily evoked by this rare instance of a man who is suffering pain, but it is evidently inadequate when confronted by the more likely case of an isolated and depressed woman who does not want to be a burden and who has at best uncertain access to adequate health care and whose own wishes are rarely elicited or heeded. When this case, the case of Mary X, is taken into account, we see that the critical issue facing Americans in end-of-life care is not the lack of autonomy.

The case of Mary X — a widow facing a progressive chronic illness, fearing dependency on her children, unable to get proper medical coverage and who therefore, without a personal physician with whom she can talk, is depressed, receives no medication or counseling and pursues P.A.S. as her only option — stands as representative of the more probable P.A.S. candidate. It demonstrates not the lack of autonomy (autonomy is, after all, only for those with power), but rather the inequities in our country, our inability to care properly for the dying and the lack of concern for the common good that presently demoralizes the American social landscape. In particular, it exposes the truth that women do not have equal rights and equal opportunities. In short, the typical case is a poignant reminder of our social failure to the aging, to women and to the poor. With that reminder, are we inclined to endorse P.A.S.?

Mary X's case raises a question that Uncle Louis's did not — what will be the social effect of a law that permits P.A.S.? Proponents for the case of Uncle Louis, being exclusively interested in individual autonomy, never entertain that question. They are only interested in the autonomous person. But proponents of the case of Mary X try to persuade us that the law that Uncle Louis wants invalidated is the same law that keeps the more common Mary X from being marginalized to death.

144 Reflection

Karen Lebacqz

Since the question to which we respond is already quite delimited, let me add one more condition: not only is the person terminally ill and requesting termination of life, but she is in enduring and intractable pain that cannot be relieved short of being under heavy and constant doses of drugs. Under these conditions, to ask the question whether active euthanasia is ever permissible seems to me a bit absurd, if not obscene. The question should be inverted: is it ever permissible *not* to use active euthanasia for one who suffers so, with no hope of recovery? We would not hesitate to put an animal out of its misery. Why, then, would we not extend the same compassion to a human being?

No, make that: the same compassion to our mother or father, our brother, our child, our friend.[1] Surely if we care about another, as Nel Noddings so forcefully asserts, we would want to prevent that other's suffering.[2]

Of course, there are all the *practical* reasons for not doing so. How do we ensure that the person truly requests euthanasia? How do we measure enduring and intractable pain? Who will effect the active euthanasia, and how can it be administered in a way that reduces or eliminates the likelihood of abuse of the system? These are not unimportant questions. But in my view, they do not undermine the central moral issue, which has to do with caring, compassion, and prevention of suffering in the face of death.

Consider a woman dying of bone cancer, the mother of one of my friends. As the disease progresses, the pain worsens. To handle the pain, she is drugged constantly and sleeps more than 20 hours out of each day. Is it better to be so drugged than to be dead? Is it different? There was a time when Catholic moral theology did not allow painkillers to be used during childbirth, ostensibly because of the importance of being in possession of one's faculties in order to face God.[3] While today we might deem the refusal of painkillers during childbirth rather cruel, the underlying principle of being in possession of one's faculties as one faces death merits attention. I am not sure that it is better to be alive and permanently in a drugged state than to be dead. Minimally, this seems to be something over which human beings should be given some choice.

I have watched my own parents sign "living wills" in order to try to retain some choice over their ends. Would I really have the courage to refuse treatment on their behalf if that came to be necessary? I'm not sure I would, for although I would want to honor their wishes, I would also have a hard time letting go of those whom I love so much. Would I then have the courage to give them something to induce death if they requested it? Would I be moved by compassion for their suffering or by revulsion at the idea that I bring about death? The questions are not easy.

Or consider my own case. My paternal grandmother died in a diabetic coma. A diabetic coma is perhaps a better way to die than some other ways, and it can be deliberately induced. Diabetes may be, in that sense, a "convenient" disease. I do not know yet whether I have inherited late-onset diabetes. If I have, I may have some options that are not open to those without convenient diseases. If my body were ravaged by disease, my spirit weary from intractable pain, my death inevitable, and my soul ready to face God, I would want to have something available to me to end my life.

That is not a decision I would make easily or lightly. I know the cautions about euthanasia — the danger that it is only a temporary depression speaking, and not the "real" person; the possibility that the patient to be killed is not in fact terminally ill; the risk that social policy supporting voluntary euthanasia would too easily turn into involuntary euthanasia. These dangers I take seriously. I belong to no organizations that advocate voluntary euthanasia, for I find them too unguarded about such dangers.

Nonetheless, I think there are circumstances in which active euthanasia is *morally* justifiable. To say it is morally justifiable is not to say that it should become social policy; that is another matter. Moreover, the situation posed here is very limited; circumstances in which patients are terminally ill and have requested that their lives be terminated, along with the further qualification that they are in enduring and intractable pain.

To sum up, I love life. I want my parents to live forever. I wish my grandmother had not died. I resist my own aging and movement toward death. And yet I am also a Christian. I know that death is not the last word, not the greatest evil. Failure to live, to care, to enact justice, to be in proper relationship — those are greater evils. Death can serve evil or it can serve the values of life. As a way of bringing about death, active euthanasia can serve evil or it can serve the values of life. When it serves the values of life, it can be morally justified.

1. See Stanley Hauerwas, "My Uncle Charlie May Not Be Much of a Person but He's Still My Uncle Charlie," in *Truthfulness and Tragedy* (Notre Dame, Ind.: Notre Dame University Press, 1977).

2. Nel Noddings, *Caring: A Feminine Approach to Ethics and Moral Education* (Berkeley and Los Angeles: University of California Press, 1984), p. 32: "The mother as one-caring . . . wants first and most importantly to relieve her child's suffering."

3. How much misogyny entered that decision is beyond the scope of this piece.

From Ron Hamel, ed., *Choosing Death: Active Euthanasia, Religion, and the Public Debate* (Philadelphia: Trinity Press International, 1991), pp. 87-88. Used by permission.

145 A Dignified Dying

Hans Küng

The Emergency

I openly concede that here I am not speaking impartially. This brings me back to my introductory comments on my lifelong reflection. It may help to show how important it is to discover the truth if here I insert a personal reminiscence which has become decisive for me. Almost exactly forty years ago, on 11 October 1954, I celebrated my first eucharist as a newly ordained priest of the Catholic Church in the crypt of St Peter's, Rome, with my family and friends. On the way there my brother, who was twenty-two at the time, had suffered a fainting fit. Nothing serious, we all thought; he was simply overtired and exhausted. After three weeks' convalescence in Italy he was taken to one of the world authorities on brain surgery of the time, to Professor Krähenbühl, in Zurich. The diagnosis was that he had an inoperable brain tumour between the cerebellum and the cortex. Periods in hospital with radiation and chemotherapy followed — but all in vain. Finally he was discharged as incurable. His condition grew worse and worse. One limb after another, one organ after another, ceased to function, a terribly slow process of dying with increasingly heavy pressure on the heart, circulation and breathing, lasting for weeks while all the time he was clearly conscious. Finally there were days of gasping until finally — almost a year to the day after the first attack — he choked on the rising fluid in his lungs.[1]

Since then I have kept asking myself whether this is the death that God gives, that God ordains. Must men and women 'submissively' accept this, too, till the end as 'God-given', 'divinely willed', even 'pleasing to God'? I still ask myself the question today, especially after, in preparation for a lecture on euthanasia,[2] at the invitation of Professor Ernst Grote, in the neurosurgical clinic of the University of Tübingen, I was able to watch for the first time the opening of a brain, quite by chance a very similar case — and again the diagnosis was that it was inoperable, despite today's amazingly precise computer-tomography, laser techniques and microsurgery. 10,000 people in Germany fall ill each year with brain tumours, and a further 10,000 have metastases in the brain.

Of course I have been familiar with the traditional arguments of theology, so to speak, from my youth.[3] They go like this:

- Human life is a 'gift of the love of God'; it is God's 'gift', I am told, and therefore beyond our control. That is correct and remains true. But something else is also true: in accordance with God's will, life is at the same time also a human task and thus made our responsibility (and not that of others). It is an autonomy based on theonomy.
- It is added that human life is solely God's 'creation'. But in accordance with the will of the creator, is it not primarily a voluntary 'creation' by parents, and so from the beginning a new experience of our time — something for which men and women are responsible?
- People must endure to their 'ordained end', it is argued in return. But my question is: What end is ordained? Does God really control the reduction of human life to purely biological life?
- 'Premature' giving back of life is said to be a human No to the divine Yes, a 'rejection of the rule of God and his loving providence'. It is tantamount to a 'violation of a divine law', an 'insult to the dignity of the human person', a 'crime against life', indeed an 'attack on the human race'. But (and truly I am not just thinking of my brother's case), what is the meaning of such lofty words in the face of a life which is definitively destroyed and in the face of intolerable suffering?

Behind these and similar arguments ('the argument from sovereignty') stands a misguided view of God based on biblical texts which are chosen one-sidedly and taken literally:[4] God as the creator who simply exercises sovereign control over human beings, his servants; their unconditional lord and owner, their absolute ruler, lawgiver, judge and basically also executioner. But not God as the father of the weak, the suffering, the lost, who gives life to human beings and cares for them like a mother, the God of the covenant who shows solidarity, who wants to have human beings, in his image, as free, responsible partners. So for the terminally ill our theological task is not a spiritualizing and mystification of suffering or even a pedagogical use of suffering ('purgatory on earth') but — in the footsteps of Jesus, who

1. As a caption for his memorial portrait we chose a sentence from the Book of Wisdom 4.13: 'Someone who has come to fulfilment in a short time has fulfilled long times.'

2. A lecture first given to the International Congress of the Society of University Neurosurgeons at the University in Tübingen in 1988 and then to the American Association of Neurological Surgeons in San Francisco in 1992.

From Hans Küng, "A Dignified Dying," in *Dying with Dignity: A Plea for Personal Responsibility,* Hans Küng and Walter Jens (New York: Continuum, 1995), 1-40. Reproduced by kind permission of Continuum International Publishing Group.

3. Cf. the Declaration of the Congregation for the Doctrine of Faith, 5 May 1980, esp. p. 452.

4. This aspect of the question has been clearly worked out by the Protestant theologian W. Neidhart, 'Das Selbstbestimmungsrecht des Schwerkranken aus der Sicht eines Theologen', in *Schriftenreihe der Schweizerischer Gesellschaft für Gesundheitspolitik* 36, Muri, Switzerland 1994.

healed the sick — one of reducing and removing suffering as far as possible. For while suffering certainly teaches people to pray, in some cases it also teaches them to curse. There are said to be theologians who fear a 'society free of suffering' — and one asks what kind of world they live in. Indeed, there are theologians who in this connection call for a 'share in Christ's suffering' — as though Jesus would have argued for the intolerable suffering of a terminally ill patient kept alive on drugs.

However, in order to avoid misunderstandings, I immediately add: in opposition to certain advocates of active help in dying like the Australian moral philosopher Peter Singer, I am by no means of the opinion that people become 'non-persons' or 'no-longer persons' as a result of an incurable illness, the weakness of old age or definitive loss of consciousness.[5] One can understand how in particular those who are seriously ill react vigorously to such a view (and occasionally, in excess, even to any discussion). My standpoint is precisely the opposite: simply because human beings are human beings and remain so to the end, even when they are terminally ill (expecting death within a foreseeable period) or dying (expecting death in a short time), they have the right not only to a dignified life but also to a dignified dying and farewell, a right which may possibly (I say possibly) be refused them by endless dependence on apparatus or drugs. This can happen when in a process of dying which can last for hours or months, even years, only a vegetable existence is possible, safeguarded by all the techniques of pharmacological 'immobilization'. Therefore *a priori* the question cannot be dismissed: what is to be done in such cases?

Doctors, above all, answer that a clear distinction must be made between active and passive help in dying. I concede that conceptually that is certainly the case. But every doctor knows that in the increasingly rapid development of today's medicine the grey areas between active and passive help in dying are increasing considerably. To ask a specific question: why should the ending of a medical measure to sustain life — for example, switching off a ventilator — be only a passive help in dying and therefore one which is allowed? Moreover, many doctors feel that switching off a machine like a ventilator is quite an active measure. In terms of effect, which is quite clearly the onset of death, stopping a positive action (switching off a machine or disconnecting a drip) can be precisely the same as performing a positive action, say, giving an overdose of morphine, and in some circumstances can even result in a much more painful death. It is often almost impossible to make a specific distinction in practice where a clear distinction must be made conceptually: the boundaries between all such terms as active and passive, natural and artificial, sustaining and ending life, are fluid. And the legal fiction, that passive help in dying is simply 'not doing something', seems to me to be a not very convincing *ad hoc* construction, if not a contradiction in terms.

So are we to condemn the numerous people

- who did not understand those American doctors who, supported by lawyers and courts, kept the unsaveable, unconscious Karen Ann Quinlan alive artificially for years and against the will of her parents;[6]
- but who, conversely, understood that Dutch woman doctor who put her semi-paralysed, depressive seventy-eight-year-old mother to sleep with an overdose of morphine and was therefore given only a token sentence;
- and also those who helped a woman author in Switzerland, hopelessly ill from cancer of the stomach, in accordance with quite definite rules of the Exit organization, to have the painless death which is allowed there?

In former centuries the issue was to protect against premature shortening of life (and this protection must also be guaranteed today against relatives greedy to inherit or irresponsible doctors or nurses). But in our time the issue is also increasingly the prevention of excessive prolongation of life which the patient thinks he or she can claim, which the relatives call for 'at any price' or the doctor forces on the dying (out of an interest in research or for ideological reasons). So what about active help in dying? Where some call this 'killing', others refer to 'compassion', 'mercy', 'grace', 'helping love'. What is the case? For a Christian who is a disciple of the merciful Jesus, at any rate there must not be just an ethic of prohibitions and sanctions. What then? With discipleship of Jesus goes an ethic of the responsible shaping of life — from beginning to end.

5. Cf. P. Singer, *Praktischer Ethik,* Stuttgart 1984; H. Kuhse and P. Singer, *Should the Baby Live? The Problem of Handicapped Infants,* Oxford 1985. Think of all the implications of Singer's terrifying remarks: 'I therefore propose that one should attach no greater value to the life of a foetus than to the life of a non-human being at a similar stage of rationality, self-awareness, capacity for reason, sensibility, etc. As no foetus is a person, no foetus has the same claim to life as a person' (*Praktische Ethik,* 162). For the life of a newborn child this means: '. . . the life of a newborn child thus has less value than the life of a pig, a dog or a chimpanzee' (169). Thus what Singer says about people with severe mental disturbances comes as no surprise: 'So it seems that, for example, the killing of a chimpanzee is worse than the killing of a person with a serious mental disturbance, who is not a person' (135). Almost any decision leading to the death of the unborn or newborn can be justified by such criteria and examples, as they have no right to life and there are always conflicting interests. For a critical discussion of Singer's view cf. H. Hegselmann and R. Merkel (eds.), *Zur Debatte über Euthanasia. Beiträge und Stellungnahmen,* Frankfurt 1991; J.-P. Wils (ed.), *Streitfall Euthanasia. Singer und der 'Verlust des Menschlichen',* Tübingen 1990. After the Holocaust, the distinction between 'fit to live' and 'unfit to live' can no longer be used neutrally in an 'innocent' way. To regard birth as the limit for the right to life and even to regard a newborn child as not a person seems to me to have no foundation in biology, to be ethically unacceptable and legally pernicious. Handicapped newborn babies and people in a coma are to be respected as human persons.

6. Cf. the account by the parents Joseph and Julia Quinlan, *Karen Ann. The Quinlans Tell Their Story,* New York 1977.

Human Responsibility Even for the End

Today we no longer have just exceptional cases, as is shown by the figures from Holland, where at least there is more truthful information than there is in Germany.[7] Nor should it be said that here I am showing too much 'feeling' for those suffering in tragic situations and sacrificing hallowed principles. As a scholar and a theologian am I to switch off all feelings? The real question is what really are the sacred principles that are to be maintained in our day.

Anyone with a humane disposition is in favour of great respect for life and its unassailable dignity. The 'Declaration on a Global Ethic' approved by the Parliament of the World's Religions in Chicago in 1993 makes the following statement about the obligation to a culture of non-violence and reverence for all life: 'In the great ancient religious and ethical traditions of humankind we find the directive: *You shall not kill!* Or in positive terms: *Have respect for life!* Let us reflect anew on the consequences of this ancient directive: all people have a right to life, safety, and the free development of personality in so far as they do not injure the rights of others. No one has the right physically or psychically to torture, injure, much less kill, any other human being. And no people, no state, no race, nor religion has the right to hate, to discriminate against, to "cleanse", to exile, much less to liquidate a "foreign" minority which is different in behaviour or holds different beliefs.'[8] All this is to be given unqualified approval. But in Chicago the as-yet-unclarified special question of help in dying, about which there is as yet no consensus in any religion, far less between religions, was rightly bracketted off. On this point, first clarification and then consensus must be struggled for. Of course any human being hopes for an easy death, without bodily torment, oppressive anxiety and degradation. But what if things turn out differently?

Today even the more conservative theologians and bishops concede at any rate, for example, by their modified position on birth control — that we are in a time of rapid change in our consciousness of values and norms, which is brought about not by the ill will of human beings but by the rapid changes in society, science, technology and also medicine. Not everything can come from the devil if today increasing direction of the processes of life is possible and is a matter of human responsibility. It makes me think when so many moral theologians who today still have problems with more active help in dying used to have similar difficulties with active, 'artificial' birth control, which they similarly interpreted and rejected as a 'no' to the sovereignty of God over life, until they were finally forced to recognize that God has made human beings responsible for the very beginning of human life — something, however, which the present Pope still does not recognize.

Would it not be consistent to assume that the same God now, more than before, had made the end of human life a human responsibility? This God does not want us to foist responsibility on him that we ourselves can and should bear. With freedom God has also given human beings the right to utter self-determination. Self-determination does not mean arbitrariness, but a conscientious decision. Self-determination also always includes responsibility for oneself, and this always has not only an individual but also a social component (respect for others). It would not be responsibility, but frivolity, arbitrariness, if for example a man in the prime of life, without a thought for wife and children, asked for help in dying because of a failure or a setback in his career. But would it also be arbitrary if a man who all his life has worked honestly and for others, yet at the end — after a clear medical diagnosis — is threatened by a tumour or perhaps years of senile dementia, total senility in old age, were to do the same thing, wanting to bid a conscious and dignified farewell to his family? In view of the question, 'In doubt does one decide for life or for the conscience?' must not respect for the conscience of the patient and his or her self-determination (even in the face of a possibly weakened freedom) have priority? Anything other than respect for conscience would seem to me to be an outdated medical paternalism. Conversely: no doctor can be obliged to undertake any medical practice against his or her conscience. But in cases of doubt doctors can be obliged to help in the search for another doctor.

Or is the patient perhaps to be comforted by doctors who are boasting of having given a woman almost one hundred years old a 'new hip' so that she can go home again and live for about another six months? Or by the fact that a severely burned woman, brought by rescue helicopter to a specialist clinic, could be kept alive another six months? To live another six months — is that good in itself? Have you ever seen an electrician who fell on to a high voltage cable (I have)? His head looked literally like a burnt cabbage (one could just recognize a displaced eye and a few teeth), and he was so seriously injured that he was unrecognizable and did not even dare to show himself to his family. Yet today he can still be kept alive indefinitely by the technical possibilities of medicine. It is not surprising that many people are afraid not only of pain and suffering but also of being imprisoned in a highly technological medical system, afraid of total dependence and loss of control over their own selves, drugged until they are dozy and sleepy, no longer thinking, no longer drinking, no longer experiencing anything.

There is no doubt about it: if someone afflicted by such a fate wants to keep his or her life, then such a per-

7. In 1991 in the Netherlands, according to the official Remmelink report, 2300 patients were given 'euthanasia' by doctors at their express wish; in a further 400 cases the doctors gave help in suicide; in about 1100 cases they ended the life of those who were 'incapable of deciding' (the number of unreported cases may be considerably higher).

8. Cf. H. Küng and K. J. Kuschel (ed.), *A Global Ethic. The Declaration of the Parliament of the World's Religions,* London and New York 1993, 25.

son is to be respected and offered every help. Truly no one should be compelled or even urged to die a day or even an hour earlier than he or she wants. But conversely, no one should be forced to go on living at all costs. The right to continued life is not a duty to continue life; the right to life is not a compulsion to live.[9] So what if a person who is terminally ill finds life intolerable, and voluntarily, stubbornly and consistently expresses his or her desire to die? That there are cases like this should not constantly be denied: there are. One hears from doctors that so many completely disfigured people have been glad to have been kept alive. But there is hardly any talk of those who in their misery throw themselves from a high window in the clinic. There are so many fearful cases where one can understand it if someone says: 'My condition is intolerable. My greatest, last, wish is to die. . . .' And how can anyone presume to decide whether another person shall live or die and seek to compel him or her to go on living and suffering? Certainly the human wish to die can only be the necessary condition for the doctor to intervene, and not the basis of the intervention. The basis can only be the well-being of the patient as he or she (and not the doctor or a third person) feels it.

One will hardly find an argument even in the Bible, which in any case knows no absolute inviolability of life, against suicide and voluntary death. In the Old Testament, the way in which Abimelech, Samson or Razis (in II Maccabees 14) kill themselves is reported in part with approval; the New Testament differs over the case of the traitor Judas. But nowhere in the Bible is suicide explicitly forbidden. Moreover, Jesus of Nazareth nowhere described sickness as a fate imposed by God, to be accepted in submission; rather, he identified with sufferers in opposition to sickness, and in many cases provided help. And if even the first king of Israel, Saul, whose kingdom failed and who, when defeated by his enemies, finally fell on his own sword,[10] is not censured anywhere, could it be that other people who in the utmost distress have ended lives which they have no longer felt to have any human dignity will find a merciful judge? Who of us would want to judge whether a suicide in a state of neurotic depression or in a situation of extraordinary oppression is an 'impulsive reaction' or 'carefully thought out'? In the early Christian centuries those Christian women who preferred death by their own hand or with the help of others to brothels were explicitly praised by church fathers like Chrysostom, Eusebius and Jerome.[11]

There is no mistaking the fact that human responsibility has taken on another dimension in connection with the end of human life, as it has with its beginning, and men and women today are in a fundamentally new situation for which one cannot derive simple recipes from the Bible. But to what extent is this a fundamentally new situation?[12] For the first time in human history, in the past century human beings have succeeded, by improving living conditions and by extraordinary progress in medicine, in most cases in delaying death, which formerly did its work within a few hours, days or at most months. It has thus become possible to extend the time between the beginning and end of a fatal illness or total senility to many years. In this way human life, which hitherto embraced the phases of ante-natal existence, childhood, adolescence, adulthood and old age (and the majority of people never reached the last two phases), has been extended by a further phase: the years of terminal illness or senility. All this is the result, not of a 'natural' development to be attributed to 'nature' or the will of God, but of an almost Promethean effort on the part of human beings, who have themselves created this new phase. However, for some people it has become an almost intolerable burden. And in the face of this completely new situation, as earlier in the question of birth control, so also in help in dying, an ethic which attempts to be both scriptural and contemporary will consider its position and attempt also to find a responsible way for the last phase of human life.

A Theologically Responsible Middle Way

Of course I am also quite clear about the pernicious consequences that a deviation from the principle of the inviolability of human life can have. I know that as in the present unsatisfactory system, so too in a future system, there can be and will be abuses: for example, social pressure on patients finally to put an end to their lives and thus make room for younger people or bring relief to family and society. And I say equally clearly that a legal limit must be put on all macabre legacy-hunting by relatives and profit-orientated aids towards dying offered by health insurance schemes, and on the exploitation of transitory depressions. Such abuses must be fought against with every means, including the law, and also be made criminal offences.

The Reformed theologian Harry M. Kuitert of Amsterdam, who I find confirms my view in a number of respects, lays down the following conditions for granting active help in dying:[13]

9. Cf. A. Eser, 'Freiheit zum Sterben — kein Recht auf Tötung', *Juristenzeitung* 41, 1986, 786-95.

10. Cf. I Samuel 31.4.

11. Cf. 'Selbsttötung', *Staatslexikon* IV, Freiburg ^{7}1988, 1154-63 (E. Seidler — H. Kindt — A. Pieper — B. Stoeckle — A. Eser).

12. This aspect has been described particularly clearly by the French theologian J. Pohier, 'Quitter la vie? Ou etre quitté par elle?', *Gérontologie et société* 58, 1991, 63-9.

13. Cf. H. M. Kuitert, *Een gewenste dood;* German, *Der gewünschte Tod. Euthanasia und humanes Sterben,* Gütersloh 1991, 65f. Cf. the criteria of the Royal Dutch Medical Association formulated as early as 1985. According to the information bulletin about 'Exit' dated 16 October 1993 (Grenchen, Solothurn Canton), this organization for help in dying based in German-speaking Switzerland stands for: 1. the right of human self-determination; 2. the right of sick people freely to decide on medical clinical care; 3. help in voluntary death for the most seriously ill or invalid. It seeks to

1. The request must come from the sick person and not from relatives or nursing staff, and must be expressed in a well-considered and consistent way to the doctor in person (the expression of a constant desire for death?).
2. The suffering of the patient must justify such a request because it is intolerable or experienced as intolerable.
3. Help in dying is to be reserved solely for the doctor, who can help towards a gentle and not a botched or painful death.
4. The doctor has first to discuss with a colleague (an external colleague? and also with the next of kin?) the seriousness of the request, the accuracy of the diagnosis of the patient's condition and the most responsible way of carrying out the measures which will end life.
5. Doctors have to make a note of their conditions (according to the new Dutch law the doctor must send a report to the coroner, but normally there will be no prosecution).

It is primarily a matter for doctors and lawyers to work out concrete guidelines to remove the manifest legal uncertainty. The Netherlands has given an example of how this can be done. Clear legal guidelines for dealing with the problem of euthanasia could also remove the anxieties of so many people in Germany, and in other countries too, and help to avoid some conflicts of conscience among doctors. Why shouldn't the elementary principle that human beings have a right to self-determination even in dying be prescribed by the law? Or might a sphere outside the law be desirable specifically for this last stage of human life, in which, in a literal and highly personal way, an individual's 'To be or not to be?' is the question?

No, legal guidelines on areas of responsibility (with reference to killing on request, help in suicide and killing without the express wish of the person concerned) seem to me to be more consistent, both ethically and legally, and, in view of the large number of undisclosed cases, to be more truthful than recourse to an extremely vague 'emergency above the law' in which active help in dying will be 'tolerated' 'in individual cases'. In the latter situation patients are dependent on the autocratic decision of the doctor and open to possibly intolerable suffering at the very point when their helplessness is at its greatest. Dying cannot in any case be declared to be a free arena for medical diagnosis, as some doctors want and some legal judgments seem to presuppose. If the patient's 'head' is at stake (and not the doctor's), doctors cannot decide in a 'well-meaning' way 'over the patient's head', when their approach, while well-meaning, may possibly have been shaped by traditional thought — patterns and notions of faith on which there has not been sufficient critical reflection.[14] A clearly documented advance directive made by the patient is also a necessary part of the regulation, in the cause of legal clarity. This should be made — and here Switzerland is also an example — quite voluntarily and protected against abuse by numerous safeguards, but then it should be unconditionally respected by the doctor, provided that it does not go against the actual will of the patient.[15] This would spare doctors conflicts of conscience.

We should also reflect that an invocation of dangers is not in itself a refutation. After all my experience as a theologian on matters relating to the rejection of birth control, I am no longer impressed when people talk of breaching of the dam or going over the precipice. Indeed, there are long-term general interests to be protected, but quite unmistakably there is also the oppressive distress of the dying of individuals. Certainly the 'living with cancer' that is recommended is possible for a while, but in some cases it can become completely intolerable. And here there should be an end to claims made particularly by theologians, but also by some doctors, that basically there are hardly any people who really want to die; that their wish to die is merely communicating in a 'disguised' way the desire for better care and human concern, so that 'a literal understanding of the request for euthanasia could only disappoint them'.[16] In any case, it

---

achieve these aims by: 1. establishing the right of every member to passive help in dying in accordance with his or her advance directive; 2. the direction of Exit hospices (with exclusively palliative care); 3. support in voluntary death for seriously ill and handicapped men and women who want to die.

14. Cf. A. Eser, 'Der Arzt im Spannungsfeld von Recht und Ethik. Zur Problematik "ärztlichen Ermessens"', in O. Marquard et al. (eds.), *Ethische Probleme des ärztlichen Alltags*, Paderborn 1988, 78-103.

15. Cf. the ten-page legal opinion by Professor M. Keller of the University of Zurich. He concludes by answering a question put to him by experts, 'Are advance directives drafted in the form which Exit proposes for its members binding on everyone, namely doctors, hospital doctors and nursing staff?': 'The patient's directive is admissible: it is also binding (on the persons mentioned). The doctor may deviate from it only if he can prove that it does not correspond to what is now in fact the will of the patient; no account should be taken of the possible or hypothetical will of the patient beside his directive. The testator can (validly) commission a third party (as an executor) to see that his directive is observed; the person so charged can execute the directive; the doctor treating the patient may not appeal to medical secrecy in connection with the person mandated.' Contrary to the expectations of those who requested it, the opinion of the Swiss Academy of Medical Sciences given by Professor Jean Guinand of Neunberg and Professor Oliver Guillod of Geneva confirmed that advance directives are binding (it can be obtained from Exit in Grenchen). There have recently also been initiatives in this direction in the Federal Republic of Germany. Thus for example by September 1994 the senior citizens' committee of Böblingen/ Württenberg had already sent out 10,000 advance directives. A newspaper article indicates that very recently a further 15,000 enquiries have been received.

16. The most recent example of such an 'ethic of life' favoured by Rome, which continues to work with pseudo-arguments completely in line with the 5 May 1980 Declaration of the Congregation of the Doctrine of Faith, is E. Schockenhoff, *Ethik des Lebens. Ein theologischer Grundriss*, Mainz 1993, 328-40: 331. At any rate, this theologian steers clear of the comparison with Nazi practice which

is said, pharmacological medicine can do everything to ensure that the wish for termination does not arise at all.

But doesn't that make the doctor master of life and death and rob patients of autonomy where they want the decision of their consciences to be taken seriously? Of course there are temporary depressive moods and cases of loveless care and a lack of visits. But in return it can be asked: aren't also many doctors afraid of this last wish for active help in dying? So don't they sometimes withhold the necessary information and avoid a clarificatory person-to-person conversation? Of course not everyone who is willing to die will reveal this desire to a doctor or a pastor whose mind is closed, but in that case — as I have heard from more than one nurse — it will be expressed to the less prejudiced sister who does not forsake them in their dying days.

Certainly doctors have conflicts of conscience over the terminally ill. But I am not convinced by those doctors who — though there are also others — openly maintain traditional principles and even emphatically reject any active help in dying, but who, in many cases where palliative therapy has come up against its undeniable limits, *secretly* increase the dose of morphine more than is necessary.[17] There is no doubt that the well-being of the sick is the supreme law. But couldn't this supreme law itself require the sick person to be spared unending terror in favour of an end without terror?

Certainly, lawyers in particular see themselves confronted with conflicts of norms (between private law and public law) and have to worry about the effects of particular changes in the legal system as a whole. But I am not convinced by those lawyers who — though there are also others — without reflecting on their ideological presuppositions formally keep to the positive law (the *ius conditum,* without concern for the *ius condendum*), and who do not even recognize that particularly in the case of help in dying the 'highest law can result in the greatest injustice'.

To conclude: certainly theologians and churchmen in particular call for a special moral sensitivity. But I am not convinced by those — though there are also others — who in the case of help in dying, as formerly in the case of abortion, immovably advance rigoristic standpoints which are not understood even by the majority of their own confession. The churches generally, and the Catholic Church in particular, are called on to take a reasonable middle way between moral rigorism and moral libertinism in order to contribute to a consensus and not polarize and divide society by extreme positions; otherwise the German Conference of Bishops, like the Dutch Conference of Bishops, will ultimately (as in the debate over abortion) end up as the great loser, because, like the Dutch bishops, it has forfeited the support not only of public opinion, but also of the other Christian churches, indeed of most of its own church members.[18] Or perhaps we too will arrive at the point reached in France, where, according to the most recent opinion poll, eighty-three per cent of the population are guided in moral questions solely by their own consciences, and only one per cent (!) by the teaching of the church?[19]

Happily, even in Catholic moral theology today there is increasingly a move away from such rigoristic standpoints and an emphasis that the ultimate criterion must not be the maximal prolongation of life in the biological sense, but the realization of human values, to which biological life is subordinate. Thus as early as 1980 the Tübingen Catholic theologian Alfons Auer stated that the traditional theological basis for the view that human life is not under our control ('relationality to God') was 'ultimately unconvincing'.[20] So not 'every human suicide (and thus not active euthanasia either)' is '*a priori* absolutely and decisively to be rejected as immoral'. In his view the problem can be 'decided only by a responsible evaluation of benefits'. Indeed, according to Auer, every human being has 'a right for his or her conscientious decision to be respected by others. It is not within the competence of ethical reflection to evaluate personal moral decisions. It has the task of making visible what is binding in the various spheres of human life and expressing this incommunicable formula.' And other theologians have expressed themselves even more clearly on this question, like the Protestant ethicists Joseph Fletcher and Harry Kuitert, and the Catholic theologians P. Sporken

is usual in Rome (the *Osservatore Romano* refused to publish a refutation by the Dutch Christian Democrat Minister of Justice, Ernst Hirsch Ballin, of the sweeping Vatican charges against the new euthanasia legislation of the Dutch Parliament).

17. According to the most recent study in the *British Medical Journal,* on the basis of their own information a third of British doctors have at some time given active help in dying. Almost half of them would be prepared to do so if active help in dying were made legal (press release of May 1994). — While this book was going to press, the report of a referendum in the US state of Oregon held on 8 November 1994 reached me; there, by a majority of 52%, medical help in suicide is allowed on certain conditions. Doctors may not give 'lethal injections', but may prescribe drugs at the request of patients. The sick persons must take these themselves. The condition here is that the patient must have asked for the fatal drug at least three times within fifteen days, once in writing in the presence of two witnesses. Moreover, two doctors need to confirm that the sick person has only six months to live and is of sound mind. Patients suffering from depressions are not to have anything prescribed for them.

18. Cf. J. Backbier and J. Mourits, 'Ist der Deich gebrochen? Die neue Euthanasiegesetzgebung in den Niederlanden', in *Herder Korrespondenz,* 1994, 3, 125-9 (Statement by the Dutch Bishops, 128). Already in the 1986 report on 'Euthanasia and Pastoral Care' produced by the synods of the two great Reformed churches of the Netherlands, the decision to have one's life ended is said in certain cases to be a responsible one.

19. The survey was carried out for the three press organs *Le Monde, La Vie* and *L'Actualité religieuse dans le monde* by three leading sociologists of religion (G. Michelat, J. Sutter and J. Potel), Cf. the summary account by A. Woodrow of *Le Monde* in *The Tablet,* 21 May 1994.

20. Cf. A. Auer, 'Probleme der Sterbehilfe aus theologischer Sicht', in Grundmann et al., *Krebsbekämpfung* II, New York 1980, 137-45: 141-3.

and A. Holderegger.[21] Karl Barth had already affirmed as an 'exceptional case' that 'not every act of self-destruction is as such suicide': 'Self-destruction does not have to be the taking of one's own life. Its meaning and contention might well be a definite if extreme form of the self-offering required of man.'[22]

So as a Christian and a theologian I feel encouraged, after a long 'consideration of the benefits', now to argue publicly for a middle way which is responsible in both theological and Christian terms: between an anti-religious libertinism without responsibility ('unlimited right to voluntary death') and a reactionary rigorism without compassion ('even the intolerable is to be borne in submission to God as given by God'). And I do this because as a Christian and a theologian I am convinced that the all-merciful God, who has given men and women freedom and responsibility for their lives, has also left to dying people the responsibility for making a conscientious decision about the manner and time of their death.[23] This is a responsibility which neither the state nor the church, neither a theologian nor a doctor, can take away.

This self-determination is not an act of arrogant defiance of God; just as the grace of God and human freedom are not exclusive, neither are God's predestination and human self-determination. In this sense, self-determination is demarcation over against others: just as no one may urge, necessitate or compel others to die, so too no one may compel them to continue to live. And is there a more personal decision than that of the terminally ill as to whether to end or not to end their suffering? If God makes the whole of life a human responsibility, then this responsibility also applies to the last phase of our lives; indeed, it applies even more to the real emergency of our lives, when it is a matter of dying. Why should this last phase of life in particular be exempted from responsibility?

21. Cf. J. Fletcher, 'The Patient's Right to Die', in A. B. Downing (ed.), *Euthanasia and the Right to Death. The Case for Voluntary Euthanasia,* London 1969, 61-70. H. M. Kuitert, *Der gewünschte Tod* (n. 13); P. Sporken, *Menschlich sterben,* Düsseldorf 1972; id., *Umgang mit Sterbenden,* Düsseldorf [2]1975. A. Holderegger, 'A Right to a Freely Chosen Death? Some Theological Considerations', *Concilium* 179, 1985, 95, writes: 'Among theologians this fundamental insight has increasingly given rise to the conviction that there is no other way than establishing the possibility of killing or suicide as one given by the creator along with the actual power of running one's own life, so as to conclude that man has to make the moral judgment of the circumstance in which it is to be regarded as justified and in which it is not.'

22. K. Barth, *Church Dogmatics* III.4, Edinburgh 1961, 410.

23. Cf. Kuitert, *Der gewünschte Tod* (n. 13), 69: 'The right to life and the right to die is the nucleus of self-determination; it is an inalienable right and includes the freedom even to decide the time and manner of our end, instead of leaving this decision to others or to the outcome of medical intervention.' On the question of suicide cf. id., *Darf ich mir das Leben nehmen?,* Gütersloh 1990. R. Garventa, *Il suicidio nell'età del nichilismo,* Milan 1994, opens up interesting aspects.

How to Die?

No false comfort, certainly not! But isn't there also an authentic, true comfort? There is not only a time to live but also a time to die, and there should not be a concern to delay this artificially or compulsively. 'For everything there is a season . . . a time to be born and a time to die,' says Koheleth, the preacher of transitoriness.[24] The truth in truthfulness — that is also my concern in this question. Here I do not want to proclaim anything from above in magisterial fashion, but merely to make my personal standpoint clear. I want to raise justified questions for reflection, which I hope will relax some of the tension in the great dispute that is already in the making, and prevent the fronts which are already developing from becoming rigid. Not least for that reason, at this point I am making a stand in the political discussion which has just started, so that this time, at least in Germany, in this question which is so serious we may avoid the party-political and church-political polarizations that made the question of abortion such a fanatical one. But that will work only if we can raise the debate to another level. To another level?

Yes, and that brings me back to the point which is decisive for me: precisely because I am convinced that death is not the end of everything, I am not so concerned about an endless prolongation of my life — certainly not under conditions which are no longer commensurate with human dignity. Precisely because I am convinced that another new life is intended for me, as a Christian I see myself given freedom by God to have a say in my dying, a say about the nature and time of my death — in so far as this is granted me. Certainly, the question of a dignified dying may not in any case be reduced to the question of active help in dying; but it may not be detached from that either. A dignified dying also includes responsibility for dying in keeping with human dignity — not out of mistrust and arrogance towards God but out of unshakeable trust in God, who is not a sadist, but the merciful God whose grace proves eternal.

Those who trust in God at the same time trust that death is not the end. In the light of the Eternal One, who alone can grant 'deep, deep eternity', the death of mortal life becomes transcendence into God's eternal life. As the old prayer for the dead in the eucharist has it, *'Vita mutatur, non tollitur'*: life is transformed, not taken away. So should I be anxiously concerned how short or long this mortal life is finally to be?

Here on the basis of my faith I am not a jot more certain about my dying than other people: in the face of the majesty of death, self-confidence is least of all appropriate. None of us knows when and how our death will come about, and each individual dies his or her own death in an ultimate solitude. No one knows what will happen at the decisive moment, whether one will die in peace and tranquillity, or in panic, with anxiety, pain and

24. Cf. Koheleth 3.1f.

crying. So I may not be certain of myself, but only of the forgiveness and grace of God in faith in Jesus Christ. But hope in this God should make my life different from a life without hope.

And it is to precisely that point that these comments have ultimately led: to a different, more serene, indeed more dignified, attitude to dying on the basis of a different attitude to God. Many men and women have gone this way before us. So if we have to break off all relations to human beings and things, then for believers, supported and helped by every medical art, and comforted (for those who wish it) by the sacraments of the church, this means a farewell to fellow men and women, an inward leave-taking, a return and homecoming to one's basic ground and origin, one's true home. It is a farewell which is perhaps not without pain and anguish, but which is said in composure and surrender, at any rate without weeping and wailing, and also without bitterness and despair. Rather, it is said in hopeful expectation, quiet certainty and (after all necessary affairs have been settled) embarrassed gratitude for all the good and not so good things that now finally and definitively — thank God — lie behind us.[25] Such a dying into God, with a sense of embarrassed gratitude, seems to me to be what we may hope for in trust: a truly dignified dying.

25. The prayer of brother Klaus von Flüe can also be understood as a dying prayer:

'My Lord and my God, take from me all that keeps me from you.
My Lord and my God, give me all that helps me towards you.
My Lord and my God, take me from myself and give me wholly to you.'

For the basic theological questions addressed in this plea see the detailed account in my book *Eternal Life?*, London and New York 1984, reissued 1991.

146 Rational Suicide and Reasons for Living

Stanley Hauerwas

1. Suicide and the Ethics of Autonomy

There is a peculiar ambiguity concerning the morality of suicide in our society. Our commitment to the autonomy of the individual at least implies that suicide may not only be rational, but a "right."[1] Yet many continue to believe that anyone attempting suicide must be sick and therefore prevented from killing themselves. This ambiguity makes us hesitant even to analyze the morality of suicide because we fear we may discover that our society lacks any coherent moral policy or basis for preventing suicide.

Therefore the very idea of "rational suicide" is a bit threatening. We must all feel a slight twinge of concern about the book soon to be published by the British Voluntary Euthanasia Society that describes the various painless and foolproof methods of suicide. But it is by no means clear why we feel uncomfortable about having this kind of book widely distributed. As Nicholas Reed, the general secretary of the Society, suggests: suicide is "more and more seen as an acceptable way for a life to end, vastly preferable to some long, slow, painful death. We're simply helping in the fight for another human right — the right to die."[2]

We think there must be something wrong with this, but we are not sure what. I suspect our unease about these matters is part of the reason we wish to deny the existence of rational or autonomous suicide. If all potential suicides can be declared ill by definition then we can prevent them ironically because the agent lacks autonomy. Therefore we intervene to prevent suicides in the name of autonomy which, if we were consistent, should require us to consider suicide a permissible moral act.

1. For example, T. Beauchamp and J. Childress (*Principles of Biomedical Ethics* [New York: Oxford University Press, 1979], p. 90) suggest, "If the principle of autonomy is strongly relied upon for the justification of suicide, then it would seem that there is a right to commit suicide, so long as a person acts autonomously and does not seriously affect the interests of others."

2. "British 'Right to Die' Group Plans to Publish Manual on Suicide," *New York Times.*

Once I was a participant in a seminar in medical ethics at one of our most prestigious medical schools. I was there to speak about suicide, but the week before the seminar had considered abortion. At that time I was told by these beginning medical students they decided it was their responsibility to perform an abortion if a woman requested it because a woman has the right to determine what she should do with her body — an ethical conclusion that they felt clearly justified on grounds of protecting the autonomy of the patient. Moreover this position, they argued, was appropriate if the professional dominance and paternalism of the medical profession was to be broken.

However, I asked them what they would do if they were attending in the Emergency Room and someone was brought in with slashed wrists with a suicide note pinned to their shirt front. First of all would they take the time to read the note to discover the state of the patient? Secondly would they say this is clearly not a medical matter and refuse to accept the patient? Or would they immediately begin to save the person's life? With the same unanimity concerning their responsibility to perform abortion they felt they must immediately begin trying to save the person's life.

The reason they gave to justify their intervention was that anyone taking their life must surely be sick. But it was not clear what kind of "sickness" was under consideration unless we define life itself as some kind of syndrome. Failing to make the case that all suicides must be sick, they then suggested they must act to save such a person's life because it was their responsibility as doctors. But again I pressed them on what right they had to impose their role-related responsibilities on those who did not seek their services and, in fact, had clearly tried to avoid coming in contact with them. They then appealed to experience, citing cases when people have recovered from suicide attempts only to be thankful they had been helped. But again such appeals are not convincing since we can also point to the many who are not happy about being saved and soon make another attempt.

Our discussion began to be more and more frustrating for all involved, so a compromise was suggested. These future physicians felt the only solution was that when a suicide came to the Emergency Room the first time, the doctor's responsibility must always be to save their life. However if they came in a second time they could be allowed to die. That kind of solution, however, is not only morally unsatisfactory, but pragmatically difficult to institutionalize. What happens if each time the person is brought to the hospital they get a different physician?

I have told this story because I think it nicely illustrates the kind of difficulties we feel when we try to get a moral handle on suicide. We feel that Beauchamp and Childress are right that if a suicide is genuinely autonomous and there are no powerful utilitarian reasons or "reasons of human worth and dignity standing in the way, then we ought to allow the person to commit suicide, because we would otherwise be violating the person's autonomy."[3]

However, I want to suggest that this way of putting the matter, while completely consistent with an ethics of autonomy, is also deeply misleading. It is misleading not only because it reveals the insufficiency of autonomy either as a basis or ideal for the moral life[4] but also it simply fails to provide an appropriate account of why any of us decides or should decide to stay alive. Indeed it is odd even to think of our willingness to live as a decision. For example Beauchamp and Childress do not explain how anyone could take account of *all* relevant variables and future possibilities in considering suicide. Indeed that seems an odd condition, for if we required it of even our most important decisions it would stop us from acting at all.

Yet by challenging this account I want clearly to distinguish my position from those who are intent to deny the possibility of rational suicide. I think that suicide can be and often is a rational decision of an "autonomous" agent, but I do not therefore think it is justified. It is extremely interesting, for example, that Augustine did not claim that suicide was irrational in criticizing the Stoic acceptance and even recommendation of suicide. Rather he pointed out that their acceptance of suicide belied their own understanding of the relation between evil and happiness and how a wise man thus should deal with adversity. Though the quote is long I think it worth providing the full text. Augustine says,

> There is a mighty force in the evils which compel a man, and, according to those philosophers, even a wise man, to rob himself of his existence as a man; although they say, and say with truth, that the first and greatest utterance of nature, as we may call it, is that a man should be reconciled to himself and for that reason should naturally shun death — that he should be his own friend, in that he should emphatically desire to continue as a living being and to remain alive in this combination of body and soul, and that this should be his aim. There is a mighty force in those evils which overpower this natural feeling which makes us employ all our strength in our endeavor to avoid death — which defeat this feeling so utterly that what was shunned is now wished and longed for, and, if it cannot come to him from some other source, is inflicted on a man by himself. There is a mighty force in those evils which make Fortitude a murderer — if indeed she is still to be called fortitude when she is so utterly vanquished by those evils that she not only cannot by her endurance keep guard over the man she has undertaken to govern and protect, but is herself compelled to

3. T. Beauchamp and J. Childress, *Principles of Biomedical Ethics*, p. 93.

4. See F. Bergman, *On Being Free* (Notre Dame: University of Notre Dame Press, 1977); and G. Dworkin, "Moral Autonomy," in *Morals, Science, and Sociality*, ed. H. Engelhardt and D. Callahan (Hastings-on-Hudson, N.Y.: Hastings Center Publications, 1978).

go so far as to kill him. The wise man ought, indeed, to endure even death with a steadfastness, but a death that comes to him from outside himself. Whereas if he is compelled, as those philosophers say, to inflict it on himself, they must surely admit that these are not only evils, but intolerable evils, when they compel him to commit this crime.

It follows from this that the life weighed down by such great and grievous ills, or at the mercy of such chances, would never be called happy, if the men who so term it, and who, when overcome by the growing weights of ills, surrender to adversity encompassing their own death — if these people would bring themselves to surrender to the truth, when overcome by sound reasoning, in their quest for the happy life, and would give up supposing that the ultimate, Supreme God is something to be enjoyed by them in this condition of mortality.[5]

The question is not, therefore, the question of whether suicide is "rational." Augustine knew well that the Stoics could provide outstanding examples of cool, unemotional, and rational suicide. He rather asks what kind of blessedness we should expect out of life. For Augustine the Stoic approval of suicide is an indication of the insufficient account they provided about what human existence should be about — namely they failed to see that the only happiness worth desiring is that which came from friendship with the true God. "Yet," he says, "these philosophers refuse to believe in this blessedness because they do not see it; and so they attempt to fabricate for themselves an utterly delusive happiness by means of a virtue whose falsity is in proportion to its arrogance."[6] So the issue is understood within a conception of life we think good and worthy.

2. The Grammar of Suicide

Before developing this line of reasoning, however, it should be pointed out that the discussion to this point has been trading on the assumption that we know what suicide is. Yet that is simply not the case. For as Beauchamp and Childress suggest, definitions of suicide such as "intentionally caused self-destruction not forced by the action of another person" are not nearly as unambiguous as they may at first seem. For example they point out when persons suffering from a terminal illness or mortal injury allow their death to occur we find ourselves reluctant to call that act "suicide," but if persons with a terminal illness take their life by active means we do refer to that act as one of suicide. Yet to only describe those acts that involved a direct action as suicide is misleading since we are not sure how we should describe cases where "a patient with a terminal condition might easily avoid dying for a long time but might choose to end his life immediately by not taking cheap and painless medication."[7]

Beauchamp and Childress suggest the reason we have difficulty deciding the meaning of suicide is that the term has an emotive meaning of disapproval that we prefer not to apply to certain kinds of ambiguous cases. The very logic of the term therefore tends to prejudice any pending moral analysis of the rightness or wrongness of suicide. As a means to try to deal with this problem they propose an "uncorrupted" definition of suicide as what occurs "if and only if one intentionally terminates one's own life — no matter what the conditions or precise nature of the intention or the causal route to death."[8]

As sympathetic as one must feel with their attempt to provide a clear and non-prejudicial account of suicide, however, the very idea of an "uncorrupted" definition of suicide distorts the very grammar of such notions. Beauchamp and Childress are quite right to point out that the notion itself cannot settle how and why suicide applies to certain kinds of behavior and not others. But what must be admitted, as Joseph Margolis has recently argued, is the culturally variable character of suicide. There are many competing views about the meaning and nature of suicide, "some religious, some not, some not even significantly so characterized. . . . There is no simple formula for designating, except trivially, an act of taking, or yielding, or making likely the end of, one's life that will count, universally, as suicide. No, some selection of acts of this minimal sort will, in accord with an interpreting tradition, construe what was done as or as not suicide; and, so judging, the tradition will provide as well for the approval or condemnation of what was done. In short, suicide, like murder itself, is an act that can be specified only in a systematic way without a given tradition; and that specification itself depends on classifying the intention of the agent. We can say, therefore, that there is no

5. Augustine, *The City of God,* trans. Henry Bettenson (Harmondsworth: Penguin, 1977), pp. 856-57.

6. Ibid., p. 857. Earlier Augustine had argued, "There were famous heroes who, though by the laws of war they could do violence to a conquered enemy, refused to do violence to themselves when conquered; though they had not the slightest fear of death, they chose to endure the enemy's domination rather than put themselves to death. They were fighting for their earthly country; the gods they worshipped were false; but their worship was genuine and they faithfully kept their oaths. Christians worship the true God and they yearn for a heavenly country; will they not have more reason to refrain from the crime of suicide, if God's providence subjects them for a time to their enemies for their probation or reformation. Their God does not abandon them in that humiliation, for he came from on high so humbly for their sake," pp. 35-36.

7. Beauchamp and Childress, *Principles of Biomedical Ethics,* p. 86.

8. Ibid., p. 87. Elsewhere Beauchamp provides a fuller account arguing suicide occurs when "a person intentionally brings about his or her own death in circumstances where others do not coerce him or her to the action, except in those cases where death is caused by conditions not specifically arranged by the agent for the purpose of bringing about his or her own death." T. Beauchamp, "Suicide," in *Matters of Life and Death,* ed. T. Regan (New York: Random House, 1980), p. 77.

minimal act of commission or omission that counts as suicide, except relative to some tradition; and, within particular traditions, the justifiability of particular suicides may yet be debatable."[9]

So the very way one understands "suicide" already involves moral judgments and requires argument. So I shall contend that if we rightly understand what life is about, suicide should be understood negatively and should not therefore be recommended as an alternative for anyone. This is not to deny that from certain perspectives suicide can be considered rational — as an institution, that is, a way of characterizing a whole range of behavior, as well as an individual act. That it can be so understood, however, reveals how little the issue turns on the question of "rationality." We must rather ask whether the tradition through which we understand the meaning and nature of suicide is true.

3. Why Suicide Is Prohibited

I have argued elsewhere that suicide as an institution must be considered morally doubtful. That conclusion is based on the religious understanding that we should learn to regard our lives as gifts bestowed on us by a gracious Creator.[10] That such an appeal is explicitly religious is undeniable, but I would resist any suggestion that the religious nature of this appeal disqualifies it from public argument. Rather it is a reminder of Margolis' contention that any account of suicide necessarily draws on some tradition. Therefore my appeal to this kind of religious presupposition is but an explicit avowal of what any account of suicide must involve — though I certainly would not contend that the only basis for disapproving suicide is religious.

It is important, however, that the significance of the shift to the language of gift be properly appreciated. For it is a challenge to our normal presumptions about the way the prohibition of suicide is grounded in our "natural desire to live." Indeed it is not even clear to me that we have a "natural desire to live," or even if we do what its moral significance entails. The very phrase "natural desire to live" is fraught with ambiguity, but even worse it seems to suggest that when a person finds they no longer have such a desire there is no longer any reason for living.

In contrast the language of gift does not presuppose we have a "natural desires to live," but rather that our living is an obligation. It is an obligation that we at once owe our Creator and one another. For our creaturely status is but a reminder that our existence is not secured by our own power, but rather requires the constant care of and trust in others. Our willingness to live in the face of suffering, pain, and sheer boredom of life is morally a service to one another as it is a sign that life can be endured as well as a source for joy and exuberance. Our obligation to sustain our lives even when they are threatened with or require living with a horrible disease is our way of being faithful to the trust that has sustained us in health and now in illness.[11] We take on a responsibility as sick people. That responsibility is simply to keep on living as it is our way of gesturing to those who care for us that we can be trusted and trust them even in our illness.

There is nothing about this position which entails that we must do everything we can do to keep ourselves alive under all conditions. Christians certainly do not believe that life is inherently sacred and therefore it must be sustained until the bitter end. Indeed the existence of the martyrs is a clear sign that Christians think the value of life can be overridden.[12] Indeed I think there is much to be said for distinguishing between preserving life and only prolonging death, but such a distinction does not turn on technical judgments about when we have in fact started dying, though it may involve such a judgment.[13] Rather the distinction is dependent on the inherited wisdom of a community that has some idea of what a "good death" entails.[14]

Such a death is one that allows us to remember the dead in a morally healthy way — that is, the manner of death does not prevent the living from remembering the manner and good of their life. To be sure we can train ourselves to remember a suicide as if the suicide said nothing about their life, but I think we would be unwise to do so. For to face the reality of a death by suicide is a reminder how often our community fails to offer the trust necessary to sustain our lives in health and illness. Suicide is not first a judgment about the agent, but a reminder that we have failed to embody as a community the commitment not to abandon one another. We fear being a burden for others, but even more to ourselves. Yet it is only by recognizing that in fact we are inescapably a burden that we face the reality and opportunity of living truthfully.

It is just such a commitment that medicine involves and why the physician's commitment to caring for the sick seems so distorted by an ethics of autonomy. Medicine is but a gesture, but an extremely significant gesture of a society, that while we all suffer from a condition that cannot be cured, nonetheless neither will we be abandoned. The task of medicine is to care even when it cannot cure.[15] The refusal to let an attempted suicide die is

9. J. Margolis, *Negativities: The Limits of Life* (Columbus: Merriall, 1975), pp. 25-26.

10. S. Hauerwas, *Truthfulness and Tragedy* (Notre Dame: University of Notre Dame Press, 1977), pp. 101-15.

11. See S. Hauerwas, "Reflections on Suffering, Death, and Medicine," *Ethics in Science and Medicine* 6 (1979): 229-37.

12. See S. Hauerwas, *Community of Character* (Notre Dame: University of Notre Dame Press, 1980).

13. S. Hauerwas, *Vision and Virtue* (Notre Dame: University of Notre Dame Press, 1974), pp. 166-86.

14. S. Hauerwas, "Religious Conceptions of Brain Death," in *Brain Death: Interrelated Medical and Social Issues,* ed. J. Korein (New York: New York Academy of Sciences, 1978), pp. 329-36.

15. S. Hauerwas, "Care," in *Encyclopedia of Bioethics,* ed. W. Reich (New York: Free Press, 1978), 1: 145-50.

only our feeble, but real, attempt to remain a community of trust and care through the agency of medicine. Our prohibition and subsequent care of a suicide draws on our profoundest assumptions that each individual's life has a purpose beyond simply being "autonomous."

4. Reasons for Living and "Rational Suicide": An Example

However, the kind of religious appeals I have made as well as this kind of talk about "purpose" can easily be misleading. For it sounds as though suicide is religiously prohibited because people who believe in God really know what life is about. But that is not the case — at least in the usual sense a phrase such as "what life is about" is understood. Indeed the very reason that living is an obligation is that we are to go on living even though we are far from figuring out what life is about. Our reason for living is not that we are sure about the ultimate meaning of life, but rather that our lives have been touched by another and through that touch we believe we encounter the very being that graciously sustains our existence.

Indeed one of the problems with discussions of "rational suicide" is they seem to be determined by the assumption that the decision to live or to die turns on whether life, and more importantly, one's particular life, has meaning or purpose. Thus, Margolis, for example, suggests that a relatively neutral understanding of the issue raised by suicide is whether the deliberate taking of one's life in order simply to end it, not instrumentally for any ulterior purpose, can ever be rational or rationally justified. He suggests a rational suicide is when a person "aims overridingly at ending his own life and who, in a relevant sense, performs the act. The manner in which he suicides may be said to be by commission or omission, actively or passively, directly or indirectly, consciously or unconsciously, justifiably or reprehensibly — in accord with the classificatory distinctions of particular traditions."[16] According to Margolis such suicide is more likely to be justified if the person "decided that life was utterly meaningless" or "sincerely believed life to have no point at all."[17]

My difficulty with such a suggestion is that I have no idea what it would mean to know that life, and in particular my life, was "utterly meaningless" or had "no point at all." In order to illustrate my difficulty about these matters let me call your attention to one of the better books about suicide — John Barth's *The Floating Opera*.[18] Barth's book consists of Todd Andrews' account of how one day in 1937 he decided to commit suicide. There was no particular reason that Andrews decided to commit suicide and that, we discover, is exactly the reason he decided to do so — namely, there is no reason for living or dying.

The protagonist has written the book to explain why he changed his mind and in the process we discover quite a bit about him. Most people would describe him as a cynic, but there is more to him than that. Andrews makes his living by practicing law in a small backwater town in the Chesapeake tidewater country. He became a lawyer because that is what his father wanted, but he is later stunned by his father's suicide. What bothered him was not that his father killed himself, but that he did so because he could not pay his debts due to the Depression.

Andrews has chosen to live free from any long-term commitments since the day in WWI when he killed a German sergeant with whom he had shared a foxhole through a terrible night of shelling. His lack of commitment extends even to his arrangement for living — he lives in a hotel room where he registers on a day to day basis. He has, however, been involved in a long-term affair with Jane Mack, his best friend's wife. Harrison Mack not only approved but actually arranged this as a further extension of their friendship. However by mutual agreement they have recently decided to end this form of their relation.[19] This is partly the result of the recent birth of Jeannie, who, even though her paternity remains unclear, has given the Macks a new sense of themselves as a couple.

Andrews also suffers from two diseases — subacute bacteriological endocarditis and chronic infection of the prostate. He was told thirty-five years ago that the former could kill him any time. The latter disease only caused him to cease living a wastrel's existence he had assumed during law school and begin what he claims is almost a saintly life. And indeed his life is in many ways

16. Margolis, *Negativities*, p. 29.

17. Ibid., p. 24.

18. J. Barth, *The Floating Opera* (New York: Avon, 1956). For a similar approach from which I have learned much see H. Nielsen, "Margolis on Rational Suicide: An Argument for Case Studies in Ethics," *Ethics* 89, no. 4 (1979): 394-400. The fact that we must resort to example when considering such matters is an important indication how easily abstract discussions of the rightness or wrongness of suicide, for which there is no substitute and must certainly be done, can as easily mislead as they can help us clarify why the suicide is rightly understood in a negative manner. Seldom are any of us sure why it is we act and do not act as we do. We may say we would rather die than live with such and such disease, but how can we be so sure that is the reason? Beauchamp and Childress' suggestion that ideally a person contemplating suicide would consider all the variables is as much a formula for self-deception as one for self-knowledge. I suspect that is why Barth's book is so helpful — namely it is only by telling a story that we come to understand how the prohibition against suicide is meant to shape the self.

19. Andrews admits that this turn of affairs made him reconsider briefly his decision to commit suicide since the Macks might interpret his suicide as caused by their decision. But he says that this lasted only a moment since it occurred to him "What difference did it make to me how they interpreted my death? Nothing, absolutely, makes any difference. Nothing is ultimately important. And that, at least partly by my own choosing, that last act would be robbed of its real significance, would be interpreted in every way but the way I intended. This fact once realized, it seemed likely to me that here was a new significance, if possible even more genuine," Barth, *The Floating Opera*, p. 224.

exemplary, for he is a man who lives his life in accordance with those convictions he thinks most nearly true.

Even though he is not a professional philosopher, Andrews is a person with a definite philosophical bent. For years he had been working on notes, suitably filed in three peach baskets, for the writing of a Humean type *Inquiry* on the nature of causation. For if Hume was right that causes can only be inferred, then his task is to shorten as much as possible the leap between what we see and what we cannot see. That is, to get at the true reasons for our actions.[20]

This becomes particularly relevant if we are to understand Andrews' decision to commit suicide. He fully admits that there are abundant psychological reasons, for those inclined for such explanations, to explain his suicide — a motherless boyhood, his murder of the German sergeant, his father's hanging himself, his isolated adulthood, his ailing heart, his growing sexual impotency, injured vanity, frustrated ambition, boredom — the kinds of things psychoanalysts identify as "real" causes.[21] But for him the only reasons that interest him in dying are philosophical. These he states in five propositions which constitute his completed *Inquiry*. They simply are:

I. Nothing has intrinsic value. Things assume value only in terms of certain ends.
II. The reasons for which people attribute value to things are always ultimately arbitrary. That is, the ends in terms of which things assume value are themselves ultimately irrational.
III. There is, therefore, no ultimate "reason" for valuing anything.
IV. Living is action in some form. There is no reason for action in any form.
V. There is, then, no "reason" for living.[22]

And so Todd Andrews decided to kill himself one day in 1937.

However before doing so he decided to go see *The Original and Unparalleled Floating Opera*, a local minstrel show on a rundown showboat. The absurdity of the show matches perfectly Andrews' view of the absurdity of life. During the performance, Andrews goes to the ship's galley, turns on the gas only to be interrupted and saved by a workman who angrily calls him a damn fool — not because he tried to take his life, but because he could have blown up the ship.

More importantly, however, just as he is recovering, the Macks, who had also been attending the opera, rush into the galley with Jeannie who had suddenly taken sick and fainted. Though appealed to for help, Andrews suggests he is no good at such things and advises the Macks to rush to the hospital. However, the local doctor arrives and advises an alcohol rub, reassuring everyone nothing is seriously wrong. In the emergency, however, and the concern Andrews felt about Jeannie, he discovers he no longer wants to commit suicide even though he could still easily jump into the Choptank river. For as he tells us, "something was different. Some qualitative change had occurred, instantly, down in the dining room. The fact is I had no reason to be concerned over little Jeannie, and yet my concern for that child was so intense, and had been so immediately forthcoming, that (I understood now) the first desperate sound of Jane's voice had snapped me out of a paralysis which there was no reason to terminate. No reason at all. Moreover, had I not, in abjuring my responsibility for Jeannie, for the first time in my life assumed it — for her, for her parents, and for myself? I was confused, and I refused to die that way. Things needed explaining; abstractions needed to be straightened out. To die now was simply out of the question, though I hated to spoil such a perfect day."[23]

Andrews suspects most philosophizing to be rationalization, but nonetheless his experience requires him to return to the propositions of his *Inquiry* to make a small revision of the fifth: V. There is then, no "reason" for living (or for suicide).[24] For now he tells us that he realized that even if values are only relative there are still relative values. "To realize that nothing has absolute value is surely overwhelming, but if one goes no further from that proposition than to become a saint, a cynic, or a suicide on principle, one hasn't gone far enough. If nothing makes any final difference, that fact makes no final difference either, and there is no more reason to commit suicide, say, than not to, in the last analysis. Hamlet's question is, absolutely, meaningless. A narrow escape."[25]

The Christian prohibition of suicide is clearly based in our assumption that our lives are not ours to do with as we please. But that prohibition is but a reminder of the kind of commitments that make suicide, which appears from certain perspectives and at particular times in our lives so rational, so wrong. It reminds us how important our commitment is to be the kind of people who can care about a sick little girl and in the process learn to care for ourselves. That kind of lesson may not give life meaning, but it is certainly sufficient to help us muddle through with enough joy to sustain the important business of living.

20. The full title is actually *An Inquiry into the Circumstances Surrounding the Self-Destruction of Thomas F. Andrews, of Cambridge, Maryland, on Ground-Hog Day, 1930 (More Especially into the Causes Therefor)*. Andrews tells us his aim is simply to learn why his father hanged himself. Andrews admits the real problem was one of "imperfect communication" between him and his father as he could find no adequate reason for his father's act. His *Inquiry*, however, became primarily a study of himself since he realized to understand imperfect communication requires perfect knowledge of each party. Andrews suggests at the end of the book if we have not understood his change of mind he is again cursed with imperfect communication — but the suggestion seems to be we have a better chance at communication than he had with his father as now at least we have Todd Andrews' story.

21. Barth, *The Floating Opera*, p. 224.

22. Ibid., pp. 238-43.

23. Ibid., p. 266.

24. Ibid., p. 270.

25. Ibid.

147 "Whose Life Is It, Anyway?" Ours, That's Whose!

Gloria Maxson

In this national year of the disabled, I take strong exception to the film *Whose Life Is It, Anyway?* for its underlying false premise; that the life of a disabled person could not be worth living, and should thus be "mercifully" terminated by suicide or euthanasia. As a chairbound victim of polio and arthritis, I strongly protest that the life I and my many disabled friends lead has genuine value in the sight of God — and humanity.

In the film, Richard Dreyfuss plays Ken, a young sculptor who has become a "quad" (quadriplegic — a person who is paralyzed in all four extremities) in a car accident, and decides in the initial period of trauma — never an auspicious time to make major decisions — that suicide is the only "rational" choice for a man severely disabled. In its one-sided argument in favor of Ken's death, the film denies the value of the lives we disabled persons live.

Whose Life Is It, Anyway? stacks the deck in favor of its position by failing to present the options available to a quadriplegic. It is shockingly untypical that Ken is kept for six months in intensive care before any rehabilitation is begun; actually, most quads have *completed* their rehabilitative training by that time. Glib doctors and social workers tell Ken he will "feel better" when his therapy starts — but it never does; nor is Ken ever taught to use such adaptive devices as reading machines and special typewriters. He is never introduced even to an electric wheelchair but is wheeled passively about, which deepens the sense of immobility and total dependency that makes him long for death.

What a difference an electric chair (covered by Medicare) has made in my own life! Gone is that awful sense of being preyed upon, the "sitting duck" syndrome that kept me weeping on the porch in driving rain, terrified to enter the house where I imagined that Something huge, mindless, nameless and malign awaited me. Now my husband says *I* am the Something mindless and malign as I careen at full tilt down our block, terrorizing the "fluffy old pussies" (Agatha Christie's phrase for little old ladies). I could have told the Ken character that if we can't have wings-at-our-heels, we can at least have wheels-at-our-hips. But no one tells him that or anything else that could alter his death wish.

Another inadequately treated aspect of Ken's trauma is his bitter sense of lost virility and conviction that he is "not a man anymore." Again, those around him fail to give him the insights provided by any good SCI (spinal cord injury) specialist, namely, that 70 per cent of quads can have normal genital intercourse, and that there are many other satisfying ways of making love, as the disabled veteran in *Coming Home* — a much more honest film — showed. No one examines Ken's sexuality to determine what sensory avenues are still open to him. Through those parts that confirm the popular assumptions about quadriplegics' sexuality, the man I saw the film with — himself a quad — kept muttering such things as: "There's more sex between the ears than between the extremities! As much warmth *north* of the Masters-Johnson line [the waistline] as *south* of it!"

We were both unnerved by Ken's insistence that death is "the only way out" since he is "dead already." The poet Robert Frost, and any of us "black-eyed ones" (Thomas Mann's phrase; the healthy-and-wealthy are "the blue-eyed ones"), could have told Ken that "the only way out is through," and to "learn what to make of a diminished thing." In the real world, any good doctor would have introduced Ken to SCI patients whose successful coping would have helped him navigate his dark passage back to life. But in the film no one helps him through the initial stages of grief and despair to self-acceptance. It is never explained to Ken that even a quadriplegic on dialysis, like himself, need not be hospitalized for life; with modern techniques and attendants, a person can live at home with the family and friends who can help him or her learn a new way of life based on "viable alternatives." All these tragic omissions strengthen Ken's case for taking his life — a case carefully manipulated by the film.

Although sculpting was Ken's life, he is not shown the many other ways his thwarted creativity could be expressed; only teaching is suggested, and he angrily rejects it. I, too, felt the awful anguish of losing my artistry with piano and guitar when my hands became crippled with arthritis. I could not have foreseen then, in the midst of my moist jeremiads, that one day I'd have an electric keyboard on which I could play melody with the two remaining, dancing fingers on my right hand, and automatic chords and rhythms with a dancing thumb on the left. Now, as I dash off "Für Elise," "Minuet in G" and "Turkish March," Beethoven no longer turns over in his grave, but sits bolt upright and bellows, "Ach Du Lieber, Meine Gloria — das ist gut!" I could not see that dark night of the soul, when all problems became "soul-sized," that I would be able to transfer my guitar skills to a large ukulele, and bawl out the same old ballads and naughty calypsos I did before. Furthermore, when I could no longer type at 90 wpm, or even handwrite, I didn't know I'd soon type with two fingers and find an orthopedic gripper that would enable me to write again, in so neat a hand my husband says it is "one of the graphic arts," and calls me "the Picasso of the ballpoint pen!"

As my friend and I viewed the film, we grew nervous on hearing the audience murmur assent to all the nihilisms about the disabled life, and remembered all the times people had said to us, "If I were you, I'd kill myself." It's just a small step from that to, "And why *don't* you?" In the audience, we sense a latent antagonism to our vulgar tenacity in preserving our lives, our precious "space" on this crowded planet — a space which may be hotly contested in the future, with elderly and ill-derly classed as expendables. Many films and plays still perpetuate the false notion that a disabled life is not worth living — a misperception that is still killing people, through suicide and misguided "mercy killings."

The film *Whose Life?* traffics in the current political mood that is dangerously cutting back vital aid to the severely disabled. At one point in the film, a character grumbles that "we are spending thousands on people like Ken, with little return, when with a few cents we could save Third World children!" How dare people force us to choose between our lives and those of Third World children! True, much money *is* wasted keeping Ken alive and hospitalized; for much less he could have been cared for at home, safely and with better results.

This film reflects the negative views about disability that are gaining wide acceptance in the many "wrongful life" suits against doctors for allowing babies born with defects to live. More hospitals now routinely offer parents of disabled babies the option of "mercy killing," even if the baby's defect is only deafness. A TV film told the story of a man who shot his quadriplegic brother on request, again reinforcing the misconception that a disabled life is worthless. *Whose Life?* purports to be an honest drama about an important social and ethical dilemma of our time, but in its shrinking from the moral obligation of treating the issue factually, the film is irresponsible. It was puzzling to hear such film critics as Gene Shalit of the "Today" show praise it as "life-affirming" — an enigmatic phrase, indeed, to use about a film that advocates suicide. To us of the black-eyed community, Mr. Shalit, "life-affirming" means body-retraining and body-retaining. Anything less is mere wordplay and sophistry.

As the film ended, my friend and I joined the crowd in the lobby to munch popcorn and chat, and received so many glances — some openly hostile — that we felt we might have to stand (sit) our ground or we'd be rushed and strung up between features! No matter what the public feels, *I* will never willingly relinquish a life that contains my husband, family, friends, a home, lobster thermidor, music and P. G. Wodehouse! Even in my handicapped childhood, I would have chosen to live. I read somewhere that all of nature's young things are valiant — they do not whine or bargain, but despite their wounds fight fiercely to live, and revel in being — and I know it is true. Perhaps I've "just compensated," as an atheistic college friend used to tell me. My reply is, "Yes, I have compensated — Christ is my compensation." For just as in my blinded early childhood I developed the "facial perception" that set every hair vibrating when someone is near, so now my nerve ends vibrate with the sense of that Presence who stands near but outside my harsh circumstances, and molds them into coherence and beauty.

Whose life is it, Ken? It's all of ours — and it should have been yours.

CHAPTER TWENTY-THREE

Accepting Death

The poet Robert Fraser's "A Modern Psalm" reminds us that medical technology has become a powerful idol. The psalm begins:

> Medical science is my shepherd; I shall not want,
> It maketh me to lie down in hospital beds;
> It leadeth me beside the marvels of technology.

The poet also reminds us of the consequences of our idolatry:

> Surely coma and unconsciousness shall follow me
> all the days of my continued breathing;
> And I will dwell in the intensive care unit forever.

Medical technology sometimes does great things for those who are ill and would die without its use. But this technology is also one way we avoid facing our mortality. The often over-zealous promises made on behalf of stem cell research, the surprising number of very old who opt for heart surgery, and the success of medical dramas on television that constantly depict people being rescued from the brink of death are just three examples of our salvific trust in medical technology. Our culture has an idolatrous trust in the power of technology in general, and of medical technology's ability to save us from our own mortality in particular.

The notion that we can master suffering and death through technology is part of the cultural context for thinking about death and dying. Another aspect of that context is the debate about assisted suicide and euthanasia, which is dealt with extensively in the previous chapter. When medical technology no longer appears able to save us from suffering and death — or worse, when that same technology appears to perpetuate our suffering and trap us in dying — we are tempted to master death by dictating the time and manner of its coming. Indeed, as of this writing, Oregon and Washington State have voter-initiated, legalized physician assisted suicide.

Still another part of the cultural context for discussing death and dying is our enthusiasm for autonomy. North Americans, especially those in the U.S., talk about their commitment to autonomy with various terms — e.g., right to privacy, self-reliance, self-expression, personal liberty, noninterference, informed consent, and so on. As Willard Gaylin and Bruce Jennings observe, the concept of autonomy is ubiquitous in our culture, where "a particularly individualistic interpretation is placed on nearly every social and moral value in American life today."[1]

This commitment to autonomy is nowhere more evident than in contemporary health care. Informed consent and end-of-life documents, such as living wills, are rooted in a commitment to autonomy. Final decision making about all medical treatment is seen to rest with the individual patient, even extending one's own autonomy via end-of-life documents into a future time when one is no longer able or competent to exercise that freedom. At the end of life, we reject but also often demand treatment in the name of personal freedom. And an individual's right to choose is the foundation for many arguments in favor of assisted suicide. Autonomy is far from the only value operative in health care, but it is always a dominant, and sometimes *the* dominant, value at work.

The essays in this section can be read as challenging our cultural context surrounding death and dying: refusing to think we can master death either through technology or through assisted suicide, and qualifying autonomy as the overriding value in end-of-life decision making. For example, Vigen Guroian's "The Case of Baby Rena" (selection 148) steadfastly refuses to entertain euthanasia or assisted suicide as licit Christian options. But neither does Guroian express undue confidence in medical technology. Instead, he insists on a common Christian distinction between killing (euthanasia, assisted suicide) and allowing to die.

Guroian challenges the logic operative in the foster parents' argument that Rena be maintained on a respirator so that they could discover God's will. Rena was obviously dying and was in constant pain. Guroian argues that "God does not need respirators to work miracles," and that only a devaluation of the physical world and God's presence within it could miss that God's will was that Baby

1. Willard Gaylin and Bruce Jennings, *The Perversion of Autonomy: Coercion and Constraints in a Liberal Society*, rev. ed. (Washington, D.C.: Georgetown University Press, 2003), p. 47.

Rena be allowed to die. In such circumstances, says Guroian, the Christian obligation is to remain present and offer care but not oppose death. Because we know that God does not abandon us even in death, we can remain present to each other without the illusion that we can master death, either through our technology or through killing.

James F. Bresnahan's "Catholic Spirituality and Medical Interventions in Dying" (selection 149) also assumes a distinction between killing and allowing to die, between aiming at death and accepting its coming. Moreover, Bresnahan challenges common understandings of autonomy. Instead of freedom through control, Bresnahan invites us to also recognize the Christian freedom of self-surrender to God, including the graced freedom to accept limitations, contradictions, and disappointments, and the freedom to hand ourselves over to God in our dying, just as in our living. For Bresnahan, this freedom means that we have a right, even a duty, to reject medical treatment that is excessively burdensome to oneself, one's loved ones, or one's community. In this context, end-of-life documents can be more than tools of a simple assertion of autonomy into the future. Instead, they can be designed as testimonies of our surrender back to God and as mechanisms for expressing love and concern for those left behind in our dying.

In "The Catholic Tradition on Forgoing Life Support" (selection 150), Kevin D. O'Rourke discusses the Catholic distinction between ordinary and extraordinary means in prolonging life, which is a helpful companion to Bresnahan. O'Rourke points us to the ultimate human good of friendship with God and the difference between killing oneself and not prolonging life. Particularly helpful is O'Rourke's clarification that factors such as the length of therapy or the cost to patient or family or community can move a medical procedure from being ordinary (morally required) to extraordinary (not morally required). Thus, the burdensomeness mentioned by Bresnahan is determined by context and is a key factor in discerning whether a given medical procedure is considered morally obligatory. Moreover, the discernment process focuses on more than the individual patient; it includes the impact of the procedure on family and community.

In "Having Enough Faith Not to Be Healed" (selection 151), John Brunt affirms palliative care as being well suited to several Christian convictions. First, death is a defeated enemy. For biblical faith, death is an enemy, not a friend, not comparable to the beauty of a shooting star. But it is a defeated enemy; Jesus Christ is the first fruits of the resurrection. Palliative care is compatible with this notion of death: neither romanticizing death nor acceding to the easier way out of assisted suicide. Second, biblical faith has an "even if" quality to it: we trust in God even when God does not fulfill our agenda or things go terribly wrong. Such faith trusts that God is at work for good in all situations, even those that are contrary to God's ultimate will. Consistent with this "even if" quality, palliative care seeks to provide care and opens space to find meaning even though death is imminent. Third, biblical faith is communal; it has a distinct "with each other" quality. Palliative care embraces elements of care beyond the physical, including a focus on relationships.

Like the other essays here, Brunt's account of the compatibility between Christian convictions and palliative care runs counter to certain elements of our cultural context. Trusting God for salvation, this account does not try to master death through technology or assisted suicide. And our society's focus on autonomy is qualified by convictions about the centrality of relationships and community to healing, even in death.

Our culture's enthusiasm for autonomy is qualified by several other essays here as well. For example, the narratives by David Schiedermayer, "House Calls on Cardinal Jackson" (selection 152), and Margaret E. Mohrmann, "God Will Find a Way" (selection 153), illustrate instances where medical treatment is continued in substantial part out of care and loyalty to the patient's family members. We fool ourselves if we think that health care is only about the patient. Schiedermayer and Mohrmann both recognize that it is sometimes appropriate to "let die," to stop resisting death. But the stories also show us that a physician's history with the patient and loyalty to the patient's family rightly influence medical decision making, sometimes even justifying continued treatment when others would view it as futile care. The stories are also important because they remind us that much of our best moral thinking requires narrative display. These stories cannot be reduced to discursive, linear arguments; their force and intelligibility would be lost. Sometimes it is only in the telling of stories that we understand why a particular patient's history or various family relationships matter in decisions of health care.

Gilbert Meilaender's essay, "Who Decides?" (selection 154), also challenges our extensive confidence in freedom and autonomy, in part by challenging the appropriateness of living wills for Christians. Meilaender suggests that living wills can be manifestations of an idolatrous desire for autonomy and self-deceptive efforts at mastery and self-control even in death. Instead, "we are to prefer the health care power of attorney to the living will. It too . . . reaches out into a future beyond the limits of our competence, but it does so in a way that recognizes and affirms dependence. It anticipates and accepts that others will have to bear some burden for us as we may for them." In contrast to a society that prioritizes freedom and independence, Meilaender affirms interconnectedness, dependency, and burden sharing.

Interconnectedness and burden sharing in end-of-life decision making are themes running throughout Curtis Freeman's "What Shall We Do with Norman? An Experiment in Communal Discernment" (selection 155). Freeman's essay revolves around an actual case of communal discernment about allowing a terminally ill member of their church to die. We are, says Freeman, embodied, social selves invited by God to lives of stewardship and service. This understanding is in sharp contrast to notions of substituted judgment, best interest, and many end-of-life documents that enshrine individualism and fail to take seriously a communal discernment that attempts to determine what one *should* will rather than what one *would* will.

In Freeman's story, there is no deep confidence in technology's ability to save. Instead, our lives are viewed as gifts from a gracious Creator. Out of this understanding, the community does not seek either to cling to the gift of Norman's life or to expedite its passage. The central question for them was how they as a community should help Norman to live with integrity and fidelity to his baptism and commitment to Christ while he was dying. Their answer, in part, is that a good death requires participation "in communities of virtue that can remember life and construe death (even the dying of noncompetents) with meaning and purpose." Freeman is here especially keen to highlight the importance of participation in communities that embody Christian hope and patience if we are to frame our dying in a thoroughly Christian way. Thus, the quality of the community in which one participates during life has direct consequences for the quality and fidelity to Christ of one's death.

The essays in this section challenge our cultural context for thinking about death and dying, including end-of-life decision making. M. Therese Lysaught's "Love Your Enemies: Toward a Christoform Bioethic" (selection 156) pushes the explicitly Christian framing of end-of-life decision making even further. Lysaught reads three stories in tandem: the Terri Schiavo case, Holy Week, and the autobiography of Joseph Cardinal Bernardin. Each story is, in its own way, an end-of-life case. Lysaught highlights the family and cultural conflict evident in the Schiavo case. This case lays bare what William F. May already noticed about the practices of medicine and bioethics: the dominant metaphors are those of conflict and war, with suffering and death as the enemy and technological medicine as the savior. The conflict that ran throughout the Schiavo case was actually augmented by the practice of bioethics. By contrast, the stories of Holy Week and Cardinal Bernardin remind us that salvation comes through Christ from the triune God, and that Christians ought to be committed to the often costly practices of forgiveness and reconciliation. Lysaught therefore suggests that a "Christoform bioethic" would focus not only on the principle of autonomy but also, more importantly, on love of enemy, forgiveness, and reconciliation. Acquiring this focus is not a simple matter; it requires the appropriate community, rituals, institutional embodiment, and lifelong practices, such as daily prayer. As with Freeman, Lysaught's piece pushes toward a lifelong, communal framing of end-of-life decision making. But Lysaught goes further in inviting us to consider the revolutionary implications of a bioethics that takes Christian convictions about love of enemy and reconciliation seriously.

Both implicitly and explicitly, the essays in this section challenge aspects of the cultural context for thinking about death and dying. Each exhibits a chastened view of technology's ability to save. Several explicitly adopt the classic Christian distinction between killing and letting die. Our culture's enthusiasm for freedom and autonomy is also challenged and qualified, sometimes by affirming the physician's role, sometimes by underlining the importance of family connections, and most often by attending in new ways to the Christian community's role in living and dying.

You are invited to consider whether these authors have gotten it right. For example, do some essays here under- or overvalue technology and the bodily life it sustains? Or do they have the balance essentially correct? And when is it appropriate to remove life-sustaining technology? Throughout these essays we have examples of both removing (Baby Rena and Norman) and maintaining (the stories by Schiedermayer and Mohrmann) such therapies. Do the essays here get it right about autonomy or do they too readily ignore the dangers of anyone other than the patient making end-of-life decisions? And do they get it right regarding end-of-life documents such as living wills? Can we reconcile Meilaender's and Freeman's critique of living wills with Bresnahan's affirmation of them? And what of palliative care and hospice? Are Brunt and Bresnahan right that such movements are particularly well-suited to Christian convictions? If so, should Christians be more known for their ready participation in these movements as both caregivers and patients? And finally, what is the role of specific Christian convictions in accepting death? Are certain convictions — for example, death as a defeated enemy, the "even if" quality of faith, the virtues of hope and patience, the call to love of enemy — so central to how Christians view the world that they should definitively mark how Christians respond to death?

While hardly espousing exactly the same positions, the authors in this chapter challenge the cultural context for thinking about death and challenge us to specifically consider how Christians should confront death. These are significant challenges indeed.

SUGGESTIONS FOR FURTHER READING

Cohen, Cynthia B., et al. "Using Our Medical Powers Appropriately." In *Faithful Living, Faithful Dying: Anglican Reflections on End of Life Care* (Harrisburg: Morehouse Publishing, 2000), pp. 39-60.

Geis, Sally B., and Donald E. Messer, eds. *How Shall We Die? Helping Christians Debate Assisted Suicide* (Nashville: Abingdon Press, 1997), pp. 13-74.

Guroian, Vigen. *Life's Living Toward Dying: A Theological and Medical-Ethical Study* (Grand Rapids: Eerdmans, 1996).

Hamel, Ronald, and Michael R. Panicola. "Must We Preserve Life?" *America* 190, no. 14 (2004): 6-13.

Hamel, Ronald P., and M. Therese Lysaught. "Choosing Palliative Care: Do Religious Beliefs Make a Difference?" *Journal of Palliative Care* 10, no. 3 (1994): 61-65.

Kelly, David F. *Medical Care at the End of Life: A Catholic Perspective* (Washington, D.C.: Georgetown University Press, 2006).

O'Rourke, Kevin D. "Reflections on the Papal Allocution Concerning Care for Persistent Vegetative State Patients." *Christian Bioethics* 12, no. 1 (2006): 83-97.

Panicola, Michael. "Catholic Teaching on Prolonging Life: Setting the Record Straight." *Hastings Center Report* 31, no. 6 (November-December 2001): 14-25.

Ryan, Rosemary. "Palliative Care and Terminal Illness." *The National Catholic Bioethics Quarterly* 1, no. 3 (Autumn 2001): 313-20.

Schiedermayer, David. "Commuting to the Valley of the Shadow of Death: What My Patients Have Taught Me about Death — and Life — by Permitting Me to Be with Them at the End." *Christianity Today* 37 (October 4, 1993): 33-34.

Sulmasy, Daniel P. "Terri Schiavo and the Roman Catholic Tradition of Forgoing Extraordinary Means of Care." *Journal of Law, Medicine, and Ethics* 33, no. 2 (Summer 2005): 359-62.

Vaux, Kenneth L., and Sara A. Vaux. *Dying Well* (Nashville: Abingdon Press, 1996).

148 The Case of Baby Rena

Vigen Guroian

The God whose love is steadfast and whose mercy is abundant would never sanction euthanasia. However humanitarian or well-meaning the motives of those who advocate or practice euthanasia might be, they cannot justify what they do. In a Christian evaluation of the rightness or wrongness of euthanasia, the euthanizers' *aim* (i.e., their specific intent to bring about the death of an individual) is more important than their *motivation* (i.e., their desire to put an end to suffering). Or, to put it another way, the fact that euthanizers mean well is less important than the fact that the result of their "good intentions" is a person's death. While Christians might acknowledge the good intentions of those who in the name of humanitarianism practice euthanasia, we are constrained to condemn the act as sinful and wrong. The aim of euthanasia is contrary to everything God intends for us and has done for us in a fallen and sinful world, which, apart from his presence and saving activity, is a cosmic cemetery.[1]

There is a difference between a God-centered humanism and a naturalistic humanitarianism, and Christians must explain and emphasize that difference as a witness to an increasingly secular and utilitarian culture. To shed light on some of the important issues involved here, I want to take an extended look at the perplexing real-life case of a fourteen-month-old infant who died a painful and tragic death at a Washington, D.C., hospital.

The story of how "Baby Rena" met her death was reported in a two-part, front-page feature in the *Washington Post* in July of 1991.

> Murray Pollack, a physician at [Washington's] Children's Hospital, felt the time had come to change the rules. His 18-month old patient, Baby Rena, was dying, a victim of AIDS and heart disease. For six weeks, ever since her arrival at the intensive-care unit in late January, she had been breathing only with the help of a respirator. She was in so much pain that Pollack kept her constantly sedated. When nurses performed even the simplest procedure, such as weighing her, her blood pressure shot up and tears streamed down her face. But

1. See Gilbert C. Meilaender, "Euthanasia and Christian Vision" [Thought 57 (December 1982): 465-75; reprinted in *On Moral Medicine*, 2nd ed., ed. Stephen E. Lammers and Allen Verhey (Grand Rapids: Eerdmans, 1998), pp. 655-62].

From Vigen Guroian, *Life's Living Toward Dying* (Grand Rapids: Eerdmans, 1996), pp. 66-80.

a tube in her throat made it impossible for her to utter a sound.[2]

Pollack had been called in to take the case after Baby Rena was brought to Children's Hospital on January 30. She died at the hospital on March 25. From the outset, Pollack judged that her case was probably "futile." In his view, keeping her on the respirator was not so much a life-saving measure as an intrusion into her dying process that intensified and prolonged her suffering. Pollack argued that he and the medical staff had "a responsibility to do what's best for Rena . . . and to give her the appropriate care — and that is not always giving her all care."[3] Pollack was not advocating mercy killing. Rather, he wanted those responsible for her care to "let go" — to let Rena die the death she was dying as well as possible — and in his judgment that called for removing her from intensive care and the respirator and providing medication to relieve her severe pain. Death would likely come sooner rather than later.

Children's Hospital requires the consent of parents or legal guardians to remove a minor from a respirator. Rena's mother had abandoned her at birth, making her a ward of the District government. She had been assigned foster parents, and while they had no legal standing in the decision, they strongly objected to Pollack's recommendations. They believed that God had told them "to take the child, and rear her in the nurture and admonition of God's word . . . and to battle the spirits of infirmity."[4] They demanded that her treatment "be motivated by a spiritual sense of obedience to God."[5] When the hospital sought the government's permission to take Rena off the respirator, the request was denied.

Baby Rena's foster parents, the pastor of their church, and their friends all played a significant role in determining the way in which she died. They all professed a Christian belief in the sanctity of life, and yet I cannot find a basis in my understanding of the Christian tradition to agree with either their reasoning or their judgment. Resources within the Christian faith lead me to believe that there are good reasons for drawing a distinction in health-care settings between directly killing people and allowing them to die. The former is euthanasia and is morally wrong; under certain circumstances, the latter is not. In fact, acquiescence in the face of an impending death may sometimes be required by Christian conscience. There are circumstances in which Christians are permitted — even duty bound — to let life ebb away in its natural course, so long as that course of action remains in accord with a corresponding duty to provide care that relieves pain and comforts the dying person.

Too often today, conscientious religious and nonreligious people alike lack the moral means to distinguish and accept such possibilities. This issue, like so many other moral controversies, tends to get framed in either/or terms: either one believes that everything possible must be done to save life or one supports euthanasia. The Baby Rena case illustrates how people get caught up in this sort of moral cul-de-sac. Religious and nonreligious antagonists tend to view one another's arguments as proof positive that they are far apart in worldview, but in fact they often stand on common ground: both their positions are rooted in secularity.

In defending a distinction between direct killing (euthanasia) and allowing to die, Paul Ramsey once observed that people in our society who hold opposite positions on euthanasia often end up defining it in the same way. Religious conviction does not seem to be a determining factor.

> The case for either of these points of view [favoring euthanasia or favoring efforts to save life at all costs] can be made only by discounting and rejecting the arguments for saving life qualifiedly but not always. In both cases, an ethics of only caring for the dying is reduced to the moral equivalent of euthanasia — in the one case, to oppose this ever, in the other case, to endorse it. Thus, the extremes meet, both medical scrupulosity and euthanasia, in rejecting the discriminating concepts of traditional medicine.[6]

Operating on the basis of a simple definition of God's sovereignty over life and an almost Manichaean identification of sickness and death with the demonic spirits, Baby Rena's foster parents were incapable of making a distinction between euthanasia and caring for Rena to the point of letting her die. Ramsey insisted that the traditional ethic (grounded in the belief that God is Creator, Lord of Life, and Redeemer) clearly holds that "letting life ebb away is *not* the same as actively encompassing a patient's life."[7] How is it that Baby Rena's foster parents, devoted religious people, failed to see and act on this important distinction? Why is it that they were held captive to the current popular meaning of euthanasia, to thinking in terms of the restrictive alternatives of either a utilitarian devaluation of life or an ethical vitalism that mystifies and absolutizes human life?

I think Alexander Schmemann had it basically right when he argued that the mark of secularism is the absence of God experienced in society and in people's lives. Vast numbers of people in our culture, religious and nonreligious alike, carry this mark of secularism in their understandings of God and the world, and this is nowhere more evident than in their attitudes toward death and dying.

Unconvinced of the existence of God or an afterlife, nonreligious secularists typically associate all value in life

2. Benjamin Weiser, "A Question of Letting Go," *Washington Post,* 14 July 1991, p. 1.

3. Benjamin Weiser, "While Child Suffered, Beliefs Clashed," *Washington Post,* 15 July 1991, p. 6.

4. Weiser, "A Question of Letting Go," p. 18.

5. Weiser, "While Child Suffered, Beliefs Clashed," p. 6.

6. Ramsey, *The Patient as Person* (New Haven: Yale University Press, 1970), p. 146.

7. Ramsey, *The Patient as Person,* p. 156.

with human agency — human projects to eliminate suffering, injustice, and the like. They refuse to explain the world "in terms of an 'other world' of which no one knows anything, and life . . . in terms of a 'survival' about which no one has the slightest idea." Rejecting religious orthodoxies that ground the value of life in terms of death and an afterlife, they explain "death in terms of life."[8]

These nonreligious secularists may differ among themselves, however, about the scale of value on which human life ought to be measured. Some hold personal existence as the only concrete value and adhere to an ethical vitalism that insists on using every means possible in all circumstances to ward off personal death. Others reason from a utilitarian framework that the value of a life is qualified by the degree of good or happiness, pleasure or fulfillment that might reasonably be expected in it. On the basis of this quality-of-life principle, they argue that some lives might not be worth living, and hence that we might properly choose to end them through physician-assisted suicide or euthanasia.

Of late, increasing numbers of individuals are claiming the right and the competence to make such decisions.[9] In this regard, Dr. Jack Kevorkian is hardly exceptional. The medical ethicist Daniel Callahan has astutely pointed out the hubris of such claims and how they can lead to an outright denial of the distinction between killing and letting die. The argument for euthanasia and the legalization of physician-assisted suicide is basically "about the centrality and validity of control," says Callahan. "By making a denial of the distinction between killing and allowing to die central to the argument, the euthanasia movement has embodied the assumption, the conceit actually, that man is now wholly in control of everything, responsible for all life and all death.[10]

On the face of it, religious people like Baby Rena's foster parents who make the "other" spiritual world the measure of all value seem to be the opposite of nonreligious secularists. They profess to assign all ultimate decisions about life and death to God rather than human beings. And yet, significantly, both camps ground their reasoning in the presupposition that the world is essentially meaningless because God is absent from it. The nonreligious secularists simply remove God from the equation on the basis of either atheistic or agnostic presumptions; people like Baby Rena's foster parents — who I believe can be fairly characterized as religious secularists — effectively act as though God is restricted to a spiritual realm and is wholly absent from this fallen and sin-ridden world. From the standpoint of the classical Christian understanding of life and death, both camps inappropriately devalue the world by presuming that God is absent from it. The nonreligious secularists look only to human endeavor for meaning and single-mindedly seek to alleviate human suffering by whatever means possible, including the facilitation of death. The religious secularists look only to the spiritual realm for meaning and single-mindedly seek to preserve human life at all costs, on the grounds that such life is a gift from God that ought to be sustained at all costs, no matter what amount of physical suffering might be involved in the process of dying.

I believe that Baby Rena's foster parents made their decisions about her welfare on the basis of this kind of secular religious worldview. Their own description of their beliefs suggests that their religion is rooted in a metaphysical and moral dualism that radically separates physical existence (this world) from spiritual existence (the other world). This body-and-spirit dualism moved otherwise loving adults to insist that a small child's extreme physical pain be prolonged.

But what does it mean to care for the spiritual well-being of a loved one who is dying if that care does not include seriously taking account of the physical pain she endures and the imminence of her death?[11] During one

8. Alexander Schmemann, *For the Life of the World: Sacraments and Orthodoxy* (Crestwood, N.Y.: St. Vladimir's Seminary Press, 1973), p. 98.

9. More than twenty years ago, Marya Mannes argued this way in *Last Rights* (New York: William Morrow, 1974). More recently, medical ethicist Margaret P. Battin has dismissed religious proscriptions of suicide and euthanasia and advocated a fundamental right of suicide (*Least Worst Death: Essays in Bioethics on the End of Life* [New York: Oxford University Press, 1994]).

10. Callahan, *What Kind of Life: The Limits of Medical Progress* (New York: Simon & Schuster, 1990), p. 242.

11. Kathleen M. Foley, a physician and professor at the Memorial Sloan-Kettering Cancer Center, has written extensively on the all-too-common failure to prescribe pain-reducing medicines and treatments to patients in advanced stages of cancer and other terminal illnesses. She argues that the growing interest in physician-assisted suicide might be more properly addressed if physicians and health-care providers were better educated in pain assessment and treatment and if patients and their families were better informed of their options. See, e.g., "The Relationship of Pain and Symptom Management to Patient Requests for Physician-Assisted Suicide," *Journal of Pain and Symptom Management* 5 (July 1991): 289-97.

Baby Rena's foster parents stood in the way of reducing her pain, but it is even more often the case that attending physicians allow their patients to suffer needlessly because they are not sufficiently well trained in assessing pain and supplying remedies. This judgment is supported by a recently published five-year study, the largest of its kind, which included the responses of over nine thousand patients in five teaching hospitals. The study was designed "to improve end-of-life decision making and reduce the frequency of a mechanically supported, painful, and prolonged death." The results were disappointing. "The phase I observation confirmed substantial shortcomings in care of seriously ill hospitalized adults. The phase II intervention failed to improve care or patient outcomes. Enhancing opportunities for more patient-physician communication, although advocated as the major method for improving outcomes," was found to be "inadequate to change established practices" ("A Controlled Trial to Improve Care for Seriously Ill Hospitalized Patients," *Journal of the American Medical Association* 274 [22/29 November 1995]: 1591). The report concluded, "We are left with a troubling situation. The picture we describe of the care of seriously ill or dying persons is not attractive. One would certainly prefer to envision that, when confronted with life-threatening illnesses, the patient and family would be included in

conversation between the hospital staff and the parents, the foster father sketched three pictures, representing Rena's body, soul, and spirit. "We see that she had AIDS," he said. "It's real, because you can see it under the microscope." He went on to thank the hospital staff for working hard to meet her medical needs — the needs of her body. But he complained that they were ignoring her spiritual side. Pointing to the third sketch, he said, "It seems to me that until the hospital really addresses the spiritual area we won't be able to defeat these various spirits of infirmity, including AIDS, that we're fighting against here." He explained his belief that the decisions about Rena needed "to be motivated by a spiritual sense of obedience to God. It's most important to find out what God desires or what God wills for Rena." At one point, a hospital social worker said, "What you're saying is that you don't want to give up on the spiritual part even though we're giving up on the physical part." The father nodded his head. He recalled an earlier occasion on which Rena had rallied after the hospital staff had given up hope. "If we give up now, we won't fully understand. . . . We won't fully know that God's word is true."[12]

The foster father spoke of the need to discover what God wants as if that wasn't already evident at the level of Baby Rena's fleshly suffering and dying. What more could the parents possibly have been waiting for to reveal God's will in the situation? As Ramsey so aptly put it, "No Biblical theologian should take umbrage at the suggestion that a pronouncement of death is a medical question." Indeed, I would broaden that to say that no Christian should take umbrage at the suggestion that judgments about when death is imminent or further medical treatment is futile are properly medical determinations. "What personal life do we know except within the ambiance of a bodily existence?"[13] God does not need respirators to work miracles, but God entrusts determinations of whether we are biologically dying to our physicians whether they themselves trust in him or not. One writer of a letter to the editors of the *Washington Post* questioned the foster parents' identification of the will of God with doing everything possible to keep Rena alive:

> I hope that people reading the article on Baby Rena do not get the impression that keeping her on the respirator was the only decision that people with faith in God could have made. . . .
>
> Having faith [sometimes] requires people to voluntarily give control over a situation to God. Although giving up control is the key to doing God's will, you still need to figure out what it is that God wants you to do — that's the hard part.[14]

Preserving the Moral Distinction Between Killing and "Letting Die"

In his remarkable little book *The Patient as Person* Paul Ramsey ruminates,

> It may be that only in an age of faith when men know that dying cannot pass beyond God's love and care will men have the courage to apply limits [to lifesaving interventions in] medical practice. It may be that only upon the basis of faith in God can there be a conscionable category of "ceasing to oppose death," making room for caring for the dying. It may also be that only an age of faith is productive of absolute limits upon the taking of the lives of terminal patients, because of the alignment of many a human will with God's care for them here and now, and not only in the there and then of his providence.[15]

Baby Rena's foster parents were far more fixed on the "there and then" of God's providence than on any sort of effort to discern the alignment of the many human wills involved in her care with God's care. As I have been suggesting, this fixation on the "there and then" and a corresponding devaluation of the "here and now" belongs to a spiritualism and otherworldliness that are the symptom and product of secularism itself, not its opposite, as those who hold such religious views typically think. This is one area in which there is no practical difference between a secularized Christianity and modern fundamentalism. Nonreligious secularism is characteristically expressed in a desacralization of human life and the experienced world; Judeo-Christian religious secularism is characteristically expressed in the breakdown of the symbolic and sacramental structures in and by which individuals and communities experience God as both transcendent over the world and wholly manifest within it. Baby Rena's foster parents made repeated appeals to God and his law, but they were unable to imagine that God's encompass-

discussions, realistic estimates of outcome would be valued, pain would be treated, and dying would not be prolonged. That is still a worthy vision" (p. 1597).

The *Washington Post* cited Joanne Lynn, the director of the Center to Improve Care of the Dying at George Washington University Medical Center, as saying that "she was dumbfounded by the finding that more than one-third of the patients [in the study] died in pain. 'We would never tolerate rates like this for postoperative infections.' " In fact, the study revealed that "more than half of the patients who died were reported by their families in moderate or severe pain during most of their final three days of life." This figure is even more staggering given that the subjects of the report were a controlled group of patients who were supposed to benefit from the initiatives implemented by the study. The report stated that the most disturbing finding was that the measures that were meant "to improve care failed to have any discernible impact" (Don Colburn, *Washington Post,* 22 November 1995, p. 10).

I believe that to some extent it is inevitable that this study would be disappointing. The crisis in the ethos of medicine and medical care runs so deep that it cannot be resolved by procedure alone.

12. Weiser, "While Child Suffered, Beliefs Clashed," p. 6.

13. Ramsey, *The Patient as Person,* p. 61.

14. "The Agonizing Decisions Surrounding Baby Rena" (letter from Monica Michelizzi), *Washington Post,* 22 July 1991, p. 10.

15. Ramsey, *The Patient as Person,* p. 156.

ing love might permit a practical ethical distinction in the "here and now" between direct killing and letting die. They could not imagine that a merciful God would sanction allowing Baby Rena to die. The Orthodox Christian tradition, on the other hand, views this sort of allowing to die as not merely permissible but actually desirable in some cases, as we noted in Chapter 3 in our consideration of the prayer for the hastening of the dying process.

The articles in the *Washington Post* did not say whether Dr. Pollack was a religious man, but when I compare his proposals for Baby Rena's medical care with those of her foster parents, I believe that his proposals were more in keeping with the classical Christian conviction that in the here and now God's care should be aligned with human reason and judgment in decisions about when life is ebbing and need not be heroically extended. In making this judgment, I am simply comparing Pollack's plea that Baby Rena be allowed to die with the foster parents' insistence that her life be prolonged at all costs; I am not unqualifiedly endorsing Pollack's ethical reasoning, because I can't know fully what that reasoning entailed. The newspaper reports suggest that Pollack based his ethical judgment on a medical determination of the futility of additional treatment and a concern for the quality of the patient's remaining life. But there is nothing in the newspaper's description of Pollack's reasoning to indicate that he never considered euthanasia a possible solution to Baby Rena's plight or that it would have violated his ethical standards to have proposed such a course of action. For Christians, the distinction between killing and letting die is key.

Daniel Callahan provides a definition that is helpful in our efforts to make this distinction:

> "Letting die" is only possible if there is some underlying disease that will serve as the cause of death. Put me on a respirator now, when I am in good health, and nothing whatever will happen if it is turned off. I cannot be "allowed to die" by having a respirator turned off if I have healthy lungs. It is wholly different, however, if a doctor gives me a muscle-relaxing injection that will paralyze my lungs. Healthy or not, those lungs will cease to function and I will die. That is what it means to "kill" someone as distinguished from "letting" someone die. Put more formally, there must be an underlying fatal pathology if allowing to die is even possible. Killing, by contrast, provides its own fatal pathology. Nothing but the action of the doctor giving the lethal injection is necessary to bring about death.[16]

It has been argued that one need not appeal to faith in God to secure this distinction within medical ethics. This is essentially Callahan's own position.[17] But on this point I side with Ramsey. In the relatively rarefied atmosphere of medical ethics, it may be possible to establish principles and rules that secure a distinction between killing and letting die without recourse to the resources of the Christian tradition. But, as Ramsey suggests, it is becoming increasingly difficult to maintain this distinction as the moral force of biblical theism diminishes in our culture. Biblically rooted theism provides us with the conviction that God, the absolute source and sustainer of our being and our Redeemer, does not abandon us in death. As St. Paul says, "Neither death, nor life, . . . nor anything else in all creation, will be able to separate us from the love of God" (Rom. 8:38-39). Biblical theism has a vision of a *summum bonum* that supports making calibrated judgments about the kind and extent of the care we owe to those who are in the last stages of dying. But this vision is not predominant in our culture. The distinction between killing and letting die is not anchored in anything; not even appeals to the principle of trust between patient and physician or the doctor's Hippocratic oath seem sufficient.

We can find evidence of this problem in one of John Updike's short stories entitled "Killing." As the story opens, a young woman named Anne is sitting with her dying father in a nursing home. A series of strokes has left him unconscious, unable to swallow or communicate. Anne has made the decision that he should be kept in the nursing home rather than moved to a hospital where he would be fed intravenously. The hospital treatment might be able to extend his life, but it would not be able to change the fact that his condition is hopeless. Wherever he will lie, death will be near at hand. The attending physician has assured Anne that she has acted wisely, but she remains plagued with guilt. She cannot shake the thought that by leaving her father in the nursing home she has in effect ordered his execution. As Updike puts it, she "realized that her decision had been to kill her father. He could not swallow. He could not drink. Abandoned he must die.[18]

Most medical ethicists agree that in certain terminal cases, when intravenous feeding might actually contribute to pain or discomfort and needlessly slow the inevitable dying process, a decision like the one Anne authorizes is morally permissible.[19] But no one seems to have communicated this to Anne. She seems to be ignorant of the medical-ethical distinction between killing and let-

16. Callahan, *The Troubled Dream of Life* (New York: Simon & Schuster, 1993), p. 77.

17. Callahan establishes this position in both *What Kind of Life* and *The Troubled Dream of Life.* See also chap. 2 of James F. Childress's *Priorities in Medical Ethics* (Philadelphia: Westminster Press, 1981).

18. Updike, "Killing," in *Trust Me* (New York: Fawcett Crest, 1987), p. 16. Updike describes the dying man as having parched lips and as exuding a putrid stench from his mouth. This is a realistic description of a patient who fails to receive the proper care in such a situation. To prevent dehydration and discomfort, caregivers must provide a regimen of oral hygiene and topical application of wetting agents or sipping fluids if the patient is conscious (see Joyce V. Zerwekh, "The Dehydration Question," *Nursing*, January 1983, pp. 47-51).

19. See Bonnie Steinbock, Joanne Lynn, James Childress, and Daniel Callahan, "Feeding the Dying Patient," *Hastings Center Report* 5 (October 1983): 13-22.

ting die. There is no indication that she has been told why withholding intravenous feeding might be appropriate in her father's case. In the end, however, it is not really likely that such information and counseling would suffice to allay Anne's anguish. Denied essential supportive relationships, she is lacerated by her conflicting love for and revulsion at her bedridden, dying father. Like so many of her contemporaries, she has been cast into a situation for which she is ill prepared. While her sentiments run deep, her moral resources are threadbare and poorly defined. And, as is the case with so many other women in our society (in which this burden more often than not falls on women), she is alone in the time of crisis. She has been abandoned by an estranged husband, and her siblings are too busy and too distant to bother to help. Nor does she have a religious community in which she might voice her feelings of guilt and find forgiveness.

In "Killing," Updike ruthlessly unmasks the desolation of modern life that we try to cover with technology, therapeutic strategies, and euphemism. More important, through the compelling character of Anne he shows us how family members who are forced to make decisions about dying loved ones are often pushed to the precipice of total despair and an exhausted embrace of the thanatos syndrome. In Anne's case, an "irrational" love for her father, a lingering legacy of guilt from a largely moribund Christian past, and the unavailability of legal physician-assisted suicide or euthanasia combine to lead her to an otherwise reasonable and probably right decision. But one has to wonder how soon her character will be superseded in our literature by a "compassionate" and "heroic" daughter who has no qualms about authorizing euthanasia for her dying father.

Conclusion

In light of the tragic story of Baby Rena, there is one practical point that I would like to stress: biblical faith does make it possible for us to make reasonable moral judgments about when our primary obligation to a patient is not to do everything possible to extend her life but rather to care for her as if she is dying. There can come a time when we should no longer seek to cure the patient but should instead turn our efforts to providing care for her in order that her death be the best possible death. Informed by a true biblical faith, we will seek to navigate a course between an absolutistic ethical vitalism on the one hand and a utilitarian ethic of "quality of life," triage, and euthanasia on the other. In the concluding chapter [of *Life's Living Toward Dying*] we will turn to an exploration of some of the finer points of a biblically informed ethic of caring for the dying.

149 Catholic Spirituality and Medical Interventions in Dying

James F. Bresnahan

Should Catholics in the United States prepare advance directives governing the kind of medical care they would want at the time of their dying? This question entails a fundamental but neglected issue of Catholic spirituality: How should Catholics and other Christians, and persons without formal religious affiliation too, prayerfully prepare for their dying within our contemporary high-technology medical culture? What attitudes and dispositions toward our inevitable dying should we seek to cultivate through prayer and reflection — given the power of modern technology to manage, delay and prolong that dying?

These questions require us to face the realities of our North American first-world culture, our way of resisting mortality and our frequently superstitious faith in technology. We must ask how we should respond to the prevailing preoccupation of many care-givers who emphasize aggressive use of cure-oriented medical treatment over the alternative medical treatment, comfort care, even when confronted with inevitable dying. How shall we respond, as well, to the proposals now being made legally to authorize assisted suicide or active euthanasia as a kind of technological "quick fix" for the kinds of suffering that accompany dying?

Finally, can we regard advance directives, the Living Will or Durable Agency for Health Care as practical measures to express these spiritual attitudes and dispositions toward dying that we have sought in prayer? Dare we regard legal provisions for specifying the kind of terminal care we want and do not want as "merely secular" and legalistic measures, perhaps even as irreligious temptations? Or can we make of such a document a personal spiritual testament?

Mandatory Information about Advance Directives

All of us will be increasingly unable to avoid these questions. As of Dec. 1, 1991, all health care institutions receiving Medicare or Medicaid funds will be required by Federal law (the Danforth provision of the Omnibus

Reprinted with permission of James F. Bresnahan and America Press, Inc., 106 West 56th Street, New York, NY 10019. Originally published in *America*'s June 29, 1991, issue.

Budget Reconciliation Act of 1990) to provide information on the law of the local jurisdiction enabling the patient to prepare advance directives for accepting or refusing medical care when the patient may have become incapable of personally authorizing or refusing a particular kind of care. This, in turn, will force all prudent physicians to discuss human dying and advance directives with their patients *before* they are admitted to a hospital or nursing facility — under penalty of finding their patients unduly alarmed or confused or even panicked by the information provided to them by the institution. The Federal law, therefore, forces us to deal with our North American disposition to avoid thinking about or discussing our dying and what it means for Christian believers to be cared for in a high-technology milieu.

The short answer to these questions about the religious meaning of human dying is familiar to all of us who are Catholics. We are to hold a crucifix. We are to pray to follow Christ in his dying. But this short answer does not reach far enough. We need to think through prayerfully all that this implies in the concrete for each one's dying under high-technology medical care. This was not necessary when medical treatment was comparatively impotent. It is necessary now.

Christian Dying as a Dying with and in Christ

We are called by the empowering grace of Christ to live our lives, each of us uniquely, in the likeness of Jesus' own life among us. As Jesus lived for others, so must we. But following the way of Jesus leads "up to Jerusalem." Finally, that is to say, we are called, each one, to die our deaths in the likeness of Jesus' own dying.

Hence we must wrestle with the religious meaning of dying. It is fundamental to our understanding of our baptism, in which we are plunged into the dying of the Lord and also into His risen life. And this same calling is equally fundamental to our regular celebration of the Eucharist, in which we relive over and over again our union with Christ's life, death and Resurrection.

The late German Jesuit theologian, Karl Rahner, in his *Theology of Death,* elaborates this spirituality of Christian dying as a manifestation of our fundamental faith. Just as we receive and respond to the gift of living a life of love in Christ's likeness, so too are we to be drawn eventually to receive and enter into the grace of sharing in the dying of Christ. Our dying, like our living, is a work of freedom under grace. In our final attitude toward death, then, we are called and empowered to replicate Jesus' own free, redeeming self-surrender to the Father. As St. Paul insists, we are to fill up in our own bodies the suffering of Christ for His body, the church. By freely accepting our dying, we come to participate personally and finally in the fullness of that redemption which Christ has prepared for us in His own passion and dying.

Spirituality of Dying and Catholic Medical Ethics

Our calling to make our dying a freely accepted fate, not just something forced upon us, is a major presupposition of current Catholic moral theology when it comes to making decisions about medical treatment in the face of death. Catholic ethicians such as Richard McCormick, S.J., John Paris, S.J., and Dennis Brodeur have eloquently expressed this moral theology in *America* (3/28/87). Less attention has been paid, however, to the roots of this moral theology in Catholic spirituality and dogmatics. Catholic moral theology rejects what Richard McCormick has called "medical vitalism," a clinging to biological existence at all costs, precisely because not only our living but also our dying is to be the object of our freedom. We are called to make decisions not only about preserving life and health but also about accepting our dying. We have to take a responsible moral stand about dying as well as living.

On the one hand, therefore, we reject the use of medical measures that are deliberately aimed at precipitating death, or that initiate a new lethal process to short-circuit a process of dying already underway from disease or injury. We rule out, therefore, the technological quick fix of lethal injection or deliberate overdose even though the subjective motivation of such acts may be to relieve suffering.

On the other hand, we affirm that measures needed to relieve suffering are always morally justified, and often morally demanded, even though death may occur sooner as a result of them — as long as we are not seeking to cause death but are trying prudently to measure the dose of analgesic to the needs of the suffering patient. And, though we reject deliberately planned, active euthanasia and assisted suicide, we strongly affirm that as death approaches we are allowed, sometimes even required, to refuse cure-oriented treatment that merely prolongs our dying.

The best Catholic moral theology thus requires us to strike a balance. We have a moral right and even in some circumstances the duty to reject "excessively burdensome" medical treatments even though death will follow from that decision. We may never simply reject our dying, and, finally, we must take responsibility for the way of our dying. The contemporary hospice movement (well described by William F. Carr in *America* 3/25/89) provides a practical expression of this moral theology of dying. This approach, of course, does not satisfy advocates of euthanasia and assisted suicide, for whom human autonomy is an absolute. At the other extreme, it is rejected as homicidal interference with God's providence by advocates of medical vitalism (who include a fringe of ultraconservative Catholics acting in the name of what they understand to be a "pro-life" ethic). Nonetheless, to many people in our society the well-known Catholic *via media* between precipitately causing death and hanging desperately onto mere biological existence appears to be utterly reasonable.

Within these moral boundaries, therefore, the Catholic moral theology of dying implies that each one of us is called to exercise responsible, discerning freedom in preparation for our dying. Each of us is to make a decision about the burdensomeness of proposed treatments and about the qualitative acceptability of the outcome of such treatments in our time of dying. Each of us must weigh burdens against benefits, not only for ourselves but for those we love and for our community. Graced freedom will be finally expressed by each one of us in our dying — Rahner's theological point. This implies that we will exercise spiritual discernment in preparing for and making this decision, a discernment that is rooted in prayerfully seeking to be ready to enter into Christ's dying when the time of death approaches for each of us.

Catholic Spirituality and Medical Ethics in Ecumenical Perspective

This Catholic rejection of excessively burdensome treatment even though death follows has been widely influential in shaping a consensus in contemporary discussions of medical ethics. The basic human wisdom of this approach is widely shared not only by other Christians, but also by those of other religious convictions and of no religious affiliation. The reasonableness of being able to refuse excessively burdensome treatment and to respond affirmatively and adequately to the needs of those who suffer while refusing to precipitate death deliberately appeals to the moral experience of many persons involved in medical care-giving. Along with Catholics they endorse a hospice approach to dying that promises spiritual and psychological support as well as pain control rather than torturously prolonging the dying process in the name of cure. And they do so because they find a reasonable approach to dying too often absent in our medical culture — too few care-givers who are well trained in the hospice technique, too few who believe that it is really "respectable" medical care.

What resonance, we may ask, does the Catholic spirituality of dying evoke in those who agree with our moral theology but do not share our specific Catholic convictions about dying with Christ? The answer will be found in our shared moral experience, in the practical wisdom contained in this spirituality. That is, those who are not Catholic or even Christian, and who do not share the explicitly Catholic spirituality of dying, but who agree with our moral practice, do so because they recognize that human mortality must be met by something other than blind protest.

What resonates is the Catholic realism about dying as a normal event of human living. The spirituality of people who are not Catholic involves a fundamental piety about the struggle of the human person to come to terms not only with living but also with dying. All of us who seek to discern and decide about the role of medical treatment at the time of dying confront dimensions of human experience common to all persons of good will. We confront the mystery of suffering, of anticipatory grief, of seeking even in this extremity to care well for those we love and will leave behind. Each of us dies in relationship to others, with concern for those whom we seek to make loving even unto the end. The "secular" piety that accepts these realities need not find a thoroughly Catholic spirituality of dying wholly strange.

Some, of course, are puzzled at the readiness of Catholic moral theology to permit, though not to inflict, death, to forgo "life-prolonging" treatments when one reasonably judges them to be excessively burdensome — even though death results. The puzzle is solved by understanding that freely submitting to death can mean dying in Christ. While life and health are to be cherished as gifts of God, a Christian's dying is also the final gift of God's calling us to be conformed to Christ. Our dying is thus seen and accepted as the final gift of redemption in Christ. While persons who are not Christian will not ordinarily see their dying in these precise terms, many do experience a basic human need to exercise their autonomy by coming to terms with the ultimate limit of mortality.

Dying with Christ and Freely Dealing with Mortality

Yet, for many, Karl Rahner's emphasis on graced freedom in entering into our dying with Christ presents a still deeper puzzle. How can we be "free" in this ultimate experience of limitation, of necessity, of unavoidable fate? Dying is what is inexorably imposed upon us by our mortal nature. We suffer death, and in faith we recognize that this reflects the mystery of human sinfulness that implicates us all — and Christ's redemptive transformation of the consequences of that sinfulness in his dying. But can we really claim to be free in what we do not, finally, control?

Christ suffered precisely this death of ours — He whom "the Father made sin though He was without sin." And Christ in his agony prayed to be delivered from the hour of His execution. Yet Jesus also states that He has come freely to "this hour." All four Gospel accounts of His passion and death underline Jesus' willing surrender of Himself in death into the hands of His Father "for us and for our salvation." So it must be possible for a follower of Jesus to join Christ's free self-surrender to dying.

In our culture generally, but especially in contemporary medical ethics, the exercise of human autonomy tends to be thought of almost exclusively as *control*. Patient autonomy is considered almost exclusively in terms of the patient's sharing control of diagnosis and treatment with the physician. Yet, in the patient/care-giver relationship there is always an element of free self-entrustment and submission to what is not and cannot be controlled. A patient's autonomy, therefore, contains an unavoidable dimension of submission, of willing self-surrender to the expert judgment and skill of the care-giver in the therapeutic alliance. Necessarily we exercise our freedom not only in controlling what is done to us but also *in submitting to it.*

In facing the advent of human dying, both patient and care-giver confront what cannot, in the end, be wholly controlled and manipulated. For all of us must die. The challenge is to live out the human meaning of this final event of life by an exercise of freedom that is not simply "in control." Pierre Teilhard de Chardin, the French Jesuit paleontologist and theologian, gives us insight into the spirituality that grasps this mystery of human freedom as not only active but also and necessarily passive.

Graced Freedom in Submission to Death

In his *Divine Milieu,* Teilhard's primary concern was to encourage Christians to see their free initiative in worldly activity as creative, as truly a "building of the earth" which has permanent significance in the fullness of human redemption. But he insists that such a positive spiritual vision of human effort would be incomplete without recognizing and accepting what he calls God's "divinization of our passivities." We are to recognize both passivities of growth and passivities of diminishment as fundamental dimensions of the finite human sharing in God's creativity.

For Teilhard, therefore, the more ready we are to embrace our worldly tasks as our share in God's work of bringing the Body of Christ to completion, the more we must be ready to exercise graced freedom in accepting limitations, contradictions and disappointments in our activity. This acceptance is no less a freedom than the achievement of freedom through control. The final, decisive passivity of diminishment by which we enter the fullness of union with Christ is death. Ultimately, as humans drawn into the cosmic mystery of the Incarnation, we must be prepared to exercise our freedom in our dying, though this will not involve control, but submission, acceptance, self-surrender.

This spiritual understanding of the freedom in dying proposed by Rahner and Teilhard resonates with the common human experiences of loss and grief. We are always being trained by the crucial events of life to ask forgiveness of those we love for our defects in serving them in love, and we are being led constantly throughout our lives to that moment when we shall make our last concern the continued living in love of those whom we must leave behind. Over and over again I have seen those dying in hospitals far more concerned for the good of those they love and are living than for their own entry into the fearful experience of death. And I have seen those who practice a hospice approach to dying enable this kind of autonomy in the dying.

Those who are experienced in the hospice way of medical care of the dying become aware of the work of love toward those left behind that is inherent in human dying. The "life review," for instance, by which the dying person comes to terms with the meaning of his or her life by telling some personal history testifies to the deep meaning of our final struggle to express ourselves even in what is imposed upon us in our dying. The dying permit themselves to be loved and cared for by dear ones and care-givers. (Sadly, Dr. Timothy Quill's patient, described recently in *The New England Journal of Medicine,* apparently refused to do this.) The faithfulness of care-givers to one who is dying anticipates each one's own hope to be faithful to those left behind at the moment of death.

Advance Directives and the Meaning of Dying

What, then, does this Christian spirituality of death lead us to do in planning for our dying in a high-technology medical culture? In an advance directive we have a means of expressing the prayerful discernment that our spirituality seeks.

Advance directives that express our desire to take free responsibility for our dying include the Living Will and the Durable Power of Attorney (or Agency) for Health Care. These are legal documents explicitly authorized by the laws of many states but also possibly effective under common law in many other states that have not yet legislated their legal status. These documents record a person's wishes about which cure-oriented medical treatments a person refuses to have initiated or continued under specified circumstances when terminally ill but possibly incompetent, that is, unable any longer to express one's wishes. They focus our thoughts and prayers on our dying as it is likely to be in this culture.

The Living Will expresses for all concerned one's wishes about terminal care — but primarily it is addressed to the physicians who attend one's dying. The Durable Power of Attorney gives similar instructions about what end-stage care one wants, but it also appoints a specified person to act on one's behalf with care-givers to carry out these wishes. Some of the language in the widely noticed 1990 Cruzan decision of the U.S. Supreme Court implies that we have a 14th Amendment right to consent to or refuse medical care right up to the time of our death even when we may have become permanently incompetent. It is widely agreed that the case would have been resolved even under the strict evidentiary requirements of Missouri had Nancy Cruzan executed either a Living Will or a Durable Power of Attorney and indicated that she would not want medically engineered nutrition and hydration to prolong her dying in a permanent vegetative state.

Since the tendency of modern high-technology medicine is to persist in so-called "life-sustaining" treatments rather than shift to care that primarily aims to relieve suffering and enable the terminal patient to interact freely with loved ones and friends, these advance directives are needed to limit those kinds of medical intervention that merely prolong dying. If I am conscious, of course, I can instruct my physician directly and personally. But should I become unconscious or even partially impaired in my ability to instruct my doctor about treatments to be foregone, I will want to have taken responsibility for the impact of my dying on those around me. And since modern medical interventions can extend my dying even in an impaired or unconscious state, advance directives are more and more needed today. Constant progress in medical techniques not only prolongs functional living but also has the effect of unduly prolonging dying. Indeed, in my experience, the success of contemporary medicine in giving us "more time" often, if not always, brings with it the burden of a more difficult and frequently more painful dying.

Planning for Dying: Control or Submission?

In this medical culture, we need to explore the spiritual meaning of advance directives as an unavoidable challenge to our prayerful reflection and prudent planning. As Catholics we need to ask ourselves how we can use these legally formulated directives to express our faith convictions and commitments. And in this post–Vatican II era, as ecumenically minded Catholics we need to ask how our understanding of the ultimate meaning of such measures may coincide or conflict with that of non-Catholics with whom we live and work and die.

To take up a theme in contemporary Christian ethical discussions, the link between moral theology and Christian spirituality is narrative, the *story* of Jesus of Nazareth and its impact on our personal and communal story. In an advance directive I can give an account of how I wish my living and my dying to take its shape from the living and dying of Jesus.

The impact of Christ's life on our own hinges on discerning what one ought to do and to be. My prayerful reflection on Christ's dying should, first of all, shape decision-making about my own dying. What burdens do I find excessive for me, beyond bounds, or only acceptable if God gives special inspiration for that? How do I wish to avoid rashness and presumption should I become unable to express myself to my care-givers? What burdens do I refuse to see imposed on those whom I love? These points can be added to the standard forms of the Living Will or Durable Power of Attorney. Suffering will be given each of us, and grace will be given to bear it, but we must each take account of the possibilities of being ourselves, or having those we care about, made subject to excessive suffering.

Second, when engaged in confronting our own mortality, our spirituality can and should shape as well our individual and communal response to others in their suffering and dying. We are called to stand faithfully by those who are dying, to relieve their suffering in all ways possible when the dying person does not forbid us to do so. The greatest fear of the dying is abandonment by loved ones or care-givers. It is true that each of us enters an utterly lonely moment in dying, a moment in which one will echo Christ's own cry, "My God, my God, why have you forsaken me?" Yet as Christians we know that the presence of Mary and John at the foot of the cross models the behavior toward the dying that we should adopt. And we have considered St. Joseph the special saint of the dying because of our well-founded assumption that Jesus and Mary stayed by him in his dying.

Catholic piety and behavior in preparation for dying and in support of the dying requires stronger emphasis in preaching than it has now. Pastors should be reflecting and praying with their congregations for the purpose of enabling them to write a Living Will or Durable Power as a personal spiritual testament. And in general, the challenge of making advance directives such as a treatment ought to lead every Catholic parish to participate actively in the hospice movement.

Faithful and appropriate care of the dying and prayerful acceptance of our own dying effectively counter the tendencies of our time to deal inappropriately with dying — both superstitious devotion to an excessively aggressive use of technology to prolong dying and that despairing resort to the technological quick fix of induced death.

150 The Catholic Tradition on Forgoing Life Support

Kevin D. O'Rourke

The phrase "ordinary and extraordinary means to prolong life" is familiar to many people inside and outside of the health-care profession. From an ethical perspective, there is general agreement that ordinary means must be used to prolong life when fatal or terminal illness threatens and extraordinary means may be forgone in the same circumstances. It sounds simple. Yet the application of these terms in clinical situations is never simple, either for people who will be making these ethical decisions or for health-care professionals, the doctors, nurses, and pastoral care advisors who will assist patients or their families in making these decisions. Theoretical, emotional, and ethical confusion often accompanies ethical decision making in these circumstances and beclouds the hearts and minds of decision makers.

This article seeks to dispel some of the reasons for confusion and difficulty in applying these terms. I shall begin with a short history concerning the development of these terms (I); then I will consider the difference between suicide, euthanasia, and allowing to die (II); the difference between comfort care and medical life support (III); the meanings of the terms *ordinary, extraordinary, proportionate,* and *disproportionate* (IV); the criteria for forgoing life support[1] (V); and when (VI) and by whom (VII) the decision to withhold or remove life support should be made. In the course of the article, I will present some variant connotations that often lead to conflicting interpretations and disparate conclusions in clinical situations.

I. Origin and Evolution of the Terms

Whether life must be pursued above all other goods and at all times was studied extensively by theologians for the first time at the University of Salamanca in Spain in the sixteenth century. Before this time, in difficult circumstances people of faith often made decisions to forgo the medical or surgical means that might prolong human life, but their decisions were more the result of necessity than of theological analysis. The sixteenth century was a time of extensive change. The New World had been discovered, and missionaries were sending back questions to the University concerning the rights of native peoples and their conquerors. Printing with moveable type had been perfected in the prior generation. On the European continent, nationalism was developing, and the Reformation and Counter-Reformation were taking place. Most significant for our purposes, medicine was starting to develop as a science. It was determined that life could be shortened or prolonged by reason of occupation, diet, medical procedures, and drugs.

A leader in the development of the theology of "death and dying" was Francisco de Vitoria, a Dominican theologian, called the Father of International Law,[2] who taught at the University of Salamanca. When commenting upon the writing of St. Thomas Aquinas, especially in regard to homicide and abstinence, he stated some theological principles that have endured to contemporary times.[3] For example:

- Human life is a great gift from God; a great good but not an absolute good, nor the ultimate good.
- Man is not the master of life, but should use all fitting means to prolong life. If the means to prolong life are not fitting or if they impose an excessive burden, they need not be utilized.
- The ultimate human good is friendship with God. All human acts should be ordered toward this ultimate end.
- God does not desire us to be interested in a long life; he wishes us to be interested in a good life.
- It is one thing to kill oneself; it is a different thing to not prolong life.

Other theologians at Salamanca followed and developed the thought of de Vitoria concerning the duties in regard to prolonging life.[4] It seems that Domingo Bañez, O.P., toward the end of the sixteenth century, coined the terms *ordinary* and *extraordinary means* to prolong life. In the ensuing centuries, the teaching of the Salamanca theologians was very important in developing moral

1. "Forgoing life support" implies withholding or removing life support. The phrase was popularized by the President's Commission for the Study of Ethical Problems in Medicine and Biomedical and Behavioral Research, *Deciding to Forego Life-Sustaining Treatment: Ethical, Medical, and Legal Issues in Treatment Decisions* (Washington, DC: United States Government Printing Office, 1983).

Originally published in the *National Catholic Bioethics Quarterly* 5.3 (Autumn 2005): 537-53.

2. Diarmaid MacCulloch, *The Reformation: A History* (New York: Viking Press, 2003), 67-68.

3. See Francisco de Vitoria, O.P., *On Homicide and Commentary on Summa theologiae IIa-IIae Q. 64 (Thomas Aquinas),* trans. John Doyle (Milwaukee, WI: Marquette University Press, 1997); Francisco de Vitoria, O.P., "Relectio de Temperantia," in *Obras: Relectiones Theologicas,* vol. 3, ed. Teofilo Ordanoz, O.P. (Madrid: Biblioteca de Autores Christianos, 1960).

4. Daniel Cronin, "The Moral Law in Regard to the Ordinary and Extraordinary Means of Conserving Life," in *Conserving Human Life,* ed. Russell E. Smith (Braintree, MA: Pope John XXIII Medical-Moral Research and Educational Center, 1989), 39.

teaching concerning the prolongation of life. The concepts mentioned above were applied to new methods in medicine and surgery, but the foundational principles were never challenged by later theologians.[5] The consensus of theologians through the centuries in regard to use and removal of life support led to the first authentic papal teaching in this regard, by Pope Pius XII in 1957.[6] This statement was followed by the *Declaration on Euthanasia* in 1980, issued by the Congregation for the Doctrine of the Faith (CDF) and approved by Pope John Paul II.[7] More recently, Pope John Paul II also spoke about the removal of life support and the care of the dying, being careful to distinguish between the removal of unnecessary life support and euthanasia.[8] Finally, the bishops of the United States have applied the teaching of the Church to issues involving Catholic hospitals and nursing homes in the *Ethical and Religious Directives (ERD)*.[9]

II. The Difference between Suicide, Euthanasia, and Allowing to Die

For Christians, and for many others as well, human life is considered to be a gift from the Creator, and the control of human life implies stewardship, not absolute autonomy. Human life may be compared to the talents given by the master to his servants, which he expects them to invest so that there will be a proper return (Mt 25:14-30). Hence, this gift of life must be used wisely and prudently to strive for the purpose of life. As Thomas Aquinas stated, "Every man has it instilled in him by nature to love his own life and whatever is directed thereto; and to do so in due measure, that is, to love these things not as placing his end therein, but as things to be used for the sake of his last end."[10] For committed Christians, the purpose of life is found in friendship with God and living with Him forever.[11] However, the time may come in a person's life when he is reasonably convinced that life is coming to an end, because of an internal threat to homeostasis and the conviction that prolonging life by additional medical treatment will not bring him closer to God. Family members or legal proxies may also be called upon to make a decision of this nature for patients who are unable to speak for themselves (see section VII below). In these circumstances one may decide that prolonging life is not the best investment of energy, time, or money that can be made in the time remaining. Seeking to prolong life in such a situation may not benefit the patient and may interfere with the pursuit of other, more important goods or duties. Hence, if further therapies to prolong life "do not offer a reasonable hope of benefit or entail an excessive burden" insofar as attaining the purpose of life is concerned, they may be refused.[12] The intention inherent in an act of this nature does not constitute suicide or euthanasia.[13] Rather, it is an act whose moral object may be accurately described as "allowing to die for legitimate reasons." When a person chooses to have life support withheld or removed in such a case, or when the decision is made by a proxy, the decision maker is not making a choice in favor of death. Rather, an indirect choice is made about when the patient will die, "taking into account the state of the sick person and his or her physical and moral resources."[14]

Suicide occurs when the intention inherent in the human act (the moral object, purpose, or *finis operis* of the act) is self-destruction. Euthanasia occurs when the intention inherent in the act is to end the life of another person, with or without the consent of the person, and the motive (or *finis operantis*) for the act is to alleviate or eliminate suffering. In euthanasia, the act of killing may be accomplished by commission or omission; that is, by performing a lethal act or by withholding some life-prolonging therapy which should be utilized. The *Declaration on Euthanasia* defines such an act in the following manner: "By euthanasia is understood an action or an omission which of itself or by intention causes death, in order that all suffering may in this way be eliminated."[15]

5. Cronin, "The Moral Law," 41.

6. Pius XII, "The Prolongation of Life: Allocution to the International Congress of Anesthesiologists" (November 24, 1957), *The Pope Speaks* 4.4 (1958): 395-398. Pope Pius XII also gave several allocutions on other medical topics. See *The Human Body: Papal Teachings* (Boston: Daughters of St Paul, 1960).

7. Congregation for the Doctrine of the Faith, *Declaration on Euthanasia* (May 5, 1980), http://www.vatican.va/roman_curia/congregations/cfaith/documents/rc_con_cfaith_doc_19800505_euthanasia_en.html.

8. John Paul II, *Evangelium vitae* (March 25, 1995) (Boston: Daughters of St. Paul, 1995), n. 65; John Paul II, "On Life-Sustaining Treatments and the Vegetative State" (March 20, 2004), *National Catholic Bioethics Quarterly* 4.3 (Autumn 2004): 574-576; John Paul II, "To the Participants in the 19th International Conference of the Pontifical Council for Pastoral Health Care" (November 12, 2004), *National Catholic Bioethics Quarterly* 5.1 (Spring 2005): 153.

9. U.S. Conference of Catholic Bishops, *Ethical and Religious Directives for Catholic Health Care Services* (Washington, DC: USCCB, 2001).

10. Thomas Aquinas, *Summa theologiae,* II-II, Q. 126.1, from Aquinas, *Summa Theologica,* trans. Fathers of the English Dominican Province (Westminster, MD: Christian Classics, 1981).

11. *Catechism of the Catholic Church,* trans. U.S. Conference of Catholic Bishops (Vatican City: Libreria Editrice Vaticana, 1994), n. 1, n. 356; see also *Summa theologiae,* II-II, Q. 23.1.

12. United States Conference of Catholic Bishops, *Ethical and Religious Directives,* nn. 56, 57.

13 I have borrowed the term "intention inherent in the act" from Elizabeth Anscombe. I believe it does away with the ambiguity which sometimes results if the term "intention" is used in regard to the moral object, and also for the goal of the agent. See G. E. M. Anscombe, *Collected Philosophical Papers,* vol. 3 (Oxford: Blackwell Publishing, 1981), 86.

14. Congregation for the Doctrine of the Faith, *Declaration on Euthanasia,* IV.

15. Ibid., II.

Clearly, whether euthanasia has occurred cannot be discerned simply from the physical result of commission or omission of a medical act. Rather, the moral object of the act must be determined. To reject additional medical efforts which do not correspond to the actual circumstances of the patient (that is, aggressive care) is not to reject life itself or the God who gave it, but is simply to reject efforts that will not help to complete the task of striving for the purpose of life. As Pope John Paul II declared:

> The refusal of aggressive treatment is neither a rejection of the patient nor of his or her life. Indeed, the object of the decision on whether to begin or to continue a treatment has nothing to do with the value of the patient's life, but rather with whether such medical intervention is beneficial for the patient.[16]

This act, which is contrary to euthanasia, is aptly described as "allowing to die for legitimate reasons." These legitimate reasons are either "no hope of benefit" or "excessive burden." Both euthanasia and allowing to die have the same physical result: death of the patient. But they have a radically different moral significance.

Pope John Paul II explained the distinction between allowing to die and euthanasia in the following manner:

> Euthanasia must be distinguished from the decision to forgo so-called "aggressive medical treatment," in other words, medical procedures which no longer correspond to the real situation of the patient, either because they are now disproportionate to any expected results or because they impose an excessive burden on the patient and his family. . . . To forgo extraordinary or disproportionate means is not the equivalent of suicide or euthanasia; it rather expresses acceptance of the human condition in the face of death.[17]

When comparing euthanasia and the elimination of pain as death approaches, the teaching authority of the Church has clarified the issue on several occasions. If analgesics are given to control or eliminate pain (intention inherent in the action), this is not an act of euthanasia, even though the medication given may indirectly shorten the patient's life.[18] This is an application of the principle of double effect. There is concern that the life of patients afflicted with terminal cancer might be shortened by the use of morphine or other analgesics, but research seems to indicate this seldom happens.[19]

16. John Paul II, "To the Participants in the 19th International Conference," n. 4.

17. John Paul II, *Evangelium vitae,* n. 65.

18. Pius XII, "To the 9th National Congress of the Italian Society of Anesthesiology" (February 24, 1957), *Acta Apostolica Sedis* 49 (1957); John Paul II, *Evangelium vitae,* n. 65; Congregation for the Doctrine of the Faith, *Declaration on Euthanasia,* III.

19. K. M. Foley, "Drug Therapy of Cancer Pain," *Pain* 18, suppl. 1 (1984): S199.

III. The Difference between Medical Therapy and Basic Health Care

Before discussing in detail the criteria for removing life support, for the sake of clarity let us distinguish those medical or surgical procedures which are employed to prolong life from those activities that furnish comfort care, sometimes called basic health care or minimal care.[20] In the former category are all medical and surgical procedures designed to combat illness and disease and alleviate pain. Usually, these procedures require the expertise of medical professionals in order to be utilized. In the latter category are those activities that may not improve the health of the patient, but which demonstrate human compassion and respect for the person. For example, people who are suffering from illness or disease, no matter what their cognitive affective function, should be bathed and kept clean and free from pain. Thirst and other effects of dehydration should be controlled insofar as possible. If they are in pain, analgesics should be administered even though health cannot be restored.

Some procedures of palliative care seem to be a combination of comfort care and medical care.[21] In recent times, different opinions have been put forward as to whether assisted nutrition and hydration (ANH) for people in a permanent vegetative state (PVS) amounts to comfort care or a medical procedure. For example, Pope John Paul II affirmed in a recent papal allocution that ANH for PVS patients is "normal care" and a "natural means of preserving life, not a medical act."[22] The Multi-Society Task Force on PVS, on the other hand, maintained that ANH is a medical procedure,[23] as did the U.S. Supreme Court.[24]

Clearly, the method by which ANH is delivered is a medical procedure, especially if installing the feeding tube involves surgery, as it often does, and if the patient must be monitored by health-care professionals in order to prevent infection and aspiration pneumonia. But the material conveyed via ANH procedures to sustain nutrition for PVS patients may be assigned fittingly to the category of basic health care, or normal comfort care. As John Connery, S.J., stated, "artificial feeding seems to be a combination of both [medical treatment and basic health care]."[25] Whatever this type of care is called, it is

20. John Paul II, "On Life-Sustaining Treatments," n. 4; see also Thomas O'Donnell, S.J., *Medicine and Christian Morality* (New York: Alba House, 1996), 65.

21. Yvonne Carter, Christina Faull, and Richard Woolf, eds., *The Handbook of Palliative Care* (London: Blackwell Publishers, 1998).

22. John Paul II, "On Life-Sustaining Treatments," n. 4.

23. Multi-Society Task Force on PVS, "Medical Aspects of the Persistent Vegetative State — Second of Two Parts," *New England Journal of Medicine* 330.22 (June 2, 1994): 1572.

24. *Cruzan v. Director, Missouri Department of Health,* 110 S. Ct. 2841 (1990).

25. John Connery, S.J., "The Ethical Standards for Withholding/Withdrawing Nutrition and Hydration," *Issues in Law and Medicine* 2.2 (September 1986): 89.

important to note that the moral norms for forgoing it are the same as those for forgoing medical care: no hope of benefit or excessive burden. For example, moving a person to prevent bed sores is basic or comfort care. But if death is imminent, there is no need to move the patient, because it would not offer hope of benefit. Or the patient may be so fragile that to move her would cause intense pain or even a fracture. Moving her may be omitted because it is an excessive burden.

It seems that the 2004 papal allocution maintains that ANH is a benefit for a person in PVS. But contrary to many statements referring to it, the allocution does not preclude the consideration of excessive burdens that might rule out the use of ANH therapy. As the Australian Catholic Bishops' Conference stated in response to the papal allocution of March 20, 2004:

> In particular cases, however, the provision of nutrition and hydration may cease to be obligatory, e.g., if the patient is unable to assimilate the material provided or if the manner of the provision itself causes undue suffering to the patient, or involves an undue burden to others.[26]

In the allocution of March 20, 2004, Pope John Paul II spoke of "the heavy human, psychological and financial burden" for the family.[27] The cost of nursing care for a PVS patient, for example, may be excessive, even though the cost of nutrition might be minimal.

IV. Comparison of Terms: *Ordinary* and *Extraordinary, Proportionate* and *Disproportionate*

For centuries, the terms *ordinary* and *extraordinary* were used for determining the use of life support. If the medical therapy was ordinary, there was a moral obligation to use it; if it was extraordinary, its use was optional. In 1980, the CDF suggested in the *Declaration on Euthanasia* that the terms *proportionate* and *disproportionate* might be more accurate than ordinary and extraordinary.[28] In order to signify the meaning of both sets of terms, the *Declaration* added:

> In any case, it will be possible to make a correct judgment as to the means by studying the type of treatment to be used, its degree of complexity or risk, its cost and the possibilities of using it, and comparing these elements with the result that can be expected, taking into account the state of the sick person and his or her physical and moral resources.[29]

It seems the main reason for the suggested change in terminology arose from the tendency to interpret the terms *ordinary* and *extraordinary* in an abstract or generic manner; that is, the decision whether a medical means to prolong life was ordinary or extraordinary was often made without reference to the condition of the patient. Using the terms in an abstract or generic sense, only the cost, usual effectiveness, availability of a medical device, and potential pain inflicted would be considered when designating a medical or surgical procedure as ordinary or extraordinary. The overall condition of the patient was not considered until after the terms of ordinary or extraordinary care had been decided. This would often result in confusing terminology. The means in question might be considered ordinary in the abstract, but this designation would be changed to extraordinary once the condition of the patient had been considered. Thus, a respirator or a feeding tube might be designated as an ordinary means to prolong life, but after consideration of the patient's condition, it might be considered extraordinary.[30]

Connery and Thomas O'Donnell, S.J., mention some theologians who used this abstract or generic form of determination, though Connery states that overall, "the sensitivities of the individual were taken into account."[31] Clearly, the more accurate designation of moral responsibility in choosing or rejecting medical or surgical procedures rests upon a diagnosis of pathology and prognosis of possible effects of medical care.

Since the *Declaration on Euthanasia* was issued, the terms *proportionate* and *disproportionate* have been used as synonyms for *ordinary* and *extraordinary* by Catholic theologians, but they have not supplanted the original terms. Hence, in this study, I shall use the terms *ordinary* and *extraordinary,* but will always insist that a determination cannot be made concerning the moral obligation to use a particular therapy until the condition of the patient and the potential effect upon the patient is known, insofar as possible. Thus, I shall use the term in the "relative sense," as indicated by O'Donnell.[32]

The tendency to use the terms *ordinary and extraordinary* in an abstract manner can still be found in the writings of some physicians and other health-care professionals, and very frequently in the conversations of people who must make decisions for loved ones concerning the use or removal of life support. Therapies which, in the abstract sense of the term, were at one time experi-

26. Bishops Committee on Doctrine and Morals (Australian Catholic Bishops' Conference), Bishops Committee for Health Care (Australia), and Catholic Health Australia, "Briefing Note on the Obligation to Provide Nutrition and Hydration" (September 3, 2004), n. 3, http://www.acbc.catholic.org.au/documents/2004090316.pdf.

27. John Paul II, "On Life-Sustaining Treatments," n. 6.

28. Congregation for the Doctrine of the Faith, *Declaration on Euthanasia,* IV; also see Benedict Ashley, O.P., and Kevin O'Rourke, O.P., *Health Care Ethics: A Theological Analysis,* 4th ed. (Washington, DC: Georgetown University Press, 1997), 420.

29. Congregation for the Doctrine of the Faith, *Declaration on Euthanasia,* IV.

30. See Gerald Kelly, "The Duty of Using Artificial Means of Preserving Life," *Theological Studies* 11 (1950): 214-216.

31. John Connery, S.J., "Prolonging Life: The Duty and Its Limits," *Catholic Mind* (October 1980): 44-57; O'Donnell, *Medicine and Christian Morality,* 55-63.

32. Thomas J. O'Donnell, *Medicine and Christian Morality,* 62.

mental or extraordinary and later became standard or ordinary care include, for example, blood transfusions and angioplasties (surgical reconstructions of blood vessels). But whether such a therapy should be utilized or may be withheld or withdrawn from a particular patient cannot be determined from the moral perspective until the condition of the patient is factored into the decision. Thus, in any oral or written discussion concerning life support, the meaning of the terms must be made clear at the beginning in order to avoid confusion later on.

V. The Criteria for Forgoing Life Support

The phrase "forgoing life support" refers to withholding and withdrawing life support. The criteria for withholding life support are the same as those for withdrawing life support that is already being utilized. In the latter case, however, the emotional response is more intense, because it usually implies that the patient will die shortly after medical therapy is withdrawn.[33]

The specific criteria for distinguishing between ordinary and extraordinary or between proportionate and disproportionate medical therapy are the hope of benefit that the therapy offers, and the burden imposed by the therapy upon the patient, the family, and the community.[34] Pope John Paul II expressed the same criteria in this way: "The possible decision either not to start or to halt a treatment will be deemed ethically correct if the treatment is ineffective or obviously disproportionate to the aims of sustaining life or recovering health."[35] In general, the benefits sought through medical care are the preservation or restoration of health and the alleviation of pain. In short, the goal of medicine is to promote optimal functioning, given the person's physical and mental capacities.[36] Medical therapy does not always result in a cure. It does not always improve or restore health or prolong life. Often it merely circumvents, abates, or alleviates an illness or disease, but does not eliminate it.

While medical care is directed primarily toward physiological or psychological functions, it often offers social or spiritual benefit indirectly. The benefit of medical care enables one to pursue the goods of life. These goods may be physical, psychological, social, or spiritual. These are proximate goods, explicitly or implicitly ordered toward the ultimate good of life, friendship with God. These proximate goods are often more prominent in the minds of persons as they evaluate hope of benefit associated with particular medical therapies. For example, when making serious medical decisions, people ponder what effects the therapies will have upon their health, their vocations, and their families.

Would this surgery improve my overall well-being and allow me a more pain-free life? Would this medicine enable me to cope with the stress of life more adequately? Will the medication or surgery enable me to return to work? Will this therapy enable my loved one, for whom I am the proxy, to regain consciousness, or will it simply prolong a comatose condition? Finally, how expensive will the medical procedure be? What other goods would the family have to forgo if we invest in this medical therapy? Thus, economic, psychic, and social goods more often are the immediate concern of decision makers. They are all included under the general category of hope of benefit. But these goods are at least implicitly ordered to a higher good. As Pope Pius XII stated in his famous declaration on life support in 1957, "Life, health, all temporal activities are in fact subordinated to spiritual ends."[37]

Burdens

The burdens of medical care might also affect the pursuit of the goods that are significant in human life; thus, the burdens might be economic, physiological, psychological, social, or spiritual. Since the sixteenth century, economic burdens, extreme pain, risk of losing life, and great subjective repugnance have been the principal burdens considered.[38] In order to justify forgoing life support, the burden must be judged to be excessive. Determining an *excessive* burden is often a difficult process. All medical care is a burden in one sense. But an excessive burden makes striving for the continuation of life, or an important good of life, a moral impossibility — or at least very difficult.[39] Certainly, some objective norms can be set for judging burden. Theologians seek to do this, presupposing a certain degree of courage (the virtue of fortitude). Thus, direct killing of oneself or another, even to avoid suffering, is prohibited. But subjective disposition must also be considered.

At one time, some moral theologians suggested that a woman of tender conscience might find it an excessive burden to consult a male physician, and thus they thought that such a woman would be excused from consulting a physician. What may seem to be an excessive burden for one person might be considered negligible by another person. As the *Declaration on Euthanasia* states, "In the final analysis, it pertains to the conscience either of the sick person, or of those qualified to speak in the sick person's name . . . to decide in the light of moral obligations and of the various aspects of the case."[40] For this reason Catholic tradition has always insisted that the

33. Ashley and O'Rourke, *Health Care Ethics,* 442.

34. United States Conference of Catholic Bishops, *Ethical and Religious Directives,* nn. 56, 57.

35. John Paul II, "To the Participants in the 19th International Conference," n. 4.

36. Henrik Blum, *Expanding Health Care Horizons: From a General Systems Concept of Health to a National Health Policy* (Oakland, CA: Third Party Publishing Company, 1983), 102.

37. Pius XII, "The Prolongation of Life," 398.

38. O'Donnell, *Medicine and Christian Morality,* 59; Connery, "The Ethical Standards," 91.

39. Cronin, "The Moral Law," 31.

40. Congregation for the Doctrine of the Faith, *Declaration on Euthanasia,* IV.

patient or the proxy has the right to make the final decision concerning the refusal of health care, as we shall see in section VII. Kevin Wildes detects a retreat from this principle in regard to some recent statements of bishops' conferences in regard to the use of ANH: "In trying to objectivize the benefits of medically assisted feeding and hydration they neglect the subjective element for determining ordinary care. The benefits of a treatment can only be determined within the context of a patient's life."[41]

Research on the burdens that people consider excessive indicates that many people would consider being paralyzed, and able to breathe only if assisted by a respirator, an excessive burden.[42] Yet many people actually in this condition adjust to their situations very well and desire to prolong life by using life support.[43] Thus, the ethical responsibility to consult the patient with regard to forgoing life support, and the need to afford these persons the proper counseling, cannot be emphasized too greatly. We shall have more to say about this factor when we consider personal and proxy decision making.

Future Burdens Considered

When discussing burdens, theologians consider not only the present burden associated with a particular medication or medical procedure, but also any future burden. As Connery says, "In assessing any particular means, it made no difference whether the burden to the patient was experienced before, during, or after the treatment."[44] For example, the burden associated with respirator-assisted breathing is considered by most people to be a minimal burden, especially if intubation is necessary for only a short time. However, the length of time that this burden might endure must also be taken into consideration. For example, a young athlete fractured the C3 vertebra in a trampoline accident. Able to breathe only with a respirator, and now quadriplegic, he was informed two weeks after the accident that this condition would last for the rest of his life. Communicating with his family through eye contact, he convinced them to ask his physicians to remove the respirator because the prospect of living the rest of his life in this condition was an overwhelming burden. The family agreed with him. Having consulted with ethicists, the physicians brought in people who were living successfully with the same disability, but he and the family persisted in their request. After a time, the physicians ceded to their request. A less dramatic forgoing of life support often happens when a dialysis patient, experiencing severe and continual fatigue, realizes that she no longer benefits sufficiently from the treatment, determines to discontinue the treatment even though, if continued, it might prolong her life for the foreseeable future.

The financial burden resulting from prolonged medical therapy can be misconstrued. For example, the materials needed for tube feeding (i.e., ANH) are inexpensive: a rubber tube and some cans of Ensure. But installing a gastrostomy tube or a tube into the vena cava (hyperalimentation) is a surgical procedure performed in a surgical suite, and long-term nursing care will be necessary for a person with these devices. These considerations are all part of the financial burden. To set these considerations aside is unrealistic.[45]

Two Criteria, or One?

Are two criteria used when evaluating medical therapy, or are benefit and burden to be combined? Connery expressed a preference for keeping them separate, because they deal with different issues. "In practice, at least, the question of benefit seems limited largely to terminal cases; burden can be an issue even in cases which are not terminal."[46] From a theoretical perspective, these are two distinct criteria, and sometimes they are different in the practical situation. For instance, a patient suffering from cancer may determine that prolonging life for another ten days may be ineffective, even though there is no serious pain or financial burden. Or drug therapy for patients with AIDS may offer hope of benefit, but some patients might deem it an excessive burden because of the expense involved.

More often, in an actual case, benefit and burden are compared to each other. The end result is a statement that the medical therapy in question is either a burden or a benefit. Some authors restrict their considerations to the benefit/burden terminology and seldom consider benefit and burden as separate criteria.[47] In the *ERD*, directives 56 and 57 distinguish between hope of benefit and excessive burden, but in directive 58 the two are combined in the discussion on the use of ANH.

Quality-of-Life Considerations

The question is often asked whether quality-of-life considerations can be used as criteria for determining whether a medical procedure offers hope of benefit or imposes an excessive burden. But in any discussion of this nature, it is necessary to realize that quality of life is an ambiguous term; it has different connotations at dif-

41. Kevin Wildes, "Ordinary and Extraordinary Means and the Quality of Life," *Theological Studies* 57.3 (September 1996): 510.

42. Bryan Jennett, "Attitudes to the Permanent Vegetative State," in *The Vegetative State: Medical Facts, Ethical and Legal Dilemmas* (New York: Cambridge University Press, 2002), 73-86.

43. See Not Dead Yet, http://www.notdeadyet.org.

44. Connery, "Prolonging Life," 45.

45. Germain Grisez, "Should Nutrition and Hydration Be Provided to Permanently Unconscious and Other Mentally Disabled Persons?" *Issues in Law and Medicine* 5.2 (Fall 1989): 168.

46. Connery, "The Ethical Standards," 47.

47. Dan W. Brock, "Death and Dying," in *Medical Ethics*, 2nd ed., ed. Robert Veatch (Boston: Jones and Bartlett, 1997), 360; J. Stuart Showalter and Brian L. Andrew, *To Treat or Not to Treat: A Working Document for Making Critical Life Decisions* (St. Louis, MO: Catholic Health Association of the United States, 1984).

ferent times.[48] In one sense, it refers to our relationship to God. In this sense, all have the same quality of life and dignity because God loves each person. This is the sense in which Pope John Paul II used the term when he spoke against quality-of-life decisions in the allocution concerning the care of PVS patients.[49]

But the term is also used to measure human function. People with impaired human function are said to have an impaired or lower quality of life. Some people have impaired human function as the result of a genetic or physical anomaly. If a person with a disability of this nature contracts a serious disease, it would be highly immoral to withhold care because of the genetic or physical disability. Consider, for example, a child with Down syndrome who has a ruptured appendix. The parents' refusal of surgery or medication to treat the ruptured appendix would be a grave violation of the child's right to life. But there is a third meaning to the term "quality of life." Judgments of this nature "rely on the discernment of the patient."[50] Some people have impaired function resulting from illness or disease, and for these people the quality of life is fittingly considered when benefits and burdens are assessed, as a document cited with approval in the papal allocution maintains.[51] Let us suppose that one's mother has cancer, which has metastasized throughout her body, and her kidneys begin to fail. Should we consider her overall condition as we decide whether dialysis will be beneficial for her?

In order to obviate the difficulties that arise from the use of the term "quality of life," Father O'Donnell suggested in a private conversation that the term "quality of function" be used whenever a question arises about withdrawing life support from a person suffering impaired function from a serious illness or disease.[52] Although it is difficult to change the terms used in regard to death and dying, this seems to be a far better alternative when discussing conditions resulting from serious pathologies.

VI. When Should the Decision to Forgo Life Support Be Made?

This is one of the more misunderstood questions in regard to forgoing life support. Since humans have a serious obligation to seek health in order to prolong life, they have a moral obligation to seek to overcome illness and disease, unless the means to accomplish this goal does not offer hope of benefit or imposes an excessive burden. When a less serious illness or disease is present, we often rely upon the natural homeostasis of the body to resist it. For example, many people do not take medicines or antibiotics if they contract a minor case of influenza, relying instead upon rest, liquids, and the natural resistance of the body to gradually restore health. However, when a more serious illness or disease threatens, one that might cause death if not eliminated or abated, the prudent person makes a decision to utilize medications or surgery to help the body overcome it, or at least to mitigate its effects.

Thus, the logical time to make decisions about utilizing the means to prolong life is when a person contracts a serious illness. Usually, the initial reaction to a serious illness will not involve a rejection of medical means due to lack of benefit or excessive burden. But in time, as the illness progresses, if the medical therapy is ineffective or becomes acutely onerous, a decision to reject medical means might be made for the reasons mentioned above. When decisions have to be made for persons unable to make decisions for themselves, proxy decision makers may decide to forgo life support for these reasons.

Often, people believe that life support, either for oneself or for another who is incapable of making healthcare decisions, must be continued until it is no longer physically possible to keep a person alive. This implies that life support cannot be removed until the fatal disease can no longer be resisted, and that death will occur within a short time, no matter what medications or medical procedures are utilized. Physicians with this mentality often assert that life support cannot be removed because the patients are not suffering from terminal illness. This seems to be the rationale underlying a recent statement of the World Federation of Catholic Medical Associations concerning patients in a vegetative state: "VS patients cannot in any way be considered terminal patients, since their condition can be stable and enduring."[53] O'Donnell states that "there is in the medical profession an ideal which demands the fighting off of pain and death until the last possible moment."[54]

The assertion that life support cannot be removed unless a terminal illness is present is contrary to the consistent tradition in Catholic moral theology. When theologians of the sixteenth century considered questions concerning the duty to prolong life, they posited cases which did not presuppose the presence of terminal illness. Moreover, in the *Declaration on Euthanasia*, the question is posed, "Is it necessary in all circumstances to have recourse to all possible remedies?"[55] Section IV of the declaration indicates that several circumstances may prompt a decision to withdraw life support before a ter-

48. James J. Walter and Thomas A. Shannon, eds., *Quality of Life: The New Medical Dilemma* (Mahwah, NJ: Paulist Press, 1990), 78-82.

49. John Paul II, "On Life-Sustaining Treatments," n. 5.

50. Kevin Wildes, "Ordinary and Extraordinary Means," 511.

51. Pontifical Council *Cor Unum*, "Question of Ethics Regarding the Fatally Ill and the Dying" (June 27, 1981), cited in John Paul II, "On Life-Sustaining Treatments," n. 4.

52. Thomas O'Donnell, S.J., personal communication, 1994.

53. See joint statement of the World Federation of Catholic Medical Associations and the Pontifical Academy for Life, "Considerations on the Scientific and Ethical Problems Related to Vegetative State," n. 4, http://www.vegetativestate.org/documento_FIAMC.htm.

54. O'Donnell, *Medicine and Christian Morality*, 67.

55. Congregation for the Doctrine of the Faith, *Declaration on Euthanasia*, IV.

minal illness is diagnosed. Guidance for withdrawing life support even before a so-called terminal illness is present is offered:

> In any case, it will be possible to make a correct judgment as to the means by studying the type of treatment to be used, its degree of complexity or risk, its cost and the possibilities of using it, and comparing these elements with the result that can be expected, taking into account the state of the sick person and his or her physical and moral resources.[56]

Furthermore, the notion that life support may be forgone only if the patient suffers from a terminal illness neglects the second criteria for forgoing life support: excessive burden.

The thought that a terminal illness must be diagnosed before life support can be withdrawn was used by the lower courts in the famous *Brophy, Conroy,* and *Cruzan* cases. But these decisions were later reversed when the higher courts considered the matter more thoroughly and determined that the key issue was not whether a terminal illness was present but rather the effect of the therapy upon the patient. Some of the judges in the lower courts maintained that if death occurred after the removal of life support, the result was homicide. But the decision of the higher courts rightly inferred that if death occurred after the removal of life support, death was not the intention inherent in the action. Rather, the cause of death was the terminal illness from which the patient suffered, not the removal of life support.[57]

Another misleading attitude maintains that life support can be withdrawn only if death is "imminent and inevitable." This phrase is used in the encyclical *Evangelium vitae,* n. 65, and is also stated in an unofficial Vatican document seeking to summarize church teaching on medical ethics.[58] Of course, if death is imminent and inevitable, this diagnosis can be factored into the decision-making process. Indeed, it makes the decision whether or not to forgo life support easier. But the statement about "imminent and inevitable" death in the encyclical does not indicate that life support can be withdrawn *only* if death is imminent and inevitable. The encyclical quotes the *Declaration on Euthanasia* as the source of its teaching. As we have seen, this document envisions life support being removed even if death is not imminent and inevitable. Unfortunately, some people purporting to speak for the Church have recently focused upon this phrase and maintain that any removal of comfort care or life support that results in death is euthanasia, unless death is imminent and inevitable. This is contrary to five hundred years of theological analysis.

56. Ibid.

57. T. O'Donnell, "Fatal Pathology: Not Removal of Life Support," *Medical-Moral Newsletter* (February 1987): 7.

58. Pontifical Council for Pastoral Assistance to Health Care Workers, *Charter for Health Care Workers* (Boston: Daughters of St. Paul, 1995), n. 120.

VII. Who Makes the Decision?

Often, it is unclear which person has the right to determine whether the means to prolong life are ordinary or extraordinary. Clearly, the physician is deeply involved in the decision. He or she must present an opinion as to whether the means in question will cure, help significantly, or have no effect upon the ailing patient. In other words, the diagnosis and prognosis are primarily the responsibility of the physician. But other circumstances, in addition to medical effectiveness, must be considered. What about expense, pain, and inconvenience? What about the spiritual condition of the patient? Only the patient or the proxy can determine these factors accurately.

For this conclusion, the Catholic tradition does not rely upon the legal right of autonomy, as does the modern teaching of bioethics. Rather, the source of this personal responsibility is the "sacred and inviolable" character of the human person.[59] Hence, the radical right to make the ethical decision concerning means to prolong life belongs to the patient. Pope Pius XII spoke to this issue:

> The rights and duties of the doctor are correlative to those of the patient. The doctor, in fact, has no separate or independent right where the patient is concerned. In general, he or she can take action only when the patient explicitly or implicitly, directly or indirectly, gives permission.[60]

The *ERD* also speaks to this issue:

> The free and informed consent of the person or the person's surrogate is required for medical treatments and procedures, except in an emergency situation when consent cannot be obtained and there is no indication that the patient would refuse consent to the treatment.
>
> Free and informed consent requires that the person or the person's surrogate receive all reasonable information about the essential nature of the proposed treatment and its benefits; its risks, side-effects, consequences, and cost; and any reasonable and morally legitimate alternatives, including no treatment at all.[61]

The number of articles and books devoted to the topic of informed consent illustrate that the right of the patient to make health-care decisions is prominent in the study of bioethics.

Proxy Consent

The most difficult situation in regard to consent arises when the patient is incapable of decision making and a proxy must make decisions.

If the patient is too young to indicate his or her wishes, or if the patient has failed to indicate the preferred ther-

59. John Paul II, *Evangelium vitae,* n. 53.

60. Pius XII, "The Prolongation of Life," 393-398.

61. U.S. Conference of Catholic Bishops, *Ethical and Religious Directives,* nn. 26, 27.

apy as death threatens, the proxy, usually a family member, acts in the *best interest of the patient.* That is, he or she, acting with the advice of the attending physician, indicates the preferred therapy, or forgoing of it, given the circumstances. In the United States, the use of advance directives, in which the patient, when competent, names a proxy (not always a family member) to make health-care decisions when he or she is not competent to do so, is recommended. These directives have been recognized as a legitimate means of preparing for future health-care needs by the U.S. bishops' conference.[62]

When acting under the guidance of an advance directive, the proxy should seek to offer *substitute judgment;* that is, to follow the previously expressed wishes of the patient if these wishes are in accord with the teaching of the Church. However, if the circumstances are not the same as those envisioned by the patient, as often happens in crisis situations, the proxy may have to act in the best interest of the patient. In all circumstances, the people assisting in care and decision making must take care to assure that dying remains a spiritual experience for the patient, rather than an expression of previous personal controversies.

Family Concerns

While families are often called upon to offer substitute or best-interest decisions when their loved ones are not able to make decisions for themselves, family decisions need not be totally altruistic. That is, it may happen that the family will have concerns of its own, which, if not taken into consideration, would inflict excessive burdens upon the family. This often is the case when nursing a comatose patient imposes a serious burden upon the family. The *ERD* implies that family concerns should be recognized when decisions about life support are being made by a patient (directives 56 and 57). Connery stated, "A patient would be free to omit a means to preserve life even if he did so to remove a burden from the family."[63] Moreover, Pius XII made two statements relevant to family decision making:

> The rights and duties of the family depend in general upon the presumed will of the unconscious patient if he is of age and *sui juris.* Where the proper and independent duty of the family is concerned, they [the family] are usually bound only to the use of ordinary means.

When discussing the removal of respirators, he added,

> Consequently, if it appears that the attempt at resuscitation constitutes in reality such a burden for the family that one cannot in all conscience impose it upon them, they can lawfully insist that the doctor should discontinue these attempts, and the doctor can lawfully comply.[64]

62. Ibid., n. 25.
63. Connery, "The Ethical Standards," 91.
64. Pius XII, "The Prolongation of Life," 399.

Finally, a statement of the U.S. Bishops' Committee for Pro-Life Activities in regard to family decisions about ANH should be kept in mind:

> We should not assume that all or most decisions to withhold or withdraw medically assisted nutrition and hydration are attempts to cause death. To be sure, any patient will die if all nutrition and hydration are withheld. But sometimes other causes may be at work — for example, the patient may be imminently dying, whether feeding takes place or not. *At other times,* although the shortening of the patient's life is one foreseeable result of an omission, the real purpose of the omission was to relieve the patient of a particular procedure that was of limited usefulness to the patient or unreasonably burdensome for the patient and the patient's family or caregivers. This kind of decision should not be equated with a decision to kill or with suicide.[65]

Of course, the family does not have a moral obligation to request withdrawal of life support if it seems to be extraordinary. The family may continue care, if it does not violate the rights of other persons or facilities associated with caring for the patient. Thus, the rights of doctors and hospitals to declare that life support should be withheld or withdrawn must be respected, even if the family does not wish to follow their advice.

Community Interest

The community is also mentioned as a stakeholder when decisions about life support are necessary.[66] People belong to small and large communities. In a small community, the expense and care that a particular therapy might impose could be a factor when decisions about life support are made, because if funds are not expended for one person, they may benefit another person. In religious communities, for example, there is usually a fund to finance health care. But this fund is not an insurance fund in the strict sense; the members of the community contribute to it. Thus, if a community member requires expensive therapy, others in the community may not have access to adequate therapy, or the contributions of individual members may have to be increased.

Recently, a friend of mine who is prominent in the field of bioethics was afflicted with a serious stroke, and refused extensive therapy, stating that he did not want to expend the funds of his community upon therapy that would have doubtful success. In other words, he determined that in his condition, and given the finances of the community, such care would not offer hope of benefit and was therefore extraordinary, even though it would have prolonged his life.

65. U.S. Bishops' Committee for Pro-Life Activities, "Nutrition and Hydration: Moral and Pastoral Reflections" (April 2, 1992), *Origins* 21.44 (April 9, 1992): 707 (emphasis added).
66. U.S. Conference of Catholic Bishops, *Ethical and Religious Directives,* nn. 56, 57.

At present, given the method of paying for health care in the United States, the larger community, the state, or the insurance company do not often become a significant factor in making decisions about forgoing life support. While the funding methods of state-sponsored health care and insurance companies are too complicated to discuss in this article, if care is withheld or removed from one person, there does not seem to be a direct benefit for another person, and the uninsured do not benefit from cost reduction for the insured. This situation could change if universal health care ever becomes a reality within the social policy in the United States.

The Purpose of Life

From the consideration of the Catholic tradition, several conclusions may be drawn. Decisions concerning hope of benefit and excessive burden should be made in view of the proximate and ultimate goals of human life. Euthanasia and allowing to die for legitimate reasons have the same physical result, but are vastly different from an ethical perspective. There is a legitimate distinction between basic health care and medical therapy, but the ethical norms governing their use are similar. Medical therapy may be withheld or withdrawn even if a terminal illness is not present, and even if death is not imminent and inevitable. The needs and goods of the patient should dominate the decisions of the proxy, but the needs and goods of the family and the community should not be ignored. And finally, dying is a spiritual experience which should help a person fulfill the purpose of life.

151 Having Enough Faith Not to Be Healed

John D. Brunt

In her book "The Dying Process," British researcher Julia Lawton quotes Ann, one of the hospice patients she studied. "I don't like the idea of lingering. If it's going to happen, let it happen. Not all this hanging on, dying inch by inch, fighting every step of the way."[1] In focusing on the dilemma of faith and fight, does faith demand fight? Is it a lack of faith to give up the fight for cure and accept palliative care? Is it a lack of faith on the part of the dying patient's loved ones to cease efforts of cure and healing and focus instead on comfort and support? Some families have been troubled by this question.

If God is an all-powerful God who can heal, then doesn't it show a lack of trust in him to give up the fight and quit trying for a cure? Before we answer this question, we need to lay some groundwork first in definitions. By "palliative care" I mean care that gives holistic nurture, comfort and support to a dying patient without continuing an attempted cure. As Andrew Billings says, "Palliative care is defined as comprehensive, interdisciplinary care of patients and families facing a terminal illness focusing primarily on comfort and support."[2] Kathleen Egan and Mary Labyak contrast palliative care with general medical care that seeks curative care and tries to reverse the disease process as medical care, while palliative care accepts the reality of impending death and involves the expert management of end stage disease symptomology as a prerequisite to providing the opportunity for patients and family to find growth, meaning, and value in the dying and bereavement experience.[3] Palliative care is then distinguished from curative care in that it's not trying to heal a person's disease. Instead, it attempts to be holistic, open to death and keeping the patient comfortable and supported in a loving way. Pallia-

1. Julia Lawton, *The Dying Process: Patients' Experiences of Palliative Care* (New York: Routledge, 2000), p. i.

2. Andrew J. Billings, "Palliative Care," *British Medical Journal,* Vol. 321, Issue 7260 (September 2, 2000), p. 555.

3. Kathleen A. Egan and Mary J. Labyak, "Hospice Care: A Model for Quality End of Life Care," in *Textbook of Palliative Nursing,* pp. 7-26, Betty Rolling Ferrell, ed. (New York: Oxford University Press, 2001), p. 9.

From John Brunt, "Having Enough Faith Not to be Healed," *Update (Loma Linda University Center for Christian Bioethics)* 18.1 (July 2002): 1-5. Used by permission of Loma Linda University Center for Christian Bioethics.

tive care is also to be distinguished from euthanasia or assisted suicide. In palliative care the goal is not to hasten death as an end, although many palliative caregivers are willing to give medications to ease pain even though they might hasten death, and are willing to avoid certain kinds of interventions that might prolong life. Some have criticized this aspect of palliative care. Julia Lawton, for instance, argues that, focusing so intently on the easing of pain, palliative caregivers forget the tragedy of other indignities of dying and believes that for some assisted suicide would be a more humane way to deal with the total experience of suffering.[4] Finally, for the purposes of this paper, when we speak of palliative care, we're not talking about the triage involved in financially based decisions not to provide services for certain illnesses within a given population. As we're defining it, palliative care does not withhold curative medical care because it is too expensive, but because it is futile or not desired by the patient. Lila Shotton defines futile care as "care that may be both incompetent and inappropriate and indeed harmful because there is no realistic chance of cure and there are side effects in the attempts at cure."[5] In summary, palliative care means giving comfort and holistic support where there is no reasonable hope that curative cure will be successful or desired.

How can you give up curative care and only comfort a loved one? Isn't God capable of healing? Shouldn't you keep doing all that you can? Shouldn't you keep going if you have faith? Some, as I said, have considered such treatments a lack of faith, and these are pastoral questions. And usually it's people of religious faith who face this issue. I will address it from my own Christian perspective in the hope that this perspective might also have relevance for those in other faith traditions. The route to an answer might seem circuitous. We are going to go in several directions before we get to the conclusion. We'll first look at the nature of death, then the nature of faith. Then, finally, we'll look at the conclusion.

First, a Biblical perspective on death. The last thirty years have seen a major paradigm shift in our understanding of death. Death has come into the open. We no longer try to hide it. Health care providers no longer try to pretend that everything is okay and avoid the subject of death. We have learned from people like Elisabeth Kübler-Ross how to deal with the various stages of response to death and be open and honest about it. However, some of this emphasis on openness to death has gone beyond the concept of facing death honestly and has tried to say that death should become a friend, to be welcomed as just another passage in life. For instance, I once heard Dr. Ross use the metaphor of a shooting star for death. She said that we enjoy the beauty of a shooting star even though we know it really is the death of a meteor. In similar fashion, we should come to see beauty in human death and consider it merely a transformation. In other death and dying literature, there exists a romanticizing of death.

However, the Bible refers to death as an enemy. Swiss theologian Oscar Cullmann, in his work titled "Immortality of the Soul: A Resurrection of the Dead," contrasted Socrates' death with Jesus' death. He pointed out that when Socrates drank the hemlock and faced death, he did it with sublime calm. Death was a friend. But when Jesus faced death, he sweated blood and prayed that this cup might pass from him.[6] In 1 Corinthians 15:26, Paul calls death the last enemy. According to Genesis 3, death was introduced as the consequence of sin, in opposition to God's original plan. This Biblical picture of death comports with our experience. It is true that sometimes death is preferable to suffering or torture. It is true that many people come to the place in old age where so much of their body is already failing that they welcome death. But it is only because evil has already taken away the qualities of vibrant life that death is so welcomed. Death is not beautiful. It is not natural. It is an enemy.

In one of the most painful moments of my life, I stood with two of my closest friends, husband and wife, at the cargo-receiving dock of the airport in Pasco, Washington. We watched in the distance as a plane approached and landed. Passengers got off, luggage was removed, and finally a large box was taken off the plane. It was placed onto one of those luggage carts and driven from the passenger terminal over to the cargo docks where we stood. This plain, white box held the body of their 25-year-old daughter who had been senselessly, brutally, randomly murdered while serving as an intern in Washington, D.C., during her first year out of college. I found absolutely nothing in this moment that bore any resemblance to watching a shooting star. If death is an enemy, shouldn't we always fight to the end?

Ah, but there is something else we should say about death. If we're faithful to the Biblical perspective, death is not only an enemy, but it is a defeated enemy. Jesus Christ is already the first fruits of the resurrection. According to Paul throughout 1 Corinthians 15, the world changed at the resurrection of Jesus Christ. We received the assurance that death would not have the last word. God will resurrect humans to a new life just as he resurrected Jesus. Yes, death is an enemy. But, it is a defeated enemy.

Viewing death as a defeated enemy does two things. First, it shows us the value of human bodily existence. Life in this world is valuable enough for God to raise the dead and resurrect bodily existence again. Second, life in this world, though valuable, is not ultimate. There is something beyond this life. Otherwise, Scripture could not tell us that there are things in life worth dying for. In Revelation 12:11, saints who remain faithful to Jesus

4. Lawton, pp. 176-181.

5. Leila Shotton, "Can Nurses Contribute to Better End-of-Life Care?" *Nursing Ethics,* Vol. 7, No. 2 (March, 2000), p. 134.

6. Oscar Cullmann, "Immortality of the Soul or Resurrection of the Dead?" in *Immortality and Resurrection: Death in the Western World: Two Conflicting Currents of Thought,* Krister Stendahl, ed. (New York: Macmillan, 1965), pp. 9-53, esp. pp. 12-20.

Christ in spite of threats of persecution are commended because they did not love their lives so much as to shrink from death. This is why Jesus could say, "For whoever wants to save his life will lose it. But, whoever loses his life for me and for the gospel will save it" (Matt. 10:39 and Matt. 16:25). Life is valuable and transcends this world. Therefore, death is an enemy, though a defeated one.

Before suggesting what this might mean for the question of whether it is a lack of faith to resort to palliative care, we must also attempt to gain a certain perspective on faith. Religious people sometimes think of faith in terms that God will act to answer all of their prayers and fulfill their agendas. After all, it was Jesus himself who said, "I tell you the truth. If you have faith as small as a mustard seed, you can say to this mountain, 'Move from here to there.' And it will. Nothing will be impossible for you" (Matt. 17:20). If one reads this passage isolated from other texts, one might easily conclude that it would be a lack of faith for the medical profession to cease curative care if nothing is impossible for God. How can we give up trying? If there is no cure, doesn't it just mean we haven't prayed with enough faith to move the mountain? But a closer look at Scripture as a whole shows a different and deeper concept of faith.

Faith does not simply believe that God will fulfill our agenda. It trusts him even when our prayers seem to go unanswered. There are numerous Biblical examples of this. Daniel 3 recounts Shadrach, Meshach and Abednego, Daniel's companions, being placed in a blazing furnace because they would not bow down to a golden statue. "O Nebuchadnezzar. We don't need to defend ourselves before you in this matter. If we are thrown into the blazing furnace, the God we serve is able to save us from it. And he will rescue us from your hand, O king. But even if he does not, we want you to know, O king, that we will not serve your gods or worship the image of gold you have set up." Notice the words "even if not." These men gave witness to a faith that continues its commitment to God even if he did not rescue them from this furnace.

Another Biblical example. After the Hebrew prophet Habakkuk had argued with God how it could possibly be just for the Babylonians, those evil people, to come and destroy Judah as God had predicted, his dialogue with God and his sense of the presence of God finally led him to submission. And he said, "Even though the fig tree does not bud, and there are no grapes on the vines. Even though the olive crops fail and the fields produce no food. Even though there are no sheep in the pen and no cattle in the stalls. Yet, I will rejoice in the LORD. I will be joyful in God my Savior" (Hab. 3:17-18).

One more Biblical example. The apostle Paul, while imprisoned in Rome awaiting trial, facing the possibility of death, wrote to the Philippians. And he said, "But even if I am being poured out like a drink offering on the sacrifice and service coming from your faith, I am glad and rejoice with all of you" (Phil. 2:17).

Notice the "even if" quality of faith in all three of these Biblical examples. The deepest Biblical faith is trusting God even if, even though. Even if he doesn't fulfill our agenda. Even if our prayers don't seem to be answered in our way. A more shallow view of faith can lead to cruelty. You see, if every person's failure to get what he or she prayed for is simply a lack of their faith, I can blame them for not having more faith. I remember a friend whose daughter was in a serious car accident. They thought she would die, but fortunately she lived. She did have some permanent damage, though amazingly small considering the severity of the accident. Some "friends," you know the kind, with whom you don't need enemies, came to them afterwards and told them that their daughter would have been healed completely if they had just been able to pray with more faith. The fact is, however, we do not have any way to answer the problem of why in some cases there is cure and in some cases there isn't. We have no way in this world of knowing the why to each of our questions. But, we do know who is with us.

Standing in front of my class several years ago, I specifically prayed for two things: that God would help them in their exam and that he would provide safety as they traveled home for Christmas vacation. God certainly answered the prayer for help on the test. I recall a bright and beautiful young woman sitting in the front row. She wrote a great essay and the "A" I gave her hardly did justice to the depth of her thought. A couple of hours later, I learned that halfway to her home in Seattle, the car she was traveling in hit ice on a freeway off-ramp, slid into another car, and she was killed instantly. She was the only one killed in the accident. I have no way of explaining why she died and the others lived.

Biblically, faith does not simply believe that God will do what we ask. It is the belief that God, according to Romans 8:28, continues to work for good in all situations, even those situations that are not good and are contrary to his ultimate will. True faith is persistent trust in God "even if" we cannot understand the tragedies of life. "Even when" we cannot answer why.

Biblical faith has a communal element to it. When Paul expresses his faith even if he is imprisoned and facing death, notice that he goes on to add, "I will be glad and rejoice with you, and I want you to rejoice with me." For Paul, faith is not an autonomous, individual trust in God. It involves a shared experience with others. True faith means joining a body with others and, as he says in both Romans 12:15 and 1 Corinthians 12:26, rejoicing with those who rejoice and weeping with those who mourn. There is this "with each other" quality of faith as well. Faith is communal. Now we're finally ready to answer the initial question. Hence, I believe there are three reasons as to why curative care can move to palliative care while remaining consistent with faith.

First, consistent with the view that death is a defeated enemy, palliative care neither romanticizes death and accepts the easy road of practices such as assisted suicide, nor avoids the subject. Rather, palliative care accepts death realistically and treats the dying patient holistically.

Second, palliative care is consistent with this "even if" quality of faith. Palliative care accepts the inevitability of death and seeks to confront that inevitability without giving up on life. It attempts to continue finding meaning and even joy in life for the dying and their families. Through its holistic approach, it seeks to face the inevitability of death without sinking into despair. It recognizes that fighting the disease is no longer sensible, but it continues to find strength and meaning in the atmosphere of nurture and support that palliative care provides. In this sense, palliative care can become a powerful example of that "even if" quality of faith, that finding meaning in God even though death is imminent. There's a skill in knowing when to fight and when not to fight. There comes a time when the decay of death has come so close that we must accept it's reality. Christians must fight death. Death is not God's will. But there comes a time not to fight. It is a time to relieve suffering and try to make the most of each day. The reason that Christians carry on medical work around the world is the belief that death is the enemy. But it is a defeated enemy.

Third, palliative care is consistent with the communal nature of faith and its holistic embrace of those elements that go beyond physical care and focus on the deeper issue of relationships, meaning, and the realm of the spirit. They are faithful to that "with each other" element of faith. I think of Grace, a member of my congregation. She was dying of cancer in an acute care hospital. Grace was a single, middle-aged woman, an only child who had no family. She had never married, and both of her parents had died. She herself had been a nurse in this very hospital and knew most of the physicians and nurses who cared for her personally. I remember one day she spoke of the care she had received in that hospital and how every physical need had been met. I quote her directly at this point, not because I approve of her language, but because I fear that without quoting her directly I wouldn't be able to share the intensity of what she said. She said, "They've all been so competent and so kind. But I wish that just once, they could be real with me and share the emotions of what is happening. I know it's hard on them." She went on to say, "I know they care. Sometimes I hear them go outside the door and cry in the hall as they leave. But I wish, just once, they could share that with me, but they never do. They're just too damn professional."

Palliative care seeks to take away this wall of impersonal professionalism and offer holistic support. It's willing to be with in the true sense of faith. Willing to rejoice with and weep with. Fighting not for cure, but for meaning. Offering no cure for the disease, but providing care for the discomfort. Always hoping for a miracle, but continuing to trust and hope even if no miracle occurs. Attempting to continue relating to the patient as a whole person with honesty, sensitivity and caring.

152 House Calls on Cardinal Jackson

David Schiedermayer

House calls are easily scheduled. You look on your pocket calendar for a time when you are not in meetings or in clinic. Over the lunch hour, maybe. You call the person you are going to see, tell him or her of your plans, then see if he or she agrees. You don't even need a secretary to make the arrangements for you. Like a rendezvous with a friend, a house call is something you'd best plan yourself. And don't forget to ask for directions.

I BEGAN VISITING Cardinal Jackson when she was seventy-three. Now she's seventy-nine. She lives in the central city of Milwaukee. If you take 27th Street north from Wisconsin Avenue, you pass Family Hospital, now out of business. You pass the businessmen cruising for prostitutes on State. You pass the porn shops, the pawn shops, the checks-cashed shops, and you turn and finally arrive at a neighborhood where a large factory provides several hundred decent jobs. Around this factory, neat little green-lawned homes prove that jobs mean life and love. Some of the homes have chain-link fences with gates in front of them. Cardinal's home has such a fence, with a little latch on the gate that you have to lift up. No drug houses on her street, but more people hanging around the corners than a suburban doc is used to, so I fumble quickly at the latch.

My 78 Dodge Colt, golden and rusted, sits by the curb. I use it for house calls because no one ever bothers to steal it or anything in it. But even if I owned a nicer car, say a pricey little Toyota, I don't think I'd be afraid to drive it in Cardinal's neighborhood. You see, there's a factory there. Things are made near her house, heavy metal parts for engines, and Cardinal's daughter married a hard-working man. He can afford to live in this part of town.

His name is Joe Brown. I've only met him once, but I always feel his presence in the house. When I thought during one of Cardinal's hospitalizations that she was going to die, I spoke to Joe, who ran the family meeting.

"I'm sorry, really sorry to tell you all this. But we think that Cardinal is now dying. Her temperature has been over 105 for more than a day, in spite of very strong antibiotics. I'm sorry to bring you this news. We're doing all

From David Schiedermayer, "House Calls on Cardinal Jackson," in *Putting the Soul Back in Medicine: Reflections on Compassion and Ethics* (Baker Publishing Group, 1994).

we can to keep her comfortable. She's getting Tylenol and pain medicines and she doesn't seem to be suffering from the fever."

"Doctor, when will it be? Do you know?"

"I don't know. But she can't go on like this. The fever is too high. It takes too much out of her, especially at her age. And then there is the pneumonia. It's not much better and could be getting worse."

"Thanks for calling us all here. The whole family in town is here. We will just wait. Does anyone have any questions?"

Of course, I was wrong about Cardinal. After a day or two she opened her eyes again. The fever resolved. She went home. Joe was puzzled by my deathbed predictions, I heard later from his wife. Cardinal had looked worse before.

When I walk up the steps — past neatly trimmed grass, yellow tulips, some Japanese yews — and knock on the door, it is always Cardinal's daughter who answers. Mrs. Brown was a nurse when I first met her. I agreed to see her mother at home. Six years have passed, six years of turning and wiping and washing Cardinal Jackson. Six years of house calls every month or two or three, six or seven hospitalizations for pneumonias which didn't respond to antibiotics. Always the nurse-daughter answers the door.

"Good morning, Mrs. Brown. How are you today? How is Mrs. Jackson? I haven't talked to you since we talked on the phone a while back."

"Good morning, doctor. How are you?"

"Okay, really okay. What a hot summer, eh? I think maybe I'm not dressed for it. And I don't have air conditioning in my car."

"Oh, yes, it's hot. And mother feels it. She's always cool, her skin seems to stay so cool, and during the summer she heats up to about right."

"Is she still having a fever?"

"Well, only about 101 axillary."

I go to the bedside, pulling out my stethoscope. "Let's listen. Hello, Mrs. Jackson. Dr. Schiedermayer. I'm just going to listen to your lungs. Look at those braids! Who did those?"

"The kids do that. Sometimes I do. Does she sound okay?"

"Yeah, alright. But she does have the gurgles."

"Same?"

"Same, yeah. But her skin looks good. Let's look at the urine in the catheter. Looks pretty clear too, doesn't it?"

Always, when I see Cardinal Jackson, I am obsessed with her eyes. They are green, humid, warm, and smoky. Her freckles, her tiny gray braids, her smooth skin. She doesn't look a day over sixty. And she has been mindless, lights-are-on-but-nobody's-home, for over ten years. But her eyes are as wild as a girl's. They cannot say all they have seen, but that is the wonder and the mystery of Cardinal Jackson's eyes.

When she was born they named girls after birds and boys after old men. She grew up in tough times, knew hard work and poverty well enough. That is why her eyes surprise even more. You would think they would be small and cold and stony from all they had seen. But they are full as the moon, luminous and sweet.

Cardinal Jackson is always in the end of the living room. The room is set up especially for her. Mrs. Jackson's bed and medical supplies have been where they are for nearly a decade now. Occasionally the TV and sofa are moved, but the bed remains fixed. I suppose there's no other way to turn it, and if it were in the other part of the room there wouldn't be room for the sofa and the TV. I turn and speak again to Mrs. Jackson's daughter.

"The urine looks as if it is flowing all right. I don't think the fever is from a urine infection, but if we need to use antibiotics we should probably use strong ones to cover urine germs also. Do you have enough potassium?"

"Yes, I think so, but I'm going to need more Tylenol. Also, will you send the copy of the order to the home-health-care office?"

"Sure. I'll check. Now, what's happening with her skin here . . ."

"A little breakdown on mother's heel. I have a dressing on it and we are using the heel protector."

"Good; let me know if it opens up. Good; it looks like it's healing. It looks okay for now. Is she having good bowel movements?"

"Oh, yes. This new tube feeding is real good for that. Real good."

"Good. Cardinal. Cardinal! I'm going to look at your hands."

"She holds them so tight. We've got that new pad in there. If we don't use it sometimes she'll scratch herself bad right on the inside of the hand there."

"It works. This kind of protector works."

"Yeah, it's working well. I keep her nails short, too, so she won't dig them in so much like before."

"Good. I'm sorry, I can't remember now. Have we given her a flu shot every year? This year?"

"Yes. The nurse came last fall."

"Okay, we'll do it again in about two months. October. Remind me. I'll try to write it down, too. Anything else?"

"Doctor, look at this."

"Hmmm. Yes, I see that."

"What is it?"

"Well, I think just a skin growth. A skin growth, but not cancer. It comes on with aging. Has it always been that big?"

"Yes, lately."

"We'll keep an eye on it. She looks good. You have been doing a good job with her. Goodbye, Cardinal! Goodbye, Mrs. Brown."

"Goodbye, Dr. S. I'll let you out. Thank you so much for coming."

"Sure. Thank you. Call me if the fever comes back. Bye!"

The door is doubly unlocked and then doubly locked

again after I leave. It's hot and miserably humid outside. A central air conditioner is humming at the side of the house.

I turn on the radio as I drive back to the hospital. I like Wisconsin Public Radio, but today they're talking about all the drive-by shootings in the inner city. The Dodge feels a bit less invincible. So I just switch over to country music. The song is about somebody's grandmother's eyes.

I DRIVE BY the factory. It's the change of shift. They still wear those blue-gray working shirts that my grandpa wore when he worked as a foreman in the paper mill. They still carry lunches in steel buckets, probably with a small thermos tucked in the upper cover. Saves the price of a cup of coffee. I drive by the girls, the porno, the booze. I think of Cardinal's green eyes. Somehow they help me keep driving, keep my eyes straight ahead.

WHEN YOU MAKE house calls, an old Wisconsin doc once told me, you should somehow find your way back to the kitchen. The kitchen is where you learn about a patient's personality and interests and religion. Kitchens are much better than most rooms, especially for learning about religion. (I have had coffee in Cardinal Jackson's kitchen; it is small but clean.)

One long glance in the fridge can be worth more than months of futile questioning about dietary compliance in the clinic. If a diabetic has high blood sugars, look at what he or she eats.

Dress modestly. Carry a black bag if you have one, a stethoscope if you don't. When you examine the patient, if dignity permits, have a family member present. Always look at the patient's hands and ask about his or her bowels. Talk to both the patient and the family members.

Keep your eyes open, but don't snoop. Don't open any drawers, but check for pets and insects and look at the art. Remember the smell of a patient's house; let it register deep in your brain, and you may be able to recall it when you talk to the patient on the phone or see the patient in the office.

Maybe keep some notes. Linger just a little while longer than you really have to. People can tell.

After making house calls to a patient, you naturally want to go to the funeral when he or she dies. In fact, when you make house calls you are kind of expected at the funeral. Don't miss a one, especially in churches where the people are so used to singing they don't use hymnals.

The old doc told me, the way things are going in medicine, doctors should make house calls whenever they can find an excuse. I have found at least three or four.

ONCE YOU HAVE dementia or some other seriously mind-destroying illness, your family usually doesn't take any more pictures of you. Even though Cardinal is beloved, this is true of her. Her last picture was taken when she was fifty-five, maybe sixty. Her smile is dignified. She is erect. She looks right at you. Her hair is a bit less gray, her eyes are always the same, but the smile says she sees the camera and knows the photographer. She doesn't know the photographer anymore. No use taking pictures. The lights, oh the green lights, are on, but nobody's home, nobody's home.

WHEN I GET BACK to the medical school I go to my office, which is near the anatomy lab. Sometimes I go over and sign out the large bucket with the preserved brains in it. I give talks at schools about the brain. The most striking thing about the preserved brain is the heaviness. It is all dead weight, more like an amputated limb than a brain. Lifting it is like picking up an unexpectedly heavy stone.

The children sit enthralled at the sight and the smell of the brain. They want me to put the brain back in the skull I bring, but I explain that the brain is not the skull's own brain. I see them struggle with the concept of human dissection and disembodiment. I am sympathetic; I struggle too. What kind of person was that skull, they ask. Was it a boy or a girl?

I can only tell them that it is good for them to take both their brains and skulls to school. One is tempted, in school, to use them well, even show them off a bit. Learn while you can, I tell them. Soon enough, the brain turns to mush. And I think of Cardinal Jackson.

Cardinal was the old kind of no-nonsense, have-fun, sing-like-an-angel Christian. Her family has been objectively blessed through it, but I wonder if they can see this as I can.

Anyway, Cardinal is now blessed. She is rocked like a baby by her daughter as if that is the normal thing to do. She is cradled, blissfully ignorant, through her slow dying and all of her leakiness. Sing it for me, the blind preacher says, when the soloist finishes the song. Sing the old song about the amazing grace of God. Please sing.

I AM ON the phone with Mrs. Brown, "Cardinal's fever is still there?"

"Yes, and now it's up to around 103, 104. The only time it goes down is right after the Tylenol."

"Well, I guess we'll have to go with antibiotics again. Did she have diarrhea with the Keflex last time?"

"Yes, quite a bit."

"Well, let's try Cipro. Didn't that work before?"

"Yes, it knocked the fever out in two or three days. And you know, doctor, that the fever didn't come back after that one for quite a while."

"Well, let's try it. I'll call it in to the pharmacy. Is she breathing pretty fast with the fever?"

"Yes, pretty fast, and even grunting a little bit. But thanks for calling me back. And can you plan a visit a bit sooner than usual?"

"Sure. I will be there tomorrow over the noon hour. Or let's make it in the morning, around eleven."

"Okay. And can you call in some more potassium and Tylenol, too?"

"Sure I can. I don't like the rapid breathing. Keep in touch. Bye."

"Goodbye."

When I lecture, the students ask me why I keep treating her. Why not just stop treating, they ask.

Why not? Six years of knowing her, that's why not. A dozen life-threatening infections, that's why not. Already a no-code (no CPR), that's why not. Already no intensive care unit treatment, that's why not. Another doctor started the feeding, and I began caring for the patient after she had been on tube feeding for four years, that's why not. I asked the daughter several times about stopping tube feeding. Shocked her each time, and she said definitely no each time, that's why not.

A socioeconomic history of discrimination and mistreatment or undertreatment, that's why not. A tradition of poor health care and nontreatment, that's why not. The need to show her somehow we're not abandoning her, that's why not. Because her daughter's a nurse, that's why not. Because her daughter loves her and thinks it's best to keep doing things just like we are, that's why not. Because I can't stand to think of the fire dying in those green eyes, that's why not.

But why not just let her die, they ask.

And I try but I really can't explain. I can't say it. I honestly can't. It just doesn't make sense to them. They just don't understand yet, but they will understand when they have a Cardinal of their own.

Dying, you want dying, I guess I should say to them. I know how to stop treatment and let dying happen. I have stood by the bedside of plenty of patients. I have seen long, slow dying.

I have witnessed the leaving, the parting, the closing.

For example.

He has cancer of the lung but is dying of the union of the tumor's appetite with his fatigue and pain and depression. I have given him pain medication and done what I could, but he has been going downhill for the last several days, blood pressure drifting lower, pulse thready, breathing irregular. Now as I stand in his room I think that death has moved in before me, slipping in the door ahead of me.

The man's eyes are already distant. The room is cold and humming. Death has been a whispering wind in his sleep, sweeping away.

So then, I should ask the students, so then are we children of the sun or of the earth? If the students will answer this question, then I will also tell them why I don't just let Cardinal Jackson die.

What is it that gives a person dignity? What is that inner grace which projects out toward the doctor so that he, despite his intellect and education and training and skills, is taken aback? Whatever it is, Cardinal has it. And she has passed it on to her daughter. It manifests itself as inner ability, as a palpable sense of self. The dignified are above reproach.

Cardinal even moans with dignity. You can't take dignity away from the dignified. They wear it too lightly.

Once, Cardinal became critically ill in the middle of the night and the paramedics took her to the nearest hospital — not mine. Another physician took care of her, and when he called me up to tell me of his treatment plans I realized that Cardinal's disease was ordinary. To him, she looked like an old demented patient with recurrent pneumonias. He just hadn't ever seen her picture. He hadn't seen her eyes. They always close when she gets very sick. It wasn't even his fault, but he took care of her like she was a vegetable. And her family knew it. After she was discharged from the hospital, her daughter called me.

"Doctor?"

"Yes, Mrs. Brown. I heard she was in the hospital. How is she doing now? How is her breathing now?"

"She's got a bit of diarrhea from what's left of the antibiotic from the hospital. But her breathing is a lot better."

"Good. But let's try stopping the antibiotic and backing down on her tube feeding a bit. Is she still at a total of five cans a day?"

"Yes. But I've been giving her a lot of water too, because I was worried about the diarrhea."

"Well, let's back down to two cans a day, just for a day or two. But keep going with the water."

"All right."

"Is it real loose?"

"Yes, pretty much. But it is brown, and I don't see any blood."

"Good. Good. Any bedsores on her butt?"

"No, we keep her pretty well turned."

One time when I made a house call, Cardinal was so sick we had to hospitalize her emergently. I drove her daughter to the hospital. I asked her whether she ever thought about Cardinal dying.

"Oh, yes, I think about it sometimes."

"This may be the time. She's breathing fifty times a minute, and I know you don't want the respirator."

"No, no respirator. Still, God will take her when he's good and ready."

"You think soon? You mean, you think he's not going to take her this time? You think . . ."

"Well, not yet. I think she'll go more quietly, at home some night."

"Hmmm. Yes."

Cardinal does not survive because of me. She is alive because her daughter is a nurse. You can't hire love like hers. Cardinal would have been slain by a bedsore years ago if she had lived in some nursing homes. I don't know the exact cost of her care, but it's probably a lot and would be a lot more if her daughter weren't her main nurse.

The weather was turning colder. To be more specific,

twelve inches of snow had fallen, and a cold sun was shining. The temperature was way below zero. I slipped through the chain-link fence and rang the doorbell.

"Hello, Mrs. Brown. What a cold day!"

"Hello, Dr. S. How are you?"

"Okay. How are you? How's Cardinal? She looks like she's resting well. And look at her hair this time!"

"Oh, she's doing pretty well, doctor. She's had a temperature of about 101, but her cough is pretty clear."

"Good. Let's see how she's doing. Her lungs sound about the same. Do you need more Tylenol?"

"Yes, I think it would be good to have some more."

"Good. Hi, Cardinal. She's really awake today. Look at these beads! How do you do this?"

"Oh, my daughter did that for Mom."

"She looks like a little girl today."

"Yes, she does." Mrs. Brown turns to a young woman who comes through the kitchen door. "Doctor S., this is my daughter, Alicia."

"Hello, Alicia. I don't think I've met you before."

"Yes, well, I've been away in the army and in school."

"Oh, what school? Far away?"

"The U."

"That's a good school. Good. What are you studying?"

"Biology."

"Oh, yeah? I studied that once or twice myself. Not always an easy topic. They can make it hard."

Mrs. Brown says proudly, "She wants to be a doctor. A pediatrician."

"Great. But it's hard. The studying is hard. They work hard. Lots of phone calls."

"I know it. But I'm doing pretty well in school."

"Well, good. I'm sure you are. Good luck. You've had plenty of practice taking care of your grandmother, here."

Both laugh. "Yes. We sure have. Yes."

Cardinal's eyes are on the ceiling. She doesn't see me when I say goodbye. But her daughter and granddaughter walk me toward the door. We talk some more about medical school. I smell Lubiderm cream. New rug. The television is on, a talk show. No change in the plaques or pictures on the walls. Something good cooking in the kitchen. I remember that smell from before: greens. Mrs. Brown unlocks the door for me, and I have time to glance back toward the bed. Cardinal Jackson is breathing slowly and steadily.

153 God Will Find a Way

Margaret E. Mohrmann

This time the call for a bed in the P.I.C.U. came from the pediatric neurologist. There was a child in intensive care at the National Institutes of Health (N.I.H.) whose parents wanted him transferred so they could be closer to their family. The child, Jermaine Rogers, now sixteen months old, initially had been admitted to our hospital several months earlier by this neurologist because the child had been losing his developmental skills. He no longer attempted to walk and had even lost the ability to sit on his own. His age-appropriate cooing and babbling efforts at language had faded into nothing more than grunts and cries. The evaluation at that time, while it yielded no definitive diagnosis, showed with certainty that he had some sort of degenerative neurological disease that could not fail to follow the course of all similar disorders, more or less swiftly to death. Jermaine's parents, in love with this much-wanted child — their second, born twenty years after the first — could not believe this, especially in the absence of a name for the disease, something they could look up in the library to make sense of the intolerable idea that their child could not be treated and would soon die. At their request, the neurologist referred them to the N.I.H. for a second opinion, and they went gladly.

They were at the N.I.H. for months, spring to fall. There the clinicians and researchers could only confirm the original impression, although they could do so with somewhat more precision. Jermaine had an as-yet-unnamed disorder of the mitochondria, the energy system, of his nerve and muscle cells. His specific version of mitochondrial failure was thus far unique but close enough to other, also rare varieties for the prognosis to be undeniable. His nerve and muscle cells, their energy supply dwindling to zero, were dying off piecemeal, their shared functions weakened then left undone. Jermaine's muscles could no longer support him, and his nerves could not tell them to do so anyway. Even without a textbook entry for the disorder, the N.I.H. physicians had a lot to tell his parents: The inescapable consequence of this deterioration was that, sooner rather than later, Jermaine's respiratory muscles would no longer do the work of breathing for him, and, before or after that happened, his heart muscles would no longer be able to pump blood. There was nothing available, or even remotely imaginable, that medicine could offer to halt the process or to replace function, once lost. A ventilator to support his breathing, when that gave out, would only prolong the inevitable, for nothing could restore the deteriorating muscles of his heart. Even a heart transplant would not begin to solve his problems. Jermaine was going to die, probably within a few months.

However, before they said any of this to his parents, Jermaine stopped breathing, and the N.I.H. physicians, despite what they knew, intubated him and attached the tube to a ventilator to breathe for him, without having discussed the ultimate futility of that move with his parents. Now the N.I.H. staff wanted to take him off the ventilator and allow him to die. Mr. and Mrs. Rogers, although they had by now heard all that the doctors wanted them to know, refused and asked that their son be transferred back to our hospital. Thus the neurologist's request for a P.I.C.U. bed.

I groaned. To give one of the precious four P.I.C.U. beds to a child with no hope of survival (that is not what intensive care is for, I muttered into the phone) but with what promised to be an extended course of dying while his parents fought any attempts to bring the inevitable closer sounded like a nightmare. What fools had put him on the ventilator in the first place? Nothing in medical ethics requires a physician to do something futile. Cowards. Researchers without an ounce of clinical sensitivity in their brains. In my anger (but in my mind only, not aloud, fortunately), I fell back on all the usual slander of "that other hospital" — the lofty status of the N.I.H. notwithstanding — even as I knew that the same thing could well have happened, probably would have happened, at my medical center. It gave me someone to blame for what I now anticipated. But, on the other hand, there were the parents to consider: they needed not to be 500 miles away from family while this tragedy played itself out. We were their home hospital, and, like it or not, we were where they should be for this last act. "Yes, you can have the bed."

Jermaine arrived the next day, much as described. I saw him briefly as I made my rounds that afternoon and heard the nurse's report about his unresponsiveness. He needed no sedation to allow the ventilator to breathe for him; he had some reflex responses but nothing else and did not appear to be uncomfortable or in pain. His parents were described by the P.I.C.U. staff as quiet, friendly people who wanted to be with their son as much as possible, but were gracious in acceding to the requirements of the unit. The nurses' comments let me know that they saw the problem as I did and were resigned to yet another long-term, hopeless boarder, of whom there had been far too many in the P.I.C.U.

We all still carried the haunting memory of Dustin, a patient who had languished in the P.I.C.U. for more than a year because his parents' lawyers insisted there was more money to be extracted from the toy manufacturer they held responsible for his strangulation if Dustin were alive and expensive than if he were dead and no longer a financial burden. He should have been allowed to die months earlier from the pervasive hypoxic damage that had left him unaware of everything but pain, but instead he had been kept alive by all extraordinary means until he finally contracted an overwhelming sepsis that killed him quickly despite treatment. The long days of caring for him and about him had taken their toll on the staff. His parents had dealt with their grief at home; they rarely came in after the first few weeks. "Dustin" became the unit's shorthand for that which was intolerable in pediatric intensive care: intense but futile labor, intense emotional attachment that has no reasonable hope of seeing the beloved child survive, intense moral distress at the staff's helplessness in the face of powerful forces — legal, economic, egotistical, pedagogical, scientific, and so many others — that seemed to care about everything but the welfare of the child and the well-being of the workers. As the nurses told me about Jermaine, I think we all saw Dustin's ghost hovering in the background.

Two days after Jermaine was admitted, the neurologist called me. "I'd like to transfer Jermaine to your service."

Oh, great, I thought, just what I need. "Why?" I asked warily.

"I just can't work with these parents," he spat out through what sounded like clenched teeth. "They simply can't accept his diagnosis and the fact that he's going to die. They won't hear of taking him off the ventilator. They won't even let me talk about it! They're some kind of religious fanatics, you know, and they have this absurd idea that God's going to step in and heal him — and we have to keep him going until God gets around to it!"

He paused, then added with much less heat, "And . . . I think there could be some bad feeling left from when he was in here before. You know, I was the one who had to give them the diagnosis first and, well, I think they just associate me with the bad news."

I'll bet, I mused. You are not exactly famous for your charming bedside manner. Let it go and think, I chastised myself. "Yes, I'll take him. Tell the parents I'll be by later this afternoon to examine him, and then I'll come talk with them."

He signed off with a brusque "Thanks."

What have I done? I wondered. But, to tell the truth, I saw myself as being good at working with "difficult" families. I was quite sure I could convince them to let us take Jermaine off the ventilator. I even remember thinking, with a satisfied snort, "I'll have him out of there by the end of the week." How stupid. Self-righteousness is a constant temptation for those who profess medicine, for whom the pressure to be right creates too many opportunities to feign unwarranted authority or unattained skills. And it can be a most effective blinder, as I learned the hard way in this case, as in others.

I examined Jermaine thoroughly and reviewed his chart. If one could disregard the ventilator attachment and his location in an I.C.U., Jermaine looked like a peacefully sleeping, healthy, beautiful toddler, with a full head of curly dark hair, long curving eyelashes, smooth and unmarked coffee-colored skin, and an easy rise and fall of his chest with each breath. But this was a child who would neither rouse from his sleep nor shake off his posture of repose. Jermaine was not brain dead, but he was certainly absent. Although he was receiving no sedating or paralyzing medications, he responded to neither verbal nor physical stimuli, with the exception of an occasional withdrawal reflex when a finger was pinched. These reflex responses were not accompanied by grimaces or any changes in his pulse rate, so they did appear to be reflexes only and not evidence of awareness of pain. His limbs were flaccid. He had been quite stable since his return to us, requiring no changes in ventilator settings and no additional oxygen. His lungs were normal — it was his chest muscles that no longer worked. His pulse was a bit fast and his blood pressure at the lower limits of normal for his age. All was as the neurologist had described.

My conversation with Jermaine's parents was a revelation. Jermaine's parents had met in college, where they were both accounting majors. After graduation they had started a small business in a town less than thirty minutes from our hospital, where they could be close to both families. Their accounting firm had been modestly successful, such that they were able to hire a replacement for Mrs. Rogers while she was with Jermaine at the N.I.H.; Mr. Rogers had stayed behind to continue running the business. Their enforced separation seemed to have been one of the major reasons for their requesting Jermaine's transfer back to us — that and the presence of their large extended family back home, plus a church community in which they were deeply involved. They had found it impossible to live through such a crisis so far from all that held them together as a family and as individuals.

They treasured their older child, now in her last year of college, but had always wanted more children. It had not seemed to be in the cards until the "miraculous" pregnancy with Jermaine happened, long after they had stopped hoping for another child. He was a beautiful, healthy baby who was precocious in his development, ready to walk at nine months, and generous in his affections. Then came the incomprehensible changes: his attention turned inward, his smiles fewer, and he showed no interest in standing up — followed by the day when he could no longer sit without support. That was the signal to them that he was not just taking a breather from his accelerated developmental course. He was moving backward, losing the skills he had already mastered so easily.

We discussed the process of diagnosis and what it had been like for them to hear the verdict. They briefly mentioned that the neurologist's abruptness had exacerbated the pain of his message, but were at pains to assure me that they had never doubted his explanations and prognosis. Their insistence on a second opinion had to do with their perception of their obligations to Jermaine, and to God, rather than with any lack of trust in the neurologist's competence or truthfulness. They understood and accepted the information he had given them, as they did the more detailed confirmation from the N.I.H. doctors — they could, in fact, tell me more about it than I had already gleaned. However, they did not believe that the medical pronouncements were the last word on Jermaine. Their faith, the central motif of their lives, assured them that God was in charge of prognoses and could effect a cure, or some other form of recovery, despite the hopeless picture presented by the medical experts. They did not know whether God *would* do so in this case — they were far from blindly optimistic — but they were quite sure the decision was God's to make and not theirs or ours.

After that first discussion, we parted amicably. I had a lot to think about. I felt great respect and admiration for their strength, their understanding, and, yes, the solidity of their belief. They were not the "fanatics" the neurologist had declared them to be, not by my understanding of the word. They were intelligent, reasonable people, facing an unfathomable grief with courage and steadfastness, while remaining faithful to the truth of their lives. I began to reconstrue my obligations as not only to care for Jermaine but also to honor his parents as they found their own way through this dreadful upheaval.

Little changed over the next few weeks, with the exception of the growing restlessness of some of my colleagues. The head of the adult medical I.C.U., the unit that got the P.I.C.U.'s "overflow" when its four beds were full, as was usually the case, called me daily to quiz me about my apparent commitment to providing futile care in the P.I.C.U. As he intoned, more than once, we are under no moral or legal obligation to provide futile care (conveniently begging the basic question of how to define *futile*). He urged me to take Jermaine off the ventilator, to let him die and free up the P.I.C.U.'s allotment of scarce resources. I understood his point all too well; I had often been the one making the same argument to other physicians with patients in the P.I.C.U. who, in my view, should not be there. Dustin's case had been a paradigm of futility and frustration. But at the same time, I continued to talk with Jermaine's parents, and I knew I could not make a unilateral decision to stop life support. There was work going on here that was not futile.

In one of my many conversations with Jermaine's parents, after we had come to know each other better, I heard more of their beliefs about God's willingness to intervene directly in people's lives, to heal just at the time when there seems no hope of healing. Because they had been so honest with me about their faith, I thought I could say something of what I believed. This was by no means a usual practice for me, but in this situation I felt sharply the mismatch between their giving and my receiving. They had been open with me, trusting that I would respect what they said and neither turn away nor try to overcome their theology with my science. I could no longer be only a blank sounding board. Tentatively, I ventured out.

"I also believe that God is involved somehow, even intensely involved, in our illnesses and our healings," I said. "But I just can't believe God plays games with us, especially about something as painful as this. I mean, if God were going to cure Jermaine, I think it would have happened long before now. I don't think God would wait until Jermaine's brain and body are so terribly damaged and you have gone through these months of agony, just to pull it out at the end so it looks like an even bigger miracle. It would have been a miracle seven months ago. Why wait?"

They nodded their understanding of my position; I suspect they had been there several times over. Mr. Rogers responded: "That may be true. You may be right. But we just don't know, do we? We don't know what God may be going to do. And our job, while we're waiting to see what he'll do, is to make sure we don't place any obstacles in his way. If we take Jermaine off that ventilator, we take away from God any chance of his acting. We can't do that."

I began to see more clearly then an idea that had been taking shape in my mind over the years I had been caring for critically ill children. There was a definite limit — its location not always distinct, but the fact of the boundary certain nonetheless — to what I could do for patients in my care. My knowledge and skill were of primary importance and had to be used well on their behalf, but, once all that could and should be done was done, the children would survive or they would not. The families, however, especially the parents, would without question outlive their child's illness. The quality of *their* survival — what the rest of their lives would be like after the critical event, with or without a surviving child — had something to do with how I worked with them during the crisis. In the case of Jermaine's parents, in particular, I realized that, although Jermaine would surely die (I still did not believe God would stage a last minute restoration), it was of central importance to his parents' future that they be able to remember that in the midst of the struggle they had remained faithful to Jermaine and to God, according to their understanding of what such fidelity required.

During that conversation, or perhaps another, I found that they were familiar with the concept of brain death. Further, were Jermaine brain dead, they would interpret that to be sufficient evidence that God did not intend to heal him, and they then would not oppose taking him off life support. That interchange led me to ask them whether there were situations other than brain death that might also count as reliable signs that Jermaine's death was within God's will. Puzzled, they asked for examples. Well, I posited, he could develop an overwhelming infection, as happens to children on ventilators and intravenous feedings, that might outstrip the power of any antibiotic we have available. Yes, they thought, that would be convincing. If the antibiotics could not stop the infection, there would be no point in doing anything more, no point in trying to resuscitate him if his heart stopped because of the sepsis.

And then, I said, there is his heart. We had talked before about the evidence we already had that Jermaine's disease was sapping the strength of his heart muscle. His rapid pulse and low-normal blood pressure had been the first indications of a heart trying harder but accomplishing less. Subsequent studies had confirmed that his heart was becoming as flabby and unresponsive to nerve impulses as had the rest of his musculature. We had put him on a medication to support his blood pressure, but it provided only slight improvement. I had not expected, nor led his parents to expect, that it would make much difference — thus, I could justify its use to myself, believing that it could not significantly prolong the inevitable but would honor his parents' desires for treatment. We had discussed the likelihood that Jermaine's death would come that way, as heart failure that we could not overcome. Now I asked if that too would count as evidence that God was not going to work a miracle for Jermaine. Yes, they nodded, certainly. They agreed that resuscitative efforts were not to be used if Jermaine's heart failed. No "code," no chest compressions, no frantic attempts to infuse energy into a heart that could no longer use it.

It was only a few days after we had that conversation that Jermaine's heart gave up the struggle. That morning his blood pressure began dropping steadily, despite the medication still flowing into his veins. His parents had not yet come in to visit. I called them at home to describe what was happening. They knew what it meant and decided to stay home and gather their family and friends around them while I kept them informed by phone. Within the hour, Jermaine's heart went into "electromechanical dissociation," a condition in which the nerves stimulate the heart appropriately, as indicated by the electrocardiogram (E.K.G.), but the heart muscle fails to respond by contracting. Despite electrical activity mimicking a normal E.K.G., there is no pulse, no pumping action by the heart, no flow of blood through the body. In Jermaine's case, this was the final degeneration. He died quietly, almost ten weeks after his return from the N.I.H.

I called his parents to tell them that Jermaine was dead. They thanked me briefly and hung up. They called back later to give information about the funeral home they had chosen. I never heard from them again, but I have never forgotten what they taught me. Nor have I ever doubted that keeping Jermaine on the ventilator was the right thing to do. Had there been any evidence that he was suffering, it would have been a different matter. I cannot be certain how things would have turned out in that event, although I imagine I would have been called on, by his parents and by my own sense of obligation, to do all possible to relieve that suffering before using it as a trumping argument for stopping his life support. Were his suffering ultimately unrelievable, I like to think they would have agreed not to force Jermaine to stay in his tortured body. They, I suspect, know the scriptures better than I: God does not test us beyond our power to endure, but always provides a way out.

I have said that I realized, in working with Jermaine's parents, that the nature of my encounters with them could have some effect on the quality of their survival of such a terrible loss. I still believe this to be true, although, as is the case with most of the families I have known, I do not know how their lives after Jermaine's death played out. I hope they have continued to find the strength and consolation, in each other and in their beliefs, that carried them through his protracted dying. Their faithfulness — to Jermaine, to God, to themselves, and to their extended families — stands as a lasting reminder to me of the complexity of what we do and whom we touch in medicine and of the truth that, in virtually every serious medical intervention, there is more than one "patient" whose life is at stake.

154 Who Decides?

Gilbert Meilaender

Our focus in the last chapter [of *Bioethics: A Primer for Christians*] was on the substance of treatment decisions — *what* we should do and what criteria governed those choices. Sometimes, however, we may wonder or argue about *who* should decide. We might, of course, simply ask our doctors to decide what is best, and there was a time not that long ago when doctors' recommendations about treatment were seldom disputed. The past few decades, however, have seen a strong rejection of medical paternalism and an increasing emphasis upon patient self-determination. The presumption now is that the patient decides what course of treatment shall be pursued.

Having taken the measure of the language of self-determination in Chapter 6, we should be wary of depicting the possibilities for treatment decisions in this way. Even fully autonomous patients, if there are such, have no absolute right to decide upon their course of treatment. If they did, physicians would simply be technicians, putting their skills (for a price) at the service of our desires. However tempted we might be by that picture, however often medical hubris or paternalism may push us toward it, we should not really want it.[1] A *patient* is something different from a *client,* and a physician is not an automobile mechanic. When he examines, handles, and even cuts upon our body, the doctor lays hold upon our person. As patients, therefore, we quite rightly should be involved in deliberations about the course of our treatment; for our person is involved. But so is the doctor's person involved as he commits himself to care for us. We should not want it any other way.

There may be times, of course, when no agreement is reached between doctor and patient, and the best we can do is withdraw from the mutual bond we have forged. Lacking agreement on the substance of the matter, we take refuge in a procedural solution that leaves both parties free to turn elsewhere. Patients need not submit to doctors' recommendations; doctors need not practice what they consider bad medicine simply because patients

1. We should not want it because it misses the *moral* truth of medicine. In this country, however, the *law* has moved increasingly in the direction of patient autonomy. Here, though, I am reflecting upon what our moral judgment as Christians ought to be when we consider the relation of patient and physician.

From Gilbert Meilaender, "Who Decides?" in *Bioethics: A Primer for Christians,* 2nd ed. (Grand Rapids: Wm. B. Eerdmans, 2005), 75-83.

want it. In a society such as ours — where substantive agreement is sometimes so lacking that a commitment to "fair procedures" is almost all we share — Christian physicians often find themselves in difficult situations. Not wishing to abandon patients who disagree with their judgments about the best course of treatment, they may feel drawn or even compelled to practice what they regard as bad medicine (which is a moral, not just a technical, category). Moreover, there is no guarantee that the medical profession itself will support Christian principles in the practice of medicine. That is already the case with respect to abortion and prenatal screening, and it may increasingly be true of assisted suicide and euthanasia. Christian care-giving institutions, such as hospices, will face similar difficulties if assisted suicide and euthanasia become legally permissible. To be sure, it is one thing to acquiesce in a patient's decision to pursue a course of treatment when the physician simply thinks there are better and wiser courses; it is another to do moral evil in the name of not abandoning one's patient. Christian physicians in our society will probably have to take increasing care to make clear to their patients from the outset their own understanding of good medical practice and the limits to which they adhere.

Incompetent Patients

Even if patients' wishes are not entirely determinative, they may quite rightly want to be involved in deliberations about their course of treatment. (Of course, that involvement may also take the form of saying what they do *not* want to know or intentionally leaving decisions to others, and we should also respect that form of involvement. Personal involvement is not demonstrated only through a concern for mastery and control.) Sometimes, however, patients are unable to participate in deliberations about treatment. This may happen for a short time due to the trauma of injury, but more difficult are cases of patients who will be incompetent to help make decisions for the entire course of their treatment — infants and young children, the severely demented, the retarded, the permanently unconscious. In these cases we are forced to ask in earnest, Who decides?

In recent years the professions of both law and medicine have recommended advance directives — either a living will or a health care power of attorney — as the best way to answer this question. In essence, it attempts to circumvent the question by having the patient, while still competent, determine and state how he wants to be treated if and when he should become incompetent.

Not all patients will have executed an advance directive, however, and, in the very nature of the case, some patients will never be able to do so (because, for example, they are infants, or have been retarded from birth). In those circumstances some have turned to what is called a "substituted judgment" standard, and, in fact, the law sometimes compels us to turn in that direction. According to this approach, we should ask what a patient would have wanted if he were able to tell us. There are, of course, different ways to try to answer such a question. We might assume that he would want what any "reasonable person" would want in his circumstances. But then we may discover that we have no agreed-upon standard of "reasonableness." The blood transfusion that seems reasonable to me will look quite different to the faithful Jehovah's Witness. The lengthy round of chemotherapy that seems choiceworthy to you may look quite undesirable to me.[2]

Taken seriously, therefore, the substituted judgment standard may direct our attention away from the hypothetical reasonable person to the actual person who is the patient. Sometimes we know (from family or friends, for example) a good bit about what this person might have wanted. Sometimes the evidence may be sketchier — when, for example, he once opined in a late-night conversation with friends, "I'd never want to be kept alive on any machines." And sometimes, of course, the patient will be one who has no "track record" of past opinions or decisions — for example, a newborn, or a person who has been profoundly retarded from birth. For such patients substituted judgment seems inappropriate, although courts have sometimes applied it. Thus, for example, in the case of Joseph Saikewicz, who had been retarded from birth and at age sixty-seven suffered from a form of leukemia for which chemotherapy was a possible treatment, the Supreme Court of Massachusetts, attempting to apply a substituted judgment standard, held that "the decision in cases such as this should be that which would be made by the incompetent person, if that person were competent, but taking into account the present and future incompetency of the individual as one of the factors which would necessarily enter into the decision-making process of the competent person."[3] The thought of an utterly hypothetical Saikewicz — who is

2. The difficulty of determining what is "reasonable" is even more troubling when the patient is a child for whom parents ordinarily make decisions. For example, Christian Scientists, who often turn to their own practitioners for faith healing rather than to standard medical practice, have sometimes been prosecuted for child neglect when they have not sought standard care for their seriously ill children. These are hard cases. No society can survive without some minimal agreement about what constitutes "reasonable" care for one's child. Indeed, the very existence of child abuse and neglect laws indicates that, and we would not permit a religious sect to revive the ancient practice of sacrificing the first-born son to God. That would fall beyond the bounds of "reasonableness" for us. Nevertheless, we ought to be reluctant to narrow too quickly our understanding of what is reasonable in approaches to medical care. Impressive as the healing powers of the medical profession are, they are not the only healing powers. To suppose that they are would, for Christians, truly be "unreasonable."

3. Supreme Judicial Court of Massachusetts, 1977. 373 Mass. 728, 370 N.E.2d.417. The case is reprinted in a variety of sources. See, for example, Thomas A. Shannon and Jo Ann Manfra, eds., *Law and Bioethics: Texts with Commentary on Major U.S. Court Decisions* (Ramsey, NJ: Paulist Press, 1982), pp. 173-92.

not the real Joseph Saikewicz at all — being given one moment of lucid rationality in which to decide whether, as the person he actually is, he would want chemotherapy is itself a *reductio ad absurdum* of the attempt to apply a substituted judgment standard in such cases.

It is only our nearly idolatrous attachment to the language of autonomy that drives us to such lengths, of course, and where the law will permit it we should not hesitate to turn from substituted judgment to an attempt simply to assess what is in the patient's *best interests.* To be sure, there is no guarantee that this language will not also lead us astray. For patients with severely diminished capacities, we may too easily be influenced by the fact that we would not desire such a life for ourselves. Instead of asking, "Is his life a benefit to him?" we need to learn to ask, "What, if anything, can we do that will benefit the life he has?" Our task is not to judge the worth of this person's life relative to other possible or actual lives. Our task is to care for the life he has as best we can. Properly applied, a best interests standard can free us from the often futile quest for what he would have wanted. It can free our energies and direct them toward the right question: Given the person he is now and has become, how can we best nourish and care for the life he has?

Advance Directives

Obviously, some of these difficulties, for some patients, can be avoided if they have expressed their treatment preferences in advance — if, that is, they have, while competent, formally stated how they wish to be treated if a day comes when they are incompetent and unable to participate in decision making. An advance directive is an attempt to extend our autonomy into a future time when we are no longer autonomous. As such, it is a product of the emphasis upon self-determination within our society over the last several decades, and it even has about it an illusory quality that attempts to give privileged status to one moment of independence in the course of an entire life that begins in dependence and, often, ends in dependence. Therefore, if they are not used with care, advance directives give rise to a kind of metaphysical self-deception.

Two forms of advance directives have been developed. What is called a "living will" was first given legal standing by the state of California in 1976. In enacting a living will I attempt to describe in advance the possible medical conditions that might overtake me in the future, and I attempt also to stipulate how I would want to be treated (or not treated) under those conditions. Developed at a time when the chief concern was the heavy hand of medical paternalism, the living will has often been conceived as an instrument for refusing treatment, for getting rid of that heavy hand. In principle, however, there is no reason why one could not use such an instrument to express a desire *for* treatment, even for all possible treatments. And, of course, the laws of any state may set limits on the treatments one can refuse or require. By contrast, a health care power of attorney attempts to say less about the future. Eschewing the attempt to predict possible medical conditions or treatments, it simply designates a proxy — one who will be authorized to participate in decision making on my behalf if I become unable to do so.[4]

There is, I think, no single "Christian" position on advance directives, but, in my judgment, we would not be wise to make use of the living will. After the U.S. Supreme Court issued its decision in the Nancy Cruzan case (in 1989), it was reported that the Society for the Right to Die received over 100,000 requests for information about living wills in less than a month. This testifies to an enormous sense of dis-ease within our culture. Even though the normal human biography begins and ends in dependence, we deeply desire independence. That is understandable, of course, and in itself quite appropriate. But it ceases to be appropriate when it invites and encourages us to live a lie. When we attempt so definitively to extend our autonomous choices into that period of life when we are no longer self-determining, we come very close to such self-deception. In part, we deceive ourselves into supposing that we can actually anticipate with precision future medical conditions and possible treatments — a supposition that physicians themselves regularly resisted until lingering guilt over medical paternalism and the onslaught of malpractice litigation led them to acquiesce more readily in anything that appeared to be a patient's decision. More important, however, is the deception that cuts more deeply into our sense of self and encourages us to approach even the grave in a spirit of mastery and control.

Moreover, a living will lets others off the hook too easily. Patients who are unable to make decisions for themselves because, for example, they are severely demented or permanently unconscious have, in a sense, become "strangers" to the rest of us. We see in them what we may one day be, they make us uneasy, and we react with ambivalence. No matter how devoted our care, our uneasiness with a loved one who has become a stranger to us may prompt us to do less than we ought to sustain her life. It is important, therefore, to structure the medical decision-making situation in such a way that conversation is forced among the doctor, other caregivers, the patient's family, and the pastor or priest. Advance directives, often with the force of legal recognition standing behind them, are designed to eliminate the need for such extended conversation. That is part of their problem, for they free us from the need to deal with the ambivalence we feel in caring for a loved one who has now become a burdensome stranger.

I realize, of course, that freeing loved ones from such burdens is supposed to be one of the benefits of a living

4. There are also mixed or combined advance directives in which one both names a proxy and provides that proxy with information about one's treatment preferences. I do not treat this as a separate alternative because, as far as I can tell, it is best described as a slightly different kind of living will.

will, but Christians ought to be wary of such language.[5] For to burden one another is, in large measure, what it means to belong to a family — and to the new family into which we are brought in baptism. Families would not have the significance they do for us if they did not, in fact, give us a claim upon each other. At least in this sphere of life we do not come together as autonomous individuals freely contracting with each other. We simply find ourselves thrown together and asked to share the burdens of life while learning to care for one another. Often, of course, we will resent such claims on our time and energy. Indeed, learning not to resent them is likely to be the work of a lifetime. If we decline to learn the lesson, however, we cease to live in the kind of community that deserves to be called a family, and we are ill prepared to live in the community for which God has redeemed us — a community in which no one stands on the basis of his rights, and all live by that shared love Christians have called charity.

I think, therefore, that we ought to prefer the health care power of attorney to the living will.[6] It too, of course, reaches out into a future beyond the limits of our competence, but it does so in a way that recognizes and affirms dependence. It anticipates and accepts that others will have to bear some burdens for us as we may for them. To medical caregivers it says simply: "Here is a person upon whom I have often been dependent for love and care in the past. Now, when I can no longer participate in decisions about my medical care, I am content to continue to be dependent upon his love and care. Talk with him about what is best for me." In the cultural circumstances in which we find ourselves, I do not think Christians can do better than this.

5. In this paragraph and the preceding one I draw upon the language of my short piece titled "I Want to Burden My Loved Ones," *First Things,* October 1991, pp. 12-14.

6. There may, of course, be some people — especially quite elderly people — for whom no close relatives remain as possible proxies. They may understandably feel driven to enact a living will. One wonders, however, whether the church could not provide better alternatives, whether a proxy within the Body of Christ could not be found.

155 What Shall We Do with Norman? An Experiment in Communal Discernment

Curtis W. Freeman

I. Introduction

Norman was seventy-nine years old and lived alone. He normally kept to himself, but for most of his life he had been actively involved in his church. Norman never married, and he was not close to any of his family. His church family (as he liked to call them) was the only family Norman knew for many years. Norman was always eccentric and usually a little on the cranky side, but it was faithfulness to his friends that was perhaps Norman's most enduring and endearing quality.

Norman always enjoyed an active life. He tried to play golf, walk, or jog every day. One Saturday afternoon while jogging he collapsed in cardiac arrest. By the time the paramedics arrived and stabilized him, he had suffered ischemia from the prolonged CPR. He was taken to the emergency room at a large public hospital where it was determined that he did not meet the criteria of total brain death, and therefore he was not "really dead." Although the neurological damage to his cerebral hemisphere had been sufficient to cause the cessation of its function, his brain stem was still intact. According to hospital policy Norman was placed in CCU where a ventilator was attached to assist his breathing, a nasogastric tube was inserted to provide nutrition, and an intravenous drip was connected to maintain hydration. He was subsequently placed in a geriatric care unit of the hospital.

Norman left no advance directives, and because no immediate family member could be located to act on his behalf the hospital continued to assist his breathing with the ventilator and to provide him with nutrition and hydration. Norman subsequently began to breathe on his own without assistance, but his condition remained unchanged. He was in a state of permanent unconsciousness, and his prognosis was grim. Later diagnosis determined that he was in a persistent vegetative state (PVS). He was unable to accept optimal feeding, and he had several persistent infections, although none of them was life-threatening. A long-time friend, an attorney and

C. W. Freeman, "What Shall We Do with Norman? An Experiment in Communal Discernment," *Christian Bioethics* 2.1 (1996): 16-41. Used by permission.

member of Norman's church family, applied for and was named as his court-appointed guardian. The attorney-friend possessed the legal authority but felt that he lacked the moral authority to make a substituted judgment. He thus turned to the collective wisdom of the church. Among this community of friends he hoped to find discernment and support. In the meantime Norman hovered precariously somewhere near the boundary between life and death.

In one sense there is nothing really unique or unusual about this story. Accounts about people who remain permanently unconscious are common in textbooks, journals, magazines, and newspapers. The issues and arguments have become familiar. But in another sense this story is quite unique and unusual because of *who* was left to make a decision on Norman's behalf and *how* that decision would be made. It was difficult to know just what sort of response to make to Norman, for to me, Norman was not merely a case or a scenario. We were friends, and I was his pastor. I added my voice to others in Norman's church family as we collectively tried to make sense of his life and his death.

Our relationship to one another and to Norman made a difference in the perspective from which we considered the issues of withdrawing and/or withholding treatment. We were not a group of physicians trying to determine what was the best treatment for this patient; nor were we a hospital ethics committee seeking an impartial viewpoint; nor were we a group of policy-wonks attempting to construct a fair set of guidelines to govern other cases like Norman's. We were a group of Christian friends searching for affirmations that lay at the heart of our faith and reached to the limits of our existence.

As we have reflected on our role in deciding whether and/or to what extent we could assist in allowing Norman to die, we were deeply troubled by the moral ambiguity of our involvement. We wanted to resist the morally questionable practice of directly causing the death of anyone — especially a friend (and a helpless, non-competent one at that). This led us as a Christian community to explore the sanctity of life in hopes that it might clear our vision to see the issues at stake and to discern a course to follow. Perhaps our initial expectations were too optimistic, but we found the discussion to be helpful.

One thing we discovered is that our understanding of the sanctity of life has changed. It is no longer an abstract principle that floats timelessly in a world of ideas. As an ethical norm it has come to make sense only within the narrative of a Creator who imbues life with sacredness. The sanctity of life is also a way of seeing things that is rooted in the common stories and the concrete practices which have shaped our shared life in Christ — a shared life that still included Norman. We further realized that the sanctity of life is not finally about life in general. It is ultimately about the sanctity of a particular life; it is about the sanctity of Norman's life.

II. Life and Sanctity in Creation

The collective wisdom of our fellowship was that Norman, incompetent though he may have been, was still a member of the human community. Our faith has taught us that human life is sacred and that we are to regard it with respect. It was, then, important to consider more closely how the sanctity of Norman's life was to shape our moral judgments about how to care for him in his dying. As Christians our understanding of the sanctity of life is situated in the story of creation. This story is paradigmatic because it *informs* our moral judgments, but more importantly because it *forms* our moral sense of selfhood (Goldberg, 1981, pp. 37-38, 176-78; Goldberg, 1985, pp. 13-19). The story provides the fundamental clues for "learning how to construe life and the world in light of such beliefs and with the images in which they are set forth" (Hartt, 1977, p. 241). The first moral task was then to become skilled in the narrative-dependent language so as to interpret and experience our world in terms of that story (Lindbeck, 1984, p. 34). It was therefore important for us to attend to the narrative practice of construing Norman's life as appropriate to God. *Were we respecting the sanctity of this life that had been entrusted to us?*

a. Life as Donation

The creation narrative of Genesis tells of how the Lord God formed the man from the dust and breathed into his nostrils the breath of life (Gen. 2:7). The Creator also planted a garden in Eden and put the man there (Gen. 2:8). This illuminating story enables us to see that human life and the world we inhabit are not of our own making (Brueggemann, 1982, p. 40). The Creator is "the Lord and giver of life," and creation is a gift of the life-giving Lord. The gracious Creator of inexhaustible donation is also the eternal Spirit of creative animation. As Nicholas Lash says, "God is given-ness, . . . and the givenness of God gives life" (Lash, 1993, p. 92). It is this givenness which lies at the center of our understanding of the sanctity of life.

The appeal to the sanctity of life, however, can easily be distorted by *idolatry*. The sanctity of life *does not mean* that we Christians regard life (even *human* life) to be sacred in itself and, therefore, to be sustained to the bitter end. Such claims to the inherent sacredness of life arise from an idolatrous impulse to worship (or reverence) the creation rather than the Creator (Rom. 1:25). Locating the sanctity of life within the story of creation is a safeguard which guides us to learn that the sacredness of human life depends on the Creator's act of blessing the goodness of life by simply giving it. Each life is thus sacred because it is a gift bestowed by a gracious Creator. That the gift of life is, as Karl Barth says, *a loan* suggests our moral responsibility is to learn what it means to hold our existence *in trust* (Barth, 1961, p. 328). We wondered what sort of gestures would signify our acknowledgment of God as Creator.

Of course, it is one thing to affirm the sanctity of life as long as the lives we and our loved ones are entrusted with enjoy minimal suffering and require little sacrifice. It is quite another matter to be faithful to the trust of existence when we become chronically ill or (like Norman) hopelessly overmastered. It is then not without reason that we should ask whether this obligation to receive life sometimes stretches our moral resources beyond the limit. But even then, perhaps especially then, we "hope against hope" (Rom. 4:18) that we will discover a graciousness at the bottom of life that enables us to receive *this* life as a gift of the life-giving Lord.

b. Life as Embodied

When the Creator breathed the breath of life into the man "he became a soul" (Gen. 2:7). It does not say that he *had* a soul. *Having a soul* is Greek; *being a soul* is Hebrew. We humans do not *have* souls; we *are* souls (Wolff, 1974, p. 10). The corollary is also true. We humans do not *have* bodies; we *are* bodies. Although we are not only our bodies, it is only through our bodies that we exist. Thus, we are to understand that the sacredness of life is embodied and that there is no existence apart from the body (Robinson, 1925, p. 366). As Paul Ramsey put the matter, to be a human means to be "an embodied soul or an ensouled body" (Ramsey, 1970, p. xiii).

Being "an embodied soul" is displayed in the restless longing for the *qualitative difference* of a spiritual life that cannot be found in the *quantitative sameness* of mere biological existence, even in a long and healthy life. The qualitative-quantitative tension in human existence is finally resolved by and fulfilled in the Christian hope of the resurrection of the body (1 Cor. 15:35-57). Being "an ensouled body" is marked by the fact that our existence has a destiny that is inextricably linked to the body. God made us to be embodied historical creatures. Unless our biological history is interrupted by accident or distorted by disease, this natural shape moves progressively from birth to death (Meilaender, 1993, p. 29). And because the gift of life comes to us only in the course of embodied existence, the sacredness of human life applies in times of sickness as well as health — in our dying as well as our living. Death stands as the final enemy which robs us of that which God calls into existence and declares to be good. Our most basic moral convictions then are to cherish life and to resist death. Thus, we are not to seek the death of ourselves or anyone else.

The embodiedness of existence can be distorted by the opposite extremes of *dualism* and *vitalism*. In dualism the body is regarded as something which is alien or foreign to the self from which the true self must be freed. It is precisely this dualistic "flight from the *particular*" that was the error of gnosticism (Williams, 1990, p. 25, Williams' emphasis). The church fathers resisted the gnostic solution of salvation *in abstract knowledge*. They maintained instead that the message of redemption is located *in historical existence*. Thus, they developed a theological tradition in which the sacred is known and experienced biologically, i.e., in a body.

Unfortunately, the endless mutations of dualism continue to exert their influence on our understanding of human existence. For example, Daniel Wikler suggests that the definition of death should be changed from total brain death to the "permanent loss of sentience" (Wikler, 1988, pp. 44-45). He argues that this revised definition would remove the moral ambiguity of withdrawing and withholding treatments which maintain PVS patients like Norman. Wikler argues that we should be prepared to declare the body to be alive but the patient not to be alive. This proposed criterion, however, separates the death of the self from the body and thus denies the embodiedness of human existence.

Baruch Brody is rightly suspicious of such efforts to pronounce the permanently unconscious patient to be "dead." Before we do so, he suggests it is important to ask whether we are prepared to bury or cremate a body that is still breathing (Brody, 1988, p. 34). Our moral discomfort at such a thought is exactly what is wrong with the dualistic accounts of human existence which abstract life and death from embodiedness. The Christian account of death remains inextricably linked to the body.

The sacredness of life can also be pushed in the other extreme direction of vitalism, which maintains that "the mere presence of a heartbeat, respiration, or brain activity is compelling reason to sustain all efforts to save the [patient's] life" ("Standards of Judgment for Treatment of Imperiled Newborns," 1987, p. 13). Thus, by vitalistic standards all withholding and withdrawing of treatment is regarded to be morally wrong. The sanctity of the entire natural history of our lives, however, does not necessarily demand that all human life must be preserved at any cost. Indeed, even Karl Barth, who vigorously resisted any form of euthanasia (active or passive) as a violation of the divine command, questioned whether the "artificial prolongation of life does not amount to human arrogance in the opposite direction" of medical fanaticism or human torture (Barth, 1961, p. 427). There is an important distinction to be maintained between *preserving life* and *prolonging death*. Vitalism does not permit this distinction. The difficult matter of moral judgment is the determination of how far we must go in resisting death without becoming vitalists.

Daniel Callahan has argued that medical technology as an ideology has seduced the sanctity of life to the vitalistic extreme so that we must "follow technology wherever it goes so long as it preserves life" (Callahan, 1994, p. 14). This seduction supplies the moral force for using technology to keep alive PVS patients like Norman. Callahan contends that PVS patients are dying and that extending their dying by artificial nutrition and hydration is "extraordinary" treatment. Allowing such a death should, therefore, be regarded as an act of *omission* rather than *commission* (Callahan, 1994, pp. 14-15).[1]

1. Callahan supports this contention by pointing out that artifi-

Gilbert Meilaender counters Callahan by arguing that even if feeding a permanently unconscious patient is considered as medical treatment it should be regarded as "ordinary" care, but Meilaender suggests that the more appropriate distinction to be maintained is between *acknowledging* death (which religious faith allows) and *choosing* or aiming for it (which Jews and Christians in particular reject). He further asserts that someone in a PVS is not a *dying patient* but is a severely *disabled person* (Meilaender, 1994, pp. 15-17; Meilaender, 1987, pp. 102-11).

Meilaender rightly observes that the distinction in moral parlance between killing and letting die is not always clear.[2] Thus, his focus on the *agent* rather than simply the *action* (or *inaction*) is helpful. Moreover, Meilaender *may be* correct that the distinction between omission and commission as a public policy would eventually collapse and thus prepare the way for the kind of direct killing advocated by the euthanasia movement. It is not clear, however, that society would lack the moral and political will to resist that temptation. Two of Meilaender's further judgments seem far less clear: (1) that PVS patients like Norman should be regarded as disabled and thus are entitled to continued treatment and (2) that those who withdraw nutrition and hydration are thereby choosing death. Regarding Meilaender's first point, his description of PVS as a severe disability stretches the limit of the term. Indeed, we wanted to resist the temptation to regard Norman as a *nonperson* who could be abandoned, but it did not seem correct to regard him as a *disabled patient* who was entitled to aggressive medical treatment. For us Norman remained a member of the human community, but it seemed better to describe him as a *dying member*. With regard to Meilaender's second point, clearly, we did *foresee* that the withdrawal of nutrition and hydration would (in the absence of a miracle) hasten Norman's death, but we did not *intend* to hasten his death. Our intention was to see that Norman was given proper care. Artificial nutrition and hydration no longer seemed to be appropriate ways to care for him.

That we attempted to maintain this distinction between *foresight* and *intention* can be clarified in the expectation of our response to the outcome of withdrawing treatment. In the event that the withdrawal of Norman's treatment hastened his death, it would not be an occasion for rejoicing that our aims were successful. Moreover, were Norman to survive "miraculously" after the removal of his nutrition and hydration we would neither regard our intentions to have been frustrated nor seek another method to secure his death.

Our conclusion (supported by medical judgment) was that Norman was dying. We did not believe that respecting the embodiedness of his life necessarily obligated us to ensure that every measure be taken to sustain his biological existence, nor were we convinced that such a course of treatment was required by the responsibility to care for the life which had been entrusted to us. In fact, we began to suspect that our most stringent duty was to assist Norman to live a different kind of life from the one that we were forcing him to live, but we wondered how Norman could live well while dying.

c. Life as Vocation

The creation narrative also makes explicit that the givenness of life carries with it the weight of moral responsibility. The Creator placed the man in the garden to till and keep it (Gen. 2:15). We are reminded of our creaturehood inasmuch as we respond to the Creator's invitation to become *stewards of* and *participants in* the creative process, and we understand that the divine call is to *service*, not to *survival*. We wondered if it were possible to think of Norman (or anyone else in a PVS) as fulfilling a creaturely vocation in any meaningful sense. We clearly wanted to reject the reduction of vocation to productivity, for we believe that the weak and vulnerable maintain their creaturehood and can fulfill a vocation even when the labor of their lives is not "productive." We thus attempted to resist the temptation to shift the standard from the *sanctity of life* to the *quality of life*. To some it might appear that the overriding moral question was "Should we let Norman die?" or "Can we help Norman die well?", but for us the troublesome question became "How can we enable Norman to live well while dying?" We could not immediately discern how (or if) we could assist Norman to answer the Creator's call to live well.

Moreover, the story makes the divine command even more present in the *permission* to eat freely in the garden and the *prohibition* to not eat of one tree, i.e., the tree of the knowledge of good and evil (Gen. 2:16-17). We may wistfully long for a world where there are no dangerous trees, only safe ones (Brueggemann, 1982, p. 45). That option, however, is not open to us. We inhabit a world where the fabric of our existence is woven together by the choices we make. To be responsible selves is to come to terms with both the freedoms *and* the limits of our existence (H. R. Niebuhr, 1963).

The choices we make and the destinies we choose will be filled with promise and fraught with tragedy. Reinhold Niebuhr observed that

---

cial nutrition and hydration were first developed as a means of helping people overcome the temporary inability to eat or swallow. Moreover, he says that the inability to eat is one of the classical symptoms of a dying body. Callahan's position seems to be supported by a recent study of end-stage cancer patients who were palliated without forced feeding or hydration. See McCann and others, 1994, pp. 1263-66. A recent report on late improvement in consciousness after a post-traumatic vegetative state, however, seems to suggest that the diagnosis of PVS is not alone sufficient to describe one as dying. See Childs and Mercer, 1996, pp. 24-25.

2. For a robust discussion of the legal, medical, religious, and philosophical problems associated with the distinction see Bonnie Steinbock and Alasdair Norcross (eds.), *Killing and Letting Die*, 2nd edition (1994).

> Christianity's view of history is tragic insofar as it recognizes evil as an inevitable concomitant of even the highest spiritual enterprises. It is beyond tragedy inasfar as it does not regard evil as inherent in existence itself but as finally under the dominion of a good God (R. Niebuhr, 1937, pp. x-xi).

Life and the choices which shape it are necessarily but not ultimately tragic. The sacredness of life presupposes that we are agents entrusted with freedom to answer the Creator's call. Our destinies are thus shaped by learning to be *responsive to* and *responsible under* the divine command. The sanctity of human life demands the exercise of our freedom to follow a vocation that is full of both terrible dangers and wonderful possibilities.

We should be careful, however, not to take the exercise of human freedom to be an intrinsic good. The goodness of moral agency like the goodness of life itself, is derivative. It, too, is part of the given. Moreover, this freedom cannot be abstracted from the natural history of our biological existence. Human freedom does not exist for itself. It serves the end of moral responsibility in history under the divine command.

Consequently, the decision whether to withdraw (e.g., nutrition and hydration) and/or withhold (e.g., antibiotics) treatment from Norman was not without moral ambiguity. Some among the community voiced concerns that "we should not keep Norman alive this way," and that "we should let him go because he has suffered long enough." But by so acting to *eliminate the suffering* we recognized it would also *eliminate the sufferer* (Hauerwas, 1986, p. 24).[3] No matter how charitable the intention, it did not go unnoticed that the termination of Norman's treatment would nonetheless be a morally unhappy act.

d. Life as Communal

Even after the gracious Creator bestowed the gift of life to the man, there is the declaration, "It is not good that a man should be alone" (Gen 2:18). So, the Creator determined to make a partner for him. First, he tried the animals, but none was found to be a suitable companion for the man. Then God took a rib from the man and made the woman. We are reminded of the other creation account in which both male and female are made in the image of the Creator (Gen. 1:27), which also suggests that we are not fully human in isolation. It is finally only in community that we find the sacredness in life which God the Creator wills and blesses.

Just as sacredness is not *inherent to* human life but only as human life is viewed as *appropriate to* God, it is also not an ontic category *within the self* but a dialogic notion *between the self and others*. In relationship with others (and the Other) we encounter the goodness of trust, fidelity, and love which sustain our existence. Even in his present state we were conscious of the uniqueness and sacredness of Norman's life as we confronted the thought that this life now ending would never come again (Job 14:12-14), but we were still puzzled about our obligations to Norman as a member of the human community.

This communal dimension of the sanctity of life serves as a check against the proclivity toward *individualism* in decision-making that has created a society of moral strangers. In the absence of advance directives, the current practice suggests that (1) surrogates should make a *substituted judgment* for an incompetent based on speculation about what the incompetent would choose were he or she competent. Lacking any direct knowledge of either performative or preferential wishes, (2) the choice should be made on the basis of what is in the *best interest* of the incompetent person (Buchanan and Brock, 1989, pp. 93-96). A strict application of the *substituted judgment standard* fails to appreciate the importance of a communal casuistry that attempts to discern *what one should will* rather than simply *what one would will*. As Karl Barth rightly reminded us, because human life belongs to God it was not theologically sufficient to say "Such and such is what Norman would have wanted." We needed to ask whether an action would be consistent with the life of service to God (Barth, 1961, pp. 397ff.).

The *best interest standard* is morally unhelpful in most cases of the permanently unconscious because it is difficult to weigh benefits and burdens (Arras, 1988, pp. 939-44). How can the beneficial or burdensome aspects of the treatment of PVS patients be meaningfully assessed if they cannot feel pain? If indeed those who permanently lack the capacity for consciousness have no experiential interests, can they be considered to have any interests other than those they had prior to unconsciousness? Those prior future-oriented interests might include what one would want should he or she become permanently unconscious (Buchanan and Brock, 1989, pp. 126-32).

More importantly, the best interest standard privatizes the moral process. As Ezekiel Emanuel has argued, the decision whether to maintain an incompetent patient also depends on the kind of life that members of the community think is good and valuable. He proposes a community-based alternative that is grounded in the notion of "informed community consent" which would grant local communities the ethical and political authority to enact their own concept of the good (Emanuel, 1987, pp. 15-20). If adopted, this communal proposal would further fragment the modern vision of health care

3. It may be questioned whether it is appropriate to speak of the "pain" or "suffering" of patients like Norman who exhibit only the autonomic functions of brain stem activity. I am open to the suggestion by Jan Van Eys that suffering is something we impute to others. If he is correct, the statement "Norman has suffered long enough" is not meaningful as a physiological or phenomenological explanation of his condition. What it requires for coherence is a sociological and, finally, theological account which displays what it means to construe Norman's life and death appropriate to God and the church. This need for a theological account seems to suggest that Christian suffering is not (or should not be) a private experience but rather represents the communal description given by friends who share a common life.

that is committed to the liberal values of modernity and with it the practice and institutions of medicine. But perhaps it would not be a bad thing to ask what it might mean to practice medicine so as to fit better with the convictions of Orthodox Jews, Catholic Christians, or Seventh-Day Adventists in addition to the beliefs of pluralists and secularists. From such a communal perspective the question is not whether it is ever permissible to sacrifice the life of a noncompetent. Rather, it is a matter of asking how we might do so without yielding to the utilitarian temptation.[4]

Were we respecting the sanctity of Norman's life with which we had been entrusted? It was the consensus of Norman's church family that if indeed he was a dying member of the human community the NG tube and IV were merely prolonging his dying. It was our judgment that respecting the sanctity of Norman's life thus permitted the withdrawal of these life-sustaining measures. The sanctity of life helped us to understand the general direction of our moral judgment, and it suggested that such extraordinary measures were not necessarily an appropriate way to care for a member of the human community. However, it was still unclear how we were best to care for our friend and brother Norman.

The sanctity of life alone was thus unhelpful in a decisive sense because it was not a matter of *whether* Norman's life was sacred but rather *how* the sanctity of his life was best to be honored.[5] Moreover, the narrative exposition of the donational, biological, vocational, and communal dimensions of human existence clarified our identification of Norman as a member of the community of God's creation. However, our most determinative relationship with Norman remained unillumined by the sanctity of life. Specifically, it did not account for his identity as a member of the community of God's new creation which we witnessed in his Christian baptism on May 9, 1926. We decided to pursue the question of Norman's claims on us and our duties toward him as a baptized Christian and fellow church member.

4. I am quite aware that by suggesting a move away from a uniform model and a move toward a truly pluralistic approach to medicine there will be some communities who will put people to death by virtue of such standards as social worth and quality of life. In the name of community as a principle some lives ironically will be judged as "not worth living." It should go without saying that this type of utilitarianism is precisely what I want to resist, both by argument and embodiment. I simply see no way given my communal premise to rule out the possibility of such a medicine grown cruel. However, in a pluralistic communitarian approach the truth of an alternative community's medical vision turns on the persuasiveness of their moral display.

5. Ronald Dworkin argues that both sides of the current moral debate about euthanasia "agree that life is sacred, [but] . . . disagree about the source and character of that sacred value and therefore about which decisions respect and which dishonor," in 'Life is sacred. That's the easy part,' 1993, p. 36. Dworkin offers an account of the sanctity of life which is rooted, not in the *instrumental* or *subjective* (personal) value of human existence, but rather in the intrinsic value of all human life, in *Life's Dominion,* 1993, p. 71. Although I obviously wish to reject Dworkin's secular version of sanctity, I nevertheless agree with his view that the issue is not whether we accept some notion of sanctity but "how life's sanctity should be understood and respected," *Life's Dominion,* p. 217.

III. Living and Dying As Christians

In view of the neopaganism of mid-twentieth-century Western culture, Emil Brunner asked,

> What does the fact of having been baptized mean for the large number of contemporary people who do not know and do not even care to know whether they have been baptized? (Brunner, 1964, p. 184).

By reminding the baptized that they were no longer to serve the interests of self, tribe, or nation, Brunner called the pagan commitments of Christians into question and urged them to consider what it might mean to live faithfully under the Lordship of Christ. Brunner's question is worth repeating to Christians who are being asked to serve the ends of modern medicine and a pluralistic public policy. It was worth repeating to Norman's church family, for it was in baptism that he became a member of the community. What did the fact of having been baptized mean for Norman, who did not know whether or not he had been baptized, and what did the fact of his baptism mean for us as a community that must remember it? The moral question at issue may be stated even more directly. *How could we as a community of discernment assist Norman to live with integrity the life which he owned in baptism?* Could we enable our Christian brother to live well as he was dying?

a. Assisting by Discernment

As we struggled to decide what to do about Norman our baptized brother and to understand our role as a community of discernment, three questions required further clarification. *What* is discernment? *Who* possesses the gift of discernment? *When* is discernment rightly exercised?

Discernment is a gift of the Holy Spirit (1 Cor. 12:10) which enables Christians to seek "the mind of the Lord" (1 Cor. 2:14-16). Discernment is the skill of knowing the direction of the gospel when one is faced with conflictual choices. It thus enables those who live under the Lordship of Christ and are guided by the leadership of the Spirit to determine the moral trajectory of one's baptismal pledge in a given instance. A recent commentator defines discernment as a "process of sorting out some matter of controversy, seeking a solution to some problem, resolving some conflict, or finding an answer to some question" (Harder, 1993, p. 17). The gift of discernment is related to the virtue of prudence, namely, that the end of human action and the means of achieving it are in keeping with reason (Pieper, 1966, p. 20). Discernment, however, seeks to maintain the end and means of moral action in keeping with the gospel. As such, discernment is more than practical rationality. It is a matter of evangelical casuistry. Discernment is not a *naturally endowed trait,* nor is it a *habitually acquired skill.* It is a *spiritually formed gift.* But who possesses it?

Discernment is formed and found in the church as a confessional community. Discernment is not a matter of individual intuition; it is a process of social reflection.[6] The confessional community becomes a discerning community by virtue of the loosing and binding keys which they have received from Christ the Lord (Mt. 16:18-19). Those who stand together under the Lordship of Christ are authorized to discern through a social process *that from which they are liberated* and *that to which they are obligated.* The power of the keys to loose and bind is the proclamation of the gospel which the confessing church is authorized to preach (Jeschke, 1988, pp. 24-30).[7] Thus, the process of discernment is limited to evangelical casuistry, that is, to judgments that follow the ethical direction of the gospel. But when is moral discernment rightly exercised?

The Reformers of the sixteenth century (Calvin, Zwingli, and the Baptists) regarded divinely authorized discernment to be correctly practiced when it followed what they called the "rule of Christ" (Mt. 18:15-18). The rule delineates a series of practical steps that facilitate the social process of discernment (Yoder, 1984, 26; Yoder, 1991, pp. 34-39; Harder, 1993, pp. 50-51; Jeschke, 1988, pp. 23-34). Balthasar Hubmaier, an early Baptist, wrote that "the one who is baptized testifies publicly that he has pledged himself to live according to the rule of Christ" (Pipkin and Yoder, 1989, p. 127).[8] Hubmaier contended that it is by virtue of this pledge that the baptized submit themselves to the loosing and binding authority of the baptizing community. The process of discernment is also aided by the Holy Spirit (Jn. 20:22-23), who guides the community into truth (Jn. 16:13). Thus, moral discernment which adheres to the pattern of the rule is performed by the community that lives together under the Lordship of Christ and the leadership of the Spirit.

The authorization of a discerning process does not, however, imply divine ratification of every church decision. Discernment can, unfortunately, be wrongly exercised in such a way that is consistent with neither the Lordship of Christ nor the leadership of the Spirit (Jeschke, 1993, pp. 168-69). Because moral decision-making within a community can be abused, the rule of Christ is often complemented by what Zwingli called the rule of Paul (1 Cor. 14:26-33). This rule is guided by the conviction that the Spirit's work is apparent in the free exercise of gifts and in the open process by which all voices of the congregation are heard.[9] Congregational consensus is both the goal and the evidence of the rule, and majority vote prevails only as a last resort (Dana, 1944, p. 228). The "democratic" and "egalitarian" assumptions underlying the spiritual process of discernment attempt to protect the community's moral judgments from rigid legalism and arbitrary authoritarianism.

In baptism Norman affirmed his solidarity with the Christ and his people. He recently reaffirmed that commitment by entrusting his spiritual well-being, again to the community. The summer before his heart attack Norman reunited with his church family (after a brief separation) and announced that he had "come back home to die." Perhaps he suspected something might happen to him. We thus regarded it to be our duty as a community of discernment to seek care for our brother which would be consistent, not with a set of universal rules or specific consequences, but with the direction of the gospel in the shared life of discipleship.

Our understanding thus far could be summarized as follows. *One,* Norman's condition was irreversible and untreatable. The artificial nutrition and hydration were not therapeutic (since there is no cure for PVS) or palliative (given that he displayed no response to pleasure or pain), nor were the antibiotics effective in the elimination or amelioration of his smoldering infections. We questioned the assumption that aggressive medical treatment was the kind of care Norman needed. *Two,* the best medical judgment suggested that Norman's condition was terminal. Perhaps it was not imminently so since his autonomic reflexes were still functioning, but the fact that he stopped eating and could not receive optimal nutrition (even by forced-feeding) was an indication of his dying. By maintaining nutrition and hydration we were only prolonging his dying. *Three,* our aim was to celebrate life as a great (but not the greatest) good and to resist death as a great (but not the greatest) evil. Nevertheless, when someone is irreversibly in the process of dying (as we believed Norman was), there comes a time when death should no longer be resisted and when it may even be wrong to resist death. We did not wish to violate the responsibility entrusted to us either by deliberately causing or by arrogantly resisting Norman's death. We came to agree with Paul Ramsey's policy of always (but only) caring for the dying, but we were still puzzled about how best to care for Norman (Ramsey, 1970). *Four,* our mo-

6. The communal process of discernment sketched out in this essay is very different from the account proposed by Gustafson, 1968, pp. 17-36. For Gustafson, discernment is the moral skill of an individual agent to make fitting judgments as to what God enables and requires. Gustafson rightly says that "the moral discernment of Christians takes place within the Christian community," ibid., p. 34. However, his account of discernment is not directly connected to such communal practices as baptism, communion, preaching, prayer, or discipleship. It remains a matter of individual intuition, whereas the congregational process described in this essay attempts to connect moral insight with ecclesiastical disciplines.

7. Jeschke shows the evangelical interpretation of the keys to be one of the chief insights of the Protestant Reformers.

8. In a letter addressed to Thomas Muentzer, Conrad Grebel argued similarly that "even an adult is not to be baptized without Christ's rule of binding and loosing," in Williams and Mergal, 1957, p. 80.

9. John Howard Yoder provides a sociological account of the discerning process according to the rules of Christ and Paul in 'The hermeneutics of peoplehood,' in Yoder, 1984, pp. 15-45.

tive was not one of humanitarian concern to do the most loving thing or to relieve suffering. Rather, we were motivated out of a covenantal responsibility to assist Norman in living with integrity the life that he owned on May 9, 1926, and which, up until his incompetency, he continued to affirm.[10]

b. Living with Integrity

The prevailing wisdom in decisions about the treatment of mentally incapable patients is guided by respect for patient autonomy. Beauchamp and Childress define this principle as the conviction that independent and intentional "actions should not be subjected to controlling constraints by others" (Beauchamp and Childress, 1994, p. 126). Although respect for patient self-determination is the first and foremost bioethical principle, they concede that its status is only *prima facie* and can be overridden by competing moral considerations. In practice, however, the goodness of human existence is too often reduced to the capacity of individuals to act independently and intentionally. Within the ethics of autonomy, noncompetents like Norman retain their moral agency through advance directives or in substituted judgments of surrogates which enact the patient's stated (or implied) wishes to refuse or to permit specific treatments. These legal instruments enshrine a previous autonomous state that is abstracted from the noncompetent's biological history and disconnected from a discerning community. The upshot is that by elevating an abstracted account of autonomy other goods are trumped and competing moral voices are effectively silenced.[11]

In one of the most definitive and influential statements of the Baptist religion, E. Y. Mullins suggested that the historical significance of Baptists is an emphasis on the competency of the soul. By defining this notion as soul competency under God, not as human self-sufficiency, he attempted to nuance the doctrine. Mullins believed the benefits of soul competency were evident both exclusively and inclusively. Soul competency "excludes all human interference . . . and every form of religion by proxy." It also includes a constellation of correlative Baptist distinctives (axioms), e.g., the priesthood of the believer and the separation of church and state. For Mullins, "religion is a personal matter between the soul and God" (Mullins, 1908, pp. 53-56). It is at this point that the Baptist heritage seems to connect with medical ethics. In an attempt to encourage the practice of advance directives, one chaplain writes that "because Baptists have long honored the principles of soul competency and the priesthood of the believer, we can deeply appreciate the principle of self-determination" (Madison, 1993, p. 3).

This apparent connection between the Baptist heritage and medical ethics is, however, a weak one. Harold Bloom argues convincingly that Mullins invented the notion of soul competency by drawing from the language of economic self-sufficiency and Emersonian self-reliance, which was then superimposed on the Baptist theme of Christian liberty (Bloom, 1992, pp. 200-217). This distorted Baptist account of human agency is akin to the familiar principle of patient autonomy in part because both draw from the secular well of the Enlightenment, but soul competency was too limited to guide our decision about Norman.

Soul competency as a motto for Baptists was meant to ensure the capacity for an unmediated and unassailable experience with God. It was not successful, however, in establishing an ecclesiastical account of corporate experience, as is attested by the curious absence of a chapter on the church in Mullins' magisterial work, *The Christian Religion in Its Doctrinal Expression* (Mullins, 1917). Soul competency simply was not robust enough to sustain the link between individual freedom and communal discernment which were mutually necessary for our deliberation about what to do with Norman. The final word of both soul competency and autonomy is that my life and my decision are my own, while the witness of the gospel is that our lives are not our own (1 Cor. 6:19-20). As James McClendon rightly observes, the doctrine of soul competency "was framed too much in terms of the rugged individualism of pre–New Deal America to do justice to the shared discipleship earlier baptists had embraced" (McClendon, 1986, p. 30).

Even in a PVS Norman remained a part of the community he joined in baptism, and he was still responsible for living his life in keeping with that baptismal pledge. Our role was to support and sustain him in those decisions which we understood to be consistent with faithful discipleship. Even though the community possessed the authority to take measures of corrective discipline against one of its members, such action was not to be pursued without hearing the voice of the member in question. Thus, an attempt was made to listen to Norman in the matter. What would he have to say to us about what we should do? Several members of the church knew that Norman had expressed a wish not to have his life artificially maintained by "machines." This declaration was decidedly ambiguous, but even a recently drafted living will which included references to such artificial devices as feeding tubes and respirators would have been an insufficient basis for decision. A single statement could not be abstracted from the life of the friend that we had grown to know well in the sixty-seven years since his baptism.[12]

10. Gilbert Meilaender distinguishes between the aim and motive of killing (and allowing to die) in Meilaender, 1987, pp. 85-89.

11. David B. Fletcher reviews several recent works which critique the priority of autonomy in bioethics and emphasize the importance of family as a moral community, in Fletcher 1993, pp. 121-24. For an account of some of the problems associated with family decisions about the termination of treatment see Areen, 1987, pp. 229-35.

12. Buchanan and Brock distinguish between *performative* statements (e.g., living wills, DNR orders, durable power of attorney for heath care, and other advance directives) and *preferential* statements (e.g., an oral utterance like "I don't ever want to be kept

The issue for us was neither the absolute end of arbitrary patient autonomy (i.e., to do what Norman wanted) nor the unjust means of coercive communal authority (i.e., to disregard his expressed wishes). Rather, we were struggling with how to assist Norman to live with integrity. Our decision would consider the character of Norman's whole life and the convictions that shaped him. Was his present condition consistent with the integrity of the life in Christ as Norman had lived it?[13] The consensus of the community was that extending Norman's existence in a PVS by means of artificial nutrition and hydration was not in keeping with his life as we had known him. However, our decision would depend, not only on *the integrity of Norman's character,* but on our understanding of *fidelity to the Christian narrative* enacted in baptism to which Norman pledged himself.

c. Dying and Rising in Baptism

If we were to discern the moral commitments implied in Norman's baptism we first needed to consider the meaning of our practice of baptism. James McClendon presents the Baptist practice with great clarity:

> Baptists first seek to proclaim the Gospel. When (and only when) hearers, whether our own children or outsiders, respond by confessing faith in Christ as Lord and savior, they are accepted as candidates, immersed in the triune name in the presence of the congregation by the minister, and (in most churches) thereby admitted to membership in the congregation as brothers [or sisters] in Christ (McClendon, 1966, p. 7).

Because "baptism is reserved for those who commit themselves to Christ in active faith" (McClendon, 1966, p. 7), the Baptist heritage seeks to give witness to a believers' church constituted by voluntary membership.[14] What did the fact of Norman's baptism signify for us as a community that must remember it in light of the gospel?

It was a sign of *his solidarity with the crucified one.* In baptism the believer is buried with Christ into his death (Rom. 6:3). The seventeenth-century Baptist Leonard Busher wrote that to be baptized is to be "dipped for dead in water" (Beasley-Murray, 1990 [1973], p. 133). Norman's baptism was the declaration of his death. The significance of his baptism was neither as an imitative reenactment of a death like Christ nor as a mediated union with him. The watery grave of baptism signified that Norman died with Christ (Beasley-Murray, 1990 [1973], pp. 132-38). It was the enactment of a solemn promise to trust God even in the darkness of death. From that point forward Norman's destiny was inescapably linked to the crucified one, who experienced and opened up the transcendence and transformation of a God that was hidden in the midst of suffering. Although we were still troubled by questions about the biological nature of death, we were reassured by our theological construal of it. A decision to withdraw life-sustaining measures from Norman would not indicate our abandonment of him to the hopelessness of the grave. Rather, it would manifest the conviction enacted in baptism, that is, the hope of finding God, as Jesus did, in the contradictions of suffering and death (Williams, 1990 [1979], pp. 180-83).

Norman's baptism was also a sign of *his union with the risen one.* Just as the baptized are united with the Lord in his death, so are they raised with him through faith in the power of God (Rom. 6:4-5; Col. 2:12). Death has been swallowed up in the victory of Christ's resurrection as the old order with its powers passed away (1 Cor. 8:54; Col. 2:15), and the believer is risen with Christ to participate in the new creation which was inaugurated with the resurrection (2 Cor. 5:17). Therefore, if anyone is "in Christ," qualitative and comparative standards no longer count in the estimate of persons as together believers participate in the new people of God (2 Cor. 5:16-17; Eph. 2:15; Gal. 3:28) (Beasley-Murray, 1990 [1973], pp. 138-43; Yoder, 1972, pp. 226-28; Yoder, 1991, pp. 38-39). Baptism, so understood, is a political act. It was with a conviction grounded in the social reality of Christ's resurrection that we still recognized Norman as our brother, and it was with a faith rooted in this shared hope that we remained confident of God's power to raise up our brother Norman.

In baptism Norman owned God's act in Christ, and in baptism his life was claimed by God (Beasley-Murray, 1990 [1973], pp. 143-46). The sacrament of baptism signified the fact that God returned Norman's life, not to him, but to the community of the new creation in which we were participants and of which we were stewards. Thus, it was through baptism that we began to understand

---

alive on machines"). Because performative statements are clear and specific acts of will, they should be given great moral weight, but even a performative act may be inconsistent with the integrity of one's life and therefore should not be an automatic trump of all other moral judgments. See Buchanan and Brock, 1989, pp. 116-17. Buchanan and Brock give five helpful "rules of thumb" for weighing preferential statements, pp. 120-21.

13. On integrity of character as an action-guiding notion see Allen Verhey, 'Integrity, humility, and heroism: May patients refuse medical treatment?' in Lammers and Verhey, 1987, pp. 467-72.

14. I have attempted to defend the catholicity of believers' baptism against the charges of sectarianism as it is meant to serve the ends of a more determinative community and not to be an end in itself. See Freeman, 1994, pp. 89-91. Stanley Hauerwas has challenged my continued use of the adjective "voluntary" because, he contends, it obscures the question of "who is policing my life when I use it." For him the question becomes "What kind of community provides a real alternative that frees me from the powers so that as I look back I can say, 'Thank God!'?" I still contend that voluntary membership preserves the important distinction between church and state. For as Brunner and Barth observed, the existence of millions of baptized pagans challenges the practice of infant baptism (Barth, 1948). The Baptist practice is consistent with the role of the church to *be* the church and of the sacrament of baptism to *identify* her sons and daughters. I would add that this close link between the believer's profession of faith and entrance into the community encourages the church to resist the tyranny of both arbitrary autonomy and unjust authority.

what it meant to receive the giftedness of Norman's life. Just as the story of creation required us to recognize that creaturely existence is itself a gift to the human community, so the narrative of the new creation obligated us to acknowledge Norman's life as a gift to the community of the baptized. He was buried with Christ in death, but he was raised to walk in new life (Rom. 6:4). Unless (and until) God gives a new life through the Holy Spirit there is nothing to receive, but because in the sacrament of baptism we acknowledged God's gift we were thereby entrusted with the responsibility to nurture and care for this life. And just as the goodness of human existence is enriched by answering the Creator's call, so Christian existence is fulfilled by following the Master's invitation (Mt. 4:19). The sanctity of life so construed was not finally about receiving life in general. It was about receiving a particular life. It was about receiving Norman's life into the community of the new creation.

Our responsibility for Norman was to assist him in living the life he embraced in baptism — a life which included a destiny that was conformed to the crucified and risen one. That was not the destiny we chose for Norman; it was the destiny he owned. We recognized with Norman that our lives are not our own to be guided by autonomy and liberty. Our existence as Christians serves the good ends of a more determinative community — God's new creation of which baptism is a sign.

We would not unjustly override Norman's freedom, nor would we directly intend his death. But it was clear to us that prolonging his dying existence in a PVS served no end that would not finally be realized in his biological death. We thus reached the consensus as a community that continuing nutrition and hydration were not appropriate ways of assisting our dying friend and brother to live the life he owned in baptism. We therefore reached the conclusion that all life-sustaining (death-prolonging) care should be withdrawn. In taking such action we were not abandoning Norman; rather, we were assisting him to claim the destiny he had already chosen — to die and rise with Christ. Moreover, we were confident that if death were to result (foreseen though unintended), even that tragedy was gain in light of the gospel (Phil. 1:21).

IV. Patience and Hope in Community

In the dedication of *The Rule and Exercise of Holy Dying* Jeremy Taylor addressed the Earl of Carbery, "My Lord, it is a great art to dye well" (Taylor, 1989, p. 6). Taylor wrote his book for Lady Carbery, but she died, as did Taylor's own wife, before it was completed. The title, however, is somewhat misleading because the rules and exercises are not addressed to the dying but to the living. One cannot learn to die well on the deathbed; one must understand holy dying as a continuation of holy living. The sick and dying person can only exercise the virtues, practice the skills, and exhibit the graces that already have been acquired. Taylor proposes three precepts that guide those who seek to cultivate the virtues necessary for dying well: (1) always expect death, (2) every day prepare for death, and above all else (3) live under the discipline of the cross (Taylor, 1989, pp. 49-52). The rules and exercises contained in *Holy Dying* share the aim of habituating the virtues of patience, faith, repentance, charity, and justice that enable one to die well.

Taylor's rules for a holy death presuppose an imminent and protracted dying, and thus they seem to preclude a sudden and unexpected event like the case of Norman. More troubling still is his assertion that the moral strength of the virtues is unavailable to "fools, children, distracted persons, lethargical, apoplectical, or any wayes senselesse and uncapable of humane and reasonable acts." The deaths of incompetently unvirtuous persons may be assisted "only by prayers" (Taylor, 1989, p. 200).

Thinking collectively about Norman has challenged our assumptions about what it means to live and die well. We concurred with Taylor's judgment that a good death is to be a holy death and that one learns to die well as one acquires the virtues to live well. Indeed, it is quite possible that the rancorous public debate on questions related to the definition of death, the criteria of personhood, and the right to die has obscured what may be the most important moral issue at stake.

Specifically, we believe the definition of a good death does not depend merely on maintaining the dignity of honoring autonomous decisions but rather on possessing the strength of acting from virtuous character. We contend against Taylor, however, that a good death is not reserved for virtuous individuals but rather for those who share life together in communities of virtue that can remember life and construe death (even the dying of noncompetents) with meaning and purpose. We were thus led to ask the question, what *kind of people must we be to give witness to the fact that we welcome life as the good gift and accept death as the mysterious work of the gracious Creator?*[15] Our answer, quite obviously, was that we must be a community of virtue, but further questions still required our attention. Which virtues would enable us to assist Norman in dying well? How should the moral shape of our character be enacted?

a. Patience to Wait

Above all we remained committed not to abandon Norman in his dying, but the process of waiting has tested the limits of our patience. We waited daily by seeing that his affairs were in order and by simply being present with him in the hospital. To watch and pray seemed simple but appropriate gestures to convey the character of our

15. I borrow this question from Hauerwas, who argues that in order to understand why abortion is a morally unhappy act for Christians we must start by asking, not "Is the fetus a child with a right to life?" but rather "What kind of people should we be to welcome children into the world?" (Hauerwas, 1981, p. 198).

faith. As a consequence we learned something about the uniquely Christian shape to the virtue of patience. Whereas the moral history of courage can be traced to success in soldiering, the Christian account of patience arises out of the witness of martyrdom. A noble death for the Greeks and Romans followed the pattern of a courageous death in battle. A good death for the Christian imitated the example of the martyr's constancy. Courage maintains moral strength when one must be prepared to face danger, especially the danger of death in warfare; patience provides sustaining grace when one must be ready to suffer for the gospel. The end of Christian patience is endurance, whereas the end of civil courage is aggression. We thus understood patience as tied to the baptismal pledge, that is, the readiness to die for Christ and one another (Rom. 6:3-4; Jn. 15:13; 1 Jn. 3:16). Christian patience is about suffering and enduring hardship for others (Hauerwas, 1993, pp. 251-60; see Aristotle, II.7 [1107b1-5] and III.6 [1115a10-24], 1941, pp. 959-60 and 974-75; St. Thomas Aquinas, II.II.124.2, 1964, 42:42-47).

We found this virtue wonderfully illustrated in a story. Henri Nouwen tells of resigning his teaching position at Harvard Divinity School to become the priest of Daybreak, "a community where mentally handicapped people and their assistants try to live together in the spirit of the Beatitudes." There his understanding of life was transformed by his friendship with a young man named Adam. Each morning Nouwen spent an hour and a half medicating, bathing, shaving, dressing, and feeding Adam. What Nouwen has learned from Adam is "that what makes us human is our heart, the center of our being, where God has hidden trust, hope, and love."

On one occasion, when Adam's parents came to visit, Nouwen asked what Adam brought to their home. His father answered, "He brought us peace." Nouwen reflects:

> I know that he is right. After months of being with Adam, I am discovering in myself an inner quiet that I did not know before. Adam is one of the most broken persons among us, but without any doubt our strongest bond. Because of Adam there is always someone home; because of Adam there is a quiet rhythm in the house; because of Adam there are moments of silence; because of Adam there are always words of affection and tenderness; because of Adam there is patience and endurance; because of Adam there are smiles and tears visible to all; because of Adam there is always time and space for forgiveness and healing. Yes, because of Adam there is peace among us (Nouwen, 1988).

Nouwen's insight provides a hint of how to receive the stranger, and in so doing to discover a friendship that the ethics of autonomy cannot provide or understand. It is not a society of moral strangers based on the equality of personhood, for those like Adam and Norman are not persons by such standards. It is rather a community rooted in grace, where the givenness of others enriches us with the life-giving Spirit. Because of Norman there is peace among us.

b. Hope against Hope

For Norman to die well he needed a community that possessed the patience to wait, but a good death also required a people whose witness remained hopeful in the face of what medical judgment regarded as futility. We found such a hope displayed in Bunyan's classic story *The Pilgrim's Progress.* After a long and arduous journey Christian and Hopeful see the Celestial City at a distance. Yet, between them and the City, there is one last obstacle — the River of Death. It is deep and wide. Its current is swift, and its waters are dark. As Christian and Hopeful stand at the river's edge, two men with shining garments and glowing faces approach them. The two strangers explain to the travelers that there is no bridge across the river and that all who enter the City must pass through these waters. Christian becomes afraid, and he asks how deep the waters are. The strangers reply, "You shall find it deeper or shallower as you believe in the king of the place." So Christian and Hopeful enter the river. Upon entering, Christian begins to sink. He cries out to his friend Hopeful, "I sink in deep waters; the billows go over my head, all [its] waves go over me." But Hopeful answers back, "Be of good cheer, my brother, I feel the bottom, and it is good" (Bunyan, 1984, p. 128). As Norman crossed over the dark waters of death, it was our duty to give voice to the hopeful witness that we too feel the bedrock on which we stand, namely, the gospel of the crucified and risen Lord.

It seemed clear enough that Norman's treatment was not of therapeutic benefit to him and that his condition was indeed medically futile, but our concern for Norman was to be a hopeful community to a dying friend. Although no treatment could cure Norman, it was still morally relevant to ask about our obligation to care for him and about his claim to a community of friends that would not abandon him in his dying. Our regard for the sanctity of life and our baptismal covenant to live and die as Christians did not obligate us to continue sustaining Norman's life artificially. There is, after all, "a time to die" (Eccl. 3:2), and we did not want to prolong his dying unnecessarily. Our commitment to Norman and his claim on us was to be a community of care in his dying.

As we tried to understand what it would mean for us to help Norman die well, we searched in the following ways. First, we attempted to be faithful in telling the story which reminded us that our lives and Norman's were part of a larger pattern that gives a purpose to our lives and our deaths (Hauerwas, 1990, p. 112). Moreover, we sought insight and illumination from saints and martyrs who display how to live and die well. Finally, and perhaps most important, we pledged to one another (and to Norman) our presence, which we have come to believe is God's way of sustaining us in the face of the tragic. As we followed this path, we hoped to discover what it meant to affirm, not just the sanctity of life generically, but the sanctity of the particular life of someone whom we knew named Norman.

V. A Concluding and Morally Unhappy Postscript

On December 15, 1993, after Norman's IV and feeding tube were removed, he was finally placed in a hospice. He died one week later. Norman's friends and church family were there for the funeral and graveside service. We will miss him very much.

References

— (1991). 'Identifying the key decision maker and making the decision,' Hastings Center Project Group on the Termination of Treatment. Reprinted in T. Mappes and J. Zembaty (eds.) (1991), *Biomedical Ethics*, 3rd ed., McGraw-Hill, New York, pp. 346-51.

— (1987). 'Standards of judgment for treatment of imperiled newborns,' *Hastings Center Report* (December), reprinted in T. Mappes and J. Zembaty (eds.) (1991), *Biomedical Ethics*, 3rd ed., McGraw-Hill, New York.

Aquinas, T. (1964). *St. Thomas Aquinas: Summa Theologiae*, Blackfriars ed., McGraw Hill, New York.

Aristotle (1941). *Nicomachean Ethics*, in *The Basic Works of Aristotle*, Richard McKeon (ed.), Random House, New York.

Areen, J. (1987). 'The legal status of consent obtained from families of adult patients to withhold or withdraw treatment,' *Journal of the American Medical Association*, 258 (10 July), pp. 229-35.

Arras, J. (1988). 'The severely demented, minimally functional patient: An ethical analysis,' *Journal of the American Geriatrics Society*, 36, reprinted in T. Mappes and J. Zembaty (eds.) (1991), *Biomedical Ethics*, 3rd ed., McGraw-Hill, New York, pp. 351-59.

Barth, K. (1948). *The Teaching of the Church Regarding Baptism*, Ernest A. Payne (trans.), SCM Press, London.

Barth, K. (1961), *Church Dogmatics*, III/4, A. T. Mackay and others (trans.), T. & T. Clark, Edinburgh.

Beasley-Murray, G. R. (1990) [1973]. *Baptism in the New Testament*, William B. Eerdmans, Grand Rapids.

Beauchamp, T., and Childress, J. (1994). *Principles of Biomedical Ethics*, 4th ed., Oxford University Press, New York.

Bloom, H. (1992). *The American Religion: The Emergence of the Post-Christian Nation*, Simon and Schuster, New York.

Brody, B. (1988). 'Ethical questions raised by the persistent vegetative patient,' *Hastings Center Report* (February-March), pp. 33-37.

Brueggemann, W. (1982). *Genesis*, John Knox Press, Atlanta.

Brunner, E. (1964). *Truth as Encounter*, T. H. L. Parker (trans.), Westminster Press, Philadelphia.

Buchanan, A., and Brock, D. (1989). *Deciding for Others: The Ethics of Surrogate Decision Making*, Cambridge University Press, New York.

Bunyan, J. (1984). *The Pilgrim's Progress*, N. H. Keeble (ed.), Oxford, New York.

Callahan, D. (1994). 'The sanctity of life seduced,' *First Things* (April), pp. 13-15.

Childs, N., and Mercer, W. (1996). 'Brief report: Late improvement in consciousness after post-traumatic vegetative state,' *The New England Journal of Medicine*, 334 (4 January), pp. 24-25.

Dana, H. E. (1944). *A Manual of Ecclesiology*, Central Seminary Press, Kansas City.

Dworkin, R. (1993). *Life's Dominion*, Alfred A. Knopf, New York.

Dworkin, R. (1993). 'Life is sacred. That's the easy part,' *The New York Times Magazine* (16 May).

Emanuel, E. (1987). 'A communal vision of care for incompetent patients,' *Hastings Center Report* (October-November), pp. 15-20.

Fletcher, D. (1993). 'The difference that family makes,' *Second Opinion* (April), pp. 121-24.

Freeman, C. (1994). 'A confession for catholic baptists,' in *Ties That Bind: Life Together in the Baptist Vision*, Gary A. Furr and Curtis W. Freeman (eds.), Smyth and Helwys, Macon, GA, pp. 83-97.

Goldberg, M. (1981). *Theology and Narrative: A Critical Introduction*, Abingdon Press, Nashville.

Goldberg, M. (1985). *Jews and Christians: Getting Our Stories Straight*, Abingdon Press, Nashville.

Gustafson, J. (1968). 'Moral discernment in the Christian life,' in *Norm and Context in Christian Ethics*, G. Outka and P. Ramsey (eds.), Charles Scribner's Sons, New York, pp. 17-36.

Harder, L. (1993). *Doors to Lock and Doors to Open*, Herald Press, Scottdale.

Hartt, J. (1977). *Theological Method and Imagination*, Seabury Press, New York.

Hauerwas, S. (1981). *A Community of Character*, University of Notre Dame Press, Notre Dame.

Hauerwas, S. (1986). *Suffering Presence*, University of Notre Dame Press, Notre Dame.

Hauerwas, S. (1990). *Naming the Silences*, William B. Eerdmans, Grand Rapids.

Hauerwas, S. (1993). 'The difference of virtue and the difference it makes: Courage exemplified,' *Modern Theology*, 9 (July).

Jeschke, M. (1988). *Discipling in the Church*, 3rd ed., Herald Press, Scottdale.

Lammers, S., and Verhey, A. (eds.) (1987). *On Moral Medicine*, William B. Eerdmans, Grand Rapids.

Lash, N. (1993). *Believing Three Ways in One God*, University of Notre Dame Press, Notre Dame.

Lindbeck, G. (1984). *The Nature of Doctrine*, Westminster Press, Philadelphia.

McCann, R., and others (1994). 'Comfort care for terminally ill patients,' *Journal of the American Medical Association*, 272 (26 October), pp. 1263-66.

McClendon, J. (1966). 'Why baptists do not baptize infants,' in *The Sacraments: An Ecumenical Dilemma*, Paulist Press, New York, pp. 7-15.

McClendon, J. (1986). *Ethics: Systematic Theology*, Abingdon, Nashville.

Madison, T. (1993). 'Advance directives (of living wills),' *Therefore . . .*, The newsletter of the Christian Life Commission of the Baptist General Convention of Texas (September).

Meilaender, G. (1987). *The Limits of Love*, The Pennsylvania State University Press, University Park.

Meilaender, G. (1993). 'Terra es animata, on having a life,' *Hastings Center Report* (July-August), pp. 25-32.
Meilaender, G. (1994). 'Response to Daniel Callahan,' *First Things* (April), pp. 15-17.
Mullins, E. Y. (1908). *The Axioms of Religion,* Judson Press, Philadelphia.
Mullins, E. Y. (1917). *The Christian Religion in Its Doctrinal Expression,* The Sunday School Board, Nashville.
Niebuhr, H. R. (1963). *The Responsible Self,* Harper and Row, New York.
Niebuhr, R. (1937). *Beyond Tragedy: Essays on the Christian Interpretation of History,* Charles Scribner's Sons, New York.
Nouwen, H. (1988). 'Because of Adam,' *Weavings* (March/April).
Pieper, J. (1966). *The Four Cardinal Virtues,* University of Notre Dame Press, Notre Dame.
Pipkin, H. W., and Yoder, J. (trans. and eds.) (1989). *Balthasar Hubmaier: Theologian of Anabaptism,* Herald Press, Scottdale.
Ramsey, P. (1970). *The Patient as Person,* Yale University Press, New Haven.
Robinson, H. W. (1925). 'Hebrew psychology,' in *The People of the Book,* Arthur S. Peake (ed.), Clarendon Press, Oxford.
Steinbock, B., and Norcross, A. (eds.) (1994). *Killing and Letting Die,* 2nd ed., Fordham University Press, New York.
Taylor, J. (1989) [1651]. *The Rule and Exercises of Holy Dying,* P. G. Stanwood (ed.), Clarendon Press, Oxford.
Wikler, D. (1988). 'Not dead, not dying? Ethical categories and persistent vegetative state,' *Hastings Center Report* (February-March), pp. 41-47.
Williams, G., and Mergal, A. (eds.) (1957). *Spiritual and Anabaptist Writers,* Westminster Press, Philadelphia.
Williams, R. (1990) [1979]. *The Wound of Knowledge,* Cowley Publications, Cambridge.
Wolff, H. (1974). *Anthropology of the Old Testament,* Margaret Kohl (trans.), Fortress Press, Philadelphia.
Yoder, J. (1972). *The Politics of Jesus,* William B. Eerdmans, Grand Rapids.
Yoder, J. (1984). *The Priestly Kingdom: Social Ethics as Gospel,* University of Notre Dame Press, Notre Dame.
Yoder, J. (1991). 'Sacrament as social process: Christ the transformer of culture,' *Theology Today* 48 (April), pp. 33-34.

156 Love Your Enemies: Toward a Christoform Bioethic

M. Therese Lysaught

On March 31, 2005, Terri Schiavo died. For the two months prior to her death, the United States watched the debacle of the fight over her life play out in the media. One could not pick up a newspaper, turn on the television, or surf a news Web site without encountering daily developments in her case. Photographs, cartoons, and images soon became iconic; one glance would tell what version of the story was leading the headlines. Like many of the "classic cases" in medical ethics, the case of Terri Schiavo gripped public consciousness in a powerful way.

Two years later the repercussions from her death and the public struggle that preceded it have certainly not died down.[1] Her name continues to incite passion. The case has caused distress within the health-care system and for Catholics trying faithfully to navigate end-of-life decisions. The number of people seeking to complete living wills remains up, while many patients and families are worried that they can no longer be morally justified in refusing or withdrawing medically assisted nutrition and hydration. On the American political scene, competing political action committees have been formed to continue to lobby both sides of her case. Her husband has formed one called TerriPAC, to enact legislation to prevent the kinds of challenges her parents presented to his decisional authority. Another, Terri's List, has been formed to help elect politicians who supported or would support her parents' bid.

In the United States it is difficult to find a person not acquainted with the case. Almost everyone has an opinion. Yet the specifics of the case are elusive. What *were* the facts? Terri Schiavo suffered an event leading to anoxia and severe brain damage in 1990; there was a financial settlement in the case; soon after that her husband began a bid to disconnect her surgically implanted feed-

1. In the interest of space, I will not include a description of the case here. It was long and complicated, and how the story was to be told was a central part of the conflict. A quick Internet search will supply any interested reader with a surfeit of stories and Web sites on the case.

From M. Therese Lysaught, "Love Your Enemies: Toward a Christoform Bioethic," in *Gathered for the Journey: Moral Theology in Catholic Perspective.* Ed. David Matzko McCarthy and M. Therese Lysaught. Grand Rapids: Wm. B. Eerdmans, 2007, pp. 307-28.

ing tube, a bid to which her parents objected; legal suit and countersuit continued for the next twelve years, with the result that 2005 witnessed both a flurry of problematic legislative moves as well as a public vigil by primarily supporters of Terri's parents during her final three months; her feeding tube was disconnected on March 18, and it took her thirteen days to die. These seem to be the agreed-upon facts.

The rest is controverted, or perhaps it is more correct to say that the two sides of the case give radically different accounts in terms of: the cause of the anoxia; her proper diagnosis; her prognosis; the motives on each side; and so on. Each side told radically different stories. In fact, on the one-year anniversary of her death, her parents and former husband both released their "tell-all" books, each offering their own narration of the long and tortured history that constitutes *Terri's Story.*[2]

In this chapter I will use the Schiavo case as a place from which to examine that field we now call "bioethics." For while the Schiavo case provides a tidy focus for this particular chapter, I would argue that much that I will say here — at least the outlines — could be transposed to the analysis of other cases and issues in bioethics.

Medical quandaries, in our secularized medical culture, are usually cast as being about particular, highly charged treatment decisions. Ought someone be allowed to "pull the plug" or not? Generally, this question is answered by bringing forward one specific principle, for example, autonomy, the inviolability of life, or utility. The principle is applied to the case in a formulaic fashion and produces an answer; the answers emerging from the various principles are then seen as incommensurable. The question is: Which principle will trump?

I would like to suggest, however, that health-care ethics is not primarily about quandaries; it is not primarily about particular, highly charged treatment decisions. Do decisions need to be made? Certainly. But treatment decisions — and their execution — constitute a small percentage of the actions and interactions that occur in health-care settings, that surround the realities of being ill, suffering, and dying. Those truly concerned with what Christian discipleship looks like in the face of illness, suffering, dying, and medicine — what we call health-care ethics — must attend at least as assiduously to the shape of their actions and interactions the bulk of the time. Christian health-care ethics, in other words, is not about isolated, rare, occasional treatment decisions; it is about the shape of the entire Christian life as lived within and around the context of medicine.

Secondly, quandaries in bioethics are often presented as opportunities for us (the viewers, or voyeurs) to weigh in on what in particular *other* people ought or ought not to decide or do in their specific crises. On the Schiavo case everyone, it seemed, had an opinion about whether or not her treatment should have been discontinued. I would suggest, however, that in this particular case especially, this was only one of the moral questions. In this case, because of the way the initial conflict was handled, because of the nature of bioethics, and because of the role of the media, an equally (if not more critical) moral issue arose.

This issue was the fomenting of enmity. I would argue that enmity became the centrally operative moral dynamic in the case. At its root, this case was not simply a conflict about treatment decisions. Rather, the case itself was fueled by a disastrous brokenness and enmity between members of Terri's family, between people she loved deeply. This was the engine that drove the case: a decade-long fracture within Terri's family, most likely with fault and conflict of interest on both sides.

What is more, the antagonism — rather than being modulated or defused by bioethics — was augmented by the discipline's inherently conflictual nature. It is not incidental that most of the "classic cases" that have shaped the field of medical ethics have been legal cases. As a result, medical ethics shares the weaknesses of the law, especially insofar as its model of decision making is essentially adversarial. Who gets to decide when those involved disagree? Whose rights trump rights or interests of others? Who *wins?* Certainly, conflict is what brings cases to the ethics committee or courtroom. But such a model fails truly to *resolve* conflict. It might move the question out of the hospital or the hospice room, thereby providing a tidy answer for the medical establishment, but rarely does it truly address or resolve the moral pain and alienation at the center of such cases.[3]

Then, familial antagonism augmented by a conflict-centered ethics was amplified by activists on both sides of the case. Media-saturated as we have become, the country seemed to take hold of the elements of the case that fit the mold of television drama, with its love for legal maneuvering *(Law and Order)* and medical theater *(ER),* both mixed with scandal. Through attempts to gain power through the media, as well as political and legal channels, activists used these avenues of discourse to shape the very *meaning* of the Schiavo case. While most Christians responded to the Schiavo case with regret and quiet dismay, sympathy and compassion — and of course, prayer — those who caught the spotlight of the media offered a response of a different sort: protest, tearful distress, outrage, civil disobedience, anger, hostility. Many a self-identified Christian was heard excoriating the opponents as agents of the culture of death, as "killers," as "murderers." One of the judges in the case, George Greer, was under the protection of armed guards and was ultimately asked to leave his Southern Baptist church.[4] Bioethicists played out the politics of the bed-

2. This is the title of one of the already many books on Terri Schiavo (by Diana Lynne, WND Books, 2005).

3. For example, in the Schiavo case the decision was made over two years. The case came to an end. And yet, twelve months later, the hostility of the family members continues.

4. "Judge in Schiavo Case Asked to Leave Church," *Christian Century,* April 19, 2005, p. 15.

side vigil in print and private conversation, alternately referring to their opponents as either "scary" or "heretics." The actions of external activists, in other words, did not provide an alternative to the media drama, but reflected the dominant environment of fear and conflict. In the public sphere, secularists and Christians alike contributed to — even fomented — hostility and enmity.

Finally, wrapped up in these layered conflicts lurked the shadow of the ultimate enemy, death. Certainly a particular way of construing death — a theology of death — lies behind contemporary conflicts in bioethics. For those who have lost an eschatological horizon, those no longer shaped by the conviction that life transcends death, life becomes the ultimate and greatest good, an end in itself. Anything that threatens this end becomes the determinative enemy.

This, then, is what I believe to be an important reading of the Schiavo case — that it was not only a story about a particular treatment decision but it was equally a story of brokenness and hostility fomented into enmity by the actions of persons external to the case, some of whom even publicly identified themselves as Christians. To see this as a crucial reading of the Schiavo case shifts our attention away from immediate considerations of treatment decisions. It suggests that the case — and perhaps bioethics itself — needs to be approached in a radically different way than we are used to. It raises different questions. And those questions will require different sorts of answers. Here, I will argue, one of the overriding questions (though, admittedly, not the only question) is how one engages one's enemies, including, in the context of medicine, the enemy death.

Death as the Enemy, Medicine as War

In my description above, I suggested that activists in this case appeared to view death as the ultimate enemy. In staking out such a position, they merely embody the deep commitments of our culture. William F. May, onetime member of the President's Council on Bioethics and longtime member of the guild of theological ethicists, makes the case that contemporary medicine has both learned to and schools us to see death as the enemy.

In his book *The Physician's Covenant,* May describes at length how military metaphors and images, how the language of war itself, pervade the practice of medicine:

> The metaphor of war dominates the modern, popular understanding of disease and determines in countless ways the medical response. We see germs, viruses, bacteria, and cancers as invaders that break the territorial integrity of the body; they seize bridgeheads and, like an occupying army, threaten to spread, dominate, and destroy the whole. . . . Victims look for help to professionals, who, acquainted with the weapons of war, can take charge of the defense. The professional needs "intelligence." And so medicine has developed diagnostic procedures, scanning devices, and early warning systems more complex than the radar equipment of World War II, to let the professional know the enemy's location and the scale of the attack. . . . As in war, the very weapons used to fight the enemy can themselves endanger those on whose behalf one wields them. . . . The hospital becomes a military compound. . . . A kind of military discipline prevails there. . . . Modern medicine has tended to interpret itself not only through the prism of war but through the medium of its modern practice, that is, unlimited, unconditional war.[5]

This language of war is ubiquitous — found within medicine itself, but equally used by the media, in scientific journals, even by bioethicists. Take, for example, the realm of medical research. In 1971 Richard Nixon launched the "War on Cancer." Thirty-five years have passed, and this war is far from over — the same metaphor was employed and developed extensively in a 2002 report on cancer research in the major scientific journal *Nature.*[6] For many, and certainly for the media, clinical medicine via biotechnology is engaged in a war against disease, disability, suffering, and death. The tools of research and the clinic are the "medical armamentarium." Those who suffer from particular illnesses are "survivors." Cures are hailed as "magic bullets." And so on . . .

The metaphor of war is used most often when a new technology needs to be sold to political and public audiences in the United States. A recent example of this is the debate on human embryonic stem cell research. An article by two prominent bioethicists — Glenn McGee and Art Caplan — exemplifies this.[7] In their article "The Ethics and Politics of Small Sacrifices in Stem Cell Research," they use at least seven war-related images in seven pages. They characterize researchers who seek to develop therapies from human embryonic stem cells as fighting a "just war," a "war against suffering," caused by the whole gamut of diseases from Parkinson's to cancer to heart disease and more. They compare the annual mortality of cancer, which might potentially be alleviated through human embryonic stem cell research, to the number of people killed "in both the Kosovo and Vietnam conflicts." They suggest that advocates of human embryonic stem cell research plan to "sacrifice embryos for a revolutionary new kind of research." They characterize Parkinson's disease as an evil "dictator" dreaming up the most nefarious "chemical war campaign." Resonating with wartime rhetoric, they note that "adults and even children are sometimes forced to give [their lives],

5. William F. May, *The Physician's Covenant: Images of the Healer in Medical Ethics* (Philadelphia: Westminster, 1983), pp. 64-66.

6. Alison Abbott, "On the Offensive," *Nature* 416 (April 4, 2002): 470-74.

7. Glenn McGee and Arthur Caplan, "The Ethics and Politics of Small Sacrifices in Stem Cell Research," *Kennedy Institute of Ethics Journal* 9, no. 2 (1999): 151-57. The quotations in this paragraph are from this article.

but only in the defense or at least interest of the community's highest ideals and most pressing interests."

But why war? How is it — to simply mention another example — that the race to map the human genome could become construed as an issue of national security (an analogy to war)?[8] How can one mount a war on something as amorphous as cancer? More importantly, what is required before someone can even start thinking about medical research and practice in terms of war?

To fight a war, as recent history reminds us all too well, requires an enemy, and for May, that enemy is death. As he notes: "death looms as supremely antihuman, the absolute, invincible enemy which, nonetheless, we must resist to affirm our humanity."[9] He argues that the vision of medicine as a practice of war and the understanding of death as the supreme enemy arise out of the broader religious consciousness of contemporary culture. In an increasingly secularized culture, people may no longer believe in God, but that does not mean that gods do not rule their lives. "The modern interpretation of disease as destructive power fits in with the religious preoccupations of our time. . . . However, the gods that enthrall modern men and women do not bless but threaten them."[10] For May, the god above all gods is death. Death and the related god of suffering are those we fear most, those that wield the most power over us.[11] Perceived as absolute evil, "the *summum malum* of violent death," he notes, "has replaced God as the effective center of religious consciousness in the modern world."[12]

These dark forces threaten us; before them we stand helpless, innocent yet powerless. Without a champion to intervene on our behalf and defend us, we have no hope. Medicine has become over the past four decades just such a champion — a redeemer. May notes that only recently has the image of physician as fighter replaced the image of physician as parent; "the goal of medicine [now] defines itself negatively and adversarially as being either to prevent suffering or to prevent death."[13] May describes the physician as "the titan who responds to the sacred by seizing power in his or her own right and doing battle with the enemy."[14] The physician is the one that wields "the retaliatory powers that modern biomedical research places at his or her disposal."[15] Medicine, in this way, becomes our savior.[16]

May highlights this language to demonstrate a larger point — that images and metaphors tell stories, compressed prototypical stories. Without words, without arguments, they encapsulate narratives in which we become located, narratives that shape our social role, our identities, indeed, the choices we make, the actions we take, and the ways we live our lives. Who we understand ourselves to be is deeply implicated in what we do. As such, images and metaphors "do not simply describe the world, they partly create and re-create the world to conform to a [particular vision of reality]."[17]

What vision of reality is being presented where death is spoken of as "god," medicine as savior? If nothing else, we are being presented with a theological vision of reality. Indeed, a "religious consciousness" lies behind modern medicine and bioethics, one deeply at odds with Christianity. And it shapes us powerfully. For in the Schiavo case we found such faulty theological convictions wielded even by some Christians. Take, for example, this theology of salvation (known in the discipline of theology by the technical term "soteriology"). Medicine was implored as the agent of salvation — able either to "save" Terri from death or to "save" her from suffering the indignity inflicted on her in sustaining her life.[18] Equally, salvation seemed to rest in the hands of the judi-

8. John Beatty, "Origins of the U.S. Human Genome Project: Changing Relationships between Genetics and National Security," in *Controlling Our Destinies: Historical, Philosophical, Ethical, and Theological Perspectives on the Human Genome Project,* ed. Phillip R. Sloan (Notre Dame, Ind.: University of Notre Dame Press, 2000), p. 141.

9. May, *The Physician's Covenant,* p. 63.

10. May, *The Physician's Covenant,* p. 31.

11. May, *The Physician's Covenant,* p. 34.

12. May, *The Physician's Covenant,* p. 67.

13. May, *The Physician's Covenant,* p. 69.

14. May, *The Physician's Covenant,* p. 33.

15. May, *The Physician's Covenant,* p. 34.

16. One might even say that "Christ the physician" (a traditional Christian image) becomes physician-as-Christ, the one who (with the help of biotechnology) fights relentlessly against the last enemy, death. As Michael West, founder of Geron, CEO of Advanced Cell Technology, and cloning advocate, notes: "We're trying *to save* the lives of our fellow human beings who have *no hope* today" (Faith Keenan, "Cloning: Huckster or Hero?" *Business Week,* July 1, 2002, pp. 86-87, emphasis added). Science has become hope for those who have no other hope. Insofar as hope is a theological virtue, this is a striking theological claim.

17. May, *The Physician's Covenant,* p. 20.

18. It is easy to slip into this account of medicine-as-savior because it is, in part, a parody of the account of salvation offered by the Christian tradition. For the Christian tradition, suffering, death, and the other forces that threaten us and fear of which dominates our lives are nothing other than what traditional theological language has referred to as "the principalities and powers." Within the Christian narrative, they are understood as enemies. For example, Saint Paul, in his impassioned exhortation on the essence of salvation, concludes: "Then comes the end, when [Christ] hands over the kingdom to God the Father, after he has destroyed every ruler and every authority and power. For he must reign until he has put all his enemies under his feet. The last enemy to be destroyed is death" (1 Cor. 15:24-26). Paul clearly regards death as the enemy. Even Christ, as portrayed here, saw death as an enemy, triumphed over it, and will ultimately *destroy* it. Here, and in the book of Revelation, we find language of a great war between Christ and the principalities and powers that rule the world, the last and greatest of which is death, an enemy that has ultimately been defeated by the cross and resurrection. The language here seems violent, even militaristic. As such, is it not appropriate to resist death, to war against it, to respond to it even with violent means if necessary? We need to take care in reading passages like 1 Cor. 15 too literally. For while Christ may well consider death an enemy, it would be out of character for the risen Christ to act violently, even toward this greatest of enemies. Christ, we believe, has triumphed over death. But as his initial victory was nonviolent, so also must be his final defeat of death.

cial system — to Governor Jeb Bush, to judges, to congresspeople were offered from both sides laments and petitions not unlike one finds in the Psalms.

For Christians, of course, salvation rests not in the hands of Jeb Bush or medical technology, but in the hands of the triune God who has acted in Jesus Christ. Jesus was not necessarily absent from the rhetoric bandied about during early 2005. Ironically, Jesus took his place on some placards proclaiming this distorted soteriology. But this Jesus was more the Jesus of Mel Gibson than, perhaps, the Jesus of the Gospels — a bloody corpus abstracted from the rest of his story. Jesus became a rhetorical tool. Some mapped Terri onto Christ, rendering her a Christ figure, the Suffering Servant of Isaiah. Judges and politicians became her betrayers, "Judas Iscariots," in the words of Operation Rescue's Randall Terry.[19]

Though more could be said, I hope it is becoming clear how, in spite of the apparent rifts between some Christians and secularists in this case, when one presses behind the surface rhetoric, one finds a remarkable degree of overlap, of substantive agreement, of ideological and theological similarity in their positions. Insofar as this theology drives their actions, it calls for a theological response.

Holy Week

But where to begin? One of the most interesting editorial cartoons published in March 2005 subtly gives us a possibility. The cartoon depicts Terri lying in a hospital bed. Superimposed over her, though not immediately obvious, is the shadow of a cross mapping itself onto her body so that she becomes the corpus. Lying at the foot of her bed is a sponge and a bottle labeled vinegar. The cartoon, in other words, trades on the not inconsequential fact that Terri's final vigil began during Holy Week.

Holy Week stands as the most important week of the liturgical year, the week when the church celebrates in time and ritual the central claim of the gospel. Here, in other words, the church enacts the normative claims of the Christian faith. Certainly Christians are called to see Christ "in the least among us," as many of the placards of the protestors proclaimed; thus, to see Christ in Terri is a move that was certainly legitimate both theologically and according to most of Christian tradition. But while Terri was "read" as Christ, a *christological* reading of her dying and death was not at the forefront of the media hype. For as Christians, we are not called to save Christ from death but rather to follow him. We are to follow him as he dies, understanding his death to mark God's victory over death. And we are called to follow him in the shape of his life. In other words, Christology is indeed normative for Christian ethics, but not as it played out in the public battles of the Schiavo case. What would public engagement in the Schiavo case have looked like had the Christians party to the vigil (although not they alone) understood Terri's death christologically or saw the primary christological agents to be *themselves* rather than Terri?

Let us briefly consider Holy Week: Beginning with Jesus' triumphal entry into Jerusalem on Passion Sunday, Christians follow him day by day, moment by moment, through his last meal with his friends; his great act of service to them as he washes their feet; his agonized decision on how to respond to the enemies he knows will soon accost him; his unjust arrest and the mockery of justice that followed; his betrayal by his friends; and his horrific walk up the road to Calvary. At the pinnacle of the story stands the crucifixion, the passion, Good Friday. Here Jesus accepts a clearly unjust death and utters the amazing words: "Father, forgive them; for they do not know what they are doing" (Luke 23:34). And through his entry into death, God vanquishes it.

As Christians follow Jesus to Calvary during Holy Week, we hold vigil, as did Terri's supporters. We watch as the one we proclaim to be God rejects hatred, violence, and even judicial resistance to the powers of the world as a way of saving his life. Jesus chastises those who suggest violence to protect him. He stands mute in the face of judicial proceedings, rather than seeking his rights or paying lawyers exorbitant amounts of money to find every last loophole to save him. He shows that his life (and therefore our lives) is not about winning against adversaries, asserting his rights, or triumphing over others. He takes the pain and brokenness, injustice and sin of the world onto his own body in order to reconcile it to God and to show us the path toward reconciliation with each other.

In contrast to us in our hyper-litigious outlook, Jesus understands faithfulness to God fundamentally to be about something else. It is not about saving his life, even his most innocent of lives. Because of Jesus' victory over death, life within the Christian tradition has never been understood as an end in itself. The passion stories speak first and foremost not about the inviolability of life — rather, they display Jesus' engagement with the principalities and powers that dominate the world and his commitment to loving his enemies, to praying for those who are persecuting him, to forgiving others as *the* exemplar of God's very character, God's very way of being in the world. And he indicates that *this* is the Way to be followed. *This* is the Christ to be imitated. This is the truth affirmed — against all expectation and "common sense" — by God in the resurrection.

The resurrection, Holy Week reminds us, is the center of the Christian story. Forgiveness and the commitment to concrete reconciliation between enemies in the here and now, even in the face of suffering and an unjust death — *this* is the story that the church retells and lives

19. Others described Terri using the language of martyrdom. Although I cannot explore it at length here, it would be equally interesting to analyze the martyrdom language used in this case, especially the differences between Christian public action in this case and the sort of Christian public action that surrounded the martyrdom of Christians in the early church or, for that matter, in the twentieth century.

again each year at Holy Week. *This* is this story that Christians retell and live again each time we celebrate the Eucharist. *This,* the church affirms, in both its liturgical life and the shape of the liturgical year, is the overarching framework within which all other Christian convictions and principles must be ordered.

Thus, I would argue that the "public" engagement of Christians in the Schiavo case rooted in the liturgical practice of Holy Week would have looked very different. Even when life is at stake, even when an innocent life is at stake, even when a life may be taken unjustly, the eucharistic center of the church requires that Christian engagement with their enemies be shaped by love, normed by commitments to reconciliation.[20] In light of this, what might it have looked like had those who kept vigil for Terri Schiavo recognized that as they journeyed with her toward her death we journeyed as a church with Jesus to his passion, had they "read" her death not according to the conflictual story of bioethics and the U.S. legal system but through the lens of the central claims of the gospel?

Christian Practices and *The Gift of Peace*

There are no better answers to these questions than those exemplars in the Christian tradition. It is in the actual lives of people trying to live the Christian life that we can find the possibility of what we might call a christoform bioethic and learn what makes such a bioethic possible. One such exemplar that I would like to focus on here is Joseph Cardinal Bernardin and his autobiography entitled (not accidentally) *The Gift of Peace.* Bernardin is an important figure for at least two reasons. First, in his life and autobiography he explicitly embodies Christian engagement with medicine and the end of life; his story is in part the story of his terminal journey with pancreatic cancer. Moreover, for a number of years he was also head of the Office of Pro-Life Activities for the National Conference of Catholic Bishops, a position from which he launched into public consciousness the phrase "the consistent ethic of life."[21] Bernardin brings together in his life the church's deep commitment to life while reading it through the lens of the gospel.

20. To be clear, I am not suggesting that the lens of Holy Week would lead us to a position that would simply "let go" or be passive in the face of threats to life or in the face of death. The question is rather of the shape of Christian engagement in the face of injustice and death.

21. Importantly, immediately prior to becoming head of the Office of Pro-Life Activities, Bernardin chaired the bishops' committee for the landmark document *The Challenge of Peace: God's Promise and Our Response.* As I have argued elsewhere, if one looks at Bernardin's life and writings as a whole, one can make an argument that the consistent ethic of life can be read as an ethic of peacemaking. See my "From the Challenge of Peace to the Gift of Peace: Rereading the Consistent Ethic of Life as an Ethic of Peacemaking," in *The Consistent Ethic of Life: Assessing Its Reception and Relevance,* ed. Tom Nairn (Maryknoll, N.Y.: Orbis, 2008), pp. 109-31.

The Gift of Peace is a deceptively simple book. On its face it seems a somewhat random series of autobiographical reflections — the story of how he was falsely accused of sexual abuse; his struggle with terminal pancreatic cancer; and a brief opening reflection on how he took up the practice of daily prayer. But he clearly includes these three stories between the covers of one book because he saw them as deeply interconnected. And it is these interconnections that are crucial to our consideration of the Schiavo case. Allow me to briefly unpack these pieces.

He begins the book — and frames the entire work — with his story of learning how to attend to prayer. He recounts that in the 1970s — then a forty-five-year-old archbishop — he was called to account by some friends for neglecting his own personal prayer life and attending too much to the doing of "good works" and the business of being archbishop. At their urging he decided to devote the first hour of his day to prayer and meditation — to simply spending time with God.

One thing this experience taught him was how deeply he wished for control, how tightly we tend "to hold onto ourselves and everything and everybody familiar to us."[22] Learning to pray for him meant learning how to "let go," to release his hold on those things that hold him in bondage, and to open himself completely to God's presence in our lives. This was no quick or easy process, but it proved absolutely crucial to his ability to face what came later. As he notes:

> I have desperately wanted to open the door of my soul as Zacchaeus [the tax collector] opened the door of his house. Only in that way can the Lord take over my life completely. Yet many times in the past I have only let him come in part of the way. I talked with him but seemed afraid to let him take over. Why was I afraid? Why did I open the door only so far and no more? . . . At times I think it was because I wanted to succeed and be acknowledged as a person who has succeeded. At other times I would become upset when I read or heard criticism about my decisions or actions. When these feelings prevailed, I wanted to control things, that is, I wanted to make them come out "right." . . . Have I feared that God's will may be different from mine and that if his will prevailed I would be criticized? . . . To come at this another way, I wonder if I refused to let the Lord enter all the way into my soul because I feared that he would insist that . . . I let go of certain things I was reluctant or unwilling to give up.[23]

This lengthy passage describes, I would guess, not only his life but also the dynamics of our lives. Equally, it captures an absolutely critical aspect of our exploration. Here we see the cardinal embark on a particular practice — the practice of prayer — a traditional Christian practice. It is through, and only through, this practice that he develops

22. Joseph Cardinal Bernardin, *The Gift of Peace* (Chicago: Loyola University Press, 1997), p. 7.

23. Bernardin, *The Gift of Peace,* pp. 7-9.

a particular disposition, attitude, skill, virtue — he names this "letting go," but we could equally call it "openness" to God and others, liberation from those things that possess us (pride, possessions, power, fear), trust in God, learning to understand God as the Lord of life, and so on. In his life he had long believed these things in theory, but he acknowledges that he had not really believed them in practice because he had not lived as if they were true.

These virtues, these dispositions prove critical for the last two major events of his life. The first of these is the false accusation of sexually abusing a seminarian. He introduces this chapter of his life with a meditation on "emptying oneself" — "emptying myself of everything — the plans I consider the largest as well as the distractions I judge the smallest — so that the Lord can really take over."[24] He quotes the Pauline hymn of the kenotic Christ ("Though he was in the form of God,/did not regard equality with God/as something to be exploited,/but emptied himself,/taking the form of a slave. . . ./he humbled himself/and became obedient to the point of death — / even death on a cross" [Phil. 2:6-8]) to convey what he means by "emptying oneself."

I will not rehearse the details of this part of the story here (I would encourage all to read it), but a few key elements are important. As with crisis situations in medicine, the accusation came out of nowhere and was devastating. His world was, in many ways, turned upside down. The accusation struck at one of the key centers of his identity — his chastity. Because he was cardinal archbishop of Chicago and well known, when the news broke millions of people heard it and most likely believed it to be true. He was angry, bewildered at who could possibly launch such a false charge against him, and deeply humiliated. "As never before," he notes, "I felt the presence of evil."[25] Here a destructive power was at work, bearing down on him, threatening everything he held valuable — his life's work, his deepest convictions, his personal reputation, his position as cardinal of Chicago.

Yet at the same time he felt equally sustained by the conviction that "the truth will make you free" (John 8:32). He knew almost tangibly the presence of the God he had come increasingly to know in prayer. And the habit of prayer he had learned through ordinary days and years now becomes crucial. Before facing hordes of reporters the day after the accusation becomes public, he prays the rosary early in the morning, meditating on the Sorrowful Mysteries, and later spends an hour by himself in prayer and meditation. While he feels very much akin to Jesus in the garden during his aloneness and agony, he equally knows that it is God's grace, strength, and presence that enable him to face the reporters, to stand calmly in the face of evil, and to speak the truth in love and peaceableness.

Moreover, from the beginning he finds himself overwhelmed with a sense of compassion for his accuser. A few days after the filing of the charges, he notes, "I felt a genuine impulse to pray with and comfort him."[26] He almost immediately writes a letter to the man, asking if he might visit him to pray with him. The man's lawyers never deliver the letter. The case eventually unravels on its own, and the charges are eventually dropped as the "evidence" proves to be fabricated. Bernardin could have simply rejoiced in his vindication, or he could have brought countercharges for defamation of character. But this is not the road he chooses. Rather, eleven months after the suit was dropped, he again tried to contact his accuser. This time he was successful. In the end, he met with him and — beyond what would be wildly unimaginable — was reconciled with him.[27] They became friends, such that six months later, when Bernardin was diagnosed with pancreatic cancer, one of the first letters he received was from his former accuser. It is a powerful story of forgiveness and reconciliation.

Bernardin makes clear that only his openness to the presence and grace of God in his life, an openness given by God and cultivated through the practice of prayer, enabled this story to unfold as it did. Through the practice of prayer Bernardin learned to love God and to let go of the god of self-love. He developed the virtues necessary to be able to love one who was clearly his enemy, a person who he said inflicted upon him the most damage, in the most vicious manner, that he had ever experienced. What does such love look like? It is nonviolent — the cardinal made clear to his advisers and attorneys at the outset of the crisis that there would be no scorched-earth countersuit to beat the enemy down. It is compassionate — it feels the pain of the other, even of the enemy. It is reconciling — it seeks not to obliterate the enemy but to overcome the enmity between them through reconciliation. It reaches out to the enemy, both to create community with the enemy and to do the work of God's love in the world.

To this extent it is christoform — Bernardin makes clear that such is the nature of Christian love, rooted in the person of Jesus. Through his practice of prayer he has come to know Jesus as a fully human person, one who both experienced pain and suffering and yet "transformed human suffering into something greater: an ability to walk with the afflicted and to empty himself so that his loving Father could work more fully through him."[28] And it is this Jesus that he meets through his practice of prayer that increasingly becomes the One who shapes his life.

This experience becomes the prelude to the final chapter of his story, the story of his struggle with terminal pancreatic cancer complicated by painful spinal stenosis.[29] In his narrative, we watch as he uses the tools of

24. Bernardin, *The Gift of Peace,* pp. 15-16.

25. Bernardin, *The Gift of Peace,* p. 23.

26. Bernardin, *The Gift of Peace,* p. 25.

27. It is not unimportant that this reconciliation involves the sacraments of reconciliation and Eucharist.

28. Bernardin, *The Gift of Peace,* p. 46.

29. Clearly, Bernardin's medical situation differed from Terri Schiavo's medical situation. Nonetheless, he is a key exemplar insofar as the objective of this chapter is to shift attention to questions

medicine to resist the growth of cancer in his body. We watch as he wins a short-lived remission, and then as the cancer returns with renewed virulence. But importantly, the autobiography of his illness is not primarily about his illness — it is instead about how his illness leads him into a new world of ministry, meeting, being present to and praying for literally hundreds of others who struggle with cancer.

It is also about how his illness leads him to a new understanding of death. The final chapter in his story he entitles "Befriending Death." As the phrase suggests, he comes to regard "death not as an enemy or threat but as a friend."[30] The reorientation is first suggested to him by his friend Henri Nouwen, who learned it during his ministry among persons with disabilities in the Daybreak Community of L'Arche. As Bernardin notes: "It's very simple. If you have fear and anxiety and you talk to a friend, then those fears and anxieties are minimized and could even disappear. If you see them as an enemy, then you go into a state of denial and try to get as far away as possible from them. People of faith who believe that death is the transition from this life to eternal life, should see death as a friend."[31] Nouwen's insight resonates with Bernardin's life, shaped as it was by practices of "letting go" and giving God Lordship over his life; of practicing forgiveness; of ministering to others who were sick and dying. Liberation from the tyranny of suffering and death, reconciliation with death, and learning to love the enemy death to the point of calling it "friend" are for Bernardin the fruits of a worshipful life lived amidst the community of the broken. This he believes is "God's special gift to us all: the gift of peace. When we are at peace, we find the freedom to be most fully who we are, even in the worst of times. . . . We empty ourselves so that God may more fully work within us. And we become instruments in the hands of the Lord."[32]

Such peace, of course, is the peace of Christ. Even though the cardinal comes to refer to death as his friend, he continues to understand his journey as one that enters into Christ's passion. As he moves into the final phase of his illness, he notes, "the cross has become my constant companion."[33] As such, Bernardin's rereading of death is clearly christoform — shaped by a Christlike self-emptying, death, and resurrection. The love he gains for this enemy death is Christian love — *agape,* God's love for us — which is embodied most completely on the cross.

beyond those of treatment decisions — to attend to the question of the shape of Christian engagement with enmity and death in the myriad of ways they come together in the context of health care.

30. Bernardin, *The Gift of Peace,* p. 126.

31. Bernardin, *The Gift of Peace,* pp. 127-28. In learning to love our enemies, do they necessarily remain such, namely, *enemies?* The gospel does not promise that if we love our enemies, such enmity will disappear. In fact, it seems to promise that habits of loving one's enemies may well multiply them or lead to crucifixion or martyrdom.

32. Bernardin, *The Gift of Peace,* p. 153.

33. Bernardin, *The Gift of Peace,* p. 129.

Here and elsewhere, loving one's enemies means forgiveness of the real injuries, pain, and suffering they cause us. It means being reconciled to the presence and reality of the other. It means foregoing the fantasy that we "win" by eliminating or defeating them with violence. It might mean that we are rightly to "resist" their attempts to have power over us, to govern our lives with fear, to determine our actions.[34]

Toward a Christoform Bioethic

Here, then, we have what I am sure is a very different approach to the case of Terri Schiavo than most analyses offer. In addition, I hope it lays the groundwork for developing a new approach to Christian (and/or "Catholic") bioethics. In the interest of summing up, let me offer four points by way of conclusion.

First, the Schiavo case should highlight for us that quite often the central *moral* issue in end-of-life cases, or perhaps even within medicine and bioethics more broadly, is the need for reconciliation. Not only do families often come into the clinical setting "fractured," but there is also nothing like a medical crisis, especially one like this — where a sudden catastrophe in the life of a vi-

34. In many ways, it ought not be surprising that Bernardin was able to embody such a counterintuitive approach to death. For importantly, he was also a first-order Franciscan oblate. This distinctive attitude of peace and reconciliation in the face of death finds a new form in the work of Saint Francis of Assisi. Saint Francis, that most popular saint of all times, is particularly noted for his deep devotion to Jesus and how closely his life conformed to that of Christ in the Gospels. Francis is often referred to as *alter Christi* — "another Christ." Two years before his death, Saint Francis retreated to a mountaintop hermitage in La Verna, Italy, where, in the course of months of intense prayer, he received the stigmata, the marks of Jesus' passion in his hands, feet, and sides. The pain of the stigmata was compounded over the next two years by additional painful conditions, including blindness. And yet he continued to be filled with joy, his enthusiasm bursting forth in one of his most classic prayers, *The Canticle of Brother Sun.* Here, as Francis praises the trinitarian God in each element of God's magnificent creation, he culminates with death: "Praised be you, my Lord, through our Sister Bodily Death, from whom no living man can escape." Francis greets death, in other words, not only as a friend but also as a sister, and what is more, as that through which God can be praised. Thus, via Francis and others, the Christian tradition acknowledges the reality of death — that it is, indeed, the greatest of human enemies — but at the same time, from the beginning and at many points thereafter, the tradition witnesses that the distinctive Christian response is to approach it by saying, "Peace be with you"; "Praise you, Lord, for our sister bodily death."

This Franciscan attitude pervaded Bernardin's life. It is reported that when Bernardin, as cardinal archbishop of Chicago, faced what he knew would be a particularly difficult or contentious meeting, he would open the meeting with Saint Francis's classic peace prayer that begins "Lord, make me an instrument of your peace. . . ." It is also not coincidental that the last initiative he started was the Catholic Common Ground Initiative designed to try to foster reconciliation among the increasingly polarized factions in the Catholic Church.

brant young woman then stretches on and on and on — to exacerbate or even create such fractures, bringing to the surface and magnifying all sorts of unresolved issues. And as is often the case, the one imperiled, about whom decisions have to be made, is the very one that helped mediate and foster the fragile family dynamic. Without her the family fragments. This, however, should not be unexpected. Families are fragile in all sorts of ways, and illness, disability, death can be extraordinary blows.

Yet this fact of brokenness and need for reconciliation are not treated as a dimension of "medical ethics" proper. Even Catholic moral theologians or Christian bioethicists — to whom the concept of "reconciliation" is more readily available than it is perhaps to secular bioethicists — proceed as if the sole question is finding the right decision maker or making the right decision. Reconciliation is portrayed as a long, messy, nonclinical process for the chaplain or the social worker; it's part of *sacramental* theology, not moral theology.

To this my response is: well, yes and no. As my analysis suggests, I do think the sacraments and the practices of the Christian life are the place to find the resources for addressing the pressing questions of theology and medicine. Consequently, I would argue that we ought to resist this too-clean distinction between sacramental and moral theology. Rather, moral theologians need to make much clearer the connection between Christian ethics and Christian worship and to demonstrate just how this connection might work.

Nor is reconciliation simply a "pastoral" rather than an "ethical" issue. It is important for more than our feelings of unity. The autonomy of choice and the sanctity of life have become the central (and often sole) moral questions in the realm of bioethics because they deal with what are considered critical human goods — freedom and life. These are considered essential components of who we are. But a truly theological anthropology, a vision of the human person rooted in the Trinity and the fullest embodiment of the image of God who was Jesus Christ, does not stop there. It does not relegate human relatedness and community to simply a "pastoral" dimension. To be in community is not simply nice but is necessary to who we are. And imperiled community is equally, if not perhaps more problematic than, imperiled autonomy. If morality and ethics are about the pursuit of central human goods under the aegis of faith, then the need for reconciliation is a central moral question.

Second, I would argue that, theologically, reconciliation must be the overarching context of all other moral and ethical analysis. Does this mean that freedom and the sanctity of life are irrelevant? Not at all. Rather, it is about the proper ordering of goods, as Augustine would say. Absent this proper ordering — this ordering of Christian commitments under the overarching context of reconciliation and forgiveness — we risk more than moral disorder; we risk — in Augustine's terms — real evil. Consequently, it is possible in the clinical setting to achieve a "legally" or "procedurally" correct decision that is a complete failure. Saint Paul reminds us that if we speak in tongues, have the gift of prophecy, give all we possess to the poor, and become martyrs, but have not love, we are nothing. Similarly, if we achieve a "procedurally correct" outcome according to the canons of bioethics — either discontinuing or continuing artificial nutrition and hydration in the Schiavo case — but have not reconciliation (which is, of course, love), what do we have?

In other words, as Bernardin's story makes clear, I do not mean to suggest that treatment decisions are completely irrelevant — when first diagnosed, he pursued treatment aggressively; when the cancer returned, he again initially chose treatment but then decided to withdraw treatment and to allow death to come. In this he embodied the long-standing wisdom of the Catholic tradition, that life is a gift to be valued but not to be pursued at all costs.

But the treatment decisions are not the focus of his account of the end of life. Instead, the focus is on how he lived in the face of death. These are the real theological-moral questions that every Christian will face. How do Catholics or Christians act in the face of death? How do we act when faced with this real evil that promises to tear apart the fabric of our lives? How do we act when faced with other people who, through their actions in end-of-life situations, become our enemies (even if they are members of our families)? On an institutional level, what would it mean to develop a decision-making process, algorithm, etc., that took the overarching goal of reconciliation seriously? What would it look like? What would the outcomes be? What would it look like for health-care institutions to name reconciliation as a "core value" and to make sure it informs their policies, practices, language, and ethos? What would it look like for Catholic moral theology or bioethics to be shaped around a commitment to reconciliation? Forty years ago the words "autonomy" and "informed consent" were foreign to the clinical setting. How different might clinical medicine look forty years hence if Christians conscientiously tried to introduce into medical ethics the language of forgiveness?

Thirdly, to be clear, forgiveness and reconciliation are not Pollyanna, touchy-feely, why-can't-we-all-just-get-along sorts of things. Rather, they are concrete practices that require continual effort and a lifetime to learn. They are not the sort of thing one will wake up one morning to and say, "Aha! I'm a forgiving person!" As Bernardin makes clear in his own story, his ability to forgive his accuser and to face death not as the end but as the opportunity for a new ministry was a gift — a gift of God, sustained by God's gracious, creative, and life-giving presence — made possible by his two-decade-long practice of daily prayer. Practices like prayer help instill in us specific virtues so crucial in crises and as we die — virtues like patience and openness to the other. Equally, they habituate us to more readily see the world not under the descriptions our culture gives us as normative (e.g., fight a lawsuit with a lawsuit) but rather under the auspices of the Christian story.

Nor are forgiveness and reconciliation best left to the initiative of individuals. So counter to our nature is it to love our enemies, to forgive them, to be reconciled with them, that it's almost impossible to do alone (those people who figure out how to, we usually call "saints"). Christianity (as well as Judaism and Islam) has set aside special rites and special times to call us to account, knowing well that, left to our own devices, we would never do it. It is too hard, especially when we are overwhelmed with the pain caused by alienation and brokenness. Forgiveness and reconciliation must be mediated by the community, by the institutions within which patients and families find themselves. These things must be intentional, they must be attended to, they must be practiced. And they must be practiced within the community of the church, both because without it they would never happen, and because without them the church itself could not be sustained, for they are its very essence.

Finally, I will grant you that love of enemy and forgiveness are far more difficult to legislate than the principle of sanctity of life or the right to autonomy. Nor are they easy to live out. But those who claim to be Christian — as did so many people in the Schiavo and other end-of-life cases — know that this is the ultimate context for all other commitments, even the Christian commitment to life. And it is our call as Christians to show that it is possible, to embody in our lives a politics not primarily of the state and federal court, not of health-care policies, nor of fear and enmity, but rather of redemption.

Action is the "test" of our belief. Do we face whatever threatens us calmly, truthfully, peaceably, as Bernardin did his accuser, relentlessly seeking reconciliation in the midst of it? Do we encounter the thing or person who threatens us as an opportunity to launch a new ministry, a new witness to Christ's presence in our lives, to create a network of prayer, friendship, and reconciliation, beyond what we ever could have imagined? Only by dwelling in the Christian story every day, in the Eucharist, and through feasts such as the triduum, can we begin to see life as a gift through which God can be glorified, enemies as those who need compassion, and death as the enemy transformed.

As we act, so we will witness. Many fear that speaking of bioethics in such resoundingly Christian terms cannot help but alienate those who do not share the Christian faith. But I disagree. The witness of Cardinal Bernardin has moved many who had little interest in faith or Christianity to see that there might be another way. Showing is always more powerful than saying. Christians, indeed, are called to minister to the brokenness of the world, but this ministry must necessarily resemble the lead of the one we claim to follow, namely, the witness of Jesus Christ, the trinitarian God incarnate. It is our call as Christians to show that it is possible, to attempt to embody this. And if we do, I bet we'd be amazed by how God's grace would heal the world.